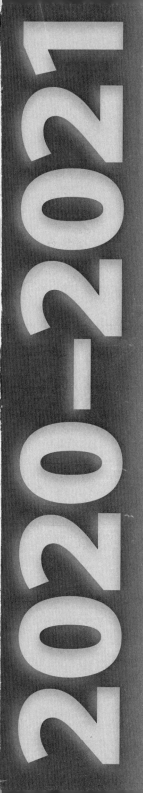

2020–2021

MW01028761

Oncology Nursing Drug Handbook

Gail M. Wilkes, MS, RN
Oncology Nursing Consultant
Kilauea, Hawaii

Margaret Barton-Burke, PhD, RN, FAAN
Mary Ann Lee Professor of Oncology Nursing
University of Missouri, St. Louis
Research Scientist
Siteman Cancer Center
St. Louis, Missouri

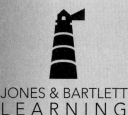

JONES & BARTLETT
LEARNING

World Headquarters
Jones & Bartlett Learning
5 Wall Street
Burlington, MA 01803
978-443-5000
info@jblearning.com
www.jblearning.com

Jones & Bartlett Learning books and products are available through most bookstores and online booksellers. To contact Jones & Bartlett Learning directly, call 800-832-0034, fax 978-443-8000, or visit our website, www. jblearning.com.

Substantial discounts on bulk quantities of Jones & Bartlett Learning publications are available to corporations, professional associations, and other qualified organizations. For details and specific discount information, contact the special sales department at Jones & Bartlett Learning via the above contact information or send an email to specialsales@jblearning.com.

Copyright © 2020 by Jones & Bartlett Learning, LLC, an Ascend Learning Company

All rights reserved. No part of the material protected by this copyright may be reproduced or utilized in any form, electronic or mechanical, including photocopying, recording, or by any information storage and retrieval system, without written permission from the copyright owner.

The content, statements, views, and opinions herein are the sole expression of the respective authors and not that of Jones & Bartlett Learning, LLC. Reference herein to any specific commercial product, process, or service by trade name, trademark, manufacturer, or otherwise does not constitute or imply its endorsement or recommendation by Jones & Bartlett Learning, LLC and such reference shall not be used for advertising or product endorsement purposes. All trademarks displayed are the trademarks of the parties noted herein. *Oncology Nursing Drug Handbook 2020–2021* is an independent publication and has not been authorized, sponsored, or otherwise approved by the owners of the trademarks or service marks referenced in this product.

There may be images in this book that feature models; these models do not necessarily endorse, represent, or participate in the activities represented in the images. Any screenshots in this product are for educational and instructive purposes only. Any individuals and scenarios featured in the case studies throughout this product may be real or fictitious, but are used for instructional purposes only.

The authors, editor, and publisher have made every effort to provide accurate information. However, they are not responsible for errors, omissions, or for any outcomes related to the use of the contents of this book and take no responsibility for the use of the products and procedures described. Treatments and side effects described in this book may not be applicable to all people; likewise, some people may require a dose or experience a side effect that is not described herein. Drugs and medical devices are discussed that may have limited availability controlled by the Food and Drug Administration (FDA) for use only in a research study or clinical trial. Research, clinical practice, and government regulations often change the accepted standard in this field. When consideration is being given to use of any drug in the clinical setting, the health care provider or reader is responsible for determining FDA status of the drug, reading the package insert, and reviewing prescribing information for the most up-to-date recommendations on dose, precautions, and contraindications, and determining the appropriate usage for the product. This is especially important in the case of drugs that are new or seldom used.

ISBN: 978-1-284-17132-7
ISSN: 1536-0024

Production Credits
VP, Product Management: Amanda Martin
Director of Product Management: Matthew Kane
Product Manager: Teresa Malmberg
Product Assistant: Melina Leon
Project Manager: Kristen Rogers
Director of Marketing: Andrea DeFronzo
Marketing Manager: Lindsay White
Production Services Manager: Colleen Lamy
VP, Manufacturing and Inventory Control: Therese Connell

Product Fulfillment Manager: Wendy Kilborn
Composition: S4Carlisle Publishing Services
Project Management: S4Carlisle Publishing Services
Cover Design: Michael O'Donnell
Text Design: Michael O'Donnell
Senior Media Development Editor: Troy Liston
Rights Specialist: John Rusk
Printing and Binding: LSC Communications
Cover Printing: LSC Communications

6048

Printed in the United States of America
23 22 21 20 19   10 9 8 7 6 5 4 3 2 1

Contents

Chapter 2   Cytoprotective Agents   **429**

Chapter 3   Molecular Targeted Therapy   455

Chapter 7   Nausea and Vomiting   1487

Chapter 8   Anorexia and Cachexia   1553

Chapter 12 Constipation   1923

Chapter 13 Diarrhea   1943

Key to Abbreviations

ABV	doxorubicin (doxorubicin HCl Adriamycin) bleomycin vincristineac
ac	*ante cibum;* before meals
ADH	antidiuretic hormone
Afib	atrial fibrillation
AIDS	acquired immunodeficiency syndrome
ALL	acute lymphocytic leukemia
ALT	alanine aminotransferase (formerly SGPT)
AML	acute myelocytic leukemia
ANC	absolute neutrophil count
ANLL	acute nonlymphocytic leukemia
APC	adenomatous polyposis coli gene
APL	acute promyelocytic leukemia
aPTT	activated partial thromboplastin time
ARDS	adult respiratory distress syndrome
ASA	acetylsalicylic acid
AST	aspartate aminotransferase (formerly SGOT)
AUC	area under curve
BBB	blood–brain barrier
BCR-ABL	mutation resulting in the formation of the Philadelphia chromosome, found in 90% of patients with CML
bid	*bis in die;* twice a day
bili	bilirubin
BMT	bone marrow transplant
BP	blood pressure
BRM	biologic response modifier
BTP	breakthrough pain
BUN	blood urea nitrogen
Ca	calcium
CAPD	continuous ambulatory periotoneal dialysis
CBC	complete blood count
CFU-GEM	colony-forming unit–granulocyte, erythrocyte, megakaryocyte, and macrophage
CHF	congestive heart failure
CLL	chronic lymphocytic leukemia
CML	chronic myelogenous leukemia
CPK	creatinine phosphokinase
CR	complete response, e.g., disappearance of all detectable tumor cells

creat	creatinine
CSF	colony-stimulating factor
CTZ	chemoreceptor trigger zone
CVA	cerebrovascular accident
CXR	chest x-ray
D_5W	5% dextrose in water
DEHP	diethylhexlphthalate
DHFR	difolate reductase
DIC	disseminated intravascular coagulation
DLCO	diffusion capacity of the lung for carbon monoxide, which reflects rate of gas transfer across the alveolar-capillary membrane
DLT	dose-limiting toxicity
DMSO	dimethyl sulfoxide
DTIC	dacarbazine
DVT	deep vein thrombosis
EBV	Epstein–Barr virus
ECHO	echocardiogram
EDTA	edetic acid, one of several salts of edetic acid used as a chelating agent
EGFRI	epidermal growth factor receptor inhibitor
EPS	extra pyramidal side effects
ESRD	end stage renal disease
FAC	fluorouracil-adriamycin-cytoxan combination chemotherapy
FOLFIRI	combination chemotherapy of folinic acid (leucovorin), 5-fluorouracil, and irinotecan
FOLFOX	combination chemotherapy of folinic acid (leucovorin), 5-fluorouracil, and oxaliplatin
FSH	follicle-stimulating hormone
FUDR-MP	5-fluoro-23-deoxyuridine-53-monophosphate
FVC	forced vital capacity
G6PD	glucose-6-phosphate dehydrogenase
GABA	gamma-aminobutyric acid
GBPS	gated blood pool scan
G-CSF	granulocyte-colony-stimulating factor
GFR	glomerular filtration rate
GGT	(SGGT) gamma-glutamine transferase
GU	genitourinary
HACA	human antichimeric antibody
HAMA	human antimurine antibody
HCC	hepatocellular cancer
HCl	hydrochloride
HCT	hematocrit
Hgb	hemoglobin
5-HIAA	5-hydroxyindoleacetic acid
HIV	human immunodeficiency virus
5-HT_2	5-hydroxytryptamine 2
5-HT_3	5-hydroxytryptamine 3

Hs	*hora somni;* at bedtime
HSV	herpes simplex virus
HUS	hemolytic uremic syndrome
ICP	intracranial pressure
ICU	intensive care unit
IFN	interferon
IL	interleukin
I/O	intake/output
IOP	intraocular pressure
IT	intrathecal
IVB	intravenous bolus
IVP	intravenous push; intravenous pyelogram
JAK	Janus kinase, part of JAK-STAT signaling pathway
LAK	lymphocyte activated killer cells
LDH	lactate dehydrogenase
LFTs	liver function tests
LH	luteinizing hormone
LHRH	luteinizing hormone-releasing hormone
LVEF	left ventricular ejection fraction
lytes	electrolytes
MAb	monoclonal antibody
MAC	mycobacterium avium complex
MAO	monoamine oxidase
MAOI	monoamine oxidase inhibitor
MAPK	mitogen-activated protein kinase pathway, aka Ras-Raf-MEK-ERK pathway
MCV	mean corpuscular volume
MI	myocardial infarction
MIU	milli international units
MOPP	mustard-oncovin-prednisone-procarbazine combination chemotherapy for Hodgkin's disease
mTOR	mammalian target of rapamycin, which coordinates cell growth, nutrient use, and angiogenesis
MTX	methotrexate
MU	milli units
NCI	National Cancer Institute
NHL	non-Hodgkin's lymphoma
NK	natural killer cells
NK1	neurokinin 1 receptor for substance P
NMDA	N-methyl-D-aspartate pain receptor
NS	normal saline
NSAIDs	nonsteroidal anti-inflammatory drugs
n/v	nausea/vomiting
OS	overall survival
OTC	over-the-counter
PACs	premature atrial contractions
PBPCs	packed red blood cells for transfusion

PCA	patient controlled analgesia
PCP	*Pneumocystis (carinii) jiroveci* pneumonia
PFS	progression-free survival
PFTs	pulmonary function tests
phos	phosphorus
plts	platelets
PDGFR	platelet-derived growth factor receptor
PI3K	phosphatidylinositol 3-kinase pathway, most frequently mutated pathway in cancer
PML	polymorphonuclear leukocyte
PR	partial response, e.g., reduction in tumor mass by 50% lasting for 3 months or longer
PRN	*pro re nata;* as needed
PSA	prostate-specific antigen
PT	prothrombin time
PTEN	phosphatase and tensin homolog
PTH	parathyroid hormone
PTT	partial thromboplastin time
PVCs	premature ventricular contractions
qid	*quater in die;* four times a day
QT	measure of the interval of time between the start of the Q wave and end of T wave; if prolonged, it can increase risk of fatal ventricular arrhythmias
RAS	protein that activates a number of pathways, such as MAPK pathway
REMS	risk evaluation and management strategy
RFTs	renal function tests
RT	radiation therapy
RUQ	right upper quadrant
SBP	systolic blood pressure
sed rate	sedimentation rate
SGOT	serum glutamic-oxalacetic transaminase
SGPT	serum glutamic-pyruvic transferase
SIADH	syndrome of inappropriate antidiuretic hormone
SNRI	serotonin and noradrenalin reuptake inhibitors
SOB	shortness of breath

SPF	skin protection factor
SSRI	selective serotonin reuptake inhibitors
SQ	subcutaneous
SSRI	selective serotonin reuptake inhibitor
STAT	signal transducers and activators of transcription protein pathway, which carries a message from the cell surface to the cell nucleus and then activates transcription of specific genes
Sx	symptom
T	temperature
T_3	triiodothyronine
T_4	thyroxine
TCA	tricyclic antidepressants
TFT	thyroid function tests
TGF	transforming growth factor beta
THC	tetrahydrocannabinol
tid	*ter in die*; three times a day
TIL	tumor-infiltrating lymphocytes
TKI	tyrosine kinase inhibitor
TLS	tumor lysis syndrome
TMP-SMX	trimethoprim-sulfamethoxazole
TNF	tumor necrosis factor
TTP/HUS	thrombotic thrombocytopenic purpura/hemolytic anemia syndrome
UA	urinalysis
ULN	upper limit of normal
US	ultrasound
UTI	urinary tract infection
VC	vomiting center
VEGF	vascular endothelial growth factor
Vfib	ventricular fibrillation
VOD	veno-occlusive disease
VS	vital signs
VSCC	voltage-sensitive calcium channel
VZV	varicella zoster virus
WHO	World Health Organization
XRT	radiation therapy

Preface

Oncology nurses provide expert nursing care to patients with cancer and their families as the patient moves along the disease trajectory from diagnosis to primary treatment and cure, or to remission, then possible relapse, and death. The nurse uses the nursing process to assess patient and family needs in high-incidence problem areas identified in the Oncology Nursing Society (ONS) standards: health promotion, patient/family education, coping, comfort, nutrition, complementary and alternative medicine, protective mechanisms, mobility, GI and urinary function, sexuality, cardiopulmonary function, oncologic emergencies, palliative and end-of-life care, and survivorship (Brandt & Wickham, 2013).

In 2003, Andrew von Eschenbach, MD, set the NCI challenge goal as the elimination of suffering and death due to cancer. He identified seven major initiatives to accomplish this goal, including development of more effective strategies for prevention and screening; early detection as well as improvement of our understanding of the molecular processes of carcinogenesis; and refinement of molecular targeted therapy (von Eschenbach, 2003). In this view, cancer becomes a chronic disease characterized by periods of exacerbations and remissions. As has been demonstrated in work on angiogenesis, malignant tumors must establish a blood supply when they reach a size of 1–2 mm in order to obtain oxygen and glucose and to remove cellular waste products. Mortality is caused by metastasis in most people with cancer, and if a malignancy is confined to 1–2 mm with a combination of chemotherapy, anti-angiogenesis drugs, and other signal transduction inhibitors, along with immune checkpoint inhibitors, then indeed, people can "live with cancer." Today, more and more is being revealed about genetic tumor-typing and identifying tumor targets that individualize cancer care, much like doing blood cultures to identify an infectious organism and tailoring antimicrobial therapy to the infectious microbe. Together, the nurse and patient, along with other members of the healthcare team and family, develop a plan of care. Because cancer, for many, is a chronic illness with periods of remission and relapse, nursing goals center around promoting self-care and empowering the patient and family to live a high-quality, meaningful life outside the hospital or office practice.

Nurses are involved in the pharmacologic management of disease (e.g., chemotherapy, including targeted molecular and immunological therapy) and of symptoms that arise during the course of illness (e.g., pain, anxiety, cachexia, diarrhea, constipation, nausea, vomiting). In addition, as patients receive more aggressive treatment, nurses are deeply involved in the management of complications of disease or treatment, such as infection. As new technologies emerge, such as new molecular and biological/immune-targeted therapies, nurses need to stay abreast of newly approved agents, their mechanisms of action, potential side effects, and issues of cost. Knowledge of cancer biology, immunology and metastases is evolving and each offers potential targets. Nurses must keep up with understanding the fundamental molecular flaws, and immune function, both to teach patients and their families, as well as to understand the mechanism of action and potential toxicities. As the paradigm moves to multitargeted oral agents, the nurse must be creative in developing strategies to promote adherence with treatment regimens and individualize patient care to enhance adherence and self-care at home. For example, nurses are working to establish the evidence base for minimization of toxicity and distress related to EGFR inhibitor rash. In addition, as the cost of cancer therapy—targeted and biological/immune therapies, in particular—skyrockets, the nurse must be able either to access resources or to refer patients and their families to resources for help. Finally, oncology nurses have long said that much of symptom management is in the domain of nursing practice, and they continue to advocate for effective management and symptom resolution. Knowledge of the drugs used in cancer care is critical for today's practicing nurse. In the past, pharmacists wrote drug books for nurses that did not address the application of the nursing process to potential drug toxicities. Today, as the science of cancer treatment is rapidly exploding, it is imperative to keep current with new, emerging therapies and nursing implications.

The Oncology Nursing Society identifies knowledge and competencies for nurses who will administer and care for individuals receiving chemotherapy, targeted therapy and immunotherapy (2017). This book is divided into sections addressing broad areas of nursing practice; individual chapters within each section present an introductory overview. Included in *Chapter 1* of this edition are chemotherapy agents, which were updated for new indications, postmarketing side effects, and warnings and precautions. Two drugs added are apalutamide (Erleade) and liposomal daunorubicin and cytarabine for injection (Vyxeos). *Chapter 2* addresses cytoprotective agents. Molecular and immunological targeted therapies have been separated as both have evolved into their own specialty. *Chapter 3* addresses the foundation of molecular targeted therapeutic agents, with a discussion of signal transduction, hallmarks of cancer, and key nursing issues in the administration of molecular targeted therapy such as QTc prolongation and risk of sudden cardiac death. This is intended to provide a framework for understanding the new agents that target molecular flaws. Many of these agents inhibit steps in the processes of carcinogenesis and metastases in the areas of signal transduction (growth receptor over expression, and mutation of signaling proteins in major signaling pathways), cell-cycle movement (cyclin-dependent kinases, apoptosis), angiogenesis, invasion, and metastases. In addition, the processes of apoptosis and ubiquitination are further explored. Drugs include the small molecules that can be taken orally and others, such as proteasome inhibitors. All chapters have been reviewed and updated. Many new drugs have been added.

Chapter 1: trifluridine/tipiracil (Lonsurf) and calaspargase pegol-mknl (Asparlas)

Chapter 2: glucarpidase (Voraxaze) and levoleucovorin (Khapzory)

Chapter 3: abemaciclib (Verzenio), acalabrutinib (Calquence), alpelisib (Piqray), binimetinib (Mektovi), copanlisib (Aliqopa), duvelisib (Copiktra), encorafenib (Braftovi), erdafitinib (Balversa), dacomitinib (Vizimpro), ivosidenib (Tibsovo), glasdegib (Daurismo), gilteritinib (Xospata), larotrectinib (Vitrakvi), and lorlatinib (Lorbrena)

Chapter 4: axicabtagene ciloleucel (Yescarta), bevacizumab-awwb (Mvasi, biosimilar), brentuximab vedotin (Adcetris), cemiplimab-rwlc (Libtayo), epoetin alfa-epbx (Retacrit), filgrastim-aafi (Nivestym), gemtuzumab ozogamicin (Mylotarg), inotuzumab ozogamicin (Besponsa), mogamulizumab-kpkc (Poteligeo), moxetumomab pasudotox-tdfk (Lumoxiti), pegfilgrastim-jmdb (Fulphila), rituximab-abbs (Truxima), tagraxofusp-erzs (Elzonris), tisagenlecleucel (Kymriah), trastuzumab-dkst (Ogivri), trastuzumab-dttb (Ontruzant), trastuzumab-pkrb (Herzuma), trastuzumab qyyp (Trazimera), and trastuzumab and hyaluronidase-oysk (Herceptin Hylecta)

Chapter 5: adalimumab-adaz (Hyrimoz), adalimumab-adbm (Cyltezo), adalimumab-atto (Amjevita), anakinra (Kineret), baricitinib (Olumiant), etanercept-szzs (Erizi), etanercept-ykro (Eticova), infliximab-abda (Renflexis), infliximab-dyyb (Inflectra), and sarilumab (Kevzara)

Chapter 11: baloxavir marboxil (Xofluza), delafloxacin (Baxdela), eravacycline (Xerava), imipenem/cilastatin sodium/relebactam (Recarbrio), letermovir (Prevymis), meropenem/vaborbactam (Vabomere), omadacycline (Nuzyra), and plazomicin (Zemdri). The antibiotics are eravacycline and omadacycline (a tetracycline); plazomicin (an aminoglycoside); imipenem (a penem antibiotic) cilastatin (a renal dehydropeptidase inhibitor) relebactam (a betalactamase inhibitor); meropenem (a penem antibacterial) vaborbactam (a beta-lactamase inhibitor); and delafloxin (a fluoroquinolone antibacterial). The antivirals include letermovir (a CMV DNA terminase complex inhibitor) and baloxavir marboxil (antiviral for the flu).

Chapter 4 addresses immunological targeted therapy, with a foundation in the immune system and how malignant cells circumvent immune surveillance. Drug categories include immune checkpoint inhibitors, CAR T-cell therapy, and genetically modified oncolytic viral therapy. Monoclonal antibodies are included in this chapter. The ASCO/NCCN guidelines on management of toxicity of immune checkpoint inhibitors (eg, irAEs) has been summarized into a reference chart in the chapter introduction. The notion of biosimilar agents is discussed in the Chapter 4 introduction, and a table of the currently available biosimilar drugs was added. Because oncology nurses are often asked to administer monoclonal antibodies and other unusual drugs to patients with autoimmune diseases, *Chapter 5*, addresses chemobiotherapy for noncancer diseases, specifically agents used in the treatment of rheumatoid arthritis. New drugs including biosimilars have been added.

In *Sections 2* (Symptom Management) and *3* (Complications), *Chapters 6, 7, 8, 9, 10, 11, 12*, and *13* have been updated. *Appendix 2* is abridged and referenced to indicate how to locate the NCI Common Toxicity Criteria of Adverse Events (CTCAE) 4.03.

All agents were updated to reflect newly approved indications. Specific drugs are described in terms of their mechanism of action, metabolism, FDA indications, dosage/range, administration, drug interactions, laboratory effects/interference, special considerations, and application of the nursing process to manage potential adverse effects. The most important and common drug side effects are discussed.

Nursing priorities in the assessment and management of EGFRI skin toxicity are discussed in terms of pathophysiology and consensus management strategies. As more targeted therapies are used that have prolongation of the QT interval in the cardiac cycle as side effects, this is discussed in detail with nursing implications. Standards may change as new scientific knowledge becomes available and as dictated by governmental regulations that affect practice. This book will be updated regularly with new drugs and nursing management strategies to reflect those changes.

The authors, editor, and publisher have made every effort to provide accurate information. However, they are not responsible for errors, omissions, or for any outcomes related to the use of the contents of this book and take no responsibility for the use of the products and procedures described. Treatment and side effects described in this book may not be applicable to all people; likewise, some people may require a dose or experience a side effect that is not described herein. Drugs and medical devices are discussed that may have limited availability, controlled by the Food and Drug Administration (FDA) for use only in a research study or clinical trial. Research, clinical practice, and government regulations often change the accepted standards in this field. When consideration is being given for use of any drug in the clinical setting, the healthcare provider or reader is responsible for determining FDA status of the drug, reading the package insert, and reviewing prescribing information for the most up-to-date recommendations on dose, precautions, and contraindications, and determining the appropriate usage for the product. This is especially important in the case of drugs that are new or seldom used.

DRUG INFORMATION sections reflect current prescribing practices in the United States, which may differ from clinical practices in Europe and the United Kingdom.

References

Brandt JM, Wickham R. *Statement on the Scope and Standards of Oncology Nursing Practice, Generalist and Advanced Practice.* Pittsburgh, PA: Oncology Nursing Society; 2013: 21–35.

Oncology Nursing Society. Education of the nurse who administers and cares for the individual receiving chemotherapy, targeted therapy and immunotherapy. October 2017. Available at https://www.ons.org/advocacy-policy/positions/education/chemotherapy-biotherapy. Accessed July 3, 2018.

von Eschenbach. Keynote presentation: *Summit Series on Cancer Clinical Trials. Executive Summary VIII: Retooling the System: Implementing Solution.* September 29–October 1, 2003.

Contributors

Catherine K. Bean, BSN, RN, BA
Tampa, FL

Deborah Berg, BSN, RN
North Londonderry, NH

Karen Ingwersen, MS, RN
Belmont, MA

Section 1
Cancer Treatment

Chapter *1*
Introduction to Chemotherapy Drugs

Traditional chemotherapy drugs interfere with cell division, leading to cell kill, called *cytocidal effects*, or failure to replicate, called *cytostatic effects* (see Figure 1.1). Unfortunately, drugs cannot discriminate between frequently dividing cells that are normal and those that are malignant. Consequently, normal cells and malignant cells/ are injured. Thus, anticipated acute side effects are found also in normal cell populations that divide frequently, i.e., bone marrow (BM), gastrointestinal (GI) mucosa, gonads, and hair follicles. Since normal cells are better able to repair themselves, these side effects are usually reversible. Depending on drug properties, delayed, longer-term toxicities may occur, which may be irreversible. Properties to be aware of include route of administration, dose, excretion, and predilection for uptake by specific organ cells. Examples of toxicities are:

- Lung toxicity from bleomycin, busulfan, and the nitrosoureas (BCNU, CCNU)
- Cardiomyopathy from the anthracyclines doxorubicin and daunorubicin, the anthracenedione mitoxantrone, as well as from the mitotic inhibitor paclitaxel
- Renal dysfunction from cisplatin and high-dose methotrexate
- Hemorrhagic cystitis (bladder) from ifosfamide and cyclophosphamide
- Neurotoxicity from the platinums, taxanes, and vinca alkaloids
- Development of second malignancies from melphalan and cyclophosphamide, either alone or when certain drugs are combined with radiotherapy

Nurses play a critical role in patient assessment, education, drug administration, and minimization of toxicities. See Table 1.1 for prechemotherapy nursing assessment guidelines. Table 1.2 describes classifications of antineoplastic drugs. Table 1.3 highlights the newly updated 2016 American Society of Clinical Oncology (ASCO)/Oncology Nursing Society (ONS) chemotherapy administration safety standards. The new standards include clarification and expansion of the previous standards (e.g., two-person verification of chemotherapy preparation processes, labeling of patient medications dispensed from the healthcare setting for administration at home, etc.) and highlight the administration of vinca alkaloids via mini-bags in institutions where intrathecal medications are administered (Neuss et al., 2017).

This 2020 edition has been updated to include newly approved drugs. This section examines antineoplastic agents and classifies them by their mechanism(s) of action. As knowledge of cancer and its treatment emerge, drugs may be reclassified, such as the anthracycline antitumor antibiotics, which now appear to work by inhibiting topoisomerase II.

As an example, the topoisomerase inhibitors cause protein-linked DNA single-strand breaks and block DNA and RNA synthesis in dividing cells, thus preventing cells from entering mitosis. To better understand the topoisomerase inhibitors, it is important to go back to the DNA helix. The entire DNA genome consists of two strands wound into a double

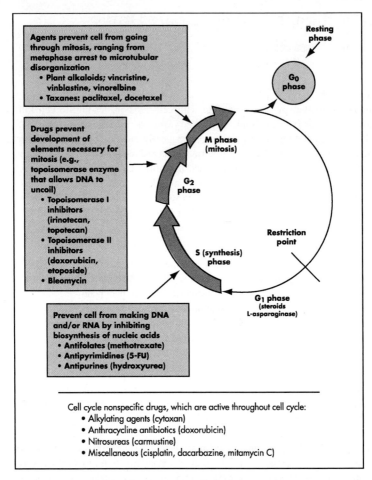

Figure 1.1   Mechanism of Action of Major Chemotherapy Drugs

helix, which measures more than 3 feet long. In order to fit into a tiny cell, it is condensed into chromosomes by torsion of the helix. During cell replication, the DNA strands that are coiled in the double helix need to unwind so that they can separate and be copied. This is made possible by the topoisomerase I and II enzymes (Chen and Liu, 1994).

Topoisomerase I relaxes tension in the DNA helix torsion by causing a transient single-strand break or nick in the DNA when it covalently bonds to the end of one of the DNA strands. The other, intact strand then passes through the break, and relaxation of the DNA helix occurs as the strands swivel at the strand break.

The topoisomerase I enzyme then reseals the cleaved strand (religation step), and the enzyme is released from the DNA strand. Transcription (copying of the strands) is then

Table 1.1   Prechemotherapy Nursing Assessment Guidelines

Potential Problems/Nursing Diagnoses	Physical Status: Assessment Parameters/Signs and Symptoms	Drug and Dose-Limiting Factors/Nursing Implications
Hematopoietic System		
1. Impaired tissue perfusion related to chemotherapy-induced anemia, leading to activity intolerance, changes in cardiopulmonary status due to compensatory changes	• Hgb (norms women, 12–14; men, 14–16) • HCT% (norms women, 36–46; men, 42–54) • Vital signs (↓BP, ↑pulse, ↑ or ↓respiration) • Pallor (face, palms, *conjunctiva*) • Fatigue or weakness • Vertigo	Hgb < 8 g HCT < 20% and blood transfusions not initiated • Consider erythropoietin growth factor support when Hgb < 10 g/dL when receiving anemia-causing chemotherapy, e.g., cisplatin for palliation; do not exceed an Hgb of 12 g/dL (NCCN, 2016)
2. Impaired immunocompetence and potential for infection related to chemotherapy-induced neutropenia, lymphopenia	• WBC (norm 4,500–9,000/mm³); ANC > 2,000/mm³ • Lymphocyte count > 500/mm³ • Pyrexia/rigor, erythema, swelling, pain any site • Abnormal discharges, draining wounds, skin/mucous membrane lesions • Productive cough, SOB, rectal pain, urinary frequency	WBC ≤ 3,000/mm³; ANC < 1,000/mm³–1,500/mm³; Fever > 38°C or 100.4°F • Hold all myelosuppressive agents (exceptions may include leukemia, lymphoma, and/or situations in which there is neoplastic marrow infiltration) • Consider growth factor support to prevent febrile neutropenia if risk > 20% • Febrile neutropenia is a medical emergency • Severe risk of infection ANC < 500 cells/mm³ • Protective precautions if actual or potential ANC < 500 cells/mm³
3. Potential for injury (bleeding) related to chemotherapy-induced thrombocytopenia	• Platelet count (150,000–400,000/mm³) • Spontaneous gingival bleeding or epistaxis • Presence of petechiae or easy bruisability • Hematuria, melena, hematemesis, hemoptysis • Hypermenorrhea • Signs and symptoms of intracranial bleeding (irritability, sensory loss, unequal pupils, headache, ataxia)	Platelet count ≤ 100,000/mm³ • Hold all myelosuppressive agents (exceptions may include leukemia, lymphoma, and/or situations in which there is neoplastic marrow infiltration) • Platelet transfusion if bleeding • Platelet precaution: platelet count < 20,000 cells/mm³

(continues)

Table 1.1 *(Continued)*

Potential Problems/Nursing Diagnoses	Physical Status: Assessment Parameters/Signs and Symptoms	Drug and Dose-Limiting Factors/Nursing Implications
Integumentary System		
1. Potential for injury related to severe sterile inflammatory rash	• EGFR inhibitor rash • Assess for risk of infection, itching, open areas *Anthracyclines such as doxorubicin	• Teach patient self-care to avoid infection, maintain hydration and skin integrity; use sunscreens and hat when outside • Discuss topical and/or systemic preventive or treatment of evolving rash • Consider doxycycline 100 mg PO bid, topical clindamycin gel, and/or steroid taper
2. Alteration in skin integrity related to alopecia	*May be partial or total alopecia	* Explore effect of hair loss on patient, and encourage verbalization of feelings * Discuss ways to facilitate coping, such as cranial prosthesis prior to losing hair, *Look Good Feel Better* American Cancer Society programs
3. Anorexia	• Lab values: Albumin and total protein • Normal weight/present weight and % of body weight loss • Normal diet pattern/changes in diet pattern • Alterations in taste sensation, dysgeusia • Early satiety	• Manage nutrition impact symptoms • Dietary teaching • Appetite stimulants as needed
4. Nausea and vomiting	• Lab values: Electrolytes • Pattern of n/v (incidence, duration, severity); hydration status • Hydration status • Antiemetic plan: Drug(s), dosage(s), schedule, efficacy: Other (dietary adjustments, relaxation techniques, environmental manipulation)	Intractable n/v × 24 h: IV hydration if unable to take oral fluids • Aggressive combination antiemesis (serotonin and NK$_1$ antagonists and dexamethasone; palonostron for severe with delayed nausea and/or vomiting; addition of aprepitant to serotonin-antagonist for highly emetogenic, moderately emetogenic with delayed nausea and vomiting)

Table 1.1 *(Continued)*

Potential Problems/Nursing Diagnoses	Physical Status: Assessment Parameters/Signs and Symptoms	Drug and Dose-Limiting Factors/Nursing Implications
5. Bowel disturbances A. Diarrhea	• Normal pattern of bowel elimination • Consistency (loose, watery/bloody stools) • Assess hydration status and ability to take fluids in • Frequency and duration (no./day and no. of days) • Antidiarrheal drug(s), dosage(s), efficacy	• Diarrheal stools × 3/24 h above baseline • Hold antimetabolites (esp. methotrexate, 5-FU); irinotecan • Teach patient self-administration of antidiarrheal medicine • Assess electrolytes, need for parenteral hydration • Antibiotic therapy for unresolved diarrhea per MD as mucositis may occur during nadir, with resulting sepsis.
B. Constipation	• Normal pattern of bowel elimination • Consistency (hard, dry, small stools) • Frequency (hours or days beyond normal pattern) • Stool softener(s), laxative(s), efficacy • Assess medication profile for opioids, antiemetics	No BM × 48 h past normal bowel patterns • Hold vinca alkaloids (vinblastine, vincristine) • Teach patient to take stool softener with serotonin-antagonist antiemetic or opioids to prevent constipation from the drug

6. Hepatotoxicity	• Lab values: LDH, ALT, AST, alk phos, bili
	• Pain/tenderness over liver, feeling of fullness
	• Increase in n/v or anorexia
	• Changes in mental status
	• Jaundice
	• High-risk factors:
	  • Hepatic metastasis
	  • Concurrent hepatotoxic drugs
	  • Viral hepatitis
	  • Graft-vs-host disease
	  • Abdominal XRT
	  • Blood transfusions
		Evidence of chemical hepatitis:
		• Hold hepatotoxic agents (esp. methotrexate, 6-MP), until differential dx established
		• Hold oxaliplatin if venous occlusive disease suspected
		• Hold or dose-reduce drugs metabolized by liver if severe liver dysfunction (e.g., docetaxel, doxorubicin, trabectedin)

(continues)

TREATMENT

Table 1.1   (Continued)

Potential Problems/Nursing Diagnoses	Physical Status: Assessment Parameters/Signs and Symptoms	Drug and Dose-Limiting Factors/Nursing Implications
Respiratory System		

Impaired gas exchange or ineffective breathing pattern related to chemotherapy-induced pulmonary fibrosis	• Lab values: PFTs CXR
	• Respirations (rate, rhythm, depth)
	• Chest pain
	• Nonproductive cough
	• Progressive dyspnea
	• Wheezing/stridor
	• High-risk factors:
	  • Total cumulative dose of bleomycin
	  • Age > 60 years
	  • Preexisting lung disease
	  • Concomitant use of other pulmonary toxic drugs
	  • Prior/concomitant XRT
	  • Smoking hx
		• Acute, unexplained onset respiratory symptoms, or worsening beyond baseline
		• Hold all antineoplastic agents until differential dx established (e.g., bleomycin, busulfan, oxaliplatin, gemcitabine)
		• Interstitial lung disease (ILD) is a class effect of EGFR antagonists (rare), e.g., cetuximab, erlotinib
		• Chemotherapy drug may be combined with EGFR antagonists (e.g., gemcitabine and erlotinib). If pulmonary symptoms develop, hold drug until ILD can be ruled out

Cardiovascular System		
Decreased cardiac output related to chemotherapy-induced: 1. Cardiac arrhythmias 2. Cardiomyopathy 3. Hypertension 4. QTc Prolongation	• Lab values: cardiac enzymes, electrolytes, ECG, ECHO, MUGA, QTc interval measurement • Vital signs • Presence of arrhythmia (irregular radial/apical pulse) • Signs sx CHF (dyspnea, ankle edema, PND, decrease in LVEF, S_3 gallop, nonproductive cough, rales, cyanosis) • Review results of cardiac ECHO or MUGA scan prior to first dose, then every 2–3 months as indicated for the specific drug, e.g., trabectedin. Discuss holding drug for LVEF < LLN with physician/NP/PA.	• Acute sx CHF and/or cardiac arrhythmia • Hypertension: risk increased in combination with bevacizumab • Hold all antineoplastic agents until differential dx established • Total dose doxorubicin > 350–550 mg/m²; also assess epirubicin, daunorubicin cumulative dose and compare to drug threshold • Risk of CHF increased when chemotherapy given with trastuzumab; hold anthracyclines, trastuzumab, paclitaxel; monitor LVEF closely and hold drug per standard

Table 1.1 *(Continued)*

Potential Problems/Nursing Diagnoses	Physical Status: Assessment Parameters/Signs and Symptoms	Drug and Dose-Limiting Factors/Nursing Implications

	• History of Congenital Long QT Syndrome, CAD, medications which prolong QTc
	• High-risk factors:
	  • Total cumulative dose anthracyclines
	  • Preexisting cardiac disease
	  • Prior/concurrent mediastinal XRT
	  • Combined anthracycline, cyclophosphamide, trastuzumab, and paclitaxel
	• LV EF < 50%; QTc > 500 msec
		• Trastuzumab should never be given **concomitantly** with doxorubicin
		• Monitor baseline and serial ejection fractions (LVEF) while receiving treatment with potentially cardiotoxic drugs; evaluate any significant ↓ in LVEF; see specific guidelines but if drop in LVEF > 10% from baseline, or lower than LLN (e.g., 50%), drug is usually held
		• Severe hypertension: hold bevacizumab until hypertension controlled
		• Hold drug if QTc ≥ 500 msec, or > 50 msec longer than baseline QTc

Genitourinary System
1. Alteration in fluid volume (excess) related to chemotherapy-induced:
  A. Glomerular or renal tubule damage
  B. Hyperuricemic nephropathy
2. Alteration in comfort related to chemotherapy-induced hemorrhagic cystitis
	• Lab values: BUN, creatinine clearance, serum creatinine, uric acid, electrolytes, urinalysis, magnesium, calcium, phosphate
	• Color, odor, clarity of urine
	• 24-hour fluid intake and output (estimate/actual)
	• Hematuria; proteinuria
	• Development of oliguria or anuria
	• High-risk factors:
	  • Preexisting renal disease
	Concurrent treatment with nephrotoxic drugs (esp. aminoglycoside antibiotics)
	• Bevacizumab: rare nephrotic syndrome
		• Hold cyclophosphamide, ifosfamide, cisplatin
		• Serum creatinine > 2.0 and/or
		• Creatinine clearance < 70 mL/min
		Hematuria
		• Hold cisplatin, streptozotocin Anuria × 24 h
		• Hold bevacizumab if patient develops nephrotic syndrome or 24-hour urine shows protein more than 2 g
		• Check BUN/creatinine before treatment
		• 24-hour urine for protein if spilling protein

(continues)

Table 1.1   *(Continued)*

Potential Problems/Nursing Diagnoses	Physical Status: Assessment Parameters/Signs and Symptoms	Drug and Dose-Limiting Factors/Nursing Implications
Nervous System		
1. Impaired sensory/motor function related to chemotherapy-induced A. Peripheral neuropathy (PN) B. Cranial nerve neuropathy C. Acute oxaliplatin neurotoxicity D. Chemotherapy-induced cognitive changes	• Paresthesias (numbness, tingling in feet, fingertips) • Trigeminal nerve toxicity (severe jaw pain) • Jaw or muscle spasm • Diminished or absent deep tendon reflexes (ankle and knee jerks) • Motor weakness/slapping gait/ataxia • Visual and auditory disturbances • Cold-induced paresthesias and dysesthesias lasting < 14 days (oxaliplatin) • Cognitive changes may be influenced by genetics, comorbidities; incidence estimated at 20% of patients receiving standard-dose chemotherapy	Presence of any neurologic signs and symptoms or worsening: • Perform brief nursing neuro exam before each treatment, focusing on symptom analysis and functional impairment; consult MD for full neuro exam if signs/symptoms or worsening of existing signs/symptoms • For progressive chronic PN (grade 2 or higher), hold vinca alkaloids, cisplatin, examethyl-melamine, oxaliplatin, procarbazine and discuss treatment plan with physician or midlevel • Acute oxaliplatin neurotoxicity: increase length of infusion time to 6 h (decreases peak serum level by 32%); teach patient to avoid cold exposure to hands/feet, oral mucosa for 1–3 days after oxaliplatin drug administration • Assess for motor/sensory changes, impact on function and ability to do ADLs prior to oxaliplatin, taxane, or cisplatin administration; hold for grades 3 and 4 toxicity (see *Appendix 2*)

Table 1.1 *(Continued)*

Potential Problems/Nursing Diagnoses	Physical Status: Assessment Parameters/Signs and Symptoms	Drug and Dose-Limiting Factors/Nursing Implications
		• Teach avoidance of cold for 1–3 days after oxaliplatin administration • Cognitive changes may appear after adjuvant therapy; assess for changes in memory, concentration, effect on work or school performance; reinforce teaching if slower ability to learn new information, following directions
2. Impaired bowel and bladder elimination related to chemotherapy-induced autonomic nerve dysfunction	• Urinary retention • Constipation/abdominal cramping and distension • High-risk factors: • Changes in diet or mobility • Frequent use of opioid analgesics • Obstructive disease process	Presence of any neurologic signs and symptoms • Hold vinca alkaloids until differential dx established

ALT = alanine aminotransferase; AST = aspartate aminotransferase; bili = bilirubin; BM = bowel movement; CHF = congestive heart failure; CXR = chest x-ray; dx = diagnosis; ECG = electrocardiogram; ECHO = echocardiogram; EGFR = epidermal growth factor receptor; 5-FU = 5-fluorouracil; hx = history; LDH = lactate dehydrogenase; LVEF = left ventricular ejection fraction; MUGA = multigated acquisition (MUGA heart scan); n/v = nausea and vomiting; PFT = pulmonary function test; 6-MP = 6-mercaptopurine; SOB = shortness of breath; sx = symptoms; XRT = radiation therapy.

Modified from Engleking C. Prechemotherapy Nursing Assessment in Outpatient Settings. *Outpatient Chemotherapy* 1998; 3(1): 10–11.

Table 1.2   Classifications of Antineoplastic Drugs

Classification	Mechanism of Action	Examples
Cell-Cycle Specific Agents		
Antimetabolites	Interfere with DNA and RNA synthesis by acting as false metabolites, which are incorporated into the DNA strand or block essential enzymes, so that DNA synthesis is prevented	Pemetrexate (Alimta) Cytosine arabinoside (ara-C, Cytosar-U) Eniluracil5-Fluorouracil (5-FU) Floxuridine (FUDR, 5-FUDR) Hydroxyurea (Hydrea) 6-Mercaptopurine (6-MP, purinethol) Methotrexate (amethopterin, Mexate, Folex) 6-Thioguanine (6-TG) Gemcitabine (Gemzar®) Fludarabine (Fludara®) Capecitabine (Xeloda®) Pralatrexate (Folotyn®) Tipiracil/trifluridine (Lonsurf®)
Mitotic Spindle Poisons		
A. Vinca Alkaloids	Crystallize microtubules of mitotic spindle causing metaphase arrest (vincristine, vinblastine, vindesine), role in blocking DNA and preventing cell division in M phase (vinorelbine)	Vincristine (VCR, Oncovin) Vinblastine (VLB, Velban) Vinorelbine (Navelbine®)
B. Epothilone	Naturally occurring microstabilizing agents similar to taxanes; bind tubulin and cause apoptotic cell death	Ixabepilone (Ixempra®)
C. Microtubule Dynamics Inhibitor	Synthetic analogue of a sea sponge product; inhibit growth phase of microtubules and sequester tubulin, causing disruption of spindle and cell death.	Eribulin (Halaven®)
D. Taxanes	Promote early microtubule assembly; prevent depolymerization, causing cell death (paclitaxel); enhance microtubule assembly and inhibit tubulin depolymerization, thus arresting cell division in metaphase (docetaxel)	Paclitaxel (Taxol®) Docetaxel (Taxotere®) Paclitaxel protein bound particles for injection (Abraxane®) Cabazitaxel (Jevtana®)
Epipodophyllotoxins	Damage the cell prior to mitosis, late S and G_2 phase; inhibit topoisomerase II	Etoposide (VP-16, Vepesid®) Teniposide (VM-26, Vumon®)
Camptothecins	Act in S phase to inhibit topoisomerase I and cause cell death	Topotecan (Hycamtin®) Irinotecan (CPT-11, Camptosar®) Irinotecan liposomal
Miscellaneous		G_1 phase: L-asparaginase (ELSPAR), prednisone G_2 phase: Bleomycin (Bleo, Blenoxane)

Table 1.2 *(Continued)*

Classification	Mechanism of Action	Examples
Alkylating Agents	Substitute alkyl group for H+ ion causing single- and double-strand breaks in DNA, as well as crosslinkages; thus, DNA strands are unable to separate during DNA replication	Bendamustine (Treanda) Busulfan (Myleran®, oral; Busulfex®, IV) Carboplatin (Paraplatin) *Carmustine (BiCNU, BCNU) Chlorambucil (Leukeran) Cisplatin (Cis-Platinum, CDDP, Platinol) Cyclophosphamide (Cytoxan, CTX, Neosar) Dacarbazine (DTIC-Dome, imidazole) Estramustine phosphate (Estracyte, Emcyt) Oxaliplatin (Eloxatin®) Ifosfamide (IFEX) *Lomustine (CCNU) Mechlorethamine hydrochloride (nitrogen mustard, mustargen, HN_2) Melphalan (Alkeran, 1-PAM, phenylalanine mustard) Oxaliplatin (Eloxatin) *Streptozocin (streptozotocin, Zanosar) Thiotepa (triethylene thiophosphoramide, TSPA) Trabectedin (Yondelis®)
Antibiotics	Use a variety of mechanisms to prevent cell division and death (DNA strand breakage, intercalation of base pairs, inhibition of RNA and DNA synthesis)	Dactinomycin (actinomycin D, Cosmegan) Daunorubicin hydrochloride (daunomycin, cerubidine) Doxorubicin hydrochloride (Adria, adriamycin) Epirubicin HCl (Ellenee) Idarubicin (Idamycin) Mithramycin (mithramycin, plicamycin) Mitomycin C (Mito, mutamycin) Mitoxantrone (Novantrone)

*Nitrosoureas (cross blood–brain barrier).

**Table 1.3   ASCO/ONS Chemotherapy Administration Safety Standards Highlights
(*See Document for Full Details)**

Standard Domain and Content

---

1. **Domain 1: Creating a Safe Environment: Staffing and General Policy**
   a) Staffing-related standards: policies and procedures and/or guidelines for verification of training and continuing education for clinical staff
   b) Informed consent is documented before beginning chemotherapy treatment.
2. **Domain 2: Treatment Planning, Patient Consent, and Education**
   a) Patients are provided with verbal and written/electronic information as part of their education before the first treatment (including patient diagnosis, goals of treatment, planned duration of treatment, potential short- and long-term adverse effects, symptoms that require immediate contact, safe handling, follow-up plans, and contact information for the healthcare setting).
   b) Oncology programs have a missed appointment policy and expectations for contact with the patient for more information and rescheduling.
   c) Patient and family education expectations.
3. **Domain 3: Ordering, Preparing, Dispensing, and Administering Chemotherapy**
   a) Standard chemotherapy regimens by diagnosis and references are defined.
   b) Chemotherapy orders are signed manually or electronically once approved by licensed independent practitioners (LIPs) who are determined to be qualified by the healthcare setting.
   c) Policy for managing chemotherapy orders that vary from the standard regimens is available with required supporting references and/or authorization by a second LIP. An exception order is documented in the medical record.
   d) The healthcare setting has a policy for chemotherapy orders that specify parameters (e.g., no verbal orders except to stop or hold chemotherapy administration; use of standardized, regimen-level preprinted or electronic forms for parenteral chemotherapy).
   e) Chemotherapy is prepared by a licensed pharmacist, pharmacy technician, physician, or RN who has documented education and competency validation for chemotherapy preparation.
   f) Specifics of independent double checks are identified: prior to drug preparation, after drug preparation, before drug administration.
   g) Policies and procedures for preparation of intrathecal medication, administration immediately after a time-out, and double-check procedure should be documented and followed.
   h) Policy for administration of vinca alkaloids by mini-bag in healthcare settings that administer IT medication(s) should be identified.
4. **Domain 4: Monitoring after Chemotherapy is Administered, Including Adherence, Toxicity, and Complications**
   a) Monitoring and assessment (e.g., protocol for life-threatening emergencies, policy/procedure to complete initial assessment of patient adherence to oral chemotherapy, patient assessment before chemotherapy, medication reconciliation)
   b) Policies that require tracking of cumulative drug doses for specific drugs; assessment of each patient's ongoing chemotherapy adherence and toxicity at each clinical encounter; and evaluation/documentation of treatment-related toxicities and communication prior to next scheduled chemotherapy administration.
   c) Chemotherapy is defined as all antineoplastic agents, parenteral and oral, and includes traditional chemotherapy and targeted agents.

Data from Neuss MN, Polovich M, McNiff K, et al. 2013 updated American Society of Oncology/Oncology Nursing Society Chemotherapy Administration Safety Standards Including Standards for the Safe Administration and Management of Oral Chemotherapy. *Oncol Nurs Forum* 2013; 40(3): 225–233.

initiated. Interestingly, topoisomerase I is found in greater concentrations in patients with cancers of the colon, non-Hodgkin's lymphoma, and some leukemias. Drugs such as topotecan and irinotecan work by inhibiting the religation or repair of the single-strand break by binding to topoisomerase I, and cells are arrested in the G_2 phase.

Topoisomerase II is also involved in the relaxation of the helix torsion, but it causes a double-strand break to allow crossing of two double-stranded DNA segments. It then causes the closing of the two DNA strand breaks. This permits assembly of chromatin, as well as condensation and decondensation of the chromosomes, and separation of the DNA in the daughter cells during mitosis. Drugs that are well known to interfere with topoisomerase II are etoposide (non-intercalator and cell cycle specific for M phase) and doxorubicin (intercalator of base pairs and cell cycle nonspecific) (Nitiss, 2009).

Descriptions of the drugs in the chapter have been updated to reflect new indications. Agents that have now been approved by the Food and Drug Administration (FDA) for use in cancer treatment have been updated.

EMERGING FRONTIERS

As our knowledge of genomics and proteogenomics grows, the promise of individualized cancer therapy increases. Although the human genome was decoded in 2003, this only opened the door to understanding each of the 20,000 different genes. As each individual—except for identical twins—has a unique genetic makeup, so too each individual with cancer has individual genetic features of the tumor. Genetic signatures have emerged showing the different types and responses of colon/rectal, breast, and lung cancers to therapy (Cowen et al., 2010). Already, microarray technology is used to identify genetic signatures within tumors that are likely to respond to given drug therapy and those that are not.

A question that has been answered is which women with node-negative, estrogen receptor-positive breast cancer should receive adjuvant chemotherapy. A report by the National Surgical Adjuvant Breast and Bowel Project revealed that a 21-gene recurrence assay is able to quantify and predict the magnitude of benefit from chemotherapy (tamoxifen compared with tamoxifen plus chemotherapy). Women with a low recurrence risk ($<18\%$) derived minimal if any benefit from chemotherapy, whereas women with high-risk tumors ($>31\%$) derived a large benefit (an absolute decrease in 10-year distant recurrence rate) of 27.6% (mean). Women with intermediate recurrence did not appear to derive a large benefit, but the study could not say that there was no benefit to receiving chemotherapy (Brufsky, 2014). As no two people have identical genetic makeups, their ability to metabolize drugs may also differ. Proteogenomics can help predict toxicity based on certain polymorphisms or different variations in a gene that is responsible for drug metabolism. Patients receiving irinotecan with a specific polymorphism have an increased risk of BM suppression. For example, tamoxifen is a prodrug, which is metabolized into its active metabolite in the liver via the cytochrome P450 CYP2D6 microenzyme system. In a recent study, women who were poor metabolizers of tamoxifen were 2.5 times more likely to have breast cancer recurrence or death than women with normal CYP2D6 (Goetz et al., 2012).

New technology has permitted a reduction in toxicity and/or increasing dosing from a number of drugs. For instance, nanotechnology to manufacture liposomal delivery vehicles for docetaxel, doxorubicin, daunorubicin, cytarabine, amphotericin, paclitaxel, and camptothecins is currently available or is being studied. The liposomal "wrapping" of water-soluble or -insoluble drugs permits the drug to be preferentially delivered to sites of infection, inflammation, or tumor. Liposomes may pass through gaps in the endothelial lining of blood capillaries within the tumor, where the drug may be unpackaged and released within the tumor. Healthy tissues, on the other hand, have capillary walls that prevent the leakage of liposomes into the tissues, so that toxicity is reduced. The targeting of liposomes for specific tissues or disease sites is accomplished by variation in the number of lipid layers, and the size, charge, and permeability of the layers. The future of nanotechnology has never been brighter, as new applications to drugs are studied. While molecular-targeted and immunologically targeted therapies continue to expand with great vigor, chemotherapy continues to play an important role in cancer care. Efforts are being made to try to find agents offering equal efficacy to parenteral chemotherapy that can improve quality of life, such as new oral antineoplastic agents, by minimizing trips to the hospital or intrusive administration techniques.

Within the last few years, interest and clinical testing of new approaches to old drugs has occurred. 5-Fluorouracil (5-FU) is an old drug that has good efficacy in colorectal cancer and other gastrointestinal cancers. However, it is limited, and increased doses are not necessarily more effective. Also, given by continuous infusion (CI), 5-FU is often more effective because, being cell cycle specific for the S phase, more malignant cells are likely to be exposed to CI of chemotherapy than if the drug is given by bolus injection.

In an effort to improve the efficacy, new oral fluoropyrimidines have been developed, along with other agents that decrease the breakdown of 5-FU, so that serum drug levels are higher and more sustained, mimicking a CI. An example of a prodrug is capecitabine (Xeloda). In an effort to reduce the toxicity of bolus 5FU/LV, de Gramont et al. (1997) showed that infusional 5FU/LV was equivalent or, in one study, superior, in efficacy but significantly less toxic. This has become the standard way to administer 5FU/LV in the United States at this time. Capecitabine is preferentially taken up by tumor cells. The drug has been approved for both the adjuvant treatment of patients with colon cancer, as well as patients with advanced metastatic breast and colorectal cancers. Capecitabine has been shown to be equivalent to 5FU/LV and is being used as a replacement in combination with oxaliplatin, irinotecan, or alone during radiotherapy. A new combination agent is trifluridine and tipiracil (Lonsurf). Trifluridine is a nucleoside metabolic inhibitor, and tipiracil is a thymidine phosphorylase inhibitor. Adding tipiracil to trifluridine increases trifluridine exposure by inhibiting its metabolism by thymidine phosphorylase. As an antimetabolite, the cell takes up trifluridine into its DNA, thinking it is uridine, and the false metabolite prevents DNA synthesis and cell proliferation. This has shown efficacy in colorectal cancer.

As the cancer treatment paradigm shifts toward the administration of oral chemotherapy as well as targeted agents, nurses must focus on patient safety, strategies to enhance adherence to prescribed therapy, and teaching patient/family to provide self-care, including notifying the provider of early toxicity. Successful treatment requires meticulous assessment of patient/family learning needs and styles, in addition to close telephone monitoring and triage of telephone calls. Other strategies may be useful in monitoring patient adherence, such as (1) giving the patients a detailed calendar showing the pill(s) to take each day/time, with small check boxes that they can check off as the dose is taken, (2) asking the patients to maintain a diary of dose administration and side effects, or (3) asking the patients to bring their pill bottles with them to each visit for a pill count. Studies are underway using electronic methods to monitor patient adherence.

Planned drug holidays in patients with advanced cancers are another changing paradigm. A number of studies in patients with advanced colorectal cancer (CRC) showed that more aggressive therapy with 5-FU, leucovorin (LV), and oxaliplatin (FOLFOX) for 6 cycles, followed by maintenance using 5-FU/LV only for 12 cycles, and then returning to FOLFOX compared with FOLFOX4 continuously resulted in similar overall survival, but with less neurotoxicity in the group receiving a period of maintenance (OPTIMOX1) (Tournigand et al., 2006); however, completely halting chemotherapy for a period of time resulted in earlier onset of progression. A similar study by Labianca et al. (2006) of patients with metastatic CRC looked at intermittent 5-FU, LV, and irinotecan (FOLFIRI) and found similar survival with less toxicity and cost in patients receiving intermittent FOLFIRI compared with those receiving continuous FOLFIRI.

Finally, national evidence-based treatment guidelines based on randomized clinical trials for patients with specific types of cancer have been promulgated, and studies are beginning to document patients who receive therapy based on these guidelines compared with those that do not have lower mortality. There is compelling evidence in the treatment of patients with colon and rectal cancer that older patients derive the same benefit from chemotherapy without greater toxicity (Cronin et al., 2006). Nurses need to advocate for older patients to consider carefully all treatment options to derive the maximal benefit.

Oncology nurses work very hard to prevent or minimize toxicity from chemotherapy agents in their patients. It is now apparent that certain patients have different abilities to metabolize certain drugs, called polymorphisms, or variability in the genes that are responsible for metabolizing the drug. For example, if a patient does not metabolize the drug as well due to a genetic factor, that patient will have more toxicity, such as neutropenia. Pharmacogenetics is an emerging field that will allow the use of knowledge of polymorphisms and drug-metabolizing enzymes to maximize the benefit and minimize the risk to patients. For example, 10% of the US population expresses the UGT1A1*28 polymorphism, which reduces the metabolism of SN-38, the active metabolite of irinotecan. This results in higher serum levels with more grades 3 and 4 neutropenia in those patients who should receive lower doses of irinotecan. Patients can be tested for this allele, or any patient who has a high bilirubin should be suspected, and a lower dose of the drug should be used initially. In addition, genetic profiling will assist in predicting responses to certain chemotherapy agents such as 5-FU/cisplatin combinations, 5-FU, oxaliplatin, and other agents.

Stimulated by the success of taxanes, epothilones were discovered, and the first, ixabepilone (Ixempra), is now FDA-approved for patients with advanced breast cancer who have progressed on paclitaxel. Epothilones are a class of natural substances that cause tubulin polymerization and stabilization similar to paclitaxel. However, these substances have activity in tumor cell lines that are resistant to paclitaxel due to mutations in beta-tubulin (Altmann, 2003). Another agent that interferes with the tumor cell in mitosis is Eribulin mesylate (Halaven), a non-taxane microtubular dynamics inhibitor, a product of a sea sponge. Although fewer chemotherapy agents are being developed that have collateral damage in normal, frequently dividing organ systems, many more targeted agents are being developed and are presented in *Chapter 5*.

Antineoplastic agents are classified by mechanism of action (see Table 1.2). Cell cycle–specific agents are most active during specific phases of the cell cycle and include antimetabolites (S or synthesis phase), vinca alkaloids (M or mitotic phase), and miscellaneous drugs. Examples of these include L-asparaginase and prednisone (G_1 phase) and bleomycin and etoposide (G_2 phase). In addition, effective drugs such as the taxanes, which have a clear mechanism of action at therapeutic doses, may in fact have an antiangiogenic effect at lower, more frequent dosing. Endothelial cells appear to be very sensitive to the taxanes.

Cell cycle-nonspecific agents can damage cells in all phases of the cell cycle and include alkylating agents (cyclophosphamide, cisplatin), antitumor/antibiotics (doxorubicin, mitomycin-C), the nitrosoureas (carmustine, lomustine), and others (dacarbazine, procarbazine) (see Table 1.2).

Antineoplastic agents are effective because they interfere with cellular metabolism and replication, resulting in cell death. When malignant cells mutate and develop mechanisms to evade programmed cell death, the tumor cells are no longer sensitive to the drug(s), and resistance emerges. Because of their mechanism of action, it is critical that nurses protect themselves when handling these drugs so that they are not exposed to the potential drug hazards. These drugs can be:

- *Mutagenic*: capable of causing a change in the genetic material within a cell that can be passed on to future cell generations
- *Teratogenic*: capable of causing damage to a developing fetus exposed to the drug; the greatest risk is during the first trimester of pregnancy when the fetal organ systems are developing
- *Carcinogenic*: capable of causing malignant change in a cell

In 1985, the Occupational Safety and Health Administration (OSHA) developed guidelines for the safe handling of antineoplastic agents. These guidelines were revised in 1995 and then again in 2004 to include all hazardous drugs (see *Appendix I*). NIOSH (2014) has updated recommendations as of March 2004 and issues periodic lists of hazardous antineoplastics. Despite nurses' knowledge about potential risks of hazardous drug (HD) exposure, studies continue to show suboptimal adherence to national guidelines (Polovich and Clark, 2012; Polovich and Martin, 2011). Callahan et al. (2016) conducted a study to identify factors associated with oncology nurses' use of HD safe-handling precautions in inpatient clinical research units. The authors found that while the nurses had high knowledge of risk and guideline recommendation, conflict of interest (participants perceived conflict between their drive to protect themselves and drive to provide medical care to patients) and perceived barriers to personal protective equipment (PPE) likely contributed to reduced adoption of PPE practices. In 2016, the U.S. Pharacopeial Convention (USP) published its own safe handling standards, known as USP 800, which are intended to improve protection of personnel and the environment when hazardous drugs are prepared or administered (USP, 2017). An in depth reply to frequently asked questions (FAQs) is found at http://www.usp.org/frequently-asked-questions/hazardous-drugs-handling-healthcare-settings (Updated October 2019). Compliance to these standards is required in July 2018 (Eisenberg, 2017).

Hormones are used in the management of hormonally sensitive cancers, such as breast and prostate cancers. The hormone changes the hormonal environment, probably affecting growth factors, so that the stimulus for tumor growth is suppressed or removed (see Table 1.4). New selective estrogen receptor modulators (SERMs) and aromatize inhibitors are being developed to improve on the demonstrated success of tamoxifen.

TREATMENT

Table 1.4   Common Hormonal Agents

Classification	Examples
Adrenocorticoids	cortisone hydrocortisone dexamethasone methylprednisone methylprednisolone prednisone prednisolone
Androgens	testosterone propionate (Neo-hombreol, Oreton)
Anti-androgens (nonsteroidal)	bicalutamide (Casodex) flutamide (Eulexin) nilutamide (Nilandron)
Androgen receptor inhibitors	enzalutamide (Xtandi)
Androgen biosynthesis inhibitors • CYP17 enzyme inhibitor (blocks other sources of androgen)	abiraterone (Zytiga®)
• Lutenizing hormone-releasing hormone analogue (LHRH analogue), LH-RH agonist	Goserelin acetate (Zoladex) Histrelin (Vantas implant) leuprolide acetate (Lupron, Lupron depot) Triptorelin (Trelstar)
Gonadatropic-releasing hormone antagonist (suppresses lutenizing hormone (LH) and follicle-stimulating hormone (FSH) and thereby decreases testes production of testosterone	Degarelix (Firmagon)
CYP17 enzyme inhibitor (blocks other sources of androgen, e.g., prostate cancer cells, adrenals)	Abiraterone (Zytiga)
Selective estrogen receptor modulators (SERMs) (Antiestrogen, nonsteroidal)	tamoxifen citrate (Nolvadex) toremifene citrate (Fareston) raloxifene (Evista)
Selective aromatase inhibitors (Antiestrogen, nonsteroidal) • Reversible	anastrozole (Arimidex) letrozole (Femara)
Selective aromatase inhibitor Antiestrogen (steroidal) • Irreversible	exemestane (Aromasin)
Antiestrogen, receptor antagonist	Fulvestrant (Faslodex)
Progesterones	medroxyprogesterone acetate (Provera, Depo-Provera) megestrol acetate (Megace, Pallace)

Lastly, as obesity becomes a national health problem, the question arises about calculating dosages accurately. Thompson et al. (2010) conducted a survey of oncologists and board-certified oncology pharmacists, via the Association of Community Cancer Centers and Board of Pharmaceutical Specialties, to determine current practices of empiric chemotherapy dose adjustments in obese patients. Of the 174 responses, 95% were returned by pharmacists, and of them, 50% practiced in academic medical centers. The most common methods used were (1) adjusted body weight in calculating BSA and (2) capping BSA. They found that indeed there was no standard of practice, but that decisions were determined based on intent to treat, degree of obesity, performance status, age, and type of medication. The American Society of Clinical Oncology (ASCO) developed clincial practice guidelines (Lyman, 2012) recommending that full weight-based cytotoxic chemotherapy doses be used, as they found no data to show increased toxicity at full weight-based dosing. They recommended further research into pharmacogenetics and the role of pharmacokinetics in obese patients.

COMPLICATIONS OF DRUG ADMINISTRATION

The most dreaded complications of antineoplastic drug administration are administering the drug to the wrong patient, administering an incorrect dose, or administering a drug via the incorrect route (e.g., IT instead of IV). For all of these reasons, it is critical that the nurse follow established safety standards. See Table 1.3 (Neuss et al., 2013; Polovich et al., 2014). In reviewing the drug profiles in this chapter, as well as *Chapters 3 and 4*, remember that the oncology nurse must double check the order against the received, prepared drug with another chemotherapy-competent RN or other professional. Many institutions require this to be an independent double check. In addition, the nurse together with another chemotherapy-competent RN must verify the patient prior to the chemotherapy-competent RN administering the drug. The patient should also be asked to verify the drug she/he is expecting to receive. The second chemotherapy-competent RN should also verify the pump settings for infusion when performing the chemotherapy double check prior to administration. If the oncology nurse is preparing the chemotherapy drug, an independent double check is required with a healthcare professional prior to mixing the drug. This means the nurse must get another competent oncology professional to independently double check the order (e.g., review the order, past chemotherapy the patient has received, cumulative dose of drugs such as doxorubicin, and relevant laboratory and testing, such as ECHO or MUGA scan results). Once the drug has been prepared and the ordered amount withdrawn in a syringe, the nurse should have another oncology nurse or pharmacist double check the amount of drug withdrawn, against the dilution and ordered amount, prior to the drug being further diluted in an infusion bag. The drug must be labeled as soon as it is prepared, either as a syringe for IVP or as an infusion bag. Intrathecal drugs should be prepared separately from other chemotherapy, identified with a specific intrathecal (IT) sticker, labeled, and placed in a container or space identified as only for IT medication. A rigorous identification process should surround the dispensing of the drug to the physician or NP/PA who is going to administer the drug, and only IT drugs should be dispensed at that time. In addition, at the bedside, there should be a "time-out" procedure. This is to prevent potentially lethal drug errors, such as IT administration of bortezomib (Velcade) or vincristine (Oncovin). It is much easier to prevent the error, because once administered, the drug cannot be taken back.

Complications include hypersensitivity reactions (HSRs) and extravasation. HSRs are mediated by an immune mechanism, IgE, and involve the release of vasoactive agents (e.g., histamine, leukotrienes, prostaglandins) by the mast cells in tissue and basophils in the blood *when exposed to a drug a second time, after prior exposure,* and thus, when the immune cells are sensitized. This results in contraction of smooth muscle and dilation of capillaries (Lenz, 2007). Patient response depends on the severity of the HSR, and ranges from rash to frank anaphylaxis. See Table 1.5. The systemic response is characterized by degrees of urticaria, rash, hypotension, more severe grade 3 bronchospasm (symptomatic, with angioedema), and grade 4 anaphylaxis, with profound vasomotor collapse. In contrast, some patients have a reaction, which may be severe, *on first exposure* to the drug. This reaction is not an immune reaction and is not mediated by IgE, but rather an *anaphylactoid* reaction, in which the drug or vehicle (e.g., Cremophor with paclitaxel) interacts with the mast cells and basophils, causing a release of the vasoactive agents; however, the end result is the same, and the nursing/medical interventions are the same whether the reaction is immune related or not. Thus, the nurse must be vigilant at all times when administering chemotherapy. Patients who have had hypersensitivity reactions to certain chemotherapy agents may be successfully desensitized and go on to complete their therapy (Feldweg et al., 2005).

All drugs can cause hypersensitivity reactions including anaphylaxis, but only a few drugs cause severe problems. These include the following:

- Paclitaxel (related to carrier vehicle solution Cremaphor)
- Docetaxel (related to delivery vehicle solution Tween)
- Cisplatin
- Carboplatin, oxaliplatin (delayed HSR, occurring around cycle 7)
- Teniposide (VumoM-26)
- Bleomycin (less common; 2% incidence in lymphoma patients)
- Cetuximab (Erbitux, discussed in *Chapter 4*), 3% incidence with most occurring on the first treatment, geographically related; may be fatal
- Rituximab (Rituxan, discussed in *Chapter 4*)
- Infliximab (Remicade, discussed in *Chapter 5*)

In addition, certain drugs can cause delayed hypersensitivity, such as carboplatin and oxaliplatin, where the patient develops a range of signs and symptoms of hypersensitivity after receiving a number of cycles of the drug, such as seven cycles of carboplatin. For nursing management of patients experiencing hypersensitivity or anaphylaxis, as recommended by the Oncology Nursing Society Practice Committee, see Table 1.5.

EXTRAVASATION

Specific chemotherapeutic drugs called *vesicants* may cause severe tissue necrosis if extravasated or inadvertently administered outside the vein. Some of these drugs have antidotes that will minimize or prevent local tissue damage. These are shown in Table 1.6. For a Standardized Nursing Care Plan for management of patients experiencing extravasation, see Table 1.7. It is imperative that the nurse be very careful when administering vesicant chemotherapy to minimize the chance of this occurring. The nurse carefully assesses the patient's response, the administration site, and patency of the IV site throughout the

Table 1.5   Management of Hypersensitivity (HSR), Anaphylactic Reaction, Cytokine Release Syndrome (CRS), and Anaphylactoid Reaction

1. Review the patient's allergy history. Patients with preexisting allergies are at increased risk.
2. Review drug(s) to be administered and risk for a reaction.
    A. **HSR (chemotherapy):** L-asparaginase, bleomycin (5% incidence in lymphoma patients), paclitaxel, docetaxel, cisplatin, carboplatin, oxaliplatin, etoposide.
    B. **HSR, CRS (biotherapy):** interferons, interleukin-2, denileukin diftitox, murine and chimeric MAbs; recognize that patients can still react to humanized and human MAbs.
3. Consider prophylactic medications with hydrocortisone and/or an antihistamine in atopic/allergic individuals. (This requires a physician's order.)
4. *Patient and family education:* Assess the patient's readiness to learn. Inform patient of the potential for an allergic reaction and instruct to report any unusual symptoms such as:
    A. Uneasiness or agitation
    B. Abdominal cramping
    C. Itching
    D. Chest tightness
    E. Light-headedness or dizziness
    F. Chills
5. Ensure that emergency equipment and medications are readily available.
6. Obtain baseline vital signs and note patient's mental status.
7. As appropriate, perform a scratch test, intradermal skin test, or test dose before administering the full dosage (this requires a physician's order). If there is no reaction, the remaining dose can be administered. If an allergic response is suspected, discontinue the test dose (unless it has been completed), maintain the intravenous line, and notify the physician.
8. For a *localized allergic response*:
    A. Evaluate symptoms; observe for urticaria, wheals, localized erythema.
    B. Administer diphenhydramine and/or hydrocortisone as per physician's order.
    C. Monitor vital signs every 15 minutes for 1 hour.
    D. Continue subsequent dosing or desensitization program according to a physician's order.
    E. If a "flare" reaction appears along the vein with doxorubicin (Adriamycin) or daunorubicin, flush the line with saline.
        a. Ensure that extravasation has not occurred.
        b. Administer hydrocortisone or diphenhydramine 25–50 mg intravenously with a physician's order, followed by a 0.9% NS flush. This may be adequate to resolve the "flare" reaction.
        c. Once the "flare" reaction has resolved, continue slow infusion of the drug.
        d. Monitor for repeated "flare" episodes. It is preferable to change the intravenous site if possible. Consider premedication with an antihistamine for subsequent cycles.
        e. Document specific observations, intervention, and patient response.
9. For a generalized allergic response, assess for the following signs or symptoms (these usually occur within the first 15 minutes of the start of the infusion or injection). Reaction can be either an *anaphylactoid (has never been exposed to the drug before) or anaphylaxis (severe hypersensitivity reaction after having received the drug before)*.
    A. Subjective signs and symptoms:
        a. Generalized itching
        b. Chest tightness
        c. Agitation
        d. Uneasiness

Table 1.5   (Continued)

  e. Dizziness
  f. Nausea
  g. Crampy abdominal pain
  h. Anxiety
  i. Sense of impending doom
  j. Desire to urinate or defecate
  k. Chills
 B. Objective signs:
  a. Flushed appearance (edema of face, hands, or feet)
  b. Localized or generalized urticaria
  c. Respiratory distress with or without wheezing
  d. Hypotension
  e. Cyanosis
  f. Difficulty speaking
10. For a *generalized allergic response:*
 A. Stop the infusion immediately and notify the physician.
 B. Maintain the intravenous line with appropriate solution to expand the vascular space, e.g., NS.
 C. If not contraindicated, ensure maximum rate of infusion if the patient is hypotensive.
 D. Position the patient to promote perfusion of the vital organs; the supine position is preferred.
 E. Monitor vital signs every 2 minutes until stable, then every 5 minutes for 30 minutes, then every 15 minutes as ordered.
 F. Reassure the patient and the family.
 G. Maintain the airway and anticipate the need for cardiopulmonary resuscitation.
 H. All medications must be administered with a physician's order.
 I. Anticipate administering the following medications for the following effects:
  a. Vasoconstriction to increase cardiac output and blood pressure, as well as bronchodilation to open the airway:
   1) epinephrine (1:1,000, 0.3–0.5 mL or 0.3–0.5 mg IM or subcutaneous q 10–15/min; or if hypotensive, 1:10,000 concentration giving 0.5–1.0 mL [0.1 mg] IVP in adults; in pediatrics, 1:1,000 0.01 mL/kg [up to 0.3 mL])
   2) dopamine 2–20 micrograms/kg/min (adults)
  b. Antihistamines to stop allergic release of histamines:
   1) diphenhydramine: 25–50 mg IVP (adults), 1 mg/kg (max 50 mg), pediatrics
   2) ranitidine 50 mg IV or famotidine 20 mg IV (adults)
  c. Bronchodilation: aminophylline 5 mg/kg IV over 30 min (adults)
  d. Anti-inflammation/bronchodilation: steroids. Hydrocortisone 100–500 mg IV (peds 1–2 mg/kg), or methylprednisolone 30–50 mg IV (peds 0.3–0.5 mg/kg), or dexamethasone 10–20 mg IVP (peds 1–2 mg/kg), or hydrocortisone 100–500 mg IV (peds 1–2 mg/kg)
11. Document the incident in the medical record according to institution policy and procedures.
12. Physician-guided desensitization may be necessary for subsequent dosing.

Data from Polovich M, Olsen M, LeFebvre KB (eds), *Chemotherapy and Biotherapy Guidelines and Recommendations for Practice.* 4th ed. Pittsburgh, PA: ONS; 2014: 163–168; Ellis AK, Day JH. Diagnosis and Management of Anaphylaxis. *Can Med Assoc J* 2003; 169(4): 307–312; Sheperd GM. Hypersensitivity Reactions to Chemotherapeutic Drugs. *Allergy Immunol* 2003; 24: 253–262.

Table 1.6   Vesicants and Irritants

		Vesicants		
Chemotherapeutic Agents	**Antidote**	**Antidote Preparation**	**Antidote and Local Care**	**Comments, Patient Monitoring, and Follow-Up**
Alkylating Agents				
Mechlorethamine (nitrogen mustard, Mustargen®)	Isotonic sodium (Na) thiosulfate	Prepare 1/6 molar solution 1. **10% Na thiosulfate** solution, mix 4 mL with 6 mL sterile water for injection. 2. **25% Na thiosulfate** solution, mix 1.6 mL with 8.4 mL sterile water. 3. Store at room temperature (15–30°C or 59–86°F).	1. Inject antidote (2 mL sodium thiosulfate solution for each mg of mechlorethamine extravasated) into subcutaneous (SC) tissue of the area of extravasation, using a 25- or 27-gauge needle (change needle with each injection). 2. Teach patient to a. apply ice for 6–12 hrs after antidote administration. b. elevate arm and hand, and to report swelling right away (peripheral extravasation).	1. Na thiosulfate neutralizes nitrogen mustard, forming thioesters, which are excreted via the kidneys. 2. Time is essential in treating extravasation. 3. Apply ice for 6–12 hours after antidote administered to minimize local reaction (Polovich et al., 2012). 4. Assess the extravasation area the next day for pain, blister formation, and desquamation; then in accordance with policy and clinical judgment. 5. Teach the patient/caregiver to monitor the extravasation site and call the practice right away if fever, chills, worsening pain, blistering, desquamation, swelling.
Trabectedin (Yondelis)	None known		1. Drug is administered via a central line only for a 24 hr CI. Although cold is nonevidence based, cold is suggested—15–20 min for at least 4 times a day × 24 hr. 2. Evidence of tissue necrosis may occur >1 week after extravasation (Janssen, 2015).	1. Assess the patency of line and insertion site at least every 4 hr during 24 hr infusion. Teach patient to call if any leakage, swelling, discomfort. Assess the extravasation area for pain, blister formation, and desquamation; then in accordance with policy and clinical judgment.

Table 1.6 *(Continued)*

Vesicants

Chemotherapeutic Agents	Antidote	Antidote Preparation	Antidote and Local Care	Comments, Patient Monitoring, and Follow-Up
				2. Teach the patient/caregiver to monitor the extravasation site and call the practice right away if fever, chills, worsening pain, blistering, desquamation, swelling.
Antitumor antibiotics				
Anthracyclines Doxorubicin (Adriamycin®) Daunorubicin (Cerubidine) Epirubicin (Ellence) Idarubicin (Idamycin)	Dexrazoxane	Drug may cause fetal harm if used during pregnancy; nursing mothers should discontinue nursing or discontinue the drug (Topotarget, 2011). Dexrazoxane **must be started within 6 hours of the extravasation.** Dose: Day 1: 1,000 mg/m^2 Day 2: 1,000 mg/m^2 Day 3: 500 mg/m^2; Maximum dose per day:	1. Apply cold pad with circulating ice water, ice pack, or Cryogel pack for 15–20 min at least 4 times a day until able to start antidote. 2. Remove ice at least 15 min prior to starting dexrazoxane. 3. DO NOT give with DMSO as this may worsen injury. 4. Use safe chemotherapy, safe handling, and administration precautions. 5. Administer IV over 1–2 hr in a large vein in the opposite arm unless contraindicated (e.g., lymphedema); in that case, use large vein distal to the extravasation site. 6. Give at about the same time each day × 3.	1. Dexrazoxane is a free-radical scavenger so protects tissue from free radical damage caused by anthracycline extravasation. Totect™ is FDA-approved for anthracycline extravasation but has been unavailable; The generic dexrazoxane has been shown to be effective (Arroyo et al., 2010). 2. Extravasations of less than 1–2 cc often will heal spontaneously. If greater than 3 cc, ulceration often results. 3. Assess the extravasation each day of dexrazoxane treatment: presence or worsening of pain, blister formation, desquamation; then in accordance with policy and clinical judgment.

(continues)

Table 1.6 *(Continued)*

		Vesicants		
Chemotherapeutic Agents	**Antidote**	**Antidote Preparation**	**Antidote and Local Care**	**Comments, Patient Monitoring, and Follow-Up**
		days 1, 2 is 2 g and on day 3 is 1 g. Dose-reduce 50% for impaired renal function (CrCl < 40 mL/min). Mix each 500 mg drug vial with 50 mL diluent, and further dilute in 1L NS. Use PPE in handling and administration of drug as it is hazardous (e.g., chemo gown and gloves). Store at room temperature (15–30°C or 59–86°F).	7. Teach patient about self-care measures and side effects of dezrazoxane: nausea, vomiting, stomatitis, BMD, elevated LFTs, burning at the infusion site.	4. Teach the patient/caregiver to elevate the affected arm/hand, to monitor the extravasation site, and to call the practice right away if fever, chills, worsening pain, blistering, desquamation, or arm/hand stiffening or swelling occurs. 5. Teach patient to protect the extravasation site from sunlight and heat. 6. Discuss frequency of assessing cbc/plt, LFTs after administering dexrazoxane with physician or NP/PA. 7. Most common adverse effects of dexrazoxane are nausea, pyrexia, injection-site pain, and vomiting. 8. If drug is given in a clinic setting, anticipate how and where dexrazoxane will be administered if the extravasation occurs on a Thursday or Friday as the drug must be given 3 days in a row.

Table 1.6 *(Continued)*

Chemotherapeutic Agents	Antidote	Vesicants		Comments, Patient Monitoring, and Follow-Up
		Antidote Preparation	Antidote and Local Care	
Other Antitumor Antibiotics				
Mitomycin (mitomycin-C, Mutamycin®)	None known		1. Apply ice pack 15–20 min at least 4 times a day, for the first 24 hours, to increase comfort at the site. 2. Elevate for 48 hours, then resume normal activity.	1. Protect from sunlight. 2. Delayed skin reactions have occurred in areas far from original IV site. 3. Assess the extravasation area the next day for pain, blister formation, desquamation, then in accordance with policy and clinical judgment. 4. Teach the patient/caregiver to elevate the affected arm/hand, to monitor the extravasation site, and to call the practice right away if fever, chills, worsening pain, blistering, desquamation, or arm/hand stiffening or swelling occurs. 5. Discuss with physician or NP/PA referral to specialists as needed (e.g., plastic/hand surgeon, OT/PT, pain management).
Anthracenedione Mitoxantrone (concentrated dose) [Novantrone]	Unknown		1. Apply ice pack 15–20 min at least 4 times a day, for the first 24 hours, to increase comfort at the site. 2. Teach patient to elevate arm/hand.	1. Antidote and local care measures unknown. 2. Ulceration rare unless concentrated dose infiltrates. 3. Drug is blue and causes blue skin discoloration.

(continues)

Table 1.6   *(Continued)*

Chemotherapeutic Agents	Vesicants			
	Antidote	Antidote Preparation	Antidote and Local Care	Comments, Patient Monitoring, and Follow-Up
				4. Assess the extravasation area for pain, blister formation, desquamation, arm or hand stiffening or swelling the next day, then in accordance with policy and clinical judgment. 5. Teach the patient/caregiver to monitor the extravasation site and call the practice right away if fever, chills, worsening pain, blistering, desquamation, or hand stiffening or swelling occurs. 6. Discuss with physician or NP/PA referral to specialists as needed (e.g., plastic/hand surgeon, OT/ PT, pain management).
Vinca alkaloids/ microtubular inhibiting agents Vincristine (Oncovin®e) Vinblastine (Velban®e) Vinorelbine (Navelbine®f) Now, vinca alkaloids are administered via mini-bag in healthcare settings that also prepare and administer IT medications (Neuss et al., 2017).	Hyaluronidase	Hyaluronidase Amphadase (bovine): Vial contains 150 units per 1 mL: use undiluted; store in refrigerator at 2–8°C (36–46°F).	1. Administer 1 mL of hyaluronidase solution as five separate injections, each containing 0.2 mL of hyaluronidase into the area of extravasation, using a 25- or 27-gauge needle (change needle with each injection).	1. Hyaluronidase is an enzyme that degrades hyaluronic acid so that extravasated drug diffuses away from site of injury and is absorbed. 2. Assess the extravasation area for pain, blister formation, desquamation, hand/ arm swelling the next day, then in accordance with policy and clinical judgment.

Table 1.6 *(Continued)*

		Vesicants	
Chemotherapeutic Agents	Antidote	Antidote Preparation	Antidote and Local Care	Comments, Patient Monitoring, and Follow-Up
		Hydase: Vial contains 150 units per 1 mL: use undiluted; store in refrigerator at 2–8°C (36–46°F). Hylenex: Vial contains 150 units per 1 mL: use undiluted; store in refrigerator at 2–8°C (36–46°F). Vitrase (bovine): Vial contains 200 units per 1 mL: Dilute 0.75 mL solution with 0.25 mL 0.9% sodium chloride (final concentration is 150 units per 1 mL); store in refrigerator at 2–8°C (36–46°F).	2. Apply warm pack for 15–20 min at least 4 times per day for the first 24–48 hours and elevate arm/hand.	3. Teach the patient/caregiver to monitor the extravasation site and call the practice right away if fever, chills, worsening pain, blistering, desquamation, arm/hand swelling or stiffness occurs.

(continues)

Table 1.6   (*Continued*)

Vesicants

Chemotherapeutic Agents	Antidote	Antidote Preparation	Antidote and Local Care	Comments, Patient Monitoring, and Follow-Up
Taxanes				
Paclitaxel (Taxol®a) Docetaxel (Taxotere®) Paclitaxel protein-bound particles for injectable suspension) (albumin-bound) [Abraxane].	None	None known	Apply ice pack for 15–20 min at least 4 times per day for the first 24 hours.	1. Paclitaxel: injection-site reactions, including those following extravasation: – are usually mild (erythema, tenderness, skin discoloration, swelling at injection site). Recall of skin reactions can occur. – more severe events have been reported (phlebitis, cellulitis, induration, skin exfoliation, necrosis, fibrosis), which may be delayed up to 7–10 days from date of extravasation (Teva, 2012). 2. Docetaxel infusion-site reactions are generally mild (hyperpigmentation, inflammation, erythema, skin dryness, extravasation, phlebitis or swelling of the arm) [Sanofi-aventis, 2015]. 3. Abraxane® may cause phlebitis, cellulitis, induration, ncecrosis, and fibrosis during or up to 7–10 days after a prolonged infusion. Recall may occur at a prior site of paclitaxel injection. Abraxane infusion should be infused over 30 minutes to reduce infusion-related adverse reactions (Celgene, 2018).

Table 1.6 *(Continued)*

Vesicants

Chemotherapeutic Agents	Antidote	Antidote Preparation	Antidote and Local Care	Comments, Patient Monitoring, and Follow-Up
				4. Assess the extravasation area the next day for pain, blister formation, desquamation, hand/arm swelling and stiffness, then in accordance with policy and clinical judgment.
				5. Teach the patient/caregiver to
				a. apply ice pack (per local care above)
				b. monitor the extravasation site and call the practice right away if fever, chills, worsening pain, blistering, desquamation, arm/hand swelling or stiffness occurs.

Irritants

Chemotherapeutic Agents	Antidote	Antidote Preparation	Antidote and Local Care	Comments, Patient Monitoring, and Follow-Up
Alkylating agents				
Bendamustine hydrochloride (Treanda®)				1. May cause erythema, marked swelling and pain; dilution in 500 mL and infusion over 1–2 hours reduces venous irritation (Watanabe et al., 2013).
Dacarbazine (DTIC)				1. May cause phlebitis.
				2. Protect drug from sunlight.
Ifosfamide Carboplatin				1. May cause phlebitis.
				2. Antidote or local care measures unknown.

(continues)

Table 1.6   *(Continued)*

			Vesicants	
Chemotherapeutic Agents	**Antidote**	**Antidote Preparation**	**Antidote and Local Care**	**Comments, Patient Monitoring, and Follow-Up**
Melphalan (Alkeran®)				1. Consider using a CL if the patient has poor venous access (GlaxoSmithKline, 2014).
Oxaliplatin (however, has vesicant potential)				1. Oxaliplatin has vesicant potential, so is best given via CL, although care must be taken as it can still extravasate from a CL. If oxaliplatin given via peripheral line, drug can be diluted in 500 mL D5W (Sanofi-aventis, 2015) and infused over 6 hours to decrease discomfort.
				2. High-dose dexamethasone can reduce inflammation in the event of extravasation (Kretzschman et al., 2003). Topical heat may reduce discomfort.
Antitumor antibiotics				
Daunorubicin citrate (DaunoXome®)				1. May cause pain or burning at IV site.
				2. Antidote or local care measures unknown.
Nitrosoureas				
Carmustine (BCNU)				1. Diluent is absolute alcohol and may cause phlebitis. Local care measures are unknown.
				2. Antidote or local care measures unknown.

Table 1.6 *(Continued)*

Chemotherapeutic Agents	Vesicants			Comments, Patient Monitoring, and Follow-Up
	Antidote	Antidote Preparation	Antidote and Local Care	
Antitumor antibiotics				
Doxorubicin liposome (Doxil®)				1. May produce redness and tissue edema. 2. Low ulceration potential. 3. If ulceration begins or pain, redness, or swelling persist, treat like doxorubicin.
Bleomycin (Blenoxane®)				1. May cause irritation to tissue. 2. Little information known.
Epipodophyllotoxin				
Etoposide (VP-16)			Apply warm pack.	1. Treatment necessary only if large amount of a concentrated solution extravasates. In this case, treat like vincristine or vinblastine. 2. May cause phlebitis, urticaria, and redness.

[a] Bristol-Myers Squibb Oncology, Princeton, NJ.
[b] Pharmacia & Upjohn Co, Kalamazoo, MI.
[c] Chiron Therapeutics, Emeryville, CA.
[d] Andria Laboratories, Dublin, OH.
[e] Eli Lilly and Co., Indianapolis, IN.
[f] Glaxo Wellcome Oncology/HIV, Research Triangle Park, NC.

Data from Lundbeck ILC. Mustargen [package insert]. Deerfield, IL. 2012; Polovich M, Olsen M, LeFebvre KB (eds), *Chemotherapy and Biotherapy Guidelines and Recommendations for Practice*, 4th ed. Pittsburgh, PA: ONS; 2014: 155–163; Polovich M, White JM, Kelleher LO. *Chemotherapy and Biotherapy Guidelines and Recommendations for Practice*, 2nd ed. Pittsburgh, PA: Oncology Nursing Society; 2005: 34; Griffin-Sobel JP. *Clin J Oncol Nurs* 2005; 9(5): 510; Sanofi-aventis US, LLC. Taxotere [package insert]. Bridgewater, NJ. December 2015; Hospira, Inc. Paclitaxel Injection [package insert]. Lake Forest, IL. July 2013; Bedford Labs. Dexrazoxane [package insert]. Bedford, OH. June 2010; TopoTarget USA. Totect [package insert]. Rockaway, NJ. November 2009; Janssen, Inc. Yondelis (trabectedin) [package insert]. Horsham, PA. October 2015.
Note: Generic dexrazoxane (Bedford Labs) and Totect® (Bedford Labs) and Totect® are reconstituted with sodium lactate. Zinecard® (dexrazoxane) must be reconstituted with sterile water.

Table 1.7   Standardized Nursing Care Plan for Management of the Patient Experiencing Extravasation

Nursing Diagnosis	Defining Characteristics	Expected Outcomes	Nursing Interventions

I. Potential alteration in skin integrity related to extravasation.	I. Vesicant drugs may cause erythema, burning, tissue necrosis, tissue sloughing.	I. Extravasation, if it occurs, is detected early with early intervention to minimize severity and extent of injury.	I. Careful technique is used during venipuncture.
			  A. Select venipuncture site away from underlying tendons and blood vessels.
			  B. Secure IV so that catheter/needle site is visible at all times.
			  C. Administer vesicant through freely flowing IV, constantly monitoring IV site, blood return, and patient response. Nurse should be thoroughly familiar with institutional policy and procedure for administration of a vesicant agent, and management of extravasation.
			  D. If vesicant drug is administered as a CI, drug must be given through a patent central line and monitored closely.

II. Potential pain at site of extravasation.	II. Vesicant drugs include:
	  A. Commercial agents
	    1. dactinomycin
	    2. daunorubicin
	    3. doxorubicin
	    4. mitomycin C
	    5. estramustine
	    6. mechlorethamine
	    7. vinblastine
	    8. vincristine
	    9. vinorelbine
	    10. idarubicin
	    11. vindesine
		II. Skin and underlying tissue damage is minimized.	II. If extravasation is suspected:
			  A. Stop drug administration.
			  B. Aspirate any residual drug and blood from IV tubing, IV catheter/needle, IV site if possible.
			  C. Instill antidote, if one exists, through needle if able to remove remaining drug in previous step. If standing orders are not available, notify MD and obtain order.
			  D. Remove needle.
			  E. Inject antidote into area of apparent infiltration, if antidote is recommended, using 25-gauge needle into subcutaneous tissue.
			  F. Apply topical cream if recommended.
			  G. Cover lightly with occlusive sterile dressing.
			  H. Apply warm or cold applications as prescribed.
			  I. Elevate arm.

Table 1.7 *(Continued)*

Nursing Diagnosis	Defining Characteristics	Expected Outcomes	Nursing Interventions
	12. epirubicin 13. esorubicin 14. cisplatin (if concentrated) 15. mitoxantrone 16. paclitaxel (if concentrated) 17. fluorouracil (if concentrated) 18. Trabectedin		J. Assess site regularly for pain, progression of erythema, induration, and for evidence of necrosis: 1. If outpatient, arrange to assess site or teach patient to and to notify provider if condition worsens. Arrange next visit for assessment of site depending on drug, amount infiltrated, extent of potential injury, and patient variables. Some vesicants, e.g., trabectedin and vincristine, may not show tissue necrosis for > 1 week after drug extravasation. 2. Discuss with MD the need for plastic-surgical consult if erythema, induration, pain, tissue breakdown occurs. 3. Assess the extravasation area the next day for pain, blister formation, and desquamation; then in accordance with policy and clinical judgment. 4. Teach the patient/caregiver to monitor the extravasation site and call the practice right away if fever, chills, worsening pain, blistering, desquamation. 5. Document monitoring plan and follow up concisely. K. When in doubt about whether drug is infiltrating, treat as an infiltration.

(continues)

Table 1.7 *(Continued)*

Nursing Diagnosis	Defining Characteristics	Expected Outcomes	Nursing Interventions
			L. Document precise, concise information in patient's medical record:
			1. Date, time
			2. Insertion site, needle size, and type
			3. Drug administration technique, drug sequence, and approximate amount of drug extravasated
			4. Appearance of site, patient's subjective response
			5. Nursing interventions performed to manage extravasation, and notification of MD
			6. Photo documentation if possible
			7. Follow-up plan
			8. Nurse's signature
			9. Institutional policy and procedure for documentation should be adhered to

III. Potential loss of function of extremity related to extravasation.

IV. Potential infection related to skin breakdown.

Data from Polovich M, Whitford JM, Olsen M (eds). *Chemotherapy and Biotherapy Guidelines and Recommendations for Practice*, 4th ed. Pittsburgh, PA: ONS; 2014: 155–163; Janssen, Inc. Yondelis (trabectedin) [package insert]. Horsham, PA. October 2015.

administration of the vesicant agent. If ever in doubt whether or not a drug is extravasating, treat it as an extravasation to minimize potential tissue damage to the patient; then, start another IV in the patient's other arm, and continue the drug administration.

When vesicants are administered as a CI, a central line (CL) is required. In addition, it is imperative that the CV insertion site be checked for signs/symptoms of extravasation regularly, and that the patient be instructed to tell the nurse immediately if leakage, stinging, or burning is felt. As many CIs of vesicant chemotherapy occur when the patient is at home, it is again imperative to instruct the patient to pay attention to any changes in sensation at the site, and to call the nurse if any discomfort, stinging, burning, or leakage is felt. A number of patients have had extravasation of drug from a huber needle dislodged from an implanted port, onto or under the surrounding skin, which then caused a necrotic ulcer and necessitated explantation of the subcutaneous port. Dexrazoxane for injection (Totect™) was approved for the treatment of doxorubicin extravasations. It works as a free radical scavenger and may inhibit topoisomerase II irreversibly (Mouridsen et al., 2007; Schulmeister, 2007). As Totect™ is not actively marketed at this time and is unavailable, the generic equivalent dexrazoxane is commonly used (ASHP, 2016). However, the drug in itself is cytotoxic, expensive, and must be administered within 6 hours of the extravasation. The drug is given as an infusion daily for 3 days.

Within the last decade, oncology nurses have been humbled by the reports of significant and lethal errors that have occurred during the chemotherapy prescription, admixing, and administration processes. It is clear that institutional and physician office practices must have a systematic review of the entire linked process and take steps to prevent the occurrence of these errors and tragic consequences through competent checks and balances. Fortunately, the series of well-publicized errors has been a "wake-up" call, and oncology nurses, pharmacists, and physicians have worked together to develop safe environments for clinical practice. The Oncology Nursing Society position paper, "Regarding the Preparation of the Professional Registered Nurse Who Administers and Cares for the Individual Receiving Chemotherapy," states that the nurse administering chemotherapy and caring for patients receiving chemotherapy should complete a chemotherapy course and clinical practicum to deliver chemotherapy safely and competently. The course topics should include history of cancer chemotherapy; drug development; principles of cancer chemotherapy; chemotherapy preparation, storage, and transport; nursing assessment; chemotherapy administration; safety precautions during chemotherapy administration; disposal/accidental exposure and spills; and, finally, institutional considerations (ONS Position Paper, 2012; Polovich, 2011; NIOSH Safe Handling of Hazardous Drugs, June 2014).

In an effort to recognize and encourage quality in the care of oncology patients, ASCO and ONS have joined together to issue "Chemotherapy Administration Safety Standards," which specify for the first time in 2008 the expected standards in providing chemotherapy to patients in the outpatient setting. These guidelines are now being applied to inpatient settings and pediatric settings (Neuss et al., 2017). See Table 1.3. Further, ASCO's Quality Oncology Practice Initiative (QOPI) ensures that these standards are supported in the oncologist-led, practice-based quality improvement program.

Finally, in the last decade, we have seen new challenges. As the frequency of cancer chemotherapy treatments has increased, so has the demand for these drugs, leading to drug shortages. In 2013, up to 83% of oncologists have experienced a drug shortage (Gogineni et al., 2013). In the study, 78% of oncologists reported treating the patient with a different drug or drug regimen, 77% substituted different drugs partway through therapy, 43% had to delay treatment, 37% had to choose among patients who need a particular drug, 29% omitted doses, 20% gave reduced doses, and 17% referred patients to another practice. Clearly, the drug shortage is interfering with high-quality cancer care in the United States.

In the past, a Drug Shortages Summit was convened by ASHP, the Institute for Safe Medication Practices (ISMP), the American Society of Anesthesiologists, and the American Society of Clinical Oncology (ASCO). The group found that in addition to increased demand for some of the drugs, fewer manufacturers are producing sterile injectables, and most are generic. Not only does this decrease the manufacture of some of the drugs, but two of the largest manufacturers of sterile injectables were forced to shut down some production lines in 2010 due to inadequate quality-control standards, further reducing supply of the products (Drug Shortages Summit Summary Report, 2010). The ASHP has been instrumental in monitoring drugs in short supply, identifying those that have been resolved, and providing guidance for hospitals and health systems. Today, the shortage is often of common generic chemotherapy drugs, forcing physicians to substitute more expensive brand name drugs or similar drugs that may not have the supporting clinical trial evidence to support it. In addition, supportive medications such as antiemetics may also be in short supply. Deciding which patient will receive a scarce chemotherapy drug raises ethical and moral issues. The drug shortage has affected both adult and pediatric cancer patients alike. Pediatric oncologists developed a guideline embracing an ethical framework for rationing scarce, potentially lifesaving drugs to children with cancer (Unguru et al., 2016). The ASHP website listing current drug shortages is available at http://www.ashp.org/Drug-Shortages/Current-Shortages.

References

AbbVie Inc. Lupron (leuprolide acetate for depot suspension) [package insert]. North Chicago, IL. January 2019.

Abraxis Bioscience LLC, Celgene Corp. Abraxane (paclitaxel-protein bound particles for injectable suspension) [package insert]. Summit, NJ. August 2018.

Actavis Pharma, Inc. Fludarabine phosphate [package insert]. Parsippany, NJ. June 2014.

Allergan USA, Inc. Trelstar (triptorelin pamoate for injectable suspension) [package insert]. Madison NJ. December 2018.

Altmann KH. Epothilone B and Its Analogues—A New Family of Anticancer Agents. *Mini Rev Med Chem* 2003 Mar; 3(2): 149–158.

Alza Pharmaceuticals and Janssen Products LP. Doxil (doxorubicin HCl liposome injection) [package insert]. Horsham, PA. April 2017.

American Society of Hospital Pharmacists. Dexrazoxane injection. Available at http://www.ashp.org /menu/DrugShortages/CurrentShortages/bulletin.aspx?id=415. Accessed August 27, 2016.

ANI Pharmaceuticals, Inc. Nilandron (nilutamide) [package insert]. Baudette, MN. December 2015.

APP Pharmaceuticals, LLC. Floxuridine for Injection, USP [package insert]. Schamburg, IL. August 2012.

APP Pharmaceuticals, LLC. Vinblastine [package insert]. Scheumburg, IL. January 2012.

Arroyo PA, Perez RU, Feijoo MAF, et al. Good Clinical and Cost Outcomes using Dexrazoxane to Treat Accidental Epirubicin Extravasation. *J Cancer Res* 2010; 6: 573–574.

Aslex Pharmaceutical Inc. Dacogen (decitabine) [package insert]. Dublin, CA. October 2014.

Aspen Global Incorporated. Leukeran (chlorambucil) [package insert]. Grand Bay, Mauritius [distributed by Prasco Labs, Mason, OH]. February 2016.

Astellas Pharma Inc. Xtandi (enzalutamide) [package insert]. Northbrook, IL. October 2016.

AstraZeneca. Arimidex (anastrazole) [package insert]. Wilmington, DE. May 2014.

AstraZeneca Pharmaceuticals, LLP. Casodex (bicalutamide) [package insert]. Wilmington, DE. November 2017.

AstraZeneca Pharmaceuticals, Inc. Faslodex (fulvestrant injection) [package insert]. Wilmington, DE. March 2019.

AstraZeneca Pharmaceuticals, LLP. Zoladex 3.6-mg (goserlin acetate implant) [package insert]. Wilmington, DE. July 2016.

AstraZeneca Pharmaceuticals, LLP. Zoladex 10.8-mg (goserlin acetate implant) [package insert]. Wilmington, DE. February 2016.

Aubert RE, Stanek EJ, Yao J, et al. Risk of Breast Cancer Recurrence in Women Initiating Tamoxifen with CYP2D6 Inhibitors. *J Clin Oncol* 2009; 27:18s (suppl; abst CRA 508).

Baxter Healthcare Corp. Cyclophosphamide [package insert]. Deerfield, IL. May 2013.

Baylin SB, Herman JG, Graff JR, et al. Alterations in DNA Methylation—A Fundamental Aspect of Neoplasia. *Adv Cancer Res* 1998; 72: 141–196.

Bedford Laboratories. VinBLAStine sulfate [package insert]. Bedford, OH, April 2014.

Bristol-Myers Squibb Co. Hydrea (hydroxyurea) [package insert]. Princeton, NJ. December 2017.

Bristol-Myers Squibb Co. Etopophos (etoposide) [package insert]. Princeton, NJ. May 2017.

Brufsky AM. Predictive and Prognostic Value of the 21-Gene Recurrence Score in Hormone Receptor-positive, Node-positive Breast Cancer. *Am J Clin Oncol* 2014; 37(4): 404–410.

Callahan A, Ames NJ, Manning ML, et al. Factors Influencing Nurses' Use of Hazardous Drug Safe -handling Precautions. *Oncol Nurs Forum* 2016; 43(3): 342–349.

Camp-Sorrell D. Chemotherapy Toxicities and Management. *Chapter 17* in Yarbro CH, Frogge MH, Goodman M. *Cancer Nursing: Principles and Practice,* 6th ed. Sudbury, MA: Jones and Bartlett Publishers; 2005; 412–458.

Caraco Pharmaceutical Laboratories, Ltd. Doxorubicin hydrochloride liposome injection for intravenous infusion [package insert]. Detroit MI, September 2012.

Celgene Corporation. Abraxane (protein-bound paclitaxel particles for injectable suspension) [package insert]. Summit, NJ. August 2018.

Celgene Corporation. Vidaza (azacitidine for injection) [package insert]. Summit, NJ. March 2016.

Centers for Disease Control and prevention (CDC). The National Institute for Occupational Safety and Health (NIOSH). NIOSH list of antineoplastic and other hazardous drugs in healthcare settings: proposed additions to the NIOSH hazardous drug list 2016. Available at https://www.cdc.gov /niosh/docs/2016-161/default.html. Accessed October 15, 2019.

Cephalon, Inc. Trisenox (arsenic trioxide) [package insert]. North Wales, PA. February 2015.

Cephalon, Inc. Treanda (bendamustine) [package insert]. North Wales, PA. March 2015.

Chen AY, Liu LF. DNA Topoisomerases: Essential Enzymes and Lethal Targets. *Annu Rev Pharmacol Toxicol* 1994; 34: 191–218.

Chen HY, et al. 5 Gene Pattern Predicts NSCLC Outcome. *New Engl J Med* 2007; 356: 11–20.

Chu E, DeVita VT. *Physicians' Cancer Chemotherapy Drug Manual 2016*. Burlington, MA. Jones and Bartlett Learning, 2016.

Connor TH, MacKenzie BA, DeBord DG, et al. *NIOSH List of Antineoplastic and Other Hazardous Drugs in Healthcare Settings 2014*. Cincinnati OH: US Department of Health and Human Services, Centers for Disease Control and Prevention, National Institute for Occupational Safety and Health, DHHS (NIOSH) Publication No. 2014-138 (Supercedes 2012-150). September 2014.

Cowen PA, Anglesio M, Etemadmoghadam D, Bowtell DL. Profiling the Cancer Genome. *Ann Rev of Genomics and Human Genetics* 2010; 11: 133–159.

Cronin DP, Harlan LC, Potosky AL, et al. Patterns of Care for Adjuvant Therapy in a Random Population-Based Sample of Patients Diagnosed with Colorectal Cancer. *Am J Gastroenterol* 2006; 101(10): 2308–2318.

Davies C, Pan H, Goodwin J, et al. Long-term Effects of Continuing Adjuvant Tamoxifen to 10 years versus Stopping at 5 years after Diagnosis of Oestrogen Receptor-positive Breast Cancer: AT-LAS, a Randomized Trial. *Lancet* 2013; 381(9869): 805–816.

Drug Shortages Summit Members. Drug Shortages Summit Summary Report, November 5, 2010. Available at https://www.ashp.org/-/media/assets/news-and-media/docs/media-story-ideas-drug-shortages-summit.ashx. Accessed October 15, 2019.

Eisai Inc. Gliadel (carmustine implant) [package insert]. Woodcliff Lake, NJ. August 2013.

Eisai Inc. Havalen (eribulin mesylate) [package insert]. Woodcliff Lake, NJ: Eisai Inc. December 2017.

Eisenberg S. Hazardous Drugs and USP 800: Implications for Nurses. *Clin J Oncol Nurs* 2017; 21(2): 179–187.

Ekholm M, Bendahl P-O, Ferno M, et al. Two Years of Adjuvant Tamoxifen Provides a Survival Benefit compared with No Systemic Treatment in Premenopausal Patients with Primary Breast Cancer: Long-term Follow-up (>25 years) of the Phase III SBII:2pre Trial. *J Clin Oncol* 2016; Published online before print May 9, 2016, doi: 10.1200/JCO.2015.65.6272; *JCO* May 9, 2016, JCO656272.

Eli Lilly and Co. Alimta (pemetrexed disodium heptahydrate injection, powder, for solution) [package insert]. Indianapolis, IN. January 2019.

Eli Lilly and Co. Gemzar (gemcitabine) [package insert]. Indianapolis, IN. December 2018.

Endo Pharmaceuticals Solutions Inc. Vantas (histrelin acetate implant) [package insert]. Malvern, PA. June 2017.

Endo Pharmaceuticals Solutions Inc. Valstar (valrubicin) [package insert]. Malvern, PA. May 2017.

Ferring Pharmaceuticals. Firmagon (degarelix) [package insert]. Parsippany, NJ. May 2017.

Fresenius Kabi USA, LLC. Cladribine injection [package insert]. Lake Zurich, IL. August 2014.

Fresenius Kabi USA, LLC. Melphalan HCl [package insert]. Lake Zurich, IL. August 2016.

Galen US Inc. DaunoXome (Liposomal daunorubicin) [package insert]. Souderton, PA. December 2011.

Genentech USA Inc. Xeloda (capecitabine) [package insert]. South San Francisco, CA. December 2016.

Genzyme Corp. Clofar (clofarabine) [package insert]. Cambridge, MA. December 2015.

GlaxoSmithKline. Arranon (nelarabine) [package insert]. Research Triangle Park, NC. December 2014.

Goetz MP, Suman V, Hoskin TL, et al. CYP2D6 Metabolism and Patient Outcome in the Austrian Breast and Colorectal Cancer Study Group Trial (ABCSG) 8. *Clin Cancer Res* 2012; doi: 10.1158/1078-0432.CCR-12-2153.

Gogineni K, Schuman KL, Emanuel EJ. Survey of Oncologists about Shortages of Cancer Drugs: Letter to the Editor. *N Engl J Med* 2013; 369(25): 2463–2463.

Griggs JJ, Mangu PB, Anderson H, et al. Appropriate Chemotherapy Dosing for Obese Adult Patients with Cancer: American Society of Clinical Oncology Practice Guideline. *J Clin Oncol* 2012; 30(13): 1553–61.

Heritage Pharmaceuticals. BiCNU (carmustine) [package insert]. Eatontown, NJ. November 2013.

Hospira, Inc. Blenoxane (Bleomycin) [package insert]. Lake Forest, IL. January 2013.

Hospira, Inc. Carboplatin injection, solution [package insert]. Lake Forest, IL. August 2015.

Hospira, Inc. Cytarabine injection, solution [package insert]. Lake Forest, IL. January 2015.

Hospira, Inc. Dacarbazine for injection [package insert]. Lake Forest, IL. January 2016.

Hospita, Inc. Methotrexate [package insert]. Lake Forest, IL. June 2018.

Hospira, Inc. Mitoxantrone for injection [package insert]. Lake Forest, IL. May 2018.

Hospira, Inc. Paclitaxel injection [package insert]. Lake Forest, IL. May 2018.

Hospira, Inc. Vincristine injection [package insert]. Lake Forest, IL. January 2017.

Ipsen Biopharmaceuticals, Inc. Onidyve (irinotecan, liposomal) [package insert]. Basking Ridge, NJ. June 2017.

Ipsen Biopharmaceuticals, Inc. Somatuline Depot (lanreotide) [package insert]. Basking Ridge, NJ. April 2019.

Janssen Pharma. Zytiga (abiraterone acetate) tablets [package insert]. Horsham, PA. April 2018.

Janssen Products LP. Yondelis (trabectedin) [package insert]. Horsham, PA. January 2019.

Janssen Products LP. Erleada (apalutamide) [package insert]. Horsham, PA. February 2018.

Jazz Pharaceuticals, Inc. Erwinasze (Asparaginase injection) [package insert]. Palo Alto, CA. March 2016.

Jazz Pharaceuticals, Inc. Daunorubicin and cytarabine liposome for injection (Vyxeos) [package insert]. Palo Alto, CA. August 2017.

Kretzschmar A, Pink D, Thuss-Patience P, et al. Extravasation of Oxaliplatin. *J Clin Oncol* 2003; 21: 4068–4069.

Labianca R, Floriani I, Cortesi E, et al. Alternating Versus Continuous "FOLFIRI" in Advanced Colorectal Cancer (ACC): A Randomized "GISCAD" Trial. *J Clin Oncol* 2006; 24(18S): 3505.

Lenz HL. Management and Preparedness for Infusion and Hypersensitivity Reactions. *Oncologist* 2007; 12: 601–609.

Lyman GH. Weight-based Chemotherapy Dosing in Obese Patients with Cancer: Back to the Future. *J Oncol Pract* 2012; 8(4e): 62–64.

Merck & Co., Inc. Temodar (temozolomide) [package insert]. Whitehouse Station, NJ. October 2017.

Mouridsen HT, Langer SW, Buter J, et al. Treatment of Anthracycline Extravasation with Savene (dexrazoxane): Results from Two Prospective Clinical Multicentre Studies. *Annals of Oncol* 2006; 18: 546–550.

Mylan Pharmaceuticals. Tamoxifen Citrate [package insert]. Morgantown, WV. April 2013.

Neuss MN, Polovich M, McNiff K, et al. 2013 Updated American Society of Oncology/Oncology Nursing Society Chemotherapy Administration Safety Standards Including Standards for the Safe Administration and Management of Oral Chemotherapy. *Oncol Nurs Forum* 2013; 40(3): 225–233.

Neuss MN, Gilmore TR, Belderson KM, et al. 2016 Updated American Society of Clinical Oncology/ Oncology Nursing Society Chemotherapy Administration Safety Standards, Including Standards for Pediatric Oncology. *Oncol Nurs Forum* 2017; 44(1): 1–13.

NextSource Biotechnology. Gleostine (lomustine) [package insert]. Miami, FL. September 2018.

Nitiss JL. Targeting DNA Topoisomerase II in Cancer Chemotherapy. *Nat Rev Cancer 2009*; 9: 338–350.

NIOSH (2014). List of Antineoplastic and Other Hazardous Drugs in Healthcare Settings. Washington, DC: Department of Health and Human Services. Available at https://www.cdc.gov/niosh /topics/hazdrug/default.html. Accessed August 27, 2016.

Novartis Pharmaceuticals Corporation. Arranon (nelarabine) [package insert]. East Hanover, NJ. November 2018.

Novartis Pharmaceuticals Corporation. Femara (lerozole) [package insert]. East Hanover, NJ. April 2018.

Novartis Pharmaceuticals Corporation. Hycamptin (topotecan) [capsules package insert]. East Hanover, NJ. September 2018.

Novartis Pharmaceuticals Corporation. Hycamptin (topotecan) [injection package insert]. East Hanover, NJ. September 2018.

Occupational Safety and Health Administration. *Controlling Occupational Exposure to Hazardous Drugs* 1995 Washington (OSHA Instruction CPL 2-2.20B).

Oncology Nursing Society Board of Directors. Pittsburgh, PA: *ONS Position Paper: Regarding the Preparation of the Professional Registered Nurse Who Administers and Cares for the Individual Receiving Chemotherapy*. Oncology Nursing Society; 2012.

Otsuka Pharmaceutical Co, Ltd. Busulfex (busulfan) injection [package insert]. Tokyo, Japan. January 2015.

Ovation Pharmaceuticals. Cosmegen (dactinomycin) [package insert]. Deerfield, IL. March 2008.

Pfizer, Inc. Emcyt (estramustine phosphate sodium) [package insert]. New York, NY. June 2007.

Pfizer, Inc. Aromasin (exemestane) [package insert]. New York, NY. May 2018.

Pfizer, Inc. Cytarabine [package insert]. New York, NY. December 2011.

Polovich M, Clark PC. Factors Influencing Oncology Nurses' Use of Hazardous Drug Safe-handling Precautions. *Oncol Nurs Forum* 2012; 39: E299–E309.

Polovich M, Martin S. Nurses' Use of Hazardous Drug Handling Precautions and Awareness of National Patient Safety Guidelines. *Oncol Nurs Forum* 2011; 38: 718–726.

Polovich M, Olsen M, LeFebvre KB. *Chemotherapy and Biotherapy Guidelines and Recommendations for Practice,* Oncology Nursing Society; 4th ed. Pittsburgh, PA: ONS; 2014: 158–162.

Polovich M, Whitford JM, Olsen M. *Chemotherapy and Biotherapy Guidelines and Recommendations for Practice,* 3rd ed. Pittsburgh, PA: ONS; 2009: 105–110.

Pro-Straken. Fareston (toremifene) [package insert]. Bridgewater, NJ. October 2012.

R-PHARMA US. Ixempra (ixabepilone) [package insert]. Princeton, NJ. January 2016.

Sagent Pharmaceuticals. Epirubicin hydrochloride injection [package insert]. Schumburg, IL. August 2017.

Sagent Pharmaceuticals. Fludararbine [package insert]. Schumburg, IL. August 2016.

Sagent Pharaceuticals. Fluorouracil [package insert]. Schumburg, IL. January 2017.

Sagent Pharmaceuticals. Vinorelbine [package insert]. Schaumburg, IL. May 2014.

Sanofi-aventis. Taxotere (docetaxel) [package insert]. Bridgewater, NJ. October 2018.

Sanofi-aventis. Eloxatin (Oxaliplatin) [package insert]. Bridgewater, NJ. October 2015.

Sanofi-aventis. Jevtana (cabazitaxel) [package insert]. Bridgewater, NJ. January 2018.

Schulmeister L. Totect™: A new Agent for Treating Anthracycline Extravasation. *Clin J Oncol Nurs* 2007; 11(3): 387–395.

Servier Pharmaceuticals, LLC. Asparlas (calaspargase pegol-mknl) injection [package insert]. Boston, MA. December 2018.

Sigma-Tau Pharmaceuticals, Inc. Depocyt (cytarabine injection, lipid complex) [package insert]. Gaithersburg, MD. December 2014.

Sigma-Tau Pharmaceuticals, Inc. Oncaspar (pegasparaginase) [package insert]. Gaithersburg, MD. May 2015.

Spectrum Pharmaceuticals, Inc. Folotyn (pralatrexte injection) [package insert]. Westminster CO, November 2016.

Spectrum Pharmaceuticals, Inc. Evomela (melphalan HCl) [package insert]. Westminster, CO. September 2017.

Talon Therapeutics Inc. Marqibo (vinCRIStine liposome). Irvine, CA. November 2016.

Taiho Oncology. Lonsurf (trifluridine and tipiracil) [package insert]. Princeton, NJ, February 2019.

TerSera Therapeutics. Zoladex (goserelin acetate) [package insert]. Lake Forest, IL. July 2017.

Teva Parenteral Medicines, Inc. Daunorubicin HCl injection [solution package insert]. Irvine, CA. December 2012.

Teva Parenteral Medicines, Inc. Zanosar (streptozocin) solution [package insert]. Irvine, CA. September 2018.

Teva Pharmaceuticals USA, Inc. Fludarabine [package insert]. North Wales, PA. September 2014.

Teva Pharmaceuticals USA, Inc. Doxorubicin HCl [package insert]. North Wales, PA. February 2014.

Teva Pharmaceuticals USA, Inc. Idarubicin HCl [injection package insert]. North Wales, PA. January 2015.

Teva Pharmaceuticals USA, Inc. Ifosfamide [package insert]. North Wales, PA. December 2015.

Teva Pharmaceuticals USA, Inc. Irinotecan [package insert] North Wales, PA. January 2015.

Teva Pharmaceuticals USA, Inc. Synribo (omacetaxine mepesuccinate) [package insert]. North Wales, PA. June 2017.

Teva Pharmaceuticals USA, Inc. Platinol (cis-platinum) [package insert]. North Wales, PA. October 2015.

Thompson LA, Lawson AP, Sutphin SD, et al. Description of Current Practices of Empiric Chemotherapy Dose Adjustment in Obese Adult Patients. *J Oncol Pract* 2010; 6(3): 141–145.

Tolmar Pharmaceuticals, Inc. Eligard (leuprolide acetate) [package insert]. Fort Collins, CO, April 2019.

Topotarget A/S. Totect (dexrazoxane) [package insert]. Copenhagen, Denmark. May 2011.

Tournigand C, Cervantes A, Figer A, et al. OPTIMOX1: A Randomized Study of FOLFOX4 or FOLFOX7 with Oxaliplatin in a Stop-and-go Fashion in Advanced Colorectal Cancer: A GERCOR Study. *J Clin Oncol* 2006; 24(3): 394–400.

Unguru Y, Fernandez CV, Bernhardt B, et al. An Ethical Framework for Allocating Scarce Life-saving Chemotherapy and Supportive Care Drugs for Childhood Cancer. *JNCI J Natl Cancer Inst* 2016; 108(6): djv392 (Commentary) doi:10.1093/jnci/djv392. Available at http://jnci.oxfordjournals.org/content/108/6/djv392.full.pdf+html. Accessed May 5, 2016.

U.S. Pharmacopeial (USP) Convention (2016). USP publishes standard on handling hazardous drugs in healthcare settings. Available at http://www.usp.org/news/usp-publishes-standard-handling-hazardous-drugs-healthcare-settings. Accessed July 17, 2017.

U.S. Pharmacopeial Convention (2017). Frequently asked questions: 800 hazardous drugs-handling in healthcare settings. Available at https://www.usp.org/frequently-asked-questions/hazardous-drugs-handling-healthcare-settings. Accessed October 15, 2019.

Watanabe H, Ikesue H, Tsujikawa T, et al. Decrease in Venous Irritation by Adjusting the Concentration of Injected Bendamustine. *Biological and Pharmaceutical Bulletin* 2013; 36: 574–578.

Drug: abiraterone acetate (Zytiga)

Class: CYP17 inhibitor.

Mechanism of Action: Abiraterone is an androgen biosynthesis inhibitor that inhibits the enzyme CYP17, which is expressed in testicular, adrenal, and prostatic tumor tissues. CYP17 is required for androgen biosynthesis. CYP17 catalyzes 2 sequential reactions: (1) conversion of pregnenolone and progesterone to derivatives, and (2) formation of DHEA (dehydroepiandrosterone) and androstenedione, which are androgen precursors of testosterone. CYP17 inhibition by abiraterone can cause increased adrenal mineralocorticoid production. Androgen-sensitive prostate cancer is sensitive to agents that decrease androgen serum levels. Androgen deprivation therapies (e.g., GnRH agonists or orchiectomy) decrease androgen production by the testes, but not the adrenals or in the tumor. It is not necessary to monitor testosterone levels, and although PSA levels may change, it does not necessarily correlate to clinical benefit.

Metabolism: Following oral administration, abiraterone acetate is hydrolyzed to abiraterone, the active metabolite. Median time to reach maximum plasma abiraterone concentrations is 2 hours. Food affects systemic exposure of the drug: low-fat meals result in 5-fold higher levels, and high-fat meals result in 17-fold higher levels of abiraterone. Therefore, drug should be taken on an empty stomach. Drug is highly protein-bound (>99%) to human plasma proteins, albumin, and alpha-1 acid gycoprotein. Neither prodrug nor drug is a substrate of P-glycoprotein (P-gp), but abiraterone acetate is an inhibitor of P-gp. No studies have been performed with other transporter proteins. There are two inactive metabolites that involve CYP3A4 and SULT2A1. The mean terminal half-life of abiraterone in plasma is 12 ± 5 hours. After oral administration, 88% is recovered in feces (55% abiraterone acetate and 22% abiraterone), and 5% in urine. Hepatic dysfunction increases systemic exposure: 1.1-fold with mild (Child–Pugh Class A), and 3.6-fold in moderate (Child–Pugh Class B), prolonging mean half-life of abiraterone to 18 hours and 19 hours, respectively. Drug has not been studied in patients with severe (Class C) hepatic dysfunction. There is no increase in systemic exposure in patients with severe renal dysfunction.

Indication: Drug is FDA-approved in combination with prednisone for the treatment of patients with (1) metastatic castration-resistant prostate cancer (CRPC); (2) metastatic high risk castration-sensitive prostate cancer (CSPC).

Contraindication: Women who are or may become pregnant. Drug should not be used in patients with baseline severe hepatic impairment (Child–Hugh Class C).

Dosage/Range:

CRPR: Abiraterone acetate 1,000 mg (two 500-mg tablets or four 250-mg tablets) orally once daily on an empty stomach (at least 1 hour before or 2 hours after a meal) with water; with prednisone 5 mg orally **twice daily**.

CSPC: Abiraterone acetate 1,000 mg (two 500-mg tablets or four 250-mg tablets) orally once daily on an empty stomach (at least 1 hour before or 2 hours after a meal) with water; with prednisone 5 mg orally **once daily.**

Patients receiving abiraterone acetate should also receive a gonadotropin-releasing hormone (GnRH) analog concurrently or should have had bilateral orchiectomy.
- Hepatic Impairment:
    - *Moderate hepatic impairment* (baseline, (Child–Pugh class B)): Reduce starting dose to 250 mg PO once daily. Monitor ALT, AST, and bilirubin before starting therapy, then weekly for the first month, every 2 weeks for the next 2 months of treatment, then monthly. If ALT and/or AST > 5× ULN or total bilirubin is >3× ULN occur in a patient with moderate hepatic impairment, discontinue drug and do not retreat with abiraterone.
    - Do not administer to patients with baseline severe hepatotoxicity (Child–Pugh class C).
    - *Patients who develop hepatotoxicity during treatment* (e.g., ALT or AST > 5 × ULN or total bilirubin > 3 × ULN): Hold drug in until recovery to baseline or AST and/or ALT ≤ 2.5 ULN and total bilirubin ≤1.5× ULN; then re-treatment may be started at a reduced dose of 750 mg once daily. Monitor serum transaminases and bilirubin at least every 2 weeks × 3 months, and monthly thereafter. If hepatotoxicity occurs at 750 mg once daily, interrupt until recovery and dose-reduce to 500 mg orally. If hepatotoxicity occurs at this dose, discontinue treatment with abiraterone.

- Permanently discontinue drug in patients who develop a concurrent elevation of ALT >3× ULN and total bilirubin > 2× ULN in the absence of biliary obstruction or other causes.
- *Dose modification for strong CYP3A4 inducers (e.g., phenytoin, carbamazepine, rifampin, rifabutin, phenobarbital):* Avoid concurrent use if possible. If must administer concurrently, increase the dose of abiraterone to twice daily (e.g., from 1,000mg once daily to twice daily). If the concomitant strong *CYP3A4* inducer is discontinued, reduce the dose back to previous dose of once a day dosing.

Drug Preparation:
- Oral, available as 250-mg (uncoated) and 500-mg (film-coated) tablets.

Drug Administration:
- Assess LFTs (ALT, AST, bilirubin) baseline before starting treatment, then every 2 weeks for first 3 months of treatment, then monthly thereafter.
- Teach patient to
  - Take once daily on an empty stomach with water, swallow whole, and do not chew or crush tablet.
  - Drug must be taken on an empty stomach, one hour before or two hours after a meal. Take one tablet of prednisone 5 mg PO twice a day, ideally with food at a different time from the abiraterone (more than 1hour before, or more than 2 hour after taking abiraterone).
  - Do not make up a missed dose of either abiraterone acetate or prednisone; rather, take the normal dose the next day and do not make up a missed dose; patient should tell the physician if he or she misses more than one dose.
  - Avoid if pregnant or may become pregnant as drug can harm a developing fetus. Women who are or may be pregnant should not handle the drug unless wearing gloves. Men receiving the drug should use a condom if having sex with a pregnant woman. The patient should use both a condom and another effective method of birth control if he is having sex with a woman of child-bearing potential. Use these precautions during and for 1 week after treatment with abiraterone.

Drug Interactions: Drug is a strong inhibitor of CYP1A2 and CYP2D6, and a moderate inhibitor of CYP2C9, CYP2C19, and CYP3A4/5. Drug is also a substrate of CYP3A4.

- Dextromethorphan (CYP2D6 substrate): 2.8-fold increase in systemic exposure.
- Strong CYP3A4 inhibitors or inducers: AVOID or use with caution, and monitor the patient closely.
- CYP2D6 substrates with a narrow therapeutic index (e.g., all tricyclic antidepressants, most SSRI antidepressants, tramadol, oxycodone, antipsychotics, beta blockers). Avoid coadministration; if must coadminister, use together cautiously and consider a dose reduction of the concomitant CYP2D6 substrate.

Lab Effects/Interference:
- Decreased testosterone and PSA levels.
- Increased ALT, AST, bilirubin, increased alkaline phosphatase.
- Hypokalemia, hypertriglyceridemia, hypercholesterolemka, hyperglycemia, hypophosphatemia.
- Anemia, lymphopenia.

Special Considerations:

- Warnings and Precautions:
  - *HTN, hypokalemia, and fluid retention due to mineralocorticoid excess:* Mineralocorticoid excess may occur due to CYP17 inhibition; use drug cautiously in patients with a history of cardiovascular disease. Safety in patients with LVEF < 50%, or NYHA class III or IV heart failure, has not been established. Correct HTN and hypokalemia before treatment. Monitor BP, serum potassium, and symptoms of fluid retention at least monthly. Control HTN and correct abnormal serum potassium before and during therapy. Use drug cautiously and monitor closely patients with heart failure, recent MI, or ventricular arrhythmia.
  - *Adrenocortical insufficiency:* Monitor for signs and symptoms of adrenal insufficiency (fatigue, lightheadedness with position change, muscle weakness, fever, weight loss, nausea/vomiting/diarrhea, changes in mood/personality, myalgias, arthralgias, headache, low BP when standing, but high BP when supine, increased bronze pigmentation of skin, urinary frequency), and discuss management with physician or midlevel practitioner. Assess patients at times when risk of adrenocortical insufficiency may be high: patients withdrawn from prednisone, who have prednisone dose reductions, or who have unusual stress. Patients may require increased corticosteroid doses before, during, and after stressful situations.
  - *Hepatotoxicity*
    - In postmarketing reports, there have been Zytiga-associated severe hepatic reactions (e.g., fulminant hepatitis, acute liver failure, and death).
    - Assess LFTs (ALT, AST, direct BR) baseline, then every 2 weeks for the first 3 months, then monthly thereafter (more frequently if the LFTs are elevated). Increases in liver enzymes may require dose interruption, dose modification, and/or dose discontinuation. Promptly assess LFTs if patient develops signs/symptoms of hepatotoxicity.
    - Patients with moderate hepatic impairment should have ALT, AST, bilirubin assessed baseline, then every week for the first month, every 2 weeks for the following 2 months of treatment, and monthly thereafter, or more frequently as needed.
    - Concurrent elevated ALT (>3× ULN) and total bilirubin (>2× ULN) in the absence of biliary obstruction: permanently discontinue abiraterone.
    - Patients who develop hepatotoxicity (ALT ± AST > 5 × ULN or total bilirubin >3× ULN) should have abiraterone stopped. Drug can be restarted at a reduced dose of 750 mg once daily following return of LFTs to patient's baseline or to AST/ALT <2.5 × ULN and total bilirubin <1.5 × ULN. Once drug is restarted, monitor the patient's LFTs at a minimum every 2 weeks for 3 months, then monthly thereafter.
  - Reinforce patient teaching that drug MUST be taken on an empty stomach, as drug systemic exposure (AUC) is 10-fold higher when taken with meals.
  - Most common side effects occurring in ≥10% of patients are fatigue, joint swelling/discomfort, hypokalemia, edema, myalgia, hot flush, diarrhea, nausea, vomiting, cough, HTN, headache, URI.
  - Most common lab abnormalities (>20%) are anemia, increased alkaline phosphatase, hypertriglyceridemia, lymphopenia, hypercholesterolemka, hyperglycemia, elevated AST and ALT, hypophosphatemia, hypokalemia.

- Drug is contraindicated in women who are or may become pregnant; drug should not be used in patients with baseline severe hepatic impairment (Child–Hugh Class C). Men with female sexual partners who are of reproductive potential should use effective contraception to prevent pregnancy.

Potential Toxicities/Side Effects and the Nursing Process

I. POTENTIAL FOR INJURY related to MINERALOCORTICOID EXCESS-INDUCED EDEMA, HTN, HYPOKALEMIA, AND STEROID-INDUCED IMMUNOSUPPRESSION

Defining Characteristics: Water retention may occur and lead to CHF, hypertension, and edema; hypokalemia may occur due to increased excretion of potassium. Osteoporosis may occur with long-term corticosteroid therapy. Steroids increase susceptibility to infections, may mask or aggravate infection, and may prolong or delay healing of injuries.

Nursing Implications: Identify patients at risk for complications associated with fluid/sodium retention (i.e., patients with preexisting cardiac, renal, hepatic dysfunction); monitor fluid and electrolyte balance and assess for imbalance. Document baseline cardiac status and monitor through therapy. Teach patients to report the following right away: dizziness, fast heartbeats, feeling faint or lightheaded, confusion, muscle weakness, pain in the legs, and swelling in legs or feet. Instruct patient to report signs/symptoms of hypokalemia (anorexia, muscle twitching, tetany); monitor electrolytes regularly and discuss abnormal values with physician. Encourage high-potassium diet, and instruct patient in safety measures as needed, such as taking prednisone with food 2 hours prior to or 1 hour after abiraterone. Teach patient to report slow healing of wounds, signs/symptoms of infection (erythema, warmth, purulence) of skin areas, as well as cough, dyspnea, signs/sympoms of URI, and burning on urination. Reinforce/teach patient hygiene measures for mouth, perineum, and skin.

II. ALTERATION IN COMFORT related to MYALGIAS, ARTHRALGIAS, FEVER, HOT FLUSH, DYSPEPSIA

Defining Characteristics: Signs and symptoms of adrenocortical insufficiency may occur: fatigue, lightheadedness with position change, muscle weakness, fever, weight loss, nausea/vomiting/diarrhea, changes in mood/personality, myalgias, arthralgias, headache, low BP when standing but high BP when supine, increased bronze pigmentation of skin, and urinary frequency. Severity and incidence is reduced with coadministration of prednisone.

Nursing Implications: Teach patient that arthralgias, myalgias, fever, discomfort may occur, and strategies to reduce discomfort. Monitor for signs and symptoms of adrenal insufficiency, and discuss management with physician or midlevel practitioner. Assess patients at times when risk of adrenocortical insufficiency may be high: patients withdrawn from prednisone, who have prednisone dose reductions, or who have unusual stress. Patients may require increased corticosteroid doses before, during, and after stressful situations.

Drug: adrenocorticoids (cortisone, dexamethasone, hydrocortisone, methylprednisolone, prednisolone, prednisone)

Class: Hormones.

Mechanism of Action: Cause lysis of lymphoid cells, which leads to their use against lymphatic leukemia, myeloma, malignant lymphoma. May also recruit malignant cells out of G_0 phase, making them vulnerable to damage caused by cell cycle phase-specific agents.

Metabolism: Metabolized by the liver, excreted in urine. Prednisone is activated by the liver in its active form, prednisolone.

Dosage/Range:
- Varies according to which preparation is used. Dexamethasone is 25 times the potency of hydrocortisone.
- Cortisone 25 mg
- Dexamethasone 0.75 mg
- Hydrocortisone 20 mg
- Methylprednisolone 4 mg
- Prednisone, prednisolone 5 mg

Drug Preparation:
- None

Drug Administration:
- Oral

Drug Interactions:
- May increase K+ loss and hypokalemia when combined with amphotericin B or potassium-depleting diuretics.
- Warfarin (Coumadin) dose may need to be increased.
- Insulin or oral hypoglycemia dose may need to be increased.
- Oral contraceptives may inhibit steroid metabolism.

Lab Effects/Interference:
- Increased Na, decreased K with hypokalemic alkalosis.
- Decreased ^{131}I uptake and protein-bound iodine concentration. May cause difficulty monitoring therapeutic response of patients treated for thyroid conditions.
- False-negative results in nitroblue tetrazolium test for systemic bacterial infections.
- May suppress reactions to skin tests.
- Corticosteroids may cause demargination of white blood cells from the vein walls, increasing WBC on testing.

Special Considerations:
- Chronic steroid use is associated with numerous side effects. Intermittent therapy is safer and, under some conditions, just as effective as daily therapy.

TREATMENT

Potential Toxicities/Side Effects and the Nursing Process

I. ALTERATION IN NUTRITION, LESS THAN BODY REQUIREMENTS, related to GASTRIC IRRITATION, DECREASED CARBOHYDRATE METABOLISM, AND HYPERGLYCEMIA

Defining Characteristics: Steroids can cause increased secretion of hydrochloric acid and decreased secretion of protective gastric mucus, which can exacerbate an existing gastric ulcer. They are insulin antagonists and may cause gluconeogenesis. In addition, steroids may increase appetite and cause weight gain.

Nursing Implications: Administer drugs with meals or an antacid. Instruct patient to report evidence of gastric distress immediately; teach patient to take steroids prior to a meal or with milk or food. Obtain baseline glucose levels and monitor periodic blood sugars throughout therapy. Teach patient to recognize signs/symptoms of hyperglycemia (polyuria, polydipsia, polyphagia), and to report these to the doctor or nurse.

II. POTENTIAL FOR INJURY related to SODIUM AND WATER RETENTION, ALTERATIONS IN FLUID AND ELECTROLYTE BALANCE, AND STEROID-INDUCED IMMUNOSUPPRESSION

Defining Characteristics: Sodium and water retention may occur and lead to CHF, hypertension, and edema in susceptible individuals; hypokalemia and hypocalcemia may occur due to increased excretion of potassium and calcium. Osteoporosis may occur with long-term therapy. Steroids increase susceptibility to infections and tuberculosis, may mask or aggravate infection, and may prolong or delay healing of injuries.

Nursing Implications: Identify patients at risk for complications associated with fluid/sodium retention (i.e., patients with preexisting cardiac, renal, hepatic dysfunction); monitor fluid and electrolyte balance and assess for imbalance. Document baseline cardiac status and monitor through therapy. Instruct patient to report signs/symptoms of hypokalemia (anorexia, muscle twitching, tetany, polyuria, polydipsia) and of hypocalcemia (leg cramps, tingling in fingertips, muscle twitching); monitor electrolytes regularly and discuss abnormal values with physician. Encourage high-potassium, high-calcium diet, and instruct patient in safety measures as needed. Teach patient to report slow healing of wounds, signs/symptoms of infection (erythema, warmth, purulence) of skin areas, as well as sore throat and burning on urination. Reinforce/teach patient hygiene measures for mouth, perineum, and skin.

III. POTENTIAL FOR INJURY related to RAPID WITHDRAWAL OF THERAPY

Defining Characteristics: Long-term therapy leads to suppression of normal adrenal function. Rapid cessation of therapy will lead to adrenal insufficiency, characterized by anorexia, nausea, orthostatic hypotension, dizziness, depression, dyspnea, hypoglycemia, and rebound inflammation (fever, myalgias, arthralgia, malaise). It can be fatal.

Nursing Implications: Discuss with physician the taper of steroids and instruct patient and family carefully. Teach patient to report symptoms of rapid withdrawal to nurse or physician.

IV.   POTENTIAL FOR BODY-IMAGE DISTURBANCE related to CUSHINGOID CHANGES

Defining Characteristics: Cushingoid state may occur with prolonged use and may be diminished by every-other-day dosing. Changes include moonface, striae, purpura, acne, and hirsutism. In addition, increased appetite from steroids may lead to weight gain.

Nursing Implications: Teach patient about potential changes and provide reassurance that they will resolve once therapy ceases; encourage patient to verbalize feelings, and provide emotional support.

V.   POTENTIAL FOR SENSORY/PERCEPTUAL ALTERATIONS related to CATARACTS OR GLAUCOMA, AND OCULAR INFECTIONS (increased risk)

Defining Characteristics: Cataracts or glaucoma may develop with prolonged steroid use; risk of ocular infections from virus or fungi is increased.

Nursing Implications: Teach patient to report signs/symptoms of eye infection, such as discharge, erythema, or visual changes; ophthalmologic exams are recommended every 2–3 months.

VI.   INEFFECTIVE COPING related to AFFECTIVE/BEHAVIORAL CHANGES

Defining Characteristics: Emotional lability, insomnia, mood swings, euphoria, and psychosis may occur, causing ineffective coping and role-relationship problems if unprepared.

Nursing Implications: Teach patient and family that affective/behavioral changes may occur and that they will resolve once therapy is discontinued. Encourage patient and family to report these changes, especially if troublesome.

VII.   IMPAIRED PHYSICAL MOBILITY related to MUSCULOSKELETAL CHANGES

Defining Characteristics: With chronic, high-dose usage, loss of muscle mass, muscle weakness (steroid myopathy), tendon rupture, osteoporosis, pathologic fractures, and aseptic necrosis of the heads of the humerus and femur can occur.

Nursing Implications: Teach patient that muscle weakness and other effects can occur with therapy and that muscle cramping may occur with discontinuation of therapy. Teach patient to report weakness, cramping, and any musculoskeletal changes. If weakness occurs, therapy may be discontinued.

Drug: altretamine (Hexalen, Hexamethylmelamine)

Class: Alkylating agent.

Mechanism of Action: The exact mechanism of action is unknown. May inhibit incorporation of thymidine and uridine into DNA and RNA, respectively, inhibiting DNA and RNA synthesis. Altretamine is believed not to act as an alkylating agent in vitro, but it may be activated to an alkylating agent in vivo. Also may act as an antimetabolite with activity in S phase.

Metabolism: Well absorbed orally, although bioavailability is variable. Protein-bound with peak plasma concentration in 1 hour. Metabolized extensively in the liver, with majority excreted in the urine. Some of the drug is excreted as respiratory CO_2. Half-life of the parent compound is 4.7–10.2 hours.

Indication: For use as a single agent in the palliative treatment of patients with recurrent ovarian cancer following first-line therapy with a cisplatin and/or alkyating agent-based combination.

Dosage/Range:
- 260 mg/m^2 daily in four equally divided doses × 14 or 21 consecutive days, repeated every 28 days.
- Discontinue for 14 or more days and restart at 200 mg/m^2 daily if any of the following occur: refractory GI intolerance, WBC < 2,000 cells/mm^3 or ANC < 1,000 cells/mm^3, platelet count < 75,000/mm^3, or progressive neurotoxicity.

Drug Preparation:
- Available in 50-mg capsules.

Drug Administration:
- Oral. Administer dose after meals and at bedtime.

Drug Interactions:
- Concurrent administration of drug with monoamine oxidase (MAO) inhibitor antidepressants may cause severe orthostatic hypotension.

Lab Effects/Interference:
- Decreased CBC.
- Increased BUN, creatinine.

Special Considerations:
- Nausea and vomiting can be minimized if patient takes dose 2 hours after meals and at bedtime.
- Nadir 3–4 weeks after treatment.

Potential Toxicities/Side Effects and the Nursing Process

I. INFECTION AND BLEEDING related to BM DEPRESSION

Defining Characteristics: Causes mild to moderate BM suppression, with nadir occurring 21–28 days after beginning treatment, and rapid recovery within 1 week of cessation of drug. Anemia occurs in 33% of patients and is moderate to severe in 9% of patients.

Nursing Implications: Assess CBC, WBC, differential, and platelet count before each cycle of drug administration, as well as for signs/symptoms of infection or bleeding. Teach patient signs/symptoms of infection and bleeding, and instruct to report them immediately. Teach self-care measures to minimize risk of infection and bleeding, including avoidance of OTC aspirin-containing medications. Assess energy and activity tolerance; discuss blood transfusion with physician as appropriate. Discuss with physician dose interruption and reduction if WBC < 2,000/mm^3, ANC < 1,000/mm^3, or platelet count < 75,000/mm^3.

II. SENSORY/PERCEPTUAL ALTERATIONS related to PERIPHERAL NEUROPATHY AND CNS EFFECTS

Defining Characteristics: Peripheral sensory neuropathy occurs in 31% of patients and is moderate to severe in 9% of patients. Paresthesia, hyperesthesia, hyperreflexia, and numbness may occur; they are reversible. CNS effects of agitation, confusion, hallucinations, depression, mood disorders, and Parkinson-like symptoms may occur, and usually are reversible. Neurologic effects are more common with continuous dosing > 3 months, rather than pulse dosing.

Nursing Implications: Assess baseline neurologic status. Teach patient that possible side effects may occur, and instruct to report them. If nerologic toxicity is severe, drug should be dose reduced, then discontinued if symptoms do not improve.

III. ALTERATION IN NUTRITION, LESS THAN BODY REQUIREMENTS, related to NAUSEA AND VOMITING, DIARRHEA, ABDOMINAL CRAMPS, ANOREXIA

Defining Characteristics: Nausea occurs in 33% of patients and is dose related. Tolerance may develop after 3 weeks of drug administration. Diarrhea and cramps may be dose limiting. Anorexia may occur.

Nursing Implications: Premedicate with antiemetics (phenothiazines are usually effective) at least initially, then as needed. Divide dose into four doses, and give 1–2 hours after meals and at bedtime. Instruct patient to report nausea/vomiting, diarrhea, abdominal cramping. Teach self-administration of prescribed antidiarrheals and self-care techniques to manage cramps (e.g., heat pads or position change). If GI side effects are refractory to symptom management, discuss interrupting dose and then dose reduction with physician.

IV.   ALTERATION IN SKIN INTEGRITY related to SKIN RASHES

Defining Characteristics: Skin rashes, pruritus, eczematous skin lesions may occur but are rare.

Nursing Implications: Assess for changes in skin color, texture, and integrity. Teach patient to report any changes in skin, and discuss measures to minimize discomfort.

V.   ALTERATION IN ELIMINATION related to RENAL DYSFUNCTION

Defining Characteristics: Elevations in BUN (9% of patients) or creatinine (7%) can occur.

Nursing Implications: Assess baseline renal status and monitor renal function studies throughout treatment.

VI.   POTENTIAL SEXUAL DYSFUNCTION related to DRUG EFFECTS

Defining Characteristics: Drug is mutagenic, carcinogenic, and teratogenic. Drug causes testicular atrophy and decreased spermatogenesis. It is unknown whether drug is excreted in human milk.

Nursing Implications: Discuss with patient and partner normal sexual patterns and anticipated dysfunction resulting from drug or disease. Provide information, emotional support, and referral for counseling as appropriate.

Drug: aminoglutethimide (Cytadren, Elipten)

Class: Adrenal steroid inhibitor.

Mechanism of Action: Causes "chemical adrenalectomy." Blocks adrenal production of steroids, reducing levels of glucocorticoids, mineralocorticoids, and estrogens. Also inhibits peripheral aromatization of androgens to estrogens.

Metabolism: Well absorbed orally. Hydroxylated in liver; undergoes enterohepatic circulation. Most of drug is excreted in urine.

Indication: For the suppression of adrenal function in selected patients with Cushing's syndrome. It does not affect the underlying disease process.

Dosage/Range:
- 750–2,000 mg PO daily in divided doses.
- 40-mg hydrocortisone daily given to replace glucocorticoid deficiencies.

Drug Preparation:
• None. Available in 250-mg tablets.

Drug Administration:
• Oral.

Drug Interactions:
• Drug enhances dexamethasone metabolism, so hydrocortisone should be used for gluco-corticoid replacement.
• Warfarin (Coumadin) dose may need to be increased.
• Alcohol potentiates drug side effects.
• May need to increase doses of theophylline, digitoxin, or medroxyprogesterone.

Lab Effects/Interference:
• Hypothyroidism: monitor TFT.
• Elevated LFTs, especially SGOT, alk phos, bili.

Special Considerations:
• Skin rash may develop within 5–7 days, lasting 8 days, often with malaise and fever (37.7–39°C [100–102°F]). If not resolved in 7–14 days, drug should be discontinued.
• Adjuvant corticosteroids need to be administered.

Potential Toxicities/Side Effects and the Nursing Process

I.   ALTERATION IN ENDOCRINE FUNCTION related to ADRENAL INSUFFICIENCY

Defining Characteristics: Drug causes reversible chemical adrenalectomy by blockade of steroid hormone production. Patient will experience signs/symptoms of adrenal insufficiency if enough replacement glucocorticoid steroids are not received. Signs/symptoms of adrenal insufficiency include hyponatremia, hypoglycemia, dizziness, and postural hypotension. In addition, possible ovarian blockade may result in virilization.

Nursing Implications: Teach patient about self-administration of hydrocortisone replacement therapy (i.e., administer in AM with breakfast), potential side effects, and tapering schedule; refer to section on adrenocorticoids. Teach patient side effects of hormone replacement and self-assessment techniques, including weekly weights and signs/symptoms of infection. Monitor electrolytes, especially Na+, K+, and Ca++. Assess for signs/symptoms of adrenal insufficiency (fatigue, anorexia, nausea, vomiting, diarrhea, weight loss, weakness, dizziness, and low blood sugar). As appropriate, explore with patient's significant other reproductive and sexuality patterns and the impact chemotherapy may have. Recognize that patient may need increased hydrocortisone and mineralocorticoid support if surgery is needed (increased stress requirement).

II.   IMPAIRED SKIN INTEGRITY related to DRUG RASH

Defining Characteristics: Area of erythema, pruritus, and unexplained dermatitis may appear within 1 week of treatment and disappear in 5–8 days. May be accompanied by malaise and low-grade fever.

Nursing Implications: Teach patient to report symptoms and to avoid scratching involved areas if rash develops. Assess skin for any changes and rash development. Consider use of Sarna cream, and use of OTC diphenhydramine.

III.   SENSORY/PERCEPTUAL ALTERATIONS related to TRANSIENT SYMPTOMS

Defining Characteristics: Transient symptoms such as drowsiness, lethargy, somnolence, visual blurring, vertigo, and ataxia may occur, as may nystagmus. Lethargy may be severe in elderly patients.

Nursing Implications: Document baseline neurologic function and general health assessment. Teach patient possible side effects, self-assessment, and to report symptoms. Discuss with physician possible dose reduction for significant symptoms.

IV.   ALTERATION IN NUTRITION related to NAUSEA/VOMITING AND ANOREXIA

Defining Characteristics: Nausea/vomiting and anorexia occur in approximately 10–13% of patients and are mild.

Nursing Implications: Initially, premedicate (and teach patient to) with antiemetics prior to drug administration. Usually symptoms subside within 2 weeks. Encourage small, frequent feedings.

V.   ALTERATION IN OXYGENATION/PERFUSION related to HYPOTENSION

Defining Characteristics: Drug may block aldosterone production leading to orthostatic or persistent hypotension. This is not usually a problem when hydrocortisone replacement is given.

Nursing Implications: Monitor BP regularly. Instruct patient to change position slowly and to report dizziness.

Drug: anastrozole (Arimidex)

Class: Nonsteroidal aromatase inhibitor.

Mechanism of Action: Inhibits the enzyme aromatase. Aromatase is one of the P450 enzymes and is involved in estrogen biosynthesis. Circulating estrogen in postmenopausal women (mainly estradiol) arises from the aromatase-mediated conversion of androstenedione (made by the adrenals) to estrone, then estrone to estradiol, in the peripheral tissues, such as adipose tissue. Anastrozole is highly selective for this enzyme and does not affect steroid synthesis, so that estradiol synthesis is potently suppressed (to undetectable levels) while cortisol and aldosterone levels are unchanged.

Metabolism: Extensively metabolized, with 85% of the drug metabolized by the liver. About 10% of the unchanged drug and 60% of the drug as metabolites are excreted in the urine within 72 hours of drug administration.

Indication: Anastrozole is an aromatase inhibitor indicated for
- Adjuvant treatment of postmenopausal women with hormone receptor-positive early breast cancer.
- First-line treatment of postmenopausal women with hormone receptor-positive or hormone receptor unknown, locally advanced, or metastatic breast cancer.
- Treatment of advanced breast cancer in postmenopausal women with disease progression following tamoxifen therapy. Patients with ER-negative disease and patients who did not respond to previous tamoxifen therapy rarely responded to anastrozole.

Contraindications: (1) women of premenopausal endocrine status, including pregnant women; (2) patients with demonstrated hypersensitivity to anastrozole or any excipient.

Dosage/Range:
- 1 mg PO daily. No dosage adjustment required for mild to moderate hepatic impairment. In the ATAC adjuvant study, the treatment duration was 5 years. The optimal duration of treatment is unknown in adjuvant patients. In patients with metastatic disease, continue until disease progression.

Drug Preparation:
- None. Available as 1-mg tablet.

Drug Administration:
- Take orally with or without food, at approximately the same time daily.

Drug Interactions:
- Tamoxifen: coadministration with anastrozole decreases anastrozole serum levels by 27%.
- Estrogen: coadministration with anastrozole may decrease anastrozole activity; do not use concurrently.
- Herbal estrogen-containing supplements: may decrease drug effect.

Lab Effects/Interference:
- Elevated GGT, especially in patients with liver metastases.
- Decreased total hip and lumbar spine bone mineral density (BMD) compared with baseline.
- Total cholesterol may be increased.

Special Considerations:
- In the large Arimidex Tamoxifen Alone or in Combination (ATAC) clinical trial, anastrozole was shown to reduce the relative risk of breast cancer recurrence by 17% over tamoxifen in hormone receptor-positive patients in the adjuvant setting.
- Well tolerated with low toxicity profile.
- Coadministration of corticosteroids is not necessary.
- Absolutely contraindicated during pregnancy. The drug showed no benefit in ER-negative women.
- Most common ($\geq$10%) adverse reactions in patients with (1) early breast cancer: hot flashes, asthenia, arthritis, pain, arthralgia, pharyngitis, HTN, depression, nausea and vomiting, rash, osteoporosis, fractures, back pain, insomnia, headache, peripheral edema, lymphedema; (2) advanced breast cancer: hot flashes, nausea, asthenia, pain, headache, back pain, bone pain, increased cough, dyspnea, pharyngitis, peripheral edema.
- Warnings and Precautions:
  - Ischemic cardiovascular events: Increased incidence of ischemic events was seen in the ATAC trial in anastrozole arm (17%) compared to tamoxifen (10%). Consider risks and benefits of anastrozole in patients with preexisting ischemic heart disease.
  - Bone effects: Patients in the anastrozole arm had a mean decrease in both LS spine and total hip BMD compared to baseline, while patients in the tamoxifen arm had a mean increase in both measures compared to baseline. Monitor BMD in patients receiving anastrozole.
  - Cholesterol: More patients receiving anastrozole had elevated serum cholesterol (9%) compared to 3.5% in the tamoxifen arm.

Potential Toxicities/Side Effects and the Nursing Process

I.   SEXUAL DYSFUNCTION related to DECREASED ESTROGEN LEVELS

Defining Characteristics: Hot flashes (12%), asthenia or loss of energy (16%), and vaginal dryness may occur.

Nursing Implications: As appropriate, explore with patient and partner patterns of sexuality and impact therapy may have. Discuss strategies to preserve sexual health. Teach patient that the vaginal dryness may be from menopause rather from the drug, and that the patient SHOULD NOT use estrogen creams. Teach patient to use lubricants.

II.   POTENTIAL ALTERATION IN CARDIAC OUTPUT related to THROMBOPHLEBITIS, ISCHEMIC CARDIOVASCULAR EVENTS

Defining Characteristics: Thrombophlebitis may occur, but is uncommon. In the ATAC trial, patients in the anastrozole arm had increased incidence of ischemic events (17%) compared to tamoxifen (10%).

Nursing Implications: Identify patients at risk. Teach patients to report/come to emergency room for pain, redness, or marked swelling in arms or legs, or if shortness of breath or dizziness occurs. Assess patient for prior ischemic heart disease, and teach patient to report any changes (such as chest pain, difficulty breathing, dizziness) immediately.

III.   ALTERATION IN COMFORT related to HEADACHES, WEAKNESS, JOINT DISORDERS

Defining Characteristics: Headaches are mild and occur in about 13% of patients. Decreased energy and weakness is common. Mild swelling of arms/legs may occur and is mild. Patients receiving anastrozole had more arthrosis, arthralgias, and arthritis.

Nursing Implications: Teach patient that headache and joint disorders are usually relieved by nonprescription analgesics and to report headaches that are unrelieved. Teach patient to elevate extremities when at rest, as needed.

IV.   POTENTIAL ALTERATION IN NUTRITION, LESS THAN BODY REQUIREMENTS, related to NAUSEA

Defining Characteristics: Nausea is mild, with a 15% incidence.

Nursing Implications: Determine baseline weight, and monitor at each visit. Teach patient that nausea may occur, and to report this. Discuss strategies to minimize nausea, including diet and dosing time.

V.   POTENTIAL ALTERATION IN BOWEL ELIMINATION related to DIARRHEA

Defining Characteristics: Diarrhea is uncommon (9% incidence) and mild.

Nursing Implications: Assess for change in bowel patterns and teach patient to report diarrhea. If diarrhea occurs, teach patient that diarrhea is usually relieved by nonprescription medications, such as loperamide HCl and Kaopectate, and to report unrelieved diarrhea.

Drug: androgens: testosterone propionate (Testex), fluoxymesterone (Halotestin), testolactone (Teslac)

Class: Hormones.

Mechanism of Action: Has stimulatory effect on red blood cells that results in an increased HCT. Other mechanism of action unknown.

Metabolism: Metabolized by the liver; excreted in the urine and feces.

Dosage/Range:
- Fluoxymesterone: 10–30 mg PO daily (3–4 divided doses).
- Testolactone: 100 mg IM 3 × weekly or 250 mg PO 4 × daily.
- Testosterone propionate: 50–100 mg IM 3 × weekly.

Drug Preparation:
- Drug comes in ready-to-use vials or tablets.

Drug Administration:
- Before IM administration, shake vial vigorously and give injection immediately to avoid solution settling.

Drug Interactions:
- Pharmacologic effects of oral anticoagulants may be enhanced; monitor patient and adjust dose.

Lab Effects/Interference:
- LFTs: possible hepatic dysfunction with long-term use.
- Increased serum Ca.
- May cause decreased total serum thyroxine (T_4) concentrations and increased T_3 and T_4.

Special Considerations:
- Fluoxymesterone may increase sensitivity to oral anticoagulants. Should be administered in divided doses because of its short action.

Potential Toxicities/Side Effects and the Nursing Process

I.   POTENTIAL FOR INJURY related to SODIUM AND WATER RETENTION, HYPERCALCEMIA, AND OBSTRUCTIVE JAUNDICE

Defining Characteristics: Sodium and water retention may occur, necessitating dose reduction or diuretic use; hypercalcemia may occur initially in patients with bony metastases and needs to be distinguished from disease progression. Obstructive jaundice has occurred with methyltesterone, fluoxymesterone, and oxymetholone.

Nursing Implications: Identify patients most at risk for injury related to sodium and water retention: patients with cardiac, renal, or hepatic dysfunction, as well as patients with low serum albumin. Teach patient about potential side effects and instruct to report any changes to physician or nurse; assess patient at each visit for signs/symptoms of fluid and electrolyte imbalance. Identify patients at risk for hypercalcemia (those with bony metastases) and monitor serum calcium during first few weeks of therapy; hypercalcemia is an indication to discontinue therapy. Teach patient and family signs/symptoms of hypercalcemia (drowsiness, increased thirst, constipation, polyuria) and to notify physician. Monitor LFTs and instruct patient and family to report signs/symptoms of GI distress, diarrhea, jaundice.

II.   POTENTIAL FOR SEXUAL DYSFUNCTION related to MASCULINIZATION

Defining Characteristics: Commonly occurs in women receiving drug for > 3 months; with prolonged use, masculinization may be irreversible. Symptoms include increased libido, deepening of voice, excessive growth of body (face) hair, acne, and clitoral hypertrophy. In men, priapism (sustained and often painful erections) and reduced ejaculatory volume may occur.

Nursing Implications: Instruct patient to report symptoms of changes in sexual health. Discuss strategies to preserve sexual health; if unacceptable, discuss alternative medications with physician.

III.   ALTERATION IN NUTRITION, LESS THAN BODY REQUIREMENTS, related to NAUSEA AND VOMITING

Defining Characteristics: Nausea may occur.

Nursing Implications: Teach patient about possible side effects and administer antiemetics as ordered. Encourage small, frequent feedings and dietary modifications as appropriate.

Drug: apalutamide (Erleada)

Class: Androgen receptor inhibitor.

Mechanism of Action: Drug binds to Androgen Receptor (AR) ligand binding domain preventing DNA binding; this leads to decreased tumor cell proliferation and apoptosis (cell death).

Metabolism: CYP2C8 and CYP3A4 microenzymes metabolize drug forming active metabolite N-desmethyl apatutamide.

Indications: Treatment of patients with non-metasatic castration-resistant prostate cancer (CRPC).

Contraindications: Pregnancy.

Dosage/Range:
- Apalutamide dose is 240 mg (four 60-mg tablets) once orally with or without food.
- Patient should receive a gonadotropin-releasing hormone (GnRH) analog concurrently or should have a bilateral orchiectomy.

Dose Modifications: If the patient experiences grade 3 or higher toxicity or an intolerable side effect, hold apalutamide until symptoms improve to ≤ grade 1 or original grade, then resume at the same dose or a reduced dose (e.g., 180 mg or 120 mg) if needed.

Drug Preparation: Oral. Available in 60-mg tablets.

Drug Administration:
- Assess patient CBC, lipid profile, and serum chemistries, especially glucose and potassium baseline and periodically during treatment. Assess BP baseline and regularly during treatment as HTN may occur.
- Assess patient risk for falls. Teach patientthat drug is associated with an increased incidence of falls and fractures. Review measures to ensure patient safety.
- Teach patient to self-administer orally once daily, with or without meals, and to swallow tablet whole at about the same time every day. If a dose is missed, take the normal dose as soon as possible on the same day, returning to the usual schedule the next day. Do not take an extra dose to make up for the missed dose.
- If the patient does not have a bilateral orchiectomy, the patient should be taught to take the GnRH analogue daily during apalutamide therapy.
- Teach patients how to make living area safer from falls (e.g., remove scatter rugs, remove clutter) as drug is associated with an increased risk for falls and fractures.
- Teach patient seizures may occur rarely, and to call MD right away if this occurs. Also, discuss activities to avoid where sudden loss of consciousness could result in harm.
- Teach patient that drug may impair fertility and not to donate sperm during therapy or for 3 months after the last dose.
- Teach patients to use effective contraception when having sex with a female partner of reproductive potential during therapy and for 3 months after last dose; also to use a condom if having sex with a pregnant woman.

Drug Interactions: Medications that are sensitive substrates of CYP3A4, CYP2C19, CYP2C9, UGT, P-gp, BCRP, or OATP1B1; concurrent use with apalutamide may result in loss of activity of these medications. See package insert.

Lab Effects/Interference:
- Anemia, leukopenia, lymphopenia.
- Hypercholesterolemia, hyperglycemia, hypertriglyceridemia, hyperkalemia.

Special Considerations:
- Most common (≥10%) adverse effects were fatigue, HTN, rash, diarrhea, nausea, weight decreased, arthralgia, falls, hot flush, decreased appetite, fracture, and peripheral edema.
- Warnings and Precautions:

- *Falls and fracture*: Assess patient for falls risk and risk of fracture. Monitor patients at risk. In clinical trials, incidence was 16% vs 9% in placebo arm, and fractures occurred in 12% in those patients receiving apalutamide vs 7% in patients treated with placebo. Median time to onset of fracture was 314 days. Ensure patient receives routine bone density assessment; discuss treatment of osteoporosis with bone targeted agents as necessary.
- *Seizure*: Rarely, seizure can occur (0.2% occurrence), which occurred 354–475 days after treatment started. Permanently discontinue if patient experiences a seizure. Teach patients to avoid activities where sudden loss of consciousness may be harmful to self or others.
- *Embryo-fetal toxicity*: Drug contraindicated in pregnancy. Teach patients to use effective contraception when having sex with a female partner of reproductive potential during therapy and for 3 months after last dose; also to use a condom if having sex with a pregnant woman.

Potential Toxicities/Side Effects and the Nursing Process

I.   ALTERATION IN COMFORT related to HOT FLUSHES, FATIGUE, ARTHRALGIA, RASH, PERIPHERAL EDEMA, FALL, FRACTURE

Defining Characteristics: Fatigue occurred in 39% of patients, arthralgia in 16%, rash in 24%, peripheral edema in 11%, fall in 16%, fracture in 12%, and hot flash in 14%.

Nursing Implications: Assess baseline comfort, and self-care measures used. Teach patient these symptoms may occur and to report them. Discuss self-care strategies to improve comfort if symptoms occur, such as use of heat and cold for musculoskeletal discomfort, leg elevation for peripheral edema, and skin care for rash. If hot flashes are severe, review common hot flash management, including wearing loose, layered clothing that can be removed when the patient becomes hot, sipping cold beverages throughout the day, sleeping with light nightclothes and a window open, avoiding triggers such as caffeine or alcohol. If the patient has peripheral edema, assess for skin integrity. Teach patient self-assessment of peripheral edema, to wear loose stockings and shoes, to keep skin moisturized to prevent cracking, and comfort measures. Teach patient to report increasing edema or related problems. Teach patient to alternate activity and rest periods to minimize fatigue and conserve energy. Teach patient strategies to reduce falls risk such as removal of scatter rugs, removal of clutter and standard falls risk reduction measures. Teach patient to report falls and potential fracture right away or to seek emergency medical care.

III.   ALTERATION IN NUTRITION, LESS THAN BODY REQUIREMENTS, related to GI DYSFUNCTION

Defining Characteristics: Nausea is most common (incidence 75%), followed by vomiting (58%), abdominal pain (58%), diarrhea (53%), constipation (28%), anorexia (23%), dyspepsia (10%), abdominal tenderness or distention (8%), and dry mouth (8%).

Nursing Implications: Assess GI, nutrition status, and presence of GI dysfunction baseline, and with each visit, administer antiemetics and teach patient self-administration. Discuss risk of serotonin antagonists to prolong QT interval, and contraindication with physician. Teach patient to report signs and symptoms, and evaluate symptom-management plan based on effectiveness of symptom control. Assess presence of pain, and discuss pharmacologic and nonpharmacologic analgesic plan with physician.

Drug: arsenic trioxide (Trisenox)

Class: Cellular poison; miscellaneous antineoplastic agent.

Mechanism of Action: Not completely understood, but drug appears to cause changes in DNA with fragmentation typical of apoptosis or programmed cell death. Drug also damages and causes degradation of the fusion protein PML/RAR alpha characteristic of acute promyelocytic leukemia. The gene responsible for the fusion protein is corrected in many cases (cytogenetic complete response), so that immature malignant myelocytic cells mature into normal white blood cells.

Metabolism: Pharmacokinetics continues to be characterized. Drug is metabolized by methylation, primarily in the liver. Arsenic is stored primarily in the liver, kidney, heart, lung, hair, and nails. Drug appears to be excreted in the urine.

Indication: Drug is indicated for induction of remission and consolidation in patients with acute promyelocytic leukemia (APL) who are refractory to, or have relapsed from, retinoid and anthracycline chemotherapy, and whose APL is characterized by the presence of the t(15;17) translocation or PML/RAR-alpha gene expression.

Contraindication: hypersensitivity to arsenic.

Dosage/Range:
Adult:
- Induction dose of 0.15 mg/kg/d IV until BM remission, not to exceed 60 doses.
- Consolidation begins 3–6 weeks after induction therapy is completed, at a dose of 0.15 mg/kg/d IV for 25 doses over a period of up to 5 weeks.
- Delay treatment for severe nonhematologic (e.g., neurologic or dermatiologic) adverse reactions until the event has resolved (e.g., ≤ grade 1).
- Dilute prior to administration.

Drug Preparation:
- Drug is available in 10 mL, single-use ampules containing 10 mg of arsenic trioxide, with a concentration of 1 mg/mL, preservative-free.
- Asceptically withdraw prescribed dose from the ampule and further dilute immediately in 100–250 mL 5% dextrose injection, USP, or 0.9% sodium chloride injection, USP.
- Drug is chemically and physically stable for 24 hours at room temperature and 48 hours when refrigerated.
- Drug does not contain any preservatives, so unused portions should be discarded.

- **Overdosage:** If symptoms of serious acute arsenic toxicity appear (seizures, muscle weakness, confusion), discontinue drug immediately and chelation therapy should be considered: dimercaprol 3 mg/kg IM q 4 hours until immediate life-threatening toxicity has subsided, then give penicillamine 250 mg PO up to qid ($\leq$1 g/day).

Drug Administration:
- Administer by IV infusion over 1–2 hours, or up to 4 hours if acute vasomotore reactions occur.

Drug Interactions:
- Unknown; do not mix with any other medications.
- Drugs that can prolong the QT interval (e.g., certain antiarrhythmics or thioridazine) or lead to electrolyte abnormalities (e.g., diuretics or amphotericin B) should be avoided if possible; otherwise, scrupulous monitoring and correction of abnormalities is critical.

Lab Effects/Interference:
- Hyperkalemia or hypokalemia.
- Hypomagnesemia.
- Hyperglycemia or hypoglycemia.
- Hypocalcemia.
- Increased hepatic transaminases ALT and AST.
- Leukocytosis.
- Anemia.
- Thrombocytopenia.
- Neutropenia.
- Disseminated intravascular coagulation (DIC).

Special Considerations:
- Warnings and Precautions:
  - Drug may cause **APL differentiation syndrome** similar to that of retinoic acid acute promyelocytic leukemia (RA-APL), which is characterized by fever, dyspnea, weight gain, pulmonary infiltrates, and pleural or pericardial effusions, with or without leukocytosis. This syndrome can be fatal, and, at the first suggestion, high-dose steroids should be instituted (dexamethasone 10 mg IV bid) for at least 3 days or longer until signs and symptoms abate. The drug manufacturer states that the majority of patients do not require termination of arsenic trioxide therapy during treatment of the syndrome (Cephalon Inc. February 2015).
  - **Cardiac Conduction Abnormalities: Torsade de Pointes, Complete Heart Block, QT Prolongation:** Drug can cause QT interval prolongation and complete atrioventricular block. Prolonged QT interval can progress to a torsades de pointes–type fatal ventricular arrhythmia. Risk factors for development of torsades de pointes are significant QT prolongation; concomitant administration of drugs that prolong the QT interval; history of torsades de pointes; preexisting QT prolongation; CHF; administration of potassium-wasting diuretics; conditions resulting in hypokalemia or hypomagnesemia, such as concurrent administration of amphotericin B. QT prolongation occurred between weeks 1–5 following arsenic infusion and then returned toward baseline by the end of 8 weeks.

- Prior to starting arsenic trioxide therapy, a 12-lead ECG should be performed and serum electrolytes (potassium, calcium, magnesium) should be assessed and any abnormalities corrected prior to starting drug. If patient is also receiving other drugs that prolong the QT interval, they should be discontinued if possible, or if not possible, the patient should receive cardiac monitoring frequently.
- Monitor ECG weekly, and more frequently if clinically unstable.
- If QTc > 500 msec, complete corrective measures and reassess the QTc with serial ECGs before starting arsenic trioxide. During therapy, maintain serum potassium concentrations > 4 mEq/L and magnesium concentrations above 1.8 mg/dL. Reassess patients who reach an absolute QT interval > 500 msec, immediately correct patient risk factors, and patient/physician should review the risk–benefit of continuing the drug.
- The patient should be hospitalized for monitoring if syncope, or rapid or irregular heart rate occurs, and serum electrolytes assessed and any abnormalities corrected. Drug should be stopped until QT interval falls below 460 msec, electrolyte abnormalities are corrected, and symptoms resolve.
- **Carcinogenesis:** Drug is a human carcinogen. Drug should not be used by pregnant or breastfeeding women. Monitor for development of second primary malignancies.
- **Embryo-fetal toxicity:** Drug is embryolethal and teratogenic. Teach female patients and males who have a female sexual partner of reproductive potential to use effective contraception during and after therapy with arsenic trioxide.
- **Laboratory Testing:** At least 2 times a week, the patient should have electrolyte, hematologic, and coagulation assessed; more frequently if abnormal during the induction phase, and at least weekly during the consolidation phase. ECGs should be done weekly; more frequently if abnormal.
- Most common side effects include leukocytosis, nausea, vomiting, diarrhea, abdominal pain, fatigue, edema, hyperglycemia, dyspnea, cough, rash, itching, headaches, and dizziness.

Potential Toxicities/Side Effects and the Nursing Process

I. ALTERATION IN OXYGENATION, POTENTIAL, related to APL DIFFERENTIATION SYNDROME

Defining Characteristics: Drug may cause APL differentiation syndrome similar to the retinoic acid acute promyelocytic leukemia (RA-APL), which is characterized by fever, dyspnea, weight gain, pulmonary infiltrates, and pleural or pericardial effusions, with or without leukocytosis. This syndrome develops in response to the differentiation of immature malignant cells into mature normal white blood cells and the increased white blood cell count. The body's response is an inflammatory reaction with fluid retention in the lining of the lungs and heart. This syndrome can be fatal, and at the first suggestion, high-dose steroids should be instituted (dexamethasone 10 mg IV bid) for at least 3 days or longer until signs and symptoms abate. The drug manufacturer states that the majority of patients do not require termination of arsenic trioxide therapy during treatment of the syndrome. The reported incidence is approximately 22%. Leucocytosis, if it occurs, at levels >10 × 10^3/μL is unrelated to baseline or peak white blood cell counts. Leukocytosis was not treated with chemotherapy, and levels were lower during consolidation than during induction.

Nursing Implications: Assess temperature and VS, oxygen saturation, cardiopulmonary status baseline and at each visit. Assess weight daily, and teach patient to report any SOB, fever, or weight gain immediately. If signs or symptoms develop, notify physician immediately and discuss obtaining CXR, cardiac echo, and focused exam. Discuss CXR, ECHO, and laboratory findings with physician. Be prepared to administer high-dose steroids (e.g., dexamethasone 10 mg IV bid 3 days or longer depending on symptom resolution). Provide pulmonary and hemodynamic support as necessary. Assess CBC, with focus on white blood cell count and presence of leukocytosis.

II. POTENTIAL ALTERATION IN CARDIAC FUNCTION related to QT PROLONGATION AND ARRHYTHMIA

Defining Characteristics: Drug can cause QT interval prolongation and complete atrioventricular block. Prolonged QT interval can progress to a torsades de pointes–type fatal ventricular arrhythmia. Risk factors for development of torsades de pointes are significant QT prolongation, concomitant administration of drugs that prolong the QT interval, history of torsades de pointes, preexisting QT prolongation, CHF, administration of potassium-wasting diuretics, and conditions resulting in hypokalemia or hypomagnesemia, such as concurrent administration of amphotericin B.

Nursing Implications: Assess baseline risk, cardiovascular status, EKG-determined QT interval, electrolyte and renal blood studies, and medications the patient is taking that may prolong QT interval, such as serotonin antagonist antiemetics. At least 2 times a week, the patient should have electrolyte, hematologic, and coagulation assessed; more frequently if abnormal during the induction phase, and at least weekly during the consolidation phase. EKGs should be done weekly and more frequently if abnormal. Discuss correction of any electrolyte abnormalities, as well as other risk factors, with physician. Any drugs that prolong the QT interval should be discontinued. If the QT interval prolongation is >500 msec, this should be corrected prior to drug administration. During arsenic trioxide therapy, serum potassium should be kept >4.0 mEq/dL and serum magnesium >1.8 mg/dL. If the QT interval exceeds 500 msec, reassessment and correction of risk factors should occur. The patient should be hospitalized for monitoring if syncope or rapid or irregular heart rate occurs, and serum electrolytes assessed and any abnormalities corrected. Drug should be stopped until QT interval falls below 460 msec, electrolyte abnormalities corrected, and symptoms resolve.

III. ALTERATION IN NUTRITION, LESS THAN BODY REQUIREMENTS, related to GI DYSFUNCTION

Defining Characteristics: Nausea is most common (incidence 75%), followed by vomiting (58%), abdominal pain (58%), diarrhea (53%), constipation (28%), anorexia (23%), dyspepsia (10%), abdominal tenderness or distention (8%), and dry mouth (8%).

Nursing Implications: Assess GI, nutrition status, and presence of GI dysfunction baseline, and with each visit, administer antiemetics and teach patient self-administration. Discuss risk of serotonin antagonists to prolong QT interval, and contraindication with physician. Teach patient to report signs and symptoms, and evaluate symptom-management plan based on effectiveness of symptom control. Assess presence of pain, and discuss pharmacologic and nonpharmacologic analgesic plan with physician.

IV. ALTERATION IN PROTECTIVE MECHANISMS, related to FEVER, ANEMIA, DIC, BLEEDING

Defining Characteristics: Fever affects 63% of patients (13% febrile neutropenia), with 38% of patients having rigors. In clinical studies, 8% of patients had hemorrhage, 20% anemia, 18% thrombocytopenia, 10% neutropenia, and 8% DIC. Patients may develop infections, and in clinical studies, most commonly these were sinusitis 20%, herpes simplex 13%, upper respiratory tract infection 13%, nonspecific bacterial 8%, herpes zoster 8%, oral candidiasis 5%, and (rarely) sepsis 5%.

Nursing Implications: At least twice a week, the patient should have electrolyte, hematologic, and coagulation assessed; more frequently if abnormal during the induction phase, and at least weekly during the consolidation phase. Monitor laboratory results, and discuss abnormalities with physician. Assess patient for fever, signs and symptoms of infection, rigors, and bleeding, and implement management plan to assure patient safety. Transfuse patient as ordered, and monitor closely.

V. ALTERATION IN COMFORT related to HEADACHE, CHEST PAIN, AND INJECTION-SITE CHANGES

Defining Characteristics: Headache occurred in approximately 60% of patients, while chest pain occurred in 25%. Injection-site reactions of pain, erythema, and edema occurred in 20%, 13%, and 10% of patients, respectively.

Nursing Implications: Assess level of comfort, and develop plan for comfort, including pharmacologic and nonpharmacologic measures. Assess effectiveness, and revise plan as needed. Assess patency of IV site and need for IV catheter change. Assess need for central line. Although not necessary for drug delivery, if patient venous access is limited, this may provide enhanced patient comfort.

VI. ALTERATION IN ACTIVITY TOLERANCE related to FATIGUE, MUSCULOSKELETAL PROBLEMS

Defining Characteristics: 63% of patients reported fatigue. In clinical studies, musculoskeletal events were arthralgias (33%), myalgias (25%), bone pain (23%), back pain (18%), neck pain (13%), and pain in limbs (13%).

Nursing Implications: Assess baseline energy and activity level, and level of comfort. Assess need for assistance with ADL and home assistance. Assess need for analgesics or local measures to relieve pain and discomfort. Teach patient self-care strategies to minimize exertion and maximize activity, such as clustering activity during shopping, alternating rest and activity periods, diet, gentle exercise. Evaluate success of plan and need for revisions.

VII. ALTERATION IN FLUID AND ELECTROLYTE BALANCE related to HYPOKALEMIA, HYPOMAGNESEMIA, HYPERGLYCEMIA, EDEMA

Defining Characteristics: Hypokalemia occurs in about 50% of patients, hypomagnesemia (45%), hyperglycemia (45%), and edema (40%). Other electrolyte abnormalities are hyperkalemia (18%), hypocalcemia (10%), hypoglycemia (8%), acidosis (5%), and increased transaminases (13–20%).

Nursing Implications: At least twice a week, the patient should have electrolyte, hematologic and coagulation assessed; more frequently if abnormal during the induction phase, and at least weekly during the consolidation phase. EKGs should be done weekly and more frequently if abnormal. Teach patient that edema may occur, and to report it. Assess patient baseline and before each treatment for weight and presence of edema. Discuss abnormalities with physician, correct as ordered, and monitor closely for signs and symptoms of imbalance.

VIII. SENSORY/PERCEPTUAL ALTERATIONS, POTENTIAL, related to PARESTHESIA, DIZZINESS, TREMOR, INSOMNIA

Defining Characteristics: Insomnia occurs in 43% of patients, paresthesia (33%), dizziness (23%), tremor (13%), seizures (8%), somnolence (8%), and (rarely) coma (5%).

Nursing Implications: Assess baseline mental and neurologic status, and monitor frequently during therapy. Assess sensory function, and teach patient to report numbness, tingling, dizziness, tremor, seizure, decrease in alertness, and changes in sleep. Assess presence of paresthesias, and motor and sensory function prior to each treatment; discuss presence or worsening with physician. Teach patient self-care strategies, including maintaining safety when walking, getting up, taking a bath, or washing dishes if unable to feel temperature changes. Teach self-care measures to manage sleep problems, and discuss possible need for sleeping medication.

IX. ALTERATION IN GAS EXCHANGE, POTENTIAL, related to COUGH, DYSPNEA, HYPOXIA, PLEURAL EFFUSION

Defining Characteristics: Cough is common, affecting 65% of patients, followed by dyspnea (53%), epistaxis (25%), hypoxia (23%), pleural effusion (20%), postnasal drip (13%), wheezing (13%), decreased breath sounds (10%), crepitations (10%), rales (crackles) (10%), hemoptysis (8%), tachypnea (8%), and rhonchi (8%).

Nursing Implications: Assess baseline pulmonary status, including breath sounds and oxygen saturation, and monitor at least daily during treatment. Teach patient that symptoms may occur and to report them. Discuss management of patients experiencing cough, dyspnea, and other symptoms with physician, and develop individualized management plan.

X. ALTERATION IN SKIN INTEGRITY, POTENTIAL, related to SKIN IRRITATION

Defining Characteristics: Dermatitis affects about 43% of patients, pruritus (33%), ecchymosis (20%), dry skin (13%), erythema (13%), hyperpigmentation (8%), and urticaria (8%).

Nursing Implications: Assess baseline skin integrity and monitor at each visit. Teach patient to report any skin changes or itching. Teach patient symptomatic local measures to manage dermatitis, itch, or other changes. If plan is ineffective, discuss other measures with physician.

Drug: asparaginase (Elspar, Erwinaze [*Erwinia chrysanthemi*], L-asparaginase)

Class: Miscellaneous agents (enzyme).

Mechanism of Action: Hydrolyzes serum asparagine, which deprives leukemia cells of the required amino acid. Normal cells are spared because they generally have the ability to synthesize their own asparagine. Cell cycle–specific for G_1 postmitotic phase. Some leukemic cells are unable to synthesize asparagine. These cells must obtain asparagine from an exogenous source, the patient's serum. Administration of the enzyme L-asparaginase causes hydrolysis of asparagine to aspartate, resulting in rapid depletion of the asparagine concentration in the patient's serum. The leukemic cells cannot synthesize protein or proliferate.

Metabolism: Metabolism of L-asparaginase is independent of renal and hepatic function. The drug is not recovered in the urine and does not appear to cross the blood–brain barrier.

Indication: As a component of a multi-agent chemotherapeutic regimen for the treatment of patients with acute lymphoblastic leukemia (ALL).

Contraindications: History of hypersensitivity to the type of asparaginase (e.g., Erwinaze, *Escherichia coli*); history of or presence of serious pancreatitis, thrombosis, or hemorrhagic events with prior L-asparaginase therapy.

Dosage/Range:
- Indicated as a component of a multi-agent chemotherapeutic regimen for treatment of patients with acute lymphoblastic leukemia (ALL).
- Erwinaze (asparaginase Erwinia chrysanthem) is indicated for patients who have developed hypersensitivity to *E. coli*–derived asparaginase.
- IM or IV varies with protocol.

- **Erwinaze:**
  - To substitute for pegaspargase: 25,000 IU/m^2 IM or IV 3 times a week (M/W/F) for 6 doses for each planned dose of pegaspargase.
  - To substitute for a dose of native *E. coli* asparaginase: 25,000 IU/m^2 IM for each scheduled dose of native *E. coli* asparaginase.

Drug Preparation:
- Erwinaze: available as vials containing 10,000 IU lyophylized powder per vial. Limit the volume of reconstituted Erwinaze as a single injection to 2 mL; if reconstituted dose to be administered is >2 mL, use multiple injection sites.
- IV injection: reconstitute with sterile water for injection or 0.9% sodium chloride injection (without preservative), and use within 8 hours of restoration.
- IV infusion: dilute with 0.9% sodium chloride injection or 5% dextrose injection and use within 8 hours, only if clear; if gelatinous particles develop, filter through a 5.0-μm filter.
- IM: 6,000–12,000 units/m^2 dose as a single agent: reconstitute to 10,000 units/mL.
- The lyophilized powder must be stored under refrigeration. The reconstituted solution must also be stored under refrigeration if it is not used immediately. The solution must be discarded 8 hours after preparation.

Drug Administration:
- Erwinaze is administered IM.
- Test dose: often ordered before first dose or after restarting drug after a break; 0.1–0.2 mL of a 20- to 250-units/mL dose (2–50 units) intradermally and observe patient for 15–30 minutes.
- Use in a hospital setting. Make preparations to treat anaphylaxis at each administration of the drug and have epinephrine, diphenhydramine, and hydrocortisone nearby. Ensure that patent IV is available before giving drugs IM.

Drug Interactions:
- Prednisone: potential additive hyperglycemic effect; monitor blood glucose levels.
- Cyclophosphamide, vincristine, 6-mercaptopurine: may increase or decrease drug's effect (CTX, VCR, 6-MP).
- 6-mercaptopurine: enhanced hepatotoxicity; monitor LFTs closely.
- Methotrexate: antagonism if administered immediately prior to methotrexate; when administered some time after methotrexate, may enhance methotrexate activity.
- Synergy with cytosine arabinoside.
- Increased hyperglycemia when given together with prednisone.
- Reduced hypersensitivity when given with 6-mercaptopurine or prednisone.
- Additive neurotoxicity when given with vincristine.
- Asparaginase, when given before vincristine, will decrease vincristine excretion, with resulting increased neurotoxicity; give vincristine 12–24 hours before asparaginase.
- Live vaccines may enhance viral replication and toxicity.
- Intravenous administration of L-asparaginase concurrently with or immediately before prednisone and vincristine administration may be associated with increased toxicity.

Lab Effects/Interference:
- Increased LFTs.
- Increased pancreatic enzymes.
- Decreased hepatically derived clotting factors.
- Interferes with thyroid function tests after first 2 days of therapy: effect lasts 4 weeks.

Special Considerations:
- Warnings and Precautions:
  - Hypersensitivity Reactions (HSR): Grades 3–4 HSRs have occurred in about 5% of patients (Erwinaze, 2016). Ensure that the drug is administered in a setting with resuscitation equipment and medicines, as well as physician/NP/PA support. Discontinue the drug if serious hypersensitivity occurs.
  - Pancreatitis: occurs in 4% of patients. If patients develop symptoms, further evaluate. If patient has severe or hemorrhagic pancreatitis characterized by abdominal pain > 72 hours, amylase elevation $\geq$ 2.0 × ULN, discontinue drug. If the patient has mild pancreatitis, hold the drug until signs/symptoms subside, and amylase level returns to normal. After resolution, resume drug.
- Glucose intolerance may occur in 5% of patients, and in some cases is irreversible; perform glucose monitoring as appropriate and treat hyperglycemia with insulin as necessary and ordered.
- Thrombosis, hemorrhage may rarely occur; discontinue drug until this is resolved. After symptoms resolve, drug may be resumed.
- Drug is derived from purified *E. coli* or *Erwinia chrysanthemi,* and if an allergic reaction occurs, the patient may try the other drug. Also, pegylated asparaginase is also available.

Potential Toxicities/Side Effects and the Nursing Process

I. POTENTIAL FOR INJURY related to HYPERSENSITIVITY OR ANAPHYLACTIC REACTIONS

Defining Characteristics: Occurs in 20–30% of patients. Increased incidence after several doses administered, but may occur with first dose. Occurs less often with IM route of administration. May be life-threatening reaction, but is usually mild.

Nursing Implications: Discuss with physician use of test dose prior to drug administration. Assess baseline vital signs and mental status prior to drug administration. Review standing orders or nursing procedure for management of anaphylaxis and be prepared to stop drug immediately if signs/symptoms occur; keep IV line open with 0.9% sodium chloride, notify physician, monitor vital signs, and administer ordered medications, which may include epinephrine 1:1,000, hydrocortisone sodium succinate, and diphenhydramine. Teach patient the potential of a hypersensitivity or anaphylactic reaction and to report any unusual symptoms immediately. *E. coli* preparation of L-asparaginase and *Erwinia carotovora* preparation are non-cross-resistant, so if an anaphylactic reaction occurs with one, the other preparation may be used. HSR with Erwinaze is 17% incidence.

II.   POTENTIAL FOR INJURY related to PANCREATITIS, HEPATIC DYSFUNCTION
       OR THROMBOEMBOLISM

Defining Characteristics: Pancreatitis occurred in 4% of patients receiving Erwinaze.
Two-thirds of patients have elevated LFTs starting within the first 2 weeks of treatment
(e.g., SGOT, bili, and alk phos). Hepatically derived clotting factors may be depressed,
resulting in excessive bleeding or blood clotting. Relatively uncommon.

Nursing Implications: Monitor SGOT, bili, alk phos, albumin, and clotting factors CPT,
PTT, fibrinogen. Teach patient of the potential of excessive bleeding or blood clotting, and
instruct to report any unusual symptoms. Serious thrombotic events have been described,
including sagittal sinus thrombosis. After a 2-week course of Erwinaze therapy, fibrinogen,
protein C activity, protein S activity, and anti-III thrombin coagulation points were decreased. Assess patient for signs/symptoms of thrombosis or bleeding. Discontinue Erwinaze for a thrombotic or hemorrhagic event until symptoms resolve, and then drug may be
resumed. Assess patients receiving Erwinaze for signs/symptoms of severe or hemorrhagic
pancreatitis: abdominal pain >72 hours, amylase elevations >2.0× ULN, and stop drug.
Drug should be discontinued if severe or hemorrhagic pancreatitis; if only moderate, drug
can be reintroduced after serum amylase returns to normal levels, and signs/symptoms
resolve.

III.   ALTERED NUTRITION, LESS THAN BODY REQUIREMENTS, related to
        NAUSEA/VOMITING, ANOREXIA, HYPERGLYCEMIA

Defining Characteristics: 50–60% of patients experience mild to severe nausea and
vomiting, starting within 4–6 hours after treatment. Anorexia commonly occurs. Hyperglycemia is a transient reaction caused by effects on the pancreas with decreased insulin
synthesis. Pancreatitis occurs in 5% of patients.

Nursing Implications: Premedicate with antiemetics and continue prophylactically for
24 hours to prevent nausea and vomiting. Encourage small, frequent meals of cool, bland
foods and liquids, as well as favorite foods, especially high-calorie, high-protein foods.
Encourage use of spices and do weekly weights. Teach patient about the potential of hyperglycemia and pancreatitis, and instruct to report any unusual symptoms (e.g., increased
thirst, urination, and appetite). Monitor serum glucose, amylase, and lipase levels periodically during treatment. Report any laboratory elevations to physician. Treat hyperglycemia
issues with diet or insulin as ordered by physician. Treat pancreatitis per physician orders.

IV.   SENSORY/PERCEPTUAL ALTERATIONS related to CHANGES IN MENTAL
       STATUS

Defining Characteristics: 25% of patients experience some changes in mental status—
commonly, lethargy, drowsiness, and somnolence; rarely coma. Predominantly seen in

adults. Malaise (feeling "blah") occurs in most patients, and generally gets worse with subsequent doses. Drug does not cross BBB.

Nursing Implications: Teach patient about the potential of CNS toxicity, and instruct to report any unusual symptoms. Obtain baseline neurologic and mental function. Assess patient for any neurologic abnormalities and report changes to physician. Discuss with patient the impact of malaise on his/her general sense of well-being and strategies to minimize the distress.

V. POTENTIAL FOR SEXUAL DYSFUNCTION related to REPRODUCTION HAZARD

Defining Characteristics: Drug is teratogenic.

Nursing Implications: As appropriate, explore with patient and partner issues of reproductive and sexual patterns and impact chemotherapy will have. Discuss strategies to preserve sexuality and reproductive health (e.g., sperm banking, contraception).

VI. INFECTION, BLEEDING, AND FATIGUE related to BM DEPRESSION

Defining Characteristics: BM depression is not common. Mild anemia may occur. Serious leukopenia and thrombocytopenia are rare.

Nursing Implications: Monitor CBC, platelet count prior to drug administration, as well as signs/symptoms of infection, bleeding, or anemia. Instruct patient in self-assessment of signs/symptoms of infection, bleeding, or anemia and to report immediately.

Drug: azacytidine for injection (Vidaza)

Class: Nucleoside metabolic inhibitor (antimetabolite).

Mechanism of Action: Azacitidine is a nucleoside metabolic inhibitor (pyrimidine nucleoside analogue) of cytidine. It is believed to cause hypomethylation of DNA and to directly kill abnormal hematopoietic cells in the BM (direct cytotoxicity). Hypomethylation may restore normal function to genes critical for cell differentiation and proliferation. Direct cytotoxicity causes the death of rapidly dividing cells, including cancer cells no longer responsive to normal growth control mechanisms, and it spares non-proliferating cells that are insensitive to the drug.

Metabolism: Rapidly absorbed following subcutaneous administration, with peak plasma level in 30 minutes. Bioavailability of subcutaneously administered drug is 89% of IV dose. 85% of the total administered dose is excreted in the urine, and < 1% in feces. Mean elimination half-life is about 4 hours in both subcutaneous and IV-administered drug.

Indication: Azacytidine is indicated for treatment of patients with myelodysplastic subtypes: (1) refractory anemia (RA) or (2) refractory anemia with ringed sideroblasts (RARS) (if accompanied by neutropenia or thrombocytopenia or requiring transfusions), (3) refractory anemia with excess blasts (RAEB), (4) refractory anemia with excess blasts in transformation (RAEB-T), and (5) chronic myelomonocytic leukemia (CMMoL).

Contraindication:
- Drug is contraindicated in patients with (1) hypersensitivity to mannitol and (2) advanced malignant hepatic tumors.

Dosage/Range:
- Initial (first) cycle: 75 mg/m^2 subcutaneous injection *or* IV infusion daily for 7 days. Premedicate for nausea and/or vomiting.
- Repeat cycles every 4 weeks for at least 4 cycles. After 2 cycles, may increase dose to 100 mg/m^2 if no beneficial effect is seen and no toxicity other than nausea and vomiting has occurred. A minimum of 4–6 cycles of treatment is recommended. Complete or partial response may require additional treatment cycles.
- Continue treatment as long as the patient continues to benefit.
- Monitor patients for hematologic response and for renal toxicity; delay or reduce dose as appropriate.

Dosage Adjustment:
- If baseline (start of treatment) WBC $\geq$ 3,000/mm^3, ANC $\geq$ 1,500/mm^3, and platelets $\geq$ 75,000/mm^3, **modify dose based on nadir counts**.
  - Nadir ANC < 500/mm^3, platelets < 25,000/mm^3—give 50% dose in the next course.
  - Nadir ANC 500–1,500/mm^3, platelets 25,000–50,000/mm^3—give 67% dose in the next course.
  - Nadir ANC > 1,500/mm^3, platelets > 50,000/mm^3—give 100% of dose.
- If baseline WBC < 3,000/mm^3, ANC < 1,500/mm^3, or platelets < 75,000/mm^3, dose **adjustments should be based on nadir and BM biopsy cellularity at time of nadir**, unless there is clear improvement in differentiation (% mature granulocytes is higher and ANC is higher than at onset of that course) at the time of the next cycle—see package insert.
- Dose modification based on renal function and serum electrolytes.
  - If unexplained decreases in serum bicarbonate < 20 mEq/L, dose-reduce 50% in next cycle.
  - If elevations of BUN or serum creatinine occur, delay next dose until values return to normal or baseline, and reduce dose by 50% in next cycle.

Drug Preparation:
- Drug is a lyophilized powder in 100-mg single-use vials.
- Reconstitute aseptically with 4 mL sterile water for injection, adding diluent slowly into the vial.
- Vigorously shake or roll the vial until a uniform suspension is achieved, which will be cloudy and contain azycitidine 25 mg/mL. Do not filter the suspension after reconstitution, as this may remove active substance.

- Preparation for immediate subcutaneous administration; divide doses greater than 4 mL equally into 2 syringes and administer within 1 hour of reconstitution at room temperature.
- Preparation for delayed subcutaneous administration: reconstituted solution may be kept in the vial or drawn in a syringe(s) and refrigerated immediately (2–8°C, 36–46°F) for later use. Doses greater than 4 mL should be divided equally using 2 syringes. It may be stored for up to 8 hours if reconstituted with unrefrigerated sterile water for injection, and up to 22 hours if reconstituted with refrigerated sterile water for injection. After removal from the refrigerator, the suspension may be allowed to equilibrate to room temperature for up to 30 minutes prior to administration.
- IV preparation: reconsititute each vial with 10 mL sterile water for injection, and vigorously shake vial until dissolved. Vigorously shake or roll the vial until all solids are dissolved. Resulting solution should be a clear solution with a concentration of 10 mg/mL. Withdraw the ordered amount, and inject into a 50- to 100-mL infusion bag of either 0.9% sodium chloride injection or Lactated Ringer's Injection. Drug is INCOMPATIBLE with 5% dextrose solutions, Hespan, or solutions containing bicarbonate.

Drug Administration:
- Assess CBC/ANC, liver chemistries, and serum creatinine before first dose. Monitor patient for hematologic response and renal toxicities. Discuss abnormalities and need for dose delay or reduction with physician.
- *Subcutaneous administration:*
  - To provide a homogenous suspension, the contents of the dosing syringe must be resuspended immediately prior to subcutaneous administration. To resuspend, vigorously roll the syringe between the palms until a uniform, cloudy suspension is achieved.
  - Suspension reconstituted with nonrefrigerated water for injection for subcutaneous administration may be stored for up to 1 hour at 25°C or for up to 8 hours between 2 and 8°C (36–46°F). When reconstituted with refrigerated 2–8°C (36–46°F) water for injection, it may be stored for 22 hours at 2–8°C (36–46°F).
- Rotate sites for each subcutaneous injection (thigh, abdomen, or upper arm), and give new injection at least 1 inch from old site, and never into areas where site is tender, bruised, red, or hard. Doses >4 mL should be divided equally into 2 syringes and injected into 2 separate sites.
- *Administer IV solution* over 10–40 minutes, so that administration is completed within 1 hour of reconstitution. Visually inspect the reconstituted vial for particulate matter and discoloration, prior to administration, whenever solution and container permit.

Drug Interactions:
- IV solution: incompatible with 5% dextrose, Hespan, solutions containing bicarbonate.
- No formal drug interaction studies have been conducted.

Lab Effects/Interference:
- Decreased ANC, platelets, red blood cell counts.
- Renal tubular acidosis.
- Increased BUN and creatinine.
- Hypokalemia.

Special Considerations:
- Most common adverse reactions (>30%) by SC route: nausea, anemia, thrombocytopenia, vomiting, pyrexia, leukopenia, diarrhea, injection-site erythema, constipation, neutropenia, and ecchymosis. Most common adverse reactions by IV route included petechiae, rigors, weakness, and hypokalemia.
- Warnings and Precautions:
  - Anemia, neutropenia, and thrombocytopenia: Monitor CBC/ANC frequently, as anemia, neutropenia, and thrombocytopenia are common. Monitor CBC/ANC for response and/or toxicity, at least prior to each dosing cycle. After cycle 1, adjust doses for subsequent cycles based on nadir counts and hematologic response.
  - Hepatotoxicity: Patients with severe, preexisting hepatic impairment are at higher risk for toxicity. Use cautiously in patients with preexisting hepatic disease, as patients with extensive liver metastases have been reported to develop coma and death. Teach patients to inform their physician if they have any underlying liver or renal disease.
  - Renal impairment: Monitor patients with renal impairment for toxicity since azacitidine and its metabolites are primarily excreted by the kidneys. Monitor elderly patient's renal function closely while receiving the drug.
  - Embryo-fetal toxicity: Azacitidine may cause fetal harm when administered to a pregnant woman. Women of childbearing potential should be apprised of the potential hazard to a fetus. Teach women of childbearing potential to use effective contraception methods to prevent pregnancy while receiving azacitidine.
  - Men should be advised not to father a child while receiving azacitidine.
- Nursing mothers should discontinue nursing or discontinue use of azacitidine, taking into consideration the importance of the drug to the mother.
- Monitor liver chemistries and serum creatinine, baseline and prior to each cycle of therapy. Azacitidine and its metabolites are primarily excreted by the kidney. Patients with renal impairment should be closely monitored for renal function and toxicity.

Potential Toxicities/Side Effects and the Nursing Process

I.   INFECTION AND BLEEDING related to BM DEPRESSION

Defining Characteristics: In clinical studies 1 and 2, incidence of leukopenia was 48.2%, neutropenia 32.3%, and febrile neutropenia 16.4%. Thrombocytopenia and anemia occurred in 65.5% and 69.5% of patients, respectively.

Nursing Implications: Monitor CBC, neutrophil, and platelet count baseline and prior to cycle, then as needed postchemotherapy; assess for signs/symptoms of infection, bleeding, and anemia. Teach patient and family signs/symptoms of infection, bleeding, and anemia, and instruct to report them to nurse or physician immediately. Teach patient to avoid aspirin-containing OTC medications.

II. ALTERATION IN NUTRITION, LESS THAN BODY REQUIREMENTS, related to NAUSEA AND VOMITING, ANOREXIA, STOMATITIS, CONSTIPATION, AND DIARRHEA

Defining Characteristics: Nausea/vomiting is dose related, and occurs in about 70.5%/54.1% of patients, respectively. This tends to be worse in the first 1–2 cycles, and increases in incidence with increasing doses. Diarrhea develops in 36.4% of patients, with incidence increasing as dose increases. Constipation occurs in about 33.6% of patients and is worse during the first 2 cycles of therapy. Anorexia affects 20% of patients, and stomatitis occurs in 7.7% of patients.

Nursing Implications: Assess nutritional and elimination status baseline, and periodically at visits. Premedicate with antiemetics before injection, and teach patient self-administration of antiemetics at home; encourage small, frequent feedings as tolerated; if severe vomiting occurs, treat with alternative antiemetics and assess for signs/symptoms of fluid and electrolyte imbalance. Monitor serum potassium, as hypokalemia may be a side effect of treatment. Assess baseline bowel elimination status. Instruct patient to report onset of diarrhea and administer antidiarrheals as ordered. If diarrhea is protracted, ensure adequate hydration, monitor total body fluid balance, and teach/reinforce perineal hygiene. Instruct patient to monitor for constipation and to use measures to prevent constipation if that is a problem. If patient has anorexia, teach patient to identify nutrient-dense foods and to eat small frequent meals, including a bedtime snack. Teach patient strategies to increase appetite, depending upon an individualized assessment. Teach patient to self-assess oral mucosa and to use a systematic cleansing of teeth/mouth after meals and at bedtime. Monitor LFTs periodically during therapy and discuss abnormalities with physician.

III. ALTERATION IN COMFORT related to PYREXIA, FATIGUE, ARTHRALGIAS, HEADACHE, AND INJECTION-SITE IRRITATION

Defining Characteristics: Pyrexia occurred in 51.8% of patients, arthralgias in 22.3%, headache in 21.8%, injection-site erythema in 35%, injection-site pain in 22.7%, injection-site bruising in 14.1%, and injection-site reaction in 13.6%. Injection-site discomfort was more pronounced during the first and second cycles of therapy.

Nursing Implications: Monitor temperature and teach patient to self-assess temperature. Teach patient that pyrexia may occur and how to self-administer antipyretics. Teach measures to reduce discomfort related to myalgias if they occur, such as application of heat and NSAIDs. Teach patient strategies to conserve energy, such as alternating activity with rest. Teach patient to rotate sites used for injection, as well as local measures to increase comfort.

Drug: bendamustine hydrochloride (Treanda)

Class: Alkylating agent; nitrogen mustard derivative.

Mechanism of Action: Bifunctional with both alkylating and purine-like (antimetabolite) action. It causes sustainable double-strand DNA breaks and induces apoptosis, resulting in cell death. It appears to also cause apoptosis-independent cell death. It differs from nitrogen mustard by a benzimidazole ring, which helps to explain why the drug is active in patients who are refractory to other alkylating agents. Drug is active in dividing as well as resting cells. The exact MOA is unknown.

Metabolism: It undergoes biotransformation in the liver into an active compound; drug's active minor metabolites gamma-hydroxybendamustine and N-desmethyl-bendamustine are formed via cytochrome P450 CYP1A2. Low plasma protein binding; terminal half-life is 3.5 hours. Excreted via the kidneys as active drug and metabolites. No clinically significant differences in gender, or in geriatric patients, were seen in the adverse-reaction profile.

Indication: FDA-indicated for the treatment of patients with (1) indolent B-cell non-Hodgkin's lymphoma that has progressed during or within 6 months of treatment with rituximab or a rituximab-containing regimen, as well as (2) patients with chronic lymphocytic leukemia (CLL). Comparative efficacy to first-line therapies in CLL other than chlorambucil unknown.

Contraindications: Patients with a known hypersensitivity to bendamustine.

CLL: 100-mg/m^2 IV infusion over 30 minutes on days 1 and 2 of a 28-day cycle, for up to 6 cycles.
- Grades 3 or higher hematologic toxicity: Dose-reduce to 50 mg/m^2 on days 1 and 2; if grades 3 or higher toxicity recurs, dose-reduce to 25 mg/m^2 on days 1 and 2.
- For nonhematologic toxicity, clinically significant grades 3 or higher, dose-reduce to 50 mg/m^2 on days 1 and 2 of each cycle.
- Dose reescalation may be considered.

Indolent B-cell NHL: 120 mg/m^2 IV infusion over 60 minutes on days 1 and 2 of a 21-day cycle, for up to 8 cycles.
- Grade 4 hematologic toxicity: Dose-reduce to 90 mg/m^2 on days 1 and 2 of each cycle; if grade 4 toxicity recurs, dose-reduce to 60 mg/m^2 on days 1 and 2 of each cycle.
- Non-hematologic grades 3–4 toxicity: Dose-reduce to 90 mg/m^2 on days 1 and 2 of each cycle; if grades 3–4 toxicity recurs, dose-reduce to 60 mg/m^2 on days 1 and 2 of each cycle.

General Dosing Considerations:
- Delay treatment for grade 4 hematologic toxicity or clinically significant grade 2 or higher non-hematologic toxicity.
- Discontinue for severe skin reactions (as Stevens-Johnson syndrome [SJS] may occur), severe infusion reactions, or anaphylactic reactions.

- Assess patient for tumor lysis syndrome (TLS), especially during cycle 1 of treatment; discuss with physician/NP/PA vigorous hydration (to maintain adequate volume status) with close monitoring of blood chemistry (i.e., potassium and uric acid levels). There may be increased risk of severe skin toxicity when allopurinol and bendamustine are given concomitantly.

Drug Preparation:
- Drug is available in two formulations:
  - (1) Solution (Treanda Injection) and (2) lyophilized powder (Treanda for Injection). Do NOT mix or combine the two formulations, as they have different drug concentrations.
  - If Treanda Injection solution is used, *do not* use devices containing polycarbonate or acrylo-nitrile-butadiene-styrene (ABS), including most closed-system transfer devices (CSTDs), adapters, or syringes. ONLY USE polypropylene syringe with a metal needle and polypropylene hub to withdraw and transfer Treanda Injection. Rationale: Treanda Injection contains *N,N*-dimethylacetamide (DMA), which is incompatible with polycarbonate and ABS, causing CSTDs, adaptors, and syringes containing polycarbonate or ABS to dissolve. This may lead to leaking, breaking of CSTD components, product contamination, and injury to patient and practitioner.
- Select formulation to administer.
  - If a closed-system transfer device or adaptor is to be used as supplemental protection during preparation, or the preparation area does not have polypropylene syringes with metal needles, *only use Treanda for Injection,* the lyophilized formulation.
  - Preparing Treanda Injection (45 mg/0.5 mL or 180 mg/2 mL solution; prepare only a single dose):
    - Use only a *polypropylene* syringe with a metal needle and polypropylene hub to withdraw and transfer the drug solution.
    - Aseptically withdraw the volume needed using a **polypropylene syringe with a metal needle and polypropylene hub,** for the calculated dose from the 90 mg/mL solution; **immediately** transfer solution to a 500-mL infusion bag of 0.9% sodium chloride injection, USP (an alternative of a 500-mL infusion bag of 2.5% dextrose/0.45% sodium chloride injection USP may be considered; no other diluents are compatible); the resulting bendamustine HCl concentration in the 500-mL bag should be within 0.2–0.7 mg/mL.
    - Visually inspect the filled syringe and the prepared infusion bag to ensure that there is no visible particulate matter prior to administration. The prepared solution should be clear, colorless to yellow.
  - **Preparing Treanda for Injection** (25 mg/vial or 100 mg/vial lyophilized powder; each vial is single use only).
    - Aseptically reconstitute each Treanda for Injection vial as follows:
    - 25-mg vial: add 5 mL sterile water for injection, USP.
    - 100-mg vial: add 20 mL sterile water for injection, USP.
    - Shake well to completely dissolve the lyophilized powder; the result should be a clear, colorless to pale yellow solution with bendamustine HCl concentration of

5 mg/mL. Visibly inspect for particulate matter, and if found, do not use. *Transfer to the infusion bag must occur within 30 min of preparation.*
- Aseptically withdraw the ordered dose and **immediately** transfer it to a 500-mL infusion bag of 0.9% sodium chloride injection, USP (an alternative 500-mL infusion bag of 2.5% dextrose/0.45% sodium chloride injection USP may be considered; no other diluents are compatible); the resulting concentration of bendamustine HCl in the bag should be within 0.2–0.6 mg/mL. Thoroughly mix the contents of the infusion bag, and again inspect for any particulate matter before administration. The solution should be clear, colorless to slightly yellow in color. Discard any unused drug.
- **Admixture Stability:** Neither formulation contains an antimicrobial preservative, so the drug admixture should be prepared as close to the time of drug administration as possible.
  - **Treanda Injection** (45 mg/0.5 mL or 180 mg/2 mL solution): Once diluted in the infusion bag (either 0.9% sodium chloride USP or 2.5% dextrose/0.45% sodium chloride injection USP), the final admixture is stable for 24 hours when refrigerated at 2–8°C (36–47°F) or for 2 hours when stored at room temperature (15–30°C [59–86°F]) and room light.
  - **Treanda for Injection** (25 mg/vial or 100 mg/vial lyophilized powder): Once diluted in the infusion bag (either 0.9% sodium chloride USP or 2.5% dextrose/0.45% sodium chloride injection USP), the final admixture is stable for 24 hours when refrigerated at 2–8°C (36–47°F) or for **3 hours** when stored at room temperature (15–30°C [59–86°F]) and room light.

Drug Administration:
- Assess ANC/CBC prior to the initiation of the next cycle of therapy: ANC $\geq 1 \times 10^9$/L and platelets $\geq 75 \times 10^9$/L.
- Administer as an IV infusion over 30–60 minutes.
- Assess for rare allergic reactions.

Drug Interactions:
- Decrease bendamustine drug exposure (AUC): CYP1A2 inducers (e.g., omeprazole); smoking may decrease plasma concentrations of bendamustine and increase plasma concentrations of the active metabolites; consider alternative drugs to avoid CYP1A2 inducers.
- Increase bendamustine drug exposure (AUC): CYP1A2 inhibitors (e.g., ciprofloxacin, fluvoxamine), which may increase plasma concentrations of bendamustine and decrease concentration of active metabolites; consider alternative drugs to avoid CYP1A2 inhibitors.
- Allopurinol: increased risk of severe skin toxicity when given concomitantly with bendamustine.

Lab Effects/Interference:
- Neutropenia, platelet counts, hemoglobin.

Special Considerations:
- Warnings and Precautions:
  - Myelosuppression: In NHL studies, 98% of patients had grades 3–4 myelosuppression. Complications included neutropenic sepsis, diffuse alveolar hemorrhage with

grade 3 thrombocytopenia, and opportunistic infection (pneumonia). Monitor ANC/ CBC and platelets closely. Nadirs usually in the third week of therapy. Discuss abnormalities with physician/NP/PA and appropriate dose delays or reductions if counts have not recovered prior to next cycle of therapy.

- Infections: Pneumonia, sepsis, septic shock have occurred. Teach patient signs/symptoms of infection and to notify the physician/NP/PA right away if infection suspected.
- Anaphlyaxis and infusion reactions: Infusion reactions occurred commonly during clinical trials, characterized by fever, chills, pruritis, and rash. Rarely, anaphylaxis occurred, especially in second and subsequent cycles of therapy; anaphylactoid reactions may also occur rarely. Monitor patient closely during infusion and discontinue drug for severe reactions. Do not rechallenge patients who have grade 3 or worse allergic-type reactions. If a patient has grades 1–2 infusion reaction, consider premedication with antihistamine(s), antipyretic, and corticosteroid agents to prevent a more severe infusion reaction in subsequent cycles. Discontinue drug if a patient has a grade 4 infusion reaction, or for a grade 3 reaction if appropriate.
- TLS: Patients with high tumor burder prior to initial cycle should be evaluated for risk of TLS, and preventative measures instituted (e.g., vigorous hydration, close monitoring of serum chemistries, e.g., potassium and uric acid levels). There may be increased risk of severe skin toxicity when allopurinol is used with bendamustine.
- Skin reactions: toxic skin reactions and bullous erythema have occurred, especially when bendamustine combined with other anticancer agents (e.g., rituximab, allopurinol). Monitor patients with skin reactions closely as once developed, the reaction may increase in intensity and progress with subsequent treatment. If reaction is severe or progressive, hold or discontinue bendamustine.
- Other malignancies: MDS, myeloproliferative disorders, AML, and bronchial carcinoma have occurred after treatment with bendamustine.
- Extravasation injury: Erythema, marked swelling, and pain have occurred after extravasation of bendamustine and may require hospitalization. Ensure excellent venous access prior to starting bendamustine infusion, and monitor infusion site closely for redness, swelling, pain, infection, and necrosis during and after administration of bendamustine (Treanda, 2015).
- Embryo-fetal toxicity: Drug can cause fetal harm. Teach women to use effective contraception while receiving bendamustine and for 3 months after therapy is stopped. Mothers should not breastfeed while receiving the drug. A decision should be made whether to discontinue nursing or to discontinue the drug, taking into account the importance of the drug to the mother.
- Renal impairment: use bendamustine cautiously, and do not use if CrCl < 40 mL/min.
- Hepatic impairment: use cautiously in patients with mild hepatic impairment; do not use the drug in patients with moderate or severe hepatic impairment.
- The most common (≥15%) nonblood-related side effects when bendamustine is given (1) for CLL: pyrexia, nausea, and vomiting, and (2) for NHL: nausea, fatigue, vomiting, diarrhea, pyrexia, constipation, anorexia, cough, headache, decreased weight, rash, and stomatitis.
- The most common blood-related side effects are lymphopenia, anemia, leukopenia, thrombocytopenia, and neutropenia.

Potential Toxicities/Side Effects and the Nursing Process

I.   INFECTION AND BLEEDING related to BM DEPRESSION

Defining Characteristics: Myelosuppression is the major toxicity, with nadir occurring during the third week after drug administration, and recovery by day 28. Grades 3–4 neutropenia affects 24–98% (NHL) with 3% febrile neutropenia. Thrombocytopenia is less common with 3% grades 3–4 and <1% of patients requiring platelet transfusions. Decreased hemoglobin affects 89% of patients with 13% grades 3–4, and 20% requiring red cell transfusions.

Nursing Implications: Monitor CBC, neutrophil, and platelet count before drug administration and postchemotherapy. Subsequent treatments require ANC $\geq 1 \times 10^9$/L and platelets $> 75 \times 10^9$/L; assess for signs/symptoms of infection, bleeding, and anemia. Teach patient/family signs/symptoms of infection, bleeding, and anemia, and instruct to report them to nurse or physician immediately. Teach patient to avoid aspirin-containing OTC medications. Teach patient to report increasing fatigue, signs of severe anemia (shortness of breath, chest pain/angina, headaches). Monitor hemoglobin/hematocrit; discuss transfusion or erythrocyte growth factor support with physician if signs/symptoms develop or hematocrit falls < 25 mg/dL. Teach patient about diet high in iron.

II.   POTENTIAL FOR INJURY related to INFUSION REACTION AND ANAPHYLAXIS

Defining Characteristics: Infusion reactions occur commonly and are characterized by fever, chills, pruritus, and rash. Fever occurs in 24% of patients and chills in 6%. Rarely, anaphylactoid and anaphylactic reactions may occur, especially on the second and subsequent cycles of therapy. Two percent of patients withdrew from therapy for hypersensitivity reactions.

Nursing Implications: Assess baseline VS and mental status before drug administration. Review standing orders or nursing procedure for patient management of anaphylaxis, and be prepared to stop drug immediately if signs/symptoms occur. Keep IV line open with 0.9% sodium chloride; notify physician, monitor VS, and administer ordered medications, which may include epinephrine 1:1,000, hydrocortisone sodium succinate, and diphenhydramine. If patients develop a grade 1 or grade 2 reaction, premedicate with antihistamines, antipyretics, and corticosteroids before subsequent cycles. Do not rechallenge, and discontinue therapy for grades 3 or 4 infusion reactions.

III.   POTENTIAL FOR INJURY related to TLS

Defining Characteristics: May develop with initial therapy if patient has a large tumor burden; results from rapid lysis of tumor cells. This usually begins 1 to 5 days after initiation of therapy and causes elevations in serum uric acid, potassium, phosphorus, and creatinine.

Nursing Implications: For patients with a high tumor burden, expect medical orders to include oral allopurinol and vigorous oral hydration prior to beginning first cycle of therapy, together with IV hydration with the first cycle of therapy. Reinforce teaching about allopurinol and the importance of adhering to therapy as directed for the first few weeks after cycle 1 therapy. Monitor baseline and daily BUN, creatinine, phosphorus, uric acid, and calcium. Monitor for renal, cardiac, neuromuscular signs/symptoms of TLS.

IV. ALTERATION IN NUTRITION, LESS THAN BODY REQUIREMENTS, related to NAUSEA AND VOMITING, DIARRHEA

Defining Characteristics: Nausea and/or vomiting are dose related and occur in 20% and 16% of patients, respectively. Grades 3–4 occur in <1% of patients. Diarrhea occurs in 9% of patients and is generally mild. Dry mouth, mucositis, stomatitis, and constipation may also occur less commonly.

Nursing Implications: Assess nutritional status baseline and before each treatment. Premedicate with antiemetics before injection, and teach patient self-administration of antiemetics at home; encourage small, frequent feedings as tolerated. If severe vomiting occurs, treat with alternative antiemetics and assess for signs/symptoms of fluid and electrolyte imbalance. Monitor serum potassium, as hypokalemia may be a side effect of treatment. Assess baseline bowel elimination status. Instruct the patient to report the onset of diarrhea and to administer antidiarrheals as ordered. If diarrhea is protracted, ensure adequate hydration, monitor total body fluid balance, and teach/reinforce perineal hygiene. Teach patient dietary modifications, such as the BRAT (bananas, rice, applesauce, toast) diet if diarrhea develops.

V. POTENTIAL FOR IMPAIRED SKIN INTEGRITY related to RASH

Defining Characteristics: Rash occurs in 8% and pruritus in 5% of patients. Rarely, toxic skin reactions and bullous exanthema can occur. Skin reactions may be progressive and increase in severity with further treatment; if this occurs, drug should be withheld or discontinued.

Nursing Implications: Teach patient about possible side effects and self-care measures. Teach patient to report rash, and then monitor patient closely for signs of increase in severity or extent. Discuss with physician symptomatic treatment of skin changes and holding or discontinuing drug if rash is progressive or more severe.

Drug: bicalutamide (Casodex)

Class: Androgen receptor inhibitor; nonsteroidal antiandrogen.

Mechanism of Action: Binds to androgen receptors in the prostate, preventing normal androgen stimulation; affinity is four times greater than that of flutamide.

Metabolism: Extensively metabolized in the liver. Decreased drug excretion in patients with moderate to severe hepatic dysfunction.

Indication: Bicalutamide (Casodex) 50 mg is indicated for use in combination therapy with a lutenizing hormone-releasing hormone (LHRH) analogue for the treatment of Stage D_2 metastatic prostate cancer. Casodex 150 mg daily is not approved for use alone or with other treatments.

Contraindications: Hypersensitivity, women, and pregnancy.

Dosage/Range:
- 50 mg PO daily.

Drug Preparation:
- None.

Drug Administration:
- Orally. Given with luteinizing hormone-releasing hormone (LHRH) analogue or as a single agent after surgical castration. Teach patient to take pill at the same time each day.

Drug Interactions:
- R-bicalutamide is an inhibitor of CYP3A4; if bicalutamide is administered with a CYP 3A4 substrate, caution should be used. For example, when coadministered with midazolam, a CYP3A4 substrate, midazolam C_{max} was increased 1.5 folds, and AUC 1.9 folds.
- Warfarin: Bicalutamide may increase anticoagulant effect; monitor PT, INR closely in patients who have been on coumarin anticoagulants who have started on bicalutamide, and adjust dose as needed.

Lab Effects/Interference:
- Increased LFTs.
- Increased BUN, WBC, Hgb.

Special Considerations:
- Use cautiously in patients with moderate to severe hepatic dysfunction. Observe closely for toxicity, as dosage adjustment may be required.
- No dose modification needed for renal dysfunction.
- Warnings and Precautions:
  - *Hepatitis:* Severe hepatic injury and fatal hepatic failure have occurred, generally within the first 3–4 months of therapy. Monitor serum transaminase levels baseline before starting drug and monitor regularly for the first 4 months of treatment, then periodically. Observe for signs/symptoms of hepatic dysfunction. Teach patient to report signs/symptoms of liver dysfunction (e.g., nausea, vomiting, abdominal pain, fatigue, anorexia, flulike symptoms, dark urine, jaundice, RUQ tenderness). If signs/symptoms occur, assess LFTs immediately, especially the ALT. If patient develops jaundice, or his ALT $> 2 \times$ ULN, immediately discontinue drug and closely follow liver function.
  - *Hemorrhage with concomitant use of coumarin anticoagulant:* PT and INR may be prolonged for days to weeks after bicalutamide is started in patients currently

receiving coumarin anticoagulants and were stable. Post-marketing, some patients had serious bleeding (e.g., intracranial, retroperitoneal, GI) requiring blood transfusion and/or administration of vitamin K. Closely monitor PT/INR and adjust the anticoagulant dose as needed.

- *Gynecomastia and breast pain*: when drug given at 150-mg dose in clinical trials, gynecomastia and breast pain was reported in 38% and 39% of patients, respectively.
- *Decreased glucose tolerance:* has occurred, manifested by diabetes or loss of glycemic control in patients with preexisting diabetes. Assess baseline serum glucose and monitor it during drug therapy.
- *Lab tests*: Monitor PSA regularly to assess response to bicalutamide. If PSA levels rise on therapy, the patient should be evaluated for disease progression. If patient has objective progression with an elevated PSA, consider continuing the LHRH analogue and witholding antiandrogen therapy may be considered.
- Most common adverse events (>10% incidence): hot flashes, pain (general, back, pelvic, abdominal), asthenia, constipation, infection, nausea, peripheral edema, dyspnea, diarrhea, hematuria, nocturia, anemia.

Potential Toxicities/Side Effects and the Nursing Process

I.   ALTERATION IN COMFORT, POTENTIAL, related to GYNECOMASTIA AND HOT FLASHES

Defining Characteristics: Gynecomastia occurs in 23% of patients, breast tenderness in 26%, and hot flashes in 9.3%.

Nursing Implications: Teach patient that these side effects may occur, and discuss measures that may offer symptomatic relief.

II.   ALTERATION IN NUTRITION, LESS THAN BODY REQUIREMENTS, related to NAUSEA, POTENTIAL

Defining Characteristics: Nausea may occur in 6% of patients.

Nursing Implications: Teach patient that nausea may occur, and instruct to report nausea. Determine baseline weight, and monitor at each visit. Discuss strategies to minimize nausea, including diet modification and time of dosing.

III.   ALTERATION IN ELIMINATION, POTENTIAL, related to CONSTIPATION OR DIARRHEA

Defining Characteristics: Incidence of constipation is 6%, while that of diarrhea is 2.5%.

Nursing Implications: Assess baseline elimination pattern. Teach patient that alterations may occur, and instruct to report them if changes do not respond to usual nonprescription management strategies (OTC medications, dietary modifications).

Drug: bleomycin sulfate (Blenoxane)

Class: Antitumor action of bleomycin; isolated from fungus *Streptomyces verticullus*. Possesses both antitumor and antimicrobial actions.

Mechanism of Action: Induces single-strand and double-strand breaks in DNA. DNA synthesis is inhibited.

Metabolism: Excreted via the renal system. About 70% is excreted unchanged in urine; 30–60 minutes after IV infusion, urine levels are 10 times the serum level.

Indication: Initial indication is for palliative therapy as single agent or in combination for (1) squamous cell carcinomas (head and neck, penis, vulva, cervix); (2) lymphomas (Hodgkin's disease, NHL); (3) testicular cancer (embryonal cell, choriocarcinoma, and teratocarcinoma); (4) malignant pleural effusion (useful as a sclerosing agent for managing malignant pleural effusion and preventing recurrent pleural effusions).

Contraindications: patients who are hypersensitive or have an idiosyncratic reaction to the drug.

Dosage/Range:
- 5–20 units/m^2 once a week.
- 10–20 units/m^2 twice a week.
- **CI:** 15 units/m^2/day × 4 days.
- Pleural space (for pleurodesis): 50–60 units in 50- to 100-mL diluent, infused into pleural space and followed by change in position every 15 minutes. Give lidocaine 100–200 mg before infusion or mix with bleomycin to maximize comfort.
- Frequency and schedule may vary according to protocol and age.
- Dose reduce patients with urinary creatinine clearance <50 mL/min, and monitor renal function closely during treatment in these patients.

Drug Preparation:
- Dilute powder in 0.9% sodium chloride or sterile water to prepare 15- or 30-unit vials.

Drug Administration:
- IV, IM, or subcutaneous doses may be administered. Some clinical trial protocols may use 24-hour infusions. There is a risk for anaphylaxis in lymphoma patients and hypotension with higher doses of drug. It may be recommended that a test dose be given before the first dose to detect hypersensitivity in patients with lymphoma.
- Dose-reduce if renal insufficiency: creatinine clearance 10–50 mL/min, decrease dose by 25%; creatinine clearance <10 mL/min, give 50% of dose.
- Maximum lifetime dose is 400 units.

Drug Interactions:
- Cisplatin: may decrease bleomycin excretion with increased toxicity due to renal dysfunction.
- Oxygen: increased risk of pulmonary toxicity; do not use FiO$_2$ 100% oxygen.

- Bleomycin decreases the oral bioavailability of digoxin, so digoxin dose may need to be increased.
- Bleomycin decreases the pharmacologic effect of phenytoin when given in combination, so phenytoin dose may need to be increased.

Lab Effects/Interference:
- None.

Special Considerations:
- Warnings and Precautions:
  - Observe patients closely and frequently during therapy. Use with extreme caution in patients with significant renal function impairment or compromised pulmonary function.
  - Pulmonary toxicities occur in 10% of patients, and 1% develop nonspecific pneumonitis, which may progress to pulmonary fibrosis and death. Pulmonary function tests (PFTs) and CXR should be obtained before each course or as outlined by protocol.
  - Severe, idiosyncratic reaction similar to anaphylaxis may occur, characterized by hypotension, mental confusion, fever, chills, and wheezing has occurred in approximately 1% of lymphoma patients, occurring after the first or second dose. Monitor patients closely.
  - Renal or hepatic toxicity beginning as a deterioration in renal or hepatic function tests may occur at any time after the drug is started.
  - Embryo-fetal toxicity: Drug may cause fetal harm. Teach women of reproductive potential to use effective contraception to avoid pregnancy. Mothers should not breastfeed while receiving bleomycin.
- Maximum cumulative lifetime dose: 400 units.
- Oxygen (FiO_2) increases risk of pulmonary toxicity.
- Reduce dose for impaired renal function (urinary creatinine clearance < 50 mL/min).
- Risk of pulmonary toxicity increased in elderly (age > 70 years old); renal impairment; pulmonary disease or prior chest XRT; exposure to high oxygen concentration (i.e., surgery); cumulative doses > 400 units lifetime.
- May cause chemical fevers up to 39.4–40.5°C (103–105°F) in up to 60% of patients. May need to administer premedications such as acetaminophen, antihistamines, or, in some cases, steroids.
- Watch for signs/symptoms of hypotension and anaphylaxis with high drug doses; physician may order test dose in patients with lymphoma.
- May cause irritation at site of injection (is considered an irritant, not a vesicant).

Potential Toxicities/Side Effects and the Nursing Process

I.   POTENTIAL FOR IMPAIRED GAS EXCHANGE related to PULMONARY TOXICITY

Defining Characteristics: Pneumonitis occurs in 10% of patients and is characterized by rales, dyspnea, infiltrate on CXR; in 1% may progress to irreversible pulmonary fibrosis.

Risk factors include age > 70, dose > 400 units (but may occur at much lower doses), and concurrent or prior radiotherapy to the chest. Slower, CI may lower the risk.

Nursing Implications: Discuss with physician the need for PFTs (including DLCO, or diffusing capacity of the lung for carbon monoxide) and CXR prior to initiating therapy and monthly during therapy. Assess pulmonary status prior to each treatment (early symptom is dyspnea, and earliest sign is fine crackles). Instruct patient to report cough, dyspnea, shortness of breath. If patient needs surgery, discuss with physician the need to use very low FiO_2 during surgery, since the lung tissue has been sensitized to bleomycin, and high concentrations of oxygen will cause further lung damage. Drug should be discontinued when/if DLCO falls below 30–35% of pretreatment value (Hospira, 2013).

II.   POTENTIAL FOR INJURY related to ANAPHYLACTOID, IDIOSYNCRATIC REACTION

Defining Characteristics: Anaphylactoid reaction may occur in 1% of lymphoma patients, characterized by hypotension, confusion, tachycardia, wheezing, and facial edema. Reaction may be immediate or delayed for several hours and may occur after the first or second drug administration.

Nursing Implications: Discuss with physician the use of test dose prior to drug administration in lymphoma patients. Assess baseline VS and mental status prior to drug administration. Review standing orders or nursing procedure for patient management of anaphylaxis, and be prepared to stop drug immediately if signs/symptoms occur. Keep IV line open with 0.9% sodium chloride; notify physician, monitor VS, and administer ordered medications, which may include epinephrine 1:1,000, hydrocortisone sodium succinate, and diphenhydramine.

III.   POTENTIAL ALTERATION IN COMFORT related to FEVER AND CHILLS, AND PAIN AT TUMOR SITE

Defining Characteristics: Fever (up to 39.4–40.5°C [103–105°F]) and chills, occurring in up to 60% of patients, begin 4–10 hours after drug administration and may last 24 hours. There appears to be tolerance with successive doses of bleomycin. Pain may occur at tumor site due to chemotherapy-induced cellular damage.

Nursing Implications: Teach patient that these side effects may occur, and assess patient during and after administration. If fever occurs, notify physician and administer ordered acetaminophen, antihistamine, or steroid. If tumor pain occurs, reassure patient and discuss with physician the use of acetaminophen as analgesic.

IV. POTENTIAL FOR IMPAIRED SKIN INTEGRITY related to ALOPECIA, SKIN CHANGES, AND NAIL CHANGES

Defining Characteristics: Dose-related alopecia begins 3–4 weeks after first dose and is reversible. Skin changes occur in 50% of patients and include erythema, rash, striae, hyperpigmentation, skin peeling of fingertips, and hyperkeratosis; these are dose related and begin after 150–200 units have been administered. Skin eruptions include a macular rash over hands and elbows, urticaria, and vesiculations. Pruritus may occur. Nail changes and possible nail loss may occur. Phlebitis at the IV site may occur.

Nursing Implications: Teach patient about possible side effects and self-care measures, including obtaining a wig or cap as appropriate prior to hair loss. Encourage patient to verbalize feelings and provide patient emotional support. Discuss with physician symptomatic treatment of skin changes. Assess IV site for phlebitis and restart IV at alternate site if phlebitis develops.

V. POTENTIAL ALTERATION IN NUTRITION, LESS THAN BODY REQUIREMENTS, related to NAUSEA AND VOMITING, ANOREXIA AND WEIGHT LOSS, AND STOMATITIS

Defining Characteristics: Nausea with or without vomiting may occur; anorexia and weight loss may occur and may continue after treatment is completed; stomatitis may occur and decrease ability and desire to eat.

Nursing Implications: Administer antiemetic prior to initial treatment and revise plan for successive treatments if no nausea/vomiting. Teach patient about possible anorexia and encourage patient to eat high-calorie, high-protein foods. Assess oral mucosa prior to drug administration; teach patient self-assessment and instruct to notify nurse or physician if stomatitis develops. Teach patient oral care prior to drug administration.

VI. POTENTIAL FOR SEXUAL DYSFUNCTION related to REPRODUCTIVE HAZARDS

Defining Characteristics: Drug is mutagenic and probably teratogenic.

Nursing Implications: Discuss with patient and partner both sexuality and reproductive goals, as well as possible impact of chemotherapy. Discuss contraception and sperm banking if appropriate.

Drug: busulfan (Myleran)

Class: Alkylating agent.

Mechanism of Action: Forms carbonium ions through the release of a methane sulfonate group, resulting in the alkylation of DNA. Acts primarily on granulocyte precursors in the BM and is cell cycle phase nonspecific.

Metabolism: Well absorbed orally; almost all metabolites are excreted in the urine. Has a very short half-life.

Indications: (Initial) Treatment of chronic granulocytic leukemia; also produces prolonged remission in polycythemia vera.

Dosage/Range:
Chronic myelogenous leukemia:
- 4–8 mg/day PO for 2–3 weeks initially, then maintenance dose of 1–3 mg/m² PO daily or 0.05 mg/kg orally daily. Dose titrated based on leukocyte counts. Drug withheld when leukocyte count reaches 15,000/µL; resume when total leukocyte count is 50,000/µL; maintenance dose of 1–3 mg daily used if remission lasts > 3 months.

High doses with BM transplantation:
- See *busulfan for injection.*

Drug Preparation:
- None.

Drug Administration:
- Available in 2-mg scored tablets given orally.

Drug Interactions:
- Combination treatment with thioguanine may cause hepatic dysfunction and the development of esophageal varices in a small number of patients.

Lab Effects/Interference:
- Decreased CBC.
- Increased LFTs.

Special Considerations:
Regular dose:
- If WBC is high, patient is at risk for hyperuricemia. Allopurinol and hydration may be indicated.
- Follow weekly CBC and platelet count initially, then monthly. Dose is decreased to maintenance level when leukocyte count falls below 50,000 mm³.
- Hyperpigmentation of skin creases may occur due to increased melanin production.
- If given according to accepted guidelines, patients should have minimal side effects.

High dose:
- See *busulfan for injection.*

TREATMENT

Potential Toxicities/Side Effects and the Nursing Process

I. POTENTIAL FOR INFECTION, BLEEDING, AND FATIGUE related to BM DEPRESSION

Defining Characteristics: The nadir is at 11–30 days following initial drug administration, with recovery in 24–54 days; however, delayed, refractory pancytopenia has occurred.

Nursing Implications: Monitor CBC, WBC differential, and platelets, initially weekly, then at least monthly. Expect drug will be interrupted if counts fall rapidly or steeply. Teach patient to self-assess for signs/symptoms of infection, bleeding, or severe fatigue, and to notify nurse or physician immediately. Teach patient to avoid aspirin-containing OTC medications.

II. POTENTIAL FOR IMPAIRED GAS EXCHANGE related to INTERSTITIAL PULMONARY FIBROSIS

Defining Characteristics: Rarely, bronchopulmonary dysplasia progressing to pulmonary fibrosis can occur, beginning 1 to many years posttherapy. Symptoms are usually delayed (occurring after 4 years) and include anorexia, cough, dyspnea, and fever. High-dose corticosteroids may be helpful, but condition may be fatal due to rapid, diffuse fibrosis.

Nursing Implications: Assess pulmonary status routinely in all patients receiving long-term therapy. Discuss plan for regular pulmonary function studies with physician.

III. POTENTIAL FOR SEXUAL AND REPRODUCTIVE DYSFUNCTION related to REPRODUCTIVE HAZARDS

Defining Characteristics: Premenopausal female patients commonly experience ovarian suppression and amenorrhea with menopausal symptoms; men experience sterility, azoospermia, and testicular atrophy. Although successful pregnancies have occurred following busulfan therapy, the drug is potentially teratogenic.

Nursing Implications: Assess patient's/partner's sexual patterns and reproductive goals. Provide information, supportive counseling, and referral as needed. Teach importance of birth control measures as appropriate.

Drug: busulfan for injection (Busulfex)

Class: Alkylating agent.

Mechanism of Action: Forms carbonium ions through the release of a methane sulfonate group, resulting in the alkylation of DNA. Acts primarily on granulocyte precursors in the BM, and is cell cycle phase nonspecific.

Metabolism: After IV administration, drug achieves equal concentrations in the plasma and CSF. Drug is 32% protein-bound, metabolized in the liver, and excreted in the urine (30%). Appears metabolites may be long lived.

Indication: For use in combination with cyclophosphamide as a conditioning regimen prior to allogeneic hematopoietic progenitor cell transplantation for chronic myelogenous leukemia (CML).

Contraindication: History of hypersensitivity to drug or its components.

Dosage/Range:
Conditioning regimen:
- Indicated in combination with cyclophosphamide prior to allogeneic hematopoietic progenitor cell transplantation for CML.
- Premedicate with anticonvulsants (e.g., benzodiazepines, phenytoin, valproic acid, or levetiracetam) and antiemetic.
- 0.8 mg/kg (IBW or actual weight, whichever is lower, or adjusted IBW) IV q 6 h × 4 consecutive days (total of 16 doses), via central venous catheter, each over 2 hours.
- Cyclophosphamide dose is given on each of 2 days as a 1-hour infusion at a dose of 60 mg/kg beginning on BMT day-3, 6 hours following the 16th dose of IV busulfan.

Drug Preparation:
- Available in a 10-mL, single-use ampule containing 60 mg (6 mg/mL). Unopened ampules must be refrigerated at 2–8°C (36–46°F).
- DO NOT USE POLYCARBONATE SYRINGES OR POLYCARBONATE FILTER NEEDLES WITH BUSULFEX.
- Aseptically open ampule, and using the 25-mm, 5-micron nylon membrane syringe filter provided, remove the ordered, calculated drug dose.
- Remove the syringe/filter, replace with a new needle, and dispense the syringe contents into a bag or syringe containing 10 times the volume of the drug, either 0.9% NS injection or 5% dextrose injection. The final concentration of drug should be ≥ 0.5 mg/mL. For example, a 70-kg patient at a dose of 0.8 mg/kg given a concentration of 6 mg/mL would require 9.3 mL (56 mg) busulfan total dose. 9.3 mL of drug × 10 = 93 mL. Adding 0.9% NS inj or D$_5$W inj, the total volume is 9.3 mL + 93 mL = 102.3 mL.
- Mix contents thoroughly.
- Ensure that this meets the recommended drug concentration, e.g., (9.3 mL × 6 mg/mL)/ 102.3 mL = 0.54 mg/mL.
- Diluted drug is stable at room temperature (25°C) for up to 8 hours, but infusion must be completed within this time. Drug diluted in 0.9% NS inj, USP, is stable refrigerated (2–8°C) for up to 12 hours, but the infusion must be completed within that time.
- Dilute in 0.9% NS injection or 5% dextrose injection to 10 times volume of drug (see example in Drug Preparation) prior to IV infusion.

Drug Administration:
- Premedicate with anticonvulsant (e.g., benzodiazepine, phenytoin) and antiemetic.
- Infuse dose over 2 hours via infusion pump. Flush line with about 5 mL of IV fluid prior to and after drug infusion.

- Drug should be administered through a central line, over 2 hours. Do NOT give as a rapid infusion.
- All patients should be premedicated with an anticonvulsant, e.g., phenytoin, as drug crosses BBB and causes seizures (see *Drug Interactions*).

Drug Interactions:
- CYP3A4 inducers: Phenytoin decreases busulfan AUC by 15%, resulting in the target dose. Use carbamazepine, nafcillin, and phenobarbital cautiously.
- Other anticonvulsants may increase busulfan AUC, increasing the risk of veno-occlusive disease or seizures. Monitor busulfan exposure and toxicity closely.
- CYP3A4 inhibitors: Itraconazole decreases busulfan clearance by up to 25% with potential significant increases in serum busulfan levels. Use ciprofloxacin, clarithromycin, erythromycin, imatinib, and verapamil cautiously.
- Acetaminophen prior to (<72 hours) or concurrent with busulfan may result in decreased drug clearance and increased serum busulfan levels.
- St. John's wort: may decrease busulfan serum level; do not use concomitantly.
- Grapefruit juice: may enhance busulfan toxicity as inhibits CYP3A4 enzymes.

Lab Effects/Interference:
- Profound myelosuppression/aplasia with decreased WBC, neutrophils, Hgb/HCT, and platelet counts.
- If liver veno-occlusive disease develops, increased serum transaminases, alk phos, and bili.
- Creatinine is elevated in 21% of patients.

Special Considerations:
- Warnings and Precautions:
  - Myelosuppression: Prolonged in all patients, with severe granulocytopenia, thrombocytopenia, and anemia. Hematopoietic progenitor cell transplantation is required to prevent potentially fatal complications. Monitor ANC/CBC and platelets until engraftments. ANC < 500/mm^3 occurred a median of 4 days after transplant in clinical studies and recovered at a median of 13 days when G-CSF was used in the majority of patients. Thrombocytopenia (<25,000/mm^3) occurred at a median of 5–6 days. Administer antibiotics, red blood cells, and platelets as ordered.
  - Seizures: Use prophylactic anticonvulsants prior to busulfan dose, and use busulfan cautiously in patients with a history of seizure disorder.
  - Hepatic Veno-Occlusive Disease (HVOD): Incidence is about 8%. Patients at risk are those receiving high dose busulfan (Busulfex dose AUC concentrations of > 1,500 μm/min); history of (1) prior RT, (2) 3+ cycles of chemotherapy, or (3) a prior progenitor cell transplant. Monitor serum transaminases, alkaline phosphatase, and bilirubin daily through BMT Day +28 to identify hepatotoxicity which may precede HVOD.
  - Embryo-fetal toxicity: Teach patients: (1) Women of reproductive potential should use effective birth control measures during and after treatment with busulfan; (2) nursing mothers should not breastfeed during therapy; (3) male patients with female sexual partners of reproductive potential should use effective contraception during and after therapy with busulfan; (4) teach females and males of reproductive potential that busulfan may cause temporary or permanent infertility.

- Cardiac tamponade: has been reported in pediatric patients. Monitor for signs/symptoms, evaluate promptly, and treat if cardiac tamponade is suspected.
- Bronchopulmonary dysplasia with pulmonary fibrosis: rare but serious complication after chemotherapy. Onset of symptoms (average) is 4 years after therapy (range 4 mo–10 yr).
- Cellular Dysplasia: Busulfan may cause cellular dysplasia in many organs (characterized by giant, hyperchromatic nuclei in lymph nodes, pancreas, thyroid, adrenal glands, liver, lungs, and BM), which may cause difficult interpretation of subsequent cytologic examinations in lungs, bladder, and uterine cervix.
- Drug clearance in obese patients may be best predicted when the busulfan dose is based on adjusted ideal body weight (AIBW).
  - Ideal body weight (IBW in kg): men = 50 + 0.91 × (height in cm 152); women = 45 + 0.91 × (height in cm 152).
  - AIBW = IBW + 0.25 × (actual body weight IBW).
- No known antidote if overdose occurs; one report says that drug is dialyzable.
- Drug is metabolized by conjugation with glutathione, so consider administration of same. Drug should only be given in combination with hematopoietic progenitor cell transplantation, as expected toxicity is profound myelosuppression.
- Drug is for adult use, and has not been studied in patients with hepatic insufficiency.

Potential Toxicities/Side Effects and the Nursing Process

I.   POTENTIAL FOR INFECTION, BLEEDING, AND ANEMIA related to BM DEPRESSION

Defining Characteristics: Myelosuppression is profound in 100% of patients. ANC < 500 cells/mm^3 occurred a median of 4 days posttransplant in 100% of patients. Following progenitor cell infusion, the median recovery of neutrophil count to ≥ 500 cells/mm^3 was day 13 when prophylactic G-CSF was given. 51% of patients experienced 1+ episodes of infection; fever occurred in 80% of patients, with chills in 33%. Thrombocytopenia (< 25,000/mm^3 or requiring platelet transfusion) occurred in 5–6 days in 98% of patients. There was a median of six platelet transfusions per patient in clinical trials. Anemia affected 50% of patients, and the median number of red blood cell transfusions on clinical trials was 4 per patient.

Nursing Implications: Assess WBC, with differential, Hgb/HCT, and platelet count prior to drug administration, and at least daily during treatment. Discuss any abnormalities with physician. Monitor continuously for signs/symptoms of infection or bleeding. Teach patient signs/symptoms of infection and bleeding, self-assessment, and to report signs/symptoms immediately. Teach self-care measures to minimize infection and bleeding, including avoidance of OTC aspirin-containing medications. Discuss with physician use of granulocyte colony-stimulating factor (G-CSF) to prevent febrile neutropenia. Transfuse platelets and red blood cells per physician order.

II. ALTERATION IN CARDIAC OUTPUT, POTENTIAL, related to TACHYCARDIA, THROMBOSIS, HYPERTENSION, VASODILATION

Defining Characteristics: Mild-to-moderate tachycardia has been noted in 44% of patients (11% during drug infusion), and, less commonly, other rhythm disturbances such as arrhythmia (5%), atrial fibrillation (2%), ventricular extrasystoles (2%), and third-degree heart block (2%). Mild-to-moderate thrombosis may occur in 33% of patients, usually associated with a central venous catheter. Hypertension has been seen in 36% of patients and grades 3–4 in 3%. Mild vasodilation (flushing and hot flashes) occurs in 25% of patients. In clinical trials, most commonly in the postcyclophosphamide phase, other less common events were cardiomegaly (5%), mild EKG changes (2%), grades 3 and 4 CHF (2%), and moderate pericardial effusion (2%).

Nursing Implications: Assess baseline cardiac status frequently during shift/care depending upon patient condition, including HR, BP, EKG, and total body fluid balance. Monitor patient for changes in cardiac function throughout treatment course, and report changes immediately. Monitor central venous lines for patency, and use scrupulous care in maintaining catheters; assess for signs/symptoms of venous thrombosis, and discuss management with physician as soon as it is discovered.

III. ALTERATION IN FLUID AND ELECTROLYTE BALANCE, POTENTIAL, related to TREATMENT, CARDIAC RESPONSE

Defining Characteristics: 79% of patients develop edema, hypervolemia, or weight increase, mild or moderate.

Nursing Implications: Assess baseline fluid volume status, weight, orthostatic vital signs, and presence/absence of edema, and assess at least daily, especially after fluid or blood product infusion. Closely monitor I/O and daily total body balance, and discuss abnormalities with physician. Assess renal status, as BUN and creatinine can become elevated in 21% of patients. Assess patient for signs/symptoms of dysuria, oliguria, and hematuria, as hemorrhagic cystitis may occur with cyclophosphamide.

IV. POTENTIAL FOR IMPAIRED GAS EXCHANGE related to DYSPNEA AND INTERSTITIAL PULMONARY FIBROSIS

Defining Characteristics: Mild or moderate dyspnea was seen in 25% of study patients, and was severe in 2% (severe hyperventilation). 5% of patients in the study developed alveolar hemorrhage and died. One patient developed nonspecific interstitial fibrosis and died from respiratory failure on BMT day +98. Other reported pulmonary events were mild or moderate, including pharyngitis (18%), hiccup (18%), asthma (8%), atelectasis (2%), pleural effusion (3%), hypoxia (2%), hemoptysis (3%), and sinusitis (3%). As with oral busulfan, pulmonary fibrosis can occur 1 to many years posttherapy, with the average onset of symptoms 4 years after therapy (range 4 mo–10 yr).

Nursing Implications: Assess pulmonary status, including breath sounds, rate, and oxygen saturation, at baseline and regularly during care. Assess for any underlying problems, such as infection, effusions, and leukemic infiltrates. Teach patient to report any dyspnea, SOB, or other change, and monitor closely. Provide oxygen and support and discuss management plan with physician and implement promptly. After therapy is completed, remind patient that pulmonary fibrosis may develop as a late effect. The patient should have long-term follow-up, and report any dyspnea or SOB, especially in the cold.

V.   POTENTIAL FOR ALTERATION IN NUTRITION, LESS THAN BODY REQUIREMENTS, related to NAUSEA/VOMITING, ANOREXIA, STOMATITIS, DIARRHEA, AND ELECTROLYTE ABNORMALITIES

Defining Characteristics: The incidence of GI toxicities is high, but manageable: nausea 98%, vomiting 95%, stomatitis 97%, diarrhea 84%, anorexia 85%, dyspepsia 44%, and mild-to-moderate constipation 38%. Grades 3–4 stomatitis occurred in 26% of patients, severe anorexia in 21%, and grades 3–4 diarrhea in 5%. Additionally, hyperglycemia was seen in 67% of patients, with grades 3–4 in 15%. Hypomagnesemia was mild/moderate in 62%, and severe in 2%; hypokalemia was mild/moderate in 62% and severe in 2%; hypocalcemia was mild/moderate in 46% and severe in 3%; hypophosphatemia was mild/moderate in 17%, and hyponatremia occurred in 2%.

Nursing Implications: Assess baseline weight, usual weight, and any changes. Assess appetite, and favorite foods. Assess baseline glucose, electrolytes, and minerals, and monitor throughout therapy. Premedicate with aggressive antiemetics (serotonin antagonist) and continue protection throughout treatment. Assess efficacy and modify regimen as needed. Assess oral mucosa and teach patient self-care strategies, including assessment, what to report, oral hygiene regimen. Encourage dietary modifications as needed. Assess bowel elimination pattern baseline and daily during therapy. Teach patient to report diarrhea, and discuss management with physician. Provide comfort measures, and teach patient scrupulous hygiene to prevent infection. Discuss abnormal lab values with physician, correct hyperglycemia, and replete magnesium, potassium, phosphate, calcium, and sodium as ordered.

VI.   POTENTIAL FOR SENSORY/PERCEPTUAL ALTERATIONS related to NEUROLOGIC TOXICITY

Defining Characteristics: Drug crosses BBB, achieving levels equivalent to plasma concentration. Neurologic changes observed in clinical testing were insomnia (84%), anxiety (75%), headaches (65%), dizziness (30%), depression (23%), confusion (11%), lethargy (7%), and hallucinations (5%). Less commonly, delirium occurred in 2%, agitation in 2%, encephalopathy in 2%, and somnolence in 2%. Despite prophylaxis with phenytoin, one patient developed seizures while receiving cyclophosphamide. Special caution should be used when patients with a history of seizure disorder or head trauma receive the drug.

Nursing Implications: Assess baseline neurologic status and continue to monitor status throughout. Closely monitor patients who have a history of seizure disorder, or head trauma for the development of seizures (seizure precautions). Teach patient to report any changes in usual patterns. Discuss any abnormalities with physician, and develop collaborative symptom-management strategies, including medications. Assess patient interest in relaxation exercises or imagery, or other techniques, and teach self-care strategies. Be prepared to manage seizures as needed.

VII. ALTERATION IN HEPATIC FUNCTION, POTENTIAL, related to VENO-OCCLUSIVE DISEASE (VOD) AND GRAFT-VERSUS-HOST DISEASE (GVHD)

Defining Characteristics: Increased bilirubin occurred in 49% of patients, and grades 3–4 hyperbilirubinemia occurred in 30% within 28 days of transplantation. This was associated with GVHD in 6 patients in clinical studies, and with VOD in 8% of patients (5). Severe increases in SGPT occurred in 7%, while mild increases in alkaline phosphatase occurred in 15% of patients. Jaundice occurred in 12%, while hepatomegaly developed in 6%. VOD is a complication of conditioning therapy prior to transplant and occurred in 8% of patients (fatal in 2 of the 5 patients).

Factors that may increase risk of veno-occlusive disease are history of XRT, more than 3 cycles of chemotherapy, prior progenitor cell transplantation, or Busulfex dose AUC concentrations of >1,500 μm/min. Use Jones' criteria to diagnose VOD hyperbilirubinemia, and two of the following: painful hepatomegaly, weight gain >5%, or ascites. GVHD developed in 18% of patients (severe 3%, mild/moderate 15%, fatal in 3 patients).

Nursing Implications: Assess hepatic function baseline and daily during treatment. Discuss any abnormalities with physician. Teach the patient to report RUQ pain, weight gain, increasing girth, or yellowing of eyes or skin.

VIII. ALTERATION IN COMFORT, POTENTIAL, related to ASTHENIA, PAIN, INJECTION-SITE INFLAMMATION, ARTHRALGIAS

Defining Characteristics: Symptoms leading to discomfort include: abdominal pain (mild/moderate 69%, severe 3%), asthenia (mild/moderate 49%, severe 2%), general pain (45%), injection-site inflammation or pain (25%), chest or back pain (23–26%), and arthralgia (13%).

Nursing Implications: Assess baseline comfort, and usual strategies to promote comfort. Teach patient to report any pain, weakness, listlessness, injection-site discomfort, or any other changes. Discuss strategies to promote comfort, such as use of heat or cold. If discomfort persists, discuss pharmacologic management to reduce symptom distress.

IX.   POTENTIAL SEXUAL DYSFUNCTION related to DRUG EFFECTS

Defining Characteristics: Similar to oral busulfan: premenopausal female patients commonly experience ovarian suppression and amenorrhea with menopausal symptoms; men experience sterility, azoospermia, and testicular atrophy. The drug is potentially teratogenic.

Nursing Implications: Assess patient's signs/symptoms and partner's patterns of sexuality and reproductive goals. Teach patient/partner about need for effective contraception and provide other information as appropriate. Provide emotional support, supportive counseling, and referral as needed.

X.   ALTERATION IN SKIN INTEGRITY, POTENTIAL, related to SKIN RASH, ALOPECIA

Defining Characteristics: Rash is common (57%) and pruritus less so (28%). Alopecia occurred in 15% of patients. Character of rash ranged from mild vesicular rash (10%), mild/moderate maculopapular rash (8%), vesiculobullous rash (10%), and exfoliative dermatitis (5%). Other skin abnormalities described were erythema nodosum (2%).

Nursing Implications: Assess baseline skin integrity, presence of rashes, itching, and repeat daily. Teach patient that skin changes may occur, and to report them. Discuss use of topical agents and antipruritic medications with physician.

Drug: cabazitaxel (Jevtana injection)

Class: Microtubule inhibitor; mitotic spindle poison.

Mechanism of Action: Drug binds to tubulin and promotes its assembly into microtubules (making the structure for mitotis) while simultaneously inhibiting its disassembly. This leads to stabilization of the microtubules so that cell division is halted because the mitotic and interphase cellular functions are inhibited. Thus, tumor cell proliferation is halted.

Metabolism: Following an IV dose of 25 mg/m^2 every 3 weeks, the mean peak serum concentration (C_{max}) was reached at the end of the 1-hour infusion. The drug binds to human serum proteins (89–92%), mainly to serum albumin and lipoproteins, and the drug is equally distributed into blood and plasma. Drug is extensively metabolized in the liver (>95%) mainly by the CYP3A4/5 isoenzymes and to a lesser extent, CYP2C8. The potential for the drug to inhibit drugs that are substrates of other isoenzymes is low, and the drug does not induce CYP isoenzymes. The drug has multiple metabolites that are excreted into the urine and feces (primary route). 2.3% of the drug is excreted intact in the urine. 80% of the drug is eliminated within 2 weeks of a dose. Mild to moderate renal dysfunction does not affect the pharmacokinetics of the drug significantly. Although not studied, hepatic impairment is likely to increase cabazitaxel concentrations. Therefore, patients with hepatic impairment should not receive the drug.

Indication: Microtubule inhibitor indicated in combination with prednisone for treatment of patients with hormone-refractory metastatic prostate cancer previously treated with a docetaxel-containing regimen.

Contraindication: In patients with (1) Neutrophil count $\leq$1,500/mm^3; (2) history of severe hypersensitivity reactions to cabazitaxel or other drugs formulated with polysorbate 80 (e.g., docetaxel, so if the patient had a hypersensitivity reaction to docetaxel, the patient should not receive this drug); (3) severe hepatic impairment (total BR > 3 × ULN); (4) pregnancy.

Dosage/Range:

- Following premedication, 20 mg/m^2 IV over 1 hour, every 3 weeks in combination with prednisone 10 mg PO administered daily throughout cabazitaxel therapy. A dose of 25 mg/ m^2 IV over 1 hour can be used in select patients at the discretion of the healthcare provider. (Sanofi-aventis, 2018).
- If patient must receive a concurrent strong CYP3A4 inhibitor, consider a 25% dose reduction of cabazitaxel (Sanofi-aventis, 2016).
- Drug manufacturer recommends the following dose modifications of cabazitaxel for adverse reactions (Sanofi-aventis, 2018):
  - Dose Level Reductions:
    - Patients receiving 20 mg/m^2 who require a dose reduction should receive a dose reduced to 15 mg/ m^2.
    - If the patient is receiving 25mg/m^2, dose should be reduced to 20 mg/m^2; one additional dose reduction to 15 mg/m^2 may be considered.

Toxicity	Dose Modification
Prolonged grade $\geq$ 3 neutropenia (>1 week) despite G-CSF	Delay treatment until neutrophil count is >1,500 cells/mm^3, then reduce dose by one dose level. Use G-CSF for secondary prophylaxis.
Febrile neutropenia or neutropenic infection	Delay treatment until improvement or resolution and until neutrophil count is >1,500 cells/mm^3, then reduce dose to 20 mg/m^2. Use G-CSF for secondary prophylaxis.
Grade $\geq$ 3 diarrhea or persistent diarrhea despite anti-diarrheals, fluid, and electrolyte replacement	Delay treatment until improvement or resolution; reduce dose by one dose level.
Grade 2 PN	Delay treatment until improvement or resolution, then reduce dose by one dose level.
Grade $\geq$ 3 PN	Discontinue cabazitaxel.

Data from Sanofi-aventis. Jevtana (cabazitaxel) [package insert]. Bridgewater, NJ. January 2018.

Dose Modification for Hepatic Impairment:

- Mild hepatic impairment (total BR > 1 to $\leq$ 1.5 × ULN or AST > 1.5 × ULN): administer cabazitaxel dose to at 20 mg/m^2 and monitor LFTs closely.

- Moderate hepatic impairment (total BR > 1.5 to ≤ 3 × ULN or AST = any): reduce cabazitaxel starting dose to 15 mg/m² based on tolerability data; efficacy of this dose is unknown.
- Severe hepatic impairment (total BR > 3 × ULN): DRUG IS CONTRAINDICATED.
- *In combination with Strong CYP3A4 Inhibitors (ketoconazole, itraconazole, clarithromycin, atazanavir, indinivir, nafazodone, nelfinavir, ritonavir, saquinavir, telithromycin, voriconazole)*: Combination not recommended as results in increased serum levels of cabazitaxel, but if necessary, reduce cabazitaxel dose by 25%.

Drug Preparation:
Requires two dilutions:
- Drug contains polysorbate 80. DO NOT USE PVC infusion containers or polyurethane infusion sets for preparation or administration of cabazitaxel (use same tubing and filter as with paxitaxel).
- Drug is supplied as a kit containing one single-use vial of cabazitaxel injection 60 mg/1.5 mL polysorbate 80, and one vial of diluent 5.7 mL (13% (w/w) ethanol in water). Both vials contain an overfill to compensate for liquid loss during preparation. The overfill ensures that after dilution with the **entire contents** of the supplied diluent, there is an initial diluted solution containing 10 mg/mL of cabazitaxel. Store at 25°C (77°F). Excursions permitted at 15–30°C (59–86°F). Do not refrigerate.

First dilution:
- Aseptically add the **entire contents** of the supplied diluent into the vial of cabazitaxel 60 mg/1.5 mL; the resulting solution contains 10 mg/mL of cabazitaxel. Inject the diluent along the wall of the drug vial slowly to decrease foaming. Remove syringe/needle and gently mix the solution followed by repeated inversions for at least 45 sec. Do not shake. Let the solution stand so the foam will dissipate, although if a little foam remains, can continue to second dilution.
- Proceed to second dilution right away, or at least within 30 minutes of initial dilution.

Second dilution:
- Aseptically withdraw the ordered dose from drug vial (10 mg/mL) into a sterile 250-mL PVC-free container of either 0.9% sodium chloride solution or 5% dextrose solution for infusion. If the dose is >65 mg of cabazitaxel, use a larger volume so that a concentration of 0.26 mg/mL cabazitaxel is not exceeded. The resulting concentration of the second dilution should be between 0.10 mg/mL and 0.26 mg/mL. Once the drug is added to the infusion bag, gently invert the bag or bottle to assure mixing.
- Inspect the bag for any particles or precipitation. If precipitation occurs, discard the solution.
- Use fully prepared solution (in 0.9% sodium chloride or 5% dextrose) within 8 hours at ambient temperature (8 hours including 1-hour infusion time), or 24 hours (including 1-hour infusion time) if refrigerated. If refrigerated and crystals appear, do not use solution.

Drug Administration:
- Assess patient: Neutrophil count must be > 1,500 cells/mm³.
- Do not use if IV bag has crystals, particulate matter, or discoloration.

- Discuss with provider use of G-CSF for patients at risk for neutropenia.
- Premedication (at least 30 minutes before dose):
  - Antihistamine (e.g., diphenhydramine 25 mg or dexchlorpheniramine 5 mg)
  - Corticosteroid (e.g., dexamethasone 8 mg or equivalent)
  - H$_2$ antagonist (e.g., ranitidine 50 mg or equivalent)
  - Antiemetic regimen
  - Administer cabazitaxel IV over 1 hour, using an inline filter of 0.22-μm nominal pore size.
- Assess for signs/symptoms of hypersensitivity reactions, especially during cycles 1 and 2.

Drug Interactions:
- Strong CYP3A inducers (e.g., phenytoin, carbamazepine, rifampin, rifabutin, rifapentin, phenobarbital, St. John's wort) probably decrease cabazitaxel concentrations; avoid coadministration.
- Strong CYP3A inhibitors (e.g., ketoconazole, itraconazole, clarithromycin, atazanavir, indinavir, nefazodone, nelfinavir, ritonavir, saquinavir, telithromycin, voriconazole) are expected to raise cabazitaxel serum concentration. AVOID coadministration. If coadministered, consider 25% dose reduction of cabazitaxel (Sanofi-aventis, 2015).
- Moderate CYP3A inhibitors: use together cautiously and monitor closely for cabazitaxel adverse effects.

Lab Effects/Interference:
- Neutropenia, thrombocytopenia, anemia common.
- Hematuria (17%).

Special Considerations:
- Most common all-grade toxicities (≥10%) were neutropenia, anemia, leukopenia, thrombocytopenia, diarrhea, fatigue, nausea, vomiting, constipation, asthenia, abdominal pain, hematuria, back pain, anorexia, peripheral neuropathy (PN), pyrexia, dyspnea, dysgeusia, cough, arthralgia, and alopecia. The most common grades 3–4 adverse reactions were neutropenia, leukopenia, anemia, febrile neutropenia, diarrhea, fatigue, and asthenia. Alopecia occurs in 10% of patients.
- Warnings and Precautions:
  - *BM suppression* (neutropenia, anemia, thrombocytopenia) may occur, and neutropenic deaths have been reported (e.g., sepsis). Grades 3–4 neutropenia occurs in 82% of patients.
    - The patient should receive the drug only if the neutrophil count is >1,500/cells mm³.
    - G-CSF recommended as primary prophylaxis in patients age > 65 years, poor performance status, precious episodes of febrile neutropenia, extensive prior RT ports, poor nutritional status, or other serious comorbidies.
    - Monitor ANC/CBC weekly during cycle 1 and before each treatment cycle so dose can be adjusted if needed.
    - Caution is recommended in patients with Hgb < 10 g/dL.

- If the patient experiences febrile neutropenia or prolonged (>1 week) neutropenia despite G-CSF, the cabazitaxel dose should be decreased to 20 mg/m^2 when the patient's ANC is > 1,500/mm^3 if initial dose is 25 mg/m^2.
- *Increased toxicity in elderly patients:* Elderly patients ≥ 65 years of age were more likely to experience a fatal outcome related to certain adverse effects, including neutropenia and febrile neutropenia. Monitor closely.
  - Elderly patients should be monitored closely during therapy to identify side effects and manage them aggressively as neutropenia and febrile neutropenia occur more frequently in the elderly.
  - Telephone calls to the patient to assess tolerance between cycles, as well as to reinforce patient teaching to minimize toxicity and to encourage calling the provider if problems occur, will help identify problems early.
- *Hypersensitivity reactions* (HSRs) can occur within minutes after starting the infusion and may be characterized by generalized rash/erythema, hypotension, and bronchospasm.
  - All patients should be premedicated prior to starting the drug infusion with corticosteroid and H2 antagonist.
  - Monitor patient closely during the infusion, especially cycles 1 and 2, and emergency equipment and medications should be readily available.
  - Discontinue immediately if HSR is observed and treat immediately as appropriate. Do not rechallenge the patient.
- *Gastrointestinal toxicity* (e.g., nausea, vomiting, diarrhea) can be severe, and patients on clinical trials have died from diarrhea and electrolyte imbalance. The trial was multi-institutional (146 institutions) and involved 26 countries.
  - Rehydrate and treat with antiemetics and antidiarrheals as needed.
  - If grade 3 or higher diarrhea, delay dose, and modify dose after symptoms have resolved.
  - Deaths due to GI hemorrhage, perforation, and neutropenic enterocolitis have occurred. Risk may be increased with neutropenia, age, steroid use, concomitant use of NSAIDs, antiplatelet therapy, anticoagulation, and prior history of pelvic radiotherapy, adhesions, and GI bleeding.
  - Assess and evaluate promptly patients who develop abdominal pain and tenderness, fever, persistent constipation, diarrhea with or without neutropenia, which may be early signs/symptoms of serious GI toxicity.
- *Renal failure* with fatal outcome has been reported in the clinical trials, so patients with new-onset renal failure should be evaluated and treated aggressively, with efforts made to determine the etiology.
  - Hematuria was reported in 17% of patients.
  - Most cases occurred in association with sepsis, dehydration, obstructive uropathy.
- *Urinary disorders including cystitis:* If the patient has previously received pelvic RT, patient is at risk for developing cystitis, radiation cystitis, and hematuria. Radiation recall cystitis may occur. Monitor patients who previously received pelvic RT closely for signs/symptoms of cystitis while receiving the drug, and interrupt or discontinue the drug if severe hemorrhagic cystitis develops. Medical and/or surgical intervention may be required, requiring nursing support.

- *Respiratory disorders* such as interstitial pneumonia/pneumonitis, ILD, and ARDS have been reported and may be fatal. Patients with underlying lung disease may be at higher risk for developing any of these events, and ARDS may occur in the infection setting.
- Interrupt cabazitaxel if new or worsening pulmonary symptoms develop.
- Closely monitor patients, especially those with underlying lung disease, and promptly evaluate patients further. Drug discontinuation must be considered for new or worsening pulmonary symptoms if diagnosis confirmed.
- *Hepatic impairment*:
  - Drug is extensively metabolized in the liver, and hepatic impairment increases the risk of severe and life-threatening complications.
  - Drug should be dose reduced in patients with mild hepatic impairment (to 20 mg/m^2), and to 15 mg/m^2 for patients with moderate hepatic impairment.
- *Embryo-fetal toxicity:*
  - If the drug is used during pregnancy, or if the patient becomes pregnant while receiving the drug, the patient should be told of the potential risk to the fetus.
  - Teach women of childbearing age to use effective contraception to avoid pregnancy. Drug crosses placental barrier in rodents, so mothers receiving the drug should not nurse their infants. A decision should be made whether to discontinue nursing or to discontinue the drug.

Potential Toxicities/Side Effects and the Nursing Process

I. POTENTIAL FOR INJURY related to HYPERSENSITIVITY OR ANAPHYLAXIS REACTIONS

Defining Characteristics: Severe hypersensitivity reactions characterized by generalized rash/erythema, hypotension, and/or bronchospasm can occur, especially during the first or second infusions. If patient experiences a severe hypersensitivity reaction, patient should not be rechallenged and drug should be discontinued. Polysorbate 80 (Tween 80) is an emulsifier that is water-soluble, which is the vehicle by which cabazitaxel is soluble in the blood. Polysorbate 80 serves a similar purpose for docetaxel. However, it may cause hypersensitivity reactions. Patients who have had a hypersensitivity reaction to polysorbate 80 should not receive the drug. If the patient had a hypersensitivity reaction to docetaxel, it is likely the patient reacted to polysorbate 80 and should not receive cabazitaxel. Cardiac arrhythmias may occur in 5% of patients; hypotension may occur in 5% of patients as well.

Nursing Implications: Ensure that patient has received premedication (e.g., antihistamine, corticosteroid, H2 receptor antagonist). Assess baseline VS and mental status prior to drug administration, especially first and second doses of the drug. Monitor VS every 15 minutes, and remain with patient during first 15 minutes of drug infusion, as most reactions occur during the first 10 minutes. Continue to monitor closely for the duration of the 1-hour infusion. Stop drug if cardiac arrhythmia (irregular apical pulse) or hypo- or hypertension occur and discuss continuance of infusion with physician. Recall signs/symptoms of anaphylaxis, and if these occur, stop drug immediately and notify physician. Subjective symptoms are generalized itching, nausea, chest tightness, crampy abdominal pain, difficulty speaking, anxiety, agitation, sense of impending doom, uneasiness, desire to urinate/defecate, dizziness, chills. Objective signs are flushed appearance; angioedema of face, neck, eyelids, hands, feet; localized or generalized urticaria; respiratory distress with or without wheezing, hypotension, cyanosis. Review standing orders or nursing procedure for patient management of anaphylaxis, and be prepared to stop drug immediately if signs/symptoms occur. Keep IV line open with 0.9% sodium chloride, notify physician, monitor VS, and administer ordered medications, which may include epinephrine 1:1,000, hydrocortisone sodium succinate, and diphenhydramine. Teach patient the potential of a hypersensitivity or anaphylactic reaction and to report any unusual symptoms immediately. The drug should be permanently discontinued in patients who have a hypersensitivity reaction.

II.   POTENTIAL FOR INFECTION AND BLEEDING related to BM DEPRESSION

Defining Characteristics: Neutropenia is common (94%), with 82% grades 3–4, and is the dose-limiting toxicity. Febrile neutropenia occurred in 7% of patients. Anemia occurs in almost all patients (98%), while thrombocytopenia is less common (48%). Pyrexia was reported by 12% of patients.

Nursing Implications: Assess baseline CBC and differential to ensure that ANC is >1,500/mm^3 and platelet count is >100,000/mm^3 prior to chemotherapy, as well as for signs/symptoms of infection or bleeding. Patients should have weekly CBC/differential and assessment for neutropenia for the first cycle. Assess need for G-CSF with cycle 1 in high-risk patients (e.g., age > 65 years, poor performance status, previous episodes of febrile neutropenia, extensive prior radiation ports, poor nutritional status, or other serious comorbidities), and discuss with physician to ensure that patient receives primary prophylaxis. Teach patient signs/symptoms of infection or bleeding and to report these immediately, and teach patient self-care measures to minimize risk of infection and bleeding. This includes avoidance of crowds, proximity to people with infections, and avoidance of OTC aspirin-containing medications. Teach patient self-administration of G-CSF as ordered to prevent severe neutropenia. Instruct patient to alternate rest and activity periods and to report increased fatigue, shortness of breath, or chest pain that might herald severe anemia. If the patient is elderly, monitor more closely both at the time of treatment and between cycles, assessing for tolerance and need for additional support.

III.   ALTERED NUTRITION, LESS THAN BODY REQUIREMENTS, related to NAUSEA AND VOMITING, DIARRHEA, CONSTIPATION, DYSGEUSIA, ANOREXIA

Defining Characteristics: Diarrhea is common (47%) and may be severe and life-threatening. Nausea and vomiting occur in 34% and 22% of patients, respectively, but are mild and preventable with antiemetics. Constipation occurs in 20% of patients, while other symptoms are less common: dyspepsia (10%), anorexia (16%), dehydration (5%), dysgeusia (11%), and weight loss (9%). Mucosal inflammation affected 6% of patients.

Nursing Implications: Premedicate patient with antiemetic. If patient develops nausea and/or vomiting, encourage small, frequent intake of cool, bland foods. Instruct patient to report nausea, and teach self-administration of antiemetic medications. If nausea/vomiting occur and are severe, assess for signs/symptoms of fluid/electrolyte imbalance. Encourage patient to report onset of diarrhea. Teach patient to self-administer antidiarrheal medications if needed. If the patient has diarrhea, ensure it is well controlled and that potential complications of dehydration and electrolyte imbalance are avoided. Give special attention to the elderly patient and follow more closely between cycles as to tolerance and remaining hydrated. Involve dietitian as needed.

IV. POTENTIAL ALTERATION IN ACTIVITY TOLERANCE related to ASTHENIA, FATIGUE, ARTHRALGIA, ANEMIA

Defining Characteristics: Fatigue affects about 37% of patients, and 20% experience asthenia. Back pain (16%), arthralgia (11%), and muscle spasms (7%) may also occur.

Nursing Implications: Assess Hgb/HCT prior to each treatment and at nadir counts. Assess patient activity tolerance and ability to do ADLs. Teach patient self-care strategies to minimize exertion and maximize activity, such as clustering activity during shopping, alternating rest and activity periods, diet, gentle exercise. Instruct patient to alternate rest and activity periods and to report increased fatigue, shortness of breath, or chest pain that might herald severe anemia.

V. SENSORY/PERCEPTUAL ALTERATIONS related to SENSORY NEUROPATHY

Defining Characteristics: Grades 1–4 PN may affect up to 13% of patients (grades 3–4 < 1%). All patients previously received docetaxel, which may cause PN. Dizziness occurs in 8% of patients, as does headache.

Nursing Implications: Assess baseline neurologic status. Instruct patient to report signs/symptoms of pins-and-needles sensation, numbness, pain, increased discomfort with certain sensations, especially in the extremities, or motor weakness. Identify patients at risk: those with history of docetaxel use or with preexisting neuropathies (ethanol- and diabetes mellitus–related). Assess sensory and motor function prior to each treatment, and if abnormality found, assess impact on patient's function, safety, independence, and quality of life. Test patient's ability to button a shirt or pick up a dime from a flat surface. If severely impacting safety or quality of life, discuss with patient and physician drug discontinuance or use of cytoprotective agent. Teach self-care strategies, including maintaining safety when walking, getting up, taking a bath, or washing dishes; discuss risk of inability to sense temperature and the need to keep extremities warm in cold weather. If PN affects function, discuss impact on quality of life with patient and physician.

Drug: calaspargase pegol-mknl (Asparlas™)

Class: Miscellaneous agents (enzyme).

Mechanism of Action: Hydrolyzes serum asparagine, which deprives leukemia cells of the required amino acid. Normal cells are spared because they generally have the ability to synthesize their own asparagine. Cell cycle–specific for G_1 postmitotic phase. Some leukemic cells are unable to synthesize asparagine. These cells must obtain asparagine from an exogenous source, the patient's serum. Administration of the enzyme L-asparaginase causes hydrolysis of asparagine to aspartate, resulting in rapid depletion of the asparagine concentration in the patient's serum. The leukemic cells cannot synthesize protein or proliferate.

Metabolism: Elimination half-life 16.1 days (mean). Drug not studied in patients with renal or hepatic impairment.

Indication: As an asparaginase specific enzyme, indicated as a component of a multi-agent chemotherapeutic regimen for the treatment of ALL in pediatric and young adult patients aged 1 month to 21 years of age.

Contraindication: Patients with (1) history of serious HSRs to pegylated L-asparaginase; (2) history of serious thrombosis during L-asparaginase therapy; (3) history of severe pancreatitis related to previous L-asparaginase treatment; (4) history of serious hemorrhagic events during previous L-asparaginase therapy; (5) severe hepatic impairment.

Dosage/Range:
- Recommended dose is 2,500 units/m² IV no more frequently than every 21 days.

Dose Modification:
- Infusion reaction or HSR: (1) grade 1: reduce infusion rate by 50%; (2) grade 2: interrupt infusion, treat symptoms as ordered, when symptoms resolve resume infusion with a 50% reduction in rate; (3) grade 3–4: discontinue calaspargase pegol-mknl.
- Hemorrhage: Grades 3–4: (1) hold calaspargase pegol-mknl; (2) evaluate for coagulopathy and consider clotting factor replacement as needed; (3) resume calaspargase pegol-mknl with the next scheduled dose if bleeding controlled.
- Pancreatitis: Grades 3–4: (1) hold calaspargase pegol-mknl for elevations in lipase or amylase >3 × ULN until enzyme levels stabilize or are declining; (2) discontinue calaspargase pegol-mknl permanently if clinical pancreatitis is confirmed.
- Thromboembolism: (1) Uncomplicated DVT: (a) hold calaspargase pegol-mknl; (b) treat with appropriate antithombotic therapy; (c) upon symptom resolution consider resuming calaspargase pegol-mknl while continuing antithrombotic therapy; (2) severe or life-threatening thrombosis: (a) discontinue calaspargase pegol-mknl permanently, (b) treat with appropriate antithrombotic therapy.

- Hepatotoxicity: (1) Total bilirubin (TBILI) > 3 × to 10 × ULN: hold calaspargase pegol-mknl until TBILI levels go down to ≤ 1.5 × ULN; (2) TBILI >10 × ULN: discontinue calaspargase pegol-mknl and do not make up for missed doses (Servier Pharma, 2018).

Drug Preparation:
- Available as 3,750 units/5 mL (750 units/mL) in a single-dose vial. Solution is colorless and clear. If particulate matter, cloudiness, or discoloration are present, discard the vial. DO NOT use if vial has been shaken or vigorously agitated, frozen, or stored at room temperature for > 48 hours.
- Dilute ordered dose of calaspargase pegol-mknl in 100 mL of 0.9% sodium chloride injection USP or 5% dextrose injection USP using sterile/asceptic technique. Discard any unused portion of the drug left in the vial. Drug should be infused immediately after preparation.
- The diluted solution can be stored up to 4 hours at room temperature (15°–25°C [59°–77°F]) or refrigerated at 2°–8°C (36°–46°F) for up to 24 hours. Protect from light. DO NOT shake or freeze.

Drug Administration:
- Women of reproductive potential: (1) assess pregnancy test results prior to starting therapy (should be negative); (2) teach patients to use highly effective *non-oral contraceptive* measures to prevent pregnancy as drug is toxic to the fetus, during therapy and for at least 3 months after the last dose of calaspargase pegol-mknl. If patient is a mother, she should not breastfeed while receiving the drug.
- Assess baseline and weekly (at least) during treatment: serum bilirubin, transaminases, glucose, and clinical evaluation for toxicity until recovery from each cycle of therapy. See dose modifications above for adverse reactions.
- Immediately after drug is diluted or stored as above, administer the drug as a 1-hour infusion into a running IV of either 0.9% sodium chloride injection USP or 5% dextrose injection USP (same as drug infusion solution). Do not infuse other drugs through the same IV line during calaspargase pegol-mknl infusion.
- IRRs, HSRs: observe patients during infusion and for 1 hour after administration. Discontinue drug if a serious HSR occurs (grade 3/4 HSRs including anaphylaxis have occurred in 7–21% of patients). Have emergency medications, resuscitation equipment, and personnel close by during the infusion and for 1-hour observation postinfusion.

Lab Effects/Interference:
- Increased ALT, AST, bilirubin
- Abnormal clotting studies
- Increased amylase, lipase

Drug Interactions:
- May decrease the efficacy of oral contraceptives.

Special Considerations:
- Most common adverse effects ($\geq 10\%$) grade 3 or higher were elevated serum transaminases and bilirubin, pancreatitis, and abnormal clotting studies.
- Longer-acting asparaginase product. Safety profile similar to pegaspargase.
- Warnings and Precautions:
  - *HSRs*: observe patients during infusion and for 1 hour after administration. Discontinue drug if serious HSR occurs.
  - *Pancreatitis*: discontinue drug if pancreatitis develops. Monitor blood glucose.
  - *Thrombosis*: discontinue drug if severe or life-threatening thrombosis occurs; administer/teach patient about prescribed anticoagulants as ordered.
  - *Hemorrhage*: discontinue drug for severe or life-threatening hemorrhage. Cause should be identified early and treated promptly.
  - *Hepatotoxicity*: Monitor LFTs baseline and regularly through recovery from cycle.

Potential Toxicities/Side Effects and the Nursing Process

I.   POTENTIAL FOR INJURY related to HYPERSENSITIVITY OR ANAPHYLACTIC REACTIONS

Defining Characteristics: Grade 3–4 HSRs including anaphylaxis occurred in 7–21% of patients during clinical trials. HSRs with asparaginase products in general include angioedema, lip swelling, eye swelling, erythema, decreased BP, bronchospasm, dyspnea, pruritis, and rash.

Nursing Implications: Assess baseline vital signs and mental status prior to drug administration. Review standing orders or nursing procedure for management of anaphylaxis and be prepared to stop drug immediately if signs/symptoms occur; keep IV line open with 0.9% sodium chloride, notify physician, maintain ABCs, monitor vital signs, and administer ordered medications, which may include epinephrine 1:1,000 IM, hydrocortisone sodium succinate IV, and diphenhydramine IV. Teach patient the potential of a hypersensitivity or anaphylactic reaction and to report any unusual symptoms immediately.

II. POTENTIAL FOR INJURY related to PANCREATITIS, HEPATOTOXICITY, HEMORRHAGE, OR THROMBOEMBOLISM

Defining Characteristics: Pancreatitis occurred in 12–16% of patients in clinical trials, with grade 3 or higher pancreatitis occurring in 18% of patients. Hemorrhagic or necrotizing pancreatitis has also been reported. LFTs are elevated in a number of patients (ALT, AST, TBILI, and direct bilirubin decreased serum albumim). Grade 3–4 elevated transaminases occurred in 52% of patients, and bilirubin was increased in 20% of patients. Hepatically derived clotting factors may be depressed, resulting in excessive bleeding or blood clotting. Thrombosis may occur in 9–12% of patients as in clinical trials. Hemorrhage related to increased PT, increased PTT, and hypofibrinogenemia have occurred.

Nursing Implications: Monitor baseline LFTs; alkaline phos; albumin; and clotting factors PT, PTT, and fibrinogen. Assess bilirubin and transaminases at least weekly during cycles of chemotherapy that include calaspargase pegol-mknl for at least 6 weeks after the last dose of calaspargase pegol-mknl. Drug should be discontinued if serious liver toxicity occurs and supportive care given. Teach patient to report bleeding, severe headache, arm or leg swelling, SOB, pain in calf or chest pain, pain in abdomen, new onset nausea and/or vomiting and any unusual symptoms. If severe abdominal pain occurs, patient should seek immediate medical attention. Serious thrombotic events have been described, including sagittal sinus thrombosis. Assess patient for signs/symptoms of thrombosis or bleeding, signs/symptoms of pancreatitis and assess serum amylase and/or lipase levels to identify early pancreatic inflammation. If pancreatitis is confirmed, drug should be permanently discontinued. See Dose Modifications for these events and drug discontinuation.

III. ALTERED NUTRITION, LESS THAN BODY REQUIREMENTS, related to NAUSEA/VOMITING, DIARRHEA, HYPERGLYCEMIA

Defining Characteristics: Drug is given as part of combination chemotherapy which often causes nausea and vomiting. Hyperglycemia is a transient reaction caused by effects on the pancreas with decreased insulin synthesis. Severe diarrhea (grades 3 and higher) occurs in 9% of patients.

Nursing Implications: Premedicate with antiemetics appropriate to combination therapy. Encourage small, frequent meals of cool, bland foods and liquids, as well as favorite foods, especially high-calorie, high-protein foods. Monitor weekly weights. Teach patient about the potential of hyperglycemia and pancreatitis, and instruct to report any unusual symptoms (e.g., increased thirst, urination, and appetite). Monitor serum glucose, amylase, and lipase levels baseline and periodically during treatment. Report any laboratory elevations to physician. Treat hyperglycemia issues with diet or insulin as ordered by physician. Treat pancreatitis per physician orders.

IV. POTENTIAL FOR SEXUAL DYSFUNCTION related to REPRODUCTION HAZARD

Defining Characteristics: Drug is teratogenic.

Nursing Implications: Before starting therapy, confirm female patients of reproductive potential are not pregnant. As appropriate, explore with patient and partner issues of reproductive and sexual patterns and impact chemotherapy/calaspargase pegol-mknl will have. Discuss strategies to preserve sexuality and reproductive health. Because of a drug interaction with oral contraceptives making them possibly ineffective, teach patient effective contraception with other methods including barrier method.

Drug: capecitabine (Xeloda, N4-pentoxycarbonyl-5-deoxy-5-fluorocytidine)

Class: Nucleoside metabolic inhibitor (fluoropyrimidine carbamate).

Mechanism of Action: Two mechanisms are involved in capecitabine activity. First, metabolites bind to thymidylate synthetase, inhibiting the formation of thymidylate, which is the necessary precursor of thymidine triphosphate, and preventing DNA synthesis. Second, the false metabolite is taken up instead of uridine triphosphate during RNA synthesis, which interferes with RNA processing and protein synthesis.

Metabolism: Absorbed from the intestinal mucosa as an intact molecule, metabolized in the liver to intermediary metabolite, and then in the liver and tumor tissue to 5-FU precursor. It is then converted through catalytic activation to 5-FU at the tumor site. Metabolites are cleared in the urine.

Indications: Capecitabine in indicated for:
- Colon and rectal cancer:
  - Adjuvant treatment of patients with Duke's C colon cancer.
  - Metastatic colorectal cancer (mCRC) as first-line monotherapy when treatment with fluoropyrimidine therapy alone is preferred.
- Metastatic breast cancer:
  - Metastatic breast cancer, in combination with docetaxel after failure of prior anthracycline-containing therapy;
- As monotherapy in patients resistant to both paclitaxel and an anthracycline-containing regimen or resistant to paclitaxel and for whom further anthracycline therapy is not indicated (e.g., has received cumulative doses of 400 mg/m^2 of doxorubicin). Resistance is defined as progressive disease while on treatment with or without an initial response, or relapse within 6 months of completing treatment with an anthracycline-containing adjuvant regimen.

Contraindications: Patients with
- Severe renal impairment (CrCl < 30 mL/min).
- Hypersensitivity.

Dosage/Range:
Monotherapy (mCRC, adjuvant colon cancer, MBC): 1,250 mg/m^2 twice daily orally for 2 weeks followed by a 1-week rest period in 3-week cycles. This is equivalent to 2,500 mg/m^2 total daily dose.

- Adjuvant treatment for patients with Dukes C colon cancer: 1,250 mg/m^2 orally twice daily (morning and evening) for 2 weeks, followed by a 1-week rest period, given as 3-week cycles for a total of 8 cycles (24 weeks or 6 months) per current Xeloda PI(12/2016).
- MBC in combination with docetaxel, the recommended dose of capecitabine is 1,250 mg/m^2 twice daily for 2 weeks followed by a 7-day rest period, combined with docetaxel at 75 mg/m^2 as a 1-hour infusion every 3 weeks. Premedication according to docetaxel labeling should be given prior to docetaxel.

- See Xeloda package insert for BSA and total dose, as well as number of tablets taken at each dose.
- Capecitabine dosage may need to be individualized to optimize patient management treatment. Toxicity due to capecitabine may be managed symptomatically, by dose interruptions and dose adjustment. Once the dose has been reduced, it should not be increased at a later time.
- Doses of capecitabine omitted for toxicity should not be replaced or restored; rather, resume planned treatment cycle.
- Reduce the dose of capecitabine by 25% in patients with moderate renal impairment (CrCl 30–50 mL/min) when used as monotherapy, or when combined with docetaxel (e.g., from 1,250 mg/m^2 to 950 mg/m^2 twice daily).
- The dose of phenytoin and the dose of coumarin-derived anticoagulants may need to be reduced when either drug is administered concomitantly with capecitabine.
- See Xeloda package insert (December 2016) for toxicity directed dose levels/modifications for toxicity, and docetaxel dose reductions in combination with capecitabine.

Drug Preparation:
- Available in 150- and 500-mg tablets.

Drug Administration:
- Teach patient to self-administer tablets (1) whole with water within 30 min after a meal; (2) not to crush or cut the tablets; (3) total daily dose is divided in half, and the patient should take a dose 12 hours apart, within 30 minutes of a meal. If the tablets must be crushed, this should be done by a professional trained in safe handling of cytotoxic drugs.
- Assess ANC/CBC baseline and ensure ANC ≥ 1,500/mm^3 and platelet count ≥100,000/mm^3 prior to the patient starting therapy. See package insert for dose interruption and modification during therapy.

Drug Interactions:
- Warfarin: Elevated PT and INR resulting in bleeding, including death; monitor INR closely and adjust warfarin dose frequently as needed during and for 1 month after capecitabine therapy.
- Phenytoin: monitor phenytoin serum level closely and decrease phenytoin dose as needed.
- Leucovorin: increases the concentration of 5-FU, so synergy and enhanced toxicity; monitor toxicity closely.
- CYP2C9 substrates: coadminister carefully and monitor patient closely.
- Food: reduces rate and extent of capecitabine absorption.

Lab Effects/Interference:
- Increased bili, alk phos.
- Decreased WBCs.

Special Considerations:
- Monitor bilirubin baseline and before each cycle, as dose modifications are necessary with hyperbilirubinemia.
- Folic acid should be avoided while taking drug.

- There are reports that patients on capecitabine who develop hand–foot syndrome (HFS) involving the fingers may lose their fingerprints, which can cause problems for patients who travel internationally.
- Most common adverse reactions ($\geq$30%) were diarrhea, HFS, nausea, vomiting, abdominal pain, fatigue/weakness, and hyperbilirubinemia.
- Nursing mothers should discontinue nursing when receiving capecitabine.
- Warnings and Precautions:
  - *Diarrhea*: can be severe; monitor patient closely and replace fluid and electrolytes to prevent dehydration. Dose-interrupt and dose-reduce for reoccurrence of grade 2 or occurrence of any grade 3 or 4 diarrhea (see package insert). Necrotizing enterocolitis (typhlitis) has been reported.
  - Coagulopathy: Patients taking warfarin or oral coumarin-derivative anticoagulants may develop altered coagulation parameters and/or bleeding.
    - Assess and monitor INR or PT closely, and make dose adjustments based on laboratory results.
    - Occurs several days to up to several months after starting capecitabine therapy; may also be seen within 1 month after drug stopped.
    - Predisposing factors: age > 60, diagnosis of cancer.
- *Cardiotoxicity:* MI, myocardial ischemia, angina, dysrhythmias, cardiac arrest, cardiac failure, sudden death, ECG changes, and cardiomyopathy have occurred, and patients with prior history of coronary heart disease may be at higher risk.
- *Dihydropyrimidine dehydrogenase deficiency (DPD)* increases risk of 5-FU toxicity (e.g., stomatitis, diarrhea, neutropenia, and neurotoxicity). Hold or permanently discontinue capecitabine if unusually severe toxicity occurs, which may indicate near complete or total absence of DPD activity.
- *Dehydration and renal failure.* Dehydration may occur and result in acute renal failure, which can be fatal.
  - Increased risk in patients with preexisting compromised renal function or who are receiving concomitant capecitabine with known nephrotoxic agents. Rapid dehydration may occur in patients with anorexia, asthenia, nausea, vomiting, or diarrhea. Prevent or correct dehydration when capecitabine is started, and monitor patients closely.
    - If grade 2 or higher dehydration occurs, capecitabine therapy should be immediately interrupted and dehydration corrected.
    - Capecitabine should not be restarted until the patient is adequately rehydrated and any precipitating causes have been corrected/controlled (and as indicated, dose modifications for the precipitating adverse event).
  - Patients with baseline moderate renal impairment require dose reduction; carefully monitor patients with mild or moderate renal impairment for adverse effects. If toxicity occurs (grades 2–4), immediately interrupt therapy and adjust dose when toxicity resolves (see package insert).
- *Embryo-fetal toxicity:* Pregnancy: drug can cause fetal harm. If capecitabine is used during pregnancy, or if a patient becomes pregnant while receiving capecitabine, apprise the patient of the potential hazard to the fetus. Teach women of reproductive potential to use effective contraception to avoid pregnancy during treatment and for 6 months after last dose.

- *Mucocutaneous and dermatologic toxicity.*
  - HFS (palmar-plantar erythrodysesthesia, chemotherapy-induced acral erythema) has occurred. Median time to onset was 79 days.
    - Grade 1 = numbness, dysesthesia/paresthesia, tingling, painless swelling or erythema of the hands and/or feet and/or discomfort that does not disrupt normal activities.
    - Grade 2 = *painful* erythema and swelling of hands and/or feet and/or discomfort affecting patient's ADLs.
    - Grade 3 = moist desquamation, ulceration, blistering or severe pain of hand and/or feet, and/or severe discomfort that causes the patient to be unable to work or perform ADLs.
    - Interrupt capecitabine for grade 2 or 3 HFS until it resolves or decreases to a grade 1.
    - Grade 3: decrease dose of capecitabine when event/HFS resolves to grade 1.
  - Severe mucocutaneous reactions: Stevens–Johnson and Toxic Epidermal Necrolysis (TEN) have occurred. Capecitabine should be permanently discontinued if the patient experiences a severe mucocutaneous reaction that appears attributable to capecitabine.
- *Hyperbilirubinemia:* may occur, and patients with liver metastases are at risk. If drug-related grades 3–4 elevations in bilirubin occur, interrupt capecitabine immediately until bilirubin decreases to ≤3.0 × ULN (see package insert for dose modifications).
- *Hematologic:* do not administer drug to patients with a baseline ANC < 1,500/mm^3 and/or platelet count of <100,000/mm^3. If unscheduled lab assessments during a treatment cycle show grade 3 or 4 neutropenia or thrombocytopenia, interrupt capecitabine therapy until recovery. See package insert.
- *Geriatric patients*: patients 80 years of age and older may experience a greater incidence of grades 3–4 adverse events. Take extra care with the elderly, monitoring the patient closely and intervening promptly to minimize toxicity.
- *Hepatic insufficiency*: monitor patients with mild to moderate hepatic dysfunction related to liver metastases closely for toxicity, and intervene promptly. The effect of severe hepatotoxicity on the metabolism and disposition of capecitabine is unknown.
- Combination with other drugs (e.g., irinotecan): has not been adequately studied.

Potential Toxicities/Side Effects and the Nursing Process

I.   POTENTIAL FOR INFECTION AND BLEEDING related to BM DEPRESSION

Defining Characteristics: Commonly causes anemia, neutropenia, and thrombocytopenia.

Nursing Implications: Assess baseline CBC, WBC with differential, and platelet count prior to chemotherapy, as well as for signs/symptoms of infection or bleeding. Teach patient signs/symptoms of infection and bleeding and instruct to report these immediately; teach patient self-care measures to minimize risk of infection and bleeding. This includes avoidance of crowds, proximity to people with infections, and avoidance of OTC aspirin-containing medications.

II.   ALTERED NUTRITION, LESS THAN BODY REQUIREMENTS, related to NAUSEA AND VOMITING, STOMATITIS, AND DIARRHEA

Defining Characteristics: Nausea and vomiting occur in 30–50% of patients. Stomatitis and diarrhea also occur in about 50% of patients. Less common with reduced doses. Abdominal pain (35%), constipation (14%), anorexia (26%), dehydration (7%) also occur. Side effects are increased in the elderly (≥80 years old). The median time to first occurrence of grades 2–4 diarrhea was 34 days, and the median duration of grades 3–4 diarrhea was 5 days.

Nursing Implications: Premedicate patient with antiemetics (phenothiazines usually effective), and continue for 24 hours, at least for first cycle. Encourage small, frequent meals of cool, bland foods. Assess oral mucosa prior to drug administration and teach patient to report changes. Teach patient oral hygiene measures and self-assessment. Instruct patient to report diarrhea, to self-administer prescribed antidiarrheal medications, and to drink adequate fluids. Moderate to severe stomatitis, diarrhea, or nausea and vomiting are indications to interrupt therapy. If grade 2, 3, or 4 diarrhea occurs, capecitabine should be interrupted immediately until diarrhea resolves or decreases in intensity to grade 1. If grade 2 diarrhea reoccurs, or occurrence of any grade 3 or 4 diarrhea, capecitabine dose should be reduced.

III.   ALTERATION IN SKIN INTEGRITY/COMFORT related to HFS

Defining Characteristics: HFS occurs in more than half of patients and is characterized by tingling, numbness, pain, erythema, dryness, rash, swelling, and/or pruritus of hands and feet. Less common with reduced doses.

Nursing Implications: Teach patient about the possibility of this side effect and instruct him or her to stop drug use and inform the physician/nurse immediately should it occur. If patient has pain, expect dose interruption, with dose reduction if this is second or subsequent episode at current dose. Teach patient self-assessment of soles of feet and palms of hands daily for erythema, pain, dry desquamation, and to report pain right away. Teach patients to avoid hot showers, whirlpools, paraffin treatments of nails, vigorous repetitive movements of hands, feet, as well as other body areas; avoid tight-fitting shoes and clothes. Teach patients to take cool showers, keep skin surfaces intact and soft with skin emollients. Studies ongoing establishing evidence base for prophylaxis or treatment: vitamin B_6, urea moisturizers, nicotine patch.

IV.   ALTERATION IN COMFORT related to FATIGUE, WEAKNESS, DIZZINESS, HEADACHE, FEVER, MYALGIAS, INSOMNIA, AND TASTE PROBLEMS

Defining Characteristics: Fatigue affects approximately 43% of patients, while 42% of patients complained of weakness. Fever was reported in 18% of patients, headache 10%, dizziness 8%, insomnia 7%, and taste problems 6%. Eye irritation was reported by 13% of patients and is related to the drug's excretion via tears.

Nursing Implications: Assess baseline comfort, and teach patient that these symptoms may occur. Teach patient strategies to manage fatigue, such as alternating rest and activity periods, and consolidating tasks. Teach patient to report fever, headache, and eye irritation, and discuss management plan with physician.

Drug: carboplatin (Paraplatin)

Class: Alkylating agent (heavy metal complex).

Mechanism of Action: A second-generation platinum analogue. The cytotoxicity is identical to that of the parent, cisplatin, and it is cell cycle phase nonspecific. It reacts with nucleophilic sites on DNA, causing predominantly intrastrand and interstrand crosslinks rather than DNA-protein crosslinks. These crosslinks are similar to those formed with cisplatin but are formed later.

Metabolism: At 24 hours, postadministration, approximately 70% of carboplatin is excreted in the urine. The mean half-life is roughly 100 minutes.

Indication:
- Initial treatment of advanced ovarian carcinoma in established combination with other approved chemotherapy agents.
- Secondary, palliative treatment of patients with ovarian carcinoma recurrent after prior chemotherapy, including patients previously treated with cisplatin.
- **Contraindications:** Patients with (1) history of severe allergic reactions to cisplatin or other platinum-containing compounds, or mannitol; (2) patients with severe BM depression or significant bleeding.

Dosage/Range:
- Dose usually given as a function of area under the curve (AUC). Since carboplatin has predictable pharmakinetics based on the drug's excretion by the kidneys, AUC dosing is recommended for this drug. This allows tailoring the drug dose precisely to the individual patient's excretion of the drug (renal function). The Calvert formula is used where total dose (mg) = target AUC × glomerular filtration rate (GFR) + 25. The GFR is approximated by the urine creatinine clearance, either estimated or actual, and can be calculated by hand. The target AUC is determined by the treatment plan depending on the type of malignancy, such as an AUC of 6 for cancer of unknown primary. Then, the dose calculation can be done by hand. Additionally, the manufacturer (Bristol-Myers Squibb Oncology) distributes a calculator to determine the dose.
- See Formula Dosing for AUC doses (Hospira, 2015).
- Recurrent ovarian cancer: as a single agent, 360 mg/m^2 IV infusion every 4 weeks.
- Advanced ovarian cancer: combination therapy with cyclophosphamide: (1) 300 mg/m^2 IV on day 1 every 4 weeks × 6 cycles or (2) 600 mg IV on day 1 every 4 weeks

× 6 cycles (Hospira, 2015). Delay drug for neutrophil count <2,000/mm^2 or platelets <100,000/mm^2.

- See package insert for dose adjustments (Hospira, 2015).
- Drug dose reduction for urine creatinine clearance <60 mL/minute.
- Autologous BM transplantation: 1,600 mg/m^2 IV in divided doses over 4 days (creatinine clearance must be more than 50 mL/min).
- Intraperitoneal: 200–650 mg/m^2 in 2-L IP (ovarian cancer).

Drug Preparation:
- Aluminum needles react with carboplatin forming a precipitate and loss of potency. DO NOT use needles or IV sets containing aluminum parts that may come into contact with the drug.
- Available as a ready-to-use sterile solution in 5 mL (50 mg), 15 mL (150 mg), 45 mL (450 mg), and 60 mL (600 mg) vials. Visually inspect, and if particulate matter observed, shake and reinspect.
- Can further dilute in 5% dextrose or 0.9% sodium chloride injection USP to as low as 0.5 mg/mL concentration.
- When further dilutes, the carboplatin injectin solution is stable for 8 hours at room temperature (25°C) because of the lack of bacteriostatic preservative. Visually inspect for particulate matter or discoloration before administration; if found, the solution should not be used.

Drug Administration:
- Administered by IV bolus over 15 minutes to 1 hour.
- May also be given as a CI over 24 hours.
- May be administered intraperitoneally in patients with advanced ovarian cancer.

Drug Interactions:
- Increases renal toxicity when combined with cisplatin.
- Increases BM depression when combined with myelosuppressive drugs.
- Avoid aluminum needles in drug handling.
- Paclitaxel, docetaxel: administer carboplatin after taxane to maximize cell kill and to minimize the risk of myelosuppression caused by decreased drug excretion.
- Phenytoin: may decrease phenytoin serum levels; monitor levels, and increase drug dose as needed.
- Warfarin: may increase warfarin effect; monitor INR frequently, and dose modify as needed.

Lab Effects/Interference:
- Increased LFTs, RFTs.

Special Considerations:
- Does not have the renal toxicity seen with cisplatin.
- Thrombocytopenia is dose-limiting toxicity and correlates with GFR.
- Monitor urine creatinine clearance.

Potential Toxicities/Side Effects and the Nursing Process

I.   POTENTIAL FOR INFECTION AND BLEEDING related to BM DEPRESSION

Defining Characteristics: Myelosuppression is dose-limiting toxicity; platelet nadir is 14–21 days, with usual recovery by day 28; WBC nadir follows 1 week later, but recovery may take 5–6 weeks. The risk of thrombocytopenia is severe, especially when the drug is combined with other myelosuppressive drugs, or if the patient has renal compromise. Anemia may occur with prolonged treatment.

Nursing Implications: Assess CBC, WBC, with differential, and platelet count prior to drug administration. Monitor for signs/symptoms of infection or bleeding. Drug dosage should be reduced if urine creatinine clearance is <60 mL/min. Drug should be held or dose reduced if absolute neutrophil count (ANC) and/or platelet count is low. Teach the patient signs/symptoms of infection and bleeding, and instruct to report them immediately if they occur. Teach self-care measures to minimize infection and bleeding. Discuss with physician use of G-CSF to prevent neutropenia in heavily pretreated patients.

II.   POTENTIAL FOR ALTERED URINARY ELIMINATION related to NEPHROTOXICITY

Defining Characteristics: The drug does not have the renal toxicity seen with cisplatin (Platinol), so that only minimal hydration is needed. However, the drug is excreted by the kidneys, and concomitant treatment with drugs causing nephrotoxicity (i.e., aminoglycoside antibiotics) can alter renal function studies. Nephrotoxicity does occur at high doses, and patients with renal dysfunction are at risk. In addition, serum electrolyte loss can occur (potassium, magnesium, rarely calcium). Monitor serum electrolytes prior to treatment and periodically after treatment. Replete electrolytes as ordered.

Nursing Implications: Assess renal function studies (i.e., urine creatinine clearance, serum blood urea nitrogen [BUN], and creatinine) prior to drug administration. Discuss drug dose modification if creatinine clearance <60 cc/min, or if other values are abnormal.

III.   POTENTIAL FOR ALTERATION IN NUTRITION, LESS THAN BODY REQUIREMENTS, related to NAUSEA/VOMITING, ANOREXIA, STOMATITIS, DIARRHEA, AND HEPATIC DYSFUNCTION

Defining Characteristics: Nausea and vomiting begin 6+ hours after administration and last for <24 hours, but may be easily prevented by available antiemetics. Anorexia occurs in 10% of patients but is usually mild, lasting 1–2 days. Diarrhea occurs in 10% of patients and is mild. Reversible hepatic dysfunction is mild to moderate, as evidenced by changes in alk phos and SGOT and, rarely, serum glutamic pyruvic transaminase (SGPT) and bili.

Nursing Implications: Premedicate with antiemetics and continue protection for 24 hours, at least for the first cycle. Encourage dietary modifications as needed. Monitor LFTs prior to and periodically during treatment.

IV. POTENTIAL FOR SENSORY/PERCEPTUAL ALTERATIONS related to NEUROLOGIC CHANGES

Defining Characteristics: Neurologic dysfunction is infrequent, but there is increased risk in patients >65 years old, or if previously treated with cisplatin and receiving prolonged carboplatin treatment.

Nursing Implications: Assess baseline neurologic status and continue to monitor status throughout treatment, looking for dizziness, confusion, PN, ototoxicity, visual changes, and changes in taste. Teach patient the potential for side effects, and to report any changes.

V. POTENTIAL SEXUAL DYSFUNCTION related to DRUG EFFECTS

Defining Characteristics: Drug is mutagenic and probably teratogenic. It is unknown whether drug is excreted in breastmilk.

Nursing Implications: Assess patient's signs/symptoms and partner's patterns of sexuality and reproductive goals. Teach patient/partner about need for contraception and provide other information as appropriate. Provide emotional support.

VI. POTENTIAL FOR INJURY related to HYPERSENSITIVITY REACTIONS

Defining Characteristics: Drug may cause allergic reactions, ranging from rash, urticaria, erythema, and pruritus to anaphylaxis; they can occur within minutes of drug administration.

Nursing Implications: Assess baseline vital signs. During drug administration, observe for signs/symptoms of hypersensitivity reaction. If signs/symptoms of anaphylaxis (tachycardia, wheezing, hypotension, facial edema) occur, stop drug immediately. Keep IV patent with 0.9% sodium chloride, notify physician, monitor VS, and be prepared to administer ordered drugs (i.e., steroid, epinephrine, or antihistamines).

Drug: carmustine (BCNU, BiCNU)

Class: Nitrosourea.

Mechanism of Action: Alkylates DNA by causing crosslinks and strand breaks in the same manner as classic mustard agents; it also carbamylates cellular proteins, thus inhibiting DNA repair. Cell cycle phase nonspecific.

Metabolism: Rapidly distributed and metabolized with a plasma half-life of 1 hour; 70% of IV dose is excreted in urine within 96 hours. Significant concentrations of drug remain in cerebrospinal fluid for 9 hours due to lipid solubility of drug.

Indications: Palliative therapy as a single agent or in established combination therapy with other chemotherapy agents in the following:

- Brain tumors.
- Multiple myeloma, in combination with prednisone.
- Hodgkin's disease, as secondary therapy with other approved drugs for patients who relapse while being treated with primary therapy, or who fail to respond to primary therapy.
- NHL: as secondary therapy in combination with other approved drugs for patients who relapse while being treated with primary therapy, or who fail to respond to primary therapy.

Contraindication: Patients with previous hypersensitivity to the drug.

Dosage/Range:
Usual:
- 150–200 mg/m^2 every 6 weeks; may be given as a single dose or divided into daily infusions such as 75–100 mg/m^2 IV on 2 successive days.
- Polifeprosan 20 with carmustine (BCNU) implant: see *polifeprosan.*

Drug Preparation (see package insert for directions for use (Heritage Pharma, 2013)):
- First, dissolve carmustine with 3 mL of supplied sterile diluent (dehydrated alcohol injection USP).
- Second, aseptically add 27 mL sterile water for injection, USP. Each mL of resulting solution contains 3.3 mg of carmustine in 10% ethanol. Solution should be colorless to yellowish, clear.
- After reconstitution as recommended, carmustine is stable for 24 hours under refrigeration (2–8°C, 36–46°F). Reconstituted vials should be examined for crystal formation prior to use. If crystals are observed, they may be redissolved by warming vial to room temperature with agitation. Protect from light.
- May be further diluted with 5% dextrose injection, USP for a 2-hour infusion.
- Vials reconstituted as directed and further diluted to a concentration of 0.2 mg/mL in 5% dextrose injection USP should be stored at room temperature, protected from light, and used within 8 hours.
- Only use GLASS containers for BiCNU administration.
- See package insert for inadvertent melting of the drug if stored improperly (Heritage Pharma, 2013).

Drug Administration:
- Assess baseline PFTs, ANC/CBC, LFTs, renal function tests, and during therapy.
- Administer as a slow IV infusion over at least 2 hours, as infusing the drug more quickly can cause pain and burning at the injection site.
- Delayed BM suppression is the major toxicity: assess ANC/CBC/platelets weekly for at least 6 weeks after the dose.

Drug Interactions:
- Cimetidine may increase myelosuppression when given concurrently. AVOID IF POSSIBLE.
- Possible increased cellular uptake of drug when administered in combination with amphotericin B.
- Carmustine may decrease the pharmacologic effects of phenytoin.
- Avoid concomitant administration of renally or hepatically toxic drugs, as these may increase carmustine-induced renal or hepatic dysfunction.

Lab Effects/Interference:
- Pulmonary, hepatic, and renal function tests.

Special Considerations:
- Drug is an irritant; avoid extravasation.
- Pain at the injection site or along the vein is common. Treat by applying ice pack above the injection site and decreasing the infusion flow rate.
- Patient may act inebriated related to the alcohol diluent and may experience flushing.

Potential Toxicities/Side Effects and the Nursing Process

I.   POTENTIAL FOR INFECTION AND BLEEDING related to BM DEPRESSION

Defining Characteristics: Delayed myelosuppression is dose-limiting toxicity and is cumulative. WBC nadir 3–5 weeks after dose and persists 1–2 weeks; platelet nadir at 4 weeks, persisting 1–2 weeks. Drug should not be dosed more frequently than once every 6 weeks.

Nursing Implications: Assess baseline CBC, WBC with differential, and platelet count prior to chemotherapy and at least weekly postchemotherapy for the first cycle. Discuss dose reductions with physician for subsequent cycles if counts are lower than normal since BM depression is cumulative. Teach patient and family self-assessment for signs/symptoms of infection and bleeding, and instruct to report them immediately. Teach self-care measures to minimize risk of infection and bleeding, including avoidance of aspirin-containing medicines.

II.   POTENTIAL FOR IMPAIRED GAS EXCHANGE related to PULMONARY FIBROSIS

Defining Characteristics: Pulmonary toxicity appears to be dose related, with risk greatest in patients receiving total doses >1,400 mg (although it can occur at lower doses). Other risk factors include patients with abnormal PFTs prior to drug administration—i.e., baseline forced vital capacity (FVC) < 70% of predicted; carbon monoxide diffusion capacity (DLCO) < 70% of predicted; or if patient is receiving concurrent cyclophosphamide or thoracic radiation. Presents as insidious cough and dyspnea, or may be the sudden onset of respiratory failure. CXR shows interstitial infiltrates. Incidence is 20–30% of patients, with a mortality of 24–80%.

Nursing Implications: Assess patient's risk and baseline pulmonary function prior to chemotherapy, as well as the results of pulmonary function testing periodically during treatment, for evidence of pulmonary dysfunction. Teach patient to report any changes in respiratory pattern.

III. ALTERATION IN NUTRITION, LESS THAN BODY REQUIREMENTS, related to NAUSEA/VOMITING AND LIVER DYSFUNCTION

Defining Characteristics: Severe nausea and vomiting may occur 2 hours after administration and last 4–6 hours. Reversible liver dysfunction, although rare, is related to subacute hepatitis and is characterized by abnormal LFTs, painless jaundice, and (rarely) coma.

Nursing Implications: Premedicate with antiemetics and continue antiemetic protection for 24 hours, at least for the first treatment. Encourage small, frequent feedings of cool, bland foods, and liquids. Infuse drug over 60–120 minutes. Monitor LFTs (SGOT, SGPT, lactic dehydrogenase [LDH], alk phos, bili) during treatment and discuss any abnormalities with physician.

IV. ALTERATION IN COMFORT related to DRUG ADMINISTRATION

Defining Characteristics: Drug diluent is absolute alcohol, so irritation may result in pain along the vein path. Thrombosis is rare, but venospasms and flushing of skin or burning of the eyes can occur with rapid drug infusion.

Nursing Implications: Administer drug only through patent IV and dilute drug in 250 mL of 5% dextrose or 0.9% sodium chloride and infuse over 1–2 hours. If pain along vein occurs, use ice packs above injection site, decrease infusion rate, or further dilute drug. If patient will receive ongoing therapy, consider venous access device.

V. ALTERED URINARY ELIMINATION related to NEPHROTOXICITY

Defining Characteristics: Increase in BUN occurs in 10% of patients and is usually reversible. However, decreased kidney size, progressive azotemia, and renal failure have occurred in patients receiving large cumulative doses over long periods.

Nursing Implications: Assess baseline renal function and monitor BUN and creatinine prior to each successive cycle. Since drug is excreted by the kidneys, drug dosage should be reduced if renal dysfunction exists. If abnormalities occur and persist, discuss discontinuing drug with physician.

VI. POTENTIAL SEXUAL DYSFUNCTION related to DRUG EFFECTS

Defining Characteristics: Drug is mutagenic and teratogenic.

Nursing Implications: Assess patient's and partner's pattern of sexuality and reproductive goals. Teach patient and partner the need for contraception as appropriate. Provide emotional support and counseling, or referral as appropriate.

VII. SENSORY/PERCEPTUAL ALTERATIONS related to OCULAR TOXICITY

Defining Characteristics: Infarcts of optic nerve fiber, retinal hemorrhage, and neuroretinitis have been associated with high-dose therapy.

Nursing Implications: Assess baseline vision and appearance of eyes. Instruct patient to report any visual changes to physician or nurse.

Drug: chlorambucil (Leukeran)

Class: Alkylating agent.

Mechanism of Action: Alkylates DNA by causing strand breaks and crosslinks in the DNA. The drug is a derivative of a nitrogen mustard.

Metabolism: Pharmacokinetics are poorly understood. It is well absorbed orally, with a plasma half-life of 1.5 hours. Degradation is slow; it appears to be eliminated by metabolic transformation, with 60% excreted in urine in 24 hours.

Indication: For the palliative treatment of patients with chronic lymphatic (lymphocytic) leukemia, malignant lymphomas including lymphosarcoma, giant follicular lymphoma, and Hodgkin's disease.

Contraindications: Patients whose disease has demonstrated a prior resistance to the drug; patients with hypersensitivity to chlorambucil (there may be cross-hypersensitivity, e.g., skin rash between chlorambucil and other alkylating agents).

Dosage/Range:
- 0.1–0.2 mg/kg/day (equals 4–10 mg /day for the average patient) initially and for short pulses for 3–6 weeks with dose carefully adjusted according to patient response, and dose must be reduced as soon as there is an abrupt fall in WBC (Aspen, 2016).
- Alternate CLL regime: intermittent, biweekly, or once monthly pulse doses. Initial single dose of 0.4 mg/kg, and doses increased by 0.1 mg/kg until control of lymphocytosis or toxicity occurs (Aspen, 2016).

Drug Preparation:
- 2-mg tablets.

Drug Administration:
- Oral.
- Laboratory testing: patients must be followed carefully with weekly ANC/CBC/platelet counts.

Drug Interactions:
- None known.

Lab Effects/Interference:
- BUN, uric acid.
- LFTs, especially alk phos and AST (SGOT).
- CBC, especially WBC with differential.

Special Considerations:
- Warnings and Precautions:
  - *Drug is carcinogenic* so should not be administered to patients other than those with CLL or malignant lymphoma. Convulsions, infertility, leukemia, secondary malignancies have occurred.
  - *Skin rash:* rarely progressing to erythema multiforme, toxic epidermal necrolysis, or SJS have been reported. Discontinue chlorambucil in patients who develop a skin reaction (Aspen, 2016).
  - *Embryo-fetal toxicity:* Teach women of childbearing potential to use effective contraception to avoid pregnancy. Mothers should not breastfeed while receiving the drug; a decision should be made whether to discontinue nursing or to discontinue the drug, taking into account the importance of the drug to the mother.
  - *Lymphopenia and neutropenia:* Commonly, patients develop a slowly progressive lymphopenia during treatment that rapidly returns to normal levels after drug therapy is completed. After the third week of treatment most patients have neutropenia, which continues for up to 10 days after the last dose. When drug is discontinued, neutrophil count rapidly returns to normal. Severe neutropenia is dose related, occurring in patients who have received a total dosage of 6.5 mg/kg or continuous-dose schedule. Patients receiving a full course of RT should not receive chlorambucil at FULL dose before 4 weeks following RT completion. If the post-RT leukocyte or platelet counts are less than normal, dose should be reduced. Persistent, low neutrophil and platelet counts or peripheral lympocytosis suggest BM infiltration. If confirmed by BM biopsy, daily dosage of chlorambucil should not be >0.1 mg/kg.
  - Avoid administration of live vaccines to immunocompromised patients.

Potential Toxicities/Side Effects and the Nursing Process

I. POTENTIAL FOR INFECTION related to BM DEPRESSION

Defining Characteristics: Neutropenia after third week of treatment lasting for 10 days after the last dose. Neutropenia and thrombocytopenia occur with prolonged use and may be irreversible occasionally (especially if high total doses are given; i.e., >6.5 mg/kg). Increased toxicity may occur with prior barbiturate use.

Nursing Implications: Assess baseline CBC, including WBC with differential, and platelet count prior to dosing, as well as weekly for the first cycle of therapy. Discuss dose reduction with physician if blood values are abnormal. Teach patient self-assessment of signs/symptoms of infection and bleeding and instruct to report them immediately. Teach self-care measures to minimize risk of infection and bleeding, including avoidance of OTC aspirin-containing medications.

II.   POTENTIAL FOR SEXUAL DYSFUNCTION related to REPRODUCTIVE HAZARD

Defining Characteristics: Drug is mutagenic, teratogenic, and suppresses gonadal function with consequent temporary or permanent sterility. Amenorrhea occurs in females, and oligospermia/azoospermia occurs in males.

Nursing Implications: Assess patient's and partner's sexual patterns and reproductive goals. Provide teaching and emotional support; encourage birth control measures as appropriate.

III.   POTENTIAL FOR ALTERATION IN NUTRITION, LESS THAN BODY REQUIREMENTS, related to NAUSEA/VOMITING, ANOREXIA/WEIGHT LOSS, AND HEPATIC DYSFUNCTION

Defining Characteristics: Nausea and vomiting are rare. Anorexia and weight loss may occur and be prolonged. Hepatotoxicity with jaundice is rare, but abnormal LFTs may occur.

Nursing Implications: Administer antiemetics as needed and instruct patient in self-administration. Suggest weekly weights and dietary instruction if patient develops anorexia and weight loss. Monitor LFTs baseline and periodically during treatment. Discuss any abnormalities with physician and consider dose modification.

IV.   POTENTIAL FOR IMPAIRED GAS EXCHANGE related to PULMONARY FIBROSIS

Defining Characteristics: Bronchopulmonary dysplasia and pulmonary fibrosis may occur rarely with long-term use.

Nursing Implications: Assess patients at risk: increased risk with cumulative dose >1 g/m^2, preexisting lung disease, concurrent treatment with cyclophosphamide or thoracic radiation. Assess pulmonary status prior to chemotherapy and at each visit, notifying physician of dyspnea. Monitor PFTs periodically for evidence of pulmonary dysfunction. Teach patient to report any changes in pulmonary pattern, such as dyspnea.

V. POTENTIAL FOR SENSORY/PERCEPTUAL ALTERATIONS related to OCULAR DISTURBANCES, CNS ABNORMALITIES

Defining Characteristics: Ocular disturbances may occur (e.g., diplopia, papilledema, retinal hemorrhage). Tremors, muscular twitching, confusion, agitation, ataxia, flaccid paresis, and hallucinations have been described. Seizures, although uncommon, have occurred in adults and children during normal dosing, as well as with overdosing.

Nursing Implications: Assess baseline neurologic status prior to treatment and at each visit. Instruct patient to report any abnormalities.

Drug: cisplatin (Platinol)

Class: Heavy metal that acts like alkylating agent.

Mechanism of Action: Inhibits DNA synthesis by forming inter- and intrastrand cross-links and by denaturing the double helix, preventing cell replication. Cell cycle phase non-specific; the chemical properties are similar to those of bifunctional alkylating agents.

Metabolism: Rapidly distributed to tissues (predominately the liver and kidneys) with less than 10% in the plasma 1 hour after infusion. Clearance from plasma proceeds slowly after the first 2 hours due to platinum's covalent bonding with serum proteins; 20–74% of administered drug is excreted in the urine within 24 hours.

Indication: Indicated for the treatment of patients with:
- Metastatic testicular tumors, with other approved chemotherapy agents, after appropriate surgical and/or radiotherapeutic procedures.
- Metastatic ovarian tumors, with other approved chemotherapy agents, after appropriate surgical and/or radiotherapeutic procedures. An established combination is cisplatin plus cyclophosphamide. Cisplatin as a single-agent is indicated as secondary therapy in patients with metastatic ovarian tumors refractory to standard chemotherapy who have not previously received cisplatinum.
- Advanced bladder cancer (transitional cell), which is no longer amenable to local treatment (e.g., surgery and/or radiotherapy), as a single agent.

Contraindicated in patients with (1) preexisting renal impairment; also should not be used in (2) myelosuppression; (3) with a hearing impairment; (4) with a history of allergic reactions to cisplatin or other platinum-containing compounds.

Dosage/Range:
- Metastatic testicular cancer: 20 mg/m^2 × 5 days per cycle, with other approved chemotherapeutic drugs
- Metastatic ovarian tumors:
  - 75–100 mg/m^2 IV on day 1 in combination with cyclophosphamide 600 mg/m^2 IV on day 1, administered sequentially, with the cycle repeated every 4 weeks.
  - As a single agent, 100 mg/m^2 IV once per cycle, repeated every 4 weeks.

- Advanced bladder cancer: Cisplatin 50–70 mg/m² IV per cycle once every 3–4 weeks, depending upon the extent of prior RT exposure and/or prior chemotherapy. For heavily pretreated patients, initial dose should be 50 mg/m² IV per cycle repeated every 4 weeks.

Drug Preparation:
- Avoid aluminum needles when administering, as precipitate will form. Ensure adequate urinary output prior to administration.
- 50-mg and 100-mg vials with aqueous solution 1 mg/1 mL. Aseptically withdraw ordered dose (call MD if dose > 100 mg/m²/cycle).
- Further dilute solution with 250 mL or more of 5% dextrose (D₅ ½ NS) sodium chloride (see package insert for preparation with 5% dextrose 0% sodium chloride, and mannitol).
- Once vial is entered, the remaining drug is stable for 28 days protected from light, or 7 days under fluorescent room light.
- Do not refrigerate.

Drug Administration (Aspen, 2016):
- Avoid aluminum needles when administering, as precipitate will form. Ensure adequate urinary output prior to administration.
- Prior to initiating and before each dose:
  - Assess serum creatinine, and proceed if it is <1.5 mg/100 mL, BUN is <25 mg/100 mL and creatinine clearance;
  - Assess CBC weekly: WBC ≥4000/mm³; platelets ≥100,000/cells³; audiogram results should be WNL.
  - Assess serum magnesium, sodium, potassium, calcium, and replete as necessary.
  - Assess LFTs baseline and during therapy.
  - Assess and document neurologic exam, and document any signs/symptoms of PN.
- Pretreatment hydration with 1–2 L of IV fluid infused for 8–12 hours prior to cisplatin dose.
- Drug should be diluted in 2 L of 5%; Dextrose in ½ or 0; normal saline containing 37.5 g of mannitol, and infused over a 6- to 8-hour period.
- Urinary output should be at least 100 mL/hour.

Drug Interactions:
- Decreases pharmacologic effect of phenytoin, so dose may need to be increased.
- Possible increase in ototoxicity when combined with loop diuretics.
- Increased renal toxicity with concurrent use of aminoglycosides, amphotericin B.
- Cisplatin reduces drug clearance of high-dose methotrexate (MTX) and standard-dose bleomycin by increasing the drugs' half-life; enhances toxicity of ifosfamide (myelosuppression) and etoposide.
- Synergy when cisplatin is combined with etoposide.
- Radiosensitizing effect.
- Sodium thiosulfate and mesna: Each directly inactivates cisplatin.

- Taxanes: Administer cisplatin *after* taxanes (paclitaxel, docetaxel) to prevent delayed taxane excretion with subsequent increased BM depression.

Lab Effects/Interference:
- Decreased Mg, Ca, phos.
- Increased creatinine, uric acid.

Special Considerations:
- Warnings and Precautions:
  - *Cumulative nephrotoxicity*, potentiated by aminoglycoside antibiotics.
  - *Severe neuropathy* may occur, especially at higher or more frequent dosing. May be irreversible, and in stocking-glove distribution, with areflexia, loss of proprioception and vibratory sensation. Loss of motor function has been reported. Elderly patients may be more susceptible.
  - *Anaphylactic-like reaction* may occur manifested by wheezing, flushing, hypotension, tachycardia. Usually occurs within minutes of starting infusion, requiring epinephrine, corticosteroids, and antihistamines.
  - *Ototoxicity:* commonly occurs, is cumulative, and may be severe. Perform audiometry testing prior to starting therapy and prior to each subsequent dose of cisplatin (Aspen, 2016).
  - *Embryo-fetal toxicity:* teach women of reproductive potential to use effective contraception to avoid pregnancy during treatment.
  - *Carcinogenesis/mutagenesis*: acute leukemia as a secondary cancer has been reported, especially when cisplatin combined with other leukemogenic agents.
  - *Injection-site reactions*: closely monitor infusion site during administration to identify early extravasation.
- Administer cautiously, if at all, to patients with renal dysfunction, hearing impairment, PN, or prior allergic reaction to cisplatin.
- Hydrate vigorously before and after administering drug. Urine output should be at least 100–150 mL/hour. Mannitol or furosemide diuresis may be needed to ensure this output.
- Drug causes potassium and magnesium wasting. Add magnesium and potassium to hydration IV prior to and following cisplatin administration. Other ideas to help increase magnesium follow.
- To help increase absorption, it is recommended that excessive milk, cheese, or other high-calcium products be limited when eating foods high in magnesium. Calcium and magnesium compete to gain entrance to the body in the intestines, so a high-calcium diet increases requirements for dietary magnesium. Foods high in magnesium are those with 100 mg or greater per 100 grams, including:

Nuts: almonds, brazil nuts, cashews, peanut butter, peanuts, pecans, walnuts
Peas and beans: red beans, split peas, white beans
Other good sources: blackstrap molasses, brewer's yeast, chocolate (bitter), cocoa (dry breakfast), cornmeal, instant coffee and tea, oatmeal, shredded wheat, wheat germ, whole wheat breads, and cereals.

Potential Toxicities/Side Effects and the Nursing Process

I.   POTENTIAL ALTERATION IN URINARY ELIMINATION related to DRUG-INDUCED RENAL DAMAGE

Defining Characteristics: Dose-limiting toxicity, which may be cumulative. The drug accumulates in the kidneys, causing necrosis of proximal and distal renal tubules. Damage to renal tubules prevents reabsorption of magnesium, calcium, potassium, with resultant decreased serum levels. Renal damage becomes most obvious 10–20 days after treatment, is reversible, and can be prevented by adequate hydration and diuresis, as well as slower infusion time. Hyperuricemia may occur due to impaired tubular transport of uric acid, but it is responsive to allopurinol. Concurrent administration of nephrotoxic agents is not recommended.

Nursing Implications: Assess renal function studies prior to administration (BUN, creatinine, 24-hour creatinine clearance) and discuss any abnormalities with physician. Assess cardiac and pulmonary status in terms of tolerance of aggressive hydration. Anticipate vigorous hydration regimen with or without forced diuresis (i.e., mannitol, lasix). The typical hydration schedule is 0.9% sodium chloride or D_5 ½ NS at 250 mL/hour × 3–5 hours prechemotherapy and 3–5 hours postchemotherapy (total hydration 3 L). Outpatient hydration of 1–2 L over 1–2 hours prechemotherapy and 1 L postchemotherapy is typical. Strictly monitor I/O and total body fluid balance. Assess for signs/symptoms of fluid overload and notify physician for supplemental furosemide or other diuretic as needed. Monitor serum electrolytes (sodium, potassium, magnesium, calcium, PO_4) and replete electrolytes as ordered by physician. Teach patient and family the need for increased oral fluids on discharge—up to 3 L or more for 5 days, posttherapy.

II.   ALTERATION IN NUTRITION, LESS THAN BODY REQUIREMENTS, related to SEVERE NAUSEA AND VOMITING, TASTE ALTERATIONS

Defining Characteristics: Nausea and vomiting may be severe and will occur in 100% of patients if antiemetics are not given. They begin 1 or more hours postchemotherapy and last 8–24 hours. Since the drug is slowly excreted over 5 days, delayed nausea and vomiting may occur 24–72 hours after dose. Taste alterations and anorexia occur with long-term use.

Nursing Implications: Premedicate with combination antiemetics (i.e., serotonin antagonist, NK1 antagonist, plus dexamethasone), especially for high-dose cisplatin, and continue antiemetics for delayed nausea and vomiting, for up to 5 days, with dopamine antagonist as needed (may use effective combination antiemesis with delayed nausea/vomiting coverage). Encourage small, frequent intake of cool, bland foods as tolerated. Infuse cisplatin over at least 1 hour to minimize emesis, since slower infusion rates decrease emesis. Taste alterations may be improved with the use of spices and zinc dietary supplementation. Refer the patient for dietary consultation as needed.

III. POTENTIAL FOR INJURY related to ANAPHYLAXIS

Defining Characteristics: Anaphylaxis has occurred, characterized by wheezing, bronchoconstriction, tachycardia, hypotension, and facial edema, in patients who have previously received the drug.

Nursing Implications: Assess baseline VS and continue to assess patient during infusion. Prior to drug administration, review standing orders or protocols for nursing management of anaphylaxis: stop infusion; keep line open with 0.9% sodium chloride; notify physician; monitor VS; be prepared to administer epinephrine, antihistamines, corticosteroids.

IV. POTENTIAL FOR SENSORY/PERCEPTUAL ALTERATIONS related to NEUROLOGIC TOXICITY

Defining Characteristics: Severe neuropathy may occur in patients receiving high doses or prolonged treatment and may be irreversible, and is seen in stocking-and-glove distribution, with numbness, tingling, and sensory loss in arms and legs. Areflexia, loss of proprioception and vibratory sense, and loss of motor function can occur. Ototoxicity, beginning with loss of high-frequency hearing, affects >30% of patients. It may be preceded by tinnitus, is dose related, and can be unilateral or bilateral. The damage results from destruction of hair cells lining the organ of Corti and is cumulative and may be permanent. Rarely, ocular toxicity has occurred, but it is reversible (optic neuritis, papilledema, cerebral blindness).

Nursing Implications: Assess baseline neurologic, motor, and sensory functions prior to drug administration. Discuss use of neuroprotector in high-risk patients. Discuss baseline audiogram with physician as appropriate. Instruct patient to report changes in function or sensation, as well as diminished hearing. Discuss with physician risks versus benefits of continuing therapy if/when symptoms develop. If severe neuropathies develop, provide teaching related to activity, emotional support, and referral to physical/occupational therapy as appropriate. Discuss use of neuroprotector in high-risk patients.

V. POTENTIAL FOR ACTIVITY INTOLERANCE related to ANEMIA

Defining Characteristics: Drug may interfere with renal erythropoietin production, resulting in late development of anemia.

Nursing Implications: Teach patient to report increasing fatigue, signs of severe anemia (shortness of breath, chest pain/angina, headaches). Monitor hemoglobin/hematocrit; discuss transfusion with physician if signs/symptoms develop or hematocrit falls <25 mg/dL or symptoms (e.g., angina). Teach patient about diet high in iron. Exogenous erythropoietin (epoetin alpha) may be helpful if treatment goal is palliation.

VI.   INFECTION AND BLEEDING related to BM DEPRESSION

Defining Characteristics: BM depression is mild with low to moderate doses, but may be significant when high doses are used, or when drug is given in combination with radiation as a radiation-sensitizer. Nadir is in 2–3 weeks, with recovery in 4–5 weeks.

Nursing Implications: Assess CBC, WBC, differential, and platelet count, as well as any signs/symptoms of infection or bleeding, prior to drug administration. Teach patient to self-assess for signs/symptoms of infection and bleeding. Teach self-care measures to minimize infection and bleeding, including avoidance of aspirin-containing medications.

VII.   POTENTIAL SEXUAL DYSFUNCTION related to DRUG EFFECTS

Defining Characteristics: Drug is mutagenic and probably teratogenic.

Nursing Implications: Assess patient's and partner's sexual patterns and reproductive goals. Provide emotional support and discuss strategies to preserve sexual and reproductive health (i.e., contraception and sperm banking).

VIII.   POTENTIAL FOR ALTERATIONS IN CARDIOVASCULAR FUNCTION related to CISPLATIN-CONTAINING COMBINATION CHEMOTHERAPY

Defining Characteristics: Angina, myocardial infarction, cerebrovascular accident, thrombotic microangiopathy, cerebral arteritis, and Raynaud's phenomenon have occurred, although they are uncommon. Combination drugs include bleomycin, vinblastine, vincristine, and etoposide.

Nursing Implications: Assess cardiopulmonary status, especially if patient has preexisting cardiac disease, both prior to and throughout treatment.

Drug: cladribine (Leustatin, 2-CdA)

Class: Nucleoside metabolic inhibitor (Antimetabolite).

Mechanism of Action: Selectively damages normal and malignant lymphocytes and monocytes that have large amounts of deoxycytidine kinase but small amounts of deoxynucleotidase. The drug, a chlorinated purine nucleoside, enters passively through the cell membrane, is phosphorylated into the active metabolite 2-CdATP, and accumulates in the cell. 2-CdATP interferes with DNA synthesis and prevents repair of DNA strand breaks in both actively dividing and normal cells. The process may also involve programmed cell death (apoptosis).

Metabolism: Drug is 20% protein-bound and is cleared from the plasma within 1–3 days after cessation of treatment.

Indication: Treatment of hairy-cell leukemia (as defined by clinically significant anemia, neutropenia, thrombocytopenia, or disease-related symptoms).

Contraindications: Patients who are hypersensitive to the drug or any of its components.

Dosage/Range:
- 0.09 mg/kg/day IV as a CI for 7 days for one course of therapy of hairy-cell leukemia.

Drug Preparation:
- Available in 10 mg/10 mL preservative-free, single-use vials (1 mg/mL), which must be further diluted in 0.9% sodium chloride injection. Once prepared, the drug should be administered promptly, or if not possible, the solution may be refrigerated up to 8 hours prior to use.
- Single daily dose: add calculated drug dose to infusion bag using a sterile 0.22-µm hydrophilic syringe filter. Infusion bag: 500 mL of 0.9% sodium chloride injection, and administer over 24 hours; repeat daily for a total of 7 days.
- Seven-day CI by ambulatory infusion pump: add calculated drug dose for 7 days to infusion reservoir using a sterile 0.22-µm hydrophilic syringe filter. Then add, again using 0.22-µm filter, sufficient sterile bacteriostatic 0.9% sodium chloride injection containing 0.9% benzyl alcohol to produce 100 mL in the infusion reservoir.
- Do not use 5% dextrose, as it accelerates degradation of drug.
- Inspect parenteral dose for particulate matter and discoloration. A precipitate may occur at low temperatures, and require resolubilization by allowing the solution to warm naturally at room temperature and by vigorously shaking. DO NOT HEAT or MICROWAVE.

Drug Administration:
- Assess ANC, CBC/platelets, LFTs, and renal function tests baseline and periodically.
- Dilute in minimum of 100 mL. DO NOT use 5% dextrose, as unstable.
- Administer as CI over 24 hours for 7 days.

Drug Interactions:
- BM-suppressing drugs: increased BM suppression.
- Live attenuated vaccines: increased risk of infection; do not administer when receiving leustatin.

Lab Effects/Interference:
- Decreased CBC, platelets.
- Increased LFTs, RFTs.

Special Considerations:
- Warnings and Precautions:
  - *Immunosuppression*: do not administer live attenuated vaccines while patient is receiving the drug.
  - *Severe BM suppression*: occurs commonly. Mean counts normalized by day 12 (platelets), week 5 (neutrophil count), and week 8 (hemoglobin). Fever $\geq$ 100°F was associated with 2/3 of patients in first month of therapy, and 47% had neutropenic fever with 32% having severe neutropenia. Patients should have ANC/CBC/platelets assessed frequently during the first 4–8 weeks, posttreatment, and meticulous patient

teaching to report signs/symptoms of infection or bleeding. After CBC recovery, BM aspiration and biopsy should be performed to confirm response to cladribine.

- *Serious infections* may occur (e.g., respiratory, pneumonia, and viral skin infections).
- *Embryo-fetal toxicity*: teach women of reproductive potential to use effective contraception to prevent pregnancy during treatment.
- *When high doses used, renal dysfunction*, and neurological impairment occurred in some patients.
- *Rare cases of TLS* have occurred in patients with high tumor burden. Discuss TLS prophylaxis with provider for patients with high-tumor burden during first treatment.
- Administer with caution in patients with renal or hepatic insufficiency.
- Embryotoxic; women of childbearing age should use effective contraception to avoid pregnancy.
- May cause impairment of fertility in men.

Potential Toxicities/Side Effects and the Nursing Process

I.   INFECTION AND BLEEDING related to BM DEPRESSION

Defining Characteristics: Neutropenia occurs in 70% of patients with nadir 1–2 weeks after infusion, recovery by weeks 4–5. Incidence of infection 28%, with 40% caused by bacterial infection of lungs and venous access sites. Prolonged hypocellularity of BM occurs in 34% of patients, and may last for at least 4 months. Infections most common in patients with pancytopenia and lymphopenia due to hairy-cell leukemia. Lymphopenia is common with decreased CD4 (helper T cells) and CD8 (suppressor T cells), with recovery by weeks 26–34. Common infectious agents are viral (20%) and fungal (20%). Thrombocytopenia occurs commonly, along with purpura (10%), petechiae (8%), and epistaxis (5%). Platelet recovery occurs by day 12, but 14% of patients require platelet support.

Nursing Implications: Monitor CBC, platelet count prior to therapy, and periodically post-therapy at expected time of nadir. Monitor for, and teach patient self-assessment of signs/symptoms of infection and bleeding. Instruct patient to call physician or nurse or go to emergency room if temperature is greater than 101°F (38.3°C) or bleeding. Transfuse platelets per physician order. DO NOT give live attenuated vaccines to patients receiving leustatin due to increased risk of infection in the setting of immunosuppression (FDA, 2012).

II.   ALTERATION IN COMFORT related to FEVER, HEADACHES

Defining Characteristics: Fever (>100°F [37.5°C]) occurs in 66% of patients during the month following treatment due either to infection (47%) or the release of endogenous pyrogen from lysed lymphocytes. Other symptoms include chills (9%), diaphoresis (9%), malaise (7%), dizziness (9%), insomnia (7%), myalgia (7%), and arthralgias (5%). Headaches occur in 22% of patients.

Nursing Implications: Assess patient for fever, chills, diaphoresis during visits; assess signs/symptoms of infection. Teach patient self-assessment, how to report this, and measures to reduce fever. Anticipate laboratory and x-ray tests to rule out infection and perform according to physician order.

III. POTENTIAL IMPAIRMENT OF SKIN INTEGRITY related to RASH

Defining Characteristics: Rash occurs in 27–50% of patients. Other symptoms include pruritus (6%), erythema (6%), injection-site reactions (erythema, swelling, pain, phlebitis).

Nursing Implications: Assess skin for any cutaneous changes, such as rash or changes at injection site, and any associated symptoms such as pruritus; discuss with physician. Instruct patient in self-care measures, including avoiding abrasive skin products and clothing; avoiding tight-fitting clothing; use of skin emollients appropriate to specific skin alteration; measures to avoid scratching involved areas. Consider venous access device if skin is at risk for reaction.

IV. FATIGUE related to ANEMIA

Defining Characteristics: Fatigue occurs in 45% of patients. Red cell recovery is by week 8, but 40% of patients require red cell transfusion.

Nursing Implications: Monitor Hgb and HCT and transfuse per physician order. Administer erythropoietin per physician order and teach patient self-administration. Teach patient about diet and instruct to alternate rest and activity; stress reduction/relaxation techniques may improve energy level.

V. ALTERATION IN ELIMINATION related to DIARRHEA, CONSTIPATION

Defining Characteristics: Diarrhea occurs in 10% of patients, while constipation occurs in 9%. Abdominal pain affects 6% of patients.

Nursing Implications: Encourage patient to report onset of change in bowel habits (diarrhea or constipation), and assess factors contributing to changes. Administer or teach patient self-administration of antidiarrheal medication or cathartic as ordered. Teach patient diet modification regarding foods that minimize diarrhea or constipation.

VI. POTENTIAL FOR IMPAIRED GAS EXCHANGE related to COUGH

Defining Characteristics: Cough affects 10%, while abnormal breath sounds occur in 11%, and shortness of breath in 7%.

Nursing Implications: Assess baseline pulmonary status, including breath sounds, presence of cough, shortness of breath. Instruct patient to report symptoms of cough, shortness of breath, other abnormalities.

VII. ALTERATION IN NUTRITION, LESS THAN BODY REQUIREMENTS, related to NAUSEA, VOMITING

Defining Characteristics: Nausea is mild and occurs in 28% of patients, while vomiting may occur in 13%. If antiemetics are required, nausea/vomiting is easily controlled by phenothiazines. Renal and hepatic function studies are rarely affected.

Nursing Implications: Premedicate with antiemetics. If nausea and/or vomiting occur, teach patient to self-administer antiemetics per physician order. Encourage small, frequent feedings of cool, bland foods and liquids. Teach patient to record diet history for 2–3 days and weekly weights. If patient has decreased appetite, assess food preferences (encourage or discourage) and suggest use of spices.

VIII. POTENTIAL ALTERATION IN CARDIAC OUTPUT related to TACHYCARDIA

Defining Characteristics: Occurs rarely, with edema and tachycardia each affecting 6% of patients.

Nursing Implications: Assess baseline cardiac status, including apical heart rate, presence of peripheral edema. Instruct patient to report rapid heartbeat or swelling of ankles.

Drug: clofarabine (Clolar)

Class: Nucleoside metabolic inhibitor; purine nucleoside antimetabolite.

Mechanism of Action: Drug inhibits DNA and DNA repair, causing cell death of both cycling and quiescent cancer cells. In addition, it breaks down the mitochondrial membranes, releasing cytochrome C and apoptosis-inducing factor, leading to programmed cell death.

Metabolism: Drug is 47% protein-bound (mostly to albumin), with a terminal half-life of 5.2 hours. 49–60% of the dose is excreted unchanged in the urine. Other nonrenal excretion is unknown.

Indication: For the treatment of pediatric patients 1–21 years old with relapsed or refractory acute lymphoblastic leukemia after at least 2 prior regimens. Indication is based on response rate.

Dosage/Range: 52 mg/m^2 IV over 2 h daily × 5, to be repeated after recovery of all baseline organ function, about q 2–6 weeks. IV hydration should be continued during the 5 days of treatment.

- Patient should receive IV hydration thoughout the 5 days of treatment to prevent TLS. For first cycle, discuss with physician need for allopurinol if hyperuricemia is likely.
- Renal and hepatic function studies should be monitored during the 5 days of drug treatment.

Drug Preparation: Drug is supplied as a 20 mg in 20-mL vial. Withdraw drug using a sterile 0.2-μm syringe filter and then further dilute with 5% dextrose injection USP or 0.9% sodium chloride injection USP prior to IV infusion. This admixture may be stored at room temperature but must be used within 24 hours of preparation.

Drug Administration: Administer IV over 2 hours; if hyperuricemia (TLS), patient should receive allopurinol, and may need urine alkalinization and aggressive hydration as well.

Drug Interactions: Concurrent administration with other renally cleared drugs may alter drug levels so should be avoided during the 5 days of treatment; avoid other hepatotoxic drugs, as well as those affecting blood pressure or cardiac function if possible during drug administration.

Lab Effects/Interference:
Drug may cause
• Severe BM depression with decreased white blood cells, neutrophils, red blood cells, and platelets.
• TLS with increased levels of potassium, phosphate, uric acid, creatinine, and changes in other electrolyte values.
• Increased hepato-biliary enzyme serum levels.

Special Considerations:
• Warnings and Precautions:
   • *Myelosuppression:* may be severe and prolonged. Monitor ANC/CBC/platelets baseline and during therapy.
   • *Hemorrhage:* may be serious and include cerebral (which may be fatal), GI, pulmonary hemorrhage. Monitor platelet count and coagulation parameters and manage per physician/PA/NP.
   • *Infections*: may be severe and include sepsis due to BM suppression. Monitor for signs/symptoms of infection, interrupt drug, and manage infections per physician/NP/PA promptly.
   • *TLS:* Treatment results in the rapid lysis of peripheral leukemia cells, increasing the risk of TLS. Discuss TLS prophylaxis with physician or NP/PA to prevent TLS.
   • *Systemic inflammatory response syndrome* (SIRS) or capillary leak syndrome may occur. Monitor and discontinue drug immediately if suspected.
   • *Venous occlusive disease of the liver*: monitor for this and discontinue drug if suspected.
   • *Hepatotoxicity:* may be severe and fatal. Monitor LFTs, as well as for signs/symptoms of hepatitis and hepatic failure. Discontinue clofarabine immediately for grade 3 or greater liver enzyme and/or bilirubin elevations.
   • *Renal toxicity:* may result in increased serum creatinine and acute renal failure. Monitor renal function and interrupt or discontinue clofarabine.
   • *Entercolitis:* may be serious and fatal, often occurring within 30 days of treatment and with combination chemotherapy. Monitor patients for signs and symptoms and treat promptly.
   • *Skin reactions*: SJS and TEN have occurred and may be fatal. Discontinue clofarabine for exfoliative or bullous rash, or if SJS or TEN is suspected.

- *Embryo-fetal toxicity:* Drug is fetotoxic, so all patients (male and female) should be taught to use effective contraceptive measures to prevent pregnancy; female patients should be cautioned not to breastfeed during treatment.
- Patients who have previously received a hematopoietic stem cell transplant may be at higher risk for hepatotoxicity.

Potential Toxicities/Side Effects and the Nursing Process

I.   INFECTION AND BLEEDING related to BM DEPRESSION

Defining Characteristics: BM depression is dose limiting. Febrile neutropenia occurs in some patients. Pyrexia affects some patients, others experience rigors. Infections include bacteremia, cellulitis, herpes simplex, oral candidiasis, pneumonia, sepsis, and staphylococcal infections.

Nursing Implications: Assess WBC, neutrophil, and platelet count, and discuss any abnormalities with physician prior to drug administration; assess for signs/symptoms of skin infections (all mucosal surfaces, body orifices) and bleeding; instruct patient in signs/symptoms of infection and bleeding, as well as to report them or come to emergency room. Teach patient self-care measures to minimize risk of infection and bleeding, including avoidance of OTC aspirin-containing medications. Assess patient's Hgb/HCT and signs/symptoms of fatigue; teach patient self-assessment and to alternate rest and activity as needed.

II.   ALTERED NUTRITION, LESS THAN BODY REQUIREMENTS, related to NAUSEA AND VOMITING, ANOREXIA, DIARRHEA, AND HEPATOTOXICITY

Defining Characteristics: Nausea and vomiting occur in some patients, and can be successfully prevented with combination antiemetics. Anorexia can occur. Diarrhea is frequent, affecting some patients. Constipation affects some patients. Hepatotoxicity and jaundice occur in some patients.

Nursing Implications: Premedicate with antiemetics depending on dose, using aggressive, combination antiemetics, and continue throughout chemotherapy. If patient develops nausea/vomiting, assess fluid and electrolyte balance and the need for replacements. Assess oral mucosa prior to chemotherapy and teach patient oral hygiene regimen and self-assessment; encourage patient to report diarrhea, discuss use of antidiarrheals with physician, and teach self-care PRN. Because patients become neutropenic, all mucosal surfaces need to be assessed for infection, and patients must be taught scrupulous perineal hygiene. Monitor LFTs prior to, during, and following therapy.

III.   IMPAIRED SKIN/MUCOSAL INTEGRITY related to RASH, ANAL INFLAMMATION/ULCERATION, ALOPECIA

Defining Characteristics: Maculopapular rash, with or without fever, myalgia, bone pain, occasional chest pain, conjunctivitis, and malaise (cytarabine syndrome) may occur.

Syndrome is not common, but occurs 6–12 hours after drug administration; corticosteroids have been helpful in treating/preventing syndrome. Mucosal inflammation and ulceration of anus/rectum may occur, especially in patients with prior hemorrhoids or history of abscesses. Alopecia occurs less frequently.

Nursing Implications: Assess baseline skin and mucous membranes prior to chemotherapy and identify patients at risk for problems. Consider including corticosteroid in antiemetic regimen, especially for high-dose therapy, and discuss with physician prophylactic use of dexamethasone eye drops to prevent conjunctivitis. Teach patient scrupulous perineal hygiene, instruct to report any rectal discomfort, and assess rectal mucosa daily with high-dose therapy. Discuss with patient potential coping strategies if alopecia occurs (i.e., wig, scarves).

IV.   ALTERATION IN COMFORT, POTENTIAL, related to EDEMA, FATIGUE, LETHARGY, PAIN

Defining Characteristics: In clinical studies, frequently occurring symptoms were: edema, fatigue, injection-site pain, pain, arthralgia, back pain, myalgia, pain in limb, dermatitis, erythema, pruritus, palmar plantar erythrodysesthesia syndrome (PPE), and flushing.

Nursing Implications: Teach patient that these symptoms may occur and to report them. Teach patient self-care measures to reduce discomfort, such as application of heat or cold for pain, arthralgias, and myalgias. Teach patient to report redness and pain on palms of hands or soles of feet as this may be PPE, and would require close monitoring and follow-up to prevent moist desquamation. Instruct patient to report any symptoms that do not resolve or improve with self-care measures.

Drug: cyclophosphamide (Cytoxan)

Class: Alkylating agent.

Mechanism of Action: Causes cross-linkage in DNA strands, thus preventing DNA synthesis and cell division. Cell cycle phase nonspecific.

Metabolism: Inactive until converted by microsomes in liver and serum enzymes (phosphamidases). Both cyclophosphamide and its metabolites are excreted by the kidneys. Plasma half-life: 6–12 hours, with 25% of drug excreted after 8 hours. Prolonged plasma half-life in patients with renal failure results in increased myelosuppression.

Indications (initial): For the treatment of patients with the following, as a single agent, or in combination with other chemotherapy: (1) malignant lymphomas, including Hodgkin's disease; (2) multiple myeloma; (3) leukemias; (4) mycosis fungoides; (5) neuroblastoma; (7) adeno-carcinoma of the ovary; (8) retinoblastoma; (9) breast cancer.

Contraindications: patients with (1) hypersensitivity to cyclophosphamide; (2) urinary outflow obstruction.

Dosage/Range:
- IV: Initial course for patients with no hematologic deficiency: 40–50 mg/kg in divided doses over 2–5 days. Other regimens include 10–15 mg/kg every 7–10 days or 3–5 mg/kg twice weekly.
- Oral: usually 1–5 mg/kg/day for both initial and maintenance dosing.

Drug Preparation:
- Available in 25- and 50-mg tablets; lyophilized powder for injection: 500-mg, 1-g, and 2-g vials.
- IV Push (direct IV injection): Dilute vials with 0.9% sodium chloride injection USP only—25 mL for 500-mg vial, 50 mL for 1 g vial, and 100 mL for 2 g; all solutions will be 20 mg/mL. (2013). Gently swirl the vial to dissolve the drug completely. Do not use sterile water for injection as it results in a hypotonic solution.
- IV infusion: reconstitute with 0.9% sodium chloride injection USP or use sterile water for injection: 500-mg vial (25 mL), 1-g vial (50 mL), and 2-g vial (100 mL) resulting in a concentration of 20 mg cyclophosphamide per mL. Further dilute to a minimum concentration of 2 mg/mL using 5% dextrose injection USP, 5% dextrose and 0.9% sodium chloride injection USP, or 0.45% sodium chloride injection USP.
- Reconstituted solution: (1) using 0.9% sodium chloride injection USP is stable for 24 hours at room temperature, 6 days if refrigerated. (2) If reconstituted with sterile water for injection USP, do not store but use immediately.
- Diluted Solutions: (1) Using 0.45% sodium chloride injection USP—stable at room temperature up to 24 hours, and refrigerated, up to 6 days; (2) using 5% dextrose injection USP, or 5% dextrose and 0.9% sodium chloride injection USP: at room temperature, up to 24 hours; refrigerated, up to 36 hours.
- Reconstituted solution for oral administration: Dissolve cyclophosphamide for injection in Aromatic Elixir, National Formulary (NF). Such preparations should be stored under refrigeration in glass containers and used within 14 days.

Drug Administration:
- Oral use: Administer in morning or early afternoon to allow adequate excretion time. Should be taken with meals.
- IV use: for doses > 500 mg, pre- and posthydration to total 500–3,000 mL is needed to ensure adequate urine output and to avoid hemorrhagic cystitis. Administer drug over at least 20 minutes for doses >500 mg.
- Test urine for occult blood.
- High-dose cyclophosphamide therapy may require catheterization and constant bladder irrigation. Mesna should be given, either as a CI or in bolus doses, around drug administration.
- Rapid infusion may result in dizziness, nasal stuffiness, rhinorrhea, sinus congestion during or soon after infusion.

Drug Interactions:
- Increases chloramphenicol half-life.
- Increases duration of leukopenia when given with thiazide diuretics.
- Increases effect of anticoagulant drugs.

- Decreases digoxin level, so dose may need to be increased.
- Potentiation of doxorubicin-induced cardiomyopathy.
- Increased succinylcholine action with prolonged neuromuscular blockage.
- Increased drug action of barbiturates; induction of hepatic microsomes.

Lab Effects/Interference:
- Increased K, uric acid secondary to tumor lysis.
- Monitor electrolytes for symptoms of SIADH.
- Decreased CBC, platelets.

Special Considerations:
- Warnings and Precautions:
  - *Myelosuppression, immunosuppression, BM failure, and infections* can result from cyclophosphamide usage. Infection may occur, including sepsis and septic shock, while latent infections can be reactivated. Monitor CBC and adjust dose as needed. Do not administer unless ANC > 1,500/mm³, platelet count > 50,000/mm³. G-CSF may be administered for primary or secondary prophylaxis depending upon patient risk. Nadir for neutrophil and platelet counts is between weeks 1 and 2, with recovery by day 20.
  - *Urinary tract and renal toxicity,* including hemorrhagic cystitis, pyelitis, ureteritis, and hematuria may occur. Discontinue drug if severe hemorrhagic cystitis occurs. Other urotoxicity may require drug interruption. Before starting therapy, ensure patient does not have any urinary tract obstruction (contraindication). Monitor urinary function. Drug should be used cautiously if at all in patients with UTIs. Aggressive hydration with forced diuresis and frequent bladder emptying can reduce frequency and severity of bladder toxicity. Mesna can also prevent severe bladder toxicity.
  - *Cardiotoxicity:* risk increased with high dose. Monitor patients closely with cardiac risk factors or preexisting cardiac disease.
  - *Pulmonary toxicity:* pneumonitis, pulmonary fibrosis, and pulmonary veno-occlusive disease have been described. Late onset pneumonitis (>6 months after start of cyclophosphamide) is associated with increased mortality, and this may happen years after treatment. Monitor patients for pulmonary toxicity.
  - *Secondary malignancies:* have occurred, including MDS, leukemia, bladder cancer, lymphomas, and sarcomas.
  - *Veno-occlusive disease liver disease:* patients receiving cytoreductive regimen, including cycleophosphamide in preparation for BM transplant together with whole-body RT, busulfan, and other agents, is a major risk factor. Other risk factors include hepatitis dysfunction, prior RT to the abdomen, poor performance status, and long-term, low-dose immunosuppressive doses of cyclophosphamide.
  - *Embryo-fetal toxicity:* Teach women of reproductive potential to use highly effective contraception to avoid pregnancy during treatment, and for up to 1 year after completion of therapy.
  - *Infertility:* Cyclophosphamide interferes with oogenesis and spermatogenesis, and development of sterility appears related to drug dose, duration of therapy, and state of gonadal function at the time of treatment. Teach patients about potential risks.
  - *Impairment of wound healing:* may occur.

- *Hyponatremia:* related to increased total body water, acute water intoxication, and a SIADH-like (syndrome of inappropriate secretion of anti-diuretic hormone) syndrome may occur.
- Monitor patients with hepatic dysfunction closely for toxicity.

Potential Toxicities/Side Effects and the Nursing Process

I.   INFECTION AND BLEEDING related to BM DEPRESSION

Defining Characteristics: Leukopenia nadir occurs days 7–14, with recovery in 1–2 weeks; thrombocytopenia is less frequent and anemia is mild. Drug is a potent immunosuppressant.

Nursing Implications: Assess CBC, WBC with differential, platelet count, and signs/symptoms of infection and bleeding prior to treatment. Teach patient signs/symptoms of infection and instruct to report them if they occur. Teach patient self-care measures to minimize infection and bleeding. Increased risk of BM depression in patients with prior radiation or chemotherapy.

II.   ALTERED URINARY ELIMINATION related to HEMORRHAGIC CYSTITIS

Defining Characteristics: Metabolites of drug, if allowed to accumulate in the bladder, irritate bladder wall capillaries, causing hemorrhagic cystitis. This occurs in 7–40% of patients, is evidenced by microscopic or gross hematuria, is common with high doses, and is preventable. Long-term drug exposure may lead to bladder fibrosis.

Nursing Implications: Monitor BUN and creatinine prior to drug dose and as drug is excreted by the kidneys. Assess for signs/symptoms of hematuria, urinary frequency, or dysuria; instruct patient to report these if they occur. Instruct patient to take in at least 3 L of fluid per day and to empty bladder every 2–3 hours, as well as at bedtime. If patient is receiving a high dose, ensure vigorous hydration prior to drug administration. Bladder irrigation per protocol. Instruct patient to take oral cyclophosphamide early in the day to prevent drug accumulation in bladder during the night.

III.   ALTERATION IN NUTRITION, LESS THAN BODY REQUIREMENTS, related to NAUSEA AND VOMITING, ANOREXIA, STOMATITIS, DIARRHEA, AND HEPATOTOXICITY

Defining Characteristics: Nausea and vomiting are dose related and begin 2–4 hours after dose, peak in 12 hours, and may last 24 hours. Anorexia is common; stomatitis, if it occurs, is mild; and diarrhea is mild and infrequent. Hepatotoxicity is rare.

Nursing Implications: Premedicate with antiemetics prior to drug administration and continue prophylactically for 24 hours, at least for the first cycle. Encourage small feedings of bland foods and liquids. Encourage favorite foods and consult dietitian regarding anorexia if needed. Assess oral mucosa prior to drug administration; teach patient self-assessment techniques and oral care. Monitor LFTs before, during, and after therapy.

IV. ALTERED BODY IMAGE related to ALOPECIA, CHANGES IN NAILS AND SKIN

Defining Characteristics: Alopecia occurs in 30–50% of patients, especially with IV dosing, but some degree of hair loss occurs in all patients. Hair loss begins after 3+ weeks; hair may grow back while on therapy, but will grow back after therapy is discontinued (may be softer in texture). Hyperpigmentation of nails and skin, as well as transverse ridging of nails (banding), may occur.

Nursing Implications: Teach patient about potential hair loss and other changes. Discuss impact of hair loss on patient and strategies to minimize it (i.e., wig, scarf, cap) prior to drug administration. Assess ongoing coping during treatment. If nail changes are distressing, discuss the use of nail polish or other measures.

V. POTENTIAL SEXUAL DYSFUNCTION related to DRUG EFFECTS

Defining Characteristics: Drug is mutagenic and teratogenic. Amenorrhea often occurs in females, and testicular atrophy, possibly with reversible oligospermia/azoospermia, occurs in males. Drug is excreted in breastmilk.

Nursing Implications: Assess patient's/partner's sexual patterns and reproductive goals. Discuss strategies to preserve sexual and reproductive health, including contraception and sperm banking, as appropriate. Mothers receiving cyclophosphamide should not breastfeed.

VI. POTENTIAL FOR INJURY related to ACUTE WATER INTOXICATION (SIADH) AND SECOND MALIGNANCY

Defining Characteristics: SIADH may occur with high-dose administration (>50 mg/kg). Prolonged therapy may cause bladder cancer and acute leukemia.

Nursing Implications: Assess patients receiving high-dose cyclophosphamide: monitor serum Na+, osmolality, and urine osmolality and electrolytes; strictly monitor I/O, total body fluid balance, and daily weight. Screen patients who are receiving prolonged cyclophosphamide therapy for secondary malignancies.

VII. ALTERATION IN CARDIAC OUTPUT related to HIGH-DOSE CYCLOPHOSPHAMIDE

Defining Characteristics: Cardiomyopathy may occur with high doses as well as hemorrhagic cardiac necrosis, transmural hemorrhage, and coronary artery vasculitis at doses of

120–240 mg/kg. The mechanism is endothelial injury with subsequent hemorrhagic necrosis. The incidence is 22%, with 11% mortality, which may be decreased by dividing the dose into two split daily infusions. The risk at standard doses is increased by coadministration of doxorubicin (Adriamycin).

Nursing Implications: Assess cardiac status, especially if patient is receiving a high dose. Discuss baseline cardiac function test (GBPS) and assess for signs/symptoms of cardiomyopathy as treatment continues. Instruct patient to report dyspnea, shortness of breath, or other changes.

VIII. POTENTIAL FOR IMPAIRED GAS EXCHANGE related to PULMONARY TOXICITY

Defining Characteristics: Rare, but may occur with prolonged, high-dose therapy or continuous, low-dose therapy. Onset is insidious and appears as interstitial pneumonitis, which may progress to fibrosis. May respond to steroids.

Nursing Implications: Assess patients receiving high-dose or continuous low-dose cyclophosphamide for signs/symptoms of pulmonary dysfunction. Discuss pulmonary function studies with physician. Assess lung sounds prior to drug administration and periodically during treatment. Teach patient to report dyspnea, cough, or any abnormalities.

Drug: cytarabine, cytosine arabinoside (ara-C, Cytosar-U)

Class: Nucleoside metabolic inhibitor (Antimetabolite).

Mechanism of Action: Incorporated into DNA, slowing its synthesis and causing defects in the linkages to new DNA fragments. Also, cells exposed to cytarabine in the S phase reinitiate DNA synthesis when the drug, a pyrimidine analogue, is removed, resulting in erroneous duplication of the early portions of the DNA strands. Most effective when cells are undergoing rapid DNA synthesis.

Metabolism: Inactivated by liver enzymes in biphasic manner: half-lives 10–15 minutes and 2–3 hours. Crosses the BBB with cerebrospinal fluid concentration of 50% that of plasma; 70% of dose excreted in urine as ara-U; 4–10% excreted 12–24 hours after administration.

Indication:
- In combination with other approved anticancer drugs for remission induction in acute nonlymphocytic leukemia of adults and pediatric patients.
- Treatment of patients with acute lymphochytic or chronic myelocytic leukemia in blast phase.
- Meningeal leukemia prophylaxis and treatment by IT administration.
- **Contraindication:** hypersensitivity to the drug.

Dosage/Range:
- Varies depending on disease.
- Leukemia: 100 mg/m^2/day IV CI × 7 days OR 100 mg/m^2 IV every 12 hours (days 1–7).
- Intrathecal: 5–75 mg/m^2 every 2–7 days until CSF is clear (must use preservative-free diluent).

Drug Preparation:
- 100-mg vials: add water with benzyl alcohol, then dilute with 0.9% sodium chloride or 5% dextrose.
- 500-mg vials: add water with benzyl alcohol, then dilute with 0.9% sodium chloride or 5% dextrose.
- For intrathecal use and high dose: use preservative-free diluent.
- Reconstituted drug is stable 48 hours at room temperature and 7 days refrigerated.

Drug Administration:
- Doses of 100–200 mg can be given subcutaneously.
- Doses less than 1 g: administer via pump over 10–20 minutes.
- Doses over 1 g: administer over 2 hours or longer.

Drug Interactions:
- May be a decreased bioavailability of digoxin when given in combination.

Lab Effects/Interference:
- Decreased CBC (neutropenia, thrombocytopenia, anemia).
- Increased LFTs, RFTs.
- Increased uric acid due to tumor lysis.

Special Considerations:
- Warnings and Precautions:
  - *Potent BM suppression*: use cautiously in, and monitor patients with preexisting drug-induced BM suppression closely.
  - *Neurological changes*: reversible cerebral and cerebellar toxicity may occur with high doses; assess for changes in handwriting and heel-toe walking.
  - *Embryo-fetal toxicity*: teach women of reproductive potential to use effective contraception to avoid pregnancy. Mothers should not breastfeed while receiving the drug.
- Thrombophlebitis, pain at the injection site, should be treated with warm compresses.
- Dizziness has occurred with too-rapid IV infusions.
- Use with caution if hepatic dysfunction exists.
- Drug is excreted in tears, requiring protection of eye conjunctiva (corticosteroid eye drops such as dexamethasone 0.1% ophthalmic drops) with high-dose therapy.

Potential Toxicities/Side Effects and the Nursing Process

I. INFECTION AND BLEEDING related to BM DEPRESSION

Defining Characteristics: BM depression is related to dose and duration of therapy. WBC depression is biphasic. After a 5-day CI at doses of 50–600 mg/m^2, WBC begins to fall within 24 hours, reaching nadir in 7–9 days, briefly rises around day 12, and begins to fall again, reaching nadir at days 15–24, with recovery within 10 days. Platelet drop begins day 5, reaching nadir at days 12–15, with recovery within 10 days. Anemia is seen frequently, with megaloblastic changes common in the BM. Potent but transient suppression of primary and secondary antibody responses occur.

Nursing Implications: Assess WBC, neutrophil, and platelet count, and discuss any abnormalities with physician prior to drug administration; assess for signs/symptoms of skin infections (all mucosal surfaces, body orifices) and bleeding; instruct patient in signs/symptoms of infection and bleeding, as well as to report them or come to emergency room. Teach patient self-care measures to minimize risk of infection and bleeding, including avoidance of OTC aspirin-containing medications. Assess patient's Hgb/HCT and signs/symptoms of fatigue; teach patient self-assessment and to alternate rest and activity as needed.

II. ALTERED NUTRITION, LESS THAN BODY REQUIREMENTS, related to NAUSEA AND VOMITING, ANOREXIA, STOMATITIS, DIARRHEA, HEPATOTOXICITY

Defining Characteristics: Nausea and vomiting occurs in 50% of patients, is dose related, and lasts for several hours. Can be successfully prevented with combination antiemetics. Anorexia commonly occurs. Stomatitis occurs 7–10 days after therapy is initiated, occurs in 15% of patients, and is dose related. May be preceded by angular stomatitis (reddened area at juncture of lips). Diarrhea is infrequent and mild. Hepatotoxicity is usually mild and reversible, but drug should be used cautiously in patients with impaired hepatic function.

Nursing Implications: Premedicate with antiemetics depending on dose, using aggressive, combination antiemetics for high-dose therapy, and continue throughout chemotherapy. If patient develops nausea/vomiting, assess fluid and electrolyte balance and the need for replacements. Assess oral mucosa prior to chemotherapy and teach patient oral hygiene regimen and self-assessment; encourage patient to report diarrhea, discuss use of antidiarrheals with physician, and teach self-care PRN. Since patients become neutropenic, all mucosal surfaces need to be assessed for infection, and patients must be taught scrupulous perineal hygiene. Monitor LFTs prior to, during, and posttherapy.

III. IMPAIRED SKIN/MUCOSAL INTEGRITY related to RASH, ANAL INFLAMMATION/ULCERATION, ALOPECIA

Defining Characteristics: Maculopapular rash, with or without fever, myalgia, bone pain, occasional chest pain, conjunctivitis, and malaise (cytarabine syndrome) may occur. Syndrome is not common, but occurs 6–12 hours after drug administration; corticosteroids have been helpful in treating/preventing syndrome. Mucosal inflammation and ulceration of anus/rectum may occur, especially in patients with prior hemorrhoids or history of abscesses. Alopecia occurs less frequently.

Nursing Implications: Assess baseline skin and mucous membranes prior to chemotherapy and identify patients at risk for problems. Consider including corticosteroid in antiemetic regimen, especially for high-dose therapy, and discuss with physician prophylactic use of dexamethasone eye drops to prevent conjunctivitis. Teach patient scrupulous perineal hygiene, instruct to report any rectal discomfort, and assess rectal mucosa daily with high-dose therapy. Discuss with patient potential coping strategies if alopecia occurs (i.e., wig, scarves).

IV. POTENTIAL FOR INJURY related to NEUROTOXICITY

Defining Characteristics: Neurotoxicity can occur at high doses. If cerebellar toxicity (characterized by nystagmus, dysarthria, ataxia, slurred speech, and/or dysdiadochokinesia or inability to make fine, coordinated movements) develops, it is an indication to terminate therapy. Onset usually 6–8 days after first dose, lasts 3–7 days. Lethargy and somnolence have resulted from rapid infusion of the drug. Incidence of CNS toxicity is 10% and may be related to total cumulative drug dose, impaired renal function, and/or age > 50 years old. Ocular toxicity may occur, characterized by injection of conjunctive, corneal opacities, decreased visual acuity. This may be a result of inhibition of DNA synthesis of corneal epithelium. Conjunctivitis occurs due to excretion of drug in lacrimal tearing and can be prevented by corticosteroid eye drops. Other visual symptoms that may occur are increased lacrimation, blurred vision, photophobia, eye pain.

Nursing Implications: Assess baseline neurologic status and cerebellar function (coordinated movements such as handwriting and gait) prior to and during therapy. Teach patient to self-assess and report changes in coordination, control of eye movement, handwriting. Monitor patient for somnolence and lethargy during infusion, and infuse drug according to established guidelines. With high-dose therapy, discuss with physician use of prophylactic corticosteroid eye drops. Assess and teach patient self-assessment of eyes and instruct to report increased lacrimation, blurred vision, photophobia, eye pain.

V. POTENTIAL FOR INJURY related to TLS

Defining Characteristics: May develop with initial therapy if patient has a large tumor burden; results from rapid lysis of tumor cells. This usually begins 1–5 days after initiation of therapy and causes elevations in serum uric acid, potassium, phosphorus, BUN, creatinine.

Nursing Implications: If this is induction therapy for a patient with acute leukemia or high tumor burden, expect medical orders to include IV hydration at 150 mL/hour with or without alkalinization, oral allopurinol, strict monitoring of I/O, daily weight, and total body fluid balance determination. Monitor baseline and daily BUN, creatinine, K+, phosphorus, uric acid, and calcium. Monitor for renal, cardiac, neuromuscular signs/symptoms of TLS.

VI.   POTENTIAL SEXUAL DYSFUNCTION related to DRUG EFFECTS

Defining Characteristics: Drug is mutagenic and probably teratogenic. Although normal babies have been delivered by mothers receiving drug in first trimester, other babies have had congenital defects. It is unknown whether the drug is excreted in breastmilk.

Nursing Implications: Discuss with patient and partner sexuality and reproductive goals and possible impact of chemotherapy. Discuss contraception and sperm banking if appropriate. Discourage breastfeeding if the mother is receiving chemotherapy.

Drug: cytarabine, liposome injection (DepoCyt)

Class: Nucleoside metabolic inhibitor (Antimetabolite).

Mechanism of Action: Drug is converted to the metabolite ara-CTP intracellularly. Ara-CTP is thought to inhibit DNA polymerase, thereby affecting DNA synthesis. Incorporation into DNA and RNA may also contribute to cytarabine cellular toxicity.

Metabolism: With systemically administered cytarabine, the drug is metabolized to an inactive compound, ara-U, and is then renally excreted. In the CSF, however, conversion to the ara-U is negligible, because CNS tissue and CSF lack the enzyme necessary for the conversion to occur. Liposomal formulation gives sustained effect over 2 weeks, with a half-life in the CSF of 100–263 hours.

Indication: For the intrathecal treatment of lymphomatous meningitis.

Contraindication: (1) hypersensitivity to cytarabine or any component of the formulation, and (2) active meningeal infection.

Dosage/Range: Indicated for the intrathecal treatment of lymphomatous meningitis only. To be given as follows:

- **Induction therapy:** DepoCyt, 50 mg, administered intrathecally (intraventricular or lumbar puncture) every 14 days for 2 doses (weeks 1 and 3).
- **Consolidation therapy:** DepoCyt, 50 mg, administered intrathecally (intraventricular or lumbar puncture) every 14 days for 3 doses (weeks 5, 7, and 9) followed by 1 additional dose at week 13.
- **Maintenance therapy:** DepoCyt, 50 mg, administered intrathecally (intraventricular or lumbar puncture) every 28 days for 4 doses (weeks 17, 21, 25, and 29).
- If drug-related neurotoxicity develops, the dose should be reduced to 25 mg. If toxicity persists, treatment with DepoCyt should be terminated.
- Dexamethasone 4 mg PO twice daily × 5 days should begin on day of liposomal cytarabine injection.

Drug Preparation:
- Drug is supplied in single-use vials containing 10 mg/mL (50 mg/5 mL) and comes as a white to off-white suspension in 5 mL of fluid, preservative-free.

- Drug is to be withdrawn immediately before use and should not be used later than 4 hours from the time of withdrawal from vial.

Drug Administration:
- DO NOT use in-line filters.
- DepoCyt should be administered directly into the CSF over 1–5 minutes, via intraventricular reservoir or by direct injection into the lumbar sac. Patients should lie flat for 1 hour after administration. Patient should be directly observed for immediate toxic reaction.
- Patients should be started on dexamethasone 4 mg bid either PO or IV for 5 days beginning on the day of DepoCyt injection.

Drug Interactions:
- No formal drug interaction studies of DepoCyt and other drugs have been done.
- Expect increased neurotoxicity if drug is administered at same time as other intrathecal, cytotoxic agents.

Lab Effects/Interference:
- DepoCyt particles are similar in size and appearance to white blood cells, so care must be taken when interpreting CSF samples.

Special Considerations:
Most frequent reactions (≥10%) include headache, nausea, vomiting, arachnoiditis, weakness, confusion, pyrexia, fatigue, constipation, back pain, abnormal gait, seizures, dizziness, lethargy, insomnia, UTI, neck pain, memory impairment, dehydration, blurred vision, decreased appetite, muscle weakness, neck stiffness.
- Warnings and Precautions:
  - *Chemical arachnoiditis* (characterized by nausea, vomiting, headache, fever within 5 days of drug administration) may occur, but incidence reduced by coadministration of dexamethasone PO.
  - *Neurotoxicity*: myelopathy and other neurological toxicity may occur.
  - *Transient elevation of CSF Protein and CSF white blood* cells may occur.
  - *Embryo-fetal toxicity*: if drug is used during pregnancy or if the patient becomes pregnant while taking the drug, the patient should be apprised of the potential harm to the fetus. Women of reproductive potential should be taught to use effective contraception while receiving the drug.

Potential Toxicities/Side Effects and the Nursing Process

I. ALTERATION IN NUTRITION, LESS THAN BODY REQUIREMENTS, related to NAUSEA AND VOMITING

Defining Characteristics: Nausea, vomiting, and headache are common, and are physical manifestations of chemical arachnoiditis.

Nursing Implications: Administer dexamethasone throughout treatment course as described above. Observe patient for at least 1 hour after administration for toxicity. Administer antiemetics as ordered. Encourage small, frequent feedings of cool, bland foods. Instruct patient to report nausea and vomiting and to self-administer antiemetics as ordered.

II.   ALTERATION IN COMFORT related to HEADACHE, NECK AND/OR BACK PAIN, FEVER, NAUSEA, AND VOMITING

Defining Characteristics: Some degree of chemical arachnoiditis is expected in about one-third of patients: incidence approaches 100% of patients when dexamethasone is NOT given with DepoCyt. Causes headache, neck pain, and/or rigidity, back pain, fever, nausea, and vomiting, which are reversible.

Nursing Implications: Instruct patient in dexamethasone self-administration and to report to physician if oral doses are not tolerated. Patients should lie flat for 1 hour after lumbar puncture and should be observed for immediate toxic reactions. Administer medications to treat pain.

Drug: dacarbazine (DTIC-Dome, dimethyl-triazeno-imidazole carboxamide)

Class: Alkylating agent.

Mechanism of Action: Appears to methylate nucleic acids (particularly DNA) causing cross-linkage and breaks in DNA strands, which inhibits RNA and DNA synthesis. Also interacts with sulfhydryl groups to inhibit protein synthesis. Generally, cell cycle phase nonspecific.

Metabolism: Thought to be activated by liver microsomes; 15% of the drug crosses the blood–brain barrier. Undergoes metabolism in liver and biliary excretion, with 18–63% of drug excreted unchanged in the urine. Plasma half-life of 0.65 hour, and terminal half-life of 5 hours.

Indication: (1) For the treatment of patients with metastatic malignant melanoma, as well as for (2) second-line treatment of patients with Hodgkin's disease when used in combination with other effective agents.

Dosage/Range:
- Malignant melanoma: 2–4.5 mg/kg/day IV × 10 days; may repeat at 4-week intervals.
- Hodgkin's disease: 150 mg/m^2 IV × 5 days, in combination with other chemotherapeutic agents, repeated every 4 weeks. Alternatively, the dose is 375 mg/m^2 IV on day 1, repeated every 15 days, in combination with other antineoplastic agents.

Drug Preparation:
- Available in 200-mg vials.
- Reconstitute with 19.7 mL of sterile water for injection USP; the resulting solution concentration is 10 mg/mL of dacarbazine, having a pH of 3.0–4.0. Aseptically withdraw the ordered dose and further dilute in 5% dextrose injection USP or sodium chloride injection USP.

- After reconstitution and prior to use, the solution in the vial may be stored at 4°C for up to 72 hours or at normal room conditions for up to 8 hours. Once further diluted, the resulting solution may be stored at 4°C for up to 24 hours or at normal room conditions for up to 8 hours.

Drug Administration:
- Assess CBC, LFTs baseline and before each cycle.
- Administer via pump over 60 minutes. IVP is not recommended as drug is very emetogenic.
- Irritant—avoid extravasation.
- Pain may occur above site: usually unrelieved by slowing IV, but may be relieved by applying warm packs to painful area. May cause venospasm; slow rate if this occurs.
- Anaphylaxis has occurred with infusion of dacarbazine.

Drug Interactions:
- Increased drug metabolism with concurrent administration of Dilantin, phenobarbital; potential increased toxicity with Imuran and 6-MP.

Lab Effects/Interference:
- Decreased CBC.
- Increased LFTs.

Special Considerations:

Most frequent adverse effects are nausea/vomiting and anorexia.
- Warnings and Precautions:
  - *BM depression*: monitor CBC/platelets closely and hold/delay drug and/or dose reduce as necessary.
  - *Hepatotoxicity may* occur and rarely is accompanied by hepatic vein thrombosis and hepatocellular necrosis
  - *Embryo-fetal toxicity*: Teach women of reproductive potential to use effective contraception during therapy. Mothers should not breastfeed their infant during treatment with dacarbazine.

Potential Toxicities/Side Effects and the Nursing Process

I. INFECTION AND BLEEDING related to BM DEPRESSION

Defining Characteristics: Nadir occurs days 14–28 following drug administration; anemia may occur with long-term treatment.

Nursing Implications: Evaluate WBC, neutrophil, and platelet count and discuss any abnormalities with physician prior to drug administration; assess for signs/symptoms of infection or bleeding; instruct patient in identifying signs/symptoms of infection and bleeding, and to report them. Teach patient self-care measures to minimize risk of infection and bleeding, including avoidance of OTC aspirin-containing medications. Assess patient's Hgb/HCT and signs/symptoms of fatigue; teach patient self-assessment and instruct to alternate rest and activity as needed.

II.   ALTERATION IN NUTRITION, LESS THAN BODY REQUIREMENTS, related to NAUSEA AND VOMITING, DIARRHEA, ANOREXIA, HEPATOTOXICITY

Defining Characteristics: Nausea/vomiting occurs in 90% of patients and is moderate to severe, beginning 1–3 hours after dose, and vomiting lasting up to 12 hours. Nausea and vomiting decrease with each consecutive day the drug is given. Preventable by aggressive combination antiemetics. Diarrhea is uncommon. Anorexia is common, occurring in 90% of patients; drug may also cause a metallic taste. Hepatotoxicity is rare, but hepatic veno-occlusive disease has been described (hepatic vein thrombosis and hepatocellular necrosis).

Nursing Implications: Premedicate with combination antiemetics and continue protection during infusions. Administer drug over at least 1 hour. Use relaxation exercises, imagery, or other techniques; teach patient exercises prior to drug treatment. Teach patient to report diarrhea and administer antidiarrheal medication as ordered, or teach patient self-administration as appropriate. Encourage small, frequent feedings of favorite foods; teach patient/caregiver to make foods ahead of time so patient will have them ready for snacks when hungry; encourage use of spices if food tastes bland; encourage patient to weigh self on a weekly basis. Monitor LFTs and discuss abnormalities with physician.

III.   ALTERATION IN COMFORT related to FLU-LIKE SYNDROME, PAIN AT INJECTION SITE

Defining Characteristics: Flu-like syndromes may occur, characterized by malaise, headache, myalgia, hypotension; may occur up to 7 days after first dose, lasting 7–21 days, and may recur with subsequent doses of drug. Drug is an irritant and may cause phlebitis of vein.

Nursing Implications: Teach patient that flu-like symptoms may occur; suggest symptom management using acetaminophen as needed; encourage fluid intake of >3 L/day and rest, as determined by healthcare team. Assess patient vein selection prior to drug administration and suggest venous access device early on if patient is to receive ongoing treatment with dacarbazine (DTIC). Administer drug in 100- to 250-mL IV fluid and infuse slowly over 1 hour. Consider premedications when drug is given peripherally and discuss with physician: hydrocortisone IVP (DTIC forms precipitate with hydrocortisone sodium succinate [Solu-Cortef] but not with hydrocortisone), lidocaine 1–2% IVP, or heparin IVP to minimize vein trauma prior to DTIC infusion. Apply heat or ice above injection site to reduce venous burning.

IV.   IMPAIRED SKIN INTEGRITY related to ALOPECIA, FACIAL FLUSHING, ERYTHEMA, URTICARIA

Defining Characteristics: Alopecia occurs in 90% of patients. Facial flushing occurs rarely and is self-limiting; erythema and urticaria may occur around injection site. High dose-related photosensitization may occur, with resulting severe reaction to sunlight (e.g., burning, pain).

Nursing Implications: Teach patient about expected hair loss; encourage patient to verbalize feelings regarding anticipated/actual hair loss and discuss strategies to minimize impact of alopecia. Encourage female patients to obtain wig prior to hair loss; ask male patients to identify how they will manage hair loss. Provide emotional support. In cold climates, encourage patient to wear cap at night to prevent loss of body heat. Teach patient receiving high-dose therapy to cover body, head, and hands when exposed to sunlight, or to avoid direct sunlight. Patient should also use sunblock.

V.   POTENTIAL FOR SENSORY/PERCEPTUAL ALTERATIONS related to FACIAL PARESTHESIA, PHOTOSENSITIVITY

Defining Characteristics: Photosensitivity may occur in bright sunlight or ultraviolet light. Facial paresthesias may occur.

Nursing Implications: Instruct patient to report facial paresthesias and in self-care measures if sensory changes occur; wear sunglasses in strong sunlight; wear sunscreens when out in the sun, as well as protective clothing, including a hat; avoid UV or strong sunlight exposure if possible.

VI.   POTENTIAL SEXUAL DYSFUNCTION related to DRUG EFFECTS

Defining Characteristics: Drug is teratogenic. It is unknown whether drug is excreted in breastmilk. Drug is probably carcinogenic.

Nursing Implications: Assess patient's and partner's patterns of sexuality and reproductive goals. Teach need for contraception and provide information and referral as appropriate. Encourage verbalization of feelings and provide emotional support. Discourage breastfeeding if patient is a lactating mother.

Drug: dactinomycin (Actinomycin D, Cosmegen)

Class: Antitumor antibiotic isolated from *Streptomyces* fungus.

Mechanism of Action: Binds to guanine portion of DNA and blocks the ability of DNA to act as a template for both DNA and RNA. At lower drug doses, the predominant action inhibits RNA, whereas at higher doses both RNA and DNA are inhibited. Cell cycle specific for G_1 and S phases.

Metabolism: Most of drug is excreted unchanged in bile and urine. There is a rapid clearance of drug from plasma (approximately 36 hours). Dose reduction in the presence of liver or renal failure may be needed.

Indication:
1. As part of combination chemotherapy and/or multi-modality treatment regimen, indicated for the treatment of patients with Wilms' tumor, childhood rhabdomyosarcoma, Ewing's sarcoma, and metastatic, nonseminomatous testicular cancer.
2. As a single agent or as part of combination chemotherapy for the treatment of patients with gestational trophoblastic neoplasia. As a component of regional perfusion, for the palliative and/or adjunctive treatment of locally recurrent or locoregional solid malignancies.

Contraindication: Hypersensitivity to any components of this drug; drug should not be given at or about the time of chickenpox infection or herpes zoster because of the risk of severe, generalized disease, which may result in death.

Dosage/Range:
- Wilms' tumor, childhood rhabdomyosarcoma, and Ewing's sarcoma: 115 mcg/kg/day IV × 5 days in various combinatinos and schedules with other chemotherapy drugs (e.g., q 3–4 weeks).
- Gestational trophoblastic neoplasia: 12 mcg/kg/da IV × 5 days as a single agent, or 500 mcg on days 1 and 2 as part of a combination regimen with etoposide, methotrexate, folinic acid, vincristine, cyclophosphamide, and cisplatin.
- Metastatic nonseminomatous testicular cancer: 1,000 mcg/m² IV on day 1 as part of a combination regimen with cyclophosphamide, bleomycin, vinblastine, and cisplatin.
- Regional perfusion in locally recurrent and locoregional solid malignancies: see pertinent literature, but doses are 50 mcg (0.05 mg)/kg for lower extremity or pelvis, and 35 mcg (0.035 mg)/kg for upper extremity.

Drug Preparation:
- Asceptically add 1.1 mL of sterile water for injection (without preservative), resulting in a concentration of 500 mcg (0.5 mg)/mL. Use preservative-free water, as precipitate may develop otherwise. Inspect for particulate matter or discoloration; drug should be clear, gold-colored.

Drug Administration:
- IV: Drug is a vesicant and should be given through a running IV of 5% dextrose or 0.9% sodium chloride injection, to avoid extravasation. Extravasation can lead to ulceration, pain, and necrosis. Be sure to check the nursing policy and procedure for administration of vesicants.
- If extravasation is suspected, follow extravasation guidelines (see *Chapter 1* narrative), and apply ice to site for 15 min qid, × 3 days.

Drug Interactions:
- None significant.

Lab Effects/Interference:
- Decreased CBC.
- Increased LFTs.
- Decreased calcium.

- Dactinomycin may interfere with the bioassay procedures for determining antibacterial drug levels.

Special Considerations:
- Warnings and Precautions:
  - *Secondary malignancies*, such as leukemia, may occur in patients who have received RT and dactinomycin. Patients should receive long-term observation as cancer survivors.
  - *Embryo-fetal toxicity*: Teach women of reproductive potential to use effective contraception to avoid pregnancy while receiving this therapy. Mothers should not breast-feed while receiving dactinomycin therapy.
  - *Veno-occlusive disease* may occur and be fatal, especially in children younger than 48 months.
  - *RT*: If drug is given with RT, or within 2 months of RT: increased GI toxicity and BM suppression. In general, drug should not be given concomitantly with RT (e.g., Wilms' tumor).
  - *Toxicity from regional perfusion* is related to drug that escapes into the systemic circulation.
  - *Labs*: Monitor renal, hepatic, and BM function baseline and prior to each cycle of therapy.
- Drug is a vesicant. Give through a running IV to avoid extravasation, which may develop into ulceration, necrosis, and pain.
- Nausea and vomiting are moderate to severe. Usually occurs 2–5 hours after administration; may persist up to 24 hours.
- Potent myelosuppressive agent: Severity of nadir is dose-limiting toxicity.
- GI toxicity: Mucositis, diarrhea, and abdominal pain.
- Skin changes: Radiation recall phenomenon. Skin discoloration along vein used for injection.
- Alopecia.
- Malaise, fatigue, mental depression.
- Contraindicated in patients with chickenpox or herpes zoster, as life-threatening systemic disease may develop.

Potential Toxicities/Side Effects and the Nursing Process

I. POTENTIAL FOR INFECTION AND BLEEDING related to BM DEPRESSION

Defining Characteristics: Myelosuppression often dose-limiting toxicity. Onset of decreasing WBC and platelets in 7–10 days, with nadir 14–21 days after dose and recovery in 21–28 days. Delayed anemia.

Nursing Implications: Assess CBC, WBC, differential, and platelet count prior to drug administration, as well as for signs/symptoms of infection and bleeding, and discuss any abnormalities with physician prior to drug administration. Instruct patient in signs/symptoms of infection and bleeding, and instruct to report this; teach patient self-care measures to minimize risk of infection and bleeding, including avoidance of OTC aspirin-containing medications. Assess patient's Hgb/HCT and signs/symptoms of fatigue; teach patient self-assessment and instruct to alternate rest and activity as needed.

II. ALTERATION IN NUTRITION, LESS THAN BODY REQUIREMENTS, related to NAUSEA/VOMITING, DIARRHEA, ANOREXIA

Defining Characteristics: Nausea/vomiting may be severe and begins 2–5 hours after dose, lasting 24 hours. Diarrhea with/without cramps occurs in 30% of patients. Anorexia occurs frequently.

Nursing Implications: Use combination antiemetics to prevent nausea and vomiting. Nausea/vomiting may be prevented by aggressive, combination antiemetics, such as serotonin antagonist plus dexamethasone. Encourage small, frequent feedings of bland foods. Encourage patient to eat favorite foods and use seasonings on foods if anorexia persists; refer to dietitian as needed.

III. ALTERATION IN MUCOUS MEMBRANES related to STOMATITIS, ESOPHAGITIS, AND PROCTITIS

Defining Characteristics: Irritation and ulceration may occur along the entire GI mucosa.

Nursing Implications: Assess baseline oral mucosa and presence of irritation along GI tract. Instruct patient in self-assessment and teach patient to report irritation; instruct regarding oral hygiene regimen.

IV. POTENTIAL IMPAIRED SKIN INTEGRITY related to RADIATION RECALL, RASH, ALOPECIA, AND DRUG EXTRAVASATION

Defining Characteristics: Recalls damage to skin from previous radiation, resulting in erythema or increased pigmentation at the radiation site. Acne-like rash and alopecia can occur in 47% of patients. Drug is a potent vesicant.

Nursing Implications: Conduct baseline skin, hair assessment. Discuss with patient impact of potential changes on body image, as well as possible coping/adaptive strategies (e.g., obtain wig prior to hair loss). When administering the drug, ensure use of a patent vein to avoid extravasation; consider the use of venous access device early. Be familiar with institution's policy and procedure for administration of a vesicant and management of extravasation.

V. ALTERATION IN COMFORT related to FLU-LIKE SYMPTOMS

Defining Characteristics: Flu-like symptoms can occur, including symptoms of malaise, myalgia, fever, depression.

Nursing Implications: Inform patient this may occur. Assess for occurrence during and after treatment. Discuss with physician symptomatic management.

VI.   POTENTIAL FOR ALTERATION IN METABOLISM related to HEPATOTOXICITY AND RENAL TOXICITY

Defining Characteristics: Hepatotoxicity is related to drug metabolism in liver; renal toxicity is related to drug excretion by kidneys.

Nursing Implications: Monitor LFTUN and creatinine. Discuss abnormalities with physician, as drug doses may need to be reduced.

VII.   POTENTIAL FOR SEXUAL DYSFUNCTION

Defining Characteristics: Drug is carcinogenic, mutagenic, and teratogenic. It is unknown if drug is excreted in breastmilk.

Nursing Implications: Assess patient's/partner's sexual patterns and reproductive goals. Provide information, supportive counseling, and referral as needed. Teach importance of birth control measures as appropriate. Discourage breastfeeding if patient is a lactating mother.

Drug: daunorubicin citrate liposome injection (DaunoXome)

Class: Anthracycline antibiotic liposome; drug is isolated from streptomycin products, in particular the rhodomycin products, and encapsulated in a liposome.

Mechanism of Action: No clearly defined mechanism. Intercalates DNA, therefore blocking DNA, RNA, and protein synthesis. Binds to DNA and inhibits DNA replication and DNA-dependent RNA synthesis. Drug is encapsulated within liposomes (lipid vesicles) and is preferentially delivered to solid tumor sites. The liposomal encapsulated drug is protected from chemical and enzymatic degradation, protein binding, and uptake by normal tissues while circulating in the blood. The exact mechanism for selective targeting of tumor sites is unknown but is believed to be related to increased permeability of the tumor neovasculature. Once delivered to the tumor, the drug is slowly released and exerts its antineoplastic action.

Metabolism: Cleared from the plasma at 17 mL/min with a small steady-state volume of distribution. As compared to standard IV daunorubicin, the liposomal encapsulated daunorubicin has higher daunorubicin exposure (plasma AUC). The elimination half-life (4.4 hours) is shorter than standard daunorubicin.

Indication: Indicated as first-line cytotoxic chemotherapy for advanced HIV-associated Kaposi's sarcoma (KS). Drug is not recommended for patients with less than advanced HIV-related KS.

Contraindications: patients who have experienced a serious hypersensitivity reaction to previous doses of DaunoXome or to any of its constituents.

Dosage/Range:
- 40 mg/m^2/day IV infusion over 60 minutes every 2 weeks.
- Reduce dose in patients with impaired hepatic or renal function:
  - Serum bilirubin 1.2–3 mg/dL: give 75% of the normal dose.
  - Serum bilirubin or serum creatinine > 3 mg/dL: give 50% of the normal dose.

Drug Preparation:
- Drug is available as 50 mg of daunorubicin base in a total volume of 25 mL (2 mg/mL).
- Visually inspect for particulate matter and discoloration (drug appears as a translucent dispersion of liposomes that scatters light, but should not be opaque or have precipitate or foreign matter present).
- Withdraw the calculated volume of drug and add to an equal volume of 5% dextrose in an infusion bag to deliver a 1:1, or 1 mg/mL solution.
- Administer immediately, or may be stored in the refrigerator at 2–8°C (36–46°F) for a maximum of 6 hours.
- Use ONLY 5% dextrose, NOT 0.9% sodium chloride or any other solution.
- Drug contains no preservatives.
- Unopened drug vials should be stored in the refrigerator at 2–8°C (36–46°F), but should not be frozen. Protect from light.

Drug Administration:
- Assess ANC/CBC; hold dose if absolute granulocyte (neutrophil) count is <750 cells/mm^3. IV infusion over 60 minutes, repeated every 2 weeks.
- Do not use an inline filter.
- Drug is an irritant, not a vesicant. Prevent extravasation.
- Dose should be reduced in patients with renal or hepatic dysfunction.

Drug Interactions:
- BM suppressant agents: increased BM depression.

Lab Effects/Interference:
- Increased LFTs, RFTs (especially if elevated prior to administration).
- Increased uric acid secondary to tumor lysis.

Special Considerations:
- Warnings and Precautions:
  - *Myelosuppression*: Primary toxicity is myelosuppression, which may be severe, associated with fever and infection. Monitor patient closely for infection, including intercurrent or opportunistic infection.
  - *Potential cardiotoxicity:* Assess patient risk factors for CHF and cardiomyopathy. Assess LVEF at total doses of daunorubicin liposome at 320 mg/m^2, and every 160 mg/m^2 after that. Patients who have previously received doxorubicin >300 mg/m^2 or

equivalent of another anthracycline, those who have preexisting cardiac disease, or have received prior RT encompassing the heart should have a baseline LVEF by ECHO or MUGA, and every 160 mg/m^2 of daunorubicin liposome.

- *Triad of back pain, flushing, and chest tightness* may occur during the first 5 minutes of the infusion and subside with interruption of the infusion and generally does not recur when the infusion is resumed at a slower rate.
- *Embryo-fetal toxicity*: teach female patients of reproductive potential to use effective contraception to avoid pregnancy while receiving the drug.
- No systematic studies of drug interactions have been conducted.
- Reduce dose in patients with hepatic or renal impairment.

Potential Toxicities/Side Effects and the Nursing Process

I. POTENTIAL FOR INFECTION AND BLEEDING related to BM DEPRESSION

Defining Characteristics: Myelosuppression can be severe and affects the granulocytes primarily. Incidence of neutropenia of 36% is similar to that of patients receiving ABV (doxorubicin, vincristine, bleomycin), which is 35%. Neutropenia with <500 cells/mm^3 occurs in 15% of patients (versus 5% in patients receiving ABV). Fever incidence is 47%. Concurrent antiretroviral and antiviral agents received for HIV infection may enhance this. Patients are immunocompromised; therefore, monitoring for opportunistic infection is essential. Platelets and RBCs are less affected.

Nursing Implications: Monitor CBC, WBC, differential, and platelet count prior to drug administration, and discuss any abnormalities with physician. Drug should not be given if ANC is <750 cells/mm^3. Assess for signs/symptoms of infection or bleeding, and instruct patient in self-assessment and to report signs/symptoms immediately. Teach patient self-care measures to minimize risk of infection and bleeding, including avoidance of OTC aspirin-containing medications. Drug dosage must be reduced if patient has hepatic dysfunction: 75% of drug dose if serum bili 1.2–3.0 mg/dL, 50% reduction if bili is >3.0 mg/dL. Drug dosage must be reduced if patient has renal impairment: creatinine >3 mg/dL, give 50% of normal dose.

II. ALTERATION IN COMFORT related to TRIAD OF BACK PAIN, FLUSHING, CHEST TIGHTNESS

Defining Characteristics: This occurs in 13.8% of patients and is mild to moderate. The syndrome resolves with cessation of the infusion, and does not usually recur when the infusion is resumed at a slower infusion rate.

Nursing Implications: Infuse drug at prescribed rate over 60 minutes. Assess for, and teach patient to report, back pain, flushing, and chest tightness. Stop infusion if this occurs, and once symptoms subside, resume infusion at a slower rate.

III. POTENTIAL FOR ALTERATION IN SKIN INTEGRITY related to ALOPECIA, CHANGES IN SKIN

Defining Characteristics: Mild alopecia occurs in 6% of patients and moderate alopecia in 2% of patients, as compared to 36% of patients receiving ABV chemotherapy. The drug is considered an irritant, NOT a vesicant. Folliculitis, seborrhea, and dry skin occur in about 5% of patients.

Nursing Implications: Teach patient that hair loss is unlikely, and to report this or any skin changes.

IV. POTENTIAL FOR ALTERATION IN NUTRITION, LESS THAN BODY REQUIREMENTS, related to NAUSEA AND VOMITING, ANOREXIA, DIARRHEA

Defining Characteristics: Mild nausea occurs in 35% of patients, moderate nausea in 16% of patients, and severe nausea in 3% of patients. Vomiting is less common, with 10% experiencing mild, 10% experiencing moderate, and 3% experiencing severe vomiting. Anorexia may occur (21%) or increased appetite may occur in <5% of patients. Diarrhea may occur in 38% of patients. Other GI problems, occurring about 5% of the time, are dysphagia, gastritis, hemorrhoids, hepatomegaly, dry mouth, and tooth caries.

Nursing Implications: Premedicate with antiemetics. Encourage small, frequent feedings of bland foods. If patient has anorexia, teach patient or caregiver to make foods ahead of time, use spices, and encourage weekly weights. Instruct patient to report diarrhea and to use self-management strategies (medications as ordered, diet modification). Instruct patient to report other GI problems.

V. POTENTIAL FOR ALTERATION IN CARDIAC OUTPUT related to CARDIAC CHANGES

Defining Characteristics: Daunorubicin may cause cardiotoxicity and CHF, but studies with liposomal daunorubicin show rare clinical cardiotoxicity at cumulative doses > 600 mg/m². However, especially in patients with preexisting cardiac disease or prior anthracycline treatment, assessment of cardiac function (history and physical) should be performed prior to each dose. In addition, testing of cardiac ejection fraction and echocardiogram should be performed at cumulative doses of 320 mg/m², 480 mg/m², and every 160 mg/m² thereafter.

Nursing Implications: Assess cardiac status prior to chemotherapy administration: signs/symptoms of CHF, quality/regularity and rate of heartbeat, results of prior tests of left ventricular ejection fraction (LVEF) or echocardiogram, if performed. Instruct patient to report dyspnea, palpitations, swelling in extremities. Maintain accurate records of total dose, and expect GBPS to be repeated periodically during treatment and the drug to be discontinued if there is a significant drop in heart function.

VI. POTENTIAL FOR ACTIVITY INTOLERANCE related to FATIGUE

Defining Characteristics: Fatigue occurs in 49% of patients.

Nursing Implications: Assess baseline activity level. Instruct patient to report fatigue and activity intolerance. Teach self-management strategies, including alternating rest and activity periods, and stress reduction.

Drug: daunorubicin hydrochloride (Cerubidine, Daunomycin HCl, Rubidomycin)

Class: Anthracycline antibiotic isolated from streptomycin products, in particular therhodomycin products.

Mechanism of Action: No clearly defined mechanism. Intercalates DNA, therefore blocking DNA, RNA, and protein synthesis. Binds to DNA and inhibits DNA replication and DNA-dependent RNA synthesis.

Metabolism: Site of significant metabolism is in the liver. Doses need to be modified in the presence of abnormal liver function. Excreted in urine and bile.

Indication: in combination with other approved anticancer drugs, (1) for remission induction in adult patients with acute nonlymphocytic leukemia (myelogenous, monocytic, erythroid), and (2) for remission induction in children and adults with acute lymphocytic leukemia.

Contraindications: patients who have shown hypersensitivity to drug. Drug should not be used in patients who have previously received the recommended maximum cumulative doses of doxorubicin or daunorubicin HCL (Teva Parenteral, 2012).

Dosage/Range:
- 30–60 mg/m^2/day IV for 3 consecutive days.
- **AML induction:** 45 mg/m^2/day IV × 3 days with cytosine arabinoside 100 mg/m^2/day IV CI × 7 days.
- Adjust dose for patients 60 years and older, e.g., daunorubicin HCL 30 mg/m^2/day on days 1, 2, 3 of the first course, and on days 1,2 of subsequent courses AND cytosine arabinoside 100 mg m^2/day IV infusion daily × 7 days for the first course (see package insert).
- Adjust dose for hepatic dysfunction (25% dose reduction [DR]), BR 1.2–3 mg/dL; 50% DR BR > 3.0 mg/dL.
- Adjust dose for renal dysfunction: serum creatinine > 3 mg%, 50% dose reduction.

Drug Preparation:
- Available in 20- and 50-mg vials for injection or 20- and 50-mg vials containing lyophilized powder.
- Add sterile water to produce liquid. Drug will form a precipitate when mixed with heparin and is incompatible with dexamethasone.

Drug Administration:
- Assess ANC/CBC, LFTs, renal function tests, and cardiac function tests baseline and before each course of treatment. Assess patient for signs/symptoms of infection.
- Initial course: Discuss TLS prophylaxis with physician/NP/PA prior to initial treatment to prevent hyperuricemia due to rapid lysis of leukemic cells. Monitor uric acid level, electrolytes, and fluid volume before and during treatment.
- IV: This drug is a potent vesicant. Give through a running IV to avoid extravasation, which can lead to ulceration, pain, and necrosis. Check individual hospital policy and procedure on administration of a vesicant. Central line recommended.
- Teach patient that urine will be red or pink colored as drug is excreted in the urine and not to be alarmed.

Drug Interactions:
- Incompatible with heparin (forms a precipitate).
- Other BM suppressive drugs: increased BM depression.
- Cyclophosphamide: concurrent administration may increase cardiotoxicity. Hepatotoxic medications, such as high-dose methotrexate, may impair liver function and increase the risk of toxicity.

Lab Effects/Interference:
- Increased bili, AST, alk phos.
- Increased uric acid secondary to tumor lysis.

Special Considerations:
- Drug is a potent vesicant. Give through running IV to avoid/minimize risk of extravasation. Central line is recommended.
- Moderate to severe nausea and vomiting occur in 50% of patients within first 24 hours.
- Causes discoloration of urine (pink to red for up to 48 hours after administration).
- Warnings and Precautions:
  - *Potent myelosuppressive* agent. Nadir occurs within 10–14 days.
  - *Cardiac toxicity*:
    - Dose limit at 400–550 mg/m^2 in adults, and 300 mg/m^2 in children > 2 years old. Monitor LVEF baseline and during treatment.
    - Patients may exhibit irreversible CHF.
    - Acute toxicity may be seen within hours after administration. This is unrelated to cumulative dose and may manifest symptoms of pump or conduction dysfunction.
    - Rarely, transient ECG abnormalities, CHF; pericardial effusion (whole syndrome referred to as myocarditis-pericarditis syndrome) may occur, which may lead to death.
  - *Toxicity of drug increased with hepatic or renal impairment.* Assess LFTs and renal function tests baseline and before each dose. Reduce dose based on extent of impairment (see Dosage)
  - *Embryo-fetal toxicity*: Teach women of reproductive potential to use effective contraception to avoid pregnancy. Mothers should not breastfeed while receiving the drug, and mothers should be advised to discontinue nursing during daunorubicin therapy.
  - *Secondary leukemias* have occurred, especially when combined with other antineoplastic agents or RT.

- Drug is a vesicant, resulting in severe local tissue necrosis.
- Dose-limiting toxicities are BM suppression and cardiotoxicity.
- Side effects include reversible alopecia, acute nausea and vomiting, mucositis occurring 3–7 days after administration, diarrhea.
- Rarely, anaphylactoid reaction, fever, and chills can occur during the infusion.

Potential Toxicities/Side Effects and the Nursing Process

I.   POTENTIAL FOR INFECTION AND BLEEDING related to BM DEPRESSION

Defining Characteristics: WBC and platelet counts begin to decrease in 7 days, with nadir 10–14 days after drug dose; recovery in 21–28 days. Dose reduction indicated with renal or hepatic dysfunction as drug is excreted by these routes.

Nursing Implications: Evaluate WBC, neutrophil, and platelet count and discuss any abnormalities with physician prior to drug administration; assess for signs/symptoms of infection and bleeding; instruct patient in signs/symptoms of infection and bleeding and to report these immediately. Teach patient self-care measures to minimize risk of infection and bleeding, including avoidance of OTC aspirin-containing medications.

II.   POTENTIAL FOR ALTERATION IN CARDIAC OUTPUT related to ACUTE AND CHRONIC CARDIAC CHANGES

Defining Characteristics: Acute effects (i.e., EKG changes, atrial arrhythmias) occur in 6–30% of patients 1–3 days after dose and are not life threatening. Chronic myofibril damage resulting in irreversible cardiomyopathy is life threatening and dose related. Cumulative dose should not exceed 550 mg/m^2 or 450 mg/m^2 if patient is receiving/has received radiation to chest or with concurrent administration of cyclophosphamide or other cardiotoxic agent. CHF may develop 1–16 months after therapy ceases if cumulative dose is exceeded.

Nursing Implications: Assess baseline cardiac status, quality and regularity of heartbeat, and baseline ECG. Patient should have baseline MUGA or other measure of left ventricular ejection fraction at baseline, and periodically during treatment. If there is a significant drop in ejection fraction, then drug should be stopped. Maintain accurate documentation of doses administered so that cumulative dose is known. Instruct patient to report dyspnea, shortness of breath, edema, orthopnea.

III.   ALTERATION IN NUTRITION, LESS THAN BODY REQUIREMENTS, related to NAUSEA AND VOMITING, STOMATITIS

Defining Characteristics: Mild nausea and vomiting on the day of therapy occur in 50% of patients and can be prevented with antiemetics. Stomatitis is infrequent but may occur 3–7 days after dose.

Nursing Implications: Premedicate with antiemetics, and continue for 24 hours for protection. Assess oral mucosa prior to chemotherapy, teach patient oral hygiene regimen and self-assessment, and encourage patient to report burning or oral irritation. Assess pain in mouth, and administer analgesics as needed and ordered.

IV.   POTENTIAL FOR IMPAIRED SKIN INTEGRITY related to ALOPECIA, HYPERPIGMENTATION OF FINGERNAILS AND TOENAILS, RADIATION RECALL, AND DRUG EXTRAVASATION

Defining Characteristics: Reversible total alopecia occurs 3–4 weeks after treatment begins; nail beds become hyperpigmented. Drug is a potent vesicant and will result in severe soft tissue damage if extravasated. Damage to skin from prior irradiation may be reactivated (radiation recall). Rash may occur, as may onycholysis (nail loosening from nail bed).

Nursing Implications: Teach patient that alopecia will occur and discuss impact hair loss will have on body image. Discuss coping strategies, including obtaining wig or cap prior to hair loss. Encourage patient to verbalize feelings and provide patient with emotional support. Drug dose may be decreased with prior irradiation; assess for skin changes from radiation recall. Hyperpigmentation of nail beds may cause body-image problem; discuss with patient and identify measures to minimize distress. Ensure that drug is administered only through a patent IV and that nurse is familiar with institution's policy for vesicant administration and management of extravasation. Manufacturer recommends aspiration of any remaining drug from IV tubing, discontinuing IV, and applying ice. Assess need for venous access device early.

V.   POTENTIAL SEXUAL DYSFUNCTION related to DRUG EFFECTS

Defining Characteristics: Drug is mutagenic and teratogenic. Drug may cause testicular atrophy and azoospermia. It is unknown whether drug is excreted in breastmilk.

Nursing Implications: Assess patient's and partner's sexual patterns and reproductive goals. Provide information, supportive counseling, and referral as needed. Male patients may wish to try sperm banking. Teach importance of birth control measures as appropriate. Women receiving the drug should not breastfeed.

VI.   POTENTIAL FOR ALTERATION IN COMFORT related to ABDOMINAL PAIN, FEVER, CHILLS

Defining Characteristics: Abdominal pain may occur but is uncommon. Fever and chills, with or without rash, occur rarely.

Nursing Implications: Assess patient for occurrence and provide symptomatic management.

Drug: Daunorubicin and cytarabine liposome for injection (Vyxeos)

Class: Liposomal combination of daunorubicin, an anthracycline topoisomerase inhibitor, and cytarabine, a nucleoside metabolic inhibitor.

Mechanism of Action: Daunorubicin and cytarabine are synergistic in a 1:5 molar ratio in killing leukemia cells. Daunorubicin has anti-mitotic and cytotoxic activity (forms complexes with DNA, inhibits topoisomerase II activity, inhibits DNA polymerase activity which affects gene expression, and produces DNA-damaging free radicals). Cytarabine is a cell cycle phase-specific anti-metabolite which prevents DNA polymerase activity. The liposome carrying both drugs is preferentially taken up by leukemic cells compared to normal bone marrow cells. Once internalized in the leukemic cell, the liposome degrades, releasing the two chemotherapeutic agents.

Metabolism: Drug has a prolonged elimination half-life of 31.5 hours for daunorubicin and 40.4 hours for cytarabine with almost all the drugs remaining in the liposome in the plasma. Once released in the cell, daunorubicin is metabolized by aldoketo reductase and carbonyl reductase enzymes to the active metabolite daunorubicinol. Cytarabine is metabolized by cytidine deaminase to its inactive **metabolite**. Daunorubicin and its active metabolite are excreted in the urine (9% of administered dose) while cytarabine and its metabolite are excreted in the urine as well (71% of administered dose). Pharmacokinetics were not significantly different when drug administered to patients with mild or moderate renal dysfunction, but were not studied in patients with severe renal dysfunction. In patients with a bilirubin ≤ 3 mg/dL, pharmacokinetics were not significantly different.

Indications: Treatment of adults with newly-diagnosed therapy-related acute myelocytic leukemia (t-AML) or AML with **myelodysplasia**-related changes (AML-MRC).

Contraindications: History of serious hypersensitivity to daunorubicin, cytarabine, or any component of the formulation.

Dosage/Range:
- Induction: 1st: daunorubicin 44 mg/m^2 and cytarabine 100 mg/m^2 liposome IV over 90 minutes on Days 1,3,5; 2nd induction if needed (patient did not achieve a response): on Days 1 and 3 for subsequent cycles of induction.
- Consolidation: Daunorubicin 29 mg/m^2 and cytarabine 65 mg/m^2 liposome IV infusion over 90 minutes Days 1 and 3.
- DO NOT interchange with other daunorubicin and/or cytarabine containing products.

Dose Modifications:
- If a planned dose is missed, administer the dose as soon as possible and adjust the dosing schedule appropriately.
- HSRs: Interrupt drug infusion immediately, and manage symptoms; see below for resuming infusion at a reduced rate or discontinue treatment based on severity.

- Mild symptoms: once symptoms resolve, reinitiate infusion at half the prior rate of infusion. Consider premedication with antihistamines and/or corticosteroids for subsequent doses.
- Moderate symptoms: Do not reinitiate infusion. For subsequent infusions, premedicate with antihistamines and/or corticosteroids prior to infusion at same rate.
- Severe, life-threatening symptoms: permanently discontinue drug, and manage symptoms and closely monitor patient until symptoms resolve.
- Cardiotoxicity: Discontinue drug if cardiac function becomes impaired, unless benefit of continuing treatment outweighs risk (Jazz Pharmaceuticals, 2017).

Drug Preparation: Use PPE and standards for preparing hazardous drugs. Dose comes in a single-use vial without preservatives; do not save any unused portions for later use.

- Available as Daunorubicin 44 mg and cytarabine 100 mg encapsulated in liposome as a lyophilized cake in a single-dose glass vial for reconstitution.
- Calculate the Vyxeos dose based on daunorubicin and individual patient's BSA.
- Calculate the number of Vyxeos vials needed based on the daunorubicin dose. Remove appropriate number of vials from refrigerator and allow to come to room temperature over 30 minutes.
- Reconstitute each vial with 19 mL of Sterile Water for Injection using a sterile syringe and immediately thereafter start a 5-minute timer.
- **Carefully swirl the contents of the vial for 5 minutes** while gently inverting the vial every 30 seconds. Do not heat, vortex, or shake vigorously. After reconstitution, allow to rest for 15 minutes.
- The reconstituted solution should be opaque, purple, with homogenous dispersion, essentially free from visible particles. After reconstitution but before final dilution, the concentration is 2.2 daynorubicin and 5 mg cytarabine in each mL of reconstituted solution.
- Gently invert each vial 5 times prior to withdrawing the ordered dose from the vial for further dilution, If the reconstituted solution is not further diluted immediately, store it in the refrigerator at 2°–8°C for up to 4 hrs.
- To calculate ordered dose of reconstituted solution:
  - [volume required (mL) = dose daunorubicin (mg/m^2) $\times$ patient's BSA (m^2) divided by 2.2 (mg/mL)] (Jazz Pharmaceuticals, 2017).
- Asceptically withdraw the calculated volume of the reconstituted product from the vials(s) with a sterile syringe and transfer it toan infusion bag contining 500 mL or 0.9% Sodium Chloride Injection, USP or 5% Dextrose Injection, USP. There may be residual product remaining in the vial which should be discarded.
- Gently invert bag to mix solution: the color will be a deep purple, translucent, homogenous dispersion and free from visible particles.
- If the diluted infusion is not used immediately, store in refrigerator at 2–8°C for up to 4 hours. Inspect bag for particulate matter and discoloration prior to administration, and do not use if found.

Drug Administration:
- Assess cardiac function, CBC/differential, chemistries, LFTs, and renal function tests before Cycle 1 of induction, and before each consolidation cycle.

- If patient does not achieve remission after 1st induction cycle, a 2nd induction cycle may be administered 2–5 weeks after the 1st if no unacceptable toxicity.
- 1st consolidation cycle given 5–8 weeks after the start of the last induction (when ANC > 0.5 Gi/L and platelet count >50 Gi/L, and no unacceptable toxicity). Adminster the 2nd consolidation cycle in patients who have NO evidence of disease progression or unacceptable toxicity,
- Adminsiter by constant IV infusion over 90 minutes using an infusion pump through a central venous catheter or a peripheral IV. Do NOT use an in-line filter.
- Flush the line after drug administration with 0.9% Sodium Chloride Injection, USP or 5% Dextrose Injection, USP.

Drug Interactions:
- If coadministered with other drugs affecting cardiac function, monitor cardiac function more frequently.
- If coadministered with other drugs affecting hepatic function, monitor hepatic function more frequently.

Lab Effects/Interference:
- Neutropenia, thrombocytopenia, anemia.
- Hyponatremia, hypokalemia, hypoalbuminemia.
- Hyperbilirubinemia, increased alanine aminotransferase.

Special Considerations:
- Most common adverse effects (>25%): hemorrhagic events, febrile neutropenia, rash, edema, nausea, mucositis, diarrhea, constipation, musculoskeletal pain, fatigue, abdominal pain, dyspnea, headache, cough, decreased appetite, arrhythmia, pneumonia, bacteremia, chills, sleep disorders, and vomiting.
- Warnings and Precautions
  - Do not interchange with other daunorubicin and/or cytarabine –containing products: drugs have different formulations, dosing, and pharmacokinetics and are NOT interchangeable eg, liposomal daunorubicin, liposomal cytarabine, daunorubin HCL for injection).
  - *Hemorrhage*: related to prolonged thrombocytopenia have occurred, including fatal CNS bleeds.Incidence of any hemorrhage was 74% (compared to 56% in control arm). Epistaxis was most common, and grade 3 hemorrhage occurred in 12% of patients. Monitor cbc closely until recovery and administer platelet transfusions as needed.
  - *Cardiotoxicity*: the anthracycline daunorubicin can cause a cumulate cardiotoxicity. Increased risk of cardiotoxicity is related to prior anthracycline exposure, concomitant use of cardiotoxic drugs, oor previous RT to mediastinum. Prior to starting induction therapy, assess ECG, and LVEF findings from ECHO or MUGA. Repeat LVEF determination prior to consolidation, and as clinically required. If patient develops cardiac dysfunction, discontinue drug unless benefits outweigh the risk. Monitor cumulative daunorubicin exposure after each cycle (see package insert).
  - *HSRs*: serious or fatal HSRs have occurred, including anaphylactic reactions. Monitor patient closely during and after infusion. See dose modification.
  - *Copper overload*: Reconstituted drug contains 5 mg/mL copper gluconate, of which 14% is elemental copper (maximal theoretical copper exposure with full treatment is

106 mg/m^2. If a patient has Wilson's disease (or other copper-related metabolic disorder, monitor total serum copper, serum non-ceruloplasmin bound copper, 24-hour urine copper levels and serial neuropsychological examinations. Use this drug in these patients only if benefits outweigh the risk. If the patient has signs/symptoms of acute copper toxicity, discontinue Vyxeos.

- *Tissue necrosis*: daunorubicin is a vesicant which can cause severe local tissue necrosis at the site of drug extravasation. Administer this drug only by the IV route, never by subcutaneous or IM routes.
- *Embryo-fetal toxicity*: drug is feto-toxic. Teach females and males with female partners of reproductive potential to use effective contraception to avoid pregnancy during treatment and for 6 months after last dose.
- Nursing mothers should not breast feed while receiving the drug or for at least 2 weeks after the last dose.
- Male fertility may be compromised by this drug treaetment.

Potential Toxicities/Side Effects and the Nursing Process

I.   POTENTIAL FOR INFECTION AND BLEEDING related to BM DEPRESSION

Defining Characteristics: Hemorrhage occurred in 70% of patients compared to 49% in the standard 7+3 chemotherapy group. Febrile neutropenia occurred in 68%, and grade 3–5 was similar between the liposomal daunorubicin/cytarabine arm and the 7+3 chemotherapy group arm.Infections occurred as bacteremia (24%), catheter/device infection (16%), URI (18%), and sepsis (11%). Because of the long elimination half-life of the drug, prolonged neutropenia occurred in 17%, and prolonged thrombocytopenia 28%. Prolonged was defined as lasting past cycle day 42 in the absence of active leukemia. Patients experienced dyspnea (32%), pneumonia (26%), chills (23%), hypotension (20%), fungal infection (18%), hypoxia (18%), pyrexia (17%), and petechiae (11%).

Nursing Implications: Evaluate CBC/differential and discuss any abnormalities with physician prior to drug administration; assess for signs/symptoms of infection and bleeding; instruct patient in signs/symptoms of infection and bleeding and to report these immediately. Assess labs and patient closely as blood counts fall. Use scrupulous aseptic technique in managing central line catheter and monitor closely for infection. Teach patient self-care measures to minimize risk of infection and bleeding, including hand-washing, staying away from people with colds, avoidance of OTC aspirin-containing medications. Teach patient to call provider right away for T>100.4°F, chills, changes in mental status, or seek emergency medical care. See patient instructions in package insert.

II.   POTENTIAL FOR ALTERATION IN CARDIAC OUTPUT related to ACUTE AND CHRONIC CARDIAC CHANGES

Defining Characteristics: Acute effects (i.e., ECG changes, atrial arrhythmias) may occur in patients receiving anthracycline chemotherapy. Chronic myofibril damage resulting in

TREATMENT

irreversible cardiomyopathy is life threatening and dose related. Cumulative dose should not exceed 550 mg/m^2 or 400 mg/m^2 if patient is receiving/has received radiation to chest or with concurrent administration of cyclophosphamide or other cardiotoxic agent. Assess cumulative dose prior to giving next dose. Arrhythmias occurred in 30% of patients and non-conduction cardiotoxicity events in 20% of patients.

Nursing Implications: Assess baseline cardiac status, quality and regularity of heartbeat, and baseline ECG. Patient should have baseline MUGA or other measure of left ventricular ejection fraction at baseline, and prior to consolidation cycles during treatment. If there is a significant drop in ejection fraction, then drug should be stopped. Maintain accurate documentation of doses administered so that cumulative dose is known. Instruct patient to report dyspnea, shortness of breath, edema, orthopnea.

III. ALTERATION IN NUTRITION, LESS THAN BODY REQUIREMENTS, related to NAUSEA AND VOMITING, MUCOSTITIS, DIARRHEA, CONSTIPATION.

Defining Characteristics: Mild nausea and vomiting occur in 47% and 24% of patients respectively, and can be prevented with antiemetics. Mucositis occurred in 44% of patients. Diarrhea/colitis affected 45%, constipation (40%), and decreased appetite 29%,

Nursing Implications: Premedicate with antiemetics, and continue for 24 hours for protection. Assess oral mucosa prior to chemotherapy, teach patient a systematic oral hygiene regimen and self-assessment, and encourage patient to report burning or oral irritation. Assess pain in mouth, and administer analgesics as needed and ordered. Monitor bowel elimination status, implement plan to prevent/manage diarrhea/constipation, and teach patient self-management of diarrhea or constipation. If the patient is neutropenic and develops diarrhea (mucositis), it can result in a point of entry for bacteria and sepsis. It is critical to monitor this toxicity effectively.

IV. POTENTIAL FOR IMPAIRED SKIN INTEGRITY related to RASH, EDEMA, PRURITIS, AND DRUG EXTRAVASATION

Defining Characteristics: Rash occurred in 54% of patients, edema in 54%, and pruritis in 15%. Non-liposomal daunorubicin is a potent vesicant and will result in severe soft tissue damage if extravasated. Damage to skin from prior irradiation may be reactivated (radiation recall). Any break in skin integrity is a potential entry point for bacteria in a neutropenic patient may lead to sepsis.

Nursing Implications: As drug is infusing over 90 minutes, infusion via a central venous catheter is recommended. The nurse should be familiar with institution's policy for vesicant administration and management of extravasation. Manufacturer of non-liposomal daunorubicin recommends aspiration of any remaining drug from IV tubing, discontinuing IV, and applying ice. Manage itching.

Drug: decitabine (Dacogen, 5-aza-2-deoxycytidine)

Class: Nucleoside metabolic inhibitor (antimetabolite); molecular/genetic modulator.

Mechanism of Action: Drug is a pyrimidine analogue and prevents DNA synthesis in the S phase, leading to cell death. Drug is incorporated into DNA and inhibits DNA methyltransferase, causing hypomethylation and cellular differentiation or apoptosis (programmed cell death). Methyltransferase is an enzyme necessary for the expression of cellular genes. The cells in tumors that have progressed or that are resistant to therapy, characteristically have DNA *hyper*methylation. Decitabine "traps" DNA methyltransferase, thus greatly reducing its activity, which results in the synthesis of DNA that is *hypo*methylated. DNA hypomethylation results in activating genes that have been silent, causing the cell to differentiate, and then to die (cell death through disorganized gene expression or extinction of clones of cells that were terminally differentiated). Research has shown that the drug modulates tumor suppressor genes, the expression of tumor antigens, other genes, and overall cell differentiation. Non-proliferating cells are relatively insensitive to the drug.

Metabolism: Biphasic distribution, with mean terminal phase elimination half-life of 0.5 ± 0.31 hours. Drug is not plasma-bound to serum proteins. Metabolism not fully characterized, but appears to involve deamination in the liver, granulocytes, intestinal epithelium, and whole blood.

Indication: Treatment of patients with myelodysplastic syndromes (MDS), including: Previously treated and untreated, *de novo* and secondary MDS of all French-American-British subtypes (refractory anemia, refractory anemia with ringed sideroblast, refractory anemia, with excess blasts in transformation, chronic myelomonocytic leukemia), and Intermediate-1, Intermediate-2, and high-risk International Prognostic Scoring System groups.

Dosage/Range:
- MDS recommended treatment for at least 4 cycles of therapy; however, a CR or PR may take more than 4 cycles.

Option 1:
- Decitabine 15 mg/m^2 IV CI over 3 hours, repeated every 8 hours for 3 days.
- Subsequent treatment cycles: Repeat initial cycle every 6 weeks for a minimum of 4 cycles. Premedicate with antiemetic.
- Dose modification: Delay next cycle until ANC is 1,000/µL and platelets are 50,000/µL, and dose-reduce as follows:
  - Recovery requiring more than 6 but less than 8 weeks: Delay drug up to 2 weeks and then temporarily reduce dose to 11 mg/m^2 every 8 hours (33 mg/m^2 per day, 99 mg/m^2 per cycle) upon restarting therapy.
  - Recovery requiring more than 8 but less than 10 weeks: Assess BM for disease progression; if no progression, delay dose up to 2 more weeks and reduce dose to 11 mg/m^2 every 8 hours (33 mg/m^2 per day, 99 mg/m^2 per cycle) upon restarting therapy; maintain or dose increase in subsequent cycles as clinically indicated.

Option 2:
- Decitabine 20 mg/m^2 IV infusion over 1 hour, repeated daily × 5 days. Repeat cycle every 4 weeks. Premedicate with antiemetic therapy.
- Dose modification: If myelosuppression is present, subsequent treatment cycles of decitabine should be delayed until there is hematologic recovery (ANC = 1,000/μL, platelets = 50,000 μL).

Non-Hematologic toxicity: If any of the nonhematologic toxicities are present, do not restart until toxicity has resolved: serum creatinine ≥ 2 mg/dL, SGPT ≥ 2 times ULN; total bilirubin ≥ 2 times ULN; active or uncontrolled infection.

Drug Preparation:
- Drug supplied for injection as a sterile lyophilized white to almost-white powder in a single-dose vial containing 50 mg of decitabine. Store vials at 25°C (77°F) with excursions up to 15–30°C (59–86°F) permitted.
- Aseptically add 10 mL sterile water for injection (USP); upon reconstitution, each mL contains approximately 5.0 mg of decitabine at pH 6.7–7.3. Immediately after reconstitution, further dilute with 0.9% sodium chloride injection, or 5% dextrose injection, to a final drug concentration of 0.1–1.0 mg/mL. Use within 15 min of reconstitution, or prepare diluted solution with cold infusion fluids (2–8°C), then store at 2–8°C (36–46°F) for up to a maximum of 4 hours until administration. Inspect for clarity, and do not use if discolored or particulate matter present.

Drug Administration:
- Assess ANC/CBC prior to each cycle, and as needed. Assess LFTs and serum creatinine prior to the start of treatment. Assess patient for signs/symptoms of infection.
- Administer antiemetic.
- Administer decitabine:
  - Option 1: IV CI over 3 hours repeated every 8 hours for 3 days, repeated every 6 weeks.
  - Option 2: IV CI over 1 hour daily for 5 days, repeat cycle every 4 weeks.

Drug Interactions:
- Does not appear to affect P450 hepatic microenzymes.

Lab Effects/Interference:
- Neutropenia, thrombocytopenia, anemia.
- Hyperglycemia, hyperbilirubinemia, hypo- or hyperkalemia, hypomagnesemia.
- Increased BUN, AST, alkaline phosphatase.

Special Considerations:
- Most common adverse reactions (≥50%) are neutropenia, thrombocytopenia, anemia, and pyrexia.
- Warnings and Precautions:
  - *Neutropenia and thrombocytopenia* may be severe. CBC and platelet counts should be performed before each dosing cycle and as indicated. Consider early institution of growth factors and/or antimicrobial agents for the prevention or treatment of infections in patients with MDS.

- *Embryo-fetal toxicity*: Drug alters DNA synthesis, and may cause fetal harm; women of childbearing potential should be advised to avoid pregnancy during treatment and for one month following completion of therapy; if pregnancy occurs, the patient should be apprised of the potential hazard to the fetus. *Men should be advised not to father a child* while receiving decitabine, and for 2 months following completion of treatment. Men with female partners of childbearing potential should use effective contraception during this time.
- *Rare*ly, serious adverse events that occurred in patients receiving decitabine, regardless of causality, included cardiac events (MI, CHF, cardiopulmonary arrest, cardiomyopathy, atrial fibrillation, supraventricular tachycardia); fungal infection, bronchopulmonary aspergillosis, mycobacterium avium complex infection; intracranial hemorrhage.
- Nursing mothers should make a decision whether to stop nursing or discontinue dacitabine, taking into account the importance of the drug to the mother's health.
- Cases of Sweet's Syndrome (acute febrile neutrophilic dermatosis) have been described in post-marketing reports.

Potential Toxicities/Side Effects and the Nursing Process

I.   POTENTIAL FOR INFECTION AND BLEEDING related to BM DEPRESSION

Defining Characteristics: Dose-limiting factor is BM suppression. In MDS studies, the incidence of neutropenia was 90%, with 29% of patients developing febrile neutropenia. Thrombocytopenia occurred in 89% of patients. Drug is extensively metabolized in the liver, and partially excreted by the kidneys. Anemia occurs in 82% of patients.

Nursing Implications: Assess baseline CBC and differential, and platelet count, renal and hepatic function tests, prior to initial and subsequent cycles of chemotherapy. Drug should be held if ANC $<$ 1,000/μL platelets, 50,000/μL, BR $>$ 2.0 times ULN, AST $>$ 2 times ULN, creatinine $>$ 2.0 mg/dL (see Dosage). Discuss with physician early use of growth factor and/or antimicrobials for prevention of infection. Assess for signs/symptoms of infection, bleeding, and fatigue. Teach patient signs/symptoms of infection or bleeding, to report these immediately, and to come to the emergency room or clinic if febrile or bleeding. Teach patient self-care measures to minimize risk of infection and bleeding. This includes avoidance of crowds and proximity to people with infections, and avoidance of OTC aspirin-containing medications.

II.   ALTERED NUTRITION, LESS THAN BODY REQUIREMENTS, related to NAUSEA AND VOMITING, STOMATITIS

Defining Characteristics: Nausea and vomiting may occur, are mild to moderate, and are preventable by antiemetic medicines. Nausea occurs in 42% of patients and vomiting in 25% of patients. Stomatitis and dyspepsia occur in 12% of patients.

Nursing Implications: Premedicate patient with antiemetic. If patient develops nausea and/or vomiting, encourage small, frequent intake of cool, bland foods. Instruct patient to report nausea, and teach self-administration of antiemetic medications. If nausea/ vomiting occur and are severe, assess for signs/symptoms of fluid/electrolyte imbalance. Teach patient to self-administer antidiarrheal medications if needed. Assess baseline oral mucous membranes. Teach patient oral assessment, hygiene measures, and to report any alterations.

III.　ALTERATION IN COMFORT related to LETHARGY, FEVER, EDEMA, PAIN, RIGORS, ARTHRALGIAS

Defining Characteristics: Pyrexia affects 53% of patients, with rigors in 22% of patients, and fatigue occurred in 46%. Peripheral edema affects 25%, arthralgias 20%, and pain 13%. Catheter-site pain, erythema, and injection-site swelling occurred in 5% of patients.

Nursing Implications: Assess comfort level, symptoms experienced at baseline and prior to each dose, then prior to each cycle. Teach patient to alternate rest and activity periods. Teach patient to report fevers > 100.5°F, rigors right away, and to come to the clinic or ED. Teach patient symptomatic management of pain. Assess catheter and injection sites to rule out infection and to manage comfort.

Drug: degarelix (Firmagon)

Class: Gonadotropin-releasing hormone (GnRH) antagonist.

Mechanism of Action: Drug binds irreversibly to GnHR receptors in the pituitary gland and reduces the release of gonadotropins, thus reducing the serum levels of luteinizing hormone (LH) and follicle-stimulating hormone (FSH); this decreases the production of testosterone by the Leydig cells in the male testes. A 240-mg dose of degarelix achieves and maintains testosterone suppression below the castration level of 50 ng/dL.

Metabolism: Administered subcutaneously, degarelix forms a depot, which slowly releases the drug. The peak serum concentration (C_{max}) occurs 2 days after administration. The drug is widely distributed in body water and is 90% serum protein-bound. Drug undergoes protein hydrolysis as it passes through the hepatobiliary system, with about 70–80% metabolized and excreted in the feces and 20–30% excreted in the urine. Drug is not a substrate, inducer, or inhibitor of the P450 microenzyme system, or of the P-glycoprotein transport system. Elimination is biphasic, and the median terminal half-life of the drug is 53 days.

Indication: Drug is indicated for the treatment of patients with advanced prostate cancer.

Contraindication: Patients with (1) known hypersensitivity to degarelix or to any product components; and (2) women who are or may become pregnant (as drug can cause fetal harm).

Caution: Long-term androgen deprivation therapy prolongs the QTc interval; a risk-benefit analysis should precede use of degarelix in patients with congenital long QT syndrome, electrolyte abnormalities, CHF, or those who are taking Class IA or Class III antiarrhythmic drugs.

Drug Dosage/Range:
- Starting dose is 240 mg, and is administered subcutaneously as two injections of 120 mg each; administer deep subcutaneously in the abdomen ONLY in two separate areas.
- Maintenance dose is 80 mg given starting 28 days after initial dose and repeated every 28 days as a deep subcutaneous injection in the abdomen (ONLY).

Drug Preparation:
- Available in 80-mg and 120-mg vials. Drug must be administered within 1 hour after addition of sterile water for injection USP. Do not shake the vials. You will need gloves, alcohol pads, a clean, flat surface to work on (e.g., table), and a sharps disposal container for used syringes and needles.
- Initial: The drug pack contains 2 sets of degarelix 120-mg vial, 2–3 mL prefilled syringes containing sterile water for injection USP, 2 vial adapter, 2 injection needles, and 2 plunger rods (see package insert image). Uncap vial and use alcohol swab to wipe the rubber stopper; attach vial adapter to the vial until the spike pushes through the rubber stopper and snaps into place.
- Prepare the prefilled syringe by screwing the plunger rod into the syringe, and attach the syringe to the vial by screwing it on to the adapter. Transfer all sterile water for injection USP to the vial. With syringe still attached, swirl gently until liquid is clear. If powder adheres to side of vial above liquid surface, tilt vial slightly but do not shake, as foam will form. Reconstitution may take up to 15 minutes but usually takes a few minutes.
- Turn vial upside down and draw up to the 3-mL mark on the syringe for injection. Always withdraw the precise volume and expel air bubbles.
- Detach syringe from vial adapter, and aseptically attach administration needle to syringe.
- Immediately after reconstitution, inject 3 mL of degarelix 120 mg slowly as a deep subcutaneous injection. Repeat reconstitution procedure for the second 120-mg vial to complete the 240-mg starting dose and choose a different injection site for the second dose.
- Maintenance dose: the pack contains 1 set of degarelix 80-mg vial, 1 prefilled syringe containing 4.2 mL sterile water for injection USP, vial adapter, plunger rod, and administration needle. Use same procedure as above, but withdraw 4 mL of prepared drug into administration syringe. Administer immediately as a single 4-mL deep subcutaneous injection.
- **Drug should be used within 1 hour of reconstitution**.

Drug Administration: See package insert for step-by-step instructions of drug prep and administration.
- Starting dose is 240 mg, and is administered subcutaneously as two injections of 120 mg (3 mL) each; administer deep subcutaneously in the abdomen in two separate areas.
- Maintenance dose is 80 mg (4 mL) given starting 28 days after initial dose and repeated every 28 days as a deep subcutaneous injection in the abdomen.

- Pinch abdominal skin to achieve a deep subcutaneous injection, and insert the needle at a 45 degree angle; gently pull back the plunger to assess if needle is in vein; if blood aspirated into the syringe, product cannot be used and a new vial should be prepared.
- AVOID areas of abdominal pressure such as under belt or waistband, or near the ribs.
- Assess for hypersensitivity reactions (HSRs), including anaphylaxis, urticaria, and angioedema. Discontinue the injection immediately if not yet completed, and provide emergency support and intervention as ordered.
- Therapeutic effect should be monitored by baseline and periodic PSA testing. If the PSA rises, serum level of testosterone should be measured.
- Document injection site(s) and patient response; rotate sites on abdomen. Teach patient not to rub area of injection.

Lab Effects/Interference:
- Decreased serum LH, FSH, testosterone levels.
- Hypercholesterolemia (3–6% of patients).
- Increased liver transaminases and GGT.
- Prolonged QTc Interval.

Drug Interactions:
- Not tested, unknown.
- Clinically significant CYP450 drug–drug interactions are unlikely.

Special Considerations:
- Warnings and Precautions:
  - *Contraindicated* in women who are or may become pregnant.
  - *Hypersensitivity reactions (HSR)* may occur, including anaphylaxis, urticaria, and angioedema. If a serious HSR occurs, discontinue drug immediately, and manage reaction as clinically indicated and ordered. Do not rechallenge patient.
  - *Effect on QT/QTc Interval*: androgen deprivation may prolong the QT interval. Physicians should do a risk/benefit analysis with patients having congenital long QT syndrome, CHF, frequent electrolyte abnormalities, and patients taking other QTc prolonging drugs. Discuss with physician/NP/PA baseline ECG, serum electrolytes, and monitoring during therapy. Replete electrolyte abnormalities as ordered.
  - *Lab Tests:* Degarelix therapy results in pituitary gonadal suppression. Monitor PSA, and if PSA increases, assess testosterone serum concentration. Lab tests of pituitary gonadotropic or gonadal function may be affected during treatment and after completion of therapy.
- Use with caution in patients with severe liver or renal dysfunction. Degarelix exposure decreases 10% and 18% in patients with mild and moderate hepatic impairment (Ferring, 2015). Serum testosterone levels should be monitored monthly until medical castration is achieved, and then serum testosterone monitoring can decrease to every-other-month monitoring. Patients with severe hepatic dysfunction have not been studied, so extreme caution should be used.
- Drug is at least as effective as leuprolide in sustaining castration testosterone levels, and achieves this reduction significantly faster.

- Drug is a new-generation GnHR receptor antagonist with low histamine-release properties, without an initial testosterone surge seen in prior-generation GnHR receptor antagonists. Direct biochemical suppression of testosterone begins on day 1 of therapy.
- Long-term androgen suppression can cause QTc prolongation, so patients with risk factors such as CHF, or who are on other drugs that prolong the QTc interval, should be monitored closely with baseline and frequent ECG and QTc measurements during treatment. Monitor serum potassium, magnesium, and calcium, and ensure values are WNL.
- Hypertension occurs rarely in 6–7% of patients; monitor BP baseline and periodically during treatment.
- Most common adverse reactions occurring in 10% or more patients: injection-site reaction (pain, erythema, swelling, induration), hot flashes, increased weight, fatigue, and increased serum levels of transaminases and gamma glutamyltransferase. Most reactions were grade 1 or 2.

Potential Toxicities/Side Effects and the Nursing Process

I.   POTENTIAL ALTERATION IN COMFORT related to CHILLS, HOT FLUSHES, INJECTION-SITE PAIN, ARTHRALGIAS, ASTHENIA, INSOMNIA, COUGH

Defining Characteristics: Constitutional symptoms such as chills occur in 3–5% of patients, dizziness (9–11%), fatigue (3–23%), hot flushes (25–48%), injection-site pain (3–18%), injection-site reactions (35–44%), arthralgias (3–6%), asthenia (5–6%), back pain (3–9%), insomnia (3–8%), and cough (3–10%). Injection-site reactions were primarily transient, mild to moderate in intensity, occurred with the starting dose, and led to few discontinuations (<1%).

Nursing Implications: Assess baseline comfort, and tell patient these symptoms may occur. Discuss self-care strategies, and teach patient to report side effects that do not resolve. Assess abdominal subcutaneous injection sites for irritation, and teach patient that warm or cold compresses following drug administration may reduce discomfort. Ensure that drug is administered in abdominal sites that are NOT under belt lines, close to the ribs, or in areas that will be under pressure.

II.   POTENTIAL ALTERATION IN NUTRITION related to CONSTIPATION, DIARRHEA, WEIGHT GAIN

Defining Characteristics: Weight gain occurs in 6–13% of patients, constipation in 3–6%, and diarrhea in 3–9% of patients.

Nursing Implications: Assess baseline nutritional status, weight, and elimination status. Teach patient that these side effects may occur and to report them.

III. POTENTIAL ALTERATION IN SEXUALITY related to ERECTILE DYSFUNCTION

Defining Characteristics: Erectile dysfunction occurs in 3–9% of patients, nocturia in 2–11%, and urinary tract infections in 1–7%.

Nursing Implications: Assess baseline sexuality and teach patient that these side effects may occur and to report them. Discuss possible management strategies with physician, and revise plan as needed.

Drug: docetaxel (Taxotere)

Class: Microtubule inhibitor, taxoid, mitotic spindle poison.

Mechanism of Action: Enhances microtubule assembly and inhibits disassembly. Disrupts microtubule network that is essential for mitotic and interphase cellular function. Drug binds to free tubulin and promotes the assembly of tubulin into stable microtubules and also prevents their disassembly. Stabilization of microtubules inhibits mitosis. At low weekly doses, drug may have antiangiogenic properties.

Metabolism: Drug is extensively protein-bound (94–97%). Triphasic elimination. Metabolism involves P450 3A (CYP3A4) isoenzyme system (in vitro testing). Fecal elimination is main route, accounting for excretion of 75% of the drug and its metabolites within 7 days; 80% of the fecal excretion occurs during the first 48 hours. Mild to moderate liver impairment (SGOT and/or SGPT > 1.5 times normal and alk phos > 2.5 times normal) results in decreased clearance of drug by an average of 27%, resulting in a 38% increase in systemic exposure (AUC).

Indications: Docetaxel is a microtubule inhibitor indicated for the treatment of

- Breast cancer: (1) as a single agent in the treatment of locally advanced or metastatic breast cancer after chemotherapy failure, and (2) with doxorubicin and cyclophosphamide as adjuvant treatment of operable, node-positive breast cancer.
- NSCLC: (1) as a single agent for the treatment of locally advanced or metastatic NSCLC after platinum therapy failure, and (2) with cisplatin for the treatment of unresectable, locally advanced, or metastatic untreated NSCLC.
- Castration-resistant prostate cancer (CRPC): with prednisone, in androgen-independent (hormone refractory) metastatic prostate cancer.
- Gastric adenocarcinoma (GC): with cisplatin and fluorouracil for untreated advanced gastric adenocarcinoma, including the gastroesophageal junction.
- Squamous cell carcinoma of the head and neck cancer (SCCHN): with cisplatin and fluorouracil for induction treatment of locally advanced SCCHN.

Contraindications: (1) hypersensitivity to docetaxel or polysorbate 80; (2) neutrophil counts < 1,500 cells/mm^3.

Dosage/Range:

- All patients must receive premedication with antiemetics, as well as appropriate hydration (prior to and after cisplatin if cisplatin given in combination). Must be administered in a clinical setting equipped to manage potential infusion complications including anaphylaxis.
- Breast Cancer: (1) adjuvant breast cancer: docetaxel 75 mg/m^2 IV administered 1 hour after doxorubicin 50 mg/m^2 IVP and cyclophosphamide 500 mg/m^2 IV q 3 weeks × 6 cycles, with G-CSF support PRN; (2) locally advanced or metastatic breast cancer: 60–100 mg/m^2 IV as a 1-hour infusion every 3 weeks, as a single agent.
- NSCLC: (1) after platinum therapy failure: 75 mg/m^2 single agent, every 3 weeks; (2) chemotherapy-naive: 75 mg/m^2 followed by cisplatinum 75 mg/m^2 IV over 30–60 min every 3 weeks.
- CRPC: docetaxel 75 mg/m^2 IV infusion over 1 hour, repeated q 21 days, in combination with prednisone 5 mg PO bid continuously.
- Advanced gastric adenocarcinoma: 75 mg/m^2 as a 1-hour infusion followed by cisplatin 75 mg/m^2 over 1–3 hours (both on day 1 only), followed by fluorouracil 750 mg/m^2 per day as a 24-hour IV infusion (days 1–5), starting at the end of cisplatin infusion. Cycle is repeated every 3 weeks. Patients must receive premedication with antiemetics and hydration prior to and following cisplatin administration.
- Head and Neck Cancer:
  - **Induction therapy followed by RT (locally advanced inoperable):** 75 mg/m^2 IV over 1 hr (day 1), followed by cisplatin 75 mg/m^2 (IV over 1 hour, day 1) followed by fluorouracil 750 mg/m^2 per day as a 24-hr IV infusion (days 1–5), starting at end of cisplatin infusion, for 4 cycles. After last cycle of chemotherapy, patients should receive RT.
  - **Induction therapy followed by chemoradiation (locally advance unresectable, low surgical cure, or organ preservation):** 75 mg/m^2 IV over 1 hr (day 1), followed by cisplatin 100 mg/m^2 IV over 30 min–3 hr, day 1, followed by fluorouracil 1,000 mg/m^2 per day as a 24-hr IV infusion (days 1–4), starting at end of cisplatin infusion, repeated every 3 weeks for 3 cycles. Following chemotherapy, patients should receive chemoradiotherapy.

Docetaxel Premedication regimen with corticosteroids:

- All patients should receive oral corticosteroids as premedication (e.g., dexamethasone 8 mg PO bid × 3 days, starting 1 day prior to docetaxel) to reduce the incidence and severity of fluid retention and hypersensitivity reactions.
- For patients HRPC receiving prednisone, the doses of oral dexamethasone are 8 mg at 12 hours, 3 hours, and 1 hour prior to docetaxel dose.

Dose reductions: See package insert.

1. Patients with **breast cancer** dosed initially at 100 mg/m^2 who experience either febrile neutropenia, ANC < 500/mm^3 for >1 week, or severe or cumulative cutaneous reactions, or other grades 3–4 nonhematologic toxicity, should have dose reduced to 75 mg/m^2. If reactions continue at the reduced dose, further reduce to 55 mg/m^2 or discontinue drug. Patients dosed initially at 60 mg/m^2 who do NOT experience febrile

neutropenia, ANC < 500/mm^3 for >1 week, nadir platelets <25,000 cells/mm^3, severe cutaneous reactions, or severe PN during drug therapy may tolerate higher drug doses and may be dose escalated. Patients who develop ≥ grade 3 PN should have drug discontinued.

2. Patients receiving **adjuvant treatment of breast cancer who** experience febrile neutropenia should receive G-CSF in all subsequent cycles; if febrile neutropenia recurs, continue G-CSF and dose-reduce docetaxel to 60 mg/m^2. Patients who develop grades 3–4, severe or cumulative cutaneous reactions, or moderate neurosensory signs and/or symptoms should have docetaxel dose reduced to 60 mg/m^2. Patients who experience grades 3–4 stomatitis, should have dose reduced to 60 mg/m^2. If patient continues to experience these reactions on the reduced dose, treatment should be discontinued.

3. Patients with **NSCLC receiving monotherapy**, dosed initially at 75 mg/m^2, who experience febrile neutropenia, ANC < 500 mg/m^2 for >1 week, severe or cumulative cutaneous reactions, or other nonhematologic toxicity grade 3 or 4 should have treatment withheld until toxicity resolves and then have dose reduced to 55 mg/m^2; patients who develop grade 3 or greater PN should discontinue docetaxel chemotherapy.

4. Patients with **NSCLC receiving combination therapy** who are initially dosed at 75 mg/m^2 in combination with cisplatin and whose platelet nadir count during the previous course of therapy is <25,000 cells/mm^3, or who develop febrile neutropenia, or serious nonhematologic toxicities should have a docetaxel dose reduction to 65 mg/m^2 in subsequent cycles. If a further dose reduction is necessary, reduce dose to 50 mg/m^2.

5. Patients with **HRPC** who experience febrile neutropenia, ANC < 500/mm^3 for >1 week, or severe or cumulative cutaneous reactions, or moderate neurosensory signs and/or symptoms during docetaxel therapy should have dose reduced from 75 mg/m^2 to 60 mg/m^2. If the same symptoms arise at the reduced dosage, the drug should be discontinued.

6. Patients with **gastric or SCCHN** receiving docetaxel in combination with cisplatin and fluorouracil must receive antiemetics and appropriate hydration.

   • G-CSF is recommended for second and subsequent cycles if the patient develops febrile neutropenia, neutropenic infection, or neutropenia lasting more than 7 days. If neutropenic fever, infection, or prolonged neutropenia occur despite G-CSF, reduce docetaxel dose from 75 mg/m^2 to 60 mg/m^2; if neutropenic complications continue to occur despite dose reduction and G-CSF, reduce dose to 45 mg/m^2. In the case of grade 4 thrombocytopenia, dose-reduce docetaxel from 75 mg/m^2 to 60 mg/m^2.

   • Retreatment with docetaxel requires that neutrophils recover to >1,500 cells/mm^3 and platelets recover to >100,000 cells/mm^3. Drug should be discontinued if toxicities persist.

   • Dose modifications of fluorouracil (5-FU): (1) **grade 3 diarrhea,** first episode, reduce 5-FU dose by 20%; second episode, reduce docetaxel dose by 20% as well; (2) If **grade 4 diarrhea** occurs, first episode reduce 5-FU and docetaxel doses by 20%; if second episode occurs, discontinue treatment; (3) **grade 3 stomatitis/mucositis**: first episode, reduce 5-FU dose by 20%; second episode, stop 5-FU only in this and all subsequent cycles; third episode, dose-reduce docetaxel by 20%; (4) **grade 4**

stomatitis/mucositis: first episode, stop 5-FU only in this and all subsequent cycles; second episode, dose-reduce docetaxel by 20%.

- **Liver Impairment**: (1) AST/ALT >2.5–≤ 5 × ULN and AP ≤2.5 × ULN or AST/ALT >1.5 to ≤5 × ULN and AP >2.5 to ≤5 × ULN, dose reduce docetaxel by 20% ; (2) AST/ALT > 5 × ULN and/or AP > 5 × ULN stop docetaxel.

- Cisplaatin dose modification for **peripheral neuropathy**: (1) grade 2: reduce cisplatin dose by 20%; (2) grade 3: discontinue cisplatin. If grade 3 toxicity, discontinue treatment.

- **Nephrotoxicity** from cisplatin: (1) serum creatinine ≥ grade 2 (>1.5 × normal value) despite adequate rehydration, determine CrCl before each subsequent cycle: (2) CrCl = ≥ 60 mL/min = full dose cisplatin; (3) CrCl = 40–60 mL/min = reduce cisplatin dose by 50% at subsequent cycle; if CrCl was >60 mg/mL at end of cycle, full cisplatin dose was reinstituted at the next cycle; if no recovery seen, cisplatin was omitted from next treatment cycle; (4) CrCl is <40 mL/minL: cisplatin dose was omitted in that treatment cycle only; if CrCl was still <40 mL/min at the end of the cycle, discontinue cisplatin; if CrCl was >40 mL/min but < 60 mL/min at end of cycle, a 50% cisplatin dose was given in the next cycle; if CrCl was >60 mL/min at end of cycle, full cisplatin dose was given at next cycle.

- **Palmar plantar erythrodysesthesia**: Grade 2 or higher, stop 5-FU until recovery, and when resume, dose of 5-FU is reduced 20%.

- **Other grade > 3 toxicities** except alopecia and anemia, delay chemotherapy for a minimum of 2 weeks from the planned infusion date until resolution to ≤ grade 1, and then therapy resumed as medically appropriate.

- See package insert for docetaxel, cisplatin, and fluorouracil dose modifications and delays.

- **Combination therapy with Strong CYP3A4 Inhibitors:** avoid using concomitant strong CYP3A4 inhibitors (e.g., ketoconazole, itraconazole, clarithromycin, atazanavir, indinavir, nefazodone, nelfinavir, ritonavir, saquinavir, telithromycin, and voriconazole). If coadministration medically necessary, consider 50% docetaxel dose reduction.

Drug Preparation (requires two dilutions prior to administration):
- Vials available as 20-mg/2-mL single-use vial, and 80-mg/8-mL and 160-mg/16-mL multi-use vials. Drug contains polysorbate 80.
- Use only a 21-gauge needle to withdraw docetaxel injection from the vial (Hospira, 2014).
- Use only glass or polypropylene or polyolefin plastic (bag) IV containers.
- Asceptically withdraw the ordered amount of docetaxel injection USP (10 mg docetaxel/mL) | with a calibrated syringe and inject into a 250 mL infusion bag or bottle of 5% dextrose or 0.9% sodium chloride to produce a final concentration of 0.3–0.74 mg/mL. If a dose > 200 mg of docetaxel is required, use a larger volume of the infusion vehicle so that a concentration of 0.74 mg/mL is not exceeded.
- Thoroughly mix by gentle manual rotation.
- Inspect for any particulate matter or discoloration, and if found, discard.

TREATMENT

- Use infusion solution immediately; solution is stable under the following conditions:
  - Docetaxel Injection USP infusion solution, if stored between 2°C and 25°C (36°F–77°F), is stable for 4 hours, in either 0.9% sodium chloride or 5% dextrose solution. Use within 4 hours.

Drug Administration:

- ANC $\geq$ 1,500 cells/m^3; BR must be $<$ ULN; AST and ALT $<$ 1.5 $\times$ ULN concomitant with alkaline phosphatase $<$ 2.5 $\times$ ULN. Assess patient's ANC and liver function studies, and if abnormal, discuss with physician. See Special Considerations.
- Use only glass or polypropylene bottles, or polypropylene or polyolefin plastic bags for drug infusion, and administer infusion ONLY through polyethylene-lined administration sets. Visually inspect infusion bottle/bag for particulate matter or discoloration prior to administration.
- Patient should receive corticosteroid premedication (e.g., dexamethasone 8 mg bid) for 3 days beginning 1 day before drug administration to reduce the incidence and severity of fluid retention and hypersensitivity reactions. See *Dosage/Range.*
- Infuse drug over 1 hour.
- Assess for severe hypersensitivity reactions (HSRs), as generalized rash/erythema, hypotension, bron chospasm or, very rarely, fatal anaphylaxis have been described, despite premedication. Immediately stop drug and provide emergency management as ordered.
- Assess need for G-CSF.

Drug Interactions:

- Radiosensitizing effect.
- Theoretically, CYP3A4 inhibitors, such as ketoconazole, erythromycin, troleandomycin, cyclosporine, terfenadine, and nifedipine, can inhibit docetaxel metabolism and result in elevated serum levels of docetaxel; use together with caution or not at all.
- Theoretically, CYP3A4 inducers, such as anticonvulsants and St. John's wort, may increase metabolism and decrease serum levels of docetaxel.
- Calcitriol (high dose, DN-101): suggested increase in patient survival without added toxicity in patients with prostate cancer (Beer et al., 2007).

Lab Effects/Interference:

- Decreased CBC.

Special Considerations:

- Administration of docetaxel in Europe is not subject to U.S. Federal Drug Administration recommendations; non-PVC containers and tubing are not required.
- Warnings and Precautions:
  - *Treatment-related mortality* increases with abdnormal liver function at higher doses and in patients with breast cancer or NSCLC who had prior platinum-based therapy and who received docetaxel at 100 mg/m^2.
  - *Hepatic impairment:* Patients treated with elevated bilirubin or abnormal transaminases plus alkaline phosphatase have an increased risk of grade 4 neutropenia, febrile neutropenia, severe stomatitis, infections, severe thrombocytopenia, severe skin toxicity, and toxic death.

- Docetaxel should not be administered to patients if bilirubin $>$ upper limit of normal (ULN) or if ALT and/or AST $> 1.5 \times$ ULN concomitant with alkaline phosphatase $> 2.5 \times$ ULN.
- LFT elevations increase risk of severe or life-threatening complications.
- Assess LFTs prior to each treatment cycle.

- *Hematologic effects*: monitor CBC/differential frequently and dose-interrupt or dose-reduce per package insert. Drug should not be administered if neutrophil counts are $<$1,500 cells/mm^3. Obtain frequent blood counts and monitor for neutropenia. Hematologic responses, febrile reactions, and rates of septic death for different regimens are dose related.

- *Severe hypersensitivity reactions (HSRs)* have occurred, including very rare fatal anaphylaxis, despite premedication with 3 days of corticosteroids. HSRs may occur within minutes of initiation of docetaxel. Assess whether patient has previously had a reaction to paclitaxel as there is cross-sensitivity. Monitor patients closely during the first and second infusions for signs and symptoms, e.g., generalized rash/erythema, hypotension, and/or bronchospasm. Discontinue drug immediately for severe HSRs (e.g., characterized by generalized rash/erythema, hypotension, and/or bronchospasm, or rarely anaphylaxis) and provide aggressive medical intervention as ordered by physician or NP/PA. Do not rechallenge patients who have had a severe HSR.

- *Entercolitis and neutropenic colitis (typhlitis):* has occurred in patients receiving docetaxel alone or in combination with other chemotherapy, despite G-CSF. Monitor patients closely from onset of any symptoms of GI toxicity, and teach patients to call their provider right away with new or worsening symptoms of GI toxicity.

- *Severe fluid retention* may occur despite dexamethasone. If the patient has preexisting effusions, closely monitor the patient for possible exacerbation of effusions. If fluid retention occurs, it begins in the lower extremities, may become generalized, and patients gain a median of 2 kg. Monitor patient weight.

- *Acute myeloid leukemia (AML) or MDS* may rarely occur after treatment with the drug.

- *Cutaneous reactions* (severe skin toxicity): localized erythema of extremities with edema, followed by desquamation, has occurred. Severe skin toxicity did not occur in clinical trials in patients who received premedication with 3-day corticosteroids.

- *Neurologic reactions*: severe neurosensory symptoms (e.g., paresthesia, dysesthesia, pain) may occur and require a dose adjustment (see package insert). If symptoms persist, the drug should be discontinued. Patients for whom follow-up data were available in clinical trials had spontaneous reversal of symptoms with a median of 9 weeks from onset. Severe peripheral motor neuropathy occurred in 4.4% of patients and was mainly distal extremity weakness.

- *Eye disorders*: cystoid macular edema (CME) has been reported. If a patient has impaired vision while on treatment, a comprehensive ophthalmologic exam should be done promptly. If CME is diagnosed, docetaxel should be discontinued, and visual impairment treated per the ophthamologist. Alternative nontaxane therapy should be considered.

- *Asthenia* may be severe (reported in 14.9% of metastatic breast cancer patients), lasting a few days to several weeks.

- *Embryo-fetal toxicity*: Drug is fetotoxic. Women of childbearing potential should use effective contraception to avoid pregnancy. If the drug is used during pregnancy or if the patient becomes pregnant while receiving the drug, the patient should be apprised of the potential hazard to the fetus. Nursing mothers should make a decision to discontinue nursing or to discontinue the drug, taking into account the importance of the drug to the mother's health.

• *Alcohol content*: cases of intoxication have been reported relating to some formulations of docetaxel-containing alcohol. Alcohol may affect the CNS. Teach patients to have someone drive them following treatment and not to use machines immediately after the infusion. Each docetaxel dose of 100 mg/m^2 delivers 1.8 g/m^2 of ethanol (e.g., if BSA 2.0 m^2 this would be 3.6 grams of ethanol. Different docetaxel products may have a different amount of alcohol.

Potential Toxicities/Side Effects and the Nursing Process

I. POTENTIAL FOR INJURY related to HYPERSENSITIVITY OR ANAPHYLAXIS REACTIONS

Defining Characteristics: Severe hypersensitivity reactions characterized by hypotension, dyspnea and/or bronchospasm, or generalized rash/erythema occurred in 2.2% (2 of 92) of patients who received 3-day dexamethasone premedication. If patient experiences a severe hypersensitivity reaction, patient should not be rechallenged with docetaxel (e.g., patients with bronchospasm, angioedema, systolic BP < 80 mmHg, generalized urticaria). Minor allergic reactions are characterized by flushing, chest tightness, or low back pain.

Nursing Implications: Ensure that patient has taken premedication (e.g., dexamethasone 8 mg bid starting 1 day prior to chemotherapy). Assess baseline VS and mental status prior to drug administration, especially first and second doses of the drug. Monitor VS every 15 minutes, and remain with patient during first 15 minutes of drug infusion, as most reactions occur during the first 10 minutes. Stop drug if cardiac arrhythmia (irregular apical pulse) or hypo- or hypertension occur and discuss continuance of infusion with physician. Recall signs/symptoms of anaphylaxis, and if these occur, stop drug immediately and notify physician. Subjective symptoms are generalized itching, nausea, chest tightness, crampy abdominal pain, difficulty speaking, anxiety, agitation, sense of impending doom, uneasiness, desire to urinate/defecate, dizziness, chills. Objective signs are flushed appearance; angioedema of face, neck, eyelids, hands, feet; localized or generalized urticaria; respiratory distress with or without wheezing, hypotension, cyanosis. Review standing orders or nursing procedure for patient management of anaphylaxis, and be prepared to stop drug immediately if signs/symptoms occur, keep IV line open with 0.9% sodium chloride, notify physician, monitor VS, and administer ordered medications, which may include epinephrine 1:1,000, hydrocortisone sodium succinate, and diphenhydramine. Teach patient the potential of a hypersensitivity or anaphylactic reaction and to report any unusual symptoms immediately. Depending upon severity of reaction, when planning subsequent treatment discuss with physician administration of antihistamine prior to docetaxel and also gradual increase in infusion rate, e.g., starting at 8-hour rate × 5 minutes, then increasing to 4-hour rate × 5 minutes, then 2-hour rate × 5 minutes, and finally 1-hour infusion rate.

II.   POTENTIAL FOR INFECTION AND BLEEDING related to BM DEPRESSION

Defining Characteristics: Neutropenia may be severe, is dose related, is the dose-limiting toxicity, and is noncumulative. Nadir is day 7, with recovery by day 15. There have been some incidences of grade 4 neutropenia (ANC < 500 mm^3) in 2,045 patients (any tumor type) with normal hepatic function. There have also been incidences of febrile neutropenia requiring IV antibiotics and/or hospitalization in some patients, and a small percentage of incidences of septic deaths. Severe thrombocytopenia was less common. However, fatal GI bleeding has been reported in patients with severe hepatic impairment who received docetaxel.

Nursing Implications: Assess LFTs, as dose generally should not be given if SGOT, SGPT, alk phos, or bili suggest moderate to severe hepatic dysfunction (see Special Considerations section). Assess baseline CBC and differential to ensure that ANC is >1,500/mm^3, and platelet count is >100,000/mm^3 prior to chemotherapy, as well as for signs/symptoms of infection or bleeding. Teach patient signs/symptoms of infection or bleeding and to report these immediately, and teach patient self-care measures to minimize risk of infection and bleeding. This includes avoidance of crowds and proximity to people with infections, and avoidance of OTC aspirin-containing medications. Teach patient self-administration of G-CSF as ordered to prevent severe neutropenia, and EPO as ordered to prevent severe anemia/transfusion requirements. Instruct patient to alternate rest and activity periods, and to report increased fatigue, shortness of breath, or chest pain that might herald severe anemia.

III.   POTENTIAL ALTERATION IN ACTIVITY TOLERANCE related to ASTHENIA, FATIGUE, MYALGIA, ANEMIA

Defining Characteristics: Fatigue, weakness, and malaise may last from a few days to several weeks, but is rarely severe enough to be dose limiting. There is some incidence of asthenia (all grades) and some incidence of anemia, with grades 3 and 4 occurring in some at doses of 100 mg/m^2 and in doses of 75 mg/m^2.

Nursing Implications: Assess Hgb/HCT prior to each treatment and at nadir counts. Assess patient activity tolerance and ability to do ADLs. Teach patient self-care strategies to minimize exertion, and maximize activity, such as clustering activity during shopping, alternating rest and activity periods, diet, gentle exercise. Teach self-administration of EPO, if ordered, to prevent severe anemia/transfusion requirements. Instruct patient to alternate rest and activity periods, and to report increased fatigue, shortness of breath, or chest pain that might herald severe anemia.

IV.   POTENTIAL ALTERATION IN FLUID BALANCE related to FLUID RETENTION

Defining Characteristics: Fluid retention is a cumulative toxicity that may occur in docetaxel-treated patients. Peripheral edema usually begins in the lower extremities and may become generalized with weight gain (2 kg average). Fluid retention is not associated with cardiac, renal, or hepatic impairment and may be minimized by use of dexamethasone 8 mg bid for 3 days beginning the day prior to therapy. Severe fluid retention may occur in up to 6.5% of patients despite premedication, and is characterized by generalized edema, poorly tolerated peripheral edema, pleural effusion requiring drainage, dyspnea at rest, cardiac tamponade, or abdominal distention (due to ascites). Fluid retention usually resolves completely within 16 weeks of last docetaxel dose (range, 0–42 weeks).

Nursing Implications: Ensure that patient takes corticosteroids as ordered to minimize the risk of developing fluid retention. Assess baseline weight and skin turgor, especially in the extremities. Assess respiratory status, including breath sounds. Instruct patient to report any alterations in breathing patterns, swelling in the extremities, and weight gain. If patient has preexisting effusion, monitor effusion closely during treatment. If fluid retention occurs, instruct patient to elevate extremities while at rest. Teach patient not to use added salt when eating or cooking. Discuss with physician use of diuretics for new-onset edema, progression of edema, and weight gain, e.g., $\geq$ 2 lb.

V. POTENTIAL IMPAIRMENT OF SKIN INTEGRITY related to RASH, ALOPECIA, NAIL CHANGES

Defining Characteristics: Maculopapular, violaceous/erythematous, and pruritic rash may occur, usually on the feet and/or hands, but may also occur on arms, face, or thorax. These localized eruptions usually occur within 1 week of last docetaxel treatment, and are reversible and usually resolve prior to next treatment. Overall, there are some patients who do experience skin problems. Palmar–plantar erythrodysesthia (HFS) may occur but can be minimized by adherence to 3-day corticosteroid premedication. Drug extravasation may cause skin discoloration, but no necrosis. Most patients on every-3-week schedules experience alopecia. Changes in nails may occur in some of patients, and may be severe in a small percentage of patients (hypo- or hyperpigmentation, onycholysis [loss of nail]).

Nursing Implications: Assess skin for any cutaneous changes, such as rash, and any associated symptoms, such as pruritus, and discuss management with physician. If patient develops severe or cumulative skin toxicity, docetaxel dose should be reduced (see Special Considerations). Instruct patient in self-care measures such as avoidance of abrasive skin products and clothing, avoidance of tight-fitting clothes, the use of skin emollients appropriate for skin problem, and measures to prevent itching. Discuss potential impact of hair loss prior to drug administration, coping strategies, and plan to minimize body-image distortion (e.g., wig, scarf, cap). Assess patient for signs/symptoms of hair loss. Assess patient's response and use of coping strategies; help patient to build on effective strategies. Teach patient self-care measures to preserve hair, such as washing hair with warm water, use of a gentle shampoo and conditioner, use of a soft-bristle brush, cutting hair short to reduce pressure on hair shaft, and use of a satin pillowcase to minimize friction on hair shaft. Teach patient to wear a wide-brimmed hat and sunglasses when outside, and to use sunscreen (at least SPF 15) on scalp when outdoors without a hat. Assess nails baseline, and teach patient to report changes. Teach patient to keep nails clean and trimmed, not to wear nail polish or imitation nails, and to wear protective gloves when doing house cleaning and gardening. Teach patient to use a nail hardener if nails appear soft, and to use Lotrimin cream if ordered. Severe skin problems require a dose reduction.

VI.   SENSORY/PERCEPTUAL ALTERATIONS related to SENSORY NEUROPATHY

Defining Characteristics: Grades 1–4 PN may affect many patients, a small percentage severe. Sensory alterations are paresthesias in a glove-and-stocking distribution, and numbness. There may be loss of sensation symmetrically, of vibration, and of proprioception. Risk is increased in patients receiving both docetaxel and cisplatin, or in patients with prior neuropathy from diabetes mellitus or alcohol. Extremity weakness or transient myalgia may also occur. Patients described spontaneous reversal of symptoms in a median of 9 weeks from onset (range 0–106 weeks).

Nursing Implications: Assess baseline neurologic status. Instruct patient to report signs/symptoms of pins-and-needle sensation, numbness, pain, increased discomfort with certain sensations, especially in the extremities, or motor weakness. Identify patients at risk: those with history of cisplatin use or with preexisting neuropathies (ethanol- and diabetes mellitus–related). Assess sensory and motor function prior to each treatment, and if abnormality found, assess impact on patient's function, safety, independence, and quality of life. Test patient's ability to button a shirt or pick up a dime from a flat surface. If severely impacting safety or quality of life, discuss with patient and physician drug discontinuance or use of cytoprotective agent. Teach self-care strategies, including maintaining safety when walking, getting up, taking bath, or washing dishes; discuss inability to sense temperature and the need to keep extremities warm in cold weather. Docetaxel should be discontinued if patient develops grade 3 or 4 PN (see NCI Common Toxicity Criteria of Adverse Effects, *Appendix II*). Grade 3 motor = objective weakness, interfering with ADLs; grade 3 sensory = sensory loss or paresthesia interfering with ADLs; grade 4 motor = paralysis; grade 4 sensory = permanent sensory loss that interferes with function.

VII.   ALTERED NUTRITION, LESS THAN BODY REQUIREMENTS, related to NAUSEA AND VOMITING, DIARRHEA, CONSTIPATION, DYSGEUSIA, ANOREXIA, STOMATITIS

Defining Characteristics: Nausea and vomiting may occur, but are mild and preventable with antiemetics. Diarrhea occurs and is mild; incidence of any grade of nausea is 33–42%, vomiting 22%, and diarrhea 22–42%. Incidence of stomatitis is 26–51% (severe 5.5%). Only 1.1% of breast cancer patients who received 3-day corticosteroid treatment developed severe mucositis.

Nursing Implications: Premedicate patient with antiemetic. If patient develops nausea and/or vomiting, encourage small, frequent intake of cool, bland foods. Instruct patient to report nausea, and teach self-administration of antiemetic medications. If nausea/vomiting occur and are severe, assess for signs/symptoms of fluid/electrolyte imbalance. Encourage patient to report onset of diarrhea. Teach patient to self-administer antidiarrheal medications if needed. Assess baseline oral mucous membranes. Ensure that patient takes 3-day corticosteroid regimen. Teach patient oral assessment, hygiene measures, and to report any alterations.

VIII. ALTERATION IN VISION, POTENTIAL, related to HYPERLACRIMATION

Defining Characteristics: Epiphora or hyperlacrimation occurs as a result of lacrimal duct stenosis. There is inflammation of the conjunctiva and ductal epithelium, which occurs chronically, especially with weekly docetaxel therapy. This appears related to cumulative dose, usually about 300 mg/m^2 and resolves after treatment is stopped. Stenosis of tear ducts is reversible.

Nursing Implications: Assess baseline vision and function of tear ducts. Teach patient that this may occur, and to report it. If this occurs, teach patient to use "artificial tears" frequently throughout day, or saline eyewash. Discuss with physician use of prophylactic steroid ophthalmic solution, such as prednisolone acetate 2 gtt bid × 3 days, beginning the day before docetaxel treatment, if patient does not have a history of herpetic eye infection. If the patient is on weekly therapy, discuss with physician treatment break × 2 weeks for symptoms to resolve, and resumption of therapy on a 3-week-on, 1-week-off schedule.

Drug: doxorubicin hydrochloride (Adriamycin)

Class: Anthracycline antibiotic isolated from streptomycin products, in particular from the rhodomycin products.

Mechanism of Action: Topoisomerase-II inhibitor; antitumor antibiotic binds directly to DNA base pairs (intercalates) and inhibits DNA and DNA-dependent RNA synthesis, as well as protein synthesis; also binds to lipid cellular membrane and disrupts cellular functions, as well as creating hydroxyl free radicals (causes cardiotoxicity in heart cells). Both actions result in programmed cell death (apoptosis). Cell cycle specific for S phase.

Metabolism: Excretion of drug predominates in the liver; renal clearance is minor. Alteration in liver function requires modification of doses, whereas with renal failure there is no need to alter doses. Terminal half-life is 20–48 hours. Drug does not cross the blood–brain barrier. Drug is excreted through urine and may discolor urine from 1 to 48 hours after administration.

Indication: (initial): (1) Use in acute lymphoblastic leukemia, acute myeloblastic leukemia, Hodgkin's lymphoma, NHL, metastatic breast cancer, metastatic Wilms' tumor, metastatic neuroblastoma, metastatic soft tissue and bone sarcomas, metastatic ovarian cancer, metastatic transitional cell bladder, metastatic thyroid and gastric carcinomas, metasatic bronchogenic cancer; (2) a component of adjuvant therapy in women with axillary lymph node involvement after resection of primary breast cancer.

Contraindications: Patients with (1) myocardial insufficiency; (2) recent MI; (3) severe persistent drug-induced myelosuppression; (4) severe hepatic impairment (BR > 5 mg/dL); (5) hypersensitivity to doxorubicin.

Dosage/Range:
- Adjuvant breast cancer: doxorubicin 60 mg/m^2 IV on day 1, in combination with cyclophosphamide, every 21 days, for 4 cycles.
- Metastatic disease, leukemia, lymphoma: 60–75 mg/m^2 IV every 21 days.
- In combination with other chemotherapy: 40–75 mg/m^2 IV every 3–4 weeks.
- Consider use of lower doxorubicin dose in the recommended dose range or longer intervals between cycles for heavily pretreated patients, elderly, or obese patients.
- Cumulative doses > 550 mg/m^2 are associated with an increased risk of cardiomyopathy.

Dose Modifications:
- Discontinue doxorubicin in paitents who develop signs/symptoms of cardiomyopathy.
- Dose-reduce for hepatic dysfunction: serum bilirubin 1.2–3 mg/dL: 50% DR; serum bilirubin 3.1–5 mg/dL: 75% dose reduction.

Drug Preparation:
- Available Doxorubicin HCl injection: vials contain 10 mg/5 mL, 50 mg/25 mL, and 200 mg/100 mL as a solution.
- Dilute doxorubicin solution or reconstituted solution in 0.9% sodium chloride injection USP or 5% dextrose injection USP. Protect from light following preparation until infusion completed.
- Storage of vials of doxorubicin following reconstitution under refrigeration can result in the formation of a gelled product. Place gelled product at room temperature for 2–4 hours to return the product to a slightly viscous, mobile solution.
- Drug will form a precipitate if mixed with heparin or 5-FU.

Drug Administration:
- This drug is a potent vesicant. Give through a patent, freely flowing IV or central line and avoid extravasation, which may lead to ulceration, pain, and necrosis. Be sure to check nursing procedure for administration of a vesicant. Administer over 3–10 minutes, visualizing the IV insertion site and asking the patient to tell you if any stinging or burning is felt. Assess for blood return every 2–5 mL of injected drug. Stop the infusion if patient complains of any discomfort, or if signs/symptoms of extravastionare seen. See extravasation NCP and antidote (dexrazoxane) administration in *Chapter 1* introduction.
- Administration as a CI: Administer via a central line only.
- Assess baseline ECHO or MUGA scan results and know LVEF, and discuss with provider frequency of retesting while patient is receiving doxorubicin.
- Assess CBC/differential and LFTs and discuss any abnormalities with physican/NP/PA. ANC must be ≥1,500 cells/m^3.

Drug Interactions:
- 5-Fluourouracil or heparin: a precipitate will form. Do not use together.
- Alkaline solutions: avoid contact as hydrolysis of doxorubicin may occur.

- Barbiturates: increased plasma clearance of doxorubicin.
- Phenytoin: reduced phenytoin levels.
- Cyclophosphamide: risk of hemorrhage and increased cardiotoxicity.
- Mitomycin: increased risk of cardiotoxicity.
- Trastuzumab: increased risk of cardiotoxicity, avoid concomitant administration.
- Paclitaxel: increased risk of cardiotoxicity; give sequentially.
- Digoxin: decreased serum levels of digoxin; avoid concomitant administration.
- Mercaptopurine: increased risk of hepatotoxicity.
- Incompatible with heparin, forming a precipitate.
- Progesterone (high doses): increased neutropenia and thrombocytopenia.
- Cyclosporine: increased toxicity, coma; do not use concurrently.

Lab Effects/Interference:
- Decreased CBC.
- Increased LFTs.
- Increased uric acid secondary to tumor lysis.

Special Considerations:
- Drug is a potent vesicant. Give through patent, running IV to avoid extravasation and tissue necrosis. Give through central line if drug is to be given by CI.
- Females and males of reproductive potential: drug may impair fertility. Counsel female and male patients on pregnancy planning and prevention.
- Nausea and vomiting are dose related, occur in 50% of patients, and begin 1–3 hours after administration.
- Causes discoloration of urine (from pink to red for up to 48 hours).
- Skin changes: May cause radiation recall phenomenon—recalls reaction in previously irradiated tissue. Vein discoloration, with increased pigmentation in black patients (skin, hard palate).
- Potent myelosuppressive agent causes GI toxicities: mucositis, esophagitis, and diarrhea.
- Secondary acute myelocytic leukemia (AML) or myelodysplastic syndrome (MDS); often refractory when results from combination chemotherapy or radiation therapy.
- Warnings and Precautions
  - *Cardiomyopathy and arrhythmias*: drug may cause myocardial damage, including acute LV failure. Risk at a cumulative dose of 300 mg/m^2 is 1–2%, at 400 mg/m^2 is 3–5%, at 450 mg/m^2 is 5–8%, and at 500 mg/m^2 is 6–20% with doxorubicin given every 3 weeks alone. Assess LVEF before initiation of doxorubicin, during and after treatment is completed. Risk is further increased when drug is combined with concomitant cardiotoxic therapy (e.g., cyclophosphamide, trastuzumab).
    - Assess LVEF before drug is initiated, and regularly during and after treatment with doxorubicin. Increase frequency of MUGA/ECHO after the cumulative dose > 300 mg/m^2, using the same method of LVEF determination each time (e.g., MUGA or ECHO).
    - Dose lifetime limit at 550 mg/m^2 and less if receiving another potentially cardiotoxic drug (e.g., cyclophosphamide) or chest RT. Patients may exhibit irreversible CHF.
    - Prior chest radiation therapy (XRT): reduce total lifetime dose to 300–350 mg/m^2.

- Concomitant cyclophosphamide administration: may limit to 450 mg/m^2.
- Acute toxicity may be seen within hours after administration. This is unrelated to cumulative dose and may manifest symptoms of pump or conduction dysfunction. Rarely, transient ECG abnormalities, CHF, pericardial effusion (whole syndrome referred to as *myocarditis–pericarditis syndrome*) may occur, which may lead to death of patient.
  - Delayed cardiotoxicity when used in children. Long-term follow-up cardiac evaluations should be done due to risk of delayed cardiotoxicity.
- *Secondary malignancy*: AML or MDS has been described rarely, generally occurring within 1–3 years of treatment.
- *Extravasation and tissue necrosis*: blistering, ulceration, and necrosis may occur following extravasation and may require wide excision and skin grafting. Use meticulous technique in administering the drug, and identify any signs/symptoms of extravasation immediately. Stop drug, aspirate any drug remaining in tubing, and treat according to ONS extravastion guidelines (see *Chapter 1*). Antidote is dexrazaxane, which must be initiated within 6 hours of the extravasation.
- *Severe myelosuppression* resulting in serious infection, septic shock, transfusion requirement, hospitalization, and death may occur. Follow cbc/differential closely and teach patient to report any signs/symptoms of infection promptly.
- *Use in hepatic impairment*: Drug dosage reductions necessary for hepatic dysfunction: 50% dose given for serum bili 1.2–2.9 mg/dL, 25% dose given for serum bili 3 mg/dL. Monitor LFTs closely.
- *TLS* may occur in patients with a high tumor burden, or with rapidly proliferating tumors. Discuss TLD prophylaxis with physician/NP/PA for initial treatment of these patients. Monitor serum uric acid levels, potassium, calcium, phosphate, and creatinine; ensure adequate hydration and elimination of 100 mL/hour, and discuss use of allopurinol to prevent hyperuricemia.
- *Radiation induced toxicity* can be increased by doxorubicin administration; radiation recall can occur in paitents who receive doxorubicin HCl after prior RT.
- *Embryo-fetal toxicity*: can cause fetal harm. Teach women of reproductive potential to use effective contraception to prevent pregnancy while receiving doxorubicin. Nursing mothers should either discontinue the drug or nursing, taking into consideration the importance of the drug to the mother.

Potential Toxicities/Side Effects and the Nursing Process

I.   POTENTIAL FOR INFECTION AND BLEEDING related to BM DEPRESSION

Defining Characteristics: WBC and platelet nadir 10–14 days after drug dose, with recovery from days 15–21. Myelosuppression may be severe but is less severe with weekly dosing.

Nursing Implications: Monitor CBC, WBC, differential, and platelet count prior to drug administration; discuss any abnormalities with physician. Assess for signs/symptoms of infection or bleeding; instruct patient in self-assessment and to report signs/symptoms immediately. Teach patient self-care measures to minimize risk of infection and bleeding, including avoidance of OTC aspirin-containing medications. Drug dosage must be reduced if patient has hepatic dysfunction: 50% reduction of drug dose if bili is 1.2–3.0 mg/dL; 75% reduction if bili is >3.0 mg/dL.

II. POTENTIAL FOR ALTERATION IN CARDIAC OUTPUT related to ACUTE AND CHRONIC CARDIAC CHANGES

Defining Characteristics: Acutely, pericarditis-myocarditis syndrome may occur during infusion or immediately after (non–life-threatening EKG changes of flat T waves, ST-segment changes, PVCs). With high cumulative doses >550 mg/m^2 (450 mg/m^2 if concurrent treatment with cardiotoxic drugs or radiation to the chest), cardiomyopathy may occur. Risk is decreased if drug given as CI.

Nursing Implications: Assess cardiac status prior to chemotherapy administration: signs/symptoms of CHF, quality/regularity and rate of heartbeat, results of prior GBPS or other test of LVEF (stop drug if 10% decrease below LLN, LVEF of 45%, or decrease in LVEF of 20% at any level). Instruct patient to report dyspnea, palpitations, swelling in extremities. Maintain accurate records of total dose; expect GBPS to be repeated periodically during treatment and the drug to be discontinued if there is a significant drop in heart function.

III. POTENTIAL FOR ALTERATION IN NUTRITION, LESS THAN BODY REQUIREMENTS, related to NAUSEA AND VOMITING, ANOREXIA, STOMATITIS

Defining Characteristics: Nausea/vomiting occurs in 50% of patients, is moderate to severe, and is preventable with combination antiemetics. Onset 1–3 hours after drug dose and lasts 24 hours. Anorexia occurs frequently, and stomatitis occurs in 10% of patients.

Nursing Implications: Premedicate with combination antiemetics and continue protection for 24 hours. If patient has a central line, slower infusion of drug over 1 hour decreases nausea/vomiting. Encourage small, frequent feedings of bland foods. Anorexia occurs frequently: teach patient or caregiver to make foods ahead of time and use spices; encourage taking weight weekly. Stomatitis occurs in 10% of patients, and esophagitis may occur in patients who have received prior radiation to the chest. Perform oral assessment prior to drug administration and during posttreatment visits. Teach patient oral hygiene and self-assessment techniques.

IV. POTENTIAL ALTERATION IN SKIN INTEGRITY related to ALOPECIA, RADIATION RECALL, NAIL AND SKIN CHANGES, AND DRUG EXTRAVASATION

Defining Characteristics: Complete alopecia occurs with doses >50 mg/m^2, occurring after therapy begins. Regrowth usually begins a few months after drug is stopped.

Hyperpigmentation of nail beds and dermal creases of hands is greatest in dark-skinned individuals. Skin damage from prior radiation may be reactivated. Adriamycin "flare" may occur during peripheral drug administration, often with urticaria and pruritus, and is due to local allergic reaction. Drug is a potent vesicant and causes SEVERE tissue destruction if drug extravasates.

Nursing Implications: Discuss with patient hair loss, anticipated impact, and strategies to decrease distress, e.g., obtaining wig prior to hair loss. Assess body disturbance from hyperpigmentation and discuss strategies to minimize this, e.g., nail polish for dark nail beds. Drug must be administered via patent IV. If flare occurs, this must be distinguished from extravasation, where there is leakage of drug into the perivascular tissue. Stop or slow drug injection and flush with plain IV solution. Wait to see whether reaction will resolve. If confirmed flare, consider diphenhydramine 25 mg IVP to resolve pruritus and/or urticaria, and then resume administration of drug slowly into freely flowing IV. Assess need for venous access device early. If drug is administered as a CI, IT MUST BE GIVEN VIA A CENTRAL LINE.

V.   POTENTIAL SEXUAL DYSFUNCTION related to DRUG EFFECT

Defining Characteristics: Drug is teratogenic, mutagenic, and carcinogenic.

Nursing Implications: Assess patient's/partner's sexual patterns and reproductive goals. Provide information, supportive counseling, and referral as needed. Teach importance of birth control measures as appropriate. Male patients may wish to use a sperm bank prior to therapy.

Drug: doxorubicin hydrochloride liposome injection (Doxil)

Class: Anthracycline antibiotic isolated from streptomycin products wrapped in a STEALTH liposome.

Mechanism of Action: Topoisomerase-inhibitor; antitumor antibiotic binds directly to DNA base pairs (intercalates) and inhibits DNA and DNA-dependent RNA synthesis, as well as protein synthesis. Cytotoxic in all phases of cell cycle but maximally in S phase. Cell cycle nonspecific. Drug is encapsulated in STEALTH liposomes, which have surface-bound methoxypolyethylene glycol to protect the liposome from detection by blood phagocytes, and thus prolong circulation time. It is believed that the liposomal-encapsulated drug is able to penetrate the tumor through abnormal capillaries (tumor neovasculature) and then, once inside the tumor, accumulates and the drug is released.

Metabolism: Slower clearance from the body than doxorubicin (0.041 L/h/m^2 vs 24–35 L/h/m^2) with resulting larger AUC than a similar dose of doxorubicin. Half-life is approximately 55 hours. Has preferential uptake in Kaposi's sarcoma tumors.

Indication: Treatment of patients with (1) ovarian cancer after failure of platinum-based chemotherapy, (2) AIDS-related Kaposi's sarcoma (KS) after failure of prior systemic chemotherapy or intolerance to such therapy, (3) multiple myeloma in combination with bortezomib in patients who have not previously received bortezomib and have received at least one prior therapy.

Contraindication: hypersensitivity reactions to doxorubicin HCl or the components of DOXIL.

Dosage/Range: DO NOT substitute doxorubicin HCl for DOXIL or vice versa.

- Metastatic carcinoma of the ovary: 50 mg/m^2 IV over 1 hour every 28 days for a minimum until disease progression or toxicity.
- Multiple myeloma in combination with bortezomib: 30 mg/m^2 IV over 1 hour on day 4 (after bortezomib dose) of a 21-day treatment cycle. Continue for 8 cycles unless disease progression or unacceptable toxicity. Bortezomib 1.3 mg/m^2 IV on days 1, 4, 8, and 11 of a 21-day cycle.
- AIDS KS: 20 mg/m^2 IV over 60 minutes once every 21 days until disease progression or unacceptable toxicity.
- *Dose-reduce for HFS, stomatitis, neutropenia, thrombocytopenia*: See package insert for dose modifications. Do not reescalate dose after dose reduction.

Drug Preparation:

- Drug is available as single-dose vials containing 20 mg/10 mL and 50 mg/25 mL doxorubicin HCl in a 2-mg/mL concentration.
- Inspect drug for any particulate matter or discoloration; drug is translucent, with red liposomal dispersion.
- Further dilute drug (dose up to 90 mg) in 250 mL 5% dextrose USP ONLY; use 500 mL 5% dextrose USP for doses > 90 mg.
- Administer at once or store diluted drug refrigerated at 2–8°C (36–46°F) and administer within 24 hours.

Drug Administration:

- DO NOT ADMINISTER as bolus injection, or undiluted solution. DO NOT administer IM OR SUBCUTANEOUSLY. DO NOT SUBSTITUTE for doxorubicin (nonliposomal).
- Inspect parenteral drug products visually for particulate matter and discoloration before administration and do not use if found.
- Assess CBC/differential, LFTs. Assess palms of hands and soles of feet for HFS, as well as any areas of persistent irritation, and ask patient to describe signs/symptoms.
- Treat if ANC ≥ 1,500 cells/mm^3 and platelets > 75,000/mm^3.
- Dose-reduce for hepatic dysfunction: 50% dose reduction for bilirubin 1.2–3.0 mg/dL; 75% dose reduction if bilirubin > 3.0 mg/dL.
- Delay next dose and dose-reduce for grades 3–4 HFS, hematologic toxicity. See package insert.
- Administer IV at an initial rate of 1 mg/min to minimize risk of infusion reaction; if no reaction, increase rate to complete administration over 1 hour. Do not rapidly flush the infusion line. Do not use inline filter.

- Monitor for infusion reactions during infusion, and stop drug if reaction; discuss management with physician or NP/PA, as drug may be resumed at a slower infusion rate if symptoms are minor.
- If extravasation suspected, do not remove needle until attempts made to aspirate extravasated fluid; do not flush the line; avoid applying pressure to the site, apply ice to the site intermittently for 15 min 4× a day for 3 days, and if extravasation in the extremity, elevate the extremity. See Extravasation NCP in *Chapter 1* introduction.

Drug Interactions:
- Doxorubicin may potentiate the toxicity of (1) cyclophosphamide-induced hemorrhagic cystitis; (2) hepatotoxicity of 6-mercaptopurine; (3) radiation toxicity to heart, mucous membranes, skin, liver.

Lab Effects/Interference:
- Decreased CBC.

Special Considerations:
- Drug is an irritant, not a vesicant.
- Acute, infusion-associated reactions may occur (10% incidence) during drug infusion, characterized by flushing, shortness of breath, facial swelling, headache, chills, back pain, chest or throat tightness, and/or hypotension.
- Infusion should be stopped. If symptoms are minor, infusion may be resumed at a slower rate, but discontinue if symptoms reoccur.
- Serious and sometimes fatal allergic/anaphylactoid-like infusion reactions have been reported.
- Emergency medications and equipment should be readily available in infusion area when drug is administered, and physician or NP/PA available to give orders for management during/after infusion.
- Assessment for cardiac toxicity similar to that for doxorubicin should be done, since limited information is available as to cardiotoxicity of liposomal doxorubicin at high cumulative doses.
  - Myocardial damage may lead to CHF and may occur as the total cumualtive dose of doxorubicin approaches 550 mg/m^2.
  - Cardiac toxicity may also occur at lower cumulative doses with mediastinal irradiation or concurrent cardiotoxic agents.
- Most common adverse reactions (20% or higher): asthenia, fatigue, fever, anorexia, nausea, vomiting, stomatitis, diarrhea, constipation, HFS, rash, neutropenia, thrombocytopenia, anemia.
- Warnings and Precautions:
  - *Cardiomyopathy*: doxorubicin can result in myocardial damage, including LV failure. Risk is proportional to cumulative dose. The relationship between cumulative liposomal doxorubicin has not been determined. Assess LVEF by ECHO or MUGA baseline, during treatment, and after treatment to detect delayed cardiotoxicity. Patient should discuss risk benefit with physician/NP/PA if the patient has preexisting cardiovascular disease.

- *Infusion-related reactions*: may occur, and sometimes be serious and life-threatening characterized by flushing, SOB, facial swelling, headache, chills, chest pain, back pain, chest tightness, throat tightness, fever, tachycardia, pruritis, rash, cyanosis, syncope, bronchospasm, asthma, apnea, and hypotension. Most occur during the initial infusion. Incidence is 11%. Ensure medications and equipment for cardiopulmonary resuscitation are immediately available as well as a physician/NP/PA to prescribe rescue medications. Start liposomal doxorubicin infusion slowly (1 mg/min) and increase rate slowly to infuse over 1 hour as tolerated. If an infusion-related reaction occurs, stop the drug until resolution, then resume at a lower infusion rate as ordered. If a serious or life-threatening reaction occurs, the drug should be permanently discontinued.
- *HFS:* Generally occurs after 2–3 cycles of therapy but may occur earlier. Incidence is about 51%. The drug should be delayed for the first episode of grade 2 or greater HFS. Discontinue drug if HFS is severe and debilitating. Grades: 1 = mild erythema, swelling, not interfering with ADLs; 2 = erythema, desquamation interfering with but not preventing normal physical activities; small blisters or ulcerations < 2 cm in diameter. 3 = blistering, ulceration or swelling interfering with walking or normal activies; cannot wear regular clothing. 4 = diffuse or local process causing infectious complications, or a bed-ridden state or hospitalization.
- *Secondary oral cancers* have been described in patients receiving liposomal doxorubicin for >1 year. They have been diagnosed while on treatment, or up to 6 years after the last dose. Patients should be examined at regular intervals for oral ulceration or oral discomfort that may be suggestive of a secondary oral cancer.
- *Embryo-fetal toxicity*: Drug can cause fetal harm when used during pregnancy. Teach women of childbearing potential to use effective contraception during treatment and for 6 months after the last dose. Nursing mothers should decide whether to discontinue nursing or discontinue the drug, taking into consideration the importance of the drug to the mother's health.

Potential Toxicities/Side Effects and the Nursing Process

I. POTENTIAL FOR INFECTION AND BLEEDING related to BM DEPRESSION

Defining Characteristics: Leukopenia occurs in 91% of patients, with anemia and thrombocytopenia ($<150,000/mm^3$) less common (55% and 60%, respectively). Neutropenia ($<2,000/mm^3$) occurred in 85% and ANC ($<500/mm^3$) occurred in 13% of patients. In ovarian cancer patients, incidence of neutropenia ($<2,000$ cells/mm^3) was 51%, but ANC <500 cells/mm^3 was only 8.3%. Thrombocytopenia ($<150,000/mm^3$) occurred in 24%, while severe ($<25,000/mm^3$) occurred in 1.1% of patients with ovarian cancer. Myelosuppression is the dose-limiting toxicity in the treatment of HIV-infected patients, possibly because of HIV disease and/or concomitant medications. Anemia may also occur.

Nursing Implications: Monitor CBC, WBC, differential, and platelet count prior to drug administration, and discuss any abnormalities with physician. Assess for signs/symptoms of infection or bleeding, and instruct patient in self-assessment and to report signs/

symptoms immediately. Teach patient self-care measures to minimize risk of infection and bleeding, including avoidance of OTC aspirin-containing medications. See drug dosage reductions in Special Considerations section.

II.   POTENTIAL FOR ALTERATION IN CARDIAC OUTPUT related to ACUTE AND CHRONIC CARDIAC CHANGES

Defining Characteristics: Experience and data are limited in the cardiotoxicity of liposomal doxorubicin at high cumulative doses. Therefore, the manufacturer recommends the adoption of cardiotoxicity warnings made for doxorubicin HCl. With high cumulative doses > 550 mg/m^2 (400 mg/m^2 if concurrent treatment with cardiotoxic drugs such as cyclophosphamide, or radiation to the chest), cardiomyopathy may occur. In clinical trials, the incidence of "possibly or probably related" cardiac-related adverse events, including cardiomyopathy, arrhythmia, heart failure, pericardial effusion, and tachycardia, was 1–5% in patients with AIDS/Kaposi's sarcoma and $<1\%$ in ovarian cancer patients. In patients with multiple myeloma, the incidence of heart failure events is similar in treatment arms (3%), with decreases in LVEF 13% in combination arm compared with 8% in the bortezomib arm alone.

Nursing Implications: Assess patient risk (history of prior anthracycline chemotherapy, history of cardiovascular disease). Assess cardiac status prior to chemotherapy administration: signs/symptoms of CHF, quality/regularity and rate of heartbeat, results of prior GBPS or other test of LVEF. Instruct patient to report dyspnea, palpitations, swelling in extremities. Maintain accurate records of total dose. Expect GBPS to be repeated periodically during treatment and the drug to be discontinued if there is a significant drop in heart function.

III.   POTENTIAL FOR INJURY related to ALLERGIC INFUSION REACTION TO LIPOSOMAL COMPONENT(S)

Defining Characteristics: During the initial infusion, patients may experience an acute reaction characterized by flushing, shortness of breath, facial swelling, headache, chills, back pain, chest or throat tightness, and/or hypotension. Incidence is 5–6%. Reactions generally resolve after the immediate termination of the infusion in several hours to a day, or in some patients, after slowing of the infusion rate. Of those patients who experienced reactions, many were able to tolerate subsequent treatment without problem; however, some patients terminated therapy with liposomal doxorubicin because of the reaction.

Nursing Implications: Assess baseline comfort, vital signs, general condition. Infuse liposomal doxorubicin at 1 mg/min to minimize risk of acute reaction. Teach patient to report signs/symptoms of reaction immediately during infusion, and assess patient frequently during initial infusion. If signs/symptoms occur, stop infusion immediately. Discuss with the physician, but anticipate that if signs/symptoms are mild, infusion will resume at slower rate, and if signs/symptoms are severe, patient may not receive additional liposomal doxorubicin.

IV. POTENTIAL ALTERATIONS IN COMFORT AND ACTIVITY related to PALMAR-PLANTAR ERYTHRODYSESTHESIA (HFS)

Defining Characteristics: Incidence is approximately 3.4% in patients receiving a dose of 20 mg/m^2 and 37% in patients with ovarian cancer (16% grades 3 and 4). Toxicity becomes dose limiting in clinical studies at doses of 60 mg/m^2, or when treatment is administered more frequently than every 3 weeks. Signs/symptoms are swelling, pain, erythema, possibly progressing to desquamation of the skin on hands and feet, and usually occur after 6 weeks of treatment. Reaction is generally mild, not requiring treatment delays. However, in some patients, reaction can be severe and debilitating, necessitating discontinuance of treatment.

Nursing Implications: Assess baseline skin of patients' hands and feet, and in women with ovarian cancer, skin under areas of pressure, such as under the breasts of women with large breasts or skin folds, before each treatment. Teach patient to report signs/symptoms of reaction (e.g., tingling or burning, redness, flaking of skin in areas of pressure such as soles of feet, under breasts in large-breasted women, small blisters, or small sores on the palms of hands or soles of feet). If signs/symptoms occur, discuss treatment, treatment delays, or discontinuance. Do not use hydrocortisone cream, as this will cause greater desquamation of skin.

V. POTENTIAL FOR ALTERATION IN NUTRITION, LESS THAN BODY REQUIREMENTS, related to NAUSEA AND VOMITING, STOMATITIS, DIARRHEA, ANOREXIA

Defining Characteristics: Nausea and/or vomiting occur in 17% and 8% of patients, respectively, are mild to moderate, and are preventable with antiemetics. Stomatitis occurs in 7% of patients. Incidence of diarrhea is 8%. Anorexia may affect 1–5% of patients.

Nursing Implications: Premedicate with antiemetic (dopamine antagonist or serotonin antagonist). Encourage small, frequent feeding of bland foods. Stomatitis occurs in 7% of patients. Perform oral assessment prior to drug administration, and during posttreatment visits. Dose reductions or delay necessary for grades 2–4 stomatitis. Teach patient oral hygiene and self-assessment techniques. Instruct patient to report diarrhea, and teach self-management strategies for diarrhea.

VI. POTENTIAL FOR ALTERATION IN SKIN INTEGRITY related to ALOPECIA, RASH, PRURITUS, AND RADIATION RECALL

Defining Characteristics: Incidence of alopecia significantly less with liposomal delivery of doxorubicin, and is about 9% in AIDS/Kaposi's sarcoma patients and 15% in women with ovarian cancer. Skin damage from prior radiation may be reactivated. Rash and itching occur in 1–5% of the patients. Rarely, significant skin reactions may occur, such as exfoliative dermatitis. Drug is an irritant, but extravasation should be avoided.

Nursing Implications: Discuss with patient low incidence of hair loss, and to report hair thinning if it occurs. At that time, discuss impact and strategies to decrease distress. Instruct patient to report skin rash or itching, and discuss significance and management with physician. Teach patient to assess for skin changes in prior irradiated sites, including mucous membranes, and to report this immediately. Assess and develop management strategies depending on site and extent. Use caution to avoid drug extravasation; if infiltration occurs, stop infusion, apply ice for 30 minutes, and restart a new IV elsewhere.

VII. POTENTIAL ALTERATION IN NUTRITION related to NAUSEA AND/OR VOMITING, STOMATITIS

Defining Characteristics: Nausea occurs in 37% (severe, grades 3–4 in 8%) of ovarian cancer patients and 17% of AIDS/Kaposi's sarcoma patients. Vomiting occurs in 22% of ovarian cancer patients and 7.8% of patients with AIDS/Kaposi's sarcoma. Stomatitis occurs in 37% of women with ovarian cancer and is severe in 7.7%; overall incidence in AIDS/Kaposi's sarcoma patients is 6.8%.

Nursing Implications: Assess baseline nutritional status. Teach patient that these side effects may occur and teach self-care measures, including self-assessment, oral hygiene regimen, and to report occurrence of symptoms. Administer antiemetic prior to chemotherapy, especially in ovarian cancer patients, and assess efficacy after treatment. Revise antiemetic regimen as needed to provide complete protection from nausea and/or vomiting. Assess oral mucosa prior to each treatment. If stomatitis develops, dose reduction should be considered.

VIII. POTENTIAL SEXUAL DYSFUNCTION related to DRUG EFFECTS

Defining Characteristics: Drug is embryotoxic. Doxorubicin has been shown to be carcinogenic and mutagenic.

Nursing Implications: Assess patient's/partner's sexual pattern and reproductive goals. Provide information, supportive counseling, and referral as needed. Teach importance of birth control measures for female patients of childbearing age. Mothers who are nursing should discontinue nursing during treatment.

IX. ACTIVITY INTOLERANCE related to ASTHENIA AND FATIGUE

Defining Characteristics: Anemia is the most common hematologic event, affecting 52.6% of women with ovarian cancer, but only 25% experienced severe anemia (Hgb < 8 g/dL). Incidence for patients with AIDS/Kaposi's syndrome overall is 55%, with 4% experiencing severe anemia. Asthenia is more common in women with ovarian cancer, affecting 33%, while patients with AIDS/Kaposi's syndrome had an incidence of 9.9%.

Nursing Implications: Assess activity tolerance and HCT/Hgb baseline and prior to each treatment. Teach patients to report any changes in energy and activity level. Teach patients self-care strategies to maximize energy use and conservation. Evaluate efficacy of strategies at each visit, and if ineffective, assist patient to problem solve other alternative solutions, such as friends, volunteers, to help with activities such as shopping, food preparation.

Drug: enzalutamide (Xtandi)

Class: Androgen receptor inhibitor.

Mechanism of Action: Drug competitively inhibits androgen binding to androgen receptors, thus stopping the androgen receptor nuclear translocation and interaction with DNA. The drug acts on different steps in the androgen receptor signaling pathway, and *in vitro,* decreases prostate cancer cell proliferation and induces cell death. This results in decreased tumor volume. The major metabolite *N*-desmethyl enzalutamide has similar activity *in vitro,* to enzalutamide. Enzalutamide has higher affinity to the androgen receptor than bicalutamide.

Metabolism: The drug is well absorbed following either a fasting or high-fat meal. Enzalutamide is 97% to 98% bound to plasma proteins (primarily albumin), while the metabolite N-desmethyl enzalutamide is 95% protein bound. Following oral administration, median time to reach maximal plasma concentration (C_{max}) is 1 hour (range 0.5 to 3 hours), and with daily dosing, enzalutamide steady state is reached by day 28, with the drug accumulation approximately 8.3-fold compared to a single daily dose. Enzalutamide is metabolized in the liver by the P450 microenzyme system (CYP2C8 and CYP3A4); CYP2C8 is primarily responsible for the formation of the active metabolite *N*-desmethyl enzalutamide. Following a single dose of radiolabeled enzalutamide, 85% of the radioactivity is recovered by 77 days post dose, with 71% excreted in the urine, and 14% in the feces. The mean terminal half-life of enzalutamide given as a single dose of 160 mg is 5.8 days (range 2.8 to 10.2 days), while that of the active metabolite is 7.8 to 8.6 days. Renal and hepatic clearance of the drug and active metabolite in healthy patients and in patients with mild to moderate renal or hepatic impairment are similar; patients with severe renal (CrCl < 30 mL/min) or hepatic (Child-Pugh Class C) impairment were not studied. Bone density remains stable.

Indication: Treatment of patients with castration-resistant prostate cancer (CRPC).

Contraindication: None.

Dosage/Range:
- 160 mg (four 40-mg capsules) orally once daily at the same time each day, with or without food.
- Patient should also receive a gonadotropin-releasing hormone (GnRH) analog concurrently or should have had a bilateral orchiectomy.

Dose Modifications:
- If a patient experiences a grade 3 or higher toxicity or intolerable side effect: hold dose for 1 week or until symptoms improve to ≤ grade 2, then resume at the same or reduced dose (120 mg or 80 mg), if warranted.

- Concomitant administration of a **strong CYP2C8 inhibitor** (e.g., gemfibrozil): avoid if possible, but if unavoidable, reduce initial dose of enzalutamide to 80 mg once daily. If the strong inhibitor is discontinued, resume enzalutamide at the dose used prior to initiation of the strong CYP2C8 inhibitor.
- Concomitant **strong CYP3A4 inducer:** Avoid coadministration if possible. If medically necessary to give both drugs concurrently, increase the dose of enzalutamide from 160 mg to 240 mg once daily. If the strong inducer is discontinued, resume enzalutamide at the dose used prior to initiation of the strong CYP3A4 inducer.

Drug Preparation: None (available as 40-mg capsules, in a bottle of 120 capsules).

Drug Administration: Oral, with or without food. Patient should be instructed to take the dose at about the same time each day, and to swallow capsules whole; do not chew, dissolve, or open the capsule. If the patient forgets a dose, it should be taken when remembered unless it is at the end of the day, in which case, the normal dose should be taken the next day. The patient should not take more than the normal dose per day.

Drug Interactions:
- Drugs that **induce CYP2C8** (e.g., rifampin): may decrease serum enzalutamide level; avoid coadministration.
- Drugs that **inhibit CYP2C8** (e.g., gemfibrozil is a strong inhibitor): increase area under the plasma curve of enzalutamide and its active metabolite, thus increasing risk of toxicity; avoid coadministration if possible, and if unavoidable, reduce dose of enzalutamide.
- Drugs that **inhibit CYP3A4** (e.g., itraconazole) increase area under the curve of enzalutamide and its active metabolite by 1.3-fold in healthy volunteers, potentially increasing toxicity. Teach patient to avoid grapefruit and grapefruit juice.
- Drugs that **induce CYP3A4** (e.g., strong inducers: carbamazepine, phenobarbital, phenytoin, rifabutin, rifampin, rifapentine; moderate inducers: bosentan, efavirenz, etravirine, modafinil, nafcillin, St. John's wort) may decrease plasma level of enzalutamide, and should be avoided by selecting another drug that does not induce CYP3A4. If medically necessary to give both drugs concurrently, increase the enzalutamide dose. Teach patients to avoid St. John's wort.
- Effect on drug-metabolizing enzymes: enzalutamide is a strong CYP3A4 inducer and a moderate CYP2C9 and CYP2C19 inducer; enzalutamide reduces plasma levels of midazolam (CYP3A4 substrate), warfarin (CYP2C9 substrate), and omeprazole (CYP2C19 substrate). Avoid concomitant administration with drugs having a narrow therapeutic window, as enzalutamide may decrease drug serum level: drugs metabolized by CYP3A4 (e.g., alfentanil, cyclosporine, dihydroergotamine, ergotamine, fentanyl, pimozide, quinidine, sirolimus, and tacrolimus), CYP2C9 (e.g., phenytoin, warfarin), and CYP2C19 (e.g., S-mephenytoin). If coadministration with warfarin is unavoidable, increase INR monitoring.

Lab Effects/Interference:
- Neutropenia (15% grades 1–4; 1% grades 3–4).
- Hematuria (6.9%).

Special Considerations:

Most common adverse reactions (≥10%) are asthenia/fatigue, back pain, decreased appetite, constipation, arthralgia, diarrhea, hot flush, peripheral edema, musculoskeletal pain, headache, upper respiratory tract infection (URI), dizziness/vertigo, dyspnea, decreased weight, HTN.

- Warnings and Precautions:
  - *Seizures:* In clinical trials, seizure occurred rarely (0.4%) in patients receiving enzalutamide 160 mg once daily, occurring from 13 to 604 days after drug initiation. All seizures resolved, and as patients were removed from the clinical trial, there is no experience re-administering the drug to these patients. Patients who had a seizure also had a higher risk through predisposing factors: use of medications that can lower seizure threshold, history of traumatic brain or head injury, CVA, TIA, Alzheimer's disease, meningioma, or leptomeningeal disease from prostate cancer.
    - Monitor patients with increased risk for seizures closely, including those taking medication that may lower seizure threshold.
    - Teach patients to avoid activities where a sudden loss of consciousness could cause serious harm to themselves or others, and to report loss of consciousness or seizure right away.
    - Discontinue drug permanently in patients who develop a seizure during treatment.
  - *Posterior reversible encephalopathy (PRES)* may rarely occur. PRES is a rare neurological disorder characterized by rapidly evolving symtpoms including seizure, headache, lethargy, confusion, blindness, and other visual and neurological disturbances with or without HTN. MRI is necessary to confirm the diagnosis. Discontinue drug permanently if this occurs.
  - *HSR*: HSR may occur, characterized by edema of the face, tongue, lip, or pharynx rarely. Teach patients to temporarily stop taking the drug if any symptom occurs and seek medical care immediately. Permanently discontinue the drug for serious HSRs.
  - *Ischemic heart disease*: Occurred more frequently in the XTANDI arm in clinical trials, 2.7% vs 1.2% in the control arm. Grades 3–4 ischemic events occurred in 1.2% in the XTANDI arm compared to 0.5% in the placebo group, and death occurred in 0.4% of XTANDI patients compared to 0.1% in the placebo arm. Monitor patient closely for signs/symptoms of ischemic heart disease, and ensure patients have excellent control of cardiovascular risk factors (e.g., HTN, diabetes, dyslipidemia). Drug should be discontinued for grade 3-4 ischemic heart disease.
  - *Falls and fractures*: Falls occurred in 10% of patients in clinical trials compared to 4% of patients in the control arm. Assess patient risk for falls and fractures and develop a plan to prevent these. Consider use of bone-targed agents.
  - *Embryo-fetal toxicity*: Safety and efficacy of drug have not been established in women. Drug is feto-toxic. Teach male patients to use a condom if having sex with a pregnant woman, and to use a condom and another effective method of birth control if the patient is having sex with a woman of reproductive potential. These precautions should be used during and for 3 months after treatment with enzalutamide.

Potential Toxicities/Side Effects and the Nursing Process

I.   POTENTIAL FOR SENSORY/PERCEPTUAL ALTERATIONS related to DIZZINESS, SPINAL CORD COMPRESSION AND CAUDA EQUINA SYNDROME, PARESTHESIA

Defining Characteristics: Although most symptoms are not common, these symptoms increase the risk for falls. The incidence of falls was 4.6% in the enzalutamide group, compared with 1.3% in the placebo group. Dizziness occurred in 9.5%, spinal cord compression/cauda equina syndrome in 7.4% (compared with 4.5% in the placebo group), paresthesia in 6.6%, mental impairment disorders (amnesia, memory impairment, cognitive disorder, attention disturbance) in 4.3%, and hypoesthesia in 4%. Seizure occurred in 0.9%. Hallucinations (visual, tactile, or undefined) occurred in 1.6% (grade 1 or 2), compared with 0.3% in the placebo group, and most occurred in patients receiving opioid analgesics. Insomnia occurred in 8.8% of patients. Asthenia/fatigue occurred in 50.6%, which also increases the risk of falls.

Nursing Implications: Assess neurologic and mental status, baseline and at visits during drug administration. Assess risk for seizures (e.g., history of seizure, medications that may lower seizure threshold, brain metastases), and advise patient to avoid any activity where sudden loss of consciousness could cause serious harm to self or others. Assess for spinal cord compression or cauda equina syndrome, as these are oncologic emergencies. Assess for back pain (e.g., constant, dull, aching, radiating, may wax and wane [crescendo pain], exacerbated by movement, unrelieved by lying down), motor weakness, and sensory impairment. Teach patient to report radicular back pain right away, change in bowel or bladder patterns, or change in sensation in lower extremities. Discuss assessment with physician, nurse practitioner (NP), or physician assistant (PA) immediately, as IV dexamethasone should be administered emergently once diagnosis is confirmed. Teach patients that although these side effects may occur uncommonly, any alterations in behavior, sensation, or perception should be reported to the physician or nurse right away. Develop a plan of care with patient and family if side effects develop to manage distress, and promote safety. Drug should be stopped if a seizure occurs, and then once resolved, the patient should discuss the risks and benefits of resuming the drug with the physician. Assess patient for insomnia, and if present, discuss strategies to promote sleep, and if ineffective, discuss with physician, NP, or PA medication to promote sleep.

II.   ALTERATION IN COMFORT related to BACK PAIN, ARTHRALGIA, MUSCULOSKELETAL PAIN AND WEAKNESS, HEADACHE, HOT FLUSHES, PERIPHERAL EDEMA

Defining Characteristics: Back pain occurred in 26.4% of patients, arthralgias in 20.5%, musculoskeletal pain 15%, and weakness 9.8%; headache in 12.1% and peripheral edema in 15.4% of patients. Vasodilation or hot flushes occurred in 20.3% of patients.

Nursing Implications: Assess baseline comfort, and self-care measures used. Teach patient these symptoms may occur and to report them. If back pain occurs, assess for possible spinal cord compression or cauda equina syndrome (see I). Discuss self-care strategies to improve comfort if symptoms occur, such as use of heat and cold for musculoskeletal discomfort, acetaminophen for headache, leg elevation for peripheral edema. If hot flashes are severe, review common hot flash management, including wearing loose, layered clothing that can be removed when the patient becomes hot, sipping cold beverages throughout the day, sleeping with light nightclothes and a window open, avoiding triggers such as caffeine or alcohol. If the patient has peripheral edema, assess for skin integrity. Teach patient self-assessment of peripheral edema, to wear loose stockings and shoes, to keep skin moisturized to prevent cracking, and comfort measures. Teach patient to report increasing edema or related problems.

III.   POTENTIAL FOR INFECTION related to NEUTROPENIA

Defining Characteristics: Grades 1–4 neutropenia occurred in 15% of patients during clinical trials, with 1% grades 3–4, compared to 6% all grades in the placebo group. URI occurred in 10.9% and lower respiratory infection in 8.5% of patients receiving enzalutamide compared to 6.5% and 4.8% respectively in the placebo group.

Nursing Implications: Assess baseline CBC, WBC, and ANC baseline and at visits during therapy, as well as for signs/symptoms of infection. Teach patient signs/symptoms of infection and instruct to report these immediately. Teach patient self-care measures to minimize risk of infection, such as avoidance of crowds, and frequent hand washing.

IV.   ALTERATION IN ELIMINATION, POTENTIAL, related to DIARRHEA

Defining Characteristics: Diarrhea occurred in 21.8% of patients.

Nursing Implications: Assess baseline bowel elimination pattern and use of laxatives or stool softeners. Teach patient that diarrhea may occur, and self-care measures to minimize diarrhea, such as to modify diet, to avoid laxatives and stool softeners, to use over-the-counter antidiarrheal medicine, and to report diarrhea that persists. If these are ineffective, discuss further pharmacological management with physician.

V.   ALTERATION IN BOWEL ELIMINATION PATTERN related to DIARRHEA

Defining Characteristics: Diarrhea occurred in 21.8% of patients and was grades 3–4 in 1.1%.

Nursing Implications: Assess baseline bowel elimination status, and teach patient that diarrhea may occur and to report it. Teach patient to manage diarrhea with loperamide if needed, and to modify diet as needed (increased fluids, BRAT diet). Teach patient that if diarrhea persists, to report it as well. Discuss management (e.g., pharmacological, assessing electrolytes, IV hydration) as needed with physician/NP/PA.

VI.   ALTERATION IN ACTIVITY related to ASTHENIA, FATIGUE

Defining Characteristics: Asthenia and fatigue were the most common side effects, affecting 50.6% of patients in clinical trials.

Nursing Implications: Assess baseline activity tolerance, weakness, and level of fatigue. Teach patient that these side effects may occur and to report them. Teach patient to alternate rest and activity periods. Teach fatigue self-care measures, such as strategies to maximize energy use and conservation while shopping, interacting with friends, and other activities.

Drug: epirubicin hydrochloride (Ellence, Farmorubicin[e], Farmorubicina, Pharmorubicin)

Class: Anthracycline antitumor antibiotic analogue (topoisomerase II inhibitor).

Mechanism of Action: Drug complexes with DNA by intercalation of planar rings between DNA base pairs; this inhibits nucleic acid (DNA and RNA) and protein synthesis. This also causes cleavage of DNA by topoisomerase II, causing cell death. Drug also prevents enzymatic separation of DNA, interfering with replication and transcription. Drug also causes the production of cytotoxic free radicals.

Metabolism: Following IV administration, drug rapidly disperses into body tissues and into red blood cells; drug is 77% bound to plasma proteins. Drug is rapidly and extensively metabolized in the liver, excreted primarily through the biliary system, and to a lesser extent in the urine. Drug clearance is reduced in elderly women (35% lower in women aged > 70 years old). Drug clearance is reduced 30% in mild hepatic dysfunction, and 50% in moderate hepatic dysfunction. Drug clearance is reduced (50%) in patients with severe renal impairment (serum creatinine > 5 mg/dL). Dose reductions should be made for patients with hepatic dysfunction and patients with severe renal dysfunction.

Indication: As a component of adjuvant therapy in breast cancer patients with evidence of axillary node involvement following resection of primary breast cancer.

Contraindications: Patients with ANC < 1,500 cells/mm^3, severe myocardial insufficiency, recent MI, severe arrhythmias, previous treatment with an anthracycline up to the maximum cumulative dose, hypersensitivity to epirubicin, other anthracyclines, or anthracenediones, or severe hepatic dysfunction.

Dosage/Range:
Starting dose as part of adjuvant therapy in patients with axillary node-positive breast cancer: 100 mg/m^2 to 120 mg/m^2 IV on day 1 of each cycle, every 3–4 weeks.

- CEF-120: cyclophosphamide 75 mg/m² PO days 1–14, epirubicin 60 mg/m² IV days 1, 8; 5-FU 500 mg/m² IV days 1–8; repeat every 28 days for 6 cycles.
- FEC-100: 5-FU 500 mg/m² IV day 1, epirubicin 100 mg/m² IV day 1; cyclophosphamide 500 mg/m² IV day 1; repeated every 21 days for 6 cycles.
- Epirubicin may be given on day 1 or in divided doses on days 1 and 8 of each cycle.
- Patients receiving epirubicin HCl injection 120 mg/m² regimen should receive prophylactic antibiotic therapy.

Dose Modifications:
- Bone Marrow (BM) dysfunction:
  - Consider lower starting dose of 75–90 mg/m² if patient heavily pretreated (e.g., with existing BM Depression (BMD) or BM infiltration by tumor).
  - If patient is receiving dose divided into days 1 and 8, day 8 dose should be 75% of day 1 dose if platelet counts are 75,000–100,000/mm³ and ANC is 1,000–1,499/mm³. If day 8 platelet counts are <75,000/mm³, ANC < 1,000, or grades 3–4 nonhematologic toxicity has occurred, omit the day 8 dose.
- Hepatic dysfunction: Bilirubin 1.2–3 mg/dL or AST 2–4 × ULN, give 50% of recommended starting dose; bilirubin > 3 mg/dL or AST > 4 × ULN give 25% of recommended starting dose.
- Renal dysfunction: Consider lower doses if serum creatinine >5 mg/dL.

Dosage adjustment after first treatment cycle based on nadir counts:
- Platelet count < 50,000/mm³, ANC < 250/mm³, neutropenic fever, or grades 3–4 nonhematologic toxicity: day 1 dose should be reduced to 75% of day 1 dose given in current cycle.
- Delay day 1 chemo in subsequent cycles until platelet count ≥ 100,000/mm³, ANC ≥ 1,500/mm³, and nonhematologic toxicities have recovered to ≤ grade 1.
- **Patients receiving dose of 120 mg/m² regimen** should also receive prophylactic antibiotic therapy with trimethoprim-sulfamethoxazole or a fluoroquinolone.

Drug Preparation:
- Drug is provided as a preservative-free, ready-to-use solution of 2 mg/mL concentration (50-mg/25-mL and 200-mg/100-mL single-use vials). Product may become gelled in the refrigerator, and will return to a slightly viscous to modile solution after 2–4 hours equilibrium at controlled room temperature (59–77°F or 15–25°C).
- Use within 24 hours of penetration of rubber stopper; discard any unused drug.
- Store unopened vials in refrigerator at 36–46°F (2–8°C).

Drug Administration:
- Drug is a vesicant, so vesicant precautions should be used (check nursing procedure for administration of a vesicant).
- ANC must be >1,500 cells/mm³, platelets > 100,000/mm³.
- Administer antiemetics prior to drug administration, as drug is emetogenic.
- Assesss LFTs, serum creatinine, and cbc/differential baseline before each cycle, as well as during epirubicin treatment as needed.

- Assess results of baseline ECHO or GBPS, and discuss with physician or NP/PA frequency of monitoring during epirubicin therapy.
- Administer via slow IVP into the tubing of a freely flowing IV infusion of 0.9% NS or 5% dextrose solution over 3–5 minutes, checking blood return every few milliliters of drug. Administration time is 15–20 minutes. If drug dose is reduced, administer drug slowly over at least 3 minutes.
- Epirubicin should not be administered with other cardiotoxic agents unless cardiac function is closely monitored. Do not give epirubicin-based therapy for up to 24 weeks after stopping trastuzumab (long half-life of trastuzumab).
- Teach patients that urine will be pink-red for the first 1–2 days following drug administration.
- Drug should never be given intramuscularly or subcutaneously.

Drug Interactions:
- Cytotoxic drugs: Additive toxicity (hematologic and gastrointestinal).
- Cardioactive drugs (e.g., calcium-channel blockers): May increase risk of congestive heart failure; use together cautiously, and monitor cardiac function closely during treatment.
- Radiation therapy: Tissue sensitization to cytotoxic effects of radiation therapy; when drug is given after prior radiation therapy, a radiation recall inflammatory reaction may occur at site of prior radiation.
- Cimetidine: Increases drug AUC by 50%, DO NOT use together. Hold cimetidine during treatment with epirubicin.
- Other drugs extensively metabolized by the liver: Changes in hepatic function caused by concomitant therapies may affect clearance of epirubicin; use together with caution, if at all, and monitor for hematologic and gastrointestinal toxicity closely during treatment.
- BM-suppressing drugs: Increased BM depression.

Lab Effects/Interference:
- Decreased white blood and neutrophil cell counts, platelet counts.

Special Considerations:
- Warnings and Precautions:
  - *Injection-related reactions*: Drug is a vesicant, and severe local tissue necrosis will occur if drug infiltrates; avoid IV sites over joints, small veins, or veins on arms that have compromised venous or lymphatic drainage.
    - Venous sclerosis may occur if injections used in the same vein.
    - Extravasation may cause local pain, severe tissue lesions, and necrosis. Be careful to avoid extravasation. AVOID extravasation.
    - Facial flushing, as well as local erythema/streaking along vein path, may indicate excessively rapid administration. This may precede local phlebitis or thrombophlebitis.
  - *Myelosuppression* is the dose-limiting toxicity, and severe myelosuppression may occur. Monitor CBC/differential closely during therapy.

- *Myocardial toxicity* (e.g., CHF) may occur during therapy (acute) or months to years after cessation of therapy (delayed), and risk increases according to dose (acute or late/delayed). Delayed cardiomyopathy is manifested by decreased LVEF and signs/symptoms of CHF. It occurs late in the treatment course, or within 2–3 months after the last dose of therapy. Assess findings of baseline ECHO or MUGA, and same test repeated during therapy prior to drug administration.
  - Cumulative doses >900 mg/m^2 should generally not be exceeded.
  - Risk increases with prior anthracycline or anthracenedione therapy, past or concurrent radiation therapy to mediastinal/pericardial area, active or history of cardiovascular disease, or concomitant use of other cardiotoxic drugs.
  - Do not administer epirubicin in combination with other cardiotoxic agents unless the patient's cardiac function is closely monitored.
- *Secondary cancers* (e.g., acute myelogenous leukemia) have been reported, and risk is increased when given in combination with other cytotoxic drugs or when doses of anthracycline chemotherapy have been escalated. The estimated risk is 0.2% at 3 years and 0.8% at 5 years. Latency period can be 1–3 years.
- *Hepatic:* Doses must be reduced in patients with hepatic dysfunction. Assess bilirubin and AST levels before and during epirubicin treatment. If values are elevated, drug clearance is slowed, raising risk of toxicity. Epirubicin dose should be reduced. Drug was not studied in patients with severe hepatotoxicity.
- *Renal:* Assess serum creatinine baseline and during therapy. If value is >5 mg/dL, dose should be reduced.
- *TLS:* Rapid lysis of tumor cells may result in hyperuricemia (TLS). Discuss TLS prevention treatment in patients at high risk at initial treatment (hyperuricemic reducing agents, hydration), and monitor lab parameters closely for evidence of TLS postinfusion.
- *Immunosuppressant effects*/Increased susceptibility to infection. Do not give patient live or live-attenuated vaccines, as serious or fatal infections may occur.
- *GI:* antiemetics are necessary to prevent nausea and vomiting as drug is emetogenic.
- *Radiation recall*: Administration of epirubicin after previous RT may induce an inflammatory recall reaction at the site or irradiation.
- *Thrombophlebitis and thromboembolism* (including pulmonary embolism) have been reported.
- *Coadministration with cimetidine:* cimetidine increases epirubicin AUC by 50%. Stop cimetidine treatment during epirubicin therapy.
- *Embryo-fetal toxicity*: drug can cause fetal harm. Teach female patients of reproductive potential to use effective contraception to prevent pregnancy.
- Nursing mothers should not breastfeed during chemotherapy treatment.
- *Male fertility and reproductive outcomes.* Males with female sexual partners of childbearing potential should use effective contraception during and after cessation of epirubicin.
- *Laboratory testing*: Assess cbc/differential, and LFTs prior to and during each cycle of therapy. Perform repeated LVEF evaluations during therapy.
- Most common adverse effects in early breast cancer patients, occurring in 10% or more patients, were leucopenia, neutropenia, anemia, thrombocytopenia, amenorrhea,

lethargy, nausea/vomiting, mucositis, diarrhea, infection, conjunctivitis/keratitis, alopecia, local toxicity, and rash/itch.

- Long-term adverse effects with an incidence of 1–2% were asymptomatic drops in LVEF, CHF, secondary leukemia.
- Geriatric use: administer drug carefully with close monitoring in patients who are 70 years or older.

Potential Toxicities/Side Effects and the Nursing Process

I.   POTENTIAL FOR INFECTION, BLEEDING, FATIGUE related to BM DEPRESSION

Defining Characteristics: WBC and platelet nadir 10–14 days after drug dose, with recovery by day 21. Leukopenia and neutropenia may be severe, especially when given with other myelosuppressive chemotherapy. Thrombocytopenia may be severe, and anemia may occur.

Nursing Implications: Monitor CBC, WBC, differential, and platelet count prior to drug administration; discuss any abnormalities with physician. Assess for signs/symptoms of infection or bleeding; instruct patient in self-assessment and to report signs/symptoms immediately. Teach patient self-care measures to minimize risk of infection and bleeding, including avoidance of company of people with colds and OTC aspirin-containing medications. Dose reduction necessary in patients with hepatic dysfunction, as decreased metabolism of drug results in increased serum levels of drug and hematologic toxicity. Patients receiving 120 mg/m^2 dose should also receive prophylactic antibiotic therapy with trimethoprim-sulfamethoxazole or a fluoroquinolone antibiotic.

II.   POTENTIAL FOR ALTERATION IN CARDIAC OUTPUT related to ACUTE AND CHRONIC CARDIAC CHANGES

Defining Characteristics: Cardiotoxicity is dose related, cumulative, and may occur during or months to years after cessation of therapy. The estimated probability of developing clinically evident CHF is 0.9% at a cumulative dose of 500 mg/m^2, 1.6% at 700 mg/m^2, and 3.3% at a cumulative dose of 900 mg/m^2. The risk of CHF increases rapidly with cumulative doses in excess of 900 mg/m^2. Risk of developing cardiotoxicity is increased by history of cardiovascular disease, prior anthracycline or anthracenedione therapy, prior or concomitant radiation therapy to mediastinum and/or pericardial area, and concomitant use of other cardiotoxic drugs. Cardiotoxicity may be acute (early) or delayed (late). Signs/symptoms of early toxicity are not usually of clinical significance, do not predict late cardiotoxicity, and usually do not require change in epirubicin therapy. These include sinus tachycardia and EKG abnormalities (nonspecific ST and T-wave changes, and, rarely, PVCs, VT, bradycardia, atrioventricular, and bundle branch block). Delayed cardiotoxicity is related to cardiomyopathy, characterized by decreased left ventricular ejection fraction (LVEF) and classic signs/symptoms of CHF (tachycardia, dyspnea, pulmonary edema, dependent edema, hepatomegaly, ascites, pleural effusion, gallop rhythm). If late cardiotoxicity occurs, it is in the late stages of treatment or within months following treatment, and is cumulative dose related.

Nursing Implications: Assess cardiac status prior to chemotherapy administration: risk factors and signs/symptoms of CHF, quality/regularity and rate of heartbeat, results of baseline and periodic prior gated blood pool scan (GBPS), multigated radionuclideangiography (MUGA), echocardiogram (ECHO), or other test of LVEF. Instruct patient to report dyspnea, palpitations, and swelling in extremities. Maintain accurate records of total dose; expect GBPS or measure of LVEF to be repeated periodically during treatment and the drug to be discontinued if there is a significant drop in heart function as evidenced by LVEF falling below normal range.

III. POTENTIAL FOR ALTERATION IN NUTRITION, LESS THAN BODY REQUIREMENTS, related to NAUSEA AND VOMITING, DIARRHEA, STOMATITIS

Defining Characteristics: Nausea/vomiting occurs in >90% of patients, can be moderate to severe especially when drug is given together with other emetogenic chemotherapy, and is preventable with combination antiemetics. Onset 1–3 hours after drug dose and lasts 24 hours. Mucositis may occur; stomatitis is most common. Esophagitis is less common but may occur, especially if patient has had prior radiotherapy to the chest. Drug dose must be reduced in patients with hepatic dysfunction; otherwise, increased gastrointestinal toxicity will occur.

Nursing Implications: Assess baseline LFTs, and discuss with physician dose reduction if abnormal. Premedicate with combination antiemetics and continue protection for 24 hours. If patient has a central line, slower infusion of drug over 1 hour decreases nausea/vomiting. Encourage small, frequent feedings of bland foods. Perform oral assessment prior to drug administration and during posttreatment visits. Teach patient oral hygiene and self-assessment techniques. Teach patient to report pain, burning sensation, erythema, erosions, ulcerations, bleeding, or oral infections.

IV. POTENTIAL ALTERATION IN SKIN INTEGRITY related to ALOPECIA, RADIATION RECALL, FACIAL FLUSHING, FLARE REACTION, NAIL/ SKIN/ORAL MUCOUS MEMBRANE HYPERPIGMENTATION, AND DRUG EXTRAVASATION

Defining Characteristics: Alopecia is universal, but is reversible, with hair regrowth in 2–3 months following cessation of therapy. Skin damage and inflammation from prior radiation may be reactivated when drug is given. Drug may cause "flare" reaction or streaking along vein during peripheral drug administration, often with facial flushing, and may be related to excessively rapid drug administration. If it occurs, slow drug administration time, flush line with plain IV solution, and slowly complete therapy. This must be distinguished from extravasation, where there is leakage of drug into the perivascular tissue. Skin and nail hyperpigmentation may occur.

Nursing Implications: Discuss with patient hair loss, anticipated impact, and strategies to decrease distress, e.g., obtaining wig prior to hair loss. Assess body disturbance from hyperpigmentation and discuss strategies to minimize this, e.g., nail polish for dark nail beds. Drug must be administered via patent IV. Local phlebitis or thrombophlebitis may follow a flare reaction, so assess vein path closely, and teach patient to report any pain, erythema, or swelling following drug administration. Drug is a potent vesicant and causes SEVERE tissue destruction if drug extravasates. Teach patient to report any stinging or burning during drug administration, and stop administration if there is any question at all. Assess need for venous access device early.

V.   POTENTIAL FOR SEXUAL DYSFUNCTION related to REPRODUCTIVE HAZARD

Defining Characteristics: Drug is genotoxic, mutagenic, and carcinogenic. In laboratory animals receiving very high doses of the drug, testicular atrophy occurred. Drug may cause irreversible amenorrhea in premenopausal women (premature menopause).

Nursing Implications: Assess patient's/partner's sexual patterns and reproductive goals. Provide information, supportive counseling, and referral as needed. Teach importance of birth control measures as appropriate. Male patients may wish to use a sperm bank, and women may wish to investigate cryopreservation of oocytes prior to therapy.

Drug: eribulin mesylate injection (Halaven)

Class: Non-taxane microtubular dynamics inhibitor, synthetic analogue of the marine natural product halichondrin B.

Mechanism of Action: Drug is a synthetic analogue of halichondrin B, a natural product found in the rare marine sponge Halichondria okadai. The drug has a unique mechanism of action to suppress microtubule growth, without shortening; it also sequesters tubulin into nonfunctional aggregates to prevent (irreversibly) the formation of the mitotic spindle during mitosis so that the cell undergoes mitotic arrest at the G_2–M phase resulting in apoptosis (programmed cell death). Drug has activity in taxane-resistant cell lines.

Metabolism: Unchanged eribulin is the major circulating species in the plasma, and eribulin is negligibly metabolized by CYP3A4 in vitro. However, it does not induce or inhibit hepatic CYP3A4 activity at clinically relevant concentrations. In addition, it does not affect the metabolism of other therapeutic agents metabolized by CYP3A4. Drug is excreted primarily unchanged in the feces (82%) and the urine (9%).

Indication: Treatment of patients with (1) metastatic breast cancer who have previously received at least 2 chemotherapeutic regimens for the treatment of metastatic disease. Prior therapy should have included an anthracycline and a taxane in either the adjuvant or metastatic setting; (2) unresectable or metatatic liposarcoma who have received a prior anthracycline-containing regimen.

Contraindications: None. Drug has not been studied in patients with severe hepatic impairment (Child–Pugh C). Drug is not recommended in patients with congenital long QT syndrome.

Dosage/Range: 1.4 mg/m^2 IV over 2–5 minutes on days 1 and 8 of a 21-day cycle.

* Recommended dose of eribulin in patients with mild hepatic impairment (Child–Pugh A) is 1.1 mg/m^2 IV over 2–5 min on days 1 and 8 of a 21-day cycle.
* Recommended dose of eribulin in patients with moderate hepatic impairment (Child–Pugh B) is 0.7 mg/m^2 IV over 2–5 min on days 1 and 8 of a 21-day cycle.
* Recommended dose of eribulin in patients with moderate (CrCl 30–49 mL/min) to severe (CrCl 15–29 mL/min) renal impairment is 1.1 mg/m^2 IV over 2–5 min on days 1 and 8 of a 21-day cycle.
* Do not mix with other drugs or administer with dextrose-containing solutions.

Dose Modifications:
* Assess for PN and CBC/ANC prior to each dose.
* Do not administer drug on day 1 or 8 if the following occurs: ANC < 1,000/mm^3, platelets < 75,000/mm^3, or patient has grade 3 or 4 non-hematologic toxicities.
* Day 8 dose may be delayed for a maximum of 1 week; if toxicities do not resolve or improve to ≤ grade 2 severity by day 15, omit the dose; if toxicities have resolved or improved to ≤ grade 2 severity by day 15, administer drug at a reduced dose and initiate the next cycle no sooner than 2 weeks later.
* If a dose has been delayed for toxicity and toxicities have recovered to grade 2 or less, resume eribulin mesylate at a reduced dose as showing in the table below.
* Do not re-escalate eribulin mesylate after it has been dose reduced.
* Recommended dose modifications:

Event Description	Recommended Dose (eribulin mesylate)
Permanently reduce the 1.4 m^2 dose for any of the following: • ANC < 500/mm^3 for >7 days • ANC < 1,000/mm^3, with fever or infection • Platelets < 25,000/mm^3 • Platelets < 50,000/mm^3, requiring transfusion • Non-hematologic grade 3 or 4 toxicities • Omission or delay of day-8 dose in previous cycle for toxicity	1.1 mg/m^2
Occurrence of any event requiring permanent dose reduction while receiving 1.1 mg/m^2	0.7 mg/m^2
Occurrence of any event requiring permanent dose reduction while receiving 0.7 mg/m^2	Discontinue eribulin mesylate injection

Data from Eisai Inc. Halaven (eribulin mesylate) [package insert]. Woodcliffe Lake, NJ: Eisai Inc. December 2017. Grading of toxicities per NCI Common Terminology Criteria for Adverse Events (CTCAE, version 3.0).

Drug Preparation: Available as 1 mg per 2 mL (0.5 mg per mL).

- Aseptically withdraw ordered dose from the single-use vial and administer, either undiluted or diluted in 100 mL 0.9% sodium chloride USP.
- Do NOT dilute in or administer drug through IV line containing dextrose solutions.
- Do NOT administer in the same IV line concurrent with other medicines.
- Store undiluted drug in the syringe for up to 4 hours at room temperature or for up to 24 hours under refrigeration (40°F or 4°C).
- Store diluted solutions containing the drug for up to 4 hours at room temperature or up to 24 hours under refrigeration (40°F or 4°C).
- Discard any unused drug remaining in the vial.
- Store vial in its original carton at 25°C (77°F); excursions permitted to 15–30°C (59–86°F); do not freeze.

Drug Administration:

- Assess patient for signs/symptoms of PN, and CBC/differential before each dose. Ensure that ANC >1,000/mm^3, platelets >75,000/mm^3, and patient has no grades 3–4 non-hematologic toxicity. If PN present, discuss with physician/NP/PA.
- Assess electrolytes including serum potassium and magnesium; ensure they are WNL before sdministering first dose, and monitor these electrolytes during therapy. Low-serum potassium and magnesium may increase the risk of ventricular arrhythmias in patients at risk for developing QTc prolongation.
- Administer IV over 2–5 minutes on days 1 and 8 of a 21-day cycle.
- Do not mix with other drugs or administer with dextrose-containing solutions.

Drug Interactions:

- Dextrose-containing solutions: do not use.

Lab Effects/Interference:

- Neutropenia, leukopenia, anemia, thrombocytopenia.
- Hypokalemia, hypocalcemia (patients with liposarcoma, leiomyosarcoma).
- Increased LFTs.

Special Considerations:

- Most commonly reported adverse events (> 25%) in patients with (1) MBC: neutropenia, anemia, asthenia/fatigue, alopecia, PN, nausea, and constipation; with (2) liposarcoma and leiomyosarcoma were fatigue, nausea, alopecia, constipation, PN, abdominal pain, and pyrexia.
- Warnings and Precautions:
  - *Neutropenia:* monitor peripheral blood cell counts and adjust dose as needed.
  - Drug is embryo-fetotoxic. Women of childbearing age should use effective contraception to avoid pregnancy during eribulin therapy and for at least 2 weeks after final dose. Nursing mothers should discontinue drug or nursing, taking into account the importance of the drug to the mother. Teach men with female partners of reproductive potential to use effective contraception during eribulin treatment and for 3.5 months after the final dose. Testicular toxicity occurs in men.
  - *PN:* monitor for signs of motor and sensory PN, and manage with dose delay and adjustment (withhold dose for grades 3 or 4 PN until resolution to grade 2 or less).

TREATMENT

• *QT prolongation* occurs rarely, and was observed at day 8 in a small number of patients. Monitor for prolonged QT intervals in patients with CHF, bradyarrhythmias, taking drugs known to prolong QT interval and electrolyte abnormalities. Do not administer drug to patients with congenital long QT syndrome. **Correct hypokalemia and hypomagnesemia** before starting drug, and monitor serum levels during treatment.

Potential Toxicities/Side Effects and the Nursing Process

I.   POTENTIAL FOR INFECTION, BLEEDING, FATIGUE related to BM DEPRESSION

Defining Characteristics: Neutropenia affected 82% of patients (all grades). Incidence of grades 3–4 neutropenia was 57%, with 5% febrile neutropenia. In Study 1, neutropenia (ANC $<$ 500/mm^3) lasting $>$1 week occurred in 12% of patients, leading to discontinuation in $<$1% of patients. Mean time to nadir was 13 days, and mean time to recovery from severe neutropenia (ANC $<$ 500/mm^3) was 8 days. Patients with elevated LFTs $>$ 3 $\times$ ULN and bilirubin $>$ 1.5 $\times$ ULN experienced a higher incidence of grade 4 neutropenia and febrile neutropenia. G-CSF was used in 19% of patients. Two patients died of complications of febrile neutropenia in Study 1. Grade 3 or higher thrombocytopenia occurred in 1% of patients. Asthenia/fatigue occurred in 54%. Incidence of anemia is 58%, and thrombocytopenia 12%. In Study 2 (patients with leiomyosarcoma, liposarcoma) severe neutropenia $>$ 1 week incidence was 12%, and 0.9% experienced febrile neutropenia, and 0.9% fatal neutropenic sepsis.

Nursing Implications: Monitor CBC, WBC, differential, and platelet count prior to each drug administration, and increase frequency in patients who develop grade 3 or 4 cytopenias. Delay administration and reduce subsequent doses in patients who experience febrile or grade 4 neutropenia lasting $>$ 7 days. Discuss utility of G-CSF in high-risk patients with physician/NP/PA. Ensure that patients with hepatic dysfunction are dosed according to the Child-Pugh Class grading scale. Assess for signs/symptoms of infection or bleeding; instruct patient in self-assessment and to report signs/symptoms immediately. Teach patient self-care measures to minimize risk of infection and bleeding, including avoidance of company of people with colds and avoidance of OTC aspirin-containing medications. Teach patient to report right away fever $>$100.5°F, chills, cough, burning or pain upon urination, or other signs/symptoms of infection. Teach patient energy-conserving activities, gentle exercise, and to report fatigue. Refer to ONS Putting Evidence into Practice (PEP) cards on fatigue. Teach patient self-care strategies to reduce fatigue and increase energy (e.g., alternating rest and activity periods, gentle exercise).

II.   SENSORY/PERCEPTUAL ALTERATIONS related to PN

Defining Characteristics: PN occurred in 31–35% of patients (8% grade 3, 0.4% grade 4). Neuropathy lasting $>$1 year occurred in 5% of patients. 22% developed new or worsening neuropathy that had not recovered within a median follow-up duration of 269 days (range 25–662 days). In Study 2, grade 3 PN occurred in 3.1% of patients. Median time to any severity was 5 months (range 3.5 months–9 months). PN lasting > 60 days occurred in 58% of patients, and 63% had not recovered at 6.4 months follow-up. PN was the most common adverse reaction resulting in discontinuation. Dizziness, dysgeusia, and headache may also occur.

Nursing Implications: Assess baseline neurologic status, including history and physical for PN. Instruct patient to report signs/symptoms of pins-and-needles sensation, numbness, burning sensation, pain, increased discomfort with certain sensations, especially in the extremities, or motor weakness. Identify patients at risk: those with history of cisplatin use or with preexisting neuropathies (ethanol- and diabetes mellitus–related). Assess sensory and motor function prior to each treatment, and if abnormality found, assess impact on patient function, safety, independence, ability to do activities of daily living (ADLs), and quality of life. Test patient's ability to button a shirt or pick up a dime from a flat surface. If impacting ability to do ADLs, safety, or quality of life, discuss with physician/midlevel. Drug should be held for grade 3 or 4 PN until resolution to grade 2 or less, then can resume with dose reduction.

III.   POTENTIAL ALTERATION IN COMFORT related to FATIGUE, PAIN, DYSPNEA, ALOPECIA, PYREXIA

Defining Characteristics: Fatigue/asthenia occurred in 54% of patients, and was grade 3 or higher in 10%. Mild or moderate joint pain occurred in 22% of patients, back pain in 16%, bone pain in 12%, and extremity pain in 11%. Alopecia occurred in 45% of patients.

Nursing Implications: Teach patient that these side effects may occur and to report them. Assess patient for occurrence of symptoms and discuss measures for symptomatic relief with physician or midlevel practitioner. Assess impact of alopecia and discuss measures to preserve body image.

IV.   POTENTIAL FOR ALTERATION IN NUTRITION, LESS THAN BODY REQUIREMENTS, related to NAUSEA AND VOMITING, DIARRHEA, CONSTIPATION, STOMATITIS

Defining Characteristics: Nausea and vomiting occur in 35% and 18% of patients, respectively, in clinical trials. Constipation occurred in 25%, and diarrhea in 18%. Mucosal inflammation occurred in 9%. Anorexia and decreased weight also occurred. Hypokalemia occurs rarely. Increased LFTs (in patients with normal baseline LFTs) may occur.

Nursing Implications: Assess baseline nutritional, fluid, and electrolyte status and monitor throughout treatment. Note pretreatment LFTs and monitor during therapy. Premedicate with antiemetics prior to drug administration and continue through treatment. Monitor daily or weekly weights. Teach patient to report unrelieved nausea, vomiting, or inability to take oral fluids.

Drug: estramustine (Estracyte, Emcyt)

Class: Alkylating agent.

Mechanism of Action: Acts as a weak alkylator at usual therapeutic concentrations. A chemical combination of mechlorethamine and estradiol phosphate, estramustine is believed to selectively enter cells with estrogen receptors, where the drug acts as an alkylating agent due to bischloroethyl side-chain and liberated estrogens. Believed to have antimicrotubule activity. Cell cycle nonspecific.

Metabolism: Well absorbed orally, metabolized in liver, partly excreted in urine. Induces a marked decline in serum calcium and phosphate levels.

Indication: For the palliative treatment of patients with metastatic and/or progressive carcinoma of the prostate.

Contraindication: Not to be taken by patients with (1) known hypersensitivity to either estradiol or to nitrogen mustard, and (2) active thrombophlebitis or thromboembolic disorders, except when the actual tumor mass is the cause of the thromboembolic phenomenon and the physician believes the benefits outweigh the risks.

Dosage/Range:
* 14 mg/kg (or one 140-mg capsule for each 22 lbs or 10 kg of body weight) orally daily in 3 or 4 divided doses. Following treatment for 30–90 days, the physician should evaluate response. Drug continues as long as the favorable response lasts. Some patients have been maintained on therapy for > 3 years, at doses ranging from 10 to 16 mg/kg/day.

Drug Preparation:
* Available in 140-mg capsules.
* Store in refrigerator (2–8°C [36–46°F]); may be stored at room temperature for 24–48 hours.

Drug Administration:
* Oral with water, at least 1 hour before or 2 hours after meals. DO NOT take with milk, milk products, or calcium-rich foods or drugs (e.g., calcium-containing antacids).

Drug Interactions:
* Drug/food: milk, milk products, and calcium-rich foods may decrease drug absorption.
* Calcium-containing antacids: may impair drug absorption; take 1 hour before, or 2 hours after drug dose.
* Synergy with vinblastine.

Lab Effects/Interference:
* Changes in Ca.
* Increased serum glucose, LDH, triglyceride levels.
* Increased LFTs, RFTs.
* May affect certain endocrine (e.g., thyroid function tests, prolactin, cortisol) and LFTs because it contains estrogen.
* Decreased testosterone serum levels.

Special Considerations:

- Avoid taking drug with milk, milk products, and calcium-rich foods (e.g., antacids), as this will delay or impair drug absorption.
- Contraindicated or to be used with great caution in patients who are children or who have thrombophlebitis or thromboembolic disorders, peptic ulcers, severe hepatic dysfunction, cardiac disease, hypertension, or diabetes. Drug may increase the risk of embolic events; physician may recommend prophylactic warfarin or aspirin.
- LFT abnormalities (transaminases, BR) have occurred; monitor LFTs baseline, during therapy, and for 2 months after the drug has been withdrawn (Pfizer, 2007).
- Precautions:
  - *Fluid retention*: may be exacerbated by drug, with new peripheral edema or exacerbation of preexisting CHF. Patients with other conditions, which may be affected by fluid retention, require close monitoring (e.g., epilepsy, migraine, renal dysfunction).
  - *Drug may be poorly metabolized in patients with impaired liver function*; administer with caution and monitor closely.
  - *Drug may influence the metabolism of calcium and phosphorus.* Use wth caution in patients with metabolic bone diseases associated with hypercalcemia or in paitents with renal insufficiency. Patients with prostate cancer and osteoblastic bone metastasis are a trisk for hypocalcemia and should have close monitoring of serum calcium levels.
  - *Gynecomastia and impotence* are known antiestrogenic effects.
  - *Allergic reactions and angioedema* at times involving the airway have been reported.

Potential Toxicities/Side Effects and the Nursing Process

I.   POTENTIAL ALTERATION IN TISSUE PERFUSION related to THROMBOPHLEBITIS, THROMBOSIS

Defining Characteristics: Increased risk of clot formation, with risk for development of thrombophlebitis, pulmonary emboli, myocardial infarction, and cerebrovascular accident.

Nursing Implications: Assess patient risk; drug is contraindicated in patients with thrombophlebitis or thromboembolic disorders, unless caused by the malignancy. Should be used cautiously in these patients, and in those patients with coronary artery disease. Drug may worsen CHF. Assess baseline cardiac and peripheral vascular status, including signs/symptoms of CHF. Monitor blood pressure and glucose tolerance during therapy. Instruct patient to report immediately any signs/symptoms, e.g., dyspnea, edema, pain, and erythema in legs.

II.   BODY-IMAGE DISTURBANCE related to GYNECOMASTIA

Defining Characteristics: Mild to moderate breast enlargement may occur, with nipple tenderness initially.

Nursing Implications: Teach patient about potential side effects; discuss potential impact on body image and comfort. Encourage patient to verbalize feelings; provide information and emotional support.

III.   POTENTIAL ALTERATION IN COMFORT related to PERINEAL SYMPTOMS, HEADACHE, RASH, URTICARIA, TRANSIENT PARESTHESIAS (IV)

Defining Characteristics: Perineal itching and pain, as well as transient paresthesias of the mouth, may occur after IV administration (investigational). Other symptoms that may accompany oral dosing are rash, pruritus, dry skin, peeling skin of fingertips, thinning hair, night sweats, lethargy, pain in eyes, and breast tenderness.

Nursing Implications: Assess patient for occurrence of symptoms and discuss measures for symptomatic relief.

IV.   POTENTIAL FOR ALTERATION IN NUTRITION, LESS THAN BODY REQUIREMENTS, related to NAUSEA AND VOMITING, DIARRHEA, HEPATIC DYSFUNCTION

Defining Characteristics: Nausea and vomiting occur at higher dosing; tolerance may develop, but dose may need to be reduced. Nausea and vomiting may be delayed but become intractable and necessitate discontinuance of the drug. Diarrhea occurs occasionally. Mild elevations in liver function tests may occur (LDH, SGOT, bili) with or without jaundice, but are usually self-limiting. Abnormal Ca++ and P levels may occur.

Nursing Implications: Assess baseline nutritional fluid and electrolyte status. Premedicate with antiemetics prior to drug administration and continue through treatment. Assess baseline LFTs and Ca++ and P levels; monitor during therapy and discuss any abnormalities with physician. Monitor daily or weekly weights.

Drug: estrogens: diethylstilbestrol (DES), ethinyl estradiol (Estinyl), conjugated estrogen (Premarin), chlorotrianisene (Tace)

Class: Hormones.

Mechanism of Action: Unknown; estrogens change the hormonal milieu of the body.

Metabolism: Metabolized mainly in the liver. Undergoes enterohepatic recirculation. DES is metabolized more slowly than natural estrogens.

Dosage/Range:
- DES: Prostate cancer: 1–3 mg PO daily; breast cancer: 5 mg PO tid.
- Diethylstilbestrol diphosphate: Prostate cancer: 50–200 mg PO tid, 0.5–1.0 g IV daily × 5 days, then 250–1,000 mg each week.
- Chlorotrianisene: 1–10 mg PO tid.
- Ethinyl estradiol: 0.5–1.0 mg PO tid.

Drug Preparation:
- None.

Drug Administration:
- Oral.

Drug Interactions:
- None significant.

Lab Effects/Interference:
- Increased Ca.
- Increased T_4 levels.
- Increased clotting factors.
- Decreased serum folate.

Special Considerations:
- Long-term dosage of DES in men has been associated with cardiovascular deaths. Maximum dose should be 1 mg tid for prostate cancer.
- Can cause inaccurate laboratory results (liver, adrenal, thyroid).
- Causes rapid rise in serum calcium in patients with bony metastases; watch for symptoms of hypercalcemia.

Potential Toxicities/Side Effects and the Nursing Process

I.   POTENTIAL FOR INJURY related to THROMBOEMBOLIC COMPLICATIONS, HYPERCALCEMIA, SODIUM AND WATER RETENTION, AND CARDIOTOXICITY

Defining Characteristics: Thromboembolic complications are infrequent but serious, and increased risk occurs with long-term use and higher doses. Hypercalcemia occurs in 5–10% of women with breast cancer metastatic to bone, appears in first 2 weeks of therapy, and is aggravated by preexisting renal disease. There is an increased risk of cardiovascular-related deaths, especially in men on high-dose estrogens for prostate cancer. Drug should be used cautiously, if at all, in patients with underlying cardiac, renal, or hepatic disease.

Nursing Implications: Assess risk (preexisting cardiac, hepatic, and renal disease), baseline cardiac, and vascular status; discuss abnormalities with physician. Monitor status during therapy. Teach patient to report signs/symptoms of edema, dyspnea, localized swelling, pain, tenderness, erythema, and CNS changes. Teach female patient signs/symptoms of hypercalcemia (drowsiness, increased thirst, constipation, increased urine output) and to report this. Monitor Ca++ level in women with metastatic breast cancer closely during first few weeks of therapy.

II.   ALTERATION IN NUTRITION, LESS THAN BODY REQUIREMENTS, related to NAUSEA AND VOMITING

Defining Characteristics: Occurs in 25% of patients; intensity is related to specific drug and dose. Tolerance occurs after a few weeks of therapy.

Nursing Implications: Inform patient that this may occur; teach self-administration of antiemetics prior to drug administration per physician order, and to take drug at bedtime to decrease nausea. Discuss with physician starting patient at low dose, with increase as tolerated.

III. ALTERATION IN MALE SEXUAL FUNCTION related to GYNECOMASTIA, LOSS OF LIBIDO, IMPOTENCE, AND VOICE CHANGE

Defining Characteristics: Gynecomastia may be prevented by pretreatment of breast with low dose of radiotherapy. Feminine characteristics disappear when therapy is stopped.

Nursing Implications: Explore with patient and partner reproductive and sexual patterns and impact that chemotherapy may have. Provide information, supportive counseling, and referral as indicated. Since alternative, superior hormonal manipulative drugs are available, discuss these with physician.

IV. POTENTIAL FOR FEMALE SEXUAL DYSFUNCTION related to BREAST TENDERNESS/ENGORGEMENT, UTERINE PROLAPSE, AND URINARY INCONTINENCE

Defining Characteristics: Breast engorgement may occur in postmenopausal women; uterine prolapse and exacerbation of preexisting uterine fibroids with possible uterine bleeding may occur, as may urinary incontinence.

Nursing Implications: Explore with patient sexual and reproductive patterns, and any impact the drug may have. Provide information, supportive counseling, and referral as needed. Discuss with physician alternative hormonal manipulative drugs as needed.

Drug: etoposide phosphate (Etopophos)

Class: Plant alkaloid, a derivative of the mandrake plant (mayapple plant).

Mechanism of Action: Inhibits DNA synthesis in S and G_2 so that cells do not enter mitosis. Causes single-strand breaks in DNA. Cell cycle specific for S and G_2 phases.

Metabolism: Etoposide is rapidly excreted in the urine and, to a lesser extent, in the bile. About 30% of drug is excreted unchanged. Binds to serum albumin (94%) and then becomes extensively tissue-bound.

Indications: Management of (1) refractory testicular tumors, in combination with other approved chemotherapy agents in patients who have already received appropriate surgical, chemotherapeutic, and radiotherapeutic therapy, (2) small-cell lung cancer, in combination with cisplatin as first-line treatment.

Contraindications: patients who have demonstrated a previous hypersensitivity reaction to etoposide, etoposide phosphate, or any other component of the formulations.

Dosage/Range:
- Refractory testicular cancer, in combination with other chemotherapy agents: 50–100 mg/m^2 IV infusion daily over 5 min to 3.5 hours days 1–5 days, or 100 mg/m^2 IV infusion over 5 min to 3.5 hours daily on days 1, 3, 5 every 3–4 weeks.
- Small cell lung cancer, in combination with cisplatin: 35 mg/m^2 IV over 5 min to 3.5 hours × 4 days or 50 mg/m^2 IV over 5 min to 3.5 hours daily × 5 days every 3–4 weeks.
- Do not administer by bolus injection.
- If renal impairment (CrCl 15-50 mL/min): give 75% of dose. If CrCl is < 15 mL/min, dose should be lowered further (Bristol-Myers Squibb, 2017). Subsequent dosing should be based on patient tolerance and clinical effect.

Drug Preparation:
- The 110-mg Etopophos vial is reconstituted with 5 mL (resulting in a concentration of 20 mg/mL) or 10 mL (resulting in a concentration of 10 mg/mL) Sterile water for injection USP, 0.9% Normal Saline for Injection USP, D$_5$ Dextrose Injection USP, bacteriostatic water for injection with benzyl alcohol, or bacteriostatic normal saline with benzyl alcohol. May be further diluted with NS or D$_5$W to up to a 0.1 mg/mL final concentration.
- For injection: 114 mg etoposide phosphate is equivalent to 100 mg etoposide.
- Storage:
  - Unopened vials should be stored under refrigeration (2–8°C, 36–46°F). Keep in box to protect from light.
  - When Etopophos is reconstituted as directed in package insert, solutions can be stored in glass or plastic containers refrigerated (2–8°C, 36–46°F) for 7 days. At controlled room temperature (20–25°C, 68–77°F) for 24 hours after reconstitution with sterile water for injection USP, 5% dextrose injection USP or 0.9% sodium chloride injection USP; or 48 hours after reconstitution with bacteriostatic water for injection with benzyl alcohol or bacteriostatic sodium chloride for injection with benzyl alcohol.
  - Etopophos solutions further diluted as directed can be stored under refrigeration or at controlled room temperature for 24 hours (Bristol-Myers Squibb, 2017).

Drug Administration:
- IV infusion: administer over 5 min to 3.5 hours IV. Do not administer IV bolus.
- Inspect for clarity of solution prior to administration.
- Use safe handling precautions.

Drug Interactions:
- Enhances warfarin action by increasing prothrombin time (PT); need to monitor INR closely.

Lab Effects/Interference:
- Increased PT, INR with patients on warfarin.
- Increased LFTs, metabolic acidosis with higher doses.

Special Considerations:
- Warnings and Precautions:
  - *Myelosupprression*: is dose-limiting toxicity. Hold drug for a platelet count <50,000/ mm³ or an ANC <500/mm³ until recover. Toxicity of rapidly infused drug in patients with impaired renal or hepatic function has not been evaluated. Toxicity of infused doses >175 mg/m² are not known.
  - *Hypersensitivity reactions*: is possible, characterized by chills, fever, tachycardia, bronchospasm, dyspnea, and hypotension. Manage symptomaticallsy after drug has been terminated. Pressor agents, corticosteroids, antihistamines or volume expanders may be needed per the physician.
  - *Embryo-fetal toxicity*: Teach women of reproductive potential to use effective contraception to prevent pregnancy during treatment and for 6 months after final dose. Males with female sexual partners of reproductive potential should use condoms during drug treatment and for at least 4 months after the final dose.
  - Infertility: may occur in male patients, with oligospermia, azoospermia, and permanent infertility. In some cases, may occur several years after the end of therapy. Female patients may develop amenorrhea; recovery of menses and ovulation is a function of age at treatment. Premature menopause may occur.
  - *Secondare leukemias:* Acute leukemia may occur rarely with or without other antineoplastic drugs in combination.
- Nadir 7–14 days after treatment.

Potential Toxicities/Side Effects and the Nursing Process

I.   POTENTIAL FOR INJURY related to ALLERGIC REACTION, HYPOTENSION, ANAPHYLAXIS DURING DRUG INFUSION

Defining Characteristics: Bronchospasm (wheezing) may occur, with or without fever, chills; hypotension may occur during rapid infusion. Anaphylaxis may occur, but is rare.

Nursing Implications: Infuse drug over at least 30–60 minutes in correct amount of IV solution (stability related to volume). Monitor temperature, vital signs prior to drug administration, and periodically during treatment. Remain with patient during first 15 minutes of infusion and assess for signs/symptoms of bronchospasm. Discontinue drug and notify physician if bronchospasm or signs/symptoms of anaphylactic-like reaction occur. Maintain patent IV, monitor VS, and have ready epinephrine, diphenhydramine, and hydrocortisone, as well as emergency equipment. Be familiar with institution's practice guidelines for management of anaphylaxis.

II.   POTENTIAL FOR INFECTION AND BLEEDING related to BM DEPRESSION

Defining Characteristics: Nadir 10–14 days after drug dose, with recovery on days 21–22. Neutropenia may be severe. Profound BM suppression when given in high doses for BM/ stem cell rescue.

Nursing Implications: Monitor CBC, WBC, differential, and platelet count prior to chemotherapy and at expected nadir. Assess for signs/symptoms of infection or bleeding prior to drug administration; instruct patient in self-assessment and to report signs/symptoms immediately. Teach patient self-care measures to minimize risk of infection and bleeding, including avoidance of OTC aspirin-containing medications.

III. ALTERED NUTRITION, LESS THAN BODY REQUIREMENTS, related to NAUSEA AND VOMITING, ANOREXIA

Defining Characteristics: Nausea and vomiting are usually mild, occurring soon after infusion. Oral dosing has higher incidence of nausea/vomiting. Anorexia is mild but may be severe with oral dosing. Severe nausea and vomiting when given in high doses, requires aggressive, maximal antiemesis. In addition, hepatitis, stomatitis, and metabolic acidosis may occur with high-dose therapy.

Nursing Implications: Premedicate with antiemetics and continue prophylactically for at least 4–6 hours after drug administration. Encourage small feedings of bland, cool foods and liquids; encourage spices as desired. Consult dietitian if anorexia is severe. Patients receiving high-dose therapy should have baseline and periodic assessment of laboratory parameters (e.g., LFTs and chemistries), as well as assessment of oral mucosa. Teach patients self-care, including oral assessment, use of oral hygiene regimen, and to report pain, burning, oral lesions.

IV. BODY-IMAGE DISTURBANCE related to ALOPECIA

Defining Characteristics: Incidence is 20–90% and is dose dependent; regrowth may occur between drug cycles.

Nursing Implications: Discuss with patient possible hair loss and potential coping strategies, including obtaining wig or cap. If hair loss is complete, instruct patient to wear cap or scarf at night to prevent loss of body heat in cold climates.

V. POTENTIAL SEXUAL DYSFUNCTION related to DRUG EFFECTS

Defining Characteristics: Drug is mutagenic and teratogenic.

Nursing Implications: Explore with patient and partner sexual patterns and reproductive goals. Teach about need for contraception as appropriate. Provide information, emotional support, and referral as needed.

VI. ALTERED SKIN INTEGRITY related to RADIATION RECALL, PERIVASCULAR IRRITATION IF DRUG INFILTRATES, AND SKIN LESIONS WITH HIGH-DOSE THERAPY

Defining Characteristics: Drug is a radiosensitizer and an irritant. Patients receiving high-dose therapy may develop bullae on the skin (similar to Stevens-Johnson syndrome).

TREATMENT

Nursing Implications: Assess skin in area of prior radiation when combined therapies are given as well as mucous membranes. Drug may need to be withheld until skin healing occurs if radiation recall results in skin breakdown. Teach patient wound-management techniques. Use careful venipuncture and infuse drug through patent IV over 30–60 minutes, diluted according to manufacturer's specifications. Teach patients receiving high-dose therapy to report any skin changes.

VII. ALTERATION IN CARDIAC OUTPUT related to RARE MYOCARDIAL INFARCTION, ARRHYTHMIAS

Defining Characteristics: Rare myocardial infarction has been reported after prior mediastinal XRT in patients receiving etoposide-containing regimens. Arrhythmias are uncommon but may occur, especially in patients with preexisting coronary artery disease.

Nursing Implications: Monitor patient during infusion and instruct patient to report any unusual sensations. Discuss any abnormalities with physician.

VIII. SENSORY/PERCEPTUAL ALTERATION related to NEUROTOXICITY

Defining Characteristics: Peripheral neuropathies may occur but are uncommon and mild.

Nursing Implications: Assess motor and sensory function prior to drug administration. Instruct patient to report any changes in sensation or function. Discuss any abnormalities with physician. Encourage patient to verbalize feelings about discomfort and sensory loss, and discuss alternative coping strategies.

Data from Dorr RT, Von Hoff DD. *Cancer Chemotherapy Handbook*, 2nd ed. Norwalk, CT: Appleton & Lange; 1994: 462.

Drug: exemestane (Aromasin)

Class: Steroidal aromatase inactivator.

Mechanism of Action: Aromatase converts adrenal and ovarian androgens into estrogen, peripherally, in postmenopausal women. Exemestane acts as a false substrate (looks like androstenedione) and binds irreversibly to the aromatase enzyme, making it inactive ("suicide inhibition"). This results in a significant decrease (up to 95%) in circulating estrogen levels in postmenopausal women without affecting other adrenal enzymes. In the absence of estrogen, the stimulus for breast cancer growth is removed.

Metabolism: Oral drug is rapidly absorbed from the GI tract, with plasma levels increased by about 40% if taken after a high-fat breakfast. Drug is extensively distributed into the tissues, and is highly protein-bound (90%). Drug is extensively metabolized in the liver by the P450 3A4 (CYP3A4) isoenzyme system, and excreted equally in urine and feces. After a single dose of 25 mg, maximal suppression of circulating estrogen occurs 2–3 days after the dose, and lasts for 4–5 days. In patients with either hepatic or renal insufficiency, the dose of exemestane was three times higher than in patients with normal liver or renal function. This does not require dosage adjustment, but studies looking at the safety of chronic dosing in these groups of patients have not been done.

Indication: For (1) adjuvant treatment of postmenopausal women with estrogen-receptor positive early breast cancer who have received 2–3 years of tamoxifen and are switched to exemestane for completion of a total of 5 consecutive years of adjuvant hormonal therapy, and (2) treatment of advanced breast cancer in postmenopausal women whose disease has progressed following tamoxifen therapy. Drug is NOT indicated for treatment of pre-menopausal women.

Contraindication: Patients with a known hypersensitivity to the drug or to its excipients.

Dosage/Range:
- 25-mg tab PO daily after a meal.

Dose Modifications:
- Concomitant use of a strong CYP3A4 inducer (e.g., rifampin or phenytoin), which will decrease serum exemestane level: Exemestane dose should be 50 mg once daily after a meal (Pfizer, 2018).

Drug Preparation:
- None. Store tablets at 77°F (25°C).

Drug Administration:
- Oral, once daily, after a meal.
- Assess 25-hydroxyvitamin D levels prior to the start of aromatase inhibitor treatment; if low, patient should receive supplemental vitamin D.
- In women receiving adjuvant therapy who have or are at risk for developing osteoporosis, assess Bone Mineral Density (BMD) baseline and during therapy, as BMD decreases with treatment over time. If osteoporosis, treat as ordered.

Drug Interactions:
- CYP3A4 inhibitors: significant drug interactions unlikely.
- CYP3A4 inducers (rifampin, phenytoin, carbamazepine, phenobarbital, St. John's wort): may significantly lower exemestane serum levels; do not use concurrently.
- Estrogen-containing medications: do not co-administer as estrogen may interfere with drug's mechanism of action.

Lab Effects/Interference:
- Lymphopenia (20% incidence).
- Elevated LFTs (AST, ALT, alk phos, GGT) rarely.

Special Considerations:
- Warnings and Precautions:
  - *Administration with estrogen-containing agents*: do not coadminister as will interfere with exemestane pharmacologic action.

- *Reductions in Bone Mineral Density (BMD):* In women receiving adjuvant therapy who have or are at risk for developing osteoporosis, assess bone densitometry baseline and during therapy, as BMD decreases with treatment over time. If a decrease in BMD occurs (osteoporosis), treat as ordered.
  - *Vitamin D assessment:* 25-hydroxy vitamin D levels should be assessed prior to starting therapy as it is often low in women with early breast cancer. If serum level low, patient should receive supplemental vitamin D.
  - *Laboratory abnormalities:* Assess for lymphocytopenia, elevated LFTs (AST, ALT, GGT, alkaline phosphatase, bilirubin), and elevated serum creatinine.
  - *Use in pre-menopausal women:* NOT indicated for use in this population
  - *Embryo-fetal toxicity:* Teach women to use effective contraception during treatment, and to continue for one month after last dose.
- Drug is excreted in maternal milk so mothers should make a decision to stop nursing or stop the drug, taking into account the importance of the drug to the mother's health.
- Drug is well tolerated, with mild to moderate side effects.
- Differs from other selective aromatase inhibitors in that drug irreversibly binds to aromatase, and androgens cannot displace drug from this enzyme. Body must synthesize new aromatase to start estrogen production again.
- Exemestane has been shown to reduce the risk for breast cancer by 65% in high-risk women, adding the drug to the breast cancer preventive agent armamentarium. In addition, the study showed a 60% reduction in invasive breast cancer plus pre-invasive ductal carcinoma in situ and fewer cases to cancer precursor lesions, including atypical ductal hyperplasia and atypical lobular hyperplasia, compared to the placebo group (Goss et al., 2011).
- Most common adverse events:
  - Early breast cancer: hot flashes, fatigue, arthralgia, headache, insomnia, increased sweating.
  - Advanced breast cancer: hot flashes, nausea, fatigue, increased sweating, increased appetite.

Potential Toxicities/Side Effects and the Nursing Process

I.   ALTERATION IN ACTIVITY related to FATIGUE

Defining Characteristics: Overall incidence in studies is 22%, while incidence considered drug-related or of indeterminate cause is 8%.

Nursing Implications: Assess baseline activity tolerance and self-care ability. Teach patient that fatigue may occur but is usually mild to moderate. Teach patient to alternate rest and activity. Teach patient to manage ADLs using energy-saving strategies, e.g., shopping, cooking. Teach patient to accept assistance from friends and family as needed.

II. ALTERATION IN COMFORT related to HOT FLASHES, INCREASED SWEATING, PAIN

Defining Characteristics: Incidence of events attributable to exemestane were hot flashes (13%) and increased sweating (4%). In total evaluation of all adverse events, all patients, pain was reported in 13%.

Nursing Implications: Assess patient baseline comfort, and incidence and tolerance of hot flashes and increased sweating. Assess whether patient has any pain, as well as effectiveness of current pain-management regimen. Teach patient self-care strategies to maximize comfort, to keep cool (e.g., light, loose clothing; fans; cool drinks) and dry (e.g., use of cornstarch after bathing, fan), and to minimize any painful discomfort (e.g., depending upon type and location of pain, OTC analgesics, application of heat, cold, Tiger Balm).

III. ALTERATION IN NUTRITION, POTENTIAL, related to NAUSEA, INCREASED APPETITE

Defining Characteristics: Nausea appeared drug-related or of indeterminate cause in 9% of patients, and 3% of patients noted an increased appetite. 8% of patients receiving drug complained of weight gain (greater than 10% of baseline). These side effects are mild to moderate if they occur.

Nursing Implications: Assess baseline nutritional status, optimal and desired weight, and any changes. Teach patient to report nausea or weight gain. Teach patient strategies to minimize nausea (e.g., dietary modification, taking drug after meals) if it occurs, and discuss with physician antiemetic medication if dietary modification not effective. If patient experiences weight gain, discuss patient interest in gentle exercising, such as progressive muscle resistance, which would encourage weight gain as lean body mass rather than fat.

IV. SENSORY/PERCEPTION ALTERATIONS, POTENTIAL, related to DEPRESSION, INSOMNIA

Defining Characteristics: While not reported as side effects considered drug-related or of indeterminate cause, depression and insomnia occurred in 13% and 11%, respectively, of patients participating in the clinical trials.

Nursing Implications: Assess baseline effect, use of effective coping strategies in dealing with disease and treatment, and usual sleep patterns. Teach patient to report changes in mood, such as depression, and difficulty falling asleep, or early awakening. If this occurs, further assess symptom, and suggest self-care strategies to minimize symptom. If nonpharmacologic measures are ineffective, discuss use of antidepressant or sleeping medication with physician, depending upon assessment.

Drug: floxuridine (FUDR, 2'-deoxy-5-fluorouridine)

Class: Nucleoside metabolic inhibitor (Antimetabolite).

Mechanism of Action: Antimetabolite (fluorinated pyrimidine) that is metabolized to 5-FU when given by IV bolus, or metabolized to 5-FUDR-MP 5-fluoro-2'-deoxyuridine-5'-monophosphate when smaller doses are given, by CI intra-arterially. FUDR-MP is four times more effective in inhibiting the enzyme thymidine synthetase than 5-FU. The inhibition prevents the synthesis of thymidine, an essential component of DNA, resulting in interruption of DNA synthesis and cell death. Other FUDR metabolites inhibit RNA synthesis. Drug is cell cycle specific, with activity during the S phase.

Metabolism: When given IV, drug is transformed to 5-FU; 70–90% of drug is extracted by liver on first pass. Metabolites are excreted by kidneys and lungs. CI decreases metabolism of drug with more of the drug being converted to the active metabolite FUDR-MP.

Indication: FDA-approved for intrahepatic arterial infusion only.

Dosage/Range:
- Intra-arterially (hepatic) by slow infusion pump: 0.1–0.6 mg/kg/day $\times$ 7–14 days.

Drug Preparation:
- Reconstitute 500-mg vial of lyophilized powder with 5-mL sterile water (100 mg/mL), then dilute with 0.9% sodium chloride or D_5W to volume appropriate for intra-arterial pump.

Drug Administration:
- INTRA-ARTERIAL infusion only.
- Usually administered by slow intra-arterial infusion using a surgically placed catheter or percutaneous catheter in a major artery.
- H_2 antagonist antihistamine (i.e., ranitidine 150 mg PO bid) administered concurrently during intra-arterial infusion to prevent development of peptic ulcer disease.

Drug Interactions:
- None significant.

Lab Effects/Interference:
- Decreased WBC, platelets.
- PT, total protein, sedimentation rate (abnormal values), BSP.
- Increased LFTs.

Special Considerations:
- Higher doses of the drug increase the risk of biliary sclerosis and fibrosis.
- Drug usually given for 14 days, then heparinized saline for 14 days to maintain line patency.
- Dose reductions or infusion breaks may be necessary depending on toxicity.

Potential Toxicities/Side Effects and the Nursing Process

I. ALTERED NUTRITION, LESS THAN BODY REQUIREMENTS, related to NAUSEA/VOMITING, ANOREXIA, STOMATITIS/ESOPHOPHARYNGITIS, DIARRHEA, GASTRITIS, HEPATIC DYSFUNCTION

Defining Characteristics: Nausea and vomiting occur infrequently and are mild; anorexia is common. Mucositis is milder than 5-FU when administered intrahepatically, but more severe when given via carotid artery. Diarrhea is mild to moderately severe. Gastritis may occur, with abdominal cramping and pain. Incidence is greater in patients receiving hepatic artery infusion. Duodenal ulcers may occur in 10% of patients, be painless, and lead to gastric outlet obstruction and vomiting. Chemical hepatitis may be severe, with increased alk phos in patients receiving drug via hepatic artery infusions.

Nursing Implications: Premedicate with antiemetics as ordered and teach patient in self-administration of prescribed antiemetics. Encourage small, frequent feedings of cool, bland foods. If intractable nausea and vomiting, severe diarrhea, or severe cramping occurs, notify physician, stop drug, and infuse heparinized saline. Teach patient oral assessment and oral hygiene regimen, and instruct to report any signs/symptoms of stomatitis, esophopharyngitis. Instruct patient to report diarrhea. Teach self-care measures, including diet modification and self-administration of prescribed antidiarrheal medication. Assess for signs/symptoms of abdominal stress, cramping prior to and during infusion. Discuss with physician use of antacids and antisecretory medications. Catheter placement should be verified prior to each infusion cycle, and inadvertent drug infusion into gastric/duodenal-supplying arteries should be investigated. Monitor LFTs prior to drug initiation, during treatment, and at end of 14-day cycle. Discuss abnormalities and dose reductions with physician. Assess patient for signs/symptoms of liver dysfunction: lethargy, weakness, malaise, anorexia, fever, jaundice, icterus.

II. POTENTIAL FOR INJURY related to INTRA-ARTERIAL CATHETER PROBLEMS

Defining Characteristics: Catheter problems that may occur include leakage, arterial ischemia or aneurysm, bleeding at catheter site, catheter occlusion, thrombosis or embolism of artery, vessel perforation or dislodged catheter, infection, and biliary sclerosis.

Nursing Implications: Assess catheter carefully prior to each cycle of therapy for patency, signs/symptoms of infection. Ensure that catheter position and patency are determined prior to each cycle of therapy; do not force flushing solution—reassess and try again. If still unsuccessful, notify physician.

III. SENSORY/PERCEPTUAL ALTERATIONS related to HFS AND OTHER CNS SYMPTOMS

Defining Characteristics: HFS occurs in 30–40% of patients (numbness, sensory changes in hands and feet). Uncommonly, cerebellar ataxia, vertigo, nystagmus, seizures, depression, hemiplegia, hiccups, lethargy, and blurred vision may occur.

Nursing Implications: Assess baseline neurologic status prior to and during therapy. Teach patient that HFS may occur and instruct to report signs/symptoms. Discuss with physician use of pyridoxine 50 mg tid to prevent HFS. Assess ability to do ADLs and level of comfort.

IV. ALTERATION IN SKIN INTEGRITY related to LOCALIZED ERYTHEMA, DERMATITIS, NONSPECIFIC SKIN TOXICITY, OR RASH

Defining Characteristics: Erythema, dermatitis, pruritus, or rash may occur.

Nursing Implications: Assess for skin changes. Assess impact on comfort and body image. Teach patient self-care.

V. POTENTIAL FOR INFECTION AND BLEEDING related to BM DEPRESSION

Defining Characteristics: Occurs rarely when FUDR is given as a single agent via continuous intra-arterial infusion.

Nursing Implications: Assess baseline WBC, neutrophil count, and platelets, during treatment and at completion of 14-day infusion. Discontinue drug infusion if WBC $< 3,500/mm^3$ or if platelet count $< 100,000/mm^3$, or per established physician orders; refill pump with heparinized saline.

Drug: fludarabine phosphate (Fludara)

Class: Antimetabolite.

Mechanism of Action: Inhibits DNA synthesis, probably by inhibiting DNA-polymerase-alpha, ribonucleotide reductase, and DNA primase.

Metabolism: Drug is rapidly converted to the active metabolite 2-fluoro ara-A when given intravenously. The drug's half-life is about 10 hours. The major route of elimination is via the kidneys, and approximately 23% of the active drug is excreted unchanged in the urine.

Indication: Indicated for the treatment of adult patients with B-cell CLL who have not responded to treatment or whose disease progressed during treatment with at least one standard alkylating agent-containing regimen, or who have progressed on prior alkylating treatment.

Contraindication: Contraindicated in patients with hypersensitivity to the drug or its components. Because drug is excreted in the urine, do not administer to patients with 24 hours creatinine clearance <30 mL/min.

Dosage/Range:
- IV: 25 mg/m^2 IV over 30 minutes daily $\times$ 5 days, repeated every 28 days.
  - IV: CrCl 50–79 mL/min-dose should be 20 mg/ m^2 IV over 30 minutes daily $\times$ 5 days, repeated every 28 days.

- IV: CrCl 30–49 mL/min-dose should be 15 mg/ m^2 IV over 30 minutes daily × 5 days, repeated every 28 days. Do not administer if CrCl is <30 mL/min.
- Delay or discontinue drug if hematologic, nonhematologic, or neurotoxicity develops.

Dose Modification:
- Administer cautiously in patients with renal insufficiency. Patients with a creatinine clearance of 30–79 mL/min should receive a dose reduction; the drug should not be given to patients with a CrCl < 30 mL/min (Teva, 2014).

Drug Preparation:
- Available as fludarabine phosphate injection USP as 50 mg/2 mL sterile solution.
- IV: Aseptically add 2 mL sterile water for injection USP to the 50-mg vial, resulting in a final concentration of 25 mg/mL. The drug may then be diluted further in 100 mL of 5% dextrose or 0.9% sodium chloride.
- Once reconstituted, the drug should be used within 8 hours as it does not contain a preservative.
- Inspect for particulate matter and discoloration.

Drug Administration:
- IV infusion over 30 minutes.
- Oral: swallow tablet whole with water; may take with or without food; do not chew or crush.

Drug Interactions:
- Pentostatin: increased risk for severe, potentially fatal pulmonary toxicity; do not administer concomitantly.
- Live vaccines should not be administered during fludarabine therapy.

Lab Effects/Interference:
- Decreased CBC.
- TLS.

Special Considerations:
- Warnings and Precautions:
  - *Dose-dependent neurologic toxicities*: overdosage (four times recommended dose) has been associated with delayed blindness, coma, and death. In postmarketing experience, neurotoxicity has been reported either earlier or later than in clinical trials (range 7–225 days). Discontinue or delay treatment if neurotoxicity develops.
  - *Bone marrow suppression*: May be severe, notably anemia, thrombocytopenia, and neutropenia. BM suppression may be cumulative. Median time to nadir was 13 days for granulocytes, and 16 days for platelets. Monitor CBC/ANC closely. Rarely, trilineage BM hypoplasia or aplasia has occurred in adult patients.
  - *Autoimmune reactions*: may be life-threatening or fatal, and although uncommon, include hemolytic anemia, thrombocytopenia/ITP, Evans syndrome (autoimmune destruction of WBC, RBC or platelets), and acquired hemophilia. Steroids may or may not be helpful. See package insert (Teva, 2014).

- *Transfusion associated graft-versus-host disease*: May be seen after transfusion of nonirradiated blood and may be fatal. All patients who are planning to receive, or who have received, fludarabine should receive irradiated blood ONLY (Sagent, 2016).
- *Pulmonary toxicity*: Do not administer in combination with pentostatin, as fatal pulmonary toxicity can occur.
- *Embryo-fetal toxicity*: Teach women of reproductive potential to use effective contraception to avoid pregnancy.
- *Male fertility and reproductive outcomes*: Males with female sexual partners of child-bearing potential should use effective barrier protection to prevent pregnancy during and after treatment with fludarabine as there may be genetic changes in the spermatozoa (Sagent, 2016).
- *Tumor lysis*: TLS may occur in patients with high tumor burden. Discuss TLS prophylaxis with physician/NP/PA prior to beginning therapy.
- *Renal impairment*: Administer cautiously in patients with renal insufficiency. Patients with a creatinine clearance of 30–79 mL/min should receive a dose reduction; the drug should not be given to patients with a CrCl < 30 mL/min (Sagent, 2016).
- *Vaccination*: Avoid vaccination with live vaccines during and after treatment with fludarabine.
- Mothers should not breastfeed their infant during drug treatment.Most common toxicities were anemia, neutropenia, thrombocytopenia: nonhematologic: fever, infections, pain, neurolocial (e.g., weakness, headache), pulmonary, nausea/vomiting, rash.

Potential Toxicities/Side Effects and the Nursing Process

I.   INFECTION AND BLEEDING related to BM DEPRESSION

Defining Characteristics: Severe and cumulative BM depression may occur; nadir, 13 days (range, 3–25 days).

Nursing Implications: Monitor CBC, platelet count prior to drug administration, as well as signs/symptoms of infection and bleeding. Instruct patient in self-assessment of signs/symptoms of infection and bleeding as well as self-care measures, including avoidance of OTC aspirin-containing medication.

II. POTENTIAL FOR ACTIVITY INTOLERANCE related to ANEMIA-INDUCED FATIGUE

Defining Characteristics: BM depression often includes red cell line.

Nursing Implications: Monitor Hgb/HCT; discuss transfusion with physician if HCT does not recover postchemotherapy. Teach patient high-iron diet as appropriate.

III.   SENSORY/PERCEPTUAL ALTERATIONS related to CNS EFFECTS, PERIPHERAL NEUROPATHIES

Defining Characteristics: Agitation, confusion, visual disturbances, and coma have oc-curred. Objective weakness has been reported (9–65%), as have paresthesias (4–12%).

Nursing Implications: Assess baseline neurologic status; monitor neurologic vital signs. Teach patient signs/symptoms and instruct to report them if they occur. Evaluate these changes with physician and discuss continuation of therapy.

IV.   POTENTIAL FOR IMPAIRED GAS EXCHANGE related to PULMONARY TOXICITY

Defining Characteristics: Pneumonia occurs in 16–22% of patients. Pulmonary hypersen-sitivity reaction characterized by dyspnea, cough, interstitial pulmonary infiltrate has been observed. Fatal pulmonary toxicity has occurred when drug is given in combination with pentostatin (Deoxycoformycin).

Nursing Implications: Instruct patient in possible side effects and to report dyspnea, cough, signs of breathlessness following exertion. Assess lung sounds prior to chemother-apy administration. DO NOT administer drug in combination with pentostatin.

V.   POTENTIAL FOR SEXUAL DYSFUNCTION related to TERATOGENICITY

Defining Characteristics: Drug is teratogenic; may cause testicular atrophy. It is unknown whether drug is excreted in breastmilk.

Nursing Implications: As appropriate, explore with patient and partner issues of repro-duction and sexuality patterns, and impact that chemotherapy may have. Discuss strategies to preserve sexual and reproductive health (sperm banking, contraception). Mothers receiv-ing drug should not breastfeed.

VI.   ALTERED NUTRITION, LESS THAN BODY REQUIREMENTS, related to NAUSEA/VOMITING, DIARRHEA

Defining Characteristics: Nausea/vomiting occurs in about 36% of patients and can be prevented with standard antiemetics; diarrhea occurs in 15% of patients.

Nursing Implications: Premedicate with antiemetics; evaluate response to emetic protec-tion. Encourage small, frequent meals of cool, bland foods and liquids. If vomiting occurs, assess for signs/symptoms of fluid/electrolyte imbalance; monitor I/O and daily weights, lab results. Encourage patient to report onset of diarrhea; teach patient to administer antidi-arrheal medication as ordered.

Drug: fluorouracil, adrucil, 5-FU, 5-fluorouracil (Fluorouracil, Adrucil, 5-FU, Efudex [topical])

Class: Pyrimidine antimetabolite.

Mechanism of Action: Acts as a "false" pyrimidine, inhibiting the formation of an enzyme (thymidine synthetase) necessary for the synthesis of DNA. Also incorporates into RNA, causing abnormal synthesis. Methotrexate given prior to 5-FU results in synergism and enhanced efficacy.

Metabolism: Metabolized by the liver; most is excreted as respiratory CO_2, remainder is excreted by the kidneys. Plasma half-life is 20 minutes.

Indication: In the treatment of patients with (1) adenocarcinoma of the colon and rectum; (2) adenocarcinoma of the breast; (3) gastric adenocarcinoma; (4) adenocarcinoma of the pancreas.

Contraindicated: In the treatment of patients in a poor nutritional state, with depressed BM function, with potentially serious infections, or those with a known hypersensitivity to the drug.

Dosage/Range:
- General (Sagent, 2016):
  - IVB or IV infusion.
- **Colon and Rectal Cancer**
  - 5-FU 400mg/m² administered as an infusional regimen in combination with leucovorin alone or in combination with leucovorin and oxaliplatin or irinotecan on day 1, followed by 2,400 mg/m² to 3,000 mg/m² IV as a continuous infusion over 46 hours every 2 weeks.
  - 5-FU inection as an IVB in combination with leucovoring is 500 mg/m² IVB on days 1, 8, 15, 22, 29, and 36 in 8-week cycles.
  - De Gramont (LV5-FU2): Day 1: Leucovorin 200 mg/m² IV over 2 hours d 1, 2; 5-FU 400 mg/m² IVB followed by 600 mg/m² IV infusion × 22 hours d 1, 2.
  - FLOX and FOLFOX regimens: See oxaliplatin.
- **Adenocarcinoma of the Breast:** 5-FU as a component of a cyclophosphamide-based multidrug regimen: 500 mg/m² or 600 mg/m² IV on days 1 and 8 every 28 days × 6 cycles.
- **Gastric Adenocarcinoma:** 5-FU as a component of a platinum-containing multi-drug regimen: 200–1,000 mg/m² IV as a continuous infusion over 24 hours. The frequency and cycle length will depend upon the dose of 5-FU and the regimen.
- **Pancreatic Adenocarcinoma**: 5-FU as an infusional regimen in combination with leucovorin or as a component of a multidrug chemotherapy regimen that includes leucovorin, e.g., 400 mg/m² IVB on Day 1, followed by 2,400 mg/m² IV as a continuous infusion over 46 hours every 2 weeks.

Dose Modifications:
- Hold 5-FU for the following: (1) angina, MI, arrthythmia, heart failure in patients without prior history of CAD or myocardial dysfunction; (2) hyperammonemic encephalopathy; (3) acute cerebellar syndrome, confusion, disorientation, ataxia, or visual disturbances; (4) grade 3–4 diarrhea; grade 2–3 PPE (hand foot syndrome); (5) grade 3–4 mucositis; (6) grade 4 myelosuppression.
- Upon resolution or improvement to grade 1 diarrhea, mucositis, myelosuppression, or PPE, resume 5-FU administration at a reduced dose.

Drug Preparation:
- No dilution required. Can be added to 0.9% sodium chloride or 5% dextrose.
- Store at room temperature; protect from light. Solution should be clear: if crystals do not disappear after holding vial under hot water, discard vial.
- Inspect solution for precipitate prior to CI.

Drug Administration:
- Assess CBC/differential before each dose, assess for signs and symptoms of HFS, diarrhea, stomatitis, chest pain prior to each dose.
- Given via IV push or bolus or, most commonly, as continuous infusion (CI); CI should be infused through a central venous access device using an infusion pump.

Drug Interactions:
- Warfarin: may increase anticoagulant effect; monitor INR closely and dose warfarin based on result.
- When given with cimetidine, there are increased pharmacologic effects of fluorouracil.
- When given with thiazide diuretics, there is increased risk of myelosuppression.
- Leucovorin causes increased 5-fluorouracil cytotoxicity.

Lab Effects/Interference:
- Decreased CBC.

Special Considerations:
- Warnings and Precautions: *Increased risk of serious or fatal adverse reactions in patients with low or absent dipyrimidine dehydrogenase (DPD) activity:* Patients with certain homozygous or certain compound heterozygous mutations in the DPD gene are at increased risk for acute early-onset toxicity and severe, life-threatening, or fatal reactions caused by 5-FU (e.g., mucositis, diarrhea, neutropenia, and neurotoxicity). If a patient developes early-onset or unusually severe toxicity, hold or permanently discontinue 5-FU until genetic testing can verify condition. These patients with impaired DPD activity should not receive 5-FU.
- *Cardiotoxicity*: Patients with coronary artery disease and receiving 5-FU as a continuous infusion are at risk for developing angina, MI/ischemia, arrhythmia, and heart failure. Hold drug if patient develops cardiotoxicity.
- *Hyperammonemic encephalopathy*: 5-FU can cause this in the absence of liver disease or other cause. Assess for signs/symptoms: altered mental status, confusion, disorientation, coma, or ataxia, in the presence of concomitant elevated serum ammonia level. Hold 5-FU for this and begin ammonia-lowering therapy.

- *Neurologic toxicity:* Acute cerebellar toxicity and other neurological events may occur, characterized by confusion, disorientation, ataxia, or visual disturbances. Hold drug if this occurs.
- *Diarrhea:* Diarrhea may be severe, and drug should be held for grade 3–4 diarrhea until it has resolved or decreased to ≤grade 1, then resume 5-FU at a reduced dose. May occur before significant bone marrow suppression so ensure patient is closely monitored as diarrhea can result in severe infection if it occurs during the nadir.
- *Palmar-plantar erythrodysesthesia (hand-foot syndrome):* Symptoms include tingling, pain, swelling, and erythema with tenderness and desquamation. Palms and soles of feet become symmetrically swollen and erythematous, possibly with desquamation, then resolving in 5–7 days. Also areas of pressure are at risk, such as if the patient sits in a wheelchair frequently—assess areas of continuous pressure. HFS occurs more commonly with CI than when given as an IVB. Onset is usually after 8–9 weeks of therapy but may occur earlier. Interrupt 5-FU for grade 2–3 HFS, and resume 5-FU at a reduced dose after HFS has resolved completely or severity is ≤grade 1.
- *Myelosuppression:* can be severe and potentially fatal (neutropenia, thrombocytopenia, anemia), Nadir is days 9–14. Assess cbc/ANC prior to each treatment cycle and PRN. Hold 5-FU until grade 4 myelosuppression resolves; resume when resolved or improved to grade 1 at a reduced dose.
- *Mucositis:* may occur, and is more likely with IVB versus CI. Hold drug for grade 3-4, and resume at a reduced dose once resolved or improved to grade 1.
- *Increased risk of elevated INR with warfarin:* Closely monitor patients receiving warfarin and 5-FU, as warfarin may require frequent dose adjustments based on PT or INR.
- *Embryo-fetal toxicity:* teach women of reproductive potential, and men with female sexual partners of reproductive potential to use effective contraception to avoid pregnancy during 5-FU therapy and for 3 months after the last 5-FU dose.
- Cutaneous side effects occur, e.g., skin sensitivity to sun, splitting of fingernails, dry flaky skin, and hyperpigmentation on face, palms of hands.
- Patients who have had adrenalectomy may need higher doses of prednisone while receiving 5-FU, or dose of 5-FU may be reduced in postadrenalectomy patients.
- Reduce dose in patients with compromised hepatic, renal, or BM function and malnutrition.

Potential Toxicities/Side Effects and the Nursing Process

I. POTENTIAL FOR INFECTION AND BLEEDING related to BM DEPRESSION

Defining Characteristics: Nadir 10–14 days after drug dose; neutropenia, thrombocytopenia are dose related. Toxicity is enhanced when combined with leucovorin calcium.

Nursing Implications: Assess baseline CBC, WBC, differential, and platelet count prior to chemotherapy, as well as for signs/symptoms of infection or bleeding. Teach patient signs/symptoms of infection or bleeding, and instruct to report these immediately; teach patient self-care measures to minimize risk of infection and bleeding. This includes avoidance of crowds and proximity to people with infections, and avoidance of OTC aspirin-containing medications.

II.   ALTERED NUTRITION, LESS THAN BODY REQUIREMENTS, related to NAUSEA AND VOMITING, STOMATITIS, AND DIARRHEA

Defining Characteristics: Nausea and vomiting occur in 30–50% of patients and severity is dose dependent. Stomatitis can be severe, with onset in 5–8 days, and may herald severe BM depression. Diarrhea can be severe, and in combination with leucovorin, calcium is the dose-limiting toxicity.

Nursing Implications: Premedicate patient with antiemetics (phenothiazines are usually effective), and continue for 24 hours, at least for the first cycle. Encourage small, frequent meals of cool, bland foods. Assess oral mucosa prior to drug administration and instruct patient to report changes. Teach patient oral hygiene measures and self-assessment. Instruct patient to report diarrhea, to self-administer prescribed antidiarrheal medications, and to drink adequate fluids. Moderate to severe stomatitis or diarrhea is an indication to interrupt therapy.

III.   ALTERATION IN SKIN INTEGRITY related to ALOPECIA, CHANGES IN NAILS AND SKIN, HFS

Defining Characteristics: Alopecia is more common with 5-day course and involves diffuse thinning of scalp hair, eyelashes, and eyebrows. Brittle nail cracking and loss may occur. Photosensitivity occurs. Chemical phlebitis may occur during CI with higher doses (pH > 8.0). Palmar plantar erythrodysesthesia syndrome (PPES or HFS) may occur.

Nursing Implications: Teach patient about possible hair loss and skin changes; discuss possible impact on body image. Assess patient's risk for hair loss and skin changes during the therapy and discuss with patient strategies to minimize distress (wig, scarf, nail polish). Instruct patient to use sunblock when outdoors. Suggest implanted venous access device for CI of 5-FU, especially if patient will receive ongoing therapy. Teach patient to report redness, swelling, peeling, or pain in the palms of the hands or soles of the feet. Assess any symptoms. Drug should be held if HFS is confirmed. Teach patient to avoid heat exposure to hands and feet as this may accelerate the syndrome.

IV.   SENSORY/PERCEPTUAL ALTERATIONS related to PHOTOPHOBIA, CEREBELLAR ATAXIA, OCULAR CHANGES

Defining Characteristics: Photophobia may occur. Occasional cerebellar ataxia may occur and will disappear once drug is stopped. Drug is excreted in tears. Ocular changes that may occur are conjunctivitis, increased lacrimation, photophobia, oculomotor dysfunction, and blurred vision.

Nursing Implications: Assess baseline neurologic status, including vision. Instruct patient to report any changes. Teach patient safety precautions as needed.

TREATMENT

Drug: flutamide (Eulexin)

Class: Antiandrogen (nonsteroidal).

Mechanism of Action: Inhibits androgen uptake or inhibits nuclear binding of androgen in target tissues or both.

Metabolism: Rapidly and completely absorbed. Excreted mainly via urine. Biologically active metabolite reaches maximum plasma levels in approximately 2 hours. Plasma half-life is 6 hours. Largely plasma-bound.

Indication: For the treatment of men with locally confined Stage B2-C, and Stage D2 metastatic prostate cancer in combination with an LHRH agonist.

* Stage B2-C: Treatment with flutamide and the LHRH agonist should start 8 weeks prior to initiating R, and continue through RT.
* Stage D2: Combination therapy should continue until progression.
* **Contraindications:** 1) patients who are hypersensitive to flutamide of any component of this preparation; 2) patients with severe hepatic dysfunction. Drug is intended for use *only* in men.

Dosage/Range:
* 250 mg (2–125 mg capsules) every 8 hours (total daily dose of 750 mg).

Drug Preparation:
* None (available in 125-mg tablets).

Drug Administration:
* Oral.

Drug Interactions:
* Alcohol: increased facial flushing.
* Warfarin: may increase risk of bleeding; monitor INR closely.

Lab Effects/Interference:
* Increased LFTs.
* Increased BUN, creatinine.
* Monitor PSA for changes.

Special Considerations:
* Warnings and Precautions:
    * Drug may cause acute hepatic failure, often (50%) within the first 3 months of treatment and is reversible after discontinuation. Teach patient to report jaundice, nausea, vomiting, abdominal (RUQ) tenderness, fatigue, and anorexia and to have liver function evaluated. Assess serum transaminase levels baseline before starting the drug, then monthly for the first 4 months of therapy, then periodically thereafter. Assess LFTs at the first sign(s) or symptoms suggestive of hepatic dysfunction (e.g., nausea, vomiting, abdominal pain, fatigure, anorexia, flu-like symptoms, hyperbilirubinuria,

jaundice, RUQ tenderness). Drug should be discontinued immediately if the patient has jaundice, or ALT is $> 2 \times$ ULN with close monitoring of LFTs until resolution.

- *Embryo-fetal toxicity:* Drug should not be used by pregnant women, as fetal harm may occur.
- Aniline toxicity: rarely methemoglobinemia, hemolytic anemia, and cholestatic jaundice has occurred. In patients with glucose-6-phosphate dehydrogenase (g-6-PD) deficiency, hemoglobin M disease, and smokers, methemoglobin level monitoring should be considered (Watson Pharma, 2011).
- Most common adverse events were hot flashes, impotence, loss of libido, and diarrhea.

Potential Toxicities/Side Effects and the Nursing Process

I.   POTENTIAL SEXUAL DYSFUNCTION related to DRUG EFFECTS

Defining Characteristics: Decreased libido and impotence can occur in 33% of patients; gynecomastia occurs in 9% of patients.

Nursing Implications: Assess patient's sexual pattern, any alterations, and patient response. Encourage patient to verbalize feelings; provide information, emotional support, and referral for counseling as available and appropriate.

II.   ALTERATION IN COMFORT related to HOT FLASHES

Defining Characteristics: Hot flashes occur commonly.

Nursing Implications: Teach patient that this may occur, and encourage patient to report symptoms. Provide symptomatic support.

III.   ALTERED NUTRITION, LESS THAN BODY REQUIREMENTS, related to DIARRHEA, NAUSEA, AND VOMITING

Defining Characteristics: Diarrhea and nausea/vomiting occur in 10% of patients.

Nursing Implications: Teach patient that these may occur, and instruct to report them. Assess for occurrence; teach patient self-administration of prescribed antidiarrheal or antiemetic medications.

Drug: fulvestrant injection (Faslodex)

Class: Estrogen receptor antagonist (down regulator).

Mechanism of Action: Fulvestrant is an estrogen receptor antagonist that binds to the estrogen receptor of cells that are dependent upon estrogen for growth, including breast cancer cells that are hormone positive. There is no agonist effect as with other antiestrogens, such as tamoxifen. In addition, the estrogen receptor is also degraded so that it is lost from the cell. Because of this, there is no chance that the hormone receptor can be stimulated by low concentrations of estrogen, as with other antiestrogens, and this theoretically reduces the development of resistance.

Metabolism: When given IM, it takes 7 days for the drug to reach maximal plasma levels, which are maintained for at least 1 month. Half-life is about 40 days, and after 3–6 monthly doses, steady-state plasma area under the curve levels are reached at 2.5 times that of a single-dose injection. Drug undergoes biotransformation similar to endogenous steroids (oxidation, aromatic hydroxylation, conjugation), and oxidative pathway is via cytochrome P450 (CYP3A4). Drug is metabolized by the liver and rapidly cleared from the plasma via the hepatobiliary route. 90% is excreted via the feces; renal excretion is < 1%. There were no pharmacokinetic differences found in the elderly and younger adults, men and women, different races, patients with renal impairment, and patients with mild hepatic impairment. However, patients with moderate to severe liver dysfunction have not been studied.

Indication: For the treatment of patients with 1) hormone receptor (HR)-positive, HER2-negative advanced breast cancer in postmenopausal women not previously treated with endocrine therapy; (2) HR-positive advanced breast cancer in postmenopausal women with disease progression following endocrine therapy; (3) HR-positive, HER2 negative advanced, or metastatic breast cancer in postmenopausal women in combination with ribociclib, as initial endocrine base therapy or following disease progression on endocrine therapy; (4) HR-positive, HER2 negative advanced, or metastatic breast cancer in combination with palbociclib or abemaciclib in women with disease progression after endocrine therapy.

Contraindication: Hypersensitivity.

Dosage/Range:
• 500 mg given IM, into the buttock (gluteal area) slowly (1–2 min per injection) as 2 (5-mL) injections, one in each buttock, on days 1, 15, 29, and once monthly thereafter.
• **Moderate hepatic impairment** (Child-Pugh Class B): 250 mg IM slowly over 1–2 minutes, as one 5-mL injection, is recommended for patients with moderate hepatic impairment, into the buttock on days 1, 15, 29, and once monthly thereafter. Drug has not been studied in patients with severe hepatic impairment (Child-Pugh class C).
• Pre/perimenopausal women treated with the combination (fulvestrant and a cyclin-dependent kinase 4/6) should also receive lutenizing hormone-releasing hormone (LHRH) agonists according to current clinical practice standards. See package inserts for palbociclib (Ibrance), abemaciclib (Verzenio), and ribociclib (Kisqali) for dosing and toxicity management.

Drug Preparation: See package insert for step-by-step preparation and administration.
• Drug available in refrigerated 5 mL prefilled syringes containing 50 mg/mL.
• Remove glass syringe barrel from tray and ensure it is undamaged.
• Remove perforated patient record label from syringe.
• Peel open safety glide needle (SafetyGlide™) outer packaging; break the seal of the white plastic cover on the syringe luer connector to remove the cover with the attached

rubber tip cap. Twist to lock the needle to Luer lock connector of the syringe. For complete instructions, refer to drug package insert.

- Remove needle sheath; remove any air from the syringe (a small gas bubble may remain).
- Visually inspect syringe for any particulate matter or discoloration before administration.

Drug Administration:
- Administer IM slowly (1–2 minutes per injection) into each buttocks [two 5-mL injections, one in each buttock], on days 1, 15, 29, and once monthly thereafter.
- Z-track administration is recommended to prevent drug leakage into subcutaneous tissue.
- Immediately activate needle protection device upon withdrawal from patient by pushing lever arm completely forward until needle tip is fully covered. Visually confirm that the lever arm has fully advanced and the needle tip is covered. Hold syringe with bevel up, and note that lever arm is up. See Figure 3 in package insert.
  - If unable to activate, drop into sharps disposal container.
  - Follow same steps for second syringe.
  - DO NOT recap contaminated needles, or remove the needle as this increases the risk of accidental needlestick and transmission of infectious disease. Keep hands behind the needle at all times during use and disposal.

Drug Interactions:
- None significant, as drug does not significantly inhibit the major CYP isoenzymes, including rifampin.
- Herbals that contain estrogen may decrease the drug effect.

Lab Effects/Interference:
- Estradiol: falsely elevated levels when measured by immunoassay, as drug has a similar structure.

Special Considerations:
- Warnings and Precautions:
  - *Risk of bleeding*: use with caution in patients with bleeding diathesis, thrombocytopenia, or on anticoagulant use.
  - *Increased exposure in paitnets with hepatic impairment*: dose reduction for patients with moderate hepatic impairment (250-mg dose). Drug has not been studied in patients with severe hepatic impairment.
  - *Injection-site reaction:* injection-site–related events include sciatica, neuralgia, neuropathic pain, and PN. Use caution when administering drug at the dorsogluteal injection site due to close proximity of underlying sciatic nerve.
  - *Embryo-fetal toxicity*: Drug should not be used during pregnancy as drug can cause fetal harm. Teach women of reproductive potential to use effective contraception to avoid pregnancy during treatment and for 1 year following last dose of fulvestrant.
  - *Immunoassay measurement of serum estradiol:* Drug is structurally similar so may interfere with estradiol measurement by immunoassay (falsely elevated levels).
- Teach mothers not to breastfeed. Nursing mothers should decide whether to discontinue nursing or discontinue the drug, taking into account the importance of the drug to the mother's health.

- Most common adverse effects occurring in > 5% of patients receiving 500-mg dose were: injection-site pain, nausea, bone pain, arthralgia, asthenia, musculoskeletal pain, cough, dyspnea, and constipation.

Potential Toxicities/Side Effects and the Nursing Process

I. **ALTERATION IN COMFORT related to INJECTION-SITE REACTION, ABDOMINAL PAIN, BACK PAIN**

Defining Characteristics: Injection-site reactions (pain and inflammation) occurred in 7% of patients receiving a single 5-mL injection (European trial) as compared to 27% of patients (North American trial) receiving two 2.5-mL injections, one in each buttock. Back and bone pain occurred in 15.8% of patients, while abdominal pain occurred in 11.8% of patients and often was associated with other gastrointestinal symptoms.

Nursing Implications: Teach patient this may occur and to report it. Consider using Z-track method, and if using two separate injections of 2.5 mL, try a single-dose injection to see if discomfort is reduced. Teach patient to report bone and/or back pain. Teach patient to use OTC analgesics such as acetaminophen or nonsteroidal anti-inflammatory drugs as appropriate to bleeding history or risk factors. Discuss alternatives with physician if ineffective in symptom management.

II. **ALTERATION IN NUTRITION, POTENTIAL, related to NAUSEA, VOMITING, CONSTIPATION, DIARRHEA**

Defining Characteristics: Nausea occurs in 26%, vomiting 13%, constipation 12.5%, diarrhea 12.3%, and anorexia 9%.

Nursing Implications: Assess baseline appetite, presence of nausea and/or vomiting, and bowel elimination pattern. Teach patient that these side effects may occur, self-care measures to minimize nausea and vomiting such as dietary modification, and to report these side effects. Discuss antiemetics with physician if dietary modification is ineffective. Teach patient to use dietary modification to relieve constipation or diarrhea and, if ineffective, to use OTC laxatives or antidiarrheal medicine. If ineffective, discuss pharmacologic management with physician.

III. **ALTERATION IN SKIN INTEGRITY, POTENTIAL, related to HOT FLASHES AND PERIPHERAL EDEMA**

Defining Characteristics: Vasodilation or hot flashes occurred in 17.7% of patients, and peripheral edema in 9% of patients.

Nursing Implications: Assess baseline skin integrity, history of hot flashes in post-menopausal patients, and presence of peripheral edema. Teach patient these side effects may occur and to report them. If hot flashes are severe, review common hot flash management including wearing loose, layered clothing that can be removed when the woman becomes hot, sipping cold beverages throughout the day, sleeping with light nightgown and window open, avoiding triggers such as caffeine or alcohol, and if ineffective, discuss use of venlafaxine (Effexor) or fluoxetine (Paxil) to reduce intensity and frequency of hot flashes (Loprinski et al., 2000). Teach patient self-assessment of peripheral edema, to wear loose stockings and shoes, to keep skin moisturized to prevent cracking, and comfort measures. Teach patient to report increasing edema or related problems.

Drug: gemcitabine hydrochloride (Gemzar, difluorodeoxycytidine)

Class: Nucleoside metabolic inhibitor (Antimetabolite).

Mechanism of Action: Inhibits DNA synthesis by inhibiting DNA polymerase activity through a process called masked chain termination. It is a prodrug, structurally similar to ara-C, needing intracellular phosphorylation. It then inhibits DNA synthesis. Cell cycle-specific for S phase, causing cells to accumulate at the G_1–S boundary.

Metabolism: Pharmacokinetics varies by age, gender, and infusion time. Half-life for short infusions ranges from 32–94 minutes, while that of long infusions ranges from 245–638 minutes. Following short infusions ($<$ 70 minutes), the drug is not extensively tissue-bound; following long infusions (70–285 minutes), the drug slowly equilibrates within tissues. The terminal half-life of the parent drug, gemcitabine, is 17 minutes. There is negligible binding to serum proteins. Drug and metabolites are excreted in the urine, with 92–98% of the drug dose recovered in the urine within 1 week. Mean systemic clearance is 90 L/h/m^2. Clearance is about 30% lower in women than in men, and also reduced in the elderly, but this does not necessarily require a dose reduction.

Indications:
- Ovarian cancer: In combination with carboplatin, for the treatment of advanced ovarian cancer that has relapsed at least 6 months after completion of platinum-based therapy.
- Breast cancer: In combination with paclitaxel, for the first-line treatment of metastatic breast cancer after failure of prior anthracycline-containing adjuvant chemotherapy, unless anthracyclines were clinically contraindicated.
- NSCLC: In combination with cisplatin for the treatment of NSCLC.
- Pancreatic cancer: As a single agent for the treatment of pancreatic cancer.

Dosage/Range:
Adults:
- **Breast cancer:** 1,250 mg/m^2 IV over 30 minutes days 1, 8 q 21 days, in combination with paclitaxel 175 mg/m^2 IV over 3 hours administered prior to gemcitabine, day 1 repeated q 21 days.
  - Day 1 ANC must be $\geq$ 1,500 $\times$ 10^6/L and a platelet count of $\geq$ 100,000 $\times$ 10^6/L prior to each cycle. If ANC $<$ 1,500/mm3 or platelets $<$ 100,000, delay treatment cycle.

- Day 8: Dose-reduce 25% for ANC 1,000–1,199/mm^3 or platelets 50,000–75,000 × 10^6/L (give 75% of the full dose).
- Day 8: Dose-reduce 50% for ANC 700–999/mm^3 and platelets ≥ = 50,000/mm^3 × 10^6/L (give 50% of full dose), but hold drug if ANC < 700/mm^3 or platelets < 50,000/mm^3 × 10^6/L.
- Hold drug if ANC < 500/mm^3 or platelets < 50,000 × 10^6/L.
- **Pancreatic cancer: Weeks 1–8:** Gemcitabine 1,000 mg/m^2 IV infusion over 30 min every week for first 7 weeks followed by 1-week rest. **After Week 8:** weekly dosing on days 1, 8, 15 of 28-day cycles.
  - Dose-reduce 25% if ANC 500–999/mm^3 or platelets 50–99,000 × 10^6/L (give 75% of full dose), and hold if ANC < 500/mm^3 or platelets < 50,000 × 10^6/L.
- **Non–small-cell lung cancer** (inoperable, locally advanced stage IIIA and IIIB or metastatic) in combination with cisplatin: **4-week cycle:** 1,000 mg/m^2 IV over 30 minutes on days 1, 8, and 15, repeat q 28 days, with cisplatin 100 mg/m^2 IV on day 1 given **after** the gemcitabine infusion; or as a **3-week cycle**, with gemcitabine 1,250 mg/m^2 IV over 30 minutes on days 1 and 8; cisplatin 100 mg/m^2 IV is given following gemcitabine infusion on day 1, repeated q 3 weeks.
  - Dose-reduce 25% if ANC 500–999/mm^3 or platelets 50–99,000 × 10^6/L (give 75% of full dose), and hold if ANC < 500/mm^3 or platelets < 50,000 × 10^6/L.
  - Dose-reduce 50% for grades 3–4 nonhematologic toxicities when gemcitabine given is with cisplatin.
- **Ovarian cancer:** 1,000 mg/m^2 IV over 30 minutes on days 1 and 8 of each 21-day cycle, together with carboplatin (AUC 4) IV on day 1 after gemcitabine administration, of each 21-day cycle.
  - Day 1: ANC must be ≥ 1,500 × 10^6/L and a platelet count of ≥ 100,000 × 10^6/L prior to each cycle. If ANC < 1,500/mm^3 or platelets < 100,000, delay treatment cycle.
  - Dose modify day 8 if ANC 1,000–1,499/mm^3 or platelets 75–99,999 × 10^6/L by giving 50% of full dose; hold dose if values are lower than this.
- **See package insert** for dose modification for myelosuppression in previous cycles.
  - **Grades 3–4 Nonhematologic Toxicity:**
  - Permanently discontinue gemcitabine for:
    - Unexplained dyspnea or other evidence of severe pulmonary toxicity
    - Severe hepatic toxicity
    - Hemolytic-uremic syndrome
    - Capillary leak syndrome
    - Posterior reversible encephalopathy syndrome

Hold gemcitabine or reduce dose by 50% for other severe (grades 3–4) nonhematological toxicity until resolved. No dose modification for alopecia, nausea, or vomiting.

Drug Preparation:
- Drug available in single-use lyophilized vials of 200 mg/10 mL and 1 g/50 mL.
- Use 0.9% sodium chloride USP without preservatives and reconstitute the 200-mg vial with 5 mL, and the 1-g vial with 25 mL. Solution should be clear, colorless to light straw-colored.

- Shake to dissolve the powder. This results in a concentration of 38 mg/mL.
- Withdraw recommended dose and further dilute in 0.9% sodium chloride injection. Final concentrations may be as low as 0.1 mg/mL.
- Discard unused portion. Inspect solution for particulate matter or discoloration and do not use if these occur.
- Stable 24 hours at room temperature (20–25°C [68–77°F]). DO NOT refrigerate, as drug crystallization may occur.

Drug Administration:
- ANC $\geq$ 1,500/mm^3 and platelets $\geq$ 100,000 $\times$ 10^6/L for day 1 treatment; assess CBC/differential, LFTs, and renal function before each cycle.
- Administer IV over 30 minutes. Infusion time > 60 minutes or dosing more frequently than weekly is associated with greater toxicity.
- Administer gemcitabine before cisplatin.
- Administer gemcitabine after paclitaxel.

Drug Interactions:
- Administer cisplatin after gemcitabine to enhance renal drug clearance; paclitaxel should be administered before gemcitabine.

Lab Effects/Interference:
- Decreased CBC.
- Increased LFTs.

Special Considerations:
- Warnings and Precautions:
  - *Schedule-dependent toxicity*: Prolongation of infusion time > 60 min or more frequent dosing than once a week increased the risk of significant hypotension, severe flu-like symptoms, myelosuppression, and asthenia. The drug half-life is influenced by the length of the infusion [the volume of distribution when the gemcitabine infusion was < 70 minutes was 50 L/m^2; when the infusion lasted longer, the volume of distribution increased to 370 L/m^2].
  - *Myelosuppression*: Manifested as neutropenia, thrombocytopenia, and anemia, is increased when gemcitabine is combined with other anti-cancer drugs. As a single agent, incidence of grades 3–4 myelosuppression was 25% for neutropenia, 8% for anemia, and 5% for thrombocytopenia.
  - *Pulmonary toxicity and respiratory failure*: Pulmonary toxicity including interstitial pneumonitis, pulmonary fibrosis, pulmonary edema, and ARDS have been reported. Onset of pulmonary symptoms may occur up to 2 weeks after the last dose of gemcitabine. Drug should be discontinued in patients with unexplained dyspnea, with or without bronchospasm, or if evidence of pulmonary toxicity.
  - *Hemolytic Uremic Sundrome (HUS)*: Although rare (incidence 0.25%), HUS can lead to renal failure and be fatal. Assess renal function before beginning gemcitabine therapy, and periodically during therapy. HUS should be considered in the differential diagnosis in paiatents who develop anemia with evidence of microangiopathic hemolysis, elevation in BR or LDH, or reticulocytosis; severe thrombocytopenia; or

evidence of renal failure (elevated serum creatinine or BUN). Gemcitabine should be permanently discontinued if patient develops HUS or severe renal impairment.

- *Hepatotoxicity*: May occur, including drug-induced liver injury. Gemcitabine in patients with concurrent liver metastases or a preexisting medical history of hepatitis, alcoholism, or liver cirrhosis can exacerbate underlying hepatic insufficiency (Eli Lillly, 2014). Assess LFTs baseline before starting the drug, and periodically during therapy.
- *Embryo-fetal toxicity*: Teach female patients of reproductive potential to use effective contraception during therapy. Mothers should not breastfeed infants while receiving the drug.
- *Exacerbation of RT Toxicity*: Drug is not indicated for administration during RT. Life-threatening mucositis, especially esophagitis, and pneumonitis occurred when gemcitabine combined with RT of chest in a study of NSCLC patients. In patients receiving nonconcurrent chemoRT (given > 7 days apart), there was excessive toxicity. Radiation recall can also occur when gemcitabine is given after prior RT.
- *Capillary leak syndrome* has been described. Discontinue gemcitabine if this occurs.
- *Posterior Reversible Encephalopathy Syndrome (PRES)*: May occur, with a presentation of headache, seizure, lethargy, HTN, confusion, blindness, and other visual and neurologic disturbances. Evaluation should include MRI, and if PRES is confirmed, gemcitabine should be discontinued.
- Dose reduction or delay required for hematologic toxicity.
- Drug can rarely cause severe pulmonary toxicity (interstitial pneumonitis, pulmonary fibrosis, pulmonary edema, adult respiratory distress syndrome), occurring up to 2 weeks following the last gemcitabine infusion. If patient develops new onset dyspnea, with or without bronchospasm, stop gemcitabine until further pulmonary evaluation can proceed; discontinue drug if related to gemcitabine.
- Hemolytic uremic syndrome (HUS) and/or renal failure have been reported rarely.
- Drug is a radiosensitizer, and radiation recall may occur.
- Monitoring labs: hepatic and renal function baseline and periodically during treatment; CBC/differential before each dose; serum creatinine, potassium, calcium, magnesium during combination with cisplatin.
- Drug may cause sedation in 10% of patients; caution patient not to drive or operate heavy machinery until it is determined whether patient develops this side effect.
- Drug may be irritating to the vein, requiring local heat; may require a central line for (long-term) administration.
- The most common adverse reactions for drug as a single agent (incidence ≥ 20%) are nausea/vomiting, anemia, hepatic transaminitis, neutropenia, increased alkaline phosphatase, proteinuria, fever, hematuria, rash, thrombocytopenia, dyspnea, and peripheral edema.

Potential Toxicities/Side Effects and the Nursing Process

I. POTENTIAL FOR INFECTION AND BLEEDING related to BM DEPRESSION

Defining Characteristics: Myelosuppression is dose-limiting toxicity. Incidence of leukopenia is 63%, thrombocytopenia 36%, and anemia 73%. Dose reductions required are shown in the Special Considerations section. Grades 3–4 thrombocytopenia are more common in the elderly, and grades 3–4 neutropenia and thrombocytopenia are more common in women (especially older women). Older women were less able to complete subsequent courses of therapy. Myelosuppression is usually short-lived with recovery within 1 week. Approximately 19% of patients require RBC transfusions.

Nursing Implications: Assess baseline CBC, WBC, differential, and platelet count prior to chemotherapy, as well as for signs/symptoms of infection or bleeding. Discuss dose reductions or delay based on neutrophil and platelet counts. Teach patient signs/symptoms of infection or bleeding, and instruct to report these immediately. Teach patient self-care measures to minimize risk of infection and bleeding. This includes avoidance of crowds, proximity to people with infections, and OTC aspirin-containing medications. Transfuse red blood cells and platelets as needed per physician order.

II.   POTENTIAL ALTERATION IN NUTRITION, LESS THAN BODY REQUIREMENTS, related to NAUSEA AND VOMITING, DIARRHEA, STOMATITIS, AND ALTERATIONS IN LFTS

Defining Characteristics: Nausea and vomiting occur in 69% of patients, and of these, < 15% are severe. Nausea and vomiting are usually mild to moderate and are easily prevented or controlled by antiemetics. Diarrhea may occur (19% incidence), as may stomatitis (11% incidence). Abnormalities in liver transaminases occur in two-thirds of patients; rarely does this require drug discontinuance.

Nursing Implications: Premedicate patient with antiemetics (phenothiazides are usually effective). Encourage small, frequent meals of cool, bland foods. Teach patient self-administration of prescribed antiemetic medications, and to drink adequate fluids. Assess oral mucosa prior to drug administration, and instruct patient to report changes. Teach patient oral hygiene measures and self-assessment. Instruct patient to report diarrhea, to self-administer prescribed antidiarrheal medications, and to drink adequate fluids. Monitor LFTs baseline and periodically during therapy. Notify physician of any abnormalities and discuss implications. Drug should be used cautiously in any patient with hepatic dysfunction.

III.   POTENTIAL ALTERATION IN COMFORT related to FLU-LIKE SYMPTOMS

Defining Characteristics: Flu-like symptoms occur in 20% of patients with first treatment dose. Transient febrile episodes occur in 41% of patients.

Nursing Implications: Encourage patient to report flu-like symptoms. Treat fevers with acetaminophen per physician. Assess for alterations in comfort, and discuss symptomatic measures. If severe, discuss drug discontinuance with physician.

IV.   IMPAIRED SKIN INTEGRITY related to ALOPECIA, RASH, PRURITUS, EDEMA

Defining Characteristics: Skin rash occurs in about 30% of patients, often within 2–3 days of starting drug. The rash is erythematous, pruritic, and/or maculopapular, and may occur on the neck and extremities. Edema occurs in about 30% of patients, and is primarily peripheral but can rarely be facial or pulmonary. Edema is reversible after drug is discontinued, and appears unrelated to cardiac, renal, or hepatic impairment. Edema is usually mild to moderate. Minimal hair loss occurs in 15% of patients, and is reversible.

Nursing Implications: Assess skin integrity and presence of rash, pruritus, alopecia, and edema prior to dosing. Assess impact of these alterations on patient, and develop plan to manage symptom distress and promote skin integrity. Instruct patient to report rash, itching; discuss treatment of rash with topical corticosteroids. Teach patient self-assessment of signs/symptoms of edema, and instruct to notify healthcare provider if swelling occurs. If severe, discuss drug discontinuance with physician.

Drug: goserelin acetate (Zoladex)

Class: Gonadotropin-releasing hormone (GnRH) agonist.

Mechanism of Action: Inhibits pituitary gonadotropin, achieving a chemical orchiectomy in 2–4 weeks. Sustained-release medication provides continuous drug diffusion from the depot into subcutaneous tissue. This permits monthly injection instead of daily.

Metabolism: Absorbed slowly for first 8 days, then more rapid and constant absorption for remaining 28 days. Time to peak concentration 12–15 days for males and 8–22 days for females.

Indication: Indicated for 3.6-mg injection every 28 days: (1) use in combination with flutamide for management of locally confined carcinoma of the prostate; (2) palliative treatment of advanced prostate cancer, (3) endometriosis; (4) palliative treatment of advanced breast cancer; (5) node positive ER/PR positive early breast cancer.

Indication for 10.8-mg implant: (1) use in combination with flutamide for management of Stage 2b-T4 (Stage B2-C) prostate cancer; (2) palliative treatment of advanced prostate cancer (3-month implant NOT indicated in women).

Contraindication: (1) hypersensitivity; (2) pregnancy.

Dosage/Range:
Adults:
- Subcutaneous: 3.6-mg dose into the anterior upper abdominal wall below the navel line every 28 days or the 10.8-mg implant every 3 months.
- Stage B2-C (locally confined) prostate cancer: In combination with RT and flutamide, treatment should be started 8 weeks prior to beginning RT and should continue during

RT. A treatment regimen using Zoladex 3.6 mg depot 8 weeks before RT, followed in 28 days by Zoladex 10.8 mg depot, can be administered. Alternatively, four injections of 3.6 mg depot can be administered at 28-day intervals, two depots preceeding, and two during RT.

- Use in advanced prostate cancer is intended for long-term administration unless clinically inappropriate.
- No dosage adjustment necessary for renal or hepatic impairment.
- Zoladex 10.8 mg implant is not indicated in women as the data are insufficient to support reliable suppression of serumestradiol.

Drug Preparation:
- Goserlin acetate 3.6-mg implant is supplied in a disposable syringe device fitted with a 16-gauge siliconized hypodermic needle with protective needle syring (SafeSystem™ Syringe) [administered every 28 days].
- Goserlin acetate 10.8-mg implant is supplied in a disposable syringe device fitted with a 14-gauge siliconized hypodermic needle with protective needle syringe [administered every 12 weeks]. You cannot aspirate to check placement. If the needle tip is in a blood vessel, you will see a flash back in the syringe chamber. You must push down on plunger until cannot depress anymore to place the implant and activate the protective sleeve when the needle is withdrawn.
- Inspect package for damage. Open foil package and inspect drug.

Drug Administration:
- Position patient comfortably with the upper part of the body slightly raised. Select site on anterior abdominal wall below the navel line and prep with an alcohol swab cleansing from the center outward. Ensure site avoids underlying inferior epigastric artery and its branches.
- Administer local anesthetic if ordered.
- Examine foil pouch and syringe for damage. Remove the syringe from the opened foil pouch and hold syringe at a slight angle to the light. Check that at least a part of the goserlin acetate implant is visible.
- Grasp the red (3.6 mg) or blue (10.8 mg) plastic safety tab, pull away from syringe, and discard. Remove needle cover. Do not attempt to remove air bubbles as this may displace the implant.
- Holding the syringe around the protective sleeve, using aseptic technique, pinch the skin of the patient's anterior abdominal wall below the navel line. With the bevel of the needle facing up, **insert the needle at a 30–45° angle to the skin**, in one deliberate motion until the protective sleeve touches the patient's skin.
- DO NOT aspirate back to check for blood; if the needle penetrates a vessel, blood will instantly be seen in the chamber. If blood is seen, withdraw the needle and inject with a new syringe elsewhere. Monitor patients for signs or symptoms of abdominal hemorrhage. Use extra care when administering goserlin acetate to patients with a low BMI and/or patients receiving full dose anticoagulation (AstraZeneca, 2016).
- Do not penetrate into muscle or peritoneum.
- To administer oserlin acetate implant and to activate the protective sleeve, grasp the barrel at the finger grip and depress the plunger until it can go no further. If the plunger is

NOT depressed fully, the protective sleeve will NOT activate. When the protective sleeve "clicks," the protective sleeve will automatically begin to slide to cover the needle. The needle does not retract.

- Withdraw needle carefully and allow the protective sleeve to slide and cover needle. Dispose of the syringe in an approved sharps collector. Apply gentle pressure bandage to site.
- Document administration and location, as well as patient response, in chart.
- In the unlikely event the goserlin acetate implant needs to be surgically removed, it may be localized by ultrasound.

Drug Interactions:
- None.

Lab Effects/Interference:
- Hypercalcemia in patients with bone metastases.
- Tests of pituitary/gonadal function may be inaccurate while on therapy due to suppression of pituitary/gonadal system.
- Hyperglycemia.
- In females, rarely: elevated AST/ALT, increased lipids (HDL, LDL, triglycerides).

Special Considerations:
- Compliance to 28-day injection schedule is important, as is the 3-month schedule.
- The most common clinically significant adverse reactions occurring in >10% of men: hot flashes, sexual dysfunction, decreased erections, and lower urinary symptoms.
- The most common adverse events for women treated with breast cancer, dysfunctional uterine bleeding or endometiosis (>20% of patients) were: hot flushes, headache, sweating, acne, emotional lability, depression, decreased libido, vaginitis, breast atrophy, seborrhea, and peripheral edema.
- Tumor flare can occur on goserlin acetate initiation for both men and women.
- Premenopausal women must use effective contraception during and for 12 weeks after treatment with the drug. Nursing mothers should stop breastfeeding or stop nursing, taking into account the importance of the drug to the mother.
- Warnings and Precautions:
  - *Tumor flare phenomenon:* Transient worsening of tumor symptoms may occur during the first few weeks of treatment; this may include ureteral obstruction and spinal cord compression. Monitor patients closely at risk for tumor flare.
  - *Hypersensitivity:* HSR and anaphylaxis have rarely been reported in the administration of GnRH agonist analogues. Monitor the patient closely during and after administration.
  - *Hyperglycemia and diabetes* may occur; monitor blood glucose level baseline, during therapy, and manage according to current standard clinical practice as ordered.
  - *Cardiovascular disease:* Men receiving GnRH analogues are at risk for MI, sudden cardiac death, and stroke. Monitor for cardiovascular disease and manage according to current clinical practice as ordered.
  - *Prolonged QT/QTc interval:* Androgen deprivation therapy may increase risk. Patients at risk for prolonged QT/QTc should review risk benefit with physician. Assess

ordered electrolytes and discuss abnormalities with provider; implement repletion of electrolytes as ordered.

- *Injection-site injury and vascular injury* have been reported including pain, hematoma, hemorrhage, hemorrhagic shock, requiring blood transfusions, and surgical intervention. Take extra care when administering drug to patients with a low BMI and/ or receiving full anticoagulation. Monitor sites for injury.

Potential Toxicities/Side Effects and the Nursing Process

I.   SEXUAL DYSFUNCTION related to DECREASED TESTOSTERONE LEVELS

Defining Characteristics: Hot flashes, sexual dysfunction, and decreased erections can occur.

Nursing Implications: Assess normal sexual pattern. Refer as needed for sexual counseling.

II.   POTENTIAL ALTERATION IN CARDIAC OUTPUT related to ARRHYTHMIA, CARDIOVASCULAR DYSFUNCTION

Defining Characteristics: Arrhythmia, cerebrovascular accident (CVA), hypertension, myocardial infarction, peripheral vascular disease, chest pain may occur in 1–5% of patients.

Nursing Implications: Assess heart rate, blood pressure, peripheral pulses. Teach patient to report palpitations, shortness of breath, chest pain, or leg pain immediately. Evaluate abnormalities with physician.

III.   SENSORY/PERCEPTUAL ALTERATION related to ANXIETY, DEPRESSION, HEADACHE

Defining Characteristics: Anxiety, depression, headache may occur ($< 5\%$).

Nursing Implications: Assess baseline effect, comfort. Instruct patient to report mood disorder. Encourage patient to verbalize feelings, provide patient with emotional support, assess efficacy of supportive care, and if needed, discuss pharmacologic management of symptoms with physician.

IV.   ALTERATION IN NUTRITION, LESS THAN BODY REQUIREMENTS, related to VOMITING, HYPERGLYCEMIA

Defining Characteristics: Vomiting may occur ($< 5\%$); also increased weight, ulcer, hyperglycemia.

Nursing Implications: Teach patient to report GI disturbances. Assess severity and discuss management with physician. Assess serum glucose, and if abnormal, discuss dietary or pharmacologic management, depending upon severity, with physician.

V. ALTERATION IN BOWEL ELIMINATION related to CONSTIPATION OR DIARRHEA

Defining Characteristics: Constipation or diarrhea may occur ($<$ 5%).

Nursing Implications: Instruct patient to report problems in elimination. Teach symptomatic management.

VI. ALTERATION IN URINARY ELIMINATION related to OBSTRUCTION OR INFECTION

Defining Characteristics: Urinary obstruction, urinary tract infection, renal insufficiency may occur.

Nursing Implications: Monitor baseline urinary elimination pattern, baseline kidney function tests, and continue to monitor through therapy. Instruct patient to report signs/symptoms of urinary tract infection (UTI).

VII. ALTERATION IN COMFORT related to FEVER, CHILLS, TENDERNESS

Defining Characteristics: Chills, fever, breast swelling, and tenderness. Also, discomfort may result from injection, as a 16-gauge needle is used to inject depot.

Nursing Implications: Instruct patient to report discomfort. Discuss strategies to increase comfort. Administer local anesthetic prior to injection of medication (per physician's order).

Drug: histrelin implant (Vantas)

Class: Gonadotropin-releasing factor (GnRH) agonist.

Mechanism of Action: Histrelin inhibits pituitary gonadotropin, achieving a chemical orchiectomy.

Metabolism: Implant delivers histrelin continuously for 12 months at 50–60 micrograms per day. Drug serum concentration 50% higher in patients with severe renal dysfunction, but this is not considered clinically significant.

Indication: Palliative treatment of patients with advanced prostate cancer.

Contraindication: Known hypersensitivity; pregnancy.

Dosage/Range:
Adults:
- Histrelin implant once every 12 months.
- Histrelin implant (50 mg) is aseptically inserted subcutaneously under skin on upper, inner arm using implant tool; at 12 months, implant must be removed before new one is implanted.

Drug Preparation:
- Keep implant refrigerated until implanted.
- Select site on upper inner arm, and follow guidelines in package insert using aseptic technique and implant tool as implantation is a surgical procedure. See precise procedures for implantation and removal, with images, in package insert (Endo, 2014).
- Implant is NOT radio-opaque, so care must be given to carefully secure the implant as directed. CT or MRI is necessary to confirm placement if it is not palpable.

Drug Administration: See package insert for implantation and removal instructions.

Drug Interactions:
- Unknown.

Lab Effects/Interference:
- Hypercalcemia in patients with bone metastases.
- Tests of pituitary/gonadal function may be inaccurate while on therapy due to suppression of pituitary/gonadal system.
- Decreased serum testosterone to below castrate levels.

Special Considerations:
- Warnings and Precautions:
  - *Transient increase in serum testosterone levels:* Initially (first week of treatment) with flare of tumor symptoms or onset of new symptoms such as bone pain, neuropathy, hematuria, or ureteral/bladder outlet obstruction.
  - *Spinal cord compression, urinary tract obstruction:* May cause paralysis or renal impairment. Monitor patients with metastatic vertebral and/or urinary tract obstruction very closely during the first few weeks of treatment and manage immediately if either occurs.
  - *Difficulty locating or removing implant*: Loss of or inability to locate or remove an inserted implant has been reported. Use caution.
  - *Hyperglycemia and diabetes* have been reported in men receiving GnRH analogues. Monitor blood glucose level and manage per current clinical guidelines, and as ordered.
  - *Cardiovascular disease*: Increased risk of MI, sudden cardiac death and stroke has been reported in men receiving androgen deprivation therapy. Monitor for cardiovascular disease and manage according to current clinical standards as ordered.
  - *Prolonged QT/QTc interval* may occur in patients receiving androgen deprivation therapy. Patients should review risks and benefits with physician if at risk.
  - *Laboratory tests:* Assess serum testosterone and PSA levels to evaluate response.
- The most common adverse reactions observed in > 5% of men: hot flashes, fatigue, implant-site reactions, testicular atrophy.
- Response to the drug should be monitored using serum concentrations of testosterone and PSA periodically, especially if the anticipated clinical or biochemical response has not been achieved.

TREATMENT

Potential Toxicities/Side Effects and the Nursing Process

I.   SEXUAL DYSFUNCTION related to DECREASED TESTOSTERONE LEVELS

Defining Characteristics: Hot flashes (66% with 2.3% severe), testicular atrophy (5.3%), gynecomastia (4.1%), decreased libido (2.3%), and erectile dysfunction (3.5%) can occur.

Nursing Implications: Assess normal sexual pattern. Encourage patient to verbalize feelings to assess impact of symptoms on sexual function; refer as needed for sexual counseling. Teach patient self-care strategies to reduce distress of hot flashes.

II.   ALTERATION IN BOWEL ELIMINATION related to CONSTIPATION

Defining Characteristics: Constipation may occur ($<$ 5%).

Nursing Implications: Instruct patient to report problems in elimination. Teach symptomatic management.

III.   ALTERATION IN URINARY ELIMINATION related to OBSTRUCTION OR INFECTION

Defining Characteristics: Urinary obstruction, urinary tract infection, renal insufficiency may occur. Renal impairment occurs in 4.7% of patients.

Nursing Implications: Monitor baseline urinary elimination pattern, baseline kidney function tests, and continue to monitor through therapy. Instruct patient to report signs/symptoms of urinary tract infection (UTI).

IV.   ALTERATION IN COMFORT related to IMPLANT SITE IRRITATION, ASTHENIA, AND INSOMNIA

Defining Characteristics: Implantation site reactions occur in at least 5.8% of patients: these include bruising, pain/soreness/tenderness after insertion or removal; rarely, erythema and swelling may occur. Asthenia occurs in about 10% of patients, and insomnia in 2.9% of patients.

Nursing Implications: Instruct patient to report discomfort. Discuss strategies to increase comfort. Teach patient to self-assess and reassure local effects will resolve. Teach patient to report any signs/symptoms of infection.

Drug: hydroxyurea (Hydrea, Droxia)

Class: Nucleoside metabolic inhibitor (Antimetabolite).

Mechanism of Action: Prevents conversion of ribonucleotides to deoxyribonucleotides by inhibiting the converting enzyme ribonucleoside diphosphate reductase. DNA synthesis is thus inhibited. Cell cycle phase specific for S phase. May also sensitize cells to the effects of radiation therapy, although the process is not clearly understood.

Metabolism: Rapidly absorbed from GI tract. Peak plasma level reached in 2 hours, with plasma half-life of 3–4 hours. About half the drug is metabolized in the liver and half is excreted in urine as urea and unchanged drug. Some of the drug is eliminated as respiratory CO_2. Crosses BBB.

Indication: (1) Resistant CML; (2) locally advanced squamous cell carcinoma of the head and neck (excluding lip) in combination with concurrent chemoradiation.

Contraindication: Patients hypersensitve to drug or its components.

Dosage/Range:
- Used alone or in conjunction with other antitumor agents or RT to treat cancer. Individualize treatment based on tumor type, disease state, response to treatment, patient risk factors, and current clinical practice standards.
- 15 mg/kg; dose should be based on patient's actual or ideal weight, whichever is less.
- Dose modifications:
    - Renal impairment: reduce dose by 50% if CrCl < 60 mL/min or with end-stage renal disease, e.g., to 7.5 mg/kg once daily. On dialysis days, give hydroxyurea after dialysis.
    - Myelosuppression: if bone marrow markedly depressed, do not start therapy; a risk if patient has had prior RT or chemotherapy.
    - Cutaneous vasculitis

Drug Preparation:
- None. Hydrea available in 500-mg capsules or Droxia in 200-mg, 300-mg, and 400-mg tablets.

Drug Administration:
- Oral.
- Teach patient to swallow capsules whole and not to open them.
- Ensure patient also has a prescription for or patient can purchase and take folic acid.
- Assess CBC at least weekly during hydroxyurea treatment; correct severe anemia before starting the drug.

Drug Interactions:
- Antiretroviral drugs (e.g., didanosine, stavudine): increased risk of pancreatitis, hepatotoxicity, PN. Do not use together.

Lab Effects/Interference:
- Decreased CBC.

- Increased BUN, creatinine, uric acid.
- Increased hepatic enzymes.
- Interference with uric acid, urea or lactic acid assays: falsely elevated results.

Special Considerations:
- Warnings and Precautions:
  - *Severe myelosuppression*: Do not start treatment if BM is markedly depressed. Generally leukopenia occurs, with thrombocytopenia and anemia less common. Monitor CBC/differential baseline and during treatment and interrupt or modify dose as needed. Recovery is usually rapid once hydroxyurea interrupted.
  - *Secondaary malignancies*: Hydroxyurea is a human carcinogen. Long-term therapy is associated with rare myeloproliferative disorders, secondary leukemia, skin cancer. Teach patients to protect themselves/skin from effects of sun (e.g., SPF, hat, long-sleeve protection). Monitor for the development of secondary malignancies.
  - *Embryo-fetal toxicity*: teach women of reproductive potential to use effective contraception to avoid pregnancy during and for 6 months after last dose. Teach male patients of reproductive potential to use effective contraception, during and for at least 1 year after the last dose of therapy.
  - *Vasculitis toxicities*: Rarely, cutaneous vasculitic toxicities such as ulceration and gangrene have occurred in patients with myeloproliferative disorders, especially if interferon therapy was received in the past or concurrently with hydroxyurea. If ulcers occur, discontinue hydroxyures, and treat vasculitic ulcers.
  - *Live vaccinations* should not be given to patients receiving hydroxyurea as the virus vaccine may potentiate the replication of the virus and/or may increase the adverse reaction due to immunosuppression. Severe infection may occur as the patient's antibody response to vaccines may be decreased.
  - *Risks associated with concomitant antiretroviral drugs* (e.g., didanosine, stavudine): Pancreatitis, hepatotoxicity, and PN.
  - *Radiation Recall:* Patients who received prior RT may have exacerbation of postirradiation erythema. Monitor these patients for skin integrity, and manage symptomatically.
  - *Macrocytosis*: May occur early in treatment, and is self-limiting. This may mask the diagnosis of pernicious anemia. Prophylactic folic acid administration is recommended.
- Hydroxyurea has a side effect of dramatically lowering the WBC in a relatively short period of time (24–48 hours). In leukemia patients endangered by the potential complication of leukostasis, this is the desired effect.
- May need to pretreat with allopurinol to protect patient from TLS.
- Dermatologic radiation recall phenomena may occur.
- In combination with radiation therapy, mucosal reactions in the radiation field may be severe and require dose interruption.
- Drug has been used in the treatment of CML in chronic phase, as a radiosensitizer (primary brain tumors, head and neck cancer, cancer of the cervix or uterus, non–small-cell lung cancer), and in sickle cell anemia.
- Drug should not be used during pregnancy or by breastfeeding mothers, as drug is excreted in breastmilk.

Potential Toxicities/Side Effects and the Nursing Process

I.　INFECTION AND BLEEDING related to BM DEPRESSION

Defining Characteristics: WBC begins to decrease 24–48 hours after beginning therapy, with nadir in 10 days and recovery within 10–30 days. Leukopenia more common than thrombocytopenia and anemia, and is dose related.

Nursing Implications: Assess CBC, WBC with differential, and platelet count prior to drug administration, as well as for signs/symptoms of infection or bleeding. Doses may need to be reduced if patient has undergone prior radiotherapy or chemotherapy. Dose must be reduced if patient has renal dysfunction. Discuss any abnormalities with physician prior to drug administration. Teach patient signs/symptoms of infection and bleeding, and instruct to report them immediately. Teach self-care measures to minimize risk of infection and bleeding, including avoidance of OTC aspirin-containing medications.

II.　ALTERED NUTRITION, LESS THAN BODY REQUIREMENTS, related to NAUSEA AND VOMITING, DIARRHEA, STOMATITIS, ANOREXIA, HEPATIC DYSFUNCTION

Defining Characteristics: Nausea and vomiting are uncommon, anorexia is mild to moderate, stomatitis is uncommon, diarrhea is uncommon, and hepatic dysfunction is rare, although abnormal LFTs may occur.

Nursing Implications: Premedicate with antiemetics as needed. Teach self-administration of prescribed medications. Instruct patient to report nausea/vomiting, diarrhea, anorexia, and stomatitis. Teach patient oral hygiene regimen and assess baseline oral mucosa. Monitor baseline LFTs, and monitor them periodically during therapy.

III.　POTENTIAL ALTERATION IN FLUID/ELECTROLYTES/RENAL ELIMINATION STATUS related to TLS

Defining Characteristics: When drug is first started in patients with high tumor burden (e.g., CML with high WBC), this often results in rapid death of a large number of malignant cells. The lysis or breakdown of these cells results in the release of intracellular contents into the systemic circulation. The resulting metabolic abnormalities are hyperkalemia, hyperphosphatemia, hypocalcemia, and hyperuricemia. If these persist, renal failure with oliguria can result.

Nursing Implications: Assess baseline chemistries, including metabolic panel, renal function. Expect that if the patient is at risk for the development of TLS, the patient will begin allopurinol 200–300 mg/m^2/day prior to therapy, and receive hydration with alkalization (e.g., 50–100 mEq bicarbonate added per liter) to deliver 3 liters/m^2/day. Assess serum potassium, phosphate, calcium, uric acid, and BUN and creatinine at least daily, and discuss any abnormalities with physician to revise current regimen. Monitor I/O, weights, and total body balance carefully, and at least daily.

IV. SENSORY/PERCEPTUAL ALTERATIONS related to DROWSINESS, HALLUCINATIONS, OTHER CNS EFFECTS

Defining Characteristics: Drug crosses the BBB, so CNS effects may occur, such as drowsiness, confusion, disorientation, headache, vertigo; symptoms last < 24 hours.

Nursing Implications: Assess baseline mental status and neurologic functioning. Instruct patient to report signs/symptoms, and reassure that they will resolve. If symptoms persist, discuss interrupting drug with physician.

V. POTENTIAL SEXUAL/REPRODUCTIVE DYSFUNCTION related to DRUG EFFECTS

Defining Characteristics: Drug is mutagenic and teratogenic. Drug is excreted in breastmilk.

Nursing Implications: Assess patient's sexual patterns and reproductive goals. Discuss with patient and partner potential toxicity and impact on sexuality. Provide information, emotional support, and referral as needed. Patient should use contraceptive measures; a mother receiving the drug should not breastfeed.

Drug: idarubicin (Idamycin, Idamycin Aspen, 4-demethoxydaunorubicin)

Class: Antitumor antibiotic.

Mechanism of Action: Inhibits topoisomerase II; forms single- and double-stranded DNA breaks. Analogue of daunorubicin. Has a marked inhibitory effect on RNA synthesis.

Metabolism: Excreted primarily in the bile and urine, with approximately 25% of the intravenous dose accounted for over 5 days. The half-life is 6–9.4 hours.

Indication: In combination with other approved anti-leukemic drugs, for the treatment of acute myeloid leukemia (AML) in adults. This includes French-British (FAB) classifications M1–M7.

Dosage/Range:
- Induction: 12 mg/m^2 daily slow IVP × 3 days in combination with ara-C 100 mg/m^2 CI × 7 days, or as cytarabine 25 mg/m^2 IVB followed by cytarabine 200 mg/m^2 CI × 5 days. If verified residual leukemia following first induction course, a second course may be administered. If the patient has severe mucositis, delay until patient has recovered from toxicity and institute a 25% dose reduction.
- The benefit of consolidation in prolonging remission duration and survival is unknown.
- Dose-reduce for renal or hepatic dysfunction. Do not administer idarubicin if bilirubin > 5 mg/dL.
- Dose reduction (25%) recommended for severe mucositis in prior course.

Drug Preparation:
- Available as a red powder.
- The drug is reconstituted with 0.9% sodium chloride injection to give a final concentration of 1 mg/1 mL. See package insert.

Drug Administration:
- Drug is a vesicant. Administer IV over 10 to 15 minutes into the sidearm of a patent, freely running IV, with constant observation of the IV insertion site.

Drug Interactions:
- Other myelosuppressive drugs: Additive BM suppression; monitor patient closely.
- Incompatible with heparin—causes precipitant.
- Probenecid and sulfinpyrazone: Drugs are uricosuric agents, and concurrent use increases risk of uric acid nephropathy.

Lab Effects/Interference:
- Decreased CBC.
- Increased LFTs, RFTs.

Special Considerations:
- Vesicant.
- Discolored urine (pink to red) may occur up to 48 hours after administration.
- Cardiomyopathy is less common and less severe than with doxorubicin and daunorubicin.
- Drug is light-sensitive.
- Warnings and Precautions:
  - *Severe BM suppressant*: Drug should not be given to patients with preexisting BM suppression induced by previous drug therapy or RT unless the benefit outweighs the risk. Patients will be at risk for infection and bleeding. Laboratory and supportive facilities that are able to rapidly manage severe hemorrhage and/or severe infection must be readily available.
  - *Myocardial toxicity* as manifested by fatal CHF, acute life-threatening arrhythmias, or other cardiomyopathies may occur. Increased risk for idarubicin-induced cardiac toxicity in patients with (1) pre-existing heart disease; (2) prior anthracycline therapy with high cumulative dose; (3) treatment with other potentially cardiotoxicic agents (e.g., trastuzumab, cyclophosphamide, paclitaxel); (4) concomitant or previous RT to the mediastinal-pericardial area; (5) anemia, BM depression, infections, leukemic pericarditis and/or myocarditis; (6) active or dormant cardiovascular diseae; (7) prior therapy with other anthracyclines or antracenediones). Carefully monitor cardiac function baseline and during treatment, especially as relates to a decrease in LVEF. Avoid the use of anthracycline-based therapy for at least 5 half-lives after discontinuation of the cardiotoxic agent.
  - *Embryo-fetal toxicity*: Advise female patients of reproductive potential of potential hazard to fetus and encourage effective contraception to avoid therapy during treatment. Mothers should not breastfeed during idarubicin therapy.
  - *Labs*: Monitor ANC/CBC, LFTs, and renal function tests baseline and closely during therapy.

- *TLS*: Discuss and implement strategies to reduce risk of TLS in patients with high tumor burden at initial therapy.
- *Extravasation injury* with tissue necrosis as drug is a vesicant. Use vesicant precautions during drug administration.
- *Geriatric use*: Patients > 60 years old undergoing induction therapy are at increased risk for CHF, serious arrthymias, chest pain, MI, and asymptomatic decline in LVEF compared to younger patients.

Potential Toxicities/Side Effects and the Nursing Process

I.   INFECTION AND BLEEDING related to BM DEPRESSION

Defining Characteristics: Hematologic toxicity is dose limiting. Leukopenia nadir 10–20 days with recovery in 1–2 weeks. Thrombocytopenia usually follows leukopenia and is mild. BM toxicity is not cumulative.

Nursing Implications: Evaluate WBC, neutrophil, and platelet count and discuss any abnormalities with physician prior to drug administration. Assess for signs/symptoms of infection or bleeding and instruct patient in signs/symptoms of infection and bleeding and to report them immediately. Suggest strategies to minimize risk of infection and bleeding, including avoidance of OTC aspirin-containing medications.

II.   ALTERATION IN CARDIAC OUTPUT related to CUMULATIVE DOSES OF IDARUBICIN

Defining Characteristics: Cardiac toxicity is similar characteristically but less severe than that seen with daunorubicin and doxorubicin; CHF due to cardiomyopathy seen after large cumulative doses.

Nursing Implications: Assess cardiac status prior to chemotherapy administration: signs/symptoms of CHF, quality/regularity and rate of heartbeat, results of prior GBPS or other test of LVEF. Teach patient to report dyspnea, palpitations, swelling in extremities. Maintain accurate records of total dose; expect GBPS to be repeated periodically during treatment and the drug to be discontinued if there is a significant drop in heart function.

III.   ALTERED NUTRITION, LESS THAN BODY REQUIREMENTS, related to NAUSEA/VOMITING, ANOREXIA, STOMATITIS, DIARRHEA, AND HEPATIC DYSFUNCTION

Defining Characteristics: Nausea/vomiting is usually mild to moderate, although it is seen to some degree in most patients; anorexia commonly occurs; stomatitis is mild; diarrhea is infrequent and mild; hepatitis is rare but may occur, and there are also disturbances in LFTs.

Nursing Implications: Premedicate with combination antiemetics and continue protection for 24 hours. If patient has a central line, slower infusion of drug over 1 hour decreases nausea/vomiting. Encourage small, frequent meals of bland foods. Anorexia occurs frequently: teach patient or caregiver to make foods ahead of time and use spices; encourage weekly weights. Stomatitis and esophagitis may occur in patients who have received prior radiation and during posttreatment visits. Teach patient oral hygiene regimen and self-assessment techniques. Encourage patient to report onset of diarrhea; administer or teach patient to self-administer antidiarrheal medications. Monitor SGOT, SGPT, LDH, alk phos, and bili periodically during treatment. Notify physician of any elevations.

IV.   ALTERATION IN SKIN INTEGRITY related to ALOPECIA, SKIN CHANGES

Defining Characteristics: Alopecia occurs in about 30% of patients after oral drug and can be partial after IV drug; begins after 3 or more weeks of starting therapy, and hair may grow back while on treatment; may be slight-to-diffuse thinning. Skin changes include darkening of nail beds, skin ulcer/necrosis, sensitivity to sunlight, skin itching at irradiated areas, radiation recall, and potential necrosis with extravasation.

Nursing Implications: Discuss with patient hair loss, anticipated impact, and strategies to decrease distress, e.g., obtaining wig prior to hair loss. Assess disturbance of body image from hyperpigmentation and discuss strategies to minimize this, e.g., nail polish. Drug must be administered via patient IV. Assess need for venous access device early. If drug administered as CI, IT MUST BE GIVEN VIA A CENTRAL LINE.

V.   POTENTIAL SEXUAL/REPRODUCTIVE DYSFUNCTION related to DRUG EFFECTS

Defining Characteristics: Gonadal function and fertility may be affected (may be permanent or transient). Reported to be excreted in breastmilk.

Nursing Implications: As appropriate, explore with patient and partner issues of reproductive and sexuality patterns and impact chemotherapy will have; discuss strategies to preserve sexuality and reproductive health (e.g., contraception, sperm banking).

Drug: ifosfamide (Ifex)

Class: Alkylating agent.

Mechanism of Action: Destroys DNA throughout the cell cycle by binding to protein and by DNA crosslinking and causing chain scission, as well as inhibition of DNA synthesis. Analogue of cyclophosphamide and is cell cycle phase nonspecific. Ifosfamide has been shown to be effective in tumors previously resistant to cyclophosphamide. Activated by microsomes in the liver.

Metabolism: Only about 50% of the drug is metabolized, with much of the drug excreted in the urine almost completely unchanged. Up to 70–86% of the drug dose is recoverable in the urine. Half-life is 13.8 hours for high doses vs 3–10 hours for lower doses.

Indication (FDA): In combination with certain other approved antineoplastic agents, for the third-line treatment of germ cell testicular cancer, together with mesna.

Drug active in cancers of lung, breast, ovary, pancreas, and stomach; Hodgkin's and NHL, acute and CLL.

Contraindication: (1) Patients with urinary outflow obstruction; (2) patients hypersensitive to the drug.

Dosage/Range:
- All doses given with 2-L hydration/day and mesna to prevent the incidence of hemorrhagic cystitis.
- 1.2 grams/m^2/day $\times$ 5 days, every 3 weeks, or after recovery from hematologic toxicity.
- CI: 1,200 mg/m^2/day $\times$ 5 days, with mesna in the same infusion bag, and continuing for 1 day after the ifosfamide infusions.
- Dose-reduce by 25–50% if serum creatinine is 2.1–3.0 mg/dL and hold if creatinine > 3.0 mg/dL.

Drug Preparation:
- Available as a powder in 1- and 3-g vials and should be reconstituted with sterile water for injection.
- Further dilute ifosfamide solution to achieve concentrations 0.6–2.0 mg/mL in 55 dextrose injection, USP; 0.9% sodium chloride injection USP; Lactated Ringer's injection USP.
- Reconstituted drug or reconstituted and further diluted solution should be refrigerated and used within 24 hours. Benzyl-alcohol-containing solutions can reduce the stability of ifosfamide.
- Parenteral products should be inspected visually for particulate matter and discoloration before administration.

Drug Administration:
- IV bolus: Administer over 30 minutes. Mesna (20% of ifosfamide dose) should be administered with ifosfamide: mesna is begun 15 minutes prior to ifosfamide and repeated at 4 and 8 hours after the ifosfamide (see drug sheet on mesna). Mesna, ascorbic acid, and mucomycin have been used to protect the bladder. Pre- and posthydration (1,500–2,000 mL/day) or continuous bladder irrigations are recommended to prevent hemorrhagic cystitis.
- CI: Administer intravenously for 5 days. Mesna is mixed with ifosfamide in equal amounts (1:1 mix). Prior to initiating CI, mesna is given IVB (10% of total ifosfamide dose). Following completion of the infusion, mesna alone should be infused for 12–24 hours to protect from delayed drug excretion activity against the bladder.

Drug Interactions:
- Activity/toxicity affected by allopurinol, chloroquine, phenothiazides, potassium iodide, chloramphenicol, imipramine, vitamin A, corticosteroids, succinylcholine.

- BM–depressant drugs: additive BM depression.
- Mesna binds to and inactivates ifosfamide metabolite, thus preventing bladder toxicity.

Lab Effects/Interference:
- Decreased CBC.
- Increased RFTs, LFTs (AST and ALT).

Special Considerations:
- Metabolic toxicity is increased by simultaneous administration of barbiturates.
- Renal function: BUN, serum creatinine, and creatinine clearance must be determined prior to treatment.
- Therapy requires the concomitant administration of a uroprotector such as mesna and pre- and posthydration; may also require catheterization and constant bladder irrigation, and/or ascorbic acid.
- Test urine for occult blood.
- Dose-limiting toxicity has been renal and bladder dysfunction.
- Warnings and Precautions:
  - *Myelosuppression, immunosuppression, and infections*: Increased risk when ifosfamide is given in combination with other chemotherapeutic/hemotoxic agents and/or RT. Risk of myelosuppression is dose dependent. Monitor CBC/differential closely during treatment, and assess for, and teach patient to assess for and report, signs/symptoms of infection or bleeding. Do not administer drug unless WBC > 2,000 cells/mm^3 and platelet count > 50,000/mm^3.
  - *CNS toxicity, neurotoxicity*: This includes somnolence, confusion, hallluciations, blurred vision, psychotic behavior, extrapyrimal symptoms, urinary incontinence, seizures, and rarely coma. This may become manifest within a few hours to a few days after first dose, and usually resolves within 48–72 hours. Monitor closely and provide supportive care until episode resolves. Recurrence after several uneventful treatments has occurred. If encephalopathy develops, drug should be discontinued. Use cautiously in patients taking other CNS affecting drugs such as sedatives, opioids. CNS toxicity may impair a patient's ability to drive an automobile or operate heavy machinery.
  - *Renal and urothelial toxicity and effects*: Drug is both nephrotoxic and urotoxic. Assess glomerylar and tubular kidney function before starting ifosfamide therapy, and during therapy. Assess for increased serum creatinine, proteinuria, hematuria. Drug may also cause an SIADH-like syndrome. Renal tubular damage may occur months or years after therapy ends; it may resolve with time, remain stable, or progress (Teva, 2015). Hemorrhagic cystitis requiring RBC transfusion has been reported. Prior to starting ifosfamide regimen, patient must be evaluated to ensure there is no urinary tract obstruction (contraindication). Patient should be assessed for hematuria prior to drug administration, and if >10 RBCs per high power field, the dose delayed until resolved. Patient should be adequately hydrated prior to ifosfamide to result in a urinary output of 100 mL/hour before starting drug; mesna must be given with ifosfamide. Drug should be used cautiously if at all in patients with a UTI.
  - *Cardiotoxicity* may occur, manifested as (1) supraventricular or ventricular arrhythmias, atrial fibrillation, pulseless ventricular tachycardia; (2) decreased QRS voltage

and ST-segment or T-wave changes; (3) toxic cardiomyopathy leading to CHF and hypotension; (4) pericardial effusion, fibrinous pericarditis, and epicardial fibrosis. Risk is dose dependent, and increased in paitents with prior or concomitant treatment with other cardiotoxic drugs or RT to the cardiac region, and possibly renal impairment. Use drug cautiously in patients with preexisting cardiac disease and monitor closely during therapy.

- *Pulmonary toxicity*: Interstitial pneumonitis, pulmonary fibrosis, and other toxicity has been reported. Monitor for signs/symptoms of pulmonary toxicity, discuss findings with physician/NP/PA, and implement orders.
- *Secondary malignancies*: Risk of myelodysplastic disease, which may progress to acute leukemia, and other malignancies (e.g., lymphoma, thyroid cancer, sarcomas) have been reported.
- *Veno-occlusive disease* has been reported.
- *Embryo-fetal toxicity*: Women of reproductive potential should use effective contraception to avoid pregnancy during therapy. Men should not father a child during therapy and for up at least 6 months after the last dose. Mothers must not breastfeed their infant during therapy as drug is excreted in breast milk.
- *Effects on fertility*: Women may develop amenorrhea, and risk of it becoming permanent increases with age. Men may develop oligospermia or azoospermia, which may be reversible after several years after cessation of therapy. Discuss prior to beginning therapy with patients, and possible banking options.
- *Anaphylactic/anaphylactoid reactions* and cross-sensitivity may occur.
- *Impairment of wound healing* may occur.

Potential Toxicities/Side Effects and the Nursing Process

I. ALTERED URINARY ELIMINATION related to HEMORRHAGIC CYSTITIS AND RENAL TOXICITY

Defining Characteristics: Symptoms of bladder irritation; hemorrhagic cystitis with hematuria, dysuria, urinary frequency; preventable with uroprotection and hydration. Symptoms of renal toxicity; increased BUN and serum creatinine, decreased urine creatinine clearance (usually reversible); acute tubular necrosis, pyelonephritis, glomerular dysfunction; metabolic acidosis.

Nursing Implications: Assess presence of RBC in urine prior to successive doses, especially if symptoms are present, as well as BUN and creatinine. Administer drug with concomitant uroprotector (e.g., mesna). Encourage prehydration: oral intake of 2–3 L/day prior to chemotherapy; posthydration: increase oral fluids to 2–3 L for 2 days after chemotherapy. If possible, administer drug in morning to minimize drug accumulation in bladder during sleep. Instruct patient to empty bladder every 2–3 hours, before bedtime, and during night when awake. Monitor urinary output and total body balance. Assess urinary elimination pattern prior to each drug dose. If rigorous regimen is adhered to, minimal renal toxicity will result. Monitor BUN and creatinine.

II.   ALTERED NUTRITION, LESS THAN BODY REQUIREMENTS, related to NAUSEA AND VOMITING, HEPATOTOXICITY

Defining Characteristics: Nausea and vomiting occur in 58% of patients; dose- and schedule-dependent, with increased severity with higher dose and rapid injection. Occurs within a few hours of drug administration and may last 3 days. Elevations of serum transaminase and alk phos may occur; usually transient and resolve spontaneously without apparent sequelae.

Nursing Implications: Premedicate with antiemetics and continue prophylactically to prevent nausea and vomiting for 24 hours at least for the first treatment. Encourage small, frequent feedings of cool, bland foods and liquids. Refer to section on nausea and vomiting. Monitor LFTs during treatment.

III.   INFECTION AND BLEEDING related to BM DEPRESSION

Defining Characteristics: Leukopenia is mild to moderate. Thrombocytopenia and anemia are rare. Dosage adjustment may be necessary when ifosfamide is combined with other chemotherapy agents. Patients at risk for BM depression include patients with impaired renal function and decreased BM reserve (BM metastases, prior XRT).

Nursing Implications: Evaluate WBC, with neutrophil, and platelet count and discuss any abnormalities with physician prior to drug administration. Assess for signs/symptoms of infection or bleeding and instruct patient in signs/symptoms of infection and bleeding, and to report them immediately; discuss strategies to minimize risk of infection and bleeding, including avoidance of OTC aspirin-containing medications. Assess patient's Hgb/HCT and signs/symptoms of fatigue; teach patient self-assessment and to alternate rest and activity as needed.

IV.   ALTERATION IN SKIN INTEGRITY related to ALOPECIA, STERILE PHLEBITIS, SKIN CHANGES

Defining Characteristics: The incidence of alopecia is 83%, with 50% experiencing severe hair loss in 2–4 weeks. Sterile phlebitis may occur at injection site; irritation occurs with extravasation. Hyperpigmentation, dermatitis, and nail ridging may occur.

Nursing Implications: Discuss with patient anticipated impact of hair loss; suggest wig, as appropriate, prior to actual hair loss. Explore with patient response to hair loss and alternative strategies to minimize distress. Carefully monitor injection site during drug administration for signs/symptoms of phlebitis, irritation, vein patency. Assess skin integrity. Assess impact of skin changes on body image. Discuss strategies to minimize distress.

V. POTENTIAL SEXUAL/REPRODUCTIVE DYSFUNCTION related to DRUG EFFECTS

Defining Characteristics: Drug is carcinogenic, mutagenic, and teratogenic. Drug is excreted in breast milk.

Nursing Implications: As appropriate, explore with patient and partner issues of reproductive and sexual patterns, and impact chemotherapy will have. Discuss strategies to preserve sexuality and reproductive health (e.g., sperm banking, contraception).

VI. SENSORY/PERCEPTUAL ALTERATIONS related to CONFUSION, ACTIVITY INTOLERANCE, FATIGUE

Defining Characteristics: Intact drug passes easily into CNS; however, active metabolites do not. Lethargy and confusion may be seen with high doses, lasting 1–8 hours, usually spontaneously reversible. CNS side effects occur in about 12% of patients treated, including somnolence, confusion, depressive psychosis, hallucinations. Less frequent side effects: dizziness, disorientation, cranial nerve dysfunction, seizures, and coma. Incidence of CNS side effects may be higher in patients with compromised renal function, as well as in patients receiving high doses. In most instances, CNS changes are reversible.

Nursing Implications: Identify patients at risk (decreased renal function) and observe closely. Assess neurologic and mental status prior to and during drug administration and on follow-up. Instruct patient to report any alterations in behavior, sensation, perception. Develop a plan of care with patient and family if side effects develop to manage distress and promote safety. Drug should be stopped if confusion, hallucinations, and coma occur.

Drug: irinotecan (Camptosar, Camptothecan-11, CPT-11)

Class: Topoisomerase I inhibitor.

Mechanism of Action: Induces protein-linked DNA single-strand breaks and blocks DNA and RNA synthesis in dividing cells, thus preventing cells from entering mitosis. The active metabolite, SN-38, prevents repair (relegation) of previous, reversible single-strand breaks in DNA by binding to topoisomerase I. Topoisomerase I is an enzyme that relaxes tension in the DNA helix torsion by initially causing this single-strand break in DNA so that DNA replication can occur. Topoisomerases I and II then work together to bring about replication, transcription, and recombination of DNA material. Topoisomerase I is found in higher-than-normal concentrations in certain malignant cells, such as colon adenocarcinoma cells and non-Hodgkin's lymphoma cells.

Metabolism: Metabolized to its active metabolite SN-38 in the liver; 11–20% of the drug is excreted in the urine, and 5–39% in the bile over a 48-hour period. Mean terminal half-life is 6 hours, while that of SN-38 is 10 hours. Drug is moderately protein-bound (30–68%), while SN-38 is highly protein-bound (95%).

Indication: Patients with metastatic cancer of the colon or rectum, whose disease has recurred or progressed following initial fluorouracil-based therapy.

Contraindication: hypersensitivity to irinotecan HCl or its excipients.

Dosage/Range:
Metastatic colorectal cancers

Single agent:
- Irinotecan 125 mg/m^2 IV over 90 minutes on days 1, 8, 11, 15, then 2-week rest.
- Irinotecan 350 mg/m^2 IV over 90 minutes on day 1 every 3 weeks.

Combination regimens:
- FOLFIRI day 1: Irinotecan 180 mg/m^2 IV over 90 minutes, at the same time as leucovorin 200 mg/m^2 IV over 2 hours through separate arms of a Y-tubing, followed by 5-FU 400 mg/m^2 IVB and then 23-hour 5-FU 1,200 mg/m^2 IV CI, days 1 and 2. Total 5-FU CI dose is 2,400 mg/m^2 over 46–48 hours. Repeat q 2 weeks.
- Douillard day 1: Irinotecan 180 mg/m^2 IV over 90 minutes, at the same time as leucovorin 200 mg/m^2 IV over 2 hours through separate arms of a Y-tubing, followed by 5-FU 400 mg/m^2 IVB and then 22-hour 5-FU 600 mg/m^2 IV CI. Day 2: Leucovorin 200 mg/m^2 IV over 2 hours and then 5-FU 400 mg/m^2 IVB and then 22-hour 5-FU 600 mg/m^2 IV CI. Repeat q 2 weeks.
- CapIri: Capecitabine 1,000 mg/m^2 po bid days 1–14; irinotecan 80 mg/m^2 IV days 1 and 8. Repeat q 22 days.

Dose Modification:
See package insert for dose modifications.

Drug Preparation:
- Store unopened vials at room temperature and protect from light. Available in 2 mL-fill vial containing 40 mg, and 5-mL fill vial containing 100 mg irinotecan HCl injection.
- Drug must be diluted before infusion. Use 5% dextrose (preferred) or 0.9% sodium chloride to a final concentration of 0.12–1.1 mg/mL. Commonly, the drug is diluted in 500 mL 5% dextrose.
- Drug should be used immediately after reconstitution as it contains no antibacterial preservative. However, if it is not possible, diluted drug is stable 24 hours at room temperature. If diluted in 5% dextrose, the drug is stable for 48 hours if refrigerated (2–8°C [36–46°F]) and protected from light.

Drug Administration:
- Administer IV bolus over 90 minutes. Drug is an irritant. If extravasation occurs, the manufacturer recommends flushing the IV site with sterile water and then applying ice.
- Do not administer irinotecan if ANC < 1,000/mm^3.
- Patient must have dose reduction as recommended; drug should not be administered if the patient is neutropenic or has diarrhea.

- All patients should receive self-care instructions on management of diarrhea, self-administration of loperamide for delayed diarrhea, and assessment of the patient's ability to purchase loperamide and ability to comply with instructions.
- Closely monitor all patients aged 65 and over, because of an increased risk of both early and late diarrhea.
- Use caution when treating patients with renal or hepatic impairment and do not administer to patients on dialysis (Teva, 2015).

Drug Interactions:
- Strong CYP3A4 inducers (e.g., phenytoin, phenobarbital, carbamazepine, or St. John's wort): may decrease drug serum and active metabolite SN-38 levels, thus reducing effectiveness; do not coadminster.
- Strong CYP3A4 inhibitors (e.g., clarithromycin, indinavir, itraconazole, ketoconazole, lopinavir, nefazodone, nelfinavir, ritonavir, saquinavir, telaprevir, voriconazole) or UGT1A1 inhibitors (e.g., ketoconazole, atazanavir gemfibrozil, indinavir): inhibits SN38 catabolism by CYP3A4 with increased serum levels and subsequent toxicity of irinotecan; do not coadminister. Discontinue strong CYP3A4 inhibitors at least 1 week prior to starting irinotecan therapy. Do not administer strong CYP3A4 or UGT1A1 inhibitors with irinotecan unless there are no therapeutic alternatives (Teva, 2015).
- 5-FU: additive or synergistic effect.

Lab Effects/Interference:
- Decreased ANC, red blood cell count, platelet count.
- UGT1A1*28* allele polymorphism occurs in 10% of population; results in decreased metabolism of SN38 and subsequent increased risk of neutropenia, other toxicities.

Special Considerations:
- Most common adverse reactions ($\geq$30%) in single agent studies are nausea, vomiting, abdominal pain, diarrhea, constipation, anorexia, neutropenia, leuckopenia and lymphopenia, anemia, sthenia, fever, decreased body weight, alopecia.
- Potential life-threatening toxicity: severe myelosuppression, and both early and late diarrhea, which are dose-limiting toxicities. Patient must have weekly assessment for toxicity.
- Warnings and Precautions:
  - *Diarrhea and cholinergic reactions*: Early diarrhea accompanied by cholinergic symptoms preventable or improved with atropine. Late diarrhea can be life-threatening and should be treated promptly with loperamide. Monitor patients with diarrhea and give fluid and electrolytes as needed. Start antibiotic therapy if patient develop ileus, fever, or severe neutropenia. Interrupt drug for severe diarrhea, and dose reduce subsequent doses.
  - *Severe myeslosuppression* may occur. Manage promptly with antibiotic support. Interrupt drug and dose reduce when toxicity resolved.
  - *Patients with reduced UGT1A1 activity*: Patients who are homozygous for the UGT1A1*28 allele (both copies of alleles) are at increased risk for neutropenia and should receive dose modification. In addition, rarely, patients may lack an enzyme necessary for drug metabolism, resulting in increased toxicity (Gilbert's syndrome, abnormal glucuronidation of bilirubin).

- *Renal impairment/renal* failure may occur rarely, probably related to volume depletion related to severe vomiting and diarrhea.
- *Pulmonary toxicity*: Interstitial pulmonary disease (IPD)–like events, including deaths, have occurred. If patient develops new or progressive dyspnea, cough, and fever, interrupt irinotecan until patient can have a pulmonary evaluation. If IPD is diagnosed, drug should be discontinued and patient treated for IPD.
- *Toxicity of the 5-day regimen*: Irinotecan should not be used in combination with a regimen of 5-FU/LV for 4–5 consecutive days every 4 weeks outside of a clinical trial. IFL (Saltz) regimen may result in increased deaths and is generally not used in the United States.
- *Embryo-fetal toxicity:* Teach women of reproductive potential to use effective contraception to avoid pregnancy during treatment. Mothers should not breastfeed infant while receiving irinotecan treatment.
- *Patients with hepatic impairment*: clinical trials did not study patients with a bilirubin > 2 mg/dL or transaminases > 3 × ULN if not liver metastases, or transaminases > 5 times × ULN if liver metastases. With weekly dosage schedule, patients with total BR levels 1–2 mg/dL have greater risk of grades 3–4 neutropenia.
- Dose reductions must be made for neutropenia and severe diarrhea, and are different for combination therapy (irinotecan/5-FU/leukovorin) and irinotecan as a single agent.

Potential Toxicities/Side Effects and the Nursing Process

I.   ALTERATION IN ELIMINATION related to DIARRHEA

Defining Characteristics: Diarrhea may be early or late. Early diarrhea is characterized by onset within 24 hours of drug dose and is mediated by cholinergic pathway(s), as the metabolite SN-38 inhibits acetylcholinesterase; diaphoresis and abdominal cramping may precede diarrhea, and may be prevented by atropine. Other cholinergic effects that may appear are salivation, lacrimation, visual disturbances, piloerection, and bradycardia. This can be managed effectively with atropine 0.25–1.0-mg IV or scopolamine. Late diarrhea occurs > 24 hours after the drug dose, can be severe, prolonged, and lead to dehydration and electrolyte imbalance; the etiology appears related to changes in intestinal mucosal epithelium that prevent the reabsorption of water and electrolytes, which are then lost during diarrhea. 88% of patients may experience late diarrhea, and 31% have severe, or grades 3–4 diarrhea. Loperamide is effective in halting late diarrhea. Irinotecan should be held for grade 3 diarrhea (7–9 stools/day, incontinence, or severe cramping) and grade 4 (> 10 stools/day, grossly bloody stool, or need for parenteral support). Once recovered, decrease drug dose at next treatment per manufacturer's guidelines and per physician's order.

Nursing Implications: Acute diarrhea: teach patient to report diarrhea, sweating, and abdominal cramping during or after drug administration. Administer atropine 0.25–1 mg IVP per physician order, unless contraindicated, to prevent diarrhea. Delayed diarrhea: teach patient self-management of diarrhea (diet, fluids, avoidance of laxatives), and to notify nurse or physician of vomiting, fever, or if signs/symptoms of dehydration occur (fainting, light-headedness, dizziness). Teaching about diet should include drinking 8–10 large glasses of fluid/day, including soup/broth, soda, Gatorade; avoiding dairy products; eating small meals often; using BRAT diet (bananas, rice, applesauce, toast); and adding other foods as tolerated, such as bland, low-fiber foods, white chicken meat without skin, scrambled eggs, crackers, or pasta without sauce. Also, teach patient to avoid foods that worsen diarrhea (fatty, fried, or greasy foods, high-fiber foods with bran, raw fruits and vegetables, popcorn, beans, nuts, chocolate). Review patient's medication profile, including OTC medicines, and teach patient to stop taking any laxatives. Teach patient to avoid cigarette smoking to promote comfort. Instruct patient to record stools, and to take loperamide, not as indicated on the medication package, but as instructed: At the first episode of late-onset diarrhea, take 4 mg (two 2-mg capsules) of loperamide, then 2 mg (1 capsule) every 2 hours until free of diarrhea for at least 12 hours. Take a 4-mg dose (two 2-mg capsules) at bedtime (Camptosar recommendations). Patient should notify doctor or nurse if diarrhea is unrelieved by loperamide taken as instructed. Assess patient's ability to purchase loperamide if impoverished, and identify other sources that can provide the medication prior to patient's discharge from clinic after drug therapy. Review patient's medication profile to ensure that the patient is not taking any cathartics. Diarrhea must be monitored closely and managed aggressively to prevent morbidity and mortality.

II. POTENTIAL FOR INFECTION, ANEMIA related to BM DEPRESSION

Defining Characteristics: Leukopenia has been noted in 63% of patients on single-dose schedules, with an overall neutropenia incidence of 54%, and grades 3–4 neutropenia occurring in 26% of patients. Thrombocytopenia is uncommon, occurring in about 3% of patients. Anemia is common (61%). Nadir is commonly on days 6–9.

Nursing Implications: Evaluate CBC, with neutrophil, and platelet count, and discuss any abnormalities with physician prior to drug administration. Refer to Special Considerations section for dosage modifications based on hematologic toxicity. Assess patient tolerance of chemotherapy and nadir blood counts, especially cycle 1. Assess for signs/symptoms of infection or bleeding; instruct patient in signs/symptoms of infection and bleeding, and to report them immediately. If febrile neutropenia develops, assess and begin antibiotic therapy ASAP. Instruct in measures to minimize risk of infection and bleeding, including avoidance of OTC aspirin-containing medications. Assess patient's Hgb/HCT and signs/symptoms of fatigue; teach patient self-assessment and to alternate rest and activity as needed.

III. POTENTIAL ALTERATION IN NUTRITION, LESS THAN BODY REQUIREMENTS, related to NAUSEA AND VOMITING, DEHYDRATION

Defining Characteristics: Moderate to severe nausea and vomiting occur in 35–60% of patients, with 17% experiencing NCI grades 3–4 nausea and 13% experiencing NCI grades 3–4 vomiting. Aggressive combination antiemetics are effective in preventing nausea/vomiting.

Nursing Implications: Premedicate with aggressive combination antiemetics, such as serotonin antagonist (dolasetron, granisetron, or ondansetron) plus dexamethasone 10-mg

IV 30 minutes prior to chemotherapy to prevent nausea and vomiting. Encourage small, frequent meals of cool, bland foods and liquids. Teach patients to monitor their fluid intake, and take daily weights if nausea/vomiting occurs. Assess for signs/symptoms of fluid and electrolyte imbalance. Teach patients self-assessment, and instruct to notify doctor or nurse if these occur. Late-onset nausea and vomiting may occur, and dopamine antagonists such as prochlorperazine are then recommended. If dehydration develops, replace fluid and electrolytes to prevent worsening dehydration and cardiovascular complications.

IV. POTENTIAL FOR IMPAIRED GAS EXCHANGE related to DYSPNEA, PULMONARY INFILTRATES, FEVER

Defining Characteristics: Pulmonary effects may occur in up to 22% of patients, ranging from transient dyspnea to pulmonary infiltrates, fever, increased cough, and decreased DLCO in a small number of patients.

Nursing Implications: Assess baseline pulmonary status, and teach patient to report any changes. Assess pulmonary status prior to each treatment and at visits between treatment. If patient develops dyspnea, discuss patient having PFTs with physician, and evaluating whether related to drug. Teach patient to manage dyspnea if it occurs, including alternating activity and rest periods.

Drug: irinotecan, liposome injection (Onivyde™)

Class: Topoisomerase inhibitor

Mechanism of Action: Topoisomerase I inhibitor encapsulated in a lipid bilayer liposome. Normally, topoisomerase I relieves the torsion strain in DNA by causing single strand breaks so the DNA can relax to be copied (unzipped). Irinotecan and its active metabolite SN-38 bind irreversibly to the topoisomerase I/DNA complex, and prevent religation of the single-strand breaks. This extends into the more lethal double-stranded DNA breaks and causes the cell to die.

Metabolism: Liposomal formulation has not been tested for metabolism, but 95% of the irinotecan remains liposomal bound. Irinotecan HCL is metabolized by esterases to form the active metabolite SN-38, and by CYP3A4-mediated oxidative metabolism. Biliary and urinary excretion of irinotecan and its metabolites ranges from 25–50% in 48 hours. Asians have 56% lower total irinotecan average steady state concentraations and 8% higher total SN-38 concentration compared to whites.

Ten percent of the population expresses the UGT1A1*28 polymorphism, which reduces the metabolism of SN-38, the active metabolite of irinotecan. This results in higher serum levels with more grades 3 and 4 neutropenia in those patients who should receive lower doses of irinotecan. Patients can be tested for this allele, or any patient who has a high bilirubin should be suspected, and a lower dose of the drug should be used initially.

Indication: Treatment of patients with metastatic adenocarcinoma of the pancreas after disease progression following gemcitabine-based therapy, in combination with fluorouracil and leucovorin. It is NOT indicated as a single agent.

Contraindication: severe hypersensitivity reaction to irinotecan liposome injection or irinotecan HCl. DO NOT substitute irinotecan liposome injection for irinotecan HCl.

Dosage Range:
- DO NOT substitute irinotecan liposome injection for other drugs containing irinotecan HCl.
- 70-mg/m^2 IV infusion over 90 min every 2 weeks.
- If patient is homozygous for UGT1A1*28, starting dose is 50-mg/m^2 IV infusion over 90 min every 2 weeks.
- No recommended dose for patients with serum bilirubin above the ULN.
- Premedicate with a corticosteroid and an antiemetic 30 min prior to giving drug.

Dose Modifications:
- Grades 3 or 4 adverse reactions:
  - Hold drug; initiate loperamide for late onset diarrhea of any severity; administer IV or subcutaneous atropine 0.25–1 mg (unless clinically contraindicated) for early onset diarrhea of any severity.
  - Upon recovery to ≤ grade 1, resume irinotecan liposome injection at: (1) 1st occurrence: 50 mg/m^2 (43 mg/ m^2 if homozygous UGT1A1*28, and no prior increase in dose); (2) 2nd 43 mg/m^2; 35 mg/m^2 if homozygous UGT1A1*28, and no prior increase in dose); (3) 3rd: discontinue drug.
- Interstitial lung disease (ILD): discontinue drug in all patients.
- Anaphylactic reaction: discontinue drug in all patients.

Drug Preparation:
- Available as 43 mg/10 mL in a single-dose vial.
- Withdraw calculated volume of drug from vial and dilute in 500 mL 5% dextrose injection USP or 0.9% sodium chloride injection USP and mix diluted solution by gentle inversion. Protect diluted drug from light.
- Administer within 4 hours of preparation when stored at room temperature or within 24 hours if stored under refrigerated conditions (2–8°C [36–46°F]). Allow diluted solution to come to room temperature prior to administration. DO NOT freeze.

Drug Administration:
- Assess ANC/CBC on days 1 and 8 of every cycle, and more frequently as indicated.
- Administer irinotecan liposome injection prior to leucovorin and fluorouracil.
- Premedicate with corticosteroid and antiemetic prior to administration of irinotecan liposome injection.
- Infuse diluted solution IV over 90 minutes. Do not use an in-line filter. Discard unused portion.
- Assess for infusion reactions (e.g., rash, urticarial, periorbital edema, pruritis), which occurred on day 1 in 3% of patients studied.

Drug Interactions:
- *Strong CYP3A4 inhibitors* (e.g., ketoconazole, clarithromycin, indinavir, itraconazole, lopinavir, nefazodone, nelfinavir, ritonavir, saquinavir, telaprevir, voriconazole) or UGT1A1 inhibitors (e.g., ketoconazole, atazanavir, gemfibrozil, indinavir): increase irinotecan or metabolite SN-38 exposure; avoid using strong or discontinue strong CYP3A inhibitors at least 1 week before starting irinotecan liposome injection.
- *Strong CYP3A4 inducers:* Avoid coadministration. Substitute nonenzyme inducing therapies at least 2 weeks prior to initiation of drug.

Lab Effects/Interference:
- Neutropenia, lymphopenia, anemia, thrombocytopenia.
- Increased ALT, hypoalbuminemia.
- Decreased serum magnesium, potassium, calcium, phosphate, and sodium; increased serum creatinine.

Special Considerations:
- Warnings and Precautions:
  - *Severe neutropenia* occurred in 20% of patients (vs 2% with 5FU/LV alone) and fatal neutropenic sepsis occurred in 0.8% in Study 1. Incidence of grades 3–4 neutropenia was higher in Asian patients (55%) compared to white patients (18%). Monitor CBC on days 1 and 8 of every cycle and as needed. Hold drug if ANC $<$ 1,500/mm^3 or if neutropenic fever occurs. Resume drug when ANC $\geq$ 1,500/mm^3. Dose-reduce for grades 3–4 neutropenia or neutropenic fever after recovery for subsequent cycles.
  - *Severe diarrhea* occurred in 13% of patients receiving combination drugs. Severe diarrhea can be life-threatening and can occur as 1) late onset occurring >24 hours after drug given, and early onset (within 24 hours) which may have symptoms of a cholinergic reaction. A patient may experience both types. Hold drug for grades 2–4 diarrhea. Start loperamide for lat onset of any severity. Administer IV or SQ atropine 0.25–1 mg for early onset diarrhea of any severity unless contraindicated. After recovery to grade 1 diarrhea, resume irinotecan liposome injection at a reduced dose.
  - *ILD*: Can be severe and fatal. Hold drug in patients with new or progressive dyspnea, cough, fever, pending diagnostic workup. Discontinue drug in patients with a confirmed diagnosis of ILD.
  - *Severe hypersensitivity reaction (HSR)* may occur, including anaphylaxis. Institute medical intervention and emergency drugs as ordered. The drug should be discontinued if the patient has a severe HSR.
  - *Embryo-fetal toxicity* is likely. Teach women of reproductive potential to use effective contraception during treatment and for at least 1 month after the final dose. Teach men with partners who are have reproductive potential to use effective contraception during treatment and for 4 months after last dose. Mothers should NOT breastfeed while receiving the drug.
- Most common adverse reactions ($\geq$20%) were diarrhea, fatigue/asthenia, vomiting, nausea, decreased appetite, stomatitis, and pyrexia.

Potential Toxicities/Side Effects and the Nursing Process

I. POTENTIAL FOR INFECTION, BLEEDING, and ANEMIA related to BM DEPRESSION

Defining Characteristics: Neutropenia has been noted in 52% of patients, anemia in 97%, and thrombocytopenia in 41%. Grades 3–4 neutropenia occurred in 20% of patients. Nadir is commonly on days 6–9. Sepsis occurred in 4% of patients, neutropenic fever/neutropenic sepsis in 3%. IV catheter-related infection occurred in 3% as did gastroenteritis. Incidence of fatigue/asthenia was 56%, 21% grades 3–4.

Nursing Implications: Evaluate CBC, with neutrophil, and platelet count, and discuss any abnormalities with physician prior to drug administration. ANC must be $\geq$ 1,500/mm^3 to receive the drug. ANC/CBC should be checked on day 1 and day 8 of each cycle. Grades 3–4 myelosuppression requires dose reduction (see dosing). Assess for signs/symptoms of infection or bleeding; instruct patient in signs/symptoms of infection and bleeding and to report them immediately. If febrile neutropenia develops, assess and begin antibiotic therapy ASAP as ordered. Instruct in measures to minimize risk of infection and bleeding, including avoidance of OTC aspirin-containing medications. Assess patient's level of energy and fatigue baseline, and during therapy, as well as Hgb/HCT. Teach patient to self-assess for signs/symptoms of fatigue; and strategies to limit energy expenditure and reduce fatigue such as alternating rest and activity, and gentle exercise as tolerated.

II. ALTERATION IN ELIMINATION related to DIARRHEA

Defining Characteristics: Diarrhea may be early or late. Early diarrhea is characterized by onset within 24 hours of drug dose and is mediated by cholinergic pathway(s), as the metabolite SN-38 inhibits acetylcholinesterase; diaphoresis and abdominal cramping may precede diarrhea, and may be prevented by atropine. Other cholinergic effects that may appear are increased salivation, lacrimation, visual disturbances, piloerection, miosis, and bradycardia. This can be managed effectively with atropine 0.25–1.0-mg IV or scopolamine. Late diarrhea occurs > 24 hours after the drug dose, can be severe, prolonged, and lead to dehydration and electrolyte imbalance; the etiology appears related to changes in intestinal mucosal epithelium that prevent the reabsorption of water and electrolytes, which are then lost during diarrhea. 43% of patients may experience late diarrhea, and 9% have severe, or grades 3–4 diarrhea. Loperamide is effective in halting late diarrhea.

Nursing Implications: Irinotecan should be held for grade 2 or higher diarrhea (increase of 4–6 stools/day over baseline or moderate increase in ostomy output compared to baseline. Teach patient to begin loperamide if late diarrhea occurs, of any severity and to notify the RN/MD or NP/PA if the diarrhea persists. Administer atropine if not contraindicated for early diarrhea. Once recovered to grade 1, decrease drug dose at next treatment per manufacturer's guidelines and per physician's order. Acute diarrhea: teach patient to report diarrhea, sweating, and abdominal cramping during or after drug administration. Administer atropine 0.25–1 mg IVP per physician order, unless contraindicated, to prevent diarrhea. Delayed diarrhea: teach patient self-management of diarrhea (diet, fluids, avoidance of laxatives), and to notify nurse or physician of vomiting, fever, or if signs/symptoms of dehydration occur (fainting, light-headedness, dizziness). Teaching about diet should include drinking 8–10 large glasses of fluid/day, including soup/broth, soda, Gatorade; avoiding dairy products; eating small meals often; using BRAT diet (bananas, rice, applesauce, toast); and adding other foods as tolerated, such as bland, low-fiber foods, white chicken meat without skin, scrambled eggs, crackers, or pasta without sauce. Also, teach patient to avoid foods that worsen diarrhea (fatty, fried, or greasy foods, high-fiber foods with bran, raw fruits and vegetables, popcorn, beans, nuts, chocolate). Review patient's medication profile, including OTC medicines, and teach patient to stop taking any laxatives. Teach patient to avoid cigarette smoking to promote comfort. Instruct patient to record stools. Discuss with physician/NP/PA of using irinotecan loperamide schedule to prevent severe diarrhea: loperamide, not as indicated on the medication package, but as follows: the patient should: At the first episode of late-onset diarrhea, take 4 mg (two 2-mg capsules) of loperamide, then 2 mg (1 capsule) every 2 hours until free of diarrhea for at least 12 hours. Take a 4-mg dose (two 2-mg capsules) at bedtime (Camptosar recommendations). Patient should notify doctor or nurse if diarrhea is unrelieved by loperamide taken as instructed. Assess patient's ability to purchase loperamide if impoverished, and identify other sources that can provide the medication prior to patient's discharge from clinic after drug therapy. Review patient's medication profile to ensure that the patient is not taking any cathartics. Diarrhea must be monitored closely and managed aggressively to prevent morbidity and mortality.

III.   POTENTIAL ALTERATION IN NUTRITION, LESS THAN BODY REQUIREMENTS, related to NAUSEA AND VOMITING, DEHYDRATION

Defining Characteristics: Nausea and vomiting occurred in 51–52% of patients, respectively, and was grades 3–4 in 8% and 11% of patients, respectively. Stomatitis occurred in 32% and was grades 3–4 in 4% of patients.

Nursing Implications: Premedicate with combination antiemetics of corticosteroid and anti-emetic, such as serotonin antagonist (dolasetron, granisetron, or ondansetron) plus dexamethasone 10-mg IV 30 minutes prior to chemotherapy to prevent nausea and vomiting. Encourage small, frequent meals of cool, bland foods and liquids. Teach patients to monitor their fluid intake and take daily weights if nausea/vomiting occurs. Assess for signs/symptoms of fluid and electrolyte imbalance. Teach patients self-assessment and instruct to notify doctor or nurse if these occur. Late-onset nausea and vomiting may occur, and dopamine antagonists such as prochlorperazine are then recommended. If dehydration develops, replace fluid and electrolytes to prevent worsening dehydration and cardiovascular complications. Assess oral mucosa and teach patient self-assessment. Teach patient systematic oral cleansing with nonalcohol-containing oral rinse, such as bicarbonate or saline solution, based on the institution standard.

Drug: ixabepilone (Ixempra)

Class: Microtubule inhibitor; Epothilone B analogue.

Mechanism of Action: Normally, cells need to have flexibility in making the structures for mitosis, such as tubulin and the microtubules; the tubulin needs to be able to polymerize and then depolymerize. Ixabepilone binds to the beta-tubulin subunits on microtubules, and strongly promotes tubulin polymerization and stabilization, similar to paclitaxel but at a different binding site; the drug causes the cell to stop cycling (mitotic arrest) at the G_2/M phase of the cell cycle and to die (cytotoxicity). The drug avoids multiple tumor-resistance mechanisms, including efflux transporters and P-glycoprotein; thus, it has effectiveness against tumors that possess these mechanisms resulting in refractoriness to taxanes, anthra-cyclines, and vinca alkaloids. Ixabepilone also has antiangiogenic activity.

Metabolism: Drug is a semisynthetic analogue of epothilone B. It is a macrolide fermen-tation product of the myxobacterium Sorangium cellulosum. Drug has linear pharmaco-kinetics, with 67–77% binding to serum proteins. Drug is extensively metabolized in the liver, primarily via oxidative metabolism by CYP3A4/5 microenzyme system (hepatic mi-crosomes). This produces > 30 inactive metabolites, which are then excreted in the urine (65%) and feces (21%). Eighty-six percent of the dose is eliminated in 7 days. The terminal half-life of the drug is 52 hours, with no accumulation in the plasma when given every 3 weeks. It is unlikely that ixabepilone affects serum levels of drugs that are substrates of CYP enzymes.

Indication:
- In combination with capecitabine for the treatment of patients with metastatic or locally advanced breast cancer in patients after failure of an anthracycle and a taxane, or whose cancer is taxane-resistant and for whom further anthracycline therapy is contraindicated.
  - Anthracycline resistance is defined as progression while on therapy or within 6 months in the adjuvant setting or 3 months in the metastatic setting.
  - Taxane resistance is defined as progression while on therapy or within 12 months in the adjuvant setting or 4 months in the metastatic setting.
- As monotherapy, for the treatment of patients with metastatic or locally advanced breast cancer after failure of an anthracycline, a taxane and capecitabine.

Contraindications: (1) hypersensitivity to drugs formulated with Cremaphor® EL; (2) baseline neutrophil count < 1,500 cells/mm^3 and platelet count < 100,000 cells/mm^3; (3) Ixabepilone in combination with capecitabine in patients with AST or ALT >2.5 × ULN or bilirubin >1 × ULN due to increased risk of toxicity and neutropenia-related death.

Dosage/Range:
- 40-mg/m^2 IV infusion over 3 hours every 21 days.
- In breast cancer, given with capecitabine 1,000 mg/m^2 PO twice daily × 14 days, re-peated every 3 weeks.
- Do not exceed maximum dose calculated at BSA 2.2 m^2.

Dose Modifications: Assess patient during treatment (physically and labs, including CBC/differential, LFTs). If patient has toxicity, treatment should be delayed until recovery. If toxicity recurs, an additional 20% dose reduction should be made.

See package insert for specific dose modifications for neuropathy, capecitabine, monotherapy, hepatic impairment, concurrent use of strong CYP3A4 inhibitors, concurrent use of strong CYP3A4 inducers, and re-treatment criteria (Bristol-Myers Squibb, 2016).

Drug Preparation:

- Available as Ixempra 15 mg for injection supplied with 8-mL diluent and Ixempra 45 mg with 23.5-mL diluent. Reconstituted solution delivers ixabepilone concentration of 2 mg/mL. This must be further diluted with lactated Ringer's injection USP to a final concentration of 0.2–0.6 mg/mL. **Drug is stable only in solution with a pH in the range of 6–9.0.** Use only the solutions specified below.
- Ixempra kit contains two vials (vial containing 16 mg drug powder [labeled 15 mg] or 47 mg [labeled 45 mg] and vial of diluent containing dehydrated alcohol). Kit must be stored in a refrigerator (2–8°C [36–46°F]) in original packaging to protect from light. Remove from refrigerator 30 minutes before mixing; this will also give time for any white precipitate in the diluent to dissolve.
- Reconstitute by aseptically withdrawing diluent and slowly injecting into vial containing Ixempra drug; gently swirl and invert vial until completely dissolved. Asceptically aspirate ordered dose (2 mg/mL) into syringe.
- Further dilute in 250-mL lactated Ringer's or 0.9% sodium chloride injection USP (pH adjusted with sodium bicarbonate injection USP (see package insert), or PLASMA-LYTE A Injection pH 7.4 may also be used. A 250-mL bag of infusion fluid is sufficient [or larger if needed to deliver a final concentration of 0.2–0.6 mg/mL]. Bag must be **DEHP-free** (e.g., non-PVC). Thoroughly mix bag by manual rotation.
- Administer via DEHP-free tubing with DEHP-free final filter 0.2–1.2 microns.
- The drug infusion must be completed within 6 hours of preparation.
- Reconstituted solution is stable for 1 hour in a syringe at room temperature and light but should be further diluted as soon as possible following reconstitution. After further dilution in one of the infusion fluids specified, the infusion must be completed within 6 hours of preparation.

Drug Administration:

- ANC must be $\geq$ 1,500 cells/mm^3 and platelets $\geq$ 100,000 cells/mm^3.
- Premedication: with an H_1 antagonist (e.g., diphenhydramine 50 mg PO) and H_2 antagonist (e.g., ranitidine 150–300 mg PO) 1 hour before chemotherapy to minimize hypersensitivity reaction.
- Administer as IV infusion over 3 hours, every 3 weeks.
- If patient has had a hypersensitivity reaction to ixabepilone in the prior cycle, add a corticosteroid (e.g., dexamethasone 20-mg IV 30 minutes or PO 60 minutes before chemotherapy) to premedications.
- If drug dose is increased to 60 mg/m^2 due to coadministration with a strong CYP3A4 inducer, infuse ixabepilone over 4 hours (R-PHARMA US, 2016).
- Drug contains dehydrated alcohol; thus, assess patient's neurologic status during and after infusion.

Drug Interactions:
- Capecitabine: synergy, so used together to increase tumor cell kill.
- Strong CYP3A4 inhibitors decrease the metabolism, thus increasing plasma level of ixabepilone and thus should be avoided (ketoconazole, itraconazole, clarithromycin, atazanavir, nefazodone, saquinavir, telithromycin, ritonavir, amprenavir, indinavir, nelfinavir, delavirdine, voriconazole, grapefruit juice); if a strong CYP3A4 inhibitor must be given concurrently, reduce ixabepilone dose to 20 mg/m^2; after the strong inhibitor is discontinued, wait 1 week (washout period) before increasing the ixabepilone dose to indicated dose.
- Strong CYP3A4 inducer (e.g., pheynytoin, carbamazepine, rifampin, rifabutin, dexamethasone, phenobarbital) increases the drug metabolism, thus decreasing the plasma concentration of ixabepilone and decreasing effectiveness. Avoid coadministration, but if this is not possible, increase ixabepilone dose. Once the patient has been maintained on a strong CYP3A4 inducer, the dose of ixabepilone may be gradually increased from 40 mg/m^2 to 60 mg/m^2 given IV over 4 hours; monitor patient carefully for toxicity. If the strong inducer is discontinued, the ixabepilone dose should be returned to the dose used before the strong CYP3A4 inducer was begun.

Lab Effects/Interference:
- Neutropenia, thrombocytopenia, anemia.

Special Considerations:
- Most common adverse effects ($\geq$ 20%) are peripheral sensory neuropathy, fatigue/asthenia, myalgia/arthralgia, alopecia, nausea, vomiting, stomatitis/mucositis, diarrhea, and musculoskeletal pain. Additional reactions (related to capecitabine) were palmar-plantar erythrodysesthesia syndrome, anorexia, abdominal pain, nail disorder, and constipation.
- Drug is 3–20 times more potent than paclitaxel; toxicity profile is similar to paclitaxel.
- Drug is able to overcome p-glycoprotein-related drug resistance.
- Use cautiously and assess frequently in patients with preexisting moderate to severe PN or diabetes mellitus.
- Warnings and Precautions:
  - *PN* was common, occurring in 63–67% of patients (all grades). Grades 3–4 PN occurred in 23% in the combination group, and 14% in the ixabepilone as monotherapy trials. For patients with grades 3–4 PN, 76–79% of patients had improvement to baseline or grade 1, 12 weeks after onset. Patients at risk are those with diabetes mellitus, or those with preexisting PN.
  - *Myelosuppression* is dose dependent, manifested as neutropenia. Grade 4 neutropenia occurred in 36% of patients receiving ixabepilone plus capecitabine, and 21% treated with ixabepilone monotherapy. Monitor ANC/CBC closely and administer ixabepilone only if ANC is $\geq$ 1,500 cells/mm^3, and platelet count $\geq$ 100,000 cells/mm^3. Patients experiencing severe neutropenia or thrombocytopenia should have dose reduction (see package insert).
  - *Hepatic impairment* increases risk of grade 4 neutropenia, febrile neutropenia, and serious adverse reactions. Dose should be reduced in patients with hepatotoxicity (see package insert). Assess baseline LFTs and monitor prior to each dose of ixabepilone.

- *Hypersensitivity reactions* may occur, stimulated by Cremaphor®. All patients should receive premedication 1 hour prior to receiving the drug. Assess the patient throughout the infusion for flushing, rash, dyspnea, bronchospasm, and teach patient to report symptoms. If a reaction occurs, interrupt the infusion but keep vein open with plain solution, assess patient vital signs ensuring airway and breathing, and discuss management with physician/NP/PA. In clinical trials, 1% of patients had a severe reaction. If the reaction is severe, such as anaphylaxis, the drug should be stopped, and aggressive supportive measures instituted as ordered (see chapter introduction).
- *Embryo-fetal toxicity*: Women of reproductive potential should be advised to use effective contraception while receiving ixabepilone. Mothers should not breastfeed their infant while receiving ixabepilone.
- *Cardiac adverse reactions* (e.g., myocardial ischemia, ventricular dysfunction) occurred rarely. Caution should be used if the patient has a history of cardiac disease. The drug should be discontinued in pateints developing cardiac ischemia or impaired cardiac function.
- *Potential for cognitive impairment from dehydrated alcohol USP excipient* used in reconstituting the drug. Assess for any CNS effects or other side effects from alcohol.

Potential Toxicities/Side Effects and the Nursing Process

I.   POTENTIAL FOR INFECTION AND BLEEDING related to BM DEPRESSION

Defining Characteristics: Myelosuppression is dose dependent, expressed primarily as neutropenia. Incidence of neutropenia is 68% with grades 3–4 54% (incidence of febrile neutropenia 3% as monotherapy and 5% when given with capecitabine, with infection occurring in 5–6% of patients, respectively). Neutropenic deaths occurred in 1.9% of patients receiving ixabepilone in combination with capecitabine, with normal hepatic function or mild hepatic dysfunction, and in 0.4% in patients receiving monotherapy. Drug is contraindicated in patients with severe hepatic dysfunction (see Special Considerations), and in patients with ANC < 1,500 cells/mm^3 or platelets < 100,000 cells/mm^3. Grades 3–4 thrombocytopenia occur in 7% (monotherapy) and 8% (combination therapy) of patients, and anemia in 8% (mono) and 10% (combination). Fatigue is common, affecting 56% (mono) and 60% (combination).

Nursing Implications: Assess baseline CBC, WBC, differential, and platelet count prior to chemotherapy, as well as signs/symptoms of infection or bleeding, and assure ANC ≥ 1,500 cells/mm^3 and platelet count ≥ 100,000 cells/mm^3. If patient experienced severe neutropenia or thrombocytopenia, discuss dose reduction with physician. Teach patient the signs/symptoms of infection or bleeding, and to report these immediately, such as temperature ≥ 100.5°F. Teach patient self-care measures to minimize risk of infection and bleeding. This includes avoidance of crowds, proximity to people with infections, and OTC aspirin-containing medications. Assess baseline activity and energy level. Teach patient that fatigue may occur, and ways to minimize exertion and energy expenditure by alternating rest and activity, and organizing chores so that they are done as efficiently as possible.

II. POTENTIAL FOR INJURY related to HYPERSENSITIVITY REACTIONS

Defining Characteristics: In studies, 1% of patients had severe hypersensitivity reactions (HSRs), including anaphylaxis. The risk of HSRs is reduced by premedication with H_1 and H_2 antagonists.

Nursing Implications: Assess baseline VS and mental status before drug administration. Administer H_1 antagonist (e.g., diphenhydramine 50 mg PO) and H_2 antagonist 30–60 minutes before starting drug. If patient has had a prior reaction, administer ordered corticosteroid (e.g., dexamethasone 20-mg IV or PO) in addition. Remain with patient during first 15 minutes of infusion, and monitor frequently during infusion. Teach patient to report any itching, rash, any new sensations or symptoms. Recall signs/symptoms of HSR. If these occur, stop drug immediately, and notify physician. Subjective symptoms are generalized itching, nausea, chest tightness, crampy abdominal pain, difficulty speaking, anxiety, agitation, sense of impending doom, uneasiness, desire to urinate/defecate, dizziness, chills. Objective signs are flushed appearance; fever, chills, bronchospasm, angioedema of face, neck, eyelids, hands, feet; localized or generalized urticaria; respiratory distress with or without wheezing, hypotension, cyanosis. Review standing orders or nursing procedure for patient management of anaphylaxis and be prepared to stop drug immediately. Notify physician. Monitor VS, and administer ordered medications, which may include epinephrine 1:1,000, hydrocortisone sodium succinate, and diphenhydramine.

III. SENSORY/PERCEPTUAL ALTERATIONS related to SENSORY NEUROPATHY

Defining Characteristics: PN is common, with sensory neuropathy affecting 62–65% of patients, and motor neuropathy affecting 10–16% of patients. It occurs early with 75% of new onset and worsening neuropathy occurring during first three cycles. Dose reduction results in improvement or no worsening in neuropathy in most patients. About 10% of patients receiving monotherapy and 23% of patients receiving combination with capecitabine developed grades 3–4 PN. Median number of cycles to onset of grades 3–4 neuropathy was four cycles in both groups, with a median time to improvement of grades 3–4 to baseline or grade 1 of 4–6 weeks for patients receiving monotherapy and 6 weeks for patients receiving combination. Neuropathy is cumulative and reversible (Vahdat et al., 2007).

Nursing Implications: Assess baseline neurologic status. Instruct patient to report signs/ symptoms of pins-and-needles sensation, numbness, burning sensation, pain, increased discomfort with certain sensations, especially in the extremities, or motor weakness. Identify patients at risk: those with history of cisplatin use or with preexisting neuropathies (ethanol- and diabetes mellitus–related). Assess sensory and motor function prior to each treatment, and if abnormality found, assess impact on patient function, safety, independence, ability to do ADLs, and quality of life. Test patient's ability to button a shirt, or pick up a dime from a flat surface. If impacting ability to do ADLs, safety, or quality of life, discuss with patient and physician drug reduction (20% for grade 2 lasting > 7 days or grade 3 lasting < 7 days). If grade 3 neuropathy lasts ≥ 7 days, the drug should be discontinued. Teach self-care strategies, including maintaining safety when walking, getting up, taking a bath, or washing dishes; discuss inability to sense temperature, and the need to keep extremities warm in cold weather. See NCI Common Toxicity Criteria Adverse Events in *Appendix II*: grade 2 motor = symptomatic weakness interfering with function but not ADLs; grade 2 sensory = sensory alteration or paresthesia interfering with function but not ADLs; grade 3 motor = objective weakness, interfering with ADLs; grade 3 sensory = sensory loss or paresthesia interfering with ADLs; grade 4 motor = paralysis; grade 4 sensory = permanent sensory loss that interferes with function.

IV.   ALTERATION IN SKIN INTEGRITY related to ALOPECIA, NAIL CHANGES

Defining Characteristics: Alopecia affects 31–48% of patients in clinical trials and is reversible; 9–24% of patients developed nail changes during clinical trials. Palmar-plantar erythrodysesthesia (HFS) occurred in 64% of patients receiving capecitabine with ixabepilone.

Nursing Implications: Discuss potential impact of hair loss prior to drug administration. Discuss coping strategies and a plan to minimize body-image distortion (e.g., wig, scarf, cap). Assess patient for signs/symptoms of hair loss. Assess patient's response and use of coping strategies, and help patient to build on effective strategies. Assess patient's fingernails and toenails, and teach patients changes may occur and to report them. Develop plan of care with patient if changes are severe. Refer to capecitabine drug sheet for the assessment, prevention, and management of palmar-plantar erythrodysesthesia.

V.   ALTERATION IN COMFORT related to ARTHRALGIAS AND MYALGIAS

Defining Characteristics: Arthralgias and myalgias affect about 39–49% of patients, and musculoskeletal pain affects 20–23% of patients.

Nursing Implications: Arthralgias and myalgias may be troublesome, and can be managed with NSAIDs, application of warmth, and other comfort measures. Some patients report that swimming is helpful in minimizing discomfort. Studies of gabapentin, glutamine, and steroids have been disappointing. Opioids may be needed if severe.

VI.   ALTERATION IN NUTRITION, LESS THAN BODY REQUIREMENTS, related to NAUSEA, VOMITING, DIARRHEA

Defining Characteristics: Nausea and vomiting occur in approximately 42–53% and 29–39% of patients, respectively. It is mild and preventable with antiemetics. Diarrhea occurs in 22–44% of patients and is mild. Drug appears to cause diarrhea by direct injury to the intestinal mucosa (necrosis of cells), causing inflammation of the bowel wall and decreased absorption. Stomatitis and mucositis occur in 29–31% of patients. Constipation occurs in 16–22% of patients.

Nursing Implications: Assess patient's nutritional status, as well as elimination status. Premedicate patient with antiemetic prior to chemotherapy and give antiemetic to take at home if needed. Encourage small, frequent meals of cool, bland foods. Instruct patient to report nausea unrelieved with antiemetics, and teach self-administration of antiemetics, as most patients will receive the drug as an outpatient. If nausea/vomiting occur and are severe, assess for signs/symptoms of fluid/electrolyte imbalance and bring to clinic for aggressive antiemesis. Encourage patient to report onset of diarrhea and to self-administer antidiarrheal medications; review dietary changes to reduce bowel irritation (e.g., avoid spicy, high-fat, high-insoluble fiber foods and increase fluids to 3 L/day). If patient develops constipation, review measures and dietary changes to relieve constipation. Assess baseline oral mucous membranes. Teach patient oral assessment and to report any alterations. Assess LFTs prior to drug administration and periodically during treatment.

Drug: lanreotide (Somatuline depot injection)

Class: Somatostatin analogue.

Mechanism of Action: As a synthetic somatostatin analogue, lanreotide has a high affinity for human somatostatin receptors, so it blocks the binding of human somatostatin to the receptors, most significantly 2 and 5. This inhibits growth hormone (GH) and insulin-like growth factor (IGF-1), as well as other endocrine, neuroendocrine, exocrine, and paracrine functions.

Metabolism: Lanreotide passively diffuses from the depot into the tissues, and enters the bloodstream. Steady state is reached after 4–5 injections (4–5 months). In renal failure, drug excretion is slowed, with a twofold increase in AUC and drug half-life. Less than 5% of the drug is excreted in the urine, and less than 0.5% in the feces; instead, the major route of excretion is believed to be biliary.

Indication: (1) Long-term treatment of patients with acromegaly who have had an inadequate response to surgery and/or radiotherapy, or are not candidates for this treatment; (2) treatment of patients with unresectable, well- or moderately differentiated, locally advanced, or metastatic gastroenteropancreatic neuroendocrine tumors (GEP-NETs) to improve progression-free survival; (3) treatment of patients with carcinoid syndrome; when used, it reduces the frequency of short-acting somatostatin analogue rescue therapy.

Dosage/Range:
- **GEP-NETS:** 120 mg deep SQ in superior external quadrant of buttock, every 4 weeks. No effect on drug clearance was seen in patients with mild to moderate renal impairment. The effect of hepatic dysfunction on drug clearance in GEP-NETS patients has not been studied. Use lanreotide in these patients cautiously and monitor closely.
- **Carcinoid syndrome:** 120 mg q 4 weeks deep SQ injection. If patients are already being treated with SOMATULINE DEPOT for GEP-NET, do not administer additional dose for carcinoid syndrome.

- **Acromegaly:** 60–120 mg deep SQ every 4 weeks, starting at a dose of 90 mg every 4 weeks for 3 months. Adjust the dose thereafter based on GH and/or IGF-1 levels. If patient has moderate to severe renal or hepatic dysfunction, the initial dose should be 60 mg every 4 weeks for 3 months; adjust the dose thereafter based on GH and/or IGF-1 levels. *Dose Modification:* See package insert for acromegaly dosage adjustment for renal or hepatic impairment.

Drug Preparation:
- Available in 60 mg/0.2 mL, 90 mg/0.3 mL, and 120 mg/0.5 mL single-use, prefilled syringes with an automatic needle guard. Solution should be white to pale yellow, semisolid in formulation.

Drug Administration:
- Administer monthly by deep subcutaneous injection in the superior external quadrant of the buttock;
- Rotate injection sites.

Drug Interactions:
- Hypoglycemic agents: May result in hypoglycemia or hyperglycemia. Monitor glucose closely, and adjust antidiabetic treatment accordingly.
- Cyclosporine: Concomitant administration may decrease the bioavailability of cyclosporine, necessitating adjustment of the cyclosporine dose.
- Drugs affecting heart rate (e.g., beta blockers): Lanreotide may decrease heart rate. If given with another drug causing a similar effect, dose adjustment of the coadministered drugs may be needed.
- Drugs metabolized by the CYP3A4 liver microenzyme system, which have a narrow therapeutic window: Use cautiously; lanreotide may slow the metabolism of the coadministered drug, resulting in increased toxicity. This reaction may be the result of interference with GH.

Lab Effects/Interference:
- Hyperglycemia or hypoglycemia
- Changes in GH and IGF-1 levels

Special Considerations:
- Warnings and Precautions:
  - *Cholelithiasis and complications of cholelithiasis:* Lanreotide slows down gallbladder motility; monitor patients for the development of cholelithiasis and gallbladder sludge. Incidence in studies was 14%. Postmarketing reports describe cholelithiasis (gallstones) with complications including cholecystitis, cholangitis, and pancreatitis.
  - *Hyperglycemia and hypoglycemia:* Lanreotide inhibits the secretion of insulin and glucagon; some patients may develop hypoglycemia or hyperglycemia. Assess blood glucose at baseline and when the dose is altered, and adjust antidiabetic medicine as needed.
  - *Cardiovascular abnormalities:* Lanreotide may cause sinus bradycardia; in all three studies, the incidence was 5.5%. Teach patients which signs and symptoms to report, and manage symptomatic bradycardia. If the patient has baseline bradycardia, use

lanreotide cautiously, and monitor closely. The drug may cause hypertension in patients with acromegaly.
- *Thyroid function abnormalities:* Thyroid function may undergo slight decreases in patients with acromegaly.
- *Monitoring laboratory tests:* Acromegaly: serum GH and IGF-1 levels are useful markers of disease and treatment effectiveness.
- Lanreotide is embryocidal in animals. It should be used during pregnancy only if the potential benefit justifies the risk to the fetus. Nursing mothers should make a decision whether to discontinue nursing or the drug, taking into account the importance of the drug to the mother.
- Most common adverse reactions (≥10%) in GEP-NET patients are abdominal pain, musculoskeletal pain, vomiting, headache, injection-site reaction, hyperglycemia, hypertension, and cholelithiasis. Most common reactions in patients with acromegaly are diarrhea, cholelithiasis, abdominal pain, nausea, and injection-site reactions.
- Dizziness may occur (incidence 9%); teach patient to change position slowly. If dizziness does occur, teach the patient not to drive a car or operate machinery.

Potential Toxicities and the Nursing Process:

I.   ALTERATION IN COMFORT related to ABDOMINAL PAIN, MUSCULOSKELETAL PAIN, HEADACHE, AND INJECTION-SITE REACTION

Defining Characteristics: In study 3 with GEP-NET patients, 34% had abdominal pain, 19% musculoskeletal pain, 16% headache, and 15% injection-site reactions.

Nursing Considerations: Assess baseline comfort, and teach patient about potential side effects. Teach patient self-assessment and management, and how to contact the provider if symptoms persist or worsen. Assess the prior injection site each month, and document site rotation. Ensure that the SQ injection is deep in the superior external quadrant of the buttock. Teach patient to report persistent discomfort, formation of induration, or mass if it develops.

II.   ALTERATION IN NUTRITION, POTENTIAL related to NAUSEA, VOMITING, CHOLELITHIASIS, OR HYPERGLYCEMIA OR HYPOGLYCEMIA

Defining Characteristics: In study 3 with GEP-NET patients, 19% had vomiting and 14% had hyperglycemia. Cholelithiasis occurred in 14% of patients.

Nursing Considerations: Assess baseline nutritional status, presence of nutritional impact symptoms, and blood glucose. Teach patient about potential side effects, self-care management strategies, and reporting persistent or unrelieved vomiting. Teach patient the signs and symptoms of hypoglycemia and hyperglycemia, and how to report them if they occur. If the patient is diabetic, assess blood glucose more frequently (e.g., at the beginning of therapy and with any dose change, and during therapy), and have patient monitor it at home with fingersticks. Discuss adjustments to antidiabetic agents as needed based on blood sugar results. Teach patient signs and symptoms of cholelithiasis, and how to report them if they occur: severe abdominal pain; pain extending beneath the right shoulder or to the back; pain that worsens after a meal (e.g., fatty or greasy foods); pain that feels sharp or dull, and crampy; pain that increases when the patient takes a deep breath; and chest pain.

Drug: letrozole (Femara)

Class: Aromatase inhibitor, nonsteroidal.

Mechanism of Action: Inhibits estrogen synthesis. Drug is a highly selective, potent agent that significantly suppresses (90%) serum estradiol levels within 14 days, without interfering with other steroid hormone synthesis. Binds to the heme group of aromatase, a cytochrome P450 enzyme necessary for the conversion of androgens to estrogens. Aromatase is thus inhibited, leading to a significant reduction in plasma estradiol, estrone, and estrone sulfate. After 6 weeks of therapy, there is 97% suppression of estradiol.

Metabolism: Rapidly and completely absorbed after oral administration, with a terminal half-life of 2 days. Steady state reached in 2–6 weeks. Metabolized in the liver and excreted in the urine.

Patients with cirrhosis and severe hepatic impairment had double the drug exposure, so dose must be reduced 50% in these patients.

Indication: (1) Adjuvant treatment of postmenopausal women with hormone receptor positive early breast cancer; (2) extended adjuvant treatment of postmenopausal women with early breast cancer who have received prior standard adjuvant tamoxifen therapy; (3) first- and second-line treatment of postmenopausal women with hormone receptor positive or unknown advanced breast cancer.

Contraindication: (1) Pregnancy; (2) known hypersensitivity to the active substance or any of the excipients.

Dosage/Range:
- 2.5 mg PO daily, without regard to meals.
  - Extended adjuvant setting: optimal treatment duration unknown. In the clinical trials, treatment was for 5 years.
  - Adjuvant treatment: discontinue drug if relapse occurs.
  - Extended adjuvant treatment of early breast cancer: Planned duration in clinical trials was 5 years; discontinue if relapse occurs.
  - 1st and 2nd line advanced breast cancer: continue until tumor progression.

Dose Modifications:
- Cirrhosis or severe hepatic dysfunction: 50% dose reduction recommended to 2.5 mg letrozole **every other day**.
- No dosage adjustment in patients with impaired renal function unless creatinine clearance is < 10 mL/min.

Drug Preparation:
- Oral; available in 2.5-mg tablets.

Drug Interactions:
- Tamoxifen: coadministration with tamoxifen decreased letrozole plasma levels by 38% but was not significant when letrozole was administered immediately after tamoxifen.

Lab Effects/Interference:
- Liver transaminases may be transiently elevated.
- Increase in total cholesterol (nonfasting, adjuvant studies).
- Rare, mild ↓ in lymphocyte and/or platelet count.
- Decrease in Bone Mineral Density (BMD).

Special Considerations:
- About 200 times more potent than aminoglutethimide.
- Most common adverse reactions (> 20%): hot flashes, arthragia, flushing, asthenia, edema, arthralgia, headache, dizziness, hypercholesterolemia, increased sweating, bone pain, musculoskeletal pain.
- Precautions and Warnings:
  - *Bone effects*: Letrozole may cause decreases in BMD. In the substudy analysis, the incidence of osteoporosis was 4.1% in letrozole arm compared to 0.3% median increase in the tamoxifen arm. In the adjuvant study, the incidence of osteoporosis was 4.1% for letrozole, and 2.7% for tamoxifen, and the incidence of bone fractures 14.7% for letrozole patients, and 11.4% for those receiving tamoxifen (Novartis, 2018). In the extended adjuvant trial, the incidence of new osteoporosis was 13.3% in the letrozole arm, and 7.8% in the placebo arm. Incidence of bone fractures was 13.3% in the letrozole arm and 7.8% in the placebo arm at a median follow-up of 62 months (Novartis, 2018). Closely monitor women with or at risk for developing osteoporosis with baseline and regularly bone densitometry. Discuss treatment or prophylaxis for osteoporosis with physician/NP/PA. Teach patient to take calcium and vitamin D daily, unless contraindicated.
  - *Hypercholesterolemia:* In the adjuvant trial, 52.3% of letrozole patients developed hypercholesterolemia, compared to 28.6% in the tamoxifen arm. Monitor serum cholesterol level baseline and regularly during treatment. Discuss abnormalities and need for lipid lowering medications with physician/NP/PA.
  - *Hepatic impairment*: Cirrhosis and severe hepatic impairment significantly increases (double) the letrozole exposure. Dose must be reduced 50% in patients (e.g., every other day dosing). Monitor LFTs baseline and regularly during treatment.
  - *Fatigue and dizziness* may occur putting patient at risk for falls and injury. Teach patients to use caution when driving or using machinery until it is known how the patient reacts to letrozole.
  - *Laboratory test abnormalities*: Transient moderate decreases in lymphocyte counts were observed, and rarely a patient developed thrombocytopenia. Monitor CBC/differential baseline and during treatment.
- *Embryo-fetal toxicity:* Letrozole may cause fetal harm when administered to pregnant women, as drug is embryotoxic and fetotoxic in lab animals. If there is exposure to

letrozole during pregnancy, the patient should be apprised of the potential hazard to the fetus. Teach patients of reproductive potential to use effective contraception during and for at least 3 weeks after last dose of letrozole. Mothers should NOT breastfeed while receiving the drug.

Potential Toxicities/Side Effects and the Nursing Process

I.   ALTERATION IN COMFORT related to HOT FLASHES, ARTHRALGIAS, MYALGIA, ARTHRITIS, SWEATING, ASTHENIA, DIZZINESS, HEADACHE, BONE PAIN, EDEMA

Defining Characteristics: Most common side effects were hot flashes/flushes (33%) and arthralgia/arthritis (25%). Less commonly myalgia, back pain, fatigue/asthenia, and dizziness can occur.

Nursing Considerations: Assess baseline comfort levels, and teach patient that this discomfort may occur. Teach patient symptomatic measures, instruct to report if symptoms are unrelieved.

II.   ALTERATION IN NUTRITION, LESS THAN BODY REQUIREMENTS, related to NAUSEA/VOMITING, HYPERCHOLESTEROLEMIA

Defining Characteristics: Nausea may occur, with vomiting less common. Hypercholesterolemia may occur in up to 52% of patients.

Nursing Implications: Determine baseline weight, and monitor at each visit. Teach patient that these side effects may occur, and instruct to report this. Discuss strategies to minimize nausea, including diet and dosing time.

Discuss baseline and periodic monitoring of total cholesterol with physician or mid-level practitioner, while patient is on therapy.

III.   POTENTIAL FOR THROMBOEMBOLIC EVENT, ENDOMETRIAL HYPERPLASIA/CANCER, FRACTURES

Defining Characteristics: Updated safety data with follow-up for 73 months showed that letrozole had lower incidences of thromboembolism (2.9% vs 4.5%), and endometrial hyperplasia/cancer (0.4% vs 2.9%) when compared to tamoxifen.

In the adjuvant trial, the incidence of bone fractures at any time after randomization was 13.8% for letrozole and 10.5% for tamoxifen. The incidence of osteoporosis was 5.1% for letrozole and 2.7% for tamoxifen. In the extended adjuvant trial, the incidence of bone fractures at any time after randomization was 13.3% for letrozole and 7.8% for placebo. The incidence of new osteoporosis was 14.5% for letrozole and 7.8% for placebo.

Nursing Implications: Discuss plan to monitor and minimize bone loss with physician, and reinforce teaching with patient, such as baseline and periodic BMD testing, as well as exercise, and daily nutritional supplementation of vitamin D and calcium. Although rare, teach patient that thromboembolism and endometrial changes may occur. Teach patient to report any new onset pain or tenderness in the calf or difficulty breathing, and to discuss annual endometrial monitoring (e.g., biopsy) with patient's gynecologist.

Drug: leuprolide acetate for depot suspension (Lupron Depot, Eligard)

Class: GnRH agonist, inhibits gonadotropin secretion.

Mechanism of Action: Leuprolide acetate is a gonadotropin-releasing hormone (GnRH) agonist that potently suppresses the secretion of gonadotropins, including follicle-stimulating hormone (FSH) and luteinizing hormone (LH) from the pituitary gland, when given continuously and in therapeutic doses. There is an initial increase in circulating LH, FSH which leads to a transient rise in gonadal steroids (testosterone and dihydrotestosterone in males, and estrone and estradiol in premenopausal females), and then a significant decrease. Continuous administration of the drug results in decreased levels of LH and FSH and, in men, testosterone is reduced to castrate levels (decrease in LH causes the Leydig cells to reduce testosterone production to castrate levels).

Metabolism: Ninety-five percent of the drug is absorbed after subcutaneous injection, with 85–100% of the drug being absorbed after IM or subcutaneous injection. Drug is slightly protein-bound (43–49%). Following administration, < 5% of the drug (parent or metabolite) is recovered in the urine.

Indication: Palliative treatment of patients with advanced prostate cancer.

Contraindication: Drug is contraindicated in (1) patients hypersensitive to the GnRH, GnRH agonists, or any of the excipients in Lupron Depot; (2) pregnancy. Safety in pediatrics has not been established (Tolmar Therapeutics, Inc., 2016).

Dosage/Range:
- For palliative treatment of prostate cancer: Depot suspension 7.5 mg for 1-month administration given IM every 4 weeks; 22.5-mg depot for 3-month administration given IM every 12 weeks; s; 30 mg IM every 4-month administration, given IM every 16 weeks; OR 45 mg for 6 monthly administration, given as a single IM ijection every 24 weeks; OR 1 mg/day subcutaneous injection (not depot).

Drug Preparation:
See package insert. 7.5-mg, 22.5-mg, 30-mg, and 45-mg injections available as a kit with prefilled dual-chamber syringe.

- Use syringes, diluent, kit provided by manufacturer. See package insert for each manufacturer for step-by-step preparation of syringes and administration. Inspect depot powder, and syringe should not be used if clumping or caking. A thin layer of powder on the syringe wall is normal; diluent should appear clear. To prepare for injection:

- Screw the white plunger into the end stopper until the stopper begins to turn.
- Hold the syringe upright. Release the diluent by SLOWLY PUSHING (6–8 sec) the plunger until the first stopper is at the blue line in the middle of the syringe barrel.
- Keep the syringe upright. Gently mix the powder thoroughly to form a uniform suspension (appears milky). If the powder adheres to the stopper or caking/clumping is present, tap the syringe with your finger to disperse. DO NOT USE if any of the powder has not gone into suspension.
- Hold the syringe upright. With the opposite hand, pull the needle cap upwards without twisting.
- Keep the syringe upright. Advance the plunger to expel the air from the syringe. Inject the entire contents of the syringe IM right after reconstitution. The suspension settles very quickly following reconstitution; therefore, the drug should be mixed and used immediately.
- Injection: 5 mg/mL; kit 5 mg/mL for 7.5-mg, 22.5-mg doses.
- Lupron Depot injection kit contains the following for the 7.5-mg kit: one prefilled dual-chambered syringe containing sterile lyophilized microspheres of leuprolide acetate in a biodegradable lactic acid polymer; needle with LuproLoc safety device; one plunger; two alcohol swabs; prescribing information. Mix with 1.0 mL of accompanying diluent. Store at controlled room temperature (25°C, 77°F), with excursions 15–30°C, 59–86°F permitted.
- Lupron Depot injection kit contains the following for the 22.5-mg depot (3 months), 30 mg (4 months), 45 mg (6 months): one prefilled dual-chambered syringe containing sterile lyophilized microspheres of leuprolide acetate in a biodegradable lactic acid polymer; needle with LuproLoc safety device; one plunger; two alcohol swabs; prescribing information. Mix with 1.5 mL of accompanying diluent. Store at controlled room temperature (25°C, 77°F), with excursions 15–30°C, 59–86°F permitted.

Drug Administration:
- See package inserts for each manufacturer for administration techniques.
- Depot is administered IM (see reconstitution above; drug should be given immediately after mixing): 7.5 mg once every month, 22.5 mg once every 3 months, 30 mg once every 4 months, 45 mg once every 6 months. Rotate sites. When administering IM, any aspirated blood would be visible just below the luer lock connection (transparent safety device) if a blood vessel is accidently penetrated. After injection, immediately activate thesafety device by pushing the arrow forward with the thumb or finger until the device is fully extended and you hear or feel a click.

Drug Interactions:
- None reported.

Lab Effects/Interference (Depot):
- Decreased: PSA, testosterone levels; total serum total protein; albumin, Hgb/Hct, WBC, phosphatase, urine specific gravity

- Increased alkaline phosphatase, uric acid, BUN/creatinine, LFTs (AST, LDH), phosphorus, platelets, total cholesterol, glucose
- Leuprolide acetate suppessed the pituitary-gonadal system. Thus, diagnostic tests of diagnostic tests of pituitary gonadotropic and gonadal function during and after leuprolide therapy may be altered.
- Pituitary-gonadal system suppression will affect pituitary gonadatoropin and gonadal function diagnostic testing during and for up to 3 months after the final treatment.

Special Considerations:
- Warnings and Precautions (AbbVie, 2014):
  - *Tumor flare:* Increased serum testosterone (about 50% above baseline) during first few weeks of treatment; Monitor serum testosterone and PSA. Monitor patients with vertebral metastatic lesions and/or with urinary tract obstruction closely during first few weeks of therapy.
    - Isolated cases of worsening of symptoms or additional signs and symptoms of prostate cancer during the first few weeks of treatment.
    - A small number of patients may experience a temporary increase in bone pain, which can be managed symptomatically.
    - Isolated cases of ureteral obstruction and spinal cord compression have been reported in patients receiving GnRH agonists, which can contribute to paralysis with or without fastal complication.
  - *Laboratory tests:* Periodically assess serum concentrations of testosterone and PSA. Generally, testosterone levels increased above baseline during the first week, declining to baseline or below by the end of the second or third week. Castration levels were generally reached within 2–4 weeks. Castration levels persisted for the duration of each treatment.
  - *Hyperglycemia and diabetes:* Hyperglycemia and an increased risk of diabetes in patients receiving GnRH analogues. Monitor blood glucose and HbA1 baseline and regularly during treatment and manage using current clinical standards.
  - *Cardiovascular disease and increased risk of MI,* sudden cardiac death, and stroke have occurred in men receiving GnRH analogues. Monitor for cardiovascular disease and manage using current clinical standards.
  - *QT/QTc interval:* Androgen deprivation therapy may prolong the QT interval. See *Chapter 3* introduction for discussion of implications of QTc prolongation. Patients with congenital long QT syndrome, CHF, frequent electrolyte abnormalities, and in patients taking drugs known to prolong the QT interval, should have a risk benefit discussion with their physician. Electrolyte abnormalities, especially serum potassium, magnesium, and calcium, should be corrected, and consider ECG and electrolyte monitoring baseline and regularly during therapy for these patients.
  - *Convulsions* have occurred in paitents with no underlying risk or history of seizures as reported postmarketing. Manage according to current clinical standards.
  - *Embryo-fetal toxicity:* Major fetal abnormalities were seen in laboratory animals. Teach pregnant women and those of reproductive potential of risk.
- Infertility may be reduced in men after treatment with leuprolide acetate.

- Ensure patient is given return appointment for next injection, e.g., 1 month, 3 months, 4 months, 6 months. Sites should be documented and rotated. For Viadur, patient has implant inserted by MD/RN once yearly.
- Initially, drug causes increased LH secretion, resulting in increased testosterone secretion and tumor flare. Usually disappears after 2 weeks.
- Studies on Viadur show that implant delivers 120 micrograms of leuprolide acetate per day over 12 months, reducing testosterone levels to castration levels within 2–4 weeks after insertion.
- Adverse reactions by formulation (> 10%):
  - 7.5 mg (1 month): general pain, hot flashes/sweats, GI disorders, edema, respiratory disorder, urinary disorder.
  - 22.5 mg (3 months): general pain, injection-site reaction, hot flashes/sweats, GI disorders, joint disorders, testicular atrophy, urinary disorders.
  - 30 mg (4 months): asthenia, flu syndrome, general pain, headache, injection-site reaction, hot flashes/sweats, GI disorders, edema, skin reaction, urinary disorders.
  - 45 mg (6 months): hot flush, injection-site pain, URI, fatigue.
- In postmarketing experience, mood swings, depression, rare suicidal ideation, and rare pituitary apoplexy (presenting as sudden headache, vomiting, visual changes, ophthalmoplegia, change in mental status, sometimes cardiovascular collapse) have been reported. Patients with pituitary apoplexy may have a pituitary adenoma, and symptoms arise within 2 weeks of the first dose, sometimes within the first hour. Changes in bone density are likely as these occur with orchiectomy or treatment with a GnRH agonist analogue. Monitor bone density in patients receiving long periods of medical castration.
- Rare reports of serious drug-induced liver injury have been documented.

Potential Toxicities/Side Effects and the Nursing Process

I.   ALTERATION IN COMFORT related to HOT FLASHES, TUMOR FLARE, EDEMA

Defining Characteristics: Headache, dizziness, and hot flashes may occur. Vasodilation most common, with 67.9% incidence. Sweating may affect 5% of patients. Tumor flare may also occur initially (bone and tumor pain, transient increase in tumor size due to transient increase in testosterone levels). Breast tenderness has been reported. Peripheral edema may occur in 8% of patients.

Nursing Implications: Inform patient that symptoms may occur, that flare reaction will subside after the initial 2 weeks of therapy. Encourage patient to report symptoms early. Develop symptom management plan with patient and physician.

II.   POTENTIAL SEXUAL DYSFUNCTION related to LIBIDO, IMPOTENCE

Defining Characteristics: Frequently causes decreased libido and erectile impotence in men. Gynecomastia occurs in 3–6.9% of patients. In women, amenorrhea occurs after 10 weeks of therapy.

Nursing Implications: As appropriate, explore with patient and significant other the issues of reproductive and sexual patterns and the impact chemotherapy may have on them. Discuss strategies to preserve sexuality and reproductive health.

III. DEPRESSION, POTENTIAL, related to DRUG EFFECT

Defining Characteristics: Depression may affect up to 5.3% of patients, and less commonly, patients may develop emotional lability, insomnia, nervousness, anxiety.

Nursing Implications: Assess baseline affect and usual coping strategies. Teach patient to report change in affect. Assess effectiveness of coping strategies, encourage patient to verbalize feelings, and provide emotional support. Assess need for referral to psychiatric nurse specialist or social worker if supportive efforts ineffective.

IV. ALTERED NUTRITION, LESS THAN BODY REQUIREMENTS, related to GI SIDE EFFECTS

Defining Characteristics: Anorexia, nausea, and vomiting may occur rarely, with an incidence of < 5%.

Nursing Implications: If patients experience symptoms, encourage small, frequent feedings of favorite foods, especially high-calorie, high-protein foods. Monitor weight weekly. Assess incidence and pattern of nausea, vomiting, or anorexia if they occur. Discuss need for antiemetic with physician and patient.

V. ALTERATION IN SKIN INTEGRITY, POTENTIAL, related to INSERTION AND REMOVAL OF 12-MONTH IMPLANT

Defining Characteristics: Insertion and removal of implant caused local site bruising (34.8%) and burning (5.6%). In general, the reactions lasted 2 weeks, and then resolved completely. In about 10% of patients, reactions lasted longer than 2 weeks, or reactions did not develop until after 2 weeks.

Nursing Implications: Assess baseline skin integrity after implant insertion or removal. Teach patient that these reactions may occur, and will resolve, usually within 2 weeks. Teach patients to use local measures to minimize feeling of burning.

Drug: lomustine (Gleostine) capsules

Class: Alkylating agent (nitrosourea).

Mechanism of Action: Nitrosourea alkylates DNA with a reactive chloroethyl carbonium ion, producing strand breaks and crosslinks that inhibit RNA and DNA synthesis. Interferes with enzymes and histidine utilization. Is cell cycle phase nonspecific.

Metabolism: Completely absorbed from GI tract. Metabolized rapidly, partly protein bound. Undergoes hepatic recirculation. Lipid soluble: crosses BBB; 75% excreted in urine within 4 days.

Indication: (1) brain tumors both primary and metastatic, in patients who have already received appropriate surgical and/or radiotherapeutic procedures; (2) Hodgkin's lymphoma, in combination with other chemotherapies, following disease progression with initial chemotherapy.

Dosage/Range:
- 130 mg/m^2 PO every 6 weeks. Round dose to nearest 5 mg. Give as a single oral dose and do not repeat for at least 6 weeks. Prescribe only ONE DOSE for each treatment cycle; DO NOT dispense entire container as overdosage may be fatal.

Dose Modifications:
- Perform weekly CBC/ANC and hold next dose for >6 weeks if needed until WBC ≥ 4,000/mm^3 and platelets are ≥100,000/mm^3.
- Nadir after prior dose (see package insert): (1) no adjustment for leukocytes/mm^3: 3,000/mm^3 and higher, and platelet counts > 75,000/mm^3; (2) reduce dose by 30% for leukocyte count 2,000–2,999/mm^3, platelet count 25,000–74,999/mm^3; (3) reduce dose by 50% for leukocyte count < 2,000/mm^3, platelet count < 25,000/mm^3.

Drug Preparation:
- Oral. Available in 10-mg (white/white), 40-mg (white/green), and 100-mg (green/green) capsules.
- Confirm the total dose prescribed by the physician and the appropriate combination of capsule strengths. Use safe handling (PPE) precautions.

Drug Administration:
- Assess ANC/CBC/differential, LFTs, PFTs or DL$_{CO}$ results prior to administering dose, if patient in the hospital or clinic.
- The drug is absorbed 30–60 minutes after administration; consequently, vomiting does not usually affect efficacy.
- Teach patient that (NextSource Biotechnology, 2018):
  - Lomustine is an anticancer drug, and patients should **wear gloves** when handling the bottle or pills. Do not open or crush the capsules.
  - In order to provide the proper dose of lomustine (Gleostine); there may be two or more different types and colors of capsules in the container dispensed by the pharmacist):
  - Only ONE dose will be prescribed and filled at a time, as an accidental overdose may be fatal.
  - The dose is repeated in 6 or more weeks.
  - Take antinausea medicine to prevent an upset stomach, 30–60 minutes before taking lomustine.
  - Take the prescribed dose of capsules in one dose.
- If your skin is exposed to the drug, wash skin area immediately with soap and water.
  - If nausea and/or vomiting occurs, it usually lasts less than 24 hours, although loss of appetite may last for several days.

- Notify physician/Np/PA if any of the following reactions occur: new or worsening cough, fever, chills, sore throat, unusual bleeding or bruising, shortness of breath, chest pain, or yellowing of eyes and skin.
- Blood counts and breathing tests will be checked frequently.

Drug Interactions:
- Myelosuppressive drugs increase hematologic toxicity; reduce dose.

Lab Effects/Interference:
- Decreased CBC.
- Increased LFTs, RFTs.

Special Considerations:
- Most common adverse reactions include delayed myelosuppression, nausea, vomiting, stomatitis, and alopecia.
- Warnings and Precautions:
  - *Delayed myelosuppression*: May be fatal. Myelosuppression is delayed, dose related, and cumulative. Thrombocytopenia is usually more severe than neutropenia. Onset is usually 4–6 weeks after dose, and persists for 1–2 weeks. Cumulative effect seen by greater severity and longer duration of cytopenias. Monitor CBC/differential for at last 6 weeks after each dose; do not give drug more frequently than every 6 weeks as the risk of cumulative myelotoxicity (very severe and prolonged) is great. Dose should be modified based on nadir blood counts.
  - *Risk of overdose:* Prescribe, dispense, and **administer only enough capsules for 1 dose,** as fatal toxicity occurs with overdose. Both physician, pharmacist, and nurse should emphasize that only 1 dose is taken every 6 weeks, and nurse and/or pharmacist should confirm the prescribed dose is present in the bottle given to the patient.
  - *Pulmonary toxicity*: Pulmonary infiltrates and/or fibrosis can occur. Assess pulmonary function tests prior to treatment and repeat frequently during treatment. Patients with a baseline < 70% of predicted forced vital vapacity (FVC) or carbon monoxide diffusing capacity (DL_{CO}) are at increased risk. Onset of pulmonary toxicity is usually after an interval of 6 months or longer from the start of therapy, with cumulative doses of lomustine usually > 1,100 mg/m^2. Permanently discontinue lomustine if the patient develops pulmonary fibrosis.
  - *Secondary malignancies*: Acute leukemia and myelodysplasia can occur with long-term use.
  - *Hepatotoxicity:* Elevated serum transaminases, alkaline phosphatase, and bilirubin can occur. Monitor LFTs baseline and regularly during treatment.
  - *Nephrotoxicity:* Lomustine can cause renal failure. Monitor renal function baseline and regularly during therapy.
  - *Embryo-fetal toxicity*: Lomustine can cause fetal harm. Advise females of reproductive potential and males with female sexual partners of reproductive potential to use effective contraception during therapy and for at least 3.5 months after last dose for men, and at least 2 weeks after last dose for women. Mothers should NOT breastfeed while receiving lomustine. Drug may cause infertility in men and women of reproductive potential.

Potential Toxicities/Side Effects and the Nursing Process

I.   INFECTION AND BLEEDING related to MYELOSUPPRESSION

Defining Characteristics: Nadir of platelets: 26–34 days, lasting 6–10 days; nadir of WBC: 41–46 days, lasting 9–14 days. Delayed and cumulative BM depression with successive dosing: recovery takes 6–8 weeks. BM depression is dose-limiting toxicity.

Nursing Implications: Drug should be administered every 6–8 weeks due to delayed nadir and recovery. Monitor CBC, platelets prior to drug administration (WBC > 4,000/mm^3 and platelets > 100,000/mm^3). Dispense only one dose at a time.

II.   ALTERATION IN NUTRITION, LESS THAN BODY REQUIREMENTS, related to NAUSEA/VOMITING, ANOREXIA, DIARRHEA

Defining Characteristics: Onset of nausea/vomiting occurs 2–6 hours after taking dose; may be severe and last up to 24 hours. Anorexia may last for several days. Diarrhea is uncommon.

Nursing Implications: Administer drug on an empty stomach at bedtime. Premedicate with antiemetic and sedative or hypnotic to promote sleep. Discourage food or fluid intake for 2 hours after drug administration. Encourage small, frequent feedings of favorite foods. Encourage high-calorie, high-protein foods; monitor weekly weights. Encourage patient to report onset of diarrhea. Administer or teach patient to self-administer antidiarrheal medication. If patient taking medicine at home, teach to take antiemetic 30–60 minutes before taking dose (all capsules as a single dose).

III. ALTERATION IN URINARY ELIMINATION related to RENAL COMPROMISE

Defining Characteristics: After prolonged therapy with high cumulative doses, tubular atrophy, glomerular sclerosis, and interstitial nephritis have occurred, leading to renal failure.

Nursing Implications: Monitor BUN, creatinine prior to dosing, especially in patients receiving prolonged or high cumulative dose therapy. If abnormalities are noted, a creatinine clearance should be determined.

IV.   POTENTIAL FOR SEXUAL DYSFUNCTION related to MUTAGENIC AND TERATOGENIC QUALITIES OF LOMUSTINE

Defining Characteristics: Drug is teratogenic, mutagenic, and carcinogenic.

Nursing Implications: As appropriate, discuss birth control measures.

V. ACTIVITY INTOLERANCE related to LETHARGY, CONFUSION

Defining Characteristics: Neurologic dysfunction may occur rarely: confusion, lethargy, disorientation, ataxia.

Nursing Implications: Perform neurologic assessment as part of prechemotherapy assessment. Assess orientation and level of consciousness, gait, activity tolerance.

Drug: mechlorethamine hydrochloride (Mustargen, nitrogen mustard, HN₂)

Class: Alkylating agent.

Mechanism of Action: Produces interstrand and intrastrand crosslinkages in DNA, causing miscoding, breakage, and failures of replication. Cell cycle phase nonspecific.

Metabolism: Undergoes chemical transformation after injection with less than 0.01% excreted unchanged in urine. Drug is rapidly inactivated by body fluids. 50% of the inactive metabolites are excreted in the urine within 24 hours.

Indication: (1) IV for the palliative treatment of Hodgkin's disease (Stages III, IV), lymphosarcoma, chronic myelocytic or CLL, polycythemia vera, mycosis fungoides, and bronchogenic carcinoma; (2) intrapleurally, intraperitoneally, or intrapericardially for the palliative treatment of metastatic carcinoma resulting in effusion.

Contraindication: In patients with known infectious disease and in patients who have previously had anaphlyactic reactions to nitrogen mustard.

Dosage/Range:
- IV: 0.4 mg/kg, or 12–16 mg/m² IV as single agent; 6 mg/m² IV days 1 and 8 of 28-day cycle with MOPP regimen.
- Topical: Dilute 10 mg in 60 mL sterile water; apply with rubber gloves.
- Intracavitary: Pleural, peritoneal, pericardial: 0.2–0.4 mg/kg.

Drug Preparation:
- Add sterile water or 0.9% sodium chloride to each vial. Wear eye and hand protection when mixing.
- Administer via sidearm or rapidly running IV.
- Drug must be used within 15 minutes of reconstitution.

Drug Administration:
- Intravenous: This drug is a potent vesicant. Give through a freely running IV to avoid extravasation, which can lead to ulceration, pain, and necrosis. Check hospital's policy and procedure for administration of a vesicant.

Drug Interactions:
- Myelosuppressive drugs: Additive hematologic toxicity; dose-reduce or monitor patient closely.
- Sodium thiosulfate: inactivates drug.

Lab Effects/Interference:
- Decreased CBC.
- Increased uric acid, RFTs.

Special Considerations:
- Drug is a vesicant. Give through a running IV to avoid extravasation. Antidote is sodium thiosulfate: dilute 4 mL sodium thiosulfate injection USP (10%) with 6 mL sterile water for injection, USP, and inject subcutaneously in area of infiltration.
- Nadir is 6–8 days after treatment.
- Side effects occur in the reproductive system, such as amenorrhea and azoospermia.
- Severe nausea and vomiting.
- Systemic toxic effects may occur with intracavitary drug administration.

Potential Toxicities/Side Effects and the Nursing Process

I. ALTERATION IN NUTRITION, LESS THAN BODY REQUIREMENTS, related to NAUSEA AND VOMITING, ANOREXIA, DIARRHEA

Defining Characteristics: Nausea and vomiting occur in ~100% of patients, within 30 minutes to 2 hours of drug administration, and up to 8 hours afterward. Nausea and vomiting can be severe, but can be prevented by the use of combination antiemetics such as serotonin antagonist (granisetron or ondansetron) and dexamethasone. Anorexia and taste distortion (metallic taste) occur commonly. Diarrhea may occur up to several days after drug administration.

Nursing Implications: Premedicate with combination antiemetics such as serotonin antagonist (granisetron or ondansetron) and dexamethasone. Continue prophylactically. Antiemetic and sedative may need to be started the evening before if patient develops anticipatory nausea and vomiting. Encourage small, frequent feedings of cool, bland foods, dry toast, crackers. Monitor I/O to detect fluid volume deficit. Notify physician of the need for more aggressive antiemetic if vomitus > 750 mL. Encourage small, frequent feedings of high-calorie, high-protein foods. Encourage use of spices for anorexia and obtain weekly weights. Encourage patient to report onset of diarrhea. Administer or teach patient to self-administer antidiarrheal medication and teach diet modifications (low residue) as appropriate.

II. INFECTION AND BLEEDING related to BM DEPRESSION

Defining Characteristics: Potent myelosuppressant with nadir 6–8 days, recovery in 4 weeks. Patients at risk for profound BM depression are those with previous extensive XRT, previous chemotherapy, or compromised BM function. Lymphocyte depression occurs within 24 hours of drug dose.

Nursing Implications: Evaluate WBC, with neutrophil, and platelet count, and discuss any abnormalities with physician prior to drug administration. Assess for signs/symptoms of infection or bleeding; instruct patient in signs/symptoms of infection and bleeding, and to notify nurse or physician if they arise. Teach patient self-care measures to minimize risk of infection and bleeding, including avoidance of OTC aspirin-containing medications. Assess patient's Hgb/HCT and signs/symptoms of fatigue; teach patient self-assessment and to alternate rest and activity as needed. Transfuse red blood cells and platelets per physician order.

III. IMPAIRED SKIN INTEGRITY related to ALOPECIA, DRUG EXTRAVASATION

Defining Characteristics: Alopecia usually occurs as diffuse thinning. Drug is a potent vesicant, causing tissue necrosis and sloughing if extravasation occurs. Thrombosis or thrombophlebitis may occur despite all precautions, and venous access device may be required. Delayed cutaneous hypersensitivity is seen with topical application.

Nursing Implications: Discuss with patient hair loss, anticipated impact, and strategies to decrease distress, e.g., obtaining wig prior to hair loss. Assess body disturbance from hyperpigmentation and discuss strategies to minimize this, e.g., nail polish. Drug must be administered via patent IV. Assess need for venous access device early. Delayed cutaneous hypersensitivity (topical application) is not an indication to stop the drug. Discuss symptomatic management with physician. If extravasation is suspected, stop drug; aspirate any residual drug and blood from IV tubing, IV catheter/needle, and IV site if possible; instill antidote, sodium thiosulfate (1/6 molar), into area of apparent infiltration as per physician orders and institutional policy and procedure; apply cold or topical medication as per physician orders and institutional policy and procedure. Assess site regularly for pain, progression of erythema, induration, and for evidence of necrosis. When in doubt about whether drug is infiltrating, TREAT AS AN INFILTRATION. Teach patient to assess site, and instruct to notify physician if condition worsens. Arrange next clinic visit for assessment of site depending on drug, amount infiltrated, extent of potential injury, and patient variables. Document in patient's record as per institutional policy. Warm packs may decrease discomfort of phlebitis. Have standing orders and sodium thiosulfate injection USP (10%) close by in the event of actual infiltration of drug; dilute sodium thiosulfate with sterile water for injection and inject subcutaneously in area of infiltration.

IV. ALTERATION IN COMFORT related to CHILLS, FEVER, DIARRHEA

Defining Characteristics: Chills, fever, diarrhea may occur after drug administration. Also weakness, drowsiness, headache may occur.

Nursing Implications: Assess patient for these symptoms during hour following treatment. Instruct patient to report these symptoms and teach self-management at home if outpatient. Provide symptomatic management per physician with acetaminophen, antidiarrheal medication.

V.   POTENTIAL SEXUAL DYSFUNCTION related to DRUG EFFECTS

Defining Characteristics: Drug is teratogenic, carcinogenic. Amenorrhea occurs in females. Impaired spermatogenesis occurs in males. If administered to pregnant patients, spontaneous abortion or fetal abnormalities may occur.

Nursing Implications: As appropriate, explore with patient and partner issues of reproductive and sexual patterns, and anticipated impact chemotherapy will have. Discuss strategies to preserve sexuality and reproductive health (sperm banking, contraception).

VI.   POTENTIAL FOR SENSORY/PERCEPTUAL ALTERATIONS related to CRANIAL NERVE INJURY

Defining Characteristics: Tinnitus, deafness, and other signs of eighth cranial nerve damage occur rarely, with high drug doses or regional perfusion techniques. Temporary aphasia and paresis occur very rarely.

Nursing Implications: Assess hearing ability, presence of tinnitus prior to drug doses. If high doses of drug are given, or regional perfusion used, schedule patient for periodic audiometry. Instruct patient to report signs/symptoms of hearing loss.

Drug: melphalan hydrochloride (Alkeran, L-phenylalanine mustard, L-PAM, L-sarcolysin)

Class: Alkylating agent.

Mechanism of Action: Prevents cell replication by causing breaks and crosslinkages in DNA strands with subsequent miscoding and breakage. Cell cycle phase nonspecific. Drug is derivative of nitrogen mustard.

Metabolism: Variable bioavailability after oral administration, especially if taken with food. Therefore, dose is titrated to WBC count; 20–50% of drug is excreted in feces over 6 days, 50% excreted in urine within 24 hours. After IV administration, parent compound disappears from plasma, with a half-life of about 2 hours.

Indications: (1) PO: for the palliative treatment of multiple myeloma, and for the palliation of nonresectable epithelial carcinoma of the ovary; (2) IV: palliative treatment of patients with multiple myeloma for whom oral therapy is not appropriate.

Contraindications: Patients whose disease has shown prior resistance to melphalan, and patients with demonstrated hypersensitivity to the drug.

Dosage/Range:
- **Multiple myeloma:** PO: Several regimens, including 0.25 mg/kg/day × 4 days, in combination with prednisone 2 mg/kg/day, repeated every 6 weeks; OR 6 mg/m^2 orally

daily $\times$ 5 days every 6 weeks for myeloma; OR 0.1 mg/kg PO $\times$ 2–3 weeks, then maintenance of 2–4 mg daily when BM has recovered.
- **IV:** 16 mg/m^2.
- Dose-reduce 50% in patients with renal insufficiency (BUN $\geq$ 30 mg/dL) IV over 15–20 minutes using vesicant precautions, every 2 weeks $\times$ 4 doses; after BM recovery, drug is given every 4 weeks.

Drug Preparation:
- Oral: Available in 2-mg tablets. Take on empty stomach.
- IV: Reconstitute 50-mg vial with 10 mL of provided diluent resulting in concentration of 5 mg/mL.Rapid addition of diluent followed by vigorous shaking until clear must be done. Immediately, further dilute in 100–150 mL to produce a final concentration to a final concentration of not greater than 0.45 mg/mL, in 0.9% sodium chloride, USP. Administer diluted product over a minimum of 15 minutes, but complete administration must occur within 60 minutes of reconstitution.

Drug Administration:
- Serious hypersensitivity reactions reported with IV administration, including anaphylaxis.
- IV drug is an irritant—avoid extravasation.
- Oral melphalan is given on an empty stomach.

Drug Interactions:
- Myelosuppressive chemotherapy: Increases hematologic toxicity; dose-reduce or monitor patient very carefully.
- Cyclosporine: Increases nephrotoxicity.
- H$_2$ blockers: may decrease oral melphalan bioavailability.

Lab Effects/Interference:
- Decreased CBC.

Special Considerations:
- Nadir is 14–21 days after treatment.
- Drug dose reductions are recommended in patients with renal compromise.
- Drug is used in regional perfusion.
- Warnings and Precautions:
  - *Marked BM suppression*, most significantly with IV melphalan. Monitor ANC/CBC baseline and prior to each dose, as well as nadir counts. Subsequent cycles of therapy should proceed only if BM has recovered as evidenced by ANC/CBC.
  - *Hypersensitivithy reactions (HSR),* including anaphylaxis, largely in patients receiving the IV formulation. Incidence is 2%. Monitor patient closely during infusion, and interrupt drug and provide ordered, emergency medical support. If a HSR occurs, related either to an oral or IV dose of melphalan, do not readminister the drug.
  - *Second malignancies*: Acute nonlymphocytic leukemia, myeloproliferative syndrome, and carcinoma have been reported.
  - *Impairment of fertility*, resulting in amenorrhea in women and reversible and irreversible testicular suppression has been reported

- *Embryo-fetal toxicity*: Women of childbearing potential should be taught to use effective contraception to avoid pregnancy during melphalan treatment. Mothers should not breastfeed while receiving the drug.

Potential Toxicities/Side Effects and the Nursing Process

I.   INFECTION AND BLEEDING related to BM DEPRESSION

Defining Characteristics: BM depression may be pronounced; leukopenia and thrombocytopenia occur 14–21 days after intermittent dosing schedules. May be delayed in onset, and cumulative with nadir extended to 5–6 weeks. Combined immunosuppression from disease (e.g., multiple myeloma) and drug may prolong vulnerability to infection. Thrombocytopenia may be persistent.

Nursing Implications: Evaluate WBC, with neutrophil, and platelet count and discuss any abnormalities with physician prior to drug administration. Assess for signs/symptoms of infection or bleeding; instruct patient in signs/symptoms of infection and bleeding, and to notify nurse or physician if they arise. Teach patient self-care measures to minimize risk of infection and bleeding, including avoidance of OTC aspirin-containing medications. Assess patient for Hgb/HCT and signs/symptoms of fatigue; teach patient self-assessment and to alternate rest and activity as needed. Transfuse packed red blood cells and platelets per physician order.

II.   ALTERATION IN NUTRITION, LESS THAN BODY REQUIREMENTS, related to NAUSEA AND VOMITING, ANOREXIA

Defining Characteristics: Nausea and vomiting are mild at low, continuous dosing; severe following high doses. Anorexia occurs rarely.

Nursing Implications: Administer drug (oral) on empty stomach. Premedicate with antiemetic (oral) 1 hour before oral dose. Use aggressive antiemetic regimen for IV Alkeran. Encourage small, frequent feedings of favorite foods, especially high-calorie, high-protein foods. Encourage use of spices and obtain weekly weights.

III.   ALTERATION IN CARDIAC OUTPUT, PERFUSION related to ANAPHYLAXIS

Defining Characteristics: Severe hypersensitivity reactions can occur with IV administration, including diaphoresis, hypotension, and cardiac arrest.

Nursing Implications: Review standing orders for management of patient in anaphylaxis and identify location of anaphylaxis kit containing epinephrine 1:1,000, hydrocortisone sodium succinate (Solu-Cortef), diphenhydramine HCl (Benadryl), aminophylline, and others. Prior to drug administration, obtain baseline vital signs and record mental status. Administer drug slowly, diluted as per physician's order. Observe for following signs/ symptoms, usually occurring within first 15 minutes of infusion. Subjective signs are generalized itching, nausea, chest tightness, crampy abdominal pain, difficulty speaking, anxiety, agitation, sense of impending doom, uneasiness, desire to urinate/defecate, dizziness, chills. Objective signs are flushed appearance (angioedema of face, neck, eyelids, hands, feet), localized or generalized urticaria, respiratory distress ± wheezing, hypotension, cyanosis. For generalized allergic reaction, stop infusion and notify physician. Place patient in supine position to promote perfusion of visceral organs. Monitor VS. Provide emotional reassurance to patient and family. Maintain patent airway and have CPR equipment ready if needed. Document incident. Discuss with physician desensitization for further dosing versus drug discontinuance.

IV.   POTENTIAL SEXUAL DYSFUNCTION related to DRUG EFFECTS

Defining Characteristics: Potentially mutagenic and teratogenic.

Nursing Implications: Encourage patient to verbalize goals about family; discuss options, such as sperm banking. As appropriate, discuss or refer for counseling about birth control measures during therapy.

V.   POTENTIAL FOR INJURY related to SECOND MALIGNANCY

Defining Characteristics: Acute myelogenous and myelomonocytic leukemias may occur after continuous long-term dosing, especially in patients with ovarian cancer and multiple myeloma. Heralded by preleukemic pancytopenia of several weeks' duration. Chromosomal abnormalities characteristic of acute leukemia.

Nursing Implications: Patients receiving prolonged continuous therapy should be closely followed during and after treatment.

VI.   POTENTIAL FOR IMPAIRED GAS EXCHANGE related to PULMONARY TOXICITY

Defining Characteristics: Rare, but may occur, especially with continued chronic dosing. Bronchopulmonary dysplasia and pulmonary fibrosis.

Nursing Implications: Assess pulmonary status for signs/symptoms of pulmonary dysfunction. Assess lung sounds prior to dosing. Instruct patient to report cough or dyspnea. Discuss PFTs to be performed periodically with physician. Long-term follow-up is important.

VII.   IMPAIRED SKIN INTEGRITY related to ALOPECIA, MACULOPAPULAR RASH, URTICARIA

Defining Characteristics: Alopecia is minimal if it occurs at all. Maculopapular rash and urticaria are infrequent.

Nursing Implications: Assess skin integrity and presence of rash, urticaria, alopecia prior to dosing. Assess impact of these alterations on patient and develop plan to manage symptom distress.

Drug: Melphalan for injection (Evomela)

Class: Alkylating agent (bischloroethylamine type, bifunctional).

Mechanism of Action: Causes interstrand cross-linking with DNA, most likely by binding at the N^7 position of guanine. Drug is active against both resting and rapidly dividing tumor cells.

Metabolism: After injection, drug is rapidly distributed with terminal elimination phase half-life of 75 min. Drug penetrates in the CSF. It binds to plasma proteins 50–90%, and serum albumin is the major binding protein (40–60% of plasma protein binding), and 30% of melphalan is irreversibly bound to plasma proteins. Drug is metabolized by chemical hydrolysis into inactive metabolites. Renal excretion of the drug is low, with 5.8–21.3% excreted in the urine.

Indication: For (1) use as a high-dose conditioning treatment prior to hematopoietic progenitor (stem) cell transplantation in patients with multiple myeloma, and (2) the palliative treatment of patients with multiple myeloma for whom oral therapy is not appropriate.

Contraindication: History of serious allergic reaction to melphalan.

Dosage/Range:
- *For conditioning treatment:* melphalan injection 100 mg/m²/day administered IV infusion over 30 minutes for 2 consecutive days (day 2 and day 3) prior to autologous stem cell transplantation (ASCT, Day 0). For patients who weigh more than 130% of their ideal body weight (IBW), BSA calculation should be based on adjusted IBW (Spectrum Pharmaceuticals, Inc, 2017).
- *For palliative treatment:* 16-mg/m² IV as a single dose infusion over 15–20 minutes at 2-week intervals for 4 doses, then after adequate recovery from toxicity, at 4-week intervals.

Dose Modification:
- Renal impairment: palliative treatment: reduce dose up to 50% in patients having a BUN ≥ 30 mg/dL.

Drug Preparation:
- Available as a 50 mg lyophilized powder, in a single-dose vial for reconstitution. Drug is highly soluble in saline.
- Use normal saline solution (0.9% sodium chloride injecton USP) (8.6 mL as directed) to reconstitute drug and make a 50 mg/10mL (5 mg/mL) nominal concentration of melphalan.

- Asceptically, use negative pressure in the vial to inject 8.6 mL 0.9% sodium chloride injection USP to reconstitute the drug, making a 50 mg/10mL solution with a concentration of 5 mg/mL. If there is no vacuum in the vial, do not use and replace with a new vial.
- Reconstituted drug is stable for 24 hours refrigerated (5°C).
- Calculate required volume (based on ordered dose) and withdraw from the vial(s). Add to 0.9% sodium chloride injection, USP infusion bag obtaining a final concentration of 0.45 mg/mL. Once diluted the admixture solution is stable for 4 hours at room temperature in addition to the 1 hour following reconstitution.

Drug Administration:
- Administer antiemetic(s) prior to melphalan infusion.
- Inspect visually for particulate matter and discoloration prior to administration, and do not use if found.
- Infuse over 30 min via a central venous catheter. Drug may cause local tissue damage if the drug extravasates. Use vesicant precautions. DO NOT administer by direct injection into a peripheral vein. Administer by injecting drug slowly into a fast-running IV infusion via a central venous access line.

Drug Interactions:
- No formal tests have been conducted.
- Cyclosporine: reports of severe renal impairment in patients treated with a single dose of melphalan (140–250 mg/m^2) followed by standard oral doses of cyclosporine.
- BCNU: IV melphalan may reduce the threshold for BCNU lung toxicity.
- Nalidixic acid: when given with IV melphalan simultaneously, incidence of severe hemorrhagic necrotic enterocolitis has been reported to increase in pediatric patients.

Lab Effects/Interference:
- Neutropenia, thrombocytopenia, anemia.
- Hypokalemia, hypophosphatemia.

Special Considerations:
- Most common adverse reactions in at least 50% of patients are: decreased neutrophil count, decreased WBC, decreased platelet count, diarrhea, nausea, fatigue, hypokalemia, anemia, and vomiting.
- Warnings and Precautions:
  - *BM suppression*: *When used as a conditioning regimen*, myeloablation occurs in all patients. **Ensure stem cells have been collected and are adequate in number** before administering drug. Once administered, there is no rescue for the BM unless stem cells are infused on day 0. *As palliative treatment*: The risk of myelosuppression depends upon prior compromise with radiation, chemotherapy, or is recovering from recent chemotherapy. Supportive care for infections, bleeding, and anemia must be available for both groups of patients.
  - *GI toxicity*: *As part of a conditioning regimen*, nausea, vomiting, diarrhea, and mucositis/oral mucositis occur in over 50% of patients. Prophylactic antiemetic must be administered prior to the drug. Provide supportive care using antiemetic and antidiarrheal medications as frequency of grades 3–4 mucositis was 13% in clinical studies.

Provide nutritional support and analgesics for patients with severe mucositis. *As palliative therapy,* nausea, vomiting, diarrhea, and oral ulceration may occur. Provide necessary supportive care for all symptoms.

- *Hepatotoxicity*: Range from abnormal LFTs to hepatitis with jaundice. Hepatic veno-occlusive disease has also been reported. Assess and monitor LFTs baseline and during treatment.
- *Hypersensitivity reactions (HSRs):* Approximately 2% of patients had acute HSR, including anaphylaxis, characterized by urticaria, pruritis, edema, and skin rash; when severe, it included tachycardia, bronchospasm, dyspnea, and hypotension. Discontinue drug in patients having serious HSRs.
- *Secondary malignancy*: Drug is known to cause chromatid or chromosome damage in humans. MDS and acute leukemias have been reported in multiple myeloma patients treated with melphalan-containing chemotherapy regimens.
- *Embryo-fetal toxicity*: Teach women of reproductive potential to use effective contraception to avoid pregnancy. If patient becomes pregnant while using the drug, advise mother of potential risk to fetus. Mothers should not breastfeed while being treated with the drug. Advise men with female sexual partners of reproductive potential to use effective contraception during and after treatment with IV melphalan as drug may damage spermatozoa and testicular tissue, resulting in possible genetal fetal abnormalities (Spectrum Pharmaceuticals, Inc, 2017).
- *Infertility*: Drug may cause ovarian function suppression in premenopausal women resulting in persistent amenorrhea (9% incidence) or testicular suppression which may or may not be reversible.

Potential Toxicities/Side Effects and the Nursing Process

I. INFECTION AND BLEEDING related to BM DEPRESSION

Defining Characteristics: BM suppression: *when used as a conditioning regimen,* myeloablation occurs in all patients. **Ensure stem cells have been collected and are adequate in number** before administering drug. Once administered, there is no rescue for the BM unless stem cells are infused on day 0. *As palliative treatment*: the risk of myelosuppression depends upon prior compromise with radiation, chemotherapy, or is recovering from recent chemotherapy. Supportive care for infections, bleeding, and anemia must be available for both groups of patients.

Nursing Implications: Evaluate WBC, with neutrophil, and platelet count and discuss any abnormalities with physician prior to drug administration. For patients receiving conditioning regimen, **ensure stem cells have been collected and are adequate in number** before administering drug. Once administered, there is no rescue for the BM unless stem cells are infused on day 0. Assess for signs/symptoms of infection or bleeding; instruct patient in signs/symptoms of infection and bleeding, and to notify nurse or physician if they arise. Teach patient self-care measures to minimize risk of infection and bleeding, including avoidance of OTC aspirin-containing medications. Assess patient for Hgb/HCT and signs/symptoms of fatigue; teach patient self-assessment and to alternate rest and activity as needed. Transfuse packed red blood cells and platelets per physician order. **Ensure patients receiving conditioning regimen receive their stem cells back on day 0 regardless of any issues.**

II. ALTERATION IN NUTRITION, LESS THAN BODY REQUIREMENTS, related to DIARRHEA, NAUSEA AND VOMITING, DECREASED APPETITE, DYSGEUSIA, DYSPEPSIA

Defining Characteristics: Nutritional impact symptoms are severe. Diarrhea occurs in 93%, nausea in 90%, vomiting in 64%, decreased appetite in 49%, constipation in 48%, mucosal inflammation in 38% (10% grades 3–4), stomatitis in 28%, dysgeusia in 28%, and dyspepsia in 26%.

Nursing Implications: Premedicate with effective antiemetic(s) at least 30 min prior to IV melphalan dose before oral dose. Use aggressive antiemetic regimen for high-dose IV melphalan. Encourage small, frequent feedings of favorite foods, especially high-calorie, high-protein foods. Encourage use of spices and obtain weekly weights. To prevent oral mucositis, consider suggesting patients suck ice chips 10 min before the infusion, during the infusion for 15 minutes, and for 10 minutes following the infusion as this has been shown to significantly reduce the incidence and intensity (grades 3–4) of oral mucositis (Battle et al., 2014; Worthington et al., 2011). Keratinocyte growth factor (Kepivance) is also recommended (Lalla et al., 2014).

III. ALTERATION IN CARDIAC OUTPUT, PERFUSION related to ANAPHYLAXIS

Defining Characteristics: Acute hypersensitivity reactions, including anaphylaxis, can occur rarely (2%) with IV melphalan. Symptoms include urticarial, pruritis, edema and skin rash, and in some patients, tachycardia, bronchospasm, dyspnea, and hypotension.

Nursing Implications: Review standing orders for management of patient in anaphylaxis and identify location of anaphylaxis kit containing epinephrine 1:1,000, hydrocortisone sodium succinate (Solu-Cortef), diphenhydramine HCl (Benadryl), aminophylline, and others. Prior to drug administration, obtain baseline vital signs and record mental status. Administer drug slowly, diluted as per physician's order. Observe for following signs/symptoms, usually occurring within first 15 minutes of infusion. Subjective signs are generalized itching, nausea, chest tightness, crampy abdominal pain, difficulty speaking, anxiety, agitation, sense of impending doom, uneasiness, desire to urinate/defecate, dizziness, chills. Objective signs are flushed appearance (angioedema of face, neck, eyelids, hands, feet), localized or generalized urticaria, respiratory distress ± wheezing, hypotension, cyanosis. For generalized allergic reaction, stop infusion and notify physician. Place patient in supine position to promote perfusion of visceral organs. Monitor VS. Provide emotional reassurance to patient and family. Maintain patent airway and have CPR equipment ready if needed. Document incident. Discuss with physician drug discontinuance if anaphylaxis occurs.

IV. POTENTIAL SEXUAL DYSFUNCTION related to DRUG EFFECTS

Defining Characteristics: Potentially mutagenic and teratogenic.

Nursing Implications: Encourage patient to verbalize goals about family; discuss options, such as sperm banking. As appropriate, discuss or refer for counseling about birth control measures during therapy for women of reproductive potential, and men who have female sexual partners of reproductive potential.

V. POTENTIAL FOR INJURY related to SECOND MALIGNANCY

Defining Characteristics: Acute myelogenous and myelomonocytic leukemias may occur after continuous long-term dosing, especially in patients with ovarian cancer and multiple myeloma. Heralded by preleukemic pancytopenia of several weeks' duration. Chromosomal abnormalities characteristic of acute leukemia.

Nursing Implications: Patients receiving prolonged continuous therapy should be closely followed during and after treatment.

VI. POTENTIAL FOR IMPAIRED GAS EXCHANGE related to PULMONARY TOXICITY

Defining Characteristics: Rare, but may occur, especially with continued chronic dosing. Bronchopulmonary dysplasia and pulmonary fibrosis.

Nursing Implications: Assess pulmonary status for signs/symptoms of pulmonary dysfunction. Assess lung sounds prior to dosing. Instruct patient to report cough or dyspnea. Discuss PFTs to be performed periodically with physician. Long-term follow-up is important.

VII. IMPAIRED SKIN INTEGRITY related to ALOPECIA, MACULOPAPULAR RASH, URTICARIA

Defining Characteristics: Alopecia is minimal if it occurs at all. Maculopapular rash and urticaria are infrequent.

Nursing Implications: Assess skin integrity and presence of rash, urticaria, alopecia prior to dosing. Assess impact of these alterations on patient and develop plan to manage symptom distress.

Drug: mercaptopurine (PURIXAN oral suspension, Purinethol, 6-MP)

Class: Nucleoside metabolic inhibitor (antimetabolite).

Mechanism of Action: Nucleoside metabolic inhibitor that is activated to form 6-thioguanine nucleotides (6-TGNs). When the cell uses 6-TGN (a false metabolite) to make nucleic acids instead of purine bases, it causes the cell's cell cycle to stop and the cell to die. The drug also has other actions. Cell cycle phase specific for S phase.

Metabolism: Absorption of oral dose is incomplete with approximately 50% bioavailability. There is bioequivalence between tablet and suspension in bioavailability, although the mean C_{max} following oral suspension was 34% higher than the tablet. Does not cross BBB. Metabolized by two major pathways: (1) thiol methylation catalyzed by the enzyme thiopurine S-methyltransferase (TPMT) to form an inactive metabolite, and (2) oxidation catalyzed by the enzyme xanthine oxidase into another inactive metabolite. Elimination half-life is about 2 hours. About 46% of the dose is excreted in the urine in the first 24 hrs. There is genetic polymorphism in the TPMT gene. About 0.3% of Caucasians and African Americans have 2 non-functional alleles (copies of the genes, called homozygous-deficient), so this metabolic pathway is inactive. Ten percent of patients have one TPMT non-functional allele (heterozygous) leading to low or intermediate TPMT activity, and 90% of patients have normal TPMT activity with two functional alleles. If TPMT is inactive (homozygous-deficient patients) or reduced (low or intermediate TPMT activity), mercaptopurine is incompletely metabolized by one pathway; if normal mercaptopurine doses are administered, there is higher risk of severe mercaptopurine toxicity. TPMT genotyping or phenotyping (red blood cell TPMT activity) helps to identify patients who are homozygous-deficient or who have low/intermediate TPMT activity. See package insert for TPMT testing details.

Indication: Mercaptopurine is indicated for the treatment of patients with ALL as a component of a combination maintenance therapy regimen; drug is not indicated for but is used to treat some patients with other cancers, Crohn's disease, and ulcerative colitis.

Dosage/Range:

Maintenance:
- Starting dose in multi-agent combination chemotherapy 1.5–2.5 mg/kg (50–75 mg/m²) for acute lymphoblastic leukemia (ALL), oral.
  - After beginning mercaptopurine, dose should be determined by periodic ANC and platelet counts.
  - Monitor serum transaminase levels, alkaline phosphatase, and bilirubin levels weekly at the beginning of therapy, then monthly. Monitor LFTs daily, more frequently in patients who are receiving other potentially hepatotoxic drugs or with preexisting liver disease.
  - Reduce dose in cases of hepatic or renal dysfunction.
  - Interrupt mercaptopurine when clinical or laboratory evidence suggests hepatotoxicity.
  - Start at low end of dosing range, patients with:
    - Elderly: greater frequency of decreased hepatic, renal, or cardiac function; other concommitant disease; other drug therapy.
    - Renal impairment: increase the dosing interval to 36–48 hours; adjust subsequent doses on efficacy and toxicity.
    - Hepatic impairment: monitor transaminases and bilirubin; monitor closely for toxity; hold or adjust the dose of mercaptopurine.
- TPMT-deficient patients: perform TPMT testing; should be considered in patients who experience severe BM toxicities.

- Homozygous-deficient patients may require a 90% dose reduction (patient receives only 10% of standard dose).
- Heterozygous TPMT-deficient patients usually tolerate recommended mercaptopurine dose, but some patients do require a dose reduction.

Avoid coadministration with allopurinol, as allopurinol inhibits xanthine oxidase; if they must be coadministered, mercaptopurine dose must be reduced by at least 25% of the normal dose.

Drug Preparation:
- Oral: tablet, none; available in 50-mg tablets.
- Oral suspension (PURIXAN, 2,000 mg/100 mL or 20 mg/mL): Shake bottle vigorously for at least 30 seconds to ensure it is well mixed; color will be pink to brown viscous oral suspension. Once opened, drug should be used within 6 weeks. Ask pharmacist to give patient oral syringe and suitable adaptor, based on patient's dosing requirement.
- Tablet has been available since 1953, but precise BSA dosing and dose adjustments are difficult with the tablet; oral suspension provides more accurate and consistent dosing.

Drug Administration:
Oral:
- Teach patient how to administer mercaptopurine using gloves. If oral suspension, demonstrate how to draw up prescribed dose in a syringe.
- If the syringe will be used for multiple use, teach patient and caregivers to (1) wash the syringe with warm, soapy water and rinse well; (2) hold the syringe under water and move the plunger up and down several times to make sure the inside of the syringe is clean; (3) ensure the syringe is completely dry before using the syringe again for dosing; (4) store the syringe in a hygienic place, along with the medicine.
- Lab tests:
  - CBS/differential, transaminases, bilirubin.
  - BM should be evaluated in patients with prolonged or repeated marrow suppression to assess leukemia status and marrow cellularity.
  - Evaluate TPMT status in patients with severe BM toxicity (clinical and/or laboratory), or repeated episodes of myelosuppression.
- Drug is cytotoxic; teach patient and caregiver to use special handling and how to dispose of hazardous waste.

Drug Interactions:
Drugs that decrease the clearance of mercaptopurine and increase drug serum levels do so by (1) inhibiting first-pass oxidative metabolism by xanthine oxidase; or by (2) inhibiting TPMT enzyme. Avoid coadministration; if drugs must be coadministered, mercaptopurine dose must be reduced.

- Allopurinol: increased BM suppression, nausea, vomiting; reduce dose to 25–35% of normal.
- Myelosuppressants (e.g., chemotherapy, trimethoprim-sulfamethoxazole): increased BMD; monitor patient closely.

- Warfarin: may decrease anticoagulant effect; monitor closely and dose based on PT or INR.
- Aminosalicylate derivatives (e.g., olsalazine, mesalamine, sulfasalazine): may inhibit TPMT. If coadministered, use the lowest dose of each drug and monitor the patient closely for BMD.

Vaccines: mercaptopurine is immunosuppressive and may impair the immune response to vaccines; there may be risk of infection with live virus vaccines.

Lab Effects/Interference:
- Decreased CBC.
- Increased LFTs.
- Increased RFTs: tumor lysis.

Special Considerations:
- Drug is hepatotoxic; reports of death associated with hepatic necrosis have been reported. Risk for hepatic injury is increased when recommended dose is exceeded. Clinical jaundice appears in the first 1–2 months of treatment, but it has been reported as early as 1 week and as late as 8 years. Anorexia, diarrhea, jaundice, and ascites may appear. Reports of jaundice resolving after drug interruption, and reappearance with rechallenge have been documented. Monitor LFTs weekly when beginning mercaptopurine, then at least monthly.
- Teach women of reproductive potential to avoid pregnancy. Drug can cause embryo-fetal toxicity. If drug is used in pregnancy or if the woman becomes pregnant while taking drug, apprise patient of potential hazard to the fetus. Drug increases risk of abortions in first trimester as well as later in the pregnancy; stillbirth was seen after the first trimester as well.
- Nursing mothers should decide whether to discontinue nursing or the drug.
- Most common (> 20%) adverse reactions in clinical trials were myelosuppression (anemia, neutropenia, lymphopenia, thrombocytopenia). Adverse reactions occurring 5–20% were anorexia, nausea, vomiting, diarrhea, malaise, rash. Rare reactions (< 5%) were urticaria, hyperuricemia, oral lesions (thrush), elevated transaminases, hyperbilirubinemia, hyperpigmentation. Delayed or late toxicities include hepatic fibrosis, hyperbilirubinemia, alopecia, pulmonary fibrosis, oligospermia, secondary malignancies.
- Drug is mutagenic in animals and humans, carcinogenic in animals, and may increase risk of secondary malignancies.
  - Rarely, hepatosplenic T-cell lymphoma has been described in adolescents and young adults receiving tumor necrosis factor (TNF) blockers and azathioprine and/or mercaptopurine, as well as those receiving mercaptopurine alone, for treatment of Crohn's disease or ulcerative colitis (FDA, 2011). Drug is NOT approved for this use.
  - Patients with RA, Crohn's disease, ankylosing spondylitis, psoriatic arthritis, and plaque psoriasis may be more likely to develop lymphoma than the general population. If patient develops splenomegaly, hepatomegaly, abdominal pain, persistent fever, night sweats, and weight loss, discuss with physician, NP/PA further evaluation.

Potential Toxicities/Side Effects and the Nursing Process

I.   POTENTIAL FOR INFECTION AND BLEEDING related to BM DEPRESSION

Defining Characteristics: Nadir varies from 5 days to 6 weeks after treatment. Leukopenia more prominent than thrombocytopenia. Blood counts may continue to fall after therapy is stopped. Drug fever may occur rarely, but other causes, such as sepsis in the setting of ALL, must be ruled out first.

Nursing Implications: Evaluate WBC, with neutrophil, and platelet count, which should be monitored closely, and discuss any abnormalities with physician prior to drug administration. Assess for signs/symptoms of infection or bleeding; instruct patient to notify nurse or physician if they arise. Teach patient self-care measures to minimize risk of infection and bleeding, including avoidance of OTC aspirin-containing medications. Assess patient's Hgb/HCT and signs/symptoms of fatigue; teach patient self-assessment and to alternate rest and activity as needed. Discuss dose modifications based on CBC/differential for severe neutropenia and thrombocytopenia.

II.   ALTERATION IN NUTRITION, LESS THAN BODY REQUIREMENTS, related to HEPATOTOXICITY, GI SYMPTOMS

Defining Characteristics: Reversible cholestatic jaundice may develop after 2–5 months of treatment. Hepatic necrosis may develop. Nausea, vomiting, anorexia, diarrhea are infrequent. Stomatitis uncommon, but appears as white patchy areas similar to thrush.

Nursing Implications: Monitor transaminases, alkaline phosphatase, and bilirubin weekly at drug initiation, then monthly during treatment. Notify physician of any elevations. Assess for signs/symptoms of hepatotoxicity, which is an indication for discontinuing treatment. Instruct patient to report GI side effects and to perform self-care measures as appropriate.

III.   POTENTIAL FOR IMPAIRED SKIN INTEGRITY related to RASH

Defining Characteristics: Skin eruptions; rash may occur.

Nursing Implications: Advise patient these changes may occur. Instruct patient in symptomatic care if distress related to skin reactions occurs.

Drug: methotrexate (Amethopterin, Mexate, Folex)

Class: Nucleoside metabolic inhibitor (Antimetabolite), folic acid antagonist.

Mechanism of Action: Blocks the enzyme dihydrofolate reductase (DHFR), which inhibits the conversion of folic acid to tetrahydrofolic acid, resulting in an inhibition of the key precursors of DNA, RNA, and cellular proteins. May synchronize malignant cells in the S phase: at high plasma levels, passive entry of the drug into tumor cells can potentially overcome drug resistance.

Metabolism: Following parenteral administration, drug is completely absorbed. Oral drug is absorbed from GI tract in a dose-dependent manner: 60% bioavailability at 30 mg/m^2 or lower doses; but at doses > 80 mg/m^2, bioavailability is significantly less (possibly due to saturation effect). Peak plasma levels are reached in 1–2 hours. Drug is 50% protein-bound; concurrent use of drugs that displace methotrexate from serum albumin should be avoided. Salicylates, sulfonamides, Dilantin, some antibacterials—including tetracycline, chloramphenicol, para-aminobenzoic acid—and alcohol should be avoided, as they will delay excretion. Plasma half-life is 2 hours; 50–100% of dose is excreted into the systemic circulation, with peak concentration 3–12 hours after administration. At high doses, drug crosses blood-brain barrier (BBB), but high CSF concentrations of drug require IT administration. After absorption, drug is metabolized via hepatic and intracellular processes; some active metabolites may be retained in tissue with prolonged drug release, so effusions should be tapped prior to administration of high doses. After oral administration, some drug is partially metabolized by intestinal flora. The drug half-life is 3–10 hours for doses < 30 mg/m^2 while the terminal half-life for high doses is 8–15 hours. Drug is principally excreted via the kidneys, and it is dose- and route-dependent. After IV drug administration, most (80–90%) of unchanged drug is excreted via the kidneys (glomerular filtration and active tubular secretion) in the urine within 24 hours. Less than 10% of drug is excreted in the bile. Toxicity is believed to be the result of high methotrexate serum levels due to delayed drug excretion (with subsequent longer time of drug exposure), caused by renal impairment, third space effusion, or other factors.

Indication:
- Cancer: (1) gestational choriocarcinoma, chorioadenoma destruens and hydatidiform mole; (2) ALL for prophylaxis of meningeal leukemia and used as maintenance therapy in combination with other chemotherapy agents; (3) meningeal leukemia; (4) alone or in combination with other anticancer agents in the treatment of breast cancer, epidermoid cancers of head and neck, advanced mycosis fungoides (cutaneous T cell lymphoma, lung cancer, particularly squamous cell and small cell types, and advanced stage NHL); (5) high doses with leucovorin rescue in combination with other chemotherapy agents in nonmetastatic osteosarcoma after surgical resection or amputation of the primary tumor.
- Rheumatoid Arthritis.
- Psoriasis.

Dosage/Range:
- Cancer.
- Oral: preferred for low doses.
- IV: Low: 10–50 mg/m^2; med: 100–500 mg/m^2; high: 500 mg/m^2 and above with leucovorin rescue.
- IM: 25 mg/m^2.
- IT: 10–15 mg/m^2 with preservative-free diluent ONLY.

- Rheumatoid Arthritis (RA), juvenile RA, psoriasis: single oral dose 7.5 mg once weekly, or divided oral doses of 2.5 mg at 12-hour intervals for 3 doses, given as a course once a week.

Drug Preparation:
- 5-, 50-, 100-, and 200-mg vials are available already reconstituted.
- Powder is available in vials without preservative for IT and high-dose administration (reconstitute with preservative-free 0.9% sodium chloride).

Drug Administration:
- 5–149 mg: slow IVP.
- 150–499 mg: IV drip over 20 minutes.
- **Higher Doses:** 500–1,500 mg or higher per m^2: infusion with leucovorin rescue.
- High Dose: 12–15 gm/m^2: Minimum dose must produce a peak serum methotrexate concentration of 1,000 micromolar (10^{-3} mol/L). Usually administered as a 4-hour infusion. Leucovorin (15 mg PO or IV) every 6 hours, beginning 24 hours after the start of the methotrexate infusion.
- Assess labs: proceed only if WBC > 1,500/mL, ANC > 200/mL, platelets > 75,000/mL, serum bilirubin < 1.2 mg/dL, SGPT < 450U; serum creatinine WNL, creatinine clearance > 60 mL/min.
- Assess patient and proceed only if: absence of mucositis, or healing of existing mucositis; any effusion, e.g., pleural, has been drained dry prior to methotrexate; well hydrated (e.g., 1 L/m^2 IV fluid over 6 hours) prior to methotrexate with bicarbonate to alkalinize urine and maintain pH > 7.0 during methotrexate and leucovorin therapy. After initial prechemotherapy hydration, continue hydration at 3 L/m^2/day during methotrexate infusion, and for 2 days after the infusion has been completed. Assess serum creatinine prior to each subsequent treatment course. If creatinine has increased by 50% or more compared to prior value, reassess and document creatine clearance > 60 mL/min (even if serum creatinine is still WNL).
- Adjust leucovorin dose based on serum methotrexate levels:
  - Normal methotrexate elimination: serum level 10 micromolar at 24 hours after administration, 1 micromolar at 48 hours, and < 0.2 micromolar at 72 hours: leucovorin dose 15 mg (PO, IM, IV) q 6 hr × 60 hr (10 doses starting 24 hours after start of methotrexate infusion).
  - Delayed late methotrexate elimination: serum methotrexate level remaining > 0.2 micromolar at 72 hours, and > 0.05 micromolar at 96 hours after administration: continue 15 mg leucovorin (PO, IM, IV) q 6 hours until methotrexate level is < 0.05 micromolar.
  - Delayed early methotrexate elimination and/or evidence of acute renal injury: serum methotrexate level of ≥ 50 micromolar at 24 hours, or ≥ 5 micromolar at 48 hours after administration; OR ≥ 100% increase in serum creatinine at 24 hours after methotrexate administration (e.g., increase from 0.5 mg/dL to 1 mg/dL or more); leucovorin 150 mg IV q 3 hours until methotrexate level is < 1 micromolar; then 15 mg IV q 3 hours until methotrexate level is < 0.05 micromolar.

Drug Interactions:
- Protein-bound drugs (aspirin, sulfonamides, sulfonylureas, phenytoin, tetracycline, chloramphenicol) increase toxicity; give together cautiously and monitor patient closely.
- NSAIDs (nonsteroidal anti-inflammatory drugs, e.g., indomethacin, ketoprofen) increased and prolonged methotrexate levels; DO NOT administer concurrently with high doses of methotrexate; monitor patients closely who are receiving moderate or low-dose methotrexate, if given concurrently. Patients with RA appear to tolerate concommitant NSAIDs and methotrexate at 7.5 mg dose.
- Cotrimoxazole increased methotrexate serum level; DO NOT use concurrently.
- Proton pump inhibitors (PPIs, omeprazole, esomeprazole, pantoprazole): elevated and prolonged methotrexate serum levels; DO NOT use concurrently with high-dose methotrexate. Ranitidine did not cause changes in methotrexate levels.
- Warfarin: anticoagulant effect may increase; monitor INR closely.
- 5-FU: enhanced antitumor effect of 5-FU when methotrexate is given 24 hours before 5-FU.
- Folic acid: may reduce antitumor effect of methotrexate; do not coadminister.
- Thymidine, leucovorin: rescues normal cells from methotrexate effect; may nullify antitumor effect if given close to the time of methotrexate; usually given 24 hours after methotrexate. High-dose leucovorin may reduce the efficacy of IT methotrexate.
- L-asparaginase: reduces methotrexate antitumor effects.
- 6-mercaptopurine (6-MP): methotrexate increases 6-MP plasma levels; if given together, adjust 6-MP dose.
- Oral antibiotics (tetracycline, non-absorbable broad spectrum) may decrease intestinal absorption of methotrexate or interfere with drug metabolism; do not coadminister when methotrexate is given orally.
- Penicillins: may increase methotrexate serum levels at any methotrexate dose; use together cautiously if at all, and monitor patient closely for toxicity.
- Theophylline: methotrexate may decrease theophylline clearance; monitor theophylline levels and adjust dose.
- Folate deficiencies (e.g., trimethoprim/sulfamethoxazole) may increase risk of BM suppression; do not coadminister.

Lab Effects/Interference:
- Decreased CBC.
- Increased LFTs, RFTs.

Special Considerations:
- High doses cross the BBB; reconstitute with preservative-free 0.9% sodium chloride.
- With high doses (12–15 g/m^2), urine should be alkalinized both before and after administration, as the drug is a weak acid and can crystallize in the kidneys at an acid pH. Alkalinize with bicarbonate; add to pre- and posthydration fluids. High doses should only be given under the direction of a qualified oncologist at an institution that can provide rapid serum methotrexate level readings and has adequate leucovorin stores if needed.

- Leucovorin rescue must be given on time per orders to prevent excessive toxicity and to achieve maximum therapeutic response (see leucovorin calcium).
- Avoid folic acid and its derivatives during methotrexate therapy. Kidney function must be adequate to excrete drug and avoid excessive toxicity. Check BUN and creatinine before each dose.

Potential Toxicities/Side Effects and the Nursing Process

I.   ALTERATION IN NUTRITION, LESS THAN BODY REQUIREMENTS, related to GI SIDE EFFECTS

Defining Characteristics: Nausea and vomiting are uncommon with low dose; more common (39%) with higher and high dose; may occur during drug administration and last 24–72 hours. Anorexia is mild. Stomatitis is a common indication for interruption of therapy: occurs in 3–5 days with high dose, 3–4 weeks with low dose; appears initially at corners of mouth. Stomatitis precedes BM depression. Diarrhea is common and is an indication for interruption of therapy, as enteritis and intestinal perforation may occur; melena, hematemesis may occur. Hepatotoxicity is usually subclinical and reversible, but can lead to cirrhosis; increased risk of hepatotoxicity when given with other agents, like alcohol; transient increase in LFTs with high dose 1–10 days after treatment—may cause jaundice.

Nursing Implications: Premedicate with antiemetics if giving high-dose methotrexate; continue prophylactically for 24 hours (at least) to prevent nausea and vomiting. Encourage small, frequent feedings of cool, bland foods and liquids. Assess for symptoms of fluid and electrolyte imbalance: monitor I/O, daily weights if administered to inpatient. Assess oral cavity every day. Teach patient oral assessment and mouth care regimens. Encourage patient to report early stomatitis. Provide pain relief measures, if indicated. Explore patient compliance to rescue; discuss increase in rescue dose if moderate GI toxicity. Assess patient for diarrhea: guaiac all stools; encourage patient to report onset of diarrhea. Administer or teach patient to self-administer antidiarrheal medications. Monitor LFTs prior to drug dose, especially with high-dose methotrexate. Assess patient prior to and during treatment for signs/symptoms of hepatotoxicity.

II.   POTENTIAL FOR INFECTION AND BLEEDING related to BM DEPRESSION

Defining Characteristics: Nadir is seen 4–7 days after drug administration, with recovery by day 14. BM depression occurs in about 10% of patients.

Nursing Implications: Monitor CBC and platelet count prior to drug administration, as well as signs/symptoms of infection or bleeding. Instruct patient in self-assessment of signs/symptoms of infection or bleeding measures to decrease risk. Administer leucovorin calcium as ordered.

III. POTENTIAL FOR ALTERATION IN URINARY ELIMINATION related to RENAL TOXICITY

Defining Characteristics: As an organic acid, methotrexate is insoluble in acid urine. At doses greater than 1 g/m^2 (i.e., high dose), drug may precipitate in renal tubules, causing acute renal tubular necrosis (ATN).

Nursing Implications: Prehydrate patient with alkaline solution for several hours prior to drug administration. Maintain high urine output with a urine pH greater than 7.0 (hydration fluid may need further alkalinization); dipstick each void. Record I/O. Monitor BUN and serum creatinine before, during, and after drug administration. Increases in these values may require methotrexate dose reductions or leucovorin dose increases.

IV. POTENTIAL FOR IMPAIRED GAS EXCHANGE related to PULMONARY TOXICITY

Defining Characteristics: Pneumothorax (high dose): rare, occurs within first 48 hours after drug administration in patients with pulmonary metastasis. Allergic pneumonitis (high dose): rare but accompanied by eosinophilia, patchy pulmonary infiltrates, fever, cough, shortness of breath. Occurs 1–5 months after initiation of treatment. Pneumonitis (low-dose) symptoms usually disappear within a week, with or without use of steroids; interstitial pneumonitis may be a fatal complication.

Nursing Implications: Assess for signs/symptoms of pulmonary dysfunction before each dose and between doses (see Defining Characteristics section). Discuss PFTs to be performed periodically with physician. Assess lung sounds prior to drug administration. Instruct patient to report cough or dyspnea.

V. POTENTIAL FOR ALTERATION IN SKIN INTEGRITY related to ALOPECIA, DERMATITIS

Defining Characteristics: Alopecia and dermatitis are uncommon. Pruritus, urticaria may occur. Photosensitivity, sunburnlike rash 1–5 days after treatment; also, patient can develop radiation recall reaction.

Nursing Implications: Assess patient for signs/symptoms of hair loss. Discuss with patient impact of hair loss and strategies to minimize distress. Instruct patient to avoid sun if possible and to stay covered or wear sunblock if sun exposure is unavoidable.

VI. POTENTIAL FOR SENSORY AND PERCEPTUAL ALTERATIONS related to CNS CHANGES

Defining Characteristics: CNS effects: dizziness, malaise, blurred vision. IT administration may increase CSF pressure. Brain XRT followed by IV methotrexate may also cause neurologic changes.

Nursing Implications: Monitor for CNS effects of drug: dizziness, blurred vision, malaise. Monitor for symptoms of increased CSF pressure: seizures, paresis, headache, nausea and vomiting, brain atrophy, fever. If IV methotrexate follows brain XRT, monitor for symptoms of increased CSF pressure.

VII. POTENTIAL FOR ALTERATIONS IN COMFORT related to PAIN

Defining Characteristics: Sometimes causes back pain during administration.

Nursing Implications: Monitor patient for back and flank pain. Slow down infusion rate if it occurs. Administer analgesics if pain occurs (must avoid aspirin-containing products, as they displace methotrexate from serum albumin).

Drug: mitomycin (mitomycin C, Mutamycin, 3 Mitozytrex)

Class: Antitumor antibiotic.

Mechanism of Action: Drug acts as alkylating agent and inhibits DNA synthesis by crosslinking of DNA. Alkylating and crosslinking mitomycin metabolites interfere with structure and function of DNA.

Metabolism: Drug is rapidly cleared by the liver. May need to modify dose in presence of liver abnormalities; 10% of drug is excreted unchanged.

Indication: In combination therapy for the treatment of disseminated adenocarcinoma of the stomach or pancreas, and as palliative treatment when other modalities have failed. Not to be used as a single-agent primary therapy.

Contraindications: Patients with thrombocytopenia, coagulation disorder, or increase in bleeding tendency due to other causes; patients hypersensitive to the drug or who have had an idiosyncratic reaction in the past.

Dosage/Range:
- 10 mg/m^2 IV every 8 weeks, with 5-FU and doxorubicin (FAM regimen).
- Bladder instillations 20–40 mg in 20–40 mL of water.
- When used as a single agent, 20-mg/m^2 IV every 6–8 weeks.
- Dose Modification: Nadir from Prior Dose (see package insert): (1) Leukocyte count > 3,000/mm^3 and platelets > 75,000/mm^3: 100% prior dose; (2) leukocyte count 2,000–2,999/mm^3 and platelets 25,000–74,999/mm^3: 70% of prior dose; (3) leukocytes < 2,000/mm^3 and platelets < 25,000/mm^3: 50% of prior dose.
- No repeat dose should be given until the leukocyte count has returned to 4,000/mm^3 and platelet count to 100,000/mm^3.
- Dose reduction required if patient has hepatic dysfunction.

Drug Preparation:
- Available in 5-mg, 20-mg, and 40-mg mitomycin vials.

- Add sterile water for injection USP in 10 mL for the 5-mg vial, 40 mL for the 20-mg vial, and 80 mL to the 40-mg vial. Shake to dissolve. If the drug does not dissolve, allow the vial to stand at room temperature until it is dissolved. Depending on vial size, dilute with sterile water to obtain concentration of 0.5 mg/mL.
- Stability: Reconstituted with sterile water for injection to a concentration of 0.5 mL/mL, drug is stable for 14 days refrigerated, and 7 days at room terperature.
- Stability of diluted drug to a concentration of 20–40 micrograms per mL, at room temperature: 0.9% sodium chloride injection= 12 hours, and in sodium lactate injection, 24 hours (see package insert).
- If heparin 1,000 units to 10,000 units in 30 mL of 0.9% sodium chloride injection is added to 5–15 mg of mitomycin, it is stable 48 hours at room temperature.

Drug Administration:
- Assess labs: do not administer drug unless leukocyte count has returned to 4,000/mm^3 and platelet count to 100,000/mm^3. See dose modificaitons for nadir counts. Assess serum creatinine and do not administer drug if serum creatinine is > 1.7 mg%.
- IV: Drug is potent vesicant. Give through the sidearm of a patent, freely running IV to avoid extravasation, which can lead to ulceration, pain, and necrosis. See *Chapter 1* introduction, *ONS Chemotherapy and Biotherapy Guidelines*, 4th edition, and consult individual hospital policy for administration of a vesicant.

Drug Interactions:
- Myelosuppressive agents: Additive toxicity if overlapping nadirs; use cautiously.

Lab Effects/Interference:
- Decreased CBC, especially WBC (neutrophils) and platelets.
- Hemolytic uremic syndrome (rare): Decreased hemoglobin, platelets, and increased creatinine.

Special Considerations:
- Warnings and Precautions:
  - *BM suppression* is common, especially thrombocytopenia and leukopenia. Monitor CBC/differential baseline and repeatedly during treatment and for at least 8 weeks following therapy. Hold drug for platelets < 100,000/mm^3, leukocyte count < 4,000/mm^3, or a progressive decline in either, and resume only when minimum levels are achieved. Myelosuppression is cumulative.
  - *Renal impairment:* Assess renal function tests and do not administer drug to patients with a serum creatinine > 1.7 mg%.
  - *Embryo-fetal toxicity*: Teach women of reproductive potential to use effective contraception to prevent pregnancy. Mothers should not breastfeed during mitomycin therapy.
  - Rarely, *hemolytic uremic syndrome* can occur (characterized by rapid fall in hemoglobin, renal failure, severe thrombocytopenia) and progress to pulmonary edema and hypotension. The risk increases as the cumulative dose exceeds 60 mg.
  - Rarely, *acute SOB and severe bronchospasm* have been reported in patients who have previously received mitomycin, or who were receiving it simultaneously, and who

were now receiving vinca alkaloids. Onset of ARDS occurred within minutes to hours after the vinca alkaloid injection.

- *ARDS:* If patient requires surgery and has received mitomycin C together with other antineoplastics, the patient is at risk for ARDS. FiO_2 should be < 50%, and fluid status should be monitored closely.

Potential Toxicities/Side Effects and the Nursing Process

I.   POTENTIAL FOR INFECTION related to MYELOSUPPRESSION

Defining Characteristics: Myelosuppression is the dose-limiting toxicity. Toxicity is delayed and cumulative. Initial nadir occurs at approximately 4–6 weeks. Usually by the third course, 50% drug modifications are necessary.

Nursing Implications: Monitor WBC, HCT, platelets prior to drug administration. Monitor patients for signs/symptoms of infection. Teach patient self-assessment. Drug dosage should be reduced or held for lower-than-normal blood values.

II.   ALTERATION IN NUTRITION, LESS THAN BODY REQUIREMENTS, related to NAUSEA, VOMITING, ANOREXIA, STOMATITIS

Defining Characteristics: Mild-to-moderate nausea and vomiting occur within 1–2 hours, lasting up to 3 days, but may be prevented by adequate premedication. Anorexia occurs commonly, and stomatitis may occur.

Nursing Implications: Premedicate with aggressive antiemetics, i.e., serotonin antagonist to prevent nausea and vomiting at least for the first treatment. Encourage small, frequent feedings of cool, bland foods and liquids. Teach patient and family member preparation of meals in advance, and encourage the use of spices when patient has little appetite. Teach patient oral assessment and oral hygiene regimen, and encourage patient to report early stomatitis.

III.   POTENTIAL FOR ACTIVITY INTOLERANCE related to FATIGUE

Defining Characteristics: Fatigue is common.

Nursing Implications: Assess baseline activity level. Teach patient to report fatigue and activity intolerance. Teach self-management strategies, including alternating rest and activity periods, as well as stress reduction.

IV.   POTENTIAL FOR IMPAIRED SKIN INTEGRITY related to DRUG EXTRAVASATION, ALOPECIA

Defining Characteristics: Extravasation of drug can cause severe tissue necrosis, erythema, burning, tissue sloughing. Delayed erythema or ulceration has been reported weeks to months after drug dose, at the injection site or distant from it, and despite the fact that there was no evidence of extravasation. Alopecia occurs frequently.

Nursing Implications: Use scrupulous IV technique to prevent extravasation of the drug. If there is doubt as to whether drug has infiltrated, treat as an infiltration, aspirate any drug in the tubing, and discontinue IV. IV line must be patent. Assess for need of venous access device early. Refer to hospital policy for management of extravasation, and see beginning of this chapter. Assess site regularly for pain, progression of erythema, induration, and evidence of necrosis. Discuss with patient hair loss, anticipated impact, and strategies to decrease distress, e.g., obtaining wig prior to hair loss.

V. POTENTIAL FOR INJURY related to HEMOLYTIC UREMIC SYNDROME

Defining Characteristics: 2% of patients may experience significant increase in creatinine unrelated to total dose or duration of therapy. Thrombotic microangiopathy may occur with anemia, thrombocytopenia. Blood transfusions may exacerbate condition. Can often be fatal.

Nursing Implications: Monitor renal function, HCT, and platelets prior to each drug dose; hold dose if serum creatinine is > 1.7 mg/dL. If renal failure occurs, hemofiltration or dialysis may be necessary. Discuss risks and benefits with physician and patient if renal insufficiency is present and blood transfusion(s) is required.

VI. POTENTIAL ALTERATION IN OXYGENATION related to INTERSTITIAL PNEUMONITIS

Defining Characteristics: Rarely, interstitial pneumonitis occurs and can be quite severe (ARDS). Signs/symptoms include nonproductive cough, dyspnea, hemoptysis, pneumonia, pulmonary infiltrates on x-ray. Incidence may be reduced by dexamethasone 20-mg IV prior to dose (Chang et al., 1986).

Nursing Implications: Assess baseline pulmonary status, and monitor prior to each drug dose. Teach patient to report dyspnea, new-onset cough, or any respiratory symptoms. Discuss abnormalities with physician, and plan for further diagnostic workup.

VII. POTENTIAL FOR INJURY related to VENO-OCCLUSIVE DISEASE OF THE LIVER AFTER BM TRANSPLANT

Defining Characteristics: Hepatic veno-occlusive disease has been reported in patients who have received mitomycin C and autologous BM transplant. Signs/symptoms are abdominal pain, hepatomegaly, and liver failure.

Nursing Implications: Assess baseline LFTs, and monitor periodically during therapy. Notify physician of any abnormalities, and discuss further diagnostic workup and management. Refer to autologous BM transplant protocol.

Drug: mitotane (Lysodren)

Class: Antihormone; adrenolytic.

Mechanism of Action: Adrenocortical suppressant with direct cytotoxic effect on mitochondria of adrenal cortical cells. Forces a drop in steroid secretion and alters the peripheral metabolism of steroids.

Metabolism: 34–45% of oral dose is absorbed from the GI tract. Metabolized partly in the liver and kidneys to a water-soluble metabolite that is then excreted in the bile and urine. Small amount of drug passes into the CSF.

Indication: In the treatment of inoperable adrenal corticoid carcinoma of both functional and nonfunctional types.

Contraindicaton: Patient who are hypersensitive to the drug.

Dosage/Range:
- Dose ranges from 2–6 g/day PO in divided doses, either 3 or 4 times a day.
- Treatment usually begins with low doses (2 g/day), and the dose is gradually increased to 9–10 g/day. If severe side effects occur, reduce the dose until the maximum tolerated dose is achieved (varies from 2–16 g/day but for most patients is 9–10 g/day).
- Treatment shuld be started in the hospital until a stable dosage regimen is achieved.
- Continue therapy as long as clinical benefit outweighs toxicity. If no clinical benefit is observed after 3 months at the maximum tolerated dose, most patients will show no response; however, 10% require longer than 3 months. Clinical effectiveness is defined as reduction in tumor mass; reduction in pain, weakness, or anorexia and reduction of signs and symptoms due to excessive steroid production.
- Reduce dose in patients with hepatic dysfunction.
- Drug should be temporarily discontinued IMMEDIATELY following shock or severe trauma, since adrenal suppression is its prime action. Exogenous steroids should be given as the depressed adrenal glands may not be able to start secreting steroids immediately.

Drug Preparation:
- None.

Drug Administration:
- Oral. Available as a 500-mg tablet. Tablets should not be crushed.
- Use safe handling precautions when handling the tablets.
- Once a stable dose has been established, teach patient self-administration of the drug, strategies to minimize toxicity, and what/when to report any changes to the provider.

Drug Interactions:
- Drug is a strong inducer of CYP3A4. Monitor patients receiving other drugs that are metabolized by CYP3A4 and may need dosage adjustment for the concomitant drug.
- Neurotoxic drugs may have additive toxicity; use cautiously.

- Warfarin: may decrease anticoagulant effect and increase in dosage requirement; monitor INR and increase dose as needed.
- Steroids: decreased steroid effect requiring increased steroid dose.
- Phenytoin, cyclophosphamide, barbiturates: assess effect and need for dose adjustment.

Lab Effects/Interference:
- None.

Special Considerations:
- Warnings and Precautions:
  - *Liver disease* other than metastatic lesions: administer drug cautiously as the metabolism of mitotane may be interefered with and drug may accumulate.
  - All possible tumor should be surgically removed from large metastatic masses before mitotane administration to minimize *possibility of infarction and hemorrhage in the tumor* due to the drug's rapid cytotoxic action.
  - *Long-term continuous administration* of high doses of mitotane may lead to brain damage and impairment of function. Assess behavior and neurological system baseline and regularly during therapy (see package insert).
  - *Adrenal insufficiency:* Assess for and institute steroid replacement in these patients (may need higher doses due to changed metabolism in exogenous steroids, e.g., mitotane).
  - Drug may cause *lethargy and somnolence;* teach patient not to operate heavy equipment or drive until the effect of the drug is known.
  - *If patient undergoes stress* (infection, trauma, shock), patient will require exogenous IV steroids.
  - *Embryo-fetal toxicity:* Teach women of reproductive potential to use effective contraception during and after mitotane treatment. Mothers should NOT breastfeed while receiving mitotane.
- Use cautiously in patients with hepatic dysfunction.

Potential Toxicities/Side Effects and the Nursing Process

I. ALTERATION IN NUTRITION, LESS THAN BODY REQUIREMENTS, related to GI SIDE EFFECTS

Defining Characteristics: Nausea and vomiting occur in 75% of patients and may be dose-limiting toxicity. Anorexia may also occur. Diarrhea occurs in 20% of patients.

Nursing Implications: Nausea and vomiting may be reduced by beginning therapy with a low dose and increasing it as tolerated. Premedicate with antiemetics to prevent nausea and vomiting; continue as needed. Encourage small, frequent meals of cool, bland foods and liquids. Inform patient that nausea and vomiting can occur; encourage patient to report onset. Encourage patient to report onset of diarrhea. Administer or teach administration of antidiarrheal medication. If diarrhea is protracted, ensure adequate hydration, monitor I/O and electrolytes, teach perineal hygiene.

II.   POTENTIAL FOR INJURY related to NEUROLOGIC TOXICITY

Defining Characteristics: Lethargy and somnolence are most common; resolve with discontinuation of therapy. Dizziness, vertigo occur in about 15% of patients. Other CNS manifestations are depression, muscle tremors, confusion, headache.

Nursing Implications: Teach the patient and family about possible neurologic toxicity; assess safety of planned activities (e.g., patient should avoid activities that require alertness). Encourage patient and family to report onset of symptoms, as they may necessitate discontinuing therapy.

III.   POTENTIAL FOR IMPAIRED SKIN INTEGRITY related to RASH

Defining Characteristics: Skin irritation or rash occurs in about 15% of patients. Sometimes resolves during treatment.

Nursing Implications: Inform patient that rash is expected and will resolve when treatment is finished. Assess skin for integrity; recommend measures to decrease irritation, if indicated.

Drug: mitoxantrone (Novantrone)

Class: Anthracenediones. Antitumor antibiotic.

Mechanism of Action: Topoisomerase II inhibitor. Inhibits both DNA and RNA synthesis regardless of the phase of cell division. Intercalates between base pairs, thus distorting DNA structure. DNA-dependent RNA synthesis and protein synthesis are also inhibited.

Metabolism: Excreted in both the bile and urine for 24–36 hours as virtually unchanged drug. Mean half-life is 5.8 hours. Peak levels achieved immediately. FDA-approved for acute nonlymphocytic leukemia in adults.

Indication: (1) For reducing neurologic disability and/or frequency of clinical relapses in patients with secondary (chronic) progressive, progressive relapsing, or worsening relapsing-remitting multiple sclerosis (MS); it is NOT indicated for treatment of patients with primary progressive MS; (2) in combination with corticosteroids as initial chemotherapy for the treatment of patients with pain related to advanced hormone-refractory prostate cancer (HRPC); (3) in combination with other approved drug(s) for the initial therapy of acute nonlymphocytic leukemia (ANLL) in adults (includes myelogenous, promyelocytic, monocytic, and erythroid acute leukemias).

Contraindications: (1) patients hypersensitive to the drug; (2) not for intrathecal use; (3) baseline ANC < 1,500 cells/mm^3 unless patient treated for acute nonlymphocytic leukemia; (3) MS patients with LVEF baseline < LLN.

Dosage/Range:
- ANLL in adults: 12 mg/m^2 IV over 5–15 minutes daily on days 1–3, in combination with cytosine arabinoside 100 mg/m^2/day days 1–7 CI for induction therapy of ANLL.
- HRPC: 12–14 mg/m^2 IV over 5–15 minutes day 1 every 21 days for prostate cancer, in combination with prednisone 5 mg PO twice a day.
- **Multiple sclerosis:** 12 mg/m^2 IV over 5–15 minutes, every 3 months, maximum lifetime dose 140 mg/m^2.
- Drug AUC is 3× greater in patients with severe hepatotoxicity. If patient has MS with severe hepatotoxicity, do not administer mitoxantrone. Otherwise cautiously administer a reduced dose and monitor closely for toxicity.

Drug Preparation:
- Available as dark-blue solution in 2-mg/mL vials: 10-mL (20-mg), 12.5-mL (25-mg), and 15-mL (30-mg) multidose vials.
- May be diluted in 5% dextrose, 0.9% sodium chloride, or 5% dextrose in 0.9% sodium chloride.
- Solution is chemically stable at room temperature for at least 48 hours.
- Intact vials should be stored at room temperature. If refrigerated, a precipitate may form. This precipitate can be redissolved when vial is warmed to room temperature.

Drug Administration:
- Assess ANC/CBC/differential. Except for ANLL, drug should not be administered if the ANC is < 1,500 cells/mm^3. Assess baseline counts, and prior to each dose, then as needed.
- ALL patients should have cardiac history/PE, ECG, and determination of LVEF (by ECHO or MUGA) baseline and repeated as needed.
- MS patients: (a) if baseline LVEF is < LLN, patient should not receive mitoxantrone; (b) reassess LVEF prior to each mitoxantrone treatment (same method) and discontinue drug if LVEF is <LLN or there is a significant decrease in LVEF during therapy; (c) maximum cumulative dose is 140 mg/m^2; (d) perform annual LVEF assessment once patient completes therapy to monitor for late cardiac toxicity.
- IV short infusion over 5–15 minutes through the sidearm of a patent, freely running infusion.
- Nonvesicant. There have been rare reports of tissue necrosis after drug infiltration.
- Never give drug SQ, IM, or intra-arterially. NOT FOR intrathecal use.
- Teach patient that s/he may experience blue-green urine for 24 hours after drug administration.

Drug Interactions:
- Myelosuppressive agents: Increased hematologic toxicity if nadir overlaps; use together cautiously.
- Incompatible with admixtures containing heparin.

Lab Effects/Interference:
- Decreased CBC.
- Decreased electrolytes.

- Increased LFTs, uric acid.
- Decreased LVEF.

Special Considerations:
- Cardiotoxicity is less than that of doxorubicin or daunorubicin, but risk increases with a cumulative dose of 140 mg/m^2 in patients without a history of prior anthracycline use, and 120 mg/m^2 if prior anthracycline treatment. Monitor LVEF, and discontinue drug if there is a 15–20% decrease in LVEF.
- Warnings and Precautions:
  - *BM suppression* may be severe, especially in patients with ANLL. Give only if ANC is ≥ 1,500 cells/mm^3 (except for ANLL). Monitor CBC/differential closely and modify dose as needed. Laboratory and supportive services must be available for frequent monitoring of hematologic and chemistries, with fast results turnaround. Ajunctive therapies as needed must be readily available such as blood transfusion, antibiotics, and close assessment during nadir period if patient becomes infected.
  - *Cardiotoxicity (CHF) may be fatal*, and may occur during therapy or months to years after last dose. Risk increases with cumulative mitoxantrone dose and may occur with or without cardiac risk factors. Risk increases with history of CV disease, RT to the mediastinal/pericardial area, prior drug therapy with anthracyclines or anthracenediones, or concurrent use with other cardiotoxic drugs. Risk was 2.6% for patients up to a cumulative dose of 140 mg/m^2.
    - Assess for cardiac signs and symptoms at each visit (H+P) and assess ECG results prior to start of drug therapy.
    - Assess results of baseline LVEF (use same test throughout, either ECHO or MUGA).
    - MS patients: see package insert for ongoing evaluation of LVEF.
  - *Secondary leukemias* (AML) have occurred in patients with MS as well as patients with cancer receiving mitoxantrone.
  - *Drug must NEVER be administered SQ, IM, intra-arterially, or intrathecally.*
  - *Embryo-fetal toxicity:* Teach women of reproductive potential to use effective contraception to prevent pregnancy. Nursing mothers must NOT breastfeed while receiving mitoxantrone as drug is excreted in breast milk.

Potential Toxicities/Side Effects and the Nursing Process

I. POTENTIAL FOR INJURY related to BM DEPRESSION

Defining Characteristics: Potent BM depression; nadir 9–10 days. Granulo–cytopenia is usually the dose-limiting toxicity, and toxicity may be cumulative. Thrombocytopenia uncommon, but can be severe when it occurs. Hypersensitivity has been reported occasionally with hypotension, urticaria, dyspnea, rashes.

Nursing Implications: Monitor WBC, HCT, platelets prior to drug administration. Instruct patient in self-assessment for signs/symptoms of infection. Drug dosage should be reduced or held for lower-than-normal blood values. Instruct patient in self-assessment of signs/symptoms of bleeding. Prior to drug administration, obtain baseline vital signs. Observe for signs/symptoms of allergic reaction. Subjective signs/symptoms: generalized itching, dizziness. Objective signs/symptoms: flushed appearance (angioedema of face, neck, eyelids, hands, feet), localized or generalized urticaria. Document incident. Discuss with physician desensitization for future dose versus drug discontinuance.

II. POTENTIAL FOR ALTERATION IN CARDIAC OUTPUT related to CARDIOTOXICITY

Defining Characteristics: CHF with decreased LVEF occurs in about 3% of patients. Increased cardiotoxicity with cumulative dose greater than 180 mg/m^2; cumulative lifetime dose must be reduced if patient has had previous anthracycline therapy.

Nursing Implications: Assess for signs/symptoms of cardiomyopathy. Assess quality and regularity of heartbeat. Baseline EKG. Instruct patient to report dyspnea, shortness of breath, swelling of extremities, orthopnea. Discuss frequency of GBPS with physician.

III. ALTERATION IN NUTRITION, LESS THAN BODY REQUIREMENTS, related to NAUSEA/VOMITING AND MUCOSITIS

Defining Characteristics: Nausea and vomiting are typically not severe and occur in 30% of patients. Mucositis is more common with prolonged dosing; occurs in 5% of patients, usually within 1 week of therapy.

Nursing Implications: Premedicate with antiemetic and continue prophylactically for 24 hours to prevent nausea and vomiting, at least for the first treatment. Encourage small, frequent feedings of cool, bland foods and liquids. Teach patient oral assessment and oral hygiene regimen. Encourage patient to report early stomatitis.

IV. POTENTIAL FOR IMPAIRED SKIN INTEGRITY related to ALOPECIA AND EXTRAVASATION

Defining Characteristics: Alopecia is mild to moderate; occurs in 20% of patients. Drug is not a vesicant. Stains skin blue without ulcers. There have been rare reports of tissue necrosis following extravasation.

Nursing Implications: Discuss with patient impact of hair loss. Suggest wig as appropriate prior to actual hair loss. Explore with patient response to actual hair loss and plan strategies to minimize distress, e.g., wig, scarf, cap. Use careful technique during venipuncture and IV administration. Administer drug through freely flowing IV, constantly monitoring IV site and patient response.

V.   POTENTIAL FOR ANXIETY related to ABNORMAL COLOR OF URINE SCLERA

Defining Characteristics: Urine will be green-blue for 24 hours. Sclera may become discolored blue.

Nursing Implications: Explain to patient changes that may occur with therapy and that they are only temporary.

VI.   POTENTIAL SEXUAL DYSFUNCTION related to DRUG EFFECT

Defining Characteristics: Drug is mutagenic and teratogenic.

Nursing Implications: As appropriate, explore with patient and partner issues of reproductive and sexuality patterns and impact chemotherapy may have. Discuss strategies to preserve sexual and reproductive health (e.g., sperm banking, contraception).

Drug: nelarabine (Arranon)

Class: Nucleoside metabolic inhibitor (Antimetabolite).

Mechanism of Action: Drug is a pro-drug of deoxyguanosine analogue of ara-G (9-α-arabinofuranosylguanine), a cytotoxic agent. It is demethylated and converted into the active 5'-triphosphate ara-GTP. Ara-GTP accumulates in leukemic blasts and enters DNA where it causes inhibition of DNA synthesis and cell death. It may have other mechanisms as well.

Metabolism: Nelarabine and ara-G are rapidly eliminated from the plasma with a half-life of about 30 minutes and 3 hours, respectively. Both are extensively distributed throughout the body, and are not substantially bound to plasma proteins. Nelarabine and ara-G are partially excreted via the kidneys, 5–10% and 20–30%, respectively.

Indication: Treatment of patients with T-cell acute lymphoblastic leukemia and T-cell lymphoblastic lymphoma whose disease has not responded to or has relapsed following treatment with at least 2 chemotherapy regimens. This use is based on induction of CRs; randomized clinical trials demonstrating increased survival or other clinical benefit have not been done.

Dosage/Range:
- *Adult:* 1,500-mg/m^2 IV over 2 hours on days 1, 3, 5, repeated every 3 weeks.
- *Pediatric:* 650-mg/m^2 IV over 1 hour on days 1, 2, 3, 4, 5, repeated every 3 weeks.
- Implement measures as ordered to prevent hyperuricemia and TLS.
- Renal or hepatic impairment: Closely monitor patients with moderate or severe renal impairment, and patients with severe hepatic impairment (total bilirubin 3 × ULN), for toxicities.

- Duration of treatment has not been determined; in clinical trials, treatment continued until disease progression, unacceptable toxicity, or patient became a candidate for a BM transplant.

Dose Modifications:
- Delay dose administration for hematologic toxicity.
- Discontinue treatment for grade 2 or higher neurologic reactions.
- No dose adjustment needed for patients with CrCl $\geq$ 50 mL/min.

Drug Preparation:
- Drug available in 250-mg vials, 5 mg/mL.
- Appropriate (undiluted) dose of nelarabine should be transferred into polyvinyl chloride (PVC) infusion bags or glass containers, and administered as a 2-hour infusion in adults and a 1-hour infusion in pediatric patients. Drug is stable for 8 hours at up to 30°C in PVC infusion bags. Drug should not be used in patients with creatinine clearance of < 50 mL/minute. Drug should be discontinued for grade 2 or higher neurotoxicity (CTCAE), and dosage should be delayed for other toxicity, including hematologic toxicity.

Drug Administration:
- Assess baseline CBC/differential, BUN, serum creatinine, full electrolyte, and chemistries.
- Assess baseline neurological status and monitor closely during treatment.
- Administer diluted drug over 2 hours for adult, and 1 hour for pediatric patients.
- Implement TLS precautions as ordered (e.g., hydration, uric acid lowering medication, assess electrolytes, and monitor closely during treatment).

Drug Interactions:
- Adenosine deaminase inhibitors (e.g., pentostatin): do not coadminster.

Lab Effects/Interference:
- *Pediatric patients:* serum transaminases, bilirubin, creatinine; $\downarrow$ serum potassium, albumin, calcium, glucose, magnesium.
- *Adults:* glucose, AST.
- *Both:* anemia, neutropenia, thrombocytopenia.

Special Considerations:
- The most common ($\geq$20%) side effects in (1) adults are anemia, thrombocytopenia, neutropenia, nausea, vomiting, constipation, fatigue, pyrexia, cough, and dyspnea; (2) pediatric patients are anemia, neutropenia, thrombocytopenia, and leukopenia. Most common (> 10%) adverse neurologic reactions were (1) adult: somnolence, dizziness, peripheral neurologic disorders, hypoesthesia, headache, and paresthesia; (2) pediatrics: headache and peripheral neurologic disorders.
- Warnings and Precautions:
  - *Severe neurologic reactions* have occurred and are dose limiting. Common signs of neurological toxicity include somnolence, headache, dysesthesias, dizziness, neuropathy (sensory and motor), cerebellar disturbances, tremor, confusion, convulsions, ataxia, paresthesia, and hypoesthesia. Severe neurotoxicity includes coma, status

epilepticus, craniospinal demyelination, or ascending neuropathy similar in presentation to Guillain–Barré syndrome. Median time to onset of first event is 5 days from start of first infusion, with a median duration of 6 days. Patients at risk for these adverse effects include patients who have previously received or are concurrently receiving intrathecal chemotherapy, or previously had craniospinal RT. Monitor patient frequently for signs/symptoms of neurologic toxicity and for at least 24 hours after completion of treatment with nelarabine. Drug should be discontinued for grade 2 or higher neurotoxicity, and patient should receive appropriate supportive care.

- *Hematologic reactions:* Neutropenia, thrombocytopenia, anemia commonly occur. Assess baseline CBC/differential and monitor closely during therapy.
- *Tumor Lysis Syndrome*: Patients should receive IV hydration as ordered for the prevention and management of hyperuricemia in patients at risk for TLS (high tumor burden, first treatment). Discuss TLS prevention plan with physician/NP/PA, including the use of medication to reduce uric acid levels in patients at risk.
- *Vaccinations:* Do not administer live vaccines to immunocompromised patients.
- *Effects on ability to drive and use machines:* Patients may experience somnolence during treatment and for several days after making it dangerous to drive or operated machinery if not fully awake. Teach patients not to drive or operate machinery that may be hazardous until somnolence has resolved.
- *Embryo-fetal toxicity*: Drug is a potent teratogen. Teach women of reproductive potential to use effective contraception to prevent pregnancy while receiving nelarabine. Teach male patients with female sexual partners of reproductive potential to use effective contraception during and for at least 3 months after last dose of nelarabine. If drug is used during pregnancy or if patient becomes pregnant while taking the drug, the patient should be warned of potential hazard to the fetus. Nursing mothers should not breastfeed while receiving the drug.
- Drug is a potent antineoplastic with potentially significant neurotoxicity, which is dose-limiting, characterized by somnolence, confusion, convulsions, ataxia, paresthesias, and hypoesthesia. Severe neurotoxicity includes coma, status epilepticus, craniospinal demyelination, or ascending neuropathy (like Guillain–Barré syndrome).

Potential Toxicities/Side Effects and the Nursing Process

I.   POTENTIAL FOR INJURY related to TLS

Defining Characteristics: May develop with initial therapy if patient has a large tumor burden; results from rapid lysis of tumor cells. This usually begins 1–5 days after initiation of therapy, and causes elevations in serum uric acid, potassium, phosphorus, BUN, creatinine.

Nursing Implications: If this is induction therapy for a patient with acute leukemia or high tumor burden, expect medical orders to include IV hydration at 150 mL/hour with urine alkalinization, allopurinol prophylaxis, strict monitoring of I/O, daily weight, and total body fluid balance determination. Monitor baseline and daily serum BUN, creatinine, potassium, phosphorus, uric acid, and calcium. Monitor for renal, cardiac, neuromuscular signs/symptoms of TLS.

II. INFECTION AND BLEEDING related to BM DEPRESSION

Defining Characteristics: In pediatric patients, BM depression is very common anemia 95% (45% grade 3), neutropenia 94% (17% grade 3), and thrombocytopenia 88% (27% grade 3). In adults, anemia affects 99% of patients (20% grade 3), thrombocytopenia 86% (37% grade 3), and neutropenia 81% (14% grade 3), and 12% had febrile neutropenia.

Nursing Implications: Assess WBC, neutrophil, and platelet count, and discuss any abnormalities with physician prior to drug administration; assess for signs/symptoms of skin infections (all mucosal surfaces, body orifices) and bleeding; instruct patient in signs/ symptoms of infection and bleeding, as well as to report them or come to the emergency room. Teach patient self-care measures to minimize risk of infection and bleeding, including avoidance of OTC aspirin-containing medications. Assess patient's Hgb/HCT and signs/symptoms of fatigue; teach patient self-assessment and to alternate rest and activity as needed.

III. POTENTIAL FOR INJURY related to NEUROTOXICITY

Defining Characteristics: Neurologic events occurred in 64% of patients. In pediatric studies, most common events were headache (17%), PN (12%, sensory and/or motor), somnolence (7%), hypoesthesia (6%), seizures (6%, including grand mal and status epilepticus), paresthesia (4%), tremor (4%). Rare grades 3–4 events were status epilepticus (1 fatal), hypertonia, and 3rd nerve paralysis. In adults, somnolence was most common (23%), followed by dizziness (21%), PN (21%, including motor and/or sensory), hypoesthesia (17%), headache (15%), paresthesia (15%), ataxia (9%), depressed level of consciousness (6%), tremor (5%), blurred vision (4%), amnesia (3%). Grade 3 events in adults were rare and included aphasia, convulsion, hemiparesis, loss of consciousness, while grade 4 events included cerebral hemorrhage, coma, intracranial hemorrhage, leukoencephalopathy.

Nursing Implications: Assess baseline neurologic status, including sedation level, blurred vision, presence of numbness or tingling, difficulty with fine motor movement, such as buttoning clothes, unsteadiness when walking, or tripping. Teach patient that serious neurologic side effects may occur. Pediatric: extreme sleepiness, seizures, coma, PN, weakness, and paralysis. Adult: sleepiness, dizziness, PN, rarely seizure, aphasia, hemiparesis, loss of consciousness. Teach patient to notify the provider/go to ED immediately if they occur. Teach adult patient not to drive or operate heavy machinery if sleepiness occurs.

IV. ALTERED NUTRITION, LESS THAN BODY REQUIREMENTS, related to NAUSEA AND VOMITING, STOMATITIS, DIARRHEA, CONSTIPATION, HEPATOTOXICITY

Defining Characteristics: Nausea and vomiting are common in adults, but less common in children (10%). In adults, nausea affects 41%, vomiting 22%, diarrhea 22%, and constipation 21%. In adults, 8% of patients developed stomatitis. Nausea and vomiting can be successfully prevented with combination antiemetics. Rarely dysgeusia can occur. Drug should be used cautiously in patients with impaired hepatic function, and the patient monitored closely for toxicity.

Nursing Implications: Premedicate with antiemetics and revise regimen based on prior response to treatment. If patient develops nausea/vomiting, assess fluid and electrolyte balance and the need for replacements. Assess oral mucosa prior to chemotherapy, and teach patient oral hygiene regimen and self-assessment; encourage patient to report diarrhea, discuss use of antidiarrheals with physician, and teach self-care PRN. Since patients become neutropenic, all mucosal surfaces need to be assessed for infection, and patients must be taught scrupulous perineal hygiene. Monitor LFTs prior to, during, and after therapy.

V. ALTERATION IN COMFORT related to FATIGUE, FEVER, ASTHENIA, EDEMA, PAIN, RIGORS, MYALGIAS

Defining Characteristics: Fatigue affects 50% of adults, and can be severe in 10%. Pyrexia affects 23% and asthenia 17%. Peripheral edema affects 15%, pain 11%, rigors 8%, myalgias 13%, arthralgias 9%, muscular weakness 8%.

Nursing Implications: Assess comfort level/symptoms experienced at baseline and prior to each dose, then prior to each cycle. Teach patient to alternate rest and activity periods to manage or prevent fatigue. Teach patient to report fevers (> 100.5°F) and rigors right away, and to come to the clinic or ED. Teach patient symptomatic management of myalgias, arthralgias (e.g., local application of heat, acetaminophen if permitted).

Drug: nilutamide (Nilandron)

Class: Antiandrogen.

Mechanism of Action: Irreversibly binds to androgen receptors and inhibits androgen binding. Unlike steroidal antiandrogens, nilutamide binds specifically to adrenal androgen receptor in the nucleus of androgen-sensitive prostate cancer cells. It does not interact with progestin or glucocorticoid receptors.

Metabolism: Following oral administration, nilutamide is rapidly and completely absorbed, with 80% plasma protein binding. Steady-state levels are achieved after about 2 weeks. Though the drug is extensively metabolized in the liver, it appears that the parent drug is the active compound. The drug is excreted in the urine as metabolites. Renal impairment does not alter the properties of the drug.

Indication: In combination with surgical castration for the treatment of metastatic prostate cancer, Stage D2.

Contraindications: Patients with:
• Severe hepatic impairment (baseline hepatic enzymes should be evaluated prior to treatment).

- Severe respiratory insufficiency.
- Hypersensitivity to nilutamide or any component of this preparation.

Dosage/Range:
- 300 mg/day orally for 30 days and then 150 mg/day.

Drug Preparation/Administration:
- Oral. Start the day of or day after surgical castration for maximal benefit.

Drug Interactions:
- Has been shown to inhibit the liver cytochrome P450 isoenzymes and may decrease the metabolism of compounds requiring these systems. Monitor patients closely for toxicity if the patient is also taking phenytoin or theophylline (Chu & DeVita, 2016).
- Warfarin: nilutamide may decrease warfarin metabolism, resulting in increased antico- agulation; monitor INR closely and the dose accordingly.
- Alcohol: rare disulfiram reaction (flushing, throbbing in head and neck, headache, dys- pnea, nausea/vomiting, sweating, chest pain, palpitation, hypotension, vertigo, uneasi- ness, and confusion).

Lab Effects/Interference:
- Causes increased liver enzymes (see below); may cause increased serum glucose.

Special Considerations:
- Most common adverse effects: Delay in ocular adaption when going from a lighted area to a darker area (alleviated by wearing tinted glasses), HTN, nausea, constipation, hot flushes, increased ALT/AST, dizziness, dyspnea, abnormal vision, UTI.
- Warnings and Precautions:
  - *Hepatitis* has been described, with rare cases of death or hospitalization related to severe liver injury reported. Monitor LFTs baseline and during therapy. If transami- nases rise to greater than 2–3 times the upper limit of normal, therapy should be discontinued.
  - *Interstitial pneumonitis* has been reported in 2% of patients. Monitor PFTs and CXR baseline and during therapy. If symptoms occur, or if interstitial pneumonitis sus- pected (CXR or 20–25% decrease in DLCO and FVC), nilutamide should be discon- tinued. Teach patient to report any new or worsening SOB. Post-marketing reports have described patients with pulmonary fibrosis, which led to hospitalization and death.
  - Rarely, *aplastic anemia* may occur.
  - *Embryo-fetal toxicity*: Do not administer to pregnant women.

Potential Toxicities/Side Effects and the Nursing Process

I. ALTERATION IN NUTRITION, LESS THAN BODY REQUIREMENTS, related to NAUSEA, ANOREXIA, CONSTIPATION, CHANGES IN LFTs

Defining Characteristics: Nausea, anorexia occur infrequently. Constipation and in- creased LFTs are common, affecting 10–50% of patients.

Nursing Implications: Teach patient to report occurrence of loss of appetite or nausea. Encourage small, frequent feedings and consider antiemetic if necessary. Teach the patient to monitor bowel status and to eat foods high in roughage and prunes, to hydrate well, and to take stool softeners as needed to prevent constipation. Monitor baseline and during treatment. Discuss change in treatment if AST, ALT increase by 2–3 times ULN.

II.   ALTERATION IN CARDIAC OUTPUT related to HYPERTENSION, ANGINA

Defining Characteristics: Angina occurs in 2% of patients; unclear whether increased incidence of hypertension (9%) due to drug alone.

Nursing Implications: Instruct patient in signs and symptoms of angina, and to report to physician if they occur. Monitor BP on follow-up visits.

III.   ALTERATION IN COMFORT related to DIZZINESS, HOT FLASHES, DYSPNEA, VISUAL CHANGES

Defining Characteristics: Hot flashes occur in 28% of patients and are the most common side effect. Dyspnea is rare but is related to interstitial pneumonitis, a serious side effect of the drug; if it occurs, it is usually during the first 3 months of treatment. Patients of Asian heritage are at risk. Many patients experience impaired adaptation to light and, less commonly, changes in color vision.

Nursing Implications: Inform patient that side effects may occur and to report dyspnea immediately to physician, as therapy must be discontinued if it occurs. Baseline chest x-ray and PFTs should be done prior to treatment; if interstitial pneumonitis is suspected, the drug should be discontinued. Patients should be discouraged from driving at night because of visual changes and may find it helpful to wear tinted glasses during the day.

Drug: omacetaxine mepesuccinate for injection (Synribo)

Class: Protein synthesis inhibitor.

Mechanism of Action: Not fully understood, but protein synthesis inhibition is independent of Bcr-Abl binding. The drug is a semisynthetic derivative from cephalotaxine, an extract from the *Cephalotaxus* leaf. Drug reduces the oncoprotein levels of Bcr-Abl, as well as Mcl-1, a member of the anti-apoptosis Bcl-2 family.

Metabolism: After subcutaneous injection, peak serum level is reached in 30 minutes, and mean half-life is about 6 hours. Drug plasma protein binding is $\leq 50\%$. Drug metabolism is primarily hydrolysis into 49-DMHHT without microsomal activity, and while elimination route is unknown, $< 15\%$ of drug is excreted unchanged in the urine.

Indication: Treatment of adult patients with chronic or accelerated phase CML with resistance and/or intolerance to two or more tyrosine kinase inhibitors.

Dosage/Range:
- **Induction dose:** 1.25 mg/m^2 administered by subcutaneous injection twice daily $\times$ 14 consecutive days in a 28-day cycle; assess weekly CBC/differential.
- **Maintenance dose:** 1.25 mg/m^2 administered by subcutaneous injection twice daily $\times$ 7 consecutive days in a 28-day cycle; assess weekly CBC/differential during initial maintenance, then every 2 weeks or as clinically indicated.

Dose Modifications:
- Monitor CBC weekly during inducation and initial maintenance cycles, then every 2 weeks and as clinically indicated.
- **Hematologic:** Grade 4 neutropenia (ANC < 500 cells/mm^3) or grade 3 thrombocytopenia (platelets < 50,000 cells/mm^3) during a cycle, delay the next cycle until ANC $\geq$ 1,000 cells/mm^3 and platelet count is $\geq$ 50,000 cells/mm^3. Also, reduce the number of treatment days by 2 the next cycle, e.g., to 5 days.
- **Other (nonhematologic) toxicity:** Interrupt or delay drug until toxicity is resolved, and manage symptomatically.

Drug Preparation:
- Drug is available in a single-use vial containing 3.5 mg of omacetaxine mepesuccinate as a preservative-free, lypholized powder.
- Reconstitute with 1 mL of 0.9% Soduim Chloride Injection USP; gently swirl until solution is clear (should take < 1 minute). The final concentration is 3.5 mg/mL omacetaxine mepesuccinate.
- Inspect solution as it should be clear and colorless, and if particulate matter or discoloration is found, do not use.
- Use within 12 hours of reconstitution when stored at room temperature [20–25°C (68–77°F)], and within 6 days if refrigerated at 2–8°C (36–46°F). Protect from light.

Drug Administration:
- Teach patient to
  - Self-administer drug subcutaneously twice daily, document location, and rotate sites, or teach caregiver.
  - Have weekly CBC/differential as above during induction and initial maintenance cycles. After initial maintenance cycles, monitor CBC/differential every 2 weeks or as clinically indicated.
  - Prepare drug, handle and store drug properly, and how to clean up accidental spillage of hazardous drug.
  - Hazardous waste disposal and spill management. (Discard used needle, syringe, vials in biohazard container; do not recap or clip used needle, do not place used equipment in household trash or recycling bin; if drug accidentally spills, keep using protective eye wear and gloves, wipe spilled liquid with absorbent pad, and wash the area with soap and water. Then place pad and gloves in biohazard container and wash hands thoroughly. Return the biohazard container to the clinic or pharmacy for final disposal.)
- Ensure patient has necessary supplies for home administration: reconstituted omacetaxine mepesuccinate for injection in prefilled syringes with capped needle for subcutaneous injection (filled with patient-specific dose), protective eyewear, gloves, appropriate

biohazard container, absorbent pad(s) for placement of administrative materials and for accidental spillage, alcohol swabs, gauze pads, ice packs or cooler for transportation of reconstituted omacetaxine mepesuccinate for injection syringes.

- If a patient or caregiver cannot be trained for some reason, the drug should be administered by a healthcare professional.
- Drug dose may need to be reduced for adverse effects, e.g., neutropenia or thrombocytopenia. Signs and symptoms of infection, bleeding, fatigue, and report them right away.

Drug Interactions: Drug is a P-glycoprotein (P-gp) substrate in vitro, but does not inhibit P-gp mediated efflux of loperamide, e.g., clinically.

Lab Effects/Interference:
- Decreased WBC, neutrophil, lymphocyte, platelet, red blood cell counts.
- Increased blood glucose.
- Increased ALT, bilirubin, creatinine, and uric acid.

Special Considerations:
Most common adverse reactions in patients with CML-chronic and accelerated phases (frequency $\geq 20\%$): thrombocytopenia, anemia, neutropenia, diarrhea, nausea, fatigue, asthenia, injection-site reaction, pyrexia, infection, and lymphopenia.

Warnings and Precautions:
- *Myelosuppression:* Severe and fatal thrombocytopenia, neutropenia, and anemia. Monitor hematologic parameters weekly during induction and initial maintenance, then every 2 weeks unless more frequently as indicated. Teach patient measures to avoid infection and to self-assess and report immediately signs/symptoms of infection.
- *Bleeding:* Monitor platelet count with CBC weekly during induction and initial maintenance, then every 2 weeks or more frequently if clinically indicated. Severe thrombocytopenia and increased risk of hemorrhage may occur; fatal cerebral hemorrhage, and severe, nonfatal GI hemorrhage has occurred. Teach patient measures to prevent bleeding, to self-assess, and report immediately signs/symptoms of bleeding. Teach patient not to take ASA, NSAIDs when platelet count is $<50,000/\text{mm}^3$.
- *Hyperglycemia:* Drug can induce glucose intolerance with grades 3 or 4 hyperglycemia in 11% of patients. Hyperosmolar, nonketotic hyperglycemia may rarely occur. Monitor blood glucose levels frequently, especially in patients with diabetes or risk factors for diabetes. Avoid using drug in patients with poorly controlled diabetes mellitus, waiting until diabetes is well controlled.
- *Embryo-fetal toxicity:* Counsel women of reproductive potential to use effective contraceptives to avoid becoming pregnant, as drug is fetotoxic.

Potential Toxicities/Side Effects and the Nursing Process

I.   POTENTIAL FOR INFECTION, BLEEDING AND FATIGUE related to BM SUPPRESSION

Defining Characteristics: Grades 3–4 thrombocytopenia occurred in 85% and 88% of patients respectively, while neutropenia occurred in 81% and 71%. Grades 3–4 anemia

TREATMENT

occurred in 62% and 80%, respectively. Three percent of patients died from myelosuppression. Fatalities from cerebrovascular hemorrhage occurred in 2% of patients.

Nursing Implications: Monitor CBC/differential and platelet count weekly during induction and initial maintenance, then every 2 weeks during later maintenance, or as clinically indicated. Teach patients to report right away signs/symptoms of infection (e.g., fever $\geq$ 100.4°F, sore throat, sputum production, difficulty breathing, painful urination) or bleeding. Teach patient to avoid OTC preparations containing aspirin, NSAIDs, or other drugs that increase the potential for bleeding.

II. ALTERATION IN NUTRITION, POTENTIAL related to DIARRHEA, NAUSEA, CONSTIPATION, VOMITING, HYPERGLYCEMIA

Defining Characteristics: Diarrhea occurred in 41% of patients, nausea 35%, constipation 14%, vomiting 12%, while hyperglycemia occurred in 10–15% and hypoglycemia 6–8%. Hyperosmolar nonketotic hyperglycemia may rarely occur.

Nursing Implications: Monitor blood glucose levels baseline and frequently during therapy, especially in patients with diabetes or risk factors for diabetes. Teach patient dietary as well as pharmacologic control of diarrhea, nausea, vomiting, or constipation.

III. ALTERATION IN COMFORT, POTENTIAL related to INJECTION-SITE REACTIONS, ARTHRALGIA, FEVER, FATIGUE, ASTHENIA, PERIPHERAL EDEMA

Defining Characteristics: Injection-site reactions occurred in 35%, fatigue in 29% (5% grades 3–4), pyrexia 25%, asthenia 23%, peripheral edema 16%, arthralgia 19%, and headache 20%.

Nursing Implications: Teach patient that these reactions may occur, and to manage them symptomatically. Assess prior injection site at each visit and rotate sites. Discuss more aggressive symptom management strategies as needed with physician or NP/PA.

Drug: oxaliplatin (Eloxatin)

Class: Alkylating agent (third-generation platinum analogue).

Mechanism of Action: Blocks DNA replication and transcription into RNA by causing intrastrand and interstrand crosslinks in DNA strands. It is cell cycle nonspecific. DNA mismatch repair enzymes are unable to repair these errors, and the cell dies. Drug may also bind to proteins in the cell nucleus and cytoplasm to further injure the cell.

Metabolism: Heavily bound (98%) to plasma proteins; following 2-hour drug infusion, 15% of drug is found in plasma and 85% in tissue or excreted in the urine; 40% of the drug binds irreversibly in red blood cells within 2–5 hours of administration.

The drug concentrates in the kidney and spleen, and is excreted as platinum-containing metabolites.

Indication: In combination with infusional 5-fluorouracil (5-FU)/leucovorin for
- Adjuvant treatment of stage III colon cancer in patients who have undergone complete resection of the primary tumor.
- Treatment of advanced colorectal cancer (CRC).

Contraindication: Known allergy to oxaliplatin or other platinum compounds.

Dosage/Range:
- FOLFOX4 every 2 weeks.
- *Day 1:* Oxaliplatin 85-mg/m^2 IV infusion in 250–500 mL D$_5$W and leucovorin 200-mg/m^2 IV infusion in D$_5$W, each over 2 hours simultaneously in separate bags using a Y-line, followed by 5-FU 400 mg/m^2 IVB over 2–4 minutes, followed by 5-FU 600 mg/m^2 in 500 mL D$_5$W as a 22-hour CI.
- *Day 2:* Leucovorin 200-mg/m^2 IV infusion over 2 hours, followed by 5-FU 400 mg/m^2 IVB over 2–4 minutes, followed by 5-FU 600 mg/m^2 in 500 mL D$_5$W as a 22-hour CI.

Dose Reduction:
Reduce the dose of oxaliplatin to 75 mg/m^2 in patients receiving **adjuvant therapy** or 65 mg/m^2 in patients with advanced CRC if:
- Persistent grade 2 neurotoxicity that does not resolve.
- After recovery from grades 3–4 GI toxicities (despite prophylactic treatment) or grade 4 neutropenia or grades 3–4 thrombocytopenia. Delay next dose until neutrophils $\geq$ 1.5×10^9/L and platelets $\geq 75 \times 10^9$/L.
- For patients with severe renal impairment (CrCl < 30 mL/min), initial recommended dose is 65 mg/m^2.
- Discontinue oxaliplatin if there are persistent grade 3 neurosensory events.

Drug Preparation:
- Available in single-use 50 mg or 100 mg oxaliplatin vials, in a preservative-free, aqueous solution (5 mg/mL) concentration.
- Further dilute in 250–500 mL of 5% dextrose injection. Never prepare a final dilution with a sodium chloride solution, or other chloride-containing solutions.
- DO NOT use chloride-containing solutions or sodium chloride.
- DO NOT use aluminum needles or infusion sets containing aluminum.

Drug Administration:
- Assess ANC/CBC, electrolytes, renal function and signs/symptoms of neuropathy, or other side effects prior to treatment.
- Administer IV infusion over 2 or more hours through central line, preferably.
- May administer over 4 hours to reduce incidence of acute neuropathy symptoms.

Drug Interactions:
- Incompatible with 5-FU and other highly alkaline solutions.
- Incompatible with chloride-containing solutions (forms precipitate).

- Physically incompatible with diazepam (forms precipitate).
- Incompatible with cefepime, cefoperazone, dantrolene.
- Nephrotoxic drugs: renal excretion of oxaliplatin could be reduced with increased serum levels of oxaliplatin.
- 5-FU: At high doses (130 mg/m^2), increases plasma levels of 5-FU by 20%.
- Bevacizumab: increased response rate and survival in metastatic CRC when combined with FOLFOX.

Lab Effects/Interference:
- Decreased CBC, especially WBC and platelets.
- Elevated LFTs.

Special Considerations:
- Most common adverse reactions ($\geq$40%) were peripheral sensory neuropathy, neutropenia, thrombocytopenia, anemea, nausea, increase in serum transaminases and alkaline phosphatase, diarrhea, emesis, fatigue, and stomatitis.
- Warnings and Precautions:
  - *Allergic reactions*: monitor for development of rash, urticarial, erythema, pruritis, bronchospasm, and hypotension
    - Anaphylaxis may rarely happen (incidence grades 3–4 is 2–3% in colon cancer patients). It can evolve within minutes of starting the infusion in ANY cycle. Emergency equipment should be close by, and a provider who can prescribe emergency medications (e.g., epinephrine, corticosteroids, and antihistamines) when the drug is given. Rechallenge is contraindicated.
    - Delayed hypersensitivity reactions (HSRs) may occur at the 7th cycle or so, similar to carboplatin.
  - *Sensory neuropathy*: PN (sensory) is dose-limiting toxicity (DLT). Two distinct neurotoxicity syndromes: acute, lasting less than 14 days, and chronic persistent PN similar to cisplatin, which is the DLT. Reduce dose or discontinue if necessary for chronic or persistent neuropathy.
    - Acute, reversible, primarily peripheral sensory neuropathy: early onset within hours or 1–2 days of dosing, that resolves within 14 days, and frequently occurs with subsequent dosing.
      - Symptoms may be precipitated by exposure to cold temperature or cold objects and include transient paresthesia, dysesthesia, hypoesthesia, jaw spasm, abnormal tongue sensation, dysarthria, eye pain, and a feeling of chest pressure. Incidence is 56% over time.
      - Acute syndrome of pharyngolaryngeal dysesthesia: incidence 1–2% grades 3–4. Characterized by subjective sensations of dysphagia or dysnea, without laryngospasm or bronchospasm (no stridor or wheezing). Avoid ice (5-FU mucositis prophylalxis) during oxaliplatin infusion as cold temperature may exacerbate acute neurological symptoms.
    - *Persistent (>14 days), primarily sensory neuropathy*, usually characterized by paresthesias, dysesthesias, hypoesthesias, and may include deficits in proprioceptions

which can interfere with ADLs (e.g., writing, buttoning, swallowing, and difficulty walking from impaired proprioception).

- Incidence 48% of study patients also receiving 5-FU/LV. Most patients progressed to grade 3 from grades 1–2. Symptoms may improve after oxaliplatin discontinued.
- Adjuvant Grading: Grade 1 = mild paresthesias, loss of DTRs; grade 2 = mild or moderate objective sensory loss, moderate paresthesias; grade 3 = severe objective sensory loss or paresthesias that interfere with function.
- Advanced CRC patient Grading: Grade 1 = resolved and did not interfere with functioning; grade 2 = interferred with function but not daily activities; grade 3 = pain or functional impairment that interferes with daily activities; grade 34 = persistent impairment that is disabling or life-threatening.

- *Reversible posterior leukoencephalopathy syndrome* (RPLS or PRES) rarely occurs (< 0.1%). Signs and symptoms include headache, altered mental functioning, seizures, abnormal vision from blurriness to blindness, may be associated with HTN. Diagnosis made by MRI.
- *Severe neutropenia:* Grades 3–4 occurred in 41–44% of patients receiving oxaliplatin/ 5-FU/LV vs 5% with 5-FU/LV alone. Complications may include sepsis and septic shock. Delay oxaliplatin until ANC ≥ 1,500 × 10^9/L. Hold drug for sepsis.
- *Pulmonary toxicity:* Rarely occurs (< 0.1%). If patient develops unexplained pulmonary symptoms such as nonproductive cough, dyspnea, crackles, or pulmonary infiltrates on imaging, discontinue oxaliplatin until interstitial lung disease or pulmonary fibrosis are excluded.
- *Hepatotoxicity:* In adjuvant clinical trials, incidence of elevation of transaminases was 57%, and of alkaline phosphatase, was 42%. Monitor LFTs. Rarely, veno-occlusive disease of the liver occurs.
- *Cardiovascular toxicity*: QTc prolongation and ventricular arrhythmias have occurred, including fatal torsades de pointes (see introduction *Chapter 3* for discussion). Correct hypokalemia and/or hypomagnesemia prior to starting oxaliplatin, and monitor and keep WNL during therapy. ECG monitoring is recommended if therapy is started in patients with CHF, bradyarrhythmias, receiving drugs known to prolong the QT interval (e.g., serotonin receptor antagonist antiemetics), and electrolyte abnormalities. AVOID oxaliplatin in patients with congenital long QT syndrome.
- *Rhabdomyolysis:* Discontinue oxaliplatin if this occyrs.
- *Embryo-fetal toxicity:* Women of reproductive potential should be apprised of the potential harm to the fetus. Teach women of reproductive potential to use effective contraception during oxaliplatin therapy.
- *Recommended laboratory tests*: CBC/differential, blood chemistries (including ALT, AST, bilirubin, creatinine) prior to each cycle. If the patient is also receiving warfarin, due to the interaction with 5-FU, the patient should have frequent monitoring and dose adjustment based on INR.

Potential Toxicities/Side Effects and the Nursing Process

I. SENSORY/PERCEPTUAL ALTERATIONS related to ACUTE SENSORY NEUROPATHY

Defining Characteristics: Acute neurotoxicity appears related to ion channelopathy. It is common, affecting many patients. It is temporary, and occurs during, within hours of, or up to 14 days following oxaliplatin administration. Often precipitated by exposure to cold and characterized by dysesthesias, transient paresthesias, or hypesthesias of the hands, feet, perioral area, and throat. Acute events can be minimized by slower infusion of oxaliplatin, increasing the infusion time from 2 to 6 hours, as this lowers peak serum levels. Studies are ongoing to determine whether glutamine can prevent these, and also studies exploring 1 g calcium/1 g magnesium IVB prior to and after the oxaliplatin infusion. Most frightening for patients is pharyngolaryngeal dysesthesia characterized by a sensation of discomfort or tightness in the back of the throat and inability to breathe. It may be accompanied by jaw pain, and is often precipitated by exposure to cold. Cramping of muscles, such as fisted hand, occurs due to prolonged action potential. Rarely, dysarthria (difficulty articulating words), eye pain, and a feeling of chest pressure can occur.

Nursing Implications: Teach patient that acute neurotoxicity can occur but is not dangerous. Teach patient to minimize occurrence by avoiding exposure to cold during and for 3–5 days after drug administration, such as wearing scarves over the face in the winter, warm gloves if going outside or reaching into the refrigerator or freezer. Teach patient to avoid exposure to cold and cold liquids, if lip paresthesias present. Teach patient to use straw if drinking cool liquids. Teach patient to avoid cold air conditioning in the car or home during the summer. Teach patient how to reassure themselves they are breathing if pharyngolaryngeal dysesthesia occurs (cup hands in front of mouth or hold mirror so that breath can be felt or seen on the mirror). Teach patient to warm area, such as fingers or toes, if they become cold; for example, running warm water over affected area may help resolve the feeling. Do not use ice chips before and during 5-FU infusions to prevent stomatitis.

II. SENSORY/PERCEPTUAL ALTERATIONS related to PERSISTENT, CHRONIC SENSORY NEUROPATHY

Defining Characteristics: Peripheral neurotoxicity affects some patients, and risk increases as cumulative doses > 800 mg/m^2. Symptoms include paresthesias, dysesthesias, hypoesthesias, in a stocking-and-glove distribution, and altered proprioception (knowing where body parts are in relation to the whole). This can become manifested as difficulty writing, walking, swallowing, and buttoning buttons. IF allowed to progress, motor pathways will become involved. When drug is stopped, symptoms may get worse, but in general, symptoms resolve in 4–6 months in many patients. Ongoing studies in patients with advanced CRC are looking at temporarily stopping the drug when grades 2 or 3 neurotoxicity occurs, continuing the 5-FU/LV as maintenance, or stopping chemotherapy drugs and resuming after 12 cycles of maintenance or when disease progression occurs. This has shown to reduce the incidence and intensity of PN (OPTIMOX trial). In the MOSAIC trial, an adjuvant trial, although some patients developed grade 3 neurotoxicity after 6 months, most patients had complete resolution of grade 3 toxicity (de Gramont et al., 2003).

Nursing Implications: Assess baseline neurologic status (sensory and motor); instruct patient to report signs/symptoms. Identify patients at risk: those with preexisting neuropathies (e.g., ethanol- and diabetes mellitus–related). Assess sensory and motor function, and monitor over time prior to each treatment, such as picking up a dime from a smooth/flat surface, buttoning shirt, and writing name. Specifically, assess whether function is impaired, as this necessitates a dose reduction. If the patient is unable to perform ADLs, this necessitates drug cessation. In either case, discuss with physician, as complete neurologic exam should be performed before treatment decision as to drug holiday or discontinuance based on grade of neurotoxicity. Assess impact on patient and quality of life.

III. POTENTIAL FOR INFECTION, BLEEDING, AND FATIGUE related to BM DEPRESSION

Defining Characteristics: Mild leukopenia, and mild to moderate thrombocytopenia occur. Febrile neutropenia is very uncommon. Anemia is common.

Nursing Implications: Assess baseline CBC, WBC, differential, and platelet count prior to chemotherapy, as well as signs/symptoms of infection, bleeding, or fatigue. Teach patient signs/symptoms of infection or bleeding, and to report these immediately. Teach patient self-care measures to minimize risk of infection and bleeding. This includes avoidance of crowds, proximity to people with infections, and OTC aspirin-containing medications. Teach energy-conserving techniques and ways to minimize fatigue, such as gentle exercise as tolerated.

IV. ALTERATION IN NUTRITION, LESS THAN BODY REQUIREMENTS, related to NAUSEA AND VOMITING, DIARRHEA, HEPATOTOXICITY

Defining Characteristics: Nausea and vomiting occur commonly and are severe if patient does not receive aggressive antiemesis. Diarrhea commonly occurs in combination with 5-FU/LV. Hepatotoxicity may occur manifested by increases in transaminases and alkaline phosphatase, whereas increases in bilirubin may be related to the concomitant 5-FU/LV, as the incidence was similar in the group receiving FOLFOX compared with patients receiving only 5-FU/LV. Liver biopsies showed peliosis, nodular regenerative hyperplasia, or sinusoidal alterations, perisinusoidal fibrosis, and veno-occlusive lesions.

Nursing Implications: Premedicate patient with aggressive combination antiemetics: serotonin antagonist (granisetron or ondansetron) and dexamethasone. Encourage small, frequent feedings of cool, bland foods. Instruct patient to report nausea, and teach self-administration of antiemetics if patient is receiving drug as an outpatient. Teach the patient to report diarrhea that does not respond to usual antidiarrheal medicine and diet modification so that more aggressive management can be instituted and prevent dehydration and electrolyte imbalance. If LFTs are significantly elevated, the drug should be stopped, and hepatic dysfunction, unexplainable by liver metastases, should be evaluated.

V. POTENTIAL FOR INJURY related to DELAYED HYPERSENSITIVITY OR ANAPHYLAXIS REACTIONS (often after 8–12 cycles of therapy)

Defining Characteristics: Delayed hypersensitivity may occur after 10–12 cycles of therapy with symptoms ranging from local rash or vague symptoms such as new onset of vomiting, to anaphylaxis and severe hypersensitivity (characterized by dyspnea, hypotension requiring treatment, angioedema, and generalized urticaria). Anecdotal reports show successful desensitization using carboplatin desensitization regimens.

Nursing Implications: Assess baseline VS and mental status prior to drug administration. If patient has symptoms, discuss premedication using corticosteroid, antihistamine, and H$_2$ antagonist as ordered. Monitor VS every 15 minutes, and remain with patient during first 15 minutes of drug infusion. Stop drug if signs/symptoms of hypersensitivity or anaphylaxis occur, and notify physician. *Subjective symptoms:* generalized itching, nausea, chest tightness, crampy abdominal pain, difficulty speaking, anxiety, agitation, sense of impending doom, uneasiness, desire to urinate/defecate, dizziness, chills. *Objective signs:* flushed appearance; angioedema of face, neck, eyelids, hands, feet; localized or generalized urticaria; respiratory distress with or without wheezing; hypotension; cyanosis. Provide fluid resuscitation for hypotension per MD order, and maintain a patent airway.

Drug: paclitaxel (Taxol)

Class: Taxoid, mitotic inhibitor.

Mechanism of Action: Promotes early microtubule assembly and prevents depolymerization necessary for normal mitosis and cell division, resulting in cell death in G$_2$ and M phases of the cell cycle.

Metabolism: Extensively protein-bound, resulting in an initial sharp decline in serum level. Metabolized primarily by hepatic hydroxylation using the P450 enzyme system. Metabolites are excreted in the bile. Less than 10% of the intact drug is excreted in the urine.

Indication: (1) First-line and subsequent treatment of patients with advanced ovarian cancer; as first line, in combination with cisplatin; (2) adjuvant treatment of node-positive breast cancer patients, administered sequentially to standard doxorubicin-containing combination chemotherapy, demonstrated effect in ER/PR negative tumors (Hospira, 2018); (3) treatment of patients with metastatic breast cancer after failure of combination chemotherapy, or relapse within 6 months of adjuvant chemotherapy (which included an anthracycline unless clinically contraindicated; (4) in combination with cisplatin, for the first-line treatment of NSCLC in patients who are not candidates for potentially curative surgery and/or RT; (5) second-line treatment of patients with AIDS-related Kaposi's sarcoma (KS).

Contraindication: (1) Patients with a history of hypersensitvity reactions to paclitaxel injection or other drugs formulated in polyoxyl 35 castor oil, NF; (2) patients with solid tumors having a baseline ANC < 1,500 cells/mm^3 or in patients with AIDS-related KS with a baseline ANC < 1,000 cells/mm^3.

Dosage/Range:
- Dose-reduce if hepatic dysfunction and monitor patients closely during therapy. Do not administer drug if patient has severe hepatic impairment.
- Breast cancer:
  - **Adjuvant treatment** of patients with LN-positive breast cancer, administered sequentially to standard doxorubicin-containing combination chemotherapy (benefit at 30 months for ER/PR negative tumors). Adjuvant node-positive breast cancer: 175 mg/m^2 IV over 3 hours, every 3 weeks, for 4 courses, administered sequentially to doxorubicin-containing combination chemotherapy.
  - **Advanced breast** cancer after failure of combination therapy for metastatic disease or relapse within 6 months of adjuvant therapy (containing an anthracycline except if not tolerated): 175 mg/m^2 IV over 3 hours, every 3 weeks; if tumor overexpresses HER2 protein, given in combination with trastuzumab.
- **Ovarian cancer:** First-line (in combination with cisplatin) and subsequent therapy for patients with advanced ovarian cancer.
- Previously *untreated* ovarian cancer: 135 mg/m^2 IV over 24 hours, followed by cisplatin 75 mg/m^2 every 3 weeks or paclitaxel 175 mg IV over 3 hours followed by cisplatin 75 mg/m^2 q 3 weeks.
- Previously treated ovarian cancer: 135-mg or 175-mg/m^2 IV over 3 hours every 3 weeks.
- **Nonsmall-cell lung cancer:** First-line treatment (in combination with cisplatin) in patients who are not candidates for surgical or radiation curative therapy: non–small-cell lung cancer (NSCLC): 135-mg/m^2 IV over 24 hours, followed by cisplatin 75 mg/m^2 repeated every 3 weeks.
- **AIDS-related Kaposi's sarcoma:** Second-line treatment: 135-mg/m^2 IV over 3 hours, repeated every 3 weeks, or 100-mg/m^2 IV over 3 hours, repeated every 2 weeks (dose intensity of 45–50 mg/m^2 per week).

Other doses:
- Less myelosuppression with 3-hour vs 24-hour infusion.
- Weekly schedule: 80–100-mg/m^2 IV weekly × 3 weeks, 1 week rest, cycle repeated every 4 weeks (Chu & DeVita, 2016).
- **Dose Modification:** see package insert for dose reductions for hepatic impairment.

Drug Preparation:
- Drug is poorly soluble in water, so is formulated using polyoxyethylated castor oil (Cremophor EL) and dehydrated alcohol.
- Further dilute in 5% dextrose, 0.9% sodium chloride, 5% dextrose and 0.9% sodium chloride injection USP, or 5% dextrose in Ringer's Injection to a final concentration of 0.3 mg/mL to 1.2 mg/mL. Solutions are physically and chemically stable for up to

27 hours at ambient temperature (approximately 25°C) and room lighting conditions. Inspect container for particulate matter and discoloration prior to administration.

Drug Administration:

- Glass or polyolefin containers MUST BE USED, and polyethylene-lined administration sets must be used. DO NOT USE polyvinylchloride containers or tubing since the polyoxyethylated castor oil (Cremophor EL) causes leaching of plasticizer diethylhexylphthalate (DEHP) from polyvinylchloride plastic into the infusion fluid. Do not use Chemo Dispensing Pin device or similar devices since the device may cause the stopper to collapse, sacrificing sterility of the paclitaxel solution.
- Inline filter of < 0.22 microns MUST be used.
- Assess vital signs baseline, and remain with patient during first 15 minutes of infusion. Monitor vital signs every 15 minutes or per hospital policy.
- **Assess CBC before each treatment:**
  - Patients with solid tumors: absolute neutrophil count (ANC) must be at least 1,500 cells/mm^3 and platelet count at least 100,000/mm^3; patients with AIDS-related Kaposi's sarcoma: ANC at least 1,000 cells/mm^3.
  - If patient has severe neutropenia (<500 cells/mm^3 for 7 days or more): dose reduce 20% for all subsequent treatments when counts recover to >1,500 neutrophils. Discuss with provider secondary prophylaxis with G-CSF.
- Assess LFTs. Assess patient for signs/symptoms of PN (e.g., numbness and tingling (paresthesias) in a stocking-glove distribution, weakness).

Premedication with corticosteroids:

- Solid tumors: Dexamethasone 20 mg PO 12 and 6 hours prior to treatment. Administer diphenhydramine 50 mg and H$_2$ antagonist (cimetidine 300 mg, famotidine 20 mg, or ranitidine 50 mg) IV 30–60 minutes prior to treatment.
- AIDS-related Kaposi's sarcoma: Dexamethasone 10 mg PO 12 and 6 hours prior to treatment; administer diphenhydramine 50 mg and H$_2$ antagonist (cimetidine 300 mg, famotidine 20 mg, or ranitidine 50 mg) IV 30–60 minutes prior to treatment.
- Administer paclitaxel IV over 3 hours via infusion controller. Monitor vital signs every 15 min × 4 (first hour).
- DO NOT give drug as a bolus, as this may cause bronchospasm and hypotension.
- Assess for hypersensitivity reaction (HSR, most often occurs during first 10 minutes of infusion) and for cardiovascular effects (arrhythmia, hypotension).
- Keep resuscitation equipment nearby. Ensure physician/NP/PA with prescriptive authority locally available to area where patient is being treated in case patient has an HSR.
- Administer paclitaxel first when given in combination with cisplatin or carboplatin. There is increased cytotoxic activity when given in this sequence.
- Teach patients who have had > 6 courses of weekly paclitaxel to avoid sun exposure on skin, finger and toe nails, as they are at increased risk for developing onycholysis which is not seen with q 3 week dosing (Chu & DeVita, 2016).

Drug Interactions:

- Cisplatin: Myelosuppression is more severe when cisplatin is administered prior to paclitaxel (due to 33% reduction in paclitaxel clearance from the plasma). Therefore, paclitaxel must be given prior to cisplatin when drugs are administered sequentially.

- Carboplatin: Possible increased cytotoxicity when given *after* taxol. Also, combination of paclitaxel and carboplatin results in less thrombocytopenia than would be expected from dose of carboplatin alone (etiology of platelet-sparing effect unknown).
- Paclitaxel is metabolized by P450 cytochrome isoenzymes CYP2C8 and CYP3A4. Potential interactions may occur, including antiretroviral protease inhibitors.
  - Use together cautiously with other drugs metabolized by this system. CYP2C8 and CYP3A4 inducers: carbamazine, phenytoin, phenobarbital, rifampin: may decrease serum level of paclitaxel and decrease effect.
  - CYP2C8 and CYP3A4 inhibitors: ethinyl estradiol, fluconazole, ketoconazole, sulfonamides, testosterone, tretinoin, ciprofloxacin, clarithromycin, doxycycline, erythromycin, grapefruit juice, St. John's wort, isoniazid, protease inhibitors, verapamil: may increase serum level of paclitaxel with increased risk of toxicity. Use together cautiously, if at all.
  - CYP3A4 substrates (e.g., midazolam, busipirone, felodipine, lovastatin, eletriptan, sildenafil, simvastatin, triazolam): use together cautiously.
  - CYP2C8 substrates (e.g., repaglinide, rosiglitazone), inhibitors (gemfibrozil) and inducers (e.g., rifampin): use together cautiously.
- Doxorubicin and liposomal doxorubicin: May have increased doxorubicin serum levels, with increased incidence of neutropenia and stomatitis when paclitaxel is administered prior to doxorubicin (due to 30–35% decrease in doxorubicin clearance, possibly due to competition for biliary excretion of both agents). Therefore, doxorubicin should be given prior to paclitaxel or sequentially rather than concomitantly.
- Doxorubicin: Increased risk of cardiotoxicity when given in combination with paclitaxel, with sharp increase in risk of congestive heart failure once cumulative dose of doxorubicin is > 380 mg/m^2 (Minotti et al., 2001). Give sequentially rather than concomitantly.
- Cyclophosphamide: Increased myelosuppression when cyclophosphamide given before paclitaxel; give sequentially rather than concomitantly.
- Patients with conduction system abnormalities and taking beta blockers, calcium-channel blockers, or digoxin; Additive bradycardia may occur; assess/monitor patients closely.
- Immunosuppressive agents, other antineoplastic agents: Additive immunosuppression may occur; assess toxicity and patient response closely.
- Use cautiously in patients with: history of diabetes mellitus, chronic alcoholism, prior history of known neurotoxic agents (e.g., cisplatin), previous history of ischemic heart disease, MI within the preceeding 6 months.

Lab Effects/Interference:
- Decreased CBC.
- Increased LFTs.

Special Considerations:
- Warnings and Precautions:
  - *Anaphylaxis and severe hypersensitivity reactions (HSRs)* characterized by dyspnea and hypotension requiring treatment, angioedema, and generalized urticarial occurred

in 2–4% of patients in clinical trials. Pretreat with corticosteroids, diphenhydramine, and H2 antagonists. However, fatal reactions have occurred despite premedication. If the patient has a severe HSR to paclitaxel, do not rechallenge.

- *BM suppression*: Do not treat patients with solid tumors who have baseline neutrophil counts < 1,500 cells/mm^3, and if patient has AIDS-related Kaposi's sarcoma, do not treat if baseline ANC is < 1,000 cells/mm^3. Monitor CBC/differential frequently during therapy. Patients should not receive subsequent cycles until ANC has recovered to > 1,500 cells/mm^3 (>1,000 cells/mm^3 for patients with KS), and platelet count > 100,000 cells/mm^3.

- *Conduction abnormalities*: Rarely, (incidence < 1%) occurs, but in some cases, a pacemaker may need to be implanted. If patient developes significant conduction abnormality during paclitaxel infusion, implement medical orders and provide continuous cardiac monitoring and ensure that cardiac monitoring occurs during subsequent therapy with paclitaxel and cardiac monitoring.

- *Embryo-fetal toxicity*: Teach women of reproductive potential to use effective contraception to avoid pregnancy while receiving paclitaxel. Mothers should not breastfeed while receiving the drug as the drug may be excreted in breast milk.

- PN: common occurrence, but severe PN is unusual and requires a 20% dose reduction for all subsequent courses.

- Hepatotoxicity: Myelotoxicity may be exacerbated in patients with serum total bilirubin > 2 × ULN. Use extreme caution when treating these patients and reduce dose (see package insert).

- Injection-site reactions: if extravasation occurs, reactions are usually mild (erythema, tenderness, skin discoloration, swelling at site). Recurrence of skin reactions at site of a previous reaction can occur. Closely monitor infusion and avoid extravasation.

- Drug has radiosensitizing effects.

- Drug is embryotoxic; avoid use in pregnancy. Women of childbearing age should use effective contraception.

- Drug may be excreted in breast milk, so breastfeeding should be avoided during drug therapy.

- Dose reductions: 20% dose reduction if severe neuropathy or severe neutropenia (ANC < 500/mm^3 for 7 or more days) develop and/or consider addition of CSF support with next cycle; 25–50% dose reduction if hepatic dysfunction (hepatic metastasis > 2 cm) occurs (Chabner & Longo, 2001); 50% or more dose reduction for moderate or severe hyperbilirubinemia or significantly increased serum transferase levels, with dose of paclitaxel not exceeding 50–75-mg/m^2 IV over 24 hours, or 75–100-mg/m^2 IV over 3 hours; if AST > 2 times upper limit of normal, patient dose should not exceed 50-mg/m^2 IV over 24 hours.

- One-hour infusion of paclitaxel as well as weekly dosing regimens are being studied/used. Lower doses, e.g., 80–100-mg/m^2 IV over 1 hour weekly × 3 with 1 week off per cycle, weekly × 6 with 2 weeks off per cycle, or weekly × 12 weeks, appear to inhibit angiogenesis, and allow for increased dose density.

Potential Toxicities/Side Effects and the Nursing Process

I.   POTENTIAL FOR INJURY related to HYPERSENSITIVITY OR ANAPHYLAXIS REACTIONS

Defining Characteristics: During clinical trials, infusion reactions occured in 20–40% of patients (e.g., generalized skinrash, flushing, erythema, hypotension, dyspnea, and/or bronchospasm), usually within the first 2–3 minutes, but generally within the first 10 minutes, The incidence of infusion reactions is markedly reduced with premedication (Chu & DeVita, 2016). Anaphylaxis and severe hypersensitivity reaction (HSR) occur in 2–4% (characterized by dyspnea, hypotension requiring treatment, angioedema, and generalized urticaria). Reaction is to Cremophor in paclitaxel preparation. Signs/symptoms include tachycardia, wheezing, hypotension, facial edema; incidence of supraventricular tachycardia with hypotension and chest pain occurs in 1–2%. Patients who have severe hypersensitivity reaction should not be rechallenged with drug. Those who have less severe reactions have received 24 hours of corticosteroid prophylaxis, and have been successfully rechallenged with drug infused at a slower rate.

Nursing Implications: Assess baseline VS and mental status prior to drug administration. Ensure that patient has taken dexamethasone premedication, and administer diphenhydramine and H_2 antagonist as ordered. Monitor VS every 15 minutes, and remain with patient during first 15 minutes of drug infusion as most reactions occur during the first 10 minutes. Continue to monitor VS q 15 minutes for the remainder of the first infusion hour. Stop drug if cardiac arrhythmia (irregular apical pulse), hypotension, or hypertension occur, and discuss continuance of infusion with physician. Recall signs/symptoms of anaphylaxis, and if these occur, stop drug immediately and notify physician. *Subjective symptoms:* generalized itching, nausea, chest tightness, crampy abdominal pain, difficulty speaking, anxiety, agitation, sense of impending doom, uneasiness, desire to urinate/defecate, dizziness, chills. *Objective signs:* flushed appearance; angioedema of face, neck, eyelids, hands, feet; localized or generalized urticaria; respiratory distress with or without wheezing; hypotension; cyanosis. Review standing orders or nursing procedure for patient management of anaphylaxis, and be prepared to stop drug immediately if signs/symptoms occur, keep IV line open with 0.9% sodium chloride, notify physician, monitor VS, and administer ordered medications, which may include epinephrine 1:1,000, hydrocortisone sodium succinate, and diphenhydramine. Teach patient the potential of a hypersensitivity or anaphylactic reaction and to immediately report any unusual symptoms.

II.   POTENTIAL FOR INFECTION AND BLEEDING related to BM DEPRESSION

Defining Characteristics: Neutropenia may be severe, especially when drug is administered via 24-hour infusion. Neutropenia is also more severe when cisplatin precedes paclitaxel in sequential administration, as it reduces paclitaxel clearance by 33%. Neutropenia is also more pronounced in patients who have received prior radiotherapy. Nadir is 7–11 days after dose with recovery in 1 week. Neutropenia is dose dependent, with severe neutropenia

(ANC < 500/mm^3) occurring in 47–67% of patients. Anemia occurs frequently, but throm-bocytopenia is uncommon.

Nursing Implications: Assess baseline CBC, WBC, differential, and platelet count prior to chemotherapy, as well as signs/symptoms of infection or bleeding. Teach patient the signs/symptoms of infection or bleeding, and to report these immediately, and teach patient self-care measures to minimize risk of infection and bleeding. This includes avoidance of crowds, proximity to people with infections, and OTC aspirin-containing medications. Administer paclitaxel PRIOR to cisplatin or carboplatin when either is given in combination with paclitaxel. Teach patient self-administration of G-CSF as ordered to prevent severe neutropenia. Transfuse red blood cells and platelets per physician order.

III.   SENSORY/PERCEPTUAL ALTERATIONS related to SENSORY NEUROPATHY

Defining Characteristics: Frequency and incidence is dose dependent but appears not to be influenced by infusion duration. Overall incidence is 60%, with 3% severe neuropathy in women with breast or ovarian cancer treated with single-agent paclitaxel, but severe neuropathy occurred in 8–13% of patients with NSCLC who also received cisplatin. Onset related to cumulative dose, with incidence after first course 27% and remainder occurring after 2–10 courses. Sensory symptoms usually resolve after 2 or more months following paclitaxel discontinuance. Sensory alterations are paresthesias in a glove-and-stocking distribution, and numbness. There may be a symmetrical loss of sensation, vibration, proprioception, temperature, and pinprick. Sensory and motor neuropathy may occur in patients receiving both paclitaxel and cisplatin. There is an increased risk for motor and autonomic dysfunction in patients with neuropathy from diabetes mellitus or alcohol ingestion prior to treatment with paclitaxel. Arthralgias and myalgias affect 60% of patients, and begin 2–3 days after treatment; they resolve in a few days; may be ameliorated by low-dose dexamethasone.

Nursing Implications: Assess baseline neurologic status. Instruct patient to report signs/symptoms of pins-and-needles sensation, numbness, pain, increased discomfort with certain sensations, especially in the extremities, or motor weakness. Identify patients at risk: those with history of cisplatin use or with preexisting neuropathies (ethanol- and diabetes mellitus–related). Assess sensory and motor function prior to each treatment, and if abnormality found, assess impact on patient function, safety, independence, and quality of life. Test patient's ability to button a shirt or pick up a dime from a flat surface. If severely impacting safety or quality of life, discuss with patient and physician drug reduction (20%) or discontinuance or use of cytoprotective agent. Teach self-care strategies, including maintaining safety when walking, getting up, taking bath, or washing dishes, and discuss inability to sense temperature and the need to keep extremities warm in cold weather. See NCI Common Toxicity Criteria Adverse Effects, *Appendix II:* grade 3 motor = objective weakness, interfering with ADLs; grade 3 sensory = sensory loss or paresthesia interfering with ADLs; grade 4 motor = paralysis; grade 4 sensory = permanent sensory loss that interferes with function.

IV.   ALTERATION IN SKIN INTEGRITY related to ALOPECIA, ONYCHOLYSIS

Defining Characteristics: Complete alopecia occurs in most patients and is reversible. Onycholysis may occur in patients receiving weekly paclitaxel, and risk increases after the sixth course.

Nursing Implications: Discuss potential impact of hair loss prior to drug administration. Discuss coping strategies and plan to minimize body-image distortion (e.g., wig, scarf, cap). Assess patient for signs/symptoms of hair loss. Assess patient's response and use of coping strategies, and help patient to build on effective strategies. If the patient is receiving weekly paclitaxel, teach fingernail care (keep clean and well manicured).

V.   ALTERATION IN NUTRITION, LESS THAN BODY REQUIREMENTS, related to NAUSEA AND VOMITING, DIARRHEA, STOMATITIS, HEPATOTOXICITY

Defining Characteristics: Nausea and vomiting occur commonly in 52% of patients and are mild and preventable with antiemetics. Diarrhea occurs in 38% of patients and is mild. Stomatitis occurs in 31% and is mild, appears to be dose- and schedule-dependent, and is more common with 24-hour infusions than 3-hour infusions. Mild increase in LFTs may occur (7% bilirubin, 22% alk phos, 19% AST). Rarely, hepatic necrosis and hepatic encephalopathy leading to death have been reported. If severe hepatic dysfunction occurs, paclitaxel dose should be reduced (see Special Considerations section).

Nursing Implications: Premedicate patient with antiemetic (either serotonin antagonist or dopamine antagonist). Encourage small, frequent meals of cool, bland foods. Instruct patient to report nausea, and teach self-administration of antiemetics if receiving drug as an outpatient. If nausea/vomiting occur and is severe, assess for signs/symptoms of fluid/electrolyte imbalance. Encourage patient to report onset of diarrhea and to self-administer antidiarrheal medications. Assess baseline oral mucous membranes. Teach patient oral assessment and to report any alterations. Assess LFTs prior to drug administration and periodically during treatment.

VI.   POTENTIAL ALTERATION IN CIRCULATION related to HYPOTENSION, ARRHYTHMIA

Defining Characteristics: Hypotension during first 3 hours of infusion in 12% of patients, and transient, asymptomatic bradycardia in 30% of patients have been reported; most often patients did not require intervention. Significant cardiovascular events (syncope, rhythm abnormalities, hypertension, and venous thrombosis) occurred in 1% of patients receiving single-agent paclitaxel, but the incidence was 12–13% in patients with NSCLC receiving cisplatin as well. Of those patients with normal baseline ECGs at the beginning of paclitaxel therapy, 14% of patients developed an abnormal ECG tracing (nonspecific repolarization abnormalities, sinus bradycardia, sinus tachycardia, premature beats). Whether or not the patient received prior anthracycline therapy did not influence these events. Prior anthracycline therapy did influence the rare incidence of CHF. Rarely, patients developed myocardial infarction, atrial fibrillation, and supraventricular tachycardia. For patients receiving doxorubicin in combination with paclitaxel, there is increased risk of CHF once the cumulative dose of doxorubicin is >380 mg/m^2 (Gianni et al., 1998). Severe conduction abnormalities have been described in <1% of patients, and required pacemaker insertion in some patients. The drug should be used cautiously in patients with coronary artery disease or prior myocardial infarction within past 6 months, as well as in patients with a history of arrhythmia who are being treated with beta blockers, calcium-channel blockers, or digoxin.

Nursing Implications: Assess baseline cardiac status, history, and risk for development of CHF. Closely monitor patient during paclitaxel infusion, especially if patient has history of hypertension, or is on cardiac medications (see Drug Interactions section). Teach patient to report any dyspnea, SOB, chest pain, or heart palpitations, or any unusual feeling. If any abnormalities occur, stop infusion as appropriate and discuss further management with physician. If patient is receiving doxorubicin and paclitaxel, discuss with physician stopping combination therapy when cumulative doxorubicin dose is 340–380 mg/m^2, and continuing paclitaxel as a single agent, as this does not increase risk of CHF (Gianni et al., 1998). If the patient develops significant conduction abnormalities, discuss medical management with physician, and expect that patient will have cardiac monitoring during subsequent paclitaxel therapy.

VII. ALTERATION IN COMFORT related to FATIGUE, ARTHRALGIAS AND MYALGIAS

Defining Characteristics: Fatigue occurs commonly, and arthralgias and myalgias affect about 44% of all patients, with 8% experiencing severe symptoms. Arthralgias and myalgias commonly occurred 2–3 days after the drug was given, and resolved within a few days.

Nursing Implications: Teach patient that fatigue may occur, and ways to minimize exertion and energy expenditure by alternating rest and activity, and organizing chores so that they are done as efficiently as possible. Arthralgias and myalgias may be troublesome, and can be managed with NSAIDs, application of warmth, and other comfort measures. Some patients report that swimming is helpful in minimizing discomfort. Studies of gabapentin, glutamine, and steroids have been disappointing. Opioids may be needed if severe.

Drug: paclitaxel protein-bound particles for injectable suspension (albumin-bound), nab-paclitaxel [Abraxane]

Class: Microtubule inhibitor. Drug (Abraxane) is paclitaxel that is formulated so that paclitaxel is bound in albumin (protein) nanoparticles; it is a mitotic inhibitor, like generic paclitaxel.

Metabolism: Paclitaxel protein-bound particles for injectable suspension (Abraxane) are highly protein bound (89–99%). The half-life is approximately 27 hours. Paclitaxel protein-bound particles for injectable suspension (Abraxane) is metabolized in the liver, primarily by CYP2C8 into 6-alpha-hydroxypaclitaxel, and by CYP3A4 into two minor metabolites. Fecal excretion was approximately 20% of the administered drug, and little drug was excreted in the urine ($< 1\%$) in clinical trials.

Indications: Indicated for the treatment of patients with
- (1) Metastatic Breast Cancer (MBC) after failure of combination chemotherapy for MBC or relapse within 6 months of adjuvant chemotherapy. Prior therapy should have included an anthracycline unless clinically contraindicated;
- (2) NSCLC, locally advanced or metastatic, as first line therapy, in combination with carboplatin, in patients who are not candidates for curative surgery or radiation therapy;
- (3) Metastatic adenocarcinoma of the pancreas as first-line treatment in combination with gemcitabine.
- (4) Atelzolizumab (Tecentriq) in combination for the treatment of patients with metastatic triple negative breast cancer (TNBC) [accelerated FDA approval].

Contraindications: (1) ANC $< 1,500$ cells/mm^3; (2) severe hypersensitivity reaction to Abraxane; (3) metastatic adenocarcinoma of the pancrease with moderate to severe hepatic impairment; (4) total bilirubin $> 5 \times$ ULN or AST $> 10 \times$ ULN regardless of indication as these patients have not been studied.

Dosage/Range:
- Paclitaxel protein-bound particles for injectable suspension (albumin-bound) is different from generic paclitaxel and cannot be substituted for it.
- Metastatic Breast Cancer (MBC) after failure of combination chemotherapy, or relapse within 6 months of adjuvant chemotherapy: 260-mg/m^2 IV infusion over 30 minutes every 3 weeks.
- NSCLC: 100-mg/m^2 IV infusion over 30 min on days 1, 8, 15 of each 21-day cycle, together with carboplatin given IV on day 1 of each 21-day cycle immediately after paclitaxel protein-bound particles for injectable suspension is given.
- Adenocarcinoma of the pancreas: 125-mg/m2 IV infusion over 30–40 minutes on days 1, 8, and 15 of each 28-day cycle. Administer gemcitabine immediately after paclitaxel protein-bound particles for injectable suspension (Abraxane) is given on days 1, 8, and 15 of each 28-day cycle.
- FDA approvals with nab-paclitaxel:
  - metastatic TNBC: Nab-paclitaxel 100 mg/m^2 IV infusion on days 1, 8, 15 with atelzolizumab 840 mg IV given on days 1 and 15 in a 28-day cycle. Give the atezolizumab first followed by nab-paclitaxel when given on the same day (Genentech, 2019).
  - metastatic squamous NSCLC: Pembrolizumab (Keytruda) in combination with carboplatin and either paclitaxel or nab-paclitaxel for first line treatment.
- Do not administer drug to patients with baseline ANC $< 1,500$ cells/mm^3. Assess CBC/differential frequently, including prior to day 1 for MBC patients, and days 1, 8, 15 for NSCLC and pancreatic cancer patients.
- Do not administer drug to patients with AST $> 10 \times$ ULN or bilirubin $> 5 \times$ ULN; do not administer drug to patients with metastatic adenocarcinoma of the pancreas who have moderate to severe hepatic impairment.

- Dose reductions or discontinuation may be needed for severe hematologic, neurologic, cutaneous, or GI toxicities (see package insert).
- Reduce starting dose in patients (other than patients with pancreatic cancer) with moderate to severe hepatic impairment (see package insert).
- No dose adjustment needed for patients with mild hepatic impairment (total BR $\leq$ 1.5 $\times$ ULN, and AST $\leq$ 10 $\times$ ULN.
  - Moderate impairment: AST $<$ 10 $\times$ ULN and bilirubin $>$1.5 to $\leq$ 3 $\times$ ULN: MBC = 200 mg/m^2; NSCLC = 80 mg/m^2; Pancreatic: not recommended
  - Severe: AST $>$ 10 $\times$ ULN and bilirubin $>$ 3 to 5 $\times$ ULN: MBC = 200 mg/m^2; NSCLC = 80 mg/m^2; pancreatic = not recommended
  - Hold drug if AST $>$ 10 $\times$ ULN or bilirubin $>$ 5 $\times$ ULN.
  - See package insert.
- Dose reduction or interruption may be needed based on severe hematologic, neurologic, cutaneous, or gastrointestinal toxicities (see package insert).

Drug Preparation:

- This drug is protein (albumin)-bound paclitaxel, and it must be distinguished from other, nonprotein-bound paclitaxel formulations, such as generic paclitaxel. Do not substitute for or with other paclitaxel formulations.
- Available in single-use 100-mg lyophilized powder vials. The vial should be reconstituted with 20 mL of 0.9% sodium chloride, USP prior to IV infusion (see package insert for specific instructions). See package insert for preparation instructions and stability information. Solution will be milky white and homogenous without visible particles. If particles or settling occurs, gently invert the reconstituted vial to ensure complete resuspension before use. Discard any unused portion.
- Calculate the exact total dosing volume of 5-mg/mL suspension ordered for the patient, and slowly withdraw the calculated amount. Inject appropriate amount into an empty, sterile IV bag (plasticized polyvinylchloride (PVC) containers, PVC- or non-PVC-type IV bag). If medical devices containing silicone oil as a lubricant to reconstitute and administer the drug may result in the formation of proteinaceous strands.
- Visually inspect the reconstituted suspension in the IV bag before administration. Do not use and discard if proteinaceous strands, particulate matter or discoloration are observed.
- Stability in the vial: If not used immediately after mixing, the reconstituted vial may be stored in refrigerator at 2–8°C (36–46°F) for up to 24 hours; it should be protected from bright light by placing it in the original carton (see package insert).
- Stability in the infusion bag: If not used immediately (preferred), may be stored in refrigerator at 2–8°C (36–46°F), protected from bright light, for a maximum of 24 hours.
- Total combined refrigerated storage time of reconstituted drug in the vial and in the infusion bag is 24 hours. This may be followed by storage in the infusion bag at ambient temperature (approximately 25°C) and lighting conditions for a maximum of 4 hours.

Drug Administration:

- Assess ANC/CBC, and LFTs. Drug is contraindicated in patients with ANC $<$ 1,500 cells/mm^3, or prior severe hypersensitivity reaction to paclitaxel protein-bound particles for injectable suspension (Abraxane). Drug should not be given to patients with AST $>$ 10 $\times$ ULN or bilirubin $>$ 5 $\times$ ULN.

- Administer only if baseline ANC is $\geq$ 1,500 cells/mm^3.
- Dose-reduce for neutropenia, neuropathy, and moderate to severe hepatic impairment. Drug is not given to patients with metastatic pancreatic cancer with moderate to severe hepatic impairment.
- The use of specialized DEHP-free solution containers and administration sets is not necessary; do not use an in-line filter.
- DO NOT substitute for other paclitaxel formulations.
- No premedication is generally required, as with generic paclitaxel.
- Administer by IV infusion over 30 minutes.
- Drug is an irritant; monitor for injection-site reactions.

Drug Interactions:
- These are the same as generic, nonprotein-bound paclitaxel.
- Paclitaxel is metabolized by P450 cytochrome isoenzymes CYP2C8 and CYP3A4. Potential interactions may occur. Use cautiously with other drugs metabolized by this system (CYP2C8 and CYP3A4):

Inducers: e.g., carbamazepine, efavirenz, nevirapine, phenytoin, rifampicin

Inhibitors: e.g., cimetidine, erythromycin, fluoxetine, gemfibrozil, indinivir, ketoconazole and other imidazole antifungals, nelfinavir, ritonavir, saquinivir
- Use caution when administering paclitaxel protein-bound particles for injectable suspension (Abraxane) together with inhibitors or inducers of either CYP2C8 or CYP3A4; avoid coadministration if possible.

Lab Effects/Interference:
- Decreased white and red cell counts, neutrophil count, platelet count.
- Increased alkaline phosphatase, AST, ALT, bilirubin.

Special Considerations:
- Drug is a Cremophor-free, protein-engineered nanotransporter of paclitaxel. No premedication for hypersensitivity is generally required prior to administration of paclitaxel protein-bound particles for injectable suspension (Abraxane).
- Drug needs no special tubing or filter.
- Most common adverse reactions for patients are (1) *metastatic breast cancer:* alopecia, neutropenia, sensory neuropathy, abnormal ECG, fatigue/asthenia, myalgia/arthralgia, AST elevation, alkaline phosphatase elevation, anemia, nausea, infections, diarrhea; (2) *NSCLC:* anemia, neutropenia, thrombocytopenia, alopecia, PN, nausea, fatigue; and (3) *adenocarcinoma of the pancreas:* neutropenia, fatigue, PN, nausea, alopecia, peripheral edema, diarrhea, pyrexia, vomiting, decreased appetite, rash, dehydration.

Paclitaxel protein-bound particles for injectable suspension (Abraxane) has the following special warnings and precautions:
- *Myelosuppression* (primarily neutropenia), which is dose dependent and a dose-limiting toxicity; monitor CBC and hold/reduce dose as needed; dose modify per package insert.
- *Sensory neuropathy* occurs frequently and may require dose reduction or treatment interruption.

- *Sepsis has occurred* in 5% of patients with or without neutropenia who received drug in combination with gemcitabine. Risk factors for severe or fatal sepsis included biliary obstruction or presence of biliary stent. If a patient becomes febrile, regardless of ANC, broad spectrum antibiotics should be initiated. For febrile neutropenia, interrupt Abraxane and gemcitabine until fever resolves and ANC ≥ 1,500, then resume at a reduced dose; see package insert.
- *Pneumonitis* has occurred in 4% of patients receiving the drug with gemcitabine. Monitor patients for signs/symptoms and interrupt drugs during evaluation of pneumonitis; if pneumonitis diagnosed, permanently discontinue treatment with both drugs.
- *Severe hypersensitivity reactions* with sometimes fatal outcomes have been reported. Do not re-challenge the patient with this drug. If a patient has had a prior HSR to another taxane, cross-hypersensitivity does exist, so monitor patient closely during initiation of nab-paclitaxel.
- *Hepatic Impairment:* Increased exposure and toxicity of nab-paclitaxel can occur in patients with hepatic impairment. The drug should not be administered to patients with metastatic adenocarcinoma of the pancreas with moderate to severe hepatic impairment. In other patients with hepatic impairment, the drug should be used cautiously. These patients are at risk for severe myelosuppression and should be monitored closely. The starting dose for patients with moderate to severe hepatic impairment should be reduced (see package insert). Monitor LFTs and administer with caution. The drug is not recommended for patients with a total BR > 5 × ULN or AST > 10 × ULN.
- *Viral transmission:* Drug contains albumin derived from human blood, which has a theoretical risk of viral transmission.
- *Embryo-fetal toxicity:* Drug can harm the fetus. Counsel women of reproductive potential to use effective contraception during and for at least 6 months after last dose, as well as men with female partners of reproductive potential, to use effective contraception to avoid pregnancy during therapy and for at least 3 months after last dose.

Potential Toxicities/Side Effects and the Nursing Process

I.   POTENTIAL FOR INFECTION AND BLEEDING related to BM DEPRESSION

Defining Characteristics: Neutropenia is dose dependent and reversible, and is a dose-limiting toxicity of paclitaxel protein-bound particles for injectable suspension. Grades 3–4 neutropenia occurred in 34% of patients with MBC, 47% in patients with NSCLC, and 38% in patients with pancreatic cancer. Infectious complications occurred in 24% of patients, with oral candidiasis, respiratory tract infection, and pneumonia the most commonly reported. Thrombocytopenia is uncommon, with bleeding reported in 2% of patients. Anemia occurred in 33% of patients and was severe in 1% of patients (Hgb < 8 g/dL). Sepsis occurred in 5% of patients with or without neutropenia, and risk of severe/ fatal sepsis was increased in patients with biliary obstruction or presence of biliary stent.

Nursing Implications: Assess baseline CBC, WBC, differential, and platelet count prior to chemotherapy, as well as signs/symptoms of infection or bleeding. Teach patient the signs/symptoms of infection or bleeding, and to report these immediately, and teach patient self-care measures to minimize risk of infection and bleeding. This includes avoidance of crowds, proximity to people with infections, and OTC aspirin-containing medications. Do not administer paclitaxel protein-bound particles for injectable suspension to patients with a baseline ANC $<$ 1,500 cells/mm^3. Assess the patient with biliary obstruction or presence of biliary stents closely for fever. If a patient becomes febrile, broad spectrum antibiotics should be started immediately regardless of ANC. If the patient develops febrile neutropenia, interrupt paclitaxel protein-bound particles for injectable suspension (Abraxane) and gemcitabine until fever resolves and ANC $\geq$ 1,500, then resume treatment at a reduced dose level (see package insert). Drug dose should be reduced for neutropenia or thrombocytopenia per package insert. Administer paclitaxel protein-bound particles for injectable suspension PRIOR to cisplatin or carboplatin when either is given in combination with paclitaxel.

II.   SENSORY/PERCEPTUAL ALTERATIONS related to SENSORY NEUROPATHY, OCULAR AND VISUAL DISTURBANCES

Defining Characteristics: Sensory neuropathy is dose related, schedule-dependent, and common in patients receiving paclitaxel protein-bound particles for injectable suspension. Incidence in patients with MBC receiving 260 mg/m^2 every 3 weeks was 71%, compared to 56% in patients receiving paclitaxel in metastatic breast cancer studies. Grade 3 neuropathy occurred in 10%, and 14/24 patients had documented improvement after a median of 22 days. No grade 4 severity has been reported in clinical trials. Incidence of PN in patients with NSCLC was 48% (compared to 64% for patients receiving paclitaxel every 3 weeks) and 54% in patients with adenocarcinoma of the pancreas. Motor or autonomic neuropathy (e.g., ileus) occurs rarely. Ocular/visual disturbances may occur in 13% of the patients, especially at doses higher than recommended; in the literature, persistent optic nerve damage related to generic paclitaxel has been reported.

Nursing Implications: Assess baseline neurologic status. Instruct patient to report signs/symptoms of pins-and-needles sensation (paresthesias), numbness, pain, increased discomfort with certain sensations (dysesthesias), especially in the extremities, or motor weakness. Identify patients at risk: those with history of cisplatin use or with preexisting neuropathies (ethanol- and diabetes mellitus–related). Assess sensory and motor function prior to each treatment, and if abnormality found, assess impact on patient function, safety, independence, and quality of life. Test patient's ability to button a shirt or pick up a dime from a flat surface. Teach self-care strategies as needed, including maintaining safety when walking, getting up, taking bath, or washing dishes; explain inability to sense temperature and the need to keep extremities warm in cold weather (see NCI Common Toxicity Criteria). Teach the patient to report any ocular or visual disturbance, and discuss management or need for ophthalmologic consultation with physician. Grade 1 or 2 PN generally do not require dose adjustment. If grades 3 or higher, hold paclitaxel protein-bound particles for injectable suspension (Abraxane) until signs/symptoms resolve/improve to $\leq$ grade 1 or 2 for patients with MBC or until resolution to $\leq$ grade 1 for patients with either NSCLC or pancreatic cancer, followed by a dose reduction for all subsequent courses of paclitaxel protein-bound particles for injectable suspension (Abraxane) [see package insert].

III. ALTERATION IN SKIN INTEGRITY related to ALOPECIA

Defining Characteristics: Alopecia occurs commonly (90% in patients with MBC studied, 56% in patients with NSCLC, and 50% in patients with adenocarcinoma of the pancreas).

Nursing Implications: Discuss potential impact of hair loss prior to drug administration. Discuss coping strategies and plan to minimize body-image distortion (e.g., wig, scarf, cap). Assess patient for signs/symptoms of hair loss. Assess patient's response and use of coping strategies, and help patient to build on effective strategies.

IV. ALTERATION IN NUTRITION, LESS THAN BODY REQUIREMENTS, related to NAUSEA/VOMITING AND DIARRHEA

Defining Characteristics: Side effects that may affect nutrition are the following, with incidences for patients with MBC, NSCLC, and adenocarcinoma of the pancreas indicated for each: nausea occurred in 30% of patients with MBC, 27% in patients with NSCLC, and 54% in patients with adenocarcinoma of pancreas; vomiting in 18%, 12%, and 36% of patients respectively; and diarrhea in 27%, 15%, and 44% of patients respectively.

Nursing Implications: Premedicate patient with antiemetic if needed. Encourage small, frequent meals of cool, bland foods. Instruct patient to report nausea, and teach self-administration of antiemetics. If nausea/vomiting occurs and is severe, assess for signs/symptoms of fluid/electrolyte imbalance. Assess bowel elimination pattern and oral mucosa baseline prior to each treatment. Teach patient to report diarrhea unrelieved with self-administered anti-diarrheal medications and adequate fluid replacement.

V. ALTERATION IN COMFORT related to FATIGUE, ARTHRALGIAS, AND MYALGIAS

Defining Characteristics: Fatigue is common, with fatigue/asthenia affecting 47% of patients with MBC, 25% of patients with NSCLC, and 59% of patients with adenocarcinoma of the pancreas. Arthralgias and myalgias affect about 44% of MBC patients, with 8% experiencing severe symptoms. Arthralgias occurred in 13% and myalgias 10% in patients with NSCLC, and 11% and 10% respectively in patients with adenocarcinoma of the pancreas. Arthralgias and myalgias commonly occurred 2–3 days after the drug was given, and resolved within a few days.

Nursing Implications: Teach patient that fatigue may occur, and ways to minimize exertion and energy expenditure by alternating rest and activity, and organizing chores so that they are done as efficiently as possible. Teach patient that arthalgias and myalgias may occur, teach self-care measures to reduce discomfort, and advise patient to report discomfort that does not resolve.

Drug: pegasparaginase (Oncaspar)

Class: Miscellaneous agent (enzyme).

Mechanism of Action: Pegasparaginase is a modified form of L-asparaginase, wherein units of monomethoxypolyethylene glycol (PEG) are covalently conjugated to L-asparaginase, forming the active ingredient PEG-L-asparaginase. The enzyme hydrolyzes serum asparagine, a nonessential amino acid for both normal and leukemic cells. Unlike normal cells, leukemic cells are unable to synthesize their own asparagine (lack the enzyme asparagine synthetase and thus require exogenous L-asparagine), resulting in cell death.

Metabolism: Unclear. Elimination half-life is significantly prolonged with pegylated formulation of 5.5–7 days, compared to Erwinia asparaginase, of 16 hours, and native *E. coli* L-asparaginase of 26–30 hours. One dose of pegylated L-asparaginase of 2,500 IU/m^2 achieves similar levels of asparagine depletion as 9 doses of native *E. coli* L-asparaginase during induction, and 6 doses during each delayed intensification phase (Oncaspar package insert, 2006).

Indication: For the treatment of patients with (1) acute lymphoblastic leukemia (ALL, as first-line treatment as part of a multi-agent chemotherapeutic regimen; (2) ALL in patients hypersensitive to asparaginase, as a component of a multi-agent chemotherapeutic regimen.

Contraindications: Patients with a history of (1) serious allergic reactions to Oncaspar; (2) serious thrombosis with prior L-asparaginase therapy; (3) pancreatitis with prior L-asparaginase therapy; (4) serous hemorrhagic events with prior L-asparaginase therapy.

Dosage/Range:
- Recommended dose is 2,500 international units/m^2 IM or IV no more frequently than every 14 days.

Drug Preparation:
- Available as a 3,750 international units/5 mL single-use vial.
- For intravenous use, reconstitute with sterile water for injection, and dilute further in 100 cc NS or D5W. If giving IM, reconstitute in no more than 2 cc NS for injection. If more than 2 cc of NS is used, more than one injection site must be used.
- Do not administer Oncaspar if the drug has been frozen, stored at room temperature (+15°C–25°C; 59°F–77°F) for > 48 hours, or if the drug has been shaken or vigorously agitated.
- After the solution has been diluted for IV use, it should be administered immediately. If that is not possible, the diluted solution should be refrigerated at 2–8°C (36–46°F) for up to 46–47 hours (48 hours from time of preparation to completion of administration). See package insert.
- Inspect solution for particulate matter and/or discoloration prior to administration; if present, do not use.

Drug Administration:
- IM is the preferred route of administration because of the lower incidence of hepatotoxicity, coagulopathy, and gastrointestinal and renal disorders, as compared with the intravenous route.
- When administered IM, the volume at the injection site should be less than or equal to 2 mL; if volume to administer is larger than 2 mL, use multiple injection sites.
- When administered IV: mix in 100 mL of sodium chloride or dextrose injection 5%, infuse over a period of 1–2 hours; piggyback into a plain infusion that is already infusing.
- Observe patient during and for 1 hour after drug administration, as anaphylaxis may occur.

Drug Interactions: No formal drug interaction studies have been performed (Sigma Tau, 2015).
- Nonsteroidal anti-inflammatory drugs (NSAIDs), aspirin, dipyridamole, heparin, warfarin, and blood-dyscrasia-causing medications: Pegasparaginase causes imbalances in coagulation factors, predisposing patients to bleeding and/or thrombosis.
- Hepatotoxic medications (increased risk of toxicity).
- **Methotrexate:** Drug antagonizes antifolate effects of MTX if given before MTX administration. If given 24 hours after MTX, its antifolate activity will be terminated at that point.
- Vaccines, both live and killed virus: Patient's antibody response to the killed vaccine may be reduced for up to 1 year by the immunosuppression brought on by pegasparaginase. Such immunosuppression may also potentiate the replication of live-virus vaccines, increase the side effects of the vaccine virus, and/or may decrease the patient's antibody response to the vaccine.

Lab Effects/Interference:
- Increased LFTs, serum glucose, BUN, uric acid, amylase, lipase.
- Decreased serum albumin, plasma fibrinogen.
- Prolonged PT.

Special Considerations:
- Warnings and Precautions:
  - *Anaphylaxis and serious allergic reactions*: Hypersensitivity reactions (HSR) occur more frequently with pegasparaginase than with other chemotherapeutic agents. Patients must be closely monitored closely for signs of allergic/anaphylactic reactions, and the nurse must remain with the patient while drug is infusing. Ensure immediate access to adverse-reaction kit, including epinephrine, and that a physician/NP/PA with prescribing privileges is close by. Drug should be discontinued in patients with serious allergic reactions.
  - *Thrombosis*: Serious thrombotic events may occur, including sagittal sinus thrombosis. Drug should be discontinued if serious thrombotic events occur.
  - *Pancreatitis:* Assess baseline pancreatic enzymes and monitor during therapy. Call physician/NP/PA to assist in evaluating patients with abdominal pain for evidence of pancreatitis. Drug should be discontinued if pancreatitis occurs.

- *Glucose intolerance* can occur and may be irreversible. Monitor serum glucose baseline and regularly during therapy.
- *Coagulaopathy:* Increased PT, increased partial thromboplastin time, and hypofibrinogenemia can occur. Monitor coagulation parameters baseline and periodically during and after drug therapy. If patient has severe or symptomatic coagulopathy, discuss and implement treatment as ordered with fresh frozen plasma to replace coagulation factors.
- *Hepatotoxicity and abnormal LFTs:* Monitor AST, ALT, direct and indirect bilirubin, alkaline phosphatase, serum albumin, and plasma fibrinogen baseline and during therapy.
- *Embryo-fetal toxicity:* It is unknown if drug causes fetal harm. The drug should be given to a pregnant woman only if clearly needed. Mothers should not breastfeed while receiving this therapy.

Potential Toxicities/Side Effects and the Nursing Process

I.   POTENTIAL FOR INJURY related to HYPERSENSITIVITY OR ANAPHYLACTIC REACTIONS

Defining Characteristics: Occurs less often with IM route of administration. May be life-threatening reaction, but is usually mild.

Nursing Implications: Discuss with physician use of test dose prior to drug administration. Assess baseline VS and mental status prior to drug administration. Review standing orders or nursing procedure for management of anaphylaxis and be prepared to stop drug immediately if signs/symptoms occur; keep IV line open with 0.9% sodium chloride, notify physician, monitor vital signs, and administer ordered medications, which may include epinephrine 1:1,000, hydrocortisone sodium succinate, and diphenhydramine. Teach patient the potential of a hypersensitivity or anaphylactic reaction and to report any unusual symptoms immediately. *E. coli* preparation of L-asparaginase and *E. carotovora* preparation are non-cross-resistant, so if an anaphylactic reaction occurs with one, the other preparation may be used.

II.   POTENTIAL FOR INJURY related to HEPATIC DYSFUNCTION OR THROMBOEMBOLISM

Defining Characteristics: Most patients have elevated LFTs starting within first 2 weeks of treatment, e.g., SGOT, bili, and alk phos. Hepatically derived clotting factors may be depressed, resulting in excessive bleeding or blood clotting. Relatively uncommon.

Nursing Implications: Monitor SGOT, bili, alk phos, albumin, and clotting factors CPT, PTT, fibrinogen. Teach patient of the potential for excessive bleeding or blood clotting, and instruct to report any unusual symptoms. Assess patient for signs/symptoms of bleeding.

TREATMENT

III.   ALTERED NUTRITION, LESS THAN BODY REQUIREMENTS, related to NAUSEA/VOMITING, ANOREXIA, HYPERGLYCEMIA

Defining Characteristics: Many patients experience mild-to-moderate nausea and vomiting. Anorexia commonly occurs. Hyperglycemia is a transient reaction caused by effects on the pancreas with decreased insulin synthesis. Pancreatitis occurs in some patients.

Nursing Implications: Premedicate with antiemetics and continue prophylactically for 24 hours to prevent nausea and vomiting. Encourage small, frequent meals of cool, bland foods and liquids, as well as favorite foods, especially high-calorie, high-protein foods. Encourage use of spices and do weekly weights. Teach patient about the potential of hyperglycemia and pancreatitis, and instruct to report any unusual symptoms: e.g., increased thirst, urination, and appetite (hyperglycemia) and abdominal or stomach pain, constipation, or nausea and vomiting (pancreatitis). Monitor serum glucose, amylase, and lipase levels periodically during treatment. Report any laboratory elevations to physician. Treat hyperglycemia issues with diet or insulin as ordered by physician. Treat pancreatitis per physician orders.

IV.   SENSORY/PERCEPTUAL ALTERATIONS related to NEUROTOXICITY

Defining Characteristics: Neurotoxicity may occur in some patients—commonly, lethargy, drowsiness, and somnolence; rarely coma. Seen more frequently in adults.

Nursing Implications: Teach patient about the potential of CNS toxicity, and instruct to report any unusual symptoms. Obtain baseline neurologic and mental function. Assess patient for any neurologic abnormalities and report changes to physician. Discuss with patient the impact of malaise on his/her general sense of well-being and strategies to minimize the distress.

V.   INFECTION, BLEEDING, AND FATIGUE related to BM DEPRESSION

Defining Characteristics: BM depression is not common. Mild anemia may occur. Serious leukopenia and thrombocytopenia are rare.

Nursing Implications: Monitor CBC, platelet count prior to drug administration, as well as signs/symptoms of infection, bleeding, or anemia. Instruct patient in self-assessment of signs/symptoms of infection, bleeding, or anemia and to report immediately.

Drug: pemetrexed (Alimta)

Class: Nucleoside metabolic inhibitor (antimetolite); Folate analogue metabolic inhibitor [multitargeted antifolate].

Mechanism of Action: Inhibits key metabolic enzymatic steps (thymidylate synthase [TS], dihydrofolate reductase [DHFR], and glycinamide ribonucleotide formyltransferase

[GARFT]) critical to pyrimidine and purine synthesis, thus preventing DNA synthesis and cell division. Drug is carried into tumor cells via reduced folate carriers, metabolized intracellularly to polyglutamated form of pemetrexed that potently inhibits purine and pyrimidine synthesis. Antitumor effect dependent upon size of cellular folate pools, so folic acid must be coadministered to increase drug efficacy and minimize toxicity. Polyglutamates accumulate in the cell, with a long cellular half-life, and increased cytotoxicity. It is active in the S phase of the cell cycle.

Metabolism: Following IV administration, peak plasma levels are achieved within 30 minutes. Drug is widely distributed in body tissues, especially liver, kidneys, small intestines, and colon. Excreted by kidneys (glomerular and tubular) into the urine, with up to 90% of the drug excreted unchanged during the first 24 hours after administration. Plasma half-life is about 3 hours, with prolonged terminal half-life of 20 hours.

Indications:
- (1) Metastatic nonsquamous NSCLC, with no EGFR or ALK genomic aberrations, initial treatment, in combination with pembrolizumab and platinum chemotherapy.
- (2) Locally advanced or metastatic nonsquamous NSCLC (a) initial treatment in combination with cisplatin; (b) as maintenance treatment of patients whose disease has not progressed after 4 cycles of platinum-based first-line chemotherapy, as a single agent; (c) after prior chemotherapy as a single-agent in patients recurrent, metastatic nonsquamous NSCLC.
- (3) Mesothelioma, unresectable or in patients otherwise not candidates for curative surgery: initial treatment in combination with cisplatin.
- Pemetrexate is **not** indicated for the treatment of patients with squamous cell NSCLC.

Dosage/Range:
- With pembrolizumab in patients with a CrCl $\geq$ 45 mL/min (calculated by Cockcroft-Gault equation): pemetrexate 500 mg/m^2 IV infusion over 10 minutes, administered after pembrolizumab and prior to platinum chemotherapy, on day 1 of each 21-day cycle.
- Combination use in nonsquamous NSCLC and mesothelioma in patients with a CrCl $\geq$ 45 mL/min: 500-mg/m^2 IV over 10 minutes on day 1 of each 21-day cycle, in combination with cisplatin 75-mg/m^2 IV over 2 hours, beginning 30 minutes after the end of the pemetrexed dose.
- Single-agent use in NSCLC, 500-mg/m^2 IV day 1 of each 21-day cycle.
- Premedication regimen and concurrent medications
  - Vitamin supplementation:
    - Folic acid 400–1,000 mcg PO daily starting **7 days before** first dose of pemetrexed, during the full course of therapy, and for 21 days after the last pemetrexed dose.
    - Vitamin B$_{12}$ 1 mg IM 1 week prior to first pemetrexed dose, then every 3 cycles thereafter (may be given same day as pemetrexed).
  - Corticosteroids: Dexamethasone 4 mg PO bid the day before, the day of, and day after pemetrexed administration.

Dose Modification: Dose reductions or discontinuation may be needed based on toxicities from the preceding cycle of therapy. These reductions are based on NCI's CTCAE:

- Assess CBC/differential prior to each cycle (day 1), at nadir (day 8) and recovery (day 15). Assess CrCl prior to each cycle. DO NOT administer pemetrexate if CrCl is <45 mL/min.
- Delay initiation of next cycle of pemetrexed until (1) recovery of nonhematologic toxicity to grade 0–2, (2) ANC is ≥ 1,500/mm^3, AND (3) platelet count is ≥100,000/mm^3. Upon recovery, modify pemetrexed dosage in the next cycle as below. See other drug information for other drugs given in combination.
- Pemetrexed dose based on toxicity in most recent treatment cycle:
  - Hematologic:
    - (a) Nadir ANC < 500 cells/mm^3, and platelet count ≥ 50,000 cells/mm^3 OR platelet count <50,000/mm^3 without bleeding: DOSE-REDUCE to 75% of previous dose;
    - (b) platelet count < 50,000/mm^3 with bleeding, DOSE REDUCE to 50% of previous dose;
    - (c) Recurrent grade 3–4 myelosuppression after 2 dose reductions: discontinue pemetrexed.
- For nonhematologic
  - (a) Any grades 3–4 toxicities EXCEPT mucositis or neurologic toxicity OR diarrhea requiring hospitalization: dose reduce to give 75% of previous dose;
  - (b) Grade 3–4 mucositis: Give 50% of previous dose of pemetrexed.
  - (c) Renal toxicity: Hold drug until CrCl is 45 mL/min or greater.
  - (d) Grade 3–4 neurologic toxicity: Permanently discontinue pemetrexed.
  - (e) Recurrent grade 3–4 non-hematologic toxicity after 2 dose reductions: Permanently discontinue pemetrexed.
  - (f) Severe and life-threatening skin toxicity: Permanently discontinue pemetrexed.
  - (b) ILD/interstitial pneumonitis: Permanently discontinue pemetrexed.
- Dose modification of ibuprofen in patients with mild to moderate renal impairment (CrCl 45 mL/min–79 ml/min) receiving pemetrexed: (1) avoid administration of ibuprofen for 2 days before, the day of, and 2 days after administration of pemetrexed.

Drug Preparation:

- Drug available in 100-mg and 500-mg vials for injection.
- Reconstitute pemetrexed 100-mg vial by adding 4.2-mL and 500-mg vial by adding 20 mL 0.9% sodium chloride for injection (preservative free), resulting in a concentration of 25 mg/mL.
- Aseptically remove ordered dose and add to 100 mL 0.9% sodium chloride for injection infusion bag.
- Stable for up to 24 hours (reconstituted and infusion solutions) refrigerated.

Drug Administration:

- Assess labs prior to each cycle, which must be: ANC ≥ 1,500 cells/mm^3, platelet count ≥ 100,000 cells/mm^3, and CrCl ≥ 45 mL/min. Patients should also be monitored for nadir and recovery, e.g., days 8 and 15 of each cycle.
- Do not administer pemetrexate if CrCl < 45 mL/min.

- Ensure patient has taken premedication prior to initial dose of pemetrexed and continuing through treatment:
  - Folic acid supplement (400 to 1,000 micrograms) PO once daily beginning 1 week prior to initial treatment, and continuing throughout treatment and 21 days posttreatment.
  - Vitamin B_{12} (1,000 micrograms) IM injections every 3 cycles, beginning 1 week prior to first treatment, and continuing throughout treatment every 3 cycles thereafter. Subsequent vitamin B_{12} injections (after the initial dose) can be given the same day as pemetexed administration.
  - Dexamethasone 4 mg PO twice daily on the day before, day of, and day after treatment to help prevent skin rash.
- Ensure that patients with mild to moderate renal insufficiency (CrCl 45–79 mL/min) have stopped NSAIDs with short elimination half-lives (e.g., diclofenac, indomethacin) at least 2 days prior to receiving pemetrexed: the day of administration and for two days following. Patients with normal renal function (CrCl $\geq$ 80 mL/min) can take NSAIDs (e.g., ibuprofen 400 mg qid), without significantly reducing pemetrexed clearance.
- Administer as a 10-minute IV infusion.

Drug Interactions:
- Nephrotoxic drugs: potentially delayed pemetrexed excretion.
- Drugs secreted by renal tubules (e.g., probenecid): potential delayed pemetrexed excretion.
- Thymidine: rescues normal cells.
- Leucovorin: decreases antitumor effect of pemetrexed; do not coadminister.
- 5-FU: may increase antitumor effect of pemetrexed.
- Ibuprofen and other NSAIDs, in people with normal renal function: 20% increase in AUC of pemetrexed, due to 20% reduction in pemetrexed clearance.
- NSAIDs (short half-lives, e.g., ibuprofen): AVOID if renal compromise (creatinine clearance < 80 mL/min), stop NSAIDs 2 days prior to pemetrexed administration, the day of administration, and for 2 days following pemetrexed administration.
- NSAIDs (long half-lives): stop NSAID 5 days before, the day of, and for 2 days following pemetrexed administration.
- If patient must continue NSAIDs, 24-hour creatinine clearance should be > 80 mL/min.
- Lactated Ringer's or Ringer's Injection USP: physical incompatibility with pemetrexed; do not use together.

Lab Effects/Interference:
- Transient increase in serum transaminases and bilirubin.

Special Considerations:
- Warnings and Precautions:
  - *Vitamin supplementation required* with oral folic acid, IM vitamin B_{12} [reduces severity of hematologic and GI toxicity]; corticosteroids day before, day of, day after. See package insert.
  - *BM Suppression*: Dose-limiting toxicity. Dose reduce based on nadir, and non-hematologic toxicity

- *Renal failure*: Drug is excreted primarily unchanged. Do not administer drug if creatinine clearance is < 45 mL/min using Cockcroft and Gault formula (estimated creatinine clearance): (140 − age in years) × actual body weight (kg); males: 72 × serum creatinine (mg/dL) = mL/min; females: estimated creatinine clearance for males × 0.85.
- *Bullous and exfoliative skin toxicity*: Serious and sometimes fatal bullous, blistering, and exfoliative skin toxicity may occur, suggestive of SJS or toxic epidermal necrolysis. Permanently discontinue the drug if severe and life-threatening bullous, blistering, or exfoliating skin toxicity occurs.
- *Interstitial pneumonitis*: Can occur and may be fatal. Hold pemetrexed for acute onset of new or progressive, unexplained pulmonary symptoms (e.g., dyspnea, cough, or fever) until diagnostic evaluation is completed. If pneumonitis is confirmed, permanently discontinue the pemetrexed.
- *Radiation recall*: Monitor patients for inflammation or blistering in areas of prior RT treatment. If radiation recall occurs, permanently discontinue pemetrexed.
- *Increased risk of toxicity with ibuprofen in patients with renal impairment*: Patients with mild to moderate renal insufficiency (CrCl 45–79 mL/min): use caution. Stop ibuprofen at least 2 days prior to administering pemetrexed, the day of pemetrexed administration, and for two days following pemetrexed administration. If ibuprofen administration cannot be avoided, assess patient frequently for toxicity, including myelosuppression and renal and GI toxicity.
- *Required laboratory monitoring*: CBC/differential and renal function tests at beginning of each cycle. Do not give pemetrexed unless ANC ≥ 1,500 cells/mm^3, platelet count ≥ 100,000 cells/mm^3, and CrCl is ≥ 45 mL/min.
- *Embryo-fetal toxicity*: Women of childbearing age should use effective birth control measures. Teach women of reproductive potential to use effective contraception during and for 6 months after last treatment dose. Teach male patients with female sexual partners of reproductive potential to use effective contraception during treatment and for 3 months after last pemetrexed dose. Women should not breastfeed an infant while receiving pemetrexed.

Potential Toxicities/Side Effects and the Nursing Process

I. POTENTIAL INFECTION, BLEEDING, AND FATIGUE related to BM DEPRESSION

Defining Characteristics: BM depression is dose-limiting toxicity. Nadir is day 8 with recovery by day 15 of each cycle. Neutropenia occurred in 58% of patients, with grade 3 (19%), and grade 4 (5%). For grades 3 and 4 neutropenia, the incidence in between patients who were fully supplemented was 24%, in contrast to patients who were never supplemented (38%). The overall incidence of thrombocytopenia is 27%, with grades 3 and 4 (4% and 1%, respectively). Anemia occurred in 33% of patients overall.

Nursing Implications: Assess baseline CBC, WBC, differential and ANC, and platelet count prior to chemotherapy as well as for signs and symptoms of infection, bleeding, or anemia. Ensure labs ANC $> 1,500$ cells/mm^3, platelets $> 100,000$ cells/mm^3, AND creatinine clearance > 45 mL/min prior to drug administration. Ensure that patient has taken vitamin supplements prior to drug administration: low-dose oral folic acid or multivitamin with folic acid daily (at least 5 daily doses of folic acid must be taken during the 7-day period prior to the first dose of pemetrexed, and dosing should continue during the full course of therapy, and for 21 days after the last drug dose; vitamin B$_{12}$ 100 micrograms IM during the week prior to cycle 1, then every 3 cycles; subsequent doses can be given on same day as pemetrexed treatment). Discuss dose reductions based on nadir counts with physician as needed. Teach patient signs/symptoms of infection, and bleeding, and instruct to report them right away. Teach measures to minimize infection and bleeding, such as avoidance of crowds and proximity to people with infection, and to avoid aspirin or NSAID-containing medications. Teach patient strategies to minimize fatigue, such as alternating rest with activity, and ways to organize shopping to minimize energy expenditure.

II. POTENTIAL ALTERATION IN NUTRITION, LESS THAN BODY REQUIREMENTS, related to NAUSEA, CONSTIPATION, ANOREXIA, DIARRHEA, STOMATITIS

Defining Characteristics: Nausea occurs in 84% of patients, vomiting 58%, constipation 44%, anorexia 35%, stomatitis/pharyngitis 28%, and diarrhea 26%, in combination with cisplatin.

Nursing Implications: Premedicate with antiemetics, and ensure patient has antiemetics to take to prevent delayed emesis from cisplatin. Teach patient and family delayed emesis regimen. Encourage small, frequent meals of cool, bland foods, and to increase fluid intake. Assess oral mucosa prior to drug administration and instruct patient to report changes. Teach patient oral hygiene measures and self-assessment. Instruct patient to report diarrhea, to self-administer prescribed antidiarrheal medications and to drink adequate fluids. Monitor LFTs baseline and periodically during therapy. Notify physician of any abnormalities and discuss implications as drug studied only in patients with elevated LFTs related to liver metastases.

III. ALTERATION IN SKIN INTEGRITY related to RASH

Defining Characteristics: Incidence of rash with or without desquamation was 22%.

Nursing Implications: Assess baseline skin integrity. Teach patient that this may occur, and to take recommended dexamethasone premedication 4 mg po bid the day before, the day of, and the day after pemetrexed administration. Teach patient potential side effects of corticosteroid administration, including difficulty sleeping, mood alterations, and depression.

IV.   POTENTIAL FOR IMPAIRED GAS EXCHANGE related to DYSPNEA

Defining Characteristics: Dyspnea was reported in 66% of patients receiving pemetrexed and cisplatin therapy; 10% had grade 3 dyspnea, and 1% had grade 4 toxicity.

Nursing Implications: Teach patient that this may occur, and to report it right away if severe or worsening. Assess baseline pulmonary status, at rest, and with activity. Assess oxygen saturation with vital signs. Discuss severe or worsening dyspnea with physician.

Drug: polifeprosan 20 with carmustine (BCNU) implant (Gliadel®)

Class: Alkylating agent.

Mechanism of Action: Wafer (copolymer) containing carmustine is implanted in the surgical cavity created when brain tumor is resected. In water, the anhydride bonds of the wafer are hydrolyzed, releasing the carmustine into the surgical cavity. The carmustine diffuses into the surrounding brain tissue, reaching any residual tumor cells, and causing cell death by alkylating DNA and RNA.

Metabolism: Unknown. Dime-sized wafer is biodegradable in brain tissue, with a variable rate. More than 70% of the copolymer degrades by 3 weeks, slowly releasing 7.7 mg of carmustine in concentrations. In some patients, wafer fragments remained up to 232 days after implantation, with almost all drug gone.

Indication: For the treatment of patients with:
• Newly diagnosed high-grade malignant glioma, as an adjunct to surgery and radiation.
• Recurrent glioblastoma multiforme (GBM) as an adjunct to surgery.

Dosage/Range:
• Each wafer contains 7.7 mg of carmustine, and the recommended dose is eight wafers, or a total dose of 61.6 mg of carmustine.

Drug Preparation:
• Drug must be stored at or below 20°C (–4°F) until time of use.
• Unopened foil packages can stay at room temperature for a maximum of 6 hours at a time. The manufacturer recommends that the treatment box be removed from the freezer and taken to the operating room just prior to surgery.
• The box and pouches should be opened just before the surgeon is ready to implant the wafers. Open the sealed treatment box and remove double foil packages, handling the unsterile outer foil packet by the crimped edge VERY CAREFULLY to prevent damage to the wafers. See product information for opening the inner foil pouch and removing the wafer with sterile technique.
• Chemotherapy precautions should be used to limit exposure to the chemotherapy: surgical instruments used to remove and implant the wafers should be kept separate from other instruments and sterile fields, and should be cleaned after the procedure according to hospital chemotherapy procedure; all personnel handling the wafers or the inner foil

pouches containing the wafers should wear double gloves, which, along with unused wafers or fragments, inner foil packages, and opened outer foil package, should be disposed of as chemotherapeutic waste.

Drug Administration:
- Neurosurgeon places eight wafers into surgical resection cavity if size and shape appropriate; wafers are placed contiguously or with slight overlapping.
- Wafer may be broken into two pieces *only* if needed.

Drug Interactions:
- Unknown but unlikely, as drug is probably not systemically absorbed.

Lab Effects/Interference:
- Unknown, but unlikely.

Special Considerations:
- Warnings and Precautions:
  - *Seizures*: Incidence 54% in study 2 experienced new or worsened seizure activity during first 5 postop days. Median time to onset to first seizure was 4 days. Optimize antiseizure therapy prior to surgery. Monitor patients for seizures following implantation.
  - *Intracranial hypertension*: 23% of patients with newly diagnosed glioma (Study 1) had increased ICP. Monitor patients for signs of increased intracranial hypertension related to brain edema, inflammation, necrosis of the brain tissue surrounding the resection.
  - *Impaired neurosurgical wound healing*, including dehiscence, delayed wound healing, subdural, subgleal, or wound effusions: Monitor patient for complications of craniotomy.
  - *Meningitis:* Monitor patient for signs of bacterial or chemical meningitis.
  - *Wafer migration*: Monitor patient for signs of obstructive hydrocephalus.
  - *Embryo-fetal toxicity*: Can cause fetal harm. Women of reproductive potential should be taught to use effective contraception to avoid pregnancy. Mothers should not breastfeed.
- Patients require close monitoring for complications of craniotomy, as intracerebral mass effect has occurred that does not respond to corticosteroid treatment; in one case, this resulted in brain herniation.
- Most common adverse effects (> 10% and between arm difference 4% or greater): (1) newly diagnosed high-grade malignant glioma: cerebral edema, asthenia, nausea, vomiting, constipation, wound healing abnormalities, depression; (2) recurrent GBM: UTI, wound healing abnormalities, fever.
- No safety or effectiveness data available for pediatric patients (Eisai, 2013).

Potential Toxicities/Side Effects and the Nursing Process

I.   POTENTIAL SENSORY/PERCEPTUAL ALTERATIONS related to SEIZURES, BRAIN EDEMA, MENTAL STATUS CHANGES

Defining Characteristics: In clinical testing, the incidence of new or worsened seizures was 19% in both the group receiving the implant and those receiving the placebo. Seizures were mild to moderate in severity. In patients with new or worsened seizures postoperatively, the group receiving the implant had a 56% incidence, with median time to first new or worsened seizure of 3.5 days, versus placebo incidence of 9%, and median time to first new or worsened seizure of 61 days. Incidence of brain edema was 4%, and there were cases of intracerebral mass effect that did not respond to corticosteroids. Other nervous system effects were hydrocephalus (3%), depression (3%), abnormal thinking (2%), ataxia (2%), dizziness (2%), insomnia (2%), visual field defect (2%), monoplegia (2%), eye pain (1%), coma (1%), amnesia (1%), diplopia (1%), and paranoid reaction (1%). Rarely ($<$ 1%), cerebral infarct or hemorrhage may occur.

Nursing Implications: Monitor neurovital signs closely postoperatively, and notify physician of any abnormalities. If intracranial pressure increases, a mass effect is suspected, and if it is nonresponsive to corticosteroids, expect the patient to be taken to surgery, with possible removal of wafer or remnants. Assess baseline mental status and regularly during postoperative care. Validate changes with family members. Discuss abnormalities with physician immediately and continue to monitor closely.

II.   POTENTIAL FOR INFECTION related to HEALING ABNORMALITIES

Defining Characteristics: Most abnormalities were mild to moderate, occurred in 14% of patients, and included cerebrospinal leaks, subdural fluid collections, subgaleal or wound effusions, and breakdown. The incidence of intracranial infection (e.g., meningitis or abscess) was 4%. Incidence of deep wound infection was 6% (same as placebo) and included infection of subgaleal space, bone, meninges, and brain tissue.

Nursing Implications: Using aseptic technique, assess postoperative wound/dressing immediately postoperatively, and regularly thereafter. Assess systematically for signs/symptoms of infection or wound breakdown. Notify physician immediately and discuss antimicrobial therapy.

III.   ALTERATION IN NUTRITION, LESS THAN BODY REQUIREMENTS, related to GI SIDE EFFECTS, ELECTROLYTE ABNORMALITIES

Defining Characteristics: Rarely, GI disturbances occurred: diarrhea (2%), constipation (2%), dysphagia (1%), gastrointestinal hemorrhage (1%), fecal incontinence (1%). Hyponatremia (3%), hyperglycemia (3%), and hypokalemia (1%) also occurred.

Nursing Implications: Assess baseline nutritional status, including electrolytes. Assess bowel elimination status and monitor nutritional and bowel elimination status closely during postoperative time. Discuss interventions for abnormalities with physician.

IV.   ALTERATION IN CIRCULATION, POTENTIAL, related to CHANGES IN BLOOD PRESSURE

Defining Characteristics: Hypertension occurred in 3% of patients, and hypotension in 1%.

Nursing Implications: Assess baseline VS and monitor closely during postoperative phase. Discuss abnormalities with physician.

V.   ALTERATION IN COMFORT related to EDEMA, PAIN, ASTHENIA

Defining Characteristics: The following occur rarely: peripheral edema (2%), neck pain (2%), rash (2%), back pain (1%), asthenia (1%), chest pain (1%).

Nursing Implications: Assess baseline comfort level and monitor closely during postoperative phase. Provide comfort measures. If ineffective, discuss symptom-management strategies with physician.

Drug: pralatrexate injection (Folotyn)

Class: Folate analogue metabolic inhibitor (antimetabolite).

Mechanism of Action: Drug is a folate analogue metabolic inhibitor. It competitively inhibits the enzyme dihydrofolate reductase; it also competitively inhibits polyglutamylation by the enzyme folylpolyglutamyl synthetase, resulting in the depletion of thymidine, and other essential biologic molecules. Thus, the cell, as it goes to divide, lacks the essential DNA building blocks, is unable to complete the synthesis phase, and dies.

Metabolism: Following IV administration of pralatrexate, the terminal half-life of the drug is 12–18 hours; the pharmokinetics do not change significantly over multiple treatment cycles, and the drug does not accumulate. The drug is 67% bound to plasma proteins and is not a substrate for P-glycoprotein-mediated transport; nor does it inhibit it. Drug does not appear to inhibit or induce the hepatic CYP450 microenzyme system. 34% of IV pralatrexate is excreted unchanged in the urine. Patients with moderate to severe renal impairment should be monitored closely, as the drug has not been studied in these patients.

Indication: For the treatment of patients with relapsed or refractory peripheral T-cell lymphoma. Indication is based on overall response rate; clinical benefit (e.g., improvement in PFS or OS has not been demonstrated).

Dose Modifications for Mucositis (NCI CTCAE version 3.0 grading) [Folotyn PI 2016]

Mucositis Grade Day of Treatment	Action	Dose Upon Recovery to ≤ Grade 1
1: Grade 2	Omit dose	Continue prior dose
2: Grade 2 recurrence	Omit dose	20 mg/m^2; if severe renal impairment, 10 mg/m^2
3. Grade 3	Omit dose	20 mg/m^2; if severe renal impairment, 10 mg/m^2
4: Grade 4	STOP THERAPY	

Dose Modifications for Hematologic Toxicities [Folotyn PI 2016]

Blood Count Day of Treatment	Duration of Toxicity	Action	Dose Upon Restart
Platelet < 50,000/mcL	1 week	Omit dose	Continue prior dose
Platelet < 50,000/mcL	2 weeks	Omit dose	20 mg/m^2 ; if severe renal impairment, 10 mg/m^2
Platelet < 50,000/mcL	3 weeks	STOP THERAPY	None
ANC 500–1,000/mcL without fever	1 week	Omit dose	Continue prior dose
ANC 500–1,000/mcL with fever or ANC < 500/mcL	1 week	Omit dose, give G-CSF or GM-CSF support	Continue prior dose with G-CSF or GM-CSF support
ANC 500–1,000/μL with fever or ANC < 500/μL	2 weeks or recurrence	Omit dose, give G-CSF or GM-CSF support	20 mg/m^2 with G-CSF or GM-CSF support; ; if severe renal impairment, 10 mg/m^2
ANC 500–1,000/μL with fever or ANC < 500/μL	3 weeks or 2nd recurrence	STOP THERAPY	None

Dose Modification for All Other Treatment-Related Toxicities (NCI CTCAE version 3.0 grading) [Folotyn PI 2016]

Toxicity Grade Day of Treatment	Action	Dose Upon Recovery ≤ Grade 2
Grade 3	Omit dose	20 mg/m^2 ; if severe renal impairment, 10 mg/m^2
Grade 4	STOP THERAPY	

Data from Allos Therapeutics, Inc. Folotyn (pralatrexate) [package insert]. Westminster, CO. May 2012.

Dosage/Range:

- 30-mg/m^2 IV push over 3–5 minutes once weekly for 6 weeks in a 7-week cycle. If patient has severe renal impairment (eGFR 15 to less than 30 mL/min/1.73 m^2) dose is 15 mg/m^2.
- Patients must also take vitamin B$_{12}$ 1 mg IM every 8–10 weeks and folic acid 1.0–1.25 mg PO daily.
- Treatment interruption or dose reduction to 20-mg/m^2 IV (10 mg/m^2 if severe renal impairment) may be needed to manage toxicity. DO NOT make up any omitted doses, and do not reescalate dose once reduced.
- Use caution and monitor closely for drug side effects in patients with decreased renal function.
- Persistent elevation of LFTs may indicate liver toxicity and require dose modification. Monitor patients' LFTs closely.
- See Folotyn package insert for dose modifications.

Drug Preparation:
- Pralatrexate is available as sterile, single-use vials at a concentration of 20 mg/mL: 20 mg pralatrexate in a 1-mL solution, or 40-mg vial in 2 mL.
- Drug should be refrigerated at 2–8°C (36–46°F) and stored in its original carton to protect from light.
- Verify that solution is a clear yellow solution without particulate matter prior to drawing up the calculated dose of pralatrexate injection. Discard any drug remaining in the vial, as the drug contains no preservatives.
- Unopened vials in the original carton are stable at room temperature for 72 hours only.

Drug Administration:
- Administer if patient assessment adequate: mucositis is grade 0 or 1; platelet count ≥ 100,000/microL for first dose, and ≥ 50,000/microL for all subsequent doses; ANC ≥ 1,000/microL. Otherwise, see dose modification tables in Folotyn package insert.
- Administer IV push over 3–5 minutes via the side port of a patent, freely flowing IV of 0.9% sodium chloride injection, USP, once weekly for 6 weeks in a 7-week cycle.
- Folic acid supplementation should begin 10 days prior to first dose of pralatrexate and continue through treatment and for 30 days after the last dose of pralatrexate.
- Vitamin B_{12} 1 mg IM should be given no more than 10 weeks before the first dose of pralatrexate and continue every 8–10 weeks. Injections during pralatrexate therapy can be given on the same day as the pralatrexate.
- Assess CBC/differenital and oral mucosa baseline and prior to administration of each dose (weekly): omit or modify dose per MD for grade 2 or higher stomatitis, DO NOT make up any omitted doses. Once a dose reduction occurs, do not reescalate.
- Assess renal and hepatic function, along with other serum chemistries, prior to the first and fourth doses of each cycle. Patients with moderate to severe renal impairment should be monitored closely both for systemic toxicity (due to increased drug exposure) and with renal function testing prior to each dose. Pralatrexate can cause LFT abnormalities. If LFTs are persistently increased, this may indicate liver toxicity and require dose modification.

Drug Interactions:
- Drugs that are renally cleared (e.g., probenecid, NSAIDs, trimethoprim/sulfamethoxazole) may decrease pralatrexate clearance with risk of increased pralatrexate toxicity.

Lab Effects/Interference:
- Hypokalemia in 15% of patients; 13% elevated liver function tests (ALT, AST).

Special Considerations:
- Warnings and Precautions:
  - *BM Suppression* (thrombocytopenia, neutropenia, anemia). Monitor CBC/differential and omit and/or reduce dose based on ANC and platelet count prior to each dose (see Dosage Modifications). Administer vitamin B_{12} and teach patient to take folic adic to reduce hematologic toxicity. Patients must receive supplements in folic acid and vitamin B_{12} during pralatrexate therapy to minimize BM suppression and mucositis.

- *Mucositis*: Monitor for mucositis weekly, and if $\geq$ grade 2, omit and/or dose reduce (see Dosage Modifications, package insert). Vitamins B_{12} and folic acid will reduce risk of mucositis.
- *Dermatologic Reactions*: Assess for development (incidence 2.1%) of skin exfoliation, ulceration, and toxic epidermal necrolysis (TEN). They may be progressive and increase in severity with further treatment, and may involve skin and subcutaneous sites of known lymphoma. If reaction severe, hold or discontinue drug.
- *TLS*: Discuss patient risk and need for TLS prophylaxis with physician/NP/PA. Provide hydration, administer hyperuricemic agent, and monitor electrolytes, serum chemistries as ordered.
- *Hepatic Toxicity*: Monitor LFTs, and omit dose until recovery if it occurs. Adjust or discontinue therapy based on severity and as ordered.
- *Risk of Increased Toxicity in the Presence of Impaired Renal Function*: Patients with moderate to severe renal impairment may be at greater risk for toxicity. Dose reduction initially and further reduction for toxicity management per package insert. Monitor patients' renal function tests and systemic toxicity and discuss dose modification with physician/NP/PA. Avoid drug administration in patients with end-stage renal disease (ESRD) including those undergoing dialysis unless potential benefit exceeds risk. See package insert.
- *Embryo-fetal toxicity*: Women of childbearing age should use effective contraception, as drug can cause fetal harm. If the patient becomes pregnant, she should be informed of potential harm to the fetus. Nursing mothers should choose between receiving the drug and not nursing or discontinuing the drug to nurse.

The most common adverse effects are mucositis (70%), thrombocytopenia (41%), nausea (40%), fatigue (26%). Common serious adverse events are pyrexia, mucositis, sepsis, febrile neutropenia, dehydration, and thrombocytopenia.

Potential Toxicities/Side Effects and the Nursing Process

I.   POTENTIAL FOR INFECTION, BLEEDING, and FATIGUE related to BM DEPRESSION

Defining Characteristics: Major dose-limiting toxicity. Thrombocytopenia occurs in 41% of patients overall, with 14% grade 3 and 19% grade 4. Anemia occurs in 34% of patients, with 17% grade 3 and 2% grade 4. Neutropenia occurs in 24% of patients, with 13% grade 3 and 7% grade 4. Pyrexia occurs in 14% of patients, fatigue in 36% of patients, and epistaxis in 26% of patients. Upper respiratory infections occur in 10% of patients.

Nursing Implications: Monitor CBC and platelet count prior to drug administration, as well as signs/symptoms of infection, bleeding, and anemia. Instruct patient in self-assessment of signs/symptoms of infection (e.g., fever, chills, cough, SOB, pain or burning on urination), bleeding (e.g., epistaxis), and anemia (e.g., fatigue and tiredness) and to report this immediately. Ensure that patient is taking folic acid and receiving vitamin B_{12}. Teach patient self-care measures to minimize risk of infection and bleeding. This includes avoidance of crowds and proximity to people with infections, and avoidance of OTC aspirin-containing medications. Administer platelet and red cell transfusions per physician order.

II. ALTERATION IN NUTRITION, LESS THAN BODY REQUIREMENTS, related to MUCOSITIS, NAUSEA, VOMITING, DIARRHEA, CONSTIPATION

Defining Characteristics: Mucositis is dose limiting and occurs in 70% of patients (17% grade 3, 4% grade 4). Nausea occurs in 40% and vomiting in 25%. Diarrhea occurs in 21%, constipation in 33%, anorexia in 15%.

Nursing Implications: Teach patient to take oral folic acid supplement as directed and emphasize that nonadherence can result in severe toxicity. Assess mucositis prior to each dose administration, and dose-reduce as directed by physician based on past grade of mucositis. Premedicate with antiemetics 30 minutes before taking procarbazine to prevent nausea and vomiting prior to drug administration and teach patient self-administration of antiemetics at home. Encourage small, frequent meals of cool, bland foods and liquids. Encourage patients to report onset of mucositis, diarrhea, constipation, and anorexia and to report if symptoms persist despite intervention for 24 hours. Teach patient to self-administer antidiarrheal medications or anticonstipation medications as appropriate, along with dietary modification.

III. POTENTIAL FOR IMPAIRED SKIN INTEGRITY related to RARE DERMATITIS REACTIONS

Defining Characteristics: Rash occurs in 15% of patients. Rarely, severe dermatologic reactions occur and can be fatal (e.g., skin exfoliation, ulceration, and toxic epidermal necrolysis [TEN]). Pruritus occurs in 14% of patients. Edema occurs in 30% of patients.

Nursing Implications: Assess patient for changes in skin, and teach patient to report them right away (e.g., rash, peeling or loss of skin, sores, or blisters). Discuss management and impact on drug administration with physician prior to administration.

Drug: procarbazine hydrochloride (Matulane)

Class: Miscellaneous agent.

Mechanism of Action: Uncertain but appears to affect preformed DNA, RNA, and protein. It is a methylhydrazine derivative and acts as an alkylating agent. Cell cycle nonspecific.

Metabolism: Metabolized to active metabolites in the liver by the P450 microenzyme system. Rapidly and completely absorbed from the GI tract with peak plasma levels within 1 hour. Procarbazine metabolites taken up by lymph nodes and BM, and cross the BBB, with peak CSF levels occurring in 30–90 minutes. Also metabolized in red blood cells and kidney. Most of the drug (5%) and metabolites (70%) are excreted in the urine. Elimination half-life is 1 hour.

Indication: in combination with other anticancer drugs for the treatment of stage III and IV Hodgkin's disease, e.g., MOPP regimen (nitrogen mustard, vincristine, procarbazine, prednisone).

Dosage/Range:
- 100 mg/m^2 orally, daily from 7–14 days every 4 weeks as part of the MOPP regimen.
- Brain tumors: 60 mg/m^2 orally every day $\times$ 14 days as part of the PCV regimen.

Drug Preparation:
- None.

Drug Administration:
- Oral.
- Available in 50-mg capsules.

Drug Interactions:
- Procarbazine is synergistic with CNS depressants. Barbiturate, antihistamine, narcotic, and hypotensive agents or phenothiazine antiemetics should be used with caution.
- Disulfiram (Antabuse)-like reaction may result if the patient consumes alcohol. Symptoms include headache, respiratory difficulties, nausea and vomiting, chest pain, hypotension, and mental status changes.
- Exhibits weak MAO (monoamine oxidase) inhibitor activity. Foods containing high amounts of tyramine should be avoided: substances such as beer, wine, cheese, brewer's yeast, chicken livers, and bananas. Consumption of foods high in tyramine in combination with procarbazine may lead to intracranial hemorrhage or hypertensive crisis.
- Levodopa, meperidine: hypertension when either is taken with procarbazine. Avoid coadministration.
- Sympathomimetics, tricyclic antidepressants: CNS excitation, hypertension, palpitations, angina, hypertensive crisis; avoid coadministration.
- Antidiabetic (sulfonylurea, insulin): potentiation of hypoglycemic effect. Monitor blood sugar closely and adjust dose as needed.
- When taken in combination with digoxin, there is a decreased bioavailability of digoxin.

Lab Effects/Interference:
- Decreased CBC.
- Increased LFTs, RFTs.

Special Considerations:
- Discontinue if CNS signs/symptoms (paresthesia, neuropathy, confusion), stomatitis, diarrhea, or hypersensitivity reaction occur.
- Patients with G$_6$PD should be monitored closely for hemolytic anemia.
- Patients may develop hypersensitivity reaction (pruritus, urticaria, maculopapular rash, flushing) responding to steroid therapy and continuation of drug. If pulmonary infiltrates develop, procarbazine should be discontinued.

Potential Toxicities/Side Effects and the Nursing Process

I.   POTENTIAL FOR INFECTION AND BLEEDING related to BM DEPRESSION

Defining Characteristics: Major dose-limiting toxicity. Thrombocytopenia occurs in 50% of patients, evidenced by a delayed onset (28 days after treatment) and lasting 2–3 weeks. Leukopenia seen in two-thirds of patients, with nadirs occurring after initial thrombocytopenia. Anemias may be due to BM depression or hemolysis.

Nursing Implications: Monitor CBC, platelet count prior to drug administration, as well as signs/symptoms of infection, bleeding, and anemia. Instruct patient in self-assessment of signs/symptoms of infection, bleeding, and anemia and to report this immediately. Dose reduction often necessary (35–50%) if compromised BM function. Platelet and red cell transfusions per physician order.

II.   ALTERATION IN NUTRITION, LESS THAN BODY REQUIREMENTS, related to NAUSEA, VOMITING, DIARRHEA

Defining Characteristics: Nausea and vomiting occur in 70% of patients and may be a dose-limiting toxicity. Diarrhea is uncommon, but rarely may be protracted and thus would be an indication for dose reduction.

Nursing Implications: Teach patient to premedicate with antiemetics 30 minutes before taking procarbazine to prevent nausea and vomiting. Encourage small, frequent meals of cool, bland foods and liquids. Minimize nausea and vomiting by dividing the total daily dosage into 3–4 doses. Also, taking the pills at bedtime may decrease the sense of nausea. May administer nonphenothiazine antiemetics. Encourage patients to report onset of diarrhea. Administer, or teach patient to self-administer, antidiarrheal medications.

III.   POTENTIAL FOR SENSORY/PERCEPTUAL ALTERATIONS

Defining Characteristics: Symptoms occur in 10–30% of patients and are seen as lethargy, depression, frequent nightmares, insomnia, nervousness, or hallucinations. Tremors, coma, convulsions are less common. Symptoms usually disappear when drug is discontinued. Crosses into CSF.

Nursing Implications: Teach patient the potential for neurotoxicity and provide early counseling about these effects. Assess patients for any symptoms of neurotoxicity. Discuss strategies with patient to preserve general sense of well-being. Obtain baseline neurologic and motor function. CNS toxicity may be manifested as reactions to other drugs, e.g., barbiturates, narcotics, and phenothiazine antiemetics.

IV. ACTIVITY INTOLERANCE related to PN

Defining Characteristics: 10% of patients exhibit paresthesias, decrease in deep tendon reflexes. Foot drop and ataxia occasionally reported. Reversible when drug is discontinued.

Nursing Implications: Obtain baseline neurologic and motor function. Assess patient for any changes in motor function, e.g., ability to pick up pencils or buttons.

V. ALTERATION IN COMFORT related to FLU-LIKE SYNDROME

Defining Characteristics: Fever, chills, sweating, lethargy, myalgias, and arthralgias commonly occur at the beginning of therapy.

Nursing Implications: Teach patient the potential for flu-like syndrome and how to distinguish from actual infection. Instruct patient to report any changes in condition.

VI. POTENTIAL FOR IMPAIRED SKIN INTEGRITY related to RARE DERMATITIS REACTIONS

Defining Characteristics: Rarely occurs as alopecia, pruritus, rash, hyperpigmentation.

Nursing Implications: Assess patient for changes in skin, nails, and hair loss. Discuss with patient impact of changes and strategies to minimize distress, e.g., wearing nail polish, long-sleeved tops, wigs, scarves, caps.

VII. POTENTIAL SEXUAL DYSFUNCTION related to DRUG EFFECTS

Defining Characteristics: Drug is teratogenic. Causes azoospermia. Causes cessation of menses, although may be reversible.

Nursing Implications: As appropriate, explore with patient and partner issues of reproductive and sexuality patterns and the impact chemotherapy may have. Discuss strategies to preserve sexual and reproductive health (e.g., sperm banking, contraception).

Drug: streptozocin (Zanosar)

Class: Alkylating agent (nitrosourea).

Mechanism of Action: A weak alkylating agent (nitrosourea) that causes interstrand cross-linking in DNA and is cell cycle phase nonspecific. Appears to have some specificity for neoplastic pancreatic endocrine cells. Glucose attached to nitrosourea appears to diminish myelotoxicity.

Metabolism: 60–70% of total dose and 10–20% of parent drug appear in urine. Drug is rapidly eliminated from serum in 4 hours, with major concentrations occurring in liver and kidneys. Drug half-life is 35 minutes. Drug metabolized in the liver, and metabolites excreted in the urine.

Indication: For the treatment of patients with metastatic islet cell carcinoma of the pancreas (functional and nonfunctional) with symptomatic disease.

Dosage/Range:
- 500-mg/m^2 IV daily × 5 days. Repeat every 6 weeks; OR
- 1,000-mg/m^2 IV weekly × 2, then dose escalate if patient has not achieved a therapeutic response. Do not exceed 1,500-mg/m^2 IV for last 4 weeks of treatment (total treatment 6 weekly treatments). Patient observation follow the 6 weekly treatments.
- Dose-reduce (DR) based on 24-hour creatinine clearance (10–50 mL/min = 25% reduction; < 10 mL/min = 50% reduction).

Drug Preparation:
- Add sterile water or 0.9% sodium chloride to vial.
- If powder or solution contacts skin, wash immediately with soap and water.
- Solution is stable 48 hours at room temperature, 96 hours if refrigerated.

Drug Administration:
- Assess CBC, LFTs, renal function weekly or each cycle.
- Administer via pump over 1 hour.
- Has also been given as CI or continuous arterial infusion into the hepatic artery.
- If local pain or burning occurs, slow infusion and apply cool packs above injection site.
- Irritant; avoid extravasation.
- Administer with 1–2 L of hydration to prevent nephrotoxicity.

Drug Interactions:
- Nephrotoxic drugs (cisplatin, aminoglycosides, amphotericin B): additive nephrotoxicity; avoid concurrent use if possible.
- Steroids: increase risk of severe hyperglycemia.
- Phenytoin: antagonism of antitumor effect; do not coadminister.
- Doxorubicin: increased half-life of doxorubicin, resulting in increased myelosuppression.

Lab Effects/Interference:
- Decreased CBC.
- Increased RFTs (especially BUN).
- Increased LFTDH.
- Changes in glucose, phosphorus, albumin serum levels.

Special Considerations:
- Warnings and Precautions:
  - *Renal toxicity*: may occur, as evidenced by azotemia, anuria, hypophosphatemia, glycosuria, and renal tubular acidosis. This is dose related and cumulative. Monitor renal function before and after each course of treatment. Assess serial urinalysis (to detect

early proteinuria and if positive, should be followed by a 24-hour urine collection for protein), BUN, serum creatinine, serum electrolytes and creatinine clearance at lest weekly during, and for 4 weeks after each treatment course. Ensure adequate hydration during treatment. Do not use drug in combination with other drugs that are nephrotoxic.

- *Injection-site reactions*: extravasation may cause tissue lesions and necrosis.
- *Caution driving or using hazardous machinery:* Patients receiving the 5-day CI may feel confused or have lethargy or depression after treatment. Teach patient to have someone else drive them home and to avoid use of potentially hazardous machinery until patient knows effect.
- Drug is an irritant; give IV short infusion over 15–30 minutes or as a 6-hour infusion.

Potential Toxicities/Side Effects and the Nursing Process

I. POTENTIAL FOR ALTERATION IN URINARY ELIMINATION related to RENAL DYSFUNCTION

Defining Characteristics: 60% of patients experience renal dysfunction. Usually transient proteinuria and azotemia, but this may progress to permanent renal failure, especially if other nephrotoxic drugs are given concurrently. Signs/symptoms include proteinuria, increased BUN, hypophosphatemia, glycosuria, renal tubular acidosis, decreased creatinine clearance. Hypophosphatemia is probably earliest sign of renal dysfunction.

Nursing Implications: Closely monitor BUN, creatinine, phosphorus, urine protein, and 24-hour creatinine clearance prior to each treatment. Monitor BUN, creatinine, pH of urine, glucose/protein of urine every shift during therapy. Discuss dose reduction with physician based on creatinine clearance. Strictly monitor I/O during therapy. Hydration per physician, but usually 2–3 L/day. Rarely, renal toxicity may present as glucosuria, hypophosphatemia, and diabetes insipidus.

II. ALTERATION IN NUTRITION, LESS THAN BODY REQUIREMENTS, related to GI SIDE EFFECTS

Defining Characteristics: Nausea and vomiting occur in up to 90% of patients, beginning 1–4 hours after drug dose, and can be significantly reduced when drug is given as CI. Nausea and vomiting may worsen during 5-consecutive-day therapy; increased severity with doses > 500 mg/m^2. 10% of patients experience diarrhea with abdominal cramping. LFTs may be elevated but normalize with time. Hepatotoxicity occurs in approximately 50% of patients. Liver enzymes increase 2–3 weeks after therapy; albumin decreases, but symptoms rarely occur. May also develop painless jaundice.

Nursing Implications: Premedicate with antiemetics and continue prophylactically for 24 hours; use aggressive antiemetics when drug is given IV over 1 hour (serotonin antagonists effective). Encourage small, frequent feedings of cool, bland foods and liquids. If patient has nausea or vomiting, discuss with physician more aggressive antiemetics. Monitor

I/O closely and replace fluids. Encourage patient to report onset of diarrhea. Administer or teach patient to self-administer antidiarrheal medications. Teach patient diet modifications. Monitor LFTs prior to each treatment (alk phos, SGOT, SGPT, albumin). Assess for signs/ symptoms of hepatic dysfunction: jaundice, yellowing of skin, sclera; orange-colored urine; white or clay-colored stools; itchy skin.

III.   ALTERATIONS IN GLUCOSE METABOLISM related to HYPOGLYCEMIA

Defining Characteristics: Appears that damage to pancreatic beta cells causes sudden release of insulin, with resulting hypoglycemia in about 20% of patients. Hyperglycemia may occur in patients with insulinomas and decreased glucose tolerance. Increased fasting or postprandial blood levels may occur.

Nursing Implications: Monitor serum glucose levels every day or more frequently as needed; check urine glucose. Assess for, and instruct patient to report, the following signs/ symptoms of hypoglycemia: muscle weakness and lethargy, perspiration, flushed feeling, restlessness, headache, confusion, trembling, epigastric hunger pains. If signs/symptoms are found, encourage patient to eat or drink high-glucose food and juice and notify physician. Hypoglycemia can be prevented with nicotinamide. Assess for signs/symptoms of hyperglycemia in patient with insulinomas and instruct patient in self-assessment.

IV.   POTENTIAL FOR INFECTION AND BLEEDING related to BM DEPRESSION

Defining Characteristics: BM depression occurs in about 9–20% of patients. Nadir 1–2 weeks after administration. Occasionally, severe leukopenia and thrombocytopenia occur. Mild anemia may occur.

Nursing Implications: Monitor CBC, platelets prior to drug administration, as well as assess for signs/symptoms of infection or bleeding. Instruct patient in self-assessment of signs/symptoms of infection or bleeding.

V.   POTENTIAL FOR INJURY related to SECONDARY MALIGNANCIES

Defining Characteristics: Drug is carcinogenic; secondary malignancies are well described.

Nursing Implications: Patients receiving prolonged therapy should be screened periodically.

Drug: tamoxifen citrate (Nolvadex, Soltamox oral solution)

Class: Antiestrogen.

Mechanism of Action: Nonsteroidal antiestrogen that competitively binds to estrogen receptors, forming an abnormal complex that migrates to the cell nucleus and inhibits DNA synthesis. Also, appears to stimulate secretion of transforming growth factor beta, which proceeds to inhibit genes that stimulate cell proliferation. Activity is cell cycle specific in mid-G$_1$ phase.

Metabolism: Drug is a prodrug, and active metabolite is produced after metabolism by CYP2D6 pathway. Well absorbed from GI tract with a high degree of protein binding and peak plasma levels in 4–6 hours. Widely distributed in body tissue, especially areas where estrogen receptors are expressed. Metabolized by P450 microenzyme system in liver (CYP3A4, CYP2D6). Undergoes enterohepatic circulation, prolonging blood levels. Excreted in feces. Elimination half-life is 7–14 days.

Indications: (1) Metastatic breast cancer (MBC) in women and men; in premenopausal women, with MBC, tamoxifen is an alternative to oophorectomy or radiation of the ovaries (estrogen positive most likely to benefit); (2) adjuvant treatment of node-positive breast cancer in women after total mastectomy or segmental mastectomy, axillary dissection, and breast irradiation (most benefit in subgroup with 4+ positive axillary lymph nodes); (3) treatment of axcillary node-negative breast cancer after total mastectomy or segmental mastectomy, axillary dissection, and breast irradiation; (4) women with ductal carcinoma in situ (DCIS) to reduce risk of invasive breast cancer; (5) to reduce the risk of breast cancer in high-risk women.
- Tamoxifen reduces the occurrence of contralateral breast cancer in patients receiving adjuvant tamoxifen for breast cancer.
- While past data support 5 years of adjuvant tamoxifen therapy, in women with early-stage breast cancer, 10 years of tamoxifen threapy further reduces the risk of recurrence and breast cancer mortality (Davies et al., 2013).

Contraindications: (1) known hypersensitivity to tamoxifen or any of its ingredients; (2) when used to reduce risk of breast cancer, drug is contraindicated in women who require concomitant coumarin-type anticoagulant therapy or in women with a history of deep vein thrombosis or pulmonary embolus.

Dosage/Range:
- 20 mg PO daily (most often, 10 mg bid).

Drug Preparation:
- Available in 10-mg tablets or oral liquid solution (10 mg/5 mL).

Drug Administration:
- Oral
- Patients receiving tamoxifen to reduce cancer risk should have tamoxifen started during menstruation; if the woman has irregular menses, then she should have a negative B-HCG immediately prior to starting tamoxifen.

Drug Interactions:
- Anticoagulants (e.g., warfarin): increased PT; monitor PT closely and reduce anticoagulant dose as needed.
- CYP3A4, -2D6 inducers (carbamazepine, glucocorticoids, phenobarbital, phenytoin, rifampin, rifamycin, nevirapine): may decrease serum level of tamoxifen. Rifampin

decreased tamoxifen AUC by 86%. Aminoglutethamide also reduces plasma level of tamoxifen and its metabolite.

- CYP3A4, -2D6 inhibitors (ciprofloxacin, clarithromycin, doxycycline, erythromycin, imatinib, diclofenac, nicardipine, nefazodone, protease inhibitors, verapamil, quinidine, cimetidine, codeine, fluoxetine, haloperidol, paroxetine, fluoxetine, sertraline, antipsychotics thioridazine, perphenazine, pimozide): may block the activation of tamoxifen as tamoxifen, is a prodrug, and must be activated into the therapeutic metabolite.
- Drugs activated by P450 system: may inhibit metabolic activation of cyclophosphamide.
- Letrozole: decreased letrozole serum levels by 37%; do not give concurrently.
- Anastrozole: coadministration decreases anastrozole plasma concentration by 27%.
- St. John's wort: decreased tamoxifen serum level; do not give concurrently.

Lab Effects/Interference:
- Decreased CBC.
- Increased LFTs.
- Increased Ca.
- Interference in lab tests such as TFTs and hyperlipidemia.

Special Considerations:
- Warnings and Precautions:
  - *Effects in metatatic breast cancer patients*: hypercalcemia may occur in patients with bone metastases, within a few weeks of starting tamoxifen therapy. If this occurs, treatment of hypercalcemia should be implemented. If severe, tamoxifen should be discontinued.
  - *Effect on uterus*: increased risk of uterine malignancies, most adenocarcinomas. Rare uterine sarcomas may also occur. Teach patients to report any abnormal vaginal bleeding, and it should be promptly evaluated. Patients should have an annual gynecological examination. Other endometrial changes include hyperplasia, polyps, and menstrual irregularity or amenorrhea.
  - *Thromboembolic effects*: Increased risk for deep vein thrombosis and pulmonary emboli. Teach patients to report new onset calf pain, redness or cellulitis in the leg, chest pain, shortness of breath.
  - *Liver cancer*: rare, but may occur. Nonmalignant rare effects that may occur include fatty liver, cholestasis, hepatitis, and hepatic necrosis.
  - *Eye effects*: ocular disturbances including corneal changes, decrement in color vision perception, retinal vein thrombosis, and retinopathy have been reported.
  - *Embryo-fetal toxicity*: women should be advised to use effective contraception (barrier or nonhormonal contraception) during and for 2 months after last tamoxifen dose, to avoid pregnancy. Patients receiving tamoxifen to reduce cancer risk should have tamoxifen started during menstruation; if the woman has irregular menses, then she should have a negative B-HCG immediately prior to starting tamoxifen.
  - *Rare decreases in formed blood cell elements*: platelets, neutrophils, rare pancytopenia.
  - *Monitoring during tamoxifen therapy*: In addition to periodic CBC/platelets counts, LFTs:

- Teach patient to seek prompt medical care if new breast lump; vaginal bleeding; menstrual irregularities, change in vaginal dischare, pelvic painor pressure; symptoms of leg swelling or tenderness, unexplained SOB; or changes in vision.
- Women taking tamoxifen to reduce breast cancer risk or receiving adjuvant therapy: breast examination, mammogram, gynecologic exam prior to statting tamoxifen; these should be repeated regularly while on therapy.
- Use cautiously in patients with abnormal liver function or history of thromboembolic disease.
- Patients should be taught to notify physician immediately if patient develops abnormal uterine bleeding, pelvic pain, pain in the legs, or breathing problems.
- One study showed that women taking tamoxifen plus an SSRI that was a moderate-to-potent inhibitor of CYP2D6 (e.g., fluoxeine [Prozac], paroxetine [Paxil], sertraline [Zoloft]) had more than double the risk of breast cancer recurrence compared to those not taking them. The following SSRIs had NO effect on breast cancer recurrence: citalopram (Celexa), escitalopram (Lexapro), mirtazapine, venlafaxine, and fluvoxamine (Luvox) (Aubert et al., 2009). Some providers recommend testing of CYP2D6 to identify poor metabolizers of tamoxifen prior to starting the drug, but this is not yet recommended by the manufacturer (Mylan, 2013).
- A Swedish study (2016) showed that 2 years of adjuvant tamoxifen resulted in a long-term survival benefit in premenopausal patients with ER-positive primary breast cancer.

Potential Toxicities/Side Effects and the Nursing Process

I.   POTENTIAL FOR SEXUAL DYSFUNCTION related to CHANGES IN MENSES, HOT FLASHES

Defining Characteristics: May cause menstrual irregularity, hot flashes, milk production in breasts, vaginal discharge, and bleeding. Symptoms occur in about 10% of patients and are usually not severe enough to discontinue therapy. Drug may cause endometrial hyperplasia, polyps, and endometrial cancer.

Nursing Implications: As appropriate, explore with patient and partner issues of reproductive and sexuality patterns and the impact drug may have on them. Discuss strategies to preserve sexual and reproductive health. Teach patient that she should be closely followed by a gynecologist for annual endometrial biopsies and to report immediately abnormal uterine bleeding, or pelvic pain.

II.   POTENTIAL FOR ALTERATION IN CIRCULATION related to THROMBOEMBOLISM

Defining Characteristics: Tamoxifen has been associated with thromboembolic events and is associated with antithrombin III deficiency.

Nursing Implications: Teach patient to minimize likelihood of developing DVT, such as to avoid sitting in the same position for long periods, especially on airplanes, and to get up and walk regularly to increase venous return from the lower extremities. Teach patient to report immediately or go to the emergency department if pain in the lower extremities develops or the patient develops abrupt onset of dyspnea, shortness of breath, or any pulmonary symptom.

III.   POTENTIAL FOR ALTERATION IN COMFORT related to FLARE REACTION

Defining Characteristics: May cause flare reaction initially (bone and tumor pain, transient increase in tumor size). Nausea, vomiting, and anorexia may occur.

Nursing Implications: Inform patient of possibility of flare reaction, signs/symptoms to be aware of, and encourage patient to report any signs/symptoms. Inform patient of possibility of nausea, vomiting, and anorexia. Encourage small, frequent meals of high-calorie, high-protein foods.

IV.   POTENTIAL FOR SENSORY/PERCEPTUAL ALTERATION related to VISUAL CHANGES

Defining Characteristics: Retinopathy has been reported with high doses. Corneal changes, cataracts, decreased visual acuity, and blurred vision have occurred. Headache, dizziness, and light-headedness are rare.

Nursing Implications: Obtain visual assessment prior to starting therapy. Encourage patient to report any visual changes and discuss evaluation by ophthalmologist depending upon symptom(s). Instruct patient to report headache, dizziness, light-headedness.

V.   POTENTIAL FOR INFECTION AND BLEEDING related to BM DEPRESSION

Defining Characteristics: Mild, transient leukopenia and thrombocytopenia occur rarely.

Nursing Implications: Monitor CBC, platelets prior to drug administration and after therapy has begun. Instruct patient in self-assessment of signs/symptoms of infection or bleeding.

VI.   POTENTIAL FOR SKIN INTEGRITY IMPAIRMENT related to RASH, ALOPECIA

Defining Characteristics: Skin rash, alopecia, peripheral edema are rare.

Nursing Implications: Assess patient for signs/symptoms of hair loss, edema, and skin rash. Instruct patient to report any of these symptoms. Discuss with patient the impact of skin changes.

VII. POTENTIAL FOR INJURY related to HYPERCALCEMIA

Defining Characteristics: Hypercalcemia uncommon.

Nursing Implications: Obtain serum calcium levels prior to therapy and at regular intervals during therapy. Instruct patient in signs/symptoms of hypercalcemia: nausea, vomiting, weakness, constipation, loss of muscle tone, malaise, decreased urine output.

Drug: temozolomide (Temodar)

Class: Alkylating agent.

Mechanism of Action: Drug is a member of the imidazotetrazine class and is the active metabolite of dacarbazine in an oral form. Drug is a prodrug, forming the metabolite monomethyl triazenoimidazole carboxamide (MTIC) when chemically degraded, and is further metabolized to 5-aminoimidazole-4-carboxamide (AIC), the active cytotoxic metabolite. Drug is lipophilic and can pass through the BBB, where it has been shown to be effective against some brain tumors, possibly because of the alkaline pH. MTIC causes alkylation of DNA and RNA strands, and DNA, RNA, and protein synthesis is inhibited.

Metabolism: Well absorbed from the GI tract following oral dose (100% bioavailability), with peak concentrations in 1 hour when taken on empty stomach. The elimination half-life is 1.8 hours. The drug is degraded into MTIC in plasma and tissues. 15% of drug is excreted unchanged in the urine. Differs from dacarbazine in that formation of MTIC does not require liver metabolism. Food decreases the rate and extent of drug absorption. IV formulation.

Indication: For the treatment of adult patients with (1) newly diagnosed glioblastoma multiforme (GBM) concomitantly with RT and then as maintenance treatment; (2) refractory anaplastic astrocytoma in patients who have experienced disease progression on a drug regimen containing nitrosurea and procarbazine.

Contraindication: known hypersensitivity to any temozolomide component or to dacarbazine (DTIC).

Dosage/Range: See package insert for dosing modification guidelines.
Refractory anaplastic astrocytoma that has failed prior chemotherapy:
- Initial dose 150 mg/m^2/day orally × 5 days, repeated every 28 days.
- Dose should be adjusted to keep ANC 1,000–1,500/mm^3 and platelet count 50,000–100,000/mm^3.

Newly diagnosed GBM concomitantly with (at the same time as) radiotherapy and then as maintenance treatment:
- 75 mg/m^2 orally, daily starting the first day of RT through the last day of RT, for 42 days (maximum 49 days), followed by initial maintenance dose of 150 mg/m^2 once

daily for days 1–5 of a 28-day cycle for 6 cycles as long as ANC $\geq$ 1,500 cells/mm^3, platelet count $\geq$ 100,000 cells/mm^3, and other toxicities (except alopecia, nausea, vomiting) are less than grade 1 (CTCAE). Interrupt drug for ANC 500–1,500 cells/mm^3, platelets < 100,000/mm^3, nonhematologic toxicity grade 2; discontinue drug for ANC < 500 cells/mm^3, platelets < 10,000 cells/mm^3, and nonhematologic toxicity grades 3–4.

- Prophylaxis for *Pneumocystis carinii* pneumonia while receiving concomitant RT and temozolomide, continuing to 4 weeks after completion of RT. All patients, especially those receiving steroids, should be observed closely for lymphopenia and PCP.
- Followed by initial maintenance dose of temozolomide 150 mg/m^2/day orally $\times$ 5 days, repeated every 28 days for 6 cycles.
  - Cycle 1: Temozolomide 150 mg/m^2 orally daily $\times$ 5, then 23 days without treatment (as long as ANC > 1,500 cells/mm^3, platelet count > 100,000 cells/mm^3, and other toxicity [except alopecia, nausea, vomiting] are less than grade 1 [CTCAE]).
  - Cycle 2–6: Temozolomide 200 mg/m^2 orally daily $\times$ 5 then 23 days without treatment, repeated for 5 more cycles (as long as ANC > 1,500 cells/mm^3, platelet count > 100,000 cells/mm^3, and other toxicity [except alopecia, nausea, vomiting] are < grade 1 [CTCAE]).
  - Monitor CBC on day 22 then weekly until ANC > 1,500 cells/mm^3, and platelets > 100,000 cells/mm^3.
  - See package insert for temozolomide maintenance treatment dose levels, and dose reductions based on nadir counts and worst CTCAE toxicity.
- IV Dose: temozolomide same dose as oral capsule formulation, given as an infusion over 90 minutes (bioequivalent to oral dose).

Drug Preparation:
- Available in oral capsules as 250 mg, 180 mg, 140 mg, 100 mg, 20 mg, and 5 mg; IV dose as an 100-mg powder for injection. Bioequivalence of IV dose and capsules established when temozolomide was infused over 90 minutes only.
- Drug is stored at room temperature, protected from light and moisture.
- IV: Available as 100-mg powder for injection. Dose is the same dose as the oral dose. Add 41 mL sterile water for injection resulting in a concentration of 2.5 mg/mL. Bring vial to room temperature prior to mixing. Gently swirl to mix, and use within 14 hours of reconstitution. Leave vial at room temperature once mixed. Aseptically withdraw ordered dose, where 40 mL per vial is 100 mg (2.5 mg/mL). Discard any remaining solution. Transfer ordered dose into an empty 250-mL PVC infusion bag, and administer via pump over 90 min.
- Dose based on nadir WBC, platelet count, as well as the counts on day of treatment.

Drug Administration:
- Give orally with full glass of water on an empty stomach. Patient should take medicine at around the same time of day each day, e.g., bedtime.
- Do not crush or dissolve capsule.

- Administer IV over 90 minutes. Shorter dosing times may result in suboptimal dosing. Flush line before and after temozolomide infusion. Do not infuse with any other medication.

Drug Interactions:
- Valproic acid: reduces temozolomide clearance by 5% but may not be clinically significant; monitor drug effect closely if used together.

Lab Effects/Interference:
- Elevated liver function tests (e.g., ALT, AST; occur in up to 40% of patients), increase in alk phos.
- Decreased WBC, Hgb, and platelet count.
- Hyperglycemia.
- Elevated renal function tests.

Special Considerations:
- Warnings and Precautions:
  - *Myelosuppression*: may produce prolonged pancytopenia, resulting in aplastic anemia (this occurred in some patients taking concomitant carbamazepine, phenytoin, sufamethoxazole/trimethoprim), Administer drug only when ANC $\geq$ 1,500 cells/mm^3, platelets $\geq$ 100,000/mm^3. Assess CBC/differential on day 22 (21 days after 1st dose) or within 48 hours of that day, and weekly until the ANC is > 1,500 cells/mm^3 and platelet count is > 100,000/mm^3. Women and the elderly are at higher risk of developing myelosuppression.
  - *MDS*: MDS and secondary malignancies, including myeloid leukemia, have been observed.
  - *Pneumocystis pneumonia*: Increased incidence of PCP when drug is given over a prolonged time. Prophylaxis is required for all patiens receiving concomitant temozolomide and RT for the 42-day regimen. Patients at risk for PCP include patients receiving steroids as well.
  - *Laboratory tests*: Laboratory monitoring: With concurrent RT, monitor CBC/ differential baseline then weekly during treatment; for 28-day treatment cycles, baseline CBC/differential, repeated on day 1 and day 22. If ANC falls < 1,500 cells/mm^3, and platelet count < 100,00 cells/mm^3, see Dosing and Dose Modification Guidelines package insert. Then assess CBC weekly until recovery of ANC to >1,500 cells/mm^3 and platelet count is > 100,000/mm^3.
  - *Severe and fatal hepatotoxicity* has been reported. Assess LFTs baseline, and midway through first cycle, prior to each subsequent cycle, and 2–4 weeks after last dose of temozolomide.
  - *Embryo-fetal toxicity:* Drug causes fetal harm. Teach women of reproductive potential to use effective contraception to avoid pregnancy. Nursing mothers should make a decision to stop nursing or to discontinue the drug, taking into account the importance of the drug to the mother's health.
  - *Infusion time*: Infusion time: study showed bioequivalence when infusion time was 90 minutes, so drug must be infused over this time.

Potential Toxicities/Side Effects and the Nursing Process

I.   POTENTIAL FOR INFECTION, BLEEDING, AND FATIGUE related to BM DEPRESSION

Defining Characteristics: Thrombocytopenia and leukopenia are dose-limiting factors and occur in grade 2 or higher 40% of the time. This does not usually require administration of G-CSF. Nadir at 21–22 days, unless using 5-day treatment schedule, where nadir is day 28–29. Recovery for platelets is 7–42 days and in shorter time for WBC. Anemia may also occur, but is infrequent and less severe. Severity of BM depression depends on dose and schedule, as well as disease process. In one trial, patients with malignant glioma had severe lymphopenia (41% grade 3 and 15% grade 4).

Nursing Implications: Assess baseline WBC, differential, platelet, and Hgb/HCT prior to chemotherapy, as well as for signs/symptoms of infection or bleeding. Teach patient signs/symptoms of infection and bleeding and to report these immediately; teach patient self-care measures to minimize risk of infection and bleeding. This includes avoidance of crowds, proximity to people with infections, and OTC aspirin-containing medications. Teach patient to report fatigue and teach measures to conserve energy, such as alternating rest and activity periods. Discuss transfusion of red blood cells as needed.

II.   ALTERED NUTRITION, LESS THAN BODY REQUIREMENTS, related to NAUSEA AND VOMITING, STOMATITIS, AND DIARRHEA

Defining Characteristics: Nausea and vomiting occur in 75% of patients, usually grades 1 or 2, and usually occurring on day 1. In one trial, using a 5-day treatment regimen, 21% had grade 3 nausea, and 23% had grade 4. Stomatitis may occur in up to 20% of patients. Diarrhea, constipation, and/or anorexia may affect up to 40% of patients.

Nursing Implications: Teach patient to self-medicate with antiemetics (serotonin antagonist effective) 1 hour prior to dose and suggest evening dosing to minimize nausea/vomiting. Encourage small, frequent feedings of cool, bland foods. Teach patient to notify provider right away if nausea/vomiting persists. Assess oral mucosa prior to drug administration and teach patient to report changes. Teach patient oral hygiene measures and self-assessment. Teach patient to report diarrhea, to self-administer prescribed antidiarrheal medications, and to drink adequate fluids. Teach patient to report constipation, and manage with stool softeners or laxatives. If patient has anorexia, teach patient to select acceptable foods and to eat small portions q 2 hours and at bedtime. Teach patient to keep a diary documenting when medications are taken and side effects and to bring in medication bottle for a pill count to evaluate ability to adhere to regimen.

III.   ALTERATION IN SKIN INTEGRITY/COMFORT related to RASH, PRURITUS, ALOPECIA

Defining Characteristics: Skin rash, itching, and mild alopecia may occur, and are mild.

TREATMENT

Nursing Implications: Teach patient about the possibility of these side effects and to notify the nurse if any develop. Discuss rash with physician if moderate or severe. Teach patient local symptom-management strategies for itch. Reassure patient that hair loss is usually thinning with mild hair loss and will grow back.

IV. ACTIVITY INTOLERANCE, POTENTIAL, related to CENTRAL NERVOUS SYSTEM EFFECTS

Defining Characteristics: Lethargy (up to 40% in patients with malignant glioma), fatigue, headache, ataxia, and dizziness may occur; in clinical testing, it was unclear whether this was due to neurologic disease (i.e., malignant glioma), concurrent other drug therapy, or temozolomide.

Nursing Implications: Assess baseline energy and activity level. Teach patients that these side effects may occur, especially if the primary diagnosis is malignant glioma. Teach patient to report them. Teach patient to alternate rest and activity periods, to use supportive device such as a cane if ataxia or dizziness occurs, and other measures to maximize activity tolerance and to prevent injury.

Drug: thioguanine (Tabloid, 6-thioguanine, 6-TG)

Class: Nucleoside metabolic inhibitor (antimetabolite); thiopurine antimetabolite.

Mechanism of Action: Converts to monophosphate nucleotides and inhibits *de novo* purine synthesis. The nucleotides are also incorporated into DNA. Cell cycle specific for S phase. Thioguanine interferes with nucleic acid biosynthesis, resulting in sequential blockage of the synthesis and utilization of the purine nucleotides.

Metabolism: Oral absorption is incomplete (30%) and variable, with a plasma half-life of 11 hours. Food may affect absorption. Drug is metabolized in the liver by deamination and methylation. Metabolites are excreted in the urine and feces.

Indication: For remission induction and remission consolidation treatment of patients with acute nonlymphocytic leukemias (not recommended during maintenance due to high risk of liver toxicity).

Dosage/Range:
- **Children and adults:** 100 mg/m^2 orally every 12 hours for 5–10 days, usually in combination with cytarabine and then 100 mg/m^2 orally every 12 hours for 5 days repeated every 4 weeks for maintenance.
- 1–3 mg/kg orally daily OR 75–200 mg/m^2/day orally in one to two divided doses $\times$ 5–7 days or until remission.

Drug Preparation:
- Available in 40-mg tablets.

Drug Administration:
• Given orally between meals; can be given as a single dose.

Drug Interactions:
• Busulfan: increased hepatotoxicity; use caution when used together; monitor patient closely during long-term therapy.
• Other hepatotoxic drugs: increased risk of hepatotoxicity.

Lab Effects/Interference:
• Decreased CBC.
• Increased LFTs.
• Increased uric acid.

Special Considerations:
• Oral dose is to be given on empty stomach to facilitate absorption.
• Dose is titrated to avoid excessive stomatitis and diarrhea.
• Thioguanine can be used in full doses with allopurinol.
• Warnings and Precautions:
  • *Myelosuppression* is dose limiting. Neutropenia preceeds thrombocytopenia, with nadir 10–14 days after dose, with recovery by day 21. Immunosuppression increases risk of bacterial, fungal, and parasitic infections. Monitor CBC/differential baseline, and closely during therapy.
  • *Mucositis and diarrhea* may occur and be severe, requiring dose reduction. Teach patients to self-assess, and report if/when it occurs. Teach self-care strategies to minimize toxicity, use systematic oral cleansing, and self-administer immodium or anti-diarrheal medication as needed.
  • *Hepatotoxicity* with increased levels of serum transaminases, serum bilirubin may occur. Veno-occlusive disease of the liver can rarely occur; monitor LFTs baseline and during treatment. Monitor LFTs baseline and during treatment.
  • *Renal function tests* may be transiently elevated. Assess baseline renal function tests, and monitor during therapy.
  • *Embryo-fetal toxicity*: teach women on reproductive potential to use effective contraception during therapy with thioguanine. Drug is mutagenic, teratogenic, and carcinogenic.

Potential Toxicities/Side Effects and the Nursing Process

I.   ALTERATION IN NUTRITION, LESS THAN BODY REQUIREMENTS, related to GI SIDE EFFECTS

Defining Characteristics: Nausea and vomiting occur commonly, especially in children, but are dose related; anorexia is rare; stomatitis is rare, but most common with high doses; hepatotoxicity is rare, but may be associated with hepatic veno-occlusive disease or jaundice.

Nursing Implications: Treat symptomatically with antiemetics. Encourage small, frequent feedings of cool, bland foods and liquids. If vomiting occurs, assess for fluid and electrolyte imbalance. Monitor I/O and daily weights if patient is hospitalized. Encourage small, frequent meals of favorite foods, especially high-calorie, high-protein foods. Encourage use of spices and obtain weekly weights. Teach oral assessment and oral hygiene regimen. Encourage patient to report early stomatitis. Provide pain relief measures, if indicated. Monitor LFTs prior to drug dose. Assess patient prior to and during treatment for signs/symptoms of hepatotoxicity. Discuss drug dose reduction if mucositis or diarrhea occurs and is severe.

II.   POTENTIAL FOR INFECTION AND BLEEDING related to BM DEPRESSION

Defining Characteristics: BM depression occurs 1–4 weeks after treatment, with nadir 10–14 days and recovery by day 21. Leukopenia and thrombocytopenia are most common. Immunosuppression may occur, with increased risk of bacterial, fungal, and parasitic infections.

Nursing Implications: Monitor CBC, platelet count prior to drug administration as well as for signs/symptoms of infection or bleeding. Instruct patient in self-assessment of signs/ symptoms of infection or bleeding. Administer platelet, red blood cell transfusions per physician's order.

III.   POTENTIAL FOR SENSORY/PERCEPTUAL ALTERATION related to LOSS OF VIBRATORY SENSE

Defining Characteristics: Loss of vibratory sensation; unsteady gait may occur.

Nursing Implications: Assess vibratory sensation, gait before each dose and between treatments. Report changes to physician. Encourage patient to report any changes.

Drug: topotecan hydrochloride for injection (Hycamtin)

Class: Topoisomerase I inhibitor.

Mechanism of Action: Topoisomerase I causes reversible single-strand breaks in DNA, which permits relaxation of DNA helix prior to DNA replication. Topotecan binds to the topoisomerase I-DNA complex, thus preventing repair (religation) of the strand breaks. When the cell tries to synthesize DNA, replication enzymes interact with the complex, and this leads to double-strand DNA breaks that cannot be repaired; thus, drug prevents DNA synthesis and replication and leads to cell death.

Metabolism: After IV administration, extensively tissue-bound, with about 35% of drug bound to plasma proteins. Crosses BBB. 30% of dose is excreted in the urine. Patients with moderate renal impairment have a 33% decrease in plasma clearance; patients with moderate impairment require a dosage adjustment. Minor metabolism by the liver, so patients with liver dysfunction do not require dose modification. The oral formulation is rapidly absorbed with peak plasma concentration occurring between 1 to 2 hours and 40% bio-availability. Drug demonstrates biexponential pharmacokinetics, and the mean terminal half-life is 3–6 hours. Drug binds to plasma proteins 35%. 57% of the oral dose (five daily doses) was recovered; 20% was excreted in the urine and 33% in the feces.

Indication (IV topotecan): Patients with (1) metastatic carcinoma of the ovary after disease progression on or after initial or subsequent chemotherapy, as a single agent; (2) small cell lung cancer (SCLC) platinim-sensitive disease in patients who progressed at least 60 days after first-line chemotherapy, as a single agent; (3) Stage IVB recurrent or persistent cervical cancer that is not amenable to curative treatment, in combination therapy with cisplatin.

Indication (PO topotecan): Treatment of patients with relapsed SCLC who have had a prior CR or PR, and who are at least 45 days from the end of 1st line chemotherapy.

Contraindication: patients with a history of severe hypersensitivity reactions to topotecan.

Dosage/Range:

Parenteral (IV) Dose:
- *Metastatic carcinoma of the ovary* after failure of initial or subsequent chemo: 1.5 mg/m^2 IV infusion over 30 minutes daily for 5 consecutive days (days 1–5) starting on day 1 of a 21-day cycle. (Some oncologists use dose of 1.25 mg/m^2, which the manufacturer says has equal efficacy.) Minimum of 4 courses as tumor response may be delayed. Median time to response is 9–12 weeks.
- *SCLC:* 1.5-mg/m^2 IV infusion over 30 minutes daily for 5 consecutive days (days 1–5) starting on day 1 of a 21-day cycle. Median time to response was 5–7 weeks.
- *Cervical cancer:* 0.75-mg/m^2 IV over 30 minutes, on days 1, 2, and 3 followed by cisplatin 50-mg/m^2 IV infusion on day 1 of a 21-day cycle.
- Verify BSA area prior to drug preparation and dispensing; recommended dosage should generally NOT exceed 4-mg IV.
- *Dose Modification for Renal Impairment*: When given as a single agent, reduce the dose to 0.75 mg/m^2/day for CrCl of 20–39 mL/min (calculated with the Cockcroft-Gault method using ideal body weight).
- *Dose Modification for Adverse Reactions*: (IV preparation)
  - *Hematologic:* DO NOT give subsequent cycles of topotecan injection until ANC recovers to >1,000/mm^3, platelets recover to >100,000/mm^3, and Hgb levels recover to ≥ 9 g/cL (with transfusion if necessary).
  - As single agent, reduce topotecan dose to 1.25 mg/m^2 day for: (a) ANC < 500/mm^3 or administer G-CSF starting no sooner than 24 hours following the last dose; (b) platelet count < 25,000/mm^3 during previous cycle.
  - In combination with cisplatin, reduce the dose to 0.6 mg/ m^2/day (and further to 0.45 mg/m^2/day if necessary) for: (a) febrile neutropenia (defined as ANC < 1,000/mm^3 with temperature of ≥38°C (100.4°F) or administer G-CSF starting no sooner than 24 hours after the last dose; (b) platelet counts <25,000/mm^3 during previous cycle.

Oral Dose:

- *SCLC*: 2.3 mg/m^2/day PO once daily × 5 consecutive days with or without food, starting on Day 1 of a 21-day cycle. Round the dose to the nearest 0.25 mg and physician should prescribe the minimum number of 1-mg and 0.25-mg capsules. Prescribe the same number of capsules for each of the 5 dosing days. The provider should NOT prescribe a replacement dose for emesis.
- *Dose Modification for Renal Impairment* (calculated with the Cockcroft-Gault method using ideal body weight): (a) CrCl 30–49 mL/min: Administer 1.5 mg/m^2/day; (b) CrCl of <30 mL/min, administer 0.6 mg/m^2/day.
- *Dose Modification for Advere Effects* (capsules):
  - *Hematologic*: DO NOT give subsequent cycles of topotecan injection until ANC recovers to >1,000/mm^3, platelets recover to >100,000/mm^3, and Hgb levels recover to ≥ 9 g/cL (with transfusion if necessary). **Reduce dose by 0.4 mg/ m^2/day for**
    - ANC < 500 cells/mm^3 associated with fever or infection or lasting ≥7d days or more; or
    - ANC 500–1,000/mm^3 lasting beyond day 21 of the treatment course; or
    - Platelet counts <25,000 cells/mm^3 during previous cycle.
  - *Diarrhea:* DO NOT administer topotecan capsules to patients with grade 3 or 4 diarrhea. After recovery to grade 1 or less, reduce dose by 0.4 mg/m^2/day for subsequent courses.

Drug Preparation:

- IV formulation available as a 4-mg vial.
- Reconstitute vial with 4 mL sterile water for injection.
- Further dilute in 0.9% sodium chloride or 5% dextrose.
- Use immediately. Reconstituted vials diluted for infusion are stable at 20–25°C (68–77°F).
- Oral topotecan: Available as 0.25-mg capsules (white to yellowish-white), and 1-mg capsules (opaque pink).

Drug Administration:

- Baseline ANC for initial course must be > 1,500/mm^3 and platelets > 100,000/mm^3 for treatment. For subsequent courses, counts must recover to ANC > 1,000/mm^3, platelets > 100,000/mm^3, and hemoglobin ≥ 9 mg/dL (with transfusion if necessary).
  - Serum creatinine must be ≤ 1.5 g/dL to administer topotecan with cisplatin.
- Ovarian and SCLC: Administer 1.5-mg/m^2 IV daily over 30 minutes, days 1–5, with cycle repeated q 21 days;
- G-CSF may be required if neutropenia develops.
- Cervical cancer: 0.75-mg/m^2 IV days 1, 2, 3 followed by cisplatin 50-mg/m^2 IV over 1 hour on day 1 of the cycle, and the cycle repeated every 21 days.
- Avoid extravasation of drug, as severe reactions have been reported.

Oral topotecan:

- To administer oral topotecan, assses cbc/differential as counts must be: ANC > 1,000/mm^3, platelets > 100,000/mm^3, and hemoglobin ≥ 9 mg/dL (with transfusion if necessary).

- Teach patient to (1) take topotecan capsules with or without food, at about the same time each day $\times$ 5; (2) not to chew, crush, or divide capsules. Do not take a replacement dose for emesis.
- Teach patient NOT to take capsules if severe (grades 3–4) diarrhea (increase or 7 or more stools a day over baseline, incontinence, or hospitalization needed, or life-threatening) and to call provider to be seen, or 911 to go to the ED for monitoring of fluid and electrolytes and management of severe diarrhea which may be fatal. Hold oral topotecan for grades 3–4 diarrhea. After recovery, the dose should be reduced to 0.4 mg/m^2/day for subsequent courses.
- Discuss need for effective contraception in women of reproductive potential during treatment and for 6 months after last dose, and men with female sexual partners of reproductive potential, during treatment and for 3 months after last dose. Discuss fertility and family planning prior to starting therapy as drug can cause infertility.

Drug Interactions:
- PO: P = glycoprotein inhibitors (e.g., cyclosporine A, elacridar, ketoconazole, ritonavir, and saquinavir) or breast cancer resistance protein (BCRP) inhibitors: increase topotecan exposure; AVOID concurrent use.
- G-CSF: can prolong duration of neutropenia, so do not initiate until day 6 of a 5-day course of therapy, or day 4 of a 3-day course (24 hours after the last dose of topotecan).
- Platinum, other cytotoxic agents: increased severity of myelosuppression. Administering cisplatin on day 1 of a 5-day course of topotecan required lower doses of each agent, compared to coadministration on day 5 of the dosing schedule of topotecan.

Lab Effects/Interference:
- Decreased CBC.
- Increased LFTs, RFTs.

Special Considerations:
- Most common adverse reactions (>5%) when given IV: (a) ovarian cancer: grade 3 or 4 neutropenia, anemia, thrombocytopenia, and febrile neutropenia; (all grades) nausea, vomiting, fatigue, diarrhea, dyspnea; (b) SCLC: grade 3 or 4 neutropenia, anemia, thrombocytopenia, and febrile neutropenia; (all grades) asthenia, dyspnea, nausea, pneumonia, abdominal pain, fatigue; (c) cervical cancer: grade 3 or 4 neutropenia, anemia, thrombocytopenia; (all grades) pain, vomiting, infection/febrile neutropenia.
- Most common adverse reactions (>5%) when given PO: SCLC: grade 3 or 4 neutropenia, anemia, thrombocytopenia; (all grades) nausea, diarrhea, vomiting, alopecia, fatigue, anorexia.
- Warnings and Precautions:
  - Parenteral (IV):
  - *BM Suppression* is dose-limiting toxicity.
    - As monotherapy, grade 4 neutropenia (ANC < 500 cells/mm^3 occurred in 78% (median duration 7 days), while in combination with cisplatin, the incidence was 48%.
    - *Thrombocytopenia* (grade 4, < 25,000 cells/mm^3) occurred in 27% of patients receiving monotherapy, with a median duration of 5 days. In combination with cisplatin, 7% of patients had grade 4 thrombocytopenia.

- Anemia: grades 3–4 (Hgb < 8 g/dL) occurred in 37% of patients.
- *Neutropenic enterocolitis*: topotecan can cause fatal typhlitis; consider this possibility if patient presents with fever, neutropenia, and abdominal pain.
- *Extravasation and tissue injury*: Drug is an irritant but may result in severe injury. Monitor IV site closely during drug administration. Administer via a large vein with freely flowing IV, and if extravasation suspected, immediately stop the administration and aspirate any remaining drug from IV tubing (see chapter introduction). Monitor IV site. Administer any remaining drug via a different IV site.

Oral topotecan:

- *Myelosuppression*: Median nadir for neutrophils and platelets is day 15. Grade 4 neutropenia most commonly occurred in cycle 1. Grade 4 neutropenia occurred in 32% of patients with a median duration of 7 days. Grade 4 thrombocytopenia occurred in 6% with a median duration of 3 days. Grade 3–4 anemia occurred in 25%.
    - Ensure first cycle of topotecan capsules are administered only to patients with a baseline ANC >1,500/mm^3 and platelet count >100,000 mm^3. Teach patient dose modifications based on nadir counts.
    - Neutropenic enterocolitis (typhlitis) may occur and be fatal. Teach patients to report abdominal pain right away and seek emergency medical care if fever and neutropenia also present.
- *Diarrhea*: May be life-threatening and require hospitalization. If it occurs at the same time as neutropenia it can result in sepsis. Incidence of diarrhea is 22%, with median time to onset of grade 2 to 4 diarrhea was 9 days. Teach patients to take antidiarrheals at the first sign of diarrhea and to report it right away. Explain dose modifications based on severity of diarrhea made by physician.

Both oral and parenteral:

- *Interstital Lung Disease (ILD)*: can occur, especially in patients with the following risk factors: history of ILD, pulmonary fibrosis, lung cancer, thoracic RT, and use of pneumotoxic drugs and/or colony stimulating factors. Monitor patients for signs/symptoms of ILD (e.g., cough, fever, dyspnea, and/or hypoxia). Discontinue drug if a new diagnosis of ILD is confirmed.
- *Embryo-fetal toxicity:* Teach women of reproductive potential to use effective contraception to avoid pregnancy during topotecan therapy and for at least 1 month after the last dose. If the drug is used during pregnancy or if the patient becomes pregnant while receiving the drug, apprise the patient of the potential hazard to the fetus. Mothers should not breastfeed while receiving topotecan therapy. Male patients with female sexual partners of reproductive potential should be taught to use effective contraception during topotecan therapy and for at least 3 months after the last dose. Drug can cause infertility in men and women. Discuss fertility and family planning prior to starting therapy.
- Extravasation and tissue injury:
- Oral formulation: Teach patient to store pills out of reach of children and pets, at con-
    ᵒm temperature, and protected from light.

Potential Toxicities/Side Effects and the Nursing Process

I.   INFECTION AND BLEEDING related to BM DEPRESSION

Defining Characteristics: IV formulation: Myelosuppression is the dose-limiting toxicity. Severe grade 4 neutropenia is seen during the first course of therapy in 60% of patients. Febrile neutropenia or sepsis may occur in up to 26% of patients. Nadir occurs on day 11. Prophylactic G-CSF is needed in 27% of courses after the first cycle. Thrombocytopenia (grade 4 with platelet count $< 25,000/mm^3$) occurs in 26% of patients. Platelet nadir occurs on day 15. Severe anemia (Hgb < 8 g/dL) occurs in 40% of patients, and transfusions were needed for 56% of patients. Oral formulation: Grades 3–4 neutropenia occurred in 61% of patients, anemia in 25%, and thrombocytopenia in 37%.

Nursing Implications: Monitor CBC and platelet count prior to drug administration as well as signs/symptoms of infection or bleeding. Assess renal function baseline and prior to each treatment. Discuss dose reductions with physician (see Special Considerations section). Instruct patient in self-assessment of signs/symptoms of infection or bleeding. Administer RBCs and platelet transfusions per physician's orders. Teach patient self-administration of G-CSF as ordered. Discuss dose modification with physician depending on severity of BM depression.

II.   ALTERATION IN NUTRITION, LESS THAN BODY REQUIREMENTS, related to NAUSEA AND VOMITING, DIARRHEA, ELEVATED LFTS

Defining Characteristics: IV formulation: Nausea occurs in 77% of patients, and vomiting in 58% without premedication with antiemetics. Diarrhea occurs in 42% of patients, while constipation occurs in 39%. Abdominal pain may occur in 33% of patients. Aspirate aminotransferase (AST, previously SGOT) and alanine aminotransferase (ALT, previously SGPT) elevations occur in 5% of patients. Oral formulation: Grades 3–4 nausea occurred in 27% of patients and vomiting in 19%. Diarrhea occurred in 14%.

Nursing Implications: Premedicate with a serotonin antagonist or dopamine antagonist antiemetic, and continue prophylactically for 24 hours to prevent nausea and vomiting, at least for the first treatment. Teach patient to take oral antiemetics 1 hour before taking oral topotecan. Encourage small, frequent feedings of cool, bland, dry foods. Assess for symptoms of fluid and electrolyte imbalance: monitor I/O and daily weights if administered to an inpatient. Teach patient oral assessment and oral hygiene regimen. Encourage patient to report early stomatitis. Provide pain relief measures if indicated (e.g., topical anesthetics). Encourage patient to report onset of diarrhea. Administer or teach patient to self-administer antidiarrheal medication. Ensure adequate hydration, monitor I/O. Monitor LFTs baseline and periodically during treatment. Discuss dose modification with physician depending on severity of diarrhea in patients receiving oral topotecan.

III.   POTENTIAL FOR HEPATOTOXICITY related to HYPOALBUMINEMIA, PREEXISTING HEPATIC INSUFFICIENCY (IV formulation)

Defining Characteristics: Evidence of increased drug toxicity in patients with low protein and hepatic dysfunction. Dose reductions may be necessary.

Nursing Implications: Monitor LFTs prior to drug dose. Assess patient prior to administering drug and during treatment for signs/symptoms of hepatotoxicity.

IV.   POTENTIAL FOR SKIN INTEGRITY IMPAIRMENT related to ALOPECIA (oral formulation)

Defining Characteristics: Alopecia occurs in 10–20% of patients.

Nursing Implications: Assess patient for signs/symptoms of hair loss. Instruct patient to report any of these symptoms. Discuss with patient the impact of skin changes.

Drug: toremifene citrate (Fareston)

Class: Estrogen agonist/antagonist; selective estrogen receptor modulator (SERM).

Mechanism of Action: Nonsteroidal estrogen antagonist: competitively binds directly to estrogen receptors in breast cancer cells, preventing estrogen from binding. Has four to five times more affinity for estrogen receptor than tamoxifen.

Metabolism: Well absorbed following oral dose. Highly protein-bound (99%). Peak serum level after single dose is 3 hours, with terminal half-life of 5–6.2 days. Extensively metabolized in the liver by the P450 enzyme system. Increased terminal half-life (decreased clearance) in patients with hepatic dysfunction to 10.9 days and 21 days for the principal metabolite. Clearance not significantly changed with renal impairment. Excreted in feces and, to a lesser extent, urine.

Indication: Treatment of postmenopausal women with estrogen-receptor positive or unknown, metastatic breast cancer.

Contraindication: Patients with known hypersensitivity to drug. Toremifene citrate should not be prescribed to patients with congenital/acquired QT prolongation (long QT syndrome), uncorrected hypokalemia, or uncorrected hypomagnesemia.

Dosage/Range:
- 60 mg orally, daily; generally continued until disease progression.
- Assess baseline CBC/LFTs; electrolytes including serum potassium, magnesemium, and calcium, and these should be reassessed periodically. Patients at risk for prolonged QTc should have an ECG baseline, which should be reassessed periodically during therapy.

Drug Preparation/Administration:
- None.

Drug Interactions:
- Drugs that decrease renal calcium excretion, e.g., thiazide diuretics: increases risk of hypercalcemia (decreased calcium excretion).
- CYP3A4 inducers (carbamazepine, phenobarbital, phenytoin, ranitidine, rifampin), and St. John's wort: may decrease toremifene serum level and effect; assess for inadequate dose, and discontinue St. John's wort.
- CYP3A4 inhibitors (ciprofloxacin, clarithromycin, doxycycline, erythromycin, isoniazid, itraconazole, propofol, verapamil, others): may increase toremifene serum level and toxicity; assess for adverse effects.
- CYP2C9 substrates with narrow therapeutic window, such as warfarin or phenytoin; co-administer with caution, and monitor patients closely (e.g., increased anticoagulation effect, dose according to INR).
- Drugs that prolong the QT-interval: additive danger of prolonged QTc and torsades de pointes.

Lab Effects/Interference:
- Decreased WBC and platelets (mild).
- Hypercalcemia.
- Increased alkaline phosphatase, bilirubin, calcium, AST.
- Prolonged QTc interval.

Special Considerations:
- Monitor CBC and LFTs baseline and periodically during treatment.
- Cataracts may develop, so patient should be taught to have eye exams by an ophthalmologist baseline and then twice yearly.
- Activity, side effects, toxicity in postmenopausal women or women with unknown receptor status appear similar.
- In general, do not use drug in patients with history of thromboembolic events or as long-term therapy in women with endometrial hyperplasia.
- Most common adverse reactions are hot flushes, sweating, nausea, and vaginal discharge.
- Warnings and Precautions:
  - *Prolongation of QTc interval*, which can result in torsades de pointes, a type of ventricular tachycardia, causing syncope, seizure, and/or sudden death.
    - Avoid use in patients with long QT syndrome, and/or uncorrected hypokalemia and hypomagnesemia. Use cautiously in patients with CHF, hepatic impairment, and electrolyte abnormalities.
    - Correct hypokalemia and hypomagnesemia if they exist, prior to starting toremifene citrate, and monitor these electrolytes throughout treatment.
    - Patients at increased risk should have an ECG baseline, including QTc interval, and as clinically indicated.
    - Patient should avoid taking drugs that prolong QTc with toremifene citrate (e.g., certain anti-arrhythmics, potent CYP3A4 inhibitors), and should discuss alternatives with their physician or NP/PA.

- *Hypercalcemia and tumor flare*: patients with bone metastases are at increased risk for this, which happens during the first few weeks of treatment.
  - Tumor flare is characterized by diffuse musculoskeletal pain and erythema, together with increased size of tumor lesions that later regress; hypercalcemia may also occur.
  - If hypercalcemia occurs, discuss management with physician or NP/PA; if severe, toremifene citrate should be discontinued.
  - Monitor patients with bony metastases closely for hypercalcemia during the first weeks of therapy.
- *Tumorgenicity:* May cause endometrial hyperplasia, and some patients have developed endometrial cancer. Patients with preexisting endometrial hyperplasia of the uterus should not receive long-term toremifene therapy.
- *Drug is approved for use in post-menopausal women.* If used by premenopausal women, the patient should be taught to use effective (nonhormonal) contraception to avoid pregnancy.
  - Use in pregnancy: drug can cause fetal harm; if the drug is used during pregnancy, or if the patient becomes pregnant while taking the drug, the patient should be apprised of the potential hazard to the fetus.
  - Nursing mothers should decide whether to discontinue nursing or to discontinue the drug, taking into account the importance of the drug to the mother's health.
- *Patients are at risk for endometrial cancer.* Teach patient to have a baseline then annual gynecology exam with endometrial biopsy. Teach patient to call provider for a gynecologic exam right away if vaginal bleeding occurs.
- *Laboratory testing*: periodic CBC, serum calcium, and LFTs should be assessed and monitored.

Potential Toxicities/Side Effects and the Nursing Process

I.   POTENTIAL FOR SEXUAL DYSFUNCTION related to MENSTRUAL IRREGULARITIES, HOT FLASHES

Defining Characteristics: Similar to tamoxifen toxicity profile. May cause menstrual irregularity, hot flashes (most common), milk production in breasts, and vaginal discharge and bleeding.

Nursing Implications: As appropriate, explore with patient and partner issues of reproductive and sexuality patterns and the impact drug may have on them. Discuss strategies to preserve sexual and reproductive health.

II.   POTENTIAL FOR ALTERATION IN COMFORT related to FLARE REACTION

Defining Characteristics: May cause flare reaction initially (bone and tumor pain, transient increase in tumor size). Nausea, vomiting, and anorexia may occur. Tremor may occur and be significant in some patients.

Nursing Implications: Inform patient of flare reaction, signs/symptoms to be aware of, and encourage patient to report any signs/symptoms. Inform patient of possibility of nausea, vomiting, and anorexia. Encourage small, frequent feedings of high-calorie, high-protein foods. Teach patients to report tremor, and discuss impact on self-care ability and comfort. If patient has brain or vertebral metastases, observe closely; any transient increase in tumor size may cause severe neurologic symptoms.

III.   POTENTIAL FOR INFECTION AND BLEEDING related to BM DEPRESSION

Defining Characteristics: Mild, transient leukopenia and thrombocytopenia occur rarely. Lowest WBC count in clinical trials was 2,500/mm^3.

Nursing Implications: Monitor CBC and platelet count prior to drug administration and after therapy has begun. Instruct patient in self-assessment of signs/symptoms of infection or bleeding.

IV.   POTENTIAL FOR SKIN INTEGRITY IMPAIRMENT related to RASH, ALOPECIA

Defining Characteristics: Skin rash, alopecia, and peripheral edema are rare.

Nursing Implications: Assess patient for signs/symptoms of hair loss, edema, and skin rash. Instruct patient to report any of these symptoms. Discuss with patient the impact of skin changes.

Drug: Trabectedin (Yondelis)

Class: Alkylating agent.

Mechanism of Action: Trabectedin is an alkylating agent that binds guanine residues in the DNA minor groove, forming adducts that bend the DNA helix towards the major groove. The formation of adducts causes changes that affect DNA binding proteins, interfering with the cell cycle and causing cell death.

Metabolism: Drug is highly protein bound (97%), and the terminal elimination half-life is 175 hours. Drug is extensively metabolized in the liver, by CYP3A predominantly, and 64% of the drug is eliminated in 24 days (58% in the feces, and 6% in urine).

Indication: Treatment of patients with unresectable or metastatic liposarcoma or leiomyosarcoma who have received a prior anthracycline-containing regimen.

Contraindication: Known hypersensitivity to trabectedin. Do not administer drug to patients with severe hepatic impairment (BR > 3–10 × ULN, with any AST and ALT).

Dosage Range:
- 1.5-mg/m^2 IV CI over 24 hours, every 3 weeks through a central veous line, until disease progression or unacceptable toxicity, in patients with normal BR and AST or ALT ≤ 2.5 × ULN.
- Premedicate with dexamethasone 20-mg IV 30 min before each infusion.
- Moderate hepatic impairment: 0.9 mg/ m^2 IV CI over 24 hours, every 3 weeks through a central veous line (Moderate is defined as BR 1.5 to 3 × ULN, and AST and ALT < 8 × ULN). Do NOT administer drug to patients with severe hepatic impairment (BR > 3 × ULN, any AST/ALT.

Dose Modification:
- Permanently discontinue drug for
  - Persistent adverse reactions requiring a delay in dosing of > 3 weeks.
  - Adverse reactions requiring dose reduction following trabectedin administered at 1.0 mg/m^2 for patients with normal hepatic function; or at 0.3 mg/m^2 in patients with pre-existing moderate hepatic impairment.
  - Severe liver dysfunction: BR 2 × ULN and AST or ALT 3 × ULN with alkaline phosphatase < 2 × ULN in the prior treatment cycle for patients with normal hepatic function at baseline
  - Exacerbation of liver dysfunction in patients with pre-existing moderate hepatic impairment.
  - Capillary Leak Syndrome (CLS)
  - Rhabdomyolysis
  - Grade 3 or 4 cardiac adverse events suggesting cardiomyopathy or for patients with an LVEF that decreases < LLN
- Once dose is reduced, the dose should not be increased in subsequent treatment cycles.
  - first dose reduction: trabectedin 1.2 mg/m^2 every 3 weeks.
  - 2nd dose reduction: trabectedin 1.0 mg/m^2 every 3 weeks.
- *See package insert* for recommended dose modifications (hematologic, hepatic, cardiac, increased creaetine phosphokinase, and other non-hematologic toxicity).

Drug Preparation:
- Available as a 1 mg sterile lyophilized powder in a single-dose vial.
- Using aseptic technique, inject 20 mL of sterile water for injection USP into the vial. Shake the vial until complete dissolution. The resulting reconstituted solution is clear, colorless to pale brownish-yellow, and contains 0.05 mg/mL of trabectedin. Inspect for particulate matter and discoloration before further dilution. Discard if particles or discoloration found.
- Immediately following reconstitution, withdraw the calculated volume of trabectedin ordered and further dilute in 500 mL of 0.9% sodium chloride USP or 5% dextrose injection USP. DO NOT mix with other drugs.
- Discard any remaining solution within 30 hours of reconstituting the lyophilized powder.
- Trabectedin diluted solution is compatible with Type I colorless glass vials polyvinylchloride (PVC) and polyethylene (PE) bags and tubing, and PE and polypropylene (PP) mixture bags, polyethersulfone (PES) in-line filters, titanium, platinum or plastic ports,

silicone and polyurethane catheters, and pumps having contact surfaces made of PVC, PE, or PE/PP.

Drug Administration:
- Assess CBC/differential: ANC $> 1,500/mm^3$, platelets $> 100,000/mm^3$. Assess LFTs, CPK (CK), and results of ECHO or MUGA.
- Drug is a vesicant; use vesicant precautions.
- Premedicate with dexamethasone 20-mg IV 30 min before each infusion. Discuss antiemetic at least for first cycle with physician/NP/PA.
- Infuse diluted solution over 24 hours through a central venous line using an infusion set with a 0.2 micron polyethersulfone (PES) in-line filter to reduce risk of exposure to adventitious pathogens that may be introduced during solution preparation.
- Complete infusion within 30 hours of initial reconstitution. Discard any unused portion of the reconstituted product or of the infusion solution.
- Assess central venous catheter access site for leakage, pain, or discomfort every 4 hours or per institutional standard.
- Teach patient to report right away if there is leakage of the drug from the catheter, or around the catheter, or if the patient notices any redness, swelling, itching, or discomfort at the infusion site at any time.
- Teach patient to avoid grapefruit juice and grapefruit while receiving the drug and not to take St. John's wort.

Drug Interactions:
- **CYP3A inhibitors: may increase trabectedin serum concentration**; avoid concomitant strong CYP3A inhibitors (e.g., oral ketoconazole, itraconazole, posaconazole, voriconazole, clarithromycin, telithromycin, indinavir, lopinavir, ritonavir, boceprevir, nelfinavir, saquinavir, telaprevir, nefazodone, conivaptan). Teach patient to avoid grapefruit and grapefruit juice. If a strong CYP3A4 inhibitor for short-term use (< 14 days) must be used, administer the strong CYP3A4 inhibitor 1 week after the trabectedin infusion, and discontinue it the day prior to the next trabectedin infusion.
- **CYP3A inducers: may decrease trabectedin serum concentration**; avoid concomitant strong CYP3A inducers (e.g., rifampin, phenobarbital, St. John's wort).

Lab Effects/Interference:
- Neutropenia, thrombocytopenia, anemia
- Increased ALT, AST, creatine phosphokinase (CPK or CK)
- Decreased LVEF.

Special Considerations:
- Warnings/Precautions:
  - *Neutropenic sepsis*: may be severe and fatal. Monitor ANC baseline and before each dose. Hold drug for grade 2 or higher neutropenia, and modify dose next treatment.
  - *Rhabdomyolysis*: may occur. Assess CPK levels prior to each dose administration. Hold drug, reduce dose, or permanently discontinue based on severity.
  - *Hepatotoxicity:* hepatotoxicity including hepatic failure may occur. Assess LFTs prior to each drug dose, and as clinically indicated. Manage elevated LFTs with treatment

interruption, dose reduction, or permanent drug discontinuation based on severity and duration of hepatotoxicity. See package insert.
- *Cardiomyopathy:* may be severe and fatal. Patients with LVEF <LLN, prior cumulative anthracycline dose of ≥ 300 mg/m2, age ≥ 65 years old, or a history of cardiovascular disease may be at increased risk. Assess LVEF baseline and every 2–3 months by ECHO or MUGA. Discontinue drug if LVEF dysfunction occurs based on severity of reaction.
- *Capillary leak syndrome (CLS)* has been reported characterized by hypotension, edema, and hypoalbuminemia, and may result in death. Monitor patient closely for signs/symptoms of CLS; discontinue drug if CLS occurs, and manage promptly using standard medical management including ICU as needed.
- *Extravasation resulting in tissue necrosis:* necrosis may occur > 1 week after extravasasation. No antidote is known, and a central venous catheter is required for 24-hour infusion. Tissue necrosis may require debridement.
- *Embryo-fetal toxicity:* Teach women of reproductive potential to use effective contraception during and for 2 months after the last dose. Teach men with a female sexual partner of reproductive potential to use effective contraception during and for 5 months after the last dose. Mothers should not breastfeed while receiving the drug.
- Most common (≥20%) adverse reactions in clinical studies are: nausea, fatigue, vomiting, constipation, decreased appetite, diarrhea, peripheral edema, dyspnea, headache.

Potential Toxicities/Side Effects and the Nursing Process

I.   INFECTION AND BLEEDING related to BM DEPRESSION

Defining Characteristics: Neutropenic sepsis can occur and be fatal. In Trial 1, incidence of grades 3–4 neutropenia was 43%. Median time to first occurrence of grades 3–4 neutropenia was 16 days (range 8–9.7 months), and median time to complete resolution of neutropenia was 13 days (range 3 da–2.3 months). Febrile neutropenia was less common. Incidence of neutropenic sepsis was 2.6% with 1.1% fatality. Incidence of neutropenia by laboratory results was 66%, anemia 96% (19% grades 3–4), and thrombocytopenia 59% (21% grades 3–4).

Nursing Implications: Monitor ANC/CBC, platelet count prior to each drug dose as well as for signs/symptoms of infection or bleeding. Instruct patient in self-assessment of signs/symptoms of infection or bleeding. Hold drug if ANC < 1,500/mm^3 on treatment day, and platelet count < 100,000/mm^3. Drug should be permanently dose reduced for life-threatening or prolonged, severe neutropenia in the preceeding cycle.

II.   POTENTIAL FOR INJURY, related to RHABDOMYOLYSIS.

Defining Characteristics: Drug can cause rhabdomyolysis and musculoskeletal toxicity. Arthralgias occurred in 15%, and myalgias in 12% of patients. Creatine phosphokinase (CPK, CK) elevations occurred in 33% of patients and was grades 3–4 in 6.4% of patients in Trial 1. Rhabdomyolysis led to death in 3 patients (0.8%). Renal failure may complicate rhabdomyolysis. The median time to first occurrence of grade 3–4 CPK elevations was 2 months, and median time to complete resolution was 14 days.

Nursing Implications: Assess CPK levels prior to each drug administration. Teach patient to report severe muscle pain or weakness right away. Hold drug for serum CPK levels > 2.5 × ULN. Permanently discontinue drug for rhabdomyolysis.

III. POTENTIAL ALTERATION IN CIRCULATION related to CARDIOMYOPATHY

Defining Characteristics: In clinical trials, cardiomyopathy including cardiac failure, CHF, decreased LVEF, diastolic dysfunction, or RV dysfunction occurred. Incidence in Trial 1 was 6% (vs 2.3% in dacarbazine arm); grades 3–4 cardiomyopathy occurred in 4% vs 1.2% in the dacarbazine arm. Median time to development of grades 3–4 cardiomyopathy was 5.3 months (range 26 days to 15.3 months).

Nursing Implications: Assess/review results of LVEF by ECHO or MUGA scan baseline and every 2–3 months during treatment. Teach patient to report new chest pain, SOB, tiredness, swelling of legs, ankles or feet, heart palpitations, or any new heart problem. Drug should be held for LVEF < LLN. The drug should be permanently discontinued for symptomatic cardiomyopathy or persistent LV dysfunction that does not recover to the LLN within 3 weeks.

IV. ALTERATION IN NUTRITION, LESS THAN BODY REQUIREMENTS, related to GI SIDE EFFECTS

Defining Characteristics: Nutritional impact symptoms are common. Nausea affected 75% (grades 3–4 in 7%), vomiting 46% (6% grades 3–4), constipation 37%, and diarrhea 35%. Appetite was decreased in 37% of patients.

Nursing Implications: Premedicate with antiemetics as needed and continue prophylactically for 24 hours to prevent nausea and vomiting, as needed and ordered. Encourage small, frequent feedings of cool, bland, dry foods. Assess for symptoms of fluid and electrolyte imbalance: monitor I/O, daily weights if administered to an inpatient. Teach patient oral assessment and oral hygiene regimen. Encourage patient to report onset of diarrhea or constipation. Administer or teach patient to self-administer antidiarrheal medication. If constipation develops, review with patient self-care measures to eliminate constipation and restore normal bowel elimination. Ensure adequate hydration; monitor I/O.

Drug: Trifluridine and tipiracil (Lonsurf)

Class: Antimetabolite; Nucleoside metabolic inhibitor.

Mechanism of Action: Trifluridine is a nucleoside metabolic inhibitor, and tipiracil is a thymidine phosphorylase inhibitor. Adding tipiracil to trifluridine increases trifluridine exposure by inhibiting its metabolism by thymidine phosphorylase. As an antimetabolite, the cell takes up trifluridine into its DNA, thinking it is uridine, and the false metabolite prevents DNA synthesis and cell proliferation. The drug has antitumor activity in *KRAS*-wild-type colorectal cancer xenografts in mice.

Metabolism: After oral dosing, the mean time to peak plasma concentration (Tmax) is 2 hours and the mean elimination half-life at steady state was 2.1 hours for trifluridine and 2.4 hours for tipiracil. Absorption following a standardized high-fat, high-calorie meal is decreased with subsequent 40% decrease in AUC and C_{max}; administration of the drug within 1 hour after completion of a meal in the morning and evening is recommended based on the observed correlation between an increased trifluridine C_{max} and the decrease in neutrophil count (Taiho, 2015).

Indication: Treatment of patients with metastatic (1) CRC who have been previously treated with fluoropyrimidine-, oxaliplatin-, and irinotecan-based chemotherapy, and anti-VEGF biological therapy, and if RAS-wild-type, an anti-EGFR therapy; (2) gstric or gastroesophageal junction (GEJ) adenocarcinoma previously treated with at least 2 prior lines of chemotherapy that included a fluoropyrimidine, a platinum, either a taxane or irinotecan, and if appropriate, HER-2/neu-targeted therapy.

Contraindication: None. Do not initiate drug in patients with baseline moderate or severe hepatic impairment.

Dosage Range:
- Recommended dose is 35 mg/m²/dose (up to maximum of 80 mg per dose) orally twice daily with food on days 1–5 and days 8–12 of each 28-day cycle until disease progression or unacceptable toxicity. See package insert for dose by BSA and number of tablets patient should take (15 mg and 20 mg tablets) [Table 1, 2019].
- Trifluridine maximum dose is 80 mg per dose. Round dose to the nearest 5 mg increment.
- Dose should be taken within 1 hour after completion of morning and evening meals.
- Baseline moderate or severe hepatic dysfunction: Do not initiate drug.
- Renal dysfunction: patients with moderate renal impairment may need a dose modification for increased toxicity.

Dose Modification:
- **Starting a cycle**: Assess ANC/CBC prior to and on day 15 of each cycle. Hold cycle until ANC ≥ 1,500/mm³ or febrile neutropenia resolved; platelet count ≥ 75,000/mm³; and grades 3–4 non-hematological adverse reactions are resolved to grades 0–1.
- **Within a treatment cycle**: hold drug for any of the following (1) ANC < 500/mm³ or (2) febrile neutropenia; (3) platelets < 50,000/mm³; or (4) grades 3–4 nonhematological adverse reaction.
  - **After recovery**, reduce dose by 5 mg/m²/dose from the previous dose level if the following occurs:
    - Febrile neutropenia
    - Uncompllicated grade 4 neutropenia (which has recovered to ≥1,500/mm³) or thrombocytopenia (which has recovered to ≥ 75,000/mm³) that results in > 1 week delay in start of next cycle.

- Non-hematologic grades 3–4 adverse reaction except for grade 3 nausea and/ or vomiting controlled by antiemetic therapy or grade 3 diarrhea responsive to anti-diarrheal medication.
- A maximum of 3 dose reductions are permitted to a minimum dose of 20 mg/m^3 twice daily. Drug should be discontinued if the patient is unable to tolerate a dose of 20 mg m^2 orally twice daily. Do not escalate drug dose after it has been reduced.
- Geriatric use: Patients aged 65 and higher had a higher incidence of grades 3–4 neutropenia and thrombocytopenia, and grade 3 anemia.
- Renal impairment: no starting dose adjustment for patients with mild or moderate renal impairment (CrCl of 30–89 mL/min); monitor for potential increased toxicity. Patients with severe renal impairment (CrCl <30 mL/min) were not studied.
- Hepatic impairment: no starting dose adjustment for patients with mild hepatic impairment. Do not administer drug to patients with baseline moderate or severe hepatic impairment (total bilirubin >1.5 × ULN and any AST).

Drug Preparation:
- Drug available in 2 dosage forms and strengths:
- 15 mg trifluridine/6.14 mg tipiracil (white tablet with 15 imprinted in gray on each side)
- 20 mg trifluridine/8.19 mg tipiracil (pale red, with 20 imprinted on both sides in gray ink).

Drug Administration:
- Assess ANC/CBC/platelets prior to each cycle and day 15. See dosing modifications in Dosage/Range section. Assess for hematologic and non-hematologic toxicity.
- Teach patient self-administration:
  - Use safe handling precautions in handling tablets (e.g., gloves), and talk to the pharmacist if medication needs to be disposed of.
  - Swallow tablet(s) whole, and do not chew.
  - Take doses within 1 hour of morning and evening meals.
  - Do not take additional doses to make up for missed or held doses (e.g., if dose is vomited or missed) but continue with the next scheduled dose.

Drug Interactions: None known.

Lab Effects/Interference:
- Neutropenia, anemia, thrombocytopenia

Special Considerations:
- Most common adverse reactions (≥10%) were anemia, neutropenia, asthenia/fatigue, nausea, thrombocytopenia, decreased appetite, diarrhea, vomiting and pyrexia.
- Warnings and Precautions:
  - *Severe myelosuppression* may occur and be life-threatening (grades 3–4) consisting of anemia (18%), neutropenia (38%), and thrombocytopenia (5%). Incidence of febrile neutropenia was 3% and 2 patients (0.2%) died from neutropenic infection/sepsis, and four other patients (0.5%) died from septic shock. Assess need for G-CSF. Obtain CBC/differential (ANC) prior to and on day 15 of each cycle and as needed. Hold drug for febrile neutropenia, grade 4 neutropenia, or platelet count < 50,000/mm^3. After recovery, reduce drug dose to next lower dosage.

- *Embryo-fetal toxicity*: Drug is feto-toxic. Advise women of reproductive potential to use effective contracption during treatment, and for at least 6 months after the last drug dose. As drug is potentially genotoxic, advise male patients with female partners of reproductive potential to use condoms during drug treatment and for at least 3 months after final dose.
- Drug should not be initiated in patients with moderate or severe hepatic impairment. Patients with mild hepatotoxicity have no recommended dose adjustment, but patients with moderate (total BR > 1.5–3 × ULN and any AST) or severe (total BR > 3 × ULN and any AST) hepatotoxicity have not been studied.
- In study 1, patients with moderate renal impairment (CrCl 30–59 mL/min had a higher incidence of gr 3 or higher adverse events and dose delays/reductions compared to patients with normal renal function (CrCl ≥ 90 mL/min) (Taiho Oncology, 2015).

Potential Toxicities/Side Effects and the Nursing Process

I. INFECTION AND BLEEDING related to BM DEPRESSION

Defining Characteristics: Neutropenia occurred in 66–67% of patients, thrombocytopenia in 32–42%, and anemia in 63–77% of patients. Severe myelosuppression may occur and be life-threatening (grades 3–4) consisting of anemia (18–19%), neutropenia (38%), and thrombocytopenia (5–6%). Incidence of febrile neutropenia was 3%; two patients (0.2%) died from neutropenic infection/sepsis, and four other patients (0.5%) died from septic shock. Incidence of infection was 23–27%. Asthenia/fatigue occurred in 52% of patients.

Nursing Implications: Monitor ANC/CBC, platelet count prior to each drug dose and day 15, as well as for signs/symptoms of infection, bleeding, and fatigue. Instruct patient in self-assessment of signs/symptoms of infection or bleeding. Assess need for G-CSF. For start of cycle, hold drug if ANC < 1,500/mm^3 or platelet count < 75,000/mm^3 or grades 3–4 toxicity that has not resolved (see package insert); during a treatment cycle, hold drug if (1) ANC < 500/mm^3 or (2) febrile neutropenia; (3) platelets < 50,000/mm^3; or (4) grades 3–4 nonhematological adverse reaction. Drug should be permanently dose reduced for life-threatening or prolonged, severe neutropenia in the preceeding cycle. Assess energy level baseline and during treatment. Discuss self-care strategies to manage fatigue and economize on energy, such as alteration of activity and rest periods, and gentle exercise.

II. ALTERATION IN NUTRITION, LESS THAN BODY REQUIREMENTS, related to GI SIDE EFFECTS

Defining Characteristics: Nutritional impact symptoms are common. Nausea affected 37–48%, decreased appetite 34–39%, diarrhea 23–32%, vomiting 25–28%, stomatitis 8% (CRC patients), and dysgeusia 7% (CRC patients).

Nursing Implications: Teach patient about side effects, and self-care measures to prevent nausea and vomiting, including ordered anti-emetic. Encourage small, frequent feedings of cool, bland, dry foods. Assess for symptoms of fluid and electrolyte imbalance: monitor

I/O, daily weights if administered to an inpatient. Teach patient oral assessment and oral hygiene regimen. Encourage patient to report onset of diarrhea, and diarrhea that does not respond to anti-diarrheal medications. Teach patient to self-administer antidiarrheal medication. Ensure adequate hydration; monitor I/O.

Drug: triptorelin pamoate (Trelstar LA, Trelstar Depot)

Class: Gonadotropin-releasing hormone (GnRH) agonist.

Mechanism of Action: Potently inhibits gonadotropin secretion, resulting in an initial surge in circulating levels of luteinizing hormone (LH), follicle-stimulating hormone (FSH), testosterone, and estradiol, and then after 2 to 4 weeks of continued drug administration, sustained decreases in LH and FSH secretion, resulting in a reduction of testosterone similar to surgical castration serum levels. This removes the hormonal stimulation from prostate cancer cells and stops the growth and proliferation of prostate cells. The drug effect is reversible following discontinuance of the drug.

Metabolism: After IM administration, the drug probably undergoes metabolism by the liver, with excretion by liver and kidneys.

Indication: For the palliative treatment of patients with advanced prostate cancer.

Contraindication: (1) Known hypersensitvity to drug or its components or other GnRH agonists, or GnRH; (2) pregnancy.

Dosage/Range:
- Trelstar depot: 3.75 mg IM once every 4 weeks.
- Trelstar LA: 11.25 mg IM once every 12 weeks.
- Trelstar LA: 22.5 mg IM every 24 weeks (6 months).

Drug Preparation: See package insert.
- Double check that the correct dose of medication is in the package.
- Using the manufacturer's Mixject system, reconstitute drug vial using prefilled syringe and vial adapter (see images in package insert). Then aspirate vial contents into the syringe, and disconnect from vial adapter. Lift up needle safety cover so that it is perpendicular to the syringe.

Drug Administration:
- Administer in large muscle and rotate sites.
- Administer Trelstar LA in buttock. After withdrawal of the needle, activate the safety mechanism.
- Monitor patients closely after first two treatments, as anaphylaxis with or without angioedema may rarely occur.
- Monitor serum testosterone levels baseline and periodically.
- Monitor patients with bony metastases or disease that could cause ureteral obstruction closely after initial treatment, as flare may cause ureteral obstruction or spinal cord

compression, depending on location of metastases. In extreme cases, orchiectomy may be required to relieve obstruction of ureters.

Lab Effects/Interference:
- Decreased serum testosterone levels.
- Chronic or continuous administration of triptorelin results in suppression of pituitary-gonadal axis; diagnostic tests of pituitary-gonadal function during treatment and after therapy ends may be misleading.

Special Considerations:
- 6-month formulation maintains > 98% of patients below castrate level at 6 and 12 months.
- Monitor drug effectiveness (serum testosterone level, PSA).
- Drug is used off-label for the treatment of patients with endometriosis, in vitro fertilization, and ovarian cancer.
- Rarely can cause pituitary apoplexy (pituitary infarction) in patients who have anadenoma, characterized by sudden headache, vomiting, visual changes, ophthalmoplegia (paralysis or weakness of the muscles that control eye movement), altered mental status, and sometimes cardiovascular collapse after the first dose (within hours to 2 weeks). Emergency medical care is required.
- Warnings and Precautions:
  - *Hypersensitivity reactions* (HSRs) including anaphylactic shock, hypersensitivity, and angioedema have been reported. If HSRs occur, discontinue drug immediately and provide supportive and symptomatic care in concert with physican and/or NP/PA.
  - *Transient increase in serum testosterone* may occur, resulting in worsening of signs and symptoms or new onset of symptoms of prostate cancer during first few weeks of treatment. These include bone pain, neuropathy, hematuria, or ureteral or bladder outlet obstruction.
  - *Metastatic vertebral lesions and Urinary tract obstruction.* If patient has metastatic vertebral lesions and/or with upper or lower urinary tract obstruction, monitor patient closely during the first few weeks of therapy Spinal cord compression and renal impairment have been reported. If spinal cord compression or renal impairment develop and cannot be managed with standard treatment, an orchiectomy should be considered.
  - *Effect on QT/QTc Interval:* Androgen deprivation therapy may prolong the QT/QTc interval, and this should be considered when physician is discussing risks and benefits with patient who has congenital long QT syndrome, CHF, frequent electrolyte abnormalities, or taking drugs that are known to prolong the QTc interval. Assess serum electrolytes baseline and periodically during therapy; discuss orders to replete any abnormal (low) serum electrolytes and then rechecking lab results.
  - *Hyperglycemia and diabetes* have been reported in men receiving GnRH agoinsts. Monitor blood glucose or HbA1c baseline and periodically, and manage appropriately.
  - *Cardiovascular diseases,* including increased risk of developing MI, sudden cardiac death, and stroke have been reported. Monitor patients for signs suggestive of cardiovascular disease, and discuss management with physician or NP/PA.

- *Laboratory tests*: Monitor serum testosterone baseline and periodically during treatment to assess response to therapy.
- *Laboratory test interactions*: Chronic or continuous administration of triptorelin suppresses the pituitary-gonadal axis. This will cause misleading results of pituitary-gonadal function.
- *Embryo-fetal toxicity*: Drug is feto-toxic. Advise pregnant patients and females of reproductive potential of the potential risk to the fetus.

Potential Toxicities/Side Effects and the Nursing Process

I.   ALTERATION IN COMFORT related to HOT FLASHES, TUMOR FLARE, LEG PAIN, EYE PAIN, HEADACHE, EDEMA

Defining Characteristics: Initially, drug causes increased LH secretion, resulting in increased testosterone secretion and tumor flare. Usually disappears after 2 weeks. Headache, dizziness, and hot flashes may occur. Vasodilation most common. Tumor flare may also occur initially (bone and tumor pain, transient increase in tumor size due to transient increase in testosterone levels). Breast tenderness has been reported. Peripheral edema, leg and eye pain, headache may occur.

Nursing Implications: Inform patient that symptoms may occur and that flare reaction will subside after the initial 2 weeks of therapy. Assess and document pain score baseline, and teach patient to report pain, especially if it is new onset of back pain that may be radicular, or pelvic pain, hematuria, or urinary retention. Encourage patient to report symptoms early. Triage symptoms, and discuss emergency management if severe symptoms develop. Develop symptom management plan with patient and physician. Monitor patients with disease near ureters or bony metastases closely after initial treatment, as ureteral obstruction and spinal cord compression have occurred.

II.   POTENTIAL SEXUAL DYSFUNCTION related to LIBIDO, IMPOTENCE

Defining Characteristics: Frequently causes decreased libido and erectile impotence in men. Gynecomastia occurs in 1–10% of patients. In women, amenorrhea occurs after 10 weeks of therapy.

Nursing Implications: As appropriate, explore with patient and significant other issues of reproductive and sexual patterns and the impact chemotherapy may have on them. Discuss strategies to preserve sexuality and reproductive health.

III.   DEPRESSION, POTENTIAL, related to DRUG EFFECT

Defining Characteristics: Depression may affect up to 5.3% of patients and, less commonly, patients may develop emotional lability, insomnia, nervousness, and anxiety.

Nursing Implications: Assess baseline affect and usual coping strategies. Teach patient to report change in affect. Assess effectiveness of coping strategies. Encourage patient to verbalize feelings, and provide emotional support. Assess need for referral to psychiatric nurse specialist or social worker if supportive efforts ineffective.

IV.   ALTERED NUTRITION, LESS THAN BODY REQUIREMENTS, related to GI SIDE EFFECTS

Defining Characteristics: Anorexia, nausea, and vomiting may occur rarely.

Nursing Implications: If patients experience symptoms, encourage small, frequent feedings of favorite foods, especially high-calorie, high-protein foods. Monitor weight weekly. Assess incidence and pattern of nausea, vomiting, or anorexia if they occur. Discuss need for antiemetic with physician and patient.

Drug: valrubicin (Valstar)

Class: Anthracycline antitumor antibiotic.

Mechanism of Action: Semisynthetic analogue of doxorubicin; drug is highly lipophilic and is made soluble in Cremophor EL. Apparently, the drug does not interact with negatively charged molecules, and thus is less irritating to bladder mucosa. Drug metabolites appear to inhibit topoisomerase II so that cellular DNA cannot replicate, thus inhibiting DNA synthesis and causing chromosomal damage and cell death.

Metabolism: Drug is well absorbed by bladder mucosa with little, if any, systemic absorption unless bladder is injured/perforated. Used for bladder instillation, and excreted unchanged in the urine (98.6%).

Indication: For intravesical therapy of BCG-refractory carcinoma *in situ* of the urinary bladder in patients for whom immediate cystectomy would be associated with unacceptable morbidity or mortality.

Contraindication: Patients with (1) known hypersensitivity to anthracyclines or polyoxy castor oil; (2) concurrent UTIs; (3) a small bladder capacity (e.g., unable to tolerate a 75 mL instillation); (4) perforated bladder or compromised bladder mucosa.

Dosage/Range:
- **Intravesicular therapy** ONLY of BCG-refractory carcinoma in situ of the urinary bladder: 800 mg q week × 6 weeks. Delay administration for at least 2 weeks after transurethral resection and/or fulguration.
- High incidence of metastases in patients receiving drug in clinical trials, probably due to delayed cystectomy. Therefore, therapy should be discontinued in patients not responding to treatment after 3 months.

Drug Preparation:
- Available as injection form, 200 mg in 5-mL vial, which should be stored in the refrigerator 2–8°C (36–46°F).
- Remove vials from refrigerator and allow to warm to room temperature without heating; dilute by adding 800 mg (20 mL) to 55 mL of 0.9% normal saline injection, USP.

Drug Administration:
- Warm drug slowly to room temperature but do not heat.
- Bladder lavage by intravesicular administration of drug (total volume of 75 mL when diluted as above), allowed to dwell for 2 hours, and then voided out.
- Non-PVC tubing and non-DEHP containers and administration sets should be used to prevent leaching of PVC into drug volume (due to Cremophor EL).

Drug Interactions:
- None known due to limited, if any, systemic absorption.

Lab Effects/Interference:
- Hyperglycemia.

Special Considerations:
- Most common adverse effects: abdominal pain, nausea, myalgia, asthenia, headache, bladder pain, cystitis, dysuria, hematuris, incontinence, urinary frequency, nocturia, urethral pain, baldder spasm, urinary retention, UTI, buring sensation on urination.
- Warnings and Precautions:
  - *Bladder evaluation* should be performed prior to intravesical instillation of drug.
  - *Delaying cystectomy* can lead to development of metastatic bladder cancer, which is lethal.
  - *If bladder perforation or compromised bladder mucosal integrity exists*, delay therapy until bladder integrity is restored. Drug should NOT be given if bladder is injured, inflamed, or perforated, as systemic absorption will occur via loss of mucosal integrity. If no CR after 3 months of therapy, consider cystectomy.
  - *Use with caution in patients with severe irritable bladder symptoms*, as drug may cause symptoms of irritable bladder (during instillation and dwell time).
  - *Bladder spasm and spontaneous discharge of valrubicin* instillate may occur.
  - *Do not administer intravesical valrubicin within 2 weeks* of transurethral resection and/or fulgaration of the bladder.
  - *Embryo-fetal toxicity:* Drug is feto-toxic. Teach women of reproductive potential to use effective contraception to avoid pregnancy during treatment and for 6 months after the final dose.
- Teach patients that urine will be red- or pink-tinged for 24 hours.
- Patients with diabetes: need to check blood glucose levels, as hyperglycemia may rarely occur with treatment (1% incidence).

Potential Toxicities/Side Effects and the Nursing Process

I. ALTERATION IN URINE ELIMINATION related to DRUG EFFECTS

Defining Characteristics: Intravesicular administration of drug is associated with signs/symptoms of bladder irritation: frequency (61% of patients), dysuria (56%), urgency (57%), bladder spasm (31%), hematuria (29%), pain in bladder (28%), incontinence (22%), cystitis (15%), and urinary tract infection (15%). Less commonly, nocturia (7%), burning on urination (5%), urinary retention (4%), pain in the urethra (3%), pelvic pain (1%).

Nursing Implications: Assess baseline urinary elimination pattern, history of signs/symptoms of bladder irritation. Teach patient that these side effects may occur and to report them. Teach patient to drink 3 L of fluid for at least 2–3 days beginning day of treatment to flush bladder. Reassure patient that signs/symptoms will resolve and to report any persistent symptoms.

II. ALTERATION IN OXYGENATION, POTENTIAL, related to RARE CARDIAC EFFECTS

Defining Characteristics: Rarely, chest pain may occur (2%), as may vasodilation (2%) or peripheral edema (1%).

Nursing Implications: Assess patient's baseline cardiac status, and history of chest pain, peripheral edema. Teach patient to report any pain, or swelling in hands or feet. If this occurs, discuss management with physician. If possible, do EKG while patient is having chest pain to see if ischemia exists. Systemic absorption is possible only if bladder mucosal surfaces are injured, so this should be considered.

III. ALTERATION IN COMFORT, POTENTIAL, related to PAIN, RASH, WEAKNESS, MYALGIA

Defining Characteristics: The following discomfort may occur: headache (4%), malaise (4%), dizziness (3%), fever (2%), rash (3%), abdominal pain (5%), weakness (4%), back pain (3%), myalgia (1%).

Nursing Implications: Assess baseline comfort level, and any pain and the usual pain relief plan. Teach patient that these problems may occur rarely and to report them if they do. Teach patient these symptoms should resolve, and to use local measures to minimize discomfort. Teach patient to report any symptoms that do not resolve or that become worse.

IV.   ALTERATION IN NUTRITION, POTENTIAL, related to NAUSEA, DIARRHEA, VOMITING

Defining Characteristics: Rarely, gastrointestinal symptoms may occur: nausea affects approximately 5% of patients, diarrhea 3% of patients, and vomiting 2% of patients.

Nursing Implications: Assess baseline nutritional status, history of nausea, vomiting, or diarrhea. Teach patient that these may occur rarely and to report them if they do. If patient does develop symptoms, teach patient to take antiemetic medication as ordered, and OTC antidiarrheal medicine. Teach patient to call right away if symptoms do not resolve.

Drug: vinblastine (Velban)

Class: Plant alkaloid extracted from the periwinkle plant (*Vinca rosea*).

Mechanism of Action: Drug binds to microtubular proteins, thus arresting mitosis during metaphase; may inhibit RNA, DNA, and protein synthesis. Cell cycle specific for M phase and active in S phase.

Metabolism: About 10% of drug is excreted in feces. Vinblastine is partially metabolized by the liver (P450 microenzyme system). Minimal amount of the drug is excreted in urine and bile. Dose modification may be necessary in the presence of hepatic failure.

Indication: For the palliative treatment of (1) generalized Hodgkin's disease (Stages III, IV), lymphocytic lymphoma (nodular and diffuse, poorly and well differentiated), histiocytic lymphoma, mycosis fungoides (advanced stages), advanced carcinoma of the testis, Kaposi's sarcoma, Letterer-Siwe disease (histiocytosis X); and (2) choriocarcinoma resistant to other chemotherapeutic agents, and breast cancer, unresponsive to appropriate endocrine surgery and hormonal therapy.

Contraindication: Patients with (1) significant granulocytopenia unless resulting from disease being treated; (2) bacterial infection must be brought under control prior to initiation of vinblastine.

Dosage/Range:
- 0.1 mg/kg; 6-mg/m^2 IV weekly: CI 1.5–2.0 mg/m^2/d in 1 L D$_5$W or NS × 5 days via central line.
- Dose-reduce (50%) for bilirubin 1.5–3 mg/dL or AST 60–180 units/L; dose-reduce 75% if bilirubin 3–5 mg/dL and hold for bilirubin > 5 mg/dL or AST > 180 units/L.

Drug Preparation:
- Available in 10-mg vials. Store in refrigerator until use. Prepared syringes containing the drug must be packaged in an overwrap that is labeled "DO NOT REMOVE COVERING UNTIL MOMENT OF INJECTION. FATAL IF GIVEN INTRATHECALLY. FOR INTRAVENOUS USE ONLY."

- In healthcare settings that prepare and administer IT medications, vinblastine **must be prepared** in a mini-bag for infusion, NOT IVP.

Drug Administration:
- IV: This drug is a vesicant. Give slow IVP over 1–2 min through the sidearm of a running IV so as to avoid extravasation, which can lead to ulceration, pain, and necrosis. Refer to individual hospital policy and procedure for administration of a vesicant. Ensure there is no confusion, as drug is fatal if given intrathecally (IT).
- IV mini-bag: if the healthcare setting prepares and administers IT medications, vinblastine must be administered via a mini-bag (Neuss et al., 2017).

Drug Interactions:
- CYP3A4 inhibitors (itraconazole, erythromycin, others): increased serum drug level of vinblastine; do not use together or assess possible toxicity and dose-reduce vinblastine.
- CYP3A4 inducers (carbamazepine, dexamethasone, phenytoin, others): decreased serum levels of vinblastine; do not use together or assess need to increase dose of vinblastine.
- St. John's wort: may increase vinblastine toxicity; do not administer concomitantly.
- Grapefruit juice: may increase vinblastine toxicity; do not administer concomitantly.
- Decreased pharmacologic effects of phenytoin when given with this drug; check phenytoin levels and dose modify based on levels.
- Increases cellular uptake of methotrexate by certain malignant cells when administered sequentially, but less so than vincristine.
- Antigout medicines: may decrease effect of vinblastine. Do not use together if possible.

Lab Effects/Interference:
- Decreased WBC.

Special Considerations:
- Drug is a vesicant; give through a running IV to avoid extravasation. However, if administered in a healthcare setting that prepares and administers IT medication, then as recommended by the manufacturer, vinblastine is diluted in a flexible plastic container and prominently labeled as indicated for IV use only. If the healthcare setting does not prepare or administer IT drugs, then the vinca alkaloid may be administered IVP (Neuss et al., 2017).
- Dose modification may be necessary in the presence of hepatic failure.
- Teach women of childbearing potential to use effective contraception to avoid pregnancy. If drug is used in pregnancy or if the patient becomes pregnant while receiving the drug, the patient should be apprised of the potential hazard to the fetus. Nurisng mothers should make a decision whether to discontinue nursing or discontinue the drug, taking into account the importance of the drug to the mother's health.
- Aspermia has been reported in men.
- Leukopenia is dose limiting, with nadir day 5–10 days after a dose, and recovery to pretreatment levels 7–14 days after treatment.
- IV administration only; drug is fatal if administered intrathecally. Prepared syringes containing the drug must be packaged in an overwrap that is labeled "DO NOT REMOVE COVERING UNTIL MOMENT OF INJECTION. FATAL IF GIVEN INTRATHECALLY. FOR INTRAVENOUS USE ONLY."

- If inadvertent IT administration of vinca alkaloids occurs, **immediate** neurosurgical intervention is necessary to prevent ascending paralysis leading to death. The competent physician should (Bedford Labs, 2014):
  - Remove as much CSF as is safely possible through lumbar access.
  - Insert epidural catheter into subarachnoid space via the intervertebral space above initial lumbar access and irrigate the CSF with lactated Ringer's solution. Fresh frozen plasma should be requested and, when available, 25 mL should be added to every 1 liter of lactated Ringer's solution.
  - Neurosurgeon should insert an intraventricular drain or catheter and continue CSF irrigation with fluid removed through the lumbar access, connected to a closed drainage system. Lactated Ringer's solution should be given by CI at 150 mL/hour or a rate of 75 mL/hour when fresh frozen plasma has been added as above.
  - Rate of infusion should be adjusted to maintain a spinal fluid protein level of 150 mg/dL.
  - The following measures have also been used, but may not be essential: gluamic acid, 10 gm, IV over 24 hours, followed by 500 mg^3 × daily by mouth for 1 month. Folinic acid has been administered IV as a 100 mg bolus and then infused at a rate of 25 mg/hr × 24 hours, then bolus doses of 25 mg every 6 hours for 1 week. Pyridoxine has been given at a dose of 50 mg every 8 hours by IV infusion over 30 min.

Potential Toxicities/Side Effects and the Nursing Process

I. POTENTIAL FOR INFECTION AND BLEEDING related to BM DEPRESSION

Defining Characteristics: May cause severe BM depression; nadir 4–10 days. Neutrophils greatly affected. In patients with prior XRT or chemotherapy, thrombocytopenia may be severe.

Nursing Implications: Monitor CBC, platelet count prior to drug administration. Assess for signs/symptoms of infection or bleeding. Instruct patient in self-assessment of signs/symptoms of infection or bleeding. Dose reduction if hepatic dysfunction: 50% if bili > 1.5 mg/dL; 75% if bili > 3.0 mg/dL. Administer red blood cell and platelet transfusions per physician's orders.

II. POTENTIAL FOR SENSORY/PERCEPTUAL ALTERATIONS related to PERIPHERAL OR CENTRAL NEUROPATHY

Defining Characteristics: Occur less frequently than with vincristine. Occur in patients receiving prolonged or high-dose therapy. Symptoms: paresthesias, PN, depression, headache, malaise, jaw pain, urinary retention, tachycardia, orthostatic hypotension, seizures. Rare ocular changes: diplopia, ptosis, photophobia, oculomotor dysfunction, optic neuropathy.

Nursing Implications: Assess sensory/perceptual changes prior to each drug dose, especially if dose is high (> 10 mg) or patient is receiving prolonged therapy. Notify physician of alterations. Discuss with patient the impact changes have had, as well as strategies to minimize dysfunction and decrease distress.

III. ALTERATION IN BOWEL ELIMINATION related to CONSTIPATION

Defining Characteristics: Constipation results from neurotoxicity (central) and is less common than with vincristine. Risk factor: high dose (> 20 mg). May lead to adynamic ileus, abdominal pain.

Nursing Implications: Assess bowel elimination pattern with each drug dose, especially if dose > 20 mg. Teach patient to promote bowel elimination with fluids (3 L/day), high-fiber, bulky foods, exercise, stool softeners. Suggest laxative if unable to move bowels at least once a day. Instruct patient to report abdominal pain.

IV. ALTERATION IN NUTRITION, LESS THAN BODY REQUIREMENTS, related to GI SIDE EFFECTS

Defining Characteristics: Nausea and vomiting rarely occur. Stomatitis is uncommon but can be severe.

Nursing Implications: Premedicate with antiemetics and continue prophylactically for 24 hours to prevent nausea and vomiting, at least for the first treatment. Encourage small, frequent feedings of cool, bland foods and liquids. Assess for symptoms of fluid and electrolyte imbalance: monitor I/O, daily weights if administered to an inpatient. Teach patient oral assessment. Teach, reinforce teaching, regarding oral hygiene regimen. Encourage patient to report early stomatitis. Provide pain relief measures if indicated (e.g., topical anesthetics).

V. POTENTIAL FOR IMPAIRED SKIN INTEGRITY related to ALOPECIA

Defining Characteristics: Alopecia is reversible and mild and occurs in 45–50% of patients receiving drug. Drug is a potent vesicant and can cause irritation and necrosis if infiltrated.

Nursing Implications: Discuss with patient the impact of hair loss. Suggest wig as appropriate prior to actual hair loss. Explore with patient response to actual hair loss and plan strategies to minimize distress (e.g., wig, scarf, cap). Careful technique is used during venipuncture and intravenous administration. Administer vesicant through freely flowing IV, constantly monitoring IV site and patient response. Nurse should be THOROUGHLY familiar with institutional policy and procedure for administration of a vesicant agent. If vesicant drug is administered as a CI, drug must be given through a PATENT CENTRAL LINE. If extravasation is suspected, stop drug administration and aspirate any residual drug and blood from IV tubing, IV catheter/needle, and IV site if possible. If drug infiltration is suspected, manufacturer suggests the following after withdrawing any remaining drug from

IV: local installation of hyaluronidase; application of moderate heat. Assess site regularly for pain, progression of erythema, induration, and evidence of necrosis. When in doubt about whether drug is infiltrating, TREAT AS AN INFILTRATION. Teach patient to assess site, and instruct to notify physician if condition worsens. Arrange next clinic visit for assessment of site depending on drug, amount infiltrated, extent of potential injury, and patient variables. Document in patient's record as per institutional policy and procedure.

VI.   POTENTIAL FOR SEXUAL DYSFUNCTION related to REPRODUCTIVE HAZARD

Defining Characteristics: Drug is possibly teratogenic. Likely to cause azoospermia in men.

Nursing Implications: As appropriate, explore with patient and partner issues of reproductive and sexuality patterns and the anticipated impact chemotherapy may have. Discuss strategies to preserve sexual health (e.g., sperm banking).

Drug: vincristine (Oncovin)

Class: Plant alkaloid extracted from the periwinkle plant (*Vinca rosea*).

Mechanism of Action: Drug binds to microtubular proteins, thus arresting mitosis during metaphase. Cell cycle specific for M phase and active in S phase.

Metabolism: The primary route for excretion is via the liver (P450 microenzyme system) with about 70% of the drug being excreted in feces and bile. These metabolites are a result of hepatic metabolism and biliary excretion. A small amount is excreted in the urine. Dose modification may be necessary in the presence of hepatic failure.

Indication: For the treatment of patients with acute leukemia. In addition, in combination with other oncolytic agents in the treatment of patients with Hodgkin's disease, NHL, rhabdomyosarcoma, neuroblastoma, and Wilms' tumor.

Contraindication: Patients with the demyelinating form of Charcot-Marie-Tooth syndrome.

Dosage/Range:
- 0.4–1.4 mg/m^2 weekly (initially limited to 2 mg per dose), weekly.
- Dose-reduce 50% if paitent has a direct serum bilirubin > 3 mg/dL.
- Dose is a vesicant; give through a running IV to avoid extravasation.
- Dose modifications may be necessary in the presence of hepatic failure.

Drug Preparation:
- Supplied in 1-mg, 2-mg, and 5-mg vials. Refrigerate vials until use. Prepared syringes containing the drug must be packaged in an overwrap that is labeled "DO NOT REMOVE COVERING UNTIL MOMENT OF INJECTION. FATAL IF GIVEN INTRATHECALLY. FOR INTRAVENOUS USE ONLY."

- To reduce potential for fatal medication errors due to incorrect route of administration, vincristine sulphate injection should be diluted in a flexible plastic container and prominently labeled as indicated for IV use only.
- When vincristine is diluted with 0.9% Sodium Chloride Injection in concentrations from 0.0015–0.08 mg/mL, the infusion bag is stable for up to 24 hours when protected from light or 8 hours under normal light at 25°C (Hospira, 2017).

Drug Administration:
- Asess CBC/differential before each dose; assess baseline serum uric acid.
- Assess for signs/symptoms of neuropathy: ability to pick up a coin, button shirt; constipation.
- IV: This drug is a vesicant. In hospitals that do not prepare or administer IT drugs, give IVP through sidearm of a running IV to avoid extravasation, which can lead to ulceration, pain, and necrosis. Use vesicant administration precautions. Refer to hospital's policy and procedure for administration of a vesicant.
- In healthcare settings that prepare and administer IT medications: Administer via IV in mini-bag (0.9% Sodium Chloride USP). Use vesicant precautions.
- Avoid spillage of drug in the eye as it may cause corneal ulceration. If it occurs, wash the eye immediately and thoroughly.

Drug Interactions:
- Neurotoxic drugs: additive neurotoxicity can occur; use cautiously.
- CYP3A4 inhibitors (itraconazole, erythromycin, others): increased serum drug level of vincristine; do not use together, or assess possible toxicity and dose-reduce vincristine.
- CYP3A4 inducers (carbamazepine, dexamethasone, phenytoin, others): decreased serum levels of vincristine; do not use together, or assess need to increase dose of vincristine.
- St. John's wort: may increase vincristine toxicity; do not administer concomitantly.
- Grapefruit juice: may increase vincristine toxicity; do not administer concomitantly.
- Phenytoin: decreased phenytoin serum levels and increased seizure activity; assess phenytoin serum levels and dose accordingly.
- Asparaginase: when given prior to vincristine, will decrease vincristine excretion, with resulting increased neurotoxicity; give vincristine 12–24 hours before asparaginase.
- Decreased bioavailability of digoxin when given with this drug.
- Increased cellular uptake of methotrexate by some malignant cells when given sequentially.
- Do not mix with other drugs that change the pH.

Lab Effects/Interference:
- Decreased WBC, platelets.
- Increased uric acid.

Special Considerations:
- Warnings and Precautions:
  - *Drug has been given INTRATHECALLY by error*, resulting in death. Ensure that vincristine is labeled "For IV use only." If the healthcare setting prepares and administers IT medication, then as recommended by the manufacturer, vincristine is diluted in a flexible plastic container and prominently labeled as indicated for IV use only. If the

healthcare setting does not prepare or administer IT drugs, then the vinca alkaloid may be administered IVP (Neuss et al., 2017).

- Drug preparation is for IV use ONLY. Use Intrathecal precautions in preparing and storing IT medications, as well as a time out at the bedside to PREVENT inadvertent IT injection that will be fatal.
- Syringes containing vincristine ust be labelled using the auxiliary sticker provided, to state "FOR INTRAVENOUS USE ONLY—FATAL IF GIVEN BY OTHER ROUTES."
- Extemporaneously prepared syringes contining this product must be packaged in an overwarp which is labeled "DO NOT REMOVE COVERING UNTIL MOMENT OF INJECTION. FATAL IF GIVEN INTRATHECALLY. FOR INTRAVENOUS USE ONLY."

- *Embryo-fetal toxicity:* Teach women of reproductive potential to use effective contraception to avoid pregnancy while receiving vincristine. Mothers should not breastfeed during vincristine therapy.
- *Acute uric acid nephropathy* has been reported.
- *Use caution when administering to patients with preexisting neuromuscular disease* and when given in combination with other neurotoxic drugs.
- *Acute SOB and severe bronchospasm* have been described after the admiinistraiton of vinca alkaloids, especially if given together with mitomycin-C. Onset is within minutes to several hours after drug is given, and may occur up to 2 weeks after the mitomycin-C dose. Maintain airway and implement emergency aggressive treatment as ordered. Discontinue drug if this occurs.
- If inadvertent IT administration of vinca alkaloids occurs, **immediate** neurosurgical intervention is necessary to prevent ascending paralysis leading to death. The competent physician should (Bedford Labs, 2014):
  - Remove as much CSF as is safely possible through lumbar access.
  - Insert epidural catheter into subarachnoid space via the intervertebral space above initial lumbar access and irrigate the CSF with lactated Ringer's solution. Fresh frozen plasma should be requested and, when available, 25 mL should be added to every 1 liter of lactated Ringer's solution.
  - Neurosurgeon should insert an intraventricular drain or catheter and continue CSF irrigation with fluid removed through the lumbar access, connected to a closed drainage system. Lactated Ringer's solution should be given by CI at 150 mL/hour or a rate of 75 mL/hr when fresh frozen plasma has been added as above.
  - Rate of infusion should be adjusted to maintain a spinal fluid protein level of 150 mg/dL.
- The following measures have also been used, but may not be essential: gluamic acid, 10 gm, IV over 24 hours, followed by 500 mg 3 times daily by mouth for 1 month. Folinic acid has been administered IV as a 100 mg bolus and then infused at a rate of 25 mg/hr × 24 hours, then bolus doses of 25 mg every 6 hours for 1 week. Pyridoxine has been given at a dose of 50 mg every 8 hrs by IV infusion over 30 min.
- Liposomal vincristine (Marqibo) is FDA-approved for treatment of patients with Philadelphia chromosome-negative acute lymphoblastic leukemia (ALL), who have relapsed at least twice or whose ALL has progressed after two or more anti-leukemia regimens.

This drug is different from vincristine (Oncovin). Drug dose is different from vincristine sulfate injection—verify drug name and dose prior to preparation and administration to avoid overdosage.

Potential Toxicities/Side Effects and the Nursing Process

I. POTENTIAL FOR SENSORY/PERCEPTUAL ALTERATIONS related to PERIPHERAL CENTRAL NEUROPATHY

Defining Characteristics: Peripheral neuropathies occur as a result of toxicity to nerve fibers: absent deep tendon reflexes, numbness, weakness, myalgias, cramping, and late severe motor difficulties. Reversal or discontinuance of therapy is necessary. Increased risk exists in elderly. Cranial nerve dysfunction may occur (rare), as well as jaw pain (trigeminal neuralgia), diplopia, vocal cord paresis, mental depression, and metallic taste.

Nursing Implications: Assess sensory/perceptual changes prior to each drug dose, e.g., presence of numbness or tingling of fingertips or toes. Assess for loss of tendon reflexes: foot drop, slapping gait. Assess for motor difficulties: clumsiness of hands, difficulty climbing stairs, buttoning shirt, walking on heels. Notify physician of alterations; discuss holding drug if loss of deep tendon reflexes occurs. Discuss with patient the impact alterations have had, and strategies to minimize dysfunction and decrease distress. Discuss with patient type of alteration: memory and sensory/perceptual changes are temporary and reversible when drug is stopped. Assess patient for signs/symptoms of nerve dysfunction before each dose. Notify physician of any changes.

II. ALTERATION IN BOWEL ELIMINATION related to CONSTIPATION

Defining Characteristics: Autonomic neuropathy may lead to constipation and paralytic ileus. A concurrent use of vincristine, narcotic analgesics, or cholinergic medication may increase risk of constipation.

Nursing Implications: Assess bowel elimination pattern prior to each chemotherapy administration. Teach patient to include bulky and high-fiber foods in diet, increase fluids to 3 L/day, and exercise moderately to promote elimination. Suggest stool softeners if needed. Teach patient to use laxative if unable to move bowels at least once every 2 days. Instruct patient to report abdominal pain.

III. POTENTIAL FOR IMPAIRED SKIN INTEGRITY related to ALOPECIA

Defining Characteristics: Complete hair loss occurs in 12–45% of patients. Both men and women are at risk for body-image disturbance. Hair will grow back. Dermatitis is uncommon. Drug is potent vesicant causing irritation and necrosis if infiltrated.

Nursing Implications: Discuss with patient anticipated impact of hair loss. Suggest wig or toupee as appropriate prior to actual hair loss. Explore with patient response to actual hair loss and plan strategies to minimize distress (e.g., wig, scarf, cap). Assess impact on patient: body image, comfort. Careful technique is used during venipuncture and intravenous administration. Administer vesicant through freely flowing IV, constantly monitoring IV site and patient response. Nurse should be THOROUGHLY familiar with institutional policy and procedure for administration of a vesicant agent. If vesicant drug is administered as a CI, drug must be given THROUGH A PATENT CENTRAL LINE. When administering the drug, if extravasation is suspected, TREAT IT AS AN INFILTRATION. Stop drug administration and aspirate any residual drug and blood from IV tubing, IV catheter/needle, and IV site if possible. Manufacturer suggests the following after withdrawing any remaining drug from IV: local installation of hyaluronidase, application of moderate heat. Assess site regularly for pain, progression of erythema, induration, and evidence of necrosis. Teach patient to assess site and notify physician if condition worsens. Arrange next clinic visit for assessment of site depending on drug, amount infiltrated, extent of potential injury, and patient variables. Document in patient's record as per institutional policy and procedure.

IV.   POTENTIAL FOR INFECTION AND BLEEDING related to BM DEPRESSION

Defining Characteristics: Rare myelosuppression, mild when it occurs. Nadir 10–14 days after treatment begins.

Nursing Implications: Monitor CBC, HCT, platelet count prior to drug administration. Dose reduction if hepatic dysfunction: 50% reduction if bili $>$ 1.5 mg/dL; 75% reduction if bili $>$ 3.0 mg/dL.

V.   POTENTIAL SEXUAL DYSFUNCTION related to IMPOTENCE

Defining Characteristics: Impotence may occur, related to neurotoxicity.

Nursing Implications: As appropriate, explore with patient and partner issues of reproductive and sexuality patterns, and impact chemotherapy may have. Discuss strategies to preserve sexual health, e.g., alternative expressions of sexuality. Reassure patient that impotency, if it occurs, is usually temporary, and reversible after drug discontinuance.

Drug: VinCRIStine sulfate LIPOSOME injection (liposome-encapsulated, Marqibo)

Class: Vinca alkaloid, liposome encapsulated.

Mechanism of Action: Drug action is the same as that of vincristine sulfate: binds to tubulin, changing tubulin polymerization equilibrium, stabilizes the mitotic spindle apparatus, and prevents chromosomes from segregating so they cannot line up on the mitotic spindle. This leads to metaphase arrest and mitosis (cell division) is prevented.

TREATMENT

Metabolism: Clearance of VinCRIStine sulfate LIPOSOME from the plasma is very slow compared to nonliposomal vincristine sulfate increasing tumor exposure to the drug (much higher AUC). Drug is largely excreted in the feces with < 8% excreted in the urine.

Indication: Treatment of patients with Philadelphia chromosome-negative (Ph-) acute lymphoblastic leukemia (ALL) in second or greater relapse or whose disease has progressed following 2 or more anti-leukemic therapies. FDA indication is based on overall response rate, and clinical benefit such as improvement in overall survival has not been verified.

Contraindication: (1) patients with demyelinating conditions, including Charcot–Marie–Tooth syndrome; (2) patients hypersensitive to vincristine sulfate or any oth the other components of Marqibo (vincristine sulfate LIPOSOME injection); (3) intrathecal administration.

Dosage/Range:
- Dose is 2.25 mg/m^2 IV over 1 hour once every 7 days.

Dose Modifications for PN:
- Grade 3 (severe symptoms, inability to do ADLs) or persistent grade 2 (moderate symptoms, limiting instrumental ADLs): interrupt vincristine sulfate LIPOSOME injection (Marqibo); if PN remains at grades 3–4, discontinue Marqibo. If the PN recovers to grades 1–2, reduce Marqibo dose to 2 mg/m^2.
- Persistent grade 2 PN after the first dose reduction to 2 mg/m^2: interrupt Marqibo for up to 7 days. If the PN increases to grades 3–4, discontinue Marqibo. If PN recovers to grade 1, reduce the Marqibo dose to 1.825 mg/m^2.
- Persistent grade 2 PN after the 2nd dose reduction to 1,825 mg/m^2: Interrupt Marqibo for up to 7 days. If the PN increases to grades 3–4, discontinue Marqibo. If PN recovers to grade 1, reduce the Marqibo dose to 1.5 mg/m^2.

Drug Preparation:
- Ensure drug is VinCRIStine sulfate LIPOSOME injection NOT vincristine sulfate (non-liposomal formulation). Ensure independent double checks and verification of orders; drugs are not interchangeable and patient will be overdosed if the wrong drug is used as doses are NOT the same.
- Marqibo administration kit. Also need access to water bath, calibrated thermometer (0–100°C), calibrated electronic timer, sterile venting needle or other suitable device equipped with a sterile 0.2 micron filter, 1 mL or 3 mL sterile syringe with needle, and a 5 mL sterile syringe with needle. The manufacturer will supply the water bath, calibrated thermometer and timer to the medical facility at the initial order of Marqibo and will replace them every 2 years. **See package insert.**
- Do NOT use water with the block heater preparation process. See package insert.
- After preparation, each single-dose vial of vincristine sulfate LIPOSOME injection containes 5 mg/31 mL (0.16 mg/mL) vincristine sulfate.
- **See labeling of medication under "Vincristine Sulfate" (previous drug in this book) for requirements to distinguish it from IT medications and prevent IT administration. Label must say NOT FOR INTRATHECAL USE.**

Drug Administration:
- Assess baseline neurological status, and prior to each treatment for signs and symptoms of sensory PN (e.g., pins and needles in a stocking-glove distribution, functional impairment of picking up a coin or buttoning a shirt); central neuropathy (e.g., constipation) and motor PN (e.g., muscle weakness). Discuss abnormalities with provider, and document so that when drug next given, any progression of signs/symptoms can be seen.
- IV administration ONLY. Ensure drug has label "NOT FOR INTRATHECAL USE. Use vesicant precautions. Administer drug through a freely flowing IV or central line. See *Chapter 1* introduction.
- Administer vincristine liposome injection 2.25-mg/m^2 (or reduced dose) IV infusion over 1 hour once every 7 days.

Drug Interactions: Same as with vincristine sulfate.

Lab Effects/Interference:
- Neutropenia, thrombocytopenia, anemia

Special Considerations:
- Most common adverse reactions ($\geq$ 30%): constipation, nausea, pyrexia, fatigue, PN, febrile neutropenia, diarrhea, anemia, decreased appetite, and insomnia.
- Warnings and Precautions:
  - *Intrathecal administration is FATAL. **For IV use only.***
  - *Extravasation causes tissue injury.* Drug is a vesicant. See *Chapter 1.*
  - *Neurological toxicity:* monitor patients for peripheral motor and sensory, central and autonomic neuropathy, and reduce, interrupt, or discontinue dosing. Patients with preexisting severe neuropathy should be treated with vincristine liposome injection only after a careful risk-benefit assessement.
  - *Myelosuppression:* Monitor CBC/differential prior to each dose. Neutropenia, thrombocytopenia, or anemia may occur; consider vincristine liposome injection dose reduction or interruption and supportive care measures.
  - *TLS*: discuss TLS risk of each patient with physician/NP/PA, plan to prophylax, and implement plan. Ensure adequate hydration, agent to lower serum uric acid, and monitor serum chemistries and renal function tests closely.
  - *Constipation, bowel obstruction, and/or paralytic ileus*: institute a prophylactic bowerl regimen to prevent potential constipation, bowel obstruction, and/or paralytic ileus.
  - *Fatigue*: can occur and may be severe.
  - *Hepatotoxicity can occur.* Monitor LFTs baseline and regularly during treatment with vincristine liposome injection. Discuss abnormalities with physician/NP/PA and treatment plan modifications.
  - *Embryo-fetal toxicity:* Teach women of reproductive potential to use effective contraception to avoid pregnancy while receiving vincristine liposome injection. Mothers should not breastfeed during VinCRIStine sulfate LIPOSOME therapy.
- Dose of vincristine liposome injection is different from vincristine sulfate injection. Be very careful NOT to use the different drugs interchangeably. Ensure independent double checks to prevent possible error and overdosage.

Potential Toxicities/Side Effects and the Nursing Process

I. POTENTIAL FOR SENSORY/PERCEPTUAL ALTERATIONS related to PERIPHERAL CENTRAL NEUROPATHY

Defining Characteristics: Peripheral neuropathies occur as a result of toxicity to nerve fibers: absent deep tendon reflexes, numbness, weakness, myalgias, cramping, and late severe motor difficulties. Reversal or discontinuance of therapy is necessary. Increased risk exists in elderly. Cranial nerve dysfunction may occur (rare), as well as jaw pain (trigeminal neuralgia), diplopia, vocal cord paresis, mental depression, and metallic taste.

Nursing Implications: Assess sensory/perceptual changes prior to each drug dose, e.g., presence of numbness or tingling of fingertips or toes. Assess for loss of tendon reflexes: foot drop, slapping gait. Assess for motor difficulties: clumsiness of hands, difficulty climbing stairs, buttoning shirt, walking on heels. Notify physician of alterations; discuss holding drug if loss of deep tendon reflexes occurs. Discuss with patient the impact alterations have had, and strategies to minimize dysfunction and decrease distress. Discuss with patient type of alteration: memory and sensory/perceptual changes are temporary and reversible when drug is stopped. Assess patient for signs/symptoms of nerve dysfunction before each dose. Notify physician of any changes.

II. ALTERATION IN BOWEL ELIMINATION related to CONSTIPATION

Defining Characteristics: Autonomic neuropathy may lead to constipation and paralytic ileus. A concurrent use of vincristine, narcotic analgesics, or cholinergic medication may increase risk of constipation.

Nursing Implications: Assess bowel elimination pattern prior to each chemotherapy administration. Teach patient to include bulky and high-fiber foods in diet, increase fluids to 3 L/day, and exercise moderately to promote elimination. Suggest stool softeners if needed. Teach patient to use laxative if unable to move bowels at least once every 2 days. Instruct patient to report abdominal pain.

III. POTENTIAL FOR IMPAIRED SKIN INTEGRITY related to ALOPECIA

Defining Characteristics: Complete hair loss occurs in 12–45% of patients. Both men and women are at risk for body-image disturbance. Hair will grow back. Dermatitis is uncommon. Drug is potent vesicant causing irritation and necrosis if infiltrated.

Nursing Implications: Discuss with patient anticipated impact of hair loss. Suggest wig or toupee as appropriate prior to actual hair loss. Explore with patient response to actual hair loss and plan strategies to minimize distress (e.g., wig, scarf, cap). Assess impact on patient: body image, comfort. Careful technique is used during venipuncture and intravenous administration. Administer vesicant through freely flowing IV, constantly monitoring IV site and patient response. Nurse should be THOROUGHLY familiar with institutional policy and procedure for administration of a vesicant agent. If vesicant drug is administered as a CI, drug must be given THROUGH A PATENT CENTRAL LINE. When administering the drug, if extravasation is suspected, TREAT IT AS AN INFILTRATION. Stop drug administration and aspirate any residual drug and blood from IV tubing, IV catheter/needle, and IV site if possible. Manufacturer suggests the following after withdrawing any remaining drug from IV: local installation of hyaluronidase, application of moderate heat. Assess site regularly for pain, progression of erythema, induration, and evidence of necrosis. Teach patient to assess site and notify physician if condition worsens. Arrange next clinic visit for assessment of site depending on drug, amount infiltrated, extent of potential injury, and patient variables. Document in patient's record as per institutional policy and procedure.

IV.   POTENTIAL FOR INFECTION AND BLEEDING related to BM DEPRESSION

Defining Characteristics: Rare myelosuppression, mild when it occurs. Nadir 10–14 days after treatment begins.

Nursing Implications: Monitor CBC, HCT, platelet count prior to drug administration. Dose reduction if hepatic dysfunction: 50% reduction if bili > 1.5 mg/dL; 75% reduction if bili > 3.0 mg/dL.

V.   POTENTIAL SEXUAL DYSFUNCTION related to IMPOTENCE

Defining Characteristics: Impotence may occur related to neurotoxicity.

Nursing Implications: As appropriate, explore with patient and partner issues of reproductive and sexuality patterns and impact chemotherapy may have. Discuss strategies to preserve sexual health, e.g., alternative expressions of sexuality. Reassure patient that impotency, if it occurs, is usually temporary and reversible after drug discontinuance.

Drug: vinorelbine tartrate (Navelbine)

Class: Semisynthetic vinca alkaloid derived from vinblastine.

Mechanism of Action: Inhibits mitosis at metaphase by interfering with microtubule assembly. Specifically, it inhibits tubulin polymerization and binds preferentially to microtubules during mitosis so that mitosis is blocked at G_2–M phase, causing cell death. Also appears to interfere with some aspects of cellular metabolism, including cellular respiration and nucleic acid biosynthesis. Cell cycle specific.

Metabolism: Slow elimination; extensive tissue binding (80% bound to plasma proteins); metabolized by the liver (P450 microenzyme system). Terminal half-life is 27–43 hours. Excreted in feces (46%) and urine (18%). The investigational oral form 60–80 mg/m^2 results in comparable serum levels to that of 25- to 30-mg/m^2 IV formulation. The drug is well absorbed following oral administration, T_{max} reached in 1.5 to 3 hours. The drug is significantly taken up by lung tissue, and has an elimination half-life of 35 to 40 hours. Bioavailability of the oral capsules is 33–43%, probably because of incomplete absorption and a first-pass effect in the liver. Vomiting 3 hours after swallowing the dose does not reduce the absorption of the drug.

Indication: Drug indicated
- In combination with cisplatin for the first-line treatment of patients with locally advanced or metastatic NSCLC.
- As a single agent for the treatment of patients with metastatic NSCLC.

Contraindications: None. However, drug should not be administered to patients with a pretreatment ANC < 1,000 cells/mm³.

Dosage/Range:
- IV:
  - **Single agent**, initial dose: 30-mg/m² IV over 6–10 minutes weekly until progression or dose-limiting toxicity.
  - **In combination with cisplatin 100 mg/m²:** Vinorelbine 25-mg/m² IV over 6–10 minutes on days 1, 8, 15, and 21 of a 28-day cycle in combination with cisplatin 100 mg/m² given on day 1 of each 28-day cycle.
  - **In combination with cisplatin 120 mg/m²:** Vinorelbine 30-mg/m² IV over 6–10 minutes once a week in combination with cisplatin 120 mg/m² given on day 1 and day 29, then every 6 weeks.

Dose Modifications:
- **Hematologic toxicity:** See package insert. If ANC on day of treatment is 1,000–1,499/mm³, give 50% of vinorelbine dose. Drug should be held if ANC < 1,000/mm³, and ANC rechecked in 1 week. If drug is held for 3 consecutive weeks because ANC < 1,000/mm³, discontinue drug.
- If patient develops neutropenic fever or sepsis or drug is held for neutropenia for 2 consecutive doses due to granulocytopenia, dose should be:
  - ANC on day of treatment: ≥ 1,500, give 75% of starting dose.
  - ANC on day of treatment: 1,000–1,499: give 37.5% of starting dose.
  - If ANC < 1,000, do not administer vinorelbine, and repeat neutrophil count in 1 week.
- *Hepatic dysfunction:* if total bilirubin is 2.1–3.0 mg/dL, give 50% of initial vinorelbine dose; if total bili is > 3.0 mg/dL, give 25% of starting vinorelbine dose.
- If patient requires dose adjustment for both hematologic toxicity and hepatic insufficiency: use the lower of the doses.
- If grade 2 or higher neurotoxicity occurs, discontinue vinorelbine.

Drug Preparation:
- Drug is available as 10 mg/mL in 1- or 5-mL vials.
- Further dilute drug in:
  - A syringe using 5% dextrose injection USP or 0.9% sodium chloride injection USP to a final concentration or 1.5–3 mg/mL or

- IV bag in 0.9% sodium chloride USP, 5% dextrose USP, 0.45% sodium chloride injection USP, 5% dextrose and 0.45% sodium chloride injection USP, Ringer's Injection USP, or Lactated Ringer's injection USP, to a final concentration of 0.5–2.0 mg/mL in an IV bag.
- Stability: Diluted vinorelbine injection may be used for up to 24 hours under normal room light when stored in polypropylene syringes or polyvinyl chloride bags at 5–30°C (41–86°F).
- Prepared syringes containing the drug must be packaged in an overwrap that is labeled "DO NOT REMOVE COVERING UNTIL MOMENT OF INJECTION. FATAL IF GIVEN INTRATHECALLY. FOR INTRAVENOUS USE ONLY."

Drug Administration:
- Assess CBC/differential, as ANC must be 1,000 cells/mm^3 or higher prior to drug administration. Assess for signs/symptoms of new or worsening motor or sensory neuropathy.
- Ensure patient has a patent IV with excellent blood return.
- Infuse diluted drug IV over 6–10 minutes into sidearm port of freely flowing IV infusion, either peripherally or via central line. Use port CLOSEST TO THE IV BAG, not the patient.
- Flush vein with at least 75–125 mL of IV fluid after drug infusion.
- Drug is a vesicant; use vesicant precautions. See *Chapter 1* introduction.
- Patients should be taught to contact their physician or NP/PA if they experience increased SOB, cough, or new pulmonary symptoms, or if they experience abdominal pain or constipation.

Drug Interactions:
- Increased granulocytopenia occurs when given in combination with cisplatin.
- Possible pulmonary reactions occur when given in combination with mitomycin C, characterized by dyspnea and severe bronchospasm. May require management with bronchodilators, corticosteroids, and/or supplemental oxygen.
- CYP3A4 inhibitors (itraconazole, erythromycin, omeprazole, fluoxetine, others): increased serum drug level of vinorelbine; do not use together or *assess possible toxicity and dose-reduce vinorelbine.*
- CYP3A4 inducers (carbamazepine, dexamethasone, phenytoin, others): decreased serum levels of vinorelbine; do not use together or assess need to increase dose of vinorelbine. Monitor phenytoin levels and dose modify depending upon levels, as levels may be low.
- Paclitaxel, docetaxel: give paclitaxel or docetaxel before vinorelbine to reduce myelosuppression (reverse sequence increases toxicity of paclitaxel or docetaxel).
- St. John's wort: may decrease vinorelbine effectiveness; do not give together.
- Grapefruit juice: inhibits CYP3A4 enzymes, which may increase toxicity of vinorelbine; do not use together.

Lab Effects/Interference:
- Decreased CBC (especially WBC).
- Increased LFTs.

Special Considerations:
- Most common adverse reactions (incidence ≥ 20%) are neutropenia, anemia, increased LFTs, nausea, vomiting, asthenia, constipation, injection-site reaction, and PN.
- Warnings and Precautions:
  - *Hepatic toxicity*: monitor LFTs baseline and regularly during treatment.
  - Severe constipation and bowel obstruction, including necrosis and perforation, can occur. Ensure patient is on an effective prophylactic bowel regimen to PREVENT constipation. Monitor for abdominal pain and constipation.
  - Drug is a potent vesicant and extravasation can result in severe tissue injury, necrosis, and/or thrombophlebitis. Use extravasation precautions when administering the drug (see *Chapter 1* introduction). Immediately stop vinorelbine if extravasation is suspected, and manage extravasation.
  - Neurologic toxicity: severe motor and sensory neuropathies can occur. Patients with history of or preexisting neuropathy are at increased risk. Monitor patient closely for new or worsening signs and symptoms of neuropathy and discuss abnormal findings with physician/NP/PA.
  - Pulmonary toxicity and respiratory failure can occur. Monitor patients closely with respiratory disorders. If patient develops unexplained dyspnea and bronchospasm, immediately interrupt vinorelbine infusion, maintain patent airway, and implement emergency medical measures as ordered by physician/NP/PA.
  - Embryo-fetal toxicity: Teach women of reproductive potential to use effective contraception to avoid pregnancy while receiving vincristine liposome injection. Mothers should not breastfeed during vinorelbine therapy.
- Use drug cautiously in patients with reduced BM reserve (e.g., prior irradiation or chemotherapy).
- Drug may cause a radiation recall reaction in patients who have had prior RT.
- Avoid contamination of the eye when administering the drug. Severe eye irritation may occur; if it does, the eye should immediately be flushed with water.

Potential Toxicities/Side Effects and the Nursing Process

I. INFECTION AND BLEEDING related to BM DEPRESSION

Defining Characteristics: Leukopenia is dose-limiting toxicity; BM depression noncumulative and short-lived (< 7 days), with nadir at 7–10 days. Use with caution in patients with history of prior radiotherapy or chemotherapy. Severe thrombocytopenia and anemia are uncommon.

Nursing Implications: Monitor CBC, ANC, HCT, and platelet count prior to drug administration, as well as for signs/symptoms of infection or bleeding. Instruct patient in self-assessment of signs/symptoms of infection or bleeding. Teach patient self-care measures, including avoidance of OTC aspirin-containing medications. Dose reduction necessary for hematologic toxicity (see Special Considerations section).

II.   POTENTIAL FOR SENSORY/PERCEPTUAL ALTERATIONS related to NEUROLOGIC TOXICITY

Defining Characteristics: Incidence of mild-to-moderate neuropathy is 25%. Paresthesias occur in 2–10% of patients, but incidence is increased if patient has received prior chemotherapy with vinca alkaloids or abdominal XRT. Decreased deep tendon reflexes occur in 6–29% of patients. Constipation may occur in 29% of patients. Neuropathy is reversible.

Nursing Implications: Assess baseline neuromuscular function, and reassess prior to drug infusion, especially in the presence of paresthesias; risk is increased if drug is given concurrently with cisplatin. Teach patient to report any changes in sensation or function. Identify strategies to promote comfort and safety.

III.   ALTERATION IN NUTRITION, LESS THAN BODY REQUIREMENTS, related to NAUSEA/VOMITING, DIARRHEA, STOMATITIS, HEPATOTOXICITY

Defining Characteristics: Incidence of nausea/vomiting increases with oral dosing; mild in IV dosing, with an incidence of 44%. Vomiting occurs in 20% of patients. Diarrhea increases with oral dosing (17% incidence). Stomatitis is mild to moderate with < 20% incidence. Transient increases in LFTs (AST) occur in 67% of patients, and are without clinical significance.

Nursing Implications: Premedicate with antiemetic, such as a serotonin antagonist, prior to drug administration. Encourage small, frequent meals of cool, bland foods and liquids. Assess for symptoms of fluid/electrolyte imbalance if patient has severe nausea and vomiting. Monitor I/O, daily weights, and lab electrolyte values. Encourage patient to report onset of diarrhea. Administer, or teach patient to self-administer, antidiarrheal medications. Teach patient oral assessment. Teach and reinforce teaching of systemic oral hygiene regimen. Instruct patient to report early stomatitis, and provide pain relief measures as needed. Assess LFTs prior to drug administration baseline and periodically during treatment. Dose modifications may be necessary for hepatic dysfunction (see Special Considerations section).

IV.   POTENTIAL FOR ALTERATION IN SKIN INTEGRITY related to ALOPECIA, EXTRAVASATION

Defining Characteristics: Gradual alopecia occurs in 10% of patients, rarely progressing to complete hair loss or requiring a wig. Severity is related to treatment duration. Drug is a moderate vesicant, primarily causing venous irritation and phlebitis; 30% of patients experience injection-site reactions commonly characterized by erythema, vein discoloration, tenderness; rarely, pain and venous irritation at sites proximal to injection site.

Nursing Implications: Discuss potential impact of hair loss prior to drug administration; also assess coping strategies, and plans to minimize body-image distortion (e.g., wig, scarf, cap). Assess patient for signs/symptoms of hair loss. Assess patient's response and use of coping strategies. Scrupulous venipuncture technique is used during venipuncture. Administer vesicant through freely flowing IV via IV port closest to IV fluid bag, not patient, and administer maximally diluted drug over 6–10 minutes (not longer). If extravasation is suspected, TREAT AS AN INFILTRATION and aspirate any remaining drug from IV tubing, locally instill hyaluronidase in area of suspected infiltration, and apply moderate heat. Assess site regularly for pain, progression of erythema, and evidence of necrosis. Document in patient's record. Schedule next clinic visit for assessment of site depending on drug, amount infiltrated, extent of potential injury, and other patient variables.

V.   POTENTIAL FOR SEXUAL/REPRODUCTIVE DYSFUNCTION related to TERATOGENICITY

Defining Characteristics: Drug is teratogenic and fetotoxic.

Nursing Implications: As appropriate, explore with patient and partner issues of reproductive and sexuality patterns and the anticipated impact chemotherapy may have. Counsel female patients of childbearing age in contraceptive options.

Chapter *2*
Cytoprotective Agents

Advances in the development of effective, new chemotherapeutic agents have been slow, although a number of excellent agents have recently been approved for use. All traditional chemotherapeutic agents work by interfering with DNA and RNA replication, and protein synthesis, causing cell death or stasis. Unfortunately, unless attached to a targeted vehicle, such as a monoclonal antibody, the chemotherapy is nonselective and also damages normal cells. Often, the dose-limiting toxicity is myelosuppression, but organ toxicity specific to the chemotherapy agent may limit the drug's usefulness. Specific organ toxicity that can occur includes neurotoxicity (e.g., cisplatin, oxaliplatin, the taxanes), cardiotoxicity (e.g., anthracyclines, alone or together with trastuzumab), bladder toxicity (e.g., high-dose cyclophosphamide, ifosfamide), and nephrotoxicity (e.g., cisplatin). Thus, both doses and duration of treatment are often limited by these organ toxicities. This can compromise optimal treatment, as well as quality of life. Similarly, radiation therapy causes cell damage (e.g., ionization causes the formation of free radicals, which, in the presence of oxygen, cause damage to DNA, leading to cell death when the cell tries to replicate). Again, normal tissue in the radiation port also is damaged, such as the bone marrow (BM) in the skull, sternum, and heads of long bones, and can lead to side effects such as BM depression, which results in the need for treatment breaks and less-than-optimal radiotherapy (RT).

In an effort to protect normal cells from treatment toxicity and to limit organ toxicities, a number of agents have been developed that offer cyto (cell) or organ protection. Agents that are currently approved for use are glucarpidase, leucovorin calcium, levoleucovorin, mesna, and dexrazoxane, a chelating agent. Amifostine has shown "broad spectrum" activity in protecting multiple organ systems, such as the kidneys, BM, and nerves. In addition, it protects the parotid glands from radiation damage. Amifostine is indicated for the reduction of cumulative nephrotoxicity from cisplatin in patients with advanced ovarian and NSCLC, as well as for reducing the incidence of moderate-to-severe xerostomia in patients with head and neck cancer whose radiation port covers the parotid glands (Sun Pharma Global, 2014). Mesna is included in this chapter because it protects the bladder from the toxic effects of high-dose cyclophosphamide and ifosfamide. Leucovorin is also a classic cytoprotectant in that it "rescues" normal cells from MTX toxicity (BM and mucosal cells). Dexrazoxane reduces the incidence and severity of anthracycline-induced cardiotoxicity (Mylan, 2015). Although Totect (dexrazoxane) has been FDA approved for the management of anthracycline extravasation, it is no longer commercially available. Many practitioners use the generic version of dexrazoxane instead (Polovich et al., 2014). Note that the dilution solution is different between that of Totect and generic dexrazoxane (Mylan, 2015), which use sodium lactate, while that of Zinecard uses sterile water for injection (Pharmacia and Upjohn, 2014).

Shortages of cytoprotective drugs or drugs that increase response, have led to many questions about substitutions or rethinking what is needed. For example, leucovorin is in very short supply, but is a necessary part of the treatment regimens FOLFOX (folinic acid, 5-FU, oxaliplatin) and FOLFIRI (leucovorin, 5-FU, irinotecan) for colorectal cancer (CRC). In reviewing the many clinical trials, the National Comprehensive Cancer Network (NCCN) recommends reconsideration of smaller doses of leucovorin (studies have shown equivalence in doses ranging from 20 mg/m^2 to 500 mg/m^2) (NCCN, v.2, 2016) or using levoleucovorin (200 mg/m^2 is equivalent to standard leucovorin 400 mg/m^2) (NCCN, v.2, 2016). Totect is not currently available, but studies have now shown that dexrazoxane (generic or Zinecard) can be used equally well (Arroyo et al., 2010; Conde-Estevez et al., 2010; American Society of Hospital Pharmacists, 2016).

Neurotoxicity is important and can greatly affect quality of life. Nurses must elicit a history and perform a physical exam to identify whether the patient has developed peripheral neuropathy from specific drug(s) or, if that has been established, whether it has progressed, whether it affects the patient's ability to do ADLs, or whether it affects the patient's safety (Wilkes, 2014). The American Society of Clinical Oncology completed a systematic review of the literature and found that there were no agents that prevent chemotherapy-induced peripheral neuropathy (CIPN) (Hershman et al., 2014). They found that many of the randomized controlled trials were small and heterogeneous and underpowered so that they were unable to detect clinically important differences, and most studies were not directly comparable as they used different measurements, instruments, and outcomes. Conflicting studies often exist, some showing potential benefit of agents and others that are negative, such as the study of amifostine and glutamine, found in this chapter. However, in terms of treating neuropathic pain, duloxetine has been shown to significantly reduce CIPN-induced pain (Smith et al., 2013). See *Chapter 9*.

References

Arroyo PA, Perez RU, Feijoo MAF, Hernandez MAC. Good clinical and cost outcomes using dexrazoxane to treat accidental epirubicin extravasation. *J Cancer Res Ther* 2010; 6: 573–574.

American Society of Hospital Pharmacists. Dexrazoxane Totect shortage. Available at http://www.ashp.org/menu/DrugShortages/CurrentShortages/bulletin.aspx?id=415. Accessed May 26, 2016.

BTG International Inc. Voraxaze (glucarpidase) [package insert]. West Conshohocken, PA. August 2018.

Conde-Estevez D, Saumell S, Salar A, Mateu-de Antonio J. Successful dexrazoxane treatment of a potentially severe extravasation of concentrated doxorubicin. *Anti-Cancer Drugs* 2010; 21: 790–794.

Hershman DL, Lacchetti C, Dworkin RH, et al. Prevention and management of chemotherapy-induced peripheral neuropathy in survivors of adult cancers: American Society of Clinical Oncology clinical practice guideline. *J Clin Oncol* 2014; 32: 1941–1967.

Mylan Institutional LLC. Dexrazoxane [package insert]. Rockford, IL. May 2015.

National Comprehensive Cancer Network. NCCN Guidelines Version 2.2016 colon cancer. Available at https://www.nccn.org/professionals/physician_gls/pdf/colon.pdf. Accessed May 26, 2016.

Olsen MM, LeFebrve KB, Brassil KJ. *Chemotherapy and immunotherapy guidelines and recommendations for practice.* Pittsburgh, PA: Oncology Nursing Society Publications, 2019.

Pharmacia and Upjohn. Zinecard (dexrazoxane) [package insert]. New York, NY. April 2014.

Smith EM, Pang H, Cirrincione C, et al. Effect of duloxetine on pain, function, and quality of life among patients with chemotherapy-induced painful peripheral neuropathy. *JAMA* 2013; 309(13): 1359–1367.

Spectrum Pharmaceuticals Inc. Khapzory (levoleucovorin) [package insert]. Irvine, CA. October 2018.

Sun Pharma Global FZE. Amifostine [package insert]. Cranbury, NJ. August 2014.

Totect Website. Totect is currently not available. Available at http://totect.com/. Accessed May 26, 2016.

Wellstat Therapeutics. Vistogard (uridine triacetate) [package insert]. West Gaithersburg, MD. December, 2015.

Wilkes GM. Peripheral Neuropathy. In Yarbro CH, Wujuk D, and Gobel BH (eds). *Cancer Symptom Management,* 4th ed. Burlington, MA: Jones & Bartlett Learning, 2014; 457–493.

Drug: allopurinol sodium (Aloprim, Zyloprim, Zurinol)

Class: Xanthine oxide se inhibitor.

Mechanism of Action: Drug inhibits xanthine oxidase, the enzyme necessary for conversion of hypoxanthine (natural purine base) to xanthine, and then xanthine to uric acid, without affecting biosynthesis of purines. This lowers serum and urinary uric acid levels.

Metabolism: Well absorbed orally and IV with comparable oxypurinol (major pharmacologic component) serum levels with the relative bioavailability of oxypurinol 100%. Time to peak serum concentration is 30–120 minutes, with half-life of allopurinol 1–3 hours and oxypurinol 18–30 hours. Drug metabolized in liver to active metabolite oxypurinol, and excreted by kidneys and enterohepatic circulation.

Indication: For the management of patients with (1) signs and symptoms of primary or secondary gout (acute attacks, tophi, joint destruction, uric acid lithiasis, and/or nephropathy); (2) leukemia, lymphoma, and malignancies who are receiving cancer chemotherapy, which causes elevations of serum and urinary uric acid levels; drug should be stopped when potential for uric acid overproduction is no longer present; and (3) recurrent calcium oxalate calculi whose daily uric acid excretion > 800 mg/day in male patients and > 750 mg/day in female patients; therapy should be assessed initially and reassessed periodically to determine that treatment continues to be beneficial and that benefits outweigh the risks.

Dosage/Range:
- Gout: 200–300 mg/day (mild) or 400–600 mg/day (moderately severe) in a single or divided doses; maximum dose, 800 mg.
- Prevention of uric acid nephropathy in cancer treatment.
  - Oral: 600–800 mg/day for 2–3 days with hydration (dose-reduce if creatinine clearance is < 60 mg/mL).
  - IV: in management of patients with leukemia, lymphoma, and solid tumors receiving cancer therapy expected to cause elevated serum and urinary uric acid levels and who cannot tolerate oral therapy.
  - Adults: 200–400 mg/m^2/day, maximum 600 mg/day as a single dose or in divided doses every 6, 8, or 12 hours; optimally begin allopurinol 24–48 hours prior to chemotherapy.

• Dose-reduce for renal dysfunction based on creatinine clearance (10–20 mL/ min = 200 mg/day; 3–10 mL/min = 100 mg/day).

Drug Preparation:
• Oral: available in 100- and 300-mg tablets.
• IV: available as 30-mL vial containing 500 mg allopurinol lyophilized powder, which is stable at room temperature (25°C, 77°F).
• Reconstitute by adding 25 mL sterile water for injection.
• The ordered dose should be withdrawn, and further diluted in 0.9% NS injection or 5% dextrose for injection to achieve a final concentration of no > 6 mg/mL.
• Store at 20–25°C (68–77°F) for up to 10 hours after reconstitution.
• Do not refrigerate reconstituted or diluted product.

Drug Administration:
• Oral: give with food or immediately after meals to decrease gastric irritation.
• IV: administer over appropriate period of time given volume of diluted drug.

Drug Interactions:
• Dicoumarol: PT may be prolonged due to prolonged half-life; monitor PT closely and adjust dose as needed.
• Mercaptopurine/azathioprine: allopurinol decreased drug metabolism, so dose of mercaptopurine or azathioprine must be reduced to 1/3 or 1/4 the usual dose, and then subsequent dose adjusted based on clinical response.
• Uricosuric agents: decrease the inhibition of xanthine oxidase by oxypurinol and increase the urinary excretion of uric acid. Avoid concomitant use.
• Ampicillin/amoxicillin: increased frequency of skin rash; use together cautiously.
• Chlorpropamide: allopurinol may prolong half-life of drug, as both drugs compete for excretion in renal tubule; monitor closely for hypoglycemia if drugs used concomitantly in a patient with renal dysfunction.
• Cyclosporin: cyclosporine levels may be increased, so drug levels should be monitored closely, and dose of cyclosporine adjusted accordingly.
• Theophylline: prolonged half-life when used together; monitor theophylline levels closely and adjust dose accordingly.

Physical incompatibilities with IV allopurinol:
• Amikacin sulfate, amphotericin B, carmustine, cefotaxime sodium, chlorpromazine HCl, cimetidine HCl, clindamycin phosphate, cytarabine, dacarbazine, daunorubicin HCl, diphenhydramine HCl, doxorubicin HCl, doxycycline hyclate, droperidol, floxuridine, gentamicin sulfate, haloperidol lactate, hydroxyzine HCl, idarubicin HCl, imipenem– cilastatin sodium, mechlorethamine HCl, meperidine HCl, metoclopramide HCl, methylprednisolone sodium succinate, minocycline HCl, nalbuphine HCl, netilmicin sulfate, ondansetron HCl, prochlorperazine edisylate, promethazine HCl, sodium bicarbonate, streptozocin, tobramycin sulfate, vinorelbine tartrate.

Lab Effects/Interference:
• Increased alk phos, AST, ALT, bili.

Special Considerations:
- Dose reduction necessary in renal dysfunction.
- Contraindicated in patients hypersensitive to drug (even mild allergic reaction).
- Use cautiously with patients on diuretics, as may decrease renal function and increase serum levels of allopurinol.
- Allopurinol hypersensitivity syndrome may occur rarely and is characterized by fever, chills, leukopenia or leukocytosis, eosinophilia, arthralgias, rash, pruritus, nausea, vomiting, renal and hepatic compromise.
- Drug MUST be discontinued immediately if rash develops; stop drug at first sign of rash.
- To prevent tumor lysis syndrome, patient should receive aggressive IV hydration with or without urine alkalinization, together with allopurinol.

Potential Toxicities/Side Effects and the Nursing Process

I. POTENTIAL SENSORY/PERCEPTUAL ALTERATIONS related to CNS EFFECTS

Defining Characteristics: Drowsiness, chills, and fever have been reported in > 10% of patients. Headaches and somnolence occur in 1–10% of patients. Rarely, seizure, myoclonus, twitching, agitation, mental status changes, cerebral infarction, coma, paralysis, and tremor can occur. If fever and chills are associated with rash, eosinophilia, nausea, and vomiting, they are most likely related to rare allopurinol hypersensitivity reaction.

Nursing Implications: Assess baseline neurologic status, including mental status, and periodically during treatment. If any abnormalities, discuss with physician right away. Teach patient to report chills, fever, drowsiness, or any changes, if they occur. If they do occur, teach patient self-management strategies and to report whether they are ineffective. If so, discuss management strategies with physician. If fever and chills are associated with rash, eosinophilia, nausea, vomiting, they are most likely related to rare allopurinol hypersensitivity reaction and should be discussed with the physician immediately drug should be discontinued.

II. ALTERATION IN SKIN INTEGRITY, POTENTIAL, related to RASH, STEVENS–JOHNSON SYNDROME

Defining Characteristics: More than 10% of patients develop maculopapular rash, often associated with urticaria and pruritus; may be exfoliative. Less common but more severe, 1–10% of patients develop Stevens–Johnson syndrome or toxic epidermal necrolysis, which may be fatal. For IV administration, local injection-site reactions may occur. Alopecia has been reported in 1–10% of patients.

Nursing Implications: Assess baseline skin integrity and intactness of scalp hair. Teach patient that rash may occur, and to report it right away, as drug must be discontinued. Teach patient self-care strategies, including skin cream to moisturize the skin and to prevent itching. Discuss drug discontinuance and management with physician. Teach patient to report any hair loss. If it occurs, discuss impact on patient, self-care strategies, and if severe, discuss drug discontinuance with physician.

Drug: amifostine for injection (Ethyol, WR-2721)

Class: Cytoprotectant; free-radical scavenger, metabolized to a free thiol.

Mechanism of Action: Drug is phosphorylated by alkaline phosphatase bound in tissue membranes, producing free thiol. Inside the cell, free thiol binds to and detoxifies reactive metabolites of cisplatin and other chemotherapeutic agents, thus neutralizing the chemotherapy drug in normal tissues so that cellular DNA and RNA are not damaged. Normal cells are protected because of differences in cell physiology (higher alkaline phosphatase concentrations and tissue pH, as well as more effective vascularity in normal cells as compared to malignant cells) and transport mechanisms that promote the preferential uptake of free thiol into normal tissues. Free thiol may also scavenge reactive free-radical reactive oxygen molecules resulting from chemotherapy or RT. Free thiol may also upregulate p53 expression, so that cells accumulate in the G_1–S cell cycle phase, enabling DNA repair.

Metabolism: Drug is rapidly metabolized to an active free-thiol metabolite and cleared from the plasma, so the drug should be administered 30 minutes prior to drug dose.

Indication: To reduce the (1) cumulative renal toxicity associated with repeated administration of cisplatin in patients with advanced ovarian cancer, (2) incidence of moderate-to-severe xerostomia in patients undergoing postoperative RT for head and neck cancer, where the radiation port includes a substantial portion of the parotid glands.

Dosage/Range:
- Chemoprotectant: 910 mg/m² in 50 mL 0.9% NS administered IV over 15 minutes, 30 minutes prior to beginning chemotherapy.
- Radioprotectant: 200 mg/m²/day IVP over 3 minutes, 15 minutes prior to standard fraction radiation therapy (1.8–2.0 Gy).

Drug Preparation:
- Available in 10-mL vials containing 500 mg of drug; store at room temperature.
- Use only 0.9% sodium chloride.
- Reconstitute vial with 9.7 mL of sterile 0.9% sodium chloride, giving a concentration of 500 mg amifostine/mL. Reconstituted solution is stable for up to 5 hours at room temperature.
- Further dilute with sterile 0.9% sodium chloride to total 50 mL.
- Stable at 5–40 mg/mL for 5 hours at room temperature, and for 24 hours if refrigerated (2–8°C).

Drug Administration:
- Hypertension medicines should be stopped 24 hours prior to drug administration.

- Ensure that patient has been adequately hydrated prior to drug administration, and keep patient in supine position. Monitor BP every 5 minutes during infusion and then as clinically indicated.
  - Administer combination antiemetics:
    - Administer IV antiemetic medication 1 hour prior, and oral antiemetic 2 hours prior to amifostine administration.
  - Generally, patients should be hydrated with 1 L 0.9% NS prior to amifostine when used as a chemoprotectant.
  - Infuse amifostine IV over 15 minutes, beginning 30 minutes prior to chemotherapy or IVP 15–30 minutes prior to RT.
  - Monitor BP baseline, during the infusion, and immediately after amifostine infusion and as needed until BP returns to baseline.
  - Interrupt amifostine if systolic BP decreases significantly compared with baseline (20 mmHg if baseline <100 mmHg; 25 mmHg if baseline 100–119 mmHg; 30 mmHg if baseline 120–139 mmHg; 40 mmHg if baseline 140–179 mmHg; ≥180 baseline, if SBP falls 50 mmHg) (Sun Pharma, 2014).
  - Resume diuretic(s) and/or antihypertensive medications 30 minutes after amifostine infusion is complete as long as patient is normotensive.

Drug Interactions:
- Antihypertensive and diuretic medications may potentiate hypotension.

Lab Effects/Interference:
- May cause hypocalcemia.

Special Considerations:
- Patients unable to tolerate cessation of antihypertensive medications are not candidates for the drug.
- Studies have shown no decrease in cisplatin drug efficacy when given with first-line therapy in ovarian cancer, and no other studies have been conducted as to tumor protection by drug.
- Effectiveness of RT has not been studied when using the drug, and it should not be used in patients receiving definitive RT, except in the context of a clinical trial.
- Offers significant protection of kidneys.
- Offers protection of BM and nerves.
- Drug has been shown to protect skin, mucous membranes, and bladder and pelvic structures against late moderate-to-severe radiation reactions.

Potential Toxicities/Side Effects and the Nursing Process

I.   ALTERATION IN NUTRITION, LESS THAN BODY REQUIREMENTS, related to NAUSEA AND VOMITING, HYPOCALCEMIA

Defining Characteristics: Incidence is frequent, and nausea and vomiting may be severe. These are preventable by using serotonin antagonist and dexamethasone. Hypocalcemia noted in trials using higher doses.

Nursing Implications: Administer serotonin antagonist (e.g., granisetron, ondansetron, or dolasetron) and dexamethasone 20 mg IV prior to amifostine. Encourage small, frequent meals of cool, bland foods, and liquids. Teach patient self-management tips and to avoid greasy or heavy foods. Instruct patient to report nausea and/or vomiting that is not resolved by antiemetics. Teach patient to maintain oral hydration as tolerated. Identify patients at risk for hypocalcemia, i.e., nephrotic syndrome and depletion from many courses of cisplatin. Check baseline calcium and albumin, and monitor during therapy. Assess for signs/symptoms of hypocalcemia. Patients may receive calcium supplements as needed.

II.   ALTERATION IN OXYGENATION related to HYPOTENSION, POTENTIAL

Defining Characteristics: Drug causes transient, reversible hypotension in 62% of patients at a dose of 910 mg/m^2. Hypotension is usually manifested by a 5- to 15-minute transient decrease in systolic BP of $\leq$ 20 mmHg. Incidence is less when dose is 740 mg/m^2, and infused over 5 minutes.

Nursing Implications: Assess patient's medication profile. Antihypertensives should be stopped 24 hours prior to drug administration. Assess baseline BP, heart rate, and hydration status. Ensure that patient is well hydrated, and per physician, administer 1 L of 0.9% NS IV prior to amifostine if needed to assure euhydration; if dehydrated, patient may require 2 L. Place patient in supine position during administration of drug, and monitor BP q 5 minutes during administration, immediately after administration, and as needed postinfusion. If the BP falls below threshold (see following table), interrupt infusion and give an IVB of 0.9% NS per physician order. If BP comes back above threshold (returns to threshold within minutes and patient is asymptomatic), then resume infusion and give full dose. If BP does not return to threshold within 5 minutes, infusion should be terminated and IV hydration fluids administered per physician, and patient placed in Trendelenburg position, if symptomatic. If BP does not return to normal in 5 minutes, dose should be reduced in next cycle. Manufacturer recommends the following thresholds for supine BP:

Systolic BP (SBP)	Threshold SBP in mmHg
< 100	< 80
100–119	75–94
120–139	90–109
140–179	100–139
$\leq$ 180	$\leq$ 130

III.   ALTERATION IN COMFORT related to FLUSHING CHILLS, DIZZINESS, SOMNOLENCE, HICCUPS, AND SNEEZING

Defining Characteristics: These effects may occur during or after drug infusion and are mild. Allergic reactions are rare, ranging from skin rash to rigors, but anaphylaxis has not been reported.

Nursing Implications: Assess comfort level, and ask patient to report these symptoms. Discuss comfort measures with patient.

Drug: dexrazoxane for injection (Totect)

Class: Anthracycline extravasation neutralizer.

Mechanism of Action: Drug is a derivative of edetic acid (EDTA) and is a metal ion chelator that protects against free-radical tissue damage from extravasated anthracycline chemotherapy. It appears that by binding iron it is unavailable for oxygen; most likely it is due to the drug's activity as a free radical scavenger. Theoretically, it may antagonize the chemotherapeutic effect of previously administered drug.

Metabolism: Biphasic elimination with mean initial elimination half-life of 30 minutes and a mean terminal half-life of 2.8 hours; 42% of the dose is excreted in the urine. No plasma protein binding of drug. Dose-reduce in patients with renal dysfunction.

Indication: Drug is indicated for the treatment of adults who have an anthracycline extravasation (e.g., doxorubicin, daunorubicin, epirubicin, idarubicin).

Dosage/Range:
- Given IV infusion for 3 consecutive days, beginning as soon as possible after anthracycline extravasation but within 6 hours of the extravasation.
- Days 1 and 2: 1,000 mg/m^2 IV infusion (max 2,000 mg).
- Day 3: 500 mg/m^2 IV infusion (max 1,000 mg).
- Dose-reduce by 50% in patients with creatinine clearances < 40 mL/min.

Drug Preparation:
- Available as a Totect kit with ten 500-mg vials of dexrazoxane HCl.
- Reconstitute drug with provided diluent (50-mL vials), forming a solution of drug 10 mg/mL. Use immediately. Note: dexrazoxane and Totect use sodium lactate diluent, while Zinecard uses sterile water for injection and has no preservatives.
- Stable 4 hours after reconstitution refrigerated.
- Store unopened vials of drug powder and diluent at room temperature and protected from light and heat.
- USE SAFE CHEMOTHERAPEUTIC AGENT HANDLING PRECAUTIONS!
- Totect (dexrazoxane) is the only FDA-approved antidote for anthracycline administration, but studies have shown that dexrazoxane is effective (Mouridsen et al., 2007). Generic dexrazoxane (Bedford Labs) and Totect are reconstituted with sodium lactate, but Zinecard (dexrazoxane) must be reconstituted with sterile water.

Drug Administration:
- Give as soon as possible following anthracycline extravasation but within 6 hours of the extravasation. Give at approximately the same time each day (e.g., 24 hours apart).
- Administer IV infusion over 1–2 hours in an area or extremity other than that with the extravasation.

- DO NOT use with other extravasation management strategies (e.g., topical dimethyl sulfoxide application), as this may worsen tissue injury.
- Remove topical cooling applications at least 15 minutes before and during drug administration.
- USE CHEMOTHERAPY personal protective equipment when preparing and administering drug.

Drug Interactions:
- None known.

Lab Effects/Interference:
- Neutropenia and thrombocytopenia.
- Increased liver function tests (LFTs).

Special Considerations:
- In two prospective European studies, dexrazoxane proved to be effective and well tolerated and prevented the need for surgical resection in 53 of 54 patients.
- DRUG REQUIRES SAFE CHEMOTHERAPEUTIC AGENT HANDLING PRECAUTIONS! Also, patient side effects include BM suppression, nausea, and vomiting, and drug is embryo-fetal toxic.
- Most common side effects are neutropenia, thrombocytopenia, fever, infusion-site reactions, nausea, and vomiting.

Potential Toxicities/Side Effects and the Nursing Process

I.   POTENTIAL FOR INJURY related to BONE MARROW DEPRESSION

Defining Characteristics: Drug may cause neutropenia and thrombocytopenia.

Nursing Implications: Monitor WBC, HCT/Hgb, and platelets baseline and monitor after injections. Instruct patient in self-assessment for signs/symptoms of infection and bleeding and how to report them. Teach patient self-care measures to minimize risk.

II.   POTENTIAL ALTERATION IN METABOLISM related to HEPATIC AND RENAL ALTERATIONS

Defining Characteristics: Possible elevations in liver function studies are reversible.

Nursing Implications: Assess hepatic and renal function tests (bili, BUN, creatinine, and alk phos), baseline and before each treatment. Notify physician of any abnormalities. Dose should be reduced 50% if 24-hour creatinine clearance is < 40 mL/min.

III.   ALTERATION IN COMFORT related to PAIN AT INJECTION SITE, FEVER

Defining Characteristics: Pain at the injection site may occur, as may fever.

Nursing Implications: Assess site during and after infusion. Instruct patient to notify nurse if discomfort arises. Apply local measures to reduce discomfort. Teach patient that fever may occur, to check temperature, and if necessary to take acetaminophen and report if the fever does not resolve.

IV. ALTERATION IN NUTRITION, LESS THAN BODY REQUIREMENTS, related to NAUSEA/VOMITING

Defining Characteristics: Nausea and vomiting may occur. Drug is an antineoplastic agent.

Nursing Implications: Assess baseline nutritional status. Premedicate before initial treatment and then give as needed for days 2 and 3. Encourage small, frequent meals and liquids. Teach patient to avoid greasy, fried, or fatty foods. Encourage patient to report onset of nausea/vomiting.

Drug: dexrazoxane for injection (Zinecard)

Class: Cardioprotector.

Mechanism of Action: Enters easily through cell membranes, but the exact mechanism of cardiac cell protection is unclear. A possible mechanism is that the drug becomes a chelating agent within the cell and interferes with iron-mediated free-radical formation that otherwise would cause cardiotoxicity from anthracyclines. Drug is a derivative of EDTA.

Metabolism: 42% of the dose is excreted in the urine. No plasma protein binding of drug.

Indication: Cytoprotective agent indicated for reducing the incidence and severity of cardiomyopathy associated with doxorubicin administration in women with metastatic breast cancer who have received a cumulative doxorubicin dose of 300 mg/m^2 and who will continue to receive doxorubicin therapy to maintain tumor control. Do not use Zinecard with doxorubicin initiation. Do not use Zinecard with nonanthracycline-containing chemotherapy regimens.

Dosage/Range:
* 10:1 ratio of dexrazoxane to doxorubicin (i.e., 500 mg/m^2 of dexrazoxane to 50 mg/m^2 of doxorubicin).
* Renal Impairment: Dose-reduce by 50% for patients with CrCl < 40 mL/min.
* Hepatic Impairment: Since a doxorubicin dose reduction is recommended in presence of hyperbilirubinemia, reduce Zinecard dose proportionately (maintain the 10:1 ratio).

Drug Preparation:
* Available in 250- or 500-mg lyophilized vials.
* Reconstitute 250-mg drug with 25 mL sterile water for injection, USP; and 500-mg vial with 50 mL sterile water for injection, USP (resulting solution will contain 10 mg/mL). Following reconstitution with sterile water for injection USP, drug in vial is stable for 30 minutes at room temperature and up to 3 hours when refrigerated 2–8°C (36–46°F). pH of diluted drug is 1.0–3.0. Discard any unused solution.

- Further dilute in Lactated Ringer's Injection USP to a concentration of 1.3–3.0 mg/mL in IV infusion bags.
- The diluted infusion solution is stable for 60 minutes at room temperature or up to 4 hours when refrigerated 2–8°C (36–46°F). pH of diluted infusion solution is 3.5–5.5.
- USE SAFE CHEMOTHERAPEUTIC AGENT HANDLING PRECAUTIONS!

Drug Administration:
- Inspect solution for particulate matter and discoloration, and if precipitate for cloudiness seen, do not use.
- Give IV infusion over 15 minutes (NOT IVP); administer doxorubicin within 30 minutes after the completion of Zinecard infusion.

Drug Interactions:
- None known.

Lab Effects/Interference:
- May increase myelosuppression of concomitant doxorubicin, with leukopenia, neutropenia, and thrombocytopenia.

Special Considerations:
- DO NOT USE Zinecard with initiation of chemotherapy, as drug may interfere with tumor response. Drug may reduce the response from 5-FU, doxorubicin, and cyclophosphamide (FAC) chemotherapy when given concurrently on the first cycle of therapy (48% response rate vs. 63% without the drug, and shorter time to disease progression) (Pharmacia and Upjohn, 2014).
- Zinecard does not completely eliminate the risk of anthracycline-induced cardiac toxicity. Monitor cardiac function baseline and periodically during anthracycline therapy to assess LVEF. If LVEF decreases, continued therapy should be carefully considered against risk of producing irreversible cardiac damage.
- Drug may increase the myelosuppression effects of chemotherapy.
- Secondary malignancies (e.g., AML and MDS) have been reported in studies of pediatric patients who have received Zinecard in combination with chemotherapy. Zinecard is not indicated for use in pediatric patients. Some adults have also developed AML or MDS when receiving Zinecard in combination with anti-cancer agents known to be carcinogenic.
- Drug can cause embryo-fetal toxicity as well as maternal toxicity if used during pregnancy. Teach female patients of reproductive potential to use highly effective contraception to avoid pregnancy.
- DRUG REQUIRES SAFE CHEMOTHERAPEUTIC AGENT HANDLING PRECAUTIONS!

Potential Toxicities/Side Effects and the Nursing Process

I.   POTENTIAL FOR INJURY related to ENHANCED BONE MARROW DEPRESSION

Defining Characteristics: Drug may increase doxorubicin-induced BM depression.

Nursing Implications: Monitor WBC, HCT/Hgb, and platelets baseline and prior to each dose. Instruct patient in self-assessment for signs/symptoms of infection and bleeding, and how to report them. Teach patient self-care measures to minimize risk.

II.   POTENTIAL ALTERATION IN METABOLISM related to HEPATIC AND RENAL ALTERATIONS

Defining Characteristics: Possible elevations in liver and renal function studies may occur. Incidence did not differ from patients who received same chemotherapy (FAC) without the protector.

Nursing Implications: Assess hepatic and renal function tests (bili, BUN, creatinine, and alk phos), baseline and prior to each treatment. Notify physician of any abnormalities.

III.   ALTERATION IN COMFORT related to PAIN AT INJECTION SITE

Defining Characteristics: Pain at the injection site may occur.

Nursing Implications: Assess site during and after infusion. Instruct patient to notify nurse if discomfort arises. Apply local measures to reduce discomfort.

Drug: glucarpidase (Voraxaze)

Class: Carboxypeptidase; recombinant bacterial enzyme that hydrolyzes the carboxyl-terminal glutamate residue from folic acid and classical antifolates such as methotrexate (MTX).

Mechanism of Action: Converts MTX to its inactive metabolites (4-deoxy-4-amino-N^{10} – methylpteroic acid (DAMPA) and glutamate. This is an alternate nonrenal pathway for eliminated excess MTX in patients with renal dysfunction during high-dose MTX treatment.

Metabolism: Glucarpidase is produced by recombinant DNA technology in genetically modified *Escherichia coli*. Plasma MTX levels in study 1 was reduced by $>/= 97\%$ and was maintained at a $>95\%$ reduction for up to 8 days. MTX concentrations within 48 hours after glucarpidase administration should be measured by a chromatographic method. Mean elimination half-life ($t_{1/2}$) is 5.6 hours.

Indication: Treatment of toxic plasma MTX concentrations (>1 micromole per liter) in patients with delayed MTX clearance due to impaired renal function.

NOT indicated in patients who have the expected MTX clearance (plasma MTX concentrations within 2 standard deviations of the mean MTX excretion curve specific for the dose of MTX administered) or those with normal or mildly impaired renal function because of the potential risk of subtherapeutic exposure to MTX.

Contraindication: None.

Dose/Range:
- Single IV injection of 50 units/kg.
- No dose adjustment recommended for renal impairment. No studies of patients with hepatic impairment have been conducted.

Drug Preparation:
- Available as lyophilized powder 1,000 units/vial.
- Reconstitute contents of the vial with 1 mL of sterile saline for injection USP.
- Roll and tilt the vial gently to mix. Do not shake.
- Inspect the vial as it should be colorless, clear, and free of particulate matter; if cloudy or with particulate matter, do not use.
- Use reconstituted glucarpidase immediately or store under refrigeration at 36–46°F (2–8°C) for up to 4 hours if not used immediately. Glucarpidase does not contain preservatives. Discard any remaining unused product as it is a single-use vial.

Drug Administration:
- Single IV bolus injection of 50 units/kg over 5 minutes. Flush IV line before and after administration of glucarpidase. Monitor patient closely for allergic reaction, including anaphylaxis.
- Do not administer leucovorin within 2 hours before or after a dose of glucarpidase.
- Continue therapy with leucovorin until the MTX concentration has been maintained below the leucovorin treatment threshold for a minimum of 3 days.
- Measurement of MTX level using immunoassays is unreliable for samples collected within 48 hours after glucarpidase administration. Use chromatographic method as DAMPA interferes with the immunoassay (BTG, 2016).
- Determine the leucovorin dose 48 hours after gluarpidase injection based on the patient's pre-glucarpidase concentration.
- Continue hydration and alkalinization of the urine as ordered.

Drug Interactions:
- Leucovorin is a substrate for glucarpidase. Do not administer leucovorin within 2 hours before or after a dose of glucarpidase (reduces leucovorin AUC by 33% and Cmax by 52%).
- Do not administer other potential exogenous substrates including reduced folates and folate antimetabolites.

Lab Effects/Interference: Reduces serum MTX level by inactivating the drug.

Special Considerations:
- Most common adverse events >1% were paresthesia, flushing, nausea and vomiting, hypotension, and headache.
- No studies have been done in humans and animals about reproductive risk. Use only in pregnancy if clearly needed.
- Warnings and Precautions:
  - Serious allergic reactions, including anaphylaxis, may occur.

TREATMENT

- Measurement of MTX level within 48 hours of glucarpidase should be performed using chromatography; using immunoassays is unreliable for samples collected within 48 hours as DAMPA interferes with the immunoassay (BTG, 2016).
- Continue leucovorin therapy until the MTX concentration has been maintained < leucovorin treatment threshold for a minimum of 3 days.
- Do not administer leucovorin within 2 hours before or after the glucarpidase dose.
- Following glucarpidase dose, for 48 hours determine the leucovorin dose based on the patient's pre-glucarpidase MTX concentration.
- Continue hydration and alkalination of the urine.
- All therapeutic proteins have a risk of immunogenicity and the formation of anti-glucarpidase antibodies which may neutralize the effect of the drug.

Potential Toxicities/Side Effects and the Nursing Process

I. POTENTIAL FOR INJURY related to ALLERGIC REACTION WITH DRUG ADMINISTRATION.

Defining Characteristics: Severe allergic reactions may occur, including anaphylaxis. Incidence of hypersensitivity was <1%, rash <1%, throat irritation or tightness <1%, and flushing was 2%.

Nursing Implications: Monitor patient closely during drug injection and afterwards for signs/symptoms of HSR. Teach patient to report any changes immediately. While reaction is unlikely, have emergency medications and personnel nearby during drug administration.

Drug: leucovorin calcium (folinic acid, Citrovorum Factor)

Class: Water-soluble vitamin in the folate group (folinic acid).

Mechanism of Action: Potentiates antitumor activity of 5-FU when given prior to or concurrently with 5-FU, ± XRT. Acts as an antidote for methotrexate (MTX) and other folic acid antagonists. Circumvents the biochemical block of the enzyme inhibitors (e.g., dihydrofolate reductase [DHFR]) to permit DNA and RNA synthesis.

Metabolism: Leucovorin is metabolized to polyglutamates that are more effective in potentiating 5-FU tumor cell kill. Metabolized primarily in the liver, 50% of the single dose is excreted in 6 hours in the urine (80–90%) and stool (8% of the dose).

Indication: (1) After high-dose MTX therapy in osteosarcoma to rescue normal cells; (2) to diminish the toxicity and counteract the effects of impaired MTX elimination and of inadvertent over-dosages of folic acid antagonists; (3) treatment of megaloblastic anemias due to folic acid deficiency when oral therapy is not feasible; (4) in combination with 5-fluorouracil (5-FU) to prolong survival in the palliative treatment of patients with advanced CRC. Drug should not be mixed in the same infusion as 5-FU, as a precipitate will form.

Contraindication: Patients with pernicious anemia and other megaloblastic anemias secondary to the lack of vitamin B_{12}.

Dosage/Range:
Advanced CRC: Either of the following regimens:
- Leucovorin 200 mg/m^2 by slow IV injection over a minimum of 3 minutes followed by 5-FU at 370 mg/m^2 IV repeated daily $\times$ 5 days, and cycle repeated every 28 days; dose-reduce 5-FU for hematologic or GI toxicity.
- Leucovorin 20 mg/m^2 IV followed by 5-FU 425 mg/m^2 repeated daily $\times$ 5 days, and cycle repeated every 28 days; dose-reduce 5-FU for hematologic or GI toxicity.
- Commonly used in FOLFOX or FOLFIRI regimens:
  - FOLFOX4 every 2 weeks:
    - Day 1: Oxaliplatin 85 mg/m^2 IV infusion in 250–500 mL D_5W and leucovorin 200 mg/m^2 IV infusion in D_5W, each over 2 hours simultaneously in separate bags using a Y-line, followed by 5-FU 400 mg/m^2 IVB over 2–4 minutes, followed by 5-FU 600 mg/m^2 in 500 mL D_5W as a 22-hour continuous infusion (CI).
    - Day 2: Leucovorin 200 mg/m^2 IV infusion over 2 hours, followed by 5-FU 400 mg/m^2 IVB over 2–4 minutes, followed by 5-FU 600 mg/m^2 in 500 mL D_5W as a 22-hour CI.
  - FOLFIRI: FOLFIRI day 1: Irinotecan 180 mg/m^2 IV over 90 minutes, at the same time as leucovorin 200 mg/m^2 IV over 2 hours through separate arms of a Y-tubing, followed by 5-FU 400 mg/m^2 IVB and then 23-hour 5-FU 1200 mg/m^2 IV CI, days 1 and 2. Total 5-FU CI dose is 2400 mg/m^2 over 46–48 hours. Repeat q 2 weeks.
  - FOLFIRI: Repeat q 2 weeks.
    - Day 1: Irinotecan 180 mg/m^2 IV over 90 minutes, at the same time as leucovorin 200 mg/m^2 IV over 2 hours through separate arms of a Y-tubing, followed by 5-FU 400 mg/m^2 IVB and then 5-FU 2400 mg/m^2 IV CI over 46–48 hours.

Leucovorin rescue after high-dose MTX therapy (12–15 g/m^2):
- DO NOT ADMINISTER LEUCOVORIN INTRATHECALLY.
- Serum creatinine and MTX levels should be determined at least once daily. Continue leucovorin administration, hydration, and urinary alkalinization (to keep urine pH of 7.0 or greater) until the MTX level is $< 5 \times 10^{-8}$ M (0.05 micromolar).
- Guidelines for leucovorin dosage and administration: Dose of drug and duration of rescue dependent on serum MTX levels.
  - *Normal MTX elimination:* Lab: serum MTX level approximately 10 micromolar at 24 hours after administration, 1 micromolar at 48 hours, and < 0.2 micromolar at 72 hours; leucovorin 10 mg/m^2 IV, PO, or IM every 6 hours $\times$ 10 doses, starting EXACTLY 24 hours after beginning of MTX infusion.
  - *Delayed late MTX elimination:* Lab: serum MTX level > 0.2 micromolar at 72 hours, and > 0.05 micromolar at 96 hours after administration; continue leucovorin 10 mg/m^2 IV, PO, or IM every 6 hours $\times$ 10 doses, until MTX level < 0.05 micromolar.
  - *Delayed early MTX elimination and/or evidence of acute renal injury:* Lab: serum MTX level of 50 micromolar or more at 24 hours, or 5 micromolar more at 48 hours after administration, OR a 100% or greater increase in serum creatinine level at 24 hours after MTX administration (e.g., an increase from 0.5 mg/mL to a level of

1 mg/dL or more); leucovorin 150 mg IV every 3 hours, until MTX level is < 1 micromolar; then 15 mg IV every 3 hours until MTX level < 0.05 micromolar. These patients likely will develop reversible renal failure and need to have continuing hydration, urinary alkalinization, close monitoring of fluid and electrolyte status, until serum MTX level is acceptable and renal failure has resolved.

Drug Preparation:
• Drug is supplied in ampules or vials.
• Reconstitute vials with sterile water for injection.
• Dilute reconstituted vials or ampules further with 5% dextrose or 0.9% sodium chloride.

Drug Administration:
• With 5-FU, in a variety of combinations: e.g., leucovorin 500 mg/m²/week for 6 weeks as a 2-hour infusion; 5-FU: 500–600 mg/m²/week for 6 weeks IVB midway through leucovorin infusion, then 2-week rest, then repeat 6-week cycle.
• High-dose MTX: Administered starting EXACTLY 24 hours after the first MTX dose is given. Dose every 6 hours for up to 10 doses; then continue per table below if MTX level unacceptable.
• First dose is given IV; others can be given IM or PO when given as MTX rescue and able to keep oral liquids down, unless otherwise indicated in table below.
• IV doses are given as boluses over 15 minutes unless otherwise specified.
• When given as a rescue dose, leucovorin must be given exactly on time in order to rescue normal cells from severe MTX toxicity.

Drug Interactions:
• 5-FU potentiation.
• Folic acid: provides folinic acid so cells can make DNA (antagonizes drug effect).
• Phenobarbital, phenytoin, primidone: decreased anticonvulsant action when leucovorin given in high doses; monitor patient closely and increase anticonvulsant dose as needed.

Lab Effects/Interference:
• None.

Special Considerations:
• It is imperative that the patient receive leucovorin on schedule to avoid fatal MTX toxicity (when given as rescue). Notify the physician if the patient is unable to take the dose orally, as it then must be administered IV.
• Usually free of side effects, but allergic and local pain may occur.

Potential Toxicities/Side Effects and the Nursing Process

I.   POTENTIAL FOR INJURY related to HYPERSENSITIVITY, DRUG INTERACTIONS

Defining Characteristics: Allergic sensitization has been reported: facial flushing, itching. Leucovorin in large amounts may counteract the antiepileptic effects of phenobarbital, phenytoin, and primidone.

Nursing Implications: Monitor patient for signs/symptoms of allergic reaction. Diphen-hydramine is effective for relieving symptoms of allergic reaction. Monitor patient for symptoms of increased seizure activity if taking anticonvulsants; monitor antiepileptic drug levels.

II.   ALTERED NUTRITION, POTENTIAL, LESS THAN BODY REQUIREMENTS, related to NAUSEA, VOMITING

Defining Characteristics: Oral leucovorin rarely causes nausea or vomiting.

Nursing Implications: Administer oral leucovorin with antacids, milk, or juice if needed.

Drug: levoleucovorin (Fusilev, D,L-leucovorin)

Class: Folate analogue.

Mechanism of Action: Drug is the pharmacologically active isomer of 5-formyl tet-rahydrofolic acid that does not require further reduction by the enzyme dihydrofolate reductase in order to use folate. Acts as an antidote for MTX and other folic acid antago-nists. Circumvents the biochemical block of the enzyme inhibitors (e.g., DHFR) to per-mit DNA and RNA synthesis. Potentiates antitumor activity of 5-FU when given before or concurrently.

Metabolism: After an IV dose of 15 mg, peak serum levels were reached in 0.9 hour. Mean terminal half-life was 5–6.8 hours.

Indications: (1) Rescue after high-dose MTX therapy in osteosarcoma; (2) diminishing the toxicity associated with overdosage of folic acid antagonists or impaired methotrexate elimination; (3) treatment of patients with metastatic CRC in combination with fluorouracil.

Drug is NOT indicated for the treatment of pernicious anemia or megaloblastic anemia secondary to lack of vitamin B12 because of the risk of progression of neurologic manifes-tations despite hematologic remission.

Contraindications: (1) patients who have had severe HSRs to leucovorin products, folic acid, or folinic acid; (2) do NOT administer intrathecally.

Dosage/Range:
- Levoleucovorin is dosed at one-half the usual dose of racemic D,L-leucovorin.
- Do NOT administer intrathecally.

Rescue after high-dose methotrexate (MTX) therapy:
- Based on an MTX dose of 12 g/m^2 administered IV infusion over 4 hours: Begin 24 hours after starting the MTX infusion, start levoleucovoring 7.5 mg (5 mg/m^2) IV infusion ev-ery 6 hours × 10 doses starting exactly 24 hours after the beginning of MTX infusion.
- Determine serum creatinine and MTX levels at least once daily.

- Continue levoleucovorin administration, hydration, and urinary alkalinization (pH $\geq$ 7.0) until MTX level $< 5 \times (10)^8$ M (0.05 micromolar).
- The levoleucovorin dose may need to be adjusted.

Clinical Situation	Laboratory Findings	Levoleucovorin Dosage/ Duration
Normal MTX elimination	Serum MTX level 10 micromolar at 24 hr after administration, 1 micromolar at 48 hr, and < 0.2 micromolar at 72 hr	7.5 mg IV q 6 hr for 60 hr (10 doses starting at 24 hr after start of MTX infusion)
Delayed late elimination	Serum MTX level > 0.2 micromolar at 72 hr, and > 0.05 micromolar at 96 hr after administration	Continue 7.5 mg IV q 6 hr until MTX level is < 0.05 micromolar
Delayed early MTX elimination and/or evidence of acute renal injury*	Serum MTX level at ≥ 50 micromolar at 24 hr, or ≥ 5 micromolar at 48 hr after MTX administration, OR $\geq 100\%$ increase in serum creatinine level at 24 hr after MTX administration (e.g., an increase from 0.5 mg/dL to a level of 1 mg/dL or more)	75 mg IV q 3 hr until MTX level is < 1 micromolar; then 7.5 mg IV q 3 hr until MTX level is < 0.05 micromolar

- Patients are likely to develop reversible renal failure so should receive levoleucovorin, continuing hydration and urinary alkalinization, and monitoring of fluid and electrolyte status until the serum MTX level has fallen to <0.05 micromolar and the renal failure has resolved (Spectrum Pharmaceuticals, Inc., 2018).

Impaired MTX Elimination or Renal Impairment:
- If MTX toxicity observed, extend levoleucovorin rescue for an additional 24 hours (total of 14 doses over 84 hours) in subsequent courses.
- Because MTX is sequestered in effusions (third spacing), effusions should be tapped dry prior to MTX administration. If MTX does accumulate in a third space (e.g., ascites, pleural effusion) or because of renal insufficiency or inadequate hydration, which delays MTX elimination, use of higher doses of levoleukovorin or prolonged administration may be needed.

Overdosage of Folic Acid Antagonists or Impaired MTX Elimination:
- Start levoleucovorin in adult and pediatric patients as soon as possible after MTX overdosage or within 24 hours of MTX administration when MTX elimination is impaired.
- As the time interval between MTX administration and levoleucovorin administration increases, levoleucovorin efficacy diminishes. Administer levoleucovorin 7.5 mg (5 mg/m^2) IV q 6 hours until serum MTX level is $< 5 \times 10^{-8}$ M (0.05 micromolar).
- Monitor serum creatinine and MTX levels at least q 24 hr; Increase the dose of levoleucovorin to 50 mg/m^2 IV every 3 hours until the MTX level is $< 10^{-8}$ MIF:
  - Serum creatinine at 24-hrs increases 50% or more compared to baseline;
  - MTX level at 24-hrs is $> 5 \times 10^{-6}$ M;
  - MTX level at 48-hrs is $> 9 \times 10^{-7}$ M

- Continue concomitant hydration (3 L per day) and urinary alkalinization with sodium bicarbonate. Adjust the bicarbonate dose to maintain urine pH at 7 or greater.

Levoleucovorin in combination with 5-FU for mCRC: examples of regimens:
- Levoleucovorin 100 mg/m² by slow IV injection over a minimum of 3 minutes, followed by 5-FU at 370 mg/m² IV, daily × 5 days, repeat cycle every 28 days; dose-reduce 5-FU or delay for hematologic and other toxicity. See 5-FU.
- Levoleucovorin 10 mg/m² by slow IV injection over a minimum of 3 minutes, followed by 5-FU at 425 mg/m² IV, daily × 5 days, repeat cycle every 28 days;
- Dose-reduce 5-FU or delay for hematologic and other toxicity. See 5-FU. Do not dose modify levoleucovorin.
- Commonly used in FOLFOX (together with 5-FU and oxaliplatin) and FOLFIRI (irinotecan and 5-FU); see drug information for oxaliplatin and irinotecan for regimens.

Drug Preparation:
- Reconstitute 175-mg and 300-mg vials with 3.6 mL and 6.2 mL respectively of sterile 0.9% sodium chloride for injection USP, resulting in a 50-mg/mL solution. Visually inspect for particulate matter and discoloration; solution should be clear, colorless to yellowish in color.
- Further dilute to concentration of 0.5–5 mg/mL in 0.9% sodium chloride USP or 5% dextrose injection USP (stable for 12 hours at room temperature).

Drug Administration:
- Administer IV infusion or IVP, not faster than 16 mL (160 mg)/min because calcium content limits speed of injection, or as a short IV infusion.

Lab Effects/Interference:
- None known.

Drug Interactions:
- 5-FU: increased toxicity.
- Trimethoprim-sulfamethoxazole (Bactrim, used to treat PCP in HIV-infected patients). Coadministration resulted in increased rates of treatment failure in one study.

Special Considerations:
- **Do not administer intrathecally**.
- Dosed at one-half the usual dose of leucovorin calcium (folinic acid citrovorum factor).
- Contraindicated in persons who have had a prior allergic reaction to folic acid or folinic acid.
- Warnings and Precautions:
  - *Increased GI toxicities with 5-FU:* When given with 5-FU weekly in older patients, has caused severe enterocolitis, diarrhea, and dehydration, resulting in death. Monitor these patients closely and assess cbc/ANC frequently. Teach patient to report diarrhea right away, take anti-diarrheal medication as directed, and to drink fluids every hour.
  - *Drug Interaction with trimethoprim-sulfamethoxazole:* Concomitant use of d,l-leucovorin with trimethoprim-sulfamethoxazole for the acute treatment of *Pneumocystis jiroveci pneumonia* in HIV patients increased treatment failure and morbidity.

Potential Toxicities/Side Effects and the Nursing Process

I. POTENTIAL FOR INJURY related to HYPERSENSITIVITY, DRUG INTERACTIONS

Defining Characteristics: Allergic sensitization has been reported: facial flushing, itching.

Nursing Implications: Monitor patient for signs/symptoms of allergic reaction. Diphenhydramine is effective for relieving symptoms of allergic reaction.

II. ALTERED NUTRITION, POTENTIAL, LESS THAN BODY REQUIREMENTS, related to NAUSEA, VOMITING

Defining Characteristics: Levoleucovorin causes vomiting in 38% of patients, stomatitis in 38%, and nausea in 19% after high-dose MTX therapy. Oral leucovorin rarely causes nausea or vomiting.

Nursing Implications: Discuss need to continue antiemetics after high-dose MTX therapy with physician. Assess oral mucosa, teach patient self-assessment and to report any abnormalities. Teach patient to rinse oral mucosa after meals and at bedtime with oral rinse, such as salt water or sodium bicarbonate solution, per institutional policy and procedure.

Drug: mesna for injection (Mesnex)

Class: Sulfhydryl.

Mechanism of Action: Used to prevent ifosfamide-induced hemorrhagic cystitis. Drug is rapidly metabolized to the metabolite dimesna. In the kidney, dimesna is reduced to mesna, which binds to the urotoxic ifosfamide and cyclophosphamide metabolites acrolein and 4-hydroxyfosfamide, resulting in their detoxification.

Metabolism: Rapidly metabolized, remains in the intravascular compartment, and is rapidly eliminated by the kidneys. The drug is eliminated in 24 hours as mesna (32%) and dimesna (33%). Majority of the dose is eliminated within 4 hours. Oral mesna has 50% bioavailability of IV dose.

Indication: As a prophylactic agent in reducing the incidence of ifosfamide-induced hemorrhagic cystitis. Not indicated to reduce the risk of hematuria due to other pathological conditions, such as thrombocytopenia.

Dosage/Range:
- Initial dose should be given IV.
- Recommended IV–IV–IV: Clinical dose 20% of the mesna dose IV bolus 15 minutes before (or at the same time as the ifosfamide), 4 and 8 hours after ifosfamide or cyclophosphamide dose. Mesna dose is 20% of ifosfamide or cyclophosphamide dose, with total daily dose 60% of the ifosfamide or cyclophosphamide dose.

- IV–oral–oral: Mesna is given as an IV bolus injection in a dosage equal to 20% of the ifosfamide dosage at the time of ifosfamide administration. Mesna tablets are given orally in a dosage equal to 40% of the ifosfamide dose at 2 and 6 hours after each dose of ifosfamide. The total daily dose of mesna is 100% of the ifosfamide dose.
- Schedules:
  - IV dosing: Ifosfamide dose is 1.2 g/m^2 IV at 0 hour, with mesna 240 mg/m^2 IV at 0 hour; mesna 240 mg/m^2 IV at 4 and 8 hours post-ifosfamide.
  - IV and oral dosing: Ifosfamide dose is 1.2 g/m^2 IV at 0 hour, with mesna 240 mg/m^2 IV at 0 hour; mesna PO 480 mg/m^2 IV at 4 and 8 hours post-ifosfamide.
  - Maintain sufficient urinary output as required for ifosfamide treatment; assess urine for blood.
- The efficacy and safety of this ratio of IV–oral–oral mesna has not been established as being effective for daily doses of ifosfamide higher than 2.0 g/m^2 for 3–5 days.
- For continuous ifosfamide infusions, mesna is mixed with ifosfamide in equal amounts (1:1 mix). Prior to initiating CI, mesna is given IVB (10% of total ifosfamide dose). Following completion of the infusion, mesna alone should be infused for 12–24 hours to protect against delayed drug excretion activity against the bladder.
- Oral mesna: Dose is 40% of ifosfamide or cyclophosphamide dose (not recommended for initial dose if the patient experiences nausea and vomiting).

Drug Preparation:
- Drug available as Mesnex injection 1 gram multidose vial (100 mg/mL), and as tablets (400 mg mesna tablets).
- Dilute mesna with 5% dextrose, 5% dextrose/0.2% Sodium Chloride Injection USP, 5% dextrose/0.33% Sodium Chloride Injection USP, 5% dextrose/0.45% Sodium Chloride Injection USP, 0.9% Sodium Chloride Injection USP, or Lactated Ringer's Injection USP to create a designated fluid concentration.
- For continuous ifosfamide infusion, mesna should be mixed together in the same infusion bag with the ifosfamide.
- Stability: Mesnex injection multidose vials may be stored and used for up to 8 days after initial puncture. Store diluted solutions at 25°C (77°F); use diluted solutions within 24 hours.
- Do not mix Mesnex with epirubicin, cyclophosphamide, cisplatin, carboplatin, or nitrogen mustard.
- The benzyl alcohol contained in Mesnex injection vials can reduce the stability of ifosfamide. Ifosfamide and mesna can be mixed in the same bag, provided the final concentration of ifosfamide is not > 50 mg/mL. Higher concentrations of ifosfamide may not be compatible with mesna and may reduce the stability of ifosfamide.

Drug Administration:
- IV: Inspect solution bag for particulate matter and discoloration; do not use if either found. Administer as IV bolus injection.
- Oral: Tablet: Patients who vomit within 2 hours of taking oral mesna should repeat the dose or receive IV mesna.

TREATMENT

Drug Interactions:
- Ifosfamide: Mesna binds to drug metabolites; it is given concurrently for bladder protection.

Lab Effects/Interference:
- Can cause false-positive result on urinalysis for ketones.

Special Considerations:
- At clinical doses, mild nausea, vomiting, and diarrhea are the only side effects expected.

Potential Toxicities/Side Effects and the Nursing Process

I. POTENTIAL FOR INJURY related to MAINTENANCE OF BLADDER MUCOSAL INTEGRITY

Defining Characteristics: Mesna uniquely concentrates in the bladder and has a very low degree of toxicity, making it the uroprotector of choice against ifosfamide-related urotoxicity.

Nursing Implications: Assess daily urinalysis. Assess for hematuria per hospital policy and procedure. Hydrate vigorously.

II. ALTERATION IN NUTRITION, LESS THAN BODY REQUIREMENTS, related to NAUSEA/VOMITING, DIARRHEA

Defining Characteristics: Nausea and vomiting are minor in incidence and severity. Diarrhea is mild if it occurs.

Nursing Implications: Assess baseline nutritional status. Usual antiemetics for ifosfamide or cyclophosphamide-induced nausea/vomiting protect against mesna contribution. Encourage small, frequent meals and liquids. Teach patient to avoid greasy, fried, or fatty foods. Encourage patient to report onset of nausea/vomiting or diarrhea.

Drug: Uridine triacetate (Vistogard oral granules)

Class: Pyrimidine analogue.

Mechanism of Action: Drug is an acetylated pro-drug of uridine. Following oral administration, uridine triacetate is deacetylated throughout the body, including the systemic circulation. Uridine competitively inhibits cell damage and cell death caused by fluorouracil.

Metabolism: Pro-drug delivers 4–6 times more uridine than if uridine itself were ingested. Maximum plasma concentrations were achieved 2–3 hours after dosing. Half-life is approximately 2–2.5 hours. Uridine is metabolized by normal pyrimidine catabolic pathways in tissue.

Indications: Emergency treatment of adult and pediatric patients (1) following a fluorouracil or capecitabine overdose regardless of the presence of symptoms, or (2) who exhibit early-onset, severe, or life-threatening toxicity affecting the cardiac system or CNS, and/or early onset, unusually severe adverse reaction (e.g., GI toxicity and/or neutropenia) within 96 hours following the end of fluorouracil or capecitabine administration.

Drug is not recommended for the nonemergent treatment of adverse reactions associated with fluorouracil or capecitabine because it may diminish the efficacy of these drugs; the safety and efficacy of Vistogard initiated > 96 hours following the end of fluorouracil or capecitabine administration have not been established (Wellstat Therapeutics, 2015).

Dosage/Range:
Adults: 10 grams (1 packet) orally every 6 hours × 20 doses without regard to meals.
- Pediatrics: 6.2 g/m² (not to exceed 10 g/dose) PO every 6 hours × 20 doses without regard to meals. See full prescribing information for BSA-based dosing.

Drug Preparation/Administration:
- *Drug must be initiated within 96 hours of overdose or symptoms.*
- Pediatrics: use a scale accurate to at least 0.1 gram or a graduated teaspoon accurate to ¼ teaspoon to measure dose.
- Teach adult patient or parent to mix each dose with 3–4 ounces of soft foods, such as applesauce, pudding, or yogurt and ingest within 30 minutes of mixing. Teach patient not to chew the granules, and to drink at least 4 ounces of water after the dose.
- If the patient vomits within 2 hours of taking a dose, give a replacement dose as soon as possible after the vomiting stops. Administer the next dose at the regularly scheduled time.
- If a patient misses a dose at the scheduled time, administer that dose of uridine triacetate as soon as possible, and administer the next dose at the regularly scheduled time.
- Administer uridine triacetate granules by NG tube or G-tube when necessary (e.g., severe mucositis, coma).
  - Prepare approximately 4 fluid ounces (100 mL) of a food starch–based thickening product in water and briskly stir until thickener has dissolved.
  - Crush contents of one full 10-gram packet of uridine triacetate granules to a fine powder.
  - Add the crushed drug to 4 ounces (100 mL) of reconstituted food starch–based thickening product. For pediatric patients receiving < 10 grams, prepare the mixture at a ratio of no > 1 g/10 mL of reconstituted food starch–based thickening produce and mix thoroughly.
  - After administration using the NG or G-Tube, flush the tube with water.

Drug Interactions: None known.

Lab Effects/Interference: None known.

Special Considerations:
* Adverse reactions (> 2%) were vomiting, nausea, diarrhea.

Potential Toxicities/Side Effects and the Nursing Process

I. KNOWLEDGE DEFICIT, POTENTIAL related to PREPARATION OF URIDINE TRIACETATE.

Defining Characteristics: Patient will need 20 doses. If hospitalized, the nurse will administer the prepared dose. If/when the patient is discharged, the parent (pediatrics) or caregiver will need to be taught how to prepare the drug.

Nursing Considerations: Assess learning style and barriers to learning and develop plan to meet requirements and avoid barriers. Prepare written instructions for the parent/caregiver and ask them to repeat verbally or provide a return demonstration of the preparation process. Ensure that parent/caregiver has the name and telephone number of a nurse or provider in case questions arise or any problems develop.

Chapter *3*
Molecular Targeted Therapy

PERSONALIZED AND PRECISION CANCER CARE AND IMPLICATIONS FOR ONCOLOGY NURSES

Today, personalized, precision, and genomic cancer care is the goal in most cancer treatment centers, and while much remains to be defined, great progress has been made. Personalized and precision cancer care depends upon analyzing the genetic makeup of a patient's tumor, so precise therapy can be tailored to treat the tumor. Two existing examples of therapy tailored to specific mutations are trastuzumab (Herceptin®), developed for HER2+ breast cancer resulting from an overexpressed and/or amplified oncogene HER2, and imatinib mesylate (Gleevec®) developed to target the *BCR-ABL* mutation and resulting leukemic tyrosine kinase protein product in chronic myelocytic leukemia (CML). Both of these therapies have revolutionized the care of cancer in these two patient populations. In 2019, American Society of Clinical Oncology (ASCO) identified the major advance of the year as advances in management of rare tumors and identified that this has been possible through the "successes of immunotherapies and targeted therapies, as well as insights into molecular diagnostics and the microbiome (ASCO Post, 2019). Traditionally, drugs are tested in specific cancers, and then if effective, approved to treat those tumors. New thinking looks at the mechanism of disease (oncologic genetic drivers) and targets the genetic abnormality or mutation directly. Drug approval based on a genetic abnormality rather than site of disease is called an agnostic indication (Schilsky, 2018). Pembrolizumab (Keyturda) and nivolumab (Optiva) are immune checkpoint inhibitors discussed in *Chapter 4* and are FDA approved for the treatment of tumors that have microsatellite instability—high (MSI-H) or DNA mismatch deficient DNA repair deficiency (dMMR). Nivolulumab is FDA approved only for CRC tumors that have MSI—H or dMMR. The third drug with an agnostic indication is larotrectinib (Vitrakvi), which is indicated for the treatment of adults and children with a neurotrophic receptor typrosine kinase (*NTRK*) gene fusion without a known acquired resistance mutation (Loxo Oncology, 2018). The *NTRK* fusion gene is found in rare tumors such as mammary analogue secretory cancer, cellular or mixed congenital mesoblastic nephrome, and infantile fibrosarcoma.

This chapter is intended to establish a foundation for understanding the cellular basis of cancer and, as targeted therapy can be subdivided into molecular targeted and immunologically targeted therapies, will review molecular targeted therapy (e.g., targeting receptors outside and inside the cell), while *Chapter 4* entitled "Immunologic Targeted Therapy" addresses the advances that have been made in immunotherapy, as well as the drugs that have a biological of action (e.g., monoclonal antibodies, immune checkpoint inhibitors, vaccines, and other therapies).

IMPORTANCE TO THE ONCOLOGY NURSE

The new millennium has brought exciting promise to patients with cancer and to their nurses. As a better understanding of the process of carcinogenesis and metastasis has emerged, with it has come identified molecular and immune flaws that can be therapeutically targeted. Vogelstein et al. (2013) describe the genomic successes in identifying a few common mutations in many cancer types that drive cancer, as well as a larger number of mutations in individual tumor types that are less commonly mutated that are passenger genes. The authors point out that most human cancers result from 2–8 sequential alterations occurring over 20–30 years which confer a selective growth advantage to the particular cell (Vogelstein et al, 2013). It is important to know which are the "driver" genes as opposed to the many "passenger genes," as therapy directed to the passenger genes would not affect tumor progression. Of the approximately 140 mutated genes that drive tumorigenesis, 2 to 8 "driver" mutations are found in each tumor. The driver genes exert their proliferation effect through at least 12 signaling pathways that regulate (1) cell fate, (2) cell survival, and (3) genome maintenance (Vogelstein et al., 2013). Signaling pathways commonly mutated control **cell survival** (TGF-β, mitogen-activated protein kinase [MAPK], STAT, PI3K, RAS, cell cycle/apoptosis); **cell fate** (NOTCH, Hedgehog, APC, chromatin modification, transcriptional regulation); and **genome maintenance** (DNA damage control) (Vogelstein et al., 2013; see Table 3.1). Driver genes that are epigenetic are not mutated, but they can also be expressed in tumors, often inactivating tumor-suppressor genes, and they can be targeted to turn the tumor-suppressor genes back on. While similar genes may be mutated in patients with specific solid tumors, each patient's tumor is still distinct from another similar tumor by virtue of specific genetic alterations and helps to explain differences in patients' experience with a similar cancer. Thus, individualized medicine requires an assessment of each patient's tumor genome as well as the patient's germline genome (Vogelstein et al., 2013).

Research scientists from different institutions and professions are working in teams to identify tumor-specific mutations and flawed signaling pathways to target, as well as targeted agents to accomplish this (Saporito, 2013). One example is the Stand Up To Cancer (SU2C) Dream Team, which is targeting the PI3K pathway that is commonly mutated in women's cancers.

For the past decades, systemic and local therapies have provided cure, disease stabilization, and palliation for many patients with cancer. However, the physical cost of these benefits was often significant and included bone marrow depression with increased risk of infection, bleeding, and nausea and/or vomiting. The "magic bullet" was always sought so that benefit could be achieved with minimal toxicity. Today, many molecularly targeted

Table 3.1   Signaling Pathways Commonly Mutated in Cancer

Pathways controlling cell survival: TGF-β, MAPK, STAT, PI3K, RAS, cell cycle/apoptosis
Pathway controlling cell fate: NOTCH, Hedgehog, APC, chromatin modification, transcriptional regulation
Pathway controlling genome maintenance: DNA damage control

Modified from Vogelstein B, Papdopoulous N, Velculescu V, et al. Cancer Genome Landscapes. *Science* 2013; 229: 1546–1558.

agents, as well as immune-targeted agents, have been FDA approved and thousands more are undergoing clinical testing.

It is important for nurses to have a sound understanding of the molecular basis of cancer, the identified and potential molecular flaws and targets, and the agents that target them. The list of molecular targeted therapies is expanding day by day, and as clinical trial data establishes their usefulness, the drugs become FDA approved. As our knowledge of carcinogenesis expands, the question arises why the immune system is unable to mount a sustained attack against the tumor-expressed antigens. In some way, malignant transformation is able to also suppress the immune response. *Chapter 4* addresses a detailed review of the immune system, how tumor cells evade immune surveillance, and ways to harness this knowledge in the development of new therapies such as immune checkpoint inhibitors to stop tumor cells from "being invisible" to the immune system. Dr. Andrew von Eschenbach, MD, former NCI director, described the future of cancer care in 2003, and it still remains true:

> Today we understand cancer as both a genetic disease and a cell signaling failure. Genes that control orderly replication become damaged, allowing the cells to reproduce without restraint. A single cell's progress from normal, to malignant, to metastatic, appears to involve a series of interactive processes, each controlled by a different gene or set of genes. These altered genes produce defective protein signals, which are, in turn, mishandled by the cell. This understanding of the biology of cancer is enabling us to design interventions to preempt the cancer's progression to uncontrolled growth.

Today, oncology nurses and their patients are moving from "one size fits all" therapies (e.g., for breast cancer) into personalized, precision cancer treatment, where patient tumor tissue is analyzed for mutations and more precise cell type, which can help categorize the tumor and direct appropriate therapy. Called "precision medicine," therapies depend on precision genomics to identify the cellular flaws that first led to tumor formation and then continue to sustain it (Jones et al., 2015). Targeted molecular and biologic/immunological therapies are the key therapies. The nurse helps patients and their families to (1) understand their potential treatment choices in concert with the oncologist/hematologist, the drug's side effects, patient's self-care requirements, and cost implications; (2) identify and intervene early when adverse effects occur, by assessing patients frequently and establishing a trust relationship so the patient calls/reports issues early, in consultation with physician or NP/PA. In this regard, the nurse also facilitates communication among the members of the oncology team, as the nurse has a regular presence in the patient's care (Rubin, 2012). The nurse must be articulate in the language of targeted therapies and be effective as a patient/family educator, as so many of the targeted therapies are oral, so that the patient takes the medicine correctly, adheres to the plan, and reports toxicity early. The nurse must understand the potential drug toxicities and their differences; for example, Epidermal Growth Factor Receptor Inhibitor (EGFRI)–induced diarrhea from erlotinib (Tarceva®) is very different in management and threat to the patient from that of ipilimumab (Yervoy®), which is immune-related and may be life-threatening. The nurse must assess the patient's ability to comply with medication self-administration instructions. For example, certain drugs must be taken on an empty stomach 1–2 hours before or 2 hours after a meal; if these directions are not followed, the bioavailability of the drug is increased many times with severe adverse events (e.g., nilotinib (Tasigna®) and erlotinib (Tarceva®)).

In order to better understand targeted molecular therapy, the nurse must understand the molecular basis of cancer. For this, it is important to recall early courses in biology and genetics. A simplified review of normal cell biology is presented, and malignant biology is discussed using Hanahan and Weinberg's 10 hallmarks of cancer (2011) as an organizing framework.

NORMAL CELL BIOLOGY

The nucleus of the cell is where the genetic material, or deoxyribonucleic acid (DNA), is located. DNA is the building block of life, an incredibly simple yet complex double helix in which each strand is made up of millions of chemical bases, and each chemical base attaches to its complementary partner to pair in a specific way (cytosine with guanine, thymine with adenosine). See Figure 3.1.

Genes are a subunit of DNA, and each gene contains a code or recipe for a specific product, such as a protein or enzyme. Scientists have now identified all the 20,000 or so protein-coding genes in the human genome. These genes can each make multiple proteins. In addition, thousands of noncoding RNA molecules have been discovered that regulate the protein coding genes (NHGRI, 2015). Genes carry the blueprint of who we are. A genome is all the DNA in a cell, and genomics is a study of genomes (NHGRI, 2015). All cells have the genetic blueprint, but only the genes we need are "turned on" or expressed, such as the color for blue eyes. The genes we don't need at the moment are "turned off." In early fetal growth, many genes are turned on, and then when the embryo develops into a baby, these genes are no longer necessary, and the genes are turned off. Unfortunately, it appears that cancer is able to turn back on a number of genes that should remain off, such as those that permit unlimited cell division and for cells to change from epithelial cells to mesenchymal cells to migrate and invade neighboring tissues. Genes code for specific proteins and are contained in a chromosome. Humans have 46 chromosomes: 22 autosomal pairs and 1 pair of sex chromosomes. As research gives us greater understanding of the small RNAs, which play such a large role in regulating gene expression and function, the knowledge about their role in cancer, as well as how to manipulate them to halt tumor cell proliferation and metastases, will enable clinicians to further individualize therapy for each patient based on the tumor's genetic fingerprint (Rothschild, 2014).

CELL SIGNALING AND SIGNAL TRANSDUCTION

PROTEIN KINASES

Signal transduction is really just sending a message from outside the cell to inside the cell, or from inside the cell to other downstream proteins, telling the cell nucleus (genes) to perform a *specific* function. Protein kinases are enzymes that are able to turn on or off the signal *and can be thought of as "on and off switches."* Phosphorylation, or the addition of a phosphate group to the tyrosine, serine, or threonine residue of a protein, turns on the signal and sends it from one protein to the next protein in a bucket brigade-like fashion. Dephosphorylation, or removing the phosphate group, shuts down or turns off the signal transduction. Thus, it can be thought of as an on and off switch for the signals which govern the cell. Tyrosine kinases add the phosphate group to the tyrosine residue of the protein,

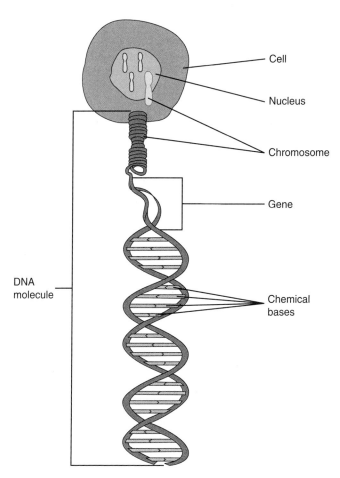

Figure 3.1   DNA: Base Pairs and Double Helix
Courtesy of National Cancer Institute.

thus turning on the signal transduction (signaling). Tyrosine kinases can be either receptor tyrosine kinases (*RTKs*) or nonreceptor tyrosine kinases (*NRTKs*). As discussed, protein kinases are key regulators of a cell's communication system, passing messages along the signaling cascade. RTKs have three sections—the extracellular portion of the receptor outside the cell to which the ligand, such as a growth factor, binds to start the message which passes through the cell membrane (transmembrane portion) to an intracellular tyrosine kinase portion inside the cell membrane, resulting in phosphorylation or sending the message to the next protein in line, like a bucket brigade. NRTKs are in the cytoplasm of the cell, and carry the message from upstream (e.g., the cell membrane or in the cytoplasm) to other proteins downstream so that the message is sent to the cell nucleus. They are not attached to a receptor. Targeted therapies that block the receptor on the outside of the cell are generally monoclonal antibodies that are too large to enter the cell and must be administered parenterally, such as trastuzumab, while drugs that target the tyrosine or serine/threonine kinases inside the cell are small molecules that can be given orally, such as tyrosine kinase inhibitors (TKIs).

Receptor Tyrosine Kinases
There are 19 families of RTKs, which are named for the growth factor or hormone that turns them on and is their ligand. These include epidermal growth factor receptor (EGFR), vascular endothelial growth factor receptor (VEGFR), platelet-derived growth factor receptor (PDGFR), insulin and insulin-like growth factor receptor (IGF-1), stem factor receptor (c-KIT), and fibroblast growth factor receptor (FGFR). When the body needs to perform a function, like making new blood vessels or new cells, it must make a specific protein that will carry out the function. The requirement message is sent to the cell as a growth factor or hormone and called a ligand. The ligand attaches to a receptor, such as RTK, on the outside of the cell membrane.

The RTK on the outside of the cell is stimulated when a ligand attaches to it. The receptor asks a neighbor receptor to pair up with it (dimerize), or the receptor can activate itself (autostimulation) to activate the receptor. Dimerization activates the phosphorylation function, which sends the message like a bucket brigade through the cell membrane and from one protein to the next, through the cytoplasm to the cell nucleus. Another way to think of this is like being in a dark room. You flip on the light switch, and the light comes on. What has happened is that the light switch is attached to a wire; when it is turned on, it sends energy in the form of electricity to the overhead light, and it is turned on. Similarly, when the ligand attaches to the receptor, after dimerization, the message goes from the receptor outside the cell, through the membrane, to inside the membrane. There, the message is attached to a tyrosine kinase, which communicates to other tyrosine kinases to carry the message through the cell to the cell nucleus like a bucket brigade. A tyrosine kinase is an enzyme that adds a phosphate group (phosphorylation), which it usually takes from ATP, the cell's energy currency, and passes it to a protein next in line, sending the message from one protein to another so the message moves "downstream" toward the cell nucleus. This is called signal transduction. RTKs are very important in sending messages telling the cell to divide, make new blood vessels such as in wound healing, and to die when the cell is old or damaged. When RTKs are mutated or overexpressed on tumor cells, they tell the cancer cells to proliferate, move, invade nearby tissue, metastasize, and to ignore programmed cell-death signals. Examples that may be mutated in cancer are the EGFR and VEGFR, which are discussed below. RTKs are often proto-oncogenes, and once mutated, they become oncogenes which stimulate the cell to continue to divide to make more cells even though the body does not need any cells. Not only are RTKs important proteins that may become mutated in cancer, so too are the individual proteins in the signaling cascade that take the message from one protein to another and ultimately to the cell nucleus where it can tell the cell to perform functions such as cell division and avoidance of apoptosis (programmed cell death). The mutated proteins in the signaling cascade can send the message to divide repeatedly through the cancer cell to the cell nucleus, without being told to do this by the cell receptor. This is a simplistic description, and there are many redundant pathways. In the following figure are examples of key proteins in signaling pathways, whose genes, which make them, can be mutated in cancer: *Ras, Raf/BRAF, MEK, MAPK,* the tumor-suppressor *PTEN,* mTOR, *PI3K,* and the antiapoptotic protein Bcl-2.

EGFR Signaling Pathway

Epidermal growth factor (EGF) stimulates cell growth, differentiation (becoming special-ized), and proliferation. For example, when you wash your hands, you slough many cells from your skin (epidermis). Although these are dead cells filled with keratin, they still need to be replaced. EGF is released and through binding to the EGFR1 on the underlying skin stem cells, stimulates the stem cells in the basal layer underneath the skin to proliferate and to migrate up to the surface (Fuchs, 2008) where the cells can replace those that have been lost during hand-washing. There are four members of the EGFR family. EGFR1 is involved in regulating the growth and development, as well as the repair of injured cells, in skin, mucosa, lungs, and colon among others. The second member is EGFR2, better known as HER (human epidermal receptor)-2, and this is important in breast tissue. EGFR3 and 4 are not well understood. All except HER-2 require a ligand to bind to the receptor to acti-vate and lead to dimerization. HER-2 does not have a ligand, but can dimerize with all the other EGFRs to activate the receptor. Once the receptor is activated, the signal (message) is sent through the membrane to the inside tyrosine kinase, from which it is sent via the Ras-Raf-MEK-MAPK and many other pathways to regulate the important cell processes of proliferation, growth and differentiation, migration, cell motility and apoptosis (pro-grammed cell death) so that when a cell has fulfilled its function or is damaged, it can be removed. See Figure 3.2.

The EGF family of receptors is very important for cell growth, differentiation, and survival. Many cancers overexpress this receptor, resulting in a more aggressive tumor

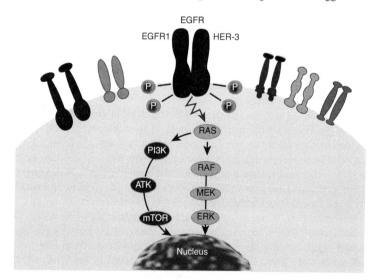

Figure 3.2   Showing EGFR Signaling

behavior with increased tendency for invasion and metastases and shorter patient survival. The HER-2-neu receptor (EGFR2) has become well known because it is amplified (more than normal copies of a gene) or overexpressed (a gene is transcribed more times than normal) in about 20% of patients with breast cancer, again conferring a poor prognosis (Tapia et al., 2006). A number of monoclonal antibodies have been developed to block the external domain of the EGFR-1 receptor (cetuximab or Erbitux®, panitumumab or Vectibix®), the external HER-2 receptor (trastuzumab or Herceptin), and the internal domains of EGFR by TKIs such as erlotinib (Tarceva, in EGFR1) and lapatinib (Tykerb®, of both EGFR1 and HER2). Today, many TKIs are multitargeted, inhibiting more than one receptor or pathway, such as lapatinib (Tykerb), which blocks both EGFR-1 and -2 receptor kinases. It may be beneficial to combine a monoclonal antibody from outside of the cell, such as trastuzumab, with a small molecule that blocks the tyrosine kinase portion inside the cell, such as lapatinib (Tykerb), which can cross the blood–brain barrier.

As one can imagine, if the EGFR is amplified (more copies of the gene than normal) or overexpressed or has other mutations, it can easily lead to cancer. EGFR has been found to be amplified or mutated in gliomas and NSCLC, while HER2 is amplified in certain breast, ovarian, and bladder cancers. Studies have shown that the leading edge of tumors often contain EGFR1 and are stimulated by EGF to invade and metastasize (Weinberg, 2014).

MAPK Pathway

The MAPK pathway is a very important signaling pathway involved in cell growth, cell proliferation, and cell differentiation. The pathway is usually turned on by growth factors outside the cell binding to RTKs. The key signaling molecule proteins in the pathway are Ras, Raf, MEK, and ERK. Once the message begins to be sent through the cell membrane, the signal travels from protein to protein, where tyrosine kinases phosphorylate then activate the next protein in line in the signaling cascade, sending the message down the pathway like a bucket brigade. Once the message reaches the cell nucleus, specific genes are transcribed (or copied as they are the recipes for a protein) onto messenger RNA (mRNA) and carried outside the nucleus to the protein factory (ribosomes on the endoplasmic reticulum). The proteins made when released will regulate the essential cell functions of cell growth, proliferation, and cell differentiation. Once the signal has been sent down the pathway, it shuts off automatically.

Unfortunately, the MAPK pathway is often dysregulated in cancer, either by abnormal expression of the proteins in the signaling cascade, or by mutations that turn on (activate) receptors downstream so that they are turned on when they should not be activated and or turned off. The proteins sending the message down the pathway are stuck in the "on" position so that the message continues to be sent time and time again. When turned on by mutation of a tyrosine kinase, or overexpression, activation can lead to increased/uncontrolled cell proliferation, avoidance of apoptosis, and resistance to chemotherapy, RT, and some targeted therapies (Weinberg, 2014). Braf is a protein made by the proto-oncogene *BRAF*, which when mutated becomes an oncogene. The proteins made by this gene then turn the "on" switch to "on" independently of any stimulation from the growth factor/RTK at the cell surface, so it keeps sending messages "downstream" so that MEK, and MAPK/ERK pathways are now always turned on, sending messages to the cell nucleus for tumor cell proliferation and survival (avoidance of apoptosis). A number of drugs have been developed to target tyrosine kinases in this pathway. While concerted efforts have been unsuccessful in finding drugs to inhibit Ras, success has been seen in targeting BRAF, an oncogenic protein made by the oncogene *BRAF* in malignant melanoma (vemurafenib, and dabrafenib). Most (90%) BRAF mutations are aV600E point mutation, which is found in some malignant melanoma as well as colon cancer tumors. This point mutation turns on the protein so that it is always signaling and stimulates MEK, which stands for MAPK/ERK kinase. MEK activates the MAPK pathway, and a MEK inhibitor has been approved, trametinib, blocking both MEK1 and MEK2. MEK also communicates through MAPK/ERK to the phosphatidylinositol-3-kinase (PI3K)-Akt/mTOR (mammalian target of rapamycin) pathways. As seen in Figures 3.2 and 3.3, MEK is central to a number of pathways.

NRTKs: Ten families of NRTKs in the cytoplasm regulate communication along key pathways, and the proteins include Jak, abl, and src. Within the cell, there are NRTKs that are key elements in sending the message through the cytoplasm of the cell, along to the nucleus, using the bucket brigade method. These can be mutated in cancer, so they turn on

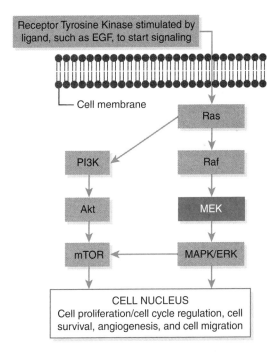

Figure 3.3   MEK: An Important Cancer Target in an Important Pathway

Modified from de Lartigue J. The MEK Junction: Protein Presents a Ripe Target for Inhibitors. Published online Thursday, October 11, 2012. Retrieved from http://www.onclive.com/publications/Oncology-live/2012 /september-2012/The-MEK-Junction-Protein-Presents-a-Ripe-Target -for-Inhibitors#sthash.xsiewpyQ.dpuf. Courtesy of OncologyLive magazine/OncLive.com.

continuously and send the message telling the cell to proliferate, invade, make new blood vessels or other malignant functions. Examples in cancer are mTOR and BCR-ABL, which are discussed below.

PI3K-Akt/mTOR Pathways

The PI3K pathway is important in regulating the cell cycle, which controls proliferation/ cell division, avoiding apoptosis as well as other functions. This pathway is mutated in a number of cancers, including aggressive prostate cancer (Toren & Zoubeidi, 2014). PI3K is a membrane-associated protein kinase, which is usually in the "off" position so signaling does not occur. When a RTK is activated, such as EGFR, it stimulates changes in the cell membrane, leading to phosphorylation, lifting the brakes off PI3K so that signaling can occur. PI3K sends signals to many proteins, most importantly Akt also known as Protein Kinase B. NRTKs can also stimulate PI3K from the cytoplasm. This leads to phosphorylation of Akt, which is also in the cell membrane, leading to phosphorylation of many proteins, including mTOR. PI3K-delta is expressed on white blood cells, but it is critical for signaling, development, migration, and survival of B lymphocytes. Idelalisib (Zydelig) is a PI3K inhibitor that stops the proliferation of malignant B lymphocytes, as well as cell signaling (B-cell receptor, CXCR4, CXCR5), which is involved in telling B lymphocytes how to migrate to the lymph nodes and bone marrow (e.g., trafficking and homing in to the lymph nodes and bone marrow). Idelalisib is FDA approved for treatment of patients with relapsed, follicular B-cell NHL or relapsed CLL (Zydelig, 2014).

This diagram shows key targets for cancer therapy and the importance of MEK in the signaling pathway. This is a simplified image but shows how the message is generated by ligand binding at the outside of the cell membrane, and the message for key normal (and malignant) cell processes is sent down via a "bucket brigade" to the tyrosine kinase proteins to the cell nucleus, thus bringing about cell proliferation, cell cycle regulation, cell survival, migration (e.g., metastasis), and angiogenesis. There is crosstalk between the RAS/MAPK/ ERK pathway and PI3K-mTOR pathway to accomplish these functions. Drugs have been FDA approved for blocking many of the pathway elements, and research continues to seek improved therapies to shut down the pathways. Unfortunately, most cancers find a way to use alternative pathways.

When mutated, Akt phosphorylates many oncogenic proteins, leading to avoidance of apoptosis and tumor cell survival. It does this by inhibiting the Bcl-2 family of antiapoptotic proteins such as BAD and BAX which keep the cancer cell from dying (Toren & Zoubeidi, 2014). This confers an aggressive phenotype, especially in aggressive prostate cancer (Toren & Zoubeidi, 2014). Akt is a very important pathway to protect from accidently being turned on, and a number of genes accomplish this. For example, the tumor-suppressor gene *PTEN* (phosphatase and tensin homologue gene) makes the protein (product) PTEN that blocks the PI3K-Akt pathway. However, the *PTEN* gene is commonly deleted or mutated in many cancers, such as prostate, breast, and bladder cancers (Papa et al., 2014), so that the Akt pathway is always turned on.

mTOR plays a central role in cell proliferation (turning on the cell cycle), cell metabolism, and regulating cell growth and angiogenesis. mTOR was named as such because rapamycin, an immunosuppressant, was able to inhibit this kinase in organ transplant patients. mTOR acts like New York's Grand Central Station, integrating multiple signals from essential pathways, such as growth factors (e.g., insulin and insulin-like growth factor), nutrients (e.g., glucose, amino acids), hormones, and stress (e.g., starvation, hypoxia, DNA damage) (Watanabe et al., 2011). It regulates protein turnover, cell growth, and differentiation, cell survival, energy balance, and the cell's response to stress. It is often dysregulated in cancer, and it is a key target (Watanabe et al., 2011). Drugs that target mTOR that are FDA approved are everolimus (Afinitor®) and temsirolimus (Torisel®). Everolimus is FDA approved to treat patients with a number of cancers, including postmenopausal women with advanced hormone receptor-positive, HER2 negative, breast cancer in combination with exemestane after failure on letrozole or anastrozole (Novartis, 2016), and temsirolimus is approved to treat patients with advanced renal cell cancer (Pfizer, 2015).

HOW DO PROTEINS CARRY OUT THE MESSAGE?

When the message ultimately arrives at the cell nucleus, it needs to tell specific genes in the DNA to carry out a function, and it does this by opening up the DNA strands where the gene is located, and transcribing the gene. Transcription means copying the gene code, which is a recipe for the specific protein, onto messenger RNA (mRNA), which is single stranded. The DNA strands separate, exposing the gene that codes for the requested enzyme or protein, and information from the gene is copied onto mRNA. The sequence of chemical bases in the gene is copied base by base onto a new strand of mRNA so that the complementary recipe is shown on the mRNA. RNA is single stranded so this is the only way to copy the gene. This piece of mRNA then travels out of the nucleus into the cytoplasm of the cell to the ribosomes, which are the cell's "protein factories." Here, the complementary copy of the protein recipe is recopied onto a ribosome by transfer RNA (tRNA) so that it is exactly like the DNA copy. Now the ribosome is told to make the specific protein. Amino acids are then assembled into a completed protein molecule. See Figure 3.4.

MUTATIONS

The body is very careful that cell birth always equals cell death so that no cell can divide unless the body needs another cell. When a cell needs to divide to make another cell (proliferation) to replace a damaged or dead cell, such as a cell lining the gastrointestinal tract, the cell's nucleus receives a message from a growth factor to divide. We know that the GI tract sloughs over 80,000,000 cells a minute during digestion, so it is easy to see why the body needs to replace used-up, dead, or damaged cells frequently. Recall the process of cell division in terms of the cell cycle, as discussed in *Chapter 1*. When each cell prepares to divide, the DNA is copied during the synthesis (S) phase to make a duplicate set of DNA so that each of the daughter cells will have identical DNA. Millions of coded genes are copied during cell division. Occasionally a mistake is made, such as when one chemical base is not correctly copied. Often this is quickly fixed, but sometimes a mutation can result in the production of an abnormal protein, enzyme, or product. Figure 3.5 shows how a mutation can lead to the production of an abnormal protein. Different types of mutations are shown in Figure 3.6. If the mutation occurs near or on a proto-oncogene or a tumor-suppressor gene, then it can potentially (1) turn on cell division when the body does not need more cells (i.e., proto-oncogene becomes a cancer-causing oncogene) or (2) silence a tumor-suppressor

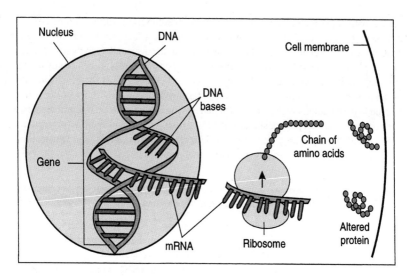

Figure 3.4 **Protein Synthesis**
Courtesy of National Cancer Institute.

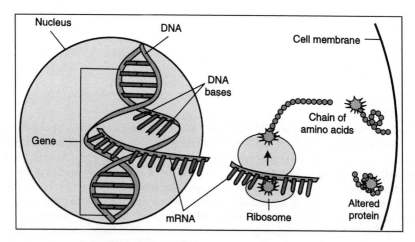

Figure 3.5 **Mutation Leading to Abnormal Protein Production**
Courtesy of National Cancer Institute.

gene so that it does not stop uncontrolled cell division. In other words, in cancer, the on-cogene is like the accelerator of a car that is stuck, driving cell division when cells are not needed, whereas the tumor-suppressor gene, when silenced, is like the brakes of a car that are failing and unable to stop the car.

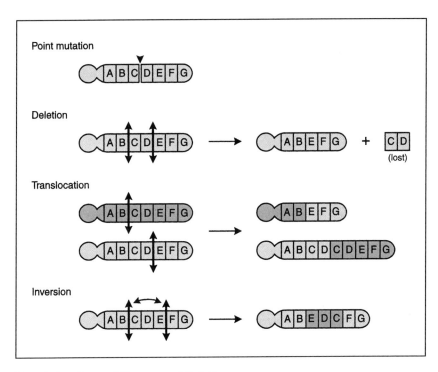

Figure 3.6   Types of Chromosomal Mutations

An example of a serious mutation is the formation of the *BCR-ABL* fusion gene and abnormal chromosome through a reciprocal translocation (exchange) between chromosome 9 and 22, forming an extra-long chromosome 9. The other chromosome is short, called the Philadelphia chromosome (Ph[1]), which contains the fused *BCR-ABL* gene, and is shown in Figure 3.7. The *ABL* gene is a proto-oncogene normally found on chromosome 9, and it encodes for a tyrosine kinase that is very tightly controlled, while the BCR (breakpoint cluster region) is on chromosome 22. The translocation is basically swapping some genes from chromosome 9 to chromosome 22, and vice versa. Once the translocation occurs, the *BCR-ABL* fusion gene now is located on chromosome 22. The new fusion gene puts a tyrosine kinase and an accelerator together so that the fusion gene encodes for an uncontrolled tyrosine kinase (an oncoprotein), causing continual cell proliferation and release of leukemic cells with the Ph[1] chromosome. The second fusion gene is *ABL-BCR,* which is located on chromosome 9 and is not involved in CML. This genetic abnormality (the creation of the Ph[1] chromosome) occurs in 90% of patients with chronic myelogenous leukemia (CML). Imatinib mesylate (Gleevec), a TKI that selectively targets this flaw, was designed specifically for this mutation, and has revolutionized the care of patients with CML. Over time, most patients develop resistance as the ATP-pocket for the tyrosine kinase changes shape, so second- and third-generation TKIs have been developed.

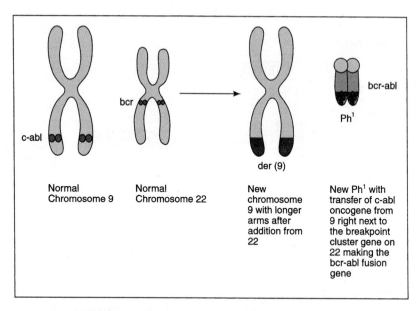

c-abl

bcr

der (9)

bcr-abl

Ph¹

| Normal
Chromosome 9 | Normal
Chromosome 22 | New
chromosome
9 with longer
arms after
addition from
22 | New Ph¹ with
transfer of c-abl
oncogene from
9 right next to
the breakpoint
cluster gene on
22 making the
bcr-abl fusion
gene |

Figure 3.7   Philadelphia Chromosome

It appears that almost all malignancies are caused by mutations in DNA; however, knowledge of epigenetic changes is evolving and helps explain why this may not always be true. Mutations in DNA can result in:

- **Gain of function:** The mutation activates one or more genes that lead to malignant transformation, such as with the *Ras, Myc, EGFR* family. This results in the speeding up of cell growth and division, which makes more cells than the body needs.
- **Loss of function:** The mutation(s) inactivate genes that control cell growth, such as the tumor-suppressor gene p53. In this case, there are no "mutation police" so that the genetic mutation is not caught, the DNA is not repaired, the cell is not destroyed which should occur if unable to repair the mutation, and the genetic flaw is perpetuated with each further cell division.

Mutations continue to be very important, and it usually takes at least four mutations to cause malignant transformation. This is shown in Figure 3.8.

Approximately 10% of these mutations are inherited or carried in the DNA of reproductive cells in individuals whose parents carry the gene, while 90% of mutations are acquired and considered sporadic. Usually, an inherited mutation does not result in cancer; rather, it increases the risk that the person will develop cancer in the course of his or her lifetime. Sporadic mutations develop during the course of one's life, due to exposure to carcinogens, and are related to relationships among and between genes and the environment. Most cancers are not inherited, although two examples of inherited vulnerability to cancer are (1) women who have mutations in the *BRCA1* and/or *BRCA2* gene (who represent 5% or so of women who develop breast cancer) and (2) individuals with hereditary polyposis in

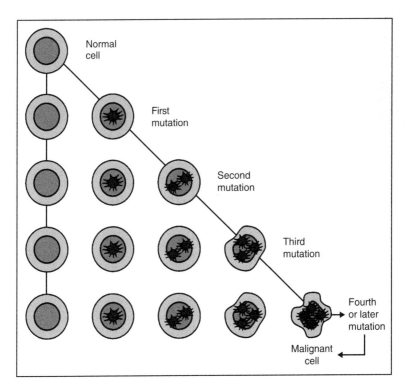

Figure 3.8   Mutations and Malignant Transformation
Courtesy of National Cancer Institute.

which one gene copy (allele) of the APC tumor-suppressor gene is silenced. *BRCA1* and *BRCA2* are DNA repair genes and are considered tumor-suppressor genes. One of these genes can be mutated not only in a few women with breast cancer but also in some patients with ovarian, pancreatic, or prostate cancer.

DNA REPAIR
O'Donovan and Livingston (2010) help us better understand the importance of BRCA1 and -2 in DNA repair of double-strand breaks. Patients with familial germline mutations in BRCA1, with resulting silencing of the gene, have 80% cumulative risk of developing breast cancer at age 70 and a risk of ovarian cancer of 30–40%. Patients with a germline mutation in BRCA2 have a cumulative risk of 50% of developing breast cancer at age 70 and between 10–15% risk of developing ovarian cancer. BRCA1 and -2 help to maintain the integrity of the genome not only by repairing DNA but also by helping to control the cell cycle at the checkpoints and regulating key mitotic or cell division steps.

The human genome is under constant stress caused from internal (e.g., reactive oxygen species, cytosine deamination resulting from metabolism) and external (e.g., UV, ionizing radiation, including cancer RT, and chemicals, including chemotherapy) stressors that damage the cell's DNA. This damage can be either single- or double-strand DNA breaks. The double-strand breaks are more toxic to the cell because there is no "normal" or correct DNA strand to serve as a repair template. If the cell cannot repair the DNA strand breaks, then the cell undergoes apoptosis as directed by the "gene police," p53. If the cell is not repaired correctly, it can lead to serious mutations or rearrangement of the chromosomes (e.g., translocations and deletions) each time the cell divides. Unfortunately, up to 50% of tumors have a mutation in the p53 gene, allowing malignant cells with significant genetic abnormalities to go through the cell cycle and divide into daughter cells.

With continued cell divisions with the unrepaired or incompletely repaired DNA, cancer may evolve. In addition, many genes on the damaged DNA are tumor-suppressor genes, so these may now be ineffective or silent. Given that within the human body, cells undergo millions of mitotic cell divisions each day to replace dead or damaged cells, it is easy to see that multiple cell divisions with damaged DNA can lead to *genomic instability and cancer*.

Thus, the cells have evolved a very sophisticated way to repair the DNA errors, especially the double-strand breaks, so that the human genome remains intact. The two major pathways to repair DNA double-strand breaks are called (1) nonhomologous end-joining (NHEJ), the primary mechanism where the ends of a double-strand break are directly religated) and (2) homologous recombination (HR, an error-free mechanism). BRCA1 and -2 repair DNA double-strand breaks by using the HR mechanism. Other repair pathways are those for single-strand DNA repair: base excision repair, nucleotide excision repair, or mismatch repair (Ford et al., 2010). If single-strand breaks or nicks are not repaired and are allowed to go through cell division, the breaks become double-strand DNA breaks. The most commonly used mechanism for DNA repair is base excision repair (BER), which refers to cutting out the damaged base or bases and replacing them (cut and patch) by using the complementary DNA as a template to synthesize the correct base or base sequence in the damaged strand (Ford et al., 2010). Remember that DNA is made up of two strands of nucleotides with a backbone of sugar and phosphate groups. The two strands are tied together by paired bases (adenine, guanine, cytosine, thymine) that attach to a sugar. A base forms a bond with another base to make a base pair: adenine always with thymine and cytosine always with guanine. The sequence of the paired bases attached to the sugar spell out the recipe or code for the protein to be made (instructions to the cell for a specific function, such as for the cell to divide). This recipe is read by mRNA and taken out to the cytoplasm to make the protein on the ribosome.

When DNA is damaged, a nuclear enzyme called poly (ADP-ribose) polymerase or PARP is activated in the nucleus of the cell. PARP1 is the most abundant member of this large family; this enzyme helps the chromatin relax, and it calls in the BER proteins to the DNA break so that they can fix it. If the double-strand break genes are damaged or nonfunctional, then the BER proteins will be their backup to repair the DNA.

Thus, if a patient has a BRCA1 or -2 mutation, PARP enzymes are critical to the survival of a cell with damaged DNA. Normally, if the damaged DNA cannot be repaired, the cell is told to die or to undergo apoptosis (programmed cell death). An important example is a cancer cell trying to recover from radiation or chemotherapy. Investigators believe that by giving chemotherapy and also blocking PARP1, they can kill the cancer cell by forcing it to undergo apoptosis. This is called *synthetic lethality,* when the cell can get along with a mutation in either of the repair pathways, but not in both pathways, which causes the cell to die (Fong et al., 2009) (Figure 3.9). Thus, PARP1 inhibition represents a new direction

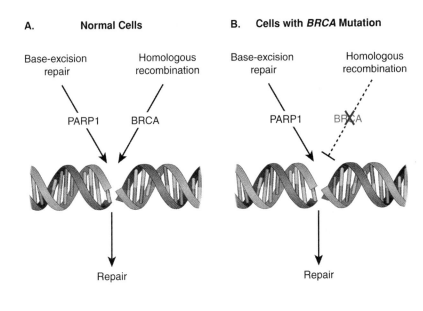

Figure 3.9   PARP Inhibitors and Synthetic Lethality
Reproduced from Wilkes GM. *Targeted Cancer Therapy: A Handbook for Nurses*. Sudbury, MA: Jones & Bartlett Publishers, 2011; 279.

in cancer drug development (Iglehart & Silver, 2009). Interestingly, PARP enzymes are "upregulated" or increased due to overexpression of the PARP1 gene in many cancers, and it is believed that this confers acquired resistance to some chemotherapy agents when the patient originally responded to the drug(s) and then, after a few treatments, no longer responds (O'Connor & Breen, 2008).

PARP inhibitors confer chemosensitization and radiosensitization. Additionally, cancer cells that do not have a functional *PTEN* tumor-suppressor gene or gene product (PTEN protein) appear sensitive to PARP inhibition because there is downregulation of a critical component of HR function (Rad51). When *PTEN* does not work (loss-of-function mutations), the cancer cell message to divide is amplified via P13K signaling, which promotes tumorigenesis (Hanahan & Weinberg, 2011). A number of aggressive cancers, including some prostate cancers, have PTEN defects, so this will be an important niche for treatment (Ana et al., 2009). Normal cells do not divide as frequently as cancer cells, and as they still have functional HR, they are relatively spared and therefore survive while the cancer cells are forced into programmed cell death. Hence, this is a selective way to kill cancer cells. At this time, three PARP inhibitors have been FDA approved: Olaparib (Lynparza®), rucaparib (Rubraca™), niraparib (Zejula™), and talazoparib (Talzenna).

MALIGNANT TRANSFORMATION: HALLMARKS OF CANCER

Ten hallmarks of cancer have been postulated by Hanrahan and Weinberg (2011) as being key to malignant transformation, invasion, and metastases. These are shown in Figure 3.10.

MALIGNANT TRANSFORMATION

How exactly does malignant transformation occur? Hanahan and Weinberg (2011) identified 10 hallmarks of cancer and targeted therapeutic approaches. These include the six original hallmarks, which are six biological capabilities acquired during the multistep process of tumorigenesis (Hanrahan & Weinberg, 2011). These biological capabilities are (1) sustaining proliferative signaling, (2) evading growth suppressors, (3) resisting cell death, (4) enabling replicative immortality, (5) inducing angiogenesis, and (6) activating invasion and metastasis. In addition, (7) reprogramming of energy metabolism (e.g., inefficient energy production using glycolysis) and (8) evasion of immune destruction which help to ensure tumor initiation, growth, invasion, and metastasis, were added. Newly added hallmarks that enable the biological capabilities as well as tumorigenesis are: (1) genome instability, which through mutations contributes genetic diversity that speeds up their acquisition and (2) inflammation, which fosters many of the hallmark capabilities.

The tumor microenvironment or stroma has gained increasing importance. Cancer cells recruit normal-appearing cells in the tumor microenvironment that contribute to malignant transformation. Signals from cells in the microenvironment may start the malignant process, and they are key figures in supporting invasion and metastases (Hanahan & Weinberg, 2011). Necrotic cell death releases proinflammatory signals into the microenvironment. Stromal cells in the microenvironment are involved in angiogenesis. It is also possible that

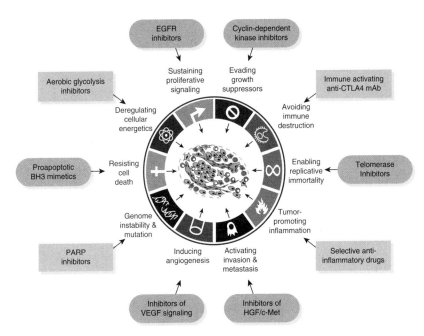

Figure 3.10   Hallmarks of Cancer
Reprinted from Hanahan D, Weinberg RA. Hallmarks of cancer: The next generation. *Cell* 2011; 144(5): 646-674.
Copyright 2011, with permission from Elsevier.

the leading edge of the tumor that is invading neighboring tissue receives signals from the microenvironment for those cells to undergo epidermal mesenchymal transition (EMT) transformation (Weinberg, 2014). Epidermal cells cannot invade and metastasize, while mesenchymal cells can migrate to different sites. Finally, the microenvironment plays an important role in helping newly landed metastatic cells make a niche and succeed to start further metastases (Hanahan & Weinberg, 2011).

GENOME INSTABILITY AND MUTATIONS, SUSTAINING PROLIFERATIVE SIGNALING, EVADING GROWTH SUPPRESSORS

Once there are mutations in both the proto-oncogene and tumor-suppressor genes, then there is no longer a balance between cell birth and cell death. Instead, there is uncontrolled cell growth. How does this happen? Again, recall the **cell cycle** as shown in Figure 3.11. Normally, the nucleus activates the cell cycle by putting the cell into cell division mode only when the stimulatory signals are greater than the inhibitory signals, e.g., the cell is big enough, there is enough nutrition to support development of the proteins to make the DNA, mitotic apparatus, etc. When this happens, levels of cyclins rise (cyclin D, followed by E, A, and B) as the cell moves through the phases of the cell cycle.

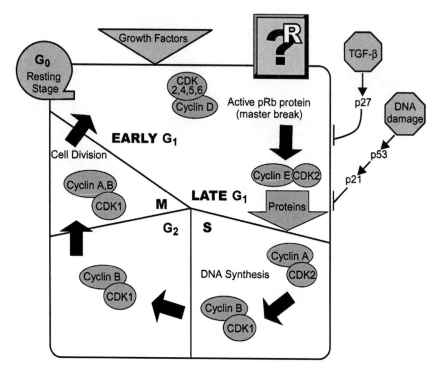

Figure 3.11   The Cell Cycle
Reproduced from Merkle CJ, Loescher LJ. The Biology of Cancer. In Yarbro CH, Frogge MH, and Goodman M (eds). *Cancer Nursing: Principles and Practice*, 6th ed. Sudbury, MA: Jones and Bartlett; 2005;15.

During the G_1 phase, the cell produces new proteins that will make DNA in preparation for cell division. The cell enlarges, and the time spent in this phase is highly variable. If division is not needed or if the cellular conditions are not right (the cell is too small or there are insufficient nutrients), then the cell goes into a resting phase called G_0. Near the end of G_1, the cell decides whether to commit to cell division, and this is called a *restriction point*. Weinberg (2014) describes this as a time when the molecular switch needs to be moved from the "off" mode to "on" mode, as follows: Cyclins D then E combine/activate CDKs, enzymes that then transfer phosphate groups from adenosine triphosphate (ATP), the energy molecule, to the retinoblastoma protein (pRB), which is the "master brake" of the cell cycle. If no phosphate groups are added to pRB, the brake keeps the cell cycle in the "off" position; however, the brake is lifted when sufficient phosphate groups are added to pRB.

Today, there are two agents that interrupt the cell cycle by blocking cyclin-dependent kinase (CDK) 4 and CDK6. Two of the most important CDKs are CDK4 and CDK 6, and these are often taken over by malignant cells. CDK inhibitors stop the cell cycle from proceeding from the G_1 phase to the S phase; thus cell proliferation is halted. Two CDK inhibitors have been FDA approved: palbociclib (Ibrance) and ribociclib (Kisqali), which are both indicated in postmenopausal women with ER-positive breast, HER2 negative, advanced or metastatic breast cancer.

When the brake on the cell cycle clock is lifted, transcription factors are released that interact with genes (turns them on or off) so that proteins are actively synthesized for moving the cell cycle through its stages. Studies have helped us better understand the role of cyclin D1 in breast cancer. Normally, the *BRCA1* gene is a tumor-suppressor gene that acts to protect against cancer by making a protein that binds to the BRCA1 docking site on the estrogen receptor. Cyclin D1 binds to the same estrogen receptor alpha as the BRCA1 protein, and it antagonizes or competes with the BCRA1 protein. Unfortunately, in 50% of breast cancer patients, cyclin D1 is overexpressed (Casimiro et al., 2012) and contributes to breast cancer tumorigenesis. This overexpression takes over the ER-alpha binding, thus negating BRCA1's repression of estrogen-responsive genes. Overexpression of cyclin D1 correlates with resistance to tamoxifen in postmenopausal women with breast cancer (Yishii et al., 2008), and to a poor prognosis in ER-alpha positive breast cancer. What complicates cyclin D1 as a target is that in some instances it confers a better prognosis in certain patients with breast cancer.

Genomic instability occurs when there are cellular mutations that are perpetuated through the cell cycle, and each resulting daughter cell may have many more mutations that the original parent cell. The mutated DNA is permitted to cycle through the cell cycle when DNA damage control is impaired through mutations of the policing *p53* ("gene police" or "guardian of the genome") or *pRB* ("guardian of the genome") genes or their protein products. Once the "gene police and genome guardian" are unable to patrol or stop the cell cycle, the tumor cells can continue to proliferate.

Well, what other factors can turn a gene on or off, besides transcription factors, which are regulated by genes that can mutate? Most mutations as discussed involve changes in DNA that silence (tumor-suppressor) or activate (oncogene) genes. Epigenetics can help explain how the environment can influence gene expression. Epigenetics refers to the fact that there is an extra layer of instructions in the chromosome that influences which genes get turned off or are silenced without altering the DNA sequence. This silencing of genes without mutational changes in DNA (that occur during cell division or mitosis) is becoming more important and has been linked to the silencing of tumor-suppressor genes in a number of malignancies. This can occur through DNA methylation and histone deacetylation (Claus & Lubbert, 2003). These two exciting areas offer new targets, and we have already seen the success of azacytidine (Vidaza®) and decitabine (Sprycel®) in the treatment of myelodysplastic syndrome (MDS). Let's take a moment to look at these mechanisms.

DNA METHYLATION

Whether or not the DNA is methylated influences gene transcription. DNA methylation means that a methyl group is added to part of the chemical structure (cytosine ring), and this methyl group sticks out into a major groove of the DNA helix so it inhibits or stops transcription of the gene located on that part of the DNA (Herman & Baylen, 2003). This occurs mostly in CpG-rich islands, as they are called, located near promoter regions of genes. At least 50% of the human genes, including housekeeping genes, have these CpG island-containing promoter regions, but they are generally unmethylated (Jones & Baylen, 2007). Hypermethylation occurs in myelodysplastic syndrome and acute leukemia, and the activity of two hypomethylating agents has led to their FDA approval for treating MDS: 5-azacitidine and decitabine, found in *Chapter 1*. These agents get into the DNA and trap methyltransferases (enzymes that help put the methyl into the DNA) on the DNA strand so that there can be no further methylation when the cell goes to divide again. However, they do not remove methyl groups from existing genes. As expected, unlike chemotherapy, which kills or stops the growth of cancer cells right away, hypomethylating agents probably require prolonged therapy to get the optimal efficacy.

HISTONE DEACETYLATION
Another exciting group of agents in the arsenal is the histone deacetylase (HDAC) inhibitor class. The chromosomal DNA is wrapped around histones, a specific type of protein. The histones determine how tightly the chromatin or DNA is wrapped: If it is tightly wrapped, the gene is turned off or silenced; if it is loosely wrapped, the gene is turned on. Imagine a coiled Slinky® toy. When the Slinky coils are on a flat surface, the coils lie tight against one another; this is analogous to the histones tightly packing the DNA so that the DNA cannot open and express the gene. The gene is thus turned off. In contrast, when the Slinky is placed on a step and slides down to the next step, the space between the Slinky rings is open; this is analogous to the histone being loosely coiled, so that the DNA is open, and the gene can be expressed or turned on.

Normally, HDACs combine with cell regulatory proteins to regulate gene transcription (copying the recipe for that gene's protein onto mRNA to be taken outside of the nucleus to the ribosome, or protein synthesis factory) and are key components of cell proliferation, angiogenesis, apoptosis, and cell differentiation. Histone deacetylators remove the acetyl groups from proteins, such as histones and transcription factors, causing the chromatin to be tightly wrapped, thus shutting off the genes. Some cancer cells have overexpression of HDACs, or they recruit extra HDACs to oncogene transcription factors, causing hypoacetylation. This results in tightening of the chromatin structure and silencing of genes, such as tumor-suppressor genes. HDAC inhibitors cause hyperacetylation, which decreases expression of oncogenes such as BCR-ABL and HER-2, stops the cell cycle, induces apoptosis, and stops angiogenesis and cell motility (George et al., 2005). HDAC inhibitors are intended to help malignant cells become normal again, since they target and accumulate in malignant cells. Examples of HDAC inhibitors are vorinostat (Zolinza®) and romidepsin (Isodax®), FDA approved for the treatment of progressive or recurrent symptoms of cutaneous T-cell lymphoma (CTCL), and belinostat (Beleodaq®), FDA approved for the treatment of patients with relapsed or refractory peripheral T-cell lymphoma (PTCL).

Tumor cells are quite clever in using alternative pathways for signal transduction of messages demanding cell proliferation, if the first pathway is blocked.

As tumor biology studies reveal key mutated genes, often drugs can be developed to target the flawed gene. For example, in acute myeloid leukemia, at least 25% of patients have a mutation in the FLT3 (FMS-like tyrosine kinase 3) gene, which makes (encodes for) an RTK that helps control proliferation, differentiation, and cell death of normal hematopoietic cells (Stirewalt & Radich, 2003). Stimulation of FLT3 receptor kinases results in activation of many downstream pathways, including PI3K/Akt (protein kinase B) and MAPK (Takahashi, 2011). Midostaurin (Rydapt) has recently been FDA approved for treatment of patients with (1) newly diagnosed FLT3 mutation-positive AML, in combination with standard chemotherapy and (2) aggressive systemic mastocytosis, systemic mastocytosis with associated hematologic neoplasm, or mast cell leukemia (Novartis, 2017).

TURNING BACK ON EMBRYOLOGIC FEATURES

Interestingly, many of the events that occur in embryogenesis are reactivated during carcinogenesis. Normally, the "software" that guides embryogenesis is turned on when needed; then when the fetus is formed, it is turned off. Apparently, however, the "software" is still present in all cells, so when the cell transforms into a malignant cell, the software can become activated again (Weinberg, 2014). To appreciate how powerful this pathway is, one must understand that the migration of embryologic tissue to the right anatomic area depends upon Hedgehog signaling. For example, the neural tissue that becomes the spinal cord has to migrate to the center of the body. The arms and legs have to form, and the fingers and toes have to be oriented perfectly so the thumb is where it should be and the baby finger in the right place. This is all dependent upon the Hedgehog signaling pathway. The Hedgehog genes code for a soluble secreted protein that ensures that the developing embryologic tissues reach the correct size, location, and cellular content. After the fetus is formed and the baby is born, the Hedgehog signaling software is largely turned off; however, the software is still in our cells. In the case of basal cell cancer formation, the Hedgehog pathway becomes reactivated and leads to malignant transformation in the skin. In fact, more than 90% of patients with basal cell cancer have mutations in one of two genes, turning the Hedgehog pathway back on. Normally, the pathway is turned off. In the resting state, the Patched (PTCH) receptor prevents the activation of the pathway by inhibiting the second protein, Smoothened (SMO). When the Hedgehog ligand is secreted, it binds to and inactivates PTCH. Without PTCH control, SMO is activated and signaling events begin, resulting in the transcription of Hedgehog target genes: those involved in cell proliferation, development, and tissue maintenance, including stem cells. The tumor microenvironment can also secrete Hedgehog ligands that support tumor growth. Vismodegib (Erivedge®) is the first Hedgehog pathway inhibitor to be FDA approved. This drug binds to and inhibits SMO, so signal transduction is shut down. A second FDA approved Hedgehog pathway inhibitor is sonidegib (Odomzo®), which is also indicated for the treatment of patients with recurrent, locally advanced basal cell carcinoma or patients who are not candidates for surgery or RT.

INDUCING ANGIOGENESIS

Many similarities exist between angiogenesis and tumor invasion and, as a result, they may have similar molecular targets. The body normally needs the ability to make new blood vessels for processes such as wound healing, female menstruation, rebuilding the endometrial lining, or making the placenta during pregnancy. The body maintains a fine balance between turning angiogenesis on and turning it off. When there are more factors favoring angiogenesis than opposing it (inhibitors), angiogenesis occurs. When cells are hypoxic or lacking oxygen, they release vascular endothelial growth factor (VEGF), also known as vascular permeability factor. VEGF initiates new blood vessel growth and causes the release of nitric oxide (NO) from the endothelial cells lining the blood vessel, which causes them to dilate. Tumors need to build new blood vessels when, as the small tumor grows, there is 2 mm or more between the nearest blood vessel and the small tumor. This is because 2 mm (the size of a pencil lead) is the diffusion distance of oxygen (Folkman, 2006). The tumor sends out VEGF to build a new blood vessel by telling the endothelial cells lining the blood vessel to proliferate and to migrate; the process is helped by other molecules. See Figure 3.12. Malignant blood vessels are flawed: they are leaky, disorganized, may have blind channels that do not connect with other vessels, and they have many different diameters so that parts of the tumor fed by narrow vessels with low blood flow remain hypoxic and resistant to chemotherapy, as chemotherapy does not reach that area.

VEGF and its receptor (VEGFR) on the endothelial cell are essential for angiogenesis. VEGF is a family of glycoproteins: VEGF-A is essential for blood vessel formation, and it is commonly referred to as VEGF (Takahashi & Shibuya, 2005). VEGF-B may be a redundant ligand; VEGF-C and VEGF-D appear to be involved with lymphangiogenesis. The VEGF ligands bind to VEGFR (receptors) 1, 2, and 3 (Flt-4), which then stimulate a signaling cascade, resulting in endothelial cell (vascular or lymphangenic) proliferation, migration, and survival. VEGFR-2 is most commonly associated with VEGF-A, but VEGFR-1 also may be linked to VEGF-A. In developing agents to target the ligand VEGF or the receptor VEGFR, some agents are selective for VEGF, like the monoclonal antibody bevacizumab (Avastin®), whereas others are oral, small-molecule TKIs that target VEGF receptors (VEGFR), such as axitinib (VEGFR-1, 2, 3). Other agents are multitargeted for VEGFR, as well as other related or unrelated targets, such as sorafenib (Nexavar®),

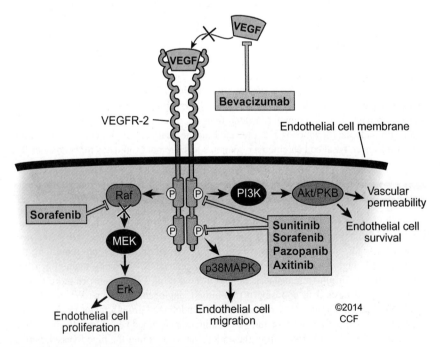

Figure 3.12   The Angiogenesis Cascade

which inhibits VEGFR-2, PDGFR-β, and Raf kinase; and sunitinib (Sutent®), which inhibits (VEGFR-1, 2, 3), stem cell factor receptor (KIT), fms-like tyrosine kinase-3 (FLT-3), colony-stimulating factor receptor type 1 (CSF-1R), and the glial cell-line-derived neurotrophic factor receptor (RET). It is becoming clear that angiogenesis occurs earlier in the malignant process, as it is necessary in the microenvironment to help selected transformed cells invade and metastasize.

The most important VEGFR appears to be VEGFR-2. When the ligand VEGF attaches to VEGFR (receptor) on the endothelial cell, the receptor dimerizes (comes together as partners with another cell surface receptor, which activates the phosphorylation message through the cell membrane), and the message for proliferation and migration of endothelial cells is sent to the endothelial cell nucleus via a tyrosine kinase bucket brigade-like system.

Antiangiogenesis agents can be divided into at least four categories based on their mechanism of action: (1) Agents that prevent VEGF from reaching their receptors on the endothelial cell (e.g., bevacizumab (Avastin), and the VEGF trap aflibercept (Zaltrap®)); (2) agents that block signaling within the endothelial cell so the nucleus of the endothelial cell never gets the message to proliferate and migrate to form the new blood vessel (e.g., small-molecule TKIs sunitinib (Sutent), sorafinib (Nexavar), cabozantinib (Cabometyx®, Cometriq®)); (3) agents that interfere with the response to hypoxia such as the mTOR inhibitors everolimus (Afinitor), temsirolimus (Torisel); and (4) agents that interfere with signals from the stroma asking for more blood vessels (e.g., thalidomide (Thalomid®), lenalidomide (Revlimid®), and pomalidomide (Pomalyst®), all immunomodulatory agents).

In the absence of antiangiogenic agents, once VEGF stimulates the endothelial cells to proliferate and migrate, the newly forming tube needs help to move through the extracellular matrix. Integrins, specifically α5β1 integrin, are proteins on the proliferating endothelial cell that act like grappling hooks to help it move toward the tumor. The sprouting endothelial tube has to migrate or move toward the tumor, and it does this by having the integrin on the endothelial cell attach to fibronectin in the extracellular matrix. The integrins then act like grappling hooks to move the new blood vessel tube to the tumor. New agents are being developed to block integrin binding so that the new blood vessel sprout cannot move toward the tumor; the proliferating endothelial cell cannot bind to fibronectin, and thus, it undergoes apoptosis (programmed cell death).

Of interest, clinical trials with bevacizumab (Avastin) showed not only the cessation of tumor angiogenesis and growth but also tumor regression, suggesting that when combined with chemotherapy, antiangiogenesis agents alter the tumor blood flow so that the chemotherapy is more effective in killing tumor cells. Thus, the mechanism of bevacizumab is thought to be twofold: blocking (1) development of new blood vessels and (2) VEGF, which is necessary for the maintenance of existing malignant blood vessels, so existing blood vessels actually normalize; this then increases blood flow within the tumor so that concomitantly administered chemotherapy can now enter the tumor more uniformly. In addition, it has been shown that there are VEGF receptors on tumor cells, and that VEGF-mediated signaling contributes to cancer stem cell function and tumor initiation (Goel & Mercurio, 2013). The VEGFR tyrosine kinases and neuropilins (NRTKs that bind VEGF and are implicated in tumor progression) are essential for mediating VEGF influence on tumor cells as they regulate the function and trafficking of growth factor receptors and integrins (Goel & Mercurio, 2013). VEGF also functions in the surrounding tumor microenvironment: (1) immune cells can express VEGFR which then allows VEGF to regulate them; (2) macrophages in the hypoxic tumor environment release VEGF, as do (3) fibroblasts in the tumor stoma (Goel & Mercurio, 2013). Thus, antiangiogenesis agents appear to directly affect tumor cells (Goel & Mercurio, 2013).

Mancuso et al. (2006) have shown in the laboratory that antiangiogenesis agents reduce the tumor blood vessels by 50–60%, but the empty sleeves of the blood vessels in the basement membrane remain, along with nonmalignant-appearing pericytes (provide strength to the new blood vessel but can also differentiate into a fibroblast, smooth muscle cell, or macrophage if needed). One day after the antiangiogenesis drug was stopped, new blood vessels sprouted in the empty sleeves in the basement membrane, connected to nearby capillaries, and by 7 days after the drug was stopped, tumors were fully revascularized and protected with tumor-related pericytes. However, when the tumor was again re-treated with an antiangiogenesis drug, the regrown vasculature regressed as much as it did the first time. This suggests that the empty sleeves of the basement membrane, as well as the pericytes, should be targeted by anticancer therapies; it also suggests that perhaps antiangiogenic drugs should be continued after tumor progression with just a change in the chemotherapy. New agents with the ability to target multiple receptors continue to be developed.

Platelet-derived growth factor (PDGF) is necessary for the pericytes, which give the newly formed blood vessel stability, much like the shingles of a house give it protection. Sorafenib (Nexavar), a multiple-targeted protein TKI, appears to block the Raf kinase step in the ras pathway, VEGFR-2, and PDGF-β.

Drugs such as bevacizumab (Avastin) neutralize VEGF, which is released by tumors to start the process of angiogenesis. This drug, in combination with chemotherapy, has produced statistically significant increased response rates, time to progression, and overall survival in patients with metastatic colon, rectal, and lung cancers. It was thought that giving patients adjuvant chemotherapy and bevacizumab for stage II/III colon cancer would prevent metastasis and increase the cure rate. However, the NSABP C-08 results reported that at 3 years, there was no statistical difference in DFS or OS. However, the patients received adjuvant chemotherapy with bevacizumab for 6 months, then bevacizumab alone for 6 months. During this time, there was a 40% reduction in disease progression that was statistically significant ($p < .0004$), which disappeared after the first year. The implication is that while this was a negative study, it may also indicate that the bevacizumab needed to be continued for 3 years to make a significant difference in DFS and as a surrogate, OS.

Normal blood vessels supply oxygen and nutrients to a cell and remove waste products. Blood vessels have an inner lining that is made up of endothelial cells that are tightly joined with their neighbors, surrounded by a basement membrane containing pericytes, which act like shingles on a house to protect the endothelial cells. Blood vessels have sensors that identify when more oxygen is needed by the tissue (e.g., oxygen and hypoxia-induced sensors or receptors). The blood vessel can then dilate to allow more blood to come to the tissue.

Hypoxia, as well as some other signals, can activate cells to release angiogenic growth factors, such as VEGF, Ang-2, FGF, and chemokines, which stimulate new blood vessel capillaries to grow from nearby existing blood vessels, a process called angiogenesis. For example, solid tumors cannot grow beyond 2 mm without building new blood vessels, as this is the diffusion distance of oxygen, so they release VEGF, among other substances, to build more blood vessels.

THE PROCESS OF ANGIOGENESIS IS USUALLY TIGHTLY CONTROLLED

• Hypoxia causes angiogenic growth factors to be released to promote new blood vessel capillary growth.

• Pericytes detach from the vessel (resulting from Ang-2 signaling).

• The growth factors bind to receptors on the endothelial cells of a nearby blood vessel, activating the endothelial cells. Once activated, the endothelial cells move away from their neighboring endothelial cells as the blood vessel dilates (VE-cadherin is responsible for the tight endothelial junctions, so VE-cadherin signaling allows the endothelial cells to loosen their junctions).

• Once activated, the endothelial cells send a signal from the cell membrane into the cell nucleus telling the nucleus (genes) to make new molecules, including enzymes, such as matrix metalloproteinases (MMPs), which dissolve tiny holes in the basement membrane of the blood vessels.

• The endothelial cells are stimulated to divide, making more endothelial cells that migrate through the holes in the basement membrane and move toward the injured tissue or malignant cells that released the growth factor, like tiny sprouting new blood vessels.

• The tip cell, at the end of the sprout, is selected (by VEGF/VEGFR, NOTCH/DLL4, neuropilin, and JAGGED1 signaling) and releases MMPs, which remodel the extracellular matrix so that the fragile blood vessel can pass through the matrix toward the tumor.

• The tip cells are guided by filopodia (cytoplasmic projections that act as small feet) as the sprout migrates toward the area where the antigenic signal came from (e.g., tumor-releasing VEGF).

• Stalk cells follow the tip cell and proliferate, extending the sprout and releasing substances like EGFL7 (EGF-like domain containing protein 7, vascular endothelial statin), which help it to bind to the extracellular matrix and also regulate the formation of the lumen of the blood vessel. Tip cells do not proliferate.

• Adhesion molecules (integrins $\alpha v\beta 3$, $\alpha v\beta 5$) act like little grappling hooks and pull the sprouting new blood vessels forward toward the tumor.

• Additional enzymes (matrix metalloproteinases, MMPs) are made that dissolve the tissue in front of the sprouting blood vessel so that it can continue to move toward the tumor. After the blood vessel moves forward, the MMPs remodel the tissue to anchor the blood vessel.

• When two tip cells of neighboring sprouts come together, the vessels fuse to form a continuous blood vessel tube or lumen.

• Extracellular matrix is used to make a basement membrane to stabilize the new vessel; endothelial cells stop proliferating, and pericytes are attached to also stabilize the new vessel (recruited by PDGFR/PDGF-B, Ang-1).

• Blood begins to flow from the parent blood vessel to the new blood vessel loops; oxygen in the blood vessel turns off the oxygen sensors in the endothelial cell and turns down angiogenic stimuli (VEGF expression), so building of the blood vessel is completed.

Table 3.2 lists agents currently FDA approved as antiangiogenic agents. In addition, altering the dose and administration schedule of some standard chemotherapy agents appears to change the mechanism of action so that the drug acts to prevent angiogenesis. As

Table 3.2   Selected Targeted Agents That Inhibit Angiogenesis

   I. Monoclonal antibodies that bind to proangiogenic growth factors or their receptors: bevacizumab (Avastin), ziv-aflibercept (Zaltrap), ramucirumab (Cyramza®).
  II. Tyrosine kinase inhibitors that block single or multiple proangiogenic growth factor receptor signals: axitinib (Inlyta®), cabozantinib capsules and tablets (Cometriq®, Cabometyx®), lenvatinib (Lenvima®), pazopanib (Votrient®), regorafenib (Stivarga®), sorafenib (Nexavar), sunitinib (Sutent), vandetanib (Caprelsa®).
 III. mTOR (mammalian target of rapamycin) inhibitors that block the response to hypoxia: everolimus (Afinitor), temsirolimus (Torisel).
  IV. Fusion Proteins: Ziv-aflibercept (Zaltrap®)
   V. Agents that may indirectly inhibit angiogenesis through mechanisms not completely understood: the immunomodulatory agents thalidomide (Thalomid), lenalidomide (Revlimid), pomalidomide (Pomalyst); Interferon alfa (Intron®, Roferon®)

The Angiogenesis Foundation, https://angio.org/learn/treatments/, accessed October 15, 2019; Chau CH, Figg WD. Antiangiogenesis Agents. Chapter 28 in DeVita VT, Lawrence TS, Rosenberg SA (eds.) *Cancer: Principles & Practice of Oncology*, 10th ed. Philadelphia, PA: Wolters Kluwer/Lippincott Williams & Wilkins, 2015.

illustrated in the complex steps of metastasis, there are many opportunities for interruption, causing the arrest of the metastatic cascade.

Drugs that inhibit angiogenesis, either by neutralizing the binding of the ligand VEGF to its receptor (e.g., bevacizumab) or by blocking signaling within the endothelial cell (e.g., sunitinib or sorafinib), or the response to hypoxia (e.g., mTOR inhibitors), may all cause (drug) class-related effects. These include hypertension, believed related to the blockade of nitric oxide, which is necessary for the walls of arterioles and other resistance vessels to relax; rare gastrointestinal perforation with unknown relationship; and bleeding events (epistaxis) with rare hemorrhage. Hypertension is usually amenable to treatment; now, angiotensin-converting enzyme (ACE) inhibitors or angiotensin II receptor blockers are preferred treatment, as they have low interaction potential with angiogenesis inhibitors, help reduce proteinuria, and prevent the expression of plasminogen-activator inhibitor-1 (which may be stimulated by angiogenesis inhibitors and increases the risk of thrombosis) (Izzedine et al., 2009; Wang & Lockhart, 2012). Maitland et al. (2010) on behalf of a consensus group made recommendations for the initial assessment, surveillance, and management of patients receiving VEGF signaling pathway inhibitors. Recommendations included controlling preexisting hypertension before initiation of a VEGF pathway inhibitor, actively monitoring BP during treatment, especially at the beginning of treatment in the first cycle, targeting a BP goal of < 140/90 (lower in patients with cardiovascular risk factors), maximizing the dose of each antihypertensive agent and adding agents based on the individual risk and comorbidities, and adding dietary and exercise interventions appropriate to the patient's clinical status. Another important issue that arises with the tyrosine protein kinases sunitinib and sorafinib is a possible reduction in left ventricular ejection fraction (LVEF).

Blockade of an angiogenesis growth factor/signaling pathway may make tumor growth worse over time, as alternate pathways for angiogenesis emerge despite the fact that theoretically, by normalizing tumor blood vessels, the tumor cells remain oxygenated, may be less likely to metastasize, and be more responsive to antitumor chemotherapy. Histidine-rich glycoproteins (HGP) are found in the tumor stroma, modulate immunity, cell adhesion, and angiogenesis and may be an excellent anticancer target (Johnson et al., 2014).

AVOIDANCE OF APOPTOSIS (PROGRAMMED CELL DEATH), ENABLING REPLICATIVE IMMORTALITY

Mutations can also occur in the genes that make important inhibitory proteins that would otherwise stop the cell cycle from progressing forward, specifically p53, pRB, p16, and p15. This is important because the cell's DNA is examined by DNA repair genes to see whether there are any mutations or mistakes and, if so, whether they can be repaired. If the DNA cannot be repaired, p53 causes the cell to go into "programmed cell death," or apoptosis. This normally eliminates any abnormal cells from the body so that the cells undergoing cell division all have intact DNA. However, in cancer, mutations often occur in the DNA repair genes as discussed under BRCA-1 and 2. Unfortunately, in over 50% of cancers, p53 is inactive (Soussi & Wiman, 2007). In some cancers, such as cervical cancer, both p53 and pRB are inactivated (Weinberg, 2014), and in SCLC and retinoblastoma, pRB is lost. Other proteins such as the cyclins or CDK, which can be synthesized in greater number, or loss of CDK inhibitors, can move the cell through the cell cycle relentlessly. Most cancers have some abnormalities in the cell cycle machinery, and each of these becomes a molecular flaw that can be targeted.

Many of the genes mutated during malignant transformation are those responsible for control of the mTOR pathway; for example, a loss of PTEN, a tumor-suppressor gene, activates mTOR signaling. mTOR is a member of the phosphatidylinositide kinase (PIK) subgroup of serine/threonine protein kinases. The other members of this family act as checkpoints in controlling DNA damage repair while mTOR controls nutrient and energy signaling and exists as two distinct complexes.

The cell cycle is responsible for cell proliferation, and CDKs regulate cells moving through the cell cycle. Cyclins regulate the activity of CDKs. mTOR controls cell proliferation by controlling cyclin D_1, which in turn controls key CDKs (4 & 6) that are responsible for moving the cell through the G_1-S restriction point. Cyclin D_1 is involved in transcribing genes, cell metabolism, and cell migration (Fu et al., 2004). Thus, malignant transformation and mutations in upstream signaling proteins can "turn on" mTOR, resulting in overexpression of Cyclin D_1 and cell proliferation in a number of cancers (breast, colon, prostate, and melanoma). Cancer cells damaged by chemotherapy are either able to repair the damaged DNA or are able to tell the cell to ignore the fact that the DNA is damaged. Normally, cells without intact DNA that cannot be repaired undergo programmed cell death (apoptosis). Activated mTOR controls p21, a gene product that stops the cell cycle so that the damaged DNA can be repaired.

Additionally, mTOR plays a central role in angiogenesis, as it controls production of hypoxia-inducible factor (HIF) proteins HIF1-α and HIF1-β. HIF is a critical transcription factor that allows the expression of genes whose products (proteins) are involved in angiogenesis, as well as cell proliferation, motility, adhesion, and survival—all qualities necessary for tumor progression and metastases (Semenza, 2003). HIF induces gene expression to produce VEGF (which stimulates endothelial cells to proliferate and migrate toward the tumor in a new tube) and angiopoietin-2 (destabilizes existing blood vessels so they can develop the tube extension in concert with VEGF and then will grow toward the tumor). Angiogenesis is tightly controlled. Hypoxia tips the balance toward angiogenesis to increase the oxygen delivered to tissues and is mediated by HIF, which is controlled by the von Hippel-Lindau (VHL) protein, a tumor-suppressor. During hypoxia, HIF is released so new blood vessels can be stimulated, and when tissue is oxygenated, HIF is rapidly broken down. In the presence of very high levels of HIF, apoptosis occurs (Semenza, 2003). When tumors subvert the upstream signaling pathways, mTOR is activated, and high levels of HIF are produced; if HVL protein is mutated or lost, HIF is not broken down, and high levels persist. This way the tumor can get the proteins and essential nutrients it needs to continue to proliferate and have adequate energy even in hypoxic conditions (Shaw, 2006). Activated mTOR also upregulates VEGF-C, which is associated with lymphangiogenesis (Kobayashi et al., 2007).

Clearly, if mTOR Complex 1 can be blocked, this theoretically will turn off cell proliferation and survival. Analogues (or "rapalogues") of rapamycin (sirolimus) are temsirolimus and everolimus. Temsirolimus (Torisel) is the first FDA-approved mTOR inhibitor and is indicated for the treatment of patients with advanced renal cell cancer, as its study endpoint of increased survival was met. Many of these patients had poor prognostic features. Everolimus (Afinitor) is FDA approved for treatment of patients with postmenopausal advanced hormone receptor-positive, HER2-negative breast cancer together with exemestane, advanced renal cell cancer, advanced pancreatic neuroendocrine tumor (PNET), and also patients with subependymal giant cell astrocytoma (SEGA). This is especially interesting because inhibition of mTOR Complex 1 primarily results in a cytostatic response rather than a cytotoxic one. It is expected that these agents may be combined with cytotoxic chemotherapy or other agents.

PI3K (phosphatidylinositide 3-kinases) is a family of intracellular signaling proteins that are important in many cell functions, such as cell migration, proliferation, differentiation, and survival. PI3K is part of the PI3K-AKT (also known as protein kinase B)-mTOR pathway. PI3K-delta is expressed on white blood cells, but it is critical for signaling, development, migration, and survival of B lymphocytes. Idelalisib (Zydelig) inhibits proliferation of malignant B lymphocytes, as well as cell signaling (B-cell receptor, CXCR4, CXCR5), which is involved in telling B lymphocytes how to migrate to the lymph nodes and bone marrow (e.g., trafficking and homing in to the lymph nodes and bone marrow). It is FDA approved for treatment of patients with (1) relapsed CLL together with rituximab, (2) relapsed follicular B-cell NHL after at least two prior systemic therapies, and (3) relapsed small lymphocytic lymphoma after at least two prior systemic therapies (Gilead, 2014).

The genes that produce p53 and pRB are also active in regulating normal cell aging or senescence, leading to programmed cell death. All somatic cells have a finite life of 50–60 doublings, after which the cell dies. At the end of the chromosomes, caps called *telomeres* count each of the cell divisions and snip off a piece of the chromosome with each division. After 50–60 divisions, the chromosome is too short to divide again. In a developing embryo, where there is rapid cell division, the chromosome is protected from being snipped off with each division by the enzyme telomerase, which replaces each snipped piece. This enzyme is not found in normal cells after the embryo develops into a fetus but is found in all tumor cells. If there is a mutation that inactivates either of these genes, the cells can use telomerase to replace each of the snipped off pieces of chromosome to become immortal. Again, telomerase becomes a molecular target. However, studies have not consistently found significant levels of telomerase in tumors.

As dividing cells progress through the cell cycle, at specific restriction points, the DNA is assessed for fidelity in copying as the DNA is replicated. If there are errors, specific repair genes attempt to correct the mistakes (mutations). If the mutation cannot be corrected, the cell is directed by p53 to undergo programmed cell death (apoptosis). Poly ADP-ribose polymerase (PARP) enzymes play a central role in DNA repair in cancer cells, and as such are considered excellent targets for therapy. These enzymes are also very important in repairing the damage from chemotherapy, which causes damage to DNA. BRCA1 and BRCA2 are also involved in repair of DNA damage from chemotherapy. Patients with mutations in BRCA1/BRCA2 depend upon PARP1 to repair DNA damage. Thus, as discussed, PARP inhibitors are being studied in patients with triple negative breast cancer, which appears to share some similar molecular features as those with BRCA1/BRCA2 mutations, and thus is also dependent upon PARP1 for repair of DNA damage.

Apoptosis is a critical process to ensure the survival of the species. It is invoked when DNA damage is not repaired, to control the cell number and proliferation during normal development, and removal of certain self-reacting lymphocytes (Ghobrial et al., 2005). Certain leukemias and lymphomas have defects in the apoptotic process so that they have immortal clones of cells, while other tumors have defects in the apoptotic regulatory pathways such as p53, nuclear factor kappa B (NFkB) or in the phosphatidylinositol-3-kinase (PI3K)/Akt pathway (Ghobrial et al., 2005). See Figure 3.13 for the extrinsic and intrinsic pathways of apoptosis.

Bcl-2 is a family of proteins that regulate apoptosis and includes proapoptotic members which encourage the cell to undergo apoptosis (Bax, Bak, Bad, Bcl-X, Bid, Bik, Bim, and Hrk) and antiapoptotic proteins which prevent apoptosis (Bcl-2, Bcl-X$_L$, Bcl-W, Mcl-1, and Bfl-1) (Ghobrial et al., 2005). The antiapoptotic proteins stop apoptosis by blocking the release of cytochrome-C from the mitochondria, while proapoptotic members promote apoptosis. Whether apoptosis occurs depends upon the balance between Bcl-2 and Bax. Bcl-2 is often overexpressed in cancer, resulting in resistance to chemotherapy and RT (Ghobrial et al., 2005).

A number of agents are being investigated that target Bcl-2 or other proteins that may suppress apoptosis. Since the antiapoptotic Bcl-2 protein inhibits apoptosis and makes the cells resistant to treatment with standard chemotherapy, drugs such as antisense oligonucleotides can theoretically disable Bcl-2 and restore responsiveness to chemotherapy. More work on Bcl-2 inhibitors has resulted in the development of a direct inhibitor of the antiapoptotic protein Bcl-2. Venetoclax (Venclexta®) has been FDA approved for the treatment of patients with CLL having a 17p (short arm of chromosome 17) deletion who have received at least one prior therapy (AbbVie, Genentech, 2018). Venetoclax is a selective small-molecule inhibitor of the Bcl-2 antiapoptotic protein and helps restore the apoptotic process by binding directly to Bcl-2 and displacing the proapoptotic proteins like BIM, thus making the mitochondrial membrane permeable and releasing cytochrome-C; this leads to activation of the caspase proenzymes and ultimately the rest of the caspase cascade, so that

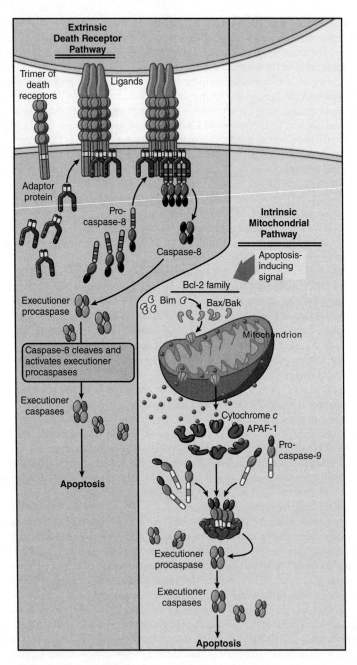

Figure 3.13   **Apoptosis**

apoptosis occurs. Overexpression of Bcl-2 has been shown in CLL cells to increase leukemic cell survival and resistance to chemotherapy (AbbVie, Genentech, 2018).

There are two apoptotic pathways leading to cell death, the extrinsic and intrinsic pathways. Both pathways ultimately join at the end using caspases (enzymes) to break apart the dying cell. As more is known about the pathophysiology of apoptosis, new drugs will emerge. Apo2L/TRAIL agents are being studied. (TRAIL stands for tumor necrosis factor (TNF)–related apoptosis-inducing ligand; it activates two cell-death pathways, resulting in apoptosis of cancer cells while normal cells are relatively resistant, and it is synergistic with chemotherapy.)

In the last decade, we have seen many new targeted agents. Bortezomib (Velcade®) is the first of the proteasome inhibitor class that is FDA approved for cancer therapy, specifically multiple myeloma, as it interferes with the interaction of the myeloma cells with the bone marrow microenvironment; and a second-generation proteasome inhibitor is approved (carfilzomib, Kyprolis®). Proteasomes are enzyme complexes that are housekeeping enzymes, which degrade or break down proteins in the cell nucleus that are no longer needed, and turn off key processes such as the cell cycle. The proteins are recycled and used again. They are found in every cell of the body. The proteasomes know which proteins to degrade because they are tagged with ubiquitin, a small protein. The ubiquitin–proteasome pathway regulates protein homeostasis within the cell. Proteasome inhibitors block this process from occurring, so the cell gets conflicting signals about cell regulation. It can be thought of as an accumulation of unwanted proteins in the cell, including the powerful proteins p53, p27, and proapoptotic Bcl-2 family members (Almond & Cohen, 2002). This causes malignant cells to undergo apoptosis or programmed cell death, while normal cells are less sensitive to this overload and can recover.

Specifically, three pathways are affected by proteasome inhibition: the cell cycle (proteins active in the cell cycle such as cyclins, CDK, and the tumor-suppressor p53 protein), apoptosis (proteins that inhibit apoptosis like XIAP, cIAP, and Bcl-2 proteins), and NFkB dependent signaling (inhibitor of this pathway is I kappa B-alpha) (Glickman & Ciechanover, 2002). Nuclear Factor (NF)-kappa B is a transcription factor that has been found to regulate a number of genes that control malignant transformation and metastases. Inactive proteins p50, p65, I kappa B-alpha, and NF-kappa B are found in the cytoplasm of the cell (outside the nucleus). When NF-kappa B is activated by carcinogens, tumor promoter factors, inflammatory cytokines, and some chemotherapy agents, I kappa B-alpha is broken down and the other two proteins move into the nucleus. They attach to DNA in the nucleus at a promoter region and activate the gene. Once NFkB is activated, it can stop apoptosis, which leads to tumor formation and resistance to chemotherapy. There is much excitement about using chemoprevention strategies to block activation of NFkB by inhibiting its signaling pathway, much as the proteasome does. In addition, it theoretically increases tumor sensitivity to chemotherapy (Bharti & Aggarwal, 2002). One such preventive approach is with nonsteroidal anti-inflammatory drugs (NSAIDs), such as aspirin. Aspirin appears to induce signal-specific I kappa-B-alpha degradation, followed by NF-kappa B nuclear translocation, leading to apoptosis, in colorectal cancer cells (Din et al., 2004).

Tumor cells also have figured out how to become invisible to the immune system, by capitalizing on a homeostatic immune mechanism to avoid autoimmune damage to the host and down regulating the activation of T-lymphocytes. These include the immune checkpoint

Programmed Death-1 (PD-1) receptors and others, which are discussed in *Chapter 4* and under the section entitled "Avoiding Immune Destruction."

ACTIVATING INVASION AND METASTASIS

First, in order to be embolized, malignant epithelial cells must overcome two types of adhesion that keeps normal cells adhering to one another and attached to the protein meshwork around it (extracellular matrix), especially in epithelial tissue. This is important because most solid cancers are epithelial, arising from the epithelial cells covering the outer layer of skin or outer layer and lining of many organs, such as the gut and lungs.

Cell-to-cell adhesion molecules keep normal cells orderly. One molecule is especially important, E-cadherin, which ensures intercellular adhesion. Early studies show that when this molecule is manipulated in cancer cells, it changes a cell from a noninvasive cell to an invasive cell capable of forming tumors. When functional E-cadherin is restored, this tendency can be reversed. Malignant cells are able to inactivate E-cadherin and are released from this requirement of cell-to-cell adhesion.

In addition, for cell survival and reproduction, normal cells must adhere to the extracellular matrix. In laboratory tests, cells in culture cannot grow unless they attach to a surface or achieve *anchorage dependence* (Ruoslahti & Reed, 1994). The molecules on the cell surface that actually do the attachment are *integrins*. Integrins must be intact for cell growth and cell division. It appears that integrins influence a protein in the cell nucleus called cyclin E-CDK2 complex (CDK), which is necessary for the cell cycle clock to move toward cell growth and division. When cells do not adhere to the extracellular matrix, the lack of integrin adherence causes inhibition of cyclin E-CDK2 in the cell nucleus; the cell cycle clock stops; and the cell commits suicide (apoptosis). Unfortunately, cancer cells are able to circumvent this process, to become *anchorage independent* so cyclin E-CDK2 stays active whether or not the cell is attached, and cells keep growing and dividing, thus avoiding programmed death. In addition, with only a few exceptions (e.g., neutrophils), normal cells cannot penetrate the underlying basement membrane on which they rest, or go through basement membranes of blood vessels (endothelial lining). Like neutrophils, malignant cells release the enzymes called *matrix metalloproteinases (MMPs)* that dissolve parts of the basement membrane, as well as the extracellular matrix, so that like a military tank, the cells can migrate away from the primary tumor and into the neighboring tissue and blood vessels for the process of metastasis.

Once in the blood vessel, it is estimated that only one cell in 10,000 is successful in setting up a new metastatic site distant from the primary tumor. As stated, it must attach to the inner lining of capillaries and dissolve holes in the blood vessel basement membrane to escape into the extravascular tissue. It appears that most cells get trapped in the nearest capillary bed they encounter after leaving the primary tumor. Metastatic cells tend to be large and easily trapped, and many secrete clotting factors that cause platelets to aggregate around them. The primary destination for venous blood from most organs is the lungs; thus, this is the most common metastatic site. Venous blood leaves the gut and goes to the liver first; the liver is the most common metastatic site for intestinal tumors. It is unclear how a metastatic niche is determined where a new tumor may begin. It is possible that a subpopulation of cells in the primary tumor has identified the characteristics needed to survive in a specific niche (Oskkarsson et al., 2014). While research has identified cancer stem cells in some solid tumors, much research continues. Cancer stem cells are likely in the primary tumor, while a second set of metastatic stem cells arises that have the following traits: stemness or the ability of self-renewal and to differentiate into different types of cancer cells, ability to make blood vessels (angiogenesis), resistance to chemotherapy and radiotherapy, have the ability to change from epithelial cell to mesenchymal cells (epithelial mesenchymal transition, or EMT) so they can move from the initial location to other body areas, and the ability to initiate a tumor in a metastatic site (Boston Biomedical, 2016). The cancer stem cells have identified dysregulated signaling pathways: JAK/STAT, Wnt/B-catein, Hedgehog, Notch, and Nanog (Boston Biomedical, 2016). The microenvironment of the metastatic site is critical, and it releases growth factors to help the newly arrived metastatic cell survive.

By studying neutrophils, normal cells that migrate where needed to fight infection, Muller et al. (2001) were able to demonstrate that chemokines, soluble substances that carry messages between cells, are responsible for directing breast cancer cells to the primary organs where breast cancer metastasizes: lymph nodes, bone marrow, lung, and liver. Chemokines are small molecules that resemble cytokines and connect with specific receptors on the cell surface, causing rearrangement of the cell's cytoskeleton. This allows cells to adhere firmly to endothelial cells (lining blood vessels) and migrate in a specific direction. Chemokines work with integrins and other proteins on the surface of the cell to direct the breast cancer cells to specific organs. The authors found that breast cancer cells have functionally active chemokine receptors. When these receptors are activated by binding with a ligand (a substance that binds to a receptor on the cell surface and that turns on signal transduction within a cell), the cell activates actin (which gives structure to a cell) polymerization with the formation of pseudopods (fake feet) that allow the cell to migrate and invade tissue. The tissues in which these ligands are overexpressed are the primary metastatic sites in breast cancer. Further, in studies, by neutralizing interactions between the chemokines and their receptors, metastases to lymph nodes and lung could be inhibited. As more is learned about the process of metastases, new agents can be developed to inhibit each of the critical steps, thus preventing the process.

REPROGRAMMING OF ENERGY METABOLISM

Most body cells use glucose for an energy source, providing a high number of ATP, the energy currency of the cell, by mitochondrial oxidative phosphorylation. If there is insufficient oxygen, for example, in hypoxic conditions, anaerobic glycolysis is normally used. Cancer cells, however, use glycolysis as their primary energy process, whether there is enough oxygen or not. Glycolysis is very inefficient, and the number of ATP generated is 18 times less than if the cancer cell used glucose as an energy source (Hanahan & Weinberg, 2011). The end product of this process is lactate. This is called the Warburg effect, after Otto Warburg who first identified this metabolic abnormality. Of course, using such an inefficient system, cancer cells need more glucose, especially as they continue to proliferate, so they increase the number of glucose receptors (GLUT1) to import more glucose into the cells (Hanahan & Weinberg, 2011). Some cancers have this metabolic energy system but also have another, for cells that are better oxygenated, which import and use the lactate as the primary energy source (Hanahan & Weinberg, 2011). As discussed in the angiogenesis section, tumor blood vessels are poorly made, with areas of hypoxia and others of oxygenation. Having two systems would be useful if the tumor cells had sections that were hypoxic and others that were better oxygenated. It has been difficult to target this hallmark. About 20% of patients with AML and 5% of patients with MDS, have genotypes containing either a mutated isocitrate dehydrogenous 1 or 2 (IDH1 or IDH2) gene, which makes an important enzyme used by the mitochondria to make energy for cellular activities (Medeiros et al., 2017). Mutated IDH1 is considered an oncogene (Vogelstein et al., 2013). The mutations cause an increase in a specific oncometabolite (R)-2-HG; (R)-2-HG inhibits chromatin-modifying histone and DNA demethylases, which then block cell differentiation so leukemic cells never mature (Medeiros et al., 2017). By releasing this blockade using IDH1 and IDH2 inhibitors, the bone marrow myeloid cells can now differentiate and mature. Enasidenib (Idhifa®) is a selective inhibitor of the mutant IDH2 enzyme which otherwise halts the leukemic cells in the blast phase (Celgene, 2017). By inhibiting the mutant enzyme, the myeloid blast cells can now proceed to differentiate into more mature, normal myeloid cells. Ivosidenib (Tibsovo®) is a selective inhibitor of the mutant IDH1 enzyme thus allowing myeloid cell differentiation to proceed (Agios, 2018).

TUMOR-PROMOTING INFLAMMATION

The relationship between cancer and chronic inflammation has been widely publicized. Inflammation is an enabling factor in tumor development (Hanrahan & Weinberg, 2011). For example, persistent infection by *Helicobacter pylori* is a causal agent of gastric cancer as well as mucosa-associated lymphoid tissue (MALT) lymphoma; human papillomavirus (HPV 16,18) has been found to cause 70% of cervical cancer cases; and hepatitis B virus can cause hepatocellular carcinoma (Grivennikov et al., 2010). As more is learned about these relationships, it appears that recurrent or persistent inflammation may induce or promote cancer through DNA damage, leading to cell proliferation in an effort to heal the area, as well as creating a stromal "soil" rich in cytokines and growth factors ideal for a malignant cell to flourish (Schottenfeld & Beebe-Dimmer, 2006). The tumor microenvironment contains many proinflammatory and inflammatory cells, as well as mediators (Crusz & Balkwill, 2015), and it appears that inflammation is important in all phases of tumorigenesis: initiation, malignant transformation, invasion, and metastasis (Grivennikov et al., 2010).

To combat cervical cancer, the FDA-approved HPV vaccines for the prevention of cervical cancer, which kills millions of women worldwide each year. Hepatitis B vaccines are used to prevent the infection, so that liver cirrhosis, liver failure, and hepatocellular cancer of the liver is prevented.

AVOIDING IMMUNE DESTRUCTION

There is great attention to the immune system now and to immunotherapeutic approaches to cancer control. Recently, with more research enhancing our understanding of how the immune system is circumvented by cancer, new drugs are being developed to target these events when the immune system's T-lymphocytes become overwhelmed or tricked by cancer cells. *Chapter 4* addresses immune surveillance and the co-opting of immune mechanisms to avoid cancer detection by the immune system. It is important for oncology nurses to be conversant about elements of the immune system so they can teach patients and their families about them. There is an urgent need, and most nurses do not have a working knowledge of the immune system.

The immune system is responsible for identifying invading microorganisms and abnormal cells that might harm the body. It uses immune surveillance to accomplish this, distinguishing self from nonself by markers on the cell surface that match the person's major histocompatibility complex (MHC) proteins, also called human leukocyte antigens (HLA). Normally, the immune system is quiet or tolerant as it encounters cells with the correct MHC proteins. However, when a microorganism invades, or a cell without the MHC protein is found, the immune system is turned on to destroy it.

Our bodies are protected by both an **innate** immune response and an **adaptive** immune response, which are both interconnected. The innate immune response is immediate, as when you get the flu. You may develop fever, malaise, and other symptoms. The innate immune response is the first line of defense, and while immediate, it is not antigen-specific, nor is there immunological memory. Of note, there are natural killer (NK) cells activated by the innate response that kill any potential target it recognizes as "nonself" that does not have an MHC protein. However, it is not antigen-specific. An antigen is any substance that can evoke an immune response and that itself subsequently reacts with the products of the response (Male, 2013).

In contrast, the adaptive immune response takes longer to evolve initially, is antigen-specific, and your body's immune system remembers the antigen, so the next time the antigen is seen, the adaptive response is much more swift and potent. In the adaptive immune system, the immune cells are able to distinguish self from nonself, to remember the "foreign" antigens to which they have been exposed (memory T and B cells), and to mount an immune attack to eliminate the foreign antigen. When the antigen is encountered again, the immune system will mount a rapid and increasingly more potent defense against the antigen. It does this by activating specific immune cells. Once an antigen is recognized as not belonging to self, dendritic cells (a type of lymphocyte) digest the foreign cell and mount a peptide fragment of the antigen on its cell surface to teach the T-lymophocyte cells to recognize the foreign antigen and to attack it. This type of cell is called an antigen-presenting cell, or APC. Key immune warriors can be activated by the dendritic cells: cytotoxic T-lymphocytes, B lymphocytes, and NK cells. First, the dendritic cell activates helper T-lymphocytes cells, which produce cytokines that activate the appropriate B lymphocyte and/or T-lymphocyte to seek and destroy the antigen(s) marked for destruction. These helper T-lymphocytes may be activated to differentiate into cytotoxic T-lymphocytes, which proliferate rapidly against the specific antigen(s) and kill the cell containing the antigen. Second, B lymphocytes can recognize APCs, and then seek and destroy the cells with this cell surface antigen. Third, NK cells can attack and destroy cells based on identifying the cell as nonself.

The three key cell types in the immune fight against cancer are B-(cell) lymphocytes, T-(cell) lymphocytes, and APCs. Cytokines allow the cells to talk to each other and orchestrate the immune reaction.

Cancer evades the immune system in a number of ways that are known today, and many other processes that are awaiting discovery. Zielinski et al. (2013) describe four ways the immune system is circumvented. First, tumors may reduce expression of the class-I MHC molecules so that they are not detected as nonself and an immune response is not activated; the tumor antigen cannot be seen by cytotoxic T-lymphocytes. Second, they can turn down (downregulate) the innate immune system's cancer-fighting NK cells. Third, they can avoid apoptosis by down-regulating Fas receptor cell surface expression so they are invisible to NK and cytotoxic T-lymphocytes. Fourth, they can promote an anti-inflammatory state favoring tumor growth through secretion of growth factors that are immunosuppressive to T-lymphocytes and macrophages.

Dunn (2006) describes a theory of immune editing that spans from immune surveillance to tumor escape. Initially, cancer cells are identified and totally eliminated. Equilibrium may occur, where cancer growth is controlled, but not all cancer cells are eliminated. Last, tumor escape occurs when the immune system is exhausted, overwhelmed, cancer cells proliferate, and metastases occurs.

Finally, cancer cells evade the immune system by suppressing immune cells locally; in the microenvironment, they can also make the immune system tolerant to the cancer antigens by co-opting the inhibitory immune checkpoints and by using immune editing described above (Schreiber et al., 2011; Zou, 2006; Pardoll, 2012). See *Chapter 4* on targeted biological/immunological therapy.

MOLECULAR TARGETED THERAPY

As personalized, genomic medicine more clearly identifies the molecular flaws in each patient's tumor, and as molecular therapy becomes available to target these flaws, regimens are individualized for each patient. Many of the targets are in genes and the proteins in the cell signaling cascade. We have seen how a cell is told to perform a function. To review, signal transduction is the communication link between and among cells, where the outside environment can tell the cell what to do, such as make more cells. Messages are sent by hormones or growth factors, called ligands, that attach to cell surface receptors (e.g., RTKs). Once the receptor dimerizes and activates phosphorylation, tyrosine kinases pass the message along from one molecule to another, like a "bucket brigade" in a signal cascade (Weinberg, 1996). This way, the message is relayed "downstream" to the cell nucleus or down specific signaling pathways to get the desired effect, such as normal cell growth, cell division, differentiation (specialization), or cell death (apoptosis). It is a precise system and has many redundant parallel pathways.

Important growth factors that initiate the message for a cell to divide are the EGF family (EGF or erB-1, erB-2 or HER-2-neu, erB-3, and erB-4), PDGF, VEGF, transforming growth factor alpha (TGF-α), and fibroblast growth factor (FGF).

Molecular targeted therapy is selective and is directed against (a) specific molecular flaw(s). The side effects are specific to the drug class and the individual drug. This is in contrast to chemotherapy, which is a systemic therapy that is nonselective and systemic in its toxicity. There is a specific language in naming molecular targeted therapies. They are generally small molecules that can be administered orally (Abramson, 2016). The suffix "tinib" refers to a kinase inhibitor (e.g., imatinib, erlotinib), while "-zomib" refers to a proteasome inhibitor (e.g., bortezomib, carfilzomib), "-ciclib" refers to a small-molecule CDK inhibitor (e.g., Palbociclib), "-rolimus" refers to an mTOR inhibitor, "-inostat" refers to a histone deacetylase inhibitor, and "-degib" refers to a Hedgehog pathway inhibitor. Table 3.3 helps to distinguish the different classes of small-molecule targeted drugs.

Table 3.3   Molecular Targeted Therapy Drugs (as of January 2019)

DRUG CLASS/DRUG	CLASS EFFECTS (embryo-fetal toxicity is a common class effect)	TARGET/INDICATIONS
ALK Inhibitor	**Class effects:** CYP3A4 drug interactions; GI symptoms; embryo-fetal toxicity; hepatotoxicity; QTc prolongation; pneumonitis.	
Alectinib (Alecensa)		RTK ALK, RET and downstream, STAT3 and AKT; ALK-positive metastatic NSCLC that has progressed or patient is intolerant of crizotinib.
Brigatinib (Alunbrig)		RTK ALK, ROS1, IGF-1R, FLT-3, as well as EGFR deletion and point mutations. Also EMLA4-ALK and NPM-ALK fusion proteins.
Ceritinib (Zykadia)		RTK ALK, IGF-1R, InsR, ROS1; ALK+metastatic NSCLC.
Crizotinib (Xalkori)		RTK ALK, ROS-1; ALK+ or ROS-1 positive metastatic NSCLC.
Loratinib (Lorbrena)		RTK ALK, ROS1, TYK1, FER, FPS; TRKA,B,C; FAK, FAK2 and ACK; ALK+ metastatic NSCLC after progression on other ALK inhibitors.
Angiogenesis Inhibitors	**Class effects:** HTN, proteinuria, bleeding/hemorrhage, impaired wound healing; embryo-fetal toxicity.	
Axitinib (Inlyta)		VEGF receptors on endothelial cells lining blood vessels; advanced RCC.
Cabozantinib (Cabometyx)		VEGF 1, 2, 3; MET, RET, ROS1, FLT-4, others. Advanced RCC, hepatocellular carcinoma previously treated with sorafenib. Diarrhea. CYP3A4 drug interactions; PPES, RPLS. Advanced RCC.
Cabozantinib\(Cometriq)		MET, HGF; VEGFR1,2,3; RET, KIT, FLT-3, others. Progressive, metastatic medullary thyroid cancer.
Levatinib (Lenvima)		VEGFR1, 2, 3; locally recurrent or metastatic progressive, RAI-refractory differentiated thyroid cancer; RCC.
Pazopanib (Votrient)		VEGFR1, 2, 3; PDGFR, FGFR; advanced RCC; advanced soft-tissue sarcoma.
Regorafenib (Stivarga)		VEGFR2, 3; PDGFR, RET, KIT, RAF; metastatic CRC; locally advanced unresectable or metastatic gastrointestinal stromal tumor (GIST), hepatocellular carcinoma previously treated with sorafenib.
Sorafenib (Nexavar)		VEGFR2, PDGF, RAF; unresectable hepatocellular cancer; advanced RCC; locally recurrent or metasatic, progressive differentiated thyroid carcinoma refractory to RAI.
Sunitinib (Sutent)		PDGFR, VEGFR 1, 2, 3; KIT, FLT-3, RET; GIST after disease progression or intolerance to Imatinib mesylate; advanced RCC; progressive, well-differentiated pancreatic neuroendocrine tumor (pNET).

(continues)

Table 3.3 (Continued)

DRUG CLASS/DRUG	CLASS EFFECTS (embryo-fetal toxicity is a common class effect)	TARGET/INDICATIONS
Vandetanib (Caprelsa)		VEGFR2, EGFR1; symptomatic or progressive medullary thyroid cancer in patients with metastatic or locally advanced unresectable disease.
Ziv-aflibercept (Zaltrap)		VEGF (recombinant fusion protein that is a decoy (VEGF trap); metastatic CRC in combination with FOLFIRI. See *Chapter 4.*
Bcl-2 Inhibitor (Restores apoptosis)	**Class effects:** TLS; embryo-fetal toxicity; neutropenia.	
Venetoclax (Venclexta)		Bcl-2; CLL with 17p deletion mutation.
BCR-ABL Kinase Inhibitors	**Class effects:** CYP3A4 drug interactions, edema, bone marrow suppression; embryo-fetal toxicity.	
Bosutinib (Bosulif)		BCR-ABL kinase, most resistant forms; adults with Ph+ CML with relapsed disease.
Dasatinib (Sprycel)		BCR-ABL kinase, other kinases including SRC; newly diagnosed Ph+ CML in chronic phase; chronic accelerated or myeloid or lymphoid blast phase Ph+ CML; Ph+ ALL.
Imatinib mesylate (Gleevec)		BCR-ABL kinase; newly diagnosed Ph+ CML in chronic phase (adult, children); Ph+ CML in blast crisis/accelerated phase/chronic phase; relapsed refractory Ph+ ADD (adults); newly diatnosed Ph+ ALL children; certain MDS in adults.
Nilotinib (Tasigna)		BCR-ABL kinase; newly diagnosed Ph+ CML in chronic phase (adult); Ph+ CML in chronic/accelerated phases (adult).
Ponatinib (Iclusig)		BCR-ABL kinase; CML in chronic/accelerated/blast phase or resistant to previous TKI therapy; Ph+ ALL resistant of intolerant to prior TKI therapy.
BRAF and MEK Inhibitors	**Class effects:** new primary malignancies, hemorrhage, HTN, eye problems including retinal vein occlusion (RVO), GI symptoms, CYP3A4 drug interactions, embryo-fetal toxicity.	
Binimetinib (Mektovi™)		Mutated *BRAF*, reversible inhibitor of MAPK/extracellular signal regulated kinase 1 (MEK1, MEK2); unresectable or metastatic melanoma with BRAF *V600E* or *V600K* mutation in combination with encorafenib.
Cobimetinib (Cotellic)— MEK inhibitor		Mutated *BRAF*, reversible inhibitor of MAPK/extracellular signal regulated kinase 1 (MEK1, MEK2); unresectable or metastatic melanoma with BRAF *V600E* or *V600K* mutation in combination with vemurafenib.
Dabrafenib (Tafinlar)— BRAF inhibitor		Mutated BRAF; unresectable or metastatic melanoma with BRAF V600E mutation.
Encorafenib (Braftovi™)		BRAF V600E mutation, as well as wilf-type BRAF and CRAF , other kinases JNK1-3, LIMK1,2,4, and STK36, in combination with binimetinib in the treatment of unresectable or metastatic melanoma with BRAF *V600E* or *V600K* mutation.

Table 3.3 *(Continued)*

DRUG CLASS/DRUG	CLASS EFFECTS (embryo-fetal toxicity is a common class effect)	TARGET/INDICATIONS
Trametinib (Mekinist)— MEK inhibitor		MEK pathway; unresectable metastatic melanoma with BRAF V600E or V600K mutation, in combination with dabrafenib.
Vemurafenib (Zelboraf)— BRAF inhibitor		Mutated BRAF; malignant melanoma with BRAF V600E mutation.
Bruton's Tyrosine kinase (BTK) inhibitor	**Class effects:** cytopenias (infection and hemorrhage); HTN; 2nd primary malignancies; TLS; embryo-fetal toxicity.	
Acalabrutinib (Calquence®)	Bruton's tyrosine kinase (signaling molecule of the B-cell antigen receptor); Mantle Cell Lymphoma (MCL).	
Ibrutinib (Imbruvica)	Bruton's tyrosine kinase (signaling molecule of the B-cell antigen receptor); MCL, CLL, CLL with 17p deletion mutation; WM.	
FLT3 kinase inhibitor (FLT: FMS-like tyrosine kinase 3)	Class effects: Nausea, vomiting, diarrhea.	
Midostaurin (Rydapt)	FLT3 wild type and mutant signaling, KIT, PDGFRα/β, VEGFR2, members of the serine/threonine kinase Protein Kinase C (PKC) family; newly diagnosed FLT3 mutation-positive AML together with standard chemotherapy; aggressive systemic mastocytosis; systemic mastocytosis with hematologic neoplasm; mast cell leukemia.	
Gilteritinib (Xospata)	FLT3 receptor signaling and proliferation in *FLT3* mutated AML cells, including *FLT3-ITD*, causing apotosis, as well as other tyrosine kinases. Adult patients with relapsed or refractory AML with a *FLT3* mutation.	
Cyclin-Dependent Kinase Inhibitor	**Class effects:** Neutropenia; embryo-fetal toxicity; CYP3A4 drug interactions; GI symptoms.	
Abemaciclib (Verzenio™)	Cyclin-dependent kinases (CDKs) 4, 6 (which allow cells to progress through G1 and S phases of cell cycle); postmenopausal women with ER+, HER2- advanced BC who have progressed on endocrine therapy or endocrine/chemotherapy (monotherapy), with fulvestrant or as a single agent.	
Palbociclib (Ibrance)	Cyclin-dependent kinases (CDKs) 4, 6 (which allow cells to progress through G1 and S phases of cell cycle); postmenopausal women with ER+, HER2- advanced BC, with letrozole or fulvestrant.	
Ribociclib (Kisqali)	CDKs 4, 6 (which allow cells to progress through G1 and S phases of cell cycle); postmenopausal women with ER+, HER2-advanced or metastatic BC, with letrozole.	
Epidermal Growth Factor Tyrosine Kinase Inhibitors, small molecule	Class toxicity: skin rash, diarrhea.	
Afatinib (Gilotrif)	Metastatic NSCLC including EGFR exon 19 deletions or exon 21 (L858R) substitution mutations.	

(continues)

Table 3.3   (Continued)

DRUG CLASS/DRUG	CLASS EFFECTS (embryo-fetal toxicity is a common class effect)	TARGET/INDICATIONS
Dacomitinib (Vizimpro)		Metastatic NSCLC with EGFR exon 19 deletion or exon 21 L858R substitution mutations, 1st line.
Erlotinib (Tarceva)		Locally advanced or metastatic NSCLC; EGFR1 including EGFR exon 19 deletions or exon 21 (L858R) substitution mutations in met NSCLC, EGFR1 in locally advanced or metastatic pancreatic cancer, together with gemcitabine.
Gefitinib (Iressa)		Metastatic NSCLC having EGFR exon 19 deletions or exon 21 (L858R) substitution mutations.
Lapatinib (Tykerb)		EGFR1, EGFR2 (HER-2); advanced or metastatic HER2+ breast cancer with capecitabine, or with letrozole.
Neratinib (Nerlynx)		EGFR1, EGFR-2 (HER2), and HER-4. Extended adjuvant treatment of adult patients with early stage, HER-2 overexpressing/amplified breast cancer, to follow adjuvant trastuzumab-based therapy.
Osimertinib (Tagrisso)		Metastatic NSCLC having EGFR T790M mutation. Tumor must be EGFR T790M mutation positive.
Fibroblast Growth Factor Receptor 1,2,3,4 Tyrosine Kinase Inhibitor	Class effects: Ocular disorders (including retinal detachment), hyperphosphatemia.	
Erdafitinib (Balversa)		FGFR 2,3 genetic mutations. Adult patients with locally advanced or metastatic urothelial carcinoma with this mutation that has progressed during or after at least 1 line of prior platinum-containing chemotherapy.
Hedgehog Pathway Inhibitors	**Class effects:** Embryo-fetal toxicity (negative pregnancy test before starting drug, effective contraception, no donation of blood, sperm); muscle spasms; risk of increased CK; GI symptoms.	
Glasdegib (Daurismo)		SMO (smoothened), a transmembrane signal transduction protein; given in combination with low dose cytarabine. Adults ≥ 75 years old with newly diagnosed AML or who co-morbidities precluding intensive induction chemotherapy.
Sonidegib (Odomzo)		SMO (smoothened), a transmembrane signal transduction protein; adults with locally advanced basal cell carcinoma, recurrent after surgery, RT or in unresectable patients.
Vismodegib (Erivedge)		SMO (smoothened), a transmembrane signal transduction protein; locally advanced or metastatic basal cell carcinoma.
Histone Deacetylase (HDAC) Inhibitors	**Class effects:** Cytopenias (infection and bleeding); hepatotoxicity; TLS; embryo-fetal toxicity; GI symptoms; drug interactions.	
Belinostat (Beleodaq)		HDAC (enzyme that prevents uncoiling of DNA strand so genes can be transcribed), so inhibition leads to cell-cycle arrest and apoptosis; relapsed or refractory peripheral T-cell lymphoma.
Panobinostat (Farydak)		HDAC; multiple myeloma, in combination with bortezomib and dexamethasone.

Table 3.3 *(Continued)*

DRUG CLASS/DRUG	CLASS EFFECTS (embryo-fetal toxicity is a common class effect)	TARGET/INDICATIONS
Romidepsin (Isodax)		HDAC; cutaneous T-cell lymphoma (CTCL); peripheral T-cell lymphoma (PTCL).
Vorinostat (Zolinza)		HDAC; cutaneous T-cell lymphoma (CTCL).
IDH1 and 2 inhibitors		Isocitrate dehydrogenase 1 and 2 (IDH2) genes make an enzyme that is found in the energy making mitochondria within the cell, and participates in making energy to fuel cell activites. It may be mutated in AML and prevent the leukemic blast cells from differentiating into mature cells. **Class effects:** Differentiation syndrome; GI toxicity; elevated bilirubin; decreased appetite nausea, vomiting, diarrhea, elevated BR, decreased appetite. IDH1: QTc prolongation.
Enasidenib (Idhifa®)		Mutated IDH2 in refractory or replapsed AML having a mutated IDH2 gene.
Ivosidenib (Tibsovo®)		Mutated IDH1 in refractory or relapsed AML having a mutated IDH1 gene.
mTOR (Mammalian Target of Rapamycin) inhibitor		**Class effects:** CYP3A4 drug interactions; pneumonitis; embryo-fetal toxicity; GI symptoms; impaired wound healing; renal failure; hyperglycemia.
Everolimus (Afinitor)		mTOR; postmenopausal adv ER+HER2-breast cancer; advanced RCC; progressive unresectable PNET (adults); renal angiomyolipoma (adults).
Temsirolimus (Torisel)		mTOR; advanced RCC.
NTRK gene fusion inhibitor		Inhibits tropomyosin receptor kinases (TRK), e.g., TRKA,B, and C. The TRK genes are encoded by the genes *NTRK1,2,3*. TRK fusion mutations are oncogenic drivers in a wide number of cancers, including papillary thyroid, NSCLC, breast, CRC and sarcomas. **Class effects:** Neurotoxicity, hepatotoxicity, embryo-fetal toxicity.
Larotrectinib (Vitrakvi)		Inhibits tropomyosin receptor kinases (TRK), e.g., TRKA,B, and C. The TRK genes are encoded by the genes *NTRK1,2,3;* pediatric and adult solid tumors with *NTRK* gene fusion, are metastatic or if surgery has high morbidity, there is no satisfactory alternative therapy is available, or patients who have progressed following treatment.
PARP [poly (ADP-ribose) polymerase] Inhibitors		**Class effects:** pneumonitis; embryo-fetal toxicity; MDS/AML transformation; CYP3A4 drug interactions.
Olaparib (Lynparza®)		PARP-1, 2, 3; germline *BRCA*-mutated advanced ovarian cancer and HER-2 negative breast cancer (actual or suspected).
Niraparib (Zejula®)		Maintenance treatment of adults with recurrent epithelial ovarian, fallopian tube, or who are in a CR or PR after platinum-based chemotherapy.
Rucaparib (Rubraca®)		PARP-1, 2, 3; germline and/or primary peritoneal cancer somatic *BRCA*-mutated advanced ovarian cancer, after 2 or more prior therapies or as maintenance therapy for recurrent ovarian, fallopian tube or primary peritoneal cancer.

(continues)

Table 3.3   (Continued)

DRUG CLASS/DRUG	CLASS EFFECTS (embryo-fetal toxicity is a common class effect)	TARGET/INDICATIONS
Talazoparib (Talzenna™)		PARP-1, 2; germline *BRCA*-mutated (*gBRCAm*) HER-2 negative locally advanced or metastatic breast cancer.
Phosphatidylinositol 3-kinase (PI3K) Inhibitor		**Class effects:** Neutropenia; severe cutaneous reactions; embryo-fetal toxicity.
Alpelisib (Piqray)		PI3K inhibitor; blocks activated mutated PIK3-α and Akt signaling which otherwise leads to malignant transformation in PIK3 mutated breast cells and breast cancer.
Copanlisib (Aliqopa™)		Phosphatidylinositol 3-kinase (PI3K) sends signals to B lymphocytes telling them where to find and attach to lymph nodes and bone marrow stroma; relapsed follicular lymphoma.
Duvelisib (Copiktra®)		Phosphatidylinositol 3-kinase (PI3K) sends signals to B lymphocytes telling them where to find and attach to lymph nodes and bone marrow stroma; adult patients with relapsed or refractory CLL or small lymphocytic lymphoma; relapsed or refractory follicular lymphoma.
Idelalisib (Zydelig®)		Phosphatidylinositol 3-kinase (PI3K) sends signals to B lymphocytes telling them where to find and attach to lymph nodes and bone marrow stroma; relapsed CLL in combination with rituximab; relapsed follicular B-cell NHL; relapsed small lymphocytic lymphoma.
Proteasome Inhibitors		**Class effects:** GI toxicity; embryo-fetal toxicity; CYP3A4 drug interactions; TLS; hepatotoxicity; thrombocytopenia.
Bortezomib (Velcade)		26S proteasome; multiple myeloma; mantle cell lymphoma.
Carfilzomib (Kyprolis)		20S proteasome; relapsed or refractory multiple myeloma in combination with dexamethasone ± lenalidomide, or as a single agent.
Ixazomib (Ninlaro)		20S proteasome (beta 5 subunit); give with lenalidomide and dexamethasone.
Tropomycin receptor kinases (TRK) Inhibitor		**Class effects:** Fatigue, nausea, dizziness, vomiting, increased AST, cough, increased ALT, constipation, diarrhea.
Larotrectinib (Vitrackvi)		Inhibits TRKA, TRKB, TRKC which are encoded by the genes for neurotrophic receptor tyrosine kinases *NTRK1, NTRK2, NTRK3*. Adult and pediatric patients with solid tumors having NTKR gene fusion without a known acquired resistance mutation, are metastatic or where surgical resection is not recommended, and no satisfactory alternative treatment.

AML: acute myeloid leukemia; BRAF: B-RAF, when mutated, becomes driver oncogene in melanoma; CRAF: RAF1; melanoma driver oncogene when mutated; GIST: gastrointestinal stromal tumor; MCL: mantle cell lymphoma; MDS: myelodysplastic syndrome; NHL: non-Hodgkin's lymphoma; NSCLC: non-small-cell lung cancer; RCC: renal cell cancer; RAI: radioactive iodine; TLS: tumor lysis syndrome; WM: Waldenstrom's macroglobulinemia; PPES: palmar-plantar erythrodysesthesia syndrome; RPLS: reversible posterior leukoencephalopathy syndrome; ALK: anaplastic lymphoma kinase.

NURSING ISSUES

CARDIOTOXICITY

Tyrosine kinases (TKs) transduce signals from the outside of, or within, the cell and send the message to the cell nucleus to stimulate or inhibit cell functions. TKIs can block receptor TKs inside the cell using small-molecule TKIs. RTKs or their ligands outside the cell are blocked using large molecules (mAbs), which prevent phosphylation; thus, this message, for cell proliferation or other survival functions, never reaches the cell nucleus. TKs in the heart are blocked as well, however, which leads to damage to myocytes and, in some individuals, altered heart function. Because cardiac function is not a clinical endpoint of the drug trials and many of the drugs are nonselective in some of their targets, it is difficult to know the exact risk and incidence of cardiotoxicity except for the well-studied trastuzumab and lapatinib. Force et al. (2007) and Mellor et al. (2011) describe our understanding of the TKI-specific cardiotoxicity. The authors point out that cardiac myocytes have a very high demand for energy (ATP) and are thus especially susceptible to agents that alter mitochondrial function.

The first and most widely studied drug is trastuzumab (Herceptin), a mAb-directed against EGFR2 (HER-2), which had an incidence of cardiotoxicity of 4–7% as a single agent, increasing to 27% when combined with an anthracycline, and manifested first as a decrease in LVEF (left ventricle pumping ability) and later as symptomatic CHF. Thus, an anthracycline chemotherapy agent should not be given at the same time as trastuzumab. Lapatinib blocks both EGFR1 and EGFR2 but in contrast only has a small risk of lowering LVEF below normal values of 50–70%. EGFR2 (HER-2) is an important pathway in cardiomyocyte development and function. In addition, HER-2 dimerizes with EGFR3 and EGFR4 RTKs and is a coreceptor for their ligands the neuregulins, which are all expressed in cardiac tissue. HER-2 (EGFR2)–EGFR4 signaling is essential to myocardial contractility in the adult. The authors hypothesize that by blocking the HER-2 receptor, dimerization does not occur, with loss of signaling leading to changes in mitochondrial membrane polarization, ATP depletion, and loss of contractility. Mitochondria are the energy factory and storehouse of ATP, the energy currency of the cell. Other factors enhancing cardiotoxicity might be mediated by ADCC, as trastuzumab is an IgG_1 mAb.

Force et al. (2007) also discuss cardiotoxicity related to TKIs. Imatinib (Gleevec) has rarely caused CHF, and in those patients, electron microscopy of the heart has shown nonspecific mitochondrial abnormalities. When cardiomyocytes are studied in culture with imatinib, there is significant damage to the mitochondria resulting in cell death and declines in ATP stores. The active myocardium uses tremendous amounts of energy in the form of ATP to contract, and if these are inadequate, the heart fails. Other hypotheses include the fact that this drug and others, like the related dasatinib, inhibit ABL, which may be protecting the heart from oxidative stress. Dasatinib has an incidence of 4% LVEF dysfunction or CHF when taken for 6 months or longer. The multitargeted TKIs sorafinib and sunitinib may cause myocardial injury as collateral effects. Patients receiving sunitinib reportedly have an 11% incidence of declines in LVEF < 50% when taken for 6 months, which may have been compounded by possible drug-induced hypothyroidism. The drug inhibits PDGFa/b, which are also expressed on cardiomyocytes and believed important in cardiomyocyte survival; however, the exact cause is unknown. Patients taking sorafinib have a 2.9% incidence of acute coronary syndrome (compared to 0.4% in the placebo arm). Sorafinib inhibits PDGFRs as well as RAF1 and BRAF, which are important in oxidative stress-induced injury. In addition, when RAF1 is deleted in a mouse heart, it develops a dilated, hypocontractile heart with fibrosed and dead cardiomyocytes; however, the actual mechanism of cardiotoxicity with these drugs is still unclear. Although there is some provocative evidence that statins may provide not only some degree of cardioprotection but also specific antitumor effects, focused research on this and other agents needs to be done to define any potential benefit or interaction (Popat & Smith, 2008). Future targeted therapy studies need to consider possible influences on the heart cells, either directly or indirectly.

QT PROLONGATION

A number of targeted anticancer agents cause prolongation of the QT interval and may be associated with sudden death. It is important to understand how prolongation of the QT interval on the EKG can be life-threatening. See Figure 3.14 for the cardiac cycle. An ECG is the capture of electrical activity in the heart over time. The QT interval measures the time or duration of ventricular activation (depolarization) and recovery (repolarization). On the ECG, the QT interval is the time from the start of the Q wave (beginning of ventricular depolarization) to the end of the T wave (ventricular repolarization). If the heart is beating rapidly, the QT interval will be short, as compared to a slower heartbeat, where the QT interval will be longer. Because this period of time is affected by how fast the heart beats, it is corrected by a mathematical formula called Bazett's formula, and the interval is called the QTc, or corrected QT interval. The QTc = QT interval divided by the square root of R-R (interval from the onset of one QRS complex to the next), measured in seconds. Occasionally, the QT correction is based on Fridericia's correction formula, with the following abbreviation (QTcF) and used in the study upon which a drug is approved (e.g., ribociclib (Kisqali)). Fortunately, the QTc is available from many Internet sources, such as Up-To-Date. The normal QTc is 0.2–0.4 seconds (or 200 to 400 ms). Normal corrected

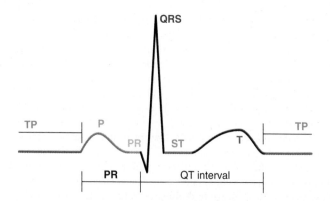

Figure 3.14   Basic Components of the ECG Complex
Reproduced from *12-Lead ECG: The Art of Interpretation*, courtesy of Tomas B. Garcia, MD.

TREATMENT

QTc intervals are < 0.44 seconds (440 ms). Since 2005, the FDA has required all drugs to be tested for their effect on the QT interval (FDA, 2005). This is because when the QTc is prolonged, it sets up a risk for tachyarrythmia, and, more worrisome, a special type of ventricular tachycardia called torsades de pointes, which on ECG looks like the ventricular beats are twisting around the isoelectric line (see Figure 3.15). This can quickly progress to ventricular fibrillation and sudden cardiac death. The risk is further increased by hypomagnesemia, hypokalemia, and hypocalcemia (Strevel et al., 2007). In addition, patients can have familial QT prolongation syndrome, or take drugs that prolong the QTc.

Table 3.4 shows selected drugs that can prolong the QTc interval. Table 3.5 shows the NCI CTCAE grading of QTc prolongation. In addition, oncology patients have co-morbidities, which increase the risk, such as older age and preexisting cardiac disease. Often they take concomitant medications that increase the risk, such as antidepressants, antiemetics, antibiotics, antihistamines, antifungals, and perhaps antipsychotics or methadone (Brell, 2010).

Oncology nurses should understand the danger of QTc prolongation and work collaboratively with physicians and midlevel practitioners to reduce the risk of adverse events. For example, although mAbs themselves do not cause QT prolongation, the mAbs cetuximab and panitumumab cause hypomagnesemia. If this becomes severe, the patient is at significant risk for torsades de pointes. Anticancer agents that are associated with increased incidence of QT prolongation include the histone deacetylase inhibitors vorinostat (Zolinza, 3.5–6%) and romidepsin (Istodax, 2–63%) and the TKIs dasatinib (Sprycel,< 1–3%), lapatinib (Tykerb, 16%), nilotinib (Tasigna, 1–10%), sunitinib (Sutent, dose dependent), and vandetanib (Vandetanib, 14%) (Yeh & Bickford, 2009; Bello et al., 2009).

As more targeted therapies are investigated and FDA approved, oncology nurses will have more agents that require monitoring of the QTc interval baseline and regularly during therapy, especially in patients with a history of cardiovascular disease or who are also taking other agents that potentially could prolong the QTc interval. In most cases, the effect of the QTc prolongation is insignificant and without sequelae. Key nursing measures, however, include (1) identifying patient's risk for prolongation of QTc over and above that conferred by the agent (e.g., hypokalemia, hypomagnesemia, congenital long QT syndrome,

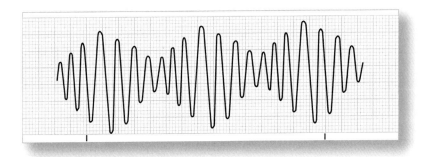

Figure 3.15   Torsades de Pointes
Reproduced from *Arrhythmia Recognition: The Art of Interpretation*, courtesy of Tomas B. Garcia, MD.

Table 3.4   Selected Drugs Increasing Risk of QTc Prolongation

Antiarrythmics: amiodarone*, bepridil*, disopyramide*, dofetilide*, dronedarone, flecainide, ibutilide*, isradipine, mibefradil, nicardipine, procainamide*, quinidine*, ranolazine, sematilide, sotalol*

Psychotropics: amitriptyline, chlorpromazine*, desipramine, doxepin, haloperidol*, lithium, mesoridazine*, olanzapine, paliperidone, pimozide*, quetiapine, risperidone, thioridazine*, sertindole, venlafaxine, ziprasidone

Antiemetics: dolasetron, droperidol, granisetron, ondansetron, palonosetron, prochlorperazine

Antimicrobials: azithromycin, chloroquine*, clarithromycin*, erythromycin*, gatifloxacin, gemifloxacin, halofantrine mefloquine*, levofloxacin, moxifloxacin, ofloxacin, pentamidine*, sparfloxacin*, spiramycin, telithromycin, voriconazole

Antihistamines: astemizole*, terfenadine*

Anticancer drugs: arsenic trioxide*, crizotinib, dasatinib, eribulin, lapatinib, nilotinib, pazopanib, romidepsin, sorafinib, sunitinib, vandetanib, vorinostat

Other drugs: alfuzosin, amantadine, atazanavir, chloral hydrate, cisapride*, dolasetron, droperidol*, felbamate, ganisetron, foscarnet, fosphenytoin, hydrochlorothiazide, indapamide, levomethadyl*, methadone*, octreotide, ondansetron, oxytocin, perflutren lipid microspheres, quinine, tacrolimus, vardenadil, vasopressin

Anticancer drugs: ceritinib, dasatinib, lapatinib, nilotinib, osimertinib, panobinostat, pazopanib, ribociclib, romidepsin, sorafenib, sunitinibm vandetanibm vemurafenib, vorinostat

*Risk of torsades de pointes

Data from Force T, et al. Cardiotoxicity of Tyrosine-Kinase Targeting Drugs. *Nat Rev Cancer* 2007; 7:332–344; Strevel EL, et al. Molecularly Targeted Oncology Therapeutics and Prolongation of the QT Interval. *J Clin Oncol* 2007; 35:3362–3372; Miranda DG, McMain CL, Smith AJ. Medication-induced QT-interval Prolongation and Torsades de Pointes. *US Pharm.* 2011; 36(2):HS-2–HS-8.

Table 3.5   National Cancer Institute CTCAE Version 4.0 Grading Criteria for QTc Prolongation

Grade	Definition
I	QTc > 450–480 msec
II	QTc > 481–500 msec or > 60 msec above baseline
III	QTc > 501 msec, on at least 2 separate ECGs.
IV	QTc > 501 msec; life-threatening signs of symptoms (e.g., arrhythmia, CHF, hypotension, shock, syncope, torsades de pointes)
V	—

Data from U.S. Department of Health and Human Services, National Institutes of Health, National Cancer Institute. Common Terminology Criteria for Adverse Events (CTCAE) Version 4.0. Published May 28, 2009 (v4.03: June 14, 2010). Available at: https://evs.nci.nih.gov/ftp1/CTCAE/CTCAE_4.03/CTCAE_4.03_2010-06-14_QuickReference_8.5x11.pdf.

taking anti-arrhythmic medications, cumulative high-dose anthracycline therapy, and history of cardiovascular heart disease) and (2) identifying and correcting hypokalemia, hypomagnesemia, and hypocalcemia, if they exist, prior to administration of the targeted agent. In addition, as ordered by the physician or midlevel practitioner, monitor ECGs with QTc calculation baseline and regularly during therapy.

A number of drug serum levels are affected by food or other interacting drugs. The nurse should review with the patient how the drug is self-administered and also what other drugs the patient is taking, either prescribed, over-the-counter (OTC), or "health food supplements." For example, with nilotinib, the drug should be taken on an empty stomach as the drug bioavailabilty is significantly increased if the drug is taken with food, with increased risk of toxicity, including QTc prolongation. The nurse should also know the specific management of patients if they develop changes in their QTc interval. For example, with nilotinib, if a patient develops a QTc of > 480 msec, the drug is withheld, the patient's serum potassium and magnesium are checked, and if below the LLN, these electrolytes are repleted, bringing them to normal limits. The patient's concomitant medications are also reviewed. If the QTc returns to < 450 msec and to within 20 msec of baseline within 2 weeks, review the medication profile for other QTc prolonging drugs and resume nilotinib at the prior dose. If the QTc is between 450 and 480 msec after 2 weeks, the nilotinib dose is reduced to 400 mg once daily. If, following dose reduction to 400 mg once daily, the QTc returns to > 480 msec, nilotinib is discontinued. An ECG with calculation of the QTc is repeated about 7 days after ANY dose adjustments (Tasigna package insert, 2015).

Although rare, if torsades de pointes does develop, the first treatment is IV magnesium sulfate 2 g, regardless of the patient's serum magnesium level (Yeh & Bickford, 2009). Defibrillation is indicated if fibrillation or sustained ventricular tachycardia occur, and overdrive transvenous pacing can be used to shorten the QTc (Yeh & Bickford, 2009). The patient's serum potassium should be maintained in the high-normal range, and any QT-prolonging medications should be discontinued, along with other drugs interfering with the patient's metabolism (Yeh & Bickford, 2009).

DRUG INTERACTIONS OF TKI

Many of the TKIs are metabolized by the P450 microenzyme system in the liver and have significant side effects with other drugs or substrates. The cytochrome P450 microenzyme system is a very important protection pathway for humans and has evolved over the millennia. It is a superfamily of isoenzymes that are found in the endoplasmic reticulum and mitochondrial membranes within cells and serve to detoxify poisons that are ingested or inhaled. They are found in the cells lining the nose, kidneys, lungs, small intestines, and liver and in the saliva. The P450 system is responsible for the metabolism of 75% of all drugs that are metabolized. Within this family, isoenzymes also synthesize estrogen and testosterone. CYP refers to cytochrome and is followed by a number, which refers to the family, then a letter, which refers to a subfamily, and then a final number, which refers to a subfamily gene. These genes regulate the proteins used to metabolize drugs. Individuals can have polymorphisms, or different copies of the gene, causing differences in how effectively liver enzymes detoxify the drugs. Sometimes this is an ethnic variation, and sometimes it is just due to an inherited gene copy. There are four classifications for how well people metabolize drugs: (1) **Ultra-rapid** metabolizers break down the drug quickly so the serum drug levels are low, and the person may need higher drug doses to get the intended drug effect; (2) **extensive** metabolizers metabolize the drug normally; (3) **intermediate** metabolizers are slightly less effective than extensive metabolizers, and the drug dose is usually effective; and (4) **poor** metabolizers break down the drug very slowly, resulting in higher serum drug levels as the drug is not completely metabolized, with more toxicity.

The CYP3A4 is the most important pathway in drug metabolism. If a drug is metabolized, it is called a **substrate**. If a drug inhibits the enzyme's activity so that the substrate is incompletely metabolized, it is called an **inhibitor**. If a drug increases the drug's metabolism, it is called an **inducer** (e.g., St. John's wort induces the CYP3A4 system, as does smoking). Induction will decrease the drug's effectiveness, making drug serum levels too low. It is very important to review a patient's medication profile while caring for a patient receiving molecular targeted therapy, and teaching the patient not to start any medication, whether OTC or prescribed, without talking with their physician, nurse, or pharmacist first.

References

Molecularly Targeted Agents (Immunologic targeted agents are shown in chapter 4, e.g., mAbs).

AbbVie Inc., and Genentech USA, Inc. Venclexta (venetoclax) [package insert]. North Chicago, IL, and South San Francisco, CA. May 2019.

Abramson, R. 2016. Overview of Targeted Therapies for Cancer. *My Cancer Genome.* Available at https://www.mycancergenome.org/content/molecular-medicine/overview-of-targeted-therapies-for-cancer/ (Updated July 12, 2016). Accessed July 29, 2016.

Agios Pharmaceuticals, Inc. Tibsovo (ivosidenib) [package insert]. Cambridge, MA. May 2019.

Almond JB, Cohen GM. The Proteasome: A Novel Target for Cancer Chemotherapy. *Leukemia* 2002; 16(4):433–443.

American Society of Clinical Oncology. *Cancer Clinical Advances of the Year 2019.* Available at https://www.ascopost.com/issues/february-10-2019/clinical-cancer-advances-2019. Accessed April 23, 2019.

Amgen and Onyx Pharmaceuticals, Inc. Kyprolis (carfilzomib) [package insert]. Thousand Oaks, CA. February 2019.

ARIAD Pharaceuticals, Inc. Iclusig (ponatinib) [package insert]. Cambridge, MA. October 2018.

ARIAD Pharmaceuticals, Inc. Alunbrig (brigatinib) [package insert]. Cambridge, MA. December 2018.

Array BioPharma, Inc. Braftovi® (encorafenib) [package insert]. Boulder, CO. January 2019.

Array BioPharma, Inc. Mektovi® (binimetinib) [package insert]. Boulder, CO. January 2019.

Ascierto PA, Kirkwood JM, Grob JJ, et al. The role of *BRAF V600* mutations in melanoma. *J Transl Med* 2012; 10:85–94. Available online at https://www.ncbi.nlm.nih.gov/pmc/articles/PMC3391993 /pdf/1479-5876-10-85.pdf. Accesssed April 15, 2019.

Astellas Pharma US, Inc. Xospata (gilteritinib) [package insert]. Northbrook, IL. November 2018.

AstraZeneca Pharmaceuticals LP. Calquence® (acalabrutinib) [package insert]. Wilmington, DE. November 2017.

AstraZeneca Pharmaceuticals LP. Caprelsa (vandetanib) [package insert]. Wilmington, DE. October 2018.

AstraZeneca Pharmaceuticals LP. Iressa (gefitinib) [package insert]. Wilmington, DE. July 2015.

AstraZeneca Pharmaceuticals LP. Lynparza (olaparib) [package insert]. Wilmington, DE. December 2018.

AstraZeneca Pharmaceuticals LP. Tagrisso (osimertinib) [package insert]. Wilmington, DE. August 2018.

Bayer HealthCare Pharmaceuticals, Inc. Aliqopa (copanlisib) [package insert]. Whippany, NJ. September 2017.

Bayer HealthCare Pharmaceuticals, Inc. Nexavar (sorafenib) [package insert]. Whippany, NJ. December 2018.

Bayer HealthCare Pharmaceuticals, Inc. Stivarga (regorafenib) [package insert]. Whippany, NJ. June 2018.

Bello CL, Mulay M, Huang X, et al. Electrocardiographic Characterization of the Qtc Interval in Patients with Advanced Solid Tumors: Pharmacokinetic-Pharmacdynamic Evaluation of Sunitinib. *Clin Cancer Res* 2009; 15(22):7045–7052.

Bharti AC, Aggarwal BB. Nuclear Factor-kappa B and Cancer: Its Role in Prevention and Therapy. *Biochem Pharmacol* September 2002; 64(5–6):883–888.

Boehringer Ingelheim Pharmaceuticals, Inc. Gilotrif (afatinib) [package insert]. Ridgefield, CT. January 2018.

Boston Biomedical. *Cancer Stem Cells: A Role in Cancer Recurrence and Metastasis.* Available at http://www.bostonbiomedical.com/. Accessed July 29, 2016.

Brell JM. Prolonged QTc Interval in Cancer Therapeutic Drug Development: Defining Arrhythmic Risk in Malignancy. *Prog Cardiovasc Dis* 2010; 53(2):164–172.

Bristol-Myers Squibb, Sprycel (dasatinib) [package insert]. Princeton, NJ. December 2018.

Casimiro MC, Crosariol M, Loro E, et al. Cyclins and Cell Cycle Control in Cancer and Disease. *Genes & Cancer* 2013. Published online February 26, 2013, as doi: 10.1177/1947601913479022.

Celgene Corporation. Idhifa (enasidenib) [package insert]. Summit, NJ. August 2017.

Celgene Corporation. Istodax (romidepsin) [package insert]. Summit, NJ. November 2018.

Chang F, Lee JT, Navolanic PM, et al. Involvement of PI3K/Akt Pathway in Cell Cycle Progression, Apoptosis, and Neoplastic Transformation: A Target for Cancer Chemotherapy. *Leukemia* 2003; 17(3): 590–603.

Chapman PB, Hauschild A, Robert C, et al. Improved Survival with Vemurafenib in Melanoma with BRAF V600E Mutation. *New Engl J Med* 2011; doi:10.1056/NEJMoa1103782 (published June 5, 2011) at NEJM.org.

Chen C, Liu Y, Cross JR, et al. Cancer-associated IDH2 Mutants Drive an Acute Myeloid Leukemia That Is Susceptible to Brd4 Inhibition. *Genes Dev* 2013; 27(18):1974-1985.

Chu CH, Figg WD. Antiangiogenesis agents. Chapter 28 in DeVita VT, Lawrence TS, Rosenberg SA (eds.) *Cancer: Principles & Practice of Oncology*, 10th ed. Philadelphia, PA: Wolters Kluwer/Lippincott Williams & Wilkins, 2015.

Claus R, Lubbert M. Epigenetic Targets in Hematopoietic Malignancies. *Oncogene* 2003; 22(42): 6489–96.

Clovis Oncology. Rubraca (rucaparib) [package insert]. Boulder, CO. April 2018.

Crusz SM, Balkwill FR. Inflammation and Cancer: Advances and New Agents. *Nat Rev Clin Oncol* 2015; 12(10):584–596. doi: 10.1038/nrclinonc.2015.105.

Deininger M, Buchdunger E, Druker BJ. The Development of Imatinib as a Therapeutic Agent for Chronic Myeloid Leukemia. *Blood* 2005; 105:2640–2653.

Din FNV, Dunlop MG, Stark LA. Evidence for Colorectal Cancer Cell Specificity of Aspirin Effects on NF Kappa B Signaling and Apoptosis. *Br J Cancer* 2004; 91:381–388.

Dunn GP, Koebel CM, Schreiber RD. Interferons, Immunity, and Immunoediting. *Nat Rev Immunol* 2006; 6(11):836–848.

Eisai Inc. Panretin (alitretinoin gel 0.1%) [package insert]. Woodcliff Lake, NJ. June 2018.

Eisai Inc. Lenvima (lenvatinib) [package insert]. Woodcliff Lake, NJ. December 2018.

Eisai Inc. Targretin (bexarotene capsules) [package insert]. Woodcliff Lake, NJ. April 2011.

Exelixis. Cabometyx (cabozantinib tablets) [package insert]. South San Francisco, CA. January 2019.

Exelixis. Cometriq (cabozantinib capsules) [package insert]. South San Francisco, CA. January 2018.

Fiorcari S, Brown WS, McIntyre BW, et al. The PI3-Kinase Delta Inhibitor Idelalisib (GS-1101) Targets Integrin-Mediated Adhesion of Chronic Lymphocytic Leukemia (CLL) Cell to Endothelial and Marrow Stromal Cells. *PLoS ONE* 2013; 8(12): e83830. doi: 10.1371/journal.pone.0083830.

Folkman J. Angiogenesis. *Ann Rev Med* 2006; 57:1–18.

Fong PC, Boss DS, Yap TA, et al. Inhibition of Poly (ADP-Ribose) Polymerase in Tumors from BRCA Mutation Carriers. *N Engl J Med* 2009; 361(2):123–134.

Force T, Krause DS, VanEtten RA. Molecular Mechanisms of Cardiotoxicity of Tyrosine Kinase Inhibition. *Nature Rev Cancer* 2007; 7:332–344.

Ford JM, Helleday T, Curtin NJ. DNA Damage Signaling and Repair in Cancer: Therapeutic Potential. *ASCO 2010 Educational Book.* Alexandria, VA: American Society of Clinical Oncology; 2010; 15(2):467–474.

Food and Drug Administration/US Department of Health and Human Services. Guidance for Industry: E14 Clinical Evaluation of QT/Qtc Interval Prolongation and Proarrhythmic Potential for Non-antiarrhythmic Drugs, October 2005. Available at http://www.fda.gov/downloads/drugs /guidancecomplianceregulatoryinformation/guidances/ucm073153.pdf. Accessed April 15, 2019.

Fuchs E. Skin stem cells: Rising to the Surface. *J Cell Biol* 2008; 180(2):273–284.

Fu M, Wang C, Li Z, et al. Minireview: Cyclin D1 Normal and Abnormal Functions. *Endocrinology* 2004; 145:5439–5447.

Gainor JF, Shaw AT. Novel Targets in Non-small Cell Lung Cancer: ROS1 and RET Fusions. *Oncologist* 2013; 18:865–875.

Genentech, Inc. Alecensa (alectinib) [package insert]. South San Francisco, CA. June 2018.

Genentech, Inc. Cotellic (cobimetinib) [package insert]. South San Francisco, CA. January 2018.

Genentech, Inc. Erivedge (vismodegib) [package insert]. South San Francisco, CA. February 2019.

Genentech, Inc. Tarceva (erlotinib) [package insert]. South San Francisco, CA. October 2016.

Genentech, Inc. Zelboraf (vemurafenib) [package insert]. South San Francisco, CA. November 2017.

Ghobrial IM, Witzig TE, Adjei AA. Targeting Apoptosis Pathways in Cancer Therapy. *CA: A Cancer J for Clin* 2005; 55:178–194.

Gilead Sciences, Inc. Zydelig (idelalisib) [package insert]. Foster City, CA. October 2018.

Glickman MH, Ciechanover A. The Ubiquitin-Proteasome Proteolytic Pathway: Destruction for the Sake of Construction. *Physiol Rev* 2002; 82(2):373–428.

Goel HL, Mercurio AM. VEGF Targets the Tumour Cell. *Nature Rev Cancer* 2013; 13:871–882.

Grivennikov SI, Greten FR, Karin M. Immunity, Inflammation, and Cancer. *Cell* 2010; 140(6):883–899. doi: 10.1016/j.cell.2010.01.025.

Gupta S, Takebe N, LoRusso P, et al. Review: Targeting the Hedgehog Pathway in Cancer. *Ther Adv in Med Oncol 2010;* 2(4):237–250.

Hanahan D, Weinberg RA. Hallmarks of Cancer: The Next Generation. *Cell* 2011; 144(5):646–674. doi: 10.1016/j.cell.2011.02.013.

Herman JG, Baylin SB. Gene Silencing in Cancer in Association with Promoter Hypermethylation. *N Engl J Med* 2003; 349(21):2042–54.

Herman R, Muchmore S. Independence Blue Cross to Cover Cancer Genome Sequencing. *Modern Healthcare* January 11, 2016. Available at http://www.modernhealthcare.com/article/20160111 /NEWS/160119985.

Iglehart JD, Silver DP. (2009). Synthetic Lethality—A New Direction in Cancer-Drug Development. *New Engl J Med* 2009; 361(2):189–191.

Infante JR, Falchook GS, Lawrence DP, et al. Phase I/II Study to Assess Safety, Pharmacokinetics, and Efficacy of the Oral MEK 1/2 Inhibitor GSK1120212 (GSK212) Dosed in Combination with the Oral BRAF Inhibitor GSK2118436 (GSK436). *J Clin Oncol* 2011; 29: (suppl; abstr CRA8503).

Ishii Y, Waxman S, Germain D. Tamoxifen Stimulates the Growth of Cyclin D1-overexpressing Breast Cancer Cells by Promoting Activation of Signal Transducer and Activator of Transcription 3. *Cancer Res* 2008; 68(3):852–860.

Izzedine H, Ederhy S, Goldwasser F, et al. Management of Hypertension in Angiogenesis Inhibitor-treated Patients. *Ann Oncol* 2009; 20:807–15.

Janssen Products, LP. Balversa (erdafitinib) [package insert]. Horsham, PA. April 2019.

Johnson LD, Goubran HA, Kotb RR. Histidine Rich Glycoprotein and Cancer: A Multi-faceted Relationship. *Anticancer Res* 2014; 34(2):593–603.

Jones PA, Baylin SB. The Epigenomics of Cancer. *Cell* 2007; 128(4):683–692.

Jones S, Anagnostou V, Lytle K, et al. Personalized Genomic Analyses for Cancer Mutation Discovery and Interpretation. *Sci Transl Med* 2015; 7(283): 283ra53. doi: 10.1126/scitranslmed.aaa7161.

Kobayashi S, Kishimoto T, Kamata S, et al. Rapamycin, a Specific Inhibitor of the Mammalian Target of Rapamycin, Suppresses Lymphangiogenesis and Lymphatic Metastases. *Cancer Sci* 2007; 98:726–733.

Kollmannsberger C, Bjarnason G, Burnett P, et al. Sunitinib in Metastatic Renal Cell Carcinoma: Recommendations for Management of Non-cardiovascular Toxicities. *Oncologist* 2011; 16: 543–553.

Kuhn DJ, Chen Q, Voorhees PM, et al. Potent activity of Carfilzomib, A Novel Irreversible Inhibitor of the Ubiquitin-proteasome Pathway, Against Preclinical Models of Multiple Myeloma. *Blood* 2007; 110(9):3281–3290.

Lacouture ME, Anadkat MJ, Bensadoun RJ, et al. Clinical Practice Guidelines for the Prevention and Treatment of EGFR Inhibitor-associated Dermatologic Toxicities. *Support Cancer Care* 2011; 19(8):1079–1095.

Ledford H, Tollefson J. Obama Proposes Cancer "Moonshot" in State of the Union Address. *Nature* (13 January 2016). doi:10.1038/nature.2016.19155. Available at http://www.nature.com/news/obama-proposes-cancer-moonshot-in-state-of-the-union-address-1.19155. Accessed May 1, 2016.

Lee J. Seeking Answers in a Genetic Code. *Modern Healthcare*. December 14, 2013. Available at http://www.modernhealthcare.com/article/20131214/MAGAZINE/312149990.

Lieberman J. Noncoding RNAs and Cancer: Knockout Punch for Cancer. *Cell* 2013; 153:9–10.

Lilly USA, LLC. Verzenio® (abemaciclib) [package insert]. Indianapolis, IN. February 2018.

Loxo Oncology, Inc. Vitrakvi (larotrectinib) [package insert]. Stamford, CT. November 2018.

Lynch TJ, Kim ES, Eaby B, et al. Epidermal Growth Factor Receptor Inhibitor-associated Cutaneous Toxicities: An Evolving Paradigm in Clinical Management. *Oncologist* 2007; 12(5): 610–621.

Maitland ML, Bakris GL, Black HR, et al. Initial Assessment, Surveillance, and Management of Blood Pressure in Paitents Receiving Vascular Endothelial Growth Factor Signaling Pathway Inhibitors. *J Natl Cancer Instit* 2010; 102:9596–9604.

Male D, Brostoff J, Roth DB, Toit IM. *Immunology,* 8th ed. Philadelphia, PA: Elsevier Saunders, 2013; 50–60.

Mancuso MR, Davis R, Norberg SM. Rapid Vascular Regrowth in Tumors after Reversal of VEGF Inhibition. *J Clin Invest* 2006; 116:2610–2621.

Medeiros BC, Fathi AT, DiNardo CD, et al. Isocitrate dehydrogenase mutations in myeloid malignancies. *Leukemia* 2017: 31:272–281.

Mellor HR, Bell AR, Valentin J-P, Roberts RRA. Cardiotoxicity Associated with Targeting Kinase Pathways in Cancer. *Toxicol Sci* 2011; 120(1):14–32.

Merck & Co., Inc. Zolinza (vorinostat) [package insert]. Whitehouse Station, NJ. December 2018.

Millennium Pharmaceuticals, Inc. Ninlaro (ixazomib) [package insert]. Cambridge, MA. November 2016.

Millennium Pharmaceuticals, Inc. Velcade (bortizemib) [package insert]. Cambridge, MA. June 2017.

Miranda DG, McMain CL, Smith AJ. Medication-induced QT-interval Prolongation and Torsades de Pointes. *US Pharm* 2011; 36(2):HS-2–HS-8.

Muller A, Homey B, Soto H. Involvement of Chemokine Receptors in Breast Cancer Metastases. *Nature* 2001; 410:50–56.

National Cancer Institute. Blue Ribbon Panel Announced to Help Guide Vice President Biden's National Cancer Moonshot Initiative. *NCI Press Release* April 4, 2016. Available at http://www.cancer.gov/news-events/press-releases/2016/blue-ribbon-panel-announced. Accessed April 30, 2016.

National Human Genome Research Institute (NHGRI). NIH Publication—15–8011, 2015. Available online at http://www.genome.gov/Pages/About/NHGRI_Brochure_2015.pdf. Accessed October 15, 2019.

Novartis Pharmaceuticals Corp. Afinitor (everolimus) [package insert]. East Hanover, NJ. April 2018.

Novartis Pharmaceuticals Corp. Farydak (panobinostat) [package insert]. East Hanover, NJ. June 2016.

Novartis Pharmaceuticals Corp. Gleevec (imatinib mesylate) [package insert]. East Hanover, NJ. September 2018.

Novartis Pharmaceuticals Corp. Kisqali (ribociclib) [package insert]. East Hanover, NJ. July 2018.

Novartis Pharmaceuticals Corp. Mekinist (trametinib) [package insert]. East Hanover, NJ. May 2018.

Novartis Pharmaceuticals Corp. Odomzo (sonidegib) [package insert]. East Hanover, NJ. September 2017.

Novartis Pharmaceuticals Corp. Piqray (alpelisib) [package insert]. East Hanover, NJ. May 2019.

Novartis Pharmaceuticals Corp. Rydapt (midostaurin) [package insert]. East Hanover, NJ. June 2018.

Novartis Pharmaceuticals Corp. Tafinlar (dabrafenib capsules) [package insert]. East Hanover, NJ. May 2018.

Novartis Pharmaceuticals Corp. Tasigna (nilotinib) [package insert]. East Hanover, NJ. July 2018.

Novartis Pharmaceuticals Corp. Tykerb (lapatinib) [package insert]. East Hanover, NJ. December 2018.

Novartis Pharmaceuticals Corp. Votrient (pazopanib) [package insert]. East Hanover, NJ. May 2017.

Novartis Pharmaceuticals Corp. Zykadia (ceritinib) [package insert]. East Hanover, NJ. March 2019.

O'Connor R, Breen L. Resistance to Chemotherapy Drugs. In Missailidis S (ed). *Anticancer Therapeutics*. New York, NY: John Wiley & Sons, 2008.

O'Donovan PJ, Livingston DM. BRCA-1 and BRCA-2: Breast/Ovarian Cancer Susceptibility Gene Products and Participants in DNA Double-Strand Break Repair. *Carcinogenesis* 2010; 31(6): 961–967.

Oskarsson T, Batlle E, Massague J. Metastatic Stem Cells: Sources, Niches, and Vital Pathways. *Cell Stem Cell* 2014; 14(3):306–321.

Papa A, Wan L, Bonora M, et al. Cancer-associated PTEN Mutants Act in a Dominant-Negative Manner to Suppress PTEN Protein Function. *Cell* 2014; 157(3):595. doi: 10.1016/j.cell.2014.03.027.

Pardoll DM. The Blockade of Immune Checkpoints in Cancer Immunotherapy. *Nat Rev Cancer* 2012; 12:252–264.

Pfizer Laboratories. Bosulif (bosutinib) [package insert]. New York, NY. October 2018.

Pfizer Laboratories. Daurismo (glasdegib) [package insert]. New York, NY. November 2018.

Pfizer Laboratories. Ibrance (palbociclib) [package insert]. New York, NY. April 2019.

Pfizer Laboratories. Inlyta (axitinib) [package insert]. New York, NY. August 2018.

Pfizer Laboratories. Lorbrena (lorlatinib)[package insert]. New York, NY. November 2018.

Pfizer Laboratories. Sutent (sunitinib) [package insert]. New York, NY. December 2018.

Pfizer Laboratories. Torisel (temsirolimus) [package insert]. New York, NY. March 2018.

Pfizer Laboratories. Vizimpro (dacomitinib) [package insert]. New York, NY. September 2018.

Pfizer Laboratories. Xalkori (crizotinib) [package insert]. New York, NY. January 2019.

Pharmacyclics LLC, and Janssen Biotech, Inc. Imbruvica (ibrutinib) [package insert]. Sunnyvale, CA and Horsham, PA. January 2019.

Popat S, Smith IE. Therapy Insight: Anthracyclines and Trastuzumab: The Optimal Management of Cardiotoxic Side Effects. *Nat Clin Pract Oncol* 2008; 5(6):324–335.

Puma Biotechnology, Inc. Nerlynx (neratinib) [Package insert]. Los Angeles, CA. June 2018.

Qiu Z, Cang Y, Goff SP. C_Abl Tyrosine Kinase Regulates Cardiac Growth and Development. *PNAS* 2010; 107(3):1136–1141.

Rini BI, Cohen DP, Lu DR. Hypertension as a Biomarker of Efficacy in Patients with Metastatic Renal Cell Cancer Treated with Sunitinib. *J Natl Cancer Inst* 2011; 103:763–773.

Rothschild SI. MicroRNA Therapies in Cancer. *Molecular and Cellular Therapies* 2014, 2:7–16.

Rubin K. Managing Immune-Related Adverse Events to Ipilimumab: A Nurse's Guide. *Clin J Oncol Nurs* 2012; 16(2):E69–E75.

Ruoslahti E, Reed JC. Anchorage Dependence, Integrins, and Apoptosis. *Cell* 1994; 77(4):477–478.

Sanofi-Aventis US LLC. Zaltrap (ziv-aflibercept) [package insert]. Bridgewater, NJ. June 2016.

Sanofi and Genzyme. Caprelsa (vandetanib) [package insert]. Cambridge, MA. October 2018.

Saporito B. The Conspiracy to End Cancer. *Time* 2013; 181(12):30–36, 38.

Schilsky RL. Tumor-agnostic Treatment for Cancer: An Expert Perspective. Available at https://www.cancer.net/blog/2018-12/tumor-agnostic-treatment-cancer-expert-perspective. Accessed April 23, 2019.

Schottenfeld D, Beebe-Dimmer J. Chronic Inflammation: A Common and Important Factor in the Pathogenesis of Neoplasia. *CA: Cancer J Clin* 2006; 56(2):69–83.

Schreiber RD, Old LJ, Smyth MJ. Cancer Immunoediting: Integrating Immunity's Roles in Cancer Suppression and Promotion. *Science* 2011; 331:1565–1570.

Semenza GL. Targeting HIF-1 for Cancer Therapy. *Nat Rev Cancer* 2003; 3(10):721–32.

Shaw RJ, Cantley LC. Ras, PI(3)K and mTOR Signaling Controls Tumour Cell Growth. *Nature* 2006; 441:424–430.

Smith EML, Pang H, Cirrincione C, et al. Effect of Duloxetine on Pain, Function and Quality of Life among Patients with Chemotherapy-induced Painful Peripheral Neuropathy: A Randomized Clinical Trial. *JAMA* 2013; 309(13):1359–1367.

Soussi T, Wiman KG. Shaping Genetic Alterations in Human Cancer: The p53 Mutation Paradigm. *Cancer Cell* 2007; 12(4):303–12.

Spectrum Pharmaceuticals, Inc. Beleodaq (belinostat) [package insert]. Irvine, CA. April 2017.

Stirewalt DL, Radich JP. The Role of FLT3 in Haematopoietic Malignancies. *Nat Rev Cancer* 2003; 3:650–665. doi: 10.1038/nrc1169.

Strevel EL, Ing DJ, Siu LL. Molecularly Targeted Oncology Therapeutics and Prolongation of the QT Interval. *J Clinc Oncol* 2007; 25(22):3362–3371.

Su F, Viros A, Milagre C, et al. RAS Mutations in Cutaneous Squamous-Cell Carcinomas in Patients Treated with BRAF Inhibitors. *N Engl J Med* 2012; 366:207–215.

Takahashi H, Shibuya M. The Vascular Endothelial Growth Factor (VEGF/VEGF Receptor System and Its Role Under Physiological and Pathological Conditions. *Clin Sci (Lond)* 2005; 109(3): 227–41.

Takahashi S. Downstream Molecular Pathways of Flt3 in The Pathogenesis of Acute Myeloid Leukemia: Biology and Therapeutic Implications. *J Hematol Oncol* 2011; 4:13–23.

Tapia C, Glatz K, Novotny H, et al. Close Association between HER-2 Amplification and Overexpression in Human Tumors of Non-breast Origin. *Modern Pathology* 2007; 20: 192–198.

Tesaro, Inc. Zejula (niraparib) [package insert]. Waltham, MA. February 2019.

Thijssen VLJL, Poirier F, Baum LG, Griffioen AW. Galectins in the Tumor Endothelium: Opportunities for Combined Cancer Therapy. *Blood* 2007; 110:2819–2827.

Toren P, Zoubeidi A. Targeting the PI3K/Akt Pathway in Prostate Cancer: Challenges and Opportunities (Review). *Int J Oncol* 2014; 45(5):1793–1801.

Verastem, Inc., Copiktra (duvelisib) [package insert]. Needham, MA. September 2018.

Vogelstein B, Papdopoulous N, Velculescu V, et al. Cancer Genome Landscapes. *Science* 2013; 229: 1546–1558.

Von Eschenbach A. *Keynote Presentation: Summit Series on Cancer Clinical Trials.* Executive summary VIII. Retooling the system, implementing solutions. Sept 29–Oct 1, 2003;1–3.

Wang T-F, Lockhart AC. Aflibercept in the Treatment of Metastatic Colorectal Cancer. *Clin Med Insights: Oncol* 2012; 6:19–30.

Watanabe R, Wei L, Huang J. mTOR Signaling, Function, Novel Inhibitors and Therapeutic Targets. *J Nucl Med* 2011; 52(4):497–500.

Weinberg RA. *The Biology of Cancer*, 2nd ed. New York, NY: Garland Science 2014; 669.

Wilkes GM. *Targeted Cancer Therapy: A Handbook for Nurses*. Sudbury, MA: Jones & Bartlett Publishers, 2011; 279.

Wood LS. Managing the Side Effects of Sorafenib and Sunitinib. *Comm Oncol* 2006; 3(9):558–562.

Wyeth Pharmaceuticals, a division of Pfizer. Torisel (temsirolimus) [package insert]. Philadelphia, PA. March 2018.

Yeh ETH, Bickford CL. Cardiovascular Complications of Cancer Therapy: Incidence, Pathogenesis, Diagnosis, and Management. *J Am Coll Cardiol* 2009; 53:2231–2247.

Yip KW, Reed JC. Bcl-2 Family Proteins and Cancer. *Oncogene* 2008; 27:6398–6406.

Zielinski C, Knapp S, Mascaux C, Hirsch F. Rationale for Targeting the Immune System through Checkpoint Molecule Blockade in the Treatment of Small-cell Lung Cancer. *Ann Oncol* 2013; 24:1170–1179.

Zou W. Regulatory T-cells, Tumor Immunity, and Immunotherapy. *Nat Rev Cancer* 2006; 6:295–307.

DRUGS

Drug: abemaciclib (Verzenio®)

Class: Kinase inhibitor: Cyclin-dependent kinase inhibitor (CDK4, CDK6).

Mechanism of Action: CDK4 and CDK6 are activated upon binding to cyclin D. The cell cycle is turned on by cyclin D1 and the cyclin-dependent kinases CDK4/6 by phosphorylation of the retinoblastoma protein (Rb), leading to cell proliferation.Abemaciclib inhibits Rb phosphorylation so the cell cycle does not get turned on, and the cell does not go from the G1 phase into the S (synthesis) phase of the cell cycle; the cell becomes "senescent" and undergoes apoptosis (cell death).

Metabolism: Steady state reached within 5 days with bid dosing. The bioavailability is 45% after oral dosing, and the median Tmax is 8 hours. High fat, high calorie meal increases AUC by 9%, and Cmax was increased by 26%. Drug level in CSF is similar to unbound plasma concentrations. The mean plasma elimination half-life is 18.3 hours. Drug is largely metabolized in the liver into several metabolites by the CYP3A4. Additional metabolites are formed through oxidation. Drug is primarily excreted in the feces (81% of dose) and 3% in urine. Elimination not affected by mild or moderate renal impairment, In patients with severe hepatic impairment, elimination half-life increased to 55 hours (compared to 20 hours in normal controls).

Indications: For the treatment of women with HR-positive, HER2-negative advanced or metastatic breast cancer:

- In combination with an aromatase inhibitor as initial endocrine-based therapy in post-menopausal women.
- In combination with fulvestrant after disease progression following endocrine therapy.
- As monotherapy after disease progression following endocrine therapy and prior chemotherapy in the metastatic setting.

Contraindications: None.

Dosage/Range: Oral with or without food, at about the same time every day.
- Recommended starting dose in combination with fulvestrant or an aromatase inhibitor: 150 mg bid. When given with fulvestrant, fulvestrant is administered on days 1, 15, and 29, then monthly.
- Recommended starting dose as monotherapy: 200 mg bid.
- Teach patient self-administration. If the patient vomits or misses a dose, take the next dose at the scheduled time. Teach patient to swallow tablets whole, and not to chew or split tablets before swallowing.
- If the patient is pre/perimenopausal and treated with abemaciclib and fulvestrant, the patient should also receive a gonadotropin-releasing hormone agonist according to current clinical practice standards.

Dose Modifications: Dose reduction by 50 mg each level: (a) if starting dose 150 mg, reduce to 100mg bid at 1st dose reduction, reduce to 50 mg bid for 2nd dose reduction; 3rd dose reduction not applicatable; (b) if starting dose is 200 mg bid, 1st dose reduction is to 150 mg bid, 2nd dose reduction is to 100 mg bid, and 3rd dose reduction is to 50 mg bid.
- Hematologic toxicity: CTCAE Grade 1 or 2: no modification; grade 3: suspend dose until toxicity resolves to ≤ grade 2, do not dose reduce; grade 3 recurrent or grades 4: suspend dose until toxicity resolves to ≤ grade 2, resume at *next lower* dose.
- Diarrhea: Grade 1: no modification; grade 2 that does not resolve within 24 hours to ≤ grade 1, suspend dose until resolution; do not dose reduce; grade 2 that persists or recurs after resuming the same dose despite maximal supportive measures: suspend dose until toxicity resolves to grade ≤ 1, resume at *next lower* dose level; grades 3 or 4 or requires hospitalization: suspend dose until toxicity resolves to ≤ grade 1, resume at *next lower* dose level.
- Hepatotoxicity: Grades 1 and 2 for ALT and AST: grade 1 (> ULN-3.0 × ULN), grade 2 (> 3.0-5.0 × ULN) without an increase in total bilirubin above 2 × ULN: no dose modification; persistent or recurrent grade 2, or grade 3 (> 5.0 – 20.0 × ULN), WITHOUT increase in total bilirubin above 2 × ULN: suspend dose until toxicity resolves to baseline or grade 1, resume at *next lower* dose level; Elevation in AST and/or ALT > 3 × ULN WITH total bilirubin > 2 × ULN in the absence of cholestasis: discontinue abemaciclib; grade 4 (> 20.0 × ULN): discontinue abemaciclib.
- Other toxicities: Grades 1 or 2: no dose modification; persistent or recurrent grade 2 toxicity that does not resolve with maximal supportive measures within 7 days to baseline or grade 1: suspend dose until toxicity resolves to ≤ grade 1, resume at *next lower* dose level; grades 3 or 4: suspend dose until toxicity resolves to ≤ grade 1, resume at *next lower* dose level.

Drug Preparation: Oral. Available in 50 mg, 100 mg, 150 mg, and 200 mg strengths.

Drug Administration:
- Monitor CBC prior to start of abemaciclib, every 2 weeks for the first 2 months, monthly for next 2 months, and a s clinically indicated. Monitor LFTs prior to start of abemaciclib, every 2 weeks × 2 months, monthly for the next 2 months, and as clinically indicated.
- Teach patient self-administration with or without food, at about the same time every day. If the patient vomits or misses a dose, take the next scheduled dose at the scheduled time.

Teach patient to swallow tablet whole, not to chew or split the tablet prior to swallowing; also do not take tablet if broken, cracked or otherwise not intact.

- Teach patient to (a) take anti-diarrheal medication at first sign of diarrhea, and to report it right away to RN/MD, and to increase oral fluid intake to at least one 8-oz glass of fluids per hour; (b) report signs/symptoms and to seek emergency medical assistance if pain in leg, redness, swelling, or feeling of warmth in leg (DVT) or difficulty breathing, rapid breathing, or sharp chest pain (PE) right away as may be DVT or PE; (c) if patient is female of reproductive potential, to use effective contraception during therapy and for at least 3 weeks after last dose of abemaciclib.

Drug Interactions:
- Strong CYP3A4 inducers: e.g., rifampin reduces effective abemaciclib dose by 67%; avoid concomitant use.
- Strong CYP3A4 Inhibitors: e.g., ketoconazole: avoid concomitant use. If needed, reduce abemaciclib dose.

Lab Effects/Interference:
- Neutropenia, anemia, thrombocytopenia.
- Increased AST, ALT, serum creatinine.

Special Considerations:
- Most common adverse effects (20%): diarrhea, neutropenia, nausea, abdominal pain, infections, fatigue, anemia, leukopenia, decreased appetite, vomiting, headache, alopecia, thrombocytopenia.
- Nursing mothers should be taught not to breastfeed while receiving the drug.
- Warnings and Precautions:
  - *Diarrhea:* Common, as affects 81%–90% of patients, grade 3 in 9%–20% of patients. Episodes have been associated with dehydration and infection. Median time to onset to first diarrhea event was 6–8 days, median duration grades 2 and 3 were 9–11 days and 6–8 days respectively. Teach patient to start anti-diarrheal therapy at 1st sign of loose stool, increase oral fluid intake and notify their provider for follow-up.If grades 3 or 4 or diarrhea that requires hospitalization, see dose modifications.
  - *Neutropenia:* Occurred in 37–46% of patients, and was grade 3 or higher (labs) in 22–32% of patients. Onset (median) was 11–33 days for grade 3 or higher neutropenia. Febrile neutropenia was rare (< 1%). Monitor CBC/differential prior to starting abemaciclib, then every 2 weeks × first 2 months, then monthly × 2, and as clinically indicated. Teach patient meaures to reduce risk of infection, and to report signs/symptoms right away. See dosing modifications.
  - *Hepatotoxicity:* Assess LFTs baseline prior to starting abemaciclib, then every 2 weeks for first 2 months, then monthly for the next 2 months, and as clinically indicated. See dose modifications.
  - *Venous thromboembolism (VTE):* Incidence was 0.6%–5%. Monitor for signs/symptoms of VTE, and teach patient to self-assess and report positive findings right away.
  - *Embryo-fetal toxicity:* Drug may cause fetal harm. Teach patients of reproductive potential to use effective contraception to avoid pregnancy during therapy and for at least 3 weeks after last drug dose.

Potential Toxicities/Side Effects and the Nursing Process

I. ALTERATION IN NUTRITION, LESS THAN BODY REQUIREMENTS, related to DIARRHEA, NAUSEA, VOMITING, CONSTIPATION, STOMATITIS, DECREASED APPETITE, INCREASED LFTs

Defining Characteristics: Diarrhea occurs in 81–90% of patients, 9–20% grade 3 across all studies. Nausea occurred in 39–64% of patients, and vomiting in 26–35% of patients. Constipation occurred in 16–17% of patients. Decreased appetite occurred in 24–45% of patients. Stomatitis affected 14–15%, and dry mouth 14% of patients. LFTs were elevated in a third of patients: ALT 13–31%, and AST in 12-30% of patients.

Nursing Implications: Assess nutritional status, bowel-elimination pattern, appetite, including LFTs (ALT, AST, bilirubin), at baseline prior to starting abemaciclib, then every 2 weeks for first 2 months, then monthly for the next 2 months, and as clinically indicated and ordered. Teach patient to report (a) start anti-diarrheal medication at the first loose stool (e.g., loperamide) right away to notify RN/MD; (b) increase oral fluids to 8 oz fluid every hour when awake to prevent dehydration if diarrhea occurs. Diarrhea may be associated with dehydration and infection: assess patient closely for both if diarrhea occurs. See dose modifications for diarrhea, hepatotoxicity. Teach the patient dietary modification if nausea and vomiting or diarrhea occur (e.g., for diarrhea, BRAT diet: bananas, rice, applesauce, and toast) and to increase oral fluids to prevent dehydration. Review high calorie high protein, small frequent feedings if patient has decreased appetite.

II. POTENTIAL FOR INJURY related to NEUTROPENIA, ANEMIA, THROMBOCYTOPENIA

Defining Characteristics: Incidence 37-46% across all studies, and grade 3 in 19-24% of patients. Anemia occurred in 22-29% and thrombocytopenia in 10-20% of patients. Infections occurred in 31-43% of patients.

Nursing Implications: Monitor CBC, absolute neutrophil count, and platelet count prior to starting abemaciclib, then every 2 weeks × first 2 months, then monthly × 2, and as clinically indicated. Teach patient meaures to reduce risk of infection, and to report signs/symptoms right away. Teach patient/family signs/symptoms of infection, bleeding, and anemia, and instruct to report them to nurse or physician immediately. Teach patient to avoid aspirin-containing OTC medications.

Drug: acalabrutinib (Calquence®)

Class: Kinase inhibitor; inhibits Bruton Tyrosine Kinase (BTK).

Mechanism of Action: Small molecule inhibitor of BTK and its active metaboliteACP-5862, so that the BTK signaling molecule of the B-cell antigen receptor (BCR) and cytokine pathways are not activated. Normally, in B-cells, BTK signaling results in activation of required pathways of B-cell proliferation, trafficking, chemotaxis, and adhesion. Blockade of BTK leads to malignant B-cell proliferation and survival (AstraZeneca, 2017).

Metabolism: Median steady state is maintained over 12 hours with prescribed dosing. Mean absolute bioavailability is 25%, and time to peak plasma concentrations (Tmax) was 0.75 hours. Food does not affect bioavailability. Drug is 97.5% bound reversibly to human plasma protein. Median terminal elimination half-life (t1/2) was 0.9 hours, and 6.9 hours for active metabolite. Drug is primarily metabolized by CYP3A4 microenzymes, and to a lesser extent by glutathione conjugation and amide hydrolysis. The active metabolite is about 50% less potent than acalabrutinib. Most (84%) of the dose is recovered in the feces, and 12% in the urine; < 1% excreted as unchanged drug.

Indications: Accelerated FDA approval for the treatment of adult patients with mantle cell lymphoma (MCL) who have received at least 1 prior therapy.

Contraindications: None.

Dosage/Range: 100 mg PO q 12 hours at approximately the same time of day, until disease progression or unacceptable toxicity.

Dose Modifications:
- *Grade 3 or higher non-hematologic toxicity, grade 3 thrombocytopenia with bleeding, grade 4 thrombocytopenia, grade 4 neutropenia lasting > 7 days:*
  - First and second *occurrence*: interrupt acalabrutinib and resume once toxicity has resolved to grade 1 or baseline level (at same dose 100 mg bid). Third *occurrence*: interrupt acalabrutinib and resume once toxicity has resolved to grade 1 or baseline level (with dose reduction to 100 mg DAILY).
  - Fourth *occurrence:* discontinue acalabrutinib.
- *Coadminsitration with a strong CYP3A inhibitor:* avoid concomitant use.
  - If inhibitor to be used short-term (e.g., anti-infective for up to 7 days), interrupt acalabrutinib.
  - If co-administered with a moderate CYP3A4 inhibitor, decrease acalabrutinib dose to 100 mg once daily.
- *Coadminsitration with a strong CYP3A inducer:* Avoid concomitant use. If must use the strong CYP3A4 inducer, increase the acalabrutinib dose to 200 mg twice daily.
- *Concomitant use with gastric acid reducing agents:*
  - Proton pump inhibitors: avoid concomitant use
  - H2 receptor antagonists: Take acalabrutinib 2 hours before taking H2-receptor antagonist.
  - Antacids: Separate dosing by at least 2 hours.

Drug Preparation: None. Available in 100 mg capsules.

Drug Administration:
- Assess CBC/differential baseline and periodically during therapy.

- Review patient medication profile for any interacting drugs (metabolized by CYP3A4). If taking PPIs, antacids or H2-receptor antagonists, see drug interactions.
- Teach patient self-admiinistration, taking the drug orally with water, with or without food, at about the same times of day. Swallow the capsule whole, without breaking or chewing the capsule. If a dose is missed by > 3 hours, skip the dose, and take the next dose at its regularly scheduled time. Do not make up a missed dose.

Drug Interactions:
- CYP3A4 inducers or inhibitors: Do not co-administer. If necessary, see dosage modification.
- Proton pump inhibitors: Avoid concomitant use.
- H2-receptor antagonists: Take acalabrutinib 2 hours prior taking the H2 receptor antagonist.
- Antacids: Separate dosing by at least 2 hours.

Lab Effects/Interference:
- Neutropenia, thrombocytopenia.
- Decreased hemoglobin.
- Increased serum creatinine (rare).

Special Considerations:
- Most common adverse effects were anemia, thrombocytopenia, headache, neutropenia, diarrhea, fatigue, myalgia, and bruising.
- Warnings and Precautions:
  - Hemorrhage: Incidence any grade was 50%. Grade 3 or higher bleeding events occurred in 2% of patients, including GI, intracranial, epistaxis. There may be increased risk in patients receiving antiplatelet inhibitors or anticoagulants. Consider holding acalabrutinib for 3–7 days pre- and post-surgery depending upon type of surgery and risk of bleeding.
  - Infection (bacterial, viral, fungal) may occur. Grade 3 or higher infections occurred in 18% of patients (most commonly pneumonia). HBV reactivation and PML have also been reported. Assess patients for signs/symptoms of infection and implement prompt antiinfective plan as ordered.
  - Cytopenias: Grades 3 or 4 neutropenia occurred in 23%, anemia (11%), and thrombocytopenia (8%). Assess CBC/differential prior to start of acalabrutinib and at least monthly as ordered during treatment.
  - Second primary malignancy: have occurred in 11% of patients, most frequently skin cancer (7% of patients). Teach patients to avoid sun exposure and to wear skin protective clothing, SPF, and a hat when outside. Teach patient to report any skin changes to their provider right away.
  - Atrial fibrillation and flutter: Overall incidence 3%, which was grade 3 in 1% of 612 patients. Monitor ECG baseline (before starting acalabrutinib) and periodically during treatment.
- Acalabrutinib is exreted into breast milk. Nursing mothers should not breast-feed while receiving the drug.

Potential Toxicities/Side Effects and the Nursing Process

I.   POTENTIAL FOR INJURY related to HEMORRAGE, CYTOPENIAS, INFECTION, FATIGUE

Defining Characteristics: While bleeding events (any) occurred in 50% of patients, serious, grade 3 or higher hemorrhage (GI, intracranial bleeding, epistaxis) occurred in 2% of patients. Bruising occurred in 21% of patients. In all acalabrutinib studies, neutropenia occurred in 36% of MCL patients (23% grade $\geq$ 3), thrombocytopenia in 44% of patients (8% grade $\geq$ 3), and decreased hemoglobin in 46% of patients, (11% grade $\geq$ 3). Hemorrhage risk may be increased in patients receiving antiplatelet or anticoagulant therapies.

Nursing Implications: Assess medication profile for interacting drugs which may increase a calabrutinib concentrations andor toxicity. Assess baseline CBC/differential prior to dosing, and at least monthly. Teach patient self-assessment of signs/symptoms of infection (e.g., T > 100.4°F, dysuria, productive cough) and bleeding (e.g., blood when brushing teeth, hematuria, nosebleed that doesn't stop within 15 mnutes, new bruising), and instruct patient to report them right away. Teach patient self-care measures to minimize risk of infection and bleeding, including avoidance of crowds, people with colds, OTC aspirin-containing and NSAID medication ns. Discuss dose interruption and modification for grade 3 or 4 toxicity with physician. Assess for fever or infection frequently, and discuss need for emergent evaluation and treatment promptly if signs or symptoms of infection are identified. Assess baseline energy level, and fatigue during thearapy. Discuss strategies to conserve energy.

II.   ALTERATION IN NUTRITION, POTENTIAL, LESS THAN BODY REQUIREMENTS, related to DIARRHEA, NAUSEA, VOMITING, CONSTIPATION

Defining Characteristics: Diarrhea affects 31% of patients, nausea 19%, constipation 15%, and vomiting 13%.

Nursing Implications: Assess baseline nutritional status and bowel-elimination status. If patient develops nausea and/or vomiting, teach patient to self-administer antiemetics 1 hour prior to each dose, and to call if nausea/vomiting persist. Discuss with physician more effective antiemetic regimen if nausea/vomiting persist. Encourage small, frequent intake of cool, bland foods as tolerated if nausea develops. Refer to dietitian as needed for meal planning. Teach patient to report diarrhea that does not respond to OTC antidiarrheal medication. Teach self-care measures of diet modification and oral fluids to 2–3 L during the waking hours. If constipation occurs, teach patient self-care measures to prevent constipation. Assess appetite, and condition of oral mucosa; teach patient self-assessment and systemic oral hygiene after meals and at bedtime.

III. ALTERATION IN COMFORT related to PAIN, HEADACHE, FATIGUE, ARTHRALGIA, AND FATIGUE

Defining Characteristics: Fatigue affected 28% of patients, abdominal pain 15%, myalgia 21%, and headache affected 39% of patients.

Nursing Implications: Teach patient that these events may occur and to report them, and teach patient strategies to conserve energy and manage symptoms. Assess baseline comfort and monitor closely during treatment. Develop plan to assure comfort depending on symptoms reported. Discuss ineffective strategies with physician/NP/PA.

Drug: afatinib (Gilotrif)

Class: Kinase inhibitor; TKI of the EGFR.

Mechanism of Action: Drug is a 4-anilinoquinazoline. It binds to the kinase domains of EGFR1, HER2, and HER4, thus irreversibly preventing the tyrosine kinase from autophosphorylation and downstream signaling to the cell nucleus. It prevents cell proliferation by inhibiting wild-type EGFR, as well in as cells expressing EGFR exon 19 deletion mutations, exon 21 L858R mutations, and some with a secondary T790 M mutation. It also inhibits proliferation in cell lines overexpressing HER2.

Metabolism: After oral dosing, time to peak afatinib plasma concentration (Tmax) is 2–5 hours. Drug is 95% protein-bound. A high-fat meal decreases AUC by 39%, and maximal concentration (Cmax) by 50%. Drug is excreted via the biliary system and the feces (85%), with 4% recovered from the urine. Elimination half-life is 37 hours with repeat dosing, and steady state is reached within 8 days. Median trough plasma concentrations are 27% higher in patients with mild renal dysfunction (Cr Cl 60–89 mL/min) and 85% higher in patients with moderate renal dysfunction (CrCl 30–59 mL/min) compared to patients with normal renal function (Cr Cl > 90 mL/min). While there is no effect on mild-to-moderate hepatic dysfunction on drug excretion, the drug has not been studied in patients with severe hepatic dysfunction.

Indications: For the treatment of patients with (1) Metastatic NSCLC whose tumor has non-resistant EGFR mutations as determined by an FDA approved test as 1st line therapy; (drug safety and efficacy are not established for other EGFR mutations) or (2) metastatic, squamous NSCLC progressing after platinum-based chemotherapy.

Dosage/Range:
- 40 mg orally once daily until disease progession or intolerance, on an empty stomach.
- Renal impairment (severe, estimated GFR 15-29 mL/min/1.73m^2): 30 mg orally, once daily

Dose Modifications:
- Hold drug for (1) any grade 3 or higher toxicity; (2) grade 2 or higher diarrhea persisting for 2 or more consecutive days while taking antidiarrheal medication; (3) grade 2

cutaneous reactions that last for > 7 days or are intolerable; and (4) grade 2 or higher renal impairment.
- Resume drug when toxicity fully resolved, returns to baseline, or improves to grade 1. Reduce dose by 10 mg less per day than the dose being taken when toxicity occurred.
- Permanently discontinue drug for (1) life-threatening bullous, blistering, or exfoliative skin lesions; (2) confirmed interstitial lung disease (ILD); (3) severe, drug-induced hepatic impairment; (4) persistent ulcerative keratitis; (5) symptomatic left ventricular dysfunction; (6) severe or intolerable adverse reactions at a dose of 20 mg per day.
- Dose Modification for Drug Interactions:
  - P-gp inhibitors: if must coadminister, reduce afatinib dose by 10 mg if not tolerated; resume the previous dose after discontinuation of P-gb inhibitor as tolerated.
  - P-gp inducers: if patient has chronic therapy with a P-gp inducer, increase afatinib dose by 10 mg as tolerated; resume previous dose 2–3 days after discontinuation of the P-gp inducer.

Drug Preparation:
- None, oral. Available in 40-mg, 30-mg, and 20-mg tablets. Store bottle at room temperature, and dispense medication in the original container to protect from exposure to high humidity and light.

Drug Administration:
- Teach patient (1) to take tablet on empty stomach, at least 1 hour before or 2 hours after a meal; (2) to not take a missed dose within 12 hours of the next dose.

Drug Interactions:
- P-glycoprotein **inhibitors** (e.g., ritonavir): administered 1 hour before afatinib increased systemic exposure by 48%; do not coadminister. Other inhibitors are cyclosporine A, ketoconazole, itraconazole, erythromycin, verapamil, quinidine, tacrolimus, nelfinavir, saquinavr, amiodarone. If must give concomitantly, reduce afatinif dose by 10 mg/day if not tolerated.
- P-glycoprotein **inducers** (e.g., rifampicin): may decrease afatinib exposure (up to 34%). Do not coadminister. Other inducers are carbamazepine, phenytoin, phenobarbital, St. John's wort. If must coadminister, increase afatinib dose by 10 mg/day as tolerated. Teach patient to avoid St. John's wort.

Lab Effects/Interference:
- Decreased serum potassium.
- Increased serum AST, ALT.

Special Considerations:
- Warnings and Precautions:
  - *Diarrhea* is common (incidence 96%, grade 3, 15%, study 1); occurs during the first 6 weeks of treatment but may be severe in 15% (grades 3–4). It may result in dehydration, with or without renal impairment, and be fatal. Renal impairment as a result of diarrhea occurred in 7% of patients in clinical trials, 2% of which were grade 3. Hold drug for grade 2 prolonged (> 48 hours) or grade 3 diarrhea (see Dose Modifications). Teach patient to take antidiarrheal medicine

(e.g., loperamide) at onset of diarrhea and to continue until no bowel movements occur for 12 hours.

- *Grade 3 bullous and exfoliative skin disorders* may occur rarely (0.2%); drug should be discontinued if life-threatening. In study 1, overall overall incidence of cutaneous reactions (rash, erythema, acneiform rash) was 90%, with grade 3 reactions 16%. Incidence of palmar-plantar erythrodysesthesia was 1.5%. Monitor patient closely for cutaneous reactions. Hold drug for grade 2 cutaneous reactions lasting > 7 days, are intolerable, or grade 3 reactions until adverse reaction resolves to grades 0–1, and resume at a reduced dose. Permanently discontinue drug for life-threatening bullous, blistering, or exfoliating lesions or if Stevens-Johnson syndrome (SJS) or toxic epidermal necrolysis (TEN) is suspected. See Dose Modifications.
- *ILD* characterized by lung infiltrates, pneumonitis, ARDS, or allergic alveolitis occurred in 1.6% of patients in clinical trials (0.4% were fatal). Risk may be higher in Asian patients (2.3%) compared to Whites. Hold drug if ILD suspected, and discontinue if ILD confirmed.
- *Hepatic toxicity:* Monitor LFTs baseline and periodically during treatment, closely monitoring patients with severe liver dysfunction. Almost 10% of patients across clinical trials had abnormalities; 0.2% were fatal. Assess LFTs baseline and periodically during therapy. Hold drug in patients with worsening LFTs, and discontinue in patients who develop severe hepatic impairment.
- *Keratitis* characterized by worsening or acute eye inflammation, lacrimation, light insensitivity, blurred vision, eye pain, and/or red eye may occur. Incidence across clinical trials was 0.7%. Hold drug if keratitis is suspected and interrupt/discontinue drug if ulcerative keratitis is confirmed. The benefits and risks of continuing treatment should be carefully discussed if keratitis is diagnosed. Use drug cautiously, if at all, in patients with a history of keratitis, ulcerative keratitis, or severe dry eye. Closely monitor patients who wear contact lenses, as this is a risk factor for keratitis and ulceration.
- *Embryo-fetal toxicity:* Drug is embryotoxic. Teach women of childbearing age to use highly effective contraception to prevent pregnancy during and for at least 2 weeks after the last dose of afatinib. Nursing mothers should discontinue drug or nursing.
- Most common side effects are diarrhea, rash/dermatitis, stomatitis, paronychia, dry skin, decreased appetite, nausea, vomiting, and pruritus.

Potential Toxicities/Side Effects and the Nursing Process

I.   ALTERATION IN ELIMINATION PATTERN related to DIARRHEA

Defining Characteristics: Diarrhea affects approximately 96% of patients with 15% of patients experiencing grade 3 diarrhea. Diarrhea usually occurs in the first 6 weeks. Six percent of patients developed renal impairment as a complication of diarrhea. Grade 2 persisting > 48 hours, or grade 3 requires drug interruption.

Nursing Implications: Assess bowel-elimination pattern baseline and regularly during therapy. Teach patient to report diarrhea; teach patient self-care strategies to manage diarrhea, such as dietary modification and self-administration of loperamide and to continue loperamide until the patient has no loose bowel movement in 12 hours; teach patient to minimize potential complications, such as dehydration and electrolyte depletion. Identify patients at risk for dehydration and follow closely, such as patients with renal insufficiency, diabetes, congestive heart failure, or the older population. Teach patient to report right away severe or persistent diarrhea. If this occurs, discuss with physician dose interruption, as well as fluid and electrolyte replacement. If diarrhea is refractory or difficult to manage, patient may become dehydrated and will be at risk for acute renal failure, which may be fatal. If the patient is dehydrated and at risk for renal impairment (e.g., preexisting renal disease, disease or medications that may lead to renal disease, advancing age), the drug should be temporarily discontinued while the patient is rehydrated. Renal function should be assessed at baseline and periodically during therapy, more closely if the patient has diarrhea and is at risk for dehydration. Hold drug for prolonged grade 2 diarrhea ($>$ 48 hours) or grade 3, or diarrhea unresponsive to therapy, until diarrhea resolves to $<$ grade 1, and reduce dose.

II.   ALTERATION IN SKIN INTEGRITY related to RASH

Defining Characteristics: As expected, because EGFR is important in skin function, this is the area of major toxicity. Rash, erythema, and caneiform rash affect 90% of patients, with an incidence of grade 3 of 16%. Incidence of grades 1–3 palmar-plantar erythrodysesthesia was 7%. Rarely, bullous, blistering, and exfoliative lesions have occurred (0.15%). Pruritus affects 21%, dry skin 31%, and paronychia 58%, with 11% grade 3 or higher.

Nursing Implications: Assess skin integrity of face, neck, arms, and upper trunk, baseline and regularly during treatment. Teach patient that rash may occur, explain the rash's usual course, and teach self-care measures for comfort. Emphasize the need to keep skin with rash clean to prevent infection. Teach patient that skin may become dry and to use skin emollients or moisturizers. Assess body image intactness; if rash develops, assess its threat to body image. Encourage patient to verbalize feelings; provide emotional support and individualize care plan to patient response. For rash management, refer to the introduction in this chapter. Teach all patients to (1) use a water-based emollient frequently during the day to prevent dryness, (2) stay hydrated, (3) avoid sun exposure and wear sun protective clothing, and (4) wear SPF 30, UVA/UVB broad spectrum. Do not use antiacne medications. Tetracycline analogues provide anti-inflammatory benefit. **Grade 1/mild rash** (localized, does not interfere with activities of daily living (ADLs), and is not infected): Goal is to preserve skin integrity, minimize discomfort, and prevent infection. Key patient teaching includes (1) use a mild soap with active ingredients that reduce skin drying, such as pyrithione zinc (Head & Shoulders); (2) consider applying aloe gel to red, tender areas; (3) report distressing tenderness, as pramoxine (lidocaine topical anesthetic) may help, (4) keep fingernails clean and trimmed; and (5) apply zinc ointment to rectal mucosa after washing. Management: maintain current drug dose, observe or give topical hydrocortisone 1% or 2.5% or clindamycin 1% gel (anti-inflammatory benefit), reassess in 2 weeks. **For grade 2/moderate**, which is generalized, mild symptoms, has minimal effect on ADLs,

- ALT or AST elevation $> 3 \times$ ULN with total bilirubin elevation $> 2 \times$ ULN in absence of cholestasis or hemolysis: permanently discontinue drug.
- Total bilirubin elevation $> 3 \times$ ULN: temporarily hold drug until recovery to baseline or to $\leq$ to $1.5 \times$ ULN, then resume at reduced dose.
- Any grade treatment-related interstitial lung disease (ILD)/pneumonitis: permanently discontinue alectinib.
- Renal Impairment: (a) Grade 3: temporarily withhold drug until serum creatinine recovers to $\leq 1.5 \times$ ULN, then resume at reduced dose; (b) grade 4 permanently discontinue alectinib.
- Symptomatic bradycardia: hold alectinib until recovery to asymptomatic bradycardia or to HR 60 bpm or greater; if contributing concomitant medication(s) identified and discontinued, or if the medication dose is adjusted, resume alectinib at previous dose once patient is asymptomatic or HR is $\geq$ 60 bpm. If no contributing concomitant medication identified, resume alectinib at reduced dose upon patient recovery of asymptomatic bradycardia or to HR $\geq$ 60 bpm.
- Bradycardia, life-threatening or requiring urgent intervention: permanently discontinue alectinib if no contributing concomitant medication(s). If other medication(s) identified or its dose adjusted, resume alectinib at a reduced dose once patient has asymptomatic bradycardia or HR $\geq$ 60 bpm. Monitor patient frequently and permanently discontinue alectinib if patient has recurrent symptomatic bradycardia.
- Elevated blood creatine phosphokinase (CPK)
  - CPK elevation $> 5 \times$ ULN: hold alectinib until recovery to baseline or to $\leq 2.5 \times$ ULN, then resume at same dose.
  - CPK elevation $> 10 \times$ ULN or 2nd occurrence of CPK elevation of $> 5 \times$ ULN: temporarily hold alectinib until recovery to baseline or to $\leq 2.5 \times$ ULN, then resume at reduced dose.

Drug Preparation: Available as 150-mg capsules.

Drug Administration:
- Monitor LFTs baseline and every 2 weeks during first 3 months of treatment, then once a month, more frequently if LFTs elevated. See dose modifications for management. Monitor renal function tests and CPK baseline and monitor CPK every 2 weeks during 1st month of treatment and in patients reporting unexplained muscle pain, tenderness or weakness. Discuss abnormalities with physician/NP/PA.
- Teach patient to (1) take capsule with food; (2) not to open or dissolve capsule contents; and (3) if dose is missed or patient vomits after taking it, take next dose at scheduled time.

Drug Interactions: None identified that require alectinib dosage adjustment.

Lab Effects/Interference:
- Increased: AST, alkaline phosphatase, CPK, bilirubin, glucose, ALT, creatinine.
- Decreased calcium, potassium, phosphate, sodium.
- Anemia, lymphopenia.

Special Considerations:
- Most common adverse effects ($\geq$ 20%) were: fatigue, constipation, edema, and myalgia.
- Warnings and Precautions:
  - *Hepatotoxicity*: Increases in hepatic transaminases and bilirubin occur primarily in the first 3 months of therapy. Monitor LFTs (including ALT, AST, total bilirubin every 2 weeks during the first 3 months of treatment, then once a month and as clinically indicated (more frequent if elevations). Hold drug and resume at a reduced dose, or permanently discontinue alectinib (see dosage).
  - *ILD/Pneumonitis*: is rare (0.4% incidence). If patient develops worsening respiratory symptoms suggestive of ILD (e.g., dyspnea, cough, fever), discuss prompt evaluation by MD/NP/PA. If ILD/pneumonitis is confirmed, hold drug immediately; if no other cause of ILD/pneumonitis is found, drug should be permanently discontinued.
  - *Renal impairment:* Incidence of renal impairment in 8% of patients. Permanently discontinue drug for grade 4 renal toxicity. Hold for grade 3 until receovery to $\leq$ 1.5 $\times$ ULN, then resume at reduced dose. Monitor serum creatinine baseline and during treatment.
  - *Bradycardia:* may occur, with about 20% experiencing a HR of < 50 bpm, and 7.5% becoming symptomatic. Monitor HR and BP regularly. There is no dose modification for asymptomatic bradycardia. If symptomatic bradycardia develops that is not life-threatening, hold alectinib until recovery to asymptomatic bradycardia, or HR $\geq$ 60 bpm and evaluate medication profile for other drugs that can reduce HR, including antihypertensives; if due to concomitant medications, resume alectinib at a reduced dose. If due to other medications, resume alectinib. If life-threatening and not due to other causes, permanently discontinue alectinib. See Dosage section.
  - *Severe myalgia and creatine phosphokinase (CPK) elevation:* Severe myalgia and CPK elevations may occur. Myalgia (musculoskeletal pain) occurs in about 26% of patients and is severe (grade 3) in about 0.7%. CPK is elevated in about 41% of patients, with grade 3 occurring in 4.0%. Median time to grade 3 CPK was 14 days in clinical studies 1 and 2. Teach patients to call providers for any unexplained muscle pain, tenderness, or weakness. Assess CPK levels every 2 weeks for the first month of treatment, then as needed to evaluate symptoms. Depending upon how severe the CPK elevation is, hold alectinib, then resume or dose modify. See Dose Modifications for management.
  - *Embryo-fetal toxicity:* Teach women of reproductive potential to use effective contraception to avoid pregnancy during therapy, and for 1 week after last alectinib dose. Women should not breast-feed while taking the drug.
  - Photosensitivity occurs in 9.9% of patients. Teach patient to avoid sun exposure and use broad-spectrum sunscreen.

Potential Toxicities/Side Effects and the Nursing Process

I. ALTERATION IN NUTRITION, POTENTIAL, LESS THAN BODY REQUIREMENTS, related to NAUSEA, VOMITING, DIARRHEA, CONSTIPATION, DYSPEPSIA, INCREASED LFTs

Defining Characteristics: Constipation occurred in 34% of patients, nausea in 18%, diarrhea in 16%, dyspepsia in 16%, and vomiting in 12%. LFT elevation occurred in 34%

Nursing Implications: Assess oral hygiene practices and status of oral mucosa, gums, and teeth baseline and regularly throughout therapy. Assess nutritional status and weight baseline and regularly during treatment. Teach patient to report stomatitis and to use a systematic cleansing regimen as determined by institutional policy. Assess baseline LFTs, and monitor LFTs and patient tolerance very closely during therapy if abnormal at baseline. If a patient develops worsening LFTs, discuss with physician dose interruption or discontinuance (see Dose Modifications). Teach patient to report irritation of lips (cheilitis) and loss of appetite.

Drug: Alectinib (Alecensa)

Class: Kinase inhibitor

Mechanism of Action: TKI targeting ALK and RET, preventing activation of downstream signaling proteins STAT3 and AKT and causing cell death of cells containing ALK (gene) fusion, amplification, or mutations. Alterations in the ALK gene that makes this tumor-specific protein have been found in 3–5% of patients with NSCLC, neuroblastoma, and rare sarcomas. The abnormality is called EMLA-ALK (echinoderm microtubule-associated protein-like 4 ALK) fusion gene, and it makes a protein product that turns on signaling for the cell to proliferate.

Metabolism: Drug reaches maximum serum concentration 4 hours after oral dosing in fed conditions, with a 37% bioavailability. Administration with a high-fat, high-calorie meal increases area under the curve (AUC) exposure by 90%. Alectinib is metabolized by CYP3A4 to its major metabolite M4, which shows a potency comparable to parent drug. M4 is subsequently also metabolized by CYP3A4. Alectinib and M4 are highly protein-bound > 99%, and cross the blood–brain barrier where CSF and serum blood concentrations are similar. M4 alone is a substrate of P-glycoprotein. Elimination half-life of alectinib is 33 hour, and for M4 is 31 hours. Drug and its metabolites were excreted in the feces (98%), with 84% unchanged alectinib, and 6% as M4. Drug has not been studied in patients with severe liver or renal impairment.

Indication(s): Treatment of patients with anaplastic lymphoma kinase (ALK)-positive, metastatic NSCLC as determined by an FDA-approved test.

Dosage/Range:
- 600 mg PO twice daily, administered with food, until disease progression or unacceptable toxicity.
- Severe hepatic impairment (Child-Pugh C) dose is 450 mg PO bid.

Dose Modifications:
- First dose reduction dose: 450 mg PO bid; 2nd dose reduction dose: 300 mg PO bid. If unable to tolerate 300 mg PO bid, discontinue alectinib.
- Elevated LFTs
  - ALT or AST > 5 × ULN with total bilirubin ≤ 2 × ULN: temporarily hold drug until recovery to baseline or ≤ 3 × ULN, then resume at reduced dose.

and no infection: Goal is to prevent infection and promote comfort. Continue EGFRI dose; use topicals (hydrocortisone 2.5% or clindamycin 1% gel) and consider adding doxycycline 100 mg PO twice daily or minocycline 100 mg PO twice daily (give antimicrobial and anti-inflammatory effect); reassess after 2 weeks. **Interrupt drug** if patient develops prolonged grade 2 cutaneous reactions (lasting > 7 days), or if intolerable. For **grades 3–4 or severe rash** (generalized, severe, has a significant impact on ADLs, and increased risk of infection): The goal is to prevent infection or identify it early to minimize complications and to promote effective coping. **Interrupt drug**. Follow institutional guidelines, e.g., treat rash with topicals (hydrocortisone 2.5%, or clindamycin 1% gel), doxycycline 100 mg PO twice daily or minocycline 100 mg PO twice daily, and methylprednisolone (Medrol dose pack); reassess after 2 weeks. Resume drug when rash improved to grade 2, at full or reduced dose (Lynch et al., 2007; Lacouture et al., 2011). If rash appears infected (exudate, vesicular formation, different appearance), obtain culture and sensitivity, treat empirically until sensitivity value determined, and/or obtain dermatology consult. Hold drug for severe rash that does not respond to medical intervention. If the drug is interrupted, afatinib can be resumed at a lower dose once skin reaction has resolved to a grade 1 or less. Teach patient to stop drug and to report the development of bullous lesions, blisters, or desquamation right away.

III. SENSORY/PERCEPTUAL ALTERATION, POTENTIAL, related to CONJUNCTIVITIS, EYE DRYNESS, KERATITIS

Defining Characteristics: Conjunctivitis and eye dryness may occur and are generally mild to moderate (grades 1 to 2). Rarely, keratitis and corneal ulceration may occur. Incidence of conjunctivitis is 11%, and keratitis is 0.8% across all studies.

Nursing Implications: Teach patient to report symptoms of keratitis (e.g., any new or worsening eye irritation, lacrimation, light sensitivity, blurred vision, eye pain, red eye) or change in visual acuity. Teach patient to use artificial tears to keep eyes lubricated. Refer patient to ophthalmologist immediately for any acute signs or symptoms, such as red eye or eye pain. Teach patient to stop drug if these occur and to report them immediately. Drug is interrupted if keratitis is suspected and if ulcerative keratitis is confirmed, drug interruption should continue or drug should be discontinued. Drug should be used cautiously in patients with a history of keratitis, ulcerative keratitis, severe dry eye, or in patients who wear contact lenses.

IV. POTENTIONAL ALTERATION IN NUTRITION, LESS THAN BODY REQUIREMENTS, related to MUCOSITIS, HEPATOTOXICITY, ANOREXIA, NAUSEA, VOMITING

Defining Characteristics: Stomatitis is common, occurring in 71% of patients receiving afatinib, with grades 3–4 occurring in 9% of patients. Cheilitis occurs in 12% of patients. Decreased appetite occurs in 19%, with 4% grades 3–4. Hepatotoxicity may occur. ALT and AST elevated in 11% and 8% of patients, respectively.

(ALT) and 51% (AST) of patients, with hyperbilirubinemia occurring in 39% of patients. Hyperglycemia affected 36% of patients.

Nursing Implications: Assess LFTs baseline and every 2 weeks for the first two months of therapy, then as ordered. Discuss elevations with MD/PA/NP. Assess baseline nutritional status and bowel-elimination status. If patient develops nausea and/or vomiting, teach patient to self-administer antiemetics 1 hour prior to each dose, and to call if nausea/vomiting is increased or persistent. Discuss with physician more effective antiemetic regimen if nausea/vomiting persist. Encourage small, frequent intake of cool, bland foods as tolerated if nausea develops. Refer to dietitian as needed for meal planning. Teach patient to report diarrhea that does not respond to OTC antidiarrheal medication or if constipation occurs that is unresponsive to fluids, laxatives, and use of high-fiber foods. Teach self-care measures of diet modification and increased oral fluids to 2–3 L during the waking hours. If constipation occurs, teach patient self-care measures to prevent constipation.

II.   ALTERATION IN COMFORT related to FATIGUE, EDEMA, ARTHRALGIA, RASH, ANEMIA

Defining Characteristics: Fatigue was the most common adverse reaction occurring in 41% of patients. Edema occurred in 30% of patients, back pain in 12% of patients, rash in 18% of patients, and anemia in 56% of patients. Weight gain occurred in 11% of patients. CPK elevation may occur. Myalgia (musculoskeletal pain) occurs in about 29% of patients, and is severe (grade 3) in about 1.2%. CPK is elevated in about 43% of patients, with grade 3 occurring in 4.6%. Median time to grade 3 CPK was 14 days in clinical studies 1 and 2.

Nursing Implications: Assess baseline parameters of weight, presence of edema, pulmonary function, red blood cell count, and monitor closely during therapy. Teach patient to monitor weight gain and edema or the development of dyspnea and to report it. Assess skin integrity baseline and frequently during treatment. Teach patient to report rash. Develop a plan to protect skin and maintain skin integrity. Assess for patient complaint of myalgia, arthralgia, weakness, and teach patient to call providers for any unexplained muscle pain, tenderness, or weakness in the first month of treatment. See Dose Modifications for management.

Drug: alitretinoin gel 0.1% (Panretin)

Class: Retinoid.

Mechanism of Action: A 9-*cis*-retinoic acid, alitretinoin is a naturally occurring, endogenous retinoid necessary for regulation of gene expression responsible for cell differentiation and replication. 9-*cis*-retinoic acid binds to and activates intracellular retinoid receptors that enable transcription of these genes. Alitretinoin has been found to inhibit the growth of Kaposi's sarcoma (KS) cells directly.

Metabolism: Drug is used topically, without any detectable plasma concentrations or metabolites.

Indication: Indicated for TOPICAL treatment of cutaneous KS lesions in patients with AIDS. It should not be used when systemic therapy for KS is necessary (> 10 KS lesions in prior month, or symptomatic lymphedema, pulmonary KS, or visceral involvement).

Contraindications: Patients with known hypersensitivity to retinoids or any product ingredients.

Dosage/Range:
- Sufficient gel applied to cover the lesion with generous coating.
- Available in 60-g tube.

Drug Preparation:
- None.
- Gel tube should be stored at room temperature.

Drug Administration:
- Use glove to apply generous coating of gel to lesions bid, avoiding surrounding skin.
- DO NOT APPLY on or near mucosal surfaces.
- Allow to dry for 3–5 minutes before covering with clothing.
- Gradually increase applications to 3–4 per day.
- If severe skin irritation develops, stop application for a few days until irritation resolves.
- DO NOT USE an occlusive dressing over gel.

Drug Interactions:
- DEET (*N, N*-diethyl-*m*-toluamide) insect repellent or products containing DEET, as gel increases DEET toxicity.
- No testing has been done to assess possible interactions between systemic antiretroviral agents, or other agents used in the systemic management of HIV infection.

Lab Effects/Interference:
- None known.

Special Considerations:
- Responses may be seen in 2 weeks, but most often take longer, rarely 14 weeks. Gel should be used as long as there is clinical benefit. Contraindicated in patients having hypersensitivity to retinoids.
- Warnings and Precautions:
  - Women of childbearing age should use effective contraception to prevent pregnancy, as it is unknown whether topical gel can modulate endogenous 9-*cis*-retinoic levels. 9-*cis*-retinoic acid is teratogenic.
- Drug SHOULD NOT BE USED by nursing mothers; mothers must discontinue nursing prior to using the drug.
- Drug may increase photosensitivity, so patients should be taught to AVOID sunlamps and to minimize sunlight exposure while receiving the drug.
- Safety testing has not been done in pediatric or geriatric (> 65 yr) populations.
- Toxicity almost exclusively related to skin reactions at the application site.

diffusion distance of oxygen) without making new blood vessels (angiogenesis). Blockade of these receptors helps to inhibit tumor growth and progression.

Metabolism: After oral dosing, bioavailability is 58%. Peak serum levels are reached in 2.5–4.1 hours, and steady state is achieved within 2–3 days of dosing. Drug solubility is pH dependent, with a higher pH resulting in lower solubility. Drug is highly protein-bound (> 99%). Plasma half-life of drug is 2.5–6.1 hours. Drug is primarily metabolized by the liver (CYP3A4/5, and to a lesser degree CYP1A2, CYP2C19, UGT1A1). Drug is excreted in the feces (41%, with 12% as unchanged drug) and urine (23%).

Indication: Drug is FDA approved for treatment of patients with advanced renal cell cancer after failure of one prior systemic therapy. FDA approved in combination with avelumab (Bavencio) for first line treatment of RCC.

Dosage/Range:
- Initial dose: 5 mg orally, twice daily 12 hours apart, with or without food; swallow tablet whole with a glass of water. If patient has moderate hepatic impairment, decrease starting dose by approximately half (Pfizer Lab, 2014).
- Dose adjustments made based on tolerability and individual safety.
  - If the patient tolerates axitinib for at least 2 consecutive weeks without adverse effects > grade 2, is normotensive, and not receiving antihypertensive medication, the dose may be increased (e.g., if increased from 5 mg twice daily, it may be increased to 7 mg twice daily, and further to 10 mg twice daily using the same criterion).
  - In combination with avelumab: axitinib dose is 5 mg PO bid (12 hours apart) with or without food, in combination with avelumab 800 mg IV infusion over 1 hour every 2 weeks. Treatment is continued until disease progression or unacceptable toxicity.
  - Some adverse drug reactions require temporary interruption or dose reduction. If dose reduction from 5 mg twice daily is required, the recommended dose is 3 mg twice daily. If additional dose reduction is required, the recommended dose is 2 mg twice daily.
- If the patient is taking a strong CYP3A4/5 inhibitor, decrease axitinib dose by approximately 50%. Subsequent doses can be increased or decreased based on safety and tolerability. If coadministration of the strong inhibitor is discontinued, the axitinib dose should be returned (after 3–5 half-lives of the inhibitor) to that used prior to the initiation of the strong CYP3A4/5 inhibitor.
- Patients with moderate hepatic impairment should start at approximately 50% of the dose, or 2.5 mg orally, twice daily. Drug has not been studied in patients with severe liver impairment.

Drug Preparation:
- None, oral. Available as 1-mg and 5-mg tablets.

Drug Administration:
- Oral. Teach patient to take tablet every 12 hours, morning and evening. Swallow tablet whole with a glass of water. Tablet may be taken with or without food.
- If the patient vomits or misses a dose, an additional dose should not be taken. The next dose should be taken at the usual time.

- Stop drug 24 hours prior to scheduled surgery.
- Prior to starting axitinib therapy:
  - Assess thyroid function tests baseline, then periodically during axitinib therapy.
  - Assess urine for protein baseline, then periodically during axitinib therapy.
  - Assess LFTs (ALT, AST, bilirubin) baseline, then periodically during axitinib therapy.
  - Assess BP; BP should be well controlled before starting axitinib.
  - If bleeding occurs and requires medical intervention, temporarily interrupt axitinib therapy.
- Drug has not been studied in patients with evidence of untreated brain metastases or recent active GI bleeding and should not be used in these patients (hemorrhagic events including fatal events have occurred).

Drug Interactions:
- Strong CYP3A4/5 inhibitors (e.g., ketoconazole, itraconazole, clarithromycin, atazanavir, indinavir, nefazodone, nelfinavir, ritonavir, saquinavir, telithromycin, and voriconazole; grapefruit or grapefruit juice): increased serum level of axitinib; avoid concurrent administration; if must give together, reduce axitinib dose by 50%.
- Strong CYP3A4/5 inducers (e.g., rifampin, dexamethasone, phenytoin, carbamazepine, rifabutin, rifapentin, phenobarbital, St. John's wort): reduced axitinib serum level: do not give concurrently. Moderate inducers (e.g., bosentan, efavirenz, etravirine, modafinil, nafcillin): may decrease serum level; avoid concurrent administration if possible.

Lab Effects/Interference:
- Decreased soluble VEGFR-2 and VEGFR-3 and increased VEGF in blood.
- Decreased hemoglobin, lymphocytes, white blood cells, platelets.
- Increased serum creatinine, glucose, lipase, amylase, ALT, ALP, sodium, potassium, TSH.
- Decreased serum bicarbonate, calcium, albumin, glucose, sodium, phosphated, T4.
- Proteinuria.

Special Considerations:
- Most common toxicities (≥ 20%) are diarrhea, HTN, fatigue, decreased appetite, nausea, dysphonia, palmar-plantar erythrodysesthesia (hand–foot syndrome [HFS]), decreased weight, vomiting, asthenia, and constipation.
- Warnings and Precautions:
  - *Hypertension*, including hypertensive crisis, has occurred. BP should be well controlled prior to starting axitinib. Monitor for hypertension and treat as needed. If hypertension is persistent despite antihypertensives, reduce axitinib dose.
  - *Arterial (TIAs, CVA, MI, retinal artery occlusion) [ATE] and venous thrombotic (PE, DVT) [VTE] events* have been observed and can be fatal. Use with caution in patients at increased risk of thrombotic events. Incidence of grades 3–4 ATEs was 1%. Incidence of VTEs was 3%, with grades 3–4 (3%). Drug should be used cautiously in patients who are at risk for or who have a history of thrombotic events. Drug has not been studied in patients who had a venous thrombotic event in the prior 6 months or arterial thrombotic event within the past 12 months.

fever, flu-like symptoms, mucosal lesions, or progressive skin rash) and to report them right away.

- *Hyperglycemia:* including ketoacidosis, was reported in 65% of patients. Grade 3 (FPG> 250–500 mg/dL) and grade 4 (FPG> 500 mg/dL) were reported in 33% and 3.9% patients, respectively. Ketoacidosis occurred in 0.7% of patients. For patients experiencing grade 2 (FPG 160–250 mg/dL) hyperglycemia, median time to first occurrence was 15 days. Almost all patients (96%) with an elevated FPG level who continued fulvestrant after stopping alpelisib had FPG return to baseline. Screening/Management: (1) before starting alpelisib, test baseline FPG, HbA1c, and optimize blood glucose; (2) monitor blood glucose and/or FPG at least once weekly × 2 weeks, then at least once every 4 weeks, and as clinically indicated; 3) monitor HbA1c every 3 months and as clinically indicated. If a patient develops hyperglycemia after starting alpelisib, (a) monitor blood glucose/FPG at least twice weekly until blood glucose/FPG decreases to normal levels; (b) during treatment with antidiabetic medication, continue monitoring at least once weekly × 8 weeks, followed by once every 2 weeks, and as clinically indicated; (c) consider consulting a diabetes practitioner for assistance with treatment of hyperglycemia and teaching patient lifestyle changes including diet. Closely monitor patients with a PMH of Type 2 diabetes. Patients with Type 1 diabetes were not studied. Teach patient signs/symptoms of hyperglycemia and to report them right away (excessive thirst, urinary frequency, voiding higher volume of urine, increased appetite with weight loss).
- *Pneumonitis:* including interstitial pneumonitis and interstitial lung disease may occur. Incidence of pneumonitis was 1.8%. If a patient develops new or worsening respiratory signs/symptoms (e.g., hypoxia, cough, dyspnea) or if pneumonitis is suspected (interstitial infiltrates on X-ray), interrupt alpelisib right away and evaluate for pneumonitis. If pneumonitis is confirmed, permanently discontinue alpelisib. Teach patients to immediately report new or worsening respiratory symptoms.
- *Diarrhea:* occurs frequently (incidence 58%) and may be severe, with dehydration and acute kidney injury. Grade 3 diarrhea occurred in 7% of patients. The median time to onset for grade 2 or 3 diarrhea was 46 days. Teach patients to report diarrhea and to start antidiarrheal therapy, increase oral fluids, and report diarrhea to their healthcare worker when it occurs. See dose modification for diarrhea.
- *Embryo-fetal toxicity:* Drug is fetotoxic. Teach women of reproductive potential, and men whose female sexual partners are of reproductive potential, to use effective contraception and condoms to prevent pregnancy during therapy with alpelisib and for one week after last dose.

Potential Toxicities/Side Effects and the Nursing Process

I.   ALTERATION IN NUTRITION, POTENTIAL, LESS THAN BODY REQUIREMENTS, related to HYPERGLYCEMIA, NAUSEA, VOMITING, DIARRHEA, STOMATITIS

Defining Characteristics: Hyperglycemia occurred in 79% of patients and was grade 3–4 in 39%. Diarrhea occurred in 58% (grade 3 in 7%), nausea in 45%, stomatitis 30%, and

---

vomiting in 27%. Weight was decreased in 27% of patients, and 36% complained of decreased appetite. Dysgeusia occurred in 18%.

Nursing Implications: Assess baseline nutritional status, weight, signs/symptoms of hyperglycemia, and bowel-elimination status. Assess baseline FBS and random blood glucose, HgbA1C, and if elevated, discuss measures to optimize blood glucose before starting alpelisib therapy. Once therapy is started, monitor blood glucose at least twice weekly until blood glucose is normal. During treatment with antidiabetic medication, monitor blood glucose at least once a week × 8 weeks, then once every 2 weeks and as clinically indicated. Teach patient lifestyle changes (e.g., gentle exercise if tolerated, diet). Assess oral mucosa. Teach patient to report signs/symptoms of hyperglycemia after treatment (e.g., increased thirst, urination, hunger with weight loss, and increased volume of urine voided). Teach patient self-care management of any antidiabetic medications (e.g., metformin). If patient develops nausea and/or vomiting, teach patient to self-administer antiemetics and administer an antiemetic prior to taking alpelisib dose. Teach patient to call if diarrhea gets worse or doesn't resolve, or if nausea/vomiting persist. Discuss with physician/NP/PA more effective antiemetic regimen if nausea/vomiting persist. Encourage small, frequent intake of cool, bland foods as tolerated if nausea develops. Refer to dietitian as needed for meal planning. Teach patient to report diarrhea that does not respond to OTC antidiarrheal medication. Teach self-care measures of diet modification and increased oral fluids to 2–3 L during the waking hours. Teach patient to self-assess oral mucosa, perform systematic oral cleansing after meals and at bedtime with normal saline or bicarbonate in water rinses, and report irritation or any lesions seen.

II.   ALTERATION IN ACTIVITY, POTENTIAL related to FATIGUE

Defining Characteristics: Fatigue occurred in 42% of patients and was grade 3 in 5%. Hgb was decreased in 42% and was grade 3 in 4.2%.

Nursing Implications: Assess patient's baseline activity level and degree of fatigue. Assess hgb baseline and during treatement. Teach patient that fatigue may occur or worsen and to report this. Teach patient to alternate rest and activity patterns and to review diet and intake of energy stores. Assess patient's family support network and their willingness to assist patient in any activities that are very tiring. Revise plan as needed.

Drug: axitinib (Inlyta)

Class: RTK inhibitor of VEGFR; angiogenesis inhibitor.

Mechanism of Action: Potent and selective inhibitor of vascular endothelial growth factor (VEGF) receptors 1, 2, 3 on the endothelial cells lining blood vessels. VEGFR inhibition prevents VEGF (ligand) from binding to the receptor on the endothelial cells, thus preventing the blood vessel endothelial cells from proliferating and migrating to form capillary tubes (angiogenesis) to send blood to the tumor. The tumor cannot grow beyond 2 mm (the

- Rash
  - Grade 1 ($<$ 10% BSA with active skin toxicity): Maintain dose. Start topical cortico-steroid treatment. Consider adding oral antihistamine to manage symptoms.
  - Grade 2: (10–30% BSA with active skin toxicity): Maintain dose; initiate or intensify topical corticosteroid and oral antihistamine treatment; consider low dose systemic corticosteroid treatment.
  - Grade 3 (e.g., severe rash not responsive to medical management, $>$ 30% BSA with active skin toxicity): Interrupt drug; initiate or intensify topical corticosteroid and oral antihistamine treatment. Once improved to $\leq$ grade 1, resume alpelisib at the same dose level for the first occurrence of rash or at next lower dose if the second occurrence.
  - Grade 4: (e.g., severe bullous, blistering, or exfoliating skin conditions; and any % of BSA with extensive superinfection, IV antibiotics indicated; life-threatening consequences): Permanently discontinue alpelisib.
- Diarrhea
  - Grade 1: Maintain dose; initiate appropriate medical therapy and monitor closely.
  - Grade 2: Initiate or intensify appropriate medical therapy and monitor as clinically indicated. Interrupt alpelisib until recovery to grade $\leq$ 1, then resume alpelisib at same dose level.
  - Grade 3 and 4: Initiate or intensify appropriate medical therapy and monitor as clinically indicated. Interrupt alpelisib until recovery to grade $\leq$ 1, then resume alpelisib at the next lower dose level.
- Other Toxicities
  - Grade 1 or 2: Maintain dose. Initiate appropriate medical therapy and monitor clinically.
  - Grade 2 or 3 pancreatitis: Interrupt alpelisib until recovery to grade $<$ 2, then resume alpelisib at the next lower dose level. ONLY ONE dose reduction permitted; if toxicity recurs, permanently discontinue alpelisib.
  - Grade 2 total bilirubin elevation: Interrupt alpelisib until recovery to grade $\leq$ 1, then resume alpelisib at the same dose level if it resolves in $\leq$ 14 days, or resume at the next lower dose level if resolved in $>$ 14 days.
  - Grade 3: Interrupt alpelisib until recovery to grade $\leq$ 1, then resume alpelisib at the next lower dose level.
  - Grade 4: Permanently discontinue alpelisib.

Drug Preparation: Available in 50-mg, 150-mg, 200-mg tablets.

Drug Administration:
- Assess baseline FBS and random blood glucose, HgbA1C, and if elevated, discuss measures to optimize blood glucose before starting alpelisib therapy. Once therapy is started, monitor blood glucose at least twice weekly until blood glucose is normal. During treatment with antidiabetic medication, monitor blood glucose at least once a week × 8 weeks, then once every 2 weeks and as clinically indicated.
- Assess baseline systems, and then for signs/symptoms of toxicity: hyperglycemia, rash, diarrhea, allergic reaction. Review patient adherence to antidiabetic regimen, if initiated, and diarrhea, skin regimens, if initiatiate, and patient responses.

- Teach patient to self-assess and report signs/symptoms of allergic reaction, hyperglycemia (increased thirst, hunger, frequent urination, blurred vision, fatigue, headache), rash, diarrhea, and any other new problem.
- Teach patient self-administration of alpelisib:
  - Take at about the same time every day.
  - Swallow tablets whole, do not chew, crush, or split prior to swallowing; Do not take if tablet is broken, cracked, or not intact.
  - If a dose is missed, take with food within the next 9 hours after the time it is usually taken; if it is late by more than 9 hours, skip that day's dose. The next day, take the drug at the usual time.
  - If the patient vomits after taking the dose, DO NOT take an additional dose on that day; resume usual dosing schedule the next day.

Drug Interactions:
- **CYP3A4 inducers:** Avoid coadminstration with a strong CYP3A4 inducer as it may decrease the efficacy of alpelisib.
- **BCRP inhibitors:** Avoid concomitant use as it may increase alpelisib serum level and increase risk of toxicity; if unavoidable, monitor patient closely for increased adverse reactions.
- **CYP2C9 substrates (e.g., warfarin):** Closely monitor patient when alpelisib is given concurrently with CYP2C9 substrates where decreases in the plasma concentration of the CYP2C9 substrate may reduce activity (e.g., coumadin).

Lab Effects/Influence:
- Decreased lymphocyte count, Hgb, platelet count, serum calcium, glucose, potassium, albumin, magnesium
- Increased aPTT, glucose, serum creatinine, GGT, ALT, lipase

Special Considerations:
- Most common adverse reactions ≥ 20% were: increased glucose, increased creatinine, diarrhea, rash, deceased lymphocyte count, increased GGT, nausea, increased ALT, fatigue, decreased Hgb, increased lipase, decreased appetite, stomatitis, vomiting, ↓weight, decreased calcium, decreased glucose, prolonged aPTT, alopecia.
- Warnings and Precautions:
  - *Severe HSRs:* have occurred, including anaphylaxis and anaphylactic shock. Symptoms included dyspnea, flushing, rash, fever or tachycardia. Incidence of grade 3 and 4 HSRs was 0.7%. Teach patients to stop the drug and to report signs/symptoms of an allergic reaction right away (e.g., flushing, rash, fever), and/or seek immediate medical assistance if severe (chest pain or trouble breathing, fast heart rate).
  - *Serious cutaneous reactions:* Stevens-Johnson syndrome (SJS, incidence 0.4%) and Erythema Multiforme (EM, incidence 1.1%) have occurred. Do not initiate therapy in patients with a PMH of SJS, EM, or TEN. If signs/symptoms of a severe cutaneous reaction occur, interrupt the drug until the reaction etiology has been clarified (by a dermatologist). If SJS, EM, or TEN is confirmed, permanently discontinue alpelisib. If it is not confirmed, alpelisib dose modification, topical corticosteroids, or oral antihistamine may be required (see dose modification). Teach patients the signs/symptoms of severe cutaneous reactions (e.g., a prodrome of

TREATMENT

Potential Toxicities/Side Effects and the Nursing Process

I. ALTERATION IN COMFORT AND SKIN INTEGRITY, POTENTIAL, related to APPLICATION SITE REACTIONS

Defining Characteristics: Toxicity begins as erythema. This may increase, and edema may develop with continued application. Most of reactions are mild to moderate, but in some patients (10%), severe reactions may occur with intense erythema, edema, and formation of vesicles. Other skin reactions occurring in > 5% of patients are rash, pain, pruritus, exfoliative dermatitis, cracking, crusting, drainage, oozing, stinging, or tingling.

Nursing Implications: Assess baseline skin integrity and condition of KS cutaneous lesions. Teach patient to apply gel only to lesions and AVOID surrounding skin, as irritation will occur. Teach patient to assess and report any changes in the lesions, such as erythema, and edema. Teach patient to reduce frequency of application if skin reaction occurs, to stop use of the gel if severe reactions occur, and to report this as soon as possible.

Drug: alpelisib (Piqray)

Class: kinase inhibitor; phosphatidylinositol-3-kinase (PI3K) inhibitor

Mechanism of Action: Mutated PIK3CA gene leads to activation of PI3K-α (kinase signaling pathway) and Akt-signaling, resulting in malignant cellular transformation and tumor formation. When the PI3K and Akt-signaling pathway is inhibited by alpelisib, reduced breast cancer growth in mice was seen. Alpelisib also increases estrogen receptor (ER) transcription in breast cancer cells (Novartis, 2019). When combined with fulvestrant there was increased anti-tumor activity in ER positive breast cancer cells.

Metabolism: Food increases drug solubility. Taking alpelisib with a high fat meal, high calorie or low fat–low calorie meal increased alpelisib AUC 73% and Cmax by 145% compared to fasting. Mean drug accumulation after oral dosing is 3 days. Median time to peak plasma concentration (Tmax) is 2–4 hours. Most (89%) of the drug is protein bound. Half life of alpelisib is 8–9 hours. Alpelisib is primarily metabolized by chemical and enzymatic hydrolysis to form the metabolite BZG791 and to a lesser extent by CYP3A4 microenzyme. Most of the drug (81%) is recovered in feces (36% unchanged, 32% the metabolite) and 14% in the urine (2% unchanged, 7.1% metabolite). Pharmacokinetics are not significantly different for patients with mild to moderate renal impairment or mild to severe hepatic impairment. Pharmacokinetics in patients with severe renal impairment was not studied.

Indication: Treatment of postmenopausal women and men with hormone receptor (HR) positive, HER2 negative, PIK3CA-mutated, advanced or metastatic breast cancer following progression on or after an endocrine-based regimen; receptor status and mutation status should be detected by FDA-approved tests. See package insert for PIK3CA mutation testing in plasma and tumor tissue. PIK3CA is the gene that is mutated, and PI3K is the kinase protein made by the gene that participates in the cell signaling.

Contraindication: Severe hypersensitivity to alpelisib or any of its components. DO not start therapy in patients who have a history of Stevens-Johnson Syndrome (SJS), Erythema Multiforme (EM), or Toxic Epidermal Necrolysis (TEN).

Dosage/Range:
- 300 mg (two 150-mg tablets) taken PO once daily **with food**; continue until disease progression or unacceptable toxicity.
- When given with fulvestrant, the recommended fulvestrant dose is 500 mg on days 1, 15, and 29 of the first cycle, then once monthly thereafter.
- For adverse reactions, consider dose interruption, dose reduction, or discontinuation.

Dose Modifications (see package insert for greater detail):
- *Dose Reduction Guidelines for Adverse Reactions:* (a) starting dose is 300 mg once daily (two 150-mg tablets); (b) first dose reduction is to 250 mg once daily (one 200-mg tablet and one 50-mg tablet); (c) second dose reduction is to 200 mg once daily (one 200-mg tablet).
- Only 1 dose reduction permitted for pancreatitis; if further dose reduction is required below 200 mg once daily, discontinue alpelisib.

Dose Modifications
- Hyperglycemia (initial antidiabetic treatment recommended is metformin)
  - Grade 1: Fasting plasma glucose (FPG)/Blood glucose (BG) > ULN-160 mg/dL or > ULN-8.9 mmol/L: Maintain dose; initiate or intensify antidiabetic treatment.
  - Grade 2: FPG/BG > 160–250 mg/dL or > 8.9–13.9 mmol/L: maintain dose; initiate or further intensify antidiabetic treatment; if FPG does not decrease to ≤ 160 mg/dL (8.9 mmol/L) within 21 days with appropriate antidiabetic treatment, reduce alpelisib dose by one dose level and follow FPG value specific recommendations.
  - Grade 3: FPG/BG > 250–500 mg/dL (13.9–27.8 mmol/L): interrupt alpelisib; initiate or intensify oral antidiabetic treatment and consider additional antidiabetic medications for 1–2 days until hyperglycemia improves. Administer IV hydration and consider appropriate treatment (e.g., intervention for electrolyte/ketoacidosis/hyperosmolar disturbances). If FPG decreases to ≤ 160 mg/dL (8.9 mmo/L) within 3–5 days under appropriate antidiabetic treatment, resume alpelisib at 1 lower dose level. If FPG does not decrease to ≤ 160 mg/dL (8.9 mmo/L) within 3–5 days with appropriate antidiabetic treatment, physician should consult an endocrine specialist with expertise in the treatment of hyperglycemia. If FPG does not decrease to ≤ 160 mg/dL (8.9 mmo/L) within 21 days following appropriate antidiabetic treatment, permanently discontinue alpelisib.
  - Grade 4: FPG/BG > 500 mg/dL (≥ 27.8 mmol/L): Interrupt alpelisib; initiate or intensify appropriate antidiabetic treatment (administer IV hydration, and assess need for treatment of electrolyte/ketoacidosis/hyperosmolar disturbances); recheck FPG within 24 hours and as clinically indicated. If FPG decreases to ≤ 500 mg/dL (27.8 mmol/L) follow FPG value specific recommendations for grade 3. If FPG value is confirmed at > 500 mg/dL (27.8 mmol/L), permanently discontinue alpelisib.

to report it. Teach patient self-care measures, including dietary modification (decreased insoluble fiber, increased soluble fiber, and increased fluid) and self-administration of OTC medicines to manage diarrhea. Teach patient to report diarrhea that does not resolve in 24 hours, or is severe, and discuss management with physician.

V.   ALTERATION IN COMFORT related to HEADACHE, ABDOMINAL PAIN, CHILLS, FEVER, FLU SYNDROME, BACK PAIN, INSOMNIA (oral capsules)

Defining Characteristics: Symptoms occur with the following incidence (300 mg/m²/day dose vs higher dose): headache (30% vs 42%), abdominal pain (11% vs 4%), chills (9% vs 13%), fever (5% vs 17%), insomnia (5% vs 11%), flulike symptoms (3% vs 13%), back pain (2% vs 11%).

Nursing Implications: Assess baseline comfort status. Teach patient that these symptoms may occur and teach self-management measures. Teach patient to report fever > 100.5°F, chills, or symptoms that persist or are severe. Discuss management with physician if these occur.

VI.   POTENTIAL ALTERATION IN SKIN INTEGRITY related to RASH, DRY SKIN, ALOPECIA, PERIPHERAL EDEMA (oral capsules), AND RASH, PRURITUS, PAIN AT GEL APPLICATION SITE (topical gel)

Defining Characteristics: Oral capsules: Symptoms occur with the following incidence (300 mg/m²/day vs higher dose): rash (17% vs 23%), exfoliative dermatitis (10.7% vs 9%), alopecia (3.6% vs 11%), and peripheral edema (13% vs 11%). Topical gel: Commonly, rash, pruritus, and pain at application site occur.

Nursing Implications: Oral capsules: Assess baseline skin integrity and extent of cutaneous lesions and teach patient to report rash right away after taking capsules, especially if peeling. Discuss drug continuance with physician if this occurs. Teach patient to use skin cream to keep skin moist, to prevent cracking and peeling, and to prevent itching as directed by the physician. Teach patient to report any hair thinning, and if it occurs, assess impact on patient's body image. Discuss measures to enhance coping, such as use of scarf, measures to protect hair follicles (e.g., gentle shampoo, avoidance of hair perms, or use of curling iron), encourage patient to verbalize feelings, and provide emotional support. Teach patient to report swelling of feet or hands, to keep skin moisturized to prevent cracking or dryness, and to report skin changes that persist or are severe. Discuss management with physician. Topical gel: Assess integrity/extent of cutaneous lesions prior to patient starting therapy. Teach patient application of topical gel on areas of lesions only. Teach patient to report rash, persistent itching, or pain at application site. Teach patient self-care measures to manage itching, or pain at application site if they occur. Discuss with physician management of rash, and if severe, discontinuance of gel.

Drug: binimetinib (Mektovi®)

Class: Kinase inhibitor; Reverible Mitogen-activated extracellular signal regulated kinase 1 (MEK) and MEK2 inhibitor.

Mechanism of Action: MEK1 and MEK2 are upstream regulators of the extracellular signal-related kinase (ERK) activity. The MAPK signaling cascade is composed of Ras, Raf, MEK, and ERK, leading to cell proliferation and resistance to apoptosis (cell death). ERK stimulates many transcription factors, which help to stimulate specific genes to make proteins to turn on cell functions like cell replication and cell survival. MAPK signaling is overactivated by cancer causing mutations like *BRAF V600* in some 50% of malignant melanoma tumors, as it turns on the MAPK system indefinitely (Ascierto et al., 2012). Strategies to block this pathway include inhibiting MEK1 and MEK2 so the message never gets to ERK, and the pathway is turned off. Binimetinib is given in combination with encoragenib as each drug targets a different kinase in the RAS/RAF/MEK/ERK pathway to stop malignant cell proliferation and to tell the cells to die (undergo apoptosis). In addition, apparently the combination of these drugs reduces the emergence of resistance to either drug in *BRAF* mutated cancer cells.

Metabolism: Bioavailability after oral dosing is at least 50%, with median time to maximal concentration (Tmax) of 1.6 hrs, and was unaffected by food ingestion. Terminal half-life of binimetinib is 3.5 hours. Metabolism is primarily by glucuronidation with UGT1A1 accounting for 61%, followed by N-dealkylation, amide **hydrolysis** and others. An active metabolite M3 is produced by CYP1A2 and CYP2C19 metabolism (represents 8.6% if binimetinib exposure). Most of the drug is excreted in the feces (62%, with 32% unchanged) and 31% excreted in the urine (6.5% unchanged drug). In patients with moderate or severe hepatitis impairment, the drug AUC increased 2-fold. No clinically significant changes in binimetinib exposure were seen in patients with severe renal impairment.

Indications: Treatment of patients with unresectable or metastatic melanoma, in combination with encorafenib, with a *BRAF V600E or V 600 K* mutation, as detected by an FDA-approved test.

Contraindications: None.

Dosage/Range:
- Confirm *BRAF V600 E or V600 K* mutation status before drug is started.
- Binimetinib 45 mg PO bid, approximately 12 hours apart, in combination with encorafenib, until disease progression or unacceptable toxicity.
- If encorafenib is permanently discontinued, discontinue binimentin.
- Moderate (total bilirubin $> 1,5$ and $\le 3 \times$ ULN and any AST) or severe hepatic impairment (total bilirubin levels $> 3 \times$ ULN and any AST): 30 mg PO twice daily (12 hours apart).

Dose Modifications:
- Dose reduction steps: (a) 1st dose reduction from 45 mg to 30 mg bid; (b) subsequent modification: permanently discontinue drug if unable to tolerate 30 mg bid.

- *Cardiomyopathy:*
  - Asymptomatic, absolute decrease in LVEF > 10% from baseline that is also below LLN: hold binimetinib for up to 4 weeks, evaluate LVEF q 2 weeks. Resume binimetinib at a reduced dose if (1) LVEF is at or above the LLN AND (2) Absolute decreae from baseline is 10% or less, AND (3) patient is asymptomatic. If the LVEF does not recover within 4 weeks, permanently discontinue binimetinib.
  - Symptomatic CHF, or absolute decrease in LVEF of > 20% from baseline thatis also < LLN: permanently discontinue binimetinib.
- *Venous thromboembolism (VTE):*
  - Uncomplicated DVT or PE: Hold binimetinib: if improves to grade 0–1, resume at a reduced dose; if no improvement, permanently discontinue binimetinib.
  - Life threatening PE: permanently discontinue binimetinib.
- *Serous retinopathy:* Symptomatic serous retinopathy/Retinal pigment epithelial detachments: hold binimetinib for up to 10 days: if improves and becomes asymptomatic, resume at the same dose; if not improved, resume at a lower dose level or permanently discontinue binimetinib.
- *Retinal vein occlusion (RVO):* any grade, permanently discontinue binimetinib.
- *Uveitis:*
  - Grade 1–3: if grade 1–2 does not respond to specific ocular therapy, or for grade 3 uveitis, hold binimetinib for up to 6 weeks. If improved, resume at same or reduced dose. If not improved, permanently discontinue binimetinib.
  - Grade 4: permanently discontinue binimetinib.
- *ILD:*
  - Grade 2: hold binimetinib for up to 4 weeks; if improved to grade 0–1, resume at a reduced dose. If not resolved in 4 weeks, permanently discontinue binimetinib.
  - Grade 3 or grade 4: permanently discontinue binimetinib.
- *Hepatotoxicity:*
  - Grade 2 AST or ALK increased: Maintain binimetinib dose; if no improvement within 2 weeks, hold binimetinib until improved to grade 0–1, or to pretreatment/baseline levels and then resume at the same dose.
  - Grade 3 or 4 AST or ALK increased: see other adverse reactions.
- *Rhabdomyolysis or Creatine Phosphokinase (CPK) Elevation:* Grade 4 asymptomatic CPK elevation or any Any grade CPK elevation with symptoms or with renal impairment: Hold binimetinib dose for up to 4 weeks: if not improved to grade 0–1 resume at a reduced dose; if not resolved within 4 weeks, permanently discontinue binimetinib.
- *Dermatologic:*
  - Grade 2: if no improvement in 2 weeks, hold binimetinib until grade 0–1; resume at same dose if 1st occurence, or reduce dose if recurrent.
  - Grade 3: Hold binimetinib until grade 0–1; resume at same dose if 1st occurrence, or reduce dose if recurrent.
  - Grade 4: permanently discontinue binimetinib.
- *Other adverse reactions (including hemorrhage):*
  - Recurrent grade 2 or 1st recurrence of any grade 3: Hold binimetinib for up to 4 weeks: if improves to grade 0–1 or to pretreatment/baseline levels, resume at a reduced dose; if no improvement, permanently discontinue binimetinib.

- 1st occurrence of any grade 4: Permanently discontinue binimetinib or hold binimetinib for up to 4 weeks: if improvement to grade 0–1 or to pretreatment/baseline
  levels, then resume at a reduced dose; if no improvement, permanently discontinue
  binimetinib.
- Recurrent grade 3: consider permanently discontinue binimetinib.
- Recurrent grade 4: permanently discontinue binimetinib.
- DO NOT dose modify (when given with encorafenib) for palmar-plantar erythrodysesthesia syndrome (PPES), non-cutaneous RAS mutation-positive malignancies, and for
  QTc prolongation (Array BioPharma, Inc., 2019).

Drug Preparation: Oral. Available as 15–mg tablets. Store at room temperature in original
bottle, keeping bottle tightly closed to protect it from moisture. Keep bottle out of reach of
children and pets.

Drug Administration:
- Teach patient self-administration of binimetinib 45 mg PO (or 30 mg if moderate or severe hepatic impairment) approximately 12 hours apart, with encorafenib, with or without food. If a dose is missed, do not take the dose within 6 hours of the next scheduled
  dose. Do not take another dose if vomiting occurs, but continue with the next scheduled
  dose.
- Assess ECHO results, LFT and CPK labs, others as ordered baseline and during therapy.

Drug Interactions: None known.

Lab Effects/Interference:
- Increased creatinine, creatine phosphokinase.
- Increased GGT, AST, ALT, alkaline phosphatase.
- Decreased serum sodium.

Special Considerations:
- Most common adverse effects (25%) in combination with encorafenib: fatigue, nausea,
  diarrhea, vomiting, abdominal pain.
- Warnings and Precautions:
  - *Cardiomyopathy:* Median time to 1st occurrence was 3.6 months. Cardiomyopathy
    resolved in 87% of patients. Assess LVEF by ECHO or MUGA scan prior to starting
    binimetinib, 1 month after starting treatment, then every 2–3 months during treat-
    ment. Patients with baseline LVEF < 50% or < LLN were studied. Monitor patients
    with cardiovascular risk factors closely during treatment. Hold, reduce dose or per-
    manently discontinue binimetinib treatment as needed. See Dose Modifications.
  - *Venous thromboembolism (VTE):* Incidence of VTE was 6%, including 3.1% of pa-
    tients that developed a PE. See dose modification. Teach patient to self-assess and
    report signs/symptoms of DVT and PE right away and/or seek emergency medical
    assistance.
  - *Ocular toxicities:*
    - *Serous retinopathy:* incidence 20%, 8% retinal detachment, and 6% macu-
      lar edema. Assess for visual signs/symptoms at each visit. Remind provider to
      perform ophthalmologic exams at regular intervals, for any new or worsening

- Theoretically, as drug is highly protein-bound, it is possible that bexarotene can displace drugs or be displaced by drugs that bind to plasma proteins (e.g., methotrexate); use together cautiously.
- Paclitaxel plus carboplatin: increased bexarotene AUC twofold.
- Bexarotene may be an inducer of CYP3A4 enzymes and reduce serum levels of the coadministered drug (e.g., atorvastin, tamoxifen, paclitaxel, oral contraceptives).
- Tamoxifen: concomitant administration of bexarotene resulted in a 35% decrease in plasma concentrations of tamoxifen.
- Atorvastin: concomitant administration of bexarotene resulted in a 50% decrease in plasma concentrations of tamoxifen.

Lab Effects/Interference:
Oral capsules:
- CA 125 assay values in patients with ovarian cancer may be increased.
- Significantly increased serum triglycerides, total cholesterol, and decreased HDL.
- Increased LFTs.
- Decreased TSH and total T_4.
- Leukopenia and neutropenia.
- Increased LDH.

Special Considerations:
Oral capsules:
- Bexarotene is contraindicated in patients: (1) with a known hypersensitivity to bexarotene or other components of the product; (2) who are pregnant or mothers who are nursing as drug is teratogenic.
  - Women of childbearing age should use effective contraception—optimally, two forms unless abstinence is chosen.
  - Effective contraception should begin 1 month, continuously, before starting the drug, continued during therapy, and for 1 month after the completion of therapy.
  - A pregnancy test should be done within 1 week prior to beginning therapy and repeated monthly during therapy. If pregnancy occurs, the drug must be stopped immediately and the woman counseled.
  - Bexarotene may reduce the plasma concentrations of oral or other systemic hormonal contraceptives (see Drug Interactions).
- Bexarotene capsules should be started on the second or third day of a normal menstrual period; no more than a one-month supply should be given so that the results of a pregnancy test are assessed, and counseling regarding avoidance of pregnancy and birth defects provided/reinforced prior to giving the prescription for the next month's bexarotene.
- Male patients with sexual partners who are pregnant, possibly pregnant, or who could become pregnant should use condoms during therapy, and for 1 month after therapy is ended.
- Patients with risk factors for pancreatitis (e.g., prior pancreatitis, uncontrolled hyperlipidemia, excessive alcohol consumption, uncontrolled diabetes mellitus, biliary tract disease, and medications known to increase triglyceride levels or to be associated with pancreatic toxicity) should generally NOT be treated with bexarotene capsules.
- Most patients have major lipid abnormalities, and one patient died of pancreatitis.

- 70% of CTCL patients who received an initial dose of $\geq$ 300 mg/m^2/day had fasting triglyceride levels > 2.5 × ULN; about 55% had values > 800 mg/dL (median 1, 200 mg/dL). Elevated serum cholesterol > 300 mg/dL occurred in 60% of patients receiving an initial dose of $\geq$ 300 mg/m^2/day, and 75% of patients receiving a higher initial dose. High-density lipoproteins (HDL) levels were reduced to < 25 mg/dL in 55% receiving an initial dose of $\geq$ 300 mg/m^2/day, and 90% of patients who received a higher initial dose. The effect on lipoproteins was reversible with drug cessation and could generally be managed with dose reduction or concomitant antilipemic therapy.
- Assess fasting blood lipid levels baseline prior to therapy, then weekly for at least the next 2–4 weeks until the lipid response is established; then assess every 8 weeks. Correct fasting lipid levels prior to starting bexarotene (triglycerides: < 400 mg/dL).
- If fasting triglycerides become elevated during therapy, start antilipemic therapy, and if necessary, dose-reduce bexarotene or drug suspended. Of patients started at 300 mg/m^2/day, 60% required antilipemic therapy; atorvastin was used in 48%; DO NOT use gemfibrozil.
- Acute pancreatitis has occurred.
- Thyroid axis alterations: clinical hypothyroidism occurs in about 50% of patients and is reversible. Hypothyroidism reported as an adverse event in 29% of patients; thyroid hormone replacement should be considered in patients with laboratory evidence of hypothyroidism.
- Baseline laboratory assessment prior to starting drug should include WBC with differential, fasting blood glucose, thyroid function tests, fasting blood lipid profile, and liver function tests.
- Patients should limit vitamin A intake to $\leq$ 15,000 international units/day to avoid possible additive toxicity.
- Drug may cause increased LFTs, and decreased T4, TSH. Treatment with thyroid hormone supplements should be considered in patients with laboratory evidence of hypothyroidism. Assess baseline thyroid function tests baseline and monitor during therapy.
- Leukopenia may occur, generally occurring 4–8 weeks after starting therapy. The incidence was 18% at the recommended initial dose, and 43% in those starting at higher doses. Incidence of grades 3–4 neutropenia was 12% and 4%, respectively. Assess WBC/ differential baseline and periodically during treatment.
- Drug may cause cataracts; patients who experience visual difficulties should have an ophthalmologic exam.
- Patients with diabetes mellitus: use caution in patients using insulin, agents enhancing insulin secretion (e.g., sulfonylureas), or insulin-sensitizers (e.g., thiazolidinedione class). Baroxetine may enhance the action of these agents and result in hypoglycemia.
- Patients should avoid direct sunlight and artificial ultraviolet light while taking bexarotene pills or gel, as severe sunburn and skin sensitivity reactions may occur due to photosensitization; patients should also wear SPF 30 or higher.
- No studies have been done with patients having hepatic dysfunction, but theoretically, hepatic dysfunction would greatly reduce metabolism/excretion and increase serum drug levels. Use cautiously, if at all, in this setting.
- Response rate in patients with cutaneous T-cell lymphoma who were refractory to one prior systemic therapy was 32%.

II.   ALTERATION IN ACTIVITY, POTENTIAL, related to HYPOTHYROIDISM (oral capsules)

Defining Characteristics: Bexarotene binds and activates retinoid $\times$ receptors, and can partner with thyroid receptor; once activated, the receptor functions as a transcription factor that regulates gene expression controlling cellular differentiation and proliferation. Drug induces reversible clinical hypothyroidism in about 50% of patients (decrease in TSH in 60% of patients, and total T_4 in 45% of patients at a dose of 300 mg/m^2/day), and hypothyroidism was reported in 29% of patients. Asthenia occurs in 29.8% of patients at a dose of 300 mg/m^2/day and in 45% of patients at higher doses.

Nursing Implications: Assess baseline thyroid function tests (TFTs) and discuss pharmacologic replacement of thyroid hormone with physician if values indicate hypothyroidism. Monitor TFTs during treatment. Teach patient that this may occur, importance of laboratory testing, fact that hypothyroidism induced by drug is reversible following discontinuance of drug, and to report signs/symptoms of hypothyroidism (e.g., weight gain, lethargy, slowed thinking, skin dryness, constipation, joint pain/stiffness). Teach patient to alternate rest and activity periods, and other measures to conserve energy.

III.   POTENTIAL FOR INFECTION related to LEUKOPENIA (oral capsules)

Defining Characteristics: Reversible leukopenia (WBC/mm^3 1,000–3,000) occurred in 18% of patients receiving dose of 300 mg/m^2/day, and in 43% of patients receiving higher doses. Patients receiving 300 mg/m^2/day had grade 3 (12%) and grade 4 (4%) neutropenia. Incidence of bacterial infection was 1.2% in patients receiving a dose of 300 mg/m^2/day (overall body infection was 13%), and bacterial infection was 13% (overall infections 22%) in patients receiving higher doses. Onset of leukopenia was 4–8 weeks. Resolution of leukopenia/neutropenia occurred in 30 days with a drug dose reduction or discontinuance in most patients (82–93%). There were rare serious adverse events associated with leukopenia/neutropenia.

Nursing Implications: Assess WBC and ANC baseline and periodically during therapy. Teach patient that leukopenia may occur and teach self-care measures, including self-assessment for infection, minimizing risk of infection, and when to notify provider. Teach patient/family signs/symptoms of infection, and how to take temperature if this is not known.

IV.   ALTERATION IN BOWEL ELIMINATION related to DIARRHEA (oral capsules)

Defining Characteristics: Diarrhea is uncommon in patients receiving dose of 300 mg/m^2/day but is more common (41%) when dose is increased.

Nursing Implications: Assess baseline elimination status and monitor throughout treatment. Teach patient that diarrhea may occur, especially if dose is > 300 mg/m^2/day, and

- *1% gel:*
  - Main side effects are rash, itching, and pain at application site.

Potential Toxicities/Side Effects and the Nursing Process

I. ALTERATION IN NUTRITION, POTENTIAL, related to ABNORMAL LIPID LEVELS, PANCREATITIS, ELEVATED LFTs, AND NAUSEA (oral capsules)

Defining Characteristics: Almost all patients experience major lipid abnormalities, including elevated fasting triglycerides (70% receiving doses of $\geq$ 300 mg/m^2/day had elevations of more than 2.5 times upper limits of normal [ULN], and 55% had values over 800 mg/dL with a median of 1,200 mg/dL), elevated cholesterol (60% of patients receiving 300 mg/m^2/day, and 75% of patients receiving doses of $\geq$ 300 mg/m^2/day), and decreased levels of the protective high-density lipoproteins (HDL) to < 25 mg/dL (55% of patients receiving a dose of 300 mg/m^2/day, and 90% of patients receiving a dose of > 300 mg/m^2/day). These values normalize after bexarotene is stopped. In most patients, either antilipemic medication or dose reduction of bexarotene allowed control over elevated levels. Rarely, patients with markedly elevated triglycerides (lowest level 770 mg/dL) can develop pancreatitis, which can be fatal. Patients with risk factors for pancreatitis should not receive the drug (e.g., history of pancreatitis, uncontrolled hyperlipidemia, uncontrolled diabetes mellitus, biliary tract disease, or medications known to increase triglyceride levels or to be associated with pancreatic toxicity). Uncommonly, patients may have elevated LFTs (5% of patients receiving an initial dose of 300 mg/m^2/day and 7% when doses of > 300 mg/m^2/day were used), but one patient developed cholestasis and died of liver failure in clinical trials. Nausea/vomiting occurs in 15%/3%, respectively, of patients receiving a dose of 300 mg/m^2/day and 7%/13% of patients receiving doses of > 300 mg/m^2/day. Anorexia affects 2% of patients receiving a dose of 300 mg/m^2/day, and 22% of patients receiving higher doses.

Nursing Implications: Assess baseline triglyceride, cholesterol, and HDL levels. If abnormal, discuss pharmacologic management plan (e.g., atorvastatin), as fasting triglyceride level should be normal before patient begins therapy. Gemfibrozil should NOT be used. Fasting triglyceride level should then be monitored weekly until the lipid response to bexarotene is known (2–4 weeks), then at 8-week intervals. Goal is to keep fasting triglyceride level < 400 mg/dL to prevent pancreatitis. If fasting triglyceride level becomes elevated during treatment, discuss with physician antilipemic medication (e.g., atorvastatin), and if no response, discuss with physician bexarotene dose reduction or drug holiday. Teach patient about importance of testing fasting triglycerides and monitoring level throughout treatment. LFTs should be assessed baseline, and after 1, 2, and 4 weeks of starting treatment; if stable, then assess every 8 weeks during treatment. Monitor serum LFTs, HDL, and discuss any abnormalities with physician (manufacturer recommends suspension or discontinuance of bexarotene if LFTs [SGOT/AST, SGPT/ALT, and bilirubin] > 3 times ULN). Assess baseline nutritional status; teach patient that nausea, vomiting, and anorexia may occur and to report them. If these occur, teach strategies to minimize occurrence, and if ineffective or symptoms are severe, discuss pharmacologic management with physician.

TREATMENT

an infection, discuss with physician or midlevel practitioner interrupting or discontinuing drug, and beginning appropriate antimicrobial treatment. Teach the patient that thrombocytopenia may occur, to avoid situations that could increase bleeding, and to report any signs or symptoms of bleeding right away. Review medication profile, and discuss discontinuance of aspirin or NSAIDs with patient and physician or NP/PA. Follow HGB/HCT and assess patient's tolerance and need for supportive measures.

II. POTENTIAL ALTERATION IN NUTRITION, LESS THAN BODY REQUIREMENTS, related to NAUSEA, VOMITING, DIARRHEA, HEPATOTOXICITY

Defining Characteristics: In clinical studies, nausea occurred in 43% of patients (grades 3–4 in 1%), vomiting in 29% (1% grades 3–4), diarrhea in 23% (2% grades 3–4), constipation in 23%, decreased appetite in 15%, and hypokalemia in 12%.

Nursing Implications: Assess baseline nutritional and elimination status, and appetite. Assess serum chemistries including renal and hepatic function, baseline and prior to each belinostat cycle. Assess patient tolerance of chemotherapy and need for premedication with antiemetics. Teach the patient to report nausea and/or vomiting that is not relieved by prescribed antiemetics. Teach patient that diarrhea or constipation may occur, dietary modifications for each problem, and to call nurse or physician for diarrhea, nausea, or vomiting that does not resolve within 24 hours with recommended OTC or prescription medicines. Notify physician of any abnormalities and discuss implications and management.

Drug: bexarotene (Targretin oral capsules and topical gel)

Class: Retinoid.

Mechanism of Action: Retinoid that selectively binds to and activates retinoid $\times$ receptors (RXRs), which have biologic activity distinct from retinoic acid receptors (RARs). The activated receptors can partner with receptor partners (e.g., retinoic acid receptors, vitamin D receptor, thyroid receptor), become activated, and then function as transcription factors that regulate the expression of genes, which control cellular differentiation and proliferation. The exact mechanism of action in cutaneous T-cell lymphoma is unknown.

Metabolism: Drug is well absorbed after oral administration, especially after a fat-containing meal, with a terminal half-life of 7 hours. Drug is highly protein-bound (> 99%). Drug appears to be metabolized by the cytochrome P450 CYP3A4 isoenzyme system in the liver, forming glucuronidated oxidative metabolites. Four metabolites are formed and are active, but it is unclear which metabolites or whether the parent drug is responsible for the efficacy of the drug. Probably excreted via the hepatobiliary system.

Indication: Bexarotene (Targretin) is indicated for the treatment of cutaneous manifestations of cutaneous T-cell lymphoma in patients who are refractory to at least one prior systemic therapy.

Contraindication: pregnancy

Dosage/Range:

Oral capsules:
- Indicated for the treatment of cutaneous manifestations of cutaneous T-cell lymphoma in patients who are refractory to at least one prior systemic therapy.
- Initial dose of 300 mg/m^2 PO per day for up to 97 weeks (maximum in clinical trials).
- Dose-reduce for toxicity to 200 mg/m^2 PO daily, then down to 100 mg/m^2 PO daily, or stop temporarily until toxicity resolves. After resolution, gradually titrate dose upward.
- Evaluate treatment efficacy at 8 weeks, and if no tumor response but the drug is well tolerated, increase dose to 400 mg/m^2 PO daily and monitor closely.
- Consider suspending or discontinuing drug if LFTs become elevated > 3 × ULN for AST, ALT, or bilirubin. Use drug cautiously in patients with hepatic insufficiency.

Topical gel:
- 1% gel indicated for the topical treatment of skin lesions in patients with early stage cutaneous T-cell lymphoma who have failed other therapies.

Drug Preparation:
- Available as 75-mg gelatin capsules in bottles of 100 capsules. The contents of the bottle should be protected from light, high temperatures, and humidity once opened.
- Store at 2–25°C (36–77°F).
- 1% gel available in tube. Store at 2–25°C (36–77°F).

Drug Administration:
- Assess:
  - Pregnancy test results, done within 1 week prior to beginning therapy and repeated monthly during therapy with oral capsule.
  - Baseline serum lipid levels must be assessed prior to initiation of therapy, and any abnormalities treated so that fasting triglycerides are normal before starting therapy.
  - LFTs baseline; then at weeks 1, 2, 4 weeks of treatment; then, if stable, every 8 weeks.
  - WBC/differential and thyroid function tests baseline, then periodically during treatment.
- Oral: single daily oral dose with a meal.
- Topical gel: apply to affected areas only (NOT entire body) as needed.

Drug Interactions:

Oral capsules:
- Presumed to be related to P450 CYP3A4 isoenzyme system metabolism.
- Inhibitors of cytochrome P450 CYP3A4 enzyme system (e.g., ketoconazole, itraconazole, erythromycin, gemfibrozil, grapefruit juice) theoretically can increase serum levels of bexarotene; DO NOT GIVE GEMFIBROZIL concomitantly with bexarotene as bexarotene levels significantly raised.
- Inducers of cytochrome P450 CYP3A4 enzyme system (e.g., rifampin, phenytoin, phenobarbital, St. John's wort) may cause a decrease in serum bexarotene concentrations. These have not been studied. If used concomitantly, assess response, and increase bexarotene accordingly. Do not give together with St. John's wort.

- Recurrence of CTCAE grade 3 or 4 adverse reaction after 2 dosage reductions: discontinue drug.
- For nausea, vomiting, diarrhea: modify dose only if duration is > 7 days with supportive management.

Drug Preparation:
- Available as a 500-mg, lyophilized powder, single-use vial for reconstitution.
- Aseptically reconstitute each vial by adding 9 mL sterile water for injection, USP so final concentration is 50 mg belinostat per mL. Swirl contents until fully dissolved. Reconstituted drug may be stored for up to 12 hours at ambient temperature (15–25°C; 59–77°F).
- Aseptically withdraw ordered amount and transfer to a 250 mL 0.9% sodium chloride for injection infusion bag. Once diluted, the drug containing bag may be stored at ambient room temperature (15–25°C; 59–77°F), for up to 36 hours, including infusion time.
- Visually inspect for particulate matter, cloudiness; if found, do not use.
- Connect infusion bag to an infusion set with a 0.22 μm inline filter and prime under the hood.

Drug Administration:
- Assess CBC/differential baseline and weekly; assess chemistries including renal and hepatic function tests prior to start of the first dose of each cycle.
- Ensure ANC $\geq 1.0 \times 10^9$/L, and platelets $\geq 50 \times 10^9$/L prior to the start of each cycle and prior to resuming treatment after treatment interruption for toxicity; ensure toxicity has recovered to grade 2 or less, and the patient has no signs/symptoms of infection.
- Drug should be discontinued in patients who have recurrent ANC nadirs $< 0.5 \times 10^9$/L and/or platelet count nadirs $< 25 \times 10^9$/L after 2 dosage reductions.
- Consider antiemetic prior to belinostat administration.
- IV infusion over 30 minutes, daily × 5, repeated every 21 days. If patient complains of infusion site pain, extend infusion time to 45 minutes.
- Based on CBC/ANC results, discuss need for dose modification with physician.

Drug Interactions:
- UGT1A1 inhibitors: drug is primarily metabolized by UGT1A1, so concomitant administration with a UGT1A1 inhibitor will increase belinostat serum levels and risk of toxicity. Do not administer with strong UGT1A1 inhibitors (e.g., atazanavir, gemfibrozil, indinavir, ketoconazole; herbals *silybum marianum, Valeriana officinalis*).
- Drug and its metabolites inhibit metabolic activities of CYP2C8, and CYP2C9. Drug coadministration with warfarin did not significantly change warfarin AUC or C_{max}.

Lab Effects/Interference:
- Thrombocytopenia, neutropenia, lymphopenia, anemia.
- Elevated LFTs, LDH.
- Hypokalemia.
- Decreased serum creatinine.
- Prolonged QT interval.

Special Considerations:
- Dose-reduce in patients with UGT1A1*28 polymorphism as this decreases belinostat metabolism and increases risk of belinostat toxicity. UGT1A1*28 polymorphism (homozygous for the UGT1A1*28 allele) is found in 20% of blacks, 10% of whites, and 2% of Asians.
- Warnings and Precautions:
  - *Thrombocytopenia, neutropenia, lymphopenia, and anemia* may occur. Base dose adjustments on ANC and platelet nadirs.
  - *Serious infections* may occur and may be fatal (e.g., pneumonia, sepsis). Do not give belinostat to patients with active infection. In addition, patients with a history of extensive or intensive chemotherapy treatment may be at greater risk of life-threatening infections.
  - *Hepatotoxicity* may occur. Monitor LFTs and discuss dose modification or hold for abnormalities. Dose-modify, interrupt, or discontinue belinostat for hepatotoxicity.
  - *Tumor lysis syndrome (TLS)* may occur in patients with advanced disease and/or a high-tumor burden. Discuss TLS prophylaxis with physician or NP/PA prior to initial dose.
  - *Gastrointestinal toxicity:* Nausea, vomiting, and diarrhea occur; manage with antiemetic and antidiarrheal medications.
  - *Embryo-fetal toxicity:* Drug is feto-toxic. Teach women of reproductive potential to use effective contraception to avoid pregnancy during treatment.
- Consider premedication with antiemetic to prevent nausea and vomiting and teach patient the use of antidiarrheals in case diarrhea develops.
- Nursing mothers should not breastfeed while receiving the drug. Nursing mothers should make a decision whether to discontinue nursing or to discontinue the drug, taking into account the importance of the drug to the mother's health.
- Drug may impair male fertility.
- Most common adverse reactions were nausea, fatigue, anemia, and vomiting.

Potential Toxicities/Side Effects and the Nursing Process

I.   POTENTIAL FOR INFECTION AND BLEEDING related to BONE MARROW SUPPRESSION

Defining Characteristics: Infections included pneumonia and sepsis. Pyrexia occurred in 37% of patients, and was grades 3–4 in 5%; cough occurred in 19%, and chills in 16%. Thrombocytopenia occurred in 16% (7% grades 3–4), and anemia occurred in 32% with 11% of patients having grades 3–4.

Nursing Implications: Assess CBC/differential and platelet counts baseline and weekly as ordered during therapy. Assess skin integrity, potential for infection, and teach patient measures to prevent infection (e.g., keeping skin intact, avoiding sources of infection, good hand-washing). Teach patient to report any signs/symptoms of infection (e.g., redness, heat, exudate on skin, temperature ≥ 100.4°F, cough, sputum production, dysuria). Assess for signs/symptoms of infection during therapy and at each visit. If a patient develops

- *Hemorrhagic events,* including fatal events, have been reported in 16% of patients, with only 1% grades 3–4. Drug has not been studied in patients with untreated brain metastases, or recent GI bleed, and should not be used in these patients. Stop drug 24 hours before scheduled surgery. If any bleeding requires medical intervention, temporarily interrupt the axitinib dose.
- *Cardiac failure* has been observed and can be fatal. Incidence in one study was 2%, with grades 3–4 cardiac failure observed in 1% of patients receiving axitinib. Monitor for signs and symptoms of cardiac failure baseline and during treatment with axitinib. Discontinuation of the drug may be required.
- *GI perforation and fistula formation* have occurred in < 1% of patients; some fatalities have occurred. Use cautiously in patients with risk for GI perforation or fistula. Monitor for symptoms of GI perforation or fistula periodically throughout axitinib treatment.
- *Thyroid dysfunction:* Hypothyroidism was reported in 19% of patients, while hyperthyroidism was reported 1%. Hypothyroidism requiring thyroid hormone replacement was also reported. Assess thyroid function before starting axitinib, and periodically during therapy. Of patients who had a TSH < 5 μ/mL before treatment, 32% had elevations of TSH to ≥ 10 μ/mL on axitinib. Monitor TSH baseline before starting axitinib, then periodically during treatment.
- *Wound-healing complications*: stop treatment with axitinib at least 24 hours prior to scheduled surgery. The decision to resume axitinib therapy after surgery should be based on clinical judgment of adequate wound healing.
- *Reversible posterior leukoencephalopathy syndrome (RPLS)* has been observed in < 1% of patients receiving axitinib. Signs/symptoms are headache, seizure, lethargy, confusion, blindness, and other visual and neurological disturbances. Mild to severe hypertension may also be present. MRI is necessary to confirm a diagnosis of RPLS. Discontinue axitinib in patients who are developing RPLS and the safety of reinitiating axitinib threrapy is unknown.
- *Proteinuria* may occur. In studies, incidence is about 11%, with 3% having grades 3–4. Assess baseline urine for protein before starting axitinib, then monitor periodically during treatment. If moderate-to-severe proteinuria occurs, reduce dose or temporarily hold drug.
- *Elevation of LFTs* has occurred (22%). Monitor ALT, AST, and bilirubin baseline prior to starting drug, then periodically during treatment. Patients with moderate hepatic dysfunction (Child-Pugh Class B) should start treatment at a 50% reduced dose. The drug has not been studied in patients with severe hepatic impairment (Child-Pugh Class C).
- *Hepatic impairment*: Drug systemic exposure is increased in patients with moderate hepatic impairment (Child-Pugh, class B) so a dose decrease is recommended when the drug is given to patients with moderate hepatic impairment.
- *Pregnancy: Drug can cause fetal harm.* Women of childbearing age/potential should be advised to use effective birth control measures to avoid pregnancy during treatment and for 1 week after the last dose. Male patients with female partners of reproductive potential should be taught to use effective contraception during and for 1 week after last drug dose.

- Nursing mothers should make the decision whether to discontinue nursing or discontinue the drug, taking into account the importance of the drug to the mother. Mothers receiving the drug should not breast-feed during treatment and for 2 weeks after the final drug dose.
- Drug can cause impaired fertility in females and males of reproductive potential.
- Drug can cause hoarseness/dysphonia: assess impact on patient, communication ability, and need for assistance.
- No starting dose adjustment in patients with preexisting mild to severe renal impairment. Caution is advised in patients with end-stage renal disease (CrCl < 15 mL/min).

Potential Toxicities/Side Effects and the Nursing Process

I.   POTENTIAL ALTERATION IN CIRCULATION related to HYPERTENSION

Defining Characteristics: Axitinib increases the incidence and severity of hypertension, a class effect of all angiogenesis inhibitors believed caused by the influence of VEGF on nitric oxide and blood vessel dilation. Overall incidence of hypertension was 40%, with 16% grades 3–4. Hypertensive crisis was reported in < 1% of patients. Median time to onset of hypertension (SBP > 150 mm Hg, DBP > 100 mm Hg) was within the first month of therapy, but starting as early as day 4. Hypertension was effectively managed with standard antihypertensive therapy, and < 1% of patients discontinued therapy due to hypertension.

Nursing Implications: Assess baseline BP prior to starting axitinib, and during treatment at each clinic visit. BP should be well controlled prior to starting axitinib. If the patient has a history of hypertension, monitor BP more closely, although hypertension develops over time. If needed, teach patient and family how to measure BP at home, and to record measurements and bring diary to clinic at each visit. Blood pressure should continue to be monitored after patient has stopped the drug. Teach patient drug administration, potential side effects, and self-care measures if prescribed antihypertensive medication, such as angiotensin-converting enzyme inhibitors, or angiotensin receptor blockers (antagonists). If patient has persistent hypertension despite standard antihypertensive therapy, the dose of axitinib should be reduced. Drug should be permanently discontinued if (1) hypertension is persistent despite antihypertensives and dose reduction, or (2) the patient develops hypertensive crisis (diastolic blood pressure > 120 mm Hg). Drug can be temporarily suspended in patients with severe hypertension until BP can be controlled with medical management. If axitinib therapy is interrupted, patients receiving antihypertensive drug(s) should be monitored closely for hypotension.

II.   ALTERATION IN COMFORT AND ACTIVITY INTOLERANCE, POTENTIAL, related to FATIGUE

Defining Characteristics: Fatigue occurs in 39% of patients, and 11% had grades 3–4 fatigue. Asthenia occurred in 21%, 5% grades 3–4. Hypothyroidism may also occur so should be evaluated.

IV.   ALTERATION IN COMFORT related to PAIN, HEADACHE, FATIGUE, MUSCLE PAIN, AND FATIGUE

Defining Characteristics: Fatigue affected 43% of patients, abdominal pain 28%, pyrexia (18%), peripheral edema (13%) of patients. Rhabdomyolysis can occur rarely, associated with increases in serum CPK (incidence 58%),

Nursing Implications: Assess baseline serum CPK and creatinine levels baseline and periodically during treatment. Teach patient to report any new muscle aches, pain, tenderness or muscle weakness right away, and discuss with provider having patient come for laboratory testing of CPK and serum creatinine if this occurs. Teach patient that fatigue, fever, edema, and abdominal pain may occur, and teach strategies to manage symptoms. Assess baseline comfort and monitor closely during treatment. Develop plan to assure comfort depending on symptoms reported. Discuss ineffective strategies with physician/NP/PA.

Drug: bortezomib (Velcade)

Class: Proteasome inhibitor.

Mechanism of Action: A reversible inhibitor of the 26S proteasome; inhibits the breakdown of ubiquinated intracellular proteins and disrupts the ubiquitin–proteasome pathway. This pathway normally regulates the intracellular concentration of specific proteins, thus controlling homeostasis. Cancer cells depend on the proteins that are available from this process to turn on the cell cycle and to make the apparatus for mitosis (cell division into two daughter cells). When the ubiquitin–proteasome pathway is disrupted, the proteins are not available, and multiple signaling pathways within the cell are disrupted, encouraging the cell to undergo apoptosis. Cell cycle movement (cell division) stops. Cells are unable to migrate, and sensitivity to chemotherapy is increased. In addition, the drug appears to downregulate the NF-kB pathway, which is necessary for cell growth, avoidance of apoptosis, and adhesion. This may restore chemosensitivity. In multiple myeloma, it interferes with cellular adhesion molecules so that tumor cells cannot bind to the bone marrow.

Metabolism: After IV administration, the drug is rapidly cleared from the plasma, with a mean elimination half-life range of 40–193 hours after multiple dosing. Drug undergoes oxidative metabolism via cytochrome P450 enzymes 3A4, 2D6, 2C19, 2C9, and 1A2. Drug is deboronated into two metabolites that are then hydroxylated into several metabolites. Unknown elimination path.

Indication: Treatment of patients with (1) multiple myeloma, including initial treatment, and (2) mantle cell lymphoma.

Dosage/Range:

- Recommended starting dose of bortezomib is 1.3 mg/m² either as an IVB (concentration 1 mg/mL) over 3 to 5 seconds or SQ (concentration 2.5 mg/mL) injection. At least 72 hours should elapse between consecutive doses of bortezomib. Ensure drug is prepared and labeled as either an **IV or SQ medication**; each route of administration has a different reconstituted concentration. Drug **cannot be administered via IT route, as it may be fatal**.

- Bortezomib retreatment may be considered for patients with multiple myeloma who had previously responded to treatment with bortezomib and who have relapsed at least 6 months after completing prior bortezomib treatment. Start at last tolerated dose.

Previously untreated multiple myeloma:
- Nine 6-week treatment cycles, given with melphalan 9 mg/m^2 and prednisone 60 mg/m^2:
  - Cycles 1–4: Twice weekly bortezomib: 1.3 mg/m^2 per dose IVB or SQ **twice weekly** (days 1, 4, 8, 11) followed by a 10-day rest period, then resume on days 22, 25, 29, and 32. Melphalan and prednisone given only on days 1–4. Cycle repeated q 6 weeks.
  - Cycles 5–9: Once weekly bortezomib: used in combination with melphalan and prednisone given on days 1–4): bortezomib is given **weekly** on days 1, 8, 22, 29. At least 72 hours must elapse between consecutive doses of bortezomib.
  - See package insert for melphalan and prednisone dosing and days.
  - Prior to beginning any cycle, platelet count should be $\geq 70 \times 10^9$/L, ANC $\geq 1.0 \times 10^9$/L, and nonhematologic toxicities should have resolved to grade 1 or baseline.
  - Consider the addition of an antiviral agent during treatment (incidence of herpes zoster was 13% in the bortezomib arm vs 5% high-dose dexamethasone arm, $p = .0002$, in the phase III APEX trial [Chanan-Khan et al., 2008]).

Previously untreated mantle cell lymphoma:
- Bortezomib is administered IV in combination with IV rituximab, cyclophosphamide, doxorubicin and oral prednisone (VcR-CAP) for 6 (3-week) treatment cycles: bortezomib 1.3 mg/m^2 on day 1, 4, 8, 11; followed by a 10-day rest period (days 12–21). At least 72 hours should elapse between consecutive doses of bortezomib.
- Bortezomib is administered first on day 1, followed by IV rituximab (375 mg/m^2) day 1 only, IV cyclophosphamide (750 mg/m^2) day 1 only, IV doxorubicin (50 mg/m^2) day 1 only, and prednisone 100 mg/m^2 PO days 1–5.
- For patients with a response first documented at cycle 6, two additional VcR-CAP cycles are recommended.
- Prior to the first day of each cycle (other than cycle 1):
  - Platelet count should be at least 100×10^9/L and ANC should be at least 1.5×10^9/L
  - Hgb should be at least 8 g/dL (at least 4.96 mmol/L)
  - Nonhematologic toxicity should have recovered to grade 1 or baseline
- Interrupt bortezomib at the onset of any grade 3 hematologic or nonhematologic toxicities excluding peripheral neuropathy (PN).

Relapsed multiple myeloma and relapsed mantle cell lymphoma:
- Bortezomib 1.3-mg/m^2 IV twice weekly $\times$ 2 weeks (days 1, 4, 8, 11) followed by a 10-day rest period (days 12–21).
  - For extended therapy of > 8 cycles, bortezomib may be given on the standard schedule or for relapsed multiple myeloma, a maintenance schedule of once weekly $\times$ 4 weeks (days 1, 8, 15, and 22, followed by a 13-day rest period on days 23–35) every 35 days.

hemorrhoids (1%). Patients with risk for brain or actual brain metastases are at risk for intracranial hemorrhage which occurred in 1.6% of patients.

Nursing Implications: Assess results of LVEF by ECHO or MUGA scan prior to starting binimetinib, 1 month after starting treatment, then every 2–3 months during treatment. Monitor patients with cardiovascular risk factors closely during treatment. Monitor BP as HTN occurred in 19% of paients. Assess for signs/symptoms of hemorrhage and VTE at each visit. Teach patient to report signs/symptoms of bleeding (e.g., headaches, dizziness, weakness, coughing up blood, black stools), and/or VTE (pain or warmth feeling calf, redness, difficulty or rapid breathing, sharp chest pain) right away and to seek emergency medical care if severe.

II.   POTENTIAL ALTERATION IN SENSORY FUNCTION related to VISUAL DISORDERS.

Defining Characteristics: Visual changes are a class effect of MEK inhibitors. Binimetinib was associated with serous retinopathy in 20% patients, with 8% retinal detachment, and 6% macular edema. Retinal vein occlusion was rare (< 0.1%). Uveitis occurred in 4% of patients.

Nursing Implications: Discuss with provider scheduling ophthalmological exam baseline and regularly during treatment. Teach patient to report any changes in vision (e.g., blurred or loss of vision, seeing colored dots, seeing halos around objects, eye pain, swelling or redness) right away for prompt evaluation, and if necessary to see emergency care if unable to see provider within 24 hours.

III.   ALTERATION IN NUTRITION, POTENTIAL, LESS THAN BODY REQUIREMENTS, related to DIARRHEA, NAUSEA, VOMITING, CONSTIPATION

Defining Characteristics: Nausea affects 41% of patients, followed by diarrhea (36%), vomiting (30%), and constipation (22%). LFTs were elevated in some patients: GGT (45%), ALT (229%), AST (27%).

Nursing Implications: Assess LFTs, nutritional and bowel-elimination status baseline and at each visit. LFTs should be assessed at least monthly, and as clinically needed. If patient develops nausea and/or vomiting, teach patient to self-administer antiemetics 1 hour prior to each dose, and to call if nausea/vomiting persist. Discuss with physician more effective antiemetic regimen if nausea/vomiting persist. Encourage small, frequent intake of cool, bland foods as tolerated if nausea develops. Refer to dietitian as needed for meal planning. Teach patient to report diarrhea that does not respond to OTC antidiarrheal medication. Teach self-care measures of diet modification and oral fluids to 2–3 L during the waking hours. If constipation occurs, teach patient self-care measures to prevent constipation. Assess appetite, and condition of oral mucosa; teach patient self-assessment and systemic oral hygiene after meals and at bedtime.

visual distrubances, and to follow new or persistent ophthalmologic findings. See Dose Modifications.

- *Retinal vein occlusion (RVO):* class effect of MEK inhibitors, although rare ($< 0.1\%$). Remind provider to perform ophthalmologic evauation immediately (or within 24 hours) if the patient reports acute vision loss or other visual disturbance. Permanently discontinue binimetinib if RVO occurs.
- *Uveitis:* Incidence pf uveitis, including iritis and iridocyclitis, was 4%. Assess for visual symptoms at each visit. Remind provider to perform ophthalmologic evauation regularly and for new or worsening visual disturbances, for any new or worsening visual distrubances, and to follow new or persistent ophthalmologic findings. See Dose Modifications.
- *Interstitial Lung Disease (ILD):* Rare (incidence 0.3%). Assess new or unexplained pulmonary symptoms or findings and rule out ILD. See Dose Modifications.
- *Hepatotoxicity:* Incidence can occur in combination therapy with encorafenib. Assess LFTs before starting binimetinib, monthly during treatment, and as clinically indicated. See Dose Modifications.
- *Rhabdomyolysis:* CPK was elevated in 58% of patients, while rhabdomyolysis was only reported in 0.1% of patients. Monitor CPK and creatinine baseline, periodically during treatment, and if patient has any signs or symptoms. Teach patient to report any signs/symptoms of new muscle pain, stiffness, weakness right away. See Dose Modifications.
- *Hemorrhage:* Incidence was 19%, and grade 3 or higher 3.2%. GI, was most common (4.2%), hematochezia (blood from anus wihout stool) 3.1%, hemorrhoidal hemorrhage 1%. Fatal intracranial hemorrhage appeared related to new or progressive brain metastases (incidence 1.6%). Assess paatients at each visit for signs/symptoms of bleeding. If patient is at risk for or has brain metastases, monitor closely. See Dose Modifications.
- *Embryo-fetal toxicity:* Drug is fetotoxic. Teach women of reproductive potential to use effective contraception during hematochezia treatment, and for at least 30 days after final binimetinib dose.
- *Risks associated with combination therapy:* See encorafenib for additional potential adverse effects when given in combination with binimetinib.

Potential Toxicities/Side Effects and the Nursing Process

I. POTENTIAL ALTERATION IN OXYGENATION related to CARDIOMYOPATHY, VTE, AND HEMORRHAGE.

Defining Characteristics: Cardiomyopathy is uncommon but can occur, with incidence 7% (grade 3, 1.6%) in the COLUMBUS trial. Median time to 1st occurrence was 3.6 months. Cardiomyopathy resolved in 87% of patients. VTE occurred in 6% of patients, including 3.1% who had PE. Hemorrhage can occur, with an incidence of 19% in the COLUMBUS trial. Most common sites were GI (4.2%), anus (hematochezia, 3.1%), and

- Doses should be separated by at least 72 hours to give normal cells a chance to recover.
- Retreatment for multiple myeloma in patients who had previously responded to bortezomib, and who relapsed at least 6 months after completing prior bortezomib therapy (alone or in combination): may retreat starting at the last tolerated dose.
  - Bortezomib 1.3 mg/m^{2}IVB or SQ twice weekly (days 1, 4, 8, 11) every 3 weeks for a maximum of 8 cycles.
  - At least 72 hours should separate consecutive doses of bortezomib.
  - Bortezomib can be given alone or in combination with dexamethasone.

Recommended starting dosage in patients with moderate or severe hepatic impairment:
- Mild (BR ≤ 1.0 × ULN, SGOT > ULN): no dose modification; if BR > 1.0–1.5 × ULN, any AST: no dose modification.
- Moderate (BR > 1.5–3 × ULN, any AST) or severe (BR > 3 × ULN, any AST): reduce starting dose to 0.7 mg/m^2 per dose during the first cycle. Consider dose escalation to 1.0 mg/m^2; or further dose reduction to 0.5 mg/m^2 may be considered based on patient tolerance.
- Dose must be individualized to prevent overdosage.
- Patients with severe preexisting PN should be treated with bortezomib only after a careful risk–benefit assessment.
  - Subcutaneous administration causes a lower incidence of PN, so subcutaneous administration of bortezomib should be considered for patients with preexisting or at high risk of PN.
- Drug dose is not modified for renal impairment, including patients requiring renal dialysis.

Dose reduction to manage adverse events:
- Bortezomib should be held at the onset of any grade 3 nonhematologic or grade 4 hematologic toxicity excluding neuropathy. Once the symptoms of toxicity have resolved, bortezomib may be restarted at a 25% reduced dose (1.3 mg/m^2 is reduced to 1 mg/m^2).

Previously untreated multiple myeloma, when given with melphalan/prednisone:
- Prolonged grade 4 neutropenia or thrombocytopenia, or thrombocytopenia with bleeding: consider 25% melphalan dose reduction next cycle.
- Platelet count ≤ 30 × 10^9/L or ANC ≤ 0.75 × 10^9/L on a bortezomib dosing day (except day 1), hold bortezomib.
- If several bortezomib doses are held consecutively due to toxicity, decrease dose of bortezomib by 1 dose level, e.g., from 1.3 mg/m^2 to 1.0 mg/m^2, or from 1 mg/m^2 to 0.7 mg/m^2.
- Grade 3 or higher nonhematological toxicity: hold bortezomib, and when resolved to grade 1 or less, resume at a dose reduced by 1 dose level. See below for dose modifications for neuropathic pain and/or PN.

Previously untreated mantle cell lymphoma, given with rituximab, cyclophosphamide, doxorubicin, prednisone:
- Any grade 3 nonhematologic toxicity or grade 4 hematologic toxicity except for PN: Hold drug at onset, and when resolved to grade 1 or less, resume at 25% dose reduction (e.g., 1.3 mg/m^2/dose reduced to 1 mg/m^2/dose; 1 mg/m^2/dose reduced to 0.7 mg/m^2/dose).

- Grade ≥ 3 neutropenia or a platelet count $\geq 25 \times 10^9$/L: Hold bortezomib for up to 2 weeks until ANC $\geq 0.75 \times 10^9$/L and a platelet count $\geq 25 \times 10^9$/L.
  - If the toxicity does not resolve, discontinue bortezomib.
  - If after holding the drug up to 2 weeks, toxicity resolves so that the ANC $\geq 0.75 \times 10^9$/L and a platelet count $\geq 25 \times 10^9$/L, resume at a dose reduced by 1 dose level (e.g., 1.3 mg/m^2/dose reduced to 1 mg/m^2/dose; 1 mg/m^2/dose reduced to 0.7 mg/m^2/dose).
  - Grade ≥ 3 nonhematologic toxicities: hold bortezomib therapy until symptoms of the toxicity have resolved to grade 2 or better. Then, reinitiate bortezomib at a dose reduced by one dose level (e.g., 1.3 mg/m^2/dose reduced to 1 mg/m^2/dose; 1 mg/m^2/dose reduced to 0.7 mg/m^2/dose).
- See prescribing information for rituximab, cyclophosphamide, doxorubicin, and prednisone for management of toxicity.

Relapsed multiple myeloma and relapsed mantle cell lymphoma:
- Hold bortezomib therapy at the onset of grade 3 nonhematologic or grade 4 hematologic toxicities excluding neuropathy, which is discussed separately. Once symptoms of toxicity have resolved, reinitiate bortezomib at a 25% reduced dose (1.3 mg/m^2 dose reduced to 1 mg/m^2 dose; 1 mg/m^2 dose reduced to 0.7 mg/m^2/dose).

Peripheral neuropathic pain, and/or peripheral sensory or motor neuropathy:
- Consider starting patient with preexisting or at high risk of PN on bortezomib given subcutaneously; patients with preexisting severe PN should be treated with bortezomib only after careful risk-benefit assessment.
- Patients experiencing new or worsening PN during bortezomib therapy may require a dose reduction and/or a less intense schedule.
  - Grade 1 without pain or loss of function (asymptomatic loss of DTRs or paresthesia): no action.
  - Grade 1 with pain or grade 2 [moderate symptoms, limiting instrumental ADLs (e.g., preparing meals, grocery or clothes shopping, using telephone, managing money)]: reduce bortezomib dose to 1 mg/m^2.
  - Grade 2 with pain or grade 3 [severe symptoms, limiting self-care ADLs (e.g., bathing, dressing and undressing, feeding self, using toilet, taking medications, not bedridden)]: withhold bortezomib therapy until toxicity resolves, then reinitiate with reduced dose of 0.7 mg/m^2 once weekly.
  - Grade 4 (life-threatening, requiring urgent intervention): discontinue drug.
  - Instrumental ADLs: preparing meals, grocery shopping, using telephone, managing money; self-care ADLs: bathing, dressing, undressing, feeding self, toileting, taking medications, not bedridden.

Drug Preparation:
- Available in single-use vials containing 3.5 mg of bortezomib sterile lyophilized powder; store unopened vials at room temperature 25°C (77°F) and protect from light.
- Drug quantity in one 3.5-mg vial may exceed the usual dose; use caution in calculating the dose to prevent overdosage.

- Use aseptic technique and reconstitute only with 0.9% sodium chloride. Inspect for particulate matter and discoloration, and, if found, do not use. Solution should be clear and colorless.
- IV: Reconstitute each vial with 3.5 mL 0.9% sodium chloride injection USP, forming a 1 mg/mL solution that should be colorless and clear (stable for 8 hours at controlled room temperature). Label as IV.
- SQ: Reconstitute each vial with 1.4 mL 0.9% sodium chloride injection USP, forming a 2.5 mg/mL solution that should be colorless and clear (stable for 8 hours at controlled room temperature). Label as SQ.
- Make certain to use the correct reconstituted concentration for the intended route, and use caution in calculating the volume to be administered. Make certain to have drawn-up volume and reconstituted vial double checked by another chemotherapy-competent professional. Formula for calculating volume are shown in the package insert (Millenium Pharmaceuticals, Inc., 2015).
- Carefully draw up prescribed amount, as drug in vial may exceed ordered dose (stable as reconstituted drug, or in a syringe including reconstituted time, for 8 hours).
- Apply VELCADE label to syringe containing drug indicating route of administration; drug CANNOT be given by the IT route.

Drug Administration:
- Assess ANC and platelet count and ensure results meet the requirements for administration (see Dosage), and that any nonhematologic toxicities have resolved to grade 1 or baseline.
- Double-check concentration and label on the syringe indicating what route is to be used.
- IV: Administer IVP over 3–5 seconds, followed by saline flush.
- SQ injection: Rotate sites for injection (thigh or abdomen), avoiding old sites (at least 1 inch away) and sites that are tender, bruised, erythematous, or indurated. Local skin irritation reported in 5% of patients, but drug is not a vesicant.
- **Bortezomib can only be administered IV or SQ. DO NOT administer intrathecally as death may result. Bortezomib should be prepared in an area separate from where IT medications are prepared.**

Drug Interactions:
- Strong CYP3A4 inhibitors (e.g., ketoconazole, ritonavir): can increase bortezomib exposure; monitor patient closely for bortezomib toxicity if drugs must be given concomitantly.
- Strong CYP3A4 inducers (e.g., rifampin, St. John's wort): can decrease bortezomib exposure; avoid concomitant use.

Lab Effects/Interference:
- Decreased neutrophil, platelet, and red blood cell counts.
- Hypoglycemia and hyperglycemia in diabetic patients.
- Increased LFTs.

Special Considerations:
- Contraindicated in patients with hypersensitivity to bortezomib, boron, or mannitol; IT administration is contraindicated; avoid use in pregnancy and teach patient not to breastfeed while receiving the drug.

- Use cautiously in patients with the following medical issues and monitor closely: hepatic dysfunction, having a history of CHF, PN, or syncope; patients receiving antihypertensive medications (additive hypotension); and patients who are dehydrated.
- Warnings and Precautions:
- *PN: Bortezomib* treatment causes a primarily sensory PN; however, cases of severe sensory AND motor PN have been reported. Patients with preexisting PN may experience worsening of PN.
  - Patients should be monitored closely for symptoms, such as burning sensation, hyperesthesia, hypoesthesia, paresthesia, discomfort, neuropathic pain, or weakness.
  - In the phase 3 relapsed multiple myeloma trial comparing bortezomib SQ to IV, incidence of ≥ grade 2 PN was 24% for SQ and 39% for IV administration. Grade ≥ 3PN occurred in 6% of SQ patients and 15% of IV patients. Patients experiencing new or worsening PN during bortezomib therapy may need a dose reduction and/or a less dose-intense schedule.
  - Improvement or resolution of PN was reported in 73% of patients who discontinued due to grade 2 PN or who had ≥ grade 3 PN in the phase 2 MM studies.
- Carefully consider risk–benefit ratio in patients with preexisting PN, and monitor closely; dose-modify or discontinue drug as needed.
  - *Hypotension:* Hypotension (postural, orthostatic, and hypotension NOS) may occur in up to 8% of patients; monitor patients receiving antihypertensive therapy, those with a history of syncope, and dehydrated patients closely.
  - *Cardiac toxicity:* Acute development or exacerbation of CHF, and new onset of decreased LVEF have occurred during bortezomib therapy, including in patients without risk factors. Closely monitor patients with risk factors for or with existing heart disease. There have been isolated cases of prolonged QT interval but it is not clear whether related to bortezomib.
  - *Pulmonary toxicity:* May occur. ARDS and acute diffuse infiltrative pulmonary disease of unknown etiology (e.g., pneumonitis, interstitial pneumonia, lung infiltration) have been observed. There are rare reports of pulmonary hypertension in the absence of left heart failure or significant pulmonary disease. If patient develops new or worsening cardiopulmonary symptoms, consider interrupting the drug; a comprehensive diagnostic evaluation should be done.
  - *Posterior reversible encephalopathy syndrome (PRES):* Rarely, PRES has occurred, characterized by seizure, hypertension, headache, lethargy, confusion, blindness, and/or other visual or other neurologic disturbance. Diagnosis is confirmed with MRI. Discontinue bortezomib if PRES develops.
  - *GI toxicity:* Nausea, diarrhea, constipation, and vomiting can occur, sometimes requiring use of an antiemetic and antidiarrheal medication. Ileus can occur; administer fluid and electrolyte replacement as needed to prevent dehydration, and interrupt bortezomib for severe symptoms.
  - *Thrombocytopenia/neutropenia:* Thrombocytopenia and neutropenia follow a cyclical pattern with nadirs occurring following the last dose of each cycle and usually recovering prior to the start of the next cycle. Mean platelet nadir in studies was 40% of baseline. CBC/platelets should be monitored frequently, and platelets assessed prior

to each dose of bortezomib. Patients who develop thrombocytopenia may require dose and schedule modification. In the VcR-CAP studies, incidence of grade 4 or higher thrombocytopenia was 32%, with 1% incidence of grade 3 and higher bleeding events. The incidence of neutropenia grade 4 and higher was 70%, incidence of febrile neutropenia grade 4 and higher was 5%, and required myeloid growth factor support in 78% of patients.

- *Tumor lysis syndrome (TLS):* May occur in patients with high-tumor burden prior to treatment. Discuss prophylaxis with provider: allopurinol and hydration.
- *Hepatic toxicity:* Acute liver failure has been reported in patients receiving polypharmacy and serious underlying medical conditions. Other reactions include hepatitis, increase in LFTs, and hyperbilirubinemia. Interrupt bortezomib therapy to assess reversibility.
- *Embryo-fetal risk:* Teach women of reproductive potential to use effective contraception during therapy, and for 2 months after last dose, to avoid pregnancy.
- Patients with diabetes may require close monitoring of blood glucose and adjustment of antidiabetic medication.
- Drug is metabolized by liver enzymes with increased drug exposure in patients with moderate or severe hepatic dysfunction, dose-reduce initially and then titrate up or down, depending upon patient response. Monitor patient closely for toxicities.
- Herpes virus infection may occur, so prophylaxis with acyclovir 400 mg PO bid is recommended during and for 3 months following completion of therapy with bortezomib; if patient has renal compromise, then the acyclovir dosage should be reduced.
- Teach patients to call provider (and give them telephone number) for dizziness, light-headedness, fainting spells, persistent headache, any changes in vision, swelling of the feet, ankles, legs, rash, shortness of breath or new cough, seizure, or increased blood glucose levels in diabetic patients.

Potential Toxicities/Side Effects and the Nursing Process

I.   POTENTIAL SENSORY/PERCEPTUAL ALTERATIONS related to SENSORY PN

Defining Characteristics: Baseline PN is common in patients with multiple myeloma. In the Relapsed multiple myeloma study, 35% of patients had new onset or aggravation of existing PN with 7% developing grade 3 PN. PN improved/resolved in 48% of patients with grade 2 or higher PN with dose adjustment or interruption, and in 73% of multiple myeloma patients who discontinued the drug. While primarily sensory, motor neuropathy can also occur. SQ injection of bortezomib resulted in grade 2 or greater PN in 24% of patients compared to 41% for those receiving IV drug.

Nursing Implications: Teach patient to report new onset or worsening of PN symptoms (numbness, pain, or burning sensation in feet or hands), any changes in sensory function (temperature sensation, knowing where body parts are in relation to the whole, etc.), functional ability (e.g., especially senses of smell and taste), and ability to carry out ADLs. Assess patient for symptoms of PN (burning sensation, hyperesthesia, hypoesthesia, paresthesia, discomfort, neuropathic pain, weakness) as well as severity of symptom(s) if they arise and potential for injury. If these are new symptoms or worsening of preexisting symptoms and patient is receiving drug IV, discuss with physician or midlevel changing to SQ administration. Teach patient measures to minimize symptoms and ensure safety. Review drug profile, and discuss with physician any potentially neurotoxic drugs that increase the risk of PN: amiodarone, antivirals, isoniazid, nitrofurantoin, or statins. If patient has neuropathic pain, discuss with physician use of duloxetine, as this has shown significant benefit in decreasing pain compared to placebo (59% vs 39%) (Smith et al., 2013).

Dose Reductions:
- Grade 1 (paresthesias +/or loss of reflexes) without pain or loss of function: no action.
- Grade 1 with pain or grade 2 (interfering with instrumental ADLs): decrease dose to 1.0 mg/m^2/dose.
- Grade 2 with pain or grade 3 (interfering with self-care ADLs): hold drug until toxicity resolves, then reinitiate with dose reduced to 0.7 mg/m^2 and change treatment schedule to once a week.
- Grade 4 (life-threatening, urgent intervention indicated): discontinue drug.

II.   POTENTIAL FOR INFECTION AND BLEEDING related to BONE MARROW DEPRESSION

Defining Characteristics: Incidences of thrombocytopenia and neutropenia were lower in the trials of multiple myeloma compared to the studies of patients with mantle cell lymphoma receiving combined therapy. In the mantle cell trial, incidence of neutropenia was 87% (83% grades 3–4), and of thrombocytopenia was 72% (57% grades 3–4). Infection incidence was 31% in the VcR-CAP arm compared to 23% in the R-CHOP arm. In the relapsed multiple myeloma study, thrombocytopenia occurred in 30% of patients (8% grades 3–4), with nadir day 11, and recovery by day 21) and neutropenia in 19% of patients (5% grade 3). Febrile neutropenia occurred in 17% of patients receiving VcR-CAP, and anemia incidence was 44%.

Nursing Implications: Assess baseline leukocyte, platelet, and Hgb/HCT and monitor before each treatment, during therapy, and more often as needed. Hold drug for grade 4 hematologic toxicity (see NCI CTCAE) and dose-reduce 25%. Assess risk for infection and integrity of skin and mucous membranes, pulmonary status, and ability to clear secretions, as well as history of past infections, baseline and prior to each treatment. Teach patient to self-assess for signs/symptoms of infection and to call provider immediately or come to the emergency room if temperature < 100.4°F, or has shaking, chills, rash, productive cough, burning on urination, or any signs/symptoms of infection or bleeding. Teach self-care strategies to minimize risk of infection and bleeding, including avoidance of OTC aspirin-containing medications.

III. ALTERATION IN NUTRITION, LESS THAN BODY REQUIREMENTS, related to NAUSEA, DIARRHEA, DECREASED APPETITE, CONSTIPATION, VOMITING, AND DEHYDRATION

Defining Characteristics: Patients in clinical studies developed these symptoms with the following incidence in the bortezomib, melphalan, and prednisone arm: nausea (39%), diarrhea (35%), constipation (23%), vomiting (26%), anorexia (19%). Diarrhea, nausea, and vomiting occur 6–24 hours after infusion. Nausea is more common in patients with multiple myeloma. Diarrhea and constipation may occur during cycles 1 and 2, and then disappear. Patients with diabetes require close monitoring of their blood glucose and may require adjustments in their antidiabetic medication.

Nursing Implications: Assess baseline weight and nutritional status, and monitor prior to each treatment. Assess glucose, electrolytes prior to each treatment to weekly, especially serum sodium and potassium; replete as necessary and teach diet high in sodium and potassium. Teach patient that serum electrolytes may be decreased and to assess for signs/ symptoms: hyponatremia (confusion, weakness, seizures), hypokalemia (muscle weakness, confusion, irregular heartbeats), hypercalcemia (constipation, thirst, confusion, muscle cramps, sleepiness), and hypomagnesemia (muscle cramps, headache, weakness). Teach patient that side effects may occur, self-care strategies, and to report them if symptoms do not resolve. Use aggressive antiemetics to prevent nausea and vomiting: serotonin antagonist IV prior to bortezomib dose and for 36 hours after each drug dose, if needed. If diarrhea develops after first treatment, teach patient to take loperamide prior to next dose of bortezomib and after every loose stool × 36 hours (not to exceed 8 tablets a day), as well as to use the BRAT diet (bananas, rice, applesauce, toast). If patient develops constipation, teach preventive self-care (stool softener, flax seed oil, milk of magnesia, prunes, or prune juice every AM to ensure BM at least every other day). Teach patient to drink 2 quarts of fluid daily, drinking 1 glass an hour while awake to prevent dehydration. Teach patient to report dizziness, light-headedness, or fainting spells, and to avoid operating heavy machinery or driving a car if these occur. Develop symptom-management plan with physician. Make referral to dietitian as appropriate. Teach diabetic patients to monitor their blood glucose closely, and discuss abnormalities and changes in their antidiabetic dose with their NP, PA, or physician.

IV. ALTERATION IN OXYGENATION, POTENTIAL, related to HYPOTENSION

Defining Characteristics: Orthostatic hypotension/postural hypotension can affect up to 13% of patients throughout therapy.

Nursing Implications: Identify patients at risk: patients with history of syncope, dehydration, or taking medications associated with hypotension. Assess baseline cardiac status, including blood pressure and heart rate, noting rhythm and rate. Teach patient to prevent injury by gradual change in position, and to report any dizziness. Teach patients to avoid dehydration, especially in warm climates. If hypotension noted, assess patient tolerance and need for intervention; discuss management with physician. Manage orthostatic/postural hypotension with adjustment of antihypertensive doses (if patient is on them), hydration, and administration of mineralocorticoids and/or sympathomimetics.

Drug: bosutinib (Bosulif)

Class: Kinase inhibitor; TKI of BCR-ABL kinase that causes CML.

Mechanism of Action: Third-generation BCR-ABL TKI. It inhibits many imatinib-resistant forms of BCR-ABL. It also inhibits the SRC family of kinases.

Metabolism: After oral dosing, peak concentration occurs in 4–6 hours. Taking the drug with a high-fat meal increases the C_{max} and AUC. Drug is highly protein-bound (94%), and is a P-gp substrate and inhibitor in vitro. Primarily metabolized by the CYP3A4 microenzyme system to inactive metabolites, mean terminal elimination time (t1/2) is 22.5 hours. Primarily excreted in the feces (91.3%) and 3% in the urine. Hepatic impairment delays excretion with increases in C_{max} and AUC 1.9–2.3 fold, respectively.

Indication: Treatment of adult patients with: (1) newly diagnosed Ph+ chronic myelogenous leukemia (CML) in chronic phase (CP) [accelerated approval]; (2) chronic, accelerated or blast phase Ph+ CML with resistance or intolerance to prior therapy.

Contraindications: Patients with a history of hypersensitivity to bosutinib as reactions have included anaphylaxis (anaphylactic shock incidence is < 0.2%).

Dosage/Range:
- *Newly diagnosed Ph+ CML-CP:* 400-mg PO once daily with food. Continue treatment until disease recurrence or intolerance.
- *Ph+ CML in CP, accelerated phase (AP) or blast phase (BP) with resistance or intolerance to prior therapy.* 500-mg PO once daily with food. Continue treatment until disease recurrence or intolerance.
- Dose escalation by increments of 100-mg once daily to a maximum of 600-mg PO daily if patient does not achieve or maintain a hematologic, cytogenetic, or molecular response and who did not have grade 3 or higher adverse reactions at the recommended starting dose.
- Dose adjustments for organ impairment (see package insert).
- Hepatic impairment baseline (mild [Child-Pugh A], moderate [Child-Pugh B], severe Child-Pugh C]): dose is 200 mg orally, daily with food, which approximates a similar AUC as 500-mg dose in patients without renal impairment (in newly diagnosed as well as recurrent/intolerant patients). There is no efficacy data for doses of 200 mg once daily.
- Preexisting (1) creatinine clearance 30–50 mL/min: Newly diagnosed 300-mg PO daily, Recurrent/intolerant patients: 400 mg PO daily; (2) severe renal impairment (CrCl < 30 mL/min): dose is 200 mg orally daily, with food, which approximates a similar

AUC as 500-mg dose in patients without hepatic impairment, in newly diagnosed patients, and 300-mg PO daily in patients who are recurrent or intolerant.

- Dose-modify for toxicity:
  - Elevated transaminases ($>$ 5 $\times$ institutional ULN): hold drug until recovery to $\leq$ = 2.5 $\times$ ULN and resume at 400 mg once daily thereafter. If recovery takes $>$ 4 weeks, discontinue drug. If transaminase elevation $\geq$ 3 $\times$ ULN occurs with elevation in bilirubin greater than 2 $\times$ ULN and alkaline phosphatase is $<$ 2 $\times$ ULN, discontinue drug. Diarrhea: grades 3–4 ($\geq$ 7 stools/day over baseline); hold drug until recovery to grade $\leq$ 1; may resume at 400 mg once daily (resistant/refractory patients).
  - Diarrhea: Grade 3–4 diarrhea (Increase of $\geq$ 7 stools/day over baseline): hold bosutinib until recovery to $\leq$ grade 1, and bosutinib may be resumed at 400 mg daily (resistant/refractory patients).
  - Other clinically significant, moderate, or severe nonhematologic toxicity, hold bosutinib until toxicity has resolved, then resume at a dose reduced 100 mg once daily. If clinically appropriate, consider reescalating bosutinib dose to the starting dose taken once daily. Doses $<$ 300 mg/day have not been studied for efficacy.
  - Myelosuppression (ANC $<$ 1,000 cells/mm^3 or platelets $<$ 50,000 cells/mm^3): hold drug until ANC $\geq$ 1,000 cells/mm^3 AND platelets $\geq$ 50,000 cells/mm^3. Resume at same dose if recovery occurs within 2 weeks. If blood counts remain low $>$ 2 weeks, upon recovery, reduce dose by 100 mg and resume treatment. If cytopenia recurs, reduce dose again by 100 mg upon recovery and resume treatment. There is no data about doses $<$ 300 mg/day.

Drug Preparation:
- Available in 100-mg and 500-mg tablets.

Drug Administration:
- Teach patient to (1) take the drug orally, daily as a single dose, with food; (2) if a dose is missed by more than 12 hours, skip the dose and take the usual dose the next day; (3) avoid concomitant use of CYP3A4 inhibitors (e.g., grapefruit products) or CYP3A4 inducers (e.g., St. John's wort).

Drug Interactions:
- *Strong CYP3A4 inhibitors* (boceprevir, clarithromycin, conivaptan, indinivair, itraconazole, ketoconazole, nefazodone, nelfinavir, posaconazole, ritonavir, saquinavir, telaprevir, telithromycin, voriconazole) *and moderate CYP3A4 inhibitors* (atazanavir, aprepitant, ciprofloxacin, crizotinib, darunavir, diltiazem, erythromycin, fluconazole, fosamprevir, grapefruit and grapefruit juice, imatinib, verapamil) **increase bosutinib plasma concentrations**; do not give concurrently.
- *Strong CYP3A4 inducers* (carbamazepine, dexamethasone, phenytoin, phenobarbital, rifabutin, rifampin, St. John's Wort) *and moderate CYP3A4 inducers* (bosetan, efavirenz, etravirine, modafinil, nafcillin) **significantly decrease bosutinib plasma concentration**; do not give concurrently.
- Proton Pump Inhibitors (PPIs) may decrease bosutinib serum levels. Avoid PPIs and consider using short-acting antacids instead.

- Substrates of p-glycoproteins (P-gp): Bosutinib may increase the plasma concentration of P-gp substrates, such as digoxin. Monitor patient closely for toxicity, and assess serum drug levels (e.g., digoxin).

Lab Effects/Interference:
- Decreased platelets, ANC, hemoglobin.
- Increased LFTs.
- Increased lipase, decreased phosphorus.

Special Considerations:
- Drug very rarely can cause hypersensitivity and anaphylaxis; then the drug is contraindicated.
- Warnings and Precautions:
  - *Myelosuppression:* Thrombocytopenia, anemia, and neutropenia occur. Monitor blood counts closely (e.g., CBC/differential, platelets): weekly for the first month, then monthly thereafter or as clinically indicated. Teach patient self-assessment for signs/symptoms of infection, bleeding, and fatigue, and to call if present. Discuss with provider dose modification (hold, dose reduce, or discontinue bosutinib)
  - *GI toxicity:* Diarrhea, nausea, vomiting, and abdominal pain occur. The median time to onset of diarrhea for newly diagnosed Ph+ CML-CP patients was 3 days, and median duration was 3 days. The median time to onset of diarrhea for resistant or intolerant patients was 2 days, and median duration 2 days. Assess for GI symptoms and manage with antidiarrheal and antiemetic medications as ordered, and fluid replacement. Teach patients to manage, and assess patient response to management strategies (e.g., medication self-administration, forcing fluids for replacement). Teach patient to call provider if symptom persists or worsens. Median time to diarrhea onset was 2 days, with a median duration of 1 day. Discuss with MD/PA/NP plan: dose interruption or reduction, or discontinuance based on toxicity.
  - *Hepatic toxicity:* may occur. Assess LFTs baseline then monthly × 3 months, then as clinically indicated; if any of the transaminases is elevated, monitor LFTs more frequently. Discuss with provider management with dose interruption, reduction, or drug discontinuance.
  - *Renal toxicity:* Decreases in estimated glomerular filtration rate have occurred during treatment. Monitor renal function baseline and during therapy, especially for patients with preexisting renal impairment or risk factors for renal dysfunction. Consider dose adjustment in patients with baseline and treatment-emergent renal impairment.
  - *Fluid retention* may rarely occur and may be manifested as pericardial effusion, pleural effusion, pulmonary edema, and/or peripheral edema. The incidence of severe edema in clinical trials was 0.4% in newly diagnosed patienets, and 5% in resistant/intolerant patients. Assess for fluid retention; discuss management with provider, including dose modification (interrupt, dose-reduce, or discontinue treatment).
  - *Embryo-fetal toxicity:* Counsel women of childbearing potential to avoid pregnancy by using effective contraception during and for at least 1 month after last dose of bosutinib. Mothers should not breastfeed while receiving the drug.
- Most common adverse events are diarrhea, nausea, thrombocytopenia, vomiting, abdominal pain, rash, anemia, pyrexia, and fatigue.

Potential Toxicities /Side Effects and the Nursing Process

I.   POTENTIAL FOR INFECTION, BLEEDING, AND FATIGUE related to BONE MARROW DEPRESSION

Defining Characteristics: Thrombocytopenia affects 84% of patients (9% grades 3–4), anemia 33%, and neutropenia 16% of patients. Fatigue occurs in 26% of patients.

Nursing Implications: Assess CBC/differential, platelet count baseline, weekly for the first month, then monthly or more frequently as needed. Teach patient to report bleeding or signs/symptoms of bleeding right away. Teach patient to self-assess for signs/symptoms of infection, bleeding, or severe fatigue. Teach patient to avoid aspirin, NSAIDs, and aspirin-containing OTC medications. Teach patient strategies to manage fatigue and conserve energy.

II.   ALTERATION IN NUTRITION, POTENTIAL, related to DIARRHEA, NAUSEA, VOMITING, ABDOMINAL PAIN, INCREASED LFTS

Defining Characteristics: Diarrhea is common, occurring in 82–84% of patients; nausea affects 46%, vomiting 37%, and abdominal pain 40%. The median time to diarrhea onset was 2 days, the median number of episodes was 3, and duration was 1 day. Decreased appetite affects 13%. Liver transaminases become elevated in 16–20% of patients.

Nursing Implications: Assess nutritional status baseline and at each visit. Teach patient that these side effects may occur, and teach self-management strategies such as antidiarrheals, antinausea medications, dietary modifications, and to report any symptoms that do not improve. Discuss prescription medication with provider to manage refractory symptoms. Teach patient tips to increase appetite (e.g., small, frequent meals, use of spices). Offer services of dietitian as appropriate. Assess and monitor LFTs baseline, then monthly × 3 months, then as clinically indicated. If transaminases become elevated, monitor LFTs more frequently.

III.   ALTERATION IN COMFORT, related to PYREXIA, EDEMA, ASTHENIA, RASH, PRURITUS, HEADACHE

Defining Characteristics: Pyrexia occurred in 22%, edema in 14%, asthenia in 11%, rash in 34%, and pruritus in 11%. Rarely edema may be manifested as pericardial effusion, pleural effusion, pulmonary edema, and or peripheral edema (incidence of severe edema 3%). Headache occurs in 20% of patients.

Nursing Implications: Teach patient that these side effects may occur. Assess baseline skin integrity, weight, presence of peripheral edema, pulmonary and cardiac status. Teach patient to report fever, swelling of legs, face or other body parts, rash, itching, shortness of breath, or any changes. Assess reported symptoms and review with patient self-care management techniques. Teach patient to weigh self at least weekly and to report increases in weight, as this may reflect edema (fluid gain). Teach patient to report right away any difficulty breathing (e.g., shortness of breath) or chest pain, and discuss evaluation with physician, NP, or PA. If rash develops, assess for allergic reaction, and other accompanying symptoms. Monitor rash and teach patient strategies to prevent infection and promote healing.

Drug: brigatinib (Alunbrig)

Classification: (Tyrosine) kinase inhibitor.

Mechanism of Action: TKI of ALK, ROS1, IGF-R1, FLT3, and EGFR deletion and point mutations. Also inhibits EMLA4-ALK, and NPM-ALK fusion proteins. By inhibiting these kinases, phosphorylation of downstream signaling proteins STAT3, AKT, ERK, and S6 does not occur, and malignant cell proliferation is blocked. Brigatinib has antitumor activity against cells with resistance to crizotinib. Drug crosses the blood–brain barrier.

Metabolism: After oral dosing, median time to peak concentration (Tmax) was 1–4 hours. Although there was a slight decrease in Cmax when brigatinib was administered with a high-fat meal, the AUC was unaffected. Drug is 66% bound to human plasma proteins. The mean plasma elimination half-life is 25 hours. Brigatinib is primarily metabolized by CYP2C8 and CYP3A4 microenzymes, although 92% of drug remains unchanged and 3.5% represents its active metabolite AP26123 (inhibits ALK with about 3X lower potency thant brigatinib). Approximately 65% of an administered dose is excreted in the feces, and 25% in the urine, with unchanged drug representing 41% in the feces, and 86% in the urine (ARIAD, 2017). The pharmakinetics of drug in patients with moderate-to-severe hepatic impairment, or with severe renal impairment, have not been studied. No dose adjustment is needed for patients with mild hepatic impairment or mild or moderate renal impairment (ARIAD, 2017).

Indications: Patients with ALK-positive metastatic NSCLC who have progressed or are intolerant to crizotinib. Indication given under accelerated approval based on tumor response rate and duration of response; continued approval may be contingent upon verification and description of clinical benefit in a confirmatory trial (ARIAD, 2017).

Contraindication: None.

Dosage Range: 90 mg orally once daily for the first 7 days. If tolerated, increase dose to 180 mg orally once daily, with or without food. Dose modification for toxicity, severe hepatic or renal impairment (see below).
* Continue treatment until disease progression or unacceptable toxicity.
* If brigatinib is interrupted for 14 days or longer for reasons other than adverse reactions, resume treatment at 90 mg once daily for 7 days before increasing dose to the previously tolerated dose.

Dose Modifications: Dose reduction levels: (a) if dose 90 mg once daily, first reduction to 60 mg once daily, second dose reduction is permanently discontinue drug; (b) if dose is

180 mg once daily, first dose reduction is to 120 mg once daily, second dose reduction to 90 mg once daily, and third dose reduction to 60 mg once daily; if unable to tolerate the 60 mg dose, the drug should be discontinued. Once patient is dose reduced for adverse reactions, do not subsequently increase the dose.

- Recommended dose modifications for adverse reactions (ILD, HTN, bradycardia, visual disturbances, creatine elevation, phosphokinase elevation, lipase/amylase elevation, hyperglycemia, other: **see package insert, table 2.**
- Dose modification if concomitant use of strong or moderate CYP3A inhibitor with brigatinib: Avoid coadministration. If coadministration with a strong CYP3A4 inhibitor cannot be avoided, reduce brigatinib daily dose by 50% (e.g., 180 mg to 90 mg, 90 mg to 60 mg). If coadministration of a moderate CYP3A4 cannot be avoided, reduce the brigatinib daily dose by approximately 40% (i.e., from 180 mg to 120 mg, 120 mg to 90 mg, or from 90 mg to 60 mg. After discontinuance of strong CYP3A inhibitor, resume brigatinib at the dose that was tolerated prior to initiating the CYP3A inhibitor.
- Dose modification for moderate CYP3A inducers: avoid coadministration. If unavoidable, increase the brigatinib daily dose in 30 mg increments after 7 days of treatment with the current brigatinib dose as tolerated, up to a maximum of twice the original brigatinib dose that was tolerated prior to initiating the moderate CYP3A4 inducer. After inducer is discontinued, resume the brigatinib dose that was tolerated before initiating the moderate CYP3A4 inducer.
- Dose modification for patients with severe hepatic impairment (Child-Pugh C): Reduce the brigatinib once daily dose by approximately 40% (i.e., from 180 mg to 120 mg, from 120 mg to 90 mg, or from 90 mg to 60 mg).
- Dose modification for patients with severe renal impairment (creatinine clearance 15–29 mL/min by Cockcroft-Gault): Reduce the brigatinib once daily dose by approximately 50% (i.e., from 180 mg to 90 mg, from 120 mg to 60 mg, or from 90 mg to 60 mg).

Drug Preparation: None. Available in 30-mg, 90-mg, and 180-mg tablets.

Drug Administration: Teach patient self-administration
- Initially, take 90 mg dose as directed for the first 7 days, then if tolerated, increase dose to 180 mg as directed once daily.
- Take tablet with or without food, swallow tablet whole, and not to crush or chew tablet. Take tablet(s) about the same time of day each day.
- If a dose is missed or vomiting occurs after taking a dose, DO NOT take an additional dose but to wait and take the next dose at the scheduled time.
- Teach patient to report right away: new or worsening breathing problem; slow heart beat; changes in vision; new (unexplained) muscle pain, tenderness or weakness; new upper abdominal pain; increased thirst, hunger, and frequency of voiding.
- Assess for signs/symptoms of adverse reactions: HR, BP baseline, at 2 weeks, and at least every month; ILD/pneumonitis: new or worsening respiratory symptoms; visual disturbance (e.g., blurred vision, diplopia, reduced visual acuity); hyperglycemia; upper abdnominal pain; monitor labs (creatine phosphokinase (CPK), amylase, lipase, glucose).

- If patient is taking medications that may alter the aPTT, monitor the patient closely and teach patient to report any bleeding.
- Teach females of reproductive potential to use effective, nonhormonal contraception during treatment and for at least 4 months after final dose. Teach males with female partners of reproductive potential to use effective contraception during treatment and for at least 3 months after last dose of brigatinib.
- Teach women who are breast-feeding NOT to breast-feed while receiving brigatinib.

Drug Interactions:
- Strong CYP3A4 inhibitor (e.g., itraconazole): increases briigatinib plasma concentrations and may increase risk of adverse reactions. Avoid concomitant administration with strong CYP3A4 inhibitors (e.g., antivirals such as indinavir); macrolide antibiotics (e.g., clarithromycin); antifungals; and conivaptan. Teach patient to avoid grapefruit juice. If concomitant administration with a strong CYP3A4 inhibitor cannot be avoided, reduce the briganitinib dose by 50% (Bayer, 2017).
- Strong CYP3A4 Inducers (e.g., rifampin): avoid coadministration as brigatinib efficacy may be reduced. Teach patient to avoid St. John's wort.
- CYP3A4 substrates: coadministration of brigatinib with CYP3A substrates can result in decreased concentrations and loss of efficacy of CYP3A substrates; hormonal contraceptives may be not be effective due to decreased drug exposure.

Laboratory Effects/Interference:
- Increased AST, ALT, alkaline phosphatase, glucose, creatine phosphokinase, lipase, amylase.
- Decreased phosphorous.
- Anemia, lymphopenia.
- Prolonged aPTT.

Special Considerations:
- Warnings and Precautions:
  - *ILD:* occurred in 3.7% in the 90 mg group, and 9.1% of patients in the 90 –> 180 mg group (at recommended dose). It occurred early in 6.4% of patients, within 9 days of starting drug, with a median onset of 2 days; grade 3 or 4 reactions occurred in 2.7% of patients. Monitor for new or worsening respiratory symptoms (e.g., dyspnea, cough) especially during the first week of treatment. Hold brigatinib if new or worsening respiratory symptoms; patient should have prompt evaluation of ILD/pneumonitis vs other causes such as pulmonary embolism, tumor progression or infectious pneumonia. If grade 1 or 2 ILD/pneumonitis, either resume brigatinib with dose reduction (see dose modification) after recovery to baseline or permanently discontinue brigatinib. If grade 3 or 4 ILD/pneumonitis, ore recurrence of grades 1–2 ILD/pneumonitis, discontinue drug permanently (ARIAD, 2017).
  - *HTN:* Reported in clinical trials (11% in 90 mg group, and 21% of 90 –> 180 mg group). Grade 3 HTN occurred in 5.9% of all patients. Ensure BP well controlled prior to starting brigatinib; monitor BP after 2 weeks, and at least monthly thereafter. Hold drug for grade 3 HTN despite optimal antihypertensive therapy, and when resolved or improved to grade 1, resume brigatinib at a reduced dose. If patient develops

grade 4 HTN, or recurrence of grade 3 HTN, consider discontinuation of brigatinib. Use brigatinib cautiously when given in combination with antihypertensive drugs that cause bradycardia.

- *Bradycardia:* HR < 60 beats per minute (bpm) occurred in 5.7% of patients in 90 mg group, and 7.6% in the 90 –> 180 mg group. Grade 2 bradycardia occurred in 1 patient in the 90 mg group (0.9%). Monitor HR and BP baseline and during treatment, and if patient is receiving a drug known to cause bradycardia that cannot be avoided, monitor closely. If the patient develops symptomatic bradycardia, hold brigatinib, and discuss with physician/NP/PA whether concomitant medication known to cause bradycardia can be changed, discontinued or dose reduced. If not, the dose of brigatinib should be reduced once symptomatic bradycardia has resolved. Brigatinib should be permanently discontinued for life-threatening bradycardia if no concomitant medication is identified.

- *Visual disturbance:* Approximately 7.3% of patients receiving 90 mg brigatinib in the ALTA (ALK in Lung Cancer Trial of AP26113) trial reported visual disturbance (e.g., blurred vision, diplopia, reduced visual acuity), and 10% of patients in the 90 –> 180 mg group. Grade 3 macular edema and cataract occurred rarely. Teach patient to report changes in vision right away. Teach patient to hold brigatinib and discuss with MD/NP/PA obtaining ophthalmologic evaluation if new or worsening visual symptoms of grade 2 or higher severity. After recovery of grade 2 or grade 3 visual disturbances to grade 1 or baseline, drug can be resumed at a reduced dose. Permanently discontinue drug if grade 4 visual disturbances.

- *Creatine phosphokinase (CPK) elevation:* Occurred in 27% of patients receiving 90-mg dose, and 48% of patients receiving 90 –> 180 mg dose. Grades 3–4 elevations occurred in 12% in the latter group. Monitor CPK baseline and during therapy. Hold brigatinib for grade 3 or 4 CPK elevations; once resolved or recovery to grade 1 or baseline, brigatinib can be resumed as same or reduced dose per package insert, Table 2.

- *Pancreatic enzyme elevation:* Amylase elevations occurred in 27% of patients at the 90-mg dose, and 39% of patients receiving the 90 –> 180 mg dose. Lipase elevations occurred in 21% of the 90-mg patients, while 45% of the 90 –> 180 mg dose experienced this. Monitor lipase and amylase baseline and during treatment. Hold brigatinib for grade 3 or 4 pancreatic enzyme elevation. Once recovered to baseline or grade 1, resume at same or reduced dose per package insert, Table 2.

- *Hyperglycemia:* 43% of patients had new or worsening hyperglycemia. Assess fasting serum glucose prior to starting brigatinib, and monitor during therapy. Discuss with MD/NP/PA management of hyperglycemia if it develops. If unable to control, hold brigatinib until controlled, and consider dose reduction of brigatinib, or permanently discontinue drug per MD.

- *Embryo-fetal toxicity:* Drug can cause fetal harm when administered to pregnant women. Teach females of reproductive potential to use effective, nonhormonal contraception during treatment and for at least 4 months after final dose. Teach males with female partners of reproductive potential to use effective contraception during treatment and for at least 3 months after last dose of brigatinib.

- Most common adverse reactions (≥ 25%): nausea, diarrhea, fatigue, cough, headache.

Potential Toxicities/Side Effects and the Nursing Process

I.   ALTERATION IN NUTRITION, POTENTIAL, LESS THAN BODY REQUIREMENTS, related to DIARRHEA, NAUSEA, VOMITING, DECREASED APPETITE, CONSTIPATION, HYPERGLYCEMIA, ELEVATED PANCREATIC ENZYMES, ELEVATED LFTS, and ABDOMINAL PAIN

Defining Characteristics: Nausea occurred in 33% (90-mg dose) to 40% (90–180 mg dose) of patients in clinical studies, and was severe in 0.9%. Diarrhea occurred in 19–38%, vomiting 24–23% (1.8% grades 3–4), constipation 15–19%, decreased appetite 15–22%, and abdominal pain in 10–17% of patients. Hyperglycemia occurred in 38–49%, with 3.6–3.7% grades 3–4. Risk may be increased in patients with diabetes, glucose intolerance, or taking corticosteroids. Lipase was increased in 21%–45% of patients, amylase 27–39% of patients, ALT 34–40% of patients, AST 38–65% of patients, alkaline phosphatase 15–29% of patients.

Nursing Implications: Assess baseline nutritional status, labs including fasting blood glucose, pancreatic enzymes, LFTs, and bowel-elimination status. Teach patient that these side effects can occur and to report them if they do not resolve. Teach patient to administer antidiarrheal medication if diarrhea occurs and to report if it does not resolve within 24 hours. Teach patient to increase oral fluid intake and to modify diet (e.g., 5–6 small meals of foods high in soluble fiber (e.g., rice, noodles, bananas, well-cooked eggs) and low in insoluble fiber (e.g., raw fruit, whole grain breads, and seeds). If patient develops nausea and/or vomiting, teach patient to self-administer antiemetics 1 hour prior to each dose and to call if nausea/vomiting persists. Discuss with physician more effective antiemetic regimen if nausea/vomiting is not improved. Encourage small, frequent intake of cool, bland foods as tolerated if nausea develops. Refer to dietitian as needed for meal planning. If constipation occurs, teach patient to increase fluid intake, self-administer laxatives, and to increase the intake of high-fiber foods. Monitor baseline and blood glucose level and discuss with physician or NP/PA the need for antihyperglycemic medication. Discuss dose interruption and dose reduction depending upon severity of symptoms. See Dose Modifications.

II.   ALTERATION IN SENSORY PERCEPTION related to VISUAL CHANGES

Defining Characteristics: In clinical trials, 7.3–10% of patients described visual disturbances including diplopia, blurred vision, reduced visual acuity, photophobia, and vitreous floaters. Signs identified include visual field defect, macular ededma, and vitreous detachment.

Nursing Implications: Assess baseline visual complaints and teach patient to report any new visual disturbances or changes in vision. Discuss with physician any abnormalities. Teach patient to report changes in vision right away. Teach patient to hold brigatinib and discuss with MD/NP/PA obtaining ophthalmologic evaluation if new or worsening visual symptoms of grade 2 or higher severity. After recovery of grade 2 or grade 3 visual

disturbances to grade 1 or baseline, drug can be resumed at a reduced dose. Permanently discontinue drug if grade 4 visual disturbances.

III. ALTERATION IN COMFORT related to FATIGUE, MYALGIA, ARTHRALGIA, HEADACHE, PN

Defining Characteristics: Fatigue occurred in 29% (90-mg group)–46% (90 –> 180-mg group), headache occurred in 28–27%, muscle spasms 12–17%, back pain 10–15%, myalgia 9.2–15%, and arthralgia 14%. Creatine phosphokinase was elevated in 27–48% of patients. PN was reported in 13% of patients.

Nursing Implications: Assess comfort and presence of discomfort and fatigue, baseline and at each visit. Assess hemoglobin/hematocrit as anemia may occur. Teach patient that these side effects may occur and to report them. Unexplained muscle pain, tenderness, or weakness should be **reported right away** as this may signal CPK elevation. Expect that the patient will be advised to come to have CPK assessed (blood test). Teach patient local comfort measures, as well as energy conservation, and discuss management plan with physician if ineffective.

Drug: cabozantinib capsules (Cometriq)

Class: Kinase inhibitor. TKI of MET and VEGFR2.

Mechanism of Action: Cabozantinib is a dual TKI of MET (stimulated by the ligand, hepatocyte growth factor, or HGF, called scatter factor), and vascular endothelial growth factor receptor 2 (VEGFR2). It also inhibits the tyrosine kinases of RET, VEGFR1, VEGFR3, KIT, TRKB, FLT-3, AXL, and TIE-2, which are involved in normal as well as cancer processes of oncogenesis, metastasis, angiogenesis, and tumor microenvironment maintenance. MET is expressed on tumor cells, endothelial cells, and on bone cells. MET is upregulated in a number of cancers (thyroid, prostate, ovarian, and breast). Stimulation of the MET receptor by its ligand hepatocyte growth factor (HGF, scatter factor) facilitates certain cancer cells becoming more aggressive, more invasive, making more blood vessels, and escaping from the initial tumor to invade and metastasize. When some cancer therapies are used to kill the majority of cancer cells in a tumor, it is believed that stimulation of the MET-signaling pathway occurs as an escape route—certain cells become more aggressive (aggressive phenotype) and escape via their new invasive and metastatic qualities. Binding of VEGF to VEGFR2 leads to endothelial cell proliferation, migration, and the formation of blood vessels that nourish the tumor and facilitate tumor embolization. When this is blocked, reduced tumor oxygenation causes increased levels of waste products, creating hypoxia. Hypoxia further upregulates MET. In some studies, use of a VEGF or VEGFR inhibitor alone can result in tumors becoming more aggressive and invasive, as MET becomes upregulated. In the laboratory, cabozantinib is a potent antiangiogenic and antitumor drug, which also reduces tumor invasiveness and metastases. The drug was designed to block MET and VEGFR2, as well to block MET-driven tumor escape. It increases tumor apoptosis, decreases tumor and endothelial cell proliferation, decreases tumor cell invasiveness and metastases; in addition, it causes a blockade of metastatic bone lesion progression and disrupts tumor vasculature.

Metabolism: Drug half-life is approximately 55 hours after consecutive oral dosing. Median time to peak plasma concentrations (T_{max}) is 2–5 hours after dosing. A high-fat meal increases C_{max} and AUC by 41% and 57%, respectively. Drug is a substrate of CYP3A4 in vitro. Drug is excreted in the feces (54%) and urine (27%).

Indication: Treatment of patients with progressive, metastatic medullary thyroid cancer.

Dosage/Range:
- 140 mg (one 80-mg and three 20-mg capsules) orally once daily on an empty stomach (no food at least 2 hours before and for at least 1 hour after taking the drug).
- DO NOT substitute COMETRIQ capsules with cabozantinib tablets as they are two different formulations and are NOT interchangeable.
- Hepatic impairment: recommended starting dose is 80 mg for patients with mild or moderate hepatic impairment. Drug is not recommended for use in patients with severe hepatic impairment.

Dose Reductions:
- Hold drug for NCI CTCAE grade 4 hematologic adverse reactions, grade 3 or greater nonhematologic adverse reactions, or intolerable grade 2 adverse reactions. Upon resolution/improvement of adverse reaction (baseline or grade 1) reduce dose as follows:
  - If previously taking 140-mg daily dose, resume at 100 mg daily (one 80-mg and one 20-mg capsule).
  - If previously taking 100 mg daily, resume treatment at 60 mg daily (three 20-mg capsules).
  - If previously taking 60 mg daily, resume at 60 mg if tolerated; otherwise, discontinue drug.
- Permanently discontinue the drug for:
  - Development of visceral perforation or fistula formation.
  - Severe hemorrhage.
  - Serious arterial thromboembolic event (e.g., MI, cerebral infarction).
  - Nephrotic syndrome.
  - Malignant hypertension, hypertensive crisis, persistent uncontrolled hypertension despite optimal medical management.
  - Osteonecrosis of the jaw.
  - Reversible posterior leukoencephalopathy syndrome.
- Patients taking strong CYP3A4 inhibitors:
  - Decrease daily dose by 40 mg (e.g., from 140 mg to 100 mg, from 100 mg to 60 mg daily).
  - After the interacting drug is discontinued, resume the dose that was used prior to initiating the CYP3A4 inhibitor 2–3 days after discontinuing the strong inhibitor.
- Patients taking strong CYP3A4 inducers:
  - Increase daily dose by 40 mg (e.g., from 140 mg to 180 mg, or from 100 mg to 140 mg daily) as tolerated.

- Once the CYP3A4 inducer is discontinued, resume the dose that was used prior to initiating the CYP3A4 inducer 2–3 days after discontinuing that drug.

Drug Preparation/Administration:
- Available in 20-mg and 80-mg capsules.
- Teach patient to take capsules on an empty stomach (no food at least 2 hours before and for at least 1 hour after taking the drug).
- Teach patient to take drug whole, not to open capsules, and not to take a missed dose within 12 hours of the next dose. Instruct patient not to drink grapefruit juice, eat grapefruit, or take St. John's wort while taking this drug.
- Stop drug at least 28 days before scheduled surgery; resume drug after surgery based on clinical judgment of adequate wound healing.

Drug Interactions: Cabozantinib is a CYP3A4 substrate.
- CYP3A4 inhibitors (strong) (e.g., atazanavir, clarithromycin, indinavir, itraconazole, ketoconazole, nelfinavir, nefazodone, saquinavir, telithromycin, ritonavir, voriconazole, grapefruit, and grapefruit juice): increase cabozantinib serum levels; do not take concomitantly. If must take concomitantly, reduce the COMETRIQ dose.
- CYP3A4 (strong) inducers, chronic exposure (e.g., carbamazepine, phenytoin, phenobarbital, rifabutin, rifampin, rifapentine, St. John's wort): decrease cabozantinib serum levels; do not take concomitantly.If must take concomitantly, increase the COMETRIQ dose.

Laboratory Effects/Interference (Incidence %):
- Increased AST (86%), ALT (86%), alkaline phosphatase (52%), bilirubin (25%).
- Lymphopenia (53%), neutropenia (35%), thrombocytopenia (35%).
- Hypocalcemia (52%), hypophosphatemia (28%), hypomagnesemia (19%), hypokalemia (18%), hyponatremia (10%).
- Proteinuria (2%).

Special Considerations:
- Most common side effects (incidence ≥ 25%) are diarrhea, stomatitis, PPES, decreased weight, decreased appetite, nausea, fatigue, oral pain, hair-color changes, dysgeusia, HTN, abdominal pain, constipation. Most common grades 3–4 side effects are fatigue (9%), HFS (13%), HTN (8%).
- Warnings and Precautions:
  - *Perforations and fistulas:* GI perforation occurred in 3% of patients, and fistula formation in 1%. Non-GI fistulas occurred in 4% (e.g., tracheal/esophageal). Monitor patients for symptoms of perforations and fistulas. Discontinue drug if perforation or fistula occurs.
  - *Hemorrhage:* severe, sometimes fatal, hemorrhage has occurred, including hemoptysis and GI hemorrhage. Incidence was 3%. Drug should not be given to patients with a recent history of hemorrhage or hemoptysis. Teach patient to report bleeding and how to manage nosebleeds. Monitor for signs and symptoms of bleeding, and stop drug if patient has severe hemorrhage.
  - *Thrombotic events* occurred at a higher incidence in cabozantinib-treated patients compared to control: venous thromboembolism (VTE): 6% vs 3%, and arterial

thromboembolism (ATE) 2% vs 0%. Discontinue drug for MI, cerebral infarction, or other serious arterial thromboembolic events.

- *Wound complications:* Stop drug at least 28 days before scheduled surgery; resume drug after surgery based on clinical judgment of adequate wound healing. Hold drug for dehiscence or complications requiring medical intervention.
- *Hypertension:* Stage 1 or 2 HTN (modified JNC criteria) occurred in 61% of patients. Monitor BP baseline prior to initiation of drug and regularly during treatment. Hold drug for HTN that is not adequately controlled with medical management; resume drug at a reduced dose when BP controlled. Discontinue drug for hypertensive crisis.
- *Osteonecrosis of the jaw (ONJ)* occurred in 1% of patients. Assess for this, and manage as directed by provider and oral surgeon. Manifested as jaw pain, osteomyelitis, osteitis, bone erosion, tooth or periodontal infection, toothache, gingival ulceration or erosion, persistent jaw pain or slow healing of the mouth or jaw after dental surgery.
  - Patient should have oral exam prior to starting drug and periodically during treatment.
  - Teach patient good oral hygiene; if patient wants to have invasive dental procedures, drug should be stopped for at least 28 days prior to scheduled surgery.
  - If ONJ occurs, discontinue drug.
- *PPES:* Occurs in 50% of patients and was severe ($\geq$ grade 3) in 13% of patients. Hold drug in patients who develop intolerable grade 2 PPES or grades 3–4 PPES until improvement to grade 1; resume drug at a reduced dose.
- *Proteinuria* was observed in 2% of patients: monitor urine protein regularly. Discontinue drug for nephrotic syndrome.
- *Reversible leukoencephalopathy syndrome (RPLS):* Occurred rarely ($<$ 1%); evaluate patient for RPLS if presenting with seizures, headache, visual disturbances, confusion, or altered mental function. Discontinue drug if patient develops RPLS.
- *Embryo-fetal toxicity:* can cause fetal harm. Counsel women of childbearing potential to use effective contraception to prevent pregnancy during and for 4 months after last dose of Cometriq. If drug is used during pregnancy, or if the patient becomes pregnant while taking the drug, patient should be apprised of the potential hazard to the fetus.
- Nursing mothers: A decision should be made whether to discontinue nursing or to discontinue the drug, taking into account the importance of the drug to the mother's health.

Potential Toxicities/Side Effects and the Nursing Process

I.   ALTERATION IN NUTRITION, POTENTIAL, LESS THAN BODY REQUIREMENTS, related to DIARRHEA, STOMATITIS, NAUSEA, VOMITING, DYSPHAGIA

Defining Characteristics: Nutritional impact symptoms are diarrhea (63%), stomatitis (51%), decreased appetite (46%), nausea (43%), oral pain (36%), dysgeusia (34%), constipation (27%), abdominal pain (27%), vomiting (24%), dysphagia (13%), dyspepsia (11%), and weight loss in 48% of patients.

Nursing Implications: Assess baseline nutritional status and bowel-elimination status. If patient develops nausea and/or vomiting, teach patient to self-administer antiemetics 1 hour prior to each dose, and to call if nausea/vomiting persist. Discuss with physician more effective antiemetic regimen if nausea/vomiting persist. Encourage small, frequent intake of cool, bland foods as tolerated if nausea develops. Refer to dietitian as needed for meal planning. Teach patient to report diarrhea that does not respond to OTC antidiarrheal medication, or if constipation occurs that is unresponsive to fluids, laxatives, and use of high-fiber foods. Teach self-care measures of diet modification and increased oral fluids to 2–3 L during the waking hours. If constipation occurs, teach patient self-care measures to prevent constipation. Monitor weight at each visit, and review nutritional impact symptoms with patient and caregiver that does cooking; assess need for referral to dietitian.

II. POTENTIAL ALTERATION IN CIRCULATION related to HTN

Defining Characteristics: Almost all patients developed elevated blood pressure. Overt HTN (stage I [systolic BP ≥ 140 mm Hg or diastolic ≥ 90 mm Hg] or II [systolic ≥ 160 mm Hg or diastolic ≥ 100 mm Hg]) occurred in 61% of patients in clinical trials, consistent with class effects of a VEGF inhibitor. Proteinuria occurred in 2% of patients.

Nursing Implications: Assess baseline circulation, including BP baseline and regularly during treatment. Discuss abnormalities with physician or midlevel practitioner. Hold drug if HTN not well controlled, and when well controlled, resume drug at a reduced dose. Drug should be discontinued for severe hypertension that cannot be controlled with antihypertensive therapy. Monitor urine for protein baseline and regularly during treatment. Discontinue drug if nephrotic syndrome occurs.

III. POTENTIAL ALTERATION IN SKIN INTEGRITY/COMFORT related to HAND-FOOT SYNDROME, HAIR CHANGES

Defining Characteristics: HFS (PPES) has been described in 50% of patients studied, characterized by redness, swelling, and pain on palms of hands and soles of feet. It was severe (grade 3 or 4) in 13% of patients. Hair-color changes (depigmentation, graying) occurred in 34% of patients.

Nursing Implications: Teach patient that this may occur and to report it. Assess at each visit palms of hands, soles of feet, and any areas of constant pressure. Teach patient to keep skin areas well moisturized and to avoid activities that cause pressure such as jogging, repeated use of palms of hands (e.g., chopping of vegetables for a long period), and activities that expose the skin of these body parts with heat (e.g., hot tub). Hold drug in patients who develop intolerable grade 2 PPES or grades 3–4 PPES until improvement to grade 1; resume drug at a reduced dose.

IV. ALTERATION IN COMFORT related to FATIGUE, ARTHRALGIAS, SENSORY SYMPTOMS

Defining Characteristics: Fatigue affected 41% of patients in clinical trials, and asthenia 21% (characterized by fatigue, malaise, and weakness). Arthralgias affected 14%, muscle spasms 12%, and musculoskeletal chest pain 9%. Sensory symptoms included headache (18%), dizziness (14%), paresthesia (7%), and peripheral sensory neuropathy (7%).

Nursing Implications: Assess comfort and presence of discomfort and fatigue, baseline and at each visit. Teach patient that these side effects may occur and to report them. Teach patient local comfort measures, as well as energy conservation, and discuss management plan with physician if ineffective.

Drug: cabozantinib tablets (Cabometyx)

Class: Kinase inhibitor. TKI of MET and VEGFR2, and others.

Mechanism of Action: Cabozantinib is a TKI of MET; vascular endothelial growth factor receptors 1, 2, and 3 (VEGF1,2,3); RET; KIT; TRKB; FLT-3; AXL; MER; TYRO3; ROS1; and TIE-2, which are involved in normal as well as cancer processes of oncogenesis, metastasis, tumor angiogenesis, drug resistance, and tumor microenvironment maintenance. MET is expressed on tumor cells, endothelial cells, and on bone cells. MET is upregulated in a number of cancers (thyroid, prostate, ovarian, and breast). Stimulation of the MET receptor by its ligand hepatocyte growth factor (HGF, scatter factor) facilitates certain cancer cells becoming more aggressive, more invasive, making more blood vessels, and escaping from the initial tumor to invade and metastasize. When some cancer therapies are used to kill the majority of cancer cells in a tumor, it is believed that stimulation of the MET-signaling pathway occurs as an escape route—certain cells become more aggressive (aggressive phenotype) and escape via their new invasive and metastatic qualities. Binding of VEGF to VEGFR2 leads to endothelial cell proliferation, migration, and the formation of blood vessels that nourish the tumor and facilitate tumor embolization. When this is blocked, reduced tumor oxygenation causes increased levels of waste products, creating hypoxia. Hypoxia further upregulates MET. In some studies, use of a VEGF or VEGFR inhibitor alone can result in tumors becoming more aggressive and invasive, as MET becomes upregulated. In the laboratory, cabozantinib is a potent antiangiogenic and antitumor drug, which also reduces tumor invasiveness and metastases. The drug was designed to block MET and VEGFR2, as well to block MET-driven tumor escape. It increases tumor apoptosis, decreases tumor, and endothelial cell proliferation, decreases tumor cell invasiveness and metastases; in addition, it causes a blockade of metastatic bone lesion progression and disrupts tumor vasculature.

Metabolism: After oral dosing, steady state reached by day 15. Median time to peak plasma concentrations (T_{max}) is 2–3 hours after dosing. The C_{max} is 19% higher with the tablets compared to the cozantinib capsules. A high-fat meal increases C_{max} and AUC by

41% and 57%, respectively. Terminal half-life is 99 hours. Cabozantinib is a substrate of CYP3A4 in vitro. Drug is excreted in the feces (54%) and urine (27%). AUC is increased by 81% and 63% in patients with mild and moderate hepatic impairment, respectively (Exelixis, 2016).

Indication: Treatment of patients with (1) advanced renal cell carcinoma (RCC); (2) hepatocellular carcinoma (HCC) previously treated with sorafenib. DO NOT CONFUSE OR SUBSTITUTE cabozantinib capsules (Cometriq) with Cabometyx tablets (Exelixis, 2019). They are NOT interchangeable.

Contraindications: None.

Dosage/Range:
- 60 mg orally, once daily, on an empty stomach (teach patient NOT to eat for at least 1 hour before and at least 2 hours after taking cabozantinib tablets). Continue therapy in patients with RCC until no clinical benefit or unacceptable toxicity, and patients with HCC until disease progression or unacceptable toxicity.
- DO NOT SUBSTITUTE cabozantinib capsules (Cometriq) with Cabometyx tablets (Exelixis, 2019).
- Mild or moderate hepatic impairment: reduce starting dose to 40 mg once daily; drug is not recommended in patients with severe hepatic impairment.

Dose Reductions:
- Stop treatment with Cabometyx at least 28 days prior to scheduled surgery, including dental surgery.
- Hold cabometyx for intolerable grade 2 adverse reactions, grade 3 or 4 adverse reactions, and osteonecrosis of the jaw. Upon resolution/improvement (e.g., return to baseline or to grade 1 reduce dose as follows:
  - If previously taking 60-mg daily dose, resume at 40 mg daily.
  - If previously taking 40 mg daily, resume treatment at 20 mg daily.
  - If previously taking 20 mg daily, resume at 20 mg if tolerated; otherwise, discontinue drug.
- Permanently discontinue the drug for:
  - Development of unmanageable fistula or GI perforation.
  - Severe hemorrhage.
  - Serious thromboembolic event (e.g., MI, cerebral infarction).
  - Hypertensive crisis or severe HTN despite optimal medical management.
  - Nephrotic syndrome.
  - Reversible posterior leukoencephalopathy syndrome.
- Patients taking strong CYP3A4 inhibitors:
  - Decrease daily dose by 20 mg (e.g., from 60 mg to 40 mg, from 40 mg to 20 mg daily).
  - After the interacting drug is discontinued, resume the dose that was used prior to initiating the CYP3A4 inhibitor 2–3 days after discontinuing the strong inhibitor.
- Patients taking strong CYP3A4 inducers:
  - Increase daily dose by 20 mg (e.g., from 60 mg to 80 mg, or from 40 mg to 60 mg daily) as tolerated.

- Once the CYP3A4 inducer is discontinued, resume the dose that was used prior to initiating the CYP3A4 inducer 2–3 days after discontinuing that drug.
- Dosage modification for patients with moderate to severe hepatic impairment:
- Reduce starting dose of Cabometyx to 30 mg once daily if moderate hepatic impairment (Child-Pugh B).
- Do not use in patients with severe hepatic impairment (Child-Pugh C).

Drug Preparation:
- Available in 20-mg, 40-mg, and 60-mg tablets.

Drug Administration:
- Teach patient to take capsules on an empty stomach (no food at least 1 hour before and for at least 2 hours after taking the drug). NEVER take the drug with food.
- Teach patient to take tablet whole, not to crush tablets, and not to take a missed dose within 12 hours of the next dose. Instruct patient not to 1) drink grapefruit juice, eat grapefruit; 2) take St. John's wort while taking this drug; and 3) not to eat foods or take nutritional supplements that inhibit cytochrome P450 metabolism; 4) do not take a missed dose within 12 hours of the next dose; 5) take tablets whole, do not chew or crush.
- Stop drug at least 28 days before scheduled surgery, including dental surgery; resume drug after surgery based on clinical judgment of adequate wound healing.
- Review patient's medication profile: identify if patient is taking drugs that strongly induce or inhibit CYP450 and if so, discuss with provider dosage modification.
- If patient has moderate hepatic impairment, dose should be modified (e.g., starting dose 40 mg once daily). If patient has severe hepatic impairment, the drug should not be prescribed for the patient.
- Teach female patients of reproductive potential that the drug is fetotoxic, and to use effective contraception to prevent pregnancy during therapy and for at least 4 months after the last drug dose. Mothers should not breast-feed while receiving the drug, or for 4 months after the last drug dose.

Drug Interactions: Cabozantinib is a CYP3A4 substrate.
- CYP3A4 inhibitors (strong) (e.g., atazanavir, clarithromycin, indinavir, itraconazole, ketoconazole, nelfinavir, nefazodone, saquinavir, telithromycin, ritonavir, voriconazole, grapefruit, and grapefruit juice): increase cabozantinib serum levels; do not take concomitantly.
- CYP3A4 (strong) inducers, chronic exposure (e.g., carbamazepine, phenytoin, phenobarbital, rifabutin, rifampin, rifapentine, St. John's wort): decrease cabozantinib serum levels; do not take concomitantly.

Laboratory Effects/Interference (Incidence %):
- Increased AST (74%), ALT (68%), alkaline phosphatase (35%), GGT (27%).
- Lymphopenia (25%), neutropenia (31%), thrombocytopenia (25%), anemia (17%).
- Hypophosphatemia (48%), hypomagnesemia (31%), hypokalemia (30%), hyponatremia (30%), hypoalbuminemia (36%), hypothyroidism (21%).
- Increased serum creatinine (58%), triglycerides (53%), hyperglycemia (37%),
- Proteinuria (2%).

Special Considerations:
- Most common side effects (incidence ≥ 25%) are diarrhea, fatigue, decreased appetite, PPE, nausea, HTN, vomiting.
- Warnings and Precautions:
  - *Perforations and fistulas:* Fistula formation occurs in 1%, and GI perforations, which may be fatal, in 1%. Monitor patients for symptoms of perforations and fistulas, including sepsis and abcess. Discontinue drug if 1) GI perforation occurs, or 2) if a fistula occurs which cannot be appropriately managed.
  - *Hemorrhage:* severe, sometimes fatal, hemorrhage has occurred, including hemoptysis and GI hemorrhage. Incidence of grade 3 to 5 hemorrhagic events was is 5% of patients. Drug should not be given to patients with a recent history of hemorrhage, including hemoptysis, hematemesis, or melena, or who are at risk for severe hemorrhage. Discontinue drug for grade 3 or 4 hemorrhage. Teach patient to report bleeding and how to manage nosebleeds. Monitor for signs and symptoms of bleeding, and stop drug if patient has severe hemorrhage.
  - *Thrombotic events:* Drug increases the risk of thrombotic events. Incidence of VTE in Cabometyx-treated patients is 7%, including 4% PE, and incidence of arterial embolic events (ATE) was 2%. Fatal thrombotic events have been described. Discontinue drug for MI, cerebral infarction, or serious ATE or VTE that require medical intervention.
  - *Hypertension and hypertensive crisis:* Drug can cause HTN and hypertensive crisis. HTN occurred in 36% of patients (17% grade 3 and < 1% grade 4). Drug should NOT be started in patients with uncontrolled HTN. Monitor BP baseline prior to initiation of drug and regularly during treatment. Hold drug for HTN that is not adequately controlled with medical management; resume drug at a reduced dose when BP controlled. Discontinue drug if severe HTN that cannot be controlled or for hypertensive crisis.
  - *Diarrhea:* Diarrhea occurred in 63% of patients with grade 3 in 11%. Hold drug in patients with intolerable grade 2 diarrhea or grades 3–4 diarrhea that cannot be managed by standard antidiarrheal treatment until improved to grade 1, then resume Cabometyx at a reduced dose.
  - *PPE:* Occurs in 44% of patients and was severe (grade 3) in 13% of patients. Hold drug in patients who develop intolerable grade 2 PPES or grade 3 PPES until improvement to grade 1; resume drug at a reduced dose.
  - *Proteinuria:* Incidence in clinical trials was 7%. Monitor urine protein of patients during Cabometyx treatment regularly. Discontinue drug if patient develops nephrotic syndrome.
  - *Osteonecrosis of the jaw (ONJ):* Incidence is rare (< 1%). Prior to starting drug, patient should have an oral exam, and periodically during therapy. Assess for ONJ: jaw pain osteomyelitis, osteitis, bone erosion, tooth or periodontal infection, toothache, gingival ulceration or erosion, persistent jaw pain or slow healing of mouth or jaw after dental surgery. Teach patient good oral hygiene, systematic cleansing at least twice a day, and to report any changes in mouth, jaw, teeth or gums. Drug should be held for at least 28 days prior to scheduled dental surgery or invasive dental procedures if possible. Hold drug if ONJ develops until complete resolution (Exelixis, 2019).

- *Wound complications:* Stop drug at least 28 days prior to scheduled surgery, and resume after surgery based on clinical judgement of adequate wound healing. Hold drug if dehiscence or wound healing complications requiring medical intervention occur.
- *Reversible leukoencephalopathy syndrome (RPLS,* a syndrome of subcortical vasogenic edema diagnosed by MRI). Evaluate patient for RPLS if presenting with seizures, headache, visual disturbances, confusion, or altered mental function. Discontinue drug if patient develops RPLS.
- *Embryo-fetal toxicity:* Can cause fetal harm. Counsel women of childbearing potential to use effective contraception to prevent pregnancy while receiving the drug and for 4 months after last dose. If drug is used during pregnancy, or if the patient becomes pregnant while taking the drug, patient should be apprised of the potential hazard to the fetus.
- Nursing mothers: A decision should be made whether to discontinue nursing or to discontinue the drug, taking into account the importance of the drug to the mother's health.

Potential Toxicities/Side Effects and the Nursing Process

I.   ALTERATION IN NUTRITION, POTENTIAL, LESS THAN BODY REQUIREMENTS, related to DIARRHEA, STOMATITIS, NAUSEA, VOMITING, DYSPHAGIA

Defining Characteristics: Nutritional impact symptoms are diarrhea (74%), stomatitis (22%), decreased appetite (46%), nausea (50%), dysgeusia (12%), constipation (25%), abdominal pain (23%), vomiting (32%), dyspepsia (12%).

Nursing Implications: Assess baseline nutritional status and bowel-elimination status. If patient develops nausea and/or vomiting, teach patient to self-administer antiemetics 1 hour prior to each dose, and to call if nausea/vomiting persist. Discuss with physician more effective antiemetic regimen if nausea/vomiting persist. Encourage small, frequent intake of cool, bland foods as tolerated if nausea develops. Refer to dietitian as needed for meal planning. Teach patient to report diarrhea that does not respond to OTC antidiarrheal medication or if constipation occurs that is unresponsive to fluids, laxatives, and use of high-fiber foods. Teach self-care measures of diet modification and increased oral fluids to 2–3 L during the waking hours. If constipation occurs, teach patient self-care measures to prevent constipation. Monitor weight at each visit, and review nutritional impact symptoms with patient and caregiver that does cooking; assess need for referral to dietitian.

II.   POTENTIAL ALTERATION IN CIRCULATION related to HTN

Defining Characteristics: Elevated blood pressure occurred in 39% of patients in clinical trials, consistent with class effects of a VEGF inhibitor. Proteinuria occurred in 12% of patients.

Nursing Implications: Assess baseline circulation, including BP baseline and regularly during treatment. Discuss abnormalities with physician or midlevel practitioner. Hold drug if HTN not well controlled, and when well controlled, resume drug at a reduced dose. Drug should be discontinued for severe hypertension that cannot be controlled with antihypertensive therapy. Monitor urine for protein baseline and regularly during treatment. Discontinue drug if nephrotic syndrome occurs.

III. POTENTIAL ALTERATION IN SKIN INTEGRITY/COMFORT related to HAND-FOOT SYNDROME, HAIR CHANGES

Defining Characteristics: HFS (PPES) has been described in 42% of patients studied, characterized by redness, swelling, and pain on palms of hands and soles of feet.

Nursing Implications: Teach patient that this may occur and to report it. Assess at each visit palms of hands, soles of feet, and any areas of constant pressure. Teach patient to keep skin areas well moisturized and to avoid activities that cause pressure such as jogging, repeated use of palms of hands (e.g., chopping of vegetables for a long period), and activities that expose the skin of these body parts with heat (e.g., hot tub). Hold drug in patients who develop intolerable grade 2 PPES or grade 3 PPES until improvement to grade 1; resume drug at a reduced dose.

IV. ALTERATION IN COMFORT related to FATIGUE, ARTHRALGIAS, SENSORY SYMPTOMS

Defining Characteristics: Fatigue affected 56% of patients in clinical trials, and asthenia 19% (characterized by fatigue, malaise, and weakness).

Nursing Implications: Assess comfort and presence of discomfort and fatigue, baseline and at each visit. Teach patient that these side effects may occur and to report them. Teach patient local comfort measures, as well as energy conservation, and discuss management plan with physician if ineffective.

Drug: carfilzomib (Kyprolis, PR-171)

Class: Proteasome inhibitor, second generation.

Mechanism of Action: Carfilzomib is a selective proteasome inhibitor. The proteasome system is a critical system that degrades and recycles proteins, which effectively turn on and off key cell functions, such as the cell cycle and cell signaling. Carfilzomib binds irreversibly to, and inhibits the chymotrypsin-like activity of, the 20S proteasome, an enzyme responsible for degrading many cellular proteins. This results in polyubiquinated proteins accumulating, which is thought to lead to cell cycle arrest, apoptosis, and inhibition of tumor growth. In lab tests, carfilzomib appeared more potent than bortezomib and demonstrated activity against multiple myeloma cells resistant to bortezomib. Carfilzomib demonstrates synergy when given with dexamethasone to enhance cell death (Kuhn et al., 2007).

Metabolism: Drug absorption is pH dependent. Drug is rapidly and extensively metabolized, probably via peptidase cleavage and hydrolysis. Half-life of drug is ≤ 1 hour on cycle 1 day 1. Elimination is believed to be extrahepatic, but the exact routes are unknown.

Indication: Treatment of patients with multiple myeloma: (1) in combination with dexamethasone or lenalidomide plus dexamethasone in patients who have relapsed or are refractory after 1–3 prior lines of therapy and (2) as a single agent in patients with relapsed or refractory disease who have received one or more lines of therapy.

Dosage/Range:
- A cycle is 28 days in length, with drug given IV on 2 consecutive days each week for 3 weeks (days 1, 2, 8, 9, 15, and 16), followed by a 2-week rest period (days 17–28).
- Calculate carfilzomib dose using actual BSA at baseline; if patient's BSA is > 2.2 m^2, calculate dose based on 2.2 m^2.

(1) Carfilzomib in combination with lenalidomide and dexamethasone
- Administer carfilzomib IV as a 10-minute infusion on 2 consecutive days, each week for 3 weeks, followed by a 12-day rest period. Each 28-day period is considered one treatment cycle. See package insert for doses of dexamethasone and lenalidomide.
- *Cycle 1* dose is 20 mg/m^2/day IV on days 1 and 2, and if well tolerated, escalate dose to a target dose of 27 mg/m^2/day on day 8 of cycle 1. Treatment is given on days 1, 2, 8, 9, 15, 16, followed by rest through days 28. Dexamethasone 40 mg is given on days 1, 8, 15, and 22, and lenalidomide 25 mg given daily days 1–21 each cycle. Continue each cycle until cycle 13. For cycle 13, and subsequent cycles, omit the day 8 and 9 doses through cycle 18. After cycle 18, discontinue carfilzomib and give only lenalidomide 25 mg PO on days 1–21, and dexamethasone 40 mg PO/IV on days 1, 8, 15, 22 of the 28-day cycles). Continue therapy until disease progression or unacceptable toxicity. Antacid and anticoagulant prophylaxis may be required with dexamethasone and lenalidomide.

(2) Carfilzomib with dexamethasone (2 regimens)
- (A) Once weekly: *Cycle 1* dose of carfilzomib is 20-mg/m^2/day IV over 30 min on day 1 and if tolerated, on day 8 dose is escalated to a target dose to 70 mg/m^2. *Cycle 2 to Cycle 9* carfilzomib dose is 70 mg/m^2 on days 1, 8, 15 of the 28-day cycle. Cycles 10 and later carfilzomib dose is 70 mg/m^2 on days 1, 8, 15 of the 28-day cycle. Dexamethasone 40 mg PO/IV is given days 1, 8, 15, and 22 of the 28-day cycle. Administer dexamethasone 30 min to 4 hours before carfilzomib.
- (B) Twice weekly: Carfilzomib is given IV as a 30-minute infusion on 2 consecutive days, each week, for 3 weeks followed by a 12-day rest period (28-day cycle).
- *Cycle 1* dose of carfilzomib is 20-mg/m^2/day IV over 30 min on days 1 and 2, and if tolerated, escalate dose to a target dose to 56 mg/m^2/day on day 8 of cycle 1. Dexamethasone 20 mg PO/IV is given days 1, 2, 8, 9, 15, 16, 22, and 23 of each 28-day cycle. Administer dexamethasone 30 min to 4 hours before carfilzomib.
- Carfilzomib dose for *Cycle 2* and later is 56 mg on days 1, 2; 8, 9; 15, 16 of each cycle.

- Treatment may be continued until disease progression or unacceptable toxicity occurs.
- If patient is on dialysis, administer drug after the dialysis procedure.

(3) Carfilzomib as Monotherapy (2 regimens)

- Carfilzomib administered IV over 10 minutes or 30 minutes dependening upon regimen.
- (A) *20/27 mg/m² regimen* by *10-minute infusion*
  - *Cycles* 1–12, administer carfilzomib as a 10-min infusion. In cycles 1–12, give carfilzomib on 2 consecutive days each week for 3 weeks (e.g., days 1, 2, 8, 9, 15, 16), followed by a 12-day rest period. From *cycle* 13 on, omit the days 8 and 9 doses of carfilzomib. Premedicate with dexamethasone 4 mg PO/IV 30 min to 4 hours prior to each dose in cycle 1. Treatment cycle is 28 days. Starting with Cycle 13, omit the days 8, 9 doses of carfilzomib. Premedicate with dexamethasone 8 mg PO or IV 30 min–4 hours before each carfilzomib in Cycle 1, then as needed to prevent infusion reactions. See package insert (Amgen and Onyx, 2017).
  - Recommended starting dose is 20 mg/m2 IV in *cycle* 1 on days 1 and 2; if tolerated, escalate the dose to 27 mg/m² on day 8 of *cycle* 1.
- (B) *20/56 mg/m²* by 30-min infusion
  - *Cycles* 1–12: administer carfilzomib IV as a 30-minute infusion on 2 consecutive days, each week for 3 weeks, followed by a 12-day rest period (e.g., days 1, 2, 8, 9, 15, 16). Initial carfilzomib dose *Cycle 1*, days 1 and 2 is 20 mg/m². If tolerated, escalate dose to 56 mg/ m² on day 8 of Cycle 1 and thereafter. *Cycles 13 and later*, omit day 8, 9 carfilzomib doses. Treatment cycle is 28 days. Premedicate with dexamethasone 8 mg PO/IV 30 min to 4 hours prior to each dose in *cycle* 1, then as needed to prevent infusion reactions. See package insert (Amgen, Onyx, 2018).
  - Recommended starting dose is 20-mg/m2 IV in *Cycle* 1 on days 1 and 2; if tolerated, escalate the dose to 56 mg/m² on day 8 of *Cycle* 1.
- Continue treatment until disease progression or unacceptable toxicity.

Dose Modifications: See package insert.

- Modify dose based on toxicity (grades 3–4 neutropenia, grade 4 thrombocytopenia, cardiac toxicity, pulmonary hypertension, pulmonary complications, hepatotoxicity, renal toxicity, PN, other toxicity). See package insert for specific dose levels and dose modifications.
- Dose level reductins for carfilzomib: (1) **carfilzomib and dexamethasone once weekly:** dose 70 mg/m²: 1st dose reduction: 56 mg m²; 2nd dose reduction: 45 mg/m²; 3rd dose reduction: 36 mg/m². **(2) carfilzomib and dexamethasone, or monotherapy (twice weekly):** dose 56 mg/m²: 1st dose reduction: 45 mg/m²; 2nd dose reduction: 36 mg/m²; 3rd dose reduction: 27 mg/m². **(3) carfilzomib, lenalidomide, and dexamethasone OR** monotherapy (twice weekly): dose 27 mg/ m²: 1st dose reduction: 20mg/m²; 2nd dose reduction: 15 mg/m².
- **Hematologic toxicity**: (1) ANC $< 0.5 \times 10^9$/L: Hold dose of carfilzomib: if recovered to $\geq 0.5 \times 10^9$/L, continue at same dose level; for subsequent drops to $< 0.5 \times 10^9$/L, follow same recommendations and consider 1 dose level reduction when restarting carfilzomib. (2) Febrile neutropenia (ANC $< 0.5 \times 10^9$/L and an oral temperature > 38.5°C on 2 consecutive readings of > 38.0°C $\times$ 2 hours): Hold dose of carfilzomib: if ANC returns to baseline and fever resolves, resume at same dose level; (3) Platelets $< 10 \times 10^9$/L or

evidence of bleeding with thrombocytopenia: Hold dose of carfilzomib; if recovered to $\geq 10 \times 10^9$/L and/or bleeding is controlled, continue at same dose level; for subsequent drops to $< 10 \times 10^9$/L, follow same recommendations and consider 1 dose level reduction when restarting carfilzomib.

- **Renal toxicity**: Serum creatinine $\geq 2 \times$ baseline or creatinine clearance is < 15 mL/min, or creatinine clearance decreases to $\leq 50\%$ of baseline, or need for hemodialysis: Hold dose and continue monitoring renal function (serum creatinine or creatinine clearance: if attributable to carfilzomib, resume when renal function has recovered to within 25% of baseline; start at 1 dose level reduction; if NOT attributable to carfilzomib, resume dosing at the physician's discretion. For end-stage renal disease patients on hemodialysis, give carfilzomib dose AFTER dialysis.
- **Other nonhematologic toxicity (severe or life-threatening)**: Hold carfilzomib until resolved or returned to baseline; consider restarting the next scheduled treatment at 1 dose level reduction.
- **Dose Modifications for Use in Hepatic Impairment**: IF mild or moderate impairment, reduce dose of carfilzomib by 25%. No dosing recommendations can be made for patients with severe hepatic impairment (Amgen, 2018).
- Dosing in Patients with End Stage Renal Disease: If the patient is on dialysis, administer carfilzomib after dialysis.

Drug Preparation:
- Drug is available in a single-use vial, as a 10-mg, a 30-mg, or 60-mg lypholyzed powder, and is refrigerated at 2–8°C, or 36–46°F. Calculate dose and number of vials needed. Patients with a BSA > 2.2 m^2 should receive a dose based on 2.2 m^2 (Amgen, Onyx, 2018). Dose adjustments do not need to be made for weight changes of $\leq 20\%$. Remove vials from refrigerator just prior to use.
  - Use a 21-gauge or larger gauge needle to aseptically reconstitute each 60-mg vial with 29-mL sterile water for injection, or 15 mL for the 30-mg vial, or 5 mL for the 10 mg vial; *slowly inject diluent onto the inside of the vial wall* to reduce foaming. There is no data to support the use of closed system transfer devices with carfilzomib (Amgen, 2018). Gently swirl or invert the vial slowly for about 1 minute, until powder is completely diluted.
  - Do not shake. If foam forms, allow vial to sit for 2–5 minutes until gone. Solution should be colorless, and if not, do not use.
  - The final solution is 2 mg/mL.
  - Draw up the calculated dose. The quantity of carfilozomib contained in one single-use vial may exceed the required dose; carefully calculate and withdraw the correct ordered dose. Carfilzomib can be administered directly by IV infusion or optionally administered in a 50 mL–100mL IV bag containing 5% Destrose Injection, USP. Use a 21-gauge needle or larger gauge needle to withdraw the ordered amount of drug. If administering via IV bag, aseptically add drawn up drug into a 50-mL or 100-mL IV bag containing 5% dextrose injection USP (based on the calculated total dose and infusion time). Do NOT give IVP or IV bolus. Discard any remaining drug in the vial. DO NOT pool unused portions from vials. Do not administer more than one dose from a vial.

- Reconstituted drug is stable, refrigerated (2–8°C, or 36–46°F): for 24 hours for vial, 24 hours for syringe, and 24 hours for IV bag (D5W); or 4 hours at room temperature in the vial, syringe, or IV bag (5% Dextrose injection, USP). Total time from reconstitution to administration should not exceed 24 hours. Vial, syringe, and IV bag are stable for 4 hours at room temperature (15–30°C or 59–86°F).

Drug Administration:
- *Hydration is required* prior to cycle 1 dosing, especially in patients at high risk for tumor lysis syndrome (TLS) or renal toxicity. Recommend oral hydration (30 mL/kg at least 48 hr prior to Cycle 1 Day 1) AND IV fluids (250–500 mL prior to each dose in Cycle 1). If needed give an additional 250–500 mL IV fluids after carfilzomib administration. Continue oral and/or IV hydration in subsequent cycles as needed. Monitor patient for fluid overload and individualize hydration to individual patient needs, especially if at risk for cardiac failure.
- *Electrolyte monitoring,* especially serum potassium should be assessed and monitored baseline and regularly during treatment.
- *Premedications:* Administer dexamethasone (recommended dose for monotherapy or combination therapy) as premedication prior to carfilzomib PO or IV at least 30 minutes but no more than 4 hours prior to all doses of carfilzomib during Cycle 1 to reduce incidence and severity of infusion reactions. If symptoms occur during subsequent cycles, reinstate dexamethasone premedication.
- Thromboprophylaxis is recommended for patients treated with carfilzomib with dexamethasone or with lenalidomide plus dexamethasone.
- Infection prophylaxis: Consider antiviral prophylaxis for patients treated with carfilzomib to decrease the risk of herpes zoster reactivation.
- Patients on hemodialysis: give carfilzomib after the hemodialysis procedure.
- Administer carfilzomib IV in a 50-mL or 100-mL IV bag of 5% Dextrose Injection USP; infuse over 10- or 30-minutes depending on regimen. See Dosage/Range.
  - Do not administer as a bolus. Flush IV line with normal saline or 5% Dextrose USP immediately before and after drug is administered. Do not mix with, or administer as an infusion with, any other medicines.
  - Monitor patient during hydration for signs/symptoms of fluid overload.

Drug Interactions:
- Dexamethasone: synergy, used in combination in multiple myeloma.

Lab Effects/Interference:
- Decreased WBC (neutropenia 21%), RBC (47%), platelets (36%). Platelet nadir day 8 with recovery by day 28.
- Increased LFTs (AST, ALT, bilirubin), increased creatinine (24%).
- Hypokalemia (13%), hypomagnesemia (13%), hyperglycemia (12%), hypercalcemia (11%), hypophosphatemia (11%), hyponatremia (10%).

Special Considerations:
- Most common adverse reactions (≥ 20% of patients) in monotherapy trials were anemia, fatigue, thrombocytopenia, nausea, pyrexia, dyspnea, diarrhea, headache, cough, peripheral edema.

- Most common adverse reactions ($\geq$ 20% of patients) in patients receiving carfilzomib in combination: anemia, neutropenia, diarrhea, dyspnea, fatigue, thrombocytopenia, pyrexia, insomnia, muscle spasm, cough, URI, hypokalemia.
- Warnings and Precautions:
  - *Cardiac toxicities:* New onset or worsening of preexisting cardiac failure has occurred (e.g., CHF, pulmonary edema, decreased LVEF) as has restrictive cardiomyopathy, myocardial ischemia, and myocardial infarction. Death due to cardiac arrest has occurred within 1 day of carfilzomib administration. Some events occurred in patients with normal baseline ventricular function. In randomized, open-label, multicenter s for combination therapies, incidence of cardiac failure was 8% (Amgen, 2018). Monitor patients for clinical signs/symptoms of cardiac failure or ischemia. Evaluate promptly if suspected. Hold carfilzomib for grade 3–4 cardiac events until recovery, and discuss with MD dose reduction based on benefit/risk assessment. See Dose Modifications. During pretreatment hydration Cycle 1, monitor patients closely for signs/symptoms of volume overload, especially if the patient is at risk for cardiac failure. Total fluid intake should be adjusted if the patient has baseline or is at risk for cardiac failure.
  - Patients aged 75 or older have an increased risk of cardiac failure compared to younger patients. Carfilzomib clinical trials excluded patients with New York Heart Association Class III and IV heart failure, recent MI, conduction anomalies, angina or arrhythmia uncontrolled by medications. Patients aged 75 and higher should have a comprehensive medical assessment including BP and fluid management PRIOR to starting carfilzomib and be monitored closely during therapy. Monitor closely for signs/symptoms of cardiac failure or ischemia and evaluate promptly. Hold carfilzomib for grade 3 or 4 cardiac adverse events until recovery, then discuss with provider whether to resume at a reduced dose (1 dose level) or stop drug.
  - *Acute renal failure:* May occur, and may be fatal. Renal insufficiency adverse events occurred in 11% of patients, and acute renal failure occurred more frequently in paitents with advanced relapsed and refractory multiple myeloma receiving carfilzomib monotherapy. Patients with baseline reduced estimated creatinine clearance had higher risk of fatal renal failure. Monitor serum creatinine and/or estimated creatinine clearance baseline and regularly through therapy. Discuss dose interruption or modification with physician/NP/PA.
  - *TLS:* Patients with multiple myeloma and a high-tumor burden are at high risk. Administer pretreatment hydration prior to cycle 1 doses and subsequent doses as needed. Discuss with provider use of uric-acid lowering drugs in patients at risk for TLS. Monitor for TLS, including uric-acid levels and treat promptly. If TLS occurs, interrupt drug until TLS resolves.
  - *Pulmonary toxicity:* Acute events such as ARDS, acute respiratory failure, and acute diffuse infiltrative pulmonary disease have occurred rarely (1%), but may be fatal. If drug-induced pulmonary toxicity occurs, discontinue carfilzomib.
  - *Pulmonary artery hypertension (PAH):* has been reported in 1% of patients. Evaluate with cardiac imaging and other tests. Hold drug for PAH until it resolves or returns to baseline and resume drug only based on a benefit/risk assessment.

- *Dyspnea:* Reported in 28% of patients, and was grades 3–4 in 4% of patients. Evaluate promptly and distinguish between cardiopulmonary symptoms. Drug should be stopped for grades 3–4 dyspnea, and when resolved, a decision should be made to restart or discontinue based on risk/benefit assessment.

- *Hypertension*, including hypertensive crisis and hypertensive emergency, have occurred. Incidence is 17%–34% when given in combination with other agents. Control HTN before starting carfilzomib. Monitor BP baseline and regularly during treatment. If HTN occurs and cannot be controlled, interrupt drug therapy and evaluate risk benefit of restarting drug.

- *Venous thrombosis*, including DVT and pulmonary embolism, has occurred. In a randomized, open-label, multicenter trial comparing carfilzomib/lenalidomide/ dexamethasone vs lenalidomide/dexamethasone, incidence was 13% in the carfilzomib arm compared to 6% in the control during the first 12 cycles of therapy. **Thromboprophylaxis is recommended for patients receiving carfilzomib/dexamethasome or carfilzomib/lenalidomide/dexamethasone, and thromboprophylaxis regimen should be based on patient's underlying risk.** As oral contraceptives or hormonal method of contraception increase the risk of thrombosis, patients should be advised to consider alternative methods of effective contraception during combination carfilzomib/dexamethasone or lenalidomide plus dexamethasone. The incidence of VTE in patients receiving carfilzomib monotherapy was 2%.

- *Infusion reactions* may occur, characterized by fever, chills, arthralgias, myalgia, facial flushing facial edema, vomiting, weakness, shortness of breath, hypotension, syncope, chest tightness or angina, may occur immediately following or up to 24 hours after drug administration. Administer dexamethasone prior to carfilzomib to reduce the incidence of infusion reactions. Teach the patient to report signs/symptoms immediately during or after treatment and to seek emergency medical care if at home and symptoms are severe.

- *Hemorrhage:* Fatal or serious hemorrhage has been reported in patients treated with carfilzomib. Hemmorrhagic events have included GI, pulmonary, intracranial and epistaxis. Bleeding can be spontaneous and has occurred in patients with normal platelet count. Patients who have signs/symptoms of blood loss should be promptly evaluated. See dose modifications in package insert (2017).

- *Thrombocytopenia* may occur. Platelet nadir occurs between days 8–15 of each 28-day cycle, with recovery by the start of a new cycle of therapy. Incidence was 32% in clinical trials. Monitor platelet count closely and hold/modify dose as appropriate. See Dose Modifications.

- *Hepatic toxicity and hepatic failure* have been reported. Monitor LFTs (AST, ALT, bilirubin) baseline and frequently during therapy. Reduce dose or hold dose based as recommended (see Dosing).

- *Thrombotic microangiopathy* has occurred, including thrombotic thrombocytopenic purpura/hemolytic uremic syndrome (TTP/HUS), and may be fatal. Monitor for signs and symptoms of TTP/HUS. Interrupt drug if suspected and discontinue if a diagnosis of TTP or HUS confirmed. If the diagnosis is excluded, restart carfilzomib.

- *Posterior reversible encephalopathy syndrome* can occur rarely. Assess for signs/symptoms (e.g., seizure, headache, lethargy, confusion, blindness, altered consciousness, and other visual and neurological disturbances, along with HTN. Consider MRI for onset of visual or neurological symptoms and discontinue drug if PRES is suspected.

- *Increased fatal and serious toxicities in combination with melphalan and prednisone in newly diagnosed transplant-ineligible patients:* Carfilzomib in combination with melphalan and prednisone is NOT indicated for this transplant ineligible patients with newly diagnosed multiple myeloma due increased fatal and serious adverse reactions (Amgen, 2018).
- *Embryo-fetal toxicity:* Drug is fetotoxic. Women of reproductive potential should use effective contraception to avoid pregnancy during carfilzomib therapy and for 6 months following last drug dose. If carfilzomib is used during pregnancy, or if the patient becomes pregnant while taking the drug, the patient should be apprised of the potential hazard to the fetus. Nursing mothers should not breast-feed while taking the drug. A decision should be made whether to discontinue nursing or to discontinue the drug, taking into account the importance of the drug to the mother's health. Teach males with female sexual partners of reproductive potential to use effective contraception during carfilzomib therapy and for 3 months after last dose.
- Most common side effects (> 30%) are fatigue, anemia, nausea, thrombocytopenia, dyspnea, diarrhea, and pyrexia.
- Herpes zoster was reactivated in 2% of patients. Consider antiviral prophylaxis in patients with a history of herpes zoster infection.

Potential Toxicities/Side Effects and the Nursing Process

I.   ALTERATION IN OXYGENATION related to DYSPNEA

Defining Characteristics: Dyspnea occurred in 28% of patients in clinical trials. Grade 3 dyspnea occurred in 4%. ARDS, acute respiratory failure, and acute diffuse infiltrative pulmonary disease have occurred.

Nursing Implications: Assess pulmonary status including breath sounds, baseline and prior to each treatment. Teach patient to report onset of or worsening of dyspnea and have patient evaluated promptly. Drug should be interrupted for severe or life-threatening dyspnea and the patient evaluated.

II.   ALTERATION IN COMFORT related to FATIGUE

Defining Characteristics: Asthenia is characterized by fatigue, malaise, and weakness. Fatigue occurred in more than half of patients.

Nursing Implications: Assess comfort and presence of discomfort and fatigue, baseline and at each visit. Teach patient that these side effects may occur and to report them. Teach patient local comfort measures, as well as energy conservation and discuss management plan with physician if ineffective.

III. ALTERATION IN NUTRITION, LESS THAN BODY REQUIREMENTS, related to NAUSEA, DIARRHEA, CONSTIPATION, HYPOKALEMIA

Defining Characteristics: Symptoms that interfere with adequate nutrition had an incidence of the following in the carfilzomib/lenalidomide/dexamethasone study: nausea occurred in 15% of patients, diarrhea 29%, constipation 17%, and lab alterations (hypokalemia 20%, hypocalcemia, 14%, and hyperglycemia 11%). Hepatic toxicity can occur, as evidenced by changes in LFTs.

Nursing Implications: Assess baseline weight and nutritional status, as well as bowel-elimination status. Teach patient that these side effects may occur and to report symptoms if uncontrolled by self-care measures. Monitor serum electrolytes and glucose, including serum potassium, before each dose and replete as needed. Monitor LFTs baseline and periodically during treatment. Teach patient self-administration of antiemetic agent, as well as antidiarrheal or cathartic as appropriate. Teach patient dietary modifications for constipation, nausea, diarrhea (e.g., small feedings with low-fat or nonspicy foods, BRAT diet: bananas, rice, applesauce, and toast). Assess efficacy of intervention and revise plan as needed.

Drug: ceritinib (Zykadia)

Class: Kinase inhibitor.

Mechanism of Action: Kinase inhibitor that targets ALK, insulin-like growth factor (IGF-1R), insulin receptor (InsR), and ROS1 (tyrosine kinase insulin receptor). Drug is most active against ALK RTK, inhibiting autophosphorylation of ALK, ALK-mediated phosphorylation of STAT (downstream signaling protein), and ALK-dependent cancer cell proliferation. Alterations in the ALK gene have been found in 3–5% of patients with NSCLC, neuroblastoma, and rare sarcomas. The abnormality is called EMLA-ALK (echinoderm microtubule-associated protein-like 4 ALK) fusion gene, and it makes a protein product that turns on signaling for the cell to proliferate. In mice, ceritinib showed dose-dependent antitumor activity against EMLA-ALK-positive NSCLC xenografts that were resistant to crizotinib. ROS1 is an RTK related to ALK, and ROS1 gene rearrangements are found in about 1–2% of patients with NSCLC (Gainor & Shaw, 2013).

Metabolism: After a single oral dose, peak plasma levels (C_{max}) occurred 4–6 hours after the dose, and steady state with daily dosing, in about 15 days. Systemic exposure (AUC) increased when administered with a meal: AUC increased 73% (C_{max} by 41%) with a high-fat meal, and 58% with a low-fat meal (C_{max} by 43%), compared to the fasting state. It is estimated that a 600 mg or higher dose taken with a meal will approximate a dose of 750 mg of ceritinib taken in a fasting state. Drug is 97% bound to human plasma proteins. The mean plasma terminal half-life (t1/2) was 41 hours. The drug is primarily metabolized by the hepatic microsomal enzyme CYP3A4, and 92.3% is excreted in the feces (68% unchanged drug) and 1.3% in the urine. Ceritinib exposure is similar in patients with normal and mild hepatic impairment, but it has not been studied in patients with moderate or severe hepatic impairment. Ceritinib exposure is similar in patients with normal and mild-to-moderate renal dysfunction. Patients with severe renal impairment (CrCl < 30 mL/min) were not studied. Drug is a substrate of the efflux transporter P-glycoprotein (P-gp).

Indications: Ceritinib (Zykadia) is indicated for the treatment of patients with ALK-positive metastatic NSCLC as determined by an FDA-approved test.

Dosage/Range:
- 450 mg orally once daily with food, until disease progression or unacceptable toxicity.
- If a dose is missed, the dose should be made up UNLESS the next dose is due within 12 hours. If vomiting occurs during the course of treatment, do not administer an additional dose and continue with the next scheduled dose.
- A recommended dose has not been determined for patients with moderate-to-severe hepatic impairment.

Dose Modifications:
- *Ceritinib dose reduction increments:* starting dose: 450-mg PO once daily with food: (1) *first dose reduction*—300-mg PO once daily with food; (2) *second dose reduction*—150-mg PO once daily with food; (3) discontinue ceritinib in patients unable to tolerate 150 mg daily with food.
- *Hepatotoxicity:*
  - ALT or AST elevation > 5 × ULN with **total bilirubin elevation** ≤ 2 × ULN: hold ceritinib until recovery to baseline or ≤ 3 × ULN, then resume certinib at the next lower dosage.
  - ALT or AST elevation > 3 × ULN with **total bilirubin elevation** > 2 × ULN (in absence of cholestasis or hemolysis): permanently discontinue ceritinib.
- *Pneumonitis/Interstitial Lung Disease (ILD),* any grade: permanently discontinue ceritinib.
  - *GI adverse events:* Severe or intolerable nausea, vomiting, or diarrhea despite optimal antiemetic or antidiarrheal therapy: Hold drug until improved, then resume at next lower dosage.
  - *Pancreatitis:* Lipase or amylase elevation > 2 × ULN; hold ceritinib and monitor serum lipase and amylase. Resume ceritinib with a 150-mg dose reduction after recovery to < 1.5 × ULN.
  - *Hyperglycemia:* Persistent hyperglycemia > 250 mg/dL despite optimal antihyperglycemic therapy: hold until hyperglycemia is adequately controlled, then resume ceritinib at the next lower dosage. If adequate hyperglycemia control cannot be achieved with optimal medical management, discontinue ceritinib.
- *Cardiac Arrhythmias:*
  - *QTc interval > 500 msec* on at least 2 separate ECGs: Hold ceritinib until QTc is < 481 msec or recovery to baseline if baseline QTc is ≥ 481 msec, then resume ceritinib at next lower dosage.
  - *QTc prolongation in combination with torsades de pointes* or polymorphic ventricular tachycardia or signs/symptoms of serious arrhythmia: Permanently discontinued ceritinib.
  - *Symptomatic bradycardia that is not life-threatening:* Hold ceritinib until recovery to asymptomatic bradycardia or to a HR of ≥ 60 bpm, evaluate concomitant medications

known to cause bradycardia, and if unable to identily another cause, resume ceritinib at the next lower dosage.

- *Clinically significant bradycardia* requiring interventions or life-threatening bradycardia in patients taking concomitant medications also known to cause bradycardia or known to cause hypotension: Hold ceritinib until recovery to asymptomatic bradycardia or to a HR of $\geq$ 60 bpm. If the concomitant medication can be adjusted or discontinued, resume ceritinib at the next lower dosage with frequent monitoring.
- *Life-threatening bradycardia* in patients who are not taking a concomitant medication also known to cause bradycardia or known to cause hypotension: Permanently discontinue ceritinib.

- *Strong CYP3A4 inhibitors:* Avoid concurrent administration. If concomitant use of a strong CYP3A4 inhibitor is unavoidable, decrease ceritinib dose by approximately 1/3, rounded to the nearest multiple of the 150-mg dosage strength. After discontinuation of a strong CYP3A4 inhibitor, resume the ceritinib dose that was taken prior to starting the strong CYP3A4 inhibitor.
- *Severe Hepatic Impairment (Child-Pugh C):* Reduce ceritinib dose by 1/3 rounded to nearest multiple of 150 mg dosage strength.
- If a dose reduction is needed due to an unlisted adverse reaction, reduce daily dose of ceritinib by 150 mg.
- Discontinue ceritinib in patients who are unable to tolerate 150 mg daily with food.

Drug Preparation: Oral. Available in both 150-mg hard gelatin capsules and 150-mg tablets.

Drug Administration:
- Assess baseline labs (LFTs, FBS, amylase, lipase) and QTc interval on ECG and regularly during therapy as ordered, with ECG with QTc interval measurement and electrolyte monitoring in patients with CHF, bradyarrhythmias, electrolyte abnormalities, or who are taking drugs known to prolong the QTc interval as ordered.
- *Teach patient to:*
  - Take prescribed dose once a day with food.
  - Avoid grapefruit and grapefruit juice during cediranib therapy.
  - Make up a missed dose of ceritinib UNLESS the next dose is within 12 hrs, then the dose should be skipped.
  - If vomiting occurs, do not administer an additional dose and continue with the next scheduled dose of ceritinib.
  - Keep medication away from children or pets.

Drug Interactions:
- CYP3A4 inhibitors (strong): increase the systemic exposure of ceritinib. Avoid coadministration with strong CYP3A4 inhibitors (e.g., some antiretrovirals like ritonavir, macrolide antibiotics like telithromycin, antifungals like ketoconazole, and nefazodone). If coadministration is unavoidable, reduce ceritinib dose by 33%, rounded to the nearest 150-mg dosage strength. In addition, avoid grapefruit and grapefruit juice, as these may inhibit CYP3A4.

- CYP3A inducers (strong): decrease systemic exposure of ceritinib. Avoid concurrent use (e.g., carbamazepine, phenytoin, rifampin, St. John's wort).
- Ceritinib may inhibit CYP3A4 and CYP2C9. Avoid concurrent use of CYP3A4 and CYP2C9 substrates, which have a narrow therapeutic window, or substrates primarily metabolized by CYP3A4 (e.g., alfentanil, cyclosporine, dihydroergotamine, ergotamine, fentanyl, pimozide, quinidine, sirolimus, tacrolimus) and CYP2C9 (e.g., phenytoin, warfarin) during treatment with ceritinib. If they must be used concurrently with ceritinib, consider dose reduction of the drug.

Lab Effects/Interference:
- Decreased Hgb, phosphate.
- Increased ALT, AST, bilirubin (total).
- Increased creatinine, glucose, lipase, amylase.

Special Considerations:
- Most common adverse reactions (incidence ≥ 25% at a dose of 450 mg PO qd with food) are diarrhea, nausea, abdominal pain, fatigue, and vomiting.
- Warnings and Precautions:
  - *Severe or persistent GI toxicity:* In clinical trials, initial dose was reduced from 750 mg to 450 mg starting dose due to diarrhea, nausea, vomiting, or abdominal pain which occurred in 95% of patients. Administer with food to reduce GI adverse reactions with 450 mg starting dose. Hold drug if symptoms are not responsive to antiemetics, antidiarrheals or fluid replacement, then when improved, resume with a dose reduction. See Dose Modifications.
  - *Hepatotoxicity:* Ceritinib can cause hepatotoxicity. Monitor LFTs (including transaminases and total bilirubin) baseline and at least monthly, and more frequently if elevated. Hold, then dose-reduce, or permanently discontinue for hepatotoxicity based on physician order. Teach patient to report these symptoms right away: fatigue, yellowing of the skin or white of the eyes, decreased appetite, itchy skin, nausea/vomiting, pain on the right side of stomach area, or if the patient bruises more easily than normal. See Dose Modifications.
  - *ILD:* Incidence up to 2.4%. Teach patients to report these symptoms right away: trouble breathing or SOB, fever, cough with or without mucus, chest pain. Monitor for signs/symptoms of ILD, and ILD occurs and if other potential causes can be excluded, ceritinib should be permanently discontinued.
  - *QTc interval prolongation:* Ceritinib can cause QTc interval prolongation, which may increase risk for ventricular tachyarrhythmias (e.g., torsades de pointes) or sudden death. Avoid use of drug in patients with congenital long QT syndrome. Monitor ECG and electrolytes in patients with CHF, bradyarrhythmias, electrolyte abnormalities, or those who are taking medications known to prolong the QTc interval. If QTc > 500 ms × 2 occasions, hold drug, then dose-reduce, or permanently discontinue ceritinib per physician order. See Dose Modifications.
  - *Hyperglycemia:* Ceritinib can cause hyperglycemia. Patients at increased risk are those with diabetes, glucose intolerance, or taking corticosteroids. Monitor fasting serum glucose prior to patient starting ceritinib therapy, and periodically after that. Initiate or optimize antihyperglycemic medications as indicated. Teach patients to

report increased thirst, increased frequency of urination, increased hunger, blurred vision, headaches, tiredness, trouble thinking or concentrating, or if breath has a fruity smell. If hyperglycemia uncontrolled, hold, then dose-reduce, or permanently discontinue drug. See Dose Modifications.

- *Bradycardia:* Ceritinib can cause bradycardia. Monitor heart rate and BP regularly. Teach patients to report right away the following symptoms: new chest pain or discomfort, dizziness or light-headedness, if you feel faint, or have abnormal heartbeats. See Dose Modification section for management.
- *Pancreatitis* may occur, with incidence < 1% in clinical trials. CTCAE grades 3–4 elevations of lipase and/or amylase occurred in 15% of patients in study 1. Monitor lipase and amylase prior to start of ceritinib therapy, and periodically after that as indicated. See Dose Modifications for management of abnormalities.
- *Embryo-fetal toxicity:* Ceritinib may cause fetal harm. Teach female patients of reproductive potential about the potential risk to a fetus and to use an effective method of contraception, both during ceritinib therapy and for 6 months after stopping the drug. Teach male patients with female partners of reproductive potential to use condoms during ceritinib therapy and for 3 months following completion of therapy. Nursing mothers should decide whether to discontinue nursing or discontinue use of the drug.

Potential Toxicities/Side Effects and the Nursing Process

I. **ALTERATION IN NUTRITION, POTENTIAL, LESS THAN BODY REQUIREMENTS, related to DIARRHEA, NAUSEA, VOMITING, DECREASED APPETITE, CONSTIPATION, HYPERGLYCEMIA**

Defining Characteristics: Diarrhea, nausea, vomiting, or abdominal pain occurred in 96% patients in clinical studies, and were severe in 14%. Diarrhea occurred in 86% (6% grades 3–4), nausea 80% (4% grades 3–4), vomiting 60% (4% grades 3–4), constipation 29%, decreased appetite 34%, and abdominal pain in 54% of patients. Dose modification was necessary for 38% of patients. Hyperglycemia occurred in 49%, with 13% grades 3–4. Risk increased in patients with diabetes, glucose intolerance, or taking corticosteroids.

Nursing Implications: Assess baseline nutritional status, labs including hyperglycemia, and bowel-elimination status. Teach patient that these side effects can occur and to report them if they do not resolve. Teach patient to administer antidiarrheal medication if diarrhea occurs and to report if it does not resolve within 24 hours. Teach patient to increase oral fluid intake and to modify diet (e.g., 5–6 small meals of foods high in soluble fiber (e.g., rice, noodles, bananas, well-cooked eggs) and low in insoluble fiber (e.g., raw fruit, whole grain breads, seeds). If patient develops nausea and/or vomiting, teach patient to self-administer antiemetics 1 hour prior to each dose and to call if nausea/vomiting persists. Discuss with physician more effective antiemetic regimen if nausea/vomiting is not improved. Encourage small, frequent intake of cool, bland foods as tolerated if nausea develops. Refer to dietitian as needed for meal planning. If constipation occurs, teach patient to increase fluid intake, self-administer laxatives, and to increase the intake of high-fiber foods. Monitor baseline and blood glucose level and discuss with physician or NP/PA the need for antihyperglycemic medication. Discuss dose interruption and dose reduction depending upon severity of symptoms. See Dose Modifications.

II.   POTENTIAL FOR ACTIVITY INTOLERANCE related to FATIGUE

Defining Characteristics: Fatigue occurred in 52% of patients and was grades 3–4 in 5%. Hemoglobin was decreased in 84% of patients (5% grades 3–4).

Nursing Implications: Assess baseline activity level and Hgb. Teach patient that fatigue may occur and may rarely be severe. Teach patient to alternate rest and activity and teach strategies to conserve energy. If fatigue is severe, discuss if family members can take over tasks that are energy-consuming, such as grocery shopping or cleaning the house. Monitor Hgb and discuss with physician or NP/PA strategies to minimize the effect of decreased Hgb if it occurs. Teach patient to report worsening fatigue.

III.   SENSORY ALTERATIONS, POTENTIAL, related to PN, VISUAL CHANGES

Defining Characteristics: Neuropathy occurred in 23% of patients and ranged from grade 1, grade 2 motor neuropathy, to grade 3 PN. Dizziness (24%) and dysgeusia (13%) were common, all grades 1 and 2. Headache occurred in 13% of patients.

Nursing Implications: Teach patient that these side effects may occur and to report them. Assess for the presence of neuropathy, comparing one side of the body to the others, focusing on the hands and feet, as PN starts at the toes and fingertips (longest axons), and then moves in a stocking-glove distribution. Discuss any positive findings with physician or NP/PA for a more focused neurological exam.

Drug: Cobimetinib (Cotellic)

Class: Kinase inhibitor; MEK1 and MEK2 inhibitor.

Mechanism of Action: Reversible inhibitor of MAPK/extracellular signal regulated kinase 1 (MEK1) and MEK2. MEK proteins regulate the extracellular signal-related kinase (ERK) pathway which leads to cell proliferation. When *BRAF V600E and V600K* mutations occur, the BRAF pathway is turned on (constitutive activation), which includes MEK1 and MEK2. By blocking MEK1 and MEK2, cell proliferation and tumor growth is turned off.

Metabolism: After oral administration, cobimetinib steady state was reached by day 9. Median time to peak plasma levels (T_{max}) was 2.4 hours. Absolute bioavailability of cobimetinib was 46% in studies. Cobimetinib is 95% bound to plasma proteins. Mean elimination half-life is 44 hr. Drug is metabolized by CYP3A oxidation and UGT2B7 glucuronidation. Most of the drug is eliminated in feces (76%, with 6.6% unchanged drug), and 17.8% eliminated in the urine (1.6% unchanged drug).

Indication(s): Treatment of patients with unresectable or metastatic melanoma with a *BRAF V600E* or *V600K* mutation, in combination with vemurafenib. Drug is NOT indicated for patients with wild-type *BRAF* melanoma.

Dosage Range:
- Confirm the patient's tumor specimen is positive for *BRAF V600E* or *V600K* mutation before patient begins therapy.
- 60 mg PO once daily for first 21 days of a 28-day cycle, until disease progression or unacceptable toxicity.

Dose Modifications: Refer to the Full Prescribing Information for vemurafenib dose modifications.
- If taking concurrent CYP3A inhibitors: Avoid concurrent administration of moderate or strong CYP3A inhibitors if possible. If the patient must take a moderate CYP3A inhibitor short term (14 days or less) and dose of cobimetinib is 60 mg, reduce *cobimetinib dose to 20 mg*; after the CYP3A inhibitor is stopped, resume previous dose of cobimetinib (60 mg). Use an alternative to a strong or moderate CYP3A inhibitor in patients who are taking cobimetinib 40 mg or 20 mg daily.
- Recommended dose reductions for cobimetinib 60-mg dose:
  - *First dose reduction:* 40 mg PO q d.
  - *Second dose reduction:* 20 mg PO q d.
  - *Subsequent modifications:* permanently discontinue cobimetinib if unable to tolerate 20 mg PO q d.
- *New primary cutaneous and noncutaneous malignancies:* no dose adjustment.
- *Hemorrhage:*
  - Grade 3 hemorrhage: hold cobimetinib for up to 4 weeks; if improved to grades 0–1, resume at the next lower dose level; if not improved within 4 weeks, permanently discontinue cobimetinib.
  - Grade 4: permanently discontinue cobimetinib.
- *Cardiomyopathy*
  - *Asymptomatic,* absolute decrease in LVEF from baseline of > 10% AND < institutional lower limit of normal (LLN): hold cobimetinib for 2 weeks; repeat LVEF. Resume at next lower dose if both 1) LVEF is at or above LLN, AND 2) absolute decrease from baseline LVEF is 10% or less. Permanently discontinue cobimetinib if ANY of the following occur: LVEF is < LLN or absolute decrease from baseline LVEF is > 10%.
  - *Symptomatic LVEF* decrease from baseline: hold cobimetinib for 4 weeks; repeat LVEF. Resume at next lower dose if all of the following are met: 1) symptoms resolve, AND 2) LVEF is at or above LLN, AND 3) absolute decrease from baseline LVEF is 10% or less. Permanently discontinue cobimetinib if ANY of the following are present: 1) symptoms persist; OR 2) LVEF is < LLN, OR 3) absolute decrease from baseline LVEF is > 10%.
- *Dermatologic Reactions:* Grade 2 (intolerable), grade 3 or 4: hold cobimetinib or reduce dose.
- *Serous retinopathy:* hold cobimetinib for up to 4 weeks; if signs/symptoms improve, resume at the next lower dose level; if not improved, or symptoms recur at the lower dose within 4 weeks, permanently discontinue drug.

- *Retinal vein occlusion:* Permanently discontinue cobimetinib.
- *LFT abnormalities and hepatotoxicity:*
  - First occurrence grade 4: hold cobimetinib for up to 4 weeks; if improved to grades 0–1, resume cobimetinib at the next lower dose level; if not improved to grades 0–1 within 4 weeks, permanently discontinue drug.
  - Recurrent grade 4: permanently discontinue cobimetinib.
- *Rhabdomyolysis and Creatine Phosphokinase (CPK) elevations:* Grade 4 CPK elevation, or any CPK elevation and myalgia: hold cobimetinib for up to 4 weeks. If improved to grade 3 or lower, resume at next lower dose level; if not improved within 4 weeks, permanently discontinue.
- *Photosensitivity:* Grade 2 (intolerable), grade 3, or grade 4: hold cobimetinib for up to 4 weeks; if improved to grades 0–1, resume at next lower dose level; if not improved within 4 weeks, permanently discontinue.
- *Other:*
  - Grade 2 (intolerable) adverse reactions or any grade 3 adverse reactions: hold cobimetinib for up to 4 weeks; if improved to grades 0–1, resume at next lower dose level; if not improved within 4 weeks, permanently discontinue.
  - First occurrence of any grade 4 adverse reaction: hold cobimetinib until adverse reaction improves to grades 0–1, then resume at the next lower dose level OR permanently discontinue cobimetinib.
  - Recurrent grade 4 adverse reaction: permanently discontinue cobimetinib.

Drug Preparation: Available as a 20-mg tablet.

Drug Administration:
- Assess baseline ECG, QTc interval baseline and during treatment, and monitor patients with increased risk for developing or worsening QTc prolongation closely. Assess electrolytes, including magnesium and potassium baseline and during therapy. Discuss correction of any abnormalities with physician/NP/PA. Assess results of ECHO or MUGA baseline, after 1 month of treatment, then every 3 months of treatment (Genentech, 2018).
- Assess LFTs baseline, then monthly during treatment or more frequently if abnormal. Discuss implications with physician/NP/PA. Assess baseline serum CPK and creatinine before patient begins treatment and monitor during treatment. Assess for signs and symptoms of severe muscle pain or myalgia, teach patient to report these right away and have serum CPK and creatinine assessed.
- Teach patient to 1) take tablet with or without food, at about the same time each day; 2) if a dose is missed or vomiting occurs after dose is taken, take the next scheduled dose (do not make up the dose); 3) report any visual disturbances right away; 4) report severe muscle pain or myalgia right away; 5) stay out of the sun as much as possible, wear protective clothing, and use a broad-spectrum UVA/UVB sunscreen (SPF ≥ 30) and lip balm when outdoors.

Drug Interactions:
- Strong or moderate CYP3A inhibitors: increase cobimetinib serum level by up to 6.7 fold (e.g., itraconazole). Avoid concurrent use. See Dose Modifications.

- Strong or moderate CYP3A4 inducers (e.g., carbamazepine, efavirenz, phenytoin, rifampin, St. John's wort): may decrease cobimetinib systemic exposure by > 80%. Avoid concurrent use.

Lab Effects/Interference:
- Anemia, lymphopenia, thrombocytopenia.
- Increased: creatinine, AST, ALT, GGT, alkaline phosphatase, creatine phosphokinase, potassium.
- Decreased phosphate, sodium, albumin, potassium, calcium.

Special Considerations:
- Most common side effects occurring in ≥ 20% of patients are: diarrhea, photosensitivity reaction, nausea, pyrexia, and vomiting. Most common grades 3–4 lab abnormalities are increased GGT, ALT, and AST; hypophosphatemia, lymphopenia, increased CPK, increased alkaline phosphatase, and hyponatremia.
- Warnings and Precautions:
  - *New primary malignancies* (cutaneous and noncutaneous) may occur. Incidence of cutaneous squamous cell was 6% (median time to detection of first was 4 months), basal cell carcinoma was 4.5% (median time to detection 4 months), and second primary melanoma (0.8%) (median time to detection 9–12 months). Patients should receive a dermatologic evaluation prior to the drug being started, then every 2 months while on therapy, and for 6 months after cobimetinib is discontinued, when administered with vemurafenib. Vemurafenib may cause noncutaneous malignancies, so patients should be monitored for signs or symptoms.
  - *Hemorrhage* may rarely occur. Incidence was 13% in trial 1. Hold cobimetinib for grade 3 hemorrhagic events and see Dose Modifications.
  - *Cardiomyopathy:* symptomatic and asymptomatic cardiomyopathy may occur with decline in LVEF. Incidence of grade 2 or 3 decrease in LVEF was 26% compared to 19% of patients who received vemurafenib alone. Median time to resolution of decreased LVEF was 3 months. Evaluate LVEF baseline, 1 month after cobimetinib initiation, then every 3 months until drug cessation (Genentech, 2015). Manage by dose interruption, decrease or drug discontinuation (see Dose Modifications).
  - *Severe dermatologic reactions:* severe rash (grades 3–4) occurred in 16% of patients in trial 1. Median time to onset of grades 3–4 rash was 11 days, and 95% of patients had complete resolution with a median time to resolution of 21 days. Manage with dose interruption, reduction, or discontinuance.
  - *Serous retinopathy* (fluid accumulation under layers of the retina) and retinal vein occlusion: incidence in trial 1 was 26%, with time to first onset 2 days–9 months, and lasting from 1 day to 15 months. Patients should have an ophthalmologic evaluation at regular intervals, and any time patient complains of new or worsening visual disturbances (Genentech, 2015). Manage with dose interruption, reduction, or cessation of drug.
  - *Hepatotoxicity:* may occur; monitor LFTs baseline and monthly during treatment or more frequently as indicated. Manage grades 3–4 abnormalities in LFTs by dose interruption, reduction, or drug cessation.

- *Rhabdomyolysis* can occur. Serum CPK and creatinine should be assessed baseline and periodically during treatment. Teach patient to report severe muscle pain or myalgia right away and assess labs.
- *Severe photosensitivity* can occur, and in trial 1 was reported in 47% of patients. Median time to first onset was 2 months, and median duration was 3 months. More than half (63%) of patients reported resolution of reactions. Teach patients to avoid sun exposure, wear protective clothing, wear SPF ($\geq$ 30) UVA/UVB broad-spectrum sunscreen and lip balm when outdoors. Manage grade 2 or higher by dose interruption, reduction, or cessation.
- *Embryo-fetal toxicity:* Teach female patients of reproductive potential to use effective contraception during treatment and for 2 months following final dose.

Potential Toxicities/Side Effects and the Nursing Process

I.   ALTERATION IN NUTRITION, POTENTIAL, LESS THAN BODY REQUIREMENTS, related to NAUSEA, VOMITING, DIARRHEA, CONSTIPATION, STOMATITIS, HEPATOTOXICITY

Defining Characteristics: In trial 1, diarrhea occurred in 60% of patients (6% grades 3–4), nausea in 41% of patients, vomiting 24%, and stomatitis occurred in 14% of patients. Abnormal liver transaminases occurred in 65–73% of patients.

Nursing Implications: Assess baseline nutritional status and bowel-elimination status. Assess LFTs. If patient develops nausea and/or vomiting, teach patient to self-administer antiemetics 1 hour prior to each dose and to call if nausea/vomiting persist. Discuss with physician/NP/PA more effective antiemetic regimen if nausea/vomiting persist. Encourage small, frequent intake of cool, bland foods as tolerated if nausea develops. Refer to dietitian as needed for meal planning. Teach patient to report diarrhea that does not respond to OTC antidiarrheal medication, or if constipation occurs that is unresponsive to fluids, laxatives, and use of high-fiber foods. Teach self-care measures of diet modification and increased oral fluids to 2–3 L during the waking hours. If constipation occurs, teach patient self-care measures to prevent constipation. Assess oral mucosa and teach patient to self-assess, to perform oral rinses after meals and at bedtime with normal saline or bicarbonate in water rinses, and to report irritation or lesions.

II   ALTERATION IN SKIN INTEGRITY, POTENTIAL, related to INCREASED RISK FOR KERATOACANTHOMA, SQUAMOUS CELL CARCINOMA, NEW MELANOMA, AND PHOTOSENSITIVITY

Defining Characteristics: Photosensitivity, rash, and rarely development of keratocanthoma (premalignant), squamous cell or basal cell carcinoma may occur. Keratocanthoma is a common low-grade skin tumor thought to originate from the hair follicle. It is often considered a form of squamous cell carcinoma. It is found in sun-exposed skin (e.g., face, forearms, and hands). It is dome-shaped, symmetrical, and surrounded by inflamed skin. There are often keratin scales and debris. It grows rapidly, and if not treated, will eventually necrose and heal with scarring. New primary melanomas may occur. Photosensitivity affects 46% of patients. Severe rash (grades 3–4) occurred in 16% of patients in trial 1. Median time to onset of grades 3–4 rash was 11 days, and 95% of patients had complete resolution with a median time to resolution of 21 days.

Nursing Implications: Patients should have a baseline dermatologic evaluation prior to beginning therapy, then every 2 months while on therapy, and continuing for 6 months after completion of drug therapy. Any suspicious lesion should be excised and biopsied, then treated as per standard of care. Drug dose is not changed. Assess patient's skin baseline and at each visit. Teach patient to stop taking the drug and call provider right away if the patient develops a severe skin reaction, such as blisters on the skin, in the mouth, fever, peeling of the skin, or redness or swelling of face, hands or soles of feet. Teach patient to self-assess skin regularly and advise provider if notice a new wart, sore, or bump that bleeds or does not heal, or a mole that changes in color. Teach patient to use strong UVA/UVB sunblock (SPF 30 or higher), lip balm, and protective clothing or to avoid exposing skin to the sun. Teach to wear a hat to protect the scalp, especially if experiencing alopecia, and to cover exposed skin with a shirt or cover. Teach patient to wear sunglasses to protect the eyes when out in the sun if it cannot be avoided. Teach the patient to report any new skin lesions on sun-exposed body parts, especially if it is growing quickly. Discuss with physician/NP/PA referral to dermatology to obtain an excisional biopsy of the lesion. For severe rash or photosensitivity reactions, discuss further management with physician: dose interruption, reduction, or discontinuance.

III.   ALTERATION IN SENSORY PERCEPTION related to VISUAL CHANGES

Defining Characteristics: The following eye disorders occurred in trial 1: chorioretinopathy 13%, retinal detachment 12%, and patients reported impaired vision (15%), serous retinopathy (fluid accumulation under layers of the retina) and retinal vein occlusion occurred in 26% of patients, with time to first onset 2 days to 9 months, and lasting from 1 day to 15 months.

Nursing Implications: Assess baseline visual complaints and teach patient to report any changes. Discuss with physician any abnormalities. Ophthalmological evaluation should be conducted baseline, periodically during treatment, and whenever patient complains of a new or worsening visual change. Teach patients to use caution when driving or operating machinery due to the risk of developing a vision disorder (Genentech, 2015). Discuss management with provider (e.g., manage with dose interruption, reduction, or cessation of drug).

Drug: copanlisib (Aliqopa)

Class: Kinase inhibitor; phosphatidylinositol-3-kinase (PI3K) inhibitor.

Mechanism of Action: Inhibits PIK-α and PIK-δ isoforms that are expressed in malignant B lymphocytes; copanlisib induces malignant cell death (apoptosis) and inhibits malignant

B cells from proliferating. It inhibits key cell-signaling pathways: B-cell receptor (BCR), CXCR12 mediated chemotaxis of malignant B-cells, and NFκB signaling in lymphoma cells (Bayer, 2017).

Metabolism: Binds to human plasma proteins 84.2% (primarily albumin), with mean terminal elimination half-life of 39.1 hours. Most (> 90%) of copanlisib is metabolized by CYP3A microsomes, and < 10% by CYP1A1. The M-1 metabolite is active and comparable to the parent drug. Copanlisib is excreted primarily in the feces (64%) and urine (15%) to a lesser degree. Approximately 50% of administered copanlisib is excreted unchanged, and 50% as metabolites. When given at a 60 mg dose, elevated plasma glucose levels increased copanlisib exposure.

Indications: Treatment of adult patients with relapsed follicular lymphoma who have received at least 2 prior systemic therapies. This is an accelerated approval based on overall response rates, and continued approval may be contingent upon verification and description of clinical benefit in a confirmatory trial (Bayer, 2017).

Contraindications: None.

Dosage/Range: 60-mg IV over 1 hour on days 1, 8, 15 of a 28-day treatment cycle (3 weeks on, 1 week off), until disease progression or unacceptable toxicity.

Dose Modifications:
- Infections:
  - Grade 3 or higher: hold copanlisib until resolution.
  - Suspected pneumocystis jiroveci pneumonia (PJP) infection of any grade: Hold copanlisib; if confirmed, treat infection until resolution, then resume copanlisib at previous dose with concomitant PJP prophylaxis.
- Hyperglycemia:
  - Predose FBS 160 mg/dL or more or random/non-fasting blood glucose ≥ 200 mg/dL: hold copanlisib until FBS is ≤ 160 mg/dL or a random non-fasting blood glucose is ≤ 200 mg/dL.
  - Predose or post-dose blood glucose 500 mg/dL or more:
    - On 1st recurrence, hold copanlisib until FBS is ≤ 160 mg/dL or a random/non-fasting blood glucose of ≤ 200 mg/dL. Then reduce copanlisib from 60 mg to 45 mg and maintain.
    - On subsequent occurrences, hold copanlisib until FBS is ≤ 160 mg/dL or a random/non-fasting blood glucose of ≤ 200 mg/dL. Then reduce copanlisib from 45 mg to 30 mg and maintain. If persistentat at 30 mg, discontinue copanlisib.
- HTN: (1) Pre-dose BP 150/90 or greater: Hold copanlisib until BP < 150/90 (SBP < 150, DBP < 90) based on 2 consecutive BP measurements at least 15 minutes apart; (2) post-dose BP 150/90 or greater (non-life threatening): if anti-hypertensive therapy is not required continue copanlisib at prior dose. If treatment is required, consider reducing copanlisib dose from 60 mg to 45 mg or from 45 mg to 30 mg. Discontinue copanlisib if BP remains uncontrolled (BP > 150/90) despite anti-hypertensive treatment; (3) post-dose elevated BP with life-threatening consequences: discontinue copanlisib.

- Non-infectious pneumonitis (NIP): (1) Grade 2: Hold copanlisib and treat NIP; if NIP recovers to grade 0-1, resume copanlisib at 45 mg; (2) if grade 2 NIP recurs, discontinue copanlisib; (3) grade 3 or higher: discontinue opanlisib.
- Neutropenia: (1) ANC 0.5–1.0 $\times$ 10^3 cells/mm^3: maintain copanlisib does; monitor ANC at least weekly; (2) ANC < 0.5 $\times$ 10^3 cells/mm^3: Hold copanlisib; monitor ANC at least weekly until ANC $\geq$ 0.5 $\times$ 10^3 cells/mm^3, then resume copanlisib at previous dose. If ANC 0.5 $\times$ 10^3 cells/mm^3 or less recurs, then reduce copanlisib dose to 45 mg.
- Severe cutaneous reaction (1) Grade 3: Hold copanlisib until toxicity resolved and reduce opanlisib dose from 60 mg to 45 mg, or from 45 mg to 30 mg; (2) life-threatening: Discontinue copanlisib.
- Thrombocytopenia: < 25 $\times$ 10^9 cells/L: Hold copanlisib; resume when platelet count returns to $\geq$ 75 $\times$ 10^9 cells/L. If recovery occurs within 21 days, reduce opanlisib from 60 mg to 45 mg or from 45 mg to 30 mg. If recovery does not occur within 21 days, discontinue copanlisib.
- Other severe and non-life-threatening toxicities: Grade 3: Hold copanlisib until toxicity is resolved and reduce copanlisib dose from 60 mg to 45 mg or from 45 mg to 30 mg.
- Use with strong CYP3A Inhibitors which increase copanlisib exposure and potential toxicity: If concomitant treatment with a strong CYP3A4 is necessary, reduce copanlisib dose to 45 mg.

Drug Preparation:
- Available as a 60-mg lyophilized solid in a single-dose vial for reconstitution and further dilution for infusion (reconstituted concentration of 15 mg/mL), For IV infusion only. Use strict aseptic and safe handling techniques.
- Reconstitute copanlisib with 4.4 mL sterile 0.9% NaCl solution resulting in a concentration of 15 mg/mL.
- Inject the measure volume through the disinfected stopper surface into the vial of copanlisib. Dissolve the lyophilized solid by gently shaking the injection vial for 30 seconds. Allow to stand for 1 minute to let bubbles rise to surface.
- If any undissolved substance is still seen, repeat the gentle shaking and settling procedure.
- Inspect for any discoloration or particulate matter: solution should be colorless to slightly yellowish.
- Once no visible particles are seen, use a sterile syringe to withdraw the ordered dose of copanlisib reconstituted solution, and further dilute in 100 mL sterile 0.9% NaCl for Injection. Mix by inversion of infusion bag.
  - 60 mg dose is 4 mL of reconstituted copanlisib.
  - 45 mg dose is 3 mL of reconstituted copanlisib.
  - 30 mg dose is 2 mL of reconstituted copanlisib.
- Use reconstituted and diluted copanlisib immediately or store the reconstituted solution in the vial, or diluted solution in the infusion bag, at 2°C–8°C (36°–46°F) for up to 24 hours before use. Allow the product to adapt to room temperature before use after removing from the refrigerator. Protect the diluted solution from direct sunlight.

Drug Administration:
- Assess patient for signs/symptoms of infection, bleeding, HTN. Hyperglycemia, HTN, and breathing problems. Assess CBC/differential, blood chemistries including blood glucose.

- Ensure blood glucose and HTN are well controlled before administering copanlisib.
- Assess BP pre and post copanlisib infusion.
- Administer copanlisib 60 mg as a 1-hour infusion on days 1, 8, 15 of a 28-day cycle (3 weeks on and 1 week off).
- Use only 0.9% sodium chloride solution; do not administer with other drugs in the infusion line.

Drug Interactions:
- CYP3A4 strong inducers: avoid concomitant administration as inducer decreases copanlisib exposure and efficacy.
- CYP3A4 strong inhibitor: avoid concomitant administration if possible as inhibitor increases copanlisib exposure and risk for potential adverse effects. If it is necessary to administer concomitantly, reduce opanlisip dose to 45 mg from 60 mg.

Lab Effects/Interference:
- Neutropenia, thrombocytopenia, decreased hemoglobin.
- Hyperglycemia, hypertriglyceridemia, hyperuricemia, increased serum lipase.
- Hypophosphatemia.

Special Considerations:
- Most common adverse effects (> 20%): hyperglycemia, diarrhea, decreased general strength and energy, HTN, leukopenia, neutropenia, nausea, lower respiratory tract infection, thrombocytopenia.
- Warnings and Precautions:
  - *Infections:* Serious, sometimes fatal, infections occurred in 19% of patients, most commonly pneumonia. Serious PJP infections occurred. Before initiating treatment, discuss with physician/NP/PA PJP prophylaxis. Monitor patient for signs/symptoms of infection and teach patient to self-assess, and report symptoms of infection right away. Hold copanlisib for grade 3 or higher infection, or in patients suspected of having PJP infection. If PJP confirmed, discuss PJP treatment, and when resolved, resume copanlisib therapy.
  - *Hyperglycemia:* Grade 3–4 (blood glucose 250 mg/dL or higher) occurs in 41% of patients probably resulting from copanlisib therapy. Blood glucose levels peak 5–8 hours post-infusion and declined to baseline in most patients.Patients with DM are at risk for developing grade 4 hyperglycemia, and should be treated with copanlisib only after their glucose is well controlled; monitor these patients very closely. Ensure blood glucose optimally controlled before each copanlisib infusion. See dose modifications.
  - *HTN:* Grade 3 HTN (SBP 160 mm Hg or greater, DBP 100 mmHg or higher) occurred in 26% of patients. Ensure optimal BP control before administering copanlisib infusion. Monitor BP pre, and post-infusion. See dose modifications.
  - *Non-infectious pneumonitis (NIP):* Occurred in 5% of patients. Assess for hypoxia, and interstitial infiltrates on XR, and teach patient to report, pulmonary symptoms such as cough, or dyspnea. If NIP occurs, hold copanlisib and administer systemic corticosteroids as ordered. See Dose Modifications.
  - *Neutropenia:* Grade 3–4 neutropenia occurred in 23% of patients, with serious neutropenic events occurring in 1.3%. Assess CBC/differential at least weekly during

copanlisib treatment. Teach patient to self-assess and report any signs/symptoms of infection (e.g., T> 100.4°F, sore throat, burning on urination). Teach patient strategies to avoid infection (e.g., handwashing). See Dose Modifications.

- *Severe cutaneous reactions:* Grades 3–4 occurred in 2.8% and 0.6% of patients respectively. Serious events were exfoliative dermatitis, exfoliative rash, pruritus, and rash. Assess patient for, and teach patient to report, rash. See Dose Modifications.
- *Embryo-fetal toxicity:* Copanlisib is feto-toxic.Teach women of reproductive potential, and males with female partners of reproductive potential, to use effective contraception during treatment and for at least 1 month after the last dose.

Potential Toxicities/Side Effects and the Nursing Process

I. ALTERATION IN NUTRITION, POTENTIAL, LESS THAN BODY REQUIREMENTS, related to HYPERGLYCEMIA, NAUSEA, VOMITING, DIARRHEA, STOMATITIS

Defining Characteristics: Hyperglycemia occurred in 54% of patients, and was grade 3 in 33%, and grade 4 in 6%. Diarrhea occurred in 36%, nausea 26%, stomatitis 14%, and vomiting 13%.

Nursing Implications: Assess baseline nutritional status, signs//symptoms of hyperglycemia, and bowel-elimination status. Assess FBS and random blood glucose. Assess oral mucosa. Teach patient to report signs/symptoms of hyperglycemia after treatment. Teach patient self-care management of any anti-diabetic medications. If patient develops nausea and/or vomiting, teach patient to self-administer antiemetics, and administer an anti-emetic prior to copanlisib infusion. Teach patient to call if nausea/vomiting persist. Discuss with physician/NP/PA more effective antiemetic regimen if nausea/vomiting persist. Encourage small, frequent intake of cool, bland foods as tolerated if nausea develops. Refer to dietitian as needed for meal planning. Teach patient to report diarrhea that does not respond to OTC antidiarrheal medication. Teach self-care measures of diet modification and increased oral fluids to 2–3 L during the waking hours. Teach patient to self-assess oral mucosa, to perform systematic oral cleansing after meals and at bedtime with normal saline or bicarbonate in water rinses, and to report irritation or any lesions seen.

II. POTENTIAL FOR INFECTION AND BLEEDING related to NEUTROPENIA AND THROMBOCYTOPENIA.

Defining Characteristics: Leukopenia occurred in 36% of patients, neutropenia, including febrile neutropenia, in 32% (grade 3 in 10% and grade 4 in 15%). Thrombocyteopenia occurred in 22% of patients (grade 3 in 7%, grade 4 in 1%). Infections occurred in 21%, primarily pneumonia, and were grade 3 in 12% and grade 4 in 2%.

Nursing Implications: Assess baseline CBC, including WBC, differential (ANC), and platelet count prior to dosing, and then as clinically indicated and ordered. Discuss dose interruption and reduction per dose modification guidelines for neutropenia and thrombocytopenia. Teach patient self-assessment of signs/symptoms of infection (e.g., T > 100.4°F, chills, burning on urination) and bleeding (including epistaxis and development of petechiae), and instruct patient to report them right away. Teach patient self-care measures to minimize risk of infection (e.g., handwashing) and bleeding, including avoidance of OTC aspirin-containing medications. Discuss dose modifications as needed based on ANC, platelet count, and presence of infection.

Drug: crizotinib (Xalkori)

Class: Kinase inhibitor; small molecule, orally bioavailable, RTK inhibitor that blocks the tumor-specific protein ALK. This is a first-in-class drug.

Mechanism of Action: Drug is a selective, ATP-competitive small-molecule inhibitor of the ALK, MET/HGF, and ROS1 (c-ros) RTKs, as well as others. By blocking the ALK RTK, crizotinib blocks tumor signaling in a number of key pathways necessary for tumor cell growth and survival. Alterations in the ALK gene that makes this tumor-specific protein have been found in 3–5% of patients with NSCLC, neuroblastoma, and rare sarcomas. The abnormality is called EMLA-ALK (echinoderm microtubule-associated protein-like 4 ALK) fusion gene, and it makes a protein product that turns on signaling for the cell to proliferate. Crizotinib competes for ATP binding with the abnormal tyrosine kinase, so the abnormal tyrosine kinase does not bind to the receptor, the pathway is not turned on, and no message is sent to the cell nucleus telling the cell to divide. Drug also inhibits *cMET*, known as hepatocyte growth factor receptor (HGFR) tyrosine kinase. cMET/HGFR is also known as scatter factor, which plays a role in metastases. ROS1 is a proto-oncogene in the insulin-receptor family and makes a protein ROS, which helps regulate cell growth and differentiation. The ROS protein is similar to the ALK protein, and both can be blocked by crizotinib. Some patients with NSCLC have ROS-1 mutations, and 1–2% have ROS1 translocations. Crizotinib serum levels may be increased in patients with severe renal impairment (cr clearance < 30 mL/min) not requiring peritoneal or hemodialysis.

Metabolism: After oral dosing, the drug bioavailability is 43%, with peak concentration in 4–6 hours. The AUC accumulated by 4- to 5.9-fold after multiple dosing, achieving steady state in 15 days, with a terminal half-life of 42 hours. There is increased systemic exposure to the drug in Asian patients but this is not clinically significant (Li et al., 2011). Drug is 91% bound to plasma proteins. Drug is predominantly metabolized by CYP3A4/5, with 63% (53% unchanged drug) excreted in the feces and 22% excreted in the urine.

Indications: Drug is indicated for the treatment of patients with (1) metastatic NSCLC that is anaplastic lymphoma kinase (ALK) positive, as detected by an FDA approved test and (2) metastatic NSCLC that is ROS1-positive. ALK and ROS-1 testing should be done by an FDA-approved test performed by laboratories with demonstrated proficiency.

Dosage/Range:
- 250 mg orally twice daily with or without food, until disease progression or patient intolerance.
- For pre-existing hepatic impairment:
  - Moderate (any AST, tpta; bilirubin > 1.5 × ULN and ≤ 3 × ULN): 200 mg orally BID.
  - Severe (any AST, bilirubin > 3 × ULN): 250 mg once daily.
- Severe renal impairment (Cr Cl < 30 mL/min) not requiring dialysis: 250 mg orally once daily.

Dose Modifications: Grade 3: hold crizotinib until recovery to grade 2 or less, then resume at the same dose schedule; grade 4: hold drug until recovery to grade 2 or less, then resume at next lower dose (except lymphopenia, unless associated with clinical events such as opportunistic infections).
- **Grades 3–4 toxicity may require the following dose level changes:**
  - First dose reduction: to 200 mg orally twice daily.
  - Second dose reduction: to 250 mg orally once daily.
  - Third/unable to tolerate crizotinib 250 mg once daily: permanently discontinue drug.
- **Hematologic (except lymphopenia, unless associated with clinical events, e.g., opportunistic infections):**
  - **Grade 3:** hold drug until recovery to grade ≤ 2, then resume at same schedule.
  - **Grade 4:** hold until recovery to grade ≤ 2, then resume at next lower dose.
- **Nonhematologic:**
  - QTc prolongation > 500 msec on at least 2 separate ECGs: hold drug until recovery to baseline or to a QTc < 481 msec, then resume drug at next lower dose.
  - QTc > 500 msec or ≥ 60 msec change from baseline with torsades de pointes or polymorphic ventricular tachycardia or signs/symptoms of serious arrhythmia: permanently discontinue drug.
  - Bradycardia (symptomatic, may be severe and medically significant, medical intervention indicated): Hold drug until recovery to asymptomatic bradycardia or to a HR ≥ 60 bpm. Evaluate concomitant medications known to cause bradycardia, as well as antihypertensive medications. If contributing concomitant medication is identified and discontinued, or its dose adjusted, resume crizotinib at previous dose upon recovery to asymptomatic bradycardia or to a HR ≥ 60 bpm. If no contributing concomitant medication is identified, or if contributing concomitant medications are not discontinued or dose modified, resume crizotinib at a reduced dose upon recovery to asymptomatic bradycardia or to a HR ≥ 60 bpm.
  - Bradycardia that is life-threatening and requires urgent intervention: Permanently discontinue crizotinib if no contributing concomitant medication is identified. If contributing concomitant medication is identified and discontinued, or its dose is adjusted, resume crizotinib at 250 mg once daily upon recovery to asymptomatic bradycardia or to a HR ≥ 60 bpm, with frequent monitoring.
  - ALT or AST > 5 × ULN with total bilirubin ≤ 1.5 × ULN: hold crizotinib until recovery to baseline or ≤ 3 × ULN, then resume at next lower dose.

- ALT or AST $> 3 \times$ ULN with concurrent total bilirubin $> 1.5 \times$ ULN (in the absence of cholestasis or hemolysis): permanently discontinue crizotinib.
- Interstitial lung disease (ILD): any grade drug-related or pneumonitis: permanently discontinue crizotinib.
- Severe visual loss (grade 4 ocular disorder): discontinue crizotinib during evaluation of severe vision loss.

Drug Preparation:
- Oral, available as 250-mg and 200-mg hard gelatin capsules.

Drug Administration:
- Teach patient to swallow capsules whole, with or without food. If a dose is missed, make up that dose unless the next dose is due within 6 hours. If vomiting occurs after taking a dose, take the next dose at the regular time. If vomiting occurs after taking a dose, take the next dose at the regular time.
- Monitor CBC with differential baseline, then monthly, as clinically indicated, assessing more frequently if grades 3–4 toxicity, or if fever or infection occurs.
- Monitor LFTs baseline then every 2 weeks for first 2 months, then monthly or as indicated during crizotinib therapy.

Drug Interactions:
- *Strong CYP3A inhibitors* increase crizotinib plasma concentrations; do not coadminister (e.g., atazanavir, clarithromycin, indinavir, itraconazole, ketoconazole, nefazodone, nelfinavir, ritonavir, saquinavir, telithromycin, troleandomycin, voricoazole). Avoid grapefruit or grapefruit juice, which may also increase plasma concentrations. Caution should be used if moderate CYP3A inhibitors are given concomitantly.
- *Strong CYP3A4 inducers:* decrease crizotinib plasma concentrations; avoid coadministration (e.g., carbamazepine, phenobarbital, phenytoin, rifabutin, rifampin, St. John's wort).
- *CYP3A substrates:* Drugs whose plasma concentrations may be altered by crizotinib: Crizotinib inhibits CYP3A. Avoid coadministration with CYP3A substrates having a narrow therapeutic window (e.g., alfentanil, cyclosporine, dihydroergotamine, ergotamine, fentanyl, pimozide, quinidine, sirolimus, and tacrolimus). If crizotinib administered with a CYP3A substrate, consider dose reduction of the CYP3A substrate to reduce its toxicity.

Lab Effects/Interference:
- Increased AST, ALT.
- Neutropenia, thrombocytopenia, lymphopenia.

Special Considerations:
- About 3–5% of patients with NSCLC have the EMLA-ALK fusion gene; they are often nonsmokers, who also do not have mutations in EGFR or KRAS gene. EMLA-ALK fusion gene is also believed to play a role in 15% of neuroblastoma in children.
- Warnings and Precautions:
    - *Hepatotoxicity:* Drug-induced hepatic toxicity with fatal outcome has occurred rarely.

- Monitor LFTs (including ALT, AST, and total bilirubin) baseline and every 2 weeks during first 2 months of crizotinib therapy, then once a month, and as clinically indicated, with more frequent assessments in patients with grades 2–4 elevations.
- If abnormalities identified, temporarily suspend, dose-reduce, or permanently discontinue drug as shown in dose modifications. Laboratory abnormalities were generally reversible on drug interruption. Transaminate elevations usually occurred within the first 2 months of therapy.
- *Interstitial lung disease (ILD)*, any grade, occurred in 2.9% of patients across all clinical trials, and 1% had grade 3 or 4. Severe, life-threatening, or fatal ILD/pneumonitis can occur. Cases generally occurred within 3 months of starting treatment. Monitor patients for pulmonary symptoms and exclude other possible causes. If ILD/pneumonitis occurs, permanently discontinue drug.
- *QTc prolongation* has occurred in 2.1% of patients across all clinical trials, especially in patients with high risk for QTc prolongation who are taking medications that can prolong the QTc. Avoid crizotinib in patients with congenital long QT syndrome. Monitor ECGs and electrolytes in patients with CHF, bradyarrhythmias, electrolyte abnormalities, or patients who are taking medications that are known to prolong the QT interval at risk baseline. Hold drug in patients who develop QTc > 500 ms on at least 2 separate ECGs until recovery to a QTc ≤ 480 msec, and then resume crizotinib at a reduced dose. Permanently discontinue drug in patients who develop QTc prolongation > 500 msec or ≥ 60 msec change from baseline with torsades de pointes or polymorphic ventricular tachycardia or signs/symptoms of serious arrhythmia. See Dose Modifications.
- *Bradycardia* occurs in 12.7% of patients and is usually asymptomatic. Full effect of drug on heart rate may not be apparent until several weeks after treatment has started. Avoid crizotinib in patients taking other agents known to cause bradycardia (e.g., beta blockers, nondihydropyridine calcium-channel blockers, clonidine, and digoxin) if possible. Monitor pulse rate and BP baseline and regularly. If symptomatic bradycardia (non-life-threatening) develops (e.g., HR < 60 bpm, dizziness, hypotension), hold drug, reevaluate the use of concomitant medications, and adjust dose once resolves to asymptomatic bradycardia or HR ≥ 60 bpm. If life-threatening bradycardia unrelated to other causes, discontinue drug. See Dose Modifications.
- *Severe visual loss*. Grade 4 visual field defect with vision loss occurred in 0.2% of patients across clinical trials. Discontinue crizotinib in patients with new onset of severe visual loss (best corrected vision < 20/200 in one or both eyes). Discuss full ophthalmological evaluation with physician/NP/PA consisting of best corrected visual acuity, retinal photographs, visual fields, optical coherence tomography (OCT) and other evaluations for new onset of severe visual loss.
- *Embryo-fetal toxicity:* Teach women of reproductive potential to use effective contraception during and for at least 45 days after the final crizotinib dose. Teach male patients with female partners of reproductive potential to use condoms during treatment with crizotinib and for 90 days after last drug dose.

- Most common adverse reactions (≥ 25%) are vision disorders, nausea, diarrhea, vomiting, edema, constipation, elevated transaminases, fatigue, decreased appetite, URI, dizziness, and neuropathy.

Potential Toxicities/Side Effects and the Nursing Process

I.   ALTERATION IN NUTRITION, POTENTIAL, LESS THAN BODY REQUIREMENTS, related to NAUSEA, VOMITING, DIARRHEA, CONSTIPATION

Defining Characteristics: In study 1, vomiting occurred in 46% of patients, diarrhea occurred in 61% of patients, constipation in 43% of patient, dysgeusia in 26%, dyspepsia in 14%, dysphagia in 10%, and abdominal pain in 26% of patients.

Nursing Implications: Assess baseline nutritional status and bowel-elimination status. If patient develops nausea and/or vomiting, teach patient to self-administer antiemetics 1 hour prior to each dose, and to call if nausea/vomiting persist. Discuss with physician more effective antiemetic regimen if nausea/vomiting persist. Encourage small, frequent intake of cool, bland foods as tolerated if nausea develops. Refer to dietitian as needed for meal planning. Teach patient to report diarrhea that does not respond to OTC antidiarrheal medication, or if constipation occurs that is unresponsive to fluids, laxatives, and use of high-fiber foods. Teach self-care measures of diet modification and increased oral fluids to 2–3 L during the waking hours. If constipation occurs, teach patient self-care measures to prevent constipation. Assess oral mucosa and teach patient to self-assess, perform oral rinses after meals and at bedtime with normal saline or bicarbonate in water rinses, and report irritation or lesions.

II.   ALTERATION IN SENSORY PERCEPTION related to VISUAL CHANGES

Defining Characteristics: In study 1, patients described vision disorders 71% of the time, including diplopia, photopsia, photophobia, photopsia, blurred vision, visual impairment, vitreous floaters, and reduced visual acuity. Changes usually started within 2 weeks of starting drug.

Nursing Implications: Assess baseline visual complaints and teach patient to report any changes. Discuss with physician any abnormalities. Ophthalmological evaluation should be considered in patients with photopsia or new or increased vitreous floaters, as these may be signs of a retinal hole or pending retinal detachment. Teach patients to use caution when driving or operating machinery due to the risk of developing a vision disorder.

III.   POTENTIAL FOR INFECTION related to BONE MARROW DEPRESSION

Defining Characteristics: In study 1, neutropenia occurred in 52% of patients, with grades 3–4 neutropenia in 11%; thrombocytopenia in 0.4%; and lymphopenia in 48% (7% grades 3–4). Fever occurred in 19% of patients, and URIs occurred in 32% of patients.

Nursing Implications: Assess baseline CBC, including WBC, differential, and platelet count prior to dosing, as well as at least weekly during first month of treatment, at least every other week for the second month of treatment, and then as clinically indicated and ordered. Discuss dose interruption and reduction as above for neutropenia and thrombocytopenia. Teach patient self-assessment of signs/symptoms of infection and instruct patient to report them right away. Teach patient self-care measures to minimize risk of infection, including avoidance of OTC aspirin-containing medications. Discuss dose reductions as needed.

IV.   ALTERATION IN COMFORT related to EDEMA, ARTHRALGIA, RASH

Defining Characteristics: In study 1, edema occurred in 49% of patients, pain in extremity 16%, and muscle spasm in 8% of patients.

Nursing Implications: Assess baseline parameters of weight, presence of edema, pulmonary function, and monitor closely during therapy. Teach patient to monitor weight gain and edema, or the development of dyspnea. Assess skin integrity baseline and frequently during treatment. Teach patient to report rash. Develop a plan to protect skin and maintain skin integrity.

Drug: dabrafenib (Tafinlar)

Class: Kinase inhibitor.

Mechanism of Action: Drug inhibits some of mutated BRAF kinases (e.g., BRAF V600E) as well as the wild-type BRAF and CRAF kinases. Mutations such as BRAF V600E can result in constituitively activated BRAF kinases that can stimulate tumor cell growth, such as melanoma.

Metabolism: After oral dosing, median time to peak plasma concentration (T_{max}) is 2 hours. Mean absolute bioavailability is 95%. If drug is administered with a high-fat mean, the C_{max} is decreased by 51%, AUC decreased by 31% and T_{max} delayed by 3.6 hours, compared to fasting state. Drug is 99.7% plasma protein-bound. Drug is primarily metabolized by liver microenzymes CYP2C8 and CYP3A4 to form hydroxy-dabrafenib, an active metabolite, which is further oxidized to form another metabolite. Most of the drug and metabolites are excreted in the bile and urine. One metabolite, desmethyl-dabrafenib, may be reabsorbed from the gut and contributes to the chemical activity. Terminal half-life of dabrafenib is 8 hours. Seventy-one percent of the drug is excreted via feces, and 23% via urine (metabolites only). Mild or moderate renal impairment and mild hepatic impairment do not effect systemic exposure of drug or its metabolites.

Indication: Drug is FDA-indicated for the treatment of patients.
• With unresectable or metastatic melanoma with *BRAF V600E* mutation, as detected by an FDA-approved test, as a single agent.

- In combination with trametinib, in unresectable or metastatic melanoma with *BRAF V600E* or *V600K* mutations, as detected by an FDA-approved test.
- Adjuvant treatment of *BRAF V600E* or *V600K* mutation-positive melanoma with lymph node involvement, after complete resection.
- Metastatic NSCLC that is *BRAF V600E* mutation positive as detected by an FDA approved test.
- *BRAF V600E* mutation-positive locally advanced or metatatic anaplastic thyroid cancer when there are no other satisfactory locoregional treatment options.
- LIMITATIONS: Not indicated for treatment of patients with wild-type *BRAF* melanoma, NSCLC, or wild-type BRAF anaplastic thyroid cancer.

Dosage/Range:
- Confirm the presence of *BRAF V600E* mutation in tumor specimens, using an FDA ap-proved test, prior to starting dabrafenib as a single agent, and *BRAF V600E or V600K* mutations in tumor specimens prior to starting combined dabrafenib and trametinib. Mu-tations must be detected by an FDA-approved test.
- 150 mg orally twice daily on an empty stomach (at least one hour prior to or two hours after a meal); take approximately 12 hours apart, taken as a single agent for unresect-able or metatatic melanoma, or in combination therapy with trametinib.for unresectable or metastatic melanoma, adjuvant treatment of melanoma, NSCLC, and for anaplastic thyroid cancer.
- Teach patient: 1) take doses approximately 12 hours apart; 2) take at least 1 hour before or 2 hours after a meal; 3) do not make up a missed dose within 6 hours of the next dose; 4) do not to open, crush, or break capsules open.

Dose Modifications: *For trametinib, review the Full Prescribing Information for dose modifications.*
- Dose reductions for dabrafenib:
  - First dose reduction: From 150 mg to 100 mg orally twice daily.
  - Second dose reduction: From 100 mg to 75 mg orally twice daily.
  - Third dose reduction: From 75 mg to 50 mg orally twice daily.
  - If unable to tolerate 50 mg twice daily, discontinue dabrafenib.
- New Primary Cutaneous Malignancies: no dose modification.
- New Primary Noncutaneous Malignancies: permanently discontinue dabrafenib in pa-tients who develop *RAS* mutation-positive noncutaneous malignancy.
- Febrile drug reaction:
  - Temperature 101.3–104°F (38.5–40°C): hold dabrafenib, until fever resolves, then resume at same or lower dose level (see previous bullet).
  - Temperature > 104°F or fever complicated by rigors, hypotension, dehydration, or renal failure: hold dabrafenib until fever resolves, then resume at a lower dose level or permanently discontinue dabrafenib.
- Cutaneous grade 2 toxicity, intolerable, or grade 3 or 4 skin toxicity: hold dabrafenib for up to 3 weeks; if improved, resume dose at a lower dose level; if not improved, perma-nently discontinue.

- Cardiac:
  - Symptomatic CHF or an absolute decrease of > 20% in LVEF from baseline that is below LLN: hold dabrafenib until LVEF improved, then resume at same dose.
- Uveitis, including iritis and iridocyclitis: If mild or moderate uveitis does not respond to ocular therapy, or for severe uveitis, hold dabrafenib for up to 6 weeks. If improved to grades 0–1, resume at the same or at a lower dose level. If not improved, permanently discontinue dabrafenib.
- Other:
  - Intolerable grade 2, or any grade 3 reactions: hold dabrafenib until adverse reaction resolves to grades 0–1, then resume at a lower dose level; if no improvement, permanently discontinue dabrafenib.
  - First occurrence of any grade 4 adverse reaction: either permanently discontinue dabrafenib or hold until reaction resolves to grades 0–1, then resume at lower dose level.
  - Recurrent grade 4 adverse reaction: permanently discontinue dabrafenib.

Drug Preparation:
- Available as 50-mg and 75-mg capsules.

Drug Administration:

Teach patient to:
- Take drug on an empty stomach, at least one hour prior to or two hours after a meal.
- Take two times a day, about 12 hours apart.
- If receiving the combination, the patient should take the trametinib once-daily dose with either the morning or evening dose of dabrafenib at the same time each day. Patient teaching pamphlet for patients taking both Taflinar (debrafenib) and Mekinist (trametinib) available at https://www.tafinlarmekinist.com.
- Teach patient (1) to take capsule whole without crushing, opening, or breaking the capsule; (2) to take a missed dose when remembered, but not if it is within 6 hours of the next scheduled dose; then just take the next scheduled dose. Do not make up the missed dose.

Drug Interactions:
- Drug is substrate of CYP3A4 and CYP2C8; metabolites are substrates of CYP3A4. Drug is substrate of human P-glycoprotein (Pgp).
- Drug is a moderate inducer of CYP3A4 and may induce other microenzymes.
- Strong inhibitors of CYP3A4 (e.g., ketoconazole, nefazodone, clarithromycin) or CYP2C8 (e.g., gemfibrozil): may increase serum level of dabrafenib; AVOID coadministration.
- Strong inducers of CYP3A4 (e.g., rifampin, phenytoin, carbamazepine, phenobarbital, St. John's wort) or CYP2C8 (e.g., rifampicin): may decrease serum level of dabrafenib; AVOID coadministration.
- Concomitant use with agents that are sensitive substrates of CYP3A4, CYP2C8, CYP2C9, CYP2C19, or CYP2B6 may result in loss of efficacy of these agents; e.g., midazolam is a CYP3A4 substrate; dabrafenib decreases midazolam C_{max} and AUC by 61% and 74%, respectively. S-Warfarin is a CYP2C9 substrate, and R-warfarin is a CYP3A4/CYP1A2 substrate so patients' INR should be closely monitored during initiation or

discontinuation of dabrafenib. Coadministration of dexamethasone and hormonal contraceptives can result in decreased serum concentrations and loss of efficacy.

Lab Effects/Interference:
- Hyperglycemia.
- Hypophosphatemia, hyponatremia, increased alkaline phosphatase.

Special Considerations:
- Drug is not approved for treatment of patients with wild-type *BRAF* melanoma. *BRAF* inhibitors can cause increased cell proliferation and tumor promotion in *BRAF* wild-type melanoma.
- Warnings and Precautions:
  - *New primary malignancies:*
    - Drug may cause the development of new *primary cutaneous malignancies* (e.g., cutaneous squamous cell carcinomas and keratocanthomas; incidence 7–11%, with median time to first squamous cell carcinoma of 2.1 months; incidence of cutaneous squamous cell carcinomas when dabrafenib is given in combination with trametinib was 3%. Incidence of basal cell carcinoma is increased in combination therapy with trametinib (incidence 3.3% vs 6% with dabrafenib alone). In NSCLC study, incidence was 3.2% with the combination, with onset to first occurrence 25 days–12.3 months.
    - If a patient developed a cutaneous squamous cell cancer while taking dabrafenib monotherapy, the patient has a 33% chance of developing 1 or more cutaneous squamous cell lesions with continued dabrafenib administration.
    - Discuss with provider the performance of dermatologic evaluations prior to starting therapy, every 2 months while on therapy, and for up to 6 months following drug discontinuance.
    - *Noncutaneous malignancies:* dabrafenib may promote growth and development of cancers with activation of *RAS* through mutation. Monitor patients for signs/symptoms of noncutaneous malignancies and permanently discontinue dabrafenib if an *RAS* mutation-positive cancer develops.
  - *Tumor promotion in* BRAF *wild-type tumors*: dabrafenib activates MAP-kinase signaling resulting in increased cell proliferation in wild-type cells when exposed to *BRAF* inhibitors. Do NOT use drug in *BRAF* wild-type melanoma or NSCLC patients.
  - *Hemorrhage,* including major hemorrhage, may occur in patients receiving the combination (incidence 19% all bleeding, and 5% serious hemorrhage, e.g., intracranial bleed); incidence is 15% with dabrafenib alone. Permanently discontinue dabrafenib and tramatinib for all grade 4 hemorrhage or any persistent grade 3 hemorrhagic events. Hold dabrafenib for grade 3 hemorrhage, and if improved, resume dabrafenib (and trametinib if the combination used) at a lower dose level.
  - *Cardiomyopathy* (defined as a decrease in LVEF $\geq$ 10% from baseline and below LLN) can occur with dabrafenib; incidence is 6% in patients receiving both dabrafenib and trametinib, compared to 2.9% with dabrafenib alone. Before beginning therapy with dabrafenib and trametinib assess LVEF (ECHO or MUGA) baseline, one month after combination started, then at 2–3 monthly intervals while on combination therapy. See Dose Modifications.

- *Serious febrile reactions:* Dabrafenib can cause serious febrile drug reactions (incidence 28% in trial 1). Serious febrile reactions and fever can become complicated by hypotension, rigors, chills, dehydration, or renal failure. The incidence and severity of fever is increased in combination dabrafenib and trametinib therapy. Hold drug if fever ≥ 101.3°F or complicated fever occurs (e.g., hypotension, rigors or chills, dehydration, or renal failure in absence of other identifiable cause). See Dose Modifications. Administer antipyretics as secondary prophylaxis when resuming dabrafenib if patient has had a prior episode. Administer corticosteroids (e.g., prednisone 10 mg qd) for at least 5 days for second or subsequent pyrexia if temperature does not return to baseline within 3 days of onset of pyrexia, or for pyrexia associated with complications such as dehydration, hypotension, renal failure, or severe chills/rigors, and there is no evidence of active infection, as ordered by physician/NP/PA (Novartis, 2015).
- *Uveitis:* Drug may cause uveitis and iritis; monitor patient baseline and regularly for visual symptoms (e.g., change in vision, photophobia, eye pain), and teach patient to report any changes. Symptomatic treatment usually involves steroid and mydriatic ophhthalmic drops. See Dose Modifications. Permanently discontinue dabrafenib for persistent grade 2 or greater uveitis of > 6 weeks' duration.
- *Serious skin toxicity:* Incidence of serious skin toxicity was 0.7% in patients receiving combined dabrafenib and trametinib therapy. If this occurs, hold dabrafenib or if toxicity is intolerable. Dabrafenib may be resumed at the next lower dose level when patient has improved within 3 weeks. See Dose Modifications. Dabrafenib causes palmar–plantar erythrodysesthesia in about 20% of patients.
- *Hyperglycemia:* Dabrafenib may cause hyperglycemia. Assess baseline serum glucose and monitor regularly during therapy as appropriate.
  - Monitor patients with diabetes very closely, as patients may need an increase in dose of or initiation of insulin or oral hypoglycemic agent.
  - Teach patients to report symptoms of hyperglycemia (e.g., polyphagia, polyuria, polydipsia).
  - Patients with Glucose-6-phosphate dehydrogenase deficiency: monitor patient closely for hemolytic anemia.
  - Embryo-fetal toxicity: Drug is fetotoxic, and dabrafenib may impair fertility in men and women of reproductive potential. Counsel women and men of reproductive potential to use effective contraception; drug may cause hormonal contraception to be ineffective, so women should use an alternative form of contraception. Nursing mothers should discontinue nursing or not take the drug. Women should avoid pregnancy during treatment and for 2 weeks after last dose of dabrafenib.
  - *Glucose-6-Phosphate Dehydrogenase Deficiency (G6PD):* Potential risk of hemolytic anemia in patients with G6PD. Monitor patients with G6PD for signs of hemolytic anemia when taking dabrafenib.
  - *Risks associated with combined treatment.* See drug information for trametinib.
  - *Embryo-fetal toxicity:* Drug is fetotoxic. Teach women of reproductive potential to use an effective non-hormonal method of contraception as drug can inactivate hormonal contraceptives, during treatment and for 2 weeks after last dose.
  - Most common side effects of dabrafenib as a single agent are hyperkeratosis, headache, pyrexia, arthralgia, papilloma, alopecia, PPES. Most common side effects

of dabrafenib in combination with trametinib are pyrexia, rash, chills, headache, arthralgia, and cough.

Potential Toxicities/Side Effects and the Nursing Process

I.   ALTERATION IN COMFORT AND HOMEOSTASIS related to FEBRILE DRUG REACTION

Defining Characteristics: Serious drug reactions (fever or fever complicated by hypotension, rigors or chills, dehydration, or renal failure without other identifiable cause) occurred in 28% of patients. Median time to initial onset was 11 days (range 1–202 days), and median duration of fever was 3 days (range 1–129 days).

Nursing Implications: Teach patient that fever may occur and to report it or the occurrence of chills, rigors, or dizziness right away. Drug should be stopped until patient discusses symptoms with physician or NP/PA. Ensure patient has a thermometer and can read it. Teach patient that dehydration can worsen this, and to make sure the patient drinks adequate fluids daily (e.g., one 8-oz glass of fluid, excluding alcohol, every hour while awake). Drug should be held for fever of 101.3°F or greater, or for chills, rigors, hypotension, or renal failure. Prophylaxis with acetaminophen may be needed when resuming drug per physician or NP/PA.

II.   ALTERATION IN SENSORY PERCEPTION related to VISUAL CHANGES

Defining Characteristics: Uveitis, including iritis, occurred in 1% of patients.

Nursing Implications: Assess baseline visual complaints and teach patient to report any changes (such as change in vision, photophobia, eye pain) right away. Discuss ophthalmic evaluation if symptoms arise. In clinical trials, symptoms were controlled with steroid and mydriatic ophthalmic drops.

III.   ALTERATION IN SKIN INTEGRITY, POTENTIAL, related to SKIN CHANGES, NEW CUTANEOUS MALIGNANCY, PPES

Defining Characteristics: Hyperkeratosis occurred in 37% of patients, alopecia in 22% of patients, PPES in 20% of patients, and rash in 17% of patients. Papilloma occurred in 27% of patients, and cutaneous squamous cell carcinoma in 7% of patients.

Nursing Implications: Teach patient that these side effects may occur and to report them. Examine skin of hands and feet, and areas of high pressure. Patient should have a dermatologic evaluation baseline starting therapy, every 2 months while on therapy, and for up to 6 months following drug discontinuance for squamous cell cancers. Teach patient to examine skin of hand, feet, areas of pressure and to report pain, edema, numbness, stinging, dysesthesias, flat blisters with a reddish halo, peeling (desquamation), painful hyperkeratotic lesions, scaly skin calluses. Teach patient to avoid hot water and to use tepid water in shower or bath; use a mild soap and to pat the area dry gently and not rub vigorously; avoid constrictive clothing; avoid prolonged pressure on feet, like jogging or long walks; avoid repetitive hand motion (e.g., raking); use skin moisturizer on hands and feet bid; and protect from the sun exposure.

Drug: dacomitinib (Vizimpro)

Class: Kinase inhibitor, EGFR.

Mechanism of Action: Reversibly inhibits EGFR kinase activity (EGFR1/HER1, HER2, and HER4), and certain EGFR activating mutations (exon 19 deletion or exon 21 L858R substitution mutation). May also have anti-tumor efficacy against intracranial tumors after oral administration.

Metabolism: After oral dosing, bioavailability is 80% and steady state is reached within 14 days. Half-life of dacomitinib is 70 hours. Drug is metabolized by the liver via oxidation and glutathione conjugation. Major metabolite with same activity as parent drug is O-desmethyl dacomitinib, formed by isoenzyme CYP2D6, and CYP3A4 contributed to minor oxidative metabolites (Pfizer, 2018). Most of drug excreted in feces (79%) and 3% in the urine.

Indication: First line treatment for patients with metastatic NSCLC having EGFR exon 19 deletion or exon 21 L858R substitution mutation in tumors, as identified by FDA-approved tests.

Contraindication: None.

Dosage/Range: 45 mg PO once daily, until disease progression or unacceptable toxicity.

Dose Modification for Adverse Effects:
- Recommended dose reduction levels: 1st dose reduction: from 45 mg to 30 mg PO qd; 2nd dose reduction: from 30 mg to 15 mg PO qd.
- *Interstitial lung disease (ILD):* Any grade: permanently discontinue dacomitinib.
- *Diarrhea:*
  - Grade 2: Hold dacomitinib until recovery to ≤ grade 1, then resume dacomitinib at same dose level; For recurrent grade 2 diarrhea: hold dacomitinib until recovery to ≤ grade 1, then resume dacomitinib at a reduced dose.
  - Grade 3 or 4: hold dacomitinib until recovery to ≤ grade 1; then resume at a reduced dose.
- *Dermatologic adverse reactions:*
- Grade 2: hold dacomitinib for persistent dermatologic adverse reactions; upon recovery to ≤ grade 1, then resume dacomitinib at same dose level. For recurrent persistent grade 2 dermatologic adverse reactions: hold dacomitinib until recovery to ≤ grade 1, then resume dacomitinib at a reduced dose.

- Grade 3 or 4: hold dacomitinib until recovery to ≤ grade 1; then resume at a reduced dose.
- *Other:* Grade 3 or 4: hold dacomitinib until recovery to ≤ grade 1; then resume at a reduced dose.

Drug Preparation:
- Available in 45-mg, 30-mg, and 15-mg tablets.
- Keep medication safely away from children and pets.

Drug Administration:

Teach patient to take dacomitinib:
- Orally, once daily with or without food.
- At about the same time of day; if a dose is vomited or missed, do not take an additional dose or make it up, rather take the next scheduled dose.
- Teach patient to use moisturizers and avoid sun (wear hat, long sleeves and long pants when outside in the sun).
- If grade 1 rash develops, teach patient use of topical antibiotics and topical steroids. If grade 2 occurs, start oral antibiotics as ordered (Pfizer, 2018).
- Teach female patients of reproductive potential to use effective contraception during and for at least 17 days after final dacomitinib dose.

Drug Interactions:
- Acid-reducing agents: PPIs (e.g., rabeprazole) decreased dacomitinib C_{max} by 51% and AUC by 39%. Do not give PPIs concomitantly. Rather, give locally acting antacids or H2 receptor antagonist where dacomitinib is administered at least 6 hours before or 10 hours after a H2-receptor antagonist.
- CYP2D6 substrates (e.g., dextromethorphan): coadministration with dacomitinib increased dextromethorphan C_{max} by 9.7 fold. Do not give concurrently with dacomitinib as minimial increases in concentration of the CYP2D6 substrate may lead to serious or life-threatening toxicities.

Lab Effects/Interference:
- Anemia, lymphopenia.
- Increased: ALT, glucose, AST, serum creatinine, Alkaline phosphatase, bilirubin.
- Decreased: serum albumin, calcium, potassium, sodium, magnesium.

Special Considerations:
- Most common adverse reactions (> 20%) were: diarrhea, rash, paronychia, stomatitis, decreased appetite, dry skin, decreased weight, alopecia, cough, pruritis.
- Teach mothers not to breast-feed while receiving the drug.
- Warnings and Precautions:
    - *ILD:* Rarely, severe and sometimes fatal ILD/pneumonitis has occurred, incidence 0.5% of patients. Monitor for pulmonary symptoms, and hold drug if ILD/pneumonitis suspected (e.g., worsening respiratory symptoms of dyspnea, cough, fever). If ILD confirmed, permanently discontinue.
    - *Diarrhea:* Can be severe, and is rarely fatal. Incidence of diarrhea was 86% in clinical trials, with grade 3 or 4 reported in 11% (0.3% fatal). Hold dacomitinib for grade 2

or higher diarrhea until recovery to ≤ grade 1, then resume at same or decreased dose level (see Dose Modifications). Teach patient to start anti-diarrheal treatment with loperamide or diphenoxylate HCL with atropine as ordered for diarrhea as soon as diarrhea occurs, and to call RN/MD if diarrhea does not respond.

- *Dermatologic adverse reactions:* Rash and exfoliative skin reactions can occur. Rash occurred in 78% in clinical trials, with grade 3–4 rash in 21% of patients. Exfoliative skin reactions occurred in 7% of patients, with 1.8% grade 3–4. Hold drug for persistent grade 2 or any grade 3–4 skin reactions until recovery to ≤ grade 1 in severity. Then drug should be resumed at same or reduced dose level (see Dose Modifications). Teach patient to avoid sun exposure as this may increase rash and exfoliation. Teach patient to use moisturizers and avoid sun (wear hat, long sleeves and long pants when outside in the sun, wear sunblock). If grade 1 rash develops, teach patient use of topical antibiotics and topical steroids. If grade 2 occurs, start oral antibiotics (Pfizer, 2018).
- *Embryo-fetal toxicity:* Drug is embryotoxic. Teach female patients of reproductive potential to use effective contraception during and for 17 days after final drug dose.

Potential Toxicities/Side Effects and the Nursing Process

I.   ALTERATION IN SKIN INTEGRITY related to RASH

Defining Characteristics: As expected, because EGFR is important in skin function, this is the area of major toxicity. Rash ranges from maculopapular to pustular on the face, neck, chest, back, and arms, affecting up to 69% of patients. Most rashes are mild to moderate, but 23% are grades 3–4. Paronychia occurred in 64% of patients (grade 3–4 in 8%), dry skin in 30%, alopecia 23%, pruritis 21%, palmar-plantar erythrodysesthesia syndrome (PPES) 15%, and dermatitis 11%.

Nursing Implications: Assess skin integrity of face, neck, arms, and upper trunk baseline, and regularly during treatment, and fingers for paronychia. Teach patient that rash may occur, its usual course, and self-care measures for comfort. Teach patient that skin may become dry and to use skin emollients or moisturizers beginning the first day of treatment. Teach patient to avoid sun exposure if possible, and to wear a sunblock, a hat, and long sleeves and long pants if going outside as the sun can increase incidence of rash. Teach patient to stay hydrated, and if itching occurs, avoid scratching as this may lead to infection. Teach patient to report it so that anti-pyritic medication can be prescribed as well as self-care measures. Teach patient self-care measures for self-care of paronychia if it develops. If rash develops, teach patient to keep skin with rash clean to prevent infection. Teach patient NOT to use anti-acne medications as the rash is a sterile, non-inflammatory rash not acne. Manufacturer recommends that the rash be managed by (1) grade 1: teach patient to apply topical antibiotics and topical steroids; (2) grade 2 or higher: teach patient to take ordered oral antibiotics (Pfizer, 2018). Assess body image intactness, and if rash develops, its threat to body image. Encourage patient to verbalize feelings, provide emotional support, and individualize care plan to patient response.

II.   ALTERATION IN ELIMINATION PATTERN related to DIARRHEA

Defining Characteristics: Diarrhea is the most common adverse effect, with an incidence of 87% (8% grade 3–4). Symptoms may be self-limited or require an antidiarrheal agent, such as loperamide. Drug should be held for grade 2 diarrhea.

Nursing Implications: Assess bowel-elimination pattern baseline and regularly during therapy. Teach patient to report diarrhea; teach patient self-care strategies to manage diarrhea such as dietary modification and self-administration of loperamide or diphenoxylate HCl with atropine sulfate as ordered, as soon as diarrhea begins; teach patient to minimize potential complications such as dehydration and electrolyte depletion by drinking fluids hourly while awake. Identify patients at risk for dehydration and follow closely, such as patients with renal insufficiency, diabetes, congestive heart failure, or the older population. Renal function should be assessed at baseline and periodically during therapy, more closely if the patient has diarrhea and is at risk for dehydration. See Dose Modifications section; drug should be held for grade 2 or higher diarrhea until recovery to grade 1 or less, and then the dose resumed or reduced.

III.   SENSORY/PERCEPTUAL ALTERATION, POTENTIAL, related to CONJUNCTIVITIS

Defining Characteristics: Conjunctivits can occur, and the incidence in clinical trials was 19%.

Nursing Implications: Teach patient to report any eye irritation, redness, pain, or change in visual acuity. Teach patient to use artificial tears to keep eyes lubricated if eyes become dry. Discuss management and need for referral to an ophthmalogist with physician/NP/PA.

IV.   POTENTIAL ALTERATION IN NUTRITION, LESS THAN BODY REQUIREMENTS, related to MUCOSITIS, DECREASED APPETITE, AND NAUSEA.

Defining Characteristics: Stomatitis was reported in 45% of patients receiving dacomitinib. Nausea occurred in 19% of patients, constipation 13%, and mouth ulceration 12%. Decreased appetite and decreased weight was reported in > 20% of patients.

Nursing Implications: Assess oral hygiene practices and status of oral mucosa, gums, and teeth baseline and regularly throughout therapy. Assess nutritional status and weight baseline and regularly during treatment. Teach patient to report stomatitis and to use a systematic cleansing regimen as determined by institutional policy. Assess baseline LFTs and monitor during therapy Teach patient to report nausea and/or vomiting and to discuss antiemetic therapy with physician or NP/PA; review instructions with patient along with diet modifications to minimize nausea and/or vomiting.

Drug: dasatinib (Sprycel)

Class: Multitargeted TKI.

Mechanism of Action: Inhibits the following kinases: BCR-ABL, SRC family (SRC, LCK, YES, FYN), c-KIT, EPHA2, and PDGFR-b. Drug forms a tighter bond with BCR-ABL kinase (300–1,000 times more potently) than imatinib mesylate (Gleevec) and binds to both active and inactive forms.

Metabolism: Drug is rapidly absorbed after oral ingestion with peak serum levels in 0.5–6 hours and an overall mean half-life of 3–5 hours. If ingested with a high-fat meal, there was a 14% increase in the mean area under the curve exposure, but this is not felt to be clinically relevant. Drug and its active metabolite bind to plasma proteins 96% and 93%, respectively. Drug is extensively metabolized by the P450 microenzyme CYP3A4. Drug is excreted in the feces (85%) and to a lesser degree the urine (4%).

Indication: Drug is indicated for the treatment of (1) newly diagnosed adults with Philadelphia chromosome-positive (Ph+) chronic myeloid leukemia (CML) in chronic phase; (2) adults with chronic, accelerated, or myeloid or lymphoid blast phase Ph+ CML with resistance or intolerance to prior therapy, including imatinib; (3) adults with Ph+ acute lymphoblastic leukemia (Ph+ ALL) with resistance or intolerance to prior therapy; (4) pediatric patients aged 1 year and older with Ph+ CML in chronic phase; and (5) pediatric patients aged 1 year and older with Ph+ALL in combination with chemotherapy.

Dosage/Range:
- Adults:
  - Chronic phase CML in adults: 100 mg PO once daily.
  - Accelerated phase CML, myeloid, or lymphoid blast phase CML, or Ph+ ALL in adults: 140 mg PO once daily.
  - Adults with CML and Ph+ ALL consider dose escalation to 140 mg once daily (chronic phase CML) or 180 mg once daily (advanced phase CML and Ph+ALL) in patients who do not achieve a hematologic or cytogenetic response at the recommended starting dosage.
- Pediatric patients in chronic phase CML and ALL, starting dose based on body weight (see package insert):
  - (a) 10–20 kg: 40 mg; (b) 20–30 kg: 60 mg; (c) 30–45 kg: 70 mg; (d) at least 45 kg: 100 mg. Tablet dosing for patients weighing < 10 kg is not recommended.
  - Recalculate the dose every 3 months or more often as necessary as the child gains weight.
  - Dose escalation in pediatric patients with chronic phase CML who do not achieve a hematologic or cytogenetic response at recommended starting dose to a maximum of 120 mg: (a) starting dose 40 mg: escalate to 50 mg/day; (b) 60 mg: escalate to 70 mg; (c) 70 mg: escalate to 90 mg; (d) 100 mg: escalate to 120 mg.
  - Pediatric patients with Ph+ ALL begin desatinib dosing on or before day 15 of induction chemotherapy, when diagnosis is confirmed and continue for 2 years (Bristol Myers Squibb, 2018).

- Administer orally, with or without a meal, once daily in the morning or evening. Teach patient to swallow tablet whole, do not crush, chew or cut. For pediatric patients having difficulty swallowing a tablet, in one clinical trial, dispersing the drug in juice resulted in a 36% lower systemic exposure. However, the effect on safety or efficacy is unknown (Bristol Myers Squibb, 2018).
- Continue dasatinib until disease progression or no longer tolerated. The effect of cessation of treatment on long-term outcome after achieving a cytogenetic response or major molecular response is unknown (Bristol-Myers Squibb, 2018).
- Use dasatinib with caution in patients with hepatic impairment.
- Dose may be increased or decreased in 20-mg increments based on individual patient response or coadministration with drugs that either increase or decrease dasatinib serum levels (see Drug Interactions).

Dose Modifications (See Package Insert for Adults and Pediatric patients):
- **Myelosuppression** is managed by dose interruption, reduction, or discontinuance. Hematopoietic growth factor has been used in patients with resistant myelosupression. See package insert for full description.
- Dose modifications for hematologic toxicity. Monitor CBC weekly for the initial 2 months and then periodically. See drug package insert. See package insert for pediatric dose adjustments for neutropenia and thrombocytopenia. If cytopenia is unrelated to leukemia, stop drug until recovery then resume; if recurs, repeat bone marrow aspirate/ biopsy. See package insert.
- **Concomitant strong CYP3A4 inducers:** CYP3A4 inducers (e.g., dexamethasone, phenytoin, carbamazepine, rifampin, rifabutin, phenobarbital) may decrease dasatinib plasma concentrations and should be avoided; St. John's wort may decrease dasatinib concentrations unpredictably and should be avoided. If a strong inducer must be coadministered with dasatinib, consider increasing dasatinib dose and monitor the patient closely for toxicity.
- **Concomitant strong CYP3A4 inhibitors:** CYP3A4 inhibitors (e.g., ketoconazole, itraconazole, atazanavir, indinavir, nefazodone, nelfinavir, ritonavir, saquinavir, telithromycin, voriconazole; also grapefruit and grapefruit juice) may increase dasatinib plasma concentrations and should be avoided. Consider an alternate drug that does not inhibit CYP3A4. If coadministration with a strong inhibitor must occur, consider decreasing dasatinib dose to 20 mg daily (if taking 100 mg a day) or 40 mg daily (if taking 140 mg daily), which approximates the AUC. However, there are no clinical data with these dose adjustments. If dasatinib is not tolerated after dose reduction, either the strong CYP3A4 inhibitor must be discontinued or dasatinib stopped until treatment with the inhibitor has ceased. When the strong inhibitor is discontinued, a washout period of approximately 1 week should occur before dasatinib dose is increased.
- **Severe nonhematological adverse reactions:** hold Sprycel until event resolves or improves. When resuming Sprycel, reduce dose depending upon the initial severity of the event.

Drug Preparation:
- None, oral. Available in 20-mg, 50-mg, 70-mg, 80-mg, 100-mg, and 140-mg tablets.

TREATMENT

Drug Administration:
- Oral, once daily. Administer once in the morning OR in the evening, with or without food; do not crush or cut.
- Assess CBC/differential weekly for the first 2 months, and then monthly, or as clinically indicated.
- Assess and discuss with physician or NP/PA correction of hypokalemia or hypomagnesemia before dasatinib administration.

Drug Interactions:
- **CYP3A4 inhibitors:** These inhibitors (e.g., ketoconazole, itraconazole, erythromycin, clarithromycin, atazanavir, indinavir, nefazodone, nelfinavir, ritonavir, saquinavir, telithromycin) may decrease metabolism of dasatinib, thus increasing serum concentrations of dasatinib; avoid coadministration, and if they must be given together, decrease dose of dasatinib. See package insert: For example, if the patient is taking dasatinib 100 mg plus a strong CYP3A4 inhibitor that cannot be changed, the dasatinib dose should be decreased to 20 mg daily; if taking dasatinib 140 mg daily, the dose should be reduced to 40 mg daily. Avoid grapefruit and grapefruit juice.
- **CYP3A4 inducers:** Rifampin decreased dasatinib serum concentrations by 81%; with others (e.g., dexamethasone, phenytoin, carbamazepine, phenobarbital, St. John's wort), avoid coadministration; if they must be given together, increase dose of dasatinib and monitor for toxicity. Patients receiving dasatinib should NOT take St. John's wort.
- **Antacids (aluminum hydroxide/magnesium hydroxide):** Decrease dasatinib AUC by 55%, as drug requires acid pH; avoid concurrent administration or administer 2 hours prior to or 2 hours after dasantinib dose.
- **H_2 blockers/PPI:** Famotidine decreases dasatinib AUC 61%; avoid concurrent administration. Consider replacing with antacids that should be taken at least 2 hours before or after dasatinib so there is no interference with absorption.
- **Simvastatin, CYP3A4 substrates**: Dasatinib is a time-dependent inhibitor of CYP3A4 and may decrease the metabolism of drugs primarily metabolized by CYP3A4, such as alfentanil, astemizole, terfenadine, cisapride, cyclosporine, fentanyl, pimozide, quinidine, sirolimus, tacrolimus, or ergot alkaloids; decreases simvastatin AUC 37%; avoid concurrent administration or administer cautiously.

Lab Effects/Interference:
- Grades 3–4 neutropenia, thrombocytopenia, and anemia.
- Hypophosphatemia, hypocalcemia.
- Elevated ALT, AST, bilirubin.
- Elevated creatinine.
- QT/QTc prolongation on EKG.

Special Considerations:
- Warnings and Precautions:
  - *Severe myelosuppression* (e.g., grades 3–4 thrombocytopenia, neutropenia, and anemia) may occur.
    - Occurrence is more frequent and occurs earlier in patients with advanced phase CML or Ph+ ALL than in chronic phase CML.

- In a trial of patients with resistance or intolerance to prior imatinib therapy and chronic phase CML, grades 3–4 myelosuppression was reported less frequently in patients receiving dasatinib 100 g once daily.
- Myelosuppression is generally reversible and manageable with dose interruption or reduction.
- Patients with chronic phase CML: Assess CBC/differential every 2 weeks for 12 weeks, then every 3 months thereafter or as clinically indicated.
- Patients with advanced phase CML or Ph+ ALL: Assess CBC/differential weekly for the first 2 months, then monthly or as clinically indicated.
- Pediatric patients with Ph+ ALL treated with dasatitinib in combination with chemotherapy, assess CBC/ANCs prior to the start of each block of chemotherapy and as clinically indicated. During consolidation blocks of chemotherapy, assess CBC/ANC every 2 days until recovery.
- *Bleeding-related events:* dasatinib can cause platelet dysfunction, in addition to thrombocytopenia. Severe central nervous system (CNS) bleeding occurred in < 1% of patients; severe GI hemorrhage occurred in 4% and generally required drug interruption and transfusions.
  - Most patients had thrombocytopenia as well.
  - Use caution if used together with other medicines that inhibit platelet function or anticoagulants.
- *Fluid retention:* Fluid retention (including ascites, edema, pleural, and pericardial effusions) can occur, which can be severe. A 5-year follow-up study of patients with chronic phase CML had an incidence of 5% grades 3–4 (Bristol-Myers Squibb, 2015).
  - If a patient develops new or worsened dyspnea on exertion or at rest, pleuritic chest pain, or dry cough suggestive of pleural effusions, evaluate by CXR and other imaging as ordered.
  - Fluid retention is manageable with supportive measures, including diuretics or short courses of steroids. Severe pleural effusions may require thoracentesis, and patient may require oxygen therapy. Consider dose reduction or treatment interruption (see Dose Modifications).
- *Cardiovascular events*: 5-year follow-up of newly diagnosed chronic phase CML patients showed cardiac ischemia events (3.9% vs imatinib 1.6%), cardiac-related fluid retention (8.5% dasatinib vs 3.9% imatinib), and conduction system abnormalities (e.g., arrhythmia and palpitations; 7% vs imatinib 5%). Monitor patients for signs/symptoms of cardiac dysfunction and discuss prompt treatment with physician.
- *Pulmonary Artery Hypertension (PAH):* Risk may be increased in developing PAH in adult and pediatric patients, which can occur early or after > 1 year of treatment. Signs/symptoms include dyspnea, fatigue, hypoxia, and fluid retention. PAH may be reversible upon discontinuation of dasatinib. Evaluate patients for underlying cardiopulmonary disease before starting dasatinib and during treatment. If PAH diagnosis is confirmed, dasatinib should be permanently discontinued.
- *Drug can cause QT interval (ventricular repolarization) prolongation.* Administer cautiously to patients who may develop prolongation of the QTc interval (hypokalemia, hypomagnesemia, congenital long QT syndrome), patients taking

anti-arrhythmic medications, or who have cumulative high-dose anthracycline therapy. Monitor and correct deficits in electrolytes (e.g., magnesium and potassium) prior to administering dasatinib.

- *Severe dermatologic reactions*: Rare cases of severe mucocutaneous dermatologic reactions, including SJS and erythema multiforme have been described. Dasatinib should be permanently discontinued if no other etiology found.
- *Tumor Lysis syndrome*: Patients with resistance to prior imatinib (primarily in advanced phase disease) who have a high-tumor burden have developed TLS. Identify patients at risk, e.g., patients with advanced stage disease and/or high-tumor burden, and ensure adequate hydration, correct uric-acid levels before starting dasatinib, and monitor electrolytes and fluid balance closely.
- *Embryo-fetal toxicity:* Drug is teratogenic and embryo-fetal toxic. Women of reproductive potential should be advised to use effective contraception to avoid pregnancy during dasatinib therapy and for at least 30 days after last drug dose. If dasatinib is used during pregnancy, or if the patient becomes pregnant while receiving the drug, patient should be apprised of potential hazard to the fetus.
- *Effects on growth and development in pediatric patients:* In pediatric trials in chronic CML after at least 2 years of treatment, bone growth and development adverse effects were reported in 5.2% of patients: epiphyses delayed fusion, osteopenia, growth retardation (1 grade 3), and gynecomastia. One case of osteopenia and one case of gynecomastia resolved on treatment. Monitor bone growth and development in pediatric patients.
- Nursing mothers should decide to discontinue nursing or discontinue the drug, taking into account the importance of the drug to the mother's health.
  - Assess patient drug profile; teach patient about possible interacting drugs, and instruct patient to tell nurse or physician before starting any OTC or herbal medications.

Potential Toxicities/Side Effects and the Nursing Process

I. POTENTIAL FOR INFECTION AND BLEEDING related to BONE MARROW DEPRESSION

Defining Characteristics: Grades 3–4 neutropenia, thrombocytopenia, and anemia are common, especially severe in patients with advanced CML or Ph+ ALL, as compared to those in chronic phase CML. Drug can cause platelet dysfunction, resulting in rare CNS or GI hemorrhage, and is most often associated with severe thrombocytopenia. Use caution if patients are also taking medications that inhibit platelet function, or anticoagulants, and monitor very closely.

Nursing Implications: Assess baseline CBC, including WBC, differential, and platelet count prior to dosing, as well as at least weekly during first month of treatment, at least every other week for the second month of treatment, and then as clinically indicated and ordered. Discuss dose interruption and reduction as above for neutropenia and thrombocytopenia. Teach patient self-assessment of signs/symptoms of infection and bleeding (including epistaxis and development of petechiae), and instruct patient to report them right away. Teach patient self-care measures to minimize risk of infection and bleeding, including avoidance of OTC aspirin-containing medications. Discuss dose reductions as needed.

II.   ALTERATION IN FLUID AND ELECTROLYTE BALANCE related to FLUID RETENTION, EDEMA

Defining Characteristics: Fluid retention is common (up to 48%). Superficial edema is most common, but pleural effusion may occur in 22% of patients. However, ascites, rapid weight gain, and pulmonary edema may develop, and in some cases, be life-threatening (pleural effusion, congestive heart failure, pulmonary hypertension, pericardial effusion, anasarca).

Nursing Implications: Assess baseline parameters of weight, presence of edema, pulmonary function, and monitor closely during therapy. Teach patient to monitor weight daily at home, and to report weight gain of 2 pounds in 1 week, development of edema, or dyspnea. Develop a plan to protect skin and maintain skin integrity and discuss the prescription of diuretics with physician or NP.

III.   ALTERATION IN NUTRITION, POTENTIAL, LESS THAN BODY REQUIREMENTS, related to NAUSEA, VOMITING, DIARRHEA

Defining Characteristics: Nausea, vomiting, diarrhea, and constipation occur.

Nursing Implications: Assess baseline nutritional status and bowel-elimination status. If patient develops nausea and/or vomiting, teach patient to self-administer antiemetics 1 hour prior to each dose and to call if nausea/vomiting persist.

Discuss with physician more effective antiemetic regimen if nausea/vomiting persist. Encourage small, frequent intake of cool, bland foods as tolerated if nausea develops. Refer to dietitian as needed for meal planning. Teach patient to report diarrhea that does not respond to OTC antidiarrheal medication. Teach self-care measures of diet modification and increased oral fluids to 2–3 L during the waking hours. If constipation, teach patient self-care measures to prevent constipation.

IV.   ALTERATION IN COMFORT related to PAIN, HEADACHE, FATIGUE, ARTHRALGIA, AND FATIGUE

Defining Characteristics: Headache, musculoskeletal pain, fatigue, myalgias/arthralgias and abdominal pain can occur.

Nursing Implications: Teach patient that these events may occur and to report them. Assess baseline comfort and monitor closely during treatment. Develop plan to assure comfort depending on symptoms reported. Discuss ineffective strategies with physician and revise plan as needed.

Drug: Duvelisib (Copiktra)

Class: Kinase inhibitor; Targets phosphatidylinositol 3-kinase PI3K-δ and PI3K-γ.

Mechanism of Action: Normal and malignant B-lymphocytes use two cell signaling pathways that are linked to malignancy: B-cell receptor signaling and CXCR12-mediated chemotaxis of malignant B-cells. Duvelisib inhibits the PI3K -δ and PI3K-γ, resulting in growth inhibition and decreased cell viability. Drug also inhibits CXCR12-induced T-cell migration, and movement of macrophages (Verastem, 2018).

Metabolism: Bioavailability after oral dosing is 42%, and median time to peak concentration (Tmax) was 1–2 hours after dosing. While there was a slight decrease in Cmax with little decrease in AUC when administered with a high fat meal, the drug can be given with or without food. Duvelisib is 98% bound to plasma proteins, and drug is metabolized primarily by cytochrome P450 CYP3A4. Elimination half-life of drug is 4.7 hours. Most (79%) of the drug is excreted in the feces (11% unchanged) and 14% excreted in the urine (< 1% unchanged).

Indications: Adult patients with (1) relapsed or refractory CLL or small lymphocytic lymphoma (SLL) after at least 2 prior therapies; (2) relapsed or refractory follicular lymphoma (FL). Accelerated approval.

Contraindication: None.

Dosage/Range:
- 25-mg capsule orally twice daily with or without food; a cycle is 28 days.
- Administer *Pneumocystis jirovecii* (PJP) prophylaxis during treatment with duvelisib; continue until the absolute CD4+ T-cell count is > 200 cells/µL. If a patient is suspected of having PJP of any grade, hold duvelisib and discontinue drug if PJP diagnosis is confirmed.
- Consider prophylactic anti-virals during duvelisib therapy to prevent cytomegalovirus (CMV) infection including CMV reactivation.

Dose Modifications:
Dose Modification Levels: (1) Initial dose: 25 mg PO bid; (2) dose reduction: 15 mg PO bid. Subsequent dose modification: discontinue duvelisib if patient unable to tolerate 15 mg PO bid.

Non-hematologic Toxicity:
- Infections:
  - Grade 3 or higher: hold duvelisib until resolved; resume at same or reduced dose.
  - Clinical CMV infectin or viremia (positive PCR antigen test): hold duvelisib until resolved; resume at same or reduced dose; if resumed, monitor patients for CMV reactivation by PCR antigen test at least monthly.
  - PJP: For suspected PJP, hold duvelisib until evaluated; if PJP confirmed, discontinue duvelisib.

- Non-infectious diarrhea or colitis:
  - Mild/moderate diarrhea (Grade 1–2 up to 6 stools per day over baseline) and responsive to anti-diarrheal agents, OR asymptomatic (grade 1) colitis: no change in dose; initiate supportive therapy with antidiarrheal agents as appropriate; monitor at least weekly until resolved.
  - Mild/moderate diarrhea (grade 1–2 up to 6 stools/day over baseline) and unresponsive to antidiarrheal agents: hold duvelisib until resolved; initiate supportive therapy with enteric acting steroids (e.g., budesonide); monitor at least weekly until resolved.
  - Abdominal pain, stool with mucus or blood, change in bowel habits, peritoneal signs OR severe diarrhea (grade 3, > 6 stools/day over baseline): hold duvelisib until resolved; initiate supportive therapy with enteric acting steroids (e.g., budesonide) or systemic steroids; monitor at least weekly until resolved; resume at reduced dose; for recurrent grade 3 diarrhea or recurrent colitis any grade, discontinue duvelisib.
  - Life-threatening: discontinue duvelisib.
- Cutaneous reactions:
  - Grade 1–2: no change in dose; initiate supportive care with emollients, anti-histamines (for pruritus) or topical steroids; monitor closely.
  - Grade 3: hold duvelisib until resolved; initiate supportive therapy with emollients, anti-histamines for pruritis, or topical steroids; monitor at least weekly until resolved; resume at reduced dose; if severe cutaneous reaction does not improve, worsens, or recurs, discontinue duvelisib.
  - Life-threatening; Stevens Johnson syndrome (SJS), TEN (toxic epidermal necrosis), DRESS (drug rash with eosinophilia and systemic symptoms). any grade: discontinue duvelisib.
- Pneumonitis without suspected infectious cause:
  - Moderate (grade 2) symptomatic pneumonitis: hold duvelisib; treat with systemic steroid therapy; if pneumonitis recovers to grade 0–1, resume duvelisib at a reduced dose; if non-infectious pneumonitis recurs or patient does not respond to steroid therapy, discontinue duvelisib.
  - Severe (grade 3) or life-threatening pneumonitis: discontinue duvelisib.
- ALT/AST elevation:
  - Grade 2: $3–5 \times$ ULN: maintain duvelisib dose; monitor at least weekly until return to $< 3–5 \times$ ULN.
  - Grade 3: $> 5–20 \times$ ULN: hold duvelisib and monitor at least weekly until return to $< 3 \times$ ULN; resume duvelisib at same dose (1st occurrence) or at a reduced dose for subsequent occurrence.
  - Grade 4 ($> 20 \times$ ULN): discontinue duvelisib.

Hematologic Toxicity:
- Neutropenia:
  - ANC 0.5–1.0 Gi/L: maintain duvelisib dose; monitor ANC at leasts weekly.
  - ANC < 0.5 Gi/L: hold duvelisib dose, monitor ANC until > 0.5 Gi/L; resume duvelisib at same dose (1st occurrence), or a reduced dose (subsequent occurrence).
- Thrombocytopenia:
  - Platelet count 25 to < 50 Gi//L (grade 3) with grade 1 bleeding: no change in dose, monitor platelet count at oesat weekly.

- Platelet count 25 to $<$ 50 Gi/L (grade 3) with grade 2 bleeding OR platelet count $<$ 25 Gi/L (grade 4): hold duvelisib; monitor platelet counts until $\geq$ 25 Gi/L and resolution of bleeding if applicable; resume duvelisib at same dose (1st occurrence) or resume at a reduced dose for subsequent occurrence.

Concomitant Use with CYP3A4 Inhibitors: Reduce duvelisib dose to 15 mg PO bid when co-administered with a strong CYP3A4 inhibitor (e.g., ketoconazole).

Drug Preparation: Available in 25 mg (white/orange) and 15 mg (pink) capsules.

Drug Administration:
- Assess patient for toxicity (infection, non-infectious diarrhea or colitis, cutaneous reactions, pneumonitis, increased LFTs, neutropenia, thrombocytopenia), and discuss abnormalities with provider.
- Teach patient self-assessment for infection and bleeding, and strategies to minimize them as well as to report T$>$ 100.4°F, chills, signs/symptoms of infection, or bleeding right away.
- Teach patient to take capsule whole, not to open, break or chew the capsule. If a dose is missed by $<$ 6 hours, take the missed dose right away; if $>$ 6 hours, wait until the next dose and take it at the usual time.

Drug Interactions:
- *Strong and moderate CYP3A inhibitors:* Coadministration with a strong inhibitor (e.g., ketoconazole) results in increase duvelisib Cmax and AUC by 1.7-fold and 4-fold respectively. Modeling suggests there is no effect on duvelisib when administered with mild or moderate CYP3A4 inhibitors. If co-administered with a strong inhibitor, reduce duvelisib dose to 15 mg bid. If co-administered with strong or moderate CYP3A4 inhibitors, monitor for duvelisib toxicity.
- *Strong and moderate CYP3A4 inducers:* Coadministration with a strong inducer (rifampin) decreased duvelisib Cmax by 66% and AUC by 82%, CYP3A4 substrates: Avoid coadministration with strong inducers.
- *CYP3A4 substrates:* coadministration with midazolam increased midazolam AUC by 3.4 fold, and Cmax by 2.2 fold. Monitor for signs of toxicities when coadministration with sensitive CYP3A4 substrates.

Lab Effects/Interference:
- Decreased wbc/ANC, lymphocytes, platelets, and red blood cells.
- Increased ALT, AST, lipase, alkaline phosphatase, serum amylase, serum potassium, creatinine.
- Decreased serum phosphorus, sodium, albumin, calcium.

Special Considerations:
- Most common adverse reactions ($\geq$ 20%): diarrhea or colitis, neutropenia, rash, fatigue, pyrexia, cough, nausea, URI, pneumonia, musculoskeletal pain, anemia.
- Nursing mothers should not breast-feed while receiving duvelisib.
- Warnings and Precautions:
  - *Infections:* Occurred in 31% of patients receiving duvelisib at the 25 mg PO bid dose, most commonly pneumonia, sepsis, and lower respiratory infections. Median time

to infection was 3 months, and 75% occurred within 6 months. Infections should be treated before a patient starts duvelisib. Teach patient to report any new or worsening signs/symptoms of infection. If grade 3 or higher infection occurs, duvelisib should be held until the infection resolves. Prevent PJP and CMV infections by prophylactic medication; continue PJP prophylaxis until the absolute CD4+ T-cell count is > 200 cells/μL. If PJP is suspected, hold duvelisib and the drug should be discontinued if PJP diagnosis is confirmed. See Dose Modifications and problem 1.

- *Diarrhea or colitis:* Diarrhea or colitis occurred in 18% of patients receiving duvelisib at 25 mg PO bid, with median time to onset of 4 months, and 75% of cases occurred by 8 months. Diarrhea or colitis lasted a median of 2 weeks (1/2 month). Teach patients to report new or worsening diarrhea. See Dose Modifications, and problem 2.
- *Cutaneous reactions:* Serious reactions occurred in 5% of patients at the 25 mg PO bid dose. Median time to onset for any cutaneous reaction was 3 months, and lasted a median of 1 month. Assess patients for pruritic, erythematous or maulo-papular skin changes. Less commonly, exanthema, desquamation, erythroderma, skin exfoliation, keratinocyte necrosis, and popular rash occurred. Teach patient to report any new or worsening skin reactions. See Dose Modifications.
- *Pneumonitis:* Serious pneumonitis without apparent infectious etiology occurred in 5% of patients receiving the 25 mg PO bid dose. Median time to onset of any grade pneumonitis was 4 months, and 75% of cases appeared within 9 months of therapy. Median duration of pneumonitis was 1 month, with 75% of cases resolving within 2 months. See Dose Modifications.
- *Hepatotoxicity:* Grade 3 AST +/or ALT elevation occurred in 8% and 2% respectively of patients receiving the 25 mg PO bid dosage. Median time to onset was 2 months. Monitor LFTs baseline and during duvelisib therapy. See Dose Modifications.
- *Neutropenia:* Grade 3–4 neutropenia occurred in 42% of patients at the 25 mg PO bid dose. Median time to onset of grade 3–4 was 2 months, and 75% of cases occurred within 4 months. Assess ANC at least every 2 weeks for the first 2 months of duvelisib therapy, then at least weekly in patients who have an ANC < 1.0 Gi/L (grade 3–4). See Dose Modifications.
- *Embryo-fetal toxicity:* Drug is feto-toxic. Teach female patients of reproductive potential, and males with female partners of reproductive potential, to use effective contraception during duvelisib therapy and for at least 1 month after last dose.

Potential Toxicities/Side Effects and the Nursing Process

I.   POTENTIAL FOR INFECTION, BLEEDING, AND FATIGUE related to BONE MARROW SUPPRESSION

Defining Characteristics: Neutropenia was common, with 34% of patients having any grade neutropenia, and 30% having grade 3 or 4 neutropenia. Most common serious infections were pneumonia, lower respiratory infection, and sepsis. Pyrexia occurred in 26% of patients and was grades 3–4 in 5%. Fatigue was reported by 29% of patients. Thrombocytopenia occurred in 17% of patients (10% grades 3–4) and anemia in 20% (11% grades 3–4) of patients. Opportunistic infections also can occur: PJP pneumonia occurred in 1% and CMV reactivation/infectin occurred in 1% of patients.

Nursing Implications: Ensure patients receive prophylactic antimicrobials to prevent PJP and CMV reactivation/infections. Assess patients for infection before starting duvelisib therapy, and if patient has signs/symptoms of infection, discuss with provider, treatment to resolution of infection before starting duvelisib. Assess CBC/differential and platelet counts baseline and at least every 2 weeks for the first 2 months of therapy as ordered during therapy. Assess CBC/differential at least weekly in patients with ANC < 1.0 Gi/L. Assess skin integrity, potential for infection, and teach patient measures to prevent infection (e.g., keeping skin intact, avoiding sources of infection, good hand-washing). Teach patient to report any signs/symptoms of infection (e.g., redness, heat, exudate on skin, temperature ≥ 100.4°F, cough, sputum production, dysuria). Assess for signs/symptoms of infection during therapy and at each visit. If a patient develops an infection, discuss with physician or midlevel practitioner interrupting or discontinuing drug, and beginning appropriate antimicrobial treatment. Teach the patient that thrombocytopenia may occur, to avoid situations that could increase bleeding, and to report any signs or symptoms of bleeding right away. Review medication profile, and discuss discontinuance of aspirin or NSAIDs with patient and physician or NP/PA. Follow HGB/HCT and assess patient's tolerance, fatigue, other symptoms, and need for supportive measures. Teach patient measures to conserve energy.

II. POTENTIAL ALTERATION IN NUTRITION, LESS THAN BODY REQUIREMENTS, related to DIARRHEA, NAUSEA, VOMITING, MUCOSITIS, HEPATOTOXICITY

Defining Characteristics: In clinical studies, diarrhea or colitis occurred in 50% of patients (23% grade 3–4). nausea occurred in 24% of patients, vomiting in 16%, mucositis in 14%, constipation in 13%, decreased appetite in 14%, and transaminase elevation in 15%. Diarrhea/colitis can be fatal and severe diarrhea/colitis occurred in 18% of patients. Median time to onset of any grade diarrhea/colitis was 4 months, and 75% of cases occurred by 8 months from start of therapy. Grade 3–4 elevation of AST/ALT occurred in 8% and 2% of patients respectively. Median time to onset of any elevation was 2 months, with a median duration of 1 month.

Nursing Implications: Assess baseline nutritional, and elimination status, and appetite. Assess serum chemistries including electrolytes and hepatic function, baseline and during therapy as ordered. Teach patient that diarrhea/colitis may occur and should be reported right away if new or worsening. See Dose Modifications. If the patient has mild or moderate diarrhea (grade 1–2, up to 6 stools/day over baseline), or is asymptomatic, patient should be taught to take antidiarrheal medications, and continue duvelisib at current dose with at least weekly monitoring until diarrhea/colitis resolves. If the diarrhea/colitis does not respond to the anti-diarrheal medication, duvelisib should be stopped and per provider, enteric acting steroids (e.g., budesonide) started with at least weekly monitoring. When diarrhea/colitis resolves, duvelisib can be resumed per provider, at a reduced dose. If the patient has abdominal pain, mucus or blood in the stool, a change in bowel habits, peritoneal signs, or severe diarrhea (Grade 3, > 6 stools/day over baseline), duvelisib should be interrupted and enteric acting steroids or systemic steroids started per physician. Patient should be evaluated for cause of diarrhea/colitis including colonoscopy, with continued at least weekly monitoring. Then, when diarrhea/colitis resolves, duvelisib can be restarted at a reduced dose per physician. If Grade 3 diarrhea/colitis recurs, duvelisib should be discontinued. Assess patient need for premedication with antiemetics. Teach the patient to report nausea and/or vomiting that is not relieved by prescribed antiemetics. Teach patient dietary modifications for each problem, and to call nurse or physician for diarrhea, nausea, or vomiting that does not resolve within 24 hours with recommended OTC or prescription medicines.

Drug: Encorafenib (Braftovi)

Class: Kinase inhibitor; Targets BRAF and CRAF.

Mechanism of Action: Encorafenib targets the RAF pathway, an important signaling pathway which is part of the MAPK pathway. When activated, the RAF-MAPK signaling pathway leads to cell proliferation and survival. In melanoma, the *BRAF (B-RAF)* gene is often mutated making the mutation *BRAF V600E*, which turns on the RAF/MEK/ERK pathway continuously, resulting in malignant cell proliferation and survival. Encorafenib inhibits BRAF V600 E to shut down this aspect of the pathway. It is given in combination with binimetinib, a MEK inhibitor, which blocks the pathway further down. Together the drugs are synergistic and help to stop tumor cell division and survival. In addition, giving the drugs together decreases the emergence of resistance in BRAF V600E mutated tumor cells.

Metabolism: Steady state is achieved within 15 days, and after oral dosing, the median Tmax is 2 hours. At least 86% of the dose is absorbed. Taking the drug with food decreases mean maximum concentration (C_{max}) by 36% but does not affect the AUC. The drug is 86% bound to human plasma proteins. The terminal half-life of the drug is 3.5 hours. Drug is primarily metabolized by N-dealkylation using CYP3A4, and to a lesser degree by CYP2C19 and CYP2D6. Drug is excreted in the feces (47%) and urine (47%).

Indications: Treatment, in combination with binimetinib, of patients with unresectable or metastatic melanoma with a *BRAF V600E* or *V600K* mutation, as detected by an FDA-approved test. Drug is NOT indicated for treatment of patients with wild-type (normal) *BRAF* melanoma.

Contraindications: None.

Dosage/Range:
- Confirm presence of *BRAF V600E* or *V600K* mutation in tumor.
- Recommended dose is 450 mg PO once daily in combination with binimetinib until disease progression or unacceptable toxicity, with or without food.

Dose Modifications:

- If binimetinib dose is held, encorafenib dose should be reduced to a maximum dose of 300 mg qd until binimetinib is resumed.
- Dose reductions: *1st dose reduction*: from 450 mg reduced to 300 mg PO qd; *2nd dose reduction:* 300 mg reduced to 200 mg po qd; *subsequent modification*: permanently discontinue if unable to tolerate 200 mg qd dose.
- *New primary malignancy:* Non-cutaneous RAS mutation-positive malignancies: permanently discontinue encorafenib.
- *Uveitis:*
  - Grade 1–3: If grade 1–2 does not respond to specific ocular therapy, or for grade 3 uveitis, hold encorafenib for up to 6 weeks; if improved, resume at same dose; if not improved, permanently discontinue encorafenib.
  - Grade 4: permanently discontinue encorafenib.
- QTc prolongation:
  - QTc (F for Fridericia's correction) $>$ 500 ms and $\leq$ 60 ms increase from baseline: Hold encorafenib until QTcF is $\leq$ 500 ms; resume at reduced dose; if more than one occurrence, permanently discontinue encorafenib.
  - QTcF $>$ 500 ms and $>$ 60 ms increase from baseline: permanently discontinue encorafenib.
- Hepatotoxicity:
  - Grade 2 AST or ALT increased: maintain encorafenib dose. If no improvement within 4 weeks, hold encorafenib until improves to grade 0-1 or to pretreatment/baseline levels and then resume at same dose.
  - Grade 3 or 4 AST or ALT increased: see other adverse reactions.
- Dermatologic:
  - Grade 2: If no improvement within 2 weeks, withhold encorafenib until grade 0-1; resume at same dose.
  - Grade 3: hold encorafenib until grade 0–1; resume at same dose if 1st occurrence, or reduce dose if recurrent.
  - Grade 4: permanently discontinue encorafenib.
- *Other adverse reactions (including hemorrhage):*
  - Recurrent grade 2 or 1st occurrence of any grade 3: hold encorafenib for up to 4 weeks. If improves to grade 0-1 or to pretreatment/baseline level, resume at reduced dose. If no improvement, permanently discontinue encorafenib.
  - First occurrence of any grade 4: permanently discontinue encorafenib or hold encoragfenib for up to 4 weeks; if improves to grade 0-1 or to pretreatment/baseline level, resume at reduced dose; if no improvement, permanently discontinue enecorafenib.
  - Recurrent grade 3: Consider permanently discontinue enecorafenib.
  - Recurrent grade 4: permanently discontinue enecorafenib.
- Dose modification for encorafenib, when given with binimetinib, is not recommended for new primary cutaneous malignancies, ocular events except ureitis, iritis, and iridocyclitis; ILD/pneumonitis; cardiac dysfunction, creatine phosphokinase (CPK) elevation; rhabdomyolysis; and venous thromboembolism. See binimetinib prescribing information for dose modifications.

- *Concomitant strong or moderate CYP3A4 inhibitors:*
  - Avoid concomitant administration of moderate or strong CYP3A4 inhibitors.
  - IF unavoidable, decrease encorafenib dose to 1/3 of encorafenib dose prior to concurrent use of strong CYP3A4 inhibitor, or 1/ 2 of encorafenib dose prior to concurrent use of moderat eCYP3A4 inhibitor.
  - After the inhibitor has been discontinued for 3–5 elimination half-lives, resume the encorafenib dose that was taken prior to starting the CYP3A4 inhibitor.

Drug Preparation: Oral. Available in 50-mg and 75-mg hard gelatin capsules. Teach patient to keep out of reach of children and pets.

Drug Administration:
- Assess QTcF baseline and regularly as ordered during treatment. Assess for changes in vision, development of any new skin lesions, or bleeding. Teach patient to report these right away.
- Teach patient to take encorafenib 450 mg PO qd, with or without food, in combination with binimetinib which is taken q 12 hours (see binimetinib). If patient misses a dose, it should not be taken within 12 hours of the next dose. The patient should not take an additional dose if vomiting occurs after the dose taken, but to wait until the next scheduled dose.
- If binimetinib is held, encorafenib dose should be reduced to a maximum dose of 300 mg qd until binimetinib is resumed.
- Teach women of reproductive potential to use effective nonhormonal contraception during therapy and for at least 2 weeks after last encorafenib dose.

Drug Interactions:
- Strong or moderate CYP3A4 inhibitors: concomitant use may increase encorafenib serum levels; avoid, and if must give concomitantly, decrease encorafenib dose (see Dose Modifications).
- Strong or moderate CYP3A4 inducers: concomitant use may decrease encorafenib serum levels; avoid, and if must give concomitantly, increase encorafenib dose (see Dose Modifications).
- Sensitive CYP3A4 substrates (e.g., hormonal contraceptives): can result in decreased substrate serum concentration and efficacy; avoid hormonal contraceptives.
- Drugs that prolong the QTc interval: avoid concurrent administration as increased risk of QTc prolongation.
- Hormonal contraceptives: encorafenib can render contraception ineffective.

Lab Effects/Interference:
- Anemia, lymphopenia, neutropenia.
- Increased creatinine, GGT, ALT, AST, glucose, alkaline phosphatase, serum magnesium.
- Hyponatremia.

Special Considerations:
- Most common adverse reactions (25%) fatigue, nausea, vomiting, abdominal pain, and arthralgia.

- Warnings and Precautions.
  - *New primary malignancies:* Cutaneous and non-cutaneous new malignancies have occurred. Cutaneous malignancies occurred in patients receiving the combination (incidence 2.6%, median time to 1st occurrence 5.8 months), and basal cell carcinoma occurred in 1.6%. The incidence in patients receiving encorafenib as a single agent was 8% and 1%, respectively, and new primary melanoma occurred in 5% of patients. Dose modification not recommended. Ensure patient has a dermatologic evaluation baseline, every 2 months during treatment, and for up to 6 months after last dose of encorafenib. Non-cutaneous malignancies may be stimulated by activation of RAS through mutation or other mechanism (Array BioPharma Inc., 2019). Monitor patients for new malignancy, and discontinue encorafenib if tumor is RAS mutation positive.
  - *Tumor promotion in BRAF wild-type tumors:* This may occur throughparadoxical activation of the MAP-kinase signaling pathway with increased proliferation of BRAF wild-type cells (Array BioPharma Inc., 2019). Ensure patient's tumor has BRAF V600E or V600K mutations before encorafenib is started.
  - *Hemorrhage:* In patients receiving combination binimetinib and encorafenib, incidence of hemorrhage was 19% (grade 3 was 3.2%), most frequently GI. Fatal intracranial hemorrhage occurred in 1.6% of patients, who also had new or progressive brain metastases. Assess for bleeding, and dose modify based on severity (see Dose Modifications).
  - *Uveitis, including iritis and iridocyclitis:* incidence was 4% in patients receiving the combination. Assess for visual symptoms at each visit, ensure physician/NP/PA perform an ophthalmologic evaluation at regular intervals, if there are new or worsening visual disturbances, and to follow any findings. Teach patient to report any changes in vision right away. Modify dose based on severity. See Dose Modifications.
  - *QTc prolongation:* encorafenib is rarely associated with a dose-dependent prolongation of the QTc interval in some patients who receive the combination (incidence 0.5%). Electrolyte abnormalities (low magnesium and potassium) theoretically increase the risk of torsades de pointes. Monitor patients who already have or who are at significant risk for development of QTc prolongation closely, including patients taking antiarrythmic medication or others known to cause QTc prolongation, or with bradyarrhythmias, severe or uncontrolled heart failure. Implement orders to correct hypomagenesemia and hypokalemia prior to start of therapy and during therapy as ordered. See Dose Modifications.
  - *Embryo-fetal toxicity:* encorafenib is fetotoxic, as is binimetinib. Teach women of reproductive potential to use effective NON-HORMONAL contraception during treatment and for 2 weeks after final dose. See Drug Interactions.
  - *Risks associated with encorafenib as a single agent:* Grade 3-4 dermatologic reactions occurred in 21% of aptients as compared to 2% in patients receiving combination encorafenib and binimetinib. Thus, if binimetinib is temporarily interrupted or permanently discontinued, reduce the dose of encorafenib (see Dosage).
  - *Risks associated with combination treatment:* See binimetinib prescribing information for additional risk of drugs in combination.

Potential Toxicities/Side Effects and the Nursing Process

I.   ALTERATION IN NUTRITION, POTENTIAL, LESS THAN BODY
      REQUIREMENTS, related to DIARRHEA, NAUSEA, VOMITING,
      CONSTIPATION

Defining Characteristics: Nausea affects 41% of patients, followed by vomiting (30%), and constipation (22%). LFTs were elevated in some patients: GGT (45%), ALT (29%), AST (27%), alkaline phosphatase (21%).

Nursing Implications: Assess LFTs, nutritional and bowel-elimination status baseline and at each visit. LFTs should be assessed at least monthly.and as clinically needed. If patient develops nausea and/or vomiting, teach patient to self-administer antiemetics 1 hour prior to each dose, and to call if nausea/vomiting persist. Discuss with physician more effective antiemetic regimen if nausea/vomiting persist. Encourage small, frequent intake of cool, bland foods as tolerated if nausea develops. Refer to dietitian as needed for meal planning. Teach patient to report diarrhea that does not respond to OTC antidiarrheal medication. Teach self-care measures of diet modification and oral fluids to 2–3 L during the waking hours. If constipation occurs, teach patient self-care measures to prevent constipation. Assess appetite, and condition of oral mucosa; teach patient self-assessment and systemic oral hygiene after meals and at bedtime.

II.   ALTERATION IN COMFORT related to PAIN, HEADACHE, FATIGUE,
       ARTHRALGIA, MYOPATHY, ABDOMINAL PAIN, AND FATIGUE

Defining Characteristics: Fatigue affected 43% of patients, abdominal pain 28%, pyrexia (18%), arthralgia (26%), myopathy (23%), headache (22%) of patients.

Nursing Implications: Assess baseline serum CPK and creatinine levels baseline and periodically during treatment. Teach patient to report any new muscle aches, pain, tenderness or muscle weakness right away, and discuss with provider having patient come for laboratory testing of CPK and serum creatinine if this occurs. Teach patient that fatigue, fever, arthralgia, myopathy, headache, and abdominal pain may occur, and teach strategies to manage symptoms. Assess baseline comfort and monitor closely during treatment. Develop plan to assure comfort depending on symptoms reported. Discuss ineffective strategies with physician/NP/PA.

Drug: Enasidenib (Idhifa)

Class: Small molecule inhibitor of isocitrate dehydrogenase 2 (IDH2) enzyme.

Mechanism of Action: IDH2 mutations may occur in AML. Blocking mutated IDH2 leads to differentiation and death of AML cells (Chen et al., 2013). As a small molecule

TREATMENT

inhibitor of IDH2 enzyme, the drug leads to decreased 2-hydroxyglutarate (2-HG) levels, reduced leukemic blast cells, and an increased percentage of mature myeloid cells (Celgene, 2017).

Metabolism: Absolute bioavailability is about 57%, with median time to T_{max} of 4 hours. Drug is 98.5% bound to human plasma protein while its metabolite AGI-16903 is 96.6% bound. The metabolite is a substrate for P-glycoprotein and BCRP. Drug has a terminal half-life of 137 hours. Metabolism appears to involve multiple CYP enzymes and multiple UGTs, as is that of the metabolite. Most of the drugs (89%) are excreted in the feces, and 11% in the urine; about 34% of unchanged drug is excreted in the feces.

Indication: Adult patients with relapsed or refractory AML with an IDH2 mutation as detected by an FDA-approved test (in blood or bone marrow).

Contraindication: None.

Dosage Range:
- 100 mg orally once daily until disease progression or unacceptable toxicity.
- Dosage modifications:
  - *Differentiation syndrome:* Administer ordered corticosteroids and perform hemodynamic monitoring.
    - Enasidenib should be interrupted for severe pulmonary symptoms that require intubation/ventilator support, and/or renal dysfunction that persists for > 48 hours after the start of corticosteroids.
    - Drug should be resumed when signs/symptoms improve to grade 2 (moderate) or lower.
  - *Noninfectious leukocytosis (WBC > 30 × 10^9/L):* Administer ordered hydroxyurea; interrupt enasidenib if leukocytosis does not improve with hydroxyurea, and resume enasidenib at 100 mg daily when WBC is < 30 × 10^9/L.
  - *Elevated bilirubin > 3 × ULN sustained for ≥ 2 weeks without elevated transaminases or other hepatic disorders:* Decrease enasidenib to 50 mg daily. Drug dose can be increased back to 100 mg daily when elevated bilirubin resolves to < 2 × ULN.
  - Other grade 3 or higher toxicities (related to treatment, including TLS): Interrupt enasidenib until toxicity resolves to ≤ grade 2 (moderate), and resume enasidenib at 50 mg daily. Drug dose can be increased back to 100 mg daily when toxicity resolves to ≤ grade 1 (mild). If grade 3 (serious) or higher toxicity occurs, discontinue enasidenib.

Drug Preparation: Available as 50-mg and 100-mg tablets.

Drug Administration:
- Assess results of pregnancy test in women of reproductive potential before patient begins therapy.
- Teach patient to take tablet:
  - Orally with or without food for a minimum of 6 months if no disease progression or unacceptable toxicity, to allow time for a clinical response.

- Take tablet at about the same time every day. Do not split or crush tablet. If a dose is missed, vomited, or not taken at the regular time, administer the dose as soon as possible on the same day, then return to the normal schedule the following day.
- Assess blood counts and chemistries for leukocytosis and TLS prior to starting drug, and monitor at least every 2 weeks × first 3 months during treatment.
- If patient is at risk for TLS, discuss prophylaxis with provider prior to patient beginning therapy. Monitor closely.
- Assess for adverse effects, and discuss with provider dose interruption or reduction.
- Assess for signs/symptoms of differentiation syndrome which is associated with rapid proliferation and differentiation of myeloid cells (Celgene, 2017): acute respiratory distress (dyspnea, hypoxia, and need for supplemental oxygen), pulmonary infiltrates, pleural effusion, renal impairment, fever, lymphadenopathy, bone pain, peripheral edema with rapid weight gain, and/or pericardial effusion. If suspected, discuss urgent management with provider (e.g., corticosteroids and close monitoring). If patient has pulmonary and/or renal dysfunction, then hospitalization is recommended for close observation and monitoring.

Drug Interactions:
- Enasidenib appears to inhibit CYP1A2, CYP2B6, CYP2C8, CYP2C9, CYP2C19, CYP2D6, CYP3A4, and UGT1A1.
- Enasidenib appears to induce CYP2B6 and CYP3A4.
- Enasidenib inhibits P-gp, BCRP, OAT1, OATP1B1, and others.
- Enasidenib may increase or decrease the concentrations of combination hormonal contraceptives.

Lab Effects/Interference:
- Increased bilirubin.
- Leukocytosis.
- Decreased calcium, potassium, and phosphorus.

Special Considerations:
- Most common (incidence ≥ 20%) adverse effects are nausea, vomiting, diarrhea, elevated bilirubin, and decreased appetite.
- Women should be advised not to breast-feed while receiving the drug.
- Warnings and precautions:
  - *Differentiation syndrome:* Incidence in clinical trials was 14%. Syndrome may be life-threatening or fatal if not treated. It is caused by rapid proliferation and differentiation of myeloid cells and can be managed by prompt administration of oral or IV corticosteroids (e.g., dexamethasone 10 mg every 12 hours), and hemodynamic monitoring. See Nursing Implications.
  - *Embryo-fetal toxicity:* Drug can cause embryo-fetal harm. Assess pregnancy status of women of reproductive potential prior to starting therapy. Teach female patients of reproductive potential and male patients with partners that are of reproductive potential to use effective contraception during therapy and for at least 1 month after the last dose.

Potential Toxicities/Side Effects and the Nursing Process

I. POTENTIAL FOR *INJURY* related to DIFFERENTIATION SYNDROME

Defining Characteristics: Syndrome is associated with rapid proliferation and differentiation of myeloid cells, and may be life-threatening and requires prompt initiation of corticosteroids and close clinical monitoring. Incidence in clinical trials was 14%. Signs and symptoms include: acute respiratory distress (dyspnea, hypoxia, and need for supplemental oxygen), pulmonary infiltrates, pleural effusion, renal impairment, fever, lymphadenopathy, bone pain, peripheral edema with rapid weight gain, and/or pericardial effusion.

Nursing Implications: If suspected, discuss urgent management with provider (e.g., corticosteroids such as dexamethasone 10 mg q 12 hours and close clinical monitoring). If patient has pulmonary and/or renal dysfunction, hospitalization is recommended for close observation and monitoring. Expect that corticosteroids will be tapered only after symptoms have resolved. Signs/symptoms may recur if corticosteroids are stopped too early. If pulmonary symptoms requiring intubation/ventilator support occur and/or renal dysfunction persist for > 48 hours after starting corticosteroids, interrupt enasidenib therapy until symptoms are no longer severe (Celgene, 2017).

II. POTENTIAL ALTERATION IN NUTRITION, LESS THAN BODY REQUIREMENTS, related to NAUSEA, VOMITING, DIARRHEA, DECREASED APPETITE, AND ELEVATED BILIRUBIN

Defining Characteristics: GI effects were common in clinical trials: nausea occurred in 50% (grade $\geq$ 3 was 5%), diarrhea 43% (grade $\geq$ 3 was 8%), and vomiting 34% (grade $\geq$ 3 was 2%). Decreased appetite affected 34% of patients, and dysgeusia affected 12% of patients. Elevated total bilirubin occurred in 81% of patients (grade $\geq$ 3 was 15%) and is believed due to drug inhibiting UGT1A1 microenzymes, and interfering with bilirubin metabolism.

Nursing Implications: Assess baseline nutritional status and bowel-elimination status. If patient develops nausea and/or vomiting, teach patient to self-administer antiemetics 1 hour prior to each dose and to call if nausea/vomiting persist. Discuss with physician more effective antiemetic regimen if nausea/vomiting persist. Encourage small, frequent intake of cool, bland foods as tolerated if nausea develops. Refer to dietitian as needed for meal planning. Teach patient to report diarrhea that does not respond to OTC antidiarrheal medication. Teach self-care measures of diet modification and increased oral fluids to 2–3 L during the waking hours.

Drug: erdafitinib (Balversa)

Class: Kinase inhibitor (fibroblast growth factor receptor inhibitor, FGFR 2,3 inhibitor).

Mechanism of Action: Proteins made by the FGFR genes are involved in many signaling pathways significant in cancer development and progression, such as regulation of cell proliferation, differentiation, and apoptosis. If FGFR is activated, it often activates RAS-MAPK and PI3K-AKT pathways. Receptors may be amplified in lung and breast cancers. Erdafitinib is a protein kinase that binds to and inhibits the enzymatic activity of FGFR 1,2,3, and 4 and also binds to RET, CSF1R, PDGFα, PDGRβ, as well as FLT4, KIT and VEGFR2 (Janssen, 2019). Erdafitinib has shown antitumor activity in a number of tumor cell lines with FGFR expression, including bladder cancer. An FDA-approved test must be used to show evidence of a FGFR 2 or FGFR 3 mutation or gene fusion within the tumor specimen.

Metabolism: After daily oral dosing, steady state was reached after 2 weeks, and median time to peak plasma concentration (t_{max}) was 2.5 hours (range 2–6 hours). High fat diet did not affect absorption. Erdafitinib is 99.8% protein bound (primarily to alfpha-1-acid glycoprotein). Mean effective half-life is 59 hours. Erdafitinib is primarily metabolized by CYP2C9 (39%) and CYP3A4 (20%). Approximately 69% of a dose can be recovered in feces (19% unchanged) and 19% in the urine (13% unchanged drug). Patients with severe renal impairment, requiring dialysis or moderate or severe hepatic impairment, were not studied).

Indication: Treatment of adult patients with locally advanced or metastatic urothelial carcinoma that has 1) susceptible FGFR 3 or FGFR 2 genetic alterations, and 2) progressed during or following at least 1 line of prior platinum-containing chemotherapy including within 12 months of neoadjuvant or adjuvant platinum-containing chemotherapy. Patients should be selected based on an FDA-approved companion diagnostic such as therascreen FGFR RGQRT-PCR kit (QIAGEN). FDA accelerated approval based on tumor response rate.

Contraindication: None.

Dosing Range:
- The inhibition of FGFR 2,3 results in increased serum phosphate levels, and initial dosing targets a serum phosphate levels of 5.5–7.0 mg/dL in early cycles (days 14–21) with continuous daily dosing.
- Teach patient to avoid concomitant agents that can change serum phosphate levels before the initial dose increase period based on serum phosphate levels (e.g., vitamin D supplements, potassium phosphate supplements, antacids, phosphate-containing enemas, or laxatives).
- Recommended starting dose is 8 mg (two 4-mg tablets) PO once daily, with a dose increase to 9 mg (three 3-mg tablets) PO once daily based on serum phosphate (PO_4) levels and tolerability at 14–21 days.
- Dose increase based on serum phosphate levels:
  - Assess serum phosphate levels 14–21 days after starting treatment.
  - Increase the dose of erdafitinib to 9 mg PO once daily if serum phosphate level is < 5.5 mg/dL and there are no ocular disorders or grade 2 or higher adverse reactions.

- Monitor serum phosphate levels monthly for hyperphosphatemia.
- Drug should be continued until disease progression or unacceptable toxicity.

Dose Modifications for Adverse Reactions:
- **Dose reduction levels (Janssen, 2019):**
  - *If dose is 9 mg a day,* first dose reduction is to 8 mg, second dose reduction is to 6 mg, third dose reduction is to 5 mg, and fourth dose reduction is to 4 mg. If a fifth dose reduction is needed, the drug should be stopped.
  - *If dose is 8 mg a day,* first dose reduction is to 6 mg, second dose reduction is to 5 mg, third dose reduction is to 4 mg, and if a fourth dose reduction is needed, drug should be stopped.
- **Dose reductions for specific adverse reactions (Grading NCI CTCAE v4.03):**
  - **Hyperphosphatemia:** All patients should restrict phosphate intake to 600–800 mg daily. If serum phosphate is > 7.0 mg/dL, discuss with provider adding an oral phosphate binder until serum phosphate level returns to < 5.5 mg/dL.
    - **5.6**–6.9 mg/dL (1.8–2.3 mmol/L): Continue erdafitinib at current dose.
    - **7.0**–9.0 mg/dL (2.3–2.9 mmol/L): Hold erdafitinib with weekly reassessments until level returns to < 5.5 mg/dL or baseline. Then erdafitinib should be restarted at same dose level. Reduce dose if hyperphosphatemia lasts > 1 week.
    - **> 9.**0 mg/dL (> 2.9 mmol/L): Hold erdafitinib with weekly reassessments until level returns to < 5.5 mg/dL or baseline. May restart erdafitinib at 1 dose level lower.
    - **> 10.**0 mg/dL (> 3.2 mmol/L) or significant alteration in baseline renal function or grade 3 hypercalcemia: Hold erdafitinib with weekly reassessments until level returns to < 5.5 mg/dL or baseline. Restart drug at 2 dose levels lower.
  - **Central Serous Retinopathy/Retinal Pigment Epithelial Detachment (CSR/RPED):**
    - Grade 1: Asymptomatic; clinical or diagnostic observation only: Withold until resolution. If resolves within 4 weeks, resume at next lower dose level. Then if no recurrence for a month, consider reescalation. If stable for 2 consecutive eye exams but not resolved, resume at the next lower dose level.
    - Grade 2: Visual acuity 20/40 or better or ≤ 3 lines of decreased vision from baseline: Hold drug until resolution; if resolves within 4 weeks, may resume at next lower dose level.
    - Grade 3: Visual acuity worse than 20/40 or > 3 lines of decreased vision from baseline: Hold until resolution. If resolves within 4 weeks, may resume 2 dose levels lower. If recurs, consider permanent discontinuation.
    - Grade 4: Visual acuity 20/200 or worse in affected eye: Permanently discontinue.
  - Other adverse reactions:
    - Grade 3: Hold erdafitinib until resolves to Grade 1 or baseline, then resume dose level lower.
    - Grade 4: Permanently discontinue.

Drug Preparation:
- Oral, available as 3-mg, 4-mg, and 5-mg tablets.
- Teach patient to store drug at room temperature between 68–77°F (20–25°C) and to store so that children and pets cannot reach the medicine.

Administration:
- Ophthalmological exam (assessment of visual acuity, slit lamp exam, fundoscopy, and optical coherence tomography) baseline, then monthly during first 4 months of treatment, then every 3 months afterwards, and at any time when visual symptoms arise.
- Assess patient history of changes in vision, eye dryness, baseline and at each visit. Teach patient to report any changes right away.
- Assess patient laboratory values, and discuss serum phosphate level with provider. Assess serum phosphate levels baseline, days 14–21, then monthly and as needed. Assess patient medication profile and identify use of any phosphate containing medications (e.g., antacids). Teach patient NOT to take any phosphate containing substances before/during the dose determination interval (days 14–21). Teach patient to restrict phosphate intake to 600–800 mg daily.
- Teach patient how to use dry eye prophylaxis with ocular demulcents as needed (e.g., artificial tears or lubricating eye gels, q 2 hours while awake).
- Review pregnancy test results of women of reproductive potential before starting therapy. Teach patients to use effective contraception during therapy and for at least 1 month after last dose. Teach male patients with female partners of reproductive potential to use effective contraception during therapy and for at least 1 month after last drug dose. If patient is a mother, teach patient not to breastfeed while receiving drug or for at least 1 month after last drug dose.
- Teach patient self-administration of the drug, with dose based on laboratory results.
  - To swallow tablets whole with or without food. If the patient vomits at any time after taking the dose, take the next dose the NEXT day. Do not make up the dose.
  - If the patient misses a dose, take it as soon as possible on the same day. Resume the regular daily dose schedule the next day. Do not make up a missed dose.
  - Teach patient restricted phosphate intake (600–800 mg daily) and diet.

Drug Interactions:
- *Strong CYP2C9 or CYP3A4 Inhibitors:*
  - Coadministration results in increased erdafitinib plasma concentrations, which may lead to increased drug-related toxicity. Consider alternative therapies not using a strong inhibitor. Example: fluconazole (strong CYP2C9 inhibitor, moderate CYP3A4 inhibitor: increased erdafitinib Cmax 121% and AUC 148%.
  - If coadministration is unavoidable, monitor patient closely for toxicity and consider dose modification (e.g., decrease the erdafitinib dose) as needed. If the strong inhibitor is discontinued, the erdafitinib dose may be increased if no drug-related toxicity.
- *Strong CYP2C9 or CYP3A4 Inducers:*
  - Coadministration of erdafitinib with strong inducers of CYP2C9 or CYP3A4 microenzymes may decrease erdafitinib serum concentrations significantly, which will lead to decreased drug efficacy. Example is rifampin, which may significantly decrease erdafitinib Cmax and AUC.
  - Avoid coadministration with either of these strong inducers.
- *Moderate CYP2C9 or CYP3A4 Inducers:*
  - Coadministration of erdafitinib with moderate inducers of CYP2C9 or CYP3A4 microenzymes may decrease erdafitinib serum concentrations, which may lead to decreased drug efficacy.

- If a moderate inducer must be coadministered at the start of erdafitinib treatment, increase the erdafitinib dose as recommended (8 mg qd with potential to increase to 9 mg qd based on serum phosphate levels on days 14–21 and tolerability).
- If a moderate inducer must be coadministered after the initial dose, increase period based on serum phosphate levels and tolerability, increase erdafitinib dose up to 9 mg qd.
- When a moderate inducer of CYP2C9 or CYP3A4 is discontinued, continue erdafitinib at the same dose, in the absence of drug-related toxicity.
- *Serum phosphate level-altering agents* may increase or decrease serum phosphate levels so that levels needed to determine initial dose (e.g., days 14–21) do not reflect erdafitinib effect. Do NOT coadminister. Examples are antacids, potassium phosphate supplements, vitamin D supplements, phosphate-containing enemas, or laxatives.
- *CYP3A4 Substrates:* coadministration may alter plasma concentrations of CYP3A4 substrate leading to loss of substrate activity or increased toxicity of the substrate. Avoid coadministration with sensitive substrates with a narrow therapeutic window.
- *OCT2 Substrates (e.g., metformin):* Coadministration may result in increased OCT2 substrate serum concentrations and potential toxicity. Consider alternative drugs or decrease the dose of OCT2 substrate based on tolerability.
- *P-glycoprotein Substrates:* Coadministration may increase the plasma concentrations of P-gp substrates, potentially leading to increased toxicity of the substrate. If coadministration is unavoidable, separate erdafitinib dose by at least 6 hours before or after administration of the P-gp substrate with a narrow therapeutic window.
- If patient is a CYO2C9 Poor Metabolizer (CYP2C9*3/*3 Genotype): Erdafitinib plasma concentrations will be higher in these patients; monitor for increased drug toxicity.

Lab Effects/Interference:
- Decreased Hgb, platelet count, leukocyte, and neutrophil counts.
- Increased phosphate (PO_4), creatinine, ALT, alkaline phosphatase, AST, calcium, potassium, fasting blood glucose.
- Decreased sodium, albumin, magnesium, phosphate.

Special Considerations:
- Most common adverse reactions ($\geq$ 20%) were increased serum phosphate, stomatitis, fatigue, increased serum creatinine, diarrhea, dry mouth, onycholysis, increased ALT, increased alkaline phosphatase, decreased sodium, decreased appetite, decreased albumin, dysgeusia, decreased Hgb, dry skin, increased AST, decreased magnesium, dry eye, alopecia, palmar-plantar erythrodysesthesia syndrome (PPES), constipation, decreased phosphate, abdominal pain, increased calcium, nausea, musculoskeletal pain.
- Warnings and Precautions:
  - *Ocular disorders:* can occur, including central serous reinopathy/retinal pigment epithelial detachment (CSR/RPED) causing visual field defects.
    - Incidence of CSR/RPED in clinical trials was 25%, with a median time to first onset of 50 days. Grade 3 CSR/RPED involving central field of vision, occurred in 3% of patients.
    - Other ocular symptoms included dry eye (28%) of patients which was grade 3 in 6% of patients. All patients should receive dry eye prophylaxis with ocular demulcents as needed.

- Ophthalmological exams: should include assessment of visual acuity, slit lamp examination, fundoscopy, and optical coherence tomography and should occur monthly during first 4 months of treatment, then every 3 months, and urgently as visual symptoms occur.
  - Hold erdafitinib if CSR occurs, and permanently discontinue if it does not resolve within 4 weeks, or if grade 4 in severity. Other ocular adverse reactions should be managed per Dose Modifications section.
- *Hyperphosphatemia:* FGFR inhibition results in increased serum phospatemia. This is useful in titrating the correct dose, but may be dangerous for the patient. Incidence was 76% of all patients, with a median time to onset for any grade of phosphatemia of 20 days (range 8–116 days) after starting erdafitinib (Janssen, 2019). A third of patients in clinical trials needed to take phosphate binders to reduce the serum phosophate level. Monitor the patient for hyperphosphatemia and use dose modifications as needed.
- *Embryo-fetal toxicity:* Drug is fetotoxic. Pregnancy testing in women with reproductive potential is recommended before starting therapy. Teach women of reproductive potential to use effective contraception during treatment and for at least 1 month after last drug dose. Teach male patients with female partners of reproductive potential to use effective contraception during treatment and for 1 month after last dose. Erdafitinib may impair fertility in females of reproductive potential. Teach mothers that they should not breast-feed while receiving the drug or for 1 month after last drug dose.

Potential Toxicities/Side Effects and the Nursing Process

I.   ALTERATION IN PERCEPTION related to OCULAR DISORDERS

Defining Characteristics: Central serous reinopathy/retinal pigment epithelial detachment (CSR/RPED) causing visual field defects. Incidence of CSR/RPED was 25% in clinical times, occurring a median of 50 days after start of therapy. Grade 3 was uncommon (3%). Other ocular symptoms included dry eye, blurred vision, increased lacrimation (tearing).

Nursing Implications: All patients should receive a comprehensive ophthalmologic exam baseline, then monthly × 4, then every 3 months, and urgently if patient complains of symptoms. The ophthalmological exam should include assessment of visual acuity, slit lamp examination, fundoscopy, and optical coherence tomography. All patients should receive dry eye prophylaxis with ocular demulcents as needed (e.g., artificial tears, hydrating or lubricating eye gels or ointments, q 2 hours while awake). Perform a nursing assessment of patient vision at each visit, and teach patient to report right away any changes in vision. Ensure that patient receives ophthalmological exams as outlined. Hold erdafitinib if CSR occurs, and permanently discontinue if it does not resolve within 4 weeks or if grade 4 in severity. Other ocular adverse reactions should be managed per Dose Modifications section.

II.   POTENTIAL INJURY related to HYPERPHOSPHATEMIA

Defining Characteristics: Inhibition of the fibroblast growth factor receptor (FGFR) results in hyperphosphatemia and is common affecting 76% of patients without a corresponding reduction in serum calcium. Median onset was 20 days (range 8–116 days). About 24% of patients experience hypophosphatemia with 22% experiencing increased serum calcium (phosphate is inversely proportional to calcium). Patients with hyperphosphatemia usually are asypmptomatic and if they had symptoms, they usually are related to the corresponding low serum calcium.

Nursing Implications: Teach patient to restrict phosphate intake to 600–800 mg daily and to NOT take any phosphate containing over-the-counter medications (e.g., antacids). Assess baseline serum phosphate and laboratory results as ordered days 14–21 when final drug dose is determined based on serum phosphate value. If patient develops hypocalcemia (not common), signs/symptoms are muscle cramps, tetany, perioral numbness, joint pain, pruritis, rash. If hyperphosphatemia is > 7.0 mg/L, discuss with provider dose modificationand need for phosphate binders to reduce serum phosphate to < 5.5 mg/dL.

III.   ALTERATION IN NUTRITION, POTENTIAL related to STOMATITIS, DIARRHEA, DRY MOUTH, CONSTIPATION, NAUSEA, VOMITING, DYSGEYSIA, DECREASED WEIGHT

Defining Characteristics: Nutritional impact symptoms are stomatitis (incidence 56%), diarrhea (47%), dry mouth (45%), constipation (28%), nausea (21%), and vomiting (13%). In addition, dysgeusia (37%) and decreased appetite can occur (38%).

Nursing Implications: Assess baseline nutritional status and bowel-elimination status. If patient develops nausea and/or vomiting, teach patient to self-administer antiemetics 1 hour prior to each dose and to call if nausea/vomiting persist. Discuss with physician more effective antiemetic regimen if nausea/vomiting persist. Encourage small, frequent intake of cool, bland foods as tolerated if nausea develops. Refer to dietitian as needed for meal planning. Teach patient to report diarrhea that does not respond to OTC antidiarrheal medication. Teach self-care measures of diet modification and increased oral fluids to 2–3 L during the waking hours. Teach self-assessment of oral mucosa and systemic cleansing after meals and bedtime. Teach patient to report oral ulcers or discomfort. Assess weight and appetite at each visit.

VI.   ALTERATION IN SKIN INTEGRITY, POTENTIAL, related to ONYCHOLYSIS, DRY SKIN, PPES, ALOPECIA, NAIL DISCOLORATION

Defining Characteristics: The incidence of skin related adverse effects were onycholysis (41%), dry skin (34%), PPES (26%), alopecia (26%), paronychia (17%), and nail discoloration (11%).

Nursing Implications: Assess patient skin and nail integrity and hair baseline and at each visit. Teach patient that adverse effects may occur and to report them. Instruct patient in self-care measures, such as avoidance of abrasive skin products and clothing, and the use of skin emollients appropriate for skin problem. Discuss potential impact of hair loss prior to drug administration, coping strategies, and plan to minimize body-image distortion (e.g., wig, scarf, cap). Assess patient for signs/symptoms of hair loss. Assess patient's response and use of coping strategies; help patient to build on effective strategies. Teach patient self-care measures to preserve hair, such as washing hair with warm water, use of a gentle shampoo and conditioner, use of a soft-bristle brush, cutting hair short to reduce pressure on hair shaft, and use of a satin pillowcase to minimize friction on hair shaft. Teach patient to wear a wide-brimmed hat and sunglasses when outside and to use sunscreen (at least SPF 15) on scalp when outdoors without a hat. Assess hands, feet, and pressure points for signs/symptoms of PPES. Initially, PPES begins as redness of palms of hands and soles of feet but may progress to drying, peeling, itching, then pain, and finally, may progress to blister formation. Teach patient to avoid hot showers and baths, use tepid water, try to minimize pressure on painful areas, and report any increase in pain, skin sloughing, or blister formation. Assess nail baseline, and teach patient to report changes. Teach patient to keep nails clean and trimmed, not to wear imitation nails, and to wear protective gloves when doing house cleaning and gardening. Teach patient to use a nail hardener if nails appear soft. If paronychia is painful, discuss with provider the use of flurandrenolide (Cordran Tape) to reduce discomfort (Lacouture, 2011).

Drug: erlotinib (Tarceva)

Class: Kinase inhibitor (epidermal growth factor receptor (HER-1/EGFR1) TKI).

Mechanism of Action: Mechanism of antitumor activity not fully characterized. Inhibits the phosphorylation of the intracellular portion of the EGFR or tyrosine kinase domain of the EGFR. Erlotinib binding affinity for EGFR exon 19 deletion or exon 21 (L858R) mutation is higher than its affinity for the wild-type (normal) receptor. This inhibits the activation of cell signaling telling the nucleus of the cell to divide, avoid programmed cell death, and release vascular endothelial growth factor (VEGF). EGFR is expressed on the cell surface of normal as well as many cancer cells.

Metabolism: Drug bioavailability is about 60% after oral administration with peak plasma concentration occurring 4 hours after ingestion. Erlotinib solubility is pH dependent, with erlotinib solubility decreasing as the pH increases. Coadministration of erlotinib with omeprazole, a PPI, decreased erlotinib exposure (AUC) and maximum concentration (C_{max}) by 46% and 61%, respectively. When erlotinib is administered 2 hours following a dose of ranitidine 300 mg (an H2 receptor antagonist), the erlotinib AUC was reduced by 33% and C_{max} by 54%; when erlotinib was administered 10 hours after the previous ranitidine evening dose and 2 hours before the ranitidine morning dose, the erlotinib AUC and C_{max} decreased by 15% and 17%, respectively.

Drug is highly protein-bound (93%). Drug is eliminated by hepatic metabolism and biliary excretion. It is primarily metabolized by the cytochrome P450 hepatic microsomal enzyme system (CYP3A4). Excretion is primarily fecal (83%, with 1% intact parent drug), with 8% excreted in the urine. Food can increase drug bioavailability by 100%. Smoking increases erlotinib clearance by 24% and decreases erotinib serum concentration.

Indications:

- Treatment of patients with metastatic NSCLC whose tumors have EGFR exon 19 deletions or exon 21 (L858R) substitution mutations, as detected by an FDA, approved test receiving first line, maintenance, or second or greater line treatment after progression following at least 1 prior chemotherapy regimen.
- First-line treatment of patients with locally advanced, unresectable, or metastatic pancreatic cancer, in combination with gemcitabine.
- Limitations of use:
  - Not recommended for use in combination with platinum-based chemotherapy.
  - Safety and efficacy have not been evaluated in patients with metastatic NSCLC whose tumors have other EGFR mutations.
- FDA approved tests for the detection of EGFR mutations in NSCLC are available at http://www.fda.gov/CompanionDiagnostics.

Dosage/Range:

- Non-small-cell lung cancer (NSCLC): 150 mg PO once daily on an empty stomach at least 1 hour before or 2 hours after meals. Treatment should continue until disease progression or unacceptable toxicity occurs.
- Pancreatic cancer: 100 mg PO once daily on an empty stomach at least 1 hour before or 2 hours after meals, in combination with gemcitabine. Treatment should continue until disease progression or unacceptable toxicity occurs.
- Dose-reduce in 50-mg decrements when necessary.

Dose Modifications (see package insert):

- **Discontinue** erlotinib for (1) interstitial lung disease (ILD); (2) severe hepatic toxicity that does not improve significantly or resolve within 3 weeks; (3) GI perforation; (4) severe bullous, blistering, or exfoliating skin conditions; (5) corneal perforation or severe ulceration.
- **Hold** erlotinib (1) during diagnostic evaluation for possible ILD; (2) for severe CTCAE grade 3 or 4 renal toxicity and consider drug discontinuance; (3) in patients without preexisting hepatic impairment for total bilirubin levels > 3 × ULN or transaminases > 5 × ULN, and discontinue eotinib if abnormal LFTs do not significantly improve or resolve within 3 weeks; (4) in patients with preexisting hepatic impairment or biliary obstruction for doubling of bilirubin or tripling of transaminases values over baseline and discontinue eotinib if abnormal LFTs do not significantly improve or resolve within 3 weeks; (5) for persistent severe diarrhea not responsive to medical management (e.g., loperamide); (6) for severe rash not responsive to medical management; (7) for keratitis of (NCI-CTC version 4.0) grades 3–4 or for grade 2 lasting > 2 weeks; (8) for acute/worsening ocular disorders such as eye pain and consider erlotinib discontinuation.

- **Drug Interaction Dose Modification:**
  - **CYP3A4 Inhibitors: Reduce erlotinib by 50-mg decrements:** if severe reactions occur with concomitant use of strong CYP3A4 inhibitors (see drug listing in Drug Interactions) or when using concomitantly an inhibitor of both CYP3A4 and CYP1A2 (e.g., ciprofloxacin), avoid concomitant use if possible.
  - **CYP3A4 Inducers/Smoking: Increase erlotinib dose by 50-mg increments as tolerated for:** (1) concomitant use with CYP3A4 inducers (see drug listing in Drug Interactions, increase dose by 50-mg increments at 2-week intervals to a maximum 450-mg dose). Avoid concomitant use if possible); (2) concurrent cigarette smoking, increase dose by 50-mg increments at 2-week intervals to a maximum of 300 mg. Immediately reduce the dose of erlotinib to the recommended dose (150 mg or 100 mg daily) upon cessation of smoking.
  - **Drugs affecting gastric pH:** (1) PPIs: avoid concomitant use of PPI if possible, as separation of dose may not eliminate the interaction, and as PPIs affect the pH of the upper GI tract for an extended period; (2) H_2 receptor antagonist: if treatment with an H_2 receptor antagonist like ranitidine is required, erlotinib must be taken 10 hours AFTER H_2 receptor antagonist dose, and at least 2 hours BEFORE the next dose of the H_2 receptor antagonist; (3) antacids: should be taken several hours before or after erlotinib.

Drug Preparation:
- Oral, available in 150-, 100-, and 25-mg tablets.

Drug Administration:
- Teach patient to (1) take dose should be taken on an empty stomach, at least 1 hour before meals or 2 hours after meals; (2) not eat grapefruit or drink grapefruit juice; (3) not take St. John's wort.
- Teach patient to report right away (1) onset or worsening of skin rash or development of bullous lesions or desquamation; (2) severe or persistent diarrhea, nausea, anorexia, or vomiting; (3) onset or worsening of unexplained shortness of breath (SOB) or cough; and (4) eye irritation. Review patient teaching insert that comes with package insert with patient and caregiver.

Drug Interactions:
- *Inducers of CYP3A4* (may increase metabolism of erlotinib and **decrease erlotinib plasma concentration): rifampin, rifabutin, rifapentine**, phenytoin, phenobarbital, St. John's wort, carbamazepine; avoid if possible; otherwise may need to increase dose of erlotinib.
- *Rifampicin* decreased erlotinib area under the curve (AUC) by 66% to 80%:
  - Use alternative drug that does not induce CYP3A4, or consider erlotinib dose escalation every 2 weeks while monitoring the patient, to a maximum dose of 450 mg. If the erlotinib dose is increased and rifampicin (or other inducer) is discontinued, reduce erlotinib dose immediately to the indicated starting dose.
- *Inhibitors of CYP3A4* (may decrease metabolism of erlotinib and **increase erlotinib plasma concentration**); strong inhibitors (e.g., atazanavir, clarithromycin, indinavir, itraconazole, ketoconazole, nefazodone, nelfinavir, ritonavir, saquinavir, telithromycin,

troleandomycin [TAO], voriconazole, or grapefruit [fruit or juice]): consider dose reduction of erlotinib if severe reactions occur.
- *Inhibitor of CYP3A4 and CYP1A2* (e.g., ciprofloxacin): consider dose reduction of erlotinib if severe reactions occur.
- *CYP1A2 Inducers:* may decrease erlotinib plasma concentrations.
- *CYP1A2 Inhibitors* (e.g., ciprofloxacin): may increase erlotinib plasma concentrations.
- Erlotinib solubility is pH dependent. Drugs that alter the pH of the upper GI tract may alter erlotinib solubility and its absorption. There is risk of low erlotinib serum levels if the drug is given in combination with drugs that change GI pH, such as omeprazole (a PPI) or ranitidine (an H_2 receptor antagonist). Avoid concomitant use of PPIs and erlotinib, as dose separation may not eliminate the drug interaction. If treatment with an H2-receptor antagonist is necessary (e.g., ranitidine), erlotinib must be taken 10 hours after the H2-receptor antagonist, and at least 2 hours before the next dose of ranitidine. Antacids should be separated by several hours from the dose of erlotinib.
- *Warfarin* increases International Normalized Ration (INR) and bleeding is possible; monitor INR and patient bleeding, and decrease warfarin dose as needed.
- Cigarette smoking reduces serum levels of erlotinib, so drug may be ineffective in smokers; teach patients to quit; it is unclear whether nicotine patches also inactivate the drug. If the patient cannot stop smoking, the erlotinib dose may be titrated upward. However, if the patient is able to stop smoking, then the dose should be immediately reduced to the indicated starting dose.

Lab Effects/Interference:
- May increase liver function tests (serum transaminases).
- May increase INR with increased potential for bleeding.

Special Considerations:
- Drug is not recommended for use in combination with platinum-based chemotherapy. The drug's safety and efficacy have not been studied as first-line treatment of metastatic NSCLC in patients whose tumors have EGFR mutations other than exon 19 deletions or exon 21 (L858R) substitutions.
- Warnings and Precautions:
  - *ILD*: Cases of serious ILD, including fatal cases, can occur with erlotinib. Incidence was 1.1% across all studies. This is a class effect of EGFR inhibitors.
    - Onset of symptoms between 5 days to > 9 months (median 39 days) after beginning erlotinib therapy.
    - Drug should be stopped immediately in patients who develop acute onset of new or progressive unexplained pulmonary symptoms, such as dyspnea, cough, and fever. Begin appropriate diagnostic workup to establish the cause.
    - If ILD is diagnosed, erlotinib should be discontinued.
    - Gemcitabine may also cause ILD. Contributing factors include concomitant/prior chemotherapy, prior radiotherapy, preexisting parenchymal lung disease, metastatic lung disease, and pulmonary infections.
  - *Acute renal failure,* renal insufficiency, and hepatorenal syndrome have been reported; some cases may be fatal.

- Renal failure may arise from exacerbation of underlying baseline hepatic impairment or severe dehydration. Incidence in NSCLC was 0.5% (vs 0.8% in control), and 1.4% in erlotinib-plus-gemcitabine arm (vs 0.4% in control).
- Monitor renal function and electrolytes during erlotinib therapy.
- Interrupt erlotinib in patients developing severe renal impairment until renal toxicity has resolved.
- *Hepatotoxicity* with or without hepatic impairment, including hepatic failure and hepatorenal syndrome, has been reported; in some cases, it may be fatal. This can occur in patients with normal hepatic function, but risk is increased in patients with baseline hepatic impairment.
- Monitor patient LFTs (transaminases, bilirubin, alkaline phosphatase) at baseline and periodically during treatment; increase monitoring frequency in patients with preexisting hepatic impairment or biliary obstruction.
- Hold erlotinib in patients without preexisting hepatic impairment for total bilirubin $> 3 \times$ ULN or transaminases $> 5 \times$ ULN.
- Hold erlotinib in patients with preexisting hepatic impairment or biliary obstruction for doubling of bilirubin or tripling of transaminase values over baseline.
- Discontinue erlotinib if abnormal LFTs meeting above criteria do not improve significantly or resolve within 3 weeks. See package insert.
- *GI perforation* may occur, and some cases may be fatal.
  - Patients at risk are those receiving concomitant antiangiogenic drug(s), NSAIDs, corticosteroids, and/or taxane-based chemotherapy, or those who have a prior history of peptic ulceration or diverticular disease.
  - Incidence in erlotinib-containing arms was 0.2% in NSCLC studies (vs 0.1% in control), and 0.4% in pancreatic studies (vs 0% in control).
  - Permanently discontinue erlotinib if GI perforation occurs.
- *Bullous, blistering, and exfoliative skin disorders* can occur, some resembling SJS/toxic epidermal necrolysis. Some cases were fatal. Incidence in erlotinib-containing arms was 1.2% in NSCLC studies (vs 0% in control), and 0.4% in pancreatic studies (vs 0% in control). Discontinue erlotinib if severe bullous, blistering, or exfoliating conditions occur.
- *Cerebrovascular accident (CVA)* was also increased (in pancreatic trial, incidence 2.5% compared to 0% in control arm). There were no CVAs in the gemcitabine/erlotinib trials.
- *Microangiopathic hemolytic anemia with thrombocytopenia* has occurred in patients with pancreatic cancer receiving erlotinib/gemcitabine (incidence 1.4% vs 0% in control).
- *Ocular disorders*: Decreased tear production, abnormal eyelash growth, keratoconjunctivitis sicca or keratitis can occur with erlotinib therapy and can lead to corneal perforation or ulceration.
  - Incidence in NSCLC studies was 17.8% in erlotinib group vs 4% in control arm, and in pancreatic cancer studies, incidence was 12.8%, vs 11.4% in control arm.
  - Interrupt erlotinib or discontinue erlotinib in patients with acute or worsening ocular disorders such as eye pain.

- *Hemorrhage in patients taking warfarin:* INR elevations and bleeding events (including hemorrhage and fatalities) associated with warfarin administration have been reported. Closely monitor patients taking warfarin or other coumarin-derivative anticoagulants, and adjust dose of warfarin accordingly.
- *Embryo-fetal toxicity:* Erlotinib can cause fetal harm. Teach women of reproductive potential to use highly effective contraception to avoid pregnancy during therapy, and for at least 1 month after the last dose of erlotinib.
  - Advise patients to contact their healthcare provider if they become pregnant, or if pregnancy is suspected, while taking erlotinib.
  - If erlotinib is used during pregnancy, or if the patient becomes pregnant while taking erlotinib, the patient should be apprised of the potential hazard to the fetus.
- Women who are nursing should decide whether to discontinue nursing or to discontinue erlotinib, taking into account the importance of the drug to the patient's health.
- Most common toxicities ($\geq 20\%$, from a pooled analysis of studies 1–4): rash, diarrhea, anorexia, fatigue, dyspnea, cough, nausea, vomiting.

Potential Toxicities/Side Effects and the Nursing Process

I.   ALTERATION IN SKIN INTEGRITY related to RASH

Defining Characteristics: As expected, because EGFR is important in skin function, this is the area of major toxicity. Rash ranges from maculopapular to pustular on the face, neck, chest, back, and arms, affecting up to 75% of patients. Most rashes are mild to moderate (Sandler et al., 2004). Typically, rash begins on days 8 through 10 of therapy, maximizing in intensity by week 2, and resolving gradually on therapy (often by week 4). Skin treatments (corticosteroids, topical clindamycin, or minocycline) have been used with varying results.

Nursing Implications: Assess skin integrity of face, neck, arms, and upper trunk baseline, and regularly during treatment. Teach patient that rash may occur, its usual course, and self-care measures for comfort. Emphasize the need to keep skin with rash clean to prevent infection and to continue taking erlotinib until told to stop by nurse or physician. Teach patient that skin may become dry and to use skin emollients or moisturizers. Assess body image intactness, and if rash develops, its threat to body image. Encourage patient to verbalize feelings, provide emotional support, and individualize care plan to patient response. For rash management, follow institutional guidelines or refer to the introduction of *Chapter 4*. Teach all patients to (1) use a water-based emollient frequently during the day to prevent dryness, (2) stay hydrated, (3) avoid sun exposure and wear SPF 30 (zinc-based). Do not use antiacne medications. Tetracycline analogues provide anti-inflammatory benefit. In general: **Grade 1/mild rash** (localized, does not interfere with ADLs, and is not infected): Goal is to preserve skin integrity, minimize discomfort, and prevent infection. Key patient teaching includes (1) use a mild soap with active ingredients that reduce skin drying, such as pyrithione zinc (Head & Shoulders), (2) consider applying aloe gel to red, tender areas, (3) report distressing tenderness, as pramoxine (lidocaine topical anesthetic) may help, (4) keep fingernails clean and trimmed, and (5) apply zinc ointment to rectal mucosa after washing. Management: maintain current drug dose, observe, or give topical hydrocortisone 1% or 2.5% or clindamycin 1% gel (anti-inflammatory benefit), reassess in 2 weeks. **For grade 2/moderate,** which is generalized, mild symptoms, and has minimal effect on ADLs, and no infection: Goal is to prevent infection and promote comfort. Continue EGFRI dose; use topicals (hydrocortisone 2.5% or clindamycin 1% gel) and consider adding doxycycline 100 mg PO twice daily or minocycline 100 mg PO twice daily (give antimicrobial and anti-inflammatory effect) and reassess after 2 weeks. **For grades 3–4 or severe rash** (generalized, severe, has a significant impact on ADLs, and increased risk of infection): The goal is to prevent infection or identify it early to minimize complications and to promote effective coping. Interrupt drug. Treat rash with topicals (hydrocortisone 2.5%, or clindamycin 1% gel), doxycycline 100 mg PO twice daily or minocycline 100 mg PO twice daily, and methylprednisolone (Medrol dose pack); reassess after 2 weeks. Resume drug when rash improved to grade 2, at full or reduced dose (Lynch et al., 2007; Lacouture et al., 2011). If rash appears infected (exudate, vesicular formation, different appearance), obtain C+S, treat empirically until sensitivity received, and/or obtain dermatology consult. Hold drug for severe rash that does not respond to medical intervention.

Teach patient to report right away the development of bullous lesions or desquamation.

II.   ALTERATION IN ELIMINATION PATTERN related to DIARRHEA

Defining Characteristics: Affects approximately 54% of patients and is mild to moderate, with only 6% of patients experiencing grade 3 diarrhea. Diarrhea usually begins weeks 3 through 4. Symptoms may be self-limited or require an antidiarrheal agent, such as loperamide. Severe diarrhea not responsive to antidiarrheal medication may require temporary dose interruption or adjustment if refractory.

Nursing Implications: Assess bowel-elimination pattern baseline and regularly during therapy. Teach patient to report diarrhea; teach patient self-care strategies to manage diarrhea such as dietary modification and self-administration of loperamide; teach patient to minimize potential complications such as dehydration and electrolyte depletion. Identify patients at risk for dehydration and follow closely, such as patients with renal insufficiency, diabetes, congestive heart failure, or the older population. If diarrhea does not resolve or is severe, discuss with physician dose interruption, as well as fluid and electrolyte replacement. If dose needs to be reduced, reduce in 50-mg increments. If diarrhea is refractory or difficult to manage, patient may become dehydrated and will be at risk for acute renal failure, which may be fatal. If the patient is dehydrated and at risk for renal impairment (e.g., preexisting renal disease, disease or medications that may lead to renal disease, advancing age), the drug should be temporarily discontinued while the patient is rehydrated. Renal function should be assessed at baseline and periodically during therapy, more closely if the patient has diarrhea and is at risk for dehydration. Hold drug for severe diarrhea that does not respond to medical intervention.

Drug: gilteritinib **651**

III. SENSORY/PERCEPTUAL ALTERATION, POTENTIAL, related to CONJUNCTIVITIS AND EYE DRYNESS

Defining Characteristics: Decreased tear production, abnormal eyelash growth, kerato-conjunctivitis, or keratitis can occur. Pooled incidence of ocular disorders in three NSCLC trials was 17.8% in the erlotinib arm, and 4% in the control arm. Incidence in erlotinib/gemcitabine arm was 12.8% and 11.4% in the control arm. Rarely, corneal ulceration or perforation may occur.

Nursing Implications: Teach patient to report any eye irritation, pain, or change in visual acuity. Teach patient to use artificial tears to keep eyes lubricated. Refer patient to ophthalmologist immediately for any acute signs or symptoms, such as red eye or eye pain. Teach patient to stop drug if these occur and to report them immediately. Drug is discontinued for corneal perforation, ulceration, or keratitis of (NCI CTCAE version 4.0) grades 3–4 or for grade 2 lasting > 2 weeks.

IV. POTENTIAL ALTERATION IN NUTRITION, LESS THAN BODY REQUIREMENTS, related to MUCOSITIS, HEPATOTOXICITY, ANOREXIA, NAUSEA, VOMITING

Defining Characteristics: Stomatitis is uncommon, occurring in 17% of patients receiving erlotinib, compared with 3% receiving placebo. Grades 3–4 occurs in < 1% of patients. It is usually mild to moderate and is generally self-limited. Anorexia affects about 52% of patients, with 8% experiencing grade 3. Hepatotoxicity may occur, especially in patients with baseline hepatic impairment.

Nursing Implications: Assess oral hygiene practices and status of oral mucosa, gums, and teeth baseline and regularly throughout therapy. Assess nutritional status and weight baseline and regularly during treatment. Teach patient to report stomatitis and to use a systematic cleansing regimen as determined by institutional policy. Assess baseline LFTs and monitor LFTs and patient tolerance very closely during therapy if abnormal at baseline. If a patient develops worsening LFTs, discuss with physician dose interruption or discontinuance (see Dose Modifications). Teach patient to report nausea and/or vomiting and to discuss antiemetic therapy with physician or NP/PA; review instructions with patient along with diet modifications to minimize nausea and/or vomiting.

Drug: gilteritinib (Xospata)

Class: Kinase inhibitor; inhibits multiple tyrosine kinases, including FMS-like tyrosine kinase 3 (FLT3).

Mechanism of Action: Acute myeloid leukemic cells may have tyrosine kinase mutations, including FLT3. About 25% of patients with AML have a FLT-3 internal tandem duplication (ITD) mutation (FLT3-ITD) which confers an aggressive course and poor prognosis.

Gilteritinib inhibits FLT3 receptor signaling and leukemic cell proliferation, and induces apoptosis in leukemic cells expressing FLT3-ITD. In patients with relapsed or refractory AML, gilteritinib quickly led to > 90% inhibition of FLT3 phosphorylation (within 24 hours after first dose), and inhibition was sustained.

Metabolism: After oral dosing, with a time to maximum concentration (T_{max}) of 4–6 hours post dose in the fasted state, and steady state is reached within 15 days. Half-life is estimated to be 113 hours. Gilteritinib is primarily metabolized by CYP3A4 microenzyme, forming metabolites M17, M16, and M10 which do not exceed 10% of the parent exposure. Most of the drug is excreted in the feces (64.5%), and 16.4% in the urine (unchanged drug and metabolites).

Indications: Treatment of adult patients with relapsed or refractory AML with FMS-like tyrosine kinase 3 (FLT3) mutation as detected by an FDA-approved test (blood or bone marrow).

Contraindications: hypersensitivity to gilteritinib or any of the excipients. Anaphylaxis has been observed in clinical trials.

Dosage/Range: 120 mg PO once daily, with or without food; treatment for a minimum of 6 months is recommended unless disease progression or unacceptable toxicity.

Dose Modification: Dose modify based on toxicity (grade 1 is mild, 2 moderate, 3 serious, grade 4 life-threatening; Astellas, 2018):
- Posterior Reversible Encephalopathy Syndrome (PRES): discontinue gilteritinib.
- QTc > 500 msec: (1) Interrupt gilteritinib; (2) resume at 80 mg when QTc interval returns to within 30 msec of baseline or ≤ 480 msec.
- QTc interval increased by > 30 msec on ECG on day 8 of cycle 1: (1) confirm with ECG on day 9; (2) if confirmed, consider dose reduction to 80 mg.
- Pancreatitis: (1) interrupt gilteritinib until pancreatitis is resolved; (2) resume gilteritinib at 80 mg.
- Other grade 3 (serious) or higher toxicity: (1) interrupt gilteritinib until toxicity resolves to grade 1; (2) resume gilteritinib at 80 mg.

Drug Preparation: Available as 40-mg tablets. Keep out of reach of children and pets.

Drug Administration:
- Assess CBC/differential and blood chemistries including CPK, baseline, at least weekly for the first month, once every other week for the second month, and once monthly for the duration of therapy. Assess ECG (QTc interval) baseline, on days 8 and 15 of Cycle 1, and prior to the start of the next 2 subsequent cycles. Discuss results with physician or NP/PA. Ensure that hypomagnesemia and hypokalemia are corrected before patient starts/continues on gilteritinib.
- Teach patient/family:
  - Take tablet with or without food at about the same time each day.
  - Do not break or crush tablets. If a dose is missed or not taken at usual time, take dose as soon as possible on the same day, and at least 12 hours prior to next scheduled dose. Return to normal schedule the following day. Do not take 2 doses within 12 hours.

- Teach female patients of reproductive potential to use effective contraception during treatment and for at least 6 months after last dose. Teach male patients of reproductive potential to use effective contraception during treatment and for at least 4 months after last dose.
- Mothers should not breastfeed while receiving the drug and for at least 2 months after last drug dose.

Drug Interactions:
- Strong CYP3A4 inhibitors increase gilteritinib exposure; avoid coadministration; if cannot avoid, monitor patient frequently for gilteritinib adverse reactions as serum level may be increased. Interrupt and dose reduce gilteritinib if serious or life-threatening toxicity occur.
- Combined P-gp and strong CYP3A4 inducers: decrease gilteritinib serum levels which may decrease gilteritinib efficacy. Avoid concomitant administration.
- Effect of gilteritinib on drugs that target $5HT_{2B}$ receptor or sigma nonspecific receptor (escitalopram, fluoxetine, sertraline): may reduce $5HT_{2B}$ drug effects; do not coadminister.

Lab Effects/Interference:
- Increased serum creatinine, glucose, triglycerides, ALT, AST, alkaline phosphatase, bilirubin, creatine kinase.
- Decreased serum calcium, albumin, phosphate, potassium, sodium.

Special Considerations:
- Most common adverse effects ($\geq 20\%$) are myalgia/arthralgia, increased serum transaminases, fatigue/malaise, fever, noninfectious diarrhea, dyspnea, edema, rash, pneumonia, nausea, stomatitis, cough, headache, hypotension, dizziness, vomiting.
- Warnings and Precautions:
  - *Posterior reversible encephalopathy syndrome (PRES):* rare occurrence, with symptoms including seizure and change in mental status. Symptoms resolved after gilteritinib was discontinued. Confirm diagnosis of PRES with brain imaging (e.g., MRI), and discontinue gilteritinib.
  - *Prolonged QTc interval:* Gilteritinib has been associated with prolonged cardiac ventricular repolarization (QT interval). Incidence in clinical trials was 1.4% patients with QTc > 500 msec, and 7% who had a increase from baseline QTc of > 60 msec. Assess ECG prior to starting gilteritinib, on days 8 and 15 of cycle 1, and prior to the start of the next 2 subsequent cycles. If QTc is > 500 msec, interrupt gilteritinib and then resume at a reduced dose (see Dose Modifications). Ensure that serum potassium and magnesium are always maintained WNL as low serum levels can increase risk of QTc prolongation and sudden death (torsades de pointes).
  - *Pancreatitis:* may occur rarely. Assess any patient closely who develops signs/symptoms of pancreatitis. Interrupt gilteritinib and resume at a reduced dose when symptoms resolve (see Dose Modifications).
  - *Embryo-fetal toxicity:* gilteritinib is fetotoxic. Teach females of reproductive potential to use effective contraception during therapy and for at least 6 months after last dose. Teach males with female sexual partners of reproductive potential to use effective contraception during therapy and for at least 4 months after last dose. Patients or

partners of patients receiving gilteritinib who become pregnant should be apprised of risk to fetus.

Potential Toxicities/Side Effects and the Nursing Process

I.   POTENTIAL RISK OF INFECTION

Defining Characteristics: Fever occurred in 35% of patients, dyspnea in 34%, cough in 25%, pneumonia in 30% (23% > grade 3), and sepsis (14% > grade 3) in 15%.

Nursing Implications: Assess patient for signs and symptoms of infection baseline and throughout treatment. Teach patient to self-assess for signs/symptoms of infection, and to report right away fever, dyspnea, productive cough, shaking chills, or any other new symptom. Ensure that patient has a thermometer at home.

II.   ALTERATION IN COMFORT related to FATIGUE, EDEMA, RASH, HYPOTENSION, HEADACHE, DIZZINESS, ABDOMINAL PAIN

Defining Characteristics: Myalgia/arthralgia occurred in 42% of patients, fatigue/malaise in 40%, edema in 34%, skin rash in 30%, hypotension in 21%, headache in 21%, and dizziness in 20% of patients.

Nursing Implications: Assess baseline comfort, and teach patient these side effects may occur. Teach self-care measures to minimize discomfort, such as alternating rest and activity for fatigue, application of warmth or hot showers for myalgias/arthralgias, self-administration of acetaminophen or other OTC analgesic based on patient characteristics. Teach patient to report dizziness and assess patient safety at home and risk for falls. Develop a falls prevention plan and discuss with patient and family. If muscle aches do not improve, discuss assessment of CK serum level.

III.   ALTERATION IN NUTRITION related to DIARRHEA, CONSTIPATION, NAUSEA, VOMITING, STOMATITIS, DECREASED APPETITE, DYSGEUSIA

Defining Characteristics: Noninfectious diarrhea occurred in 34% of patients, constipation in 27%, nausea in 27%, stomatitis in 26%, and vomiting in 20%. Dysgeusia was reported by 11% and loss of appetite in 15% of patients.

Nursing Implications: Assess baseline nutritional status, bowel elimination status, appetite, and integrity of oral mucosa. Teach patient that these side effects may occur and self-management techniques. Teach patient oral assessment, and systematic oral cleansing. Teach patient to report onset of oral lesions or pain in the mouth. Teach dietary modifications based on symptom. Discuss medication for nausea and/or vomiting with provider and teach patient self-administration.

Drug: glasdegib (Daurismo)

Class: Hedgehog pathway inhibitor.

Mechanism of Action: Glasdegib binds to and inhibits Smoothened, a transmembrane protein involved in hedgehog signal transduction.

Metabolism: Following oral dosing, absolute bioavailability is 77%, with median time to peak concentration (T_{max}) at steady state of 1.3–1.8 hours. Glasdegib is 91% bound to human plasma proteins and has a half-life ot 17.4 hours. Drug is primarily metabolized by CYP3A4 pathway, and to a lesser extent by CYP2C8 and UGT1A9. Almost half of the dose (49%) is excreted in the urine (17% unchanged), and 42% is excreted in the feces (20% unchanged).

Indications: In combination with low-dose cytarabine, for the treatment of newly–diagnosed AML in adults aged 75 or higher or who have comorbidities that preclude use of intensive induction chemotherapy. Limitations: drug has not been studied in patients with severe renal impairment or moderate to severe hepatic impairment.

Contraindications: None.

Dosage/Range: 100 mg PO qd on days 1–28 in combination with cytarabine 20 mg SQ twice daily on days 1–10 of each 28-day cycle unless unacceptable toxicity or loss of disease control, for a minimum of 6 cycles to allow time for a clinical response.

Dose Modification:
- QTc interval prolongation on at least 2 separate ECGs:
  - QTc interval $>$ 480 ms to 599 ms: (1) assess electrolyte levels and supplement as clinically needed; (2) review and adjust concomitant medications with known QTc interval prolonging effects; (3) monitor ECGs at least weekly $\times$ 2 weeks following resolution of QTc prolongation to $\leq$ 480 ms.
  - QTc interval $>$ 500 ms: (1) assess electrolyte levels and supplement as clinically needed; (2) review and adjust concomitant medications with known QTc interval prolonging effects; (3) interrupt glasdegib; (4) resume glasdegib at a reduced dose of 50 mg qd when QTc returns to within 30 ms of baseline or $\leq$ 480 ms; (5) monitor ECGs at least weekly $\times$ 2 weeks following resolution of QTc prolongation; (6) consider re-escalating dose of glasdegib to 100 mg daily if an alternative etiology for the QTc prolongation can be identified.
  - QTc interval prolongation with life-threatening arrhythmia: discontinue glasdegib permanently.
- Hematologic toxicity:
  - Platelets $<$ 10 Gi/L for $>$ 42 days in absence of disease: discontinue glasdegib and low-dose cytarabine permanently.
  - Neutrophil count $<$ 0.5 Gi/L for $>$ 42 days in absence of disease: discontinue glasdegib and low-dose cytarabine permanently.

- Non-hematologic toxicity:
    - Grade 3: (1) interrupt glasdegib and/or low dose cytarabine until symptoms reduce to mild or return to baseline; (2) resume glasdegib at the same dose level or at a reduced dose of 50 mg qd; (3) resume low-dose cytarabine at the same dose level, or at a reduced dose of 15 mg or 10 mg; (4) if toxicity recurs, discontinue glasdegib and low-dose cytarabine; (5) if toxicity is attributable to glasdegib only, cytarabine may be continued.
    - Grade 4: discontinue glasdegib and low-dose cytarabine permanently.

Drug Preparation: Available in 100-mg and 25-mg tablets. Teach patient to keep out of reach of children and pets.

Drug Administration:
- Assess results of pregnancy test of female patients of reproductive potential prior to starting glasdegib therapy.
    - Teach these patients to use effective contraception during treatment and for at least 30 days after last dose.
    - Teach male patients with female partners of reproductive potential or who are pregnant, that drug can be passed in the semen, and to use effective contraception during treatment with glasdegib and for at least 30 days after the last dose. Teach male patient that drug may impair fertility in men of reproductive potential and they should seek advice on fertility preservation before starting glasdegib therapy.
    - Teach women not to breast-feed while receiving glasdegib and for at least 30 days after the last dose.
- Teach patients not to donate blood or blood products while taking glasdegib and for at least 30 days after the last dose.
- Assess CBC/differential, electrolyes, renal and hepatic function baseline and at least once weekly for the first month. Monitor electrolytes and renal function once monthly throughout therapy. Assess creatine kinase levels before starting glasdegib, then as clinically indicated (e.g., if muscle symptoms). Monitor ECG baseline, about 1 week after starting glasdegib, and then once monthly for the next 2 months; assess QTc interval baseline, then any prolongation with therapy. Repeat ECG if abnormal, and increase frequency of ECG monitoring as needed.
- Assess medication profile for medications which are strong CYP3A4 inhibitors or medications that prolong QTc interval. If identified, discuss alternative medications with pharmacist and physician/NP/PA.
- Teach patient/family, or administer glasdegib with or without food, at about the same time each day.
    - Do not split or crush tablets.
    - If dose is vomited, do not give a replacement dose; wait until next scheduled dose.
    - If a dose is missed or not taken at the usual time, administer the dose as soon as possible and **at least 12 hours prior to the next scheduled dose**. Return to the normal schedule the following day. Do not administer 2 doses of glasdegib withint 12 hours.

TREATMENT

Drug Interactions:
- Strong CYP3A4 inhibitors: coadministration increases glasdegib plasma concentrations which may increase risk of adverse reactions; consider alternative therapies that are not strong CYP3A4 inhibitors. Monitor for increased risk of adverse reactions including QTc prolongation.
- Strong CYP3A4 inducers: coadministration decreases glasdegib plasma concentrations which may reduce glasdegib effectiveness; do not co-administer.
- QTc interval prolonging drugs: coadministration may increase risk of QTc prolongation and life-threatening arrhythmias; avoid co-administration or replace with alternative drug; if co-admininistration is unavoidable, monitor patients for increased risk of QTc-prolongation and ensure serum magnesium and potassium are WNL throughout therapy.

Lab Effects/Interference:
- Increased serum creatinine, AST, ALT, bilirubin, alkaline phosphatase, potassium, CPK.
- Decreased serum sodium, magnesium, potassium.
- With low dose cytarabine, anemia, neutropenia, thrombocytopenia.

Special Considerations:
- Most common adverse reactions (≥ 20%) were anemia, fatigue, hemorrhage, febrile neutropenia, musculoskeletal pain, nausea, edema, thrombocytopenia, dyspnea, decreased appetite, dysgeusia, mucositis, constipation, rash.
- Warnings and Precautions:
  - *Embryo-fetal toxicity:* Drug is embryotoxic, fetotoxic, and teratogenic. Female patients of reproductive potential should have a negative pregnancy test prior to starting glasdegib, and be instructed to use effective contraception during and for at least 30 days after the last drug dose. Teach male patients with female partners of reproductive potential or a pregnant partner, to use effective contraception during and for at least 30 days after last drug dose. Patients should be taught not to donate blood during treatment or for at least 30 days after last dose as blood may be given to a pregnant patient.
  - *QTc interval prolongation:* Patients can develop prolonged QTc interval (prolonged ventricular repolarization), ventricular arrhythmias including ventricular tachycardia, and fibrillation resulting in sudden death especially if serum magnesium and potassium are low. During clinical trials, 5% of patients had a QTc interval > 500 ms, and 4% had an increase from baseline QTc > 60 ms. Monitor ECGs and serum electrolytes closely. Concomitant use of other drugs which prolong the QTc interval and CYP3A4 inhibitors may further increase the risk of QTc prolongation and should be avoided. In patients with congenital long QT syndrome, CHF, electrolyte abnormalities, or those taking other QTc prolonging medications will require more frequent ECG monitoring. If the patient's QTc interval is > 500 ms, interrupt glasdegib, and discontinue drug permanently if patient with prolonged QTc interval has signs or symptoms of life-threatening arrhythmia (see Dose Modifications).
- Drug may impair male fertility in men of reproductive potential irreversibly. Teach patient how to find information about fertility preservation prior to starting treatment as appropriate.

Potential Toxicities/Side Effects and the Nursing Process

I.   ALTERATION IN SEXUALITY/REPRODUCTION related to POTENTIAL TERATOGENICITY

Defining Characteristics: Glasdegib is teratogenic, embryotoxic, and fetotoxic, causing embryo-fetal death and severe birth defects. Drug may be excreted in the semen. Drug can also be passed through blood transfusions to pregnant patients.

Nursing Implications: Assess reproductive status, sexual activity, and birth control measures used for both men and women. Teach male patients to use highly effective contraception, even after vasectomy, during sexual intercourse with female partners of reproductive potential or who are pregnant, while receiving therapy and for at least 30 days after the last dose. Ensure that women have had a negative pregnancy test before starting the drug. Teach women to use highly effective contraception measures prior to starting therapy, and to continue using it for at least 30 days after last dose of glasdegib. Mothers should not nurse while receiving glasdegib and for at least 30 days after last dose. Patients of reproductive potential may develop impaired fertility and should be counseled about fertility preservation prior to starting therapy as appropriate. Teach patients not to donate blood while taking glasdegib and for at least 30 days after the last drug dose.

II.   POTENTIAL FOR INFECTION, BLEEDING AND FATIGUE related to BONE MARROW SUPPRESSION

Defining Characteristics: Low-dose cytarabine, with which glasdegib is given, is myelosuppressive. Anemia occurred in 43% (was ≥grade 3 in 41%), febrile neutropenia 31% (31% ≥grade 3), and thrombocytopenia in 30% of patients (30% ≥grade 3). Hemorrhage occurred in 36% of patients and was severe in 6%. Pneumonia occurred in 19% (15% ≥grade 3). Fatigue was common and affected 36% of patients.

Nursing Implications: Assess baseline WBC, differential, absolute neutrophil counts, platelets baseline, and monitor at least once weekly for the 1st month. Assess skin integrity, potential for infection, and teach patient measures to prevent infection (e.g., keeping skin intact, avoiding sources of infection, good hand-washing). Teach patient to report any signs/symptoms of infection (e.g., redness, heat, exudate on skin, temperature ≥ 100.4°F, cough, sputum production, dysuria). Assess for signs/symptoms of infection during therapy and at each visit. If a patient develops an infection, discuss with physician or midlevel practitioner interrupting or discontinuing drug and beginning appropriate antimicrobial treatment. See Dose Modifications.

III.   ALTERATION IN CIRCULATION, POTENTIAL related to QTc PROLONGATION AND ARRTHYMIA DEVELOPMENT

Defining Characteristics: Glasdegib can prolong QTc interval, the period of ventricular repolarization. If the serum magnesium and/or potassium are low, then this increases the risk for ventricular arrthymia development. Ventricular tachycardia (torsades de pointes and ventricular fibrillation can result in sudden death. In the clinical trials, QTc was closely monitored so that arrthymia did not develop. Five percent of patients developed QTc interval > 500 ms and 4% had an increase from baseline QTc of > 60 ms. Normal QTc interval is 0.2–0.4 seconds (200–400 millisec or ms) but vary on whether male or female, and heart rate. The c in QTc indicates it is corrected for the variable of heart rate. CTCAE indicate that grade I is QTc > 450–480 ms, grade 2 QTC > 481–500 ms, grade 3 QTc > 501 ms on at least 2 separate ECGs, and grade 4 QTc > 501 ms with life-threatening symptoms (arrhythmia, CHF, hypotension, shock, syncope, torsades de pointes). See *Chapter 4* introduction for a fuller discussion.

Nursing Implications: Review patient's medication profile to identify strong CYP3A4 inhibitors or drugs causing QTc prolongation; if found, discuss with pharmacist and physician/NP/PA alternative drugs to decrease risk of QTc prolongation once glasdegib is started. Assess baseline ECG (QTc interval), serum electrolytes. If ECG has prolonged QTc, expect to recheck ECG a second time. Obtain orders to correct abnormal magnesium or potassium serum levels prior to starting glasdegib. Monitor electrolytes and renal function once monthly throughout therapy or more frequently if abnormal QTc. Monitor ECG approximately 1 week after starting glasdegib, and then once monthly for the next 2 months for QTc prolongation beyond baseline interval during therapy.

IV.   POTENTIAL ALTERATION IN NUTRITION related to DYSGEUSIA, NAUSEA, DIARRHEA, CONSTIPATION, NAUSEA, VOMITING, DECREASED APPETITE, HEPATOTOXICITY

Defining Characteristics: Nutritional impact symptoms may occur. Incidence of dysgeusia was 21%, nausea 29%, decreased appetite 21%, constipation 20%, abdominal pain 19%, diarrhea 18%, and vomiting. Elevations in LFTs occurred; increased AST in 28%, serum bilirubin in 25%, ALT in 24%, and alkaline phosphatase increased in 23% of patients.

Nursing Implications: Assess nutritional status, weight, bowel-elimination status pattern baseline and at each visit. Assess LFTs baseline and as ordered. Teach patient self-care measures: to take OTC antidiarrheal or anticonstipation medication as needed; to take antinausea medicine as prescribed; to modify diet for diarrhea, constipation, nausea or vomiting; high-calorie, high-protein foods frequently in small amounts if decreased taste, appetite and/or weight loss; taste stimulation strategies for altered taste. Teach patient to report any symptoms that do not resolve or improve with the established plan. To increase appetite, encourage patients to use a small plate, small portions and not to fill the plate with food; take antiemetic 30 minutes prior to eating, if nausea, and to eat small, frequent meals. Arrange dietary consultation if available and needed. Note trends in weight and discuss with provider if significant.

Drug: everolimus (Afinitor)

Class: mTOR inhibitor.

Mechanism of Action: Everolimus inhibits mTOR, so it reduces tumor cell division, growth of blood vessel, and cell metabolism. mTOR is an intracellular serine-threonine kinase protein that regulates cell proliferation and angiogenesis. It is found in the cytoplasm and turns on and off the translation of signals that tell the cell's protein factory (ribosomes) to make proteins. Proteins control all the cell functions. Proteins that activate mTOR are growth signals from EGF, insulin-like growth factor (IGF), and VEGFs. Proteins that stop mTOR activity are tuberous sclerosis complex (TSC) 1 and 2, and if there are not enough nutrients to support more cells, mTOR activity is blocked. As an mTOR inhibitor, everolimus interferes with the central regulation of tumor cell division, metabolism, and angiogenesis. Blocking this important protein results in cell cycle arrest and cell death. mTOR is also a very important component of the P13K/AKT signaling pathway that is often dysregulated in solid tumors, as it plays a role in cell cycle regulation, and it also suppresses apoptosis (Chang et al., 2003).

Specifically, everolimus binds to an intracellular protein, FKBP-12, a protein-folding chaperone, thus inhibiting mTOR kinase activity. Everolimus also reduces the activity of downstream effectors of mTOR, which are involved in protein synthesis, inhibits the expression of HIF-1, and reduces expression of vascular endothelial growth factor (VEGF). Through these actions, everolimus reduces cell proliferation, angiogenesis, and glucose uptake (Novartis, 2016).

Drug is also used as an immunosuppressant to prevent transplanted organ rejection; it reduces incidence of chronic allograft vasculopathy in heart transplant patients (drug name Certican). Drug is a proliferation signal inhibitor and inhibits the proliferation and clonal expansion of antigen-activated T-cells, which are stimulated by cytokines IL-2 and IL-5. Cells are arrested in the G1 phase of the cell cycle.

Metabolism: Peak serum concentrations achieved in 1–2 hours after oral dosing, with steady state reached within 2 weeks with once-daily dosing. mTOR inhibition is complete after a 10-mg oral daily dose. In clinical studies, a high-fat meal reduced AUC by 16%, but the manufacturer recommends the dose be given without regard to meals. Plasma binding is about 74%. Drug is a substrate of CYP3A4 and PgP (P-glycoprotein). Everolimus is mainly metabolized by CYP3A4 in the liver and to some extent in the intestinal wall and is a substrate for the multidrug efflux pump P-glycoprotein. It is metabolized into six metabolites, which have less activity than the intact drug. The mean elimination half-life of everolimus is 30 hours, with 80% of drug excreted in the feces, and 5% in the urine. Moderate hepatic dysfunction (Child-Pugh Class B) doubles the AUC, so dose should be reduced in these patients. Oral clearance of the drug is 20% higher in African American patients compared to Caucasian, and Japanese patients had, on average exposures, a higher drug exposure compared to non-Japanese. The implications of ethnic differences are unknown.

Indications:
Afinitor (everolimus) tablets are indicated for the treatment of:
- Postmenopausal women with advanced hormone receptor-positive, HER2-negative, breast cancer (advanced HR+ BC) in combination with exemestane, after failure of treatment with letrozole or anastrozole.
- Adults with progressive neuroendocrine tumors of pancreatic origin (PNETs) and adults with progressive, well-differentiated, nonfunctional neuroendocrine tumors (NETs) of GI

origin or lung origin that are unresectable, locally advanced, or metastatic. Everolimus is NOT indicated for the treatment of patients with functional carcinoid tumors.
- Adults with advanced renal cell carcinoma (RCC) after failure of treatment with sunitinib or sorafenib.
- Adults with renal angiomyolipoma and tuberous sclerosis complex (TSC), not requiring immediate surgery.

Afinitor (everolimus) tablets and Disperz are indicated for the treatment of:
- Pediatric and adult patients with tuberous sclerosis complex (TSC) who have subependymal giant cell astrocytoma (SEGA) that requires therapeutic intervention but cannot be curatively resected.

Afinitor (everolimus) Disperz is indicated for the treatment of:
- Adjunctive treatment of adult and pediatric patients aged 2 years and older with TSC-associated partial-onset seizures.

Dosage/Range:
- Everolimus (Afinitor) is available in two dosage forms: Afinitor tablets (for all indications) and tablets for oral suspension (Afinitor Disperz, for treatment of patients with SEGA and TSC).
- See package insert for dose adjustment and management recommendations for adverse reactions.

Patients with HR+ BC (HER2-negative), advanced NET, advanced RCC, or renal angiomyolipoma with (TSC):
- 10 mg once daily at the same time every day, consistently with or without food. Swallow tablet whole with a glass of water; do not crush or break tablets.
- If the patient has hepatic impairment, reduce the everolimus dose as serum exposure of everolimus is increased.
- Mild impairment (Child-Pugh Class A): 7.5 mg PO daily for patients with; the dose may be decreased to 5 mg if not well tolerated.
- Moderate hepatic impairment (Child-Pugh Class B): 5 mg PO daily for patients with the dose may be decreased to 2.5 mg if not well tolerated.
- Severe hepatic impairment (Child-Pugh Class C): if the desired benefit outweighs the risk, 2.5 mg PO daily for patients. Do not exceed dose of 2.5 mg PO daily.
- Dose adjustments should be made if a patient's hepatic (Child-Pugh) status changes during treatment.
- Avoid concomitant use of strong CYP3A4/PgP inhibitors (e.g., ketoconazole, itraconazole, clarithromycin, attazanavir, nefazodone, saquinavir, telithromycin, ritonavir, indinavir, nelfinavir, voriconazole).
  - If moderate inhibitors of CYP3A4 and/or P-glycoprotein (PgP) are required (e.g., amprenavir, fosamprenavir, aprepitant, erythromycin, fluconazole, verapamil, diltiazem), reduce the everolimus dose to 2.5 mg once daily; if tolerated, consider increasing to 5 mg once daily.
  - If the moderate inhibitor is discontinued, allow a washout period of 2–3 days before the everolimus dose is increased. The everolimus dose should be returned to the dose used prior to starting the moderate CYP3A4/PgP inhibitor.

- Avoid concomitant strong CYP3A4/PgP inducers (e.g., phenytoin, carbamazepine, rifampin, rifabutin, rifapentine, phenobarbital).
  - If coadministration with a strong CYP3A4 inducer is required, consider doubling the everolimus daily dose in 5-mg increments or less.
  - If the strong CYP3A4 drug is discontinued, allow a washout period of 3–5 days before the everolimus dose is returned to the original dose used before start of the strong CYP3A4 inducer.
- AVOID coadministration with St. John's wort, as herbal may decrease everolimus AUC unpredictably.
  - Management of severe or intolerable adverse reactions may require temporary dose interruption (with or without a dose reduction) or discontinuation. If a dose reduction is needed, suggested dose is approximately 50% lower than the daily dose previously administered (Novartis, 2018).
  - See package insert for (Table 2) dose adjustment and management recommendations for adverse reactions (Novartis, April 2018).
  - Continue treatment until disease progression or unacceptable toxicity occurs.

Subependymal Giant Cell Astrocytoma (SEGA) with TSC:
- Recommended starting dose:
  - 4.5 mg/m^2 once daily; adjust dose to attain trough concentration of 5–15 ng/mL. Use serum concentration to guide subsequent dosing.
  - Severe hepatic impairment (Child-Pugh C) or requiring *moderate CYP3A4 and/or PgP inhibitors*, reduce the starting dose of Afinitor tablets or Afinitor Disperz by 50% to 2.5 mg/m^2 once daily. If further dose reduction is necessary for toxicity when at the lowest dose, administer every other day. See package insert for full discussion.
- Assess serum trough concentration two weeks after starting therapy, after a change in dose, a change in coadministration of CYP3A4 and/or PgP inducers or inhibitors, a change in hepatic function, or a change in dosage form between Afinitor tablets and Afinitor Disperz.
- Avoid concomitant use of strong CYP3A4/PgP inhibitors. If concomitant use of moderate CYP3A4/PgP inhibitors (e.g., amprenavir, fosamprenavir, aprepitant, erythromycin, fluconazole, verapamil, diltiazem) is required:
  - Reduce Affinitor tablet or Disperz dose by 50%. Administer every other day if dose reduction is required for patients receiving the lowest available strength, and maintain trough concentration 5–15 ng/mL.
  - Assess everolimus trough concentrations approximately 2 weeks after dose reduction.
  - When the moderate inhibitor is discontinued, resume the Afinitor dose that was used before starting the inhibitor 2–3 days after discontinuation. Assess everolimus trough concentrations approximately 2 weeks later.
- Avoid the concomitant use of strong CYP3A4/PgP inducers. If concomitant use of strong inducers of CYP3A4 is required (no alternatives available), double the dose of Afinitor to 9 mg/m^2 once daily. Round to the nearest strength of Afinitor tablets or Disperz.
  - Assess everolimus trough concentration 2 weeks after doubling dose and adjust dose as necessary to maintain a trough concentration of 5–15 ng/mL.

- If the strong CYP3A4/PgP inducer is discontinued, return the Afinitor tablet or Afinitor Disperz dose to that used before starting the strong CYP3A4/PgP inducer. Assess everolimus trough concentrations approximately 2 weeks later. See package insert.
- If dose reduction is required for patients receiving the lowest available strength, administer every other day.
- Once a stable dose is attained, monitor trough concentrations every 3–6 months in patients with changing body surface area, or every 6–12 months in patients with stable BSA for the duration of treatment.
- Temporarily interrupt or permanently discontinue Afinitor tablets or Disperz for severe or intolerable adverse reactions. See package insert for dose modifications for toxicity.
  - If dose reduction required when reinitiating therapy, reduce dose by approximately 50%.
  - If the patient is receiving the lowest available strength, administer every other day.

Recommended Dosage for TSC-Associated Partial Onset Seizures: Afinitor Disperz 5 mg/m^2 once daily until disease progression or unacceptable toxicity.
- Monitor whole blood trough concentrations and titrate dose to attain trough conentrations of 5 nanograms (ng)/mL–15 ng/mL.
- Time therapeutic drug monitoring at (1) 1–2 weeks after initiation of afinitor disperz; (2) 1–2 weeks after any dose modification; (3) 1–2 weeks after a switch between Afinitor and Afinitor Disperz; (4) 2 weeks after initiation or discontinuation of P-gp and moderate CYP3A4 inhibitor; (5) 2 weeks after initiation or discontinuation of P-gp and strong CYP3A4 inhibitor; (6) 2 weeks after change in hepatic function; (7) every 3–6 months on a stable dose with changing BSA; (8) every 6–12 months on a stable dose and stable BSA.

Dose Modification for Adverse Effects: See package insert for (Table 2) dose adjustment and management recommendations for adverse reactions (Novartis, April 2018). Hepatic impairment: (1) breast cancer, NET, RCC, or TSC-associated renal angiomyolipoma patients: reduce dose; (2) TSC-associated SEGA or TSC-associated partial-onset seizures with severe hepatic impairment: reduce starting dose and adjust dose to attain target trough concentrations.

Drug Preparation:
- Afinitor Oral, tablets available in 2.5-mg, 5-mg, 7.5-mg, and 10-mg tablets with no score.
- Afinitor Disperz (tablets for oral suspension): 2-mg, 3-mg, 5-mg tablets for oral suspension, no score.

Drug Administration:
- Do not combine the 2 dosage forms (Afinitor tablets and Afinitor Disperz). Use one dosage form or the other.
- Teach patients to AVOID grapefruit, grapefruit juice, and any other nutritional supplements that inhibit cytochrome P450 or PgP activity. Patient should NOT take St. John's wort.
- Tablets: Orally, once daily at the same time of day, either consistently with or without food. The patient should swallow tablet whole with a glass of water, and tablets should not be crushed or chewed.

- Afinitor Disperz (Afinitor tablets for oral suspension) for patients with SEGA and TSC, in conjunction with therapeutic drug monitoring.
  - Wear gloves to avoid contact with everolimus when preparing suspension.

Using an oral syringe:
- Place prescribed dose of Afinitor Disperz into a 10-mL syringe. DO NOT exceed a total of 10 mg per syringe. Use an additional syringe if higher doses are required. Do not break or crush tablets.
- Draw about 5 mL of water and 4 mL of air into the syringe. Place the filled syringe into a container (tip up) for 3 minutes, until the Afinitor Disperz tablets are in suspension. Gently invert the syringe 5 times immediately prior to administration.
- After administration of the prepared suspension, draw 5 mL of water and 4 mL of air into the same syringe, swirling the contents to suspend the remaining particles. Administer the entire contents of the syringe.

Using a small drinking glass:
- Place the prescribed dose of Afinitor Disperz into a small drinking glass (maximum 100 mL), containing 25 mL of water. Do not exceed a total of 10 mg per syringe. Use an additional glass if higher doses are required. Do not break or crush tablets.
- Allow 3 minutes for suspension to occur. Stir the contents gently with a spoon, immediately prior to drinking.
- After administration of the prepared suspension, add 25 mL of water and stir with the same spoon to resuspend remaining particles; administer the entire contents of the glass.
- Disperse tablet completely in glass of water (~30 mL) by gently stirring immediately before drinking dose; rinse glass with same volume of water, and swallow the rinse completely to ensure that the entire dose is taken. Anyone who prepares the suspension for another person should wear gloves to avoid possible contact with the medicine. Take the suspension at about the same time each day, with or without food.
- Administer immediately after preparation; discard if not used within 60 minutes.
- Administer suspension orally, once daily at the same time every day, consistently with or without food.
- Monitor renal function, blood glucose, lipids, and hematologic parameters baseline and periodically during therapy.
- Drug is contraindicated in patients who are hypersensitive to the drug or other mTOR inhibitors (e.g., rapamycin derivative).
- Hypersensitivity reactions may include anaphylaxis, dyspnea, flushing, chest pain, or angioedema.

Drug Interactions:
- Everolimus is a substrate of CYP3A and also a substrate and moderate inhibitor of P-glycoprotein multidrug efflux pump. It is also a competitive inhibitor of CYP3A4 and a mixed inhibitor of CYP2D6.

HR+ BC, RCC, TSC:
- Coadministration with strong CYP3A4 inhibitors (e.g., ketoconazole, itraconazole, voriconazole, clarithromycin, nafazodone, saquinavir, telithromycin, ritonavir, indinavir, nelfinavir, voriconazole): AVOID.
- Coadministration with moderate CYP3A4 and/or PgP inhibitors (e.g., amprenavir, fosamprenavir, aprepitant, erythromycin, fluconazole, verapamil, diltiazem): AVOID; if unavoidable, see dosage and assessment after dose changes in Dosage section. If the interacting drug is discontinued, a washout period of 2–3 days should occur before the everolimus dose is increased to the dose prior to initiation of the moderate CYP3A4 and/or PgP inhibitor.
- Coadministration with strong CYP3A4 inducer (e.g., phenytoin, carbamazepine, rifampin, rifabutin, rifapentine, phenobarbital): AVOID; if unavoidable, see dosage and assessment after dose, in Dosage section.
- Grapefruit and grapefruit juice: AVOID; do not take while receiving everolimus.
- St. John's wort can increase the metabolism of everolimus and thus lower drug serum levels; do not use together.
- Inhibitors of P-glycoprotein may decrease the efflux of everolimus from intestinal cells and increase everolimus blood concentrations, so it should be avoided (e.g., ketoconazole, quinidine, erythromycin, verapamil, probenecid, cimetidine). Do NOT co-administer.
- Everolimus is a competitive inhibitor of CYP3A4 and of CYP2D6 microsomal pathways, so that drugs metabolized via these pathways may have higher serum levels; if the drug has a narrow therapeutic window, monitor for side effects or decrease dose of interacting drug.

Lab Effects/Interference:
- Increased creatinine, urinary protein, blood glucose, lipids (hyperlipidemia, hypertriglyceridemia).
- Decreased hemoglobin, lymphocytes, platelets, neutrophils.

Special Considerations:
- Most common adverse reactions (incidence ≥ 30%) include:
  - HR+ BC, advanced PNET, advanced RCC: stomatitis, infections, rash, fatigue, diarrhea, edema, abdominal pain, nausea, fever, asthenia, cough, headache, decreased appetite.
  - Renal angiomyolipoma with TSC: stomatitis.
  - SEGA with TSC: stomatitis, URI.
- Warnings and Precautions:
  - *Noninfectious pneumonitis:* Noninfectious pneumonitis is a class effect of rapamycin derivatives and may occur in up to 19% of patients (up to 4% grade 3, 0.2% grade 4); monitor patients for clinical symptoms and consider noninfectious pneumonitis in the differential (e.g., hypoxia, pleural effusion, cough, dyspnea when other causes have been excluded). Pneumonitis has been reported even when patient is receiving a reduced dose of everolimus. Teach patient to report any new or worsening respiratory symptoms right away. If symptoms occur:
    - Few or no symptoms but with radiological changes suggestive of noninfectious pneumonitis: continue everolimus therapy without dose alteration.

- Moderate symptoms: consider dose interruption until symptoms improve; consider corticosteroid therapy if needed. When symptoms improve, may introduce everolimus at 50% lower than the previous daily dose.
  - Grade 3: interrupt drug until resolution to ≤ grade 1; corticosteroids may be indicated. When this occurs, may reintroduce everolimus at 50% lower than the previous daily dose, depending upon the individual clinical circumstances.
  - Grade 4: discontinue everolimus. Corticosteroids may be needed to manage clinical symptoms.
- *Infections:* Everolimus is immunosuppressive, and patients may be at increased risk for developing bacterial, fungal, viral, or protoloan infections, including opportunistic infections, localized, and systemic infections (e.g., pneumonia, mycobacterial infections). Incidence of grade 3–4 infections was 10% and 3% respectively (Novartis, 2018).
  - Invasive fungal infections such as aspergillosis or candidiasis and viral infections (including reactivation of hepatitis B virus) have been reported, and some severe infections have been fatal.
  - Patients should complete treatment of preexisting invasive fungal infections prior to starting everolimus.
  - Monitor patients closely for signs/symptoms and treat promptly with appropriate antimicrobials. If an invasive systemic fungal infection is diagnosed, interruption or discontinuation of everolimus should be considered, and the infection treated with antifungal therapy.
- *Severe HSRs:* may include anaphylaxis, dyspnea, flushing, chest pain, and angioedema (swelling of airway/tongue, with or without respiratory impairment. Incidence of grade 3 is 1%. Assess for, and teach patient to report/seek emergency care: anaphylaxis, dyspnea, flushing, chest pain, angioedema, and stop drug if these occur. Permanently discontinue drug if clinically significant hypersensitivity develops.
- *Angiogedema with concomitant use of Angiotensin-Converting Enzyme (ACE) Inhibitors*: patients taking ACE inhibitors may be at increased risk (e.g., swelling of airways or tongue, with or without respiratory compromise). Incidence was 6.8% in patients receiving everolimus, compared to 1.3% in the control arm with an ACE inhibitor (Novartis, 2016).
- *Stomatitis, oral ulceration*: mouth ulcers, stomatitis, and oral mucositis are common (incidence 44–78% across clinical trials). Grade 3 or 4 stomatitis occurred in 4–9% of patients.
  - Teach patient to use systematic oral rinsing and topical treatments (excluding alcohol, hydrogen peroxide, iodine or thyme-containing mouth rinses, which can harm the mucosa).
  - Do not use antifungal agents unless an oral fungal infection has been diagnosed.
- *Renal failure*: renal failure, including acute renal failure, has occurred and some cases have been fatal. Monitor renal function tests (BUN, urinary protein, or serum creatinine) baseline and periodically during treatment; patients with additional risk factors should be assessed more frequently. Elevations of serum creatinine and proteinuria may occur.
- *Impaired wound healing*: increased risk of wound-related complications, such as wound dehiscence, wound infection, incisional hernia, lymphocele, seroma, which may require surgical intervention. Monitor patient closely and use caution in the perioperative period.

- *Geriatric patients*: in HR+ BC patients, the incidence of death from any cause within 28 days of the last everolimus dose was 6% in patients age 65 or older, compared to 2% in those younger than age 65. Thirty-three percent of patients age ≥ 65 permanently discontinued the drug due to adverse reactions, compared to 17% in patients < 65 years of age. Monitor elderly patients closely and ensure appropriate dose reductions are made for adverse effects.
- *Metabolic disorders:* Incidence of hyperglycemia was 75%, hypercholesterolemia 86%, and hypertriglyceridemia 73%.
  - Non-diabetic patients: monitor FBS and lipid profile prior to starting drug, and annually thereafter.
  - Diabetic patients: monitor FBS and lipid profile baseline and frequently during therapy; monitor lipids baseline and annually thereafter unless elevated. Discuss with physician/NP/PA optimal control of glucose and lipids before starting drug. If grade 3–4 metabolic events occur, drug should be held or permanently discontinued based on severity (see package insert).
- *Myelosuppression:* Anemia, lymphopenia, neutropenia, an dthrombocytopenia may occur. Grade 3 lab abnormalities occurred in 16%, and grade 4 in 2%. Monitor CBC/differential baseline, then every 6 months for the first year, then annually.
- *Drug-drug interactions* can be significant. AVOID coadministration with strong CYP3A4/PgP inhibitors; dose-reduce everolimus if coadministered with a moderate CYP3A4/PgP inhibitor; and a dose increase is recommended if coadministered with a strong CYP3A4/PgP inducer.
- *Hepatic impairment* increases systemic exposure to everolimus, and dose must be reduced. See dosage.
- *Risk of infection or reduced immune response with vaccinations:* Avoid live vaccines, and teach patient to avoid close contact with individuals who have received live vaccines (e.g., intranasal influenza, measles, mumps, rubella, oral polio, BCG, yellow fever, varicella, and TY21a typhoid vaccines). Pediatric patients should complete the recommended childhood series of vaccinations according to the American Council on Immunization Practices (ACIP) before starting the drug (accelerated vaccination schedule may be appropriate).
- *Embryo-fetal toxicity:* Teach females of reproductive potential to use effective contraception to avoid pregnancy during treatment and for 8 weeks after the last dose of everolimus. Advise male patients with female partners of reproductive potential to use effective contraception during treatment with the drug and for 4 weeks after last drug dose.
- Nursing mothers: A decision should be made to discontinue the nursing or to discontinue the drug, taking into account the importance of the drug to the mother's health.

Potential Toxicities/Side Effects and the Nursing Process

I.   POTENTIAL FOR INFECTION related to IMMUNOSUPPRESSION

Defining Characteristics: Everolimus is immunosuppressive and increases risk for opportunistic infections. Infections may be localized or systemic and include pneumonia, other bacterial infections, and invasive fungal infections (e.g., aspergillosis, candidiasis).

Incidence is approximately 37%, with 7% grade 3 and 3% grade 4. Cough occurs in 30% of patients, pyrexia in 20%, and dyspnea in 24%. In addition, some patients may experience neutropenia (14%).

Nursing Implications: Assess baseline WBC, lymphocyte, and neutrophil counts and monitor frequently during therapy. Assess skin integrity, potential for infection, and teach patient measures to prevent infection (e.g., keeping skin intact, avoiding sources of infection, good hand-washing). Teach patient to report any signs/symptoms of infection (e.g., redness, heat, exudate on skin, temperature ≥ 100.4°F, cough, sputum production, dysuria). Assess for signs/symptoms of infection during therapy and at each visit. If a patient develops an infection, discuss with physician or midlevel practitioner interrupting or discontinuing drug and beginning appropriate antimicrobial treatment. If the patient is receiving therapy for a preexisting invasive fungal infection, the patient should complete therapy before starting therapy with everolimus. If during everolimus therapy a diagnosis of systemic fungal infection is made, discontinue everolimus and treat with appropriate antifungal therapy.

II.   POTENTIAL ALTERATION IN NUTRITION, LESS THAN BODY REQUIREMENTS, related to STOMATITIS, HYPERGLYCEMIA, HYPERTRIGLYCERIDEMIA, HYPOPHOSPHATEMIA, INCREASED SERUM CREATININE, ANOREXIA, NAUSEA, VOMITING, DIARRHEA

Defining Characteristics: In clinical studies, oral mucositis (e.g., stomatitis, mouth ulcers) affected 44% of patients (compared with 7% placebo) with advanced RCC, and 86% of SEGA patients. In general, this is grade 1 or 2. Six percent of PNET developed grades 3–4. Hyperglycemia, hypercholesteremia, and hypophosphatemia have been reported. mTOR is involved in insulin signaling, which possibly explains the hypertriglyceridemia and hyperglycemia. Drug can also increase serum creatinine. Anorexia occurs in 25% of patients. Diarrhea occurs in about 30% of patients, nausea in 26%, and vomiting in 20%.

Nursing Implications: Assess baseline oral mucosa, nutritional status, and appetite. Assess fasting serum triglycerides, cholesterol, phosphate, glucose, BUN, and serum creatinine baseline and during treatment with the drug. Teach the patient to report signs/ symptoms of hyperglycemia (polyuria, polydipsia, polyphagia). Discuss with physician correction of lipids, triglycerides, and glucose if baseline tests are abnormal, prior to beginning everolimus therapy. Assess oral mucosa prior to drug administration, as well as ability to eat and drink at each visit; instruct patient to self-assess and report changes, including the appearance of white patches (candida), pain, and inability to eat or drink. Teach patient oral hygiene measures and self-assessment and to avoid alcohol- or peroxide-containing mouthwashes. Antifungal agents should not be used unless fungal infection has been diagnosed. If oral mucositis is painful, or candida is present, discuss prescription of topical analgesics and anti-candidiasis oral treatment. Discuss appropriate antiemetics (e.g., prochlorperazine) and antidiarrheal (e.g., loperamide) medicines if patient develops these symptoms. Teach patient to notify physician/nurse if oral ulcers occur, if excessive thirst occurs, or any increase in volume or frequency of urination occurs. In addition, call nurse or physician for diarrhea, nausea, or vomiting that does not resolve within 24 hours with recommended OTC medicines. Notify physician of any abnormalities, and discuss implications and management.

III.   ALTERATION IN SKIN INTEGRITY, POTENTIAL, related to RASH

Defining Characteristics: Rash has been reported in 29% of patients. In addition, pruritus was reported in 14% and dry skin in 13% of patients on clinical trials.

Nursing Implications: Assess patient skin integrity, including nails baseline and regularly during treatment. Teach patient self-assessment and local comfort measures, including the use of water-based emollients. Teach patient to report skin changes and, if self-care is ineffective, to discuss plan with physician, especially if severe.

IV.   ALTERATION IN COMFORT AND ACTIVITY TOLERANCE, POTENTIAL, related to ASTHENIA, ANEMIA

Defining Characteristics: Asthenia, weakness (affects 33% vs 23%), fatigue 31%, and anemia (92% overall, with 12% grade 3 and 1% grade 4, compared to placebo all grades 79% and 5% grade 3). Headache affects 19%.

Nursing Implications: Assess baseline CBC, Hgb, comfort, and activity tolerance, and reassess during treatment, asking patient to identify what activities now unable to do, sleep habits, and also state of mind. Discuss alternating rest and activity periods and also possibility of other family members or friends assisting with energy-consuming responsibilities to increase energy reserve. Teach patient to report increasing fatigue, signs of severe anemia (shortness of breath, chest pain/angina, headaches). Monitor hemoglobin/hematocrit; discuss transfusion with physician if signs/symptoms develop or hematocrit falls < 25 mg/dL. Teach patient about diet high in iron.

Drug: gefitinib (Iressa)

Class: Kinase inhibitor; TKI of EGFR.

Mechanism of Action: Reversibly inhibits kinase activity in EGFR unmutated (wild-type) and some EGFR mutated (exon 19 deletion or exon 21 point mutation L858R) cancer cells. It also inhibits insulin-like growth factor (IGF) and PDGF signaling.

Metabolism: After oral dosing, peak plasma level occurs 3–7 hours after dosing and is not influenced by food intake. It is extensively distributed throughout the body, and is 90% protein-bound. Drug is a substrate for membrane transport P-glycoprotein (P-gp), but this does not influence drug absorption. Gefitinib is extensively metabolized by the liver, predominantly by CYP3A4. Elimination half-life is 48 hours after IV administration, and steady state is reached in 10 days. Drug and its metabolites are excreted in feces (86%) and to a lesser degree, urine (< 4%). Drug exposure (AUC) is increased by 40% in patients with mild hepatic impairment, 263% if moderate impairment, and 166% in patients with severe impairment. If the patient has a CYP2D6 poor metabolizer phenotype, the patient is at risk for increased gefitinib AUC, and patient should be monitored closely for toxicity. Coadministration with a strong CYP3A4 inducer (e.g., rifampin) reduced gefitinib AUC by 83% while coadministration of a CYP3A4 inhibitor (e.g., itraconazole), increased mean gefitinib AUC by 80%. Drugs affecting gastric pH (e.g., sodium bicarbonate, pH above 5.0) decreased the gefitinib AUC by 47%.

Indication: First-line treatment of metastatic NSCLC that has the following EGFR mutations: exon 19 deletions or exon 21 (L858R) substitution mutations. Safety and efficacy have not been established in patients with metastatic NSCLC whose tumors have mutations other than those for which the indication was given.

Dosage/Range: Recommended dose is 250 mg PO once daily without regard to food intake.

Dose Modifications: Withhold drug for up to 14 days for (NCI CTCAE)

- Acute or worsening pulmonary symptoms (e.g., dyspnea, cough, fever).
- Grade 2 or higher increases in AST and/or ALT.
- Grade 3 or higher diarrhea.
- Severe or worsening ocular disorders (e.g., keratitis).
- Grade 3 or higher skin reactions.

Permanently discontinue drug for
- Confirmed interstitial lung disease (ILD).
- Severe hepatic impairment.
- GI perforation.
- Persistent ulcerative keratitis.

Drug Preparation: None. Drug tablets should be stored at room temperature 68–77°F (20–25°C). If the patient has difficulty swallowing, the tablet should be placed in 4–8 ounces of water and stirred for about 15 minutes until it dissolves.

Drug Administration:
- Teach patient (1) to take tablet once daily with or without food, OR if taking the dissolved tablet in water, or if difficult or unable to swallow the tablet, (2) have the patient immediately drink the solution containing the dissolved tablet or administer the dose through a nasogastric (NG) tube. Rinse the container used to dissolve the tablet with an additional 4–8 ounces of water and have the patient drink it immediately or administer it through the NG tube. (3) Do NOT take a missed dose within 12 hours of the next dose.
- Assess ALT and AST baseline and frequently during therapy.
- Assess for side effects, including changes in vision, and teach patient to report visual changes right away.

Drug Interactions:
- CYP3A4 inducers: will increase gefitinib metabolism and decrease the gefitinib plasma concentration. If patient must take a strong CYP3A4 inducer (e.g., rifampicin, phenytoin, or tricyclic antidepressants) concomitantly, the gefitinib dose should be increased to 500 mg daily.
- CYP3A4 inhibitors: will decrease gefitinib metabolism and increase the gefitinib plasma concentration. If the patient must take a strong inhibitor (e.g., ketoconazole, itraconazole) concomitantly, monitor patients closely for adverse reactions.
- Drugs affecting gastric pH: Drugs increasing gastric pH (e.g., PPIs, histamine H_2-receptor antagonists, antacids) may decrease gefitinib plasma concentration. Avoid concomitant administration of PPIs. If a PPI is required, the patient should be taught to administer gefitinib 12 hours after the last dose or 12 hours before the next dose of the PPI. If an H_2-receptor antagonist or antacid is required, the patient should take gefitinib 6 hours after or before an H_2-receptor antagonist or antacid.
- Warfarin: increased risk for bleeding and hemorrhage. Monitor INR or prothrombin time closely and teach patient to report any bleeding right away.

Lab Effects/Interference:
- Increased AST, ALT
- Proteinuria

Special Considerations:
- Most common adverse reactions occurring in > 20% of patients, and greater than placebo were skin reactions and diarrhea. Drug should be interrupted for up to 14 days for NCI CTCAE grade 3 or higher diarrhea, or grade 3 or higher skin reactions. Drug should be resumed when toxicity fully resolves or improves to Grade 1.
- Warnings and Precautions:
  - *ILD:* Hold drug for worsening pulmonary symptoms (e.g., dyspnea, cough, fever), and discontinue drug if ILD confirmed.
  - *Hepatotoxicity:* Monitor during therapy; hold drug for worsening liver function (e.g., grade 2 or higher in ALT and/or AST), and discontinue gefitinib if severe.
  - *GI perforation:* Occurs rarely (0.1%); discontinue drug if it occurs.
  - **Severe or persistent diarrhea:** Incidence of grade 3/4 toxicity 3%. Hold drug for up to 14 days for grade 3 or higher diarrhea.
  - *Ocular disorders including keratitis* (e.g., corneal erosion, aberrant eyelash growth, conjunctivitis, blephritis and dry eye) may occur. Incidence of conjunctivitis, blepharitis, and dry eye was 6%. Rarely (0.1%), drug should be interrupted for severe or worsening ocular disorders.
  - *Bullous and exfoliative skin disorders* (e.g., toxic epidermal necrolysis, SJS, erythema multiforme) have rarely occurred (0.08%). Interrupt or discontinue drug for severe blistering or exfoliating skin disorders.
  - *Embryo-fetal toxicity:* Drug is fetotoxic. Teach women to use effective contraception during drug therapy and for 2 weeks after last dose. Nursing women should discontinue breastfeeding, or discontinue the drug.
- Nutritional impact symptoms may occur with the following incidences: diarrhea (29%), decreased appetite (17%), vomiting (14%), and stomatitis (7%).

Potential Toxicities/Side Effects and the Nursing Process

I.   ALTERATION IN SKIN INTEGRITY related to RASH

Defining Characteristics: Forty-seven percent of all patients developed skin reactions, which included acne-like rash, dermatitis, drug eruption, erythema, folliculitis, maculo-papular rash, and xeroderma. Of these 2% experienced a grade 3 or 4 reaction. Five percent of patients experienced nail disorders, including onycholysis and paronychia.

Nursing Implications: Assess skin integrity of face, neck, arms, and upper trunk baseline and regularly during treatment. Teach patient that rash may occur, its usual course, and self-care measures for comfort. Emphasize the need to keep skin with rash clean to prevent infection and to continue taking gefitinib until told to stop by nurse or physician. Teach patient that skin may become dry, and to use skin emollients or moisturizers. Assess body image intactness, and if rash develops, its threat to body image. Encourage patient to verbalize feelings, provide emotional support, and individualize care plan based on patient response. For rash management, follow institutional guidelines and refer to the introduction in *Chapter 4*. Teach all patients to (1) use a water-based emollient frequently during the day to prevent dryness, (2) stay hydrated, (3) avoid sun exposure and wear SPF 30 (zinc-based). Do not use antiacne medications. Tetracycline analogues provide anti-inflammatory benefit. Management may include: **Grade 1/mild rash** (localized, does not interfere with ADLs, and is not infected): Goal is to preserve skin integrity, minimize discomfort, and prevent infection. Key patient teaching includes (1) use a mild soap with active ingredients that reduce skin drying, such as pyrithione zinc (Head & Shoulders); (2) consider applying aloe gel to red, tender areas; (3) report distressing tenderness, as pramoxine (lidocaine topical anesthetic) may help; (4) keep fingernails clean and trimmed; and (5) apply zinc ointment to anal mucosa after washing. **Management: maintain current drug dose, observe or give topical hydrocortisone 1% or 2.5%, or clindamycin 1%** gel (anti-inflammatory benefit), reassess in 2 weeks. **Grade 2/moderate rash** (generalized, mild symptoms, and minimal effect on ADLs, no infection): Goal is to prevent infection and promote comfort. Continue EGFRI dose; use topicals (hydrocortisone 2.5% or clindamycin 1% gel) and consider adding doxycycline 100 mg PO twice daily or minocycline 100 mg PO twice daily (gives antimicrobial and anti-inflammatory effect) and reassess after 2 weeks. **Grades 3–4 or severe rash** (generalized, severe, has significant impact on ADLs, and increased risk of infection): The goal is to prevent infection or identify infection early to minimize complications and to promote effective coping. Drug should be held for severe rash, CTCAE grade 3 (papules and/or pustules covering > 30% BSA, which may be associated with symptoms of pruritis or tenderness; limiting self-care ADL; associated with local superinfection with oral antibiotics indicated) or higher, for up to 14 days. Teach patient to interrupt drug as ordered. Treat rash with topicals (hydrocortisone 2.5%, or clindamycin 1% gel), doxycycline 100 mg PO bid or minocycline 100 mg PO bid, and methylprednisolone (Medrol dose pack); reassess after 2 weeks (Lacouture et al., 2011; Lynch et al., 2007). If rash appears infected (exudate, vesicular formation, different appearance), obtain C+S, treat empirically until sensitivity received, and/or discuss with provider obtaining dermatology consult.

Teach patient to report any peeling or blistering of skin as bullous and exfoliative skin disorders, such as SJS, may rarely occur; drug should be discontinued in these patients. Teach patients that nail disorders may occur and to report them.

II.   ALTERATION IN ELIMINATION PATTERN related to DIARRHEA

Defining Characteristics: Diarrhea was reported in 29% of patients in clinical studies, and was severe in 3%. Diarrhea may occur within 14 days of starting gefitinib, is usually mild to moderate, and well managed with antidiarrheal medications like loperamide (Shah, 2005). Proteinuria occurred in 35% of patients and was grade 3/4 in 4.7% (AstaZeneca, 2015).

Nursing Implications: Assess bowel-elimination pattern baseline and regularly during therapy. Teach patient to report diarrhea; teach patient self-care strategies to manage diarrhea such as dietary modification and self-administration of loperamide; teach patient to minimize potential complications such as dehydration and electrolyte depletion. Identify patients at risk for dehydration and follow closely, such as patients with renal insufficiency, diabetes, CHF, or the elderly. If diarrhea does not resolve or is CTCAE grade 3 or higher (grade 3 is an increase of 7 or more stools/day over baseline; incontinence; hospitalization indicated; severe ostomy output compared to baseline; limiting self-care ADL), drug should be interrupted for up to 14 days (AstraZeneca, 2015). Discuss with provider lab assessment, fluid and electrolyte replacement, hydration, and further management. If diarrhea is refractory or difficult to manage, this will increase the patient's risk for dehydration and risk for acute renal failure, especially if elderly or if the patient has preexisting renal disease.

Drug: ibrutinib (Imbruvica)

Class: Kinase inhibitor; Bruton's tyrosine kinase (BTK) inhibitor.

Mechanism of Action: Inhibits BTK, an important NRTK that signals messages through the B-cell lymphocyte antigen receptor (BCR), as well as cytokine receptor pathways. BCR signaling is essential for B-cell development and survival. BCR is believed to be oncogenic in mantle cell lymphoma (MCL) and chronic lymphocytic leukema (CLL), and BTK regulates cell proliferation and cell survival (Hendriks et al., 2014). BCR is composed of immunogobulins that recognize foreign antigens; when bound to the antigen, pathways are activated for B-cell lymphocyte trafficking, chemotaxis, and survival (Pharmacyclics, Inc., 2014). BTK is a key mediator regulating B-lymphocyte apoptosis, adhesion, cell migration, and homing (Pharmacyclics, Inc., 2014). Ibrutinib blocks BCR, resulting in inhibition of malignant B-cell lymphocyte proliferation, cell migration, adhesion to the microenvironment, and survival.

Metabolism: Drug is absorbed with median maximal plasma concentrations (T_{max}) reached in 1–2 hours. If taken with food, drug exposure is twofold greater compared to a fasting state. Drug is 97.3% reversibly bound to plasma proteins. Ibrutinib is metabolized by P450 microenzymes in the liver, CYP3A4 and, to a lesser degree, CYP2D6 into a few metabolites, including the active metabolite, PCI-45227. Ibrutinib affinity for BTK active sites is 15 times that of the active metabolite. Ibrutinib half-life is 4–6 hours. The drug is excreted mainly as metabolites in the stool (80%), with < 10% excreted in the urine. Moderate hepatic impairment increases drug exposure 6 times (Child-Pugh Class B).

Indication: Ibrutinib is FDA approved for treatment of patients with:
- Mantle cell lymphoma (MCL), who have received at least one prior therapy. Accelerated approval was based on overall response rate and data on improved survival or symptom control have not been shown.
- Chronic lymphocytic leukemia (CLL)/Small lymphocytic lymphoma (SLL).
- CLL/SLL with 17p deletion.
- Waldenstrom's macroglobulinemia (WM).
- Marginal zone lymphoma (MZL) who require systemic therapy and have received at least one prior anti-CD20-based therapy. Accelerated approval.
- Chronic graft versus host disease (cGVHD) after failure of one or more lines of systemic therapy.

Dosage/Range:
- Ibrutinib is given PO once daily at about the same time each day, with a glass of water. Capsule should not be opened, broken or chewed, and tablets should not be cut, crushed, or chewed.
- MCL and MZL: 560 mg orally once daily until disease progression or unacceptable toxicity.
- CLL/SLL and WM: 420 mg orally once daily. When ibrutinib is given with bendamustine and rituximab (administered every 28 days for up to 6 cycles) for the treatment of CLL/SLL, the ibrutinib dose is 420 mg once daily, while the other 2 drugs are given every 28 days for up to 6 cycles.
- cGVHD: 420 mg orally once daily until cGVHD progression, recurrence of an underlying malignancy, or unacceptable toxicity. Drug should be discontinued if the patient no longer requires therapy for cGVHD.

Dose Modifications (see package insert):
- Recommended modifications: Interrupt ibrutinib for any grade 3 or greater non-hematological adverse effect, grade 3 or greater neutropenia with infection, fever, or grade 4 hematologic toxicities. Once toxicity symptom(s) have resolved to grade 1 or baseline (recovery), drug may be reinitiated at the starting dose. If toxicity recurs, reduce dose by 140 mg/day. A 2nd dose reduction of 140 mg may be considered as needed. If toxicity persists or recurs after 2 dose reductions, discontinue ibrutinib.
- Dose reductions:
  - *First toxicity occurrence:* MCL, MZL: restart after recovery at standard dose of 560 mg daily; CLL/SLL, WM, and cGVHD after recovery: restart at standard dose of 420 mg daily.
  - *Second occurrence:* MCL, MZL: restart at 420 mg daily; CLL/SLL, WM, and cGVHD: after recovery: restart at 280 mg daily.

TREATMENT

- *Third occurrence:* MCL, MZL: restart at 280 mg daily; CLL/SLL, WM, and cGVHD after recovery: restart at 140 mg daily.
- *Fourth occurrence:* permanently discontinue ibrutinib.

Dose Modifications with CYP3A Inhibitors (see package insert for dosage modifications):

- Avoid concomitant administration with strong (or moderate CYP3A4 inhibitors. If strong CYP3A4 inhibitors (e.g., antifungals, antibiotics) must be used short term ($\leq$ 7 days), consider interrupting ibrutinib until the CYP3A4 is no longer needed. Chronic use of concomitant strong CYP3A4 inhibitors (e.g., boceprevir, indinavir, nefazodone, nelfinavir, ritonavir, saquinavir, telaprevir) is not recommended. Monitor patients receiving concomitant strong or moderate CYP3A4 inhibitors closely for toxicity. *After discontinuation of CYP3A inhibitor, resume previous ibrutinib dose.*
- *B-cell malignancy:*
  - If moderate CYP3A4 inhibitor, (e.g., voriconazole 200 mg BID or posaconazole suspension 100 mg QD, 100 mg BID, or 200 mg BID): ibrutinib dose is 140 mg; modify dose as recommended.
  - If posaconazole suspension 200 mg TID or 400 mg BID, posaconazole IV 300 mg QD, or posaconazole delayed-release tablets 300 mg QD: Reduce ibrutinib dose to 70 mg once daily; interrupt dose as recommended.
  - Other strong CYP3A inhibitors: avoid coadministration. If these inhibitors used short term (e.g., anti-infectives for 7 or less days), interrupt ibrutinib.
- *cGVHD*
  - If moderate CYP3A inhibitor: 420 mg QD. Modify dose as recommended.
  - If Voriconazole 200 mg BID or posaconazole suspension 100 mg QD, 100 mg BID, or 200 mg BID: Reduce imbrutinib dose to 280 mg daily; modify dose as recommended.
  - If posaconazole suspension 200 mg TID or 400 mg BID, posaconazole IV 300 mg QD, or posaconazole delayed-release tablets 300 mg QD: Reduce ibrutinib dose to 140 mg once daily; interrupt dose as recommended.
  - Other strong CYP3A inhibitors: avoid coadministration. If these inhibitors used short term (e.g., anti-infectives for 7 or less days), interrupt ibrutinib.
- Hepatic impairment: (1) Mild liver impairment recommended dose is 140 mg qd; (2) moderate liver impairment (Child-Pugh class B): 70 mg qd. Do not administer drug to patients with severe hepatic impairment (Child-Pugh class C).

Preparation:

- Capsules: 70-mg and 140-mg capsules.
- Tablets: 140 mg, 280 mg, 420 mg, 560 mg.

Drug Administration:

- Teach patient to swallow capsule whole, not to open, break, or chew capsule, and to take with water. Drug should be taken at about the same time each day. Teach patient to avoid grapefruit products and Seville oranges.
- Teach patient if a dose is missed, it can be taken when remembered on the same day, then resume normal schedule the next day; do not make up a missed dose.

Drug Interactions:
- CYP3A Inhibitors: increase the serum ibritinib levels, increasing toxicity. Do not coadminister strong inhibitors and reduce ibritinib dose to 140 mg if coadministered with a moderately strong inhibitor. See Dose Modifications.
- CYP3A Inducers: decrease ibritinib serum levels and reduce efficacy; avoid strong CYP3A inducers (e.g., St. John's wort).
- Antiplatelet or anticoagulant therapy: increased risk of bleeding; monitor patients closely, as well as appropriate labs.

Lab Effects/Interference:
- Neutropenia, thrombocytopenia, anemia.
- Increased serum creatinine, uric acid.

Special Considerations:
- Most common side effects (incidence ≥ 25%) in patients with B-cell malignancies (MCL, CLL, WM) were thrombocytopenia, diarrhea, neutropenia, anemia, fatigue, musculoskeletal pain, bruising, nausea, URI, and rash.
- Warnings and Precautions:
  - *Hemorrhage and bleeding:* Up to 3% of patients in studies had grade ≥ 3 bleeding events (e.g., intracranial hemorrhage including subdural hematoma, GI bleed, hematuria, and postprocedural hemorrhage). Overall bleeding of any grade, including bruising, occurred in about 44% of patients treated with ibrutinib. Patients receiving antiplatelet or anticoagulant therapies may be at increased risk of bleeding. Consider benefit of withholding ibrutinib 3–7 days prior to and after surgery based on type of surgery and risk of bleeding.
  - *Infections (bacterial, viral, fungal):* Grade 3 or greater infections occurred in 24% of patients. Consider prophylaxis according to standard of care for patients at risk for opportunistic infections. Monitor patients closely and evaluate for fever and infections, and treat appropriately.
  - Progressive multifocal leukoencephalopathy (PML) has occurred and *Pneumocystis jirovecii* pneumonia (PJP). Evaluate patients for fever and treat infections promptly, as ordered.
  - Infection may occur and may be fatal. Grade ≥ 3 infection occurred in 25% of MCL and 35% of CLL patients. Monitor patients closely for infection and treat with antimicrobials as indicated. Teach patients to report fever, signs/symptoms of infection right away.
  - *Cytopenias:* Myelosuppression is common, and grade 3–4 cytopenias, including neutropenia, occurred in 23% of patients, thrombocytopenia in 8%, and anemia in 3%. Monitor blood counts baseline and monthly.
  - *Cardiac Arrhythmias:* Fatal and serious cardiac arrhythmias have occurred. Ventricular tachyarrythmias (grade 3 or higher) occurred in 0.2% of patients, and grade 3 or higher atrial fibrillation and atrial flutter in 4%. At risk are patients with cardiac risk factors, HTN, acute infections and a past history of atrial fibrillation. Monitor patients at risk. Document rhythm on ECG if patient complains of palpitations, light-headedness, has a new irregular apical pulse, or new-onset dyspnea. Discuss

management with provider who should discuss risks and benefits of continuing ibritinib. See dose modification in package insert.

- *HTN* occurred in 12% of patients in studies, with median time to onset of 5.9 months. Grade 3 or greater HTN occurred in 5% of patients. Monitor patients for new-onset HTN or HTN that is not controlled after beginning imbrutinib. Teach patient about ordered antihypertensive medication(s) and monitor effectiveness.
- *Second primary malignancies* have been described in 10% of patients treated with ibritinib in clinical trials. Four percent were nonskin carcinomas. Most frequent, second primary malignancy was nonmelanoma skin cancer).
- *Tumor lysis syndrome (TLS)* may occur, especially those patients with a high tumor burden. Monitor patients closely for TLS if at risk, and implement medical orders to reduce the risk (e.g., hydration, medication to reduce uric acid).
- *Embryo-fetal toxicity:* Teach women of childbearing potential to use effective contraception to avoid pregnancy during therapy, and for 1 month after last dose. If pregnancy occurs while taking the drug, advise patient of potential hazards to fetus.

Potential Toxicities/Side Effects and the Nursing Process

I. POTENTIAL FOR INFECTION AND BLEEDING related to BONE MARROW DEPRESSION

Defining Characteristics: Neutropenia occurred in 47% of MCL patients (29% grade $\geq$ 3), thrombocytopenia in 57% of patients (17% grade $\geq$ 3), and decreased hemoglobin in 41% of patients, (9% grade $\geq$ 3). Neutropenia occurred in 54% of CLL patients (27% grade $\geq$ 3), thrombocytopenia in 71% (10% grade $\geq$ 3), and decreased hemoglobin in 44%. Hemorrhage risk may be increased in patients receiving antiplatelet or anticoagulant therapies.

Nursing Implications: Assess baseline CBC, including WBC and differential and platelet count prior to dosing, and at least monthly. Teach patient self-assessment of signs/symptoms of infection (e.g., T > 100.4°F, dysuria, productive cough) and bleeding (including bruising), and instruct patient to report them right away. Teach patient self-care measures to minimize risk of infection and bleeding, including avoidance of crowds, people with colds, OTC aspirin-containing medications. Discuss dose interruption and modification for grade 3 toxicity with physician. Assess for fever or infection frequently, and discuss need for emergent evaluation and treatment promptly if signs or symptoms of infection are identified.

II. ALTERATION IN NUTRITION, POTENTIAL, LESS THAN BODY REQUIREMENTS, related to DIARRHEA, NAUSEA, VOMITING, CONSTIPATION

Defining Characteristics: Diarrhea affects 51–63% of patients, nausea 21–31%, constipation 23–25%, vomiting 19–23%, stomatitis 21%, and decreased appetite 21%.

Nursing Implications: Assess baseline nutritional status and bowel-elimination status. If patient develops nausea and/or vomiting, teach patient to self-administer antiemetics 1 hour prior to each dose, and to call if nausea/vomiting persist.

Discuss with physician more effective antiemetic regimen if nausea/vomiting persist. Encourage small, frequent intake of cool, bland foods as tolerated if nausea develops. Refer to dietitian as needed for meal planning. Teach patient to report diarrhea that does not respond to OTC antidiarrheal medication. Teach self-care measures of diet modification and oral fluids to 2–3 L during the waking hours. If constipation occurs, teach patient self-care measures to prevent constipation. Assess appetite, and condition of oral mucosa; teach patient self-assessment and systemic oral hygiene after meals and at bedtime.

III.   ALTERATION IN COMFORT related to PAIN, HEADACHE, FATIGUE, ARTHRALGIA, AND FATIGUE

Defining Characteristics: Fatigue affected 41% of patients, peripheral edema 35%, musculoskeletal pain 37% of patients, arthralgias 11% of patients, and abdominal pain affected 24% of patients.

Nursing Implications: Teach patient that these events may occur and to report them, and teach patient strategies to conserve energy. Assess baseline comfort and monitor closely during treatment. Develop plan to assure comfort depending on symptoms reported. Discuss ineffective strategies with physician.

Drug: idelalisib (Zydelig)

Class: Kinase inhibitor; first-in-class PI3K-delta kinase inhibitor (phosphatidylinositol 3-kinase), a kinase that is expressed by normal and malignant B cells.

Mechanism of Action: PI3K-delta kinase is found in normal and malignant B lymphocytes. Idelalisib inhibits a number of signaling pathways, including that of the B-cell receptor (BCR), CXCR4, and CXCR5, which help the B lymphocytes navigate to lymph nodes and bone marrow. Idelalisib inhibits chemotaxis and adhesion. Fiorcari et al. (2013) found that idelalisib inhibited chronic lymphocytic leukemia (CLL) cell adhesion to the endothelial and bone marrow stromal cells that is integrin-mediated. This prevents cell proliferation and results in apoptosis.

Metabolism: After oral administration in a fasting state, T_{max} (median) was seen at 1.5 hours; when administered with a high-fat meal, the idelalisib AUC increased 1.4-fold. However, drug may be given without regard to food. Drug is highly protein-bound (> 84%). Drug is metabolized into its principal metabolite GS-563117 in the liver by aldehyde oxidase and CYP3A, with minor metabolism by UGT1A4. The metabolite is not active against PI3K-delta. Terminal elimination half-life is 8.2 hours. Approximately 78% of the drug is excreted in the feces and 14% in the urine. Drug dose does not require modification if renal dysfunction, but patients with hepatic dysfunction require close monitoring and dose modification for toxicity.

Indication:
- For the treatment of:
  - Relapsed CLL, in combination with rituximab, in patients for whom rituximab alone would be considered appropriate therapy due to other comorbidities.
  - Relapsed follicular B-cell non-Hodgkin's lymphoma (FL), in patients who have received at least 2 prior systemic therapies.
  - Relapsed small lymphocytic lymphoma (SLL), in patients who have received at least 2 prior systemic therapies.
  - Limitation of use: Idelalisib is not indicated for, and is not recommended for, first-line treatment of any patient. Idelalisib is not indicated nor recommended in combination with bendamustine and/or rituximab for the treatment of FL (Gilead, 2018).
  - Accelerated approval for use in FL and SLL based on overall response rate. Improvement in paient survival or disease related symptoms has not been established. Further confirmatory trials may be required for continued approval for these indications (Gilead, 2018).
- Contraindicated in patients with a history of serious allergic reactions, including anaphylaxis and toxic epidermal necrolysis.

Dosage/Range:
- Recommended starting dose, 150 mg orally, twice daily, tablet swallowed whole, and with or without food.
- Idelalisib should be continued until disease progression or unacceptable toxicity.

Dose Modifications:
- See specific recommendations in Table 1, package insert (Gilead, 2018). For other severe or life-threatening toxicities related to idelalisib, hold drug until toxicity has resolved. If resuming idelalisib after a dose interruption, reduce the dose to 100 mg twice daily. Recurrence of the severe or life-threatening toxicity upon rechallenge requires permanent discontinuation of idelalisib.
- **Pneumonitis:** Discontinue idelalisib for any severity of symptomatic pneumonitis.
- **ALT/AST elevation:**
  - $> 3-5 \times$ ULN: Maintain dose; monitor ALT/AST at least weekly until $\leq 1 \times$ ULN.
  - $> 5-20 \times$ ULN: Hold drug; monitor at least weekly until ALT/AST is $\leq 1 \times$ ULN; then may resume idelalisib at 100 mg bid.
  - $> 20 \times$ ULN: Permanently discontinue idelalisib.
- **Bilirubin elevation:**
  - $> 1.5-3 \times$ ULN: Maintain dose; monitor bilirubin at least weekly until $\leq 1 \times$ ULN.
  - $> 3-10 \times$ ULN: Hold drug; monitor at least weekly until bilirubin is $\leq 1 \times$ ULN; then may resume idelalisib at 100 mg bid.
  - $> 10 \times$ ULN: Permanently discontinue idelalisib.
- **Diarrhea:**
  - Moderate (CTCAE, increase of 4–6 stools/day over baseline): Maintain dose; monitor patient at least weekly until resolved.
  - Severe or requiring hospitalization (CTCAE, increase of ≥ 7 stools/day over baseline): Hold drug; monitor patient at least weekly until resolved; then may resume idelalisib at 100 mg bid.
  - Life-threatening: Permanently discontinue idelalisib.

- **Neutropenia:**
  - ANC 1.0 to < 1.5 Gi/L: Maintain idelalisib dose.
  - ANC 0.5 to < 1.0 Gi/L: Maintain idelalisib dose; monitor ANC at least weekly.
  - ANC < 0.5 Gi/L: Interrupt idelalisib; monitor ANC at least weekly until ANC ≥ 0.5 Gi/L; then may resume idelalisib at 100 mg bid.
- **Thrombocytopenia:**
  - Platelets 50 to < 75 Gi/L: Maintain idelalisib dose.
  - Platelets 25 to < 50 Gi/L: Maintain idelalisib dose; monitor platelet count at least weekly.
  - Platelets < 25 Gi/L: Interrupt idelalisib; monitor platelet count at least weekly, and may resume idelalisib at 100 mg bid when platelet count ≥ 25 Gi/L.
- Infections:
  - Grade 3 or higher sepsis or pneumonia: interrupt idelalisib dose until infection has resolved.
  - Evidence of CMV infection or viremia: interrupt idelalisib in patients with evidence of CMV infection of any grade or viremia (positive PCR or antigen test) until infection has resolved. If drug is resumed, monitor patients by PCR or antigen test for CMV reactivation at least monthly.
  - Evidence of PJP infection: interrupt drug if PJP is suspected (any grade); permanently discontinue idelalisib if PJP infection is confirmed.
- Lymphocytosis: no dose modification as this is likely a pharmacologic effect of the drug, and without other clinical findings, should not be considered progressive disease.
- **For other severe or life-threatening toxicities** related to idelalisib, hold drug until toxicity is resolved; then if resuming the drug, dose should be reduced to 100 mg bid. If severe or life-threatening idelalisib-related toxicity recurs, idelalisib should be permanently discontinued.

Drug Preparation:
- Drug is available in 150-mg and 100-mg tablets.
- Drug is FDA approved with a Risk Evaluation and Mitigation Strategy (REMS) that includes a communication plan to ensure that healthcare providers likely to prescribe Zydelig are fully informed about the risks shown in the black boxed warning (FDA, 2014).

Drug Administration:
- Teach patient to take idelalisib with or without food, to swallow the tablet whole, and to take at about the same time of day each day.
  - If a dose is missed by < 6 hours, the patient should take the missed dose right away and then the next dose as usual.
  - If a dose is missed by > 6 hours, the patient should skip the missed dose and take the next dose at the usual time.
- Teach female patients of childbearing potential to use effective contraception to avoid pregnancy while taking the drug and for at least 1 month after last dose of idelalisib.
- Assess CBC/differential and platelet counts baseline and at least every 2 weeks for the first 3 months of therapy and at least weekly in patients with ANC < 1.0 Gi/L.

- Assess ALT and AST every 2 weeks for the first 3 months of treatment, then every 4 weeks for the next 3 months, then every 1–3 months thereafter. If AST or ALT rises above 3 × ULN, monitor ALT/AST weekly until resolved. Hold idelalisib if AST or ALT is > 5 × ULN, and continue to monitor AST, ALT, and total bilirubin weekly until the abnormality is resolved.
- Assess for signs/symptoms of serious toxicity: diarrhea, cough, dyspnea, hypoxia, new or worsening abdominal pain, chills, fever, nausea/vomiting, rash, allergic reaction, signs/symptoms of infection or bleeding.
- Discuss need for dose modification with physician based on symptoms or laboratory data as needed. The optimal and safe dosing regimen for patients who receive treatment for longer than several months is unknown (Gilead, 2014).

Drug Interactions:
- CYP3A inducers: avoid coadministration with strong CYP3A inducers (e.g., rifampin, phenytoin, carbamazepine, St. John's wort), as this may lower serum level of idelalisib (e.g., 75% reduction in idelalisib AUC) and negate drug effectiveness.
- CYP3A inhibitors: may increase drug serum level and increase toxicity. If patient is taking a strong CYP3A inhibitor with idelalisib, assess patient for signs/symptoms of idelalisib toxicity; dose should be modified according to dose modification guidelines.
- CYP3A substrates: idelalisib is a strong CYP3A inhibitor: avoid coadministration of CYP3A substrates, as this may increase the sensitive substrate serum level up to fivefold.

Lab Effects/Interference:
- Neutropenia, thrombocytopenia.
- Elevated ALT, AST, bilirubin.
- Hypertriglyceridemia.
- Hyperglycemia.

Special Considerations:
- Black Boxed Warnings:
  - *Hepatotoxicity:* fatal and/or serious hepatotoxicity occurred in 18% of patients taking idelalisib as monotherapy, and 16% in patients taking it with rituximab or unapproved combination therapies. Avoid concurrent use of idelalisib and other hepatotoxic drugs.
  - Elevations > 5 × ULN have occurred, usually during the first 12 weeks of treatment, and were reversible with dose interruption. When drug was resumed at a lower dose, 26% had recurrent AST/ALT elevations.
  - Monitor hepatic function prior to and during treatment every 2 weeks for first 3 months, every 4 weeks for the next 3 months, then every 1–3 months. Interrupt and then dose-reduce or discontinue drug. If ALT or AST increase to > 3 × ULN, monitor weekly until resolved. Hold idelalisib if ALT or AST increase to > 5 × ULN and continue to monito AST, ALT and total bilirubin weekly until abnormality has resolved.
  - See Dose Modifications for monitoring frequency with abnormal values.
  - Teach patient to report right away yellowing of skin or conjunctiva, easy bruising, abdominal pain, or bleeding.
- *Severe diarrhea or colitis:* fatal and/or serious diarrhea or colitis (grade 3 or higher) occurred in 14% of idelalisib-only treated patients, and in 20% of patients receiving

combination with rituximab or other unapproved combination therapies. Avoid concurrent use with other drugs which can cause diarrhea.
- Review patient medication profile and avoid concurrent use of drugs that cause diarrhea. Idelalisib-related diarrhea does not respond well to antimotility agents.
- In clinical trials, diarrhea resolved in 1 week to a month after idelalisib was stopped. In some cases, corticosteroids were required.
- Teach patient to report immediately an increase in the number of stools/day above baseline, or by 6 or more.
- *Pneumonitis:* fatal and serious pneumonitis may occur. Incidence in clinical trials was 4%. Time to onset was < 1 month to 15 months.
    - Monitor patient for pulmonary symptoms (e.g., cough, dyspnea, hypoxia; bilateral interstitial infiltrates); or ≥ 5% decrease in oxygen saturation.
    - If these occur, interrupt drug until the etiology is determined. If pneumonitis is confirmed, idelalisib therapy should be discontinued and the patient treated with corticosteroids.
    - Teach patient to report immediately any new or worsening respiratory symptoms (e.g., cough, dyspnea).
- *Infections:* Fatal and/or serious infections occurred in 21% of patients receiving idelalisib monotherapy, and 48% when given in combination with rituximab or unapproved regimens. Most common were pneumonia, sepsis, and febrile neutropenia.
    - Treat infections BEFORE starting idelalisib.
    - Serious or fatal *Pneumocystis jirovecii* pneumonia or cytomegalovirus (CMV) occurred in < 1%. Discuss PJP prophylaxis with provider. Interrupt idelalisib if PJP infection (any grade) is confirmed.
    - Interrupt idelalisib for CMV positive PCR or antigen test until the infection has resolved; if drug is resumed, monitor the patient by PCR or antigen test for CMV reactivation at least monthly.
- *Intestinal perforation*: fatal and serious intestinal perforation can occur.
    - This may occur during moderate or severe diarrhea.
    - Teach patient to report immediately new or worsening abdominal pain, chills, fever, nausea/vomiting and to seek medical care right away.
    - Idelalisib should be permanently discontinued if intestinal obstruction occurs.
- *Severe cutanous reactions* may occur (e.g., grade ≥ 3 cutaneous reactions, such as dermatitis exfoliative, rash, rash erythematous, rash generalized, rash macular, rash macula-papular, rash papular, rash pruritus, exfoliative rash). Monitor patient closely and discontinue drug if a severe cutaneous reaction occurs. Fatal cases of SJS and toxic epidermal necrolysis (TEN) have occurred. Interrrupt idelalisib if SJS or TEN is suspected, and permanently discontinue if confirmed.
- *Anaphylaxis:* Monitor patient for severe allergic reactions and anaphylaxis; discontinue idelalisib if it occurs and provide emergency supportive care. Teach patient to seek emergency medical care right away if patient has difficulty breathing, feels faint, chest pain, or other symptoms of an anaphylactic or serious allergic reaction.
- *Neutropenia:* Grade 3 or 4 neutropenia occurred in 25% of patients receiving monotherapy, and 58% in patients receiving rituximab or unapproved combinations. Monitor blood counts at least every 2 weeks for the first 6 months, then at least weekly in patients with an ANC < 1.0 Gi/L. Teach patient to report any signs or symptoms of infection right away.

- *Embryo-fetal toxicity:* Advise women of reproductive potential to use effective contraception to prevent pregnancy while taking idelalisib, and for 1 month after the last drug dose. If the drug is used during pregnancy, or if the patient becomes pregnant while taking the drug, the patient should be apprised of the potential risk to the fetus. Mothers taking the drug should NOT breast-feed. A decision should be made to discontinue nursing or to discontinue taking the drug.
- Patients age 65 and older with indolent NHL or CLL had a higher incidence of serious adverse reactions and a higher incidence of death compared to younger patients. Monitor patients age 65 and older closely during therapy.
- Most common adverse effects (incidence ≥ 20%) are diarrhea, pyrexia, fatigue, nausea, cough, pneumonitis, abdominal pain, chills, and rash.

Potential Toxicities/Side Effects and the Nursing Process

I.   POTENTIAL FOR INFECTION AND BLEEDING related to BONE MARROW SUPPRESSION

Defining Characteristics: Neutropenia was common, with 25% of indolent NHL patients and 37% of CLL patients having grade 3 or 4 neutropenia. Infections included pneumonia, bronchitis, sinusitis, UTI and sepsis. Pyrexia occurred in 35–37% of patients and was grades 3–4 in 3–5%; cough, and chills were reported. Thrombocytopenia and anemia also occurred.

Nursing Implications: Assess CBC/differential and platelet counts baseline and at least every 2 weeks for the first 3 months of therapy as ordered during therapy. Assess CBC/differential weekly in patients with ANC < 1.0 Gi/L. Assess skin integrity, potential for infection, and teach patient measures to prevent infection (e.g., keeping skin intact, avoiding sources of infection, good hand-washing). Teach patient to report any signs/symptoms of infection (e.g., redness, heat, exudate on skin, temperature ≥ 100.4°F, cough, sputum production, dysuria). Assess for signs/symptoms of infection during therapy and at each visit. If a patient develops an infection, discuss with physician or midlevel practitioner interrupting or discontinuing drug, and beginning appropriate antimicrobial treatment. Teach the patient that thrombocytopenia may occur, to avoid situations that could increase bleeding, and to report any signs or symptoms of bleeding right away. Review medication profile, and discuss discontinuance of aspirin or NSAIDs with patient and physician or NP/PA. Follow HGB/HCT and assess patient's tolerance, fatigue, other symptoms, and need for supportive measures.

II.   POTENTIAL ALTERATION IN NUTRITION, LESS THAN BODY REQUIREMENTS, related to NAUSEA, VOMITING, DIARRHEA, HEPATOTOXICITY, RARE INTESTINAL PERFORATION

Defining Characteristics: In clinical studies, nausea occurred in 25–29% of patients, vomiting in 13–15%, diarrhea in 21–47% (2–14% grades 3–4), constipation in 23%, decreased appetite in 15%, and hypokalemia in 12%. Diarrhea can be fatal and severe diarrhea occurred in 14% of patients. Hypertriglyceridemia, hyperglycemia, and increases in AST and ALT occurred in $> 30\%$ of patients. Fatal and serious intestinal perforation can occur.

Nursing Implications: Assess baseline nutritional, and elimination status, and appetite. Assess serum chemistries including glucose, triglycerides, and hepatic function, baseline and during therapy as ordered. Assess patient tolerance of chemotherapy and need for pre-medication with antiemetics. Teach the patient to report nausea and/or vomiting that is not relieved by prescribed antiemetics. Teach patient (1) that diarrhea or constipation may occur, (2) dietary modifications for each problem, and (3) to call nurse or physician for diarrhea, nausea, or vomiting that does not resolve within 24 hours with recommended OTC or prescription medicines. If patient develops severe diarrhea or colitis, teach patient to stop the drug and to notify physician right away. Drug dose should be interrupted, and then reduced, or drug discontinued per physician. Teach patient to call physician and be prepared to seek emergency care right away if the patient develops severe abdominal pain, with or without fever, as intestinal perforation may occur.

Drug: imatinib mesylate (Gleevec)

Class: Kinase Inhibitor; protein TKI of BCR-ABL tyrosine kinase.

Mechanism of Action: Inhibits abnormal tyrosine kinase created by the Philadelphia chromosome (BCR-ABL) in CML, thus preventing cell proliferation and causing apoptosis in BCR-ABL positive cell lines (NPTK inhibitor). Drug also inhibits RTKs for PDGF. Inhibits c-Kit receptor called SCFR tyrosine kinases as well, which has resulted in marked responses in GIST (gastrointestinal stromal tumors). Fifteen to 85% of GISTs have Kit mutations that result in constitutively active kinases; imatinib mesylate selectively inhibits this mutated tyrosine kinase.

Metabolism: Well absorbed after oral administration with 98% bioavailability and C_{max} in 2–4 hours after dosing. Elimination half-life of imatinib is 18 hours, and 40 hours for primary active metabolite N-desmethyl derivative. Drug is 95% protein-bound. It is metabolized via CYP3A4 hepatic cytochrome P450 enzyme system, with 81% of the dose eliminated in 7 days, primarily via fecal route (68%) and, to a lesser degree, urinary (13%). Twenty-five percent of drug dose is excreted unchanged in feces and urine.

Indication: Treatment of
- Newly diagnosed adult and pediatric patients with Ph+ CML in chronic phase.
- Patients with Ph+ CML in blast crisis (BC), accelerated phase (AP), or in chronic phase (CP) after failure of interferon alpha therapy.
- Adult patients with relapsed or refractory Ph+ acute lymphoblastic leukemia (Ph+ ALL).
- Pediatric patients with newly diagnosed Ph+ ALL in combination with chemotherapy.
- Adult patients with myelodysplastic/myeloproliferative diseases (MDS/MPD) associated with PDGFR gene rearrangements as determined by an FDA-approved test.

- Adult patients with aggressive systemic mastocytosis (ASM), without the D816V c-Kit mutation as determined by an FDA approved test, or c-Kit mutational status is unknown.
- Adult patients with hypereosinophilic syndrome (HES) and/or chronic eosinophilic leukemia (CEL) who have FIP1L1-PDGFRα fusion kinase (mutational analysis or FISH demonstration of CHIC2 allele deletion), and for patients with HES and/or CEL who are FIP1L1- PDGFRα negative or unknown.
- Adult patients with unresectable, recurrent, and/or metastatic dermatofibrosarcoma protuberans (DFSP).
- Patients with Kit (CD117)-positive unresectable and/or metastatic malignant GISTs.
- Adjuvant treatment of adult patients following complete gross resection of Kit (CD117)-positive GIST.

Dosage/Range:
- Ph+ CML
  - Adults, CP: 400 mg/day PO as a single dose.
  - Adults, AP or BC: 600 mg/day.
  - Adult patients with Ph+ CML-CP, -AP, and -BC: consider dose escalation if no severe adverse drug reaction, no severe nonleukemia-related neutropenia or thrombocytopenia, when (1) disease has progressed, (2) failure to achieve a satisfactory hematologic response after at least 3 months of treatment, (3) failure to achieve a cytogenetic response after 6–12 months of treatment, or (4) loss of a previously achieved hematologic or cytogenetic response.
    - CP: increase dose from 400 mg/day to 600 mg/day.
    - AC, BC: increase dose from 600 mg/day to 800 mg/day (givn as 400 mg twice daily).
  - Pediatrics, CP: 340 mg/m²/day (not to exceed 600 mg).
- Ph+ ALL
  - Adults with Ph+ ALL: 600 mg/day.
  - Pediatric patients with Ph+ ALL: 340 mg/m²/day (not to exceed 600 mg/day).
- Adults with MDS/MPD: 400 mg/day.
- Adults with ASM: Determine D816V c-Kit mutation; if mutation negative, dose is 400 mg/day; if c-Kit mutational status is unknown or unavailable, consider treatment with imatinib dose of 400 mg/day if not responding satisfactorily to other treatments. For ASM associated with eosinophilia, a clonal hematological disease related to the FIP1L1-PDGFRα fusion kinase: starting dose is 100 mg/day; may increase dose to 400 mg/day if no adverse drug reactions and patient does not appear to respond to the lower dose.
- Adults with HES/CEL: 100 mg/day or 400 mg/day. If FIP1L1-PDGFRα fusion kinase: starting dose is 100 mg/day; may increase dose to 400 mg/day if no adverse drug reactions and patient does not appear to respond to the lower dose.
- Adults with DFSP: 800 mg/day.
- Adults with metastatic and/or unresectable (CD117+) GIST: 400 mg/day; may increase dose up to 800 mg/day (400 mg twice daily) if needed (e.g., showing clear signs of symptoms of disease progression, with no severe adverse drug reactions).
- Adults receiving adjuvant therapy × 36 mo for (CD117+) GIST: 400 mg/day.

Dose Modification:
- Hepatic impairment: patients with mild or moderate impairment do not require a dose adjustment. Recommended dose for patients with severe hepatic impairment is 300 mg/day. A 25% decrease in the recommended dose is suggested (see package insert).
- Renal impairment: reduced dose in moderate renal impairment.
    - Moderate renal impairment (CrCl = 20–39 mL/min): 50 % decrease in recommended starting dose, with future doses increased as tolerated; doses > 400 mg/day are not recommended.
    - Mild renal impairment (CrCl = 40–59): doses > 600 mg/day are not recommended.
    - Severe renal impairment: use with extreme caution; a dose of 100 mg/day has been used (see package insert).
- Concomitant **strong** CYP3A4 inducers (e.g., dexamethasone, phenytoin, carbamazepine, rifampin, rifabutin, rifampacin, phenobarbital): avoid. If must coadminister, increase the dose of imatinib by at least 50% and carefully monitor clinical response.

Dose modifications for nonhematologic toxicity (see package insert April 2017).

Drug modifications for hematologic toxicity (see package insert, April 2017).

Drug Preparation:
- Available in scored 100-mg and 400-mg tablets.

Drug Administration: Teach patient to
- Administer dose orally, once daily (unless the total dose is 800 mg, which is given as 400 mg twice daily), with a meal and a large glass of water.
- Give children with CML and Ph+ ALL, the daily dose once-daily, or it can be split into two: one portion dosed in the morning and one in the evening with a meal and large glass of water. There is no experience with imatinib in children < 1 years old.
- If patient is unable to swallow, dissolve drug in water or apple juice if the patient has difficulty swallowing. Dissolve the required tablet(s) in a glass of water or apple juice: use 50 mL for a 100-mg tablet, and 200 mL for the 400-mg tablet; stir with a spoon and administer immediately after drug dissolves.
- Give doses of 800 mg and above: use 400-mg tablets to reduce exposure to iron.
- Take the dose as soon as possible if they miss a dose, unless it is almost time for their next dose, in which case they should not take it. Do not take a double dose. Take tablet(s) with a meal and a large glass of water. Teach patients to avoid grapefruit and grapefruit juice and not to take St. John's wort.
- Assess CBC/differential weekly for first month, biweekly for the second month, then as clinically indicated, or periodically, e.g., every 2–3 months. Assess LFTs baseline, then monthly or as clinically indicated.

Drug Interactions:
- *CYP3A4 inhibitors* (ketoconazole, itraconazole, clarithromycin, atazanavir, indinavir, nefazodone, nelfinavir, ritonavir, saquinavir, telithromycin, voriconazole; grapefruit or grapefruit juice) may increase imatinib plasma concentrations; do not coadminister.
- *CYP3A4 inducers* (dexamethasone, phenytoin, carbamazepine, rifampin, phenobarbital; also oxcarbamazepine, fosphenytoin, primidone; St. John's wort) may increase metabolism of imatinib, so imatinib serum levels are reduced. Avoid concomitant use and find alternative agents. Use together cautiously; when used with dexamethasone, phenytoin,

carbamazepine, phenobarbital, rifabutin or rifampin, or other strong inducers, increase imatinib dose by 50%. Doses up to 1,200 mg/day (600 mg bid) have been given to patients receiving concomitant strong CYP3A4 inducers (Novartis, 2015). Patients should not take St. John's wort if taking imatinib.
- *CYP3A4 substrates* with a narrow therapeutic window (e.g., simvastatin, alfentanil, cyclosporine, diergotamine, ergotamine, fentanyl, pimozide, quinidine, sirolimus, tacrolimus; as well as triazolo-benzodiazepines, dihydropyridine calcium-channel blockers, certain HMG-CoA reductase inhibitors) increased serum levels of substrate. For example, imatinib decreases simvastatin metabolism with simvastatin serum levels **increased** 2–3.5 times. Do not administer together, as drug has a narrow therapeutic window. If necessary to coadminister, monitor patient closely for toxicity and reduce dose of substrate as needed.
- *Other CYP3A4 substrates:* eletriptan (Relpax). Do not administer eletriptan within 72 hours of imatinib. Monitor vital signs closely.
- Warfarin: do not give together with imatinib, as imatinib inhibits warfarin metabolism by CYP2C9 and CYP3A4 enzymes. Use low molecular heparin or standard heparin instead.
- Acetaminophen: systemic exposure expected to increase when coadministered with imatinib mesylate.
- Imatinib mesylate inhibits CYP2D6; when coadministering imatinib with drugs that are a substrate of CYP2D6 having a narrow therapeutic window, use caution and monitor patients closely for toxicity.

Lab Effects/Interference:
- Neutropenia, thrombocytopenia.
- Elevated hepatic transaminases (SGOT/AST, SGPT/ALT), bilirubin, serum creatinine.
- Decreased thyroid function tests (e.g., TSH) in patients who have had thyroidectomy.

Special Considerations:
- Most common adverse reactions with an incidence of ≥ 30% were edema, nausea, vomiting, muscle cramps, musculoskeletal pain, diarrhea, rash, fatigue, and abdominal pain.
- Warnings and Precautions:
  - *Fluid retention and edema:* drug often causes edema that may be severe in some patients. There is increased risk in patients at higher drug doses and in the elderly (< 65 years). Weigh patients regularly and manage unexpected rapid weight gain by drug interruption and diuretics. Pleural effusion, pericardial effusion, pulmonary edema, and ascites have been reported.
  - *Hematologic toxicity:* Drug is associated with neutropenia, thrombocytopenia, and anemia. Blood counts should be assessed weekly for the first month, biweekly for the second month, and then periodically thereafter (e.g., every 2–3 months) as clinically indicated. In CML, occurrence depends upon stage of disease and is more frequent in patients with accelerated phase CML or blast crisis and requires closer monitoring in this group. Manage bone marrow depression with dose reduction or dose interruption, and rarely, drug discontinuation. See package insert.
  - *CHF and left ventricular dysfunction* have been reported, and while rare (0.9–1.4%), are more frequent in patients with advanced age or comorbidities including previous medical history of cardiac disease. Monitor patients carefully if they have cardiac

disease, cardiac risk factors, or history of renal failure. Discuss with physician evaluation of patient with signs/symptoms of cardiac or renal failure.
- *Hepatotoxicity,* sometimes severe, can occur.
  - Cases of liver failure or injury requiring liver transplants have been reported in both short-term and long-term use of imatinib.
  - See Dosage for initial and dose reductions, if hepatic impairment, and package insert.
  - Liver function tests (LFTs) should be monitored baseline and monthly or as clinically indicated.
- *Hemorrhage:* May occur rarely in CML patients, and in one open-label trial of patients with unresectable/metastatic GIST, the incidence was 12.9%. GI tumors may be the source of GI bleeds in patients with GIST. Monitor patients for GI symptoms at the start of therapy. Rare reports, including fatalities, of GI perforation have been made.
- *Gastrointestinal disorders:* In order to reduce GI irritation, the patient should take the imatinib dose with food and a large glass of water. Rarely, GI perforation has occurred.
- *Hypereosinophilic cardiac toxicity:* Patients at risk are those with HES/CEL, and in patients with MDS/MPD or ASM associated with high eosinophil levels. Assess ECHO and serum troponin levels. See package insert for management.
- *Dermatologic toxicities:* bullous dermatologic reactions (e.g., SJS, erythema multiforme) have been reported. Assess any rash, and if bullous, discuss prompt drug interruption and confirmation of dermatology diagnosis.
- *Hypothyroidism* in patients taking levothyroxin replacement after thyroidectomy; monitor TSH levels closely in these patients.
- *Drug is embryo-fetal toxic:* Sexually active women of reproductive potential should be taught to use highly effective contraception to avoid pregnancy and continue for 14 days after stopping the drug. If the drug is used during pregnancy or if the patient becomes pregnant while taking the drug, the patient should be apprised of the potential hazard to the fetus.
- *Tumor lysis syndrome (TLS)* may occur in patients with CML, GIST, ALL, and eosinophilic leukemia receiving imatinib mesylate, and it may be fatal. Patients at risk are those with a high proliferative rate or high-tumor burden prior to treatment. Monitor these patients closely and discuss TLS prophylaxis with physician. Correct clinically significant dehydration and treat high uric-acid levels before starting imatinib mesylate.
- *Impairments related to driving and using machinery:* Teach patients that they may experience dizziness, blurred vision, or somnolence while taking imatinib and should use caution when driving a car or operating machinery.
- *Renal toxicity:* renal creatinine clearance may decline during treatment. Monitor renal function tests baseline, and regularly during treatment; identify those patients at greatest risk: those with pre-existing renal dysfunction, diabetes mellitus, HTN, or CHF.
- Because patients are treated for many years, consider potential long-term toxicities (e.g., liver, kidney, cardiac), as well as immunosuppression.

- Nursing mothers should decide whether to discontinue nursing or discontinue the drug as up to 10% of the mother's drug and its metabolites are excreted in human milk. Mothers should not breast-feed and should either discontinue the drug or nursing, taking into consideration the importance of imatinib to the mother's health.

Potential Toxicities/Side Effects and the Nursing Process

I. POTENTIAL FOR INFECTION AND BLEEDING related to BONE MARROW DEPRESSION

Defining Characteristics: Neutropenia and thrombocytopenia were common, especially in patients who received higher doses, and in patients with advanced stages of disease (blast crisis and accelerated phase). Median duration of neutropenia was 2–3 weeks, and thrombocytopenia from 3–4 weeks. Dose needs to be held and reduced as stated in the package insert. Fever affected 14% (chronic phase) to 38% (accelerated phase) of patients. Hemorrhage (CNS and GI) was treated in 13% (chronic phase) to 48% (accelerated phase) of patients.

Nursing Implications: Assess baseline CBC, including WBC and differential and platelet count prior to dosing, as well as at least weekly during first month of treatment, at least every other week for the second month of treatment, and then as clinically indicated and ordered. Discuss dose interruption and reduction as above for neutropenia and thrombocytopenia with physician/NP/PA. Teach patient self-assessment of signs/symptoms of infection (e.g., T $\geq$ 100.4°F, dysuria, productive cough) and bleeding (including epistaxis and development of petechiae), and instruct patient to report them right away. Teach patient self-care measures to minimize risk of infection and bleeding, including avoidance of OTC aspirin-containing medications.

II. POTENTIAL ALTERATION IN CIRCULATION related to CONGESTIVE HEART FAILURE

Defining Characteristics: The Abelson tyrosine kinase (ABL) protein is necessary for the general health and maintenance of cardiac muscles, especially the mitochondria (Qiu et al., 2009). Although rare (0.7%), Kerkela et al. reported that 10 patients developed CHF between 1–14 months after starting the drug; although patients had an average LVEF of 56%, on repeat testing, the average LVEF was 25%. Patients with hypereosinophilic infiltration of the myocardium are at risk of cardiogenic shock and left ventricular dysfunction, and it is reversible with systemic steroids, circulatory support strategies, and holding the drug.

Nursing Implications: Patients at risk (e.g., advanced age, cardiac comorbidities) should have determination of their LVEF baseline and periodically while receiving the drug. Assess baseline cardiac status, history, and risk for development of CHF. Closely monitor patient while receiving imatinib mesylate, especially if patient has history of hypertension or is on cardiac medications. Teach patient to report any dyspnea, SOB, chest pain, or heart palpitations, or any unusual feeling. If any abnormalities occur, teach patient to stop drug and to call the physician or nurse immediately.

III.   ALTERATION IN FLUID AND ELECTROLYTE BALANCE related to FLUID RETENTION, EDEMA, AND HYPOKALEMIA

Defining Characteristics: Fluid retention is common (52% chronic phase and 67% accelerated phase patients), especially in the elderly, and primarily reflects periorbital and lower extremity edema. However, pleural effusions, ascites, rapid weight gain, and pulmonary edema may develop, and in some cases, may be life-threatening (e.g., pleural effusion, congestive heart failure, renal failure, pericardial effusion, and anasarca). Hypokalemia was reported to occur in 2–12% of patients.

Nursing Implications: Assess baseline parameters of weight, presence of edema, pulmonary function, and monitor closely during therapy. Teach patient to monitor weight daily at home and to report weight gain of 2 pounds in 1 week, development of edema, or dyspnea. Teach the patient comfort measures for periorbital edema, such as ice packs, and self-administration of diuretics as ordered. Discuss with physician drug dose modification or interruption if severe fluid retention occurs.

IV.   ALTERATION IN NUTRITION, POTENTIAL, LESS THAN BODY REQUIREMENTS, related to NAUSEA, VOMITING, DIARRHEA, HEPATOTOXICITY

Defining Characteristics: Nausea affected 68% of patients with accelerated phase, and 55% with chronic phase; vomiting affected 54% and 28%, respectively. Diarrhea affected 54%, while constipation affected 13%. Dyspepsia affected about 19%.

Nursing Implications: Teach patient to self-administer antiemetics 1 hour prior to each dose, and to call if nausea/vomiting develop. Discuss with physician more effective antiemetic regimen if nausea/vomiting develop. Encourage small, frequent intake of cool, bland foods as tolerated if nausea develops. Refer to dietitian as needed for meal planning. Assess bowel-elimination pattern baseline and at each visit. Teach patient to report diarrhea or constipation that does not respond to antidiarrheal or anticonstipation medications. Teach dietary modifications as appropriate. Monitor LFTs baseline and periodically during therapy. Hold therapy if LFTs become abnormal (see Special Considerations).

V.   ALTERATION IN COMFORT related to MUSCLE CRAMPS, MUSCULOSKELETAL (BONE) PAIN, HEADACHE, FATIGUE, ARTHRALGIA, AND ABDOMINAL PAIN

Defining Characteristics: Muscle cramps are common, affecting 25–46% of patients. Musculoskeletal pain affects 27–37% of patients, headache 24–29% of patients, fatigue 33% of patients, rash 32% of patients, and arthralgias 26% of patients. In clinical studies, abdominal pain affected 20% of patients with chronic phase, and 26% of patients in blast crisis.

Nursing Implications: Teach patient that these events may occur and to report them. Assess baseline comfort, and monitor closely during treatment. Develop plan to assure comfort, depending on symptoms reported. For cramps, suggest drinking tonic water and taking calcium gluconate, and if ineffective, discuss with physician the prescription of quinine; for the management of bone pain, suggest NSAIDs as appropriate. Discuss ineffective strategies with physician and revise plan as needed.

VI. ALTERATION IN SKIN INTEGRITY related to RASH

Defining Characteristics: Rash may occur. In clinical studies, 32% of patients with accelerated phase, and 36% of patients in chronic phase CML reported rash. Ten percent of patients complained of pruritus.

Nursing Implications: Teach patient that rash may occur and to report it. Assess patient skin integrity, baseline and regularly, during treatment. Teach patient local comfort measures. Discuss rash and management plan with physician, especially if severe.

Drug: ivosidenib (Tibsovo)

Class: Small molecule inhibitor of isocitrate dehydrogenase 1 (IDH1) enzyme.

Mechanism of Action: IDH1 mutations may occur in AML which result in increased levels of 2-hydroxyglutarate (2-HG) levels in leukemic cells which prevent the blast cells from differentiating to mature myeloid cells. Blocking mutated IDH enzymes leads to differentiation and death of AML cells (Chen et al., 2013). As a small molecule inhibitor of IDH1 enzyme, the drug leads to decreased 2-hydroxyglutarate (2-HG) levels, induces differentiation so that there are a reduced number of leukemic blast cells, and an increased percentage of mature myeloid cells (Agios, 2018).

Metabolism: After oral dosing, median time to Cmax is about 3 hours, and steady state plasma level is reached within 14 days. Taking drug with a high-fat mean, the Cmax is increased by 98% and AUC by 25%. Ivosidenib is primarily metabolized by CYP3A4 microenzymes. Terminal drug half-life is 93 hours. Most of the drug (77%) is excreted in the feces (67% unchanged drug) and 17% excreted in the uringe (10% unchanged drug).

Indication: Adult patients with AML with a susceptible IDH1 mutation as detected by an FDA-approved test with (1) newly diagnosed AML who are ≥ 75 years or who have comorbidities that preclude use of intensive induction chemotherapy; or (2) relapsed or refractory AML. If a patient is initially without the mutation at diagnosis, upon relapse, the patient should be retested as mutation may emerge during treatment and at relapse.

Contraindication: None.

Drug Dosage/Range:
- Ivosidenib 500 mg PO qd for a minimum of 6 months, unless disease progression or unacceptable toxicity. Administer with or without food, BUT not with a high-fat meal.
- Treatment for a minimum of 6 months will allow time for a clinical response.
- Drug has not been studied in patients with preexisting severe renal or hepatic impairment. In these patients, the risks and potential benefits must be reviewed before starting treatment with ivosidenib (Agios, 2019).

Dose Modifications due to toxicity:
- Differentiation syndrome:
    - If suspected, patient should receive systemic corticosteroids and hemodynamic monitoring until symptom resolution and for a minimum of 3 days
    - Interrupt ivosidenib if severe signs +/or symptoms persist for > 48 hours after initiation of systemic corticosteroids.
    - Resume ivosidenib when signs and symptoms improve to grade 2 (moderate) or lower.
- Noninfectious leukocytosis $> 25 \times 10^9$/L or an absolute increase in total WBC of $> 15 \times 10^9$/L from baseline:
    - Initiate treatment with hydroxyurea as per standard institutional practices, and leukapheresis if clinically indicated.
    - Taper hydroxyurea only after leukocytosis improves or resolves.
    - Interrupt ivosidenib if leukocytosis is not improved with hydroxyrea, and then resume ivosidenib at 500 mg PO daily when leukocytosis has resolved.
- QTc interval > 480 msec – 500 msec:
    - Monitor and supplement electrolyte levels as clinically indicated.
    - Review and adjust concomitant medications with known QTc interval prolonging effects.
    - Interrupt ivosidenib.
    - Restart ivosidenib at 500 mg PO qd after the QTc interval returns to ≤ 480 msec.
    - Monitor ECGs at least weekly × 2 weeks following resolution of QTc prolongation.
- QTc interval > 500 msec:
    - Monitor and supplement electrolyte levels as clinically indicated.
    - Review and adjust concomitant medications with known QTc interval prolonging effects.
    - Interrupt ivosidenib.
    - Resume ivosidenib at a reduced dose of 250 mg qd when QTc interval returns to within 30 msec of baseline or ≤ 480 msec.
    - Monitor ECGs at least weekly × 2 weeks following resolution of QTc prolongation.
    - Consider re-escalating the dose of ivosidenib to 500 mg PO qd if an alternative etiology for QTc prolongation can be identified.
- QTc interval prolongation with signs/symptoms of life-threatening arrhythmia: discontinue ivosidenib permanently.
- Guillain-Barre syndrome: discontinue ivosidenib permanently.
- Other grade 3 (severe) or higher toxicity (life-threatening) considered related to treatment:
    - Interrupt ivosidenib until toxicity resolves to grade 2 or lower.

- Resume ivosidenib at 250 mg PO qd; may increase to 500 mg PO qd if/when toxicity resolves to grade 1 (mild) or lower.
- If grade 3 or higher toxicity recurs, discontinue ivosidenib.

Dose Modification for Us with Strong CYP3A4 Inhibitors: Reduce ivosidenib dose to 250 mg PO qd; if strong inhibitor is discontinued, increase the ivosidenib dose (after at least 5 half-lives of the strong inhibitor) to the full dose of 500 mg PO qd.

Drug Preparation: Available as 250 mg tablet.

Drug Administration:
- Assess (1) CBC/ANC and blood chemistries baseline and at least once a week for 1st month, once every other week for the 2nd month, then monthly for the duration of therapy; (2) blood creatine phosphokinase weekly for 1st month of therapy; (3) ECG at least once weekly for first 3 weeks of therapy, then at least monthly for duration of therapy. Assess serum electrolytes, and ensure they are WNL, especially serum magnesium, calcium, and potassium, as low levels increase the risk of venrtricular arrhythmias with QTc prolongation.
- Assess tolerance of ivosidenib (signs/symptoms of differentiation syndrome, diarrhea, nausea, vomiting, mucositis, constipation, abdnomian pain, fatigue, fever, arthralgia, dyspnea, decreased appetite). Assess medication profile to identify any potential QTc prolonging medications, and discuss changes with provider.
- Teach patient to take ivosidenib:
  - With or without food, but NOT with a high-fat meal as it increases ivosidenib concentration.
  - At about the same time every day.
  - Do not to split or crush tablets.
  - If a dose is vomited, do not take another dose, but wait until the next scheduled dose is due.
  - If the dose is missed or not taken at the usual time, take the dose as soon as possible and at least 12 hours before the next scheduled dose. Return to normal dose the next day. DO NOT take 2 doses within 12 hours.

Drug Interactions (see Section 7.1 of package insert for more detailed discussion):
- Strong or moderate CYP3A4 inhibitors: concurrent use increases ivosidenib plasma concentrations and risk of QTc prolongation; reduce ivosidenib dose with strong inhibitors. Monitor patients for increased risk of QTc interval prolongation. Ensure serum electrolytes are assessed frequently and maintained at normal values.
- Strong CYP3A4 inducers: concurrent use decreases ivosidenib plasma concentrations; avoid concomitant use with ivosidenib.
- Sensitive CYP3A4 substrates: avoid concomitant use with ivosidenib as the substrate drug efficacy may be diminished (e.g., itraconazole, ketoconazole, hormonal contraceptives).
- QTc prolonging drugs: avoid concomitant use with ivosidenib; if must co-administer, monitor patients very closely for increased risk of QTc interval prolongation. Ensure serum electrolytes are assessed frequently and maintained at normal values, especially serum magnesium, calcium, and potassium.

Lab Effects/Interference:
* Decreased Hgb, serum sodium, magnesium, potassium, phosphate.
* Increased AST, ALT, serum creatinine, bilirubin, uric acid.

Special Considerations:
* Most common adverse effects (incidence $\geq$ 20%): fatigue, leukocytosis, arthralgia, diarrhea, dyspnea, edema, nausea, mucositis, QTc prolongation on ECG; rash, pyrexia, cough, and constipation.
* Mothers should not breast-feed while taking ivosidenib.
* Warnings and Precautions:
   * *Differentiation syndrome:* In the clinical trial, differentiation syndrome occurred in 19% of patients with 79% of patients recovering after treatment or dose interruption of ivosidenib. Differentiation syndrome occurs with a rapid proliferation and differentiation of myeloid cells, characterized by noninfectious leukocytosis, peripheral edema, fever, dyspnea, pleural effusion, hypotension, hypoxia, pulmonary edema, pneumonitis, pericardial effusion, rash, fluid overload, TLS, and increased serum creatinine. Onset occurred day 1 to up to 3 months after beginning ivosidenib. If differentiation syndrome is suspected, the patient should receive dexamethasone 10 mg IV every 12 hours (or equivalent) with hemodynamic monitoring until improvement (Agios, 2018). If concomitant noninfectious leukocytosis occurs, the patient should be treated with hydroxyurea or leukopheresis to reduce the WBC. Once symptoms resolve, the corticosteroid and hydroxyurea should be tapered over a minimum of 3 days (Agios, 2018). If the patient's signs and symptoms are severe and persist for > 48 hours after starting corticosteroids, ivosidenib should be interrupted until signs/symptoms are no longer severe.
   * *QTc interval prolongation:* QTc prolongation and ventricular arrhythmias (including Ventricular Fibrillation) may occur with ivosidenib treatment. During the clinical trial, 9% of patients had a QTc prolongation > 500 msec, and 14% of patients had an increase in QTc > 60 msec over baseline. If a patient is also taking medications that can prolong the QTc (e.g., anti-arrhythmic medicatioins, fluoroquinolones, triazole anti-fungals, 5-HT3 receptor antagonists, drugs which inhibit CYP3A4) should have frequent ECG and electrolye monitoring. If the patient also has a condition which might contribute such as congenital long QTc syndrome, CHF, electrolyte abnormalities, more frequent monitoring should occur. Ivosidenib should be interrupted if the QTc increases to > 480 msec and < 500 msec. If the increase is > 500 msec, the dose should be interrupted and dose reduced when ivosidenib is resumed. If a patient develops QTc prolongation with a life-threatening arrhythmia, ivosidenib should be discontinued.
   * *Guillain-Barre syndrome:* Rare occurrence of Guillian-Barre affected < 1% of patients in the clinical study. Monitor patients for onset of new signs/symptoms of motor and/or sensory neuropathy (e.g., unilateral or bilateral weakness, sensory alterations, paresthesias, or dyspnea). Drug should be permanently discontinued if the patient develops Guillain-Barre syndrome.

Potential Toxicities/Side Effects and the Nursing Process

I. POTENTIAL FOR INJURY related to DIFFERENTIATION SYNDROME

Defining Characteristics: Syndrome is associated with rapid proliferation and differentiation of myeloid cells, and may be life-threatening. It requires prompt initiation of corticosteroids and close clinical monitoring. Incidence in clinical trials was 19%. Signs and symptoms include: acute respiratory distress (dyspnea, hypoxia, and need for supplemental oxygen), pulmonary infiltrates, pleural effusion, renal impairment, fever, lymphadenopathy, bone pain, peripheral edema with rapid weight gain, and/or pericardial effusion.

Nursing Implications: If suspected, discuss urgent management with provider (e.g., corticosteroids such as dexamethasone 10 mg q 12 hours and close clinical monitoring). If patient has pulmonary and/or renal dysfunction, hospitalization is recommended for close observation and monitoring. Expect that corticosteroids will be tapered only after symptoms have resolved. Signs/symptoms may recur if corticosteroids are stopped too early. If pulmonary symptoms requiring intubation/ventilator support occur and/or renal dysfunction persist for > 48 hours after starting corticosteroids, interrupt ivosidenib therapy until symptoms are no longer severe (Agios, 2018).

II. POTENTIAL ALTERATION IN NUTRITION, LESS THAN BODY REQUIREMENTS, related to NAUSEA, VOMITING, DIARRHEA, DECREASED APPETITE, AND MUCOSITIS

Defining Characteristics: GI effects were common in clinical trials: nausea occurred in 31% (grade ≥ 3 was 1%), diarrhea 34% (grade ≥ 3 was 2%), and vomiting 18% (grade ≥ 3 was 1%). Mucositis occurred in 28% (grade ≥ 3 was 3%), Decreased appetite affected 18% of patients, and constipation affected 20% of patients. Electrolyte abnormalities occurred: decreased serum soldium (39%) of patients), decreased magnesium (38%), potassium decreased 31%) which can increase the risk of ventricular arrhythmias with QTc prolongation.

Nursing Implications: Assess baseline nutritional status, bowel-elimination status, and serum electrolytes. If patient develops nausea and/or vomiting, teach patient to self-administer antiemetics 1 hour prior to each dose and to call if nausea/vomiting persist. Discuss with physician more effective antiemetic regimen if nausea/vomiting persist. Encourage small, frequent intake of cool, bland foods as tolerated if nausea develops. Refer to dietitian as needed for meal planning. Teach patient to report diarrhea that does not respond to OTC antidiarrheal medication. Teach self-care measures of diet modification and increased oral fluids to 2–3 L during the waking hours. Discuss with provider and implement orders to replete electrolytes so that values are WNL.

III.   ALTERATION IN COMFORT related to FATIGUE, EDEMA, FEVER, ARTHRALGIA, MYALGIA, COUGH, DYSPNEA

Defining Characteristics: Fatigue occurred in 39% of patients, edema 32%, fever 23%, arthralgia 36%, myalgia 18%, cough 22%, dyspnea 13%, and pleural effusion 13%.

Nursing Implications: Assess baseline comfort level, pulmonary and fluid status baseline and regularly during treatment. Assess for edema, weight patient, and monitor at each visit. Teach patient that these side effects may occur, and to report them if they persist. If cough, edema, weight gain, and dyspnea occur, evaluate patient for differentiation syndrome and discuss abnormalities with provider. Discuss with patient self-care measures to relieve discomfort, and teach patient to report if the symptoms do not resolve. Revise plan and discuss pharmaceutical management with provider.

Drug: ixazomib (Ninlaro)

Class: Proteasome inhibitor; third-generation, oral proteasome inhibitor.

Mechanism of Action: Reversible proteasome inhibitor, which preferentially binds and inhibits the chymotrypsin-like activity of the beta-5 subunit of the 20S proteasome. This leads to apoptosis of multiple myeloma cells. Drug has synergy with lenalidomide and dexamethasone.

Metabolism: Drug is best absorbed on an empty stomach. Median time to peak plasma concentration is 1 hour. Mean absolute bioavailability is 58%. A high-fat meal decreased AUC by 28% and C_{max} by 69%. Ixazomib is 99% protein-bound. The drug's terminal half-life is 9.5 days. Drug is metabolized by CYP microenzymes and non-CYP-proteins. At higher doses than those used clinically, CYP3A4 metabolized 42% of the drug, followed by CYP1A2 (26%) and others. Approximately 62% of a dose is excreted in the urine ($<$ 3.5% unchanged), and 22% in the feces.

Indications(s): In combination with lenalidomide and dexamethasone for the treatment of patients with multiple myeloma who have received at least one prior therapy.

Dosage/Range:
- Recommended starting doses: 28-day (4 weeks) treatment cycle:
  - Ixazomib: 4 mg PO on days 1, 8, and 15 [3 mg PO if mod-severe hepatic impairment or severe renal impairment].
  - Lenalidomide: 25 mg PO on days 1–21.
  - Dexamethasone: 40 mg PO on days 1, 8, 15, and 22.
- Concomitant medications: discuss with provider antiviral prophylaxis to reduce risk of herpes zoster reactivation.

Dose Modifications:
- Dose reductions: Recommended starting dose 4 mg (except 3 mg in patients with moderate or severe hepatic impairment, severe renal or end-stage renal disease requiring

dialysis); first dose reduction to 3 mg; second dose reduction to 2.3 mg; next dose reduction: discontinue drug.

- Thrombocytopenia ($< 30,000/mm^3$): Hold ixazomib and lenalidomide until platelet count $\geq 30,000/mm^3$. After recovery, resume lenalidomide at the next lower dose according to its prescribing information, and resume ixazomib at its most recent dose. If platelet count falls to $< 30,000/mm^3$ again, hold ixazomib and lenalidomide until platelet count $\geq 30,000/mm^3$. Following recovery, resume ixazomib at the next lower dose and resume lenalidomide at its most recent dose.

- Neutropenia (ANC $< 500/mm^3$): Hold ixazomib and lenalidomide until ANC is at least 500/mm^3. Consider adding granulocyte-colony stimulating factor (G-CSF) as per clinical guideline. Following recovery, resume lenalidomide at next lower dose according to its prescribing information and resume ixazomib at its most recent dose. If ANC falls to $< 500/mm^3$, hold ixazomib and lenalidomide until ANC is at least $500/mm^3$. Following recovery, resume ixazomib at the next lower dose, and resume lenalidomide at its most recent dose.

- Nonhematologic toxicities:
  - Rash, grades 2–3: hold lenalidomide until rash recovers to grade 1 or lower. Following recovery, resume lenalidomide at the next lower dose according to its prescribing information. If grades 2–3 rash recurs, hold ixazomib and lenalidomide until rash recovers to grade 1 or lower. Following recovery, resume ixazomib at the next lower dose and resume lenalidomide at its most recent dose. If grade 4 rash, discontinue treatment regimen.
  - PN:
    - Grade 1 (with pain) or grade 2: Hold ixazomib until PN recovers to grade 1 or lower without pain or patient's baseline. Following recovery, resume ixazomib at its most recent dose.
    - Grade 2 with pain or grade 3: Hold ixazomib until recovery to patient's baseline or grade 1 or lower; after recovery, resume ixazomib at the next lower dose.
    - Grade 4: Discontinue treatment regimen.
  - Other grade 3 or 4 nonhematologic toxicities: Hold ixazomib until recovery to grade 1 or lower or patient's baseline. If attributable to ixazomib, resume ixazomib at the next lower dose following recovery.

Drug Preparation: Available as 4-mg, 3-mg, and 2.3-mg capsules.

Drug Administration:

- Assess CBC/differential: Prior to starting a new cycle of therapy, assess ANC (must be at least $1,000/mm^3$), platelet count (must be at least $75,000/mm^3$), and any nonhematologic toxicities which should be recovered to baseline or grade 1 or lower.

- Teach patient to (1) take dose at least 1 hour before or at least 2 hours after food; (2) take at approximately the same time each week (3 weeks out of 4); (3) swallow the capsule whole and do not crush, chew, or open the capsule; (4) if a dose is delayed, or missed, take the dose only if the next scheduled dose is more than 72 hours away (DO NOT take within 72 hours of the next scheduled dose); (5) if vomiting occurs after taking a dose, do not repeat the dose; resume taking the drug at the next scheduled time.

- Concomitant medications: Discuss with provider antiviral prophylaxis to reduce risk of herpes zoster reactivation.

Drug Interactions:
• Strong CYP3A Inducers: Avoid concomitant administration of ixazomib with strong inducers (e.g., rifampin, carbamazepine, St. John's wort).

Lab Effects/Interference: Thrombocytopenia, neutropenia

Special Considerations:
• Most common (≥ 20% incidence) adverse reactions in clinical studies were: diarrhea,
constipation, thrombocytopenia, PN, nausea, peripheral edema, vomiting, and back pain.
• Warnings and Precautions:
  • *Thrombocytopenia:* Nadir occurs between days 14–21 of each 28-day cycle, with
  recovery to baseline by the start of the next cycle. Monitor platelet count at least
  monthly during treatment, or more frequently as needed during the first 3 cycles.
  Manage with dose modifications and platelet transfusion per MD.
  • *GI toxicities:* Diarrhea, constipation, nausea, and vomiting may occur. (See Nursing
  Implications below.) Adjust dose for diarrhea constipation, nausea, and vomiting as
  needed per MD.
  • *PN:* PN was primarily sensory, with motor symptoms reported < 1%. Adjust dose as
  needed per MD.
  • *Peripheral edema:* Principally grades 1 or 2. Assess for fluid retention.
  • *Cutaneous reactions* may occur, most commonly maculopapular and macular rash.
  Monitor patient for rash and discuss dose modification with MD.
  • *Hepatotoxicity:* Drug-induced liver injury, hepatic steatosis, hepatits cholestatic, and
  hepatotoxicity have rarely been reported. Monitor hepatic enzymes baseline and regularly and adjust dose for grades 3–4 per MD.
  • *Embryo-fetal toxicity:* Ixazomib is embryo-fetal toxic. Teach women of reproductive
  potential to use effective contraception during therapy and for 90 days (3 months)
  after the last dose, to avoid pregnancy. Mothers should not nurse while receiving the
  drug: discontinue nursing.
• Eye disorders (e.g., blurred vision, dry eye, conjunctivitis) have been reported, with an
incidence of 26% compared to the placebo arm which had 16%. Assess for and teach
patient to report any eye changes.

Potential Toxicities/Side Effects and the Nursing Process

I.   POTENTIAL FOR INFECTION AND BLEEDING related to BONE MARROW DEPRESSION

Defining Characteristics: Thrombocytopenia occurred in 78% of patients (26% grades
3–4) compared to the control arm (placebo plus lenalidomide and dexamethasone) which
was 54% (11% grades 3–4). Neutropenia occurred in 67% of patients (26% grades 3–4)
compared to the control arm which had 66% incidence with 30% grades 3–4.

Nursing Implications: Assess baseline ANC and platelet count, monitor before each treatment, during therapy, and more often as needed. Assess risk for infection and integrity of
skin and mucous membranes, pulmonary status, and ability to clear secretions, as well as

TREATMENT

history of past infections, baseline and prior to each treatment. Teach patient to self-assess for signs/symptoms of infection or bleeding and to call provider immediately or come to the emergency room if temperature < 100.4°F or has shaking chills, rash, productive cough, burning on urination, or any signs/symptoms of infection or bleeding. Teach self-care strategies to minimize risk of infection and bleeding, including avoidance of OTC aspirin-containing medications.

II.   ALTERATION IN NUTRITION, LESS THAN BODY REQUIREMENTS, related to NAUSEA, DIARRHEA, CONSTIPATION, VOMITING, HEPATOTOXICITY

Defining Characteristics: Symptoms that interfere with adequate nutrition were common. Diarrhea occurred in 42% (compared to 36% in control arm), constipation in 34% (vs 25%), nausea in 26% (vs 21%), and vomiting in 22% (vs 11%). Hepatic toxicity can occur, as evidenced by changes in LFTs.

Nursing Implications: Assess baseline weight and nutritional status, as well as bowel-elimination status. Teach patient that these side effects may occur and to report symptoms if uncontrolled by self-care measures. Monitor LFTs baseline and periodically during treatment. Teach patient self-administration of antiemetic agent, as well as antidiarrheal or cathartic as appropriate. Teach patient dietary modifications for constipation, nausea, diarrhea (e.g., small feedings with low-fat or nonspicy foods, BRAT diet: bananas, rice, applesauce, and toast). Assess efficacy of intervention, and revise plan as needed. Teach patient to report symptoms that persist, worsen, or do not resolve. Discuss revised plan with NP/PA/MD.

III.   POTENTIAL SENSORY/PERCEPTUAL ALTERATIONS related to SENSORY PN

Defining Characteristics: PN was primarily sensory, with < 1% motor neuropathy. Incidence was 28% with 2% grades 3–4, compared to the placebo arm which had an incidence of 21% with 2% grades 3–4.

Nursing Implications: Teach patient to report new onset or worsening of PN symptoms (numbness, pain, or burning sensation in feet or hands), any changes in sensory function (temperature sensation, knowing where body parts are in relation to the whole, etc.), functional ability (e.g., especially senses of smell and taste), and ability to carry out ADLs. Assess patient for symptoms of PN (burning sensation, hypersthesia, hypoesthesia, paresthesia, discomfort, neuropathic pain, weakness) as well as severity of symptom(s) if they arise and potential for injury. If these are new symptoms or worsening of preexisting symptoms, discuss with MD/PA/NP dose modifications.

Drug: lapatinib (Tykerb)

Class: Kinase inhibitor; 4-anilinoquinazoline kinase inhibitor of the intracellular tyrosine kinase domains of EGFR1 (ErbB1) and EGFR2 (ErbB2) domains.

Mechanism of Action: Drug inhibits tyrosine kinases of both human epidermal growth factor receptor (EGFR or) HER-1 and (EGFR-2 or) HER-2-neu, leading to arrest of cell growth and/or apoptosis in tumor cells that depend upon ErbB1 and ErbB2 cell signaling. Normally, HER-2 dimerizes with other members of the HER family, including HER-1. The message is then sent repeatedly via the tyrosine kinases to the cell nucleus telling the cell to divide. In 20% of patients with breast cancer, HER-2-neu is overexpressed, leading to increased cell proliferation, invasiveness, and conferring a poor prognosis associated with reduced survival. By blockading the tyrosine kinases, the message for repeated cell division is halted. Crosses the blood–brain barrier.

Metabolism: After oral ingestion, drug undergoes incomplete and variable absorption. Initial serum concentration identifiable in 15 minutes (median). Peak concentrations achieved in 4 hours, with steady state reached in 6–7 days of single daily dosing. Dividing the dose results in a twofold higher exposure at steady state. When given with food, systemic exposure is increased threefold higher (low-fat diet) or fourfold higher (high-fat diet). Drug is highly protein-bound (> 99%). Drug is a substrate for the transporter proteins, breast cancer-resistance protein (BCRP), and P-glycoprotein, and yet, lapatinib is also able to inhibit these efflux transporters. Drug is extensively metabolized by the CYP3A4 and CYP3A5 microenzyme system. Terminal half-life of the drug is 14.2 hours and with daily dosing is 24 hours. Drug is eliminated by the liver (P450 system) with about 27% recoverable from feces and less than 2% from the urine. Drug is not dialyzable due to high-protein binding.

Indications: Lapatinib is indicated in combination with:
- Capecitabine, for the treatment of patients with advanced or metastatic breast cancer whose tumors overexpress HER-2 and have received prior therapy, including an anthracycline, a taxane, and trastuzumab. (Limitation of use: Patients should have disease progression on trastuzumab prior to initiation of lapatinib/capecitabine treatment.) Patients should have disease progression on trastuzumab prior to starting treatment with lapatinib together with capecitabine.
- Letrozole, for the treatment of postmenopausal women with hormone receptor-positive, metastatic breast cancer that overexpresses the HER-2 receptor for whom hormonal therapy is indicated.
- Lapatinib in combination with an aromatasa inhibitor has not been compared to a trastuzumab-containing chemotherapy regimen for the treatment of metastatic breast cancer.

Dosage/Range:
- Advanced or metastatic breast cancer: 1,250 mg orally (5 tablets) once daily PO on days 1–21 continuously, at least 1 hour before or 1 hour after a meal, in combination with capecitabine, 2,000 mg/m^2/day PO bid on days 1–14, administered orally (in 2 doses with food or within 30 min of after food, approximately 12 hours apart), repeated every 21 days.
- Hormone receptor-positive, HER-2+ metastatic breast cancer: 1,500 mg PO (6 tablets) once daily, continuously in combination with letrozole (e.g., 2.5 mg once daily).
- Lapatinib should be taken at least 1 hour before or 1 hour after a meal. The dose should be taken all at once, not divided.

Dose Modifications (see package insert):

- *Decrease in LVEF:* Discontinue drug in patients with a decreased LVEF that is grade 2 or higher (NCI CTCAE v3), and in patients with an LVEF that drops below the institution's LLN (ILLN). Wait a minimum of 2 weeks, and if the LVEF returns to normal and the patient is asymptomatic, drug may be restarted at a reduced dose of 1,000 mg/day in combination with capecitabine and a dose of 1,250 mg/day in combination with letrozole.

- *Preexisting severe hepatic impairment:* Reduce dose, as systemic exposure to lapatinib (AUC) increased 14% in patients with moderate and 63% in patients with severe preexisting hepatic dysfunction. Thus, patients with severe hepatic impairment (Child-Pugh Class C) should be reduced as follows:
  - HER-2+ metastatic BC indication: Reduce from 1,250 mg/day to 750 mg/day.
  - Hormone receptor-positive, HER-2+ BC indication: Reduce 1,500 mg/day to 1,000 mg/day as this estimates a normal AUC; however, there are no clinical data to support this.
  - Discontinue and do not restart drug if patient develops severe changes in liver function tests while receiving lapatinib.

- *Diarrhea:* Interrupt lapatinib for NCI CTCAE grade 3 or grade 1 or 2 with complicating features (e.g., moderate-to-severe abdominal cramping, grade 2 or higher nausea and/or vomiting, decreased performance status, fever, sepsis, neutropenia, frank bleeding, or dehydration).
  - Lapatinib can be reintroduced at a lower dose (e.g., 1,000 mg/day reduced from 1,250 mg/day, 1,250 mg/day reduced from 1,500 mg/day) when diarrhea resolves to grade 1 or less.
  - Permanently discontinue drug for grade 4 diarrhea.

- Drug Interactions: *Strong CYP3A4 inhibitors*: Avoid concomitant administration. If avoidance of the drug is not possible, reduce lapatinib dose to 500 mg orally per day, and when interacting drug discontinued, allow 1 week washout period before adjusting lapatinib dose up to 1,250 mg/day. Teach patients NOT to drink grapefruit juice or eat grapefruit to avoid increased serum lapatinib levels.

- Drug Interactions: *Strong CYP3A4 inducers*: Avoid coadministration. If unavoidable, and must give both together, gradually titrate dose of lapatinib up to 4,500 mg/day (from 1,250 mg in HER-2+ metastatic BC) or to 5,500 mg/day (from 1,500 mg in hormone receptor-positive HER-2 BC) based on tolerability; if interacting drug is discontinued, resume original indicated dose.

- *Other toxicities:* Discontinue or interrupt drug if patient develops grade 2 or higher toxicities (NCI CTCAE). Resume at 1,250 mg/day or 1,500 mg/day (original standard dose) when improvement to grade 1 or less; for recurrent toxicity, restart at a lower dose of 1,000 mg/day (in combination with capecitabine) or 1,250 mg/day in combination with letrozole.

- Drug is contraindicated in patients with known hypersensitivity such as anaphylaxis to the drug or any of its components.

Drug Preparation:

- Oral. Available in 250-mg tablets.

Drug Administration:
Assess patient:
- Assess baseline LVEF (ECHO or MUGA) results prior to starting lapatinib, and periodically during therapy.
- Assess LFTs baseline and every 4–6 weeks during treatment.
- Assess serum potassium and magnesium; discuss plan for repletion of electrolytes if hypokalemia, hypomagnesemia occur, so that levels are repleted prior to lapatinib administration.

Teach patient:
- If taking the lapatinib/capecitabine regimen, drugs are taken in a 21-day cycle. Lapatinib is taken one time a day on days 1–21. Teach schedule for capecitabine (usually twice a day days 1–14) but per physician order.
  - Take lapatinib in a single dose 1 hour before or 1 hour after a meal.
  - Take capecitabine in two divided doses about 12 hours apart with food or within 30 minutes of a meal.
  - Make a schedule for the patient to illustrate the correct self-administration times of these 2 agents.
- If taking the letrozole/lapatinib regimen, to take letrozole as a single dose without regard to food or meals. Do not divide dose. May take with lapatinib dose.
  - Do not eat/drink grapefruit products or take St. John's wort.

Drug Interactions:
- Capecitabine: additive benefits.
- Drugs metabolized by the CYP3A4 and CYP2C8 microenzyme system: lapatinib inhibits CYP3A4 and CYP2C8 (e.g., midazolam, paclitaxel, digoxin); monitor for toxicity of drug coadministered with lapatinib, especially if narrow therapeutic window. If necessary, dose of concomitant drug may need to be reduced.
- Lapatinib inhibits p-glycoprotein (transport system); if given with drugs that are substrates of p-glycoprotein, assess for toxicity resulting from increased substrate concentration, especially if there is a narrow therapeutic window.
- Midazolam (CYP3A4 substrate): increased AUC midazolam 45% when given PO, and 22% when given IV.
- Paclitaxel (CYP2C8 and P-gp substrate): paclitaxel AUC increased 23% (24-hour exposure).
- Digoxin (P-gp substrate): increased digoxin AUC 2.8-fold. Monitor baseline digoxin serum level prior to starting lapatinib, and throughout coadministration. If serum digoxin level is > 1.2 ng, digoxin dose should be reduced by half.
- Inhibitors of CYP3A4 (atazanavir, clarithromycin, grapefruit or grapefruit juice, indinavir, itraconazole, ketoconazole, nelfinavir, nefazodone, ritonavir, saquinavir, telithromycin, voriconazole): do not coadminister.
- Inducers of CYP3A4 (carbamazepine, dexamethasone, phenobarbital, phenytoin, rifabutin, rifampin, rifapentine, St. John's wort): do not coadminister.
- Solubility of lapatinib is pH dependent, but coadministration with PPI esomeprazole did not reduce lapatinib steady-state level significantly.

Lab Effects/Interference:

- Increased BR, AST, ALT.
- QT/QTc prolongation.
- Decreased LVEF.
- Decreased WBC, ANC, platelet count when coadministered with capecitabine.

Special Considerations:

- Warnings and Precautions:
- *Decreased LVEF:* More than 57% of patients in clinical trials had a decrease in LVEF in first 12 weeks of treatment. Assess LVEF in all patients before starting lapatinib to ensure patient's baseline is within institutional normal limits. Continue to evaluate during therapy to ensure that LVEF does not decline below ILLN.
- *Hepatotoxicity* can occur (ALT or AST > 3 × ULN and total bilirubin > 2 ULN), occurring days to months after start of therapy, and may be fatal.
  - Monitor LFTs baseline and every 4–6 weeks during treatment and as clinically indicated. Discontinue and do not restart lapatinib if patients experience severe changes in LFTs.
  - If patient has severe preexisting hepatic impairment, dose-reduce drug. Discontinue and do not restart lapatinib if patients experience severe hepatotoxicity.
- *Diarrhea:* ***may*** be severe, and deaths have been reported. Of patients who develop diarrhea, about half experience it within 6 days of starting therapy
  - Diarrhea usually lasts 4–5 days, and is low-grade. Grades 3–4 occurs in < 10% and < 1% of patients, respectively.
  - Key to management is early identification: teach patients to report any change in bowel patterns immediately and to take antidiarrheal agent (e.g., loperamide) after the first unformed stool.
  - Severe diarrhea may require oral or IV fluid and electrolyte replacement, antibiotic therapy (e.g., fluoroquinolones, especially if diarrhea persists > 24 hours, there is fever, or grades 3–4 neutropenia), as well as interruption or discontinuation of lapatinib therapy.
- *Patients with severe hepatic impairment:* Reduce dose should be considered; if patient develops severe hepatotoxicity while on therapy, discontinue lapatinib and do not rechallenge the patient with lapatinib.
- *Interstitial Lung Disease (ILD):* Drug has been associated with ILD and pneumonitis due to EGFR blockade (EGF is necessary for repair of injured lung tissue). Monitor for pulmonary symptoms characteristic of ILD/pneumonitis (e.g., dyspnea, cough, fever). Discontinue lapatinib if patients experience grade 3 or greater pulmonary symptoms indicative of ILD/pneumonitis.
- *QTc Prolongation*: Lapatinib may prolong the QTc interval in some patients.
  - Consider ECG and electrolyte monitoring, especially in patients who have or may develop prolongation of the QTc (patients with hypokalemia, hypomagnesemia, congenital long QT syndrome, taking anti-arrhythmic medications or other drugs that lead to QT prolongation, and cumulative high-dose anthracycline therapy). Correct hypokalemia or hypomagnesemia before lapatinib administration.

- Ensure that hypomagnesemia or hypokalemia is corrected prior to lapatinib administration.
- *Severe cutaneous reactions*: Severe reactions such as life-threatening erythema multiforme, SJS, or toxic epidermal necrolysis (e.g., progressive skin rash often with blisters or mucosal lesions) may rarely occur (Novartis, 2015). If suspected, lapatinib should be discontinued.
- *Embryo-fetal toxicity:* Drug can cause fetal harm. Teach women of childbearing potential to use effective contraception to avoid pregnancy during treatment and for at least 1 week after last dose. Teach male patients with female partners of reproductive potential to use effective contraception during therapy and for at least 1 week after final dose. If the drug is used in pregnancy, or if the patient becomes pregnant while on the drug, the patient should be apprised of the potential hazard to the fetus.
- The most common side effects (> 20%):
  - Lapatinib together with capecitabine were diarrhea, nausea, vomiting, palmar–plantar erythrodysesthesia, rash, and fatigue.
  - Lapatinib together with letrozole: diarrhea, rash, nausea, fatigue.

Potential Toxicities/Side Effects and the Nursing Process

I.   ALTERATION IN CIRCULATION, POTENTIAL, related to LEFT VENTRICULAR DYSFUNCTION, QT PROLONGATION, EPISTAXIS

Defining Characteristics: Rarely, patients may develop a decrease in left ventricular ejection fraction (LVEF) to below the institutional lower limit of normal (ILLN). Sixty percent of the time this occurs within the first 9 weeks of treatment. QT prolongation may occur; administer with caution in patients with prolonged or who may develop prolonged QTc (those having hypokalemia, hypomagnesemia, or taking other drugs that prolong the QTc, cumulative high-dose anthracycline therapy). Bleeding may occur, primarily epistaxis (11% incidence).

Nursing Implications: Assess baseline and periodic LVEF tests, as well as assess patients for any signs or symptoms of congestive heart failure. Identify patients at risk for further decrease in LVEF or development of prolonged QTc. Correct electrolyte abnormalities (e.g., magnesium, potassium) before starting lapatinib, and monitor periodically during therapy. If LVEF falls below ILLN, the drug should be stopped for at least 2 weeks until the LVEF is above the ILLN. Discuss any abnormalities with physician or NP. Teach patient bleeding may occur and to come to ED/notify physician/NP right away if bleeding (e.g., epistaxis) does not resolve in 15 minutes with local pressure and cooling.

II.   ALTERATION IN NUTRITION, LESS THAN BODY REQUIREMENTS, related to DIARRHEA, NAUSEA, VOMITING, STOMATITIS, DYSPEPSIA, INCREASED LFTs

Defining Characteristics: Diarrhea occurs in 65% of patients, 13% grade 3, and 1% grade 4, compared to patients receiving capecitabine alone (40% with 10% grade 3). If diarrhea precedes or occurs during nadir when coadministered with capecitabine, the patient is at risk for sepsis. Diarrhea generally occurs early, often within 6 days of starting the drug; it lasts 4–5 days, and is generally mild. Nausea occurs in 44% with 2% grade 3, whereas vomiting affected 26% of patients, with 2% grade 3. Capecitabine primary side effects include diarrhea, nausea, and vomiting. Stomatitis affected 14% and dyspepsia 11%. In combination with capecitabine, which causes some elevation of LFTs, BR was elevated in 45% of patients (4% grade 3), AST in 49% of patients, and ALT in 37% of patients. One percent of patients may develop severe hepatotoxicity, which was fatal in some instances.

Nursing Implications: Assess nutritional status, bowel-elimination pattern, and appetite, including LFTs, at baseline and repeated periodically during treatment. Teach patient to report right away any change in bowel-elimination pattern. Teach patient to take loperamide. Teach patient to report any change in bowel-elimination patterns right away. Teach patient to be proactive, and to take antidiarrheal agents (e.g., loperamide) after the first unformed stool, if it occurs. Severe diarrhea requires aggressive support as needed with oral or IV hydration, electrolyte replacement, antibiotics (e.g., fluoroquinolones, especially if diarrhea persists beyond 24 hours, the patient is febrile, or has grade 3 or 4 neutropenia). Drug should be interrupted (or discontinued) until diarrhea resolves. LFTs should be repeated every 4–6 weeks during treatment. Inform patient these side effects may occur. Teach self-administration of antinausea and antidiarrheal medications (e.g., loperamide) according to protocol and to notify provider if symptoms persist so that the dose can be interrupted per protocol. Teach the patient dietary modification if nausea and vomiting or diarrhea occur (e.g., for diarrhea, BRAT diet: bananas, rice, applesauce, and toast) and to increase oral fluids to prevent dehydration. Consult dietitian to see patient for dietary counseling for anorexia. Discuss any abnormalities with physician or NP.

III.   ALTERATION IN COMFORT related to PALMAR-PLANTAR ERYTHRODYSESTHESIA (PPE), RASH, FATIGUE

Defining Characteristics: PPE is a dose-limiting side effect of capecitabine. The incidence is 53% with 12% grade 3. Acneform rash is characteristic of EGFRIs and is usually mild to moderate. A rash occurred in 28% of patients and dry skin in 10%. Fatigue is common.

Nursing Implications: Assess patient's baseline comfort, and teach that these symptoms may occur. Assess skin integrity (especially sun-exposed skin and palms of hands, soles of feet) baseline and during therapy. Teach symptom-management strategies to minimize discomfort. Teach patient to notify nurse or physician if fatigue or rash is severe, or does not resolve with local management. Discuss dose interruption or delay with physician or NP.

Teach patient about PPE: This side effect may occur, and instruct patient to stop drug and call physician/nurse immediately should it occur. If patient has pain, expect dose interruption, with dose reduction if this is the second or subsequent episode at current dose. Teach patient self-assessment of soles of feet and palms of hands daily for erythema, pain, and dry desquamation and to report pain right away. Teach patients to avoid hot showers, whirlpools, paraffin treatments of nails, vigorous repetitive movements of hands and feet, as well as other body areas; avoid tight-fitting shoes and clothes. Teach patients to take cool showers and keep skin surfaces intact and soft with skin emollients. Studies ongoing establishing evidence base for prophylaxis or treatment: vitamin B_6, urea moisturizers, nicotine patch.

Teach patient about EGFRI rash: (Refer also to the Introduction to *Chapter 4*.) Do not use antiacne medications. Tetracycline analogues provide an anti-inflammatory benefit. Teach all patients to (1) use a water-based emollient frequently during the day to prevent dryness, (2) stay hydrated, (3) avoid sun exposure and wear SPF 30 (UVA/UVB). Follow institutional guidelines. In general, **for grade 1 or mild rash (localized, does not interfere with ADLs, and is not infected):** The goal is to preserve skin integrity, minimize discomfort, and prevent infection. Key patient teaching includes to (1) use a mild soap with active ingredients that reduce skin drying such as pyrithione zinc (Head & Shoulders), (2) consider aloe gel for red, tender areas, (3) report distressing tenderness as pramoxine (lidocaine topical anesthetic may help), (4) keep fingernails clean and trimmed, and (5) apply zinc ointment to rectal mucosa after washing. Management: maintain current drug dose; observe or give topical hydrocortisone 1% or 2.5% or clindamycin 1% gel (anti-inflammatory benefit); reassess in 2 weeks. **For grade 2 or moderate rash (generalized, with mild symptoms, and minimal effect on ADLs, and is not infected):** The goal is to prevent infection and promote comfort. Continue EGFRI dose; use topicals (hydrocortisone 2.5% or clindamycin 1% gel) or consider pimecrolimus cream (immunomodulator) and add doxycycline 100 mg PO twice daily or minocycline 100 mg PO twice daily (give antimicrobial and anti-inflammatory effect) and reassess after 2 weeks. **For grades 3–4 or severe rash (generalized, severe, has a significant impact on ADLs, and increased risk of infection):** The goal is to prevent infection or identify it early to minimize complications and maximize patient coping with side effects. Hold drug until rash improves, and treat rash with topicals (hydrocortisone 2.5% or clindamycin 1% gel or pimecrolimus cream, doxycycline 100 mg PO twice daily or minocycline 100 mg PO twice daily, and methylprednisolone, Medrol dose pack); reassess after 2 weeks and interrupt or discontinue drug if rash worsens (Lynch et al., 2007). If rash appears infected (exudate, vesicular formation, different appearance), obtain C+S, treat empirically until sensitivity received, and/or obtain dermatology consult. Discuss dose modification with a physician.

Drug: lenvatinib (Lenvima)

Class: Multi-kinase inhibitor (antiangiogenic).

Mechanism of Action: Lenvatinib is a receptor kinase inhibitor of vascular endothelial growth factor: VEGFR1 (FLT1), VEGFR2 (KDR), and VEGFR3 (FLT4). The drug also inhibits fibroblast growth factor (FGF) 1–4, PDGFR-α, KIT, and RET. This blockade has been shown to interrupt angiogenesis, tumor growth, and cancer progression.

Metabolism: Following oral administration, peak plasma concentration (T_{max}) occurs 1–4 hours after dosing; when given with food, there is a delay in rate of absorption and T_{max} of 2–4 hours. The drug is highly protein-bound (98–99%) and is metabolized by CYP3A enzymes (primarily CYP3A4 and aldehyde oxidase). The terminal elimination half-life of lenvatinib is approximately 28 hours.

TREATMENT

Indications: Treatment of patients with (1) locally recurrent or metastatic, progressive, radioactive iodine–refractory differentiated thyroid cancer (DTC); (2) advanced renal cell cancer (RCC), in combination with everolimus, following one prior antiangiogenic therapy; (3) 1st line treatment of patients with unresectable hepatocellular carcinoma (HCC).

Dosage/Range:
- Recommended dose (take until disease progression or unaceptable toxicity):
  - DTC: 24 mg orally, once daily until disease progression or unacceptable toxicity.
  - RCC: 18 mg lenvatinib, together with 5 mg everolimus, orally, once daily.
  - HCC: 12 mg for patients who weigh ≥ 60 kg OR 8 mg for patients weighing < 60 kg.
- Severe renal (ClCr < 30 mL/min, Cockcroft-Gault equation) or hepatic impairment (Child-Pugh C): reduce dose to 14 mg once daily for patients with DTC, and to 10 mg once daily for RCC patients.

Dose Modifications (see package insert August 2018):
- Dose modification for persistent and intolerable or grade 2 adverse reactions or grade 3 adverse reactions or grade 4 laboratory abnormalities:
  - DTC: *1st dosage reduction* to: 20 mg once daily; *2nd dosage reduction* to 14 mg once daily; *3rd dosage reduction* to 10 mg once daily.
  - RCC: *1st dosage reduction* to: 14 mg once daily; *2nd dosage reduction* to 10 mg once daily; *3rd dosage reduction* to 8 mg once daily. When administering lenvatinib with everolimus, reduce the lenvatinib dose first, and then the everolimus dose for adverse reactions of both drugs. See everolimus prescribing information for dose modification information.
  - HCC: (1) Actual weight 60 kg or greater: *1st dosage reduction* to: 8 mg once daily; *2nd dosage reduction* to 4 mg once daily; *3rd dosage reduction* to 4 mg every other day; (2) actual weight < 60 kg: *1st dosage reduction* to: 4 mg once daily; *2nd dosage reduction* to 10 mg once daily; *3rd dosage reduction* to 4 mg every other day; *3rd dosage reduction*: discontinue drug.

Specific Dose Modifications for Adverse Reactions:
- *Hypertension (HTN):* Grade 3: Hold drug for grade 3 HTN that persists despite optimal antihypertensive therapy; resume at a reduced dose when HTN is controlled at ≤ grade 2; grade 4: permanently discontinue drug. Serious complications of poorly controlled HTN have been reported.
- *Cardiac dysfunction:* Grade 3: Withhold drug until resolved to grades 0–1 or baseline, then resume at a reduced dose or discontinue based on severity and persistence of toxicity. Grade 4: Discontinue drug.
- *Arterial thrombotic event (ATE):* Any grade: Discontinue lenvatinib.
- *Hepatotoxicity:* Grade 3 or 4: Hold lenvatinib until resolved to grades 0–1 or baseline. Either resume at a reduced dose or discontinue based on severity and persistence. Permanently discontinue drug for hepatic failure.
- *Renal failure or impairment:* Incidence of impairment was 14% and 7% in patients with HCC in two clinical trials. Grade 3–5 renal impairment/failure occurred in 3% in patients with differentiated thyroid cancer, and 2% in patients with HCC. Promptly manage diarrhea or dehydration/hypovolemia. Hold drug and resume at a reduced dose for renal

failure or impairment based on severity, and resume drug at a reduced dose or discontinue permanently as ordered.

- *Proteinuria:* 2 g or greater proteinuria in 24 hr: Hold drug until ≤ 2 grams of proteinuria per 24 hours and resume at a reduced dose; permanently discontinue lenvatinib for nephrotic syndrome.
- Diarrhea: Incidence was 49% in studies, with a grade 3 incidence of 6%. When drug administered with everolimus (RCC study), incidence of diarrhea was 81% with Grade 3 in 19% of patients. Diarrhea should be identified promptly and managed to prevent hypovolemia and electrolyte imbalance. Hold lenvatinib and resume drug at a reduced dose when patient recovers or the drug should be permanently discontinued based on severity.
- *Gastrointestinal (GI) perforation:* Any grade: permanently discontinue.
- *Fistula formation: Grade 3 or 4:* permanently discontinue.
- *QT prolongation:* Greater than 500 ms or greaeter than 60 ms increase from baseline: Hold drug until improves to ≤ 480 ms or baseline; resume at a reduced dose.
- *Hypocalcemia:* Grade 3-4 hypocalcemia occurred in 9% of patients receiving lenvatinib. In two-thirds of cases, hypocalcemia improved or resolved after calcium supplementation with or without dose modification. Monitor serum calcium levels baseline and at least monthly and replace calcium as needed during lenvatinib therapy. Hold drug and resume at reduced dose upon recovery or permanently discontinue based on severity.
- *Reversible posterior leukoencephalopathy syndrome (RPLS):* Any grade: Hold drug until RPLS is fully resolved; then resume at a reduced dose or discontinue drug based on severity and persistence of neurologic symptoms.
- *Hemorrhagic events:* Serious hemorrhagic events can occur, including fatal bleeding. Most commonly seen were epistaxis and hematuria. Serious tumor related bleeding can occur, including fatal hemorrhage, as reported in clinical trials and post-marketing reports. Carotid artery hemorrhage was seen in patients with anaplastic thyroid carcinoma more commonly than in other tumor types. Physicians should consider the risk of severe or fatal hemorrhage associated with tumor invasion or infiltration of major blood vessels (e.g., carotid artery), when discussing the risk and benefit with patients of lenvatinb therapy. If hemorrhage occurs, the drug should be held, then resume at a reduced dose when patient has recovered, or discontinued based on severity.
- *Impairment of TSH suppression/thyroid dysfunction:* Monitor thyroid function before lenvatinib is started (baseline) and at least monthly during treatment. Hypothyroidism should be treated according to standard of care.
- *Wound healing complications:* can occur, including fistula formation and wound dehiscence. Drug should be held for at least 6 days prior to scheduled surgery. Resume drug after surgery when adequate wound healing is seen. If wound healing complications occur, drug should be permanently discontinued.
- *Embryo-fetal toxicity:* Drug is fetotoxic and teratogenic. Teach women of reproductive potential to use effective contraception during lenvatinib therapy and for at least 30 days after the last dose.
- *Other adverse reactions:* Persistent or intolerable grade 2 or 3 or grade 4 laboratory abnormality: Hold lenvatinib until it resolves to grades 0–1 or baseline; resume drug at at a reduced dose; grade 4: permanently discontinue.

TREATMENT

Drug Preparation: Available as 4-mg and 10-mg capsules. Keep at room temperature and out of the reach of children and pets.

Drug Administration:

- Assess BP baseline prior to treatment, then after 1 week, then every 2 weeks for the first 2 months, then at least monthly thereafter. Discuss HTN management prior to the patient starting therapy when BP control is documented, or if HTN occurs during therapy.
- Assess patient for signs and symptoms of cardiac dysfunction, ATE, development of neurologic symptom(s), and bleeding. Teach patient to report SOB, chest pain, bleeding, or any abnormality right away.
- Assess renal function tests and LFTs at baseline before starting therapy, then every 2 weeks for the first 2 months, then at least monthly during therapy.
- Assess serum electrolytes at baseline and during treatment and correct any abnormalities. If the patient has congenital long QT syndrome, CHF, or bradyarrhythmia or is taking drugs known to prolong the QT interval, monitor the ECG at baseline and during therapy for QT-interval prolongation.
- Assess patient urine dipstick for protein before starting therapy, then periodically during therapy. If dipstick is 2+ or higher, the patient should stop lenvatinib and the provider should evaluate a 24-hour urine sample for protein.
- Assess serum calcium at baseline and at least monthly for hypocalcemia; discuss dose interruption and calcium replacement with the provider if it occurs. TSH at baseline and monthly; discuss thyroid replacement adjustment with the provider if TSH is elevated.
- Teach females of reproductive potential to use effective contraception during therapy and for at least 2 weeks after stopping the drug. Women should discontinue breastfeeding while taking the drug.
- Teach the patient to self-administer the ordered dose (1) for DTC patients, 24 mg as two 10-mg capsules and one 4-mg capsule, orally once daily with or without food; and (2) for RCC patients, 18 mg as one 10-mg capsule, and two 4-mg capsules, orally once daily with or without food, together with 5 mg everolimus. Teach the patient to (1) take the medication at the same time every day; (2) if a dose is missed and cannot be taken within 12 hours, skip that dose, and take the next dose at the usual time; (3) swallow capsules whole. If the patient has difficulty swallowing the capsules, the capsules can be dissolved in a small glass of liquid; measure 1 tablespoon (T) of water or apple juice and put the capsules into the liquid without breaking or crushing them. Leave the capsules in the liquid at least 10 minutes, then stir for at least 3 minutes. The patient should drink the mixture, and afterwards, add 1 T of water or apple juice to the glass, swirl the contents a few times, and then drink the additional liquid.

Drug Interactions:

- No dose adjustment is recommended if coadministered with CYP3A, P-glycoprotein, and breast BCRP inhibitors, or with CYP3A or P-glycoprotein inducers.

Lab Effects/Interference:

- Increased serum creatinine, ALT, AST, or lipase
- Decreased serum calcium or potassium
- Decreased platelet count

- Abnormal TSH
- Prolonged QT interval on ECG

Special Considerations:
- Most common adverse reactions were HTN, fatigue, diarrhea, arthralgia/myalgia, decreased appetite, decreased weight, nausea, stomatitis, headache, vomiting, proteinuria, palmar–plantar erythrodysesthesia (PPE) syndrome, abdominal pain, and dysphonia.
- Most common serious adverse reactions were pneumonia (4%), HTN (3%), and dehydration (3%).
- A dose reduction was necessary for 68% of patients due to adverse reactions.
- Warnings and Precautions:
  - *Hypertension (HTN):* HTN may occur, and serious complications of poorly controlled HTN have been reported. Assess BP prior to therapy. If HTN found, discuss management with physician/NP/PA to initiate or adjust medical management to control BP. HTN should be controlled prior to levatinib therapy. Monitor BP after 1 week, then every 2 weeks for the first 2 months, then at least monthly during treatment. Hold drug for grade 3 HTN that persists despite optimal antihypertensive therapy; resume at a reduced dose when HTN is controlled at ≤ grade 2; discontinue drug for life-threatening HTN.
  - *Cardiac dysfunction:* Serious and fatal cardiac dysfunction can occur. Grade 3 or higher dysfunction across all clinical trials was 3% (cardiomyopathy, L/R ventricular dysfunction, CHF, cardiac failure, ventricular hypokinesia, decreased right or LVEF or > 20% from baseline. Monitor patients for clinical symptoms/signs of cardiac dysfunction. Withhold drug for grade 3 cardiac dysfunction until resolved to grades 0–1 or baseline, then either resume at a reduced dose or discontinue based on severity and persistence of toxicity. Discontinue drug for grade 4 events.
  - *Arterial thrombotic event (ATE):* Incidence alone or with everolimus was 2%, 2% in HCC studies, and 5% in patients with DTC; grade 3–5 ATE across all studies was 2–3%. Discontinue lenvatinib if an ATE occurs.
  - *Renal failure and impairment:* Renal impairment was reported in 14% of lenvatinib-treated patients, and was grade 3 or higher in 3%, while the incidence was 18% in RCC patients (10% grades 3–4). The major risk factor in clinical studies was dehydration/hypovolemia due to diarrhea and vomiting (Eisai, 2016). Aggressive management of diarrhea and GI symptoms should start for grade 1 events. Withhold drug for grades 3–4 renal failure/impairment until resolved to grades 0–1 or baseline; then resume at a reduced dose or discontinue lenvatinib based on severity and persistence of toxicity.
  - *Hepatotoxicity:* Monitor LFTs before starting lenvatinib, then every 2 weeks for the first 2 months, and at least monthly during therapy. Monitor patients with HCC closely for hepatic failure, including hepatic encephalopathy. Hold lenvatinib for grade 3 or greater liver impairment until resolved to grades 0–1 or baseline. Either resume at a reduced dose or discontinue based on severity and persistence. Discontinue drug for hepatic failure.
  - *Proteinuria:* Occurs in 26% (HCC)–34% (DTC) of patients and is grade 3 in 6–11% (Eisai, 2018). Assess for proteinuria before starting lenvatinib, and periodically

during therapy. If urine dipstick proteinuria is ≥ 2+, obtain 24-hour urine protein. Withhold drug for proteinuria ≥ 2 g/24 hr, and resume at a reduced dose when urinary protein < 2 g/24 hr. Discontinue lenvatinib for nephrotic syndrome.

- *Diarrhea:* In study 2 in RCC, diarrhea occurred in 81% of patients, and was grades 3–4 in 19% of patients. Incidence in DTC and HCC patients was 49%, and grade 3 in 6%. Begin prompt medical management for diarrhea, and monitor closely for dehydration. Interrupt levatinib for grades 3–4 diarrhea. If grade 3 diarrhea, once it resolves to grade 1 or baseline, resume at a reduced dose. Permanently discontinue levatinib for grade 4 diarrhea despite medical management. See Dose Modifications.
- *Gastrointestinal (GI) perforation and fistula formation:* Incidence in study 1 was 2%, compared to 0.8% in the placebo arm (DTC) while in study 2, grade 3 or higher GI perforation, abscess or fistula in RCC patients was 2%. Fistulae (e.g., GI, broncho-pleural, trachea-esophageal, cutaneous, pharyngeal, female genital tract) and GI perforations have occurred. Pneumothorax has been reported. Fistulae, GI perforation, and pneumothorax may be associated with tumor regression or necrosis. Patients at risk are those who have had prior surgery or RT. Discontinue drug for GI perforation or life-threatening fistula.
- *QT prolongation:* Incidence in study 1 was 9%, with grade 3 or greater occurring in 2% of patients, while in the RCC patients, incidence was 11% with QT prolongation > 500 msec was 6% (Eisai, 2017). Monitor ECGs of patients with congenital long QT syndrome, CHF, bradyarrhythmias, or those taking drugs known to prolong the QT interval, including Class Ia and III antiarrhythmics. Monitor and correct electrolyte abnormalities in **all** patients. Monitor ECGs in patients with congenital long QT syndrome, CHF, bradyarrhythmias, or who are taking drugs known to prolong QTc. Withhold drug for grade 3 QT-interval prolongation > 500 ms; resume at a reduced dose (see first bullet, or package insert) when QT-interval prolongation resolves to baseline.
- *Hypocalcemia:* In study 1, 9% of patients receiving lenvatinib experienced grade 3 or higher hypocalcemia, and most patients responded to replacement calcium, and dose interruption and dose reduction. In study 2 (RCC patients), 6% of patients experienced grade 3 or higher hypocalcemia. Monitor serum calcium baseline and at least monthly and replace calcium as necessary during treatment with lenvatinib. Monitor ECG if hypocalcemia occurs, and interrupt and adjust dose of lenvatinib as necessary based on severity, presence of ECG changes, and persistence of hypocalcemia.
- *Reversible posterior leukoencephalopathy syndrome (RPLS):* Although rare, RPLS has occurred. If patient has symptoms, the diagnosis should be confirmed with MRI. Withhold drug until RPLS is fully resolved; then resume at a reduced dose or discontinue drug based on severity and persistence of neurologic symptoms.
- *Hemorrhagic events:* In study 1 (DTC), hemorrhagic events (e.g., epistaxis) occurred in 35% of patients receiving lenvatinib compared to 18% in the placebo group. In study 2 (RCC) incidence of hemorrhagic events was 34% (vs 26% in control), and grade 3 or higher events occurred in 8% of patients. Serious tumor-related bleeding may occur and be fatal. Grade 3 or higher hemorrhage was reported in 2% of patients. Prior to prescribing lenvatinib, the degree of tumor invasion/infiltration of major blood vessels (e.g., carotid artery) should be considered, as the risk of severe

hemorrhage associated with tumor shrinkage/necrosis. Hold lenvatinib for grade 3 hemorrhage until it resolves to grades 0–1. Either resume the drug at a reduced dose or the drug should be discontinued based on severity and persistence of hemorrhage. Drug should be discontinued in patients with grade 4 hemorrhage.

- *Impairment of TSH Suppression/Thyroid dysfunction:* Monitor TSH levels baseline and at least monthly throughout treatment. Treat hypothyroidism per standard medical practice to maintain an euthyroid state.
- *Wound healing complications:* Complications, including fistula formation and wound dehiscence have occurred. Hold drug for at least 6 days prior to scheduled surgery. Resume after surgery once adequate sound healing has occurred based on clinical judgment. Permanently discontinue drug if a patient develops wound healing complications.
- *Embryo-fetal toxicity:* Teach women of reproductive potential to use effective contraception during treatment to prevent pregnancy, and for at least 30 days after the last drug dose.

Potential Toxicities/Side Effects and the Nursing Process

I.   POTENTIAL ALTERATION IN CIRCULATION related to HYPERTENSION, HEMORRHAGE, CARDIAC DYSFUNCTION, AND ARTERIAL THROMBOEMBOLIC EVENTS

Defining Characteristics: Lenvatinib increases the incidence of hypertension—a class effect of all angiogenesis inhibitors that is believed to be caused by the influence of VEGF on nitric oxide and blood vessel dilation, which is now blocked. HTN occurred in 73% of patients (all grades) and was severe (grade 3) in 44%; fewer than 1% of patients had grade 4 HTN. Less commonly, cardiac dysfunction (decreased left or right ventricular function, cardiac failure, or pulmonary edema) occurred in 7% (compared to 2% in the placebo group), and ATE in 5% (2% in the placebo group). Hemorrhagic events occurred in 35% of patients (18% in the placebo group), most commonly epistaxis.

Nursing Implications: Assess baseline BP prior to, then after 1 week, then every 2 weeks for the first 2 months, then at least monthly during treatment. Discuss antihypertensive therapy with the provider as needed. Teach the patient about drug administration, potential side effects, and self-care measures if prescribed antihypertensive medication, such as angiotensin-converting enzyme inhibitors, beta blockers, diuretics, and calcium-channel blockers. Lenvatinib should be temporarily suspended in patients with severe hypertension until BP can be controlled with medical management. The drug should be withheld for grade 3 HTN despite optimal antihypertensive therapy, and resumed at a reduced dose when HTN is well controlled. It should be permanently discontinued if the patient develops hypertensive crisis (diastolic blood pressure > 120 mm Hg) or life-threatening HTN. Monitor the patient for signs and symptoms of cardiac decompensation (e.g., dyspnea, pedal edema); discuss the need for ECHO with the provider if signs and symptoms are found. Teach the patient to report the following conditions immediately and go to ED: severe chest pain or pressure; pain in the arms, back, neck, or jaw; shortness of breath; numbness or weakness on one body side; trouble talking; sudden severe headache; or sudden visual changes. Teach the patient that epistaxis may occur, and to report immediately/come to the emergency room for severe and persistent nose bleeds; vomiting blood; red or black stools; coughing up blood or clots; and heavy or new-onset vaginal bleeding in women.

II. ALTERATION IN NUTRITION, POTENTIAL, related to NAUSEA, VOMITING, OR DIARRHEA

Defining Characteristics: Diarrhea occurred in 67% of patients and was of grades 3–4 severity in 9%. Nausea occurred in 47%, stomatitis in 41%, vomiting in 36%, constipation in 31%, oral pain in 25%, dry mouth in 17%, and dyspepsia in 13%. Dysgeusia occurred in 18%. Weight was decreased in 51%, and appetite decreased in 54% of patients receiving lenvatinib.

Nursing Implications: Assess nutritional status at baseline and at each visit. Teach the patient that these side effects may occur, and teach self-management strategies such as use of antidiarrheals and antinausea medications, dietary modifications; teach the patient to report any symptoms that do not improve. Discuss prescription medication with the provider if the patient experiences refractory symptoms. Teach the patient tips to increase appetite (e.g., small, frequent meals; use of spices). Offer the services of a dietitian as appropriate.

III. ALTERATION IN RENAL FUNCTION related to NEPHROTIC SYNDROME, POTENTIAL

Defining Characteristics: Renal impairment occurred in 14% of patients compared to 2% of patients receiving placebo, and was related to dehydration/hypovolemia due to diarrhea and vomiting. Proteinuria occurred in 34% of patients.

Nursing Implications: Assess baseline renal function and presence of protein in urine (1+ or greater by dipstick), and monitor prior to each treatment. Discuss any abnormalities with the physician. Patients with 2+ or higher proteinuria by urine dipstick should stop the drug, and be asked to collect a 24-hour urine sample for protein analysis. The drug should be held for proteinuria ≥ 2 g/24 hr, and resume when proteinuria < 2 g/24 hr. Monitor patients closely if they develop moderate-to-severe proteinuria until improved or resolved. The drug should be discontinued if the patient develops nephrotic syndrome.

IV. ALTERATION IN COMFORT related to FATGUE, ARTHRALGIA/MYALGIA, HEADACHE, PALMAR–PLANTAR ERYTHRODYSESTHESIA, AND RASH

Defining Characteristics: Fatigue is common, occurring in 67% of patients, as are arthralgias and myalgias, occurring in 62% of patients. Headache occurred in 38%, palmar–plantar erythrodysesthesia in 32% (but was grade 3 in only 3.4%), rash in 21%, and peripheral edema in 21%. Alopecia was not common, occurring in 12% of patients.

Nursing Implications: Teach the patient that fatigue is common and offer strategies to manage it, such as alternating rest and activity. Teach the patient that arthralgias and myalgias may occur, and offer strategies to manage them (e.g., acetaminophen or ibuprofen, frequent rest periods, application of heat, massage). Teach the patient that palmar–plantar erythrodysesthesia (PPE) syndrome may occur and should be reported. Assess baseline skin integrity, including the soles of the feet and the palms of the hands. Teach the patient to self-assess all skin areas, and to report rash, as well as redness, swelling, and/or pain anywhere, but particularly on the soles of the feet and the palms of the hands. Teach the patient to avoid activities that increase blood flow in the hands and feet, such as hot showers and baths, and to take tepid showers to reduce the likelihood and severity of HFS. Teach the patient to avoid constrictive clothing and repetitive movements that can irritate the opposing skin. Teach the patient to use skin emollients to prevent skin from drying and cracking starting on day 1 of therapy, followed by wearing cotton gloves or socks to keep the emollient close to the skin until absorbed. Teach the patient to elevate the hands and feet when sitting or lying down; apply ice packs or cool compresses indirectly to the hands or feet for up to 20 minutes; gently pat the skin dry after bathing or washing; and avoid contact with laundry detergents or cleaning products with strong chemicals. Teach patient to call if pain develops or if the area (palms of hands, soles of feet, areas of pressure) becomes swollen, and discuss management with the provider.

Drug: Larotrectinib (Vitrakvi)

Classification: Kinase inhibitor; Tropomyosin receptor kinase (TRK) inhibitor of TRK A, B, and C, which are encoded by genes *NTRK 1, 2, and 3.*

Mechanism of Action: Larotrectinib inhibits the TRK protein which is encoded by the neurotrophic receptor tyrosine kinase *(NTRK)* gene (1,2,3); NTRK1 gene provides the recipe for the manufacturing of a protein essential for neurons, especially those involved in transmitting pain, temperature and touch. NTRK2 gene makes proteins important in the growth and maturation of neurons; and NTRK3 gene makes a tyrosine kinase that stimulates the MAPK pathway and turns on cell division and survival among others cell functions. When the *NTRK* gene is mutated by fusing with another gene, it has been shown to drive oncogenesis, leading to TRK fusion cancers such as almost all infantile fibrosarcomas, and many thyroid cancers, high grade pediatric gliomas, and a small percentage of lung and colon cancers. By inhibiting the tyrosine kinases associated with this fusion mutation, cell proliferation and survival is stopped. However, the drug does not work in cells with point mutations in the TRK domain that confer acquired resistance.

Metabolism: Drug has 34% oral bioavailability, and the AUC was reduced 35% when taken with a high-fat meal. Drug is 70% protein bound to human plasma proteins. Larotrectinib achieves peak plasma levels (C_{max}) 1 hour after dosing, with a half-life of 2.9 hours, and steady state is reached in 3 days. The drug is primarily metabolized by the hepatic microenzyme CYP3A4. Excretion is primarily fecal (58%, with 5% unchanged drug), and 39% (20% unchanged drug) is excreted in the urine. The AUC is increased 1.5-fold in patients with end stage renal disease, and 1.3-fold increase in patients with mild hepatic impairment, 2-fold increase with moderate impairment, and 3.2-fold increase with severe hepatic impairment.

Indications (accelerated): Treatment of adult and pediatric patients with solid tumors that:

1. Have a *NTRK* gene fusion without a known acquired resistance mutation; and
2. Are metastatic or where surgical resection is likely to result in severe morbidity; and
3. Have no satisfactory alternative treatments or that have progressed following treatment.

Contraindications: None.

Dosage/Range: Patient must have a *NTRK* gene fusion present.
- Patients with BSA at least 1.0 m^2: 100 mg PO bid;
- Pediatric patients with BSA < 1.0 m^2: 100 mg/m^2 PO bid.

Dose Modification:
- Reduce starting dosage by 50% in patients with moderate (Child-Pugh B) to severe (Child-Pugh C) hepatic impairment.
- Grade 3–4 adverse reactions: 1) withhold larotrectinib until adverse reaction improves to baseline or grade 1; resume at the next dosage modification if resolution occurs within 4 weeks; 2) permanently discontinue larotrectinib if an adverse reaction does not resolve within 4 weeks.
- Dosage Modification: 1st (BSA at least 1.0 m^2) = 75 mg PO bid, (BSA < 1.0 m^2) = 75 mg/m^2 PO bid; 2nd (BSA at least 1.0 m^2) = 50 mg PO bid, (BSA < 1.0 m^2) = 50 mg/m^2 PO bid; 3rd (BSA at least 1.0m^2) = 100 mg PO qd, (BSA < 1.0 m^2) = 25 mg/m^2 PO bid.
- Dosage modification for drug interactions:
  - Coadministration with Strong CYP3A4 Inhibitor: If unavoidable, decrease larotrectinib dpse by 50%, and after inhibitor has been discontinued for 3–5 elimination half-lives, resume larotrectinib dose taken prior to starting the CYP3A4 inhibitor.
  - Coadministration with Strong CYP3A4 Inducers: if unavoidable, double the larotrectinib dose; after inducer has been discontinued for 3–5 elimination half-lives, resume larotrectinib dose taken prior to starting the CYP3A4 inducer.

Drug Preparation:
- Available as 25-mg and 100-mg capsules, and an oral solution 20 mg/mL.

Drug Administration:
- Assess patient for signs/symptoms of neurotoxicity, fatigue, and GI symptoms during treatment. Monitor LFTs baseline and every 2 weeks for 1st month, then monthly. Discuss abnormalities with provider.
- Assess medication profile for strong CYP3A4 inducers or inhibitors as dose will need to be modified.
- Teach patient or caregiver:
  - Capsule or oral solution can be used interchangeably.
  - Do not make up a missed dose within 6 hours of the next scheduled dose.
  - If vomiting occurs after taking a dose, take the next scheduled dose at the scheduled time.
  - Swallow capsules whole with water; do not chew or crush capsules.

- Oral solution: (1) store the glass bottle of oral solution in the refrigerator; discard any unused oral solution remaining 90 days after opening the bottle; (2) prior to preparing oral dose for administration, read the Instructions for Use that come with the bottle.
- To report signs/symptoms of infection, fever, and dizziness right away. Assess patient risk for falls, and home safety.
- Teach patient to avoid St. John's Wort, grapefruit, or grapefruit juice as it can increase serum drug levels.
- Teach effective contraception to females who are able to become pregnant during treatment and for at least 1 week after last dose; males with female partners who are able to become pregnant to use effective contraception during treatment and for at least 1 week after last drug dose.
- Do not breast-feed while receiving the drug and for at least 1 week after final dose.

Drug Interactions:
- Strong CYP3A4 inhibitors (e.g., itraconazole): increase larotrectinib AUC 4.3-fold, and C_{max} by 2.8-fold; avoid coadministration and if this can not be avoided, reduce larotrectinib dose
- Strong CYP3A4 inducer (e.g., rifampin): decrease larotrectinib AUC by 81%, and C_{max} by 71%; avoid coadministration and if this can not be avoided, increase larotrectinib dose.
- Sensitive CYP3A4 substrates (e.g., midazolam): increase both the AUC (1.7-fold) and C_{max} (by 1.7-fold); avoid coadministration of the sensitive CYP3A4 substrate.
- St. John's wort, grapefruit, or grapefruit juice: increase drug serum levels, do NOT take while receiving drug.

Lab Effects/Interference:
- Increased ALT, AST, alkaline phosphatase.
- Decreased serum albumin, anemia, neutropenia.

Special Considerations:
- Most common(≥ 20%) adverse effects are fatigue, nausea, dizziness, vomiting, anemia, increased AST, cough, increased ALT, constipation and diarrhea. The most common serious adverse reactions (≥ 2%) were pyrexia, diarrhea, sepsis, abdominal pain, dehydration, cellulitis, and vomiting.
- Warnings and Precautions:
    - *Neurotoxicity:* Incidence 53%, with most occurring within first 3 months of therapy. Grade 3 neurological adverse effects: delirium (2%), dysarthria (1%), dizziness (1%), gait disturbance (1%), paresthesias (1%). Grade 4 encephalopathy was rare (grade 4). Teach patients not to drive or operate hazardous machinery until they know the neurological adverse effects they will experience. Hold or discontinue drug based on severity. If drug held, reduce the dose when resumed.
    - *Hepatotoxicity:* Incidence 45%, with median time to onset of increased AST or ALT was 2 months. Monitor LFTs every 2 weeks during first month of treatment, then monthly, and as clinically indicated. Hold or permanently discontinue therapy based on severity; if drug is held, dose modify after drug is resumed.

- *Embryo-fetal toxicity:* Drug is fetotoxic. Teach females of reproductive potential to use effective contraception during and for at least 1 week following the last dose of treatment. Teach male patients with female sexual partners of reproductive potential to use effective contraception during and for at least 1 week following the last dose of treatment.

Potential Toxicities/Side Effects and the Nursing Process

I.   ALTERATION IN NUTRITION, POTENTIAL, related to NAUSEA, VOMITING, CONSTIPATION, DIARRHEA, HEPATOTOXICITY

Defining Characteristics: Nausea occurred in 29% of patients, vomiting 26%, constipation 23%, and diarrhea 22%. Thirteen percent of patients had decreased appetite. Increased ALT occurred in 45%, AST 45%, increased alkaline phosphatase in 30% of patients.

Nursing Implications: Assess nutritional status at baseline and at each visit. Assess LFTs baseline, every 2 weeks for the first month, then monthly. Teach the patient that these side effects may occur, and teach self-management strategies such as use of antinausea/vomiting medications, antidiarrheals (diarrhea) or cathartics (constipation); dietary modifications for each symptom; teach the patient to report any symptoms that do not improve or worsen. Discuss prescription medication with the provider if the patient experiences refractory symptoms. Offer the services of a dietitian as appropriate.

II.   ALTERATION IN ACTIVITY, POTENTIAL related to FATIGUE, ANEMIA, DIZZINESS

Defining Characteristics: Fatigue occurred in 27% of paitents, and was grade 3–4 in 3% of patients. Dizziness occurred in 28% and anemia in 42% of patients. Ten percent of patients had falls.

Nursing Implications: Assess baseline activity and energy. Asssess hematocrit and hemoglobin baseline and throught therapy. Assess patient home safety and risk for falls. Teach patient to report fatigue, and dizziness. Teach patient safety interventions to manage dizziness, and strategies to manage energy deficits such as teaching alternating rest with activity, asking for help from family members to do chores. Teach patient to notify provider ASAP if dizziness worsens or the patient falls.

Drug: Lorlatinib (Lorbrena)

Class: Kinase inhibitor; multi-kinase inhibitor.

Mechanism of Action: Inhibits ALK and ROS1 kinases, as well as other kinases. Has activity against a variety of ALK mutant forms, including those in tumors progressing on crizotinib or other ALK inhibitors.

Metabolism: The mean absolute bioavailability after oral dosing is 81%, and time to median Tmax was 1.2–2 hours. Lorlatinib is 66% bound to plasma proteins, and plasma half-life is 24 hours after a single dose. Lorlatinib is primarily metabolized by CYP3A4, and UGT1A4, and to a lesser degree by CYP2C8, CYP2C19, CYP3A5, and UGT1A3. Of the circulating drug, after metabolism, 21% becomes the biologically inactive metabolite M8. Drug is excreted in the urine (48%) and feces (41%).

Indication: Treatment of patients with ALK+ NSCLC whose disease has progressed on (1) crizotinib and at least one other ALK inhibitor for metastatic disease; or (2) alectinib as the first ALK inhibitor therapy for metastatic disease; or (3) ceritinib as the first ALK inhibitor therapy for metastatic disease (Accelerated Approval).

Contraindications: Concurrent administration with strong CYP3A inducers.

Dosage/Range: 100 mg PO qd, with or without food, until disease progression or unacceptable toxicity.

Dose Modifications:
- Dose reductions: Usual dose 100 mg PO qd. (1) First dose reduction= lorlatinib 75 mg PO qd; (2) 2nd dose reduction = 50 mg PO qd.
- *CNS Effects:* (1) Grade 1: continue at same dose or hold the dose until recovery to baseline; resume lorlatinib at same or reduced dose; (2) grade 2 OR grade 3: Hold dose until grade 0–1, then resume at a reduced dose; (3) grade 4: permanently discontinue lorlatinib.
- *Hyperlipidemia:* Grade 4 hypercholesterolemia or grade 4 hypertriglyceridemia: (1) hold lorlatinib until recovery of hypercholesterolemia and/or hypertriglyceridemia to ≤ grade 2; resume lorlatinib at the same dose; (2) if severe hypercholesterolemia and/or hypertriglyceridemia recurs, resume lorlatinib at a reduced dose.
- *Atrioventricular (AV) block:*
    - (1) hold hypercholesterolemia and/or hypertriglyceridemia until PR interval is < 200 ms; resume lorlatinib at a reduced dose.
    - (2) first occurrence of complete heart block: (1) hold lorlatinib until pacemaker placed or PR interval is < 200 ms; (2) if a pacemaker is placed, resume lorlatinib at the same dose; if no pacemaker placed, resume lorlatinib at a reduced dose.
- Interstitial Lung Disease (ILD)/pneumonitis: Any grade: permanently discontinue lorlatinib.
- Other adverse reactions: (1) Grade 1 or grade 2: continue lorlatinib at same or reduced dose; (2) grade 3 or 4: hold lorlatinib until symptoms resolve to ≤ grade 2 or baseline, and resume lorlatinib at a reduced dose.
- Concomitant use of Strong CYP3A Inducers: Lorlatinib is contraindicated with strong CYP3A inducers. Discontinue strong CYP3A inducer for 3 plasma half-lives of the strong CYP3A inducer before starting lorlatinib. Avoid concomitant administration of lorlatinib with moderate CYP3A inducers.
- Concomitant use of Strong CYP3A Inhibitors: do not co-administer. If unavoidable, reduce the lorlatinib starting dose from 100 mg PO qd to 75 mg PO qd. If a patient has had

a dose reduction to 75 mg PO qd, reduce lorlatinib to 50 mg PO qd. If the strong CYP3A inhibitor is discontinued, increase the lorlatinib dose (after 3 plasma lives or the strong CYP3A inhibitor) to the dose used before starting the strong inhibitor.

Drug Preparation: Oral. Available as 100-mg and 25-mg tablets.

Drug Administration:
- Assess ECG for AV interval baseline and as ordered during therapy. Assess CBC/differential, LFTs, glucose. chemistries including lipid profile baseline and as ordered during therapy. Verify negative pregnancy status in female patients of reproductive potential prior to starting lorlatinib.
- Teach patient/family to:
  - Swallow tablets whole; do not chew, crush or split tablets. Do not take if tablet is broken, cracked, or otherwise not intact.
  - Take lorlatinib at the same time each day. If a dose is missed, take the missed dose unless the next dose is due within 4 hours. Do not take 2 doses at the same time to make up for a missed dose.
  - If patient vomits after ingesting lorlatinib, do not take an additional dose but continue with the next scheduled dose
  - Teach female patients of reproductive potential to use effective contraception during and for at least 6 months after last dose; teach males with female sexual partners of reproductive potential to use effective contraception during and for at least 3 months after the last lorlatinib dose. Teach mothers not to breast-feed while receiving lorlatinib and for 7 days after final lorlatinib dose.
  - Teach male patients of reproductive potential that lorlatinib may impair fertility transiently.
  - Teach patient to report signs of symptoms of bleeding (thrombocytopenia incidence is 23%).

Drug Interactions:
- Strong CYP3A inducers: reduce the serum concentration of lorlatinib significantly making lorlatinib ineffective. Contraindicated: do **not** co-administer. Avoid moderate CYP3A inducers as well.
- Strong CYP3A inhibitors: increase serum concentration of lorlatinib; avoid coadministration. If unavoidable, reduce lorlatinib dose.
- CYP3A substrates: avoid concomitant use of lorlatinib where minimal concentration changes may result in serious therapeutic failure.
- Hormonal contraceptives: lorlatinib can inactivate hormonal contraceptives; teach woman to use non-hormonal contraceptive measures.

Lab Effects/Interference:
- Increased cholesterolemia, triglyceridemia, serum glucose, AST, ALT, alkaline phosphatase, amylase, potassium, lipase.
- Decrreased serum albumin, phosphorus, magnesium.
- Anemia, thrombocytopenia, lymphopenia.

Special Considerations:
- Most common adverse effects (≥ 20%): edema, peripheral neuropathy, cognitive effects, dyspnea, fatigue, weight gain, arthralgia, mood effects, diarrhea.
- Warnings and Precautions:
  - *Risk of serious hepatotoxicity with concomitant use of strong CYP3A inducers:* Strong CYP3A inducers are contraindicated. Discontinue the strong CYP3A inducer for 3 plasma half-lives of the strong CYP3A inducer before starting lorlatinib. Avoid concomitant administration with a moderate CYP3A inducer; if must be administered, monitor AST, ALT and bilirubin 48 hours after starting lorlatinib and at least 3 times during the first week of starting lorlatinib. If persistent grade 2 or higher hepatotoxicity occur, discontinue either the lorlatinib or the moderate CYP3A inducer.
  - *CNS Effects:* A variety of symptoms may occur: seizure, hallucinations, changes in cognitive function and/or mood (including suicidal ideation), and changes in speech, mental status, and sleep. Median onset to first symptom was 1.2 months. Only 1.5% of patients had to permanently discontinue the drug for a CNS effect, while 9% required temporary discontinuation and 8% a dose reduction. See Dose Modifications.
  - *Hyperlipidemia:* Grade 3–4 cholesterolemia or triglyceridemia occurred in 17% of patients. Median time to onset was 15 days. Most (80%) of patients required lipid lowering agents. Initiate or titrate the lipid lowering drug dose in patients with hypercholesterolemia. Assess serum cholesterol and triglycerides baseline and 1–2 months after starting lorlatinib, and then periodically. See Dose Modifications.
  - *Atrioventricular block (AVB):* PR interval prolongation and AVB can occur in patients receiving lorlatinib. In clinical trials, 1% of patients developed AVB and 0.3% Grade 3 AVB requiring a pacemaker implantation. Assess ECG baseline and periodically during lorlatinib therapy. See Dose Modifications.
  - *Interstitial lung disease (ILD)/pneumonitis:* In clinical trials, ILD/pneumonitis occurred in 1.5% of patients, including 1.2% with grade 3–4, Teach patient to report right away worsening respiratory symptoms such as dyspnea, cough, fever. Drug should be interrupted as ILD/pneumonitis is investigated, and lorlatinib should be permanently discontinued if a diagnosis of ILD/pneumonitis is confirmed.
  - *Embryo-fetal toxicity:* Drug is feto-toxic. Confirm female patients of reproductive potential are not pregnant before starting lorlatinib therapy, and teach them to use effective non-hormonal contraception during and for at least 6 months after last lorlatinib dose. Teach male patients with female sexual partners of reproductive potential to use effective contraception during lorlatinib therapy and for at least 3 months after last dose.

Potential Toxicities/Side Effects and the Nursing Process

I. ALTERATION IN SENSORY PERCEPTION related to CNS EFFECTS

Defining Characteristics: Incidence of CNS symptoms included mood effects (23%), peripheral neuropathy (47%), cognitive effects (27%), headache (18%), dizziness (16%), speech effects (12%), sleep effects (10%).

Nursing Implications: Assess baseline neurological status, including mood, cognition and speech. Assess home safety through interview. Teach patient side effects may occur and to report them right away. Discuss dose interruption or reduction based on severity with physician/NP/PA. Teach patient self-care measures including fall prevention, and revise plan as needed.

II. ALTERATION IN NUTRITION, POTENTIAL, LESS THAN BODY REQUIREMENTS, related to NAUSEA, VOMITING, DIARRHEA, CONSTIPATION, HYPERCHOLESTEROLEMIA, HYPERTRIGLYCERIDEMIA, HYPERGLYCEMIA, INCREASED LFTs

Defining Characteristics: Diarrhea occurred in 23% of patients, nausea in 18%, constipation in 15%, and vomiting in 12%. Hypercholesterolemia occurred in 96% of patients, and hypertriglyceridemia in 90%. LFT elevation occurred in 37% (AST) and 28% (ALT) of patients. Hyperglycemia affected 52% of patients.

Nursing Implications: Assess baseline nutritional status and bowel-elimination status. Assess baseline labs including lipids, glucose, LFTs. Assess lipids 1 and 2 months after starting lorlatinib, and as ordered as patients are started/titrated on lipid lowering agents. Discuss elevations with MD/PA/NP. If patient develops nausea and/or vomiting, teach patient to self-administer antiemetics 1 hour prior to each dose, and to call if nausea/vomiting is increased or persistent. Discuss with physician more effective antiemetic regimen if nausea/vomiting persist. Encourage small, frequent intake of cool, bland foods as tolerated if nausea develops. Refer to dietitian as needed for meal planning. Teach patient to report diarrhea that does not respond to OTC antidiarrheal medication or if constipation occurs that is unresponsive to fluids, laxatives, and use of high-fiber foods. Teach self-care measures of diet modification and increased oral fluids to 2–3 L during the waking hours. If constipation occurs, teach patient self-care measures to prevent constipation. If hyperglycemia occurs, discuss management with physician/NP/PA, and teach patient signs/symptoms of hyper/hypoglycemia.

III. ALTERATION IN COMFORT related to FATIGUE, EDEMA, ARTHRALGIA, MYALGIA, RASH, ANEMIA

Defining Characteristics: Fatigue occurred in 26% of patients. Edema occurred in 57% of patients with weight gain in 24%, back pain in 13% of patients, rash in 14% of patients, and anemia in 52% of patients. Arthralgias occurred in 23%, myalgia (musculoskeletal pain) in about 17% of patients.

Nursing Implications: Assess baseline parameters of weight, presence of edema, pulmonary function, red blood cell count, and monitor closely during therapy. Teach patient to monitor weight gain and edema or the development of dyspnea and to report it. Assess skin integrity baseline and frequently during treatment. Teach patient to report rash. Develop a plan to protect skin and maintain skin integrity. Assess for patient complaint of myalgia, arthralgia, weakness, and teach patient to call providers for worsening symptoms.

Drug: Midostaurin (Rydapt)

Classification: kinase inhibitor; multi-kinase inhibitor.

Mechanism of Action: Small molecule that inhibits multiple RTKs, including wild-type FLT3, FLT3 mutant kinases (ITD and TKD), KIT (wild-type and D816V mutant), PDGFR α/β, VEGFR2 and members of the serine/threonine protein kinase C (PKC) family. When FLT3 receptor signaling is inhibited, cell proliferation of AML cells stops, and apoptosis is induced in leukemic cells expressing ITD and TKD mutant FLT3 receptors, or overexpressing wild-type FLT3 and PDGF receptors. Drug also inhibits KIT signaling, cell proliferation, histamine release, and induces apoptosis in mast cells.

Metabolism: After oral dosing, steady state is reached in 28 days. Taking medication with food increases AUC 1.2–1.6 fold. Midostauring is primarily metabolized by CYP3A4 into two active major metabolites. Midostaurin and its major active metabolites CGP62221 and CGP52421 are > 99.8% bound to plasma proteins. Mean terminal half-life is 21 hours for midostaurin, 32 hours for CGP62221, and 482 hours for CGP52421. Most of the drug and metabolites are excreted in the feces (95%) and 5% in the urine.

Indications: 1) In combination with standard cytarabine and daunorubicin induction and cytarabine consolidation chemotherapy, for the treatment of adult patients with newly diagnosed acute myeloid leukemia (AML) who are FLT3 mutation positive, as detected by a FDA approved test. It is not indicated as a single agent induction therapy; 2) treatment of adults with aggressive systemic mastocytosis (ASM), systemic mastocytosis with associated hematological neoplasm (SM-AHN), or mast cell leukemia (MCL).

Contraindication: Hypersensitivity to midostaurin or any of the excipients. Hypersensitivity reactions have occurred including dyspnea, flushing, chest pain, angioedema, and anaphylaxis.

Dosage Range:
- AML: 50 mg orally twice daily with food on days 8–21 of each cycle of induction with cytarabine and daunorubicin, and on days 8–21 of each cycle of consolidation with high-dose cytarabine.
- ASM, SM-AHN, MCL: 100 mg orally twice daily with food. Continue therapy until disease progression or unacceptable toxicity. Monitor patient for toxicity at least weekly for the first 4 weeks, every other week for the next 8 weeks, and then monthly thereafter while on treatment.
  - Dose modification for patients with systemic mastocytosis
    - ANC $< 1 \times 10^9$/L attributed to midostaurin in patients without MCL, or ANC $< 0.5 \times 10^9$/L attributed to midostaurin in patients with baseline ANC $0.5 - 1.5 \times 10^9$/L: Interrupt midostaurin until ANC $\geq 1 \times 10^9$/L, then resume

TREATMENT

midostaurin at 50 mg twice daily, and if tolerated, increase to 100 mg twice daily. Discontinue midostaurin if low ANC persists > 21 days and is suspected to be related to midostaurin.

- Platelet count < 50×10^9/L attributed to midostaurin in patients without MCL, or platelet count < 25×10^9/L attributed to midostaurin in patients with baseline platelet count of 25–75 × 10^9/L: Interrupt midostaurin until platelet count ≥ 50×10^9/L, then resume midostaurin at 50 mg twice daily, and if tolerated, increase to 100 mg twice daily. Discontinue midostaurin if low platelet count persists > 21 days and is suspected to be related to midostaurin.
- Hgb < 8 g/L attributed to midostaurin in patients without MCL, or life-threatening anemia attributed to midostaurin in patients with baseline Hgb 8–10 g/L: Interrupt midostaurin until Hgb ≥ 8 g/L, then resume midostaurin at 50 mg twice daily, and if tolerated, increase to 100 mg twice daily. Discontinue midostaurin if low Hgb persists > 21 days and is suspected to be related to midostaurin.
- Grades 3–4 nausea and/or vomiting despite optimal antiemetic therapy: Interrupt midostaurin for 3 days (6 doses), then resume midostaurin at 50 mg twice daily, and if tolerated, i Interrupt midostaurin until Hgb ≥ 8 g/L, then resume midostaurin at 50 mg twice daily, and if tolerated, increase to 100 mg twice daily. increase to 100 mg twice daily.
- Other grades 3–4 nonhematologic toxicities: Interrupt midostaurin until event has resolved to ≤ grade 2, then resume midostaurin at 50 mg twice daily, and if tolerated, increase to 100 mg twice daily.

Drug Preparation: None. Available in 25 mg capsules.

Drug Administration:
- Teach patient to:
  - Administer antiemetic 1 hour prior to drug dose to minimize nausea/vomiting.
  - Administer orally with food, twice daily, at approximately 12-hour intervals.
  - If a dose is missed or vomited, do not make up the dose; take the next dose at the usual scheduled time.
- Assess CBC/differential, ANC. Verify pregnancy status of female patients of reproductive potential within 7 days before starting therapy.
- Discuss ECG with provider for patients taking concurrently any medication that can prolong the QT interval.

Drug Interactions:
- Strong CYP3A4 inhibitors: may increase serum levels of midostaurin and its active metabolites; **do not give concurrently**; if necessary, monitor closely for increased toxicity. For example, coadministration of ketoconazole increases AUC of midostaurin by 10.4 times, and CGP62221 by 3.5 times. Teach patients to avoid grapefruit juice.
- Strong CYP3A4 inducers: decrease serum levels of midostaurin and its active metabolites; **do not give concurrently**. For example, rifampicin decreases AUC midostaurin by 96% and CGP62221 by 92%. Teach patient not to take St. John's wort.

Laboratory Effects/Interference:
- Neutropenia, thrombocytopenia, anemia.
- Hyperglycemia, increased serum creatinine, increased ALT, hypernatremia, hypocalcemia.
- aPTT prolonged.
- QT prolongation.

Special Considerations:
- Most common adverse effects (≥ 20%): (1) AML: febrile neutropenia, nausea, mucositis, vomiting, headache, petechiae, musculoskeletal pain, epistaxis, device-related infection, hyperglycemia, URI; (2) ASM, SM-AHN, MCL: nausea, vomiting, diarrhea, edema, musculoskeletal pain, abdominal pain, fatigue, URI, constipation, pyrexia, headache, dyspnea.
- QT prolongation may occur in patients with advanced SM (11%). Assess patients' medication profile for co-administered drug(s) that can increase the QTc interval, and monitor these patients closely with baseline and ongoing ECGs that document the QTc interval. Discuss management of prolonged QTc with provider.
- Warnings and Precautions:
  - *Embryo-fetal toxicity:* Drug is feto-toxic. Verify pregnancy status of women of reproductive potential within 7 days prior to starting midostaurin therapy. Teach female patients of reproductive potential to use effective contraception to prevent pregnancy during therapy and for at least 4 months after last dose.
  - *Pulmonary toxicity:* ILD and pneumonitis have occurred in patients receiving midostaurin as monotherapy or chemotherapy. Monitor patients for pulmonary symptoms; drug should be discontinued in patients having signs/symptoms without an infectious etiology.

Potential Toxicities/Side Effects and the Nursing Process

I.   POTENTIAL FOR BLEEDING, INFECTION, ANEMIA, AND FATIGUE related to BONE MARROW SUPPRESSION

Defining Characteristics: In patients with AML, febrile neutropenia occurred in 83%, while incidence was 81% in patients receiving placebo and chemotherapy. Petechiae were observed in 36% of patients. Device-related infection was 24%, URI 20%. Epistaxis occurred in 28%. In patients with Advanced SM, fatigue occurred in 34%, fatigue in 34%, epistaxis 12%. URI occurred in 30%, UTI in 16%, pneumonia in 10%, and herpes infection in 10%. Dyspnea and cough also occurred.

Nursing Implications: Evaluate CBC/differential, hemoglobin/hematocrit, and platelets at baseline, then follow closely as ordered and needed prior and nadir times of chemotherapy. Discuss any abnormalities with the physician/NP/PA. Assess for signs and symptoms of infection, bleeding, and fatigue. Teach the patient about signs and symptoms of infection and bleeding, and to report them immediately. Teach the patient self-care measures to minimize the risk of infection and bleeding, including avoidance of OTC aspirin-containing medications. Teach the patient self-assessment of fatigue and to alternate rest and activity as needed. See Dosage Modifications for neutropenia, thrombocytopenia, anemia.

II.   ALTERATION IN NUTRITION, POTENTIAL, related to NAUSEA, VOMITING, STOMATITIS; DIARRHEA or CONSTIPATION

Defining Characteristics: Of AML patients, nausea occurred in 83%, vomiting 61%, mucositis in 66% (11% grade 3), not significantly different from patients receiving placebo and chemotherapy. Hyperglycemia occurred in 20%. In the patients with advanced SM, 82% had nausea (6% grade 3/4), 6*% vomiting (6%), 54% diarrhea (8%), 34% abdominal pain, constipation in 29%, and GI hemorrhage in 14% (9%).

Nursing Implications: Assess nutritional status at baseline and at each visit. Teach the patient that these side effects may occur, and teach self-management strategies such as oral self-assessment, use of antidiarrheals and antinausea medications, systematic oral hygiene and cleansing, and dietary modifications. Teach the patient to report any symptoms that do not improve, as well as changes in oral mucosa. Discuss prescription medication with the provider if the patient experiences refractory symptoms. Teach the patient tips to increase appetite (e.g., small, frequent meals; use of spices) and manage painful mucositis. Offer the services of a dietitian as appropriate.

III.   ALTERATION IN COMFORT related to ARTHRALGIA/MYALGIA, HEADACHE, DIZZINESS, EDEMA, AND INSOMNIA

Defining Characteristics: In AML clinical trials, musculoskeletal pain occurred in 33%, arthralgia in 14%, headache in 46%, insomnia 12% while in the advanced SM trials, musculoskeletal pain affected 35%, arthralgia 19%, edema 40%, headache 26%, dizziness 13%.

Nursing Implications: Assess the patient's baseline level of comfort. Teach the patient that these side effects may occur, and teach self-management strategies. Teach the patient to report symptoms that do not improve. If this occurs, discuss with the physician/NP/PA prescription medication for refractory symptoms. Teach patient to change position slowly if dizziness develops and to ask for support to prevent falling if dizziness continues. Report dizziness that does not improve.

Drug: Neratinib (Nerlynx)

Classification: Kinase inhibitor; EGFR-1,2,4 TKI.

Mechanism of Action: By blocking EGFR-1,2,and 4, drug reduces EGFR and HER-2 autophosphoryation; this prevents activation of the downstream signaling pathways MAPK and AKT, so the malignant cell nucleus does not divide.is not told to divide and proliferate. Thus tumor growth and proliferation is inhibited.

Metabolism: Neratinib and its major active metabolites (M3, M6, M7) peak 2–8 hours after oral administration. Food increases Cmax and the AUC. The drug should be taken with food. Neratinib is tightly bound to human plasma proteins (> 99%). Mean elimination half-life range is 7–17 hours, and steady state is reached by day 21. Drug is metabolized primarily by liver microenzymes CYP3A4, and to a lesser degree by Flavin-containing monooxygenase (FMO). Neratinib is excreted primarily in the feces (97.1%), with urinary excretion only accounting for 1.13% (Puma Biotechnology Inc., 2017).

Indication: For the extended adjuvant treatment of adult patients with early stage HER-2 overexpressed/amplified breast cancer, following adjuvant trastuzumab based therapy.

Contraindication: None.

Dosage Range: 240 mg (6 tablets) orally once daily with food, continuously for 1 year. Antidiarrheal prophylaxis should begin with the first neratinib dose.and continue at least until past the 2nd cycle (56 days) of treatment.
- Weeks 1–2 (days 1–14): loperamide 4 mg tid
- Weeks 3–8 (days 15–56): loperamide 4 mg bid
- Weeks 9–52 (days 57–365): loperamide 4 mg PRN (not to exceed 16 mg per day)

Severe Hepatic Impairment: reduce starting dose to 80 mg.

Dose Modification for Adverse Reactions: See package insert.
- Recommended starting dose = 240 mg daily
  - 1st dose reduction = 200 mg daily
  - 2nd dose reduction = 160 mg daily
  - 3rd dose reduction = 120 mg daily
- General toxicities:
  - Dose interruption and/or dose reduction may be required. Discontinue neratinib if patient does not recover to grades 0–1 from treatment-related toxicity, for toxicities that result in a treatment delay > 3 weeks, or if patient cannot tolerate a dose of 120 mg daily.
  - Grade 3: hold drug until recovery to grade ≤ 1 or baseline within 3 weeks of stopping treatment. Resume drug at the next lower dose level.
  - Grade 4: discontinue drug permanently.
- Diarrhea: manage aggressively with antidiarrheal medication, dietary modification, and dose modification.
  - Grade 1 (↑ of < 4 stools/day > baseline); grade 2 (↑ of 4–6 stools/day > baseline) lasting < 5 days; grade 3 (↑ of ≥ 7 stools/day > baseline; incontinence; hospitalization indicated; limiting self-care ADLs) lasting < 2 days: (1) adjust antidiarrheal treatment; (2) dietary modifications; (3) ↑ fluid intake to 2 L/day to prevent dehydration; (4) once event resolves to ≤ grade 1 or baseline, start loperamide 4 mg with each subsequent neratinib dose administration.
  - Any grade with complicated features (e.g., dehydration, fever, hypotension, renal failure, or grade 3/4 neutropenia); grade 2 diarrhea lasting ≥ 5 days; grade 3 diarrhea lasting > 2 days: (1) Interrupt neratinib treatment; (2) dietary modifications; (3) ↑ fluid intake to 2 L/day to prevent dehydration; (4) if diarrhea resolves to grades 0–1 in longer than 1 week, then resume neratinib at reduced dose; (5) once event resolves to ≤ grade 1 or baseline, start loperamide 4 mg with each subsequent neratinib dose administration.

TREATMENT

- Permanently discontinue neratinib for (1) grade 4 diarrhea (life-threatening, requires urgent intervention) or (2) diarrhea that recurs to grade 2 or higher at a neratinib dose of 120 mg/day.
- Dose Modification for Hepatic Impairment: reduce starting dose to 80 mg once daily in patients with severe hepatic impairment (Child-Pugh C); no modifications recommended for patients with mild-to-moderate impairment (Child-Pugh A or B).
- Dose Modification for Hepatotoxicity: Assess LFTs, alkaline phosphatase baseline, then monthly for first 3 months of neratinib therapy, then as indicated. Reassess LFTs in patients with grade 3 diarrhea or if patient has any signs/symptoms of hepatotoxicity (e.g., worsening of fatigue, nausea, vomiting, RUQ tenderness, fever, rash, eosinophilia).
  - Grade 3 ALT ($>$ 5–20 × ULN) OR grade 3 biliruin ($>$ 3–10 × ULN): hold neratinib until recovery to $\leq$ grade 1; evaluate alternative causes; resume neratinib at next lower dose level if recovery to $\leq$ grade 1 occurs within 3 weeks; if grade 3 ALT or bilirubin occurs again despite 1 dose Proton Pump Inhibitorsreduction, permanently discontinue drug.
  - Grade 4 ALT ($>$ 20 × ULN) OR grade 4 bilirubin ($>$ 10 × ULN): permanently discontinue neratinib and evaluate alternative causes.

Drug Preparation: None. Drug available as 40 mg neratinib tablets. Teach patients to store at room temperature and to keep out of reach of children or pets.

Drug Administration:
- Assess LFTs, alkaline phosphatase results; Assess pregnancy test in female patients of reproductive potential; assess medication profile for medications that can interact with neratinib (e.g., gastric acid inhibitors, CYP3A4 inhibitors or inducers). See drug interactions.
- Teach female patients of reproductive potential to use effective contraception during therapy and for 1 month after last dose, and male patients with female partners of reproductive potential to use effective contraception during therapy and for 3 months after last dose of neratinib.
- Teach patient self-administration of neratinib and antidiarrheals:
  - Take daily dose (e.g., 240 mg = 6 tablets) orally once daily with food.
  - Take at about the same time of day, and swallow whole (do not crush, chew, or split tablet).
  - If a dose is missed, do not replace dose; resume neratinib with the next scheduled daily dose.
  - Take loperamide prophylaxis: (1) weeks 1–2 (days 1–14): take 4 mg three times daily; (2) weeks 3-8 (days 15–56): take loperamide 4 mg twice daily; (3) weeks 9–52 (days 57–365): take 4 mg loperamide as needed (not to exceed 16 mg per day)
  - Goal is 1–2 bowel movements per day.
    - Call HCP if you have $>$ 2 BMs per day, or have diarrhea that does not go away.
    - Call HCP **right away** if diarrhea is severe, or if you have diarrhea along with weakness, dizziness, or fever.
- To manage your diarrhea, your dose of neratinib may need to be changed or interrupted.

Drug Interactions:
- Gastric acid reducing agents: (1) PPIs: avoid concomitant use with neratinib; (2) H_2-receptor antagonists: take neratinib at least 2 hours BEFORE the next dose of the H_2-receptor antagonist or 10 hours AFTER the H_2-receptor antagonist; (3) antacids: separate dosing of neratinib by 3 hours after antacids.
- Strong (e.g., ketoconazole) or moderate (e.g., aprepitant, ciprofloxacin) CYP3A4 inhibitors: increased risk for toxicity; avoid concomitant use. Teach patients not to drink grapefruit juice or eat the fruit.
- Strong (e.g., rifampin, phenytoin) or moderate (e.g., efavirenz) CYP3A4 inducers: avoid concomitant use. Teach patients not to take St. John's wort.
- P-glycoprotein (P-gp) substrates (e.g., dabigatran, fexofenadine): monitor for adverse reactions of narrow therapeutic agents that are P-gp substrates when used concomitantly with neratinib.

Laboratory Effect/Interference: Increased LFTs, alkaline phosphatase.

Special Considerations:
- Most common adverse reactions ($> 5\%$) were diarrhea, nausea, abdominal pain, fatigue, vomiting, rash, stomatitis, decreased appetite, muscle spasms, dyspepsia, elevated AST or ALT, nail disorder, dry skin, abdominal distention, decreased weight, UTI.
- Warnings and Precautions:
  - *Diarrhea:* Teach patient to administer prophylactic antidiarrheals starting with first neratinib dose and through cycle 2 (day 56), to prevent severe diarrhea and resulting dehydration, hypotension, and renal failure. In clinical trials (ExteNET), in the neratinib arm, 95% of patients had diarrhea, 40% grade 3, and 0.1% grade 4. Incidence in most patients was the first month (93%), with a median time to onset of grade 3 or higher diarrhea at 8 days, and a median cumulative duration of grade 3 or higher diarrhea of 5 days. Monitor patients for diarrhea and treat aggressively. If severe diarrhea with dehydration occurs, give fluid and electrolytes as ordered, interrupt drug, and decrease subsequent dose of neratinib. Evaluate alternative causes of grade 3 or 4 diarrhea, or complicated diarrhea, such as infection.
  - *Hepatotoxicity:* In clinical trials, up to 10% of patients had an increase in transaminases. Assess baseline total bilirubin, AST ALT and alkaline phosphatase before starting neratinib, then monthly for the first 3 months of therapy, then every 3 months while on treatment and as clinically indicated. Assess these labs if patient develops grade 3 diarrhea, or signs/symptoms of hepatotoxicity (e.g., worsening fatigue, nausea, vomiting, RUQ tenderness, fever, or eosinophilia).
  - *Embryo-fetal toxicity:* Neratinib can cause fetal harm: (1) female patients of reproductive potential: (a) assess pregnancy test prior to the patient starting neratinib; (b) teach to use effective contraception during and for 1 month after last neratinib dose. (2) Teach male patients with female sexual partners of reproductive potential to use effection contraception during treatment and for 3 months after the last dose.
- Teach nursing mothers not to breast-feed while receiving neratinib, and for 1 month after last dose.

Potential Toxicities/Side Effects and the Nursing Process

I. ALTERATION IN NUTRITION, LESS THAN BODY REQUIREMENTS, related to DIARRHEA, NAUSEA, VOMITING, STOMATITIS, DYSPEPSIA, INCREASED LFTs

Defining Characteristics: In clinical trials, diarrhea occurred in most (95%) of patients, 40% grade 3, and 0.11% grade 4, compared to patients receiving placebo (34% with 2% grade 3). Most patients developed diarrhea in the first month (93%), with a median time to onset of grade 3 or higher diarrhea at 8 days, and a median cumulative duration of grade 3 or higher diarrhea of 5 days. Loperamide prophylaxis was effective in preventing severe diarrhea. Nausea occurs in 43% with 2% grade 3, whereas vomiting affected 26% of patients, with 3% grade 3. Stomatitis affected 14% and dyspepsia 10%. Decreased appetite occurred in 12% of patients. Elevated ALT occurred in 9% and AST in 7%. Abdominal pain occurred in 36% of patients.

Nursing Implications: Diarrhea can be severe, and requires loperamide prophylaxis; if diarrhea develops, it should be aggressively managed. *Ensure patient is able to buy the loperamide and has it before the patient starts neratinib.* Assess nutritional status, bowel-elimination pattern, and appetite, at baseline and repeated periodically during treatment. Assess LFTs baseline, monthly during first 3 months, then every 3 months and as needed. Teach patient how to take loperamide starting at the first dose of neratinib (see Drug Administration) and continuing through cycle 2 (day 56). Goal is for patient to have 1–2 BMs per day. Teach patient to report if s/he has > 2 BMs in 1 day or if diarrhea does not stop. Report to HCP **right away** if severe diarrhea develops, or if the patient has weakness, dizziness, or fever with diarrhea. Severe diarrhea requires aggressive support as needed with oral or IV hydration, electrolyte replacement, drug interruption, and intervention as ordered. If patient develops grade 3 diarrhea, LFTs should be assessed. Teach patient dietary modification to minimize dietary effect on diarrhea. Teach patient to drink a full glass of fluid every hour (goal 2 liters a day). Inform patient nausea and vomiting may occur. Teach self-administration of antinausea medications. Teach the patient dietary modification if nausea and vomiting or diarrhea occur (e.g., for diarrhea, BRAT diet: bananas, rice, applesauce, and toast) and to increase oral fluids to prevent dehydration. Consult dietitian to see patient for dietary counseling for decreased appetite. Discuss any abnormalities with physician or NP.

II. ALTERATION IN COMFORT related to EGFR-inhibitor RASH, FATIGUE

Defining Characteristics: Fatigue affected 27% of patients. Rash affected 18%, dry skin 6%, nail disorder 8%, and skin fissures 2%. Acneform rash is characteristic of EGFRIs and is usually mild to moderate.

Nursing Implications: Assess patient's baseline comfort, and teach that these symptoms may occur. Assess skin integrity (especially sun-exposed skin) baseline and during therapy. Teach symptom-management strategies to minimize discomfort. Teach patient to notify nurse or physician if fatigue or rash is severe, or does not resolve with local management. Discuss dose interruption or delay with physician or NP. *Teach patient about EGFRI rash.* Teach patient NOT to use antiacne medications. Tetracycline analogues provide an anti-inflammatory benefit. Teach all patients to (1) use a water-based emollient frequently during the day to prevent dryness, (2) stay hydrated, (3) avoid sun exposure and wear SPF 30 (UVA/UVB). Follow institutional guidelines. In general, for grade 1 or mild rash (localized, does not interfere with ADLs, and is not infected): The goal is to preserve skin integrity, minimize discomfort, and prevent infection. Key patient teaching includes to (1) use a mild soap with active ingredients that reduce skin drying such as pyrithione zinc (Head & Shoulders), (2) consider aloe gel for red, tender areas, (3) report distressing tenderness as pramoxine (lidocaine topical anesthetic may help), (4) keep fingernails clean and trimmed, and (5) apply zinc ointment to rectal mucosa after washing. Management: maintain current drug dose; observe or give topical hydrocortisone 1% or 2.5% or clindamycin 1% gel (anti-inflammatory benefit); reassess in 2 weeks. For grade 2 or moderate rash (generalized, with mild symptoms, and minimal effect on ADLs, and is not infected): The goal is to prevent infection and promote comfort. Continue EGFRI dose; use topicals (hydrocortisone 2.5% or clindamycin 1% gel) or consider pimecrolimus cream (immunomodulator) and add doxycycline 100 mg PO twice daily or minocycline 100 mg PO twice daily (give antimicrobial and anti-inflammatory effect) and reassess after 2 weeks. For grades 3–4 or severe rash (generalized, severe, has a significant impact on ADLs, and increased risk of infection): The goal is to prevent infection or identify it early to minimize complications and maximize patient coping with side effects. Hold drug until rash improves, and treat rash with topicals (hydrocortisone 2.5% or clindamycin 1% gel or pimecrolimus cream, doxycycline 100 mg PO twice daily or minocycline 100 mg PO twice daily, and methylprednisolone, Medrol dose pack); reassess after 2 weeks and interrupt or discontinue drug if rash worsens (Lynch et al., 2007). If rash appears infected (exudate, vesicular formation, different appearance), obtain C+S, treat empirically until sensitivity received, and/or obtain dermatology consult. Discuss dose modification with a physician.

Drug: nilotinib (Tasigna)

Class: Kinase Inhibitor; BCR-ABL kinase inhibitor, second generation.

Mechanism of Action: Ph+ CML is caused by a reciprocal mutation involving two chromosomes in the bone marrow (genetic material is exchanged between chromosomes 9 and 22), creating the Philadelphia chromosome. This mutation creates the fusion gene BCR-ABL on chromosome 22, which codes for a BCR-ABL fusion protein; the ABL gene expresses a membrane tyrosine kinase, while the BCR gene is an oncogene. Thus, the tyrosine kinase is always "turned on" continually stimulating cell division and resulting in CML. BCR-ABL causes cell proliferation, decreased adhesion/increased migration, inhibition of apoptosis, degradation of regulatory proteins, and prevention of DNA repair. The BCR portion of the BCR-ABL fusion protein is a protein kinase that turns on cell proliferation signals that create the excessive production of white blood cells (leukemia); however, the binding site is sometimes blocked (inactive) and sometimes active and able to bind to ATP. When a patient progresses on imatinib, it is because BCR-ABL is reactivated through a number of processes, such as amplification of BCR-ABL gene expression, or over 30 point mutations in the BCR-ABL kinase domain so that the drug cannot bind (Deininger et al., 2005). Nilotinib is a designer drug that is highly specific for and binds very tightly to the ATP-binding site of ABL (more selective and 30 times more potent an inhibitor than imatinib mesylate). The drug is active against 32 of the 33 most common BCR-ABL mutations causing imatinib resistance. The drug also inhibits the KIT and PDGFR-A proteins found in patients with GIST.

Metabolism: The drug is metabolized via the cytochrome P450 microenzyme system in the liver (CYP3A4). A high-fat diet greatly increases drug bioavailability (82%), and thus, the drug must be given on an empty stomach. Peak concentrations reached 3 hours after drug administration. Serum protein binding is 98%. Elimination half-life with daily dosing is 17 hours, and steady state is reached by day 8. Metabolism occurs by oxidation and hydroxylation. Metabolites are not pharmacologically active. More than 90% of administered dose is eliminated within 7 days primarily via the feces. Age, weight, gender, and ethnicity do not significantly affect pharmacokinetics.

Indications: FDA-indicated for the treatment of
- Adult and pediatric patients aged ≥ 1 year of age with newly diagnosed Ph+ CML in chronic phase (CP).
- Adult patients with Ph+ CML-CP and accelerated phase (AP) who are resistant to or intolerant to prior therapy that included imatinib.
- Pediatric patients aged ≥ 1 year of age with Ph+ CML-CP resistant or intolerant to prior tyrosine kinase inhibitor (TKI) therapy.

Contraindications: Patients with hypokalemia, hypomagnesemia, or long QT syndrome. Do Not administer to patients with hypokalemia, hypomagnesemia, or long QT syndrome.

Dosage/Range:
- Nilotinib should be taken twice daily at approximately 12-hour intervals and MUST be taken on an empty stomach. No food should be eaten for at least 2 hours **before** the dose and for at least 1 hour **after** the dose is taken. Capsule must be swallowed whole with water.
- *Newly diagnosed Ph+ CML* in chronic phase (CP): 300 mg PO twice daily. *Resistant or intolerant Ph+ CML* (accelerated [AP]) or CP: 400 mg orally twice daily.
- *Recommended pediatric dose:* Newly diagnosed Ph+ CML-CP or Ph+ CML-CP resistant or intolerant to prior TKI therapy: 230 mg/m^2 PO twice daily, rounded to nearest 50 mg dose (maximum single dose is 400 mg). See package insert for combining different nilotinib strengths.
- Eligibility for discontinuation of treatment after a sustained molecular response (MR4.5)—see package insert section 2.2.
    - Eligible newly diagnosed adult patiients with Ph+ CML-CP who have (1) received nilotinib for a minimum of 3 years, (2) have achieved a sustanced molecular response (MR4.5), (3) maintained a molecular response for 1 year prior to discontinuation of therapy; (4) confirmed expression of typical BCR-ABL transcripts; (5) no history of AP or BC; (6) no history of prior attempts of treatment-free remission discontinuation that resulted in relapse. Must continue to be monitored for possible loss of molecular remission after treatment stops.

- Patients with Ph+ CML-CP resistant or intolerant to imatinib who have (1) received nilotinib for at least 3 years, (2) been treated with imatinib only prior to nilotinib; (3) achieved a sustained molecular response (MR4.5); (4) MR4.5 is sustained for a minimum of 1 year immediately prior to discontinuing therapy; (5) confirmed expression of typical BCR-ABL transcripts; (6) no history of AP or BC; (7) no history of prior attempts of treatment free remission discontinuation that resulted in relapse. Monitor patient closely for loss of MR after discontinuation (see below).
- Monitoring after treatment discontinuation: Assess BCR-ABL transcript levels and CBC/differential q month × 1 year, then every 6 weeks for the second year, then every 12 weeks thereafter.
- Reinitiation of treatment in patients who lose molecular response after nilotinib discontinuance. See package insert section 2.3:
  - Newly diagnosed patients who lose Major Molecular Response (MMR) must reinitiate nilotinib therapy within 4 weeks at the dose level prior to discontinuation. Assess BCR-ABL transcript levels monthly until MMR is reestablished and every 12 weeks thereafter.
  - Patients resistant or intolerant to prior therapy (including imatinib) with confirmed loss of MR4.0 (2 consecutive measures separated by at least 4 weeks showing loss of MR4.0) or loss of MMR must reinitiate treatment within 4 weeks at dose level prior to discontinuing therapy.
  - Once nilotinib reinitiated, monitor BCR-ABL transcript levels monitored monthly until previous MMR or MR 4.0 is reestablished, then every 12 weeks thereafter.
- An ECG should be repeated 7 days after any dose adjustment.
- Dose adjustment may be required for hematologic and nonhematologic toxicities and drug interactions (see below).
- If clinically indicated, nilotinib may be given in combination with: hematopoietic growth factors (e.g., erythropoietin or G-CSF), hydroxyurea, or anagrelide.
- Nilotinib is contraindicated in patients with hypokalemia, hypomagnesemia, or long QT syndrome.

Dosage Modifications:
- *Hepatic impairment (at baseline):* consider alternative therapies, and if must administer nilotinib, reduce dose:
  - *Newly diagnosed Ph+ CML in CP:* Mild (Child-Pugh Class A), moderate (Child-Pugh Class B), or severe (Child-Pugh Class C): Reduce dosage to 200 mg twice daily; increase dosage to 300 mg twice daily based on tolerability.
  - Resistant or intolerant Ph+ CML in CP or AP: (1) Mild (Child-Pugh Class A) or moderate (Child-Pugh Class B): Reduce dosage to 300 mg twice daily; increase dosage to 400 mg twice daily based on tolerability; (2) severe ((Child-Pugh Class C): Reduce dosage to 200 mg twice daily. Increase to 300 mg twice daily and then to 400 mg twice daily based on tolerability.
- *Concomitant Strong CYP 3A4 Inhibitors:* Avoid concurrent administration.
  - If must take interacting drug, interrupt nilotinib; if must be coadministered, dose-reduce nilotinib to 300 mg once daily (resistant or intolerant Ph+ CML) or to 200 mg once daily (newly diagnosed Ph+ CML in CP).

- If the strong CYP3A4 inhibitor is discontinued, a washout period should be allowed before nilotinib is adjusted upward to the indicated dose. Monitor patient closely for prolonged QTc interval.
- Concomitant *Strong CYP 3A4 Inducers:* Do not coadminister, as increasing nilotinib dose will not compensate for loss of drug exposure. Teach patients NOT to take St. John's wort as this will decrease nilotinib serum level.
- QTc Prolongation: QTc > 480 msec on ECG:
  - Withhold nilotinib, assess serum electrolyte level, and if serum potassium and magnesium are < LLN, replete.
  - Review concomitant medications taken and reinforce taking medication on empty stomach.
  - Resume drug within 2 weeks at prior dose if QTc returns to < 450 msec and to within 20 msec of baseline.
  - If QTcF is between 450 msec and 480 msec after 2 weeks, reduce dose to 400 mg PO once daily in adults, and to 230 mg/m^2 in pediatric patients.
  - If following dose reduction, QTc returns to > 480 msec, nilotinib should be permanently discontinued.
  - An ECG should be repeated 7 days after any dose adjustment.
- Neutropenia and Thrombocytopenia:
  - For Adult patients with newly diagnosed Ph+ CML in CP at 300 mg twice daily, and resistant or intolerant Ph+ CML in CP or AP at 400 mg twice daily:
    - If ANC < 1.0 × 10^9/L and/or platelet count < 50 × 10^9/L: Stop nilotinib and monitor blood counts;
    - Resume within 2 weeks at prior dose if ANC > 1.0 × 10^9/L and platelets > 50 × 10^9/L;
    - If blood counts remain low for > 2 weeks, reduce the dose to 400 mg once daily.
  - For pediatric patients with newly diagnosed Ph+ CML in CP at 230 mg/m^2 twice daily, OR resistant or intolerant Ph+ CML in CP at 230 mg/m^2 twice daily:
    - If ANC < 1.0 × 10^9/L and/or platelet count < 50 × 10^9/L: Stop nilotinib and monitor blood counts;
    - Resume within 2 weeks at prior dose if ANC > 1.5 × 10^9/L and/or platelets > 75 × 10^9/L;
    - If blood counts remain low for > 2 weeks, reduce the dose to 230 mg/m^2 once daily.
    - If event occurs after dose reduction, consider discontinuing nilotinib.
- Selected nonhematologic lab abnormalities:
  - Elevated serum lipase or amylase ≥ grade 3: (1) Adults: Hold nilotinib, and monitor serum lipase or amylase; resume at 400 mg once daily if serum lipase or amylase returns to ≤ grade 1. Assess serum lipase levels monthly or as clinically indicated; (2) pediatric patients: Interrupt nilotinib until the event returns to ≤ grade 1; resume treatment at 230 mg/m^2 *once* daily if prior dose was 230 mg/m^2 *twice* daily; discontinue nilotinib if prior dose was 230 mg/m^2 once daily.

- Elevated bilirubin $\geq$ grade 3 (adults) or $\geq$ grade 2 (pediatrics): Hold nilotinib and monitor bilirubin until bilirubin returns to $\leq$ grade1. (1) Adult: resume at 400 mg once daily if serum bilirubin returns to $\leq$ grade 1; Pediatrics: resume at 230 mg/m^2 once daily if prior dose was 230 mg/m^2 twice daily; discontinue nilotinib if prior dose was 230 mg/m^2 once daily and recovery to $\leq$ grade 1 takes longer than 28 days.
- Elevated hepatic transaminases $\geq$ grade 3: withhold nilotinib and monitor hepatic transaminases until returns to $\leq$ grade 1; (1) Adults: resume at 400 mg once daily if hepatic transaminases return to $\leq$ grade 1; (2) Pediatric: resume at 230 mg/m^2 once daily if prior dose was 230 mg/m^2 twice daily; discontinue nilotinib if prior dose was 230 mg/m^2 once daily and recovery to $\leq$ grade 1 takes longer than 28 days.
- If other clinically significant moderate or severe nonhematologic toxicity develops (including medically severe fluid retention), hold nilotinib until toxicity resolves; (1) Adults: resume at 400 mg once daily if previous dose with 300 mg twice daily in newly diagnosed patients with CML-CP or 400 mg twice daily if resistant or intolerant CML-CP and CML-AP; discontinue nilotinib if prior dose was 400 mg once daily. Once toxicity has resolved, if clinically appropriate, consider escalating dose back to 300 mg (newly diagnosed Ph+ CML in CP) or 400 mg (resistant or intolerant Ph+ CML in CP and Ph+ CML in AP) twice daily; (2) pediatric patients: resume treatment at resume at 230 mg/m^2 once daily if prior dose was 230 mg/m^2 twice daily; discontinue nilotinib if prior dose was 230 mg/m^2 once daily; once toxicity resolves, if clinically appropriate, consider re-escalation of dose to 230 mg/m^2 twice daily.

Drug Preparation:
- Oral.
- Available in 50-mg, 150-mg, and 200-mg hard capsules.

Drug Administration:
- Assess patient's medication profile for possible interacting drugs. Teach patients NOT to eat grapefruit, drink grapefruit juice, or take St. John's wort, as these will affect nilotinib serum levels.
- Administer capsules whole on an empty stomach (2 hours after eating any food, and after taking nilotinib, wait at least 1 hour before eating any food) with a glass of water. Drink only water for 1 hour after drug administration. This is a critical point of patient education.
- If the patient is unable to swallow capsules, the contents of each capsule may be dispersed in one teaspoon (NO MORE than this) of applesauce (pureed apple) and taken immediately (within 15 min) and not stored for future use.
- If a dose is missed, the patient should NOT make up the dose but rather resume taking the next prescribed daily dose.
- Therapy is continued until disease progression or unacceptable toxicity.
- Lab monitoring: **CBC/differential** baseline, then every 2 weeks for the first 2 months, and then monthly; ECG to monitor **QTc** baseline, 7 days after first dose, and then periodically, as well as after any dose adjustments; monitor QTc closely in patients with liver impairment or receiving strong CYP3A4 inhibitors; **electrolytes:** baseline and correct

prior to starting drug, especially serum magnesium and potassium; monitor magnesium, potassium, calcium, phosphorus, sodium; monitor **serum lipase and glucose** baseline and monthly or as clinically indicated, especially in patients with a history of pancreatitis who require close monitoring; monitor **LFTs** baseline and monthly or as clinically indicated.

Drug Interactions:
* Nilotinib is a competitive inhibitor of CYP3A4, CYP2C8, CYP2C9, CYP2D6, and UGT1A1 in vitro, potentially increasing the concentrations of drugs eliminated by these enzymes; studies suggest nilotinib may induce CYP2B6, CYP2C8, and CYP2C9, and decrease the concentrations of drugs eliminated by these enzymes (e.g., single dose of nilotinib given with midazolam, a CYP3A4 substrate, increased midazolam exposure by 30%). A single dose of nilotinib given to healthy subjects did not change the pharmacokinetics and pharmacodynamics of warfarin, a CYP2C9 substrate. Use caution when nilotinib is given with substrates for these enzymes have a narrow therapeutic index.
* Nilotinib inhibits human P-glycoprotein. If nilotinib is given with drugs that are substrates of P-gp, increased concentrations of the substrate are likely, and the patient should be monitored closely. In addition, nilotinib is a substrate of P-gp. If nilotinib is administered with drugs that inhibit p-gp, increased concentrations of nilotinib are likely, and should be coadministered very cautiously.
* *CYP3A4 (strong) inhibitors* (e.g., atazanavir, clarithromycin, grapefruit or grapefruit juice, indinavir, itraconazole, ketoconazole, nefazodone, nelfinavir, ritonavir, saquinavir, telithromycin, voriconazole) may increase nilotinib plasma concentrations; do not coadminister. If administration of an interacting drug is necessary, interrupt nilotinib therapy; if continued coadministration is necessary, consider nilotinib dose reduction and monitor patient closely for prolongation of the QT interval. Ketoconazole in healthy subjects at 400 mg once daily × 6 days, increase nilotinib AUC threefold. Teach patient to avoid grapefruit or grapefruit juice.
* *CYP3A4 (strong) inducers* (e.g., carbamazepine, dexamethasone, phenytoin, phenobarbital, rifabutin, rifampicin, rifapentin, St. John's wort) may increase metabolism of nilotinib so that nilotinib serum levels are reduced. For example, rifampicin at 600 mg daily × 12 days reduces nilotinib AUC by approximately 80%; avoid concurrent use. Teach patient not to take St. John's wort if taking nilotinib.
* Drugs that affect gastric pH: Nilotinib's solubility is pH dependent, with decreased solubility at higher pH. Drugs such as PPIs that may increase gastric pH, may decrease nilotinib solubility and reduce its bioavailability. Do not use together if possible, and if they must be coadministered, use caution. If an H_2 blocker or antacid is necessary, separate doses between it and nilotinib by at least several hours.
* Drugs prolonging QTc (e.g., anti-arrhythmic drugs such as amiodarone, disopyramide, procainamide, quinidine, and sotalol; chloroquine, clarithromycin, haloperidol, methadone, moxifloxacin, and pimozide): do not use together, as will increase risk of prolonged QTc and sudden death. If treatment with any of these agents is required, interrupt nilotinib therapy. If interruption is not possible, monitor patient closely for prolongation of QT interval.

- Drugs that inhibit drug transport systems: nilotinib is a substrate of the efflux transporter P-glycoprotein (P-gp). If nilotinib is administered with a drug that inhibits P-gp, increased serum levels of nilotinib will likely result; use together cautiously.

Lab Effects/Interference:
- Increased LFTs—AST, ALT, alkaline phosphatase, BR (total)—transient.
- Increased serum creatinine, BUN, lipase (transient), glucose, amylase, CPK, LDH (uncommon), parathyroid hormone.
- Decreased serum calcium, magnesium, phosphate, potassium, sodium.
- Decreased neutrophils, platelet count, red blood cell count.
- QTc prolongation.

Special Considerations:
- Imatinib is successful in treating patients with Ph+ CML (CP, AP, and blast phases) and inducing a complete cytogenic response in 80% of patients; however, 10% will develop resistance by amplification, mutations, additional chromosomal mutations (Ault, 2007). Nilotinib can induce major cytogenetic response in 52% of patients after 6 months in imatinib-resistant or intolerant patients.
- Patient teaching about self-administration every 12 hours on an empty stomach is critical to prevent increased toxicity, and to avoid interacting drugs.
- Most common nonhematologic adverse reactions in all patient groups, occurring in 20% or more patients, were: nausea, rash, headache, fatigue, pruritus, vomiting, diarrhea, cough, constipation, arthralgia, nasopharyngitis, pyrexia, and night sweats. Hematologic adverse reactions include myelosuppression: thrombocytopenia, neutropenia, and anemia.
- Warnings and Precautions:
  - *Myelosuppression:* Grades 3–4 thrombocytopenia, neutropenia, and anemia can occur. Assess CBC baseline and every 2 weeks for the first 2 months, then monthly. Hold dose to reverse myelosuppresion, and patient may require a dose reduction.
  - *QTc Prolongation:* Drug prolongs QTc interval (ventricular repolarization), and sudden deaths have been reported. Prolongation of the QT interval can result in torsades de pointes, a type of ventricular tachycardia that can cause syncope, seizure, and/ or death. See the Introduction to *Chapter 4* for full discussion of QT prolongation and sudden death. Patients must have an ECG as follows: before starting the drug, 7 days after starting the drug, with any dose changes, and regularly during nilotinib therapy. Do not give drug to patients with hypokalemia, hypomagnesemia, or long QT syndrome.
    - Before starting nilotinib therapy, assess electrolytes, calcium, and magnesium levels, and correct hypokalemia and/or hypomagnesemia before starting nilotinib. Monitor electrolytes throughout nilotinib therapy.
    - Significant prolongation of QT interval can occur when nilotinib is taken with (1) food (inappropriately), (2) strong CYP3A4 inhibitors, and/or (3) medicinal products known to prolong the QT interval. DO NOT take nilotinib with food or these interacting drugs.
    - Nilotinib is contraindicated in patients with (1) long QT syndrome; (2) hypokalemia and/or hypomagnesemia.

- *Sudden deaths* have been reported rarely in 0.3% of patients; ventricular repolarization abnormalities may have contributed.
- *Cardiac and arterial vascular occlusive events* have occurred in 9.3% of patients on 300 mg bid dose, and 15.2% of patients on a 400 mg bid dose, after a median of 60 months on therapy. These events included ischemic heart disease-related events, peripheral arterial occlusive disease, and ischemic cerebrovascular events. Teach patients to seek immediate medical attention if they develop acute signs or symptoms of cardiovascular events. Assess patients for signs/symptoms of cardiovascular events.
- *Pancreatitis and elevated serum lipase:* patients at risk are those with a previous history of pancreatitis. If the patient develops an elevated serum lipase together with abdominal symptoms, drug should be interrupted and patient evaluated for pancreatitis. Assess serum lipase monthly or as clinically indicated.
- *Hepatotoxicity:* nilotinib may cause elevations in LFTs. Grade 3–4 elevations in bilirubin, AST, and ALT were reported more frequently in pediatric than adult patients. Monitor bilirubin, AST/ALT, alkaline phosphatase; assess baseline, monthly, or as clinically indicated during treatment. Nilotinib exposure is increased and a dose reduction is recommended in patients with impaired hepatic function, and their QT interval (on ECG) should be followed closely for evidence of prolongation.
- *Electrolyte abnormalities:* Nilotinib can cause hypophosphatemia, hypokalemia, hyperkalemia, hypocalcemia, and hyponatremia. Correct electrolyte abnormalities prior to starting nilotinib therapy, and monitor closely during therapy.
- *Drug interactions:* avoid CYP3A4 inhibitors or anti-arrhythmic drugs (e.g., amiodarone, disopyramide, procainamide, quinidine, sotalol) and other drugs that may prolong QT interval (e.g., chloroquine, clarithromycin, haloperidol, methadone, moxifloxacin, pimozide). Should coadministration of any of these drugs be medically necessary, interrupt nilotinib therapy. If this is not possible, monitor patients for prolongation of QT interval.
- *Food effects:* nilotinib bioavailability is increased with food, so nilotinib MUST NOT be taken with food; rather, teach patients no food should be consumed for at least 2 hours before and 1 hour after the dose is taken. Teach patients also to avoid grapefruit and grapefruit juice, and other foods known to inhibit CYP3A4 (e.g., noni juice, pomegranate juice). Teach patient to tell nurse or physician before taking ANY OTC medicine, vitamin, or mineral; be sure to tell nurse or physician all medications that patient is taking and whether he or she has had any trouble digesting lactose in the past.
- *Hepatic impairment:* nilotinib exposure is increased in patients with mild to severe hepatic impairment, so a lower starting drug dose must be used.
- *Tumor lysis syndrome* (TLS) can occur in patients with resistant or intolerant CML who have malignant disease progression with high WBC and/or dehydration. Assess, discuss TLS prophylaxis (e.g., hydration, uric-acid correction) with physician prior to starting nilotinib therapy, and monitor these patients. Nilotinib can cause hypophosphatemia, hypokalemia, hyperkalemia, hypocalcemia, and hyponatremia.
- *Hemorrhage:* Grade 3 or 4 hemorrhage can rarely occur (0.7% at 300 mg bid, and 1.4% at 400 mg bid).
- *Total gastrectomy:* Nilotinib drug absorption (exposure) is reduced in patients who have had a total gastrectomy. Patients require more frequent monitoring and may require a dose increase or alternative therapy.

- *Lactose:* Nilotinib capsule contains lactose so drug is not recommended for patients with galactose intolerance, severe lactase deficiency with a severe degree of intolerance to lactose-containing products or of glucose-galactose malabsorption.
- *Monitoring of laboratory tests:* CBC every 2 weeks for first 2 months, then monthly; chemistry panels including electrolytes, calcium, magnesium, LFTs, lipid profile, and glucose baseline and periodically; ECGs baseline, 7 days after initiation, and periodically, as well as following dose adjustments. See package insert for discussion.
- *Embryo-fetal toxicity:* Teach women of childbearing age to use effective contraception while receiving the drug, and for at least 14 days after last dose, as fetal harm can occur. If the drug is used during pregnancy, or if the patient becomes pregnant while taking the drug, the patient should be apprised of the potential hazard to the fetus. Mothers should not breast-feed; a decision should be made whether to discontinue nursing or to discontinue nilotinib, taking into consideration the importance of the drug to the mother's health.
- *Fluid retention:* Severe fluid retention occurred in 3.9% of patients taking nilotinib 300 mg bid, and 2.9% of patients taking 400 mg bid. Effusions can occur, including pleural, pericardial and ascites. Monitor patients for signs of severe fluid retention (e.g., unexpected rapid weight gain or swelling), and symptoms (e.g., SOB), and discuss treatment with physician/NP/PA.
- *Effects on growth and development in pediatric patients:* Long-term effects of prolonged nilotinib therapy are unknown. Monitor growth and development in patients receiving BCR-ABL TKI therapy.
- *Embryo-fetal toxicity:* Drug is fetotoxic. Teach female patients of reproductive potential to use effective contraception during treatment and for at least 14 days after the last drug dose.
- *Monitoring BCR-ABL transcript levels:* sensitivity of test must be at least MR4.5.
- (1) In patients who discontinue nilotinib therapy, monitor transcript levels monthly × 1 year, then every 6 weeks for the 2nd year, then every 12 weeks thereafter; if a loss of a major molecular response (MMR) occurs off therapy, patients should reinitiate therapy within 4 weeks; if the patient does not achieve a MMR after 3 months of reinstituted nilotinib, BCR-ABL kinase domain mutation testing should be performed;
- (2) Monitoring after reinitiation of nilotinib after loss of MMR: Monitor CBC, BCR-SABL transcripts every 4 weeks until achieve a MMR, then every 12 weeks.

Potential Toxicities/Side Effects and the Nursing Process

I. POTENTIAL FOR INFECTION AND BLEEDING related to NEUTROPENIA AND THROMBOCYTOPENIA

Defining Characteristics: Grades 3–4 neutropenia occurred in 28% of patients in chronic phase and 37% of patients with accelerated phase; thrombocytopenia in 28–37% of patients; anemia in 8–23% of patients. Febrile neutropenia occurred in < 10% of patients with accelerated phase CML. Sepsis can occur. Common infections were folliculitis, URI, herpes, candidiasis, pneumonia, UTI, and gastroenteritis.

Nursing Implications: Assess baseline CBC, WBC, differential, and platelet count before initiating therapy, then every two weeks for the first 8 weeks of treatment, and then monthly. Assess for signs/symptoms of infection or bleeding. Teach patient the signs/symptoms of infection or bleeding and to report these immediately, and teach patient self-care measures to minimize risk of infection and bleeding. This includes avoidance of crowds, proximity to people with infections, and OTC aspirin-containing medications. Discuss need for blood product support or growth factors with physician or NP.

II. ALTERATION IN CIRCULATION, POTENTIAL, related to QTc PROLONGATION

Defining Characteristics: Patients may develop QT prolongation on EKG. Do NOT administer to patients with prolonged or who may develop prolonged QTc (hypokalemia, hypomagnesemia, other drugs that prolong the QTc). Prolonged QTc in the setting of low magnesium and hypokalemia sets the stage for torsades de pointes, with ventricular tachycardia, fibrillation, and sudden cardiac death possible.

Nursing Implications: Assess baseline QTc interval. Identify patients at risk for development of prolonged QTc (congenital long QTc) syndrome, prolonged QTc > 450 msec, taking antiarrhythmics or other drugs that can prolong the QTc interval (hypokalemia, hypomagnesemia, concomitant CYP3A4 strong inhibitors). Correct electrolyte abnormalities (e.g., magnesium, potassium) before starting nilotinib and monitor periodically during therapy. Hypokalemia and hypomagnesemia in the setting of prolonged QTc may lead to torsades de pointes, ventricular fibrillation, and sudden cardiac death. QTc must be assessed baseline, 7 days after drug initiation, and periodically after that, as well as after any dosage adjustments. Teach patient to correctly take nilotinib on an empty stomach to avoid increased drug serum levels and to avoid any drugs that may interact with nilotinib, until discussion with the physician, NP, PA, or nurse. Teach patient to report feeling lightheaded, faint, or an irregular heartbeat right away. Patients with hepatic impairment should have a dose reduction to avoid increased serum levels of nilotinib. See Introduction to *Chapter 5* for more complete discussion on determining the QTc interval.

III. ALTERATION IN SKIN INTEGRITY related to RASH, PRURITUS, EDEMA

Defining Characteristics: Rash may occur. In clinical studies, 33% of patients reported rash (2% grades 3–4); 29% of patients complained of pruritus. Peripheral edema occurred in 11% of patients.

Nursing Implications: Teach patient that rash may occur and to report it. Assess patient skin integrity baseline and regularly during treatment. Teach patient local comfort measures. Teach patient self-application of topical steroids to rash or, if prescribed, systemic steroids (Ault, 2007). Discuss rash and management plan with physician, especially if severe. Teach patient to report any weight increase, swelling of the ankles, feet, or face, and any difficulty breathing or shortness of breath.

IV.   POTENTIAL ALTERATION IN NUTRITION related to NAUSEA, DIARRHEA, VOMITING, CONSTIPATION, HEPATOTOXICITY, PANCREATITIS

Defining Characteristics: Nausea affected 31% of patients (1% grades 3–4), and vomiting affected 21% (< 1% grades 3–4). Diarrhea affected 22% (3% grades 3–4), whereas constipation affected 20%. Hepatotoxicity characterized by transient and reversible increase in LFTs. Grades 3–4 lipase increased in 15–17% of patients and glucose in 11% of patients. The largest increase in bilirubin was found in patients with (TA)7 (TA)7 genotype (UGT1A1*28).

Nursing Implications: Teach patient to self-administer antiemetic 1 hour before each dose if needed and to call if nausea/vomiting develop/persist. Discuss with physician more effective antiemetic regimen if nausea/vomiting develop despite antiemetics. Encourage small, frequent intake of cool, bland foods as tolerated if nausea develops. Refer to dietitian as needed for meal planning. Assess bowel-elimination pattern baseline and at each visit. Teach patient to report diarrhea or constipation that does not respond to antidiarrheal or anticonstipation medications. Teach dietary modifications as appropriate. Monitor LFTs, serum, lipase, and glucose baseline and periodically during therapy. Discuss abnormalities with physician. Teach patient to report any abdominal pain with nausea or vomiting.

V.   POTENTIAL ALTERATION IN COMFORT related to HEADACHE, FATIGUE, ARTHRALGIA, MYALGIA

Defining Characteristics: In clinical studies, headache affected 30% of patients (3% grades 3–4). Arthralgias affected 18% of patients (2% grades 3–4) and myalgias 14% (2% grades 3–4). Bone pain and muscle spasms affected 11% of patients.

Nursing Implications: Teach patient that these events may occur and to report them. Assess baseline comfort and monitor closely during treatment. Develop plan to assure comfort depending on symptoms reported. If appropriate, suggest analgesics, the application of heat or cold, for control of myalgias and arthralgias. Discuss ineffective strategies with physician and revise plan as needed.

Drug: Niraparib (Zejula)

Classification: Poly (ADP-ribose) polymerase (PARP) inhibitor.

Mechanism of Action: Niraparib is an inhibitor of poly (ADP-ribose) polymerase (PARP) enzymes PARP-1 and PARP-2, which are important in the repair of damaged DNA. By blocking this repair pathway, tumor cells cannot repair their DNA damage, so undergo apoptosis (programmed cell death). Niraparib is active in tumors with or without deficiencies of the DNA repair gene *BRCA 1/2*.

Metabolism: After oral dosing, absolute bioavailability is 73%, and peak plasma concentration (C_{max}) is reached within 3 hours. A high-fat meal ingested before dosing did not affect pharmacokinetics. Niraparib is 83% bound to human plasma proteins; the mean drug half-life is 36 hrs ($t_{1/2}$). Drug is primarily metabolized by carboxylesterases to form a major inactive metabolite. Drug is excreted in urine (47.5%) and feces (38.8%), with 11% and 19% unchanged drug in the urine and feces, respectively. No dose adjustment is necessary for patients with mild or moderate renal impairment (CrCl > 30 mL/min) or patients with mild hepatic impairment.

Indications: Maintenance treatment of adult patients with recurrent epithelial ovarian, fallopian tube, or primary peritoneal cancer who are in a complete or partial response to platinum-based chemotherapy.

Contraindication: None.

Dosage Range:
- Recommended dose is 300 mg PO (3–100 mg capsules) once daily with or without food.
- Continue therapy until disease progression or unacceptable toxicity.
- Dose Modifications:
  - Dose levels: starting dose 300 mg/day; first dose level (reduction) to 200 mg/day; second dose level (reduction) to 100 mg a day (1–100 mg capsule); if further dose reduction needed, discontinue niraparib.
  - Platelet count < 100,000/μL: *first occurrence:* hold niraparib for a maximum of 28 days, and monitor CBC weekly until platelet count ≥ 100,000/μL; resume niraparib at same or reduced dose level; if platelet count is < 75,000/μL, resume at decreased dose level. *Second occurrence:* hold niraparib for a maximum of 28 days, and monitor CBC weekly until platelet count ≥ 100,000/μL; resume niraparib at a reduced dose level; if platelets do not recover within 28 days of treatment interruption, or if the patient has already undergone a dose reduction to 100 mg once daily, discontinue drug.
  - Neutrophil < 1000/μL or Hgb < 8 g/dL: Hold niraparib for a maximum of 28 days, and monitor CBC/differential weekly until neutrophil count ≥ 1,500/μL or Hgb returns to ≥ 9 g/dL; resume niraparib at a reduced dose level; Discontinue niraparib if neutrophils or hgb have not returned to acceptable levels within 28 days of dose interruption, or if patient already as undergone dose reduction to 100 mg once daily.
  - Hematologic adverse reaction requiring transfusion: Patients with platelet count ≤ 10,000/μL, consider platelet transfusion. If other risk factors such as coadministration of anticoagulation or antiplatelet drugs, consider interrupting these drugs and/or transfusion at a higher platelet count. Resume niraparib at a reduced dose level.
  - Nonhematologic CTCAE ≥ *grade 3* where prophylaxis is not feasible or adverse reaction persists despite treatment: hold niraparib for a maximum of 28 days or until resolution of AE; resume niraparib at a reduced dose level (up to 2 dose reductions are permitted). CTCAE ≥ *grade 3 lasting > 28 days while patient is receiving niraparib at 100 mg/day:* discontinue niraparib.
  - MDS or AML (MDS/AML) is confirmed: discontinue niraparib.

Drug Preparation: Available in 100- capsules.

Drug Administration:
- Assess CBC baseline and weekly for the first month, then monthly for the next 11 months, then periodically during treatment.
- Assess HR and BP baseline, and monthly for first year, then periodically during treatment. Discuss any abnormalities and need for antihypertensive therapy with MD or PA/NP.
- Assess pregnancy test prior to initiating drug in females of reproductive potential. Teach patients to take effective contraceptive medication to avoid pregnancy during therapy and for 6 months after the last dose.
- Teach patients how to self-administer the capsule at the same time of day, with or without food; capsules should be swallowed whole; if a dose is missed or if the patient vomits after taking the daily dose, take the dose the next day at the regular time, DO NOT make up a dose. Teach patient to consider dosing at bedtime to reduce nausea, with or without an antiemetic medication.
- Teach mothers not to breast-feed an infant during therapy and for 2 weeks after the last dose.
- Teach patient to tell healthcare provider before taking any OTC medications, vitamins, or herbal supplements.

Drug Interactions: No significant interactions known.

Lab Effects/Interference:
- Decreased hgb, platelet count, ANC.
- Increase in AST, ALT.

Special Considerations:
- Most common adverse reactions ($\geq$ 10%): thrombocytopenia, anemia, neutropenia, leukopenia, palpitations, nausea, constipation, vomiting, abdominal pain/distention, mucositis/stomatitis, diarrhea, dyspepsia, dry mouth, fatigue/asthenia, decreased appetite, UTI, elevated AST/ALT, myalgia, back pain, arthralgia, headache, dizziness, dysgeusia, insomnia, anxiety, nasopharyngitis, dyspnea, cough, rash, HTN.
- Patients should start treatment no later than 8 weeks after their most recent platinum-containing regimen. Niraparib should be taken until disease progression or intolerable adverse effects.
- Although not indicated for male patients, drug may decrease fertility in male patients.
- Warnings and Precautions
  - *Myelodysplastic Syndrome/Acute Myeloid Leukemia (MDS/AML):* In one clinical study, incidence was 1.4% compared to 1.1% in patients receiving placebo. Overall incidence is 0.9%. Onset of MDS/AML varied from < 1 month to 2 years, and patients had received prior platinum-chemotherapy. Drug should be discontinued if MDS/AML diagnosis confirmed.
  - *Bone Marrow Suppression:* Grade 3 or higher thrombocytopenia was reported in 29% of patients, anemia in 25%, and neutropenia 20%. Niraparib should NOT be started until patients have recovered from hematologic toxicity from previous chemotherapy. CBC should be assessed baseline, then weekly for the first month, then monthly

for next 11 months, then periodically after that. See dose modifications for interruption and dose reductions; if hematologic toxicities do not recover after a 28-day interruption, stop niraparib and consult an hematologist for further evaluation (e.g., bone marrow analysis, blood sample for cytogenetics).

- *Cardiovascular Effects:*
  - *HTN and hypertensive crisis* have occurred. Incidence of HTN was 20%, and Grades 3–4 HTN occurred in 9% of patients (vs 2% in the placebo arm). Monitor BP and HR monthly for the first year, and periodically after that.
  - Closely monitor patients with cardiovascular disorders, especially coronary insufficiency, cardiac arrhythmias, HTN. New-onset HTN should be managed with antihypertensive medications, and niraparib dose adjusted if needed. Changes in HR and BP may be related to pharmacological inhibition of the dopamine transporter (DAT), norepinephrine transporter (NET) and serotonin transporter (SERT) (Tesaro Inc, 2017).
- *Embryo-fetal toxicity:* Drug is genotoxic, targets actively dividing cells so is likely teratogenic and/or causes embryo-fetal death. Consider pregnancy test in female patients of reproductive potential prior to starting niraparib. Teach patients to take effective contraception to avoid pregnancy while receiving the drug, and for 6 months after last dose.

Potential Toxicities/Side Effects and the Nursing Process

I. POTENTIAL FOR BLEEDING, INFECTION, ANEMIA, AND FATIGUE related to BONE MARROW SUPPRESSION

Defining Characteristics: In clinical trials, grade 3 or higher thrombocytopenia occurred in 29% of patients, anemia in 25% of patients, and neutropenia in 20% of patients. Fatigue/asthenia occurred in 57% of patients and was severe (grades 3–4) in 8%. MDS/AML occurred in 0.9% in clinical studies. In laboratory studies, hgb was decreased in 85% of patients platelets decreased in 72%, and neutrophil count decreased in 53% of patients.

Nursing Implications: Evaluate CBC/differential, hemoglobin/hematocrit, and platelets at baseline, then weekly for first month, monthly for the next 11 months, then periodically during treatment. Discuss any abnormalities with the physician/NP/PA. The drug should not be started until resolution of myelosuppression from prior therapy has occurred (≤ grades 0–1). Assess for signs and symptoms of infection, bleeding, and fatigue. Teach the patient about signs and symptoms of infection and bleeding, and to report them immediately. Teach the patient self-care measures to minimize the risk of infection and bleeding, including avoidance of OTC aspirin-containing medications. Teach the patient self-assessment of fatigue and to alternate rest and activity as needed. If prolonged myelosuppression occurs, interrupt the drug and monitor CBC/differential weekly until recovery. If recovery (grades 0–1) has not occurred by 28 days, refer the patient to a hematologist for evaluation, including bone marrow analysis and cytogenetic study. The drug should be discontinued if a diagnosis of MDS/AML is confirmed.

II.   ALTERATION IN NUTRITION, POTENTIAL, related to NAUSEA, VOMITING, OR DIARRHEA

Defining Characteristics: Nausea was common in clinical trials (74%); constipation affected 40% of patients, vomiting 34%, abdominal pain/distention 33% (less than placebo), decreased appetite 25%, mucositis/stomatitis 20%, diarrhea 20%, dyspepsia 18%, dysgeusia and dry mouth 10%.

Nursing Implications: Assess the patient's nutritional status at baseline and at each visit. Teach the patient that these side effects may occur, and teach self-management strategies such as use of antinausea medications, and OTC medications to manage/prevent constipation and diarrhea. Discuss dietary modifications and teach patient to report any symptoms that do not improve. Discuss prescription medications with the provider if there is a need to manage refractory symptoms. Teach the patient tips to increase appetite (e.g., small, frequent meals, use of spices). Offer the services of a dietitian as appropriate.

III.   ALTERATION IN COMFORT related to ARTHRALGIA/MYALGIA, HEADACHE, DIZZINESS, BACKACHE, AND INSOMNIA

Defining Characteristics: In clinical trials, myalgias occurred in 19% of patients, back pain in 18%, arthralgias in 13%, headache in 26%, dizziness in 18%, and insomnia in 27% of patients.

Nursing Implications: Assess the patient's baseline level of comfort. Teach the patient that these side effects may occur, and teach self-management strategies. Teach the patient to report symptoms that do not improve. If this occurs, discuss with the physician/NP/PA prescription medication for refractory symptoms. Teach patient to change position slowly if dizziness develops and to ask for support to prevent falling if dizziness continues. Report dizziness that does not improve.

Drug: olaparib (Lynparza)

Class: Poly (ADP-ribose) polymerase (PARP) inhibitor.

Mechanism of Action: Drug inhibits PARP enzymes PARP 1, 2, and 3, which play important roles in DNA transcription, cell-cycle regulation, and DNA repair. This results in disruption of cancer cell processes and cell death, especially in *BRCA*-mutated tumor cells.

Metabolism: Rapid absorption after oral dosing, with peak plasma concentrations occurring 1–3 hours after the patient takes the dose. Taking the drug with a high-fat meal slows the rate of absorption but does not significantly change the extent of absorption. Olaparib is approximately 82% protein-bound and is extensively metabolized by (primarily) CYP3A4. Its terminal plasma half-life is 11.9 ± 4.8 hours, with 15% of the drug being excreted in urine and 6% in feces.

Indication: Treatment of patients with: (A) *ovarian cancer*: (1) maintenance treatment of adult patients who are in remission from first line platinum-based therapy, with suspected or actual *BRCA*-mutated (germline or somatic) advanced epithelial ovarian, fallopian tube, or primary peritoneal cancer who are in CR or PR from platinum-based chemotherapy; (2) maintenance treatment of adult patients with with recurrent epithelial ovarian, fallopian tube, or primary peritoneal cancer, who are in CR or PR from platinum-based chemotherapy; (3) treatment of adult patients with advanced *BRCA*-mutated ovarian cancer after 3 or more lines of chemotherapy [actual or suspected germline *BRCA*-mutation (*gBRCAm*)]; (B) *breast cancer*: patients with actual or suspected germline *BRCA*-mutated HER-2 negative metastatic breast cancer, after chemotherapy in the neoadjuvant, adjuvant or metastatic setting; patients who had hormone receptor positive breast cancer should have been treated with prior endocrine therapy (or be considered inappropriate for endocrine therapy).

Patients should be selected based on an FDA-approved companion diagnostic test for *BRCA-* mutations.

Dosage/Range:
- Olaparib is available as tablets (100 mg and 150 mg).
- Recommended dose is 300mg orally [(2) 150-mg tablets], taken twice daily orally, with or without food, for a total daily dose of 600 mg. The 100-mg tablet is for use if the dose is reduced.
  - 1st line maintenance of *BRCA*-mutated advanced ovarian cancer: Continue treatment until disease progression, unacceptable toxicity, or completion of 2 years of treatment: if CR, stop treatment; if evidence of disease at 2 years, treatment can be continued per healthcare provider if patient can derive further benefit.
  - Maintenance treatment of recurrent ovarian cancer, advanced *gBRCA*-mutated ovarian cancer, and *gBRCA*-mutated HER-2 negative metastatic breast cancer: Continue until disease progression or unacceptable toxicity occurs.
  - Patients with mild renal impairment (CLcr 51–80 mL/min) do not require dose adjustment.
- Moderate renal impairment (CRcl 31–50 mL/min): recommended dose is 200 mg (two 100-mg tablets), orally twice a day or a total daily dose of 400 mg. The drug has not been studied in patients with severe renal impairment or end-stage renal disease (CRcl ≤ 30 mL/min).
- Dose modifications for use with CYP3A inhibitors: avoid concomitant use of strong or moderate CYP3A inhibitors and consider alternative agents with less CYP3A inhibition.
  - If a strong CYP3A inhibitor must be co-administered, reduce olaparib dose to 100 mg twice daily (total daily dose of 200 mg).
  - If a moderate CYP3A inhibitor is co-administered, reduce the oliparib dose to 150 mg (one 150 mg tablet) twice daily (total daily dose of 300 mg).
- Dose modifications to manage toxicity:
  - Interrupt dose or reduce dose to 250 mg (one 150-mg and one 100-mg tablet) twice daily (total 500 mg daily dose).
  - If further dose reduction is necessary, reduce to 200 mg (two 100-mg tablets) taken twice daily (total daily dose of 400 mg).

Drug Preparation: Available as 100-mg and 150-mg tablets. Store at room temperature and keep out of the reach of children and pets.

Drug Administration:
- Teach the patient self-administration with or without food;
  - Swallow tablets whole; do not chew, divide, or dissolve tablet.
  - If a dose is missed, the patient should take their next dose at the scheduled time and not make up the dose.
  - Teach female patients of reproductive potential: teach to use effective contraception during treatment and for 6 months after last drug dose; teach male patients with female partners of reproductive potential or who are pregnant, to use effective contraception during therapy and for 3 months after last drug dose. Women should NOT breast-feed while receiving the drug.
- Review patient medication profile to identify CYP3A inhibitors; if strong or moderate CYP3A inhibitors are found, discuss dose reduction with provider. If CYP3A inducers are identified, discuss dose modification with provider. Teach patient to avoid eating/drinking grapefruit (juice); and not to take St. John's wort.
- Assess CBC/differential at baseline and monthly thereafter. The drug should not be started until resolution of myelosuppression from prior therapy occurs (grades 0–1).
- If prolonged myelosuppression occurs, interrupt the drug and monitor CBC/differential weekly until recovery. If recovery (grades 0–1) has not occurred by 4 weeks, refer the patient to a hematologist for evaluation, including bone marrow analysis and cytogenetic study. The drug should be discontinued if MDS/AML is confirmed.

Drug Interactions:
- CYP3A inhibitors may increase olaparib serum levels: *Avoid coadministration* with strong **inhibitors** (e.g., itraconazole, telithromycin, clarithromycin, ketoconazole, voriconazole, nefazodone, posaconazole, ritonavir, lopinavir/ritonavir, indinavir, saquinavir, nelfinavir, boceprevir, telaprevir) and **moderate inhibitors** (e.g., amprenavir, aprepitant, atazanavir, ciprofloxacin, crizotinib, darunavir/ritonavir, diltiazem, erythromycin, fluconazole, fosamprenavir, imatinib, verapamil). See the dose modification if the drug must be coadministered with olaparib. Teach the patient to avoid grapefruit and Seville oranges while taking olaparib, as these foods may also increase olaparib serum levels and toxicity.
- CYP3A4 inducers may decrease olaparib serum levels: *Avoid* concomitant administration of **strong inducers** (e.g., rifampicin, phenytoin, carbamazepine, St. John's wort), as this may decrease the serum level of olaparib by as much as 87%. Avoid coadministration with **moderate inducers** (e.g., bosentan, efavirenz, etravirine, modafinil, nafcillin), but if it is unavoidable, assess for decreased olaparib efficacy.
- Anticancer drugs: Potentiation and prolongation of myelosuppression.

Lab Effects/Interference:
- Increased: serum creatinine, rbc mean corpuscular volume (MCV)
- Decreased: hemoglobin (Hgb), lymphocyte count, ANC, platelet count

Special Considerations:
- Most common adverse reactions in 10% or more of patients in clinical trials: nausea, fatigue/asthenia, anemia, vomiting, abdominal pain, dizziness, diarrhea, neutropenia, leukopenia, nasopharyngitis/URI/influenza, respiratory tract infection, arthralgia/myalgia, dysgeusia, headache, dyspepsia, decreased appetite, constipation, stomatitis.

- Most common laboratory abnormalities ($\geq$ 25%): decrease in Hgb, increase in MCV, decrease in lymphocytes, decrease in leukocytes, decrease in ANC, increase in serum creatinine, decrease in platelets.
- Warnings and Precautions:
  - *Myelodysplastic syndrome (MDS)/AML:* May occur and be fatal. Incidence in a one-arm study and in a RCT was < 1.5%. MDS/AML was diagnosed in patients receiving the drug for less than 6 months to more than 2 years. All patients had prior chemotherapy with platinum agents and/or other DNA-damaging agents. Some patients had more than one primary malignancy, or of bone marrow dysplasia. Most cases were fatal. Monitor baseline CBC/differential at baseline before beginning therapy and at least monthly. Do not start olaparib until patients have recovered from hematologic toxicity related to prior chemotherapy ($\leq$ grade 1). If the hematologic toxicity is prolonged, interrupt olaparib and monitor CBC/ANC weekly until recovery. If after 4 weeks, the hematologic toxicity has not improved to grades 0–1, the patient should be evaluated by a hematologist, including bone marrow analysis and cytogenetics. Discontinue the drug if MDS/AML is confirmed.
  - *Pneumonitis* may occur and be fatal. If the patient presents with new or worsening respiratory symptoms (e.g., dyspnea, fever, cough, wheezing) or abnormality is seen on x-ray, interrupt the olaparib therapy and discuss further evaluation with the provider. Discontinue the drug if pneumonitis is confirmed.
  - *Embryo-fetal toxicity:*
    - Teach women of reproductive potential to use effective contraception during therapy and for 6 months after the last drug dose to avoid pregnancy.
    - Teach male patients with female partners of reproductive potential or who are pregnant to use effective contraception during treatment and for 3 months following last dose of olaparib.
- Nursing mothers should discontinue breast-feeding or discontinue the drug.

Potential Toxicities/Side Effects and the Nursing Process

I. POTENTIAL FOR BLEEDING, INFECTION, ANEMIA, AND FATIGUE related to BONE MARROW SUPPRESSION

Defining Characteristics: In clinical trials, 25–32% of patients experienced neutropenia (7–8% grades 3–4), 26–30% thrombocytopenia (3% grades 3–4), 56% lymphopenia, 25–34% anemia, and 57–85% an elevation in mean corpuscular volume. In addition, 26–43% of patients developed nasopharyngitis or URI. Anemia was common (90%), with 15% of cases being grades 3–4. Fatigue/asthenia occurred in 66% of patients and was severe (grades 3–4) in 8%.

Nursing Implications: Evaluate CBC/differential, hemoglobin/hematocrit, MCV, and platelets at baseline and then monthly. Discuss any abnormalities with the physician/NP/PA. The drug should not be started until resolution of myelosuppression from prior therapy has occurred (grades 0–1). Assess for signs and symptoms of infection, bleeding, and fatigue. Teach the patient about signs and symptoms of infection and bleeding, and to report them immediately. Teach the patient self-care measures to minimize the risk of infection and bleeding, including avoidance of OTC aspirin-containing medications. Teach the patient self-assessment of fatigue and to alternate rest and activity as needed. If prolonged myelosuppression occurs, interrupt the drug and monitor CBC/differential weekly until recovery. If recovery (grades 0–1) has not occurred by 4 weeks, refer the patient to a hematologist for evaluation, including bone marrow analysis and cytogenetic study. The drug should be discontinued if MDS/AML is confirmed.

II.   ALTERATION IN NUTRITION, POTENTIAL, related to NAUSEA, VOMITING, OR DIARRHEA

Defining Characteristics: Nausea was common in clinical trials (65–75%), as was vomiting (32–43%), diarrhea (28–31%), dyspepsia (25%), decreased appetite (22–25%), and dysgeusia (21%).

Nursing Implications: Assess the patient's nutritional status at baseline and at each visit. Teach the patient that these side effects may occur, and teach self-management strategies such as use of antidiarrheals, antinausea medications, and dietary modifications and to report any symptoms that do not improve. Discuss prescription medications with the provider if there is a need to manage refractory symptoms. Teach the patient tips to increase appetite (e.g., small, frequent meals, use of spices). Offer the services of a dietitian as appropriate.

III.   ALTERATION IN COMFORT related to ARTHRALGIA/MYALGIA, HEADACHE, OR BACKACHE

Defining Characteristics: In clinical trials, arthralgias and musculoskeletal pain occurred in 21–32% of patients (4% grades 3–4), myalgia in 22–25%, back pain in 25%, and headache in 25%.

Nursing Implications: Assess the patient's baseline level of comfort. Teach the patient that these side effects may occur, and teach self-management strategies. Teach the patient to report symptoms that do not improve. If this occurs, discuss with the physician/NP/PA prescription medication for refractory symptoms.

Drug: osimertinib (Tagrisso)

Class: Kinase inhibitor; EGFR TKI.

Mechanism of Action: Osimertinib binds irreversibly to mutated forms of the EGF receptor (EGFR): those with T790M, L858R, and exon 9 deletion. Osimertinib blocks the EGFR in NSCLC cancer cells with these mutations, so the messages to divide, make new blood vessels, and invade are not sent to the cancer cell nucleus. In the laboratory, osimertinib also inhibited activity of HER2, HER3, and other receptors.

Metabolism: After oral administration, steady state is reached in 15 days of dosing. The median time to C_{max} was 6 hours, and the C_{max} increased 14% after ingesting with a high-fat, high-calorie meal. The mean half-life is 48 hours. The drug is metabolized by oxidation (primarily CYP3A) and dealkylation. There are two metabolites that represent 10% of the active drug. Drug is primarily excreted via feces (68%) with 14% excreted in the urine. There are no data about effect of severe renal impairment or moderate or severe hepatic impairment on drug serum levels.

Indication(s): Treatment of patients with metastatic NSCLC having 1) As first line, epidermal growth factor receptor (EGFR) exon 19 deletions or exon 21 L858R mutations, as detected by an FDA-approved test; 2) EGFR T790M mutations as detected by an FDA approved test, whose disease has progressed on or after EGFR TKI therapy.

Dosage Range:
- Confirm the presence of EGFR exon 19 deletions or exon 21 L858R mutations, or T790M mutation in patient tumor specimen prior to starting osimertinib therapy.
- 80 mg PO once daily, with or without food, until disease progression or unacceptable toxicity.

Dose Modifications:
- ILD/Pneumonitis: permanently discontinue osimertinib.
- Cardiac:
  - QTc interval > 500 msec on at least 2 separate ECGs: Hold osimertinib until QTc interval is < 481 msec or recovery to baseline; if QTc ≥ 481 msec, then resume osimertinib at a 40-mg dose.
  - QTc interval prolongation with signs/symptoms of life-threatening arrhythmia: permanently discontinue osimertinib.
  - Symptomatic CHF: permanently discontinue osimertinib.
- Grade 3 or higher adverse reaction: hold osimertinib for up to 3 weeks; if improvement to grades 0–2 within 3 weeks, resume at 80 mg or 40 mg qd; if no improvement within 3 weeks, permanently discontinue osimertinib.
- If coadministration with a strong CYP3A4 inducer is unavoidable, increase osimertinib dose to 160 mg qd. When the strong CYP3A4 inducer is discontinued, wait 3 weeks, then resume the osimertinib 80-mg qd dose.

Drug Preparation: Available as 80-mg and 40-mg tablets.

Drug Administration:
- Assess results of pregnancy test for female patients of reproductive potential before starting therapy. Teach females of reproductive potential to use effective contraception during and for 6 weeks after final drug dose. Teach male patients with female sexual partners of reproductive potential to use effective contraception during treatment and for 4 months after the final dose.

- Assess CBC/differential, and teach patient to report signs/symptoms of infection or bleeding right away.
- Assess ECHO or GBPS results of LVEF in patients with cardiac risk factors prior to starting therapy, and periodically during therapy. If a patient develops cardiac symptoms while receiving therapy, discuss ECHO or GBPS testing with provider.
- If patient has a history or risk of QTc prolongation, assess ECG findings; assess electrolyte status, especially serum magnesium and potassium, and discuss repletion if results are abnormal with MD/ NP or PA.
- Teach patient to (1) take tablet as prescribed; (2) if a dose is missed, do not make up the dose and take the next dose as scheduled; (3) if difficulty swallowing, disperse tablet in 2 oz (about 60 mL) noncarbonated water only and stir until tablet is completely dispersed; swallow right away then fill the glass with 120–240 mL water and drink that to obtain any residual drug. If administer via NG tube is necessary, dissolve in 15 mL noncarbonated water and then use an additional 15 mL of water to transfer any residues to the syringe. Administer the resulting 30 mL of liquid via NG tube, then flush NG tube with 15 mL water. Do not crush, heat, or ultrasonicate during preparation.

Drug Interactions:
- Strong CYP3A Inhibitors: avoid concurrent administration if possible. If no alternative, monitor patient closely for signs and symptoms of osimertinib toxicity.
- Strong CYP3A Inducers: avoid concomitant administration as osimertinib plasma concentrations may be decreased.
- Drugs sensitive substrates of CYP3A, BCRP, or CYP1A2 with narrow therapeutic indices (e.g., fentanyl, cyclosporine, quinidine, ergot alkaloids, phenytoin, carbamazepine): avoid concomitant administration as osimertinib may increase or decrease serum plasma concentrations of these drugs.

Lab Effects/Interference:
- Hyponatremia, hypermagnesemia.
- Lymphopenia, thrombocytopenia, anemia, neutropenia.

Special Considerations:
- Most common adverse effects occurring in ≥ 25% of patients were diarrhea, rash, dry skin, and nail toxicity.
- Warnings and Precautions:
  - *Interstitial Lung Disease (ILD)/Pneumonitis:* has occurred in 3.9% of patients. Hold drug if ILD/pneumonitis suspected (e.g., patient presents with worsening of respiratory symptoms, such as dyspnea, cough, fever) and evaluate. Osimertinib should be permanently discontinued if ILD/pneumonitis diagnosed.
  - *QTc interval prolongation:* Uncommon. Monitor ECGs and electrolytes in patients who have a history or risk for QTc prolongation (e.g., congenital long QTc syndrome, CHF, electrolyte abnormalities) or who are taking medications that prolong the QTc interval. If QTc prolongation occurs, hold osimertinib, the resume at a reduced dose or permanently discontinue drug. See Dose Modifications.
  - *Cardiomyopathy* (defined as cardiac failure, chronic cardiac failure, CHF, pulmonary edema, or decreased ejection fraction): Has occurred in 2.6% of patients. Decrease in

LVEF > 10% and a drop to < 50% occurred in 3.9% of paitents. Assess LVEF baseline by echocardiogram (ECHO) or multigated acquisition (MUGA) scan in patients with cardiac risk factors prior to starting therapy, and in patients who develop relevant cardiac signs or symptoms during treatment. If patient develops symptomatic CHF, permanently discontinue osimertinib.

- See Dose Modifications for further discussion.
- *Keratitis:* Occurs rarely (0.7% of patients); Make referral to ophthalmologist right away for evaluation of signs/symptoms suggestive of keratitis (eye inflammation, lacrimation, light sensitivity, blurred vision, eye pain, and/or red eye).
- *Embryo-fetal toxicity:* Verify pregnancy status of female patients of reproductive potential prior to starting drug.Teach women of reproductive potential to use effective contraception to prevent pregnancy during treatment with osimertinib and for 6 weeks after last dose. Teach male patients who have partners of reproductive potential to use effective contraception during and for 4 months after last dose of osimertinib. Mothers should not breast-feed while receiving the drug.

Potential Toxicities/Side Effects and the Nursing Process

I. POTENTIAL FOR BLEEDING, INFECTION, AND FATIGUE related to BONE MARROW SUPPRESSION

Defining Characteristics: In studies 1 and 2, lymphopenia occurred in 63% of patients (grades 3–4 in 3.3%), thrombocytopenia in 54% (grades 3–4, 1.2%), anemia in 44%, and neutropenia in 33% (grades 3–4, 3.4%). Pnemonia occurred in 4% of patients and cough in 14%. Fatigue occurred in 14%.

Nursing Implications: Evaluate CBC/differential, hemoglobin/hematocrit, and platelets at baseline and at each visit. Discuss any abnormalities with the physician/NP/PA. Assess for signs and symptoms of infection, bleeding, and fatigue. Teach the patient about the signs and symptoms of infection and bleeding, and to report them immediately. Teach the patient self-care measures to minimize the risk of infection and bleeding, including avoidance of OTC aspirin-containing medications. Teach the patient self-assessment of fatigue and to alternate rest and activity as needed. Discuss dose modification for grade 3 or higher neutropenia.

II. ALTERATION IN CIRCULATION, POTENTIAL, related to LEFT VENTRICULAR DYSFUNCTION, QT PROLONGATION

Defining Characteristics: Rarely, patients may develop a decrease in left ventricular ejection fraction (LVEF) > 10% of baseline, to < 50% (incidence 2.4% in studies 1 and 2). QTc interval prolongation may occur rarely, especially in those with a long interval QTc (congenital) or taking medications that prolong the QTc.

Nursing Implications: Assess results of LVEF baseline and every 3 months (by ECHO or MUGA scan), as well as assess patients for any signs or symptoms of CHF. Identify patients at risk for further decrease in LVEF or development of prolonged QTc. Correct electrolyte abnormalities (e.g., magnesium, potassium) before starting osimertinib, and monitor periodically during therapy. If patient at risk for prolonged QTc (e.g., congenital prolonged QTc or taking medications that prolong QTc interval e.g., fentanyl, patient should have an ECG baseline (measure QTc) and monitor through therapy. If LVEF falls > 10% and is < 50%, hold osimertinib. If QTc > 500 msec, on two separate ECGs, hold osimertinib. See Dose Modifications. If patient develops symptomatic CHF or persistent asymptomatic LV dysfunction that does not resolve in 4 weeks, osimertinib should be permanently discontinued.

III.   ALTERATION IN NUTRITION, LESS THAN BODY REQUIREMENTS, related to DIARRHEA, NAUSEA, DECREASED APPETITE, CONSTIPATION, and STOMATITIS

Defining Characteristics: In study 1 and 2, diarrhea occurred in 42% of patients, 1% grades 3–4; nausea occurred in 17%; decreased appetite in 16%; constipation in 15%; and stomatitis in 12%.

Nursing Implications: Assess nutritional status, bowel-elimination pattern, and appetite, at baseline and at each visit during treatment. Teach patient that these side effects may occur, and strategies to self-manage. Teach patient to report any symptoms that do not resolve with self-care measures. Teach the patient dietary modification if nausea or diarrhea occur (e.g., for diarrhea, BRAT diet: bananas, rice, applesauce, and toast) and to increase oral fluids to prevent dehydration. Consult dietitian to see patient for dietary counseling for decreased appetite if severe. Discuss any abnormalities with physician or NP.

Drug: palbociclib (Ibrance)

Class: Kinase inhibitor; CDK inhibitor.

Mechanism of Action: Palbociclib inhibits CDK 4 and 6, which stops the cell cycle from proceeding from the G_1 phase to the S phase; thus cell proliferation is halted in ER-positive breast cancer cells. When combined with antiestrogens, palbociclib increased growth arrest and inhibition of ER-positive tumor growth to a greater extent than occurred with either drug alone.

Metabolism: After oral administration, the peak plasma concentration (C_{max}) is reached in 6–12 hours; however, oral bioavailability is 46% (after a dose of 125 mg). Steady state is reached within 8 days. C_{max} is increased by administration of the drug with food. Palbociclib binds to human plasma proteins (about 85%), and undergoes hepatic metabolism, primarily by CYP3A and SULT2A1 (sulfotransferase 2A1) pathways. Almost all of a dose (91.6%) is excreted in 15 days, with 74.1% recovered in the feces and 17.5% in the urine, primarily as metabolites.

Indication: For the treatment of hormone receptor (HR)-positive, human epidermal growth factor receptor 2 (HER-2)-negative advanced or metastatic breast cancer together with:
- An aromatase inhibitor as initial endocrine-based therapy in postmenopausal women or in men, OR
- Fulvestrant in patients with disease progression following endocrine therapy.

Dosage/Range:
- With food, in combination with letrozole (2.5 mg PO once daily continuously, or fulvetrant 500 mg administered on days 1, 15, 29 then once monthly.
- Starting dose: Palbociclib 125 mg orally, once daily with food, for 21 days, followed by 7 days off treatment (28-day cycle). Administer the recommended dose of an aromatase inhibitor when given with palbociclib (see the Full Prescribing Information for the aromatase inhibitor). When given with fulvestrant, the recommended dose of fulvestrant is 500 mg administered on days 1, 15, 29, and monthly thereafter (see Full Prescribing Information for fulvestrant).
- Pre/perimenopausal women treated with palbociclib plus fulvestrant should also be treated with luteinizing hormone-releasing hormone (LHRH) agonist according to current clinical practice standards.
- Interrupt or reduce palbociclib dose as needed based on patient safety and tolerability.

Dose Modifications:
- First dose reduction from 125 mg to a dose of 100 mg/day; second dose reduction from 100 mg to a dose of 75 mg/day.
- **Neutropenia**: Grade 3 (ANC $<$ 1,000–500/mm^3):
  - Day 1 of cycle: hold palbociclib, repeat CBC monitoring within 1 week. When recovered to grade $\leq$ 2 (ANC 1,000 –$<$ 1,500/mm^3), start the next cycle at the same dose.
  - Day 15 of first 2 cycles: If grade 3 on day 15, continue palbociclib at current dose to complete cycle and repeat CBC day 21.
  - If grade 4 on day 22, see grade 4 dose modification. Consider dose reduction in cases of prolonged ($>$ 1 week) recovery from grade 3 neutropenia or recurrent grade 3 neutropenia in subsequent cycles.
- Grade 3 neutropenia with fever (ANC $<$ 1,000–500/mm^3 + fever $\geq$ 38.5°C and/or infection): Hold palbociclib until recovery to grade $\leq$ 2. Resume at *next lower dose.*
- Grade 4 neutropenia: Hold palbociclib until recovery to grade $\leq$ 2; resume at *the next lower dose.*
- Nonhematologic toxicity: Grade 1 or 2: No dose adjustment needed. Grade $\geq$ 3 (persisting despite medical therapy): Withhold until symptoms resolve to grade $\leq$ 1; or grade $\leq$ 2 if not considered a safety risk for the patient; resume palbociclib at the *next lower dose.*
- If the drug must be coadministered with a strong CYP3A inhibitor, decrease the palbociclib dose to 75 mg. If the strong inhibitor is discontinued, increase the palbociclib dose to that used prior to adding the strong CYP3A inhibitor once 3–5 half-lives of the inhibitor have passed.
- Dose modification for hepatic impairment: 1) Mild or moderate hepatic impairment (Child-Pugh class A, B); 2) severe impairment (Child-Pugh class C): palbociclib 75 mg once daily for 21 consecutive days followed by 7 days off treatment (28-day cycle).

- Please refer to Ibrance package insert (April 2019). See the individual manufacturer's prescribing information for aromatase inhibitor and fulvestrant.

Drug Preparation: Oral. Available as 125-mg, 100-mg, and 75-mg hard gelatin capsules. Store at room temperature, and keep out of the reach of children and pets.

Drug Administration:
- Monitor CBC/ANC prior to start of palbociclib therapy and at the beginning of each cycle, as well as on day 15 of the first two cycles, and as clinically indicated. If the patient develops a MAXIMUM grade 1 (ANC < LLN–1,500/mm^3) or 2 (ANC 1,000–1,500/mm^3) neutropenia, in the first 6 cycles, monitor CBC/ANC for subsequent cycles every 3 months, prior to the beginning of the cycle and as clinically indicated.
- Teach the patient to take the drug at approximately the same time each day with food. If a dose is missed or vomited, the patient should not take an additional dose but rather resume dosing at the next scheduled time.
- Teach the patient to swallow the capsule whole; not to chew, crush, or open the capsule, and not to take the capsule if it is broken or cracked.

Drug Interactions:
- CYP3A inhibitors: Increase plasma concentrations of palbociclib (e.g., itraconazole increases C_{max} by 34% and AUC by 87%). Avoid concurrent use with strong CYP3A inhibitors; if such use cannot be avoided, decrease the palbociclib dose.
- CYP3A4 inducers: Decrease plasma concentration of palbociclib (e.g., rifampin decreases C_{max} by 70% and by AUC 85%). Avoid concurrent use with strong and moderate inducers.
- CYP3A substrates: For example, concomitant use of midazolam and palbociclib, increased the midazolam C_{max} by 37%, and AUC by 61%. If the substrate is sensitive and has a narrow therapeutic window, consider dose reduction of the substrate.
- Gastric pH-elevating medications: If the patient is fasting, a PPI given concomitantly reduces C_{max} by 80% and AUC by 62%. If the PPI is given to a patient who is eating, there is no significant interaction.

Lab Effects/Interference: Decreased ANC, WBC, lymphocyte count, hemoglobin, and platelet count.

Special Considerations:
- Most common adverse reactions ($\geq$ 10%): neutropenia, leukopenia, infections, fatigue, nausea, anemia, stomatitis, headache, diarrhea, thrombocytopenia, constipation, alopecia, vomiting, rash, and decreased appetite.
- Warnings and Precautions:
  - *Neutropenia:* Monitor CBC/ANC at baseline and prior to each cycle, as well as on day 14 of the first 2 cycles, and as clinically indicated. Neutropenia was the most frequent adverse reaction in studies 1 and 2. Incidence was 80% and 83%, respectively. Incidence of grade 3 or higher was 62% with letrozole, and 66% with fulvestrant. The median time to the first episode of any neutropenia was 15 days and median duration of neutropenia grade $\geq$ 3 was 7 days. Interrupt the dose, reduce the dose, or delay it if the patient develops grade 3 or 4 neutropenia. Monitor CBC/differential prior to

starting palbociclib therapy, at the beginning of each cycle as well as on day 15 of the first 2 cycles, then as clinically indicated. Monitor the patient closely for infection and give medical treatment promptly. Teach the patient to report fever or, or other signs/symptoms of infection immediately.

- *Embryo-fetal toxicity:* Palbociclib can cause fetal harm. Teach women of reproductive potential to use effective contraception to avoid pregnancy during therapy and for at least 3 weeks after the last dose.

Potential Toxicities/Side Effects and the Nursing Process

I. POTENTIAL FOR BLEEDING, INFECTION, AND FATIGUE related to BONE MARROW SUPPRESSION

Defining Characteristics: Neutropenia was the most common adverse effect, and incidence of grade 3 or higher was 62% with letrozole, and 66% with fulvestrant. The median time to the first episode of any neutropenia was 15 days and median duration of neutropenia grade $\geq$ 3 was 7 days. Thirty-five percent developed anemia with letrozole, and 30% with fulvestrant; and 17% and 23% developed thrombocytopenia respectively. Infections occurred in 31% and 47% patients, respectively. Fatigue and asthenia developed in 41% and 8–13% of patients.

Nursing Implications: Evaluate CBC/differential, hemoglobin/hematocrit, and platelets at baseline and prior to each 28-day cycle, and on day 14 of the first 2 cycles. Discuss any abnormalities with the physician/NP/PA. Assess for signs and symptoms of infection, bleeding, and fatigue. Teach the patient about the signs and symptoms of infection and bleeding, how to take a temperature and to report them, including fever, immediately. Teach the patient self-care measures to minimize the risk of infection and bleeding, including avoidance of OTC aspirin-containing medications. Teach the patient self-assessment of fatigue and to alternate rest and activity as needed. Discuss dose modification for grade 3 or higher neutropenia.

II. ALTERATION IN NUTRITION, POTENTIAL, related to NAUSEA, VOMITING, DIARRHEA, OR STOMATITIS

Defining Characteristics: Stomatitis (aphthous stomatitis, cheilitis, glossitis, glossodynia, mouth ulceration, mucosal inflammation) occurred in 25% of patients. Nausea affected 25%, and vomiting 15%. Diarrhea affected 12% and was severe (grade 3) in 4%.

Nursing Implications: Assess the patient's nutritional status at baseline and at each visit. Assess the oral mucosa for intactness and oral health habits. Teach the patient that these side effects may occur and teach self-management strategies such as systematic oral cleansing and oral assessment, use of antidiarrheals and antinausea medications, and dietary modifications, and to report any symptoms that do not improve. Discuss prescription medication with the provider if necessary to manage refractory symptoms. Teach the patient tips to increase appetite (e.g., small, frequent meals, use of spices). Offer the services of a dietitian as appropriate.

Drug: panobinostat capsules (Farydak)

Class: Histone deacetylase (HDAC) inhibitor.

Mechanism of Action: Inhibits HDAC enzyme activity so acetyl groups are not removed from some proteins surrounding DNA. As a result, there is increased acetylation of histone proteins, which relax the DNA helix and permit transcription of genes, such as tumor-suppressor genes, that are otherwise turned off by tight coiling of the DNA strands. The drug causes tumor cells to die (cell-cycle arrest and apoptosis). It is more cytotoxic to tumor cells compared to normal cells.

Metabolism: Panobinostat is 21% bioavailable after oral dosing and reaches its peak concentration about 2 hours after it is taken. The drug is extensively metabolized, primarily through CYP3A, but with minor contributions via the CYP2D6 and CYP2C19 pathways. Its terminal half-life is 37 hours, and metabolites are excreted in the urine and feces. In one study, hepatic impairment increased AUC (mild, by 43%, and moderate, by 105%) in patients receiving panobinostat compared to patients with normal hepatic function.

Indication: For the treatment of patients with multiple myeloma, who have received at least two prior regimens, including bortezomib and an immunomodulatory agent, in combination with bortezomib and dexamethasone. The drug's accelerated approval was based on PFS; continued approval may require verification and description of clinical benefit in confirmatory trials (Novartis, 2016).

Dosage/Range:
- 20 mg orally, once every other day for 3 doses per week (days 1, 3, 5, 8, 10, 12) in weeks 1 and 2 of each 21-day cycle, for 8 cycles.
- Consider continuing treatment for an additional 8 cycles (9–16) if the patient shows clinical benefit, unless unresolved severe or medically significant toxicity occurs.
- Cycles 1–8: Recommended bortezomib dose is 1.3 mg/m^2 on days 1, 4, 8, and 11; dexamethasone dose is 20 mg orally on a full stomach on days 1, 2; 4, 5; 8, 9; and 11, 12 of the 21-day cycle.
- Cycles 9–16: Panobinostat on days 1, 3, 5, 8, 10, 12 of the 21-day cycle; bortezomib on days 1 and 8; and dexamethasone on days 1, 2, and 8, 9 of the 21-day cycle.
- Hepatic impairment: reduce starting dose to 15 mg in patients with mild hepatic impairment, and to 10 mg in patients with moderate impairment; avoid use in patients with severe hepatic impairment. Monitor patients frequently so dose can be further adjusted for toxicity.
- If the patient is taking concomitant strong CYP3A inhibitors (e.g., boceprevir, clarithromycin, conivaptan, indinavir, itraconazole, ketoconazole, lopinavir/ritonavir), reduce the starting dose to 10 mg.

Dose Modifications:
- Dose and/or schedule modification may be needed to manage toxicity. Manage toxicity by treatment interruption and/or dose reductions. If dose reduction is needed, reduce the panobinostat dose in increments of 5 mg. If dosing is less than 10 mg given 3 times/week,

discontinue the drug. Keep the same treatment regimen (3-week treatment cycle) when reducing the dose. See package inserts for bortezomib and dexamethasone.

- *Thrombocytopenia:*
  - **Plt < 50 × 10⁹/L (grade 3):** Maintain panobinostat and bortezomib doses and monitor platelet counts at least weekly.
  - **Plt < 50 × 10⁹/L (grade 3) with bleeding:** Interrupt panobinostat until Platelet count ≥ 50 × 10⁹/L, monitor platelet counts at least weekly, and then restart at a reduced dose. Hold bortezomib until platelet count ≥ 75 × 10⁹/L; if only one dose was omitted prior to correction of these levels, restart bortezomib at the same dose. If 2 or more consecutive doses were omitted, or within the same cycle, bortezomib should be restarted at a reduced dose. See Farydak package insert (Novartis, 2016).
  - Discontinue panobinostat treatment if thrombocytopenia does not improve despite recommended dose adjustments or if repeated platelet transfusions are required.
- Neutropenia:
  - **ANC 0.75–1.0 × 10⁹/L (grade 3):** Maintain panobinostat and bortezomib doses.
  - **ANC 0.5–0.75 × 10⁹/L (grade 3; 2 or more occurrences):** Interrupt panobinostat dose until ANC ≥ 1.0 × 10⁹/L, then restart at the same dose; maintain the bortezomib dose.
  - **ANC < 1.0 × 10⁹/L (grade 3) with febrile neutropenia (any grade):** Interrupt panobinostat until febrile neutropenia resolves, and ANC ≥ 1.0 × 10⁹/L, then restart at a reduced dose. Hold bortezomib until febrile neutropenia resolves and ANC ≥ 1.0 × 10⁹/L; if only one dose was omitted prior to correction of these levels, restart bortezomib at the same dose. If 2 or more consecutive doses were omitted, or within the same cycle, bortezomib should be restarted at a reduced dose. See Farydak package insert (Novartis, 2016).
  - **ANC < 0.5 × 10⁹/L (grade 4):** Interrupt panobinostat until ANC ≥ 1.0 × 10⁹/L, then restart at a reduced dose. Hold bortezomib until febrile neutropenia resolves and ANC ≥ 1.0 × 10⁹/L; if only one dose was omitted prior to correction of these levels, restart bortezomib at the same dose. If 2 or more consecutive doses were omitted, or within the same cycle, bortezomib should be restarted at a reduced dose. See Farydak package insert (Novartis, 2016).
  - Grade 3 or grade 4 neutropenia: Consider dose reduction and/or the use of growth factors (e.g., G-CSF).
  - Discontinue panobinostat if neutropenia does not improve with dose modification or C-GSFs, or in case of severe infection.
- Anemia (Hgb < 8 g/dL): Interrupt panobinostat until Hgb ≥ 10 g/dL, then restart at a reduced dose.
- Diarrhea:
  - **Moderate** (4–6 stools/day, grade 2): Interrupt panobinostat until the diarrhea is resolved, then restart it at the same dose. Consider interrupting bortezomib until resolved, and then restarting it at the same dose.
  - **Severe** (≥ 7 stools/day, requiring IV fluids or hospitalization, grade 3): Interrupt panobinostat until the diarrhea is resolved, then restart it at a reduced dose. Interrupt bortezomib and then restart it at a reduced dose when the diarrhea is resolved.
  - **Life-threatening (grade 4):** Permanently discontinue both panobinostat and bortezomib.

- Start antidiarrheal medicine (e.g., loperamide) at the first sign of abdominal cramping, loose stools, or onset of diarrhea.
- Nausea or vomiting:
  - **Severe nausea (grade 3 or 4):** Interrupt panobinostat until the nausea is resolved, then restart it at a reduced dose.
  - **Severe/life-threatening vomiting (grade 3 or 4):** Interrupt panobinostat until the vomiting is resolved, then restart it at a reduced dose.
  - Consider and administer prophylactic antiemetics if needed.
  - See Farydak package insert for other adverse drug reaction management.

Drug Preparation: Available as 10-mg, 15-mg, and 20-mg capsules.

Drug Administration:
- Assess CBC/ANC before the patient starts treatment; verify baseline platelet count is $\geq$ 100×10^9/L, and ANC $\geq 1.5 \times 10^9$/L. Monitor CBC weekly or more often as clinically indicated.
- Assess ECG prior to the start of therapy and repeat during therapy as clinically indicated. Verify QTc is less than 450 msec prior to starting panobinostat therapy. If the QTc increases to 480 msec or longer, therapy should be interrupted. Correct any electrolyte abnormalities. If QT prolongation does not resolve permanently, the drug should be permanently discontinued. In the clinical trial, ECGs were monitored at baseline, and then before each cycle for the first 8 cycles.
- Assess serum electrolytes, including potassium and magnesium, at baseline, and then monitor them during therapy. Correct abnormal electrolyte levels before treatment. During the clinical trial, monitoring was performed prior the start of each cycle, at day 11 of cycles 1–8, and at the start of each cycle for cycles 9–16.
- Teach the patient about the medication schedule—that is, on which days to take panobinostat and dexamethasone, and when to come into the clinic for bortezomib.
- Teach the patient to take the drug orally on the scheduled day at about the same time, with or without food. The patient should swallow the capsule whole with a cup of water; he or she should not open, crush, or chew the capsule. If the patient misses a dose, it can be taken up to 12 hours after the specified dose time. If vomiting occurs, the patient should *not* repeat the dose, but rather take the next scheduled dose at the planned time.

Drug Interactions:
- Panobinostat is a CYP3A substrate, and it inhibits CYP2D6. It is also a P-glycoprotein (P-gp) transporter system substrate.
- Strong CYP3A4 inhibitors: Increase serum level of panobinostat; avoid concomitant use, or decrease the panobinostat dose. Teach the patient to avoid star fruit, pomegranate juice, and grapefruit or grapefruit juice. Reduce the dose of panobinostat to 10 mg if co-administered with a strong CYP3A inhibitor (e.g., boceprevir, clarithromycin, conivaptan, indinivir, itraconazole, ketoconazole, lopinavir/ritonavir, nefazodone, nelfinavir, posaconazole, ritonavir, saquinavir, telaprevir, telithromycin, voriconazole).
- Strong CYP3A4 inducers: Decrease serum level of panobinostat by as much as 70%; avoid concomitant use.

TREATMENT

- CYP2D6 substrates: Panobinostat may increase the C_{max} and AUC of sensitive substrates by 80% and 60%, respectively (e.g., atomoxetine, desipramine, dextromethorphan, metoprolol, nebivolol, perphenazine, tolterodine, venlafaxine); it may have the same effect on CYP2D6 substrates with a narrow therapeutic window (e.g., thioridazine, pimozide). Avoid coadministration. If panobinostat and a CYP2D6 substrate must be coadministered, monitor the patient closely for toxicity.
- Drugs that prolong the QT interval (e.g., anti-arrhythmic medicines such as amiodarone, disopyramide, procainamide, quinidine, and sotalol; other drugs such as chloroquine, halofantrine, clarithromycin, methadone, moxifloxacin, bepridil, and pimozide): If antiemetic agents that prolong the QT interval are used (e.g., dolasetron, ondansetron, tropisetron), monitor the ECG and QTc frequently.

Lab Effects/Interference:
- Decreased serum phosphate, potassium, and sodium
- Increased serum creatinine
- Thrombocytopenia, lymphopenia, leucopenia, neutropenia, and anemia
- Prolonged QTc interval

Special Considerations:
- Most common adverse effects occurring in 20% or more of patients in clinical trials: diarrhea, fatigue, nausea, vomiting, peripheral edema, decreased appetite, and pyrexia.
- Warnings and Precautions:
  - *Diarrhea:* Severe diarrhea occurred in 25% of patients, while diarrhea of any grade occurred in 68% of patients. Monitor and begin antidiarrheal therapy at the first sign of diarrhea, interrupt the drug, and then reduce the dose or discontinue the drug. See the Dose Modifications section.
  - *Myelosuppression* may be severe, with grades 3–4 thrombocytopenia observed in 67% of patients receiving panobinostat compared to 31% of control patients; severe neutropenia occurred in 34% (compared to 11% of controls). Assess the patient's baseline CBC, and then monitor it weekly during treatment and more frequently in the elderly.
  - *Cardiac toxicities:* Severe and fatal cardiac ischemic events, severe arrhythmias, and ECG changes may occur; arrhythmias may be exacerbated by electrolyte abnormalities.
    - Obtain an ECG baseline and periodically during treatment; assess serum electrolytes at baseline and periodically during treatment. Replete electrolytes promptly. Do not start therapy in patients with a QTc interval > 450 msec or with clinically significant baseline ST-segment T-wave abnormalities.
    - If the QTc interval ≥ 480 msec, the drug should be interrupted and electrolyte abnormalities corrected. If the QTc prolongation does not resolve, discontinue the drug.
    - The drug should not be given to patients who have had a recent MI or have unstable angina.
  - *Hemorrhage* can occur (GI, pulmonary) with thrombocytopenia; monitor the platelet count and give transfusions as needed.

- *Infections:* Localized and systemic infections (e.g., pneumonia; bacterial, invasive fungal, and viral infections) may occur. Severe infections occurred in 31% of patients. Drug should not be administered to patients with active infections. Monitor for signs/symptoms of infection during treatment, and if confirmed, interrupt treatment and institute antimicrobial therapy promptly.
- *Hepatotoxicity:* Monitor hepatic enzymes and total bilirubin at baseline and during treatment; adjust the drug dose as needed if LFTs become abnormal and follow closely until LFT values normalize or return to baseline.
- *Embryo-fetal toxicity:* The drug can cause fetal harm: Teach females of reproductive potential to use effective contraception to avoid pregnancy during and for at least 3 month after last drug dose. Teach sexually active men to use condoms while on treatment and for 6 months after the last drug dose.

Potential Toxicities/Side Effects and the Nursing Process

I.   ALTERATION IN PATTERN related to DIARRHEA

Defining Characteristics: Diarrhea occurred in 68% of patients (compared to 48% in the control arm), and was severe in 25%. Diarrhea can occur at any time during treatment.

Nursing Implications: Assess the patient's bowel-elimination pattern at baseline and then regularly during therapy. Review the patient's medication profile and teach the patient not to take stool softeners or laxative medications while receiving panobinostat. Assess and monitor patient hydration and electrolyte status (e.g., serum potassium, magnesium, phosphate) at baseline and then at least weekly during therapy. Discuss measures to correct dehydration and electrolyte disturbances with the provider, and implement steps to rehydrate the patient and correct electrolyte abnormalities as soon as possible. Ensure the patient has antidiarrheal medication (e.g., loperamide) on hand prior to starting panobinostat capsules and understands the self-administration directions, including use at the first sign of abdominal cramping, loose stools, or onset of diarrhea. Teach the patient to increase oral fluids to 1 glass every hour while awake as tolerated, and to make dietary modifications to lessen diarrhea. Teach the patient to stop the drug and call the nurse or provider at the onset of moderate diarrhea (4–6 stools/day), as the drug should be interrupted in such a case; the dose should be reduced if severe diarrhea occurs.

II.   POTENTIAL FOR BLEEDING, INFECTION, AND FATIGUE related to THROMBOCYTOPENIA, NEUTROPENIA, AND ANEMIA

Defining Characteristics: Bone marrow suppression may be severe. Thrombocytopenia occurs in 97% of patients, and neutropenia in 75%. In clinical trial of patients with relapsed multiple myeloma, grades 3–4 thrombocytopenia occurred in 67% of patients compared to 31% in the control group and required dose interruption or reduction in 31% of patients. In addition, nearly one-third (33%) required platelet transfusion. Severe thrombocytopenia can lead to life-threatening hemorrhage. Grades 3–4 hemorrhage occurred in 4% of patients receiving panobinostat.

Neutropenia was severe in 34% of patients compared to 11% of the control group, and 13% of patients had growth factor support. Severe infections occurred in 31% of patients; in some cases, they resulted in death.

Fatigue was common, affecting 60% of patients and was severe in 25% of patients. Anemia occurred in 62% of patients, and was grades 3–4 in severity in 18%.

Patients with mild and moderate hepatic impairment should have their doses reduced, and the drug should not be used in patients with severe impairment.

Nursing Implications: Assess the patient's baseline WBC, ANC, platelet, and Hgb/Hct; monitor these values at least weekly during treatment, and more frequently if needed in patients older than age 65. Discuss dose modifications based on the CBC/ANC results with the provider. Ensure that the patient does not have an active infection when beginning panobinostat treatment. Assess the patient for signs and symptoms of bleeding and/or infection. If the patient develops an infection, discuss urgent treatment with the provider, to consist of anti-infectives, as well as interruption or discontinuance of panobinostat. Teach the patient to report bleeding, increased bruising, dizziness or weakness, sweats or chills, flulike symptoms, shortness of breath, blood in sputum, increased severe fatigue, and development of any sores or areas of inflammation on the skin.

Assess the patient's activity level and fatigue at baseline and monitor them during therapy. Teach the patient to report increasing fatigue and review strategies to reduce fatigue, such as alternating rest and activity periods and engaging in gentle exercises. Assess the patient's sleep quality and rest while taking dexamethasone, as this agent can cause insomnia.

III.   ALTERATION IN OXYGENATION, REDUCED, related to CARDIAC ISCHEMIC EVENTS, ARRHYTHMIAS, AND ECG CHANGES

Defining Characteristics: Arrhythmias occurred in 12% of patients compared to 5% in the control arm of the clinical study, while cardiac ischemic events occurred in 4% of patients. This drug is not recommended in patients with a history of a recent MI or unstable angina. Abnormalities noted on ECG included ST-segment depression, T-wave abnormalities, and prolonged QT interval. Electrolyte abnormalities may exacerbate cardiac arrhythmias. Electrolyte disturbances seen in the clinical trial included hypokalemia (52%), hypophosphatemia (63%), hyponatremia (49%), and hypocalcemia (67%).

Nursing Interventions: Assess the patient's ECG and serum electrolytes at baseline before therapy begins, and then periodically during treatment. QTc must be less than 450 msec prior to the patient beginning the drug, and the drug should be interrupted if the QTc increases to 480 msec or longer during treatment. If QTc prolongation does not resolve with correction of electrolytes, permanently discontinue panobinostat. The drug also should not be given if the ECG shows significant baseline ST-segment or T-wave abnormalities. Discuss prompt repletion of electrolytes once an abnormality is detected. In the clinical trial, ECGs were performed at baseline and prior to the start of each cycle for the first 8 cycles. Serum electrolytes were assessed at baseline and prior to the start of each cycle, at day 11 of cycles 1–8, and at the start of each of cycles 9–16.

Drug: pazopanib (Votrient)

Class: Kinase inhibitor (multi-TKI).

Mechanism of Action: Drug is a multi-TKI of vascular endothelial growth factor receptor (VEGFR-1, VEGFR-2, VEGFR-3), PDGFR (α, β), fibroblast growth factor receptor (FGFR)-1 and -3, cytokine receptor (Kit), interleukin-2 receptor inducible T-cell kinase (Itk), leukocyte-specific protein tyrosine kinase (Lck), and transmembrane glycoprotein RTK (c-Fms).

Metabolism: After oral administration, pazopanib is well absorbed with peak concentrations reached 2–4 hours after the dose. If tablet is crushed, the area under the curve (AUC) is increased by 46% with increased bioavailability and rate of absorption. Drug should not be crushed. Drug systemic exposure is increased when pazopanib is taken with food, so should be dosed at least 1 hour before or 2 hours after a meal. Drug is highly bound to plasma proteins. Pazopanib is probably a substrate for P-glycoprotein (Pgp). It is primarily metabolized by the liver microenzyme CYP3A4, with a minor contribution by CYP1A2 and CYP2C8. Drug has a half-life of 30.9 hours after drug administration, and it is eliminated primarily via feces and to a lesser degree the kidney ($< 4\%$). Drug clearance from the body is reduced 50% if the patient has moderate hepatic impairment, so a maximum drug dose should be 200 mg PO once daily in these patients.

Indication:
- Treatment of patients with
  - Advanced renal cell carcinoma (RCC).
  - Advanced soft-tissue sarcoma (STS) who have received prior chemotherapy.
  - The efficacy of the drug in the treatment of patients with adipocytic STS or GISTs has not been demonstrated.
  - Safety and effectiveness in pediatric patients has not been established, and the drug is not indicated for use in pediatric patients.

Dosage/Range:
- 800 mg PO once daily without food (at least 1 hour prior to or 2 hours after a meal). Do not exceed the 800-mg dose.
- Baseline moderate hepatic impairment: 200 mg orally once daily without food (as above).
- Do not administer to patients with preexisting severe hepatic impairment (total bilirubin $> 3 \times$ ULN with any level of ALT).

Dose Modifications:
- RCC: initial dose reduction should be to 400 mg, and additional dose decrease or increase should be in 200-mg increments, based on individual tolerability.
- In STS, a decrease or increase should be in 200-mg increments, based on individual tolerability.
- Hepatic impairment:
  - Mild impairment: no dose adjustment.

- Moderate hepatic impairment: consider alternatives to pazopanib; if unavailable, reduce dose to 200 mg PO once daily.
- Drug should not be used in patients with severe hepatic impairment (total bilirubin > 3 × ULN and any level of ALT).
- Patients with isolated ALT elevations between 3 × ULN and 8 × ULN may be continued on pazopanib with weekly monitoring of LFTs until ALT returns to grade 1 or baseline.
- Patients with isolated ALT elevations of > 8 × ULN should have dose interrupted until ALT returns to grade 1 or baseline. If the potential benefit for reinitiating treatment outweighs the risk for hepatotoxicity, then reintroduce drug at a reduced dose of no more than 400 mg once daily, and assess LFTs weekly for 8 weeks. Following reintroduction of pazopanib, if ALT elevations > 3 × ULN recur, then pazopanib should be permanently discontinued.
- If ALT elevations > 3 × ULN occur concurrently with bilirubin elevations > 2 × ULN, pazopanib should be permanently discontinued. Patients should be monitored until resolution. Drug is a UGT1A1 inhibitor: mild, indirect (unconjugated) hyperbilirubinemia may occur in patients with Gilbert's syndrome. Patients with only a mild indirect hyperbilirubinemia, known as Gilbert's syndrome, and elevation in ALT > 3 × ULN should be managed as outlined for isolated ALT elevations.
- Patient taking concomitant strong *CYP3A4 inhibitor*: reduce dose of pazopanib to 400 mg PO once daily; if toxicity develops, further reduce dose of pazopanib if adverse effects occur.
- Patients taking strong *CYP3A4 inducers*: do not use together; if must use chronic CYP3A4 inducer (e.g., rifampin), pazopanib should not be used in these patients.
- Refractory HTN: if despite antihypertensive therapy and dose reduction, HTN is severe and persistent, discontinue pazopanib.

Drug Preparation:
- Pazopanib is available as 200-mg tablets. The drug should be stored at room temperature (59–86°F; 15–30°C) and kept out of reach of children or pets.

Drug Administration:
- Administer full dose orally on an empty stomach (at least 1 hour prior to or 2 hours after a meal). Teach patient that drug should NOT be crushed or chewed, as this increases the bioavailability and systemic exposure (and toxicity). If a dose is missed, it should not be taken if it is less than 12 hours until the next dose.
- Teach patient to avoid grapefruit and grapefruit juice.
- Interrupt drug 7 days prior to scheduled surgery.
- Assess LFTs baseline before starting pazopanib and at weeks 3, 5, 7, and 9; thereafter at months 3 and 4, then regularly as clinically indicated.

Drug Interactions:
- CYP3A4 inhibitors increase pazopanib serum level and risk for toxicity.
  - Avoid concurrent administration with strong CYP3A4 inhibitors (e.g., ketoconazole, ritonavir, clarithromycin, grapefruit juice).
  - If must coadminister, reduce dose of pazopanib.

- CYP3A4 inducers decrease pazopanib serum level and effectiveness;
  - Avoid concurrent administration of strong inducers such as rifampin.
  - If this is not avoidable and chronic dosing of a strong inducer is necessary, do not administer pazopanib.
- Other drugs with a narrow therapeutic window that are metabolized by CYP3A4, CYP2D6, or CYP2C8: do not coadminister, as this will inhibit the other drug's metabolism and increase risk of adverse events.
- Simvastatin: concurrent administration increases risk of ALT elevations. Use dose modification if ALT is elevated or an alternative to pazopanib.
- Chemotherapy: increased toxicity. Drug is not approved for combination therapy. However, clinical trials combining pazopanib with pemetrexed and lapatinib resulted in fatal toxicities (pulmonary hemorrhage, GI hemorrhage, sudden death). Do not combine drug with chemotherapy.
- Drugs that increase the gastric pH: Avoid concurrent administration. Consider short-acting antacids instead of PPIs or H2 receptor antagonists. Separate antacid and pazopanib dosing by several hours.

Lab Effects/Interference:
- Increased serum transaminase levels, bilirubin, alkaline phosphatase: assess liver chemistries baseline and follow closely during therapy. Interrupt as needed with dose reduction for moderate hepatic toxicity or drug discontinuance for severe hepatotoxicity.
- Hypothyroidism with increased TSH in 27% of patients; monitor thyroid function tests baseline and prior to therapy.
- Proteinuria (9%): assess baseline and during therapy.
- Serum magnesium decreased: 26%, assess and replete. Increased potassium (16%); decreased albumin (34%) and sodium (31%).
- Lipase increased (27% in some studies).
- Glucose: elevated in 41%, decreased in 17%.
- Leukopenia (44%), lymphocytopenia (43%), thrombocytopenia (36%), neutropenia (33%).
- EKG: QT prolongation ($\geq$ 500 msec); assess baseline EKG and repeat during therapy as needed; correct any serum magnesium and potassium abnormalities.

Special Considerations:
- Warnings and Precautions:
  - *Hepatic toxicity and impairment:* Severe and fatal hepatotoxicity has been observed; monitor hepatic function and interrupt, reduce, or discontinue drug as recommended.
    - Transaminase elevations occur early in treatment course (92.5% occurred in first 18 weeks).
    - Assess liver chemistry baseline prior to starting treatment, then at weeks 3, 5, 7, and 9; then at months 3 and 4, and as clinically indicated.
    - If the patient has isolated ALT elevations between 3 $\times$ ULN and 8 $\times$ ULN, continue therapy with weekly monitoring of liver function until ALT returns to grade 1 or baseline. Concomitant use of pazopanib and simvastatin increases the risk of ALT elevations and should be used cautiously if at all, with very close monitoring.

- Interrupt therapy if the ALT is $> 8 \times$ ULN until the ALT returns to grade 1 or baseline; if the benefit outweighs the risk of resuming therapy, reintroduce the dose at 400 mg PO once daily and assess liver function tests at least weekly for 8 weeks. If the ALT becomes elevated $> 3 \times$ ULN after pazopanib is reintroduced, permanently discontinue pazopanib.
- If the ALT elevation $> 3 \times$ ULN occurs at the same time as the bilirubin is elevated $> 2 \times$ ULN, pazopanib should be permanently discontinued. Continue to monitor patient until resolution.
- Pazopanib is a UGT1A1 inhibitor; mild, indirect (unconjugated) hyperbilirubinemia may occur if the patient has Gilbert's syndrome. Patients with only a mild indirect hyperbilirubinemia, known Gilbert's syndrome, and elevations in ALT $> 3 \times$ ULN should be managed as isolated ALT elevation.
- *Prolongation of QT interval (> 500 msec)* occurs rarely (2%) with torsades de pointes (atypical ventricular tachycardia that can change to ventricular fibrillation and sudden death) occurring $< 1\%$.
  - Use pazopanib cautiously in patients with a history of QT prolongation, in patients taking antiarrythmic drugs or other medications that can prolong the QT interval such as methadone, and those with relevant preexisting cardiac disease.
  - Assess ECG baseline and correct serum abnormalities of magnesium and potassium prior to administering pazopanib. Monitor QTc intervals (ECG) and electrolytes (magnesium, calcium, potassium) periodically during therapy. Electrolytes should be maintained within normal limits (WNL) during pazopanib therapy.
- *Cardiac dysfunction:* Cardiac events have occurred rarely (0.6%), such as decreased LVEF and CHF, and is likely exacerbated by uncontrolled hypertension.
  - BP should be monitored and managed promptly using antihypertensive therapy and dose modification (interruption and reinitiation at a reduced dose based on clinical judgment).
  - Monitor patients carefully for clinical signs or symptoms of CHF. Baseline and periodic evaluation of LVEF is recommended in patients at risk for cardiac dysfunction, including those who have received previous anthracycline exposure.
  - In clinical trials, HTN may have exacerbated cardiac dysfunction. BP should be monitored and managed promptly using combination antihypertensive agents and dose modification (interruption and reinitiation at a reduced dose based on clinical judgment.
- As with other VEGFR inhibitors, there are class effects:
  - *Hemorrhage:* Hemorrhagic events may occur (all grades 13%, RCC-22%, STS and death in 0.9%, RCC). Most common hemorrhagic events in RCC were hematuria, epistaxis, hemoptysis, and rectal hemorrhage; and in STS, were epistaxis, mouth hemorrhage, and anal hemorrhage. Do not administer the drug to patients with a history of hemoptysis, cerebral hemorrhage, or clinically significant GI hemorrhage in the prior 6 months, as the drug has not been studied in this population.
  - *Arterial thrombotic events:* MI, angina, ischemic stroke, and transient ischemic attack have occurred. Use caution in patients who are at risk for these events, and do not use the drug in patients who have had an event within the previous 6 months, as the drug has not been studied in this population.

- *Venous thrombotic events:* Venous thrombosis, fatal pulmonary embolus (PE) have occurred. Monitor patients for signs and symptoms of VTE and PE.
- *Reversible posterior leukoencephalopathy syndrome (RPLS)* has been reported and may be fatal. Monitor for signs/symptoms including headache, seizure, lethargy, confusion, blindness, and other visual and neurological disturbances. Patients may also have mild-to-moderate hypertension. MRI should be done to rule out RPLS. If the patient develops RPLS, the drug should be discontinued.
- *GI perforation and fistula formation* occur rarely (0.9%). Fatal fistula occurred in two patients (0.3%). Assess and monitor patients for signs and symptoms of GI perforation or fistula. Do not administer the drug in patients with a history of hemoptysis, cerebral or clinically significant GI hemorrhage in the past 6 months.
- *Hypertension (SBP > 150 mm Hg, or DBP > 100 mm Hg):* BP should be well controlled prior to the patient starting pazopanib. Incidence is 40%, with grade 3 in 4–7% of patients. HTN occurs early in treatment (40% by day 9 and 90% within the first 18 weeks). Monitor BP baseline and within one week of starting treatment, then frequently during therapy. If HTN is persistent despite antihypertensive therapy, dose-reduce pazopanib. If despite antihypertensive therapy AND dose reduction, HTN is severe and persistent, discontinue pazopanib. If hypertensive crisis develops, discontinue pazopanib.
- *Delayed wound healing:* Stop pazopanib therapy at least 7 days prior to scheduled surgery and resume after the surgical wound has fully healed. Discontinue drug if wound dehiscence develops.
- *Proteinuria:* Occurs in 9% of patients (all), with < 1% grades 3 and 4. Assess baseline urinalysis and monitor during treatment for proteinuria. If indicated, follow-up with a 24-hour urine protein. Interrupt pazopanib therapy and dose-reduce for 24-hour urine protein ≥ 3 grams/24 hr; discontinue for repeat episodes despite dose reductions.
- *Hypothyroidism:* has been reported in 7% of patients. Assess baseline thyroid function tests and monitor as needed. Diagnosis made on simultaneous rise of TSH and decline of T4.
- *Thrombotic microangiopathy (TMA),* including thrombocytopenic purpura (TTP), and hemolytic uremic syndrome (HUS) have been reported when pazopanib is used as monotherapy, in combination with bevacizumab, and in combination with topotecan; drug is not indicated for these combinations. Monitor for signs/symptoms of TMA and permanently discontinue pazopanib if patient develops TMA.
- *Interstitial lung disease (ILD)/pneumonitis* has occurred and can be fatal. Incidence of ILD/pneumonitis was 0.1%. Monitor patients for pulmonary symptoms. Pazopanib should be discontinued in patients developing ILD or pneumonitis.
- Drug should not be given concomitantly with chemotherapy (e.g., pemetrexed) or other targeted therapy (e.g., lapatinib), as there is increased toxicity and mortality.
- *Serious infections:* Have occurred with or without neutropenia. Monitor patient for signs/symptoms of infection and teach patient to report signs and symptoms. Consider drug interruption or discontinuance for serious infections.
- *Embryo-fetal toxicitiy:* In animal studies, drug is teratogenic, embryotoxic, fetotoxic, and abortifacient. Women of childbearing potential should be counseled to use effective birth control measures to avoid becoming pregnant during treatment and for at

least 2 weeks after the last drug dose. If the drug is used during pregnancy, or if the patient becomes pregnant while using the drug, the patient should be apprised of the potential hazard to the fetus. Mothers who are nursing should make a decision either to stop nursing or to discontinue pazopanib, taking into account the importance of the drug to the mother's health.

- *Increased toxicity with other cancer therapy:* Pazopanib is not indicated in combination with other agents. Clinical trials of pemetrexed and lapatinib were terminated early because of increased toxicity and mortality.
- *Increased toxicity in developing organs:* Pazopanib is not indicated for treatment of pediatric patients as it may have severe effects on organ growth and maturation (early postnatal development).

- Most common side effects (incidence $\geq$ 20%): (1) in patients with advanced RCC: diarrhea, HTN, hair-color changes (depigmentation), nausea, anorexia, and vomiting; (2) advanced STS: fatigue, diarrhea, nausea, decreased weight, HTN, decreased appetite, hair-color changes (depigmentation), vomiting, tumor pain, dysgeusia, headache, musculoskeletal pain, myalgia, GI pain, and dyspnea.

Potential Toxicities/Side Effects and the Nursing Process

I. POTENTIAL ALTERATION IN CIRCULATION related to HYPERTENSION, CARDIAC ISCHEMIA, OR MYOCARDIAL INFARCTION

Defining Characteristics: Hypertension (SBP $\geq$ 150, DBP $\geq$ 100 mm Hg) occurred in 47% of patients studied and occurred early in the course of treatment (40% by day 9, and 90% occurred during the first 18 weeks). In general, it is easily controlled with antihypertensive drugs. Grade 3 HTN was reported in 4–7% of patients. Arterial embolic events occurred in 3% of patients and were severe in 2.3% of patients.

Nursing Implications: Assess baseline blood pressure, and again after starting the drug, within 1 week; and frequently thereafter to ensure BP is controlled. If the BP is slightly elevated, assess weekly and discuss antihypertensive therapy with physician or NP. HTN should be well controlled prior to initiating pazopanib. Increased BP should be promptly treated with standard antihypertensive agents, and dose reduction or interruption of pazopanib. Pazopanib should be discontinued if hypertensive crisis occurs, or if HTN is severe despite antihypertensive therapy and dose reduction. If a patient develops cardiac ischemia and/or infarction while receiving the drug, discuss drug discontinuance with the physician. The drug should not be used in patients with a history of cardiac ischemia (angina), ischemic stroke, or TIA. If the patient is at risk for these events, monitor the patient closely during therapy.

II. ALTERATION IN NUTRITION, LESS THAN BODY REQUIREMENTS, related to DIARRHEA, NAUSEA, ANOREXIA, VOMITING, CONSTIPATION

Defining Characteristics: Diarrhea occurs in 52% of patients, nausea 26%, vomiting 21%, anorexia 22%, and dysgeusia 8%. Weight loss occurred in 9% of patients. Elevation of liver function test AST occurs in 53% of patients, while elevation in BR occurred in

36%. Hepatotoxicity may be severe and is potentially fatal. Glucose is increased in 41%, phosphorus decreased in 34%, sodium decreased in 31%, magnesium decreased in 26%, and glucose decreased in 17%.

Nursing Implications: Assess nutrition status, weight, bowel-elimination status, serum chemistries including liver function tests baseline and periodically during treatment. AST and BR must be assessed at least once every 4 weeks for the first 4 months of treatment or as clinically indicated. Continue assessments periodically after this time during therapy. Teach patient to report any changes that suggest liver toxicity right away: yellowing of skin or whites of eyes, dark urine, tiredness, nausea or vomiting, loss of appetite, pain on the right side of abdomen, easy bruisability. Teach patient self-care strategies to manage diarrhea, such as about dietary modifications (BRAT diet: bananas, rice, applesauce, and toast) and to avoid raw fruits, vegetables, whole grain breads and cereals, and seeds. Teach about soluble fiber, which absorbs fluid: applesauce, bananas, canned fruit, orange sections, boiled potatoes, white rice, products made with white flour, oatmeal, cream of rice, cream of wheat, and farina. Teach to increase oral fluids to 8–10 glasses of nonalcoholic fluids a day to prevent dehydration. Teach to increase dose-dense calories and fluid in the diet and strategies to increase appetite. Teach patient how to manage nausea, vomiting, and diarrhea by self-administration of OTC medications or prescribed medications, dietary modifications, and increased hydration. Involve nutritionist as needed to minimize symptoms. Teach patient to report symptoms that do not improve or that persist despite interventions. Teach patient signs of hyperglycemia and to report increased thirst, increased voiding, and increased hunger so that blood sugar can be evaluated.

III.   ALTERATION IN CIRCULATION related to HEMORRHAGE, POTENTIAL

Defining Characteristics: Hemorrhage occurred in 16% of patients.

Nursing Implications: Teach patient to report any episodes of bleeding right away, such as hemoptysis. Drug is not indicated for patients with a history of hemoptysis, cerebral hemorrhage, or clinically significant GI hemorrhage within the prior 6 months. If bleeding occurs, have patient evaluated by the physician or nurse practitioner.

IV.   ALTERATION IN BODY IMAGE, POTENTIAL, related to HAIR-COLOR CHANGES, HFS, SKIN DEPIGMENTATION, ALOPECIA

Defining Characteristics: Hair-color changes occur in 38% of patients, alopecia in 8%, palmar-plantar erythrodysesthesia (HFS, acral erythema) in 6%, rash in 8%, and skin depigmentation in 3% of patients.

Nursing Implications: Assess baseline skin integrity, including soles of feet and palms of hands, hair color and intactness, and teach patient that these symptoms may occur. If the patient develops calluses on the feet, suggest applying topical exfoliating agents such as Kerasal (OTC) or Keralac (prescription) on the calluses ONLY. Teach patient to self-assess all skin areas and to report rash, as well as redness, swelling, and/or pain anywhere, particularly the soles of feet and the palms of hands. Teach patient to avoid activities that increase blood flow in the hands and feet, such as hot showers and baths, and to take tepid showers to reduce likelihood and severity of HFS. Teach patient to avoid constrictive clothing and repetitive movements that can irritate the opposing skin. Teach patient to use skin emollients to prevent skin from drying and cracking. Discuss dose modification with physician or NP if patient has pain or desquamation. Assess effect of hair-color changes or hair loss. Encourage patient to verbalize feelings and provide emotional support. If needed, involve social worker in supportive counseling. Encourage patient to use scarves or hats as appropriate and to attend supportive educational sessions such as Look Good . . . Feel Better (ACS).

V.   POTENTIAL FOR INFECTION AND BLEEDING related to NEUTROPENIA AND THROMBOCYTOPENIA

Defining Characteristics: Neutropenia occurred in 34% and thrombocytopenia in 32% of patients in clinical trials.

Nursing Implications: Assess baseline blood counts and platelets. Teach patient to report fever and signs/symptoms of infection or bleeding right away. Assess medication profile and OTC medications taken. Teach patient to avoid OTC medications containing NSAIDs or aspirin. Teach patient to talk to nurse or physician before beginning any OTC medications.

Drug: ponatinib (Iclusig)

Class: Kinase inhibitor (multiple).

Mechanism of Action: Drug inhibits tyrosine kinase activity of ABL, BCR-ABL, as well as mutant forms; also inhibits VEGFR, PDGFR, FGFR, KIT, RET, TIE2, and FLT3 kinases.

Metabolism: Peak concentrations are achieved within 6 hours after oral dosing, and they are not influenced by food intake. Aqueous solubility of ponatinib is pH dependent, with lower solubility in higher pH environments. Drug is highly protein-bound ($> 99\%$) to plasma proteins. Drug is metabolized by CYP3A4 and to a lesser degree CYP2C8, CYP2D6, and CYP3A5, as well as by esterases and/or amidases. Mean terminal half-life is about 24 hours, and primary excretion is via the feces (87%).

Indication: The treatment of adult patients with:
- CML in chronic phase (CP), accelerated phase (AP), or blast phase (BP) or blast phase whose disease for whom no other TKI therapy is indicated.
- T315I-positive CML (chronic phase, accelerated phase, or blast phase) or T315I-positive Ph+ ALL.
- Ponatinib is not indicated and is not recommended for the treatment of patients with newly diagnosed chronic phase CML.

Dosage/Range:
- Optimal dose has not been established.
- Recommended initial dose: 45 mg orally once daily with or without food. Consider reduced dose for patients with chronic phase (CP) CML and accelerated phase (AP) CML who have achieved a major cytogenetic response. Continue treatment until disease progression or unacceptable toxicity.
- Dose in patients with hepatic impairment is 30 mg PO daily.
- If patient does not have a response by 3 months consider discontinuing the drug.
- See website for REMS program, with safety updates for indications, safety, and dosing considerations.

Dose Modifications:
- **Myelosuppression:** ANC $< 1.0 \times 10^9$/L or thrombocytopenia (platelets $< 50 \times 10^9$/L that are unrelated to leukemia).
- First occurrence: interrupt ponatinib and resume initial dose of 45 mg daily after recovery of ANC $\geq 1,500$ cells/mm^3 and platelets $\geq 75,000$ cells/mm^3.
- Second occurrence: interrupt ponatinib and resume at 30 mg daily after recovery of ANC $\geq 1,500$ cells/mm^3 and platelets $\geq 75,000$ cells/mm^3.
- Third occurrence: interrupt ponatinib and resume at 15 mg daily after recovery of ANC $\geq 1,500$ cells/mm^3 and platelets $\geq 75,000$ cells/mm^3.

Nonhematologic adverse reactions:
- Modify the dose or interrupt therapy.
- Do not restart ponatinib in patients with arterial or venous occlusive reactions unless patient benefit exceeds risk of recurrent arterial or venous occlusions, and no other treatment options exist.
- For adverse events other than ischemia, do not restart ponatinib until the serious event has resolved, or the potential benefit of resuming therapy is judged to outweigh the risk.

Hepatotoxicity:
- Elevated liver transaminases $> 3 \times$ ULN (grade 2 or higher): *if occurs at 45-mg dose:* interrupt dose, monitor LFTs, resume at 30-mg dose after recovery to $< 3 \times$ ULN ($\leq$ grade 1); *if occurs at 30-mg dose:* interrupt drug and resume at 15 mg after recovery to $\leq$ grade 1; *if occurs at 15-mg dose,* discontinue ponatinib.
- Elevation of AST or ALT $\geq 3 \times$ ULN concurrent with elevation in bilirubin $> 2 \times$ ULN and alkaline phosphatase $< 2 \times$ ULN: discontinue ponatinib.

Pancreatitis and elevated lipase:
- Asymptomatic grade 1 or 2 elevation of serum lipase: consider interruption or dose reduction of ponatinib.
- Asymptomatic grade 3 or 4 elevation of lipase ($> 2 \times$ ULN) or asymptomatic radiologic pancreatitis (grade 2 pancreatitis): *if occurs at 45-mg dose:* interrupt dose and resume at 30 mg after recovery to $\leq$ grade 1 ($< 1.5 \times$ ULN); *if occurs at 30 mg dose:* interrupt drug and resume at 15 mg after recovery to $\leq$ grade 1; *if occurs at 15-mg dose,* discontinue ponatinib.
- Symptomatic grade 3 pancreatitis: *if occurs at 45-mg dose*, interrupt drug, and resume at 30 mg after complete resolution of symptoms and recovery of lipase elevations to

≤ grade 1; *if occurs at 30-mg dose*, interrupt drug and resume at 15-mg dose after complete resolution and after recovery of lipase elevation to ≤ grade 1; *if occurs at 15-mg dose,* discontinue ponatinib.
- Grade 4 pancreatitis: discontinue ponatinib.

Use with strong CYP3A4 inhibitors: reduce dose to 30 mg orally, once a day.
Hepatic Impairment: (Child-Pugh A,B,C) Recommended starting dose is 30 mg once daily.

Drug Preparation:
- Available in 15-mg, 30-mg, and 45-mg tablets.

Drug Administration:
- Assess lab tests baseline and:
  - CBC/differential every 2 weeks for 3 months, then monthly and as clinically indicated.
  - Serum lipase baseline and monthly during therapy.
  - LFTs at least monthly; more frequently if patient has history of pancreatitis or alcohol abuse.
- Monitor patient for fluid retention; discuss drug interruption, reduction, or discontinuance with physician if fluid retention found.
- Monitor patient's BP, and discuss management of HTN with physician.
- Teach patient to take ponatinib with or without food, and to swallow the tablet whole. Teach patients not to crush or dissolve tablets and not to take two doses at the same time to make up for a missed dose.
- Teach patient that ponatinib contains 121 mg of lactose monohydrate in a 45-mg daily dose.
- Assess risk for tumor lysis syndrome (TLS) and ensure adequate hydration, correction of uric-acid levels prior to initial dose; highest risk in patients with advanced disease and high-tumor burden (e.g., CML-AP, CML-BP, Ph+ ALL).
- Temporarily interrupt therapy at least one week prior to major surgery, as drug may interfere with wound healing; resume when wound has healed (based on clinical judgment).
- See patient teaching under Special Considerations.

Drug Interactions:
- Drug is a substrate of CYP3A4/5 and to a lesser extent CYP2C8 and CYP2D6. Drug also inhibits the P-glycoprotein (P-gp), ATP-binding G2 (ABCG2, also known as BCRP), and bile salt export pump (BSEP) transporter systems.
- Strong CYP3A4 inhibitors (e.g., ketoconazole): increased ponatinib serum concentration with increased risk of drug toxicity; avoid concomitant administration; if must give together, reduce ponatinib drug dose.
- Strong CYP3A4 inducers (e.g., rifampin): decreased ponatinib serum concentration, with decreased drug effect; avoid concomitant administration unless potential benefit outweighs risk of possible ponatinib underexposure, and monitor for reduced effectiveness.
- pH modifying drugs (e.g., PPIs, H2 blockers, antacids): may reduce ponatinib bioavailability; avoid if possible; if must coadminister, assess for signs of decreased ponatinib effectiveness.
- Drugs that are substrates of the P-gp (e.g., aliskiren, ambrisentan, colchicine, dabigatran, etexilate, digoxin, everolimus, fexofenadine, imatinib, lapatinib, maraviroc, nilotinib,

posaconazole, ranolazine, saxagliptin, sirolimus, sitagliptin, tolvaptan, topotecan) or ABCG2 (e.g., methotrexate, mitoxantrone, imatinib, irinotecan, lapatinib, rosuvastatin, sulfasalazine, topotecan) transport system: have not been studied so concomitant administration should be avoided.

Lab Effects/Interference:
- Neutropenia, thrombocytopenia, anemia.
- Increased serum lipase, amylase.
- Increased or decreased glucose; decreased phosphorus; increased or decreased calcium; increased or decreased sodium; increased or decreased potassium; decreased bicarbonate; increased calcium; increased creatinine.
- Increased triglycerides.
- Increased LFTs, alkaline phosphatase, decreased albumin.

Special Considerations:
- Black box warnings: Arterial occlusion, venous thromboembolism, heart failure, hepatotoxicity. See Warnings and Precautions below.
- Warnings and Precautions:
  - *Arterial thrombosis* (occlusion): cardiovascular, cerebrovascular, and peripheral vascular thrombosis, including fatal MI and stroke, have occurred. Serious arterial thrombArterial occlusion has occurred in at least 35% of treated patients ponatinib (MI, stroke, stenosis of large brain arteries, severe peripheral vascular diseases requiring urgent revascularization procedures. Patients with cardiovascular risk factors are at increased risk for developing arterial thromboses, but occurred in patients with no risk factors. Interrupt and consider drug discontinuation if the patient develops an ATE (Inclusig, 2017).
  - *Venous thromboembolism:* occurred in 6% of patients: DVT, PE, portal vein thrombosis, and retinal vein thrombosis. Monitor for signs/symptoms of VTE. Consider dose modification or drug discontinuation if the patient develops a serious VTE.
  - *Hepatotoxicity:* hepatotoxicity, liver failure, and death have occurred in ponatinib-treated patients. Ponatinib may cause elevated ALT, AST, or both. Monitor hepatic function baseline, then at least monthly or as clinically indicated. Interrupt ponatinib if hepatotoxicity is suspected, dose-reduce or discontinue drug as clinically indicated.
  - *Heart failure* was a serious side effect in 9% of patients. Monitor patients for signs/symptoms of new or worsening heart failure or LV dysfunction; if it occurs, interrupt ponatinib and treat appropriately; if serious, discontinue ponatinib.
  - *HTN* occurred in 67% of patients requiring treatment (SBP $\geq$ 140 mm Hg, or DBP $\geq$ 90 mm Hg on at least one occasion), with 2% experiencing symptomatic HTN (confusion, headache, chest pain, or SOB). Monitor and manage HTN to normalize BP; interrupt, dose-reduce, or stop ponatinib if HTN not medically controlled.
  - *Pancreatitis:* clinical pancreatitis occurred in 6% of patients; lipase elevation requiring treatment occurred in 41% of patients. If patients with elevated lipase develop abdominal pain/symptoms, stop drug and evaluate for pancreatitis. Monitor serum lipase every 2 weeks for the first 2 months and then monthly thereafter, or as clinically

rtebral, middle cerebral arteries). Peripheral arterial occlusive events occurred in
ncluded fatal mesenteric artery occlusion and life-threatening peripheral artery
Patients have developed digital or distal extremity necrosis, requiring amputa-
ous thromboembolism (VTE) occurred in 5% of ponatinib-treated patients and
DVT, PE, superficial thrombophlebitis, and retinal vein thrombosis.
and serious heart failure or left ventricular dysfunction occurred in 5% of patients.
arrhythmias may occur: bradycardia (occurred in 1% of patients, e.g., complete
ock requiring pacemaker, sick sinus syndrome, atrial fibrillation with bradycardia
ses) or supraventricular tachyarrhythmias (occurred in 5%, atrial fibrillation was
st common, with other patients developing atrial flutter, supraventricular tachycar-
atrial tachycardia). Hemorrhage occurs in about 2–11% of patients, most commonly
nts with grades 3–4 thrombocytopenia.

ng Implications: Assess baseline BP, cardiac status, and risk for bleeding baseline
ring treatment. Assess BP frequently if elevated, and teach patient to monitor at home
propriate. If BP elevated, the patient should receive antihypertensive therapy, and if
ult to control, the drug should be stopped until the BP is well controlled. If BP is not
to be medically controlled, ponatinib should be interrupted, dose reduced, or stopped.
itor patients for signs/symptoms of heart failure, and discuss treatment with physician,
ding interruption of ponatinib. If heart failure is serious, drug discontinuation must be
sidered. Teach patient to report right away (1) severe headaches, (2) light-headedness,
iness or fainting, (3) changes in vision or eye pain, (4) changes in breathing, (5) chest
comfort, (6) onset of chest pain, (7) pain in the leg or leg swelling, (8) weakness on one
e of the body, (9) speech problems, (10) changes in skin color of temperature of fingers
oes, and (11) palpitations, dizziness. Anticipate performing ECG if patient reports chest
n, new-onset SOB, or symptoms suggesting fast or slow heartbeat. Discuss treatment
ergently with physician or NP/PA.

V.   ALTERATION IN ACTIVITY AND COMFORT related to FLUID RETENTION, HEADACHE, FEVER, PAIN, DYSPHONIA, RASH

Defining Characteristics: Fluid retention occurred in 23% of patients receiving ponatinib
and was serious in 3% of patients (e.g., brain edema that was fatal, pericardial effusion,
pleural effusion, ascites). The most common fluid retention events were peripheral edema
(16%), pleural effusion (7%), and pericardial effusion (3%). Rash occurred in 34–54% of
patients, arthralgias in 1–26%, myalgia in 0–22%, pain in 1–15%, and muscle spasms in
0–13% of patients. Headache occurred in 3–39% of patients.

Nursing Implications: Assess patient weight, skin turgor, baseline and at each visit for
evidence of peripheral edema, and teach patients to self-assess for the development of
swelling of feet or hands, or any changes in breathing and to report findings. If peripheral
edema develops, teach patient to do daily weight tracking and to report any increases.
Teach patient to report any changes in breathing right away. Discuss drug interruption,
dose reduction, or discontinuance. Assess skin integrity and presence of rash baseline, and
at each visit; teach patient that rash may occur and to report it. Assess rash and discuss

indicated. Consider additional monitoring in patients with a history of pancreatitis or
alcohol abuse. Interrupt or dose-reduce as needed. Do not consider resuming ponatinib until complete resolution of symptoms and serum lipase is < 1.5 × ULN.

- *Increased toxicity in newly diagnosed chronic phase (CP) CML:* Risk of serious adverse reactions was double compared to single agent imatinib. Ponatinib is not indicated for this patient population and is not recommended for use in newly diagnosed
CML-CP patients.
- *Neuropathy***:** Peripheral and cranial neuropathy may occur, and incidence of peripheral neuropathy was 20%. Most common symptoms were paresthesias, hypoesthesia,
dysgeusia, muscular weakness, hyperesthesia. Cranial neuropathy occurred in 2% of
patients.
- *Ocular toxicity:* Serious ocular toxicities leading to blindness or blurred vision have
occurred. Retinal toxicities include macular edema, retinal vein occlusion, and retinal
hemorrhage (incidence 2%). Ensure patient has a comprehensive eye exam at baseline, and periodically during treatment. See package insert.
- *Hemorrhage* occurred in 28% of patients (serious in 6%); most hemorrhagic events
occurred in patients with grade 4 thrombocytopenia, but not all. Interrupt drug for
serious or severe hemorrhage and evaluate.
- *Fluid retention* can occur and is serious in 4% of patients. Most commonly, peripheral
edema occurred in 17%, pleural effusion in 8%, and pericardial effusions in 4%. Once
case of brain edema was fatal. Monitor for fluid retention, manage patients clinically,
and interrupt, dose-modify, or discontinue drug as clinically indicated.
- *Cardiac arrhythmias* may occur; incidence is 19%. With 7% grade 3 or higher:
symptomatic bradyarrhythmias that may require a pacemaker (1%), supraventricular
tachyarrhythmias (5%, atrial fibrillation most common). Teach patient to report immediately palpitations and dizziness, or slow heartbeat along with fainting, dizziness,
or chest pain.
- *Myelosuppression* incidence is 59%, while severe myelosuppression (grades 3–4)
occurred in 50% of patients, especially patients with CML-AP, CML-BP, and Ph+
ALL, compared to patients with CML-CP. Adjust drug dose as recommended. Monitor CBC, differential, platelet count every 2 weeks for 3 months and then monthly as
clinically indicated. Interrupt drug for ANC < 1,000 cells/mm^3 or thrombocytopenia
< 50,000 cells/mm^3; monitor CBC/differential baseline then at least every 2 weeks
for the first 3 months, then monthly or as clinically indicated. See Dose Modifications
and Iclusig package insert.
- *Tumor lysis syndrome (TLS)* rarely occurred in patients with advanced disease
(AP-CML, BP-CML, or Ph+ ALL). Hyperuricemia occurred in 7% of patients (majority CP-CML). In patients with advanced disease, ensure patient has adequate hydration and treat high uric acid prior to starting ponatinib.
- *Reversible posterior leukoencephalopathy syndrome (RPLS):* has been reported.
HTN is often present, and diagnosis made by MRI. Monitor for signs/symptoms (seizure, headache, decreased alertness, altered mental functioning, vision loss, other
visual or neurological abnormalities). If RPLS is diagnosed, interrupt ponatinib, and
resume only once RPLS is resolved, and if benefit continues to outweigh risk.

- *Compromised wound healing and GI perforation:* Based on drug's mechanism of action, this toxicity is possible. Interrupt ponatinib for at least 1 week prior to major surgery. Drug should be resumed when evidence of adequate wound healing is seen.
- *Embryo-fetal toxicity:* Advise women of reproductive potential to use effective contraception during and for 3 weeks after last dose, to avoid pregnancy. If drug is used during pregnancy, or if the patient becomes pregnant while taking the drug, apprise the patient that the drug can cause fetal harm.
- Most common ($\geq$ 20%) side effects were HTN, rash, abdominal pain, rash, constipation, fatigue, headache, dry skin, arterial occlusion, HTN, arthralgia, nausea, diarrhea, lipase increased, vomiting, myalgia, pain in extremity, and pyrexia. Hematologic adverse effects included thrombocytopenia, anemia, neutropenia, lymphopenia, and leukopenia.
- Patient teaching key points: Teach patients to contact their physician right away for symptoms suggestive of (1) a blood clot (e.g., chest pain, SOB, weakness on one side of the body, speech problems, leg pain, or swelling); (2) CHF or arrhythmias (e.g., SOB, chest pain, palpitations, dizziness, or fainting); (3) hepatotoxicity (e.g., yellowing of the eyes or skin, "tea-colored" urine, drowsiness); (4) new or worsening of existing HTN (e.g., headache, dizziness, chest pain, SOB); (5) pancreatitis (e.g., new-onset or worsening nausea, vomiting, abdominal pain, or discomfort); (6) hemorrhage (e.g., unusual bleeding or easy bruising); (7) fluid retention (e.g., leg swelling, abdominal swelling, weight gain, SOB); (8) low blood counts and risk for infection and bleeding (e.g., fever, signs/symptoms of infection, bleeding). Teach patients to notify their doctor if they are planning to have a surgical procedure or had recent surgery, as drug may interfere with wound healing. Teach female patients of reproductive potential to use effective contraception to avoid pregnancy, as drug can cause embryo-fetal toxicity.

Potential Toxicities/Side Effects and the Nursing Process

I.   POTENTIAL FOR INFECTION, BLEEDING, AND FATIGUE related to BONE MARROW SUPPRESSION

Defining Characteristics: Myelosuppression is common in all patients. Grades 3–4 thrombocytopenia occurred in 36–57% of patients, and grades 3–4 neutropenia occurred in 24–63% of patients. Febrile neutropenia occurred rarely (1–25%, depending upon state of disease). Sepsis occurred in 1–22% (highest in patients with Ph+ ALL). Most common infections were pneumonia (3–13%), UTI (7–12%), URIs (1–11%), nasopharyngitis (0–12%), and cellulitis (0–11%). Anemia occurred in 9–55% of patients. Fatigue and asthenia occurred in 3–39% of patients.

Nursing Implications: Monitor CBC differential, platelet count every 2 weeks for first 3 months, then monthly or as clinically indicated. Teach patients to report signs/symptoms of infection (e.g., fever > 100.4°F, sore throat, sputum production, difficulty breathing, dysuria) or bleeding. Teach patients to avoid OTC aspirin, NSAIDs, preparations containing aspirin or NSAIDs, or other drugs that increase the risk of bleeding. Teach patient energy conservation strategies, organization of activities to reduce fatigue, and gentle exercises.

II.   ALTERATION IN NUTRITION, POTENTIAL, related DIARRHEA, CONSTIPATION, MUCOSITIS, RARE GI HEPATOTOXICITY

Defining Characteristics: Constipation occurs in 2–47% of of patients, nausea 1–32%, vomiting 2–24% of patients, oral mu orrhage occurred in 11–21% of patients, decreased appetite 8 loss. LFTs are abnormal in many patients: increased AST (41% (19%), increased alkaline phosphatase (37%), decreased albumin abnormalities: increased glucose (58%), decreased phosphorus (5 (52%), increased lipase (41%), decreased sodium (29%), decreased sium decreased (16%), potassium increased (15%), sodium increas decreased (11%), increased creatinine (7%), increased calcium (5% increased amylase (3%).

Nursing Implications: Assess nutritional status baseline and at each tory results, especially LFTs (baseline and at least monthly). Monitor for the first 2 months, then monthly or as clinically indicated. Discuss physician, NP, or PA, and understand dose interruption or modification ing information. Teach patient that nutritional impact symptoms may o them. Discuss with patient self-care management strategies to manage diarrhea, and mucositis if they occur. Teach patient systematic oral clea and at bedtime and to report any sores or pain. Discuss dietary modifica If patient develops persistent diarrhea, discuss with physician, NP/PA; la serum potassium and need for repletion, as well as hydration. Discuss phar agement of symptoms as needed. Teach patient to report right away or to cal abdominal pain or GI bleeding.

III.   POTENTIAL ALTERATIONS IN CIRCULATION related to HTN, HEMORRHAGE, CHF, ARTERIAL, AND VENOUS THROMBOEMBOL

Defining Characteristics: HTN is a class-related effect of antiangiogene Treatment-emergent HTN occurred in 67% of ponatinib-treated patients. Two clinical trials had symptomatic HTN, such as hypertensive crisis. Patients may r gent clinical intervention for HTN-associated confusion, headache, chest pain, of breath. Of patients with baseline BP WNL (SBP < 140, DBP < 90 mm Hg), veloped treatment-emergent HTN: 49% had Stage 1 (SBP $\geq$, or DBP $\geq$ 90 mm H developed Stage 2 HTN (SBP $\geq$ 160 mm Hg, or DBP $\geq$ 100 mm Hg). Of patien Stage 1 HTN at baseline, 61% developed Stage 2 HTN.

Arterial occlusion and thrombosis occurred in at least 20% of patients, and some rienced more than one type. Patients have required revascularization procedures. Ca vascular occlusion, such as MI, and coronary artery occlusion occurred in 12%, wi without CHF. Cerebrovascular occlusion, including fatal stroke, occurred in 6%; drug cause stenosis over multiple segments in major arterial vessels supplying the brain (e

management with physician, NP, or PA. Teach patient that arthralgias, myalgias, headache, or other symptoms may occur, and discuss self-care strategies to manage them. If they persist, discuss pharmacologic management with physician, NP, or PA.

Drug: regorafenib (Stivarga)

Class: Kinase inhibitor (multi-kinase inhibitor).

Mechanism of Action: Drug inhibits multiple RTKs, and the serine/threonine-specific Raf kinase. This theoretically blocks angiogenesis and tumor microenvironment maintenance (inhibiting VEGFR2-TIE2, VEGFR3, PDGFR) and tumor cell proliferation (inhibiting RET, KIT, BRAF). KIT and PDGFR-α are important kinases that drive GIST.

Metabolism: After oral dosing of 160 mg, peak plasma level is reached in a median of 4 hours. Tablets are 69% bioavailable compared to 83% when given as an oral solution. A high-fat meal increases the drug's mean AUC by 48% compared to the fasted state, while taken with a low-fat meal the AUC increases only 36%. Drug is highly protein-bound to plasma proteins (99.5%). Regorafenib is metabolized by CYP3A4 and UGT1A9 into the active metabolites M-2 and M-5, which are also highly protein-bound. The mean elimination half-life of regorafenib is 28 hours; the half-life of M-2 is 25 hours; and the half-life of M-5 is 51 hours. The drug is primarily excreted in the feces (71%), and less so in the urine (19%), with 90% of the drug eliminated in 12 days.

Indication: Treatment of patients with
• Metastatic CRC (mCRC), previously treated with fluoropyrimidine-, oxaliplatin-, and irinotecan-based chemotherapy, an anti-VEGF therapy, and if *RAS*-wild type, an anti-EGFR therapy.
• Locally advanced unresectable or metastatic gastrointestinal stromal tumor (GIST), previously treated with imatinib mesylate and sunitinib maleate.
• Hepatocellular carcinoma previously treated with sorafenib.

Dosage/Range:
• 160 mg (four 40-mg tablets) orally once daily, for the first 21 days of a 28-day cycle. Take drug with a low-fat meal (see Drug Administration), at the same time of day.
• Do not begin regorafenib unless BP is adequately controlled.

Dose Modifications:
• If dose modifications are required, make adjustments in 40-mg increments (1 tablet). The lowest dose is 80 mg daily.
• Interrupt drug for:
    • NCI CTCAE grade 2 hand–foot skin reaction (HFSR) or palmar-plantar erythro-dysesthesia syndrome, (PPES) that is recurrent or does not improve within 7 days despite dose reduction; grade 3 HFSR: interrupt drug for a minimum of 7 days.
    • Symptomatic grade 2 HTN.
    • Any grade 3 or 4 adverse reaction.
    • Worsening infection of any grade.

- Dose-reduce regorafenib to 120 mg:
  - First occurrence of grade 2 HFSR of any duration.
  - After recovery of any grade 3 or 4 adverse reaction.
  - Grade 3 ALT/AST elevation; resume only if the potential benefit outweighs the risk of hepatotoxicity.
- Dose-reduce regorafenib to 80 mg:
  - For any re-occurrence of grade 2 HFSR at the 120-mg dose.
  - After recovery of any grade 3 or 4 adverse reaction at the 120-mg dose (except hepatotoxicity or infection).
- Discontinue drug permanently for:
  - Failure to tolerate 80-mg dose.
  - Any occurrence of AST or ALT $> 20 \times$ ULN.
  - Any occurrence of AST or ALT $> 3 \times$ ULN with concurrent bilirubin $> 2 \times$ ULN.
  - Re-occurrence of AST or ALT $> 5 \times$ ULN, despite dose reduction to 120 mg.
  - For any grade 4 adverse reaction; only resume if the potential benefit outweighs the risks.
- Stop drug before surgery, and resume after wound healing. Discontinue drug for wound dehiscence.
- HTN: temporarily or permanently discontinue drug for severe or uncontrolled HTN.
- Hold drug for new or acute cardiac ischemia/infarction and resume only after resolution of acute ischemic events.
- Discontinue drug if reversible posterior leukoencephalopathy syndrome (RPLS) occurs.
- Discontinue drug if GI perforation or fistulae develop.

Drug Preparation:
- None, oral. Available in 40-mg film-coated tablets. Tablets should be kept in the bottle, not put into daily or weekly pill boxes, and any remaining tablets should be discarded 28 days after opening the bottle. The bottle should be kept tightly closed.

Drug Administration:
- Teach the patient to take with a low-fat meal that contains < 600 calories and $< 30\%$ fat. Take at the same time every day. Teach patient to take a missed dose on the **same** day, as soon as they remember, and that they **must not** take two doses on the same day to make up for a dose missed on the previous day. Teach patient to take the dose daily for the first 21 days of each 28-day cycle.
- Meal example: 2 slices white toast with 1 T low-fat margarine and 1 T jelly, 8 oz skim milk (319 calories and 8.2 g fat); or 1 c cereal, 8 oz skim milk, 1 slice toast with jam, apple juice, and 1 cup of coffee or tea (520 calories, 2 g fat).
- Monitor BP weekly for the first 6 weeks of treatment, then every cycle, or more frequently, as indicated.

Drug Interactions:
- Strong CYP3A4 inducers (e.g., carbamazepine, phenytoin, phenobarbital, rifampin, St. John's wort): decreased serum levels of regorafenib but increased mean exposure of M-5 metabolite; avoid concomitant use.

- Strong CYP3A4 inhibitors (e.g., clarithromycin, grapefruit or grapefruit juice, itraconazole, ketoconazole, posaconazole, telithromycin, voriconazole): increased mean regorafenib serum level, and decreased exposure of metabolites M-2 and M-5. Avoid concomitant administration.

Lab Effects:
- Increased AST (65%), ALT (45%), bilirubin (45%).
- Anemia (79%), thrombocytopenia (41%), lymphopenia (54%), neutropenia (3%).
- Hypocalcemia (59%), hypokalemia (26%), hyponatremia (30%), hypophosphatemia (57%).
- Increased INR (24%), lipase (46%), amylase (26%).

Special Considerations:
- Warnings and Precautions:
  - *Hepatoxicity:* Severe and sometimes fatal hepatotoxicity occurred in clinical trials. In most cases, liver dysfunction occurred during first 2 months of therapy.
    - Monitor LFTs baseline prior to starting therapy, and at least every 2 weeks for the first 2 months of treatment. Monitor LFTs monthly thereafter or more frequently as indicated.
    - If the patient develops increased LFTs, monitor LFTs weekly until improved to $<$ 3 $\times$ ULN or baseline.
    - Temporarily hold and then dose-reduce or permanently discontinue regorafenib, depending upon severity and persistence as manifested by elevated LFTs or hepatocellular necrosis.
  - *Infection:* Increased risk of infection in patients receiving drug (32%, all grades) vs 17% in control arm. Most common infections were UTI, nasopharyngitis, mucocutaneous and systemic fungal infections, and pneumonia. Hold drug for grade 3 or 4 infection, or worsening infection of any grade. Resume regorafenib at the same dose following resolution of infection (Bayer, 2017).
  - *Hemorrhage:* Incidence overall was 18.2% vs 9.5% in placebo arm. Fatal hemorrhagic events occurred in 0.7% of patients (CNS, respiratory, GI or GU systems). Permanently discontinue drug in patients with severe or life-threatening hemorrhage. Monitor INR levels more frequently in patients receiving warfarin, as INR may become excessively elevated.
  - *Dermatological toxicity:* Increased incidence of toxicity in skin and subcutaneous tissues occurred in 71.9% of patients receiving regorafenib vs 25.5% of patients receiving placebo, including HFSR, and severe rash requiring dose modification.
    - HFSR incidence 53%, most often appearing first cycle of treatment. Incidence of HFSR was higher across all clinical trials in Asian patients treated with regorafenib.
    - Incidence of grade 3 HFSR was 16% vs $<$ 1%, grade 3 rash 3% vs $<$ 1%; and severe reactions: SJS occurred in $<$ 0.1%, erythema multiforme in $<$ 0.1%, and toxic epidermal necrosis in 0.02% of patients when drug given as a single agent.
    - Hold drug, reduce the dose, or permanently discontinue drug depending upon severity and persistence of dermatologic toxicity. Institute supportive measures for symptomatic relief (Bayer, 2017).

- *HTN:* Incidence was 30–59% in Studies 1 and 2. Hypertensive crisis occurred in 0.2% across all clinical trials (0% in placebo groups). Onset of HTN was within the first cycle of therapy.
  - Do not start regorafenib therapy until BP is well controlled.
  - Monitor BP weekly for the first 6 weeks of treatment, then every cycle, or more frequently as indicated.
  - Temporarily or permanently withhold drug for severe or uncontrolled HTN.
- *Cardiac ischemia and infarction:* occurred more frequently than in placebo (0.9% vs 0.2%), in RCTs. Hold drug in patients that develop new or acute onset cardiac ischemia or infarction. Resume regorafenib only after resolution of acute cardiac ischemic events if the potential benefits outweigh the risks of further cardiac ischemia.
- *Reversible posterior leukoencephalopathy syndrome (RPLS)* may occur. It is a syndrome of subcortical vasogenic edema, diagnosed by MRI. If a patient presents with seizures, headache, visual disturbances, confusion, or altered mental function, discuss patient evaluation for RPLS with physician. Drug should be discontinued if the diagnosis of RPLS is confirmed.
- *GI perforation or fistula* occurred in 0.6% of patients across all clinical trials. Permanently discontinue drug if either of these events occur.
- *Wound-healing complications:* no studies have been conducted, but VEGFR inhibitors can impair wound healing. Stop drug at least 2 weeks prior to scheduled surgery. Resumption of drug after surgery should be based on adequate wound healing. Discontinue the drug if wound dehiscence occurs.
- *Embryo-feto toxicity:* Drug is embryo-fetal toxic. Counsel women of childbearing potential and men to avoid pregnancy and to use highly effective contraception during therapy and for 2 months after drug is discontinued. If the drug is used in pregnancy, or if the patient becomes pregnant while receiving the drug, the patient should be apprised of the potential hazard to the fetus. Nursing mothers should make a decision to discontinue nursing or to discontinue the drug, taking into account the importance of the drug to the patient's health.
- Most common side effects ($\geq$ 20%) are pain (including GI and abdominal pain), asthenia/fatigue, HFSR, diarrhea, decreased appetite/food intake, HTN, mucositis, dysphonia, infection, weight loss, rash, nausea, hyperbilirubinemia, fever.
- In the CORRECT study, patients with advanced mCRC who had progressed on all other standard therapies were randomized to receive regorafenib or placebo. Those in the regorafenib arm had improved OS (6.4 mo vs 5 mo control). Disease control rate was 44% compared to 15% in the placebo group. Drug appears to be more effective in stabilizing disease and delaying progression than marked tumor shrinkage (Grothey et al., 2012).
- In the GRID study, patients with advanced GIST who had progressed after imatinib and sunitinib therapy had significantly greater PFS (60% at 3 mo, 38% at 6 mo, compared to 11% and 0% in the control arm). Disease control for patients in the regorafenib arm was 4.8 mo compared to 0.9 mo (p < 0.001) in the control arm (Demetri et al., 2012).

Potential Toxicities/Side Effects and the Nursing Process

I. ALTERATION IN NUTRITION, POTENTIAL, related to NAUSEA, VOMITING, DIARRHEA, MUCOSITIS, HYPOTHYROIDISM, HEPATOTOXICITY, POSSIBLE GI PERFORATION OR FISTULA

Defining Characteristics: Diarrhea occurs in 47% of patients, mucositis in 40%, nausea 20%, and vomiting 17% of patients. Hypothyroidism affects 18%, and decreased appetite and food intake 31%. Weight loss occurred in 14% of patients. LFTs are abnormal in many patients: Increased AST (65%), ALT (45%), bilirubin (45%), and INR is increased in 14% of patients. Hypokalemia occurs in 26% of patients. GI perforation or fistula is rare (0.6–2.1%).

Nursing Implications: Assess baseline nutritional status, lab findings especially LFTs (transaminases and bilirubin) and serum potassium. LFTs should be assessed at least every 2 weeks during the first 2 months of treatment, then monthly or more frequently as needed. Discuss abnormalities with physician, NP, or PA, and understand dose interruption or modifications per prescribing information (see Dose Modifications above). Teach patient that nutritional impact symptoms may occur and to report them. Discuss with patient self-care strategies to manage nausea, vomiting, diarrhea, and mucositis if they occur. Teach patient systematic oral cleansing after meals and at bedtime and to report any sores or pain. Discuss dietary modifications to minimize symptoms experienced. If patient has diarrhea that persists, discuss with physician, NP, or PA the need for lab testing of serum potassium, as well as replacement therapy and hydration. If symptoms persist, discuss pharmacological management with physician, NP, or PA. Although rare, GI perforation or fistula may occur. Teach patient to come to the emergency room and to report severe pain in the abdomen, swelling in the abdomen, and high fever right away.

II. POTENTIAL ALTERATION IN CIRCULATION related to HYPERTENSION, HEMORRHAGE, CHF

Defining Characteristics: HTN is a class-related side effect of antiangiogenesis agents. As the kidney is made up of many capillaries, there may be protein leakage (proteinuria). HTN occurs in 59% of patients, and is grade 3 or higher in 28%. Proteinuria occurs in 60% of patients. Hemorrhage occurs in about 11% of patients and is severe in 4%, affecting respiratory, GI, and genitourinary tracts. Rarely, patients receiving regorafenib had increased risk of myocardial ischemia and MI (1.2% vs 0.04% in controls).

Nursing Implications: Assess baseline BP, cardiac status, and risk for bleeding baseline and during treatment. Patient should have BP assessed weekly for the first 6 weeks, then checked regularly. If elevated, the patient should receive antihypertensives, and the drug should be stopped until the BP is well controlled. Assess urine protein, and if 2+ or greater, discuss obtaining 24-hour urine for protein with provider. Usually drug is held for urine protein > 2 g/24 hours, and resumed after the urine protein is less than that. Teach patient to report severe headaches, light-headedness, or changes in vision. Teach patient to report any changes in breathing, chest discomfort, or the onset of chest pain. Discuss with provider need for ECG, and be prepared to obtain the ECG. Hold drug in patients who develop new or acute onset cardiac ischemia or infarction. Assess platelet count, and INR in patients receiving warfarin. Teach patient to report any signs/symptoms of bleeding. Monitor INR levels closely in patients receiving warfarin, and dose based on INR per physician, NP, or PA. Regorafenib should be discontinued in patients with severe hemorrhage.

III.   ALTERATION IN SKIN INTEGRITY AND COMFORT related to HFSR, RASH

Defining Characteristics: Drug causes skin and subcutaneous tissue reactions including HFSR, also known as PPE, and severe rash, which require dose modifications. The incidence of HFSR in clinical trials was 45%, with grade 3–4 HFSR occurring in 17–21% of patients in clinical trials. Rash affected 26% of patients, in which 6% were grade 3 or 4. HFSR may involve palms of hands, soles of feet, and other areas that are exposed to friction, such as knees when chronically rubbing together (e.g., in a wheelchair). Most cases appeared during the first treatment cycle, and patients often present with painful blisters, which over weeks to months are replaced by thick, hyperkeratotic areas similar to calluses (Lacouture, 2011). Rash may be severe, and rarely erythema multiforme, SJS, and toxic epidermal necrolysis have occurred.

Nursing Implications: Assess baseline skin integrity, including soles of feet and palms of hands, and teach patient that these symptoms may occur and to report them. If patient has calluses, they should be trimmed or removed. Teach patient to (1) self-assess for erythema, swelling, blisters, and pain on skin surfaces, and to report them; (2) avoid activities that increase blood flow to the hands and feet, such as hot showers and baths, and to take tepid baths and showers; (3) avoid constrictive clothing and repetitive movements that can irritate the opposing skin; (4) use skin emollients to prevent skin from drying and cracking starting on day 1 of therapy, and to use lotion and therapeutic socks (available from the drug manufacturer) until the lotion is absorbed; (5) elevate hands and feet when sitting down and to apply cool compresses to hands or feet if swollen; (6) gently pat skin dry after bathing and use mild soap. Assess grade of HFSR and teach patient to stop using drug and to call provider if pain is felt, as this may mean drug therapy should be interrupted. See Dose Modifications.

IV.   POTENTIAL FOR INFECTION related to LYMPHOPENIA

Defining Characteristics: Lymphopenia occurred in 54% of patients in clinical trials, and neutropenia in 3%. Infection occurred in 31% of patients, was grade 3 or higher in 9% of patients, and fever occurred in 28% of patients.

Nursing Implications: Assess patient's CBC/differential baseline and during treatment. Teach patient strategies to avoid infection and self-assessment for signs/symptoms of infection, as well as to report signs/symptoms of infection (e.g., T > 100.4°F, productive cough, dysuria, dyspnea). Assess patient for presence of intact mucous membranes and skin, as these are portals for infection.

TREATMENT

V. ALTERATION IN ACTIVITY AND COMFORT related to ASTHENIA, HEADACHE, FEVER, PAIN, DYSPHONIA

Defining Characteristics: Asthenia/fatigue occurred in some patients during clinical trials, and was grade 3 or higher in some patients. Pain occurred in some and fever in others. Anemia occurred in some patients, and was grade 3 or higher in a few patients. Headache occurred in some and dysphonia in some patients.

Nursing Implications: Teach patient that these symptoms may occur and how to manage them, such as alternating rest and activity, energy-conserving measures, gentle exercise. If symptoms persist, discuss prescription pharmacologic management with physician, NP, or PA.

Drug: ribociclib (Kisqali)

Class: Kinase inhibitor; CDK inhibitor.

Mechanism of Action: CDK 4,6 are activated upon binding to D-cyclins and this complex regulates cell cycle progression (proliferation) through phosphorylation of the retinoblastoma protein (pRB). Ribociclib inhibits CDK 4 and 6, which stops the cell cycle from proceeding from the G_1 phase to the S phase; thus cell proliferation is halted in ER-positive breast cancer cells. When combined with an antiestrogen, ribociclib increased growth arrest and inhibition of ER-positive tumor growth to a greater extent than occurred with either drug alone.

Metabolism: After oral administration, Cm (peak plasma level) is reached in 1–4 hrs, and steady state is reached after 8 days. Food does not affect absorption or peak plasma concentrations. Ribociclib binds to human plasma proteins (about 70%), and undergoes extensive hepatic metabolism, primarily by CYP3A. Unchanged drug is found in the feces (17%) and urine (12%). Patients with mild hepatic impairment (Child-Pugh Class A) were able to metabolize ribociclib adequately, while those with moderate (class B) or severe (class C) had < two-fold increase in mean drug exposure. Mild-to-moderate renal impairment did not affect pharmacokinetics, but the effect in patients with severe impairment is unknown (Novartis, 2017).

Indications: In combination with (1) an aromatase inhibitor for the treatment of pre/perimenopausal or postmenopausal women with hormone receptor (HR)-positive, human epidermal growth factor receptor 2 (HER-2)-negative advanced or metastatic breast cancer as initial endocrine-based therapy; or (2) fulvestrant for the treatment of postmenopausal women with HR-positiveHER-2-negative advanced or metastatic breast cancer as initial endocrine-based therapy or following disease progression on endocrine therapy.

Contraindications: None. Drug should NOT be given together with tamoxifen.

Dosage/Range:
- Ribociclib 600 mg (three 200-mg tablets) taken orally, once daily for 21 consecutive days, followed by 7 days off (28-day cycle), with or without food, in combination with an

aromatase inhibitor as recommended in the full prescribing information, or fulvestrant 500 mg administered on days 1, 15, 29, and once monthly thereafter (see fulvestrant full prescribing information).

• Pre/perimenopausal women treated with the combination should also receive a luteinizing hormone-releasing hormone (LHRH) agonist according to current clinical practice standards.

• Interrupt or reduce ribociclib dose as needed based on patient safety and tolerability.

Dose Modifications:

• Dose levels: Starting dose 600 mg: First dose reduction is to a dose of 400 mg/day (two 200-mg tablets); second dose reduction is to a dose of 200 mg/day (1-tablet). If a further dose: reduction is needed below 200 mg/day, discontinue drug. See full prescribing information for the aromatase inhibitor or fulvestrant for information about dose modifications of these drugs.

• *Neutropenia*
  • Neutropenia: Grade 3 (ANC $<$ 1,000–500/mm^3): Interrupt drug until recovery to grade $\leq$ 2; resume ribociclib at the same dose level. If toxicity recurs at grade 3, dose interrupt until recovery, then resume ribociclib at the next lower dose level.
  • Grade 3 neutropenia with fever (ANC $<$ 1,000–500/mm^3 + fever $\geq$ 38.5°C [single episode of fever $>$ 38.3°C or $>$ 38°C for more than 1 hr] and/or infection): Interrupt ribociclib until recovery to grade $\leq$ 2. Resume at *next lower dose*.
  • Grade 4 neutropenia: Hold ribociclib until recovery to grade $\leq$ 2; resume at *the next lower dose level*.

• *Hepatobiliary Toxicity:*
  • AST and/or ALT elevations from baseline (prior to starting therapy) WITHOUT increase in total bilirubin and without cholestasis
  • Grade 1 ($<$ ULN-3 $\times$ ULN): no dose adjustment.
  • Grade 2 ($>$ 3–5 $\times$ ULN): If baseline $<$ grade 2: interrupt ribociclib until recovery to $\leq$ baseline grade, then resume ribociclib at the same dose level. If grade 2 recurs, resume ribociclib at next lower dose level. If baseline is at grade 2, no dose interruption.
  • Grade 3 ($>$ 5–20 $\times$ ULN): dose interruption until recovery to $\leq$ baseline grade, then resume at next lower dose level. If grade 3 recurs, discontinue ribociclib.
  • Grade 4 ($>$ 20 $\times$ ULN): discontinue ribociclib.

• *ECGs with QTcF $>$ 480 msec:* [Uses Fridericia's correction formula rather than Bazett's which is QTc(B)]
  • Interrupt ribociclib therapy; if QTcF prolongation resolves to $<$ 481 msec, resume treatment at the same dose level.
  • If QTcF $\geq$ 481 msec recurs, interrupt dose until QTcF resolves to $<$ 481 msec; then resume ribociclib at next lower dose level.

• *ECGs with QTcF $>$ 500 msec:* [Uses Fridericia's correction formula rather than Bazett's which is QTc(B)]
  • Interrupt ribociclib therapy if QTcF $>$ 500 msec on at least 2 separate ECGs within same visit.
  • If QTcF prolongation resolves to $<$ 481 msec, resume treatment at the next lower dose level.

TREATMENT

- Permanently discontinue ribociclib if QTcF interval prolongation is either > 500 msec or > 60 msec change from baseline AND associated with any of the following: Torsades de pointes (see Nursing Considerations introduction *Chapter 3*), polymorphic ventricular tachycardia, unexplained syncope, or signs/symptoms of serious arrhythmia.
- *Dose Modifications and Management of Other Toxicities:*
  - **Grades 1–2:** no dose adjustment; initiate appropriate medical intervention and monitor as clinically appropriate;
  - **Grade 3:** Interrupt ribociclib therapy until recovery to grade ≤ 1 then resume ribociclib at same dose level. If grade 3 recurs, resume ribociclib at the next lower dose level.
  - **Grade 4:** discontinue ribociclib.
- *Hepatic Impairment:* No dose adjustment necessary for mild hepatic impairment (Child-Pugh Class A). Patients with moderate or severe hepatic impairment (Child–Pugh Class B, C) should start at 400 mg PO once daily.
- *Renal Impairment:* No dose adjustment necessary for mild or moderate renal impairment Patients with severe renal impairment should start at 200 mg PO once daily.
- *Strong CYP3A4 Inhibitor Coadministration:* **Avoid coadministration.** *If* the drug **must** be coadministered with a strong CYP3A inhibitor, decrease the ribociclib dose to 400 mg PO qd. If the strong inhibitor is discontinued, increase the palbociclib dose to that used prior to adding the strong CYP3A inhibitor once 5 half-lives of the inhibitor have passed.
- Please refer to Kisqali package insert (Novartis, March 2017). See the manufacturer's prescribing information for letrozole.

Drug Preparation: Oral. Available as 200-mg tablets. Store at room temperature, and keep out of the reach of children and pets.

Drug Administration:
- Assess laboratory parameters:
  - Monitor CBC/ANC prior to start of ribociclib, every 2 weeks for the first 2 cycles, at the beginning of each subsequent 4 cycles, and as clinically indicated.
  - Monitor serum electrolytes including potassium, calcium, phosphorous, magnesium PRIOR to starting ribociclib therapy, at the beginning of the first 6 cycles, and as clinically indicated. Correct any deficiencies before administering drug,
  - Monitor LFTs before start of ribociclib, every 2 weeks for the first 2 cycles, at the beginning of each subsequent 4 cycles, and as clinically indicated.
  - Monitor ECGs prior start of ribociclib, with repeat at approximately day 14 of cycle 1, and at the beginning of the second cycle, and then as clinically indicated. If the patient develops QTcF prolongation at any time, increase ECG monitoring frequency.
- Teach the patient to take ribociclib at approximately the same time each morning with letrozole dose days 1–21 of each cycle with or without food, and continue letrozole ONLY on days 22–28. If a dose is missed or vomited, the patient should not take an additional dose but rather resume dosing at the next scheduled time.
- Teach the patient to swallow the tablet whole; not to chew, crush, or open the capsule and not to take the capsule if it is broken or cracked. Patient should NOT take the tablet if it is broken, cracked, or not intact.

Drug Interactions:

- CYP3A inhibitors: Increase plasma concentrations of ribociclib (e.g., ritonavir increases C_{max} 3.2-fold). Avoid concurrent use with strong CYP3A inhibitors (e.g., boceprrevir, clarithromycin, conivaptan, grapefruit juice, indinavir, itraconazole, ketoconazole, lopinavir/ritonavir, nafazodone, nelfinavir, posaconazole, ritonavir, saquinavir, and voriconazole); if such use cannot be avoided, decrease the ribociclib dose.
- CYP3A4 inducers: Decrease plasma concentration of ribociclib (e.g., rifampin decreases C_{max} by 80%). Avoid concurrent use with strong and moderate inducers (e.g., phenytoin, rifampin, carbamazepine, St. John's wort).
- CYP3A substrates with narrow therapeutic index: For example, concomitant use of midazolam and ribociclib, increased the midazolam C_{max} 3.8-fold. If the substrate is sensitive and has a narrow therapeutic window (e.g., alfentanil, cyclosporine, dihydroergotamine, ergotamine, everolimus, fentanyl, pimozide, quinidine, sirolimu, tactrolimus), consider dose reduction of the substrate.
- Drugs that prolong QT interval (e.g., tamoxifen, antiarrhythmia drugs like amiodarone, dispyramide, procainamide, quinidine and sotalol; other drugs like chloroquine, halofantrine, clarithromycin, haloperidol, methadone, moxifloxacin, bepridil, pimozide, ondansetron): avoid coadministration.

Lab Effects/Interference:

- Decreased ANC, leukocytes, RBCs, platelets, lymphocytes, serum phosphorous, serum potassium
- Increased LFTs, (alanine aminotransferase, aspartate aminotransferase), creatinine

Special Considerations:

- Most common adverse reactions ($\geq$ 10%): neutropenia, nausea, fatigue, diarrhea, leukopenia, alopecia, vomiting, constipation, headache, and back pain. Alopecia occurs in 33% of patients.
- Warnings and Precautions:
  - *QT prolongation:* Do not use drug in patients with significant risk of developing QTc prolongation including patients with
  - (1) long QT syndrome, (2) uncontrolled or significant cardiac disease including recent MI, CHF, unstable angina, and bradyarrhythmias; (3) electrolyte abnormalities. Assess patient medication profile, and avoid coadministration with drugs known to prolong the QTc interval and/or strong CYP3A inhibitors, as this may lead to prolongation of the QTcF interval. Monitor ECGs/QTc baseline (drug must be started in patients ONLY if QTcF is < 450 msec), repeat ECG at day 14 of cycle 1, at the beginning of cycle 2, then as clinically indicated. Assess serum electrolytes (including serum potassium,c alcium, phosphorous, and magnesium) prior to starting treatment, at the beginning of the first 6 cycles, and as clinically indicated. Correct any abnormalities before starting iinitial and subsequent treatments. See Dose Modifications section.
  - *Increased QT prolongation with concomitant use of tamoxifen:* Ribociclib is not indicated for use with tamoxifen as significantly more patients developed QTc prolongation when receiving a combination including tamoxifen.
  - *Hepatobiliary toxicity:* Increased serum transaminases (ALT, AST) may occur; in Study 1, incidence of grade 3 or 4 increases in ALT were 10% and AST, 7%. Median

time to onset was 85 days, and median time to resolution (≤grade 2) was 22 days. Assess LFTs baseline, and monitor every 2 weeks for the first 2 cycles, at the beginning of each subsequent 4 cycles, and as clinically indicated. See dosage modification section.

- *Neutropenia:* Monitor CBC/ANC at baseline and prior to each cycle, as well as on day 14 of the first 2 cycles (every 2 weeks), at the beginning of each subsequent 4 cycles, and as clinically indicated. Neutropenia was the most frequent adverse reaction with an incidence of 74%, with grade 3/4 neutropenia in 58% of patients receiving ribociclib and aromatase inhibitor or fulvestrant. The median time to the grade 2 or higher neutropenia was 16 days. The median time to resolution of grade 3 or higher neutropenia was 12 days. Incidence of febrile neutropenia was 1%. Interrupt the dose, reduce the dose, or delay the dose as needed (See Dose Modifications section). Monitor the patient closely for infection and give medical treatment promptly. Teach the patient to report fever or chills immediately.

- *Embryo-fetal toxicity:* Ribociclib can cause fetal harm. Teach women of reproductive potential to use effective contraception to avoid pregnancy during therapy and for at least 3 weeks after the last dose.

Potential Toxicities/Side Effects and the Nursing Process

I.   POTENTIAL FOR INFECTION AND FATIGUE related to BONE MARROW SUPPRESSION

Defining Characteristics: Neutropenia was the most common adverse effect with 75% incidence, and occurrence of grade 3 was 50% with letrozole. The median time to the first episode of any neutropenia was 16 days and median time to resolution in patients with grade 3 was 15 days. Eighteen percent developed anemia with letrozole. Infections (UTI) occurred in 11%. Fatigue developed in 37% of patients.

Nursing Implications: Evaluate CBC/ANC prior to start of ribociclib, every 2 weeks for the first 2 cycles, at the beginning of each subsequent 4 cycles, and as clinically indicated. Discuss any abnormalities with the physician/NP/PA. Assess for signs and symptoms of infection and fatigue. Teach the patient about the signs and symptoms of infection, how to take a temperature and to report any abnormality, including fever, immediately. Teach the patient self-care measures to minimize the risk of infection, including avoidance of OTC aspirin-containing medications. Teach the patient self-assessment of fatigue and to alternate rest and activity as needed. Discuss dose modification for grade 3 or higher neutropenia.

II. ALTERATION IN NUTRITION, POTENTIAL, related to NAUSEA, VOMITING, DIARRHEA, STOMATITIS, or HEPATOBILIARY TOXICITY

Defining Characteristics: Nausea affected 52% of patients, diarrhea 35%, vomiting 29%, constipation 25%, stomatitis 12% and abdominal pain 11%. Decreased appetite occurred in 19% of patients. Abnormal liver function tests occurred in 18% of patients (8% grade 3, 2% grade 4).

Nursing Implications: Assess the patient's nutritional status at baseline and at each visit. Assess LFTs baseline, every 2 weeks for the first 2 cycles, at the beginning of each subsequent 4 cycles, and as clinically indicated. Discuss abnormalities with MD/PA/NP. Assess the oral mucosa for intactness and oral health habits. Teach the patient that these side effects may occur and teach self-management strategies such as use of antidiarrheals and antinausea medications, systematic oral cleansing and oral assessment, and dietary modifications, and to report any symptoms that do not improve. If diarrhea is severe, assess electrolytes especially serum potassium and replete as ordered. Discuss prescription medication with the provider if necessary to manage refractory symptoms. Teach the patient tips to increase appetite (e.g., small, frequent meals, use of spices). Offer the services of a dietitian as appropriate.

III.   ALTERATION IN CIRCULATION, POTENTIAL, related to QTc PROLONGATION

Defining Characteristics: Patients may develop QT prolongation on ECG. Do NOT administer to patients with prolonged QTc ($>$ 450 msec) or who may develop prolonged QTc (hypokalemia, hypomagnesemia, other drugs in combination that prolong the QTc). Prolonged QTc in the setting of low magnesium and hypokalemia sets the stage for torsades de pointes, with ventricular tachycardia, fibrillation, and sudden cardiac death possible.

Nursing Implications: Assess baseline QTc interval, with repeat at approximately day 14 of cycle 1, at the beginning of the second cycle, and then as clinically indicated. If the patient develops QTcF prolongation at any time, increase ECG monitoring frequency. Assess serum electrolytes including potassium, calcium, phosphorous, magnesium PRIOR to starting ribociclib therapy, at the beginning of the first 6 cycles, and as clinically indicated. Identify patients at risk for development of prolonged QTc (e.g., congenital long QTc syndrome, prolonged QTc $>$ 450 msec, taking antiarrhythmics or other drugs that can prolong the QTc interval (hypokalemia, hypomagnesemia, concomitant CYP3A4 strong inhibitors). Correct electrolyte abnormalities (e.g., magnesium, potassium) as ordered before starting ribociclib and monitor periodically during therapy. Hypokalemia and hypomagnesemia in the setting of prolonged QTc may lead to torsades de pointes, ventricular fibrillation, and sudden cardiac death. QTc must be assessed baseline, Monitor ECGs/QTc baseline (drug must be started in patients ONLY if QTcF is $<$ 450 msec), repeat ECG at day 14 of cycle 1, at the beginning of cycle 2, then as clinically indicated. See Dose modification section. Teach patient to report feeling lightheaded, faint, or an irregular heartbeat right away. Patients with hepatic impairment should have a dose reduction to avoid increased serum levels of ribociclib. See Introduction to *Chapter 4* for more complete discussion on determining the QTc interval.

Drug: romidepsin for injection (Istodax)

Class: Histone deacetylase (HDAC) inhibitor.

Mechanism of Action: Romidepsin catalyzes the removal of acetyl groups from acetylated lysine residues in histones, resulting in the modulation of gene expression. HDACs also deacetylate nonhistone protein transcription factors. Romidepsin causes acetylated histones to accumulate and induces cell cycle arrest and apoptosis in some cancer cell lines. The antineoplastic mechanism has not been fully characterized.

Metabolism: The drug is highly protein-bound after IV injection (92–94%). It undergoes extensive metabolism in the liver, primarily by the CYP3A4 system, with minor metabolism by CYP3A5, CYP1A1, CYP2B6, and CYP2C19. The terminal half-life is about 3 hours, and there is no accumulated drug with repeated dosing. Mild hepatic impairment does not affect pharmacokinetics, but moderate and severe liver impairment have not been studied. Patients with mild, moderate, or severe renal impairment did not have changes in pharmacokinetics, but patients with end-stage renal impairment have not been studied.

Indication: FDA approved for the treatment of adults with:
- Cutaneous T-cell lymphoma (CTCL) who have received at least one prior systemic treatment.
- Peripheral T-cell lymphoma (PTCL) who have received at least one prior therapy; accelerated approval based on response rate as clinical benefit (e.g., increased OS) has not been demonstrated.

Dosage/Range:
- 14-mg/m^2 IV infusion over 4 hours on days 1, 8, 15 of a 28-day cycle. Repeat cycles every 28 days as long as patient continues to derive benefit and tolerates the drug.
- Discontinue or interrupt drug (with or without dose reduction to 10 mg/m^2) to manage treatment side effects. Reduce starting dose in patients with moderate or severe hepatic impairment: (1) if moderate (bilirubin $> 1.5 \times$ ULN to $\leq 3 \times$ ULN): romidepsin dose is 7 mg/m^2; (2) if severe, e.g., bilirubin $> 3 \times$ ULN, romidepsin dose is 5 mg/m^2.

Dose Modifications:
- **Nonhematologic toxicities** (excluding alopecia):
  - Grades 2–3: Delay drug until toxicity improves to $\leq$ grade 1 or baseline; then restart at 14 mg/m^2.
  - If grade 3 toxicity recurs, delay until toxicity improves to $\leq$ grade 1 or baseline, then permanently dose-reduce to 10 mg/m^2.
  - Grade 4 toxicity: Delay until toxicity improves to $\leq$ grade 1 or baseline, then permanently dose-reduce to 10 mg/m^2.
  - Discontinue drug if grades 3–4 toxicities recur after dose reduction.
- **Hematologic toxicities:**
  - Grades 3–4 neutropenia or thrombocytopenia: Delay until cytopenia returns to ANC $\geq 1.5 \times 10^9$/L and/or platelet count returns to $\geq 75 \times 10^9$/L or baseline; then resume at 14 mg/m^2.
  - Grade 4 febrile ($\geq 38.5°C$) neutropenia or thrombocytopenia that requires platelet transfusion: Delay until cytopenia returns to $\leq$ grade 1 or baseline; then permanently dose-reduce to 10 mg/m^2.
- **Dosage in patients with hepatic impairment:** Patients with moderate or severe hepatic impairment or with end-stage renal disease should be treated with caution. Starting dose modification for patients with hepatic impairment: (1) if moderate (bilirubin $> 1.5 \times$ ULN to $\leq 3 \times$ ULN): romidepsin dose is 7 mg/m^2; (2) if severe, e.g., bilirubin $> 3 \times$ ULN, romidepsin dose is 5 mg/m^2.

Drug Preparation:
- Use recommended practices for the safe handling of hazardous drugs.
- Drug must be reconstituted with the supplied diluent and further diluted with 0.9% Sodium Chloride Injection, USP before IV infusion. Romidepsin and diluent vials contain overfill to ensure the recommended dose volume can be withdrawn at a concentration of 5 mg/mL.
- Drug is supplied as a kit with (1) sterile, lyophilized powder in a single-use 10 mg single use vial containing 11 mg romidepsin and 22 mg of bulking agent, povidone, USP, and (2) one sterile single dose vial containing 2.4 mL of diluent (2.2 mL deliverable volume) of 80% propylene glycol, USP, and 20% dehydrated alcohol, USP).
    - Each 10 mg single dose vial must be reconstituted with 2.2 mL of the supplied diluent.
    - Aseptically withdraw 2.2 mL from supplied diluents vial, and slowly inject it into the romidepsin for injection vial. Swirl until contents are completely dissolved. The reconstituted solution contains romidepsin 5 mg/mL in a deliverable volume of 2 mL. The reconstituted solution is chemically stable for up to 8 hours at room temperature.
    - Calculate volume of ordered dose, and extract the ordered dose of romidepsin from the vial(s), using aseptic technique. Further dilute romidepsin in 500 mL 0.9% sodium chloride injection, USP before infusion. Infuse over 4 hours.
- The diluted solution is compatible with polyvinyl chloride (PVC), ethylene vinyl acetate (EVA), polyethylene (PE) infusion bags and glass bottles; it is chemically stable for up to 24 hours when stored at room temperature. Prepared solution should be inspected for visible particulate matter and discoloration, and administered as soon as possible after dilution as possible.

Drug Administration:
- Infuse IV over 4 hours.
- Solution is chemically stable for at least 24 hours stored at room temperature, but it should be administered as soon after dilution as possible. Diluted solution is compatible with polyvinyl chloride (PVC), ethylene vinyl acetate (EVA), polyethylene (PE) infusion bags, as well as glass bottles.
- Visually inspect for particulate matter and discoloration prior to administration.

Drug Interactions:
- Coumadin/Coumadin derivatives: romidepsin may cause prolongation of PT and elevation of INR. Monitor PT and INR closely in patients receiving this combination.
- Romidepsin is metabolized by CYP3A4. Strong CYP3A4 inhibitors may increase the serum level of romidepsin. Drugs that are strong inhibitors of the CYP3A4 enzyme include atazanavir, clarithromycin, indinavir, itraconazole, ketoconazole, nefazodone, nelfinavir, ritonavir, saquinavir, telithromycin, and voriconazole. Avoid combination if possible, but if romidepsin is initially coadministered with a strong CYP3A4 inhibitor, monitor the patient closely for romidepsin side effects, and follow dose modifications for toxicity.
- Drugs that induce the CYP3A4 enzymes (e.g., carbamazepine dexamethasone, phenobarbital, phenytoin, rifampin, rifabutin, rifapentine) may decrease the serum level of romidepsin and should be avoided if possible. Coadministration with rifampin increased romidepsin exposure by 80%, AUC and C_{max} by 60%, possibly by rifampin inhibition

of an unknown hepatic intake process. Patients should NOT take rifampin together with romidepsin. St. John's wort should also not be taken with romidepsin.
- Drugs that inhibit drug transport systems: romidepsin is a substrate of the efflux transporter P-glycoprotein (P-gp) so that drugs that inhibit P-glycoprotein may result in increased serum levels of romidepsin when coadministered. If they are coadministered, caution should be exercised.

Lab Effects/Interference:
- Hypomagnesemia, hypokalemia, hypocalcemi, hypoalbuminemia, hyponatremia, hypophosphatemia.
- Hyperglycemia, hypermagnesemia, hyperuricemia, hyperbilirubinemia.
- Anemia, thrombocytopenia, neutropenia, lymphopenia.
- Increased AST, ALT.
- ECG ST–T-wave changes, QTc prolongation.

Special Considerations:
- The most common adverse reactions are neutropenia, lymphopenia, thrombocytopenia, infections, nausea, fatigue, vomiting, anorexia, anemia, and ECG T-wave changes.
- Warning and Precautions:
  - *Myelosuppression:* Thrombocytopenia, neutropenia, lymphopenia, and anemia can occur; monitor CBC/platelets/ANC baseline, prior to each cycle, and during treatment as indicated.
  - *Infections:* Fatal and serious infections can occur (e.g., pneumonia, sepsis, viral reactivation of Epstein Barr and hepatitis B viruses) during treatment and for up to 30 days after the end of treatment. Patients at risk may be those with a history of prior monoclonal antibody therapy directed against lymphocyte antigens, and patients with bone marrow involvement by tumor.
  - *ECG Changes:* T-wave, ST-segment changes. Patients with congenital long QT syndrome, those with a history of significant cardiovascular disease, and patients taking anti-arrhythmic drugs can develop QTc prolongation (time of ventricular contraction and relaxation) with risk of ventricular arrhythmias. These patients should have an ECG baseline and periodically during treatment.
  - If serum magnesium and potassium are low, this increases the risk for torsades de pointes, a type of ventricular tachycardia that can deteriorate into ventricular fibrillation.
  - **Prior to romidepsin administration, ensure that serum magnesium, calcium, phosphorus, and potassium are WNL.**
  - *Tumor lysis syndrome (TLS):* rarely occurs (1% incidence in patients with CTCL and 2% in paitents with Stage III/IV PTCL). Discuss with physician/NP/PA TLS prophylaxis in patients with high-tumor burden, and monitor closely.
  - *Embryo-fetal toxicity:* Drug may cause fetal harm, so pregnancy should be avoided. Teach female patients of reproductive potential to use effective contraception during therapy and for at least 1 month after last dose. Teach male patients with female sexual partners of reproductive potential to use effective contraception during therapy and for at least 1 month after the last drug dose. If romidepsin is used during pregnancy, or if the patient becomes pregnancy during therapy, the patient should be apprised of potential harm to the fetus. Nursing mothers: a decision should be made whether to

discontinue nursing or discontinue the drug, taking into account importance of the drug to the mother's health.

Potential Toxicities/Side Effects and the Nursing Process

I.   POTENTIAL FOR INFECTION, BLEEDING, AND FATIGUE related to NEUTROPENIA, THROMBOCYTOPENIA, AND ANEMIA

Defining Characteristics: The highest incidence of anemia was 72% (16% grades 3–4), thrombocytopenia 65% (14% grades 3–4), and neutropenia 57% (27% grades 3–4). Infections occurred in up to 54% of patients, with pyrexia (23%). Serious and sometimes fatal infections, including pneumonia and sepsis, have been reported in clinical trials. These infections can occur during or within 30 days after treatment, and risk may be higher in patients who have had extensive or intensive chemotherapy.

Nursing Implications: Monitor CBC, platelet count; assess at baseline, prior to each treatment, and periodically as indicated. Ensure that dose modifications are performed as indicated in dosage section. Assess for signs and symptoms of infection, bleeding, fatigue, and anemia. Teach patients to self-assess for signs and symptoms of infection, bleeding, and anemia and to call their nurse or physician right away if they occur, or to go to the emergency room. Ensure that the patient has a thermometer at home and that the patient and a family member can read the number and verbally repeat to call if the temperature is 100.4°F or higher. In addition, patients should be taught to report cough, shortness of breath, significant fatigue, chest pain, burning with urination, flulike symptoms, muscle aches, or worsening skin problems. Assess patient medication profile and any OTC medications such as those containing aspirin or NSAIDs that would increase the risk of bleeding. Instruct patient to avoid these drugs and not to begin any OTC medications without first discussing with nurse or physician. Teach patient to alternate rest and activity periods if feeling fatigued and to organize shopping and chores in a way to minimize energy expenditures.

II.   POTENTIAL ALTERATION IN CIRCULATION related to CHANGES IN ECG T-WAVE/ST-SEGMENT AND QTc PROLONGATION, HYPOTENSION

Defining Characteristics: ECG ST and T-wave changes occurred in up to 63% of patients. Prolongation of the QTc interval occurred and in rare instances led to drug discontinuation. Ventricular and supraventricular arrhythmias also were reported. Hypotension may occur in up to 23% of patients. Low serum potassium and magnesium increase the risk of arrhythmia in patients with prolonged QTc intervals.

Nursing Implications: Do baseline assessment of cardiac status, including drug profile and possible drugs that may prolong the QT interval. If a patient has risk factors (such as congenital long QT syndrome, significant cardiovascular disease, or taking anti-arrhythmic medications), ensure that baseline ECG with QTc interval has been done and that it is done periodically during treatment. Assess baseline electrolytes, especially serum potassium and magnesium, and ensure levels are WNL before administering romidepsin. Identify patients at risk for developing QTc prolongation, such as patients on anti-arrhythmic agents and patients with hypomagnesemia or hypokalemia. Replete magnesium and potassium as ordered.

III. ALTERATION IN NUTRITION, LESS THAN BODY REQUIREMENTS, related to NAUSEA, DIARRHEA, ANOREXIA, DEHYDRATION, VOMITING, DYSGEUSIA, HYPERGLYCEMIA, HYPOALBUMINEMIA

Defining Characteristics: In clinical trials, these side effects occurred with the following frequency: nausea 56–86% (6% grades 3–4), vomiting 34–52% (5–10% grades 3–4), anorexia 23–54% (< 1–4% grades 3–4), diarrhea 20–36%, dysgeusia 15–40%, constipation 12–40%, hyperglycemia 2–51%, hypoalbuminemia < 1–48%.

Nursing Implications: Assess weight, bowel-elimination status, baseline nutritional status, and glucose level along with other labs, and monitor during therapy. Teach patient that symptoms can occur and ways to minimize these effects, such as self-administration of antinausea, anticonstipation, and antidiarrheal medications and to report symptoms that do not resolve with established plan. Assess for taste disturbances, and teach dietary modifications to minimize impact. Teach patient to identify nutritionally dense (high calories and protein in the smallest amount) foods and to keep them handy in the refrigerator. Teach patient to eat small, frequent meals and to have a bedtime snack. Teach patient that goal is to take in at least 2 quarts of fluid a day and to try to drink a glass of fluid every hour while awake. Closely monitor those patients at risk for dehydration (e.g., elderly patients). Teach patient signs and symptoms of hyperglycemia (e.g., excessive thirst, frequent urination) and to report them. Discuss any abnormalities with a physician.

Drug: rucaparib (Rubraca)

Class: Poly (ADP-ribose) polymerase (PARP) inhibitor.

Mechanism of Action: Drug inhibits PARP enzymes PARP 1, 2, and 3, which play important roles in DNA transcription, cell-cycle regulation, and DNA repair. This results in disruption of cancer cell processes with DNA damage and cell death, especially in *BRCA*-mutated tumor cells.

Metabolism: Rapid absorption after oral dosing, with maximum plasma concentration (Tmax) reached in 1.9 hours. The mean absolute bioavailability was 36% (range (30–45%). Taking the drug with a high-fat meal slows the rate of absorption, and significantly raises Cmax (20%), AUC (38%), and delays Tmax by 2.5 hours as compared to fasting. Rucaparib is approximately 70% protein-bound and is metabolized primarily by the hepatic microenzyme CYP2D6 and to a lesser extent CYP1A2 and CYP3A4. Its terminal plasma half-life is 17–19 hours. Patients with mild (CrCl 60–89 mL/min) and moderate (CrCl 30–59 mL/min) renal failure had a 15% and 32% higher steady-state AUC, respectively.

Patients with mild hepatic impairment (total BR ≤ ULN, AST > ULN or total BR 1–1.5 times ULN and any AST) had no pharmacologic difference form patients with normal hepatic function (Clovis Oncology, 2016).

Indication: Treatment of 1) patients with recurrent ovarian, fallopian tube, or primary peritoneal cancer who are in a CR or PR after platinum-based chemotherapy, as maintenance therapy; 2) adult patients with *BRCA*-mutated ovarian, fallopian tube or primary peritoneal cancer after 2 or more chemotherapy regimens.

Dosage/Range:
- When used for the 2nd indication, confirm that the patient has a deleterious *BRCA* mutation (germline and/or somatic), as determined by an FDA-approved test.
- 600 mg (two 300-mg tablets) taken orally twice daily, with or without food, until disease progression or unacceptable toxicity occurs.
- Dose modifications to manage toxicity:
  - Consider interruption of therapy or dose reduction.
    - Starting dose 600 (two 300-mg tablets).
    - First dose reduction: 500 mg twice daily (one 300-mg and one 200-mg tablet)
    - Second dose reduction: 400 mg twice daily (two 200-mg tablets)
    - Third dose reduction: 300 mg twice daily (one 300-mg tablet)

Drug Preparation: Available as 200-mg, 250-mg, and 300-mg tablets. Store at room temperature and keep out of the reach of children and pets.

Drug Administration:
- Teach the patient self-administration: Take rucaparib twice daily, about 12 hours apart, with or without food.
  - If a dose is missed, or the patient vomited after taking the dose, teach the patient to omit it and to take the next dose at its scheduled time. Do not take an extra dose to make up for the missed dose.
  - Teach patient to wear sunscreen and cover exposed skin when going outside in the sun, as rucaparib may cause photosensitivity.
- Assess CBC/differential at baseline and monthly thereafter. The drug should not be started until resolution of myelosuppression from prior therapy occurs (grades 0–1). Serum creatinine, cholesterol, and LFTs (AST, ALT) should be assessed baseline and periodically during therapy.
- If prolonged myelosuppression occurs, interrupt the drug and monitor CBC/differential weekly until recovery. If recovery (grades 0–1) has not occurred by 4 weeks, refer the patient to a hematologist for evaluation, including bone marrow analysis and cytogenetic study. The drug should be discontinued if MDS/AML is confirmed.
- Teach women of reproductive potential to use effective contraception during therapy and for 6 months after the last dose of rucaparib. Female patients should not breastfeed while taking the drug, or for 6 months after last dose.

Drug Interactions: Unknown.
- Rucaparib is a substrate of P-gp and BCRP but not of renal uptake or hepatic transporters.

- Rucaparib effect on other drugs has not been studied in humans.
- Anticancer drugs: Potentiation and prolongation of myelosuppression.

Lab Effects/Interference:
- Increased: serum creatinine, ALT, AST, cholesterol.
- Decreased: hemoglobin, lymphocyte count, ANC, platelet count.

Special Considerations:
- Most common adverse reactions in 20% or more of patients in clinical trials: nausea, fatigue (including asthenia), vomiting, anemia, abdominal pain, dysgeusia, constipation, decreased appetite, diarrhea, thrombocytopenia, dyspnea.
- Most common laboratory abnormalities of patients with ovarian cancer treated with rucaparib were increased creatinine (92%), increase in ALT (74%), increase in AST (73%), increase in cholesterol (30%); decreased hemoglobin 67% (23% grade 3/4), decreased platelets (39%, 6% grade 3/4), and decrease in ANC (35%, 10% grade 3/4).
- Warnings and Precautions:
  - *Myelodysplastic syndrome (MDS)/AML:* May occur and be fatal. Incidence was 1.1%; however all patients had previously received platinum and other DNA-damaging agents. Time to onset after beginning rucaparib was from 1 month to 28 months. Monitor baseline CBC/differential at baseline before beginning therapy and at least monthly. Rucaparib should not be initiated until complete hematologic recovery caused by prior chemotherapy (≤grade 1). If prolonged hematologic toxicity occurs on treatment, interrupt therapy and monitor CBC/differential weekly; if hematologic recovery to grade 1 or less does not occur after 4 weeks, refer to a hematologist for bone marrow analysis, cytogenetic study, and further investigations. Discontinue the drug if MDS/AML is confirmed.
  - *Embryo-fetal toxicity:* Teach women of reproductive potential to use effective contraception during therapy and for 6 month after the drug is discontinued and to avoid pregnancy.
  - Nursing mothers should discontinue breast-feeding or discontinue the drug.

Potential Toxicities/Side Effects and the Nursing Process

I. POTENTIAL FOR BLEEDING, ANEMIA, AND FATIGUE related to BONE MARROW SUPPRESSION

Defining Characteristics: In clinical trials, 21% of patients experienced thrombocytopenia (5% grades 3–4), and 44% anemia (25% grade 3/4). Neutropenia occurred in 15%, pyrexia in 11%, and febrile neutropenia in 1% of patients. Fatigue/asthenia occurred in 66% of patients and was severe (grades 3–4) in 8%. In laboratory studies, 35% of patients had a decrease in ANC, with 10% grade 3/4.

Nursing Implications: Evaluate CBC/differential, at baseline and then monthly. Discuss any abnormalities with the physician/NP/PA. The drug should not be started until resolution of myelosuppression from prior therapy has occurred (grades 0–1). Assess for signs and symptoms of infection, bleeding, and fatigue. Teach the patient about signs and symptoms of infection, bleeding and fatigue, and to report them immediately. Teach the patient self-care measures to minimize the risk of infection, and bleeding, including avoidance of OTC aspirin-containing medications. Teach the patient self-assessment of fatigue and to alternate rest and activity as needed. If prolonged myelosuppression occurs, interrupt the drug and monitor CBC/differential weekly until recovery. If recovery (grades 0–1) has not occurred by 4 weeks, refer the patient to a hematologist for evaluation, including bone marrow analysis and cytogenetic study. The drug should be discontinued if MDS/AML is confirmed.

II.   ALTERATION IN NUTRITION, POTENTIAL, related to NAUSEA, VOMITING, CONSTIPATION OR DIARRHEA

Defining Characteristics: Nausea was common in clinical trials (77%), as was vomiting (46%), constipation (40%), diarrhea (34%), decreased appetite (39%), and dysgeusia (39%). Abdominal pain occurred in 32% of patients.

Nursing Implications: Assess the patient's nutritional status at baseline and at each visit. Teach the patient that these side effects may occur, and teach self-management strategies such as use of antinausea medications, prevention of constipation, self-administration of antidiarrheals, and dietary modifications. Teach patient and caregiver to report any symptoms that do not improve or persist. Discuss prescription medications with the provider if there is a need to manage refractory symptoms. Teach the patient tips to increase appetite (e.g., small, frequent meals, use of spices). Offer the services of a dietitian as appropriate.

Drug: sonidegib (Odomzo)

Class: Hedgehog pathway inhibitor.

Mechanism of Action: The Hedgehog pathway is vital during embryogenesis. In the embryo the Hedgehog pathway is responsible for cell proliferation and cell differentiation into specialized cells and organs, as well as tissue migration to the correct anatomical position within the developing embryo. For example, this pathway is critical to ensuring that the spinal cord ends up in the correct place, that the developing fetus has five fingers on each hand, five toes on each foot, and that the anatomical part is heading in the correct direction (tissue polarity). The Hedgehog pathway also plays a role in cell differentiation, stem cell maintenance, and wound healing in the adult. The Hedgehog gene codes for the sonic hedgehog (SHH) protein, which will bind to a specific cell membrane receptor complex to turn on signal transduction leading to cell proliferation. The receptor complex on the cell membrane is made up of two proteins: patched (PTCH) 1, which binds the ligand SHH, and smoothened (SMO), which turns on the actual signal transduction to activate the target genes controlling cell proliferation. Normally this pathway is almost shut down after the fetus is formed. If the PTCH1 gene becomes mutated, then the PTCH1 protein cannot bind to SMO, releasing SMO to send unlimited messages to the target genes so that unregulated cell proliferation occurs along with angiogenesis. Mutations in PTCH1, PTCH2, SMO, and another gene can occur in basal cell carcinoma (BCC). UV exposure mutates PTCH1 and is thought to be responsible for 70% of BCCs (von Gorlin syndrome). Another 10–20% of BCCs appear to be due to mutations in SMO, leading to unregulated signaling to the genes responsible for cell proliferation. Thus in BCC, the Hedgehog pathway becomes turned on without regulation, resulting in malignant transformation and growth. Hedgehog signaling from the tumor to the stroma (surrounding tissue that stimulates tumor growth) increases tumorigenesis (Gupta et al., 2010). Sonidegib binds to and inhibits SMO, the transmembrane protein that is necessary for activation of Hedgehog signal transduction. By inactivating SMO, the pathway is turned off.

Metabolism: After oral administration, $< 10\%$ of the dose is absorbed, and in fasting conditions, the median time to peak concentration (T_{max}) was 2–4 hours. Steady state is achieved in about 4 months after starting the drug. A high-fat meal increases exposure to sonidegib (AUC, C_{max}). Drug is highly bound to human plasma proteins. Elimination half-life ($t_{1/2}$) is about 28 days. Drug is primarily metabolized by CYP3A, and the drug and metabolites are eliminated via the hepatic route. Of the absorbed dose, 70% is excreted in the feces, and 30% in the urine. Mild hepatic dysfunction and mild or moderate renal impairment did not affect drug exposure. In a cross study comparison, AUC appears to be 1.7 fold higher in Japanese healthy subjects compared to Western (Whites and Blacks) subjects.

Indication: Treatment of adult patients with locally advanced basal cell carcinoma that has recurred following surgery or RT, or those who are not candidates for surgery or RT.

Dosage/Range: 200 mg PO once daily taken on an empty stomach, at least 1 hour before or 2 hours after a meal. Continue drug until disease progression or unacceptable toxicity.

- **Verify the pregnancy status of females of reproductive potential prior to beginning sonidegib. Drug should not be given to pregnant patients.**
- Assess baseline serum creatine kinase (CK) levels and renal function before starting sonidegib therapy, periodically during therapy, and as clinically needed.
- Interrupt sonidegib for
  - Severe or intolerable musculoskeletal adverse reactions.
  - First occurrence of serum CK elevation between 2.5–$10 \times$ ULN.
  - Recurrent serum CK elevation between 2.5–$5 \times$ ULN.
- Resume sonidegib at 200 mg when signs/symptoms resolve.
- Permanently discontinue drug for
  - Serum CK elevation $> 2.5 \times$ ULN with worsening renal function.
  - Serum CK elevation $> 10 \times$ ULN.
  - Recurrent serum CK elevation $> 5 \times$ ULN.
  - Recurrent severe or intolerable musculoskeletal adverse reactions.

Drug Preparation: Available as a 200-mg capsule.

Drug Administration:
- Verify that female patients of reproductive potential **are not** pregnant. Teach patient to use effective contraception during therapy and for 20 months following last dose.

- Teach male patients to use condoms with a pregnant partner or a female partner of reproductive potential during treatment and for at least 8 months after last dose to prevent semen exposure that may contain the drug.
- Teach patients not to donate blood or blood products while taking sonidegib and for 20 months following last dose as blood may be given to a woman with reproductive potential.
- Assess serum creatine kinase (CK) and renal function tests prior to starting drug in all patients, and to report any new unexplained muscle pain, spasms, tenderness, weakness, or myalgias right away.
- Teach patient how to take drug (1) take on an empty stomach, 1 hour before or 2 hours after a meal, and (2) if a dose is missed, resume dosing with the next scheduled dose.

Drug Interactions:
- CYP3A inhibitors: can increase sonidegib peak serum concentration; do not give concomitantly with strong (e.g., saquinavir, telithromycin, ketoconazole, itraconazole, voriconazole, posaconazole, nefazodone) or moderate (e.g., atanzavir, diltiazem, fluconazole) inhibitor. If a moderate CYP3A inhibitor must be coadministered, administer the moderate CYP3A4 inhibitor for < 14 days and monitor closely for adverse reactions, especially in the musculoskeleton.
- CYP3A4 inducers: may decrease sonidegib peak serum levels (e.g., carbamazepine, efavirenz, modafinil, phenobarbital, phenytoin, rifabutin, rifampin, St. John's wort). Avoid concomitant administration of strong or moderate CYP3A4 inducers.
- Acid reducing agents: concomitant administration of PPIs or H_2- may decrease the mean sonidegib steady-state AUC by 34%.

Lab Effects/Interference:
- Increased serum creatinine, serum creatine kinase (CK), glucose, lipase, AST, ALT, amylase
- Anemia, lymphopenia

Special Considerations:
- Most common adverse reactions occurring in ≥ 10% of patients were muscle spasms, alopecia, dysgeusia, fatigue, nausea, musculoskeletal pain, diarrhea, decreased weight, decreased appetite, myalgia, abdominal pain, headache, pain, vomiting, pruritis.
- Warnings and Precautions:
  - *Embryo-fetal toxicity (also black box warning):* Drug can cause severe birth defects or embryo-fetal death.
    - Ensure, and verify using pregnancy testing, thatfemale patients of reproductive potential are NOT pregnant when starting the drug, and that they understand the mportance of using effective contraception during and after drug therapy for at least 20 months.
    - Ensure male patients understand to use condoms with female partners while receiving the drug, and for at least 8 months after last dose to prevent drug exposure to the female via semen. Mothers should not breast-feed while receiving the drug, and for at least 20 months afterwards.
    - Teach patients not to donate blood or blood products during treatment and for at least 20 months after the last dose.

- *Musculoskeletal adverse reactions:* These reactions may be accompanied by serum CK elevations, a class effect of Hedgehog pathway inhibitors. Obtain serum CK and creatinine levels prior to starting therapy, periodically during therapy, and as clinically indicated. Interrupt drug temporarily if musculoskeletal reactions.
  - Muscle spasms most frequent (54%), followed by musculoskeletal pain (32%), and myalgia (19%). Increased serum CK levels occurred in 61% (grade 3–4, 8%).
  - Serum CK is monitored as rhabdomyolysis may occur, defined as serum CK $>$ 10 $\times$ baseline value with concurrent 1.5 $\times$ or greater increase in serum creatinine above baseline value.
  - Assess serum creatinine and CK levels baseline during treatment, and periodically. Teach patient to report any new unexplained muscle pain, tenderness, or weakness during treatment, right away. If a patient has musculo-skeletal adverse reactions with concurrent serum CK elevations $>$ 2.5 $\times$ ULN, assess serum creatinine and CK **at least weekly** until resolution of clinical signs and symptoms. Discuss dose modification with provider based on severity.
- Alopecia occurs in 53% of patients. Fatigue occurs in 41%, headache in 15%, and itching in 10%. Amenorrhea lasting for at least 18 months may occur in premenopausal women (Novartis, 2017).
- Nutritional impact symptoms may occur: Dysgeusia occurs in 46% of patients, nausea in 39%, diarrhea in 32%, decreased weight in 30%, decreased appetite in 23%, and vomiting in 11% of patients.

Potential Toxicities/Side Effects and the Nursing Process

I. ALTERATION IN SEXUALITY/REPRODUCTION related to POTENTIAL TERATOGENICITY

Defining Characteristics: Drug is teratogenic, embryotoxic, and fetotoxic, causing embryo-fetal death and severe birth defects. Drug may be excreted in the semen. Drug can also be passed through blood transfusions to pregnant patients. In clinical studies 2/14 premenopausal women receiving either a 200 mg or 800 mg daily dose developed amenorrhea that lasted for at least 18 months.

Nursing Implications: Assess reproductive status, sexual activity, and birth control measures used for both men and women. Teach male patients to use condoms with spermicide, even after vasectomy, during sexual intercourse with female partners while receiving therapy and for at least 8 months after the last dose. Ensure that women have had a negative pregnancy test within 7 days of starting the drug. Teach women to use highly effective contraception measures that have $<$ 1% risk of failure prior to starting therapy, and to continue using it for at least 20 months after last dose of sonidegib. Teach female patients to notify their providers immediately if they become pregnant while taking the drug or within 20 months after the last drug dose, and male patients to notify provider if his female partner becomes pregnant while taking sonidegib or within 8 months of the last drug dose. Nursing mothers should either discontinue sonidegib or discontinue nursing. Teach patients not to donate blood while taking sonidegib and for 20 months after the last drug dose.

II.   ALTERATION IN COMFORT related to MUSCULOSKELETAL ADVERSE EFFECTS

Defining Characteristics: Musculoskeletal adverse reactions are common. Muscle spasms occur in 54% of patients, and are grade 3 in 3%. Musculoskeletal pain affects 32%, and myalgia 19% of patients. Elevation in serum creatine kinase (CK) may occur, and rhabdomyolysis defined as serum CK increase $> 10 \times$ baseline value with a concurrent increase of $1.5 \times$ or greater increase in serum creatinine above baseline, occurs rarely (0.2%). Musculoskeletal pain and myalgia usually preceded increase in serum CK values. The median time to onset of grade 2 or higher serum CK elevations was 12.9 weeks, and median time to resolution to $\leq$ grade 1 was 12 days. Medical intervention was necessary in 29% of patients (magnesium supplementation, muscle relaxants, analgesics, or opioids) including 5% who required IV hydration or hospitalization. Incidence of increased serum creatinine was 92% but remained in the normal range in 76% of patients. Increased CK occurred in 61% and was grades 3–4 in 8%.

Nursing Implications: Teach patient that musculoskeletal adverse events may occur and to report right away any new or unexplained muscle pain, tenderness, or weakness during treatment or that persists after discontinuing sonidegib. Discuss with provider need for magnesium, muscle relaxants, and/or analgesics, and teach patient self-care strategies. Assess baseline serum CK and creatinine levels before initial dose of sonidegib, during treatment, and if patient reports muscle symptoms. If patient has musculoskeletal adverse reactions and concurrent serum CK elevations $> 2.5 \times$ ULN, assess serum creatinine and CK levels at least weekly. Discuss with provider temporary dose interruption or discontinuation based on severity of musculoskeletal symptoms and CK elevations.

III.   POTENTIAL ALTERATION IN NUTRITION related to DYSGEUSIA, NAUSEA, DIARRHEA, DECREASED APPETITE, WEIGHT LOSS, VOMITING

Defining Characteristics: Nutritional impact symptoms may occur. Incidence of dysgeusia was 46%, nausea 39%, diarrhea 32%, and vomiting 11%. Decreased weight occurred in 30% of patients, and decreased appetite in 23%. Hyperglycemia occurred in 51%.

Nursing Implications: Assess nutritional status, weight, and bowel-elimination status pattern baseline and at each visit. Teach patient self-care measures: to take OTC antidiarrheal medication as needed; to take antinausea medicine as prescribed; to modify diet if diarrhea (foods to decrease motility, fluids to reverse dehydration); high-calorie, high-protein foods frequently in small amounts if decreased taste, appetite and/or weight loss; taste stimulation strategies for altered taste. Teach patient to report any symptoms that do not resolve or improve with the established plan. To increase appetite, encourage patients to use a small plate, small portions and not to fill the plate with food; take antiemetic 30 minutes prior to eating, if nausea, and to eat small, frequent meals. Arrange dietary consultation if available and needed. Note trends in weight and discuss with provider if significant.

IV.   ACTIVITY INTOLERANCE, POTENTIAL, related to FATIGUE, ASTHENIA, HEADACHE, ABDOMINAL PAIN

Defining Characteristics: Fatigue occurs in 41% of patients, abdominal pain in 18%, headache in 15%, and pain in 14%.

Nursing Implications: Assess baseline activity and energy level, and teach patient this symptom may occur. Assess patient's activity patterns, and suggest ways to conserve energy.

V.   ALTERATION IN BODY IMAGE, POTENTIAL, related to ALOPECIA, PRURITIS

Defining Characteristics: Alopecia occurs in 53% of patients, and pruritis in 10%.

Nursing Implications: Assess baseline skin itching and hair distribution on scalp. Teach patient that alopecia may occur. Encourage patient to get a wig (cranial prosthesis) prior to starting therapy as appropriate. Assess effect of hair loss on patient's body image. Encourage patient to verbalize feelings and provide emotional support. If needed, involve social worker in supportive counseling. Encourage patient to use scarves and hats as appropriate and to attend supportive educational sessions such as ACS Look Good Feel Better programs if available. Teach patient self-care strategies for pruritis, and to report it if it persists. Teach patient not to scratch because it may impair skin integrity.

Drug: sorafenib (Nexavar)

Class: Kinase inhibitor; multiple-targeted TKI, antiangiogenesis agent.

Mechanism of Action: Drug inhibits a number of tyrosine kinases, including Raf kinase, an enzyme in the RAS pathway (RAS is mutated in about 20–30% of solid tumors), as well as RTKs VEGFR-2 and PDGFR-b, thus preventing cell proliferation and angiogenesis. First, sorafenib inhibits the signaling cascade in the RAS pathway, blocking uncontrolled cell growth from either excessive stimulation of the RAS pathway, or through mutations of RAS and RAF proteins. In addition, sorafenib inhibits angiogenesis by preventing the message from vascular endothelial growth factor (VEGF), telling endothelial cells to proliferate and migrate, from reaching the cell nucleus (signal transduction), and angiogenesis is prevented. It also inhibits the message that would be sent to the cell nucleus when the ligand PDGF attaches to its receptor PDGFR-b; PDGF is necessary for pericytes around the blood vessels to provide external structure during angiogenesis and to regulate capillary blood flow.

Metabolism: After oral administration, mean relative bioavailability is 38–49%, peak plasma levels in 3 hours, and mean elimination half-life of 25–48 hours. Steady-state plasma concentrations reached in 7 days with multiple doses. When drug is given with a high-fat meal, bioavailability is reduced 29% compared to that in a fasted state. Drug is highly protein-bound (99.5%). Drug is metabolized by liver P450 microenzyme system, mediated by CYP3A4, with glucuronidation mediated by UGT1A9. There are eight metabolites of the drug. Following oral dose, 96% of the drug was recovered in 14 days, with 77% of the dose excreted in the feces, and 19% in the urine.

Indication: Indicated for the treatment of patients with
- Advanced renal cell cancer (RCC).
- Unresectable hepatocellular carcinoma (HCC).
- Differentiated thyroid carcinoma (DTC), which is locally recurrent, metastatic, or progressive, and refractory to radioactive iodine treatment.

Contraindications: Sorafenib is contraindicated in (1) patients with known severe hypersensitivity to sorafenib or any other component of Nexavar, and (2) in combination with carboplatin and paclitaxel in patients with squamous cell NSCLC.

Dosage/Range:
- For patients with (1) RCC, (2) HCC, and (3) DTC:
  - 400 mg (two 200-mg tablets) PO bid taken without food, at least 1 hour before or 2 hours after a meal (total daily dose of 800 mg), until patient is no longer clinically benefiting from drug or toxicity is unacceptable. Total daily dose is 800 mg.
  - Temporarily interrupt sorafenib before major surgical procedures.
  - When dose reduction is indicated, reduce to a single 400-mg PO dose daily; if further reduction needed, change to 400-mg PO every other day.

Dose Modifications (see package insert):
- Permanent discontinuation of sorafenib for (1) grade 2 and above cardiac ischemia +/or infarction; grade 4 CHF; (2) grade 2 and above hemorrhage requiring medical intervention; (3) grade 4 severe or persistent HTN despite adequate antihypertensive therapy; (4) GI perforation (any grade); (5) severe drug-induced liver injury (DILI, see package insert) (Bayer, 2018); (6) grade 4 nonhematological toxicity.
  - *Cardiovascular events:* CHF: (a) grade 3: interrupt sorafenib until ≤ grade 1, and resume 1 dose level; (b) grade 4 CHF: discontinue drug.
  - *HTN:* (a) grade 2 asymptomatic, diastolic pressure 90–99 mm Hg: treat with antihypertensive therapy. Continue sorafenib dosing as scheduled and closely monitor BP; (b) grade 2 symptomatic/persistent OR grade 2 symptomatic increase by > 20 mm Hg (diastolic) or > 140/90 mm Hg if previously within normal range OR (c) grade 3: interrupt sorafenib until symptoms resolve and diastolic BP < 90 mm Hg. Treat with antihypertensives; reduce dose to one dose level when sorafenib resumed. If needed, reduce another dose level.
  - *QTc Prolongation:* Monitor electrolytes and ECG; if QTc is > 500 msec or for an increase from baseline of 60 msec or greater: interrupt sorafenib, correct electrolye abnormalities (magnesium, potassium, calcium), and discuss with provider when/if to resume therapy.
  - *Nonhematological toxicities:* (a) Grade 2: treat on time, and decrease one dose level; (b) grade 3: first occurrence: interrupt until ≤ grade 2, then resume with dose reduced one dose level; no improvement within 7 days, or second or third occurrence: interrupt sorafenib until ≤ grade 2, then resume with a dose decrease 2 dose levels; fourth

occurrence: interrupt until ≤ grade 2, and resume sorafenib with a dose decrease of 3 dose levels; (c) grade 4: permanently discontinue sorafenib.
- *Dose levels for HCC and RCC requiring dose reduction:* Usual dose 400 mg PO bid; first dose level: reduce from 400 mg bid to 400 mg once daily; second dose level: reduce to 400 mg every other day.
- *Dose levels for DTC requiring dose reduction:* Usual dose 400 mg PO bid. first dose level: reduce to 600 mg qd [400 mg and 200 mg 12 hours apart (e.g., two 200-mg tablets then 12 hours later one 200-mg tablet)]. Second dose level reduction to 400 mg daily (200 mg tablet twice daily); third dose level reduction to 200 mg once daily.
- *Skin toxicity HCC, RCC, and DTC* (e.g., Hand Foot Skin Reaction, HFSR):
  - Grade 1: numbness, dysesthesia, paresthesia, tingling, painless swelling, erythema, or discomfort of hands or feet that does not disrupt patient's normal activities: continue treatment at current dose and consider topical treatment for symptomatic relief.
  - *Grade 2:* painful erythema and swelling of hands or feet and/or discomfort affecting ADLs: (1) first occurrence: continue sorafenib, consider topical therapy for symptomatic relief; for HCC and RCC patients, no dose change; for DTC patients, decrease sorafenib dose to 600 mg daily; (2) no improvement within 7 days or second or third occurrence: interrupt sorafenib until toxicity resolves to grades 0–1 (HCC, RCC) or to grade 1 for DTC patients; then for patients with HCC or RCC, resume sorafenib at a reduced dose by one dose level (400 mg daily or 400 mg every other day), and for DTC patients, if sorafenib resumed, decrease dose to next level. Fourth occurrence: discontinue sorafenib.
  - *Grade 3:* moist desquamation, ulceration, blistering or severe pain in hands or feet, or severe discomfort, cannot do ADLs or work: (1) **first occurrence**, interrupt sorafenib until toxicity resolves to grade 0-1 (HCC, RCC) or grade 1 (DTC). Resume sorafenib at a dose reduced by one dose level (e.g., HCC, RCC: 400 mg qd or 400 mg every other day). DTC see schema above for dose reduction by one level. **Second occurrence**: interrupt sorafenib until toxicity resolves to grade 0–1 (HCC, RCC) or grade 1 (DTC). Resume sorafenib at a dose reduced by one dose level (e.g., HCC, RCC: 400 mg qd or 400 mg every other day), and by 2 dose levels in DTC patients (see schema above for dose reduction by level). **Third occurrence:** discontinue sorafenib.

Dose Reductions DTC:
- First dose reduction: Decrease from 400-mg bid to a 600-mg total daily dose (e.g., 400 mg PO then 200 mg 12 hours later (2 tablets and then 1 tablet 12 hours later, either dose can come first).
- Second dose reduction: 400-mg daily dose taken as 200 mg twice daily.
- Third dose reduction: 200 mg once daily.
- For patients with grades 2–3 dermatologic toxicity, once patient toxicity has resolved to grade 0–1, after at least 28 days of treatment at a reduced dose, the sorafenib dose can be increased one dose level from the reduced dose. It is estimated about 50% of patients will be able to tolerate the increased dose without recurrent grade 2-3 toxicity (Bayer, 2019).
- No dose reduction for renal dysfunction (mild, moderate, or severe [not requiring dialysis]).
- Hepatic dysfunction: no dose modification necessary for mild or moderate impairment, but patients with severe impairment have not been studied.

Drug Preparation:
- None, oral.
- Drug is available in 200-mg tablets.

Drug Administration:
- Teach patient to (1) take without food, at least 1 hour before or 2 hours after a meal; (2) not make up a missed dose; skip the dose and take the next scheduled dose as scheduled.
- Monitor BP weekly × 6 during first weeks of therapy. HTN should be well controlled.
- Drug should be temporarily interrupted prior to a major surgical procedure. Decision when to resume drug is based on clinical judgment of adequate wound healing.

Drug Interactions:
- CYP3A4 inhibitors (e.g., ketoconazole): none.
- CYP isoform-selective substrates (e.g., midazolam, omeprazole, dextromethorphan): none.
- CYP2C9 substrates (e.g., warfarin): monitor INR regularly.
- CYP3A4 inducers (e.g., carbamazepine, dexamethasone, phenobarbital, phenytoin, rifampin, St. John's wort) are expected to increase the metabolism of sorafenib and decrease sorafenib serum concentration. If they must be coadministered, consider an increase in sorafenib dose, and monitor closely for toxicity.
- CYP2B6 and CYP2C8 substrates: sorafenib inhibits the metabolism of these substrates, thus increasing serum levels. Avoid concomitant administration.
- Warfarin: INR may be elevated. Monitor INR and dose warfarin accordingly.

Lab Effects/Interference:
- Increased lipase (41%), amylase (30%).
- Decreased phosphate (45%).
- Lymphopenia (23%), neutropenia (5%), anemia (44%), thrombocytopenia (12%).
- May prolong QTc on ECG.
- Increased bilirubin, transaminases, INR.
- Low TSH.

Special Considerations:
- Drug is well tolerated with most common side effects (incidence ≥ 20%) being diarrhea, fatigue, infection, alopecia, HFSR, rash, weight loss, decreased appetite, nausea, GI and abdominal pain, hypertension, and hemorrhage.
- Warnings and Precautions:
    - *Risk of cardiac ischemia and/or infarction:* In HCC study, incidence 2.7% compared to placebo arm where incidence was 1.3% (Bayer, 2018). In RCC study incidence was 2.9% (vs 0.4%), and in DTC study, incidence was 1.9% (vs 0%). Drug should be temporarily or permanently discontinue if cardiac ischemia and/or infarction develop.
    - *Risk of hemorrhage:* If bleeding necessitates medical intervention, consider permanent drug discontinuation. To reduce the risk of bleeding in DTC, prior to treatment with sorafenib, tracheal, bronchial, and esophageal tumor infiltration should be locally treated.
    - *Risk of HTN:* Monitor BP weekly during the first 6 weeks of sorafenib therapy, then monitor and treat HTN if it develops. HTN is usually mild to moderate, occurs early

in the course of treatment, and is effectively managed with standard anti-HTN therapy. If HTN is severe or persistent despite standard antihypertensive therapy, consider temporary or permanent drug discontinuance.

- *Risk of dermatologic toxicities:* HFSR and rash are most common, usually grades 1–2, and appear during the first 6 weeks of therapy. Management strategies include topical therapies for symptomatic relief, temporary treatment interruption and/or dose modification. If severe or persistent, permanent drug discontinuation should occur. There have been reports of severe dermatologic toxicities, including Stevens-Johnson Syndrome (SJS), and toxic epidermal necrolysis (TEN), which may be life-threatening. Discontinue sorafenib if SJS or TEN occur.
- *Risk of GI perforation:* Occurs infrequently, and occurs in < 1% of patients. Patients should be taught to go to the ED immediately if they develop severe abdominal pain, with or without nausea, vomiting, or constipation, and the provider should be notified. Sorafenib should be discontinued if a GI perforation occurs.
- *Warfarin:* Infrequent bleeding with elevations in INR have been reported. Monitor patients closely if taking Coumadin while receiving sorafenib for changes in prothrombin time (PT), INR, or bleeding. Teach patients to report any signs/symptoms of bleeding.
- *Wound-healing complications:* Sorafenib should be temporarily interrupted before major surgical procedures, and the drug resumed after adequate wound healing has occurred.
- *Increased mortality observed* when administered in combination with carboplatin/paclitaxel and gemcitabine/cisplatin in squamous cell lung cancer identified in a subset analysis. The use of sorafenib in patients with squamous cell NSCLC receiving carboplatin/paclitaxel is contraindicated. Sorafenib in patients with squamous cell NSCLC receiving gemcitabine/cisplatin is not recommended. Sorafenib is not FDA approved for treatment of patients with NSCLC.
- *Risk of QT interval prolongations:* Sorafenib can prolong the QT/QTc interval and increase the risk for ventricular arrhythmias. Monitor ECG for prolonged QTc intervals in patients with CHF, bradyarrhythmias, drugs known to prolong the QTc (e.g., methadone), and electrolyte abnormalities. Do not use sorafenib for patients with congenital long QT syndrome. Monitor electrolytes and correct abnormalities (e.g., magnesium, potassium, calcium). Interrupt sorafenib if QTc is > 500 msec or for an increase from baseline of 60 msec or more (Bayer, 2017).
- *Drug-induced hepatits* (defined as elevated transaminase levels > 20 × ULN or transaminases with significant clinical sequelae (e.g., elevated INR, ascites, death, or requiring transplantation) may occur rarely. It is characterized by liver damage with significant increases in transaminases, which may result in hepatic failure and death (Bayer, 2017). Monitor LFTs baseline prior to starting therapy and regularly thereafter. If other causes are excluded (e.g., viral hepatitis, progressive malignancy), then discontinue sorafenib.
- *Embryo-fetal risk:* Drug is teratogenic and embryo-fetal toxic. Verify the pregnancy status of women of reproductive potential before starting the drug. Women of childbearing potential should use effective contraception to avoid pregnancy, or if the patient becomes pregnant while receiving the drug, patient should be apprised of

potential hazard to the fetus. Women should not breast-feed while receiving the drug. Teach female patients of reproductive potential to use effective contraception during therapy and for at least 6 months after last dose, and male patients with female sexual partners of reproductive potential to use effective contraception during therapy and for 3 months after the last dose of sorafenib.

- *Impairment of TSH Suppression in DTC:* DTC patients had a baseline TSH < 0.5 m U/L, but on sorafenib therapy, 41% of patients had an elevated TSH compared to 16% receiving placebo. In the study, the median maximal TSH was 1.6 mU/L and 25% had TSH levels > 4.4 mU/L. Monitor TSH levels baseline, then monthly in patients with DTC, and adjust thyroid replacement medication as needed.
- Drug may rarely cause osteonecrosis of the jaw (seen in post-marketing reports).

Potential Toxicities/Side Effects and the Nursing Process

I.   POTENTIAL ALTERATION IN CIRCULATION related to HYPERTENSION, CARDIAC ISCHEMIA, MYOCARDIAL INFARCTION OR QT PROLONGATION WITH VENTRICULAR ARRHYTHMIAS

Defining Characteristics: Hypertension occurred in 9–41% of patients studied. Rarely, hypertensive crisis, myocardial ischemia and/or infarction occurred. In the HCC group receiving sorafenib, the incidence of cardiac ischemia/infarction was 2.7% (1.3% in placebo group), and in the RCC group receiving sorafenib, the incidence was 2.9% (0.4% in placebo group). Drug can rarely prolong QT/QTc interval and increase risk of ventricular arrhythmias, including torsades de pointes.

Nursing Implications: Review cardiac history. Assess baseline blood pressure, and monitor weekly during the first 6 weeks of treatment. Discuss antihypertensive therapy with physician or NP. If hypertension is severe and refractory to maximal antihypertensive therapy, drug should be interrupted or discontinued. If a patient develops cardiac ischemia and/or infarction while receiving the drug, discuss drug interruption or discontinuance with the physician. If the patient has cardiac ischemia or has had an infarction, discuss the risks and benefits before beginning therapy. Drug should be avoided in patients with congenital long QT interval. Document baseline QTc in patients with CHF, bradyarrhythmias, taking other drugs known to prolong the QT interval such as antiarrhythmics, and patients with electrolyte imbalances, such as magnesium and potassium. Correct hypomagnesemia, hypokalemia and hypocalcemia in the patients and monitor ECG throughout treatment.

II.   ALTERATION IN SKIN INTEGRITY AND COMFORT related to HFS, RASH, POTENTIAL

Defining Characteristics: Erythema is common. Rash or skin desquamation occurred in 40% of patients, and HFS (acral erythema) in 30% of patients compared to 16% and 7% of patients, respectively, receiving placebo. HFS is generally grades 1–2, and appears during the first 6 weeks of treatment. Alopecia occurred in 27% of patients, pruritus in 19%, and dry skin in 11%. Areas of hyperkeratosis may occur on the soles of the feet, forming calluses (Wood, 2006). Rarely, folliculitis, eczema, erythema multiforme occurs. There have been reports of severe dermatologic toxicity (e.g., SJS and toxic epidermal necrolysis (TEN)), which may be life-threatening.

Nursing Implications: Assess baseline skin integrity, including soles of feet and palms of hands, and teach patient that these symptoms may occur. If the patient develops calluses on the feet, suggest applying topical exfoliating agents such as Kerasal (OTC) or Keralac (prescription) on the calluses ONLY. Teach patient to self-assess all skin areas and to report rash, as well as redness, swelling, and/or pain anywhere, particularly the soles of feet and palms of hands. Teach patient to avoid activities that increase blood flow in the hands and feet, such as hot showers and baths, and to take tepid showers to reduce likelihood and severity of HFS. Teach patient to avoid constrictive clothing and repetitive movements that can irritate the opposing skin. Teach patient to use skin emollients to prevent skin from drying and cracking starting on day 1 of therapy, followed by wearing cotton gloves or socks to keep the emollient close to the skin until absorbed. Teach patient to elevate hands and feet when sitting or lying down; apply ice packs or cool compresses indirectly to hands or feet for up to 20 minutes; gently pat skin dry after bathing or washing; and avoid contact with laundry detergents or cleaning products with strong chemicals.

After assessment, discuss dose modification with physician or NP if grade 2 (PAIN) or 3 (see Dose Modifications section and package insert).

Grade 1: Numbness, dysesthesia, paresthesia, tingling, painless swelling, erythema, or discomfort of the hands or feet that does not disrupt ADLs; no change, use topical therapy for symptomatic relief.

Grade 2: Painful erythema and swelling of the hands or feet and/or discomfort affecting ADLs: First occurrence, continue therapy and use local symptomatic treatment; if no improvement within 7 days, or second or third occurrence, interrupt therapy until grades 0–1, then resume with dose reduction by one dose level, either 400 mg daily or every other day; if fourth occurrence, discontinue drug.

Grade 3: Moist desquamation, ulceration, blistering or severe pain of the hands or feet, or severe discomfort that causes the patient to be unable to work or do ADLs: first or second occurrence, interrupt until toxicity resolves to grades 0–1; then decrease dose by one dose level (400 mg daily or every other day); third occurrence: discontinue drug.

Discontinue drug if SJS or TEN are suspected.

III.   ALTERATION IN NUTRITION, LESS THAN BODY REQUIREMENTS, related to DIARRHEA, NAUSEA, ANOREXIA, VOMITING, CONSTIPATION

Defining Characteristics: Diarrhea occurs in 43% of patients, constipation 15%, nausea 23%, vomiting 16%, and anorexia 16%.

Nursing Implications: Assess nutrition status, bowel-elimination status baseline and periodically during treatment. Involve nutritionist as needed to minimize symptoms, such as

BRAT diet for patient with diarrhea (e.g., bananas, rice, applesauce, and toast); increase dose-dense calories and fluid in the diet, and strategies to increase appetite. Teach patient how to manage nausea, vomiting, diarrhea, and constipation, including self-administration of OTC medications or prescribed medications, dietary modifications, and increased hydration. Teach patient to report symptoms that do not improve or that persist despite interventions.

IV.   ALTERATION IN CIRCULATION related to HEMORRHAGE, POTENTIAL

Defining Characteristics: Hemorrhage occurred in 15% of patients as compared to 8% in the placebo arm. In patients with hepatocellular carcinoma, 2.4% of patients bled from esophageal varices (compared to 4% in control group). Incidence of grades 3–4 bleeding was 2% and 0%, respectively.

Nursing Implications: Teach patient to report any episodes of bleeding right away. If bleeding requires medical intervention, discuss drug discontinuation with the physician.

V.   POTENTIAL FOR INFECTION AND BLEEDING related to NEUTROPENIA AND THROMBOCYTOPENIA

Defining Characteristics: Neutropenia occurred in 5% of patients, anemia in 44% of patients, and thrombocytopenia in 12% of patients in clinical trials.

Nursing Implications: Assess baseline blood counts and platelets. Teach patient to report fever, and signs/symptoms of infection or bleeding right away. Assess medication profile and OTC medications taken. Teach patient to avoid OTC medications containing NSAIDs or aspirin. Teach patient to talk to nurse or physician before beginning any OTC medications.

Drug: sunitinib malate (Sutent)

Class: Kinase inhibitor; multitargeted TKI.

Mechanism of Action: Drug has both antitumor and antiangiogenesis activity and inhibits multiple RTKs that are involved in tumor growth, angiogenesis, and metastatic cancer progression. It inhibits PDGFRs (α and β), vascular endothelial growth factor receptors (VEGFR-1, -2, -3), stem cell factor receptor (KIT), fms-like tyrosine kinase-3 (FLT-3), CSF-1R, and the glial cell-line–derived neurotrophic factor receptor (RET).

Metabolism: After oral ingestion, maximal plasma concentrations are reached within 6–12 hours, regardless of food intake. Drug and primary metabolite bind to plasma protein 90–95%. Drug is metabolized by the cytochrome P450 enzyme CYP3A4 to produce its primary metabolite, which is then itself metabolized by CYP3A4. Terminal half-life of sunitinib and its primary metabolite are 40–60 hours and 80–110 hours, respectively. Drug is primarily excreted via the feces.

Indication: Drug is FDA approved for the treatment of patients with
- Gastrointestinal stromal tumor (GIST) after disease progression on or intolerance to imatinib mesylate.
- Advanced renal cell carcinoma (RCC).
- Adjuvant treatment of adult patients with RCC having a high risk of recurrence following nephrectomy.
- Progressive, well-differentiated pNET when disease is unresectable, locally advanced, or metastatic.

Dosage/Range:
- GIST and advanced RCC: 50 mg orally once daily, with or without food, for 4 weeks, followed by 2 weeks off, in a 6-week cycle.
- RCC Adjuvant therapy: 50 mg orally once daily × 4 weeks, with or without food, followed by 2 weeks off (6-week cycle),
- pNET: 37.5 mg orally once daily, with or without food, continuously, without a scheduled off-treatment period (Pfizer, 2018).

Dose Modifications:
- Dose-interrupt and/or dose-modify in 12.5-mg increments or decrements based on individual tolerance and safety. Maximum dose in pNET study was 50 mg daily. In the adjuvant RCC study, minimum dose administered was 37.5 mg (Bayer, 2017).
- Dose-interrupt and/or reduce in patients without signs/symptoms of CHF who have an LVEF < 50% and > 20% below baseline or below the LLN if no baseline obtained. Discontinue drug if patient has clinical manifestations of CHF.
- If coadministration with *strong CYP3A4 inhibitors* (e.g., ketoconazole) may increase serum sunitinib levels, so dose reduction is necessary: Reduce sunitinib dose to a minimum of 37.5 mg (GIST and RCC) or 25 mg (pNET). Avoid coadministration with a strong CYP3A4 inhibitor if possible and select an alternate coadministration medication is recommended.
- If coadministration with *strong CYP3A4 inducer (e.g., rifampin)* is necessary, which may decrease sunitinib serum level: Increase sunitinib dose to a maximum of 87.5 mg (GIST and RCC) or 62.5 mg (pNET) daily if coadministration is unavoidable. If the dose is increased, monitor patient carefully for toxicity. Avoid coadministration if possible.

Drug Preparation:
- None, oral tablet. Take with or without food.
- Available as 12.5-mg, 25-mg, 37.5-mg, and 50-mg hard gelatin capsules.

Drug Administration:
- Teach patient self-administration: (1) take with or without food; (2) not to open capsule; (3) avoid grapefruit juice or fruit; (4) if a dose is missed, take it as soon as remembered. If it is close to the time of your next dose, do not take it but take the next scheduled dose. Do not take more than 1 dose of sunitinib at a time.
- Laboratory monitoring:
  - CBC with platelet count, serum chemistries, including phosphate and LFTs at the beginning of each treatment cycle. Repeat lab tests as clinically indicated.
  - Assess baseline thyroid function, as acquired hypothyroidism may occur.

- Assess baseline ECHO results; if cardiac risk factors, monitor the ECHO periodically, as well as assess for signs/symptoms of CHF.
- Patient should have a baseline ECG with calculation of QTc interval, and this should be monitored during therapy. Frequency of monitoring should increase if the patient is taking an interacting drug with increased risk of toxicity.
- Assess female patients of reproductive potential pregnancy status prior to starting sunitinib therapy as drug is fetotoxic. Teach patient to use effective contraception during sunitinib therapy and for at least 4 weeks after the final dose. Teach male patients with female sexual partners of reproductive potential to use effective birth control measures during therapy for 7 weeks after last sunitinib dose.

Drug Interactions:
- CYP3A4 inhibitors (e.g., atazanavir, clarithromycin, indinavir, itraconazole, ketoconazole, nelfinavir, nefazodone, ritonavir, saquinavir, telithromycin, voriconazole, grapefruit or grapefruit juice): Increase plasma level of sunitinib; do not give together, or dose-reduce sunitinib if used concurrently.
- CYP3A4 inducers (e.g., carbamazepine, dexamethasone, phenobarbital, phenytoin, rifabutin, rifampin, rifapentine, St. John's wort): Decrease plasma level of sunitinib by 23–46%; do not give together, or increase dose of sunitinib if given concurrently.

Lab Effects/Interference:
- Decreased lymphocyte (38%), neutrophil (53%), red blood cell (26%), and platelet counts (38%). Elevated serum lipase (25%) and amylase (17%).
- Elevated AST/ALT (39%), alkaline phosphatase (24%), total bilirubin (16%), indirect bilirubin (10%).
- Elevated serum creatinine (12%), uric acid (15%).
- Decreased phosphate (9%), increased or decreased potassium (6%, 12%), increased or decreased sodium (10%, 6%).
- Decreased thyroid function (acquired hypothyroidism).
- QT/QTc prolongation on ECG.

Special Considerations:
- Most common adverse reactions (≥ 20%) are fatigue, asthenia, fever, diarrhea, nausea, mucositis/stomatitis, vomiting, dyspepsia, abdominal pain, constipation, hypertension, peripheral edema, rash, HFS, skin discoloration, dry skin, hair-color changes, altered taste, headache, back pain, arthralgia, extremity pain, cough, dyspnea, anorexia, and bleeding.
- Patient should have CBC with platelet count, serum chemistries, including phosphate and liver function tests at the beginning of each treatment cycle; check baseline thyroid function, as acquired hypothyroidism may occur. In addition, patients should have a baseline ECHO, and if cardiac risk factors, the ECHO should be monitored periodically, as well as assessment for signs/symptoms of CHF. Patient should have a baseline ECG with calculation of QTc interval, and this should be monitored during therapy. Frequency of monitoring should increase if the patient is taking an interacting drug, with increased risk of toxicity.

- Warnings and Precautions:
  - *Hepatotoxicity:* is rare (incidence $<$ 1%), but may result in liver failure or death. Observe patient for signs/symptoms of liver failure (jaundice, elevated LFTs with encephalopathy, coagulopathy, and/or renal failure). Assess LFTs before starting the drug, during each treatment cycle, and as clinically indicated. Interrupt drug for grades 3–4 hepatotoxicity, and if unresolved, permanently discontinue drug. Drug should NOT be restarted if patient subsequently experiences severe changes in LFTs or has other signs/symptoms of liver failure. Patient safety with ALT or AST $>$ 2.5 $\times$ ULN or if liver metastases, $>$ 5.0 $\times$ ULN has not been established (Pfizer, 2017).
  - *Cardiovascular events:* Heart failure, cardiomyopathy, myocardial ischemia, and MI have been reported, some fatal. Incidence in studies was 3% of CHF (no patient was receiving adjuvant sunitinib). Discontinue sunitinib in patients with clinical manifestations of CHF; interrupt and/or reduce dose in patients without clinical evidence of CHF but do have an ejection fraction of $>$ 20% but $<$ 50% below baseline or below LLN if baseline LVEF was not obtained (Pfizer, 2018).
    - Use sunitinib cautiously in patients who are at risk for or who have a history of these events. Patients should be carefully monitored for clinical signs and symptoms of CHF while receiving sunitinib, and LVEF should be monitored baseline and periodically during therapy.
    - In patients without cardiac risk factors, a baseline LVEF should be considered.
    - Drug may cause adrenal insufficiency, so patients who are experiencing stress (e.g., surgery, trauma, severe infection) should be monitored closely.
  - *QT interval prolongation and torsade de pointes:* Drug may prolong QTc interval (drug interval for depolarization and repolarization of the heart).
    - It is dose dependent, and torsades de pointes or ventricular tachycardia has occurred in $<$ 0.1% of patients.
    - Use drug cautiously in patients at risk for prolonged QT intervals (patients with a history of QT prolongation, who are taking antiarrhythmics, with a preexisting cardiac disease, bradycardia, or electrolyte disturbance).
    - Monitor patient electrolytes and ECG baseline and during treatment, and replete electrolytes to normal values (especially potassium and magnesium).
    - If the patient is also receiving concomitant treatment with a strong CYP3A4 inhibitor that can increase sunitinib plasma concentrations, consider dose reduction of sunitinib and use caution, assessing for QTc prolongation by ECG baseline and regularly during therapy.
  - *Hypertension:* Monitor for HTN and treat with standard antihypertensive medications. If severe HTN, interrupt sunitinib until HTN controlled.
  - *Hemorrhagic events and viscus perforation:* Epistaxis is most common, but GI, respiratory, tumor, urinary tract, and brain hemorrhages have been reported. Across studies, the incidence of hemorrhagic events was 30%. Rarely, GI perforation has occurred. Tumor-related hemorrhage may occur suddenly, and if a pulmonary tumor (metastatic), may pesent as hempysis or pulmonary hemorrhage. Sunitinib is NOT approved for use in patients with lung cancer. Monitor patients with serial CBCs and PE if patient develops hemorrhage.

- *Tumor Lysis Syndrome (TLS):* Identify patients with RCC or GIST with high-tumor burden and discuss TLS prophylaxis (e.g., hydration, correction of uric acid, and monitoring of renal and electrolytes) with physician/NP/PA, and monitor patient closely.
- *Thrombotic Microangiopathy (TMA):* TMA, including thrombotic thrombocytopenic purpura (TTP) and hemolytic uremic syndrome (HUS) have been reported in patients receiving sunitinib alone and also sunitinib and bevacizumab. If TMA occurs, sunitinib should be discontinued promptly, as reversal of TMA has been observed after drug discontinuation.
- *Dermatologic toxicities:* Rarely, severe cutaneous reactions have occurred such as erythema multiforme (EM), Stevens-Johnson Syndrome (SJS), and toxic epidermal necrolysis (TEN). If patient develops signs or symptoms of EM, SJS, or TEN (e.g., progressive skin rash, with blisters or mucosal lesions), sunitinib treatment should be discontinued; If SJS or TEN is diagnosed, sunitinib must NOT be restarted. Necrotizing fasciitis has also been reported, including sites such as the perineum, and secondary to fistula formation; the drug should be discontinued in these patients.
- *Thyroid dysfunction:* Assess baseline thyroid function studies before starting treatment and monitor throughout treatment. Assess patient for signs/symptoms of hypo or hyperthyroidism and thyroiditis and if found, discuss with provider laboratory confirmation and monitoring. If hypo-, hyperthyroid, or thyroiditis occurs, discuss with physician/NP/PA standard medical management.
- *Hypoglycemia:* Sunitinib treatment can result in symptomatic hypoglycemia (incidence 0%–10% across clinical studies). Patients with pre-existing diabetes mellitus are at increased risk. Assess baseline blood glucose and monitor during therapy and after therapy is completed/discontinued; monitor patients with diabetes closely, as antidiabetic drug dose may need to be modified.
- *Wound healing:* Therapy should be temporarily interrupted in patients undergoing major surgical procedures due to risk of delayed wound healing. Ensure complete wound healing prior to resuming drug after major surgery; discuss with physician.
- *Osteonecrosis of the jaw* may rarely occur with sunitinib therapy. Consider completing preventive dentistry prior to starting drug. Avoid dental procedures while receiving sunitinib therapy if possible. Patients at risk include those receiving bisphosphonates and those with dental disease.
- *Proteinuria and nephrotic syndrome* have been reported. Assess urinalysis for protein baseline and periodically during treatment, with a 24-hour urine collection for protein if proteinuria occurs.
  - Interrupt sunitinib and dose-reduce for 24-hour urine protein $\geq$ 3 grams.
  - Discontinue sunitinib in patients with nephrotic syndrome or repeat episodes of urine protein $\geq$ 3 grams despite dose reductions.
  - The safety of continued sunitinib therapy in patients with moderate-to-severe proteinuria is unknown.
- *Embryo-fetal toxicity:* Drug is teratogenic and embryo-fetal toxic. Women of childbearing potential should be advised to use effective contraception to avoid pregnancy during therapy and for 4 weeks after final sunitinib dose. Women should not breastfeed while receiving the drug. Teach male patients with female sexual partners of reproductive potential to use effective contraception during therapy and for 7 weeks after final sunitinib dose.

Potential Toxicities/Side Effects and the Nursing Process

I. ALTERATION IN CIRCULATION, POTENTIAL, related to LEFT VENTRICULAR DYSFUNCTION, HEMORRHAGE

Defining Characteristics: Fifteen percent of patients had a decrease in left ventricular ejection fraction (LVEF) to below the lower limit of normal (LLN). Some patients (18–37%) developed bleeding events: epistaxis was most common. Less commonly, patients experienced rectal, gingival, upper GI, genital, wound bleeding, and tumor hemorrhage (NSCLC, squamous histology). Rarely, patients on clinical trials had myocardial ischemia, and one patient experienced a fatal myocardial infarction while on treatment. Rarely, GI complications including GI perforation have occurred in patients with intra-abdominal malignancies treated with sunitinib.

Nursing Implications: Assess baseline and periodic LVEF tests, as well as assess patients for any signs or symptoms of congestive heart failure. Ensure patient has a baseline determination of LVEF and that patients with cardiac disease have the determination repeated regularly during therapy. Discuss any abnormalities with physician or NP. Patients with CHF prior to starting therapy should begin sunitinib at a reduced dosage. Teach patient to perform daily weights at home and to report a weight gain of 5 lbs. or more, as well as any signs or symptoms of dyspnea or bleeding right away. Teach patient that nosebleeds may occur, and to apply pressure and hold the head down; if nosebleed does not stop within 15 minutes, patient should go to ED and call physician.

II. ALTERATION IN CIRCULATION, POTENTIAL, related to QTc PROLONGATION

Defining Characteristics: Patients may develop QT prolongation on EKG. Do NOT administer to patients with prolonged QTc or who may develop prolonged QTc (hypokalemia, hypomagnesemia, hypocalcemia, other drugs that prolong the QTc). Prolonged QTc in the setting of low magnesium and hypokalemia sets the stage for torsades de pointes, with ventricular tachycardia, fibrillation, and sudden cardiac death possible.

Nursing Implications: Assess patient's drug profile to ensure that the patient is not taking any drugs that may increase the QTc interval. Assess baseline QTc interval. Identify patients at risk for development of prolonged QTc (congenital long QTc) syndrome, prolonged QTc > 450 msec, taking antiarrhythmics or other drugs that can prolong the QTc interval (hypokalemia, hypomagnesemia, concomitant CYP3A4 strong inhibitors). Correct electrolyte abnormalities (e.g., magnesium, calcium, potassium) before starting vandetanib and monitor periodically during therapy. Hypokalemia, hypocalcemia, and hypomagnesemia in the setting of prolonged QTc may lead to torsades de pointes, ventricular fibrillation, and sudden cardiac death. QTc must be assessed baseline, and periodically during therapy. Following any dose reduction for QT prolongation, or any dose interruptions > 2 weeks, QT assessment should be conducted as previously described. If the patient has diarrhea, serum electrolytes and EKGs will need to be assessed more frequently, and electrolytes repleted. Because of the long half-life of 50–100 hours of sunitinib and its principal metabolite, a prolonged QT interval may take a few weeks to resolve. Serum potassium level should be maintained at 4 mEq/L or higher (within normal range) and serum magnesium and calcium kept WNL. Teach patient to correctly take sunitinib as prescribed, and to avoid any drugs that may interact with it, until discussion with the physician, NP, PA, or nurse. See Introduction to *Chapter 5* for a full discussion of assessing the QT (QTc) interval in patients receiving drugs that may increase the risk of serious complications.

III.   POTENTIAL ALTERATION IN CIRCULATION related to HYPERTENSION

Defining Characteristics: Hypertension occurred in 15–28% of patients being studied, compared to 11% receiving placebo. Rarely, hypertensive crisis, myocardial ischemia, and/or infarction occurred. Rarely on clinical trials, patients presented with seizures and radiologic evidence of reversible posterior leukoencephalopathy syndrome RPLS (hypertension, headache, decreased alertness, altered mental functioning, and visual loss). In patients with metastatic RCC, sunitinib-associated hypertension is associated with improved clinical outcomes without HTN-associated adverse events (Rini et al., 2011).

Nursing Implications: Assess baseline blood pressure, and monitor weekly during the first treatment cycle. Discuss antihypertensive therapy with physician or NP. If hypertension is severe (SBP > 200 mm Hg, DBP > 100 mm Hg), or refractory to maximal antihypertensive therapy, drug should be interrupted until BP controlled, or discontinued. If RPLS occurs, the drug should be interrupted.

IV.   ALTERATION IN SKIN INTEGRITY AND COMFORT related to SKIN DISCOLORATION, HFS, RASH, DEPIGMENTATION OF HAIR

Defining Characteristics: Rash affected 14% of patients, skin discoloration (yellow color) 30%, and HFS 14%. HFS differs from classic chemotherapy induced HFS in that the lesions are localized and hyperkeratotic. Changes may present as painful, symmetrical erythematous and edematous areas on palms and soles, ± paresthesias (Kollmannsberger et al., 2011). Preexisting sole hyperkeratosis may increase risk of developing painful lesions that restrict mobility. Hair-color changes occurred in 7% of patients: when on the drug for 4 weeks, the hair is depigmented (white), while pigment returns on the 2-week break off treatment, giving the hair a zebra-like appearance. Alopecia occurred in 5% of patients.

Nursing Implications: Assess baseline skin integrity, including soles of feet and palms of hands, and teach patient that these symptoms may occur. If patient has hyperkeratotic areas, discuss with physician/midlevel referral to podiatrist for evaluation/potential callus removal. Teach patient to self-assess all skin areas and to report rash, as well as redness, swelling, and/or pain anywhere, particularly the soles of feet and palms of hands. Teach patient to moisturize skin on soles of feet, palms of hands frequently and to wear thick cotton socks and avoid constrictive footwear, hot water, and excessive friction. Teach to avoid activities that increase blood flow in the hands and feet, such as hot showers and baths, and to take tepid showers to reduce likelihood and severity of HFS. Teach patient to avoid constrictive clothing and repetitive movements that can irritate the opposing skin. Teach patient to use skin emollients to prevent skin from drying and cracking. As needed, discuss with physician/midlevel, prescription of symptomatic medications: topical or systemic analgesics, pregabalin, steroid creams, dermabond (Kollmannsberger et al., 2011). Discuss with physician/midlevel dose modifications if grade 2 (dose interruption, usually for 3 days), and restart at same dose or dose reduction.

V. ALTERATION IN BOWEL-ELIMINATION STATUS related to DIARRHEA, CONSTIPATION

Defining Characteristics: Diarrhea occurs in 40% of patients, constipation 20%. Diarrhea may be irregular, with diarrhea occurring on a few days, alternating with days of normal bowel movements.

Nursing Implications: Assess bowel-elimination status, baseline and periodically during treatment. Teach patient how to manage diarrhea including self-administration of OTC medications (e.g., Imodium) or prescribed medications; avoidance of stool softeners and some fiber supplements, magnesium-containing antacids; dietary modifications (avoid spicy, fatty foods, caffeine, fruit); and increased hydration. Involve nutritionist as needed to minimize symptoms, such as BRAT diet for patient with diarrhea (i.e., bananas, rice, applesauce, and toast); increase dose-dense calories and fluid in the diet, and strategies to increase appetite. If patient develops constipation, teach self-care strategies to prevent it (stool softeners, increased fluids, fruits, and vegetables). Teach patient to report symptoms that do not improve or that persist despite treatment.

VI. POTENTIAL FOR INFECTION AND BLEEDING related to NEUTROPENIA AND THROMBOCYTOPENIA

Defining Characteristics: Neutropenia occurred in 39–45% of patients, anemia 25–37% of patients, and thrombocytopenia 18–19% of patients in clinical trials.

Nursing Implications: Assess baseline blood counts and platelets. Teach patient to report fever, and signs/symptoms of infection or bleeding right away. Assess medication profile and OTC medications taken. Teach patient to avoid OTC medications containing NSAIDs or aspirin. Teach patient to talk to nurse or physician before beginning any OTC medications.

VII. ALTERATION IN NUTRITION, LESS THAN BODY REQUIREMENTS, related to NAUSEA, STOMATITIS

Defining Characteristics: Patients developed nausea (31%), vomiting (24%), stomatitis (29%), and anorexia (33%). Other changes that may occur are taste changes, dry mouth, indigestion, and anorexia.

Nursing Implications: Assess nutritional status, integrity of oral mucosa baseline and periodically during treatment. Teach patient that these side effects may occur and to report them. Teach patient self-administration of antiemetics prior to administration of drug if nausea or vomiting has occurred. Teach patient other self-care strategies, such as to eat small, frequent meals; avoid foods that are sweet, fried, or fatty; avoid bad smells; and drink small amounts of fluids frequently. Teach patient to report persistent or continued nausea and/or vomiting. Assess efficacy and discuss change in antiemetic drug with physician if regimen ineffective. Teach patient to assess oral mucosa regularly, use oral hygiene regimen such as sodium bicarbonate in water after meals and at bedtime, and report signs/symptoms of stomatitis. Teach patient diet modification to minimize oral discomfort, such as avoiding hot, spicy, or acidic foods; eating small pieces of cool or cold foods; using a straw for drinking liquids.

Drug: talazoparib (Talzenna)

Class: PARP (poly [ADP-ribose] polymerase) inhibitor.

Mechanism of Action: Talazoparib inhibits PARP enzymes, including PARP1 and 2, which are important for DNA repair. Drug is believed to kill breast cancer cells having defective DNA repair genes (BRCA1 and BRCA2) by blocking the fall back DNA repair pathway, the PARP pathway. This results in DNA damage, decreased cell proliferation, and apoptosis.

Metabolism: Maximum time to peak serum drug level is 1–2 hours after oral dosing, with 74% drug binding to plasma proteins. Mean terminal plasma half-life is 90 hours. Drug metabolism does not involve hepatic routes, but is mono-oxidation, dehydrogenation, cysteine conjugation of mono-desfluoro-talazoparib and glucuronide conjugation. Drug is excreted primarily in the urine [68.7% (54.6% unchanged)] with 19.7% in the feces (13.6% unchanged).

Indications: Treatment of adult patients with deleterious or suspected deleterious germline breast cancer susceptibility gene (BRCA) mutation, HER2 negative, locally advanced or metastatic breast cancer using an FDA approved test to confirm germline BRCA mutations.

Contraindications: None.

Dosage/Range: 1 mg PO qd, with or without food, until disease progression or unacceptable toxicity. See below for patients with renal impairment or coadministration with P-glycoprotein (P-gp) inhibitors.

Dose Modification:
- Dose reduction levels: Starting dose: talazoparib 1 mg (one 1-mg capsule) once daily. (1) 1st dose reduction: 0.75 mg (three 0.25-mg capsules) once daily; (2) 2nd dose reduction: 0.5 mg (two 0.25-mg capsules) once daily; (3) 3rd dose reduction: 0.25 mg (one 0.25-mg capsule) once daily.

- Dose Modifications:
  - Hemoglobin < 8 g/dL: Hold talazoparib until Hgb ≥ 9 g/dL, resume talazoparib at a reduced dose;
  - Platelet count < 50,000/μL: Hold talazoparib until platelet count ≥ 75,000/μL, resume talazoparib at a reduced dose;
  - Neutrophil count (ANC) < 1000/μL: Hold talazoparib until ANC ≥ 1,500/μL, resume talazoparib at a reduced dose;
  - Non-hematologic grade 3 or 4: Hold talazoparib until ≤ grade 1; consider recuming talazoparib at a reduced dose or discontinue.
- Patients with renal failure (CrCl 30-59 mL/min as talazoparib clearance is decreased by 37.1%) = dose is 0.75 mg once daily.
- Use with P-glycoprotein (P-gp) inhibitors (e.g., amiodarone, carvedilol, clarithromycin, itraconazole, verapamil): increased talazoparib exposure by 45%; reduce talazoparib dose to 0.75 mg once daily; when the P-gp inhibitor is discontinued, increase the talazoparib dose after 3-5 half-lives of the P-gp inhibitor) to usual dose.

Drug Preparation: Available as a 1-mg and 0.25-mg capsule. Keep out of reach of children and pets.

Drug Administration:
- Assess medication profile for important P-gp and BCRP inhibitors with pharmacist, and if found, discuss implications with provider.
- Assess CBC/differential, glucose, renal function, LFTs baseline, and monitor during therapy. Verify negative pregnancy test in females of reproductive potential.
- Assess patient body image and provider resources for a cranial prosthesis (e.g., wig) as appropriate.
- Teach patient/family:
  - Swallow hard capsule whole; do not open or dissolve it.
  - Take capsule at about the same time every day.
  - If patient vomits or misses a dose, do not take an additional dose. The next prescribed dose should be taken at the usual time.
  - Potential side effects, self-management techniques, and when to call the provider (including the telephone number, on-call number).
  - Signs and symptoms of infection and bleeding to self-assess for, and to report right away. Make sure patient has a thermometer at home. Teach measures to minimize the risk of infection and bleeding.
  - Fatigue self-care techniques.
  - Effective contraception for women of reproductive potential during and for at least 7 months after the last talazoparib dose.
  - Effective contraception for men with female partners of reproductive potential and pregnant partners to use effective contraception during therapy and for at least 4 months after the last talazoparib dose.

Drug Interactions:
- P-gp inhibitors (certain ones): reduce talazoparib dose and monitor for potential increased talazoparib adverse reactions.

- Breast Cancer Resistance Protein (BCRP) transporter inhibitors: monitor for potential increased talazoparib adverse reactions.

Lab Effects/Interference:
- Decreased Hgb, leukocytes, neutrophils, platelets, serum calcium.
- Increased serum glucose, AST, ALT, alkaline phosphatase.

Special Considerations:
- Most common adverse effects ($\geq$ 20%) in clinical trials were: fatigue, anemia, nausea, neutropenia, headache, thrombocytopenia, vomiting, alopecia, diarrhea, decreased appetite.
- Alopecia may occur in 25% of patients. Assess body image and need for resources for cranial prosthesis (e.g., wig) if needed.
- Warnings and Precautions:
  - *Myelodysplastic syndrome (MDS)/AML):* rare, 0.3% incidence in 2 patients who had also received prior chemotherapy with cisplatinum agents and/or other DNA damaging agents or RT. Ensure that the patient's bone marrow has recovered from previous chemotherapy before starting talazoparib. Monitor baseline CBC/differential then monthly. If prolonged hematologic toxicity from talazoparib , interrupt talazoparib and monitor CBC/differential weekly until recovery. If not recovered in 4 weeks, a hematologist should evaluate the patient for possible MDS/AML, including a bone marrow analysis and blood sample for cytogenetics. Drug should be discontinued if a diagnosis of MDS or AML is confirmed.
  - *Myelosuppression:* talazoparib may impair hematopoiesis and can cause anemia, neutropenia, and thrombocytopenia. Grade 3 or higher anemia occurred in 39% of patients, neutropenia in 21% and thrombocytopenia in 15%. Ensure complete hematologic recovery from prior therapy before starting talazoparib. Assess CBC/differential baseline then monthly.
  - *Embryo-fetal toxicity:* Talazoparib is feto-toxic. Verify negative pregnancy status of women of reproductive potential before starting the drug. Teach (1) effective contraception for women of reproductive potential during and for at least 7 months after the last talazoparib dose; (2) effective contraception for men with female partners of reproductive potential or pregnant partners to use effective contraception during therapy and for at least 4 months after the last talazoparib dose.

Potential Toxicities/Side Effects and the Nursing Process

I.   POTENTIAL FOR INFECTION, BLEEDING, ANEMIA, AND FATIGUE related to BONE MARROW SUPPRESSION

Defining Characteristics: In clinical trials, 35% of patients experienced neutropenia (–18% grades 3–4), 27% thrombocytopenia (11% grades 3–4), and 53% anemia (38% grade 3 and 1% grade 4). Fatigue/asthenia occurred in 62% of patients and was severe (grades 3–4) in 8%.

Nursing Implications: Evaluate CBC/differential, hemoglobin/hematocrit, and platelets at baseline and then monthly. Discuss any abnormalities with the physician/NP/PA. The drug should not be started until resolution of myelosuppression from prior therapy has occurred (grades 0–1). Assess for signs and symptoms of infection, bleeding, and fatigue. Teach the patient about signs and symptoms of infection and bleeding, and to report them immediately. Teach the patient self-care measures to minimize the risk of infection and bleeding, including avoidance of OTC aspirin-containing medications. Teach the patient self-assessment of fatigue and to alternate rest and activity as needed. If prolonged myelosuppression occurs, interrupt the drug and monitor CBC/differential weekly until recovery. If recovery (grades 0–1) has not occurred by 4 weeks, refer the patient to a hematologist for evaluation, including bone marrow analysis and cytogenetic study. The drug should be discontinued if a diagnosis of MDS or AML is confirmed.

II.   ALTERATION IN NUTRITION, POTENTIAL, related to NAUSEA, VOMITING, DECREASED APPETITE, OR DIARRHEA

Defining Characteristics: Nutritional impact symptoms occurred in clinical trials with nausea affecting 49% of patients, vomiting (25%), diarrhea (22%), and decreased appetite (21%).

Nursing Implications: Assess the patient's nutritional status at baseline and at each visit. Teach the patient that these side effects may occur, and teach self-management strategies such as use of antidiarrheals, antinausea medications, and dietary modifications and to report any symptoms that do not improve. Discuss prescription antiemetic medications with the provider if there is a need to manage refractory symptoms. Teach the patient tips to increase appetite (e.g., small, frequent meals, use of spices). Offer the services of a dietitian as appropriate.

III.   ALTERATION IN COMFORT related to HEADACHE

Defining Characteristics: In clinical trials, headache occurred in 33% of patients.

Nursing Implications: Assess the patient's baseline level of comfort. Teach the patient that headache may occur, and teach self-management strategies, including self-administration of acetaminophen. Teach the patient to report symptoms that do not improve. If this occurs, discuss with the physician/NP/PA prescription medication for refractory symptoms.

Drug: temsirolimus (Torisel)

Class: Kinase inhibitor; mTOR inhibitor.

Mechanism of Action: Drug binds to the intracellular protein FKBP-12, and the protein-drug complex inhibits mTOR (or FKBP 12) kinase that is responsible for cell division. mTOR is also responsible for sensing the nutrients in the cell's environment and also for organizing actin, trafficking of the membrane, insulin secretion, protein degradation, protein kinase C signaling, and tRNA synthesis. Inhibition of the kinase makes the cell think it is starving and it stops growing (arrests cell growth in G1 phase of the cell cycle). This reduces the levels of HIFs and VEGF. As more is learned about the function of this pathway, it appears that rapamycin and mTOR inhibitors affect only some of mTOR functioning.

Metabolism: The drug is metabolized by the P450 microenzyme system in the liver (CYP3A4) into five metabolites. Sirolimus is the active metabolite. Metabolites are primarily excreted in the feces (82% within 14 days). Mean half-lives of temsirolimus and sirolimus were 17.3 hours and 54.6 hours, respectively. Patients with baseline bilirubin $> 1.5 \times$ ULN have an increased risk of grades 3–4 adverse effects and death.

Indication: For the treatment of advanced renal cell cancer.

Contraindication: Drug is contraindicated in patients with bilirubin $> 1.5 \times$ ULN.

Dosage/Range:
- 25-mg IV over 30–60 minutes once weekly until tumor progression or intolerable toxicity.
  - Pretreat with diphenhydramine 25–50-mgIV or equivalent 30 minutes before dose as ordered.

Dose Modifications:
- Hold temsirolimus for ANC $< 1,000/mm^3$, platelet count $< 75,000/mm^3$, or NCI CT-CAE grade 3 or greater adverse reactions. Once toxicities have resolved to grade 2 or less, may restart temsirolimus at a dose reduced by 5 mg/233 k to a dose no lower than 15 mg/week (Wyeth, 2015).
- Hepatic Impairment: dose-reduce in patients with mild hepatic impairment (BR > 1–$1.5 \times$ ULN or AST $>$ ULN but BR $\leq$ ULN): Reduce dose to 15 mg/week. Drug contraindicated in patients with a bilirubin $> 1.5 \times$ ULN.
- Concomitant strong CYP3A4 inhibitors: avoid; if must be coadministered, reduce temsirolimus dose to 12.5 mg/week. If the strong inhibitor is discontinued, allow a washout period of one week before adjusting the temsirolimus dose back to dose used before initiation of strong CYP3A4 inhibitor.
- Concomitant strong CYP3A4 inducers: avoid; if must be coadministered, raise temsirolimus dose from 25 mg/week up to 50 mg/week. If the strong inducer is discontinued, return to the temsirolimus dose used prior to starting the strong inducer.

Drug Preparation:
- Temsirolimus is supplied as a Torisel kit containing temsirolimus vial (25 mg/mL) and diluent vial containing 1.8 mL (with overfill).
- Before preparation, store in the refrigerator at 2–8°C (36–46°F) and protect from light.
- During preparation, protect from excessive room light and sunlight. Inspect product for particulate matter and decolorization before administration.
- Do not use bags or tubing containing the plasticizer DEHP [di(2-ethylhexyl) phthalate], which may leach DEHP from the PVC infusion bags or sets into IV solution and be administered into the patient.

TREATMENT

- Step 1: Inject 1.8 mL of supplied diluent into vial that together with an overfill of 0.2-mL results in a 10-mg/mL solution.
- Invert vial to mix, and allow air bubbles to subside. This vial is stable for 24 hours at controlled room temperature. ALWAYS combine temsirolimus injection with the supplied diluent BEFORE adding to infusion bag. Direct addition of drug to aqueous solution will result in precipitation of the drug.
- Step 2: Withdraw ordered drug amount from vial [prepared in step 1 (e.g., 2.5 mL for a temsirolimus dose of 25 mg)], and further dilute into an infusion bag containing 250 mL of 0.9% sodium chloride injection. Use an IV container such as glass, polyolefin, or polyethylene. Invert bag or bottle to mix but do not shake, as this will cause foaming. Protect IV bag containing temsirolimus from excessive room light and sunlight.
- Do not add drug directly to aqueous infusion solutions as it will cause drug precipitation. Always combine with diluent first, before adding to infusion solution. Use of 0.9% Sodium Chloride USP is recommended as drug has not been studied in other IV solutions.
- Inspect the solution for particulate matter and discoloration prior to administration.
- Drug must be used within 6 hours from the time that temsirolimus is first added to 0.9% Sodium Chloride Injection, USP.
- Drug contains polysorbate 80, which increases the rate of DEHP extraction from PVC.

Drug Administration:
- Check CBC weekly, and chemistries every other week. Hold for ANC < 1,000 cells/mm^3, platelet count < 75,000 cells/mm^3, or grade 3 or higher toxicity (NCI CTCAE). Assess baseline LFTs, as dose is reduced in patients with impaired hepatic function.
- Drug should be stored in bottles (glass, polypropylene) or plastic IV bags (polypropylene, polyolefin) that do not contain DEHP. The drug should be administered through a non-DEHP, nonpolyvinylchloride (non-PVC) tubing with appropriate filter. An administration set that does not contain DEHP with an inline filter < 5 microns, such as a polyethylene-lined administration set with an inline polyether sulfone filter with a pore size < 5 microns, should be used. Do not use bags or tubing containing the plasticizer DEHP [di(2-ethylhexyl) phthalate], which may leach from the PVC infusion bags or sets into IV solution and be administered into the patient.
- Administer the final diluted drug solution within 6 hrs from the time that temsirolimus is first added to the 0.9% sodium chloride injection, USP.
- Premedicate with 25–50 mg diphenhydramine 30 minutes before temsirolimus dose.
- After premedication, administer temsirolimus IV over 30–60 minutes once a week via an infusion pump (preferred).
- Monitor for hypersensitivity/infusion reactions (e.g., flushing, chest pain, dyspnea, hypotension, apnea, loss of consciousness, hypersensitivity, anaphylaxis) that may rarely occur, and which most often occurs very early in the first infusion, but may also occur in subsequent infusions.
  - Monitor patient closely. If a reaction occurs, stop the drug immediately, and keep vein open with a plain IV solution (e.g., 0.9% sodium chloride).
  - Have emergency equipment nearby. If stable, observe the patient for 30–60 minutes, depending upon severity of reaction.

- Physician/NP/PA may decide to resume the drug after the administration of an H1-receptor antagonist (e.g., diphenhydramine) if not already administered and/or H2 receptor antagonist (e.g., IIV famotidine 20 mg or IV ranitidine 50 mg), 30 minutes before resuming the infusion.
- Resume infusion at a slower rate (e.g., up to 60 minutes).
- A benefit-risk assessment must be done prior to continuing temsirolimus therapy if severe or life-threatening reaction occurs.
- Teach patient not to eat/drink grapefruit or grapefruit juice, and not to take St. John's wort as these interfere with temsirolimus serum levels.
- Teach female patients of reproductive potential, and male patients with female sexual partners of reproductive potential, to use effective contraception during therapy, and for at least 3 months after the final dose.

Drug Interactions:
- Strong CYP3A4 inhibitors (e.g., atazanavir, clarithromycin, indinavir, itraconazole, ketoconazole, nelfinavir, nefazodone, ritonavir, saquinavir, telithromycin, voriconazole, grapefruit juice); do not coadminister or reduce temsirolimus dose.
- Strong CYP3A4 inducers (carbamazepine, dexamethasone, phenobarbital, phenytoin, rifabutin, rifampin, rifampacin, St. John's wort): do not coadminister or consider dose adjustment if medically necessary to coadminister.
- Interactions with drugs metabolized by CYP2D6: no clinically significant effect anticipated.
- Sunitinib: Grades 3–4 dose-limiting toxicities.

Lab Effects/Interference:
- Hyperglycemia, hypertriglyceridemia, hypophosphatemia; elevated AST, alkaline phosphatase, and serum creatinine; decreased potassium.
- Neutropenia, thrombocytopenia, anemia, lymphopenia.

Special Considerations:
- Use with caution, if at all, in patients with hypersensitivity to drug, sirolimus, or polysorbate 80.
- Warnings and Precautions:
  - *Hypersensitivity infusion reactions:*
    - May be characterized by flushing, chest pain, dyspnea, hypotension, apnea, loss of consciousness, hypersensitivity, and anaphylaxis.
    - May occur very early in first infusion, but also may occur with subsequent infusions.
    - Monitor patient throughout the infusion; if a severe infusion reaction occurs, interrupt the infusion, and provide appropriate supportive care as ordered.
    - If a patient develops a hypersensitivity reactions (HSR), stop the infusion, and observe the patient for at least 30–60 minutes, depending upon severity of HSR. Physician may order the drug infusion resumed with administration of an H1-receptor antagonist if not previously administered, and/or a H2-receptor antagonist (e.g., IV famotidine 20 mg) approximately 30 minutes prior to restarting the temsirolimus infusion. Resume the infusion at a slower rate (up to 60 minutes).

- If the patient has a severe or life-threatening reaction, a benefit-risk assessment should be done prior to continuing temsirolimus therapy.
- *Hepatic impairment:*
  - Patients with baseline bilirubin $> 1.5 \times$ ULN had greater toxicity than patients with lower baseline bilirubin, and grade 3 and higher adverse events occurred more frequently in patients with bilirubin $> 1.5 \times$ ULN, including death.
  - Dose should be reduced in patients with mild hepatic impairment (see Dosage/Range).
- *Hyperglycemia/glucose intolerance*, occurs commonly with 89% having at least one episode of elevated serum glucose during clinical trials and 26% of patients reporting hyperglycemia as an adverse event.
  - This may necessitate an increase in the dose of, or initiation, of insulin and/or oral hypoglycemic agent therapy.
  - Monitor serum glucose baseline, and during treatment. Teach patients to report excessive thirst or increased volume or frequency of urination.
- *Infections* may occur as temsirolimus may be immunosuppressive. Observe patients carefully for occurrence of infections, including opportunistic infections (e.g., pneumocystis jiroveci pneumonia, PJP). If patient receiving concomitant use of corticosteroids or other immunosuppressive agents, consider PJP prophylaxis.
- *Interstitial lung disease (ILD)* may occur, and some cases may be fatal.
  - Patients may be asymptomatic or minimally symptomatic with infiltrates seen on CT or CXR.
  - Symptomatic patients may have dyspnea, cough, hypoxia, fever.
  - Teach patient to report any new or worsening respiratory symptoms right away.
  - Patient should undergo baseline radiographic assessment by lung CT scan or chest radiograph prior to starting temsirolimus therapy. Follow these assessments periodically even if patient has no clinical respiratory symptoms.
  - Patients should be followed closely for clinical respiratory symptoms:
  - If clinically significant symptoms develop, consider holding temsirolimus until after recovery of symptoms and radiologic improvement related to pneumonitis.
  - Discuss medical management with physician or NP/PA. Empiric treatment with corticosteroids and/or antibiotics may be considered.
  - Opportunistic infections such as PJP should be considered in the differential diagnosis, and if the patient requires corticosteroids, PJP prophylaxis should also be considered.
- *Hyperlipidemia* occurs commonly and may require the initiation of, or increase in dose of, the patient's current lipid-lowering agent. Assess serum triglycerides and cholesterol baseline and during temsirolimus therapy.
- *Wound-healing complications:* drug has been associated with abnormal wound healing. Use drug cautiously in perioperative period. Ensure that wound is well healed before giving drug.
- *Bowel perforation* occurs rarely and may be fatal. Teach patients to report worsening abdominal pain and bloody stools right away and to come to the emergency department for immediate evaluation.

- *Renal failure* has occurred, and cases of rapidly progressive and sometimes fatal renal failure have been reported.
- *Intracerebral hemorrhage:* patients with CNS tumors (primary or metastatic) and/or receiving anticoagulation therapy may be at increased risk of intracerebral bleeding during temsirolimus therapy.
- *Coadministration with inducers or inhibitors of CYP3A metabolism:* avoid coadministration, and if medically necessary to coadminister, adjust temsirolimus dose. Teach patients NOT to eat grapefruit or drink grapefruit juice and NOT to take St. John's wort.
- *Concomitant use of temsirolimus with sunitinib:* resulted in dose-limiting toxicities (grades 3–4 erythematous maculopapular rash, gout/cellulitis requiring hospitalization).
- *Vaccinations:* avoid live vaccines (e.g., intranasal influenza, measles, mumps, rubella, oral polio, BCG, yellow fever, varicella, and TY21a typhoid) during temsirolimus therapy.
- *Proteinuria and nephrotic syndrome:* may occur. Monitor urine protein prior to start of temsirolimus therapy, and repeat periodically during therapy. Discontinue drug if patient develops nephrotic syndrome.
- *Embryo-fetal toxicity:*
  - Drug is likely to cause fetal harm. If drug is used in pregnancy, or if the patient becomes pregnant while receiving the drug, the patient should be apprised of the potential hazard to the fetus.
  - Teach women of reproductive potential to use reliable contraception to avoid pregnancy during treatment and for 3 months after last dose.
  - Teach men with partners of childbearing potential to use reliable contraception during therapy, and to continue this for 3 months after the last temsirolimus dose.
- Most common ($\geq$ 30%) side effects are rash, asthenia, mucositis, nausea, edema, anorexia.
- Most common lab abnormalities ($\geq$ 30%) were: anemia, hyperglycemia, hyperlipidemia, hypertriglyceridemia, lymphopenia, elevated alkaline phosphatase, elevated serum creatnine, hypophosphatemia, thrombocytopenia, elevated AST, and leukopenia.
- Elderly patients are more likely to experience diarrhea, edema, and pneumonia.

Potential Toxicities/Side Effects and the Nursing Process

I. POTENTIAL FOR INJURY related to INFUSION-RELATED REACTIONS AND HYPERSENSITIVITY

Defining Characteristics: The incidence of hypersensitivity is uncommon, as most patients received premedication with diphenhydramine.

Nursing Implications: Administer premedication with diphenhydramine. Stop the infusion right away if the patient has a reaction; monitor VS and O_2 saturation for at least 30–60 minutes depending on the severity of the reaction. Discuss the addition of an H_2 antagonist 30 minutes prior to resuming the infusion to prevent further hypersensitivity with physician. Ensure that medications necessary for the management of hypersensitivity/ anaphylaxis are readily available (e.g., epinephrine, antihistamines, corticosteroids). Assess baseline VS and monitor frequently during the infusion, as specified by the infusion. Be prepared to provide emergency support as necessary (including IV saline, epinephrine, antihistamines, bronchodilators). If/when symptoms resolve, resume the infusion at 50% of the rate of the previous infusion, as directed by the physician.

II. POTENTIAL FOR INFECTION AND BLEEDING related to NEUTROPENIA AND THROMBOCYTOPENIA

Defining Characteristics: Incidence of decreased neutrophils was 19% (grades 3–4 5%), platelets 40% (1%), hemoglobin 94% (20%), and lymphocytes 53% (16%). Grade 3 or 4 neutropenia occurred in 7% of patients, thrombocytopenia in 5%, and anemia in 9% of patients in clinical trials comparing doses 75–250 mg weekly. Drug is immunosuppressive, and thus, patients are at risk for opportunistic infections.

Nursing Implications: Assess baseline blood counts and platelets. Teach patient to report fever, and signs/symptoms of infection or bleeding right away. Assess medication profile and OTC medications taken. Teach patient to avoid OTC medications containing NSAIDs or aspirin. Teach patient to talk to nurse or physician before beginning any OTC medications.

III. POTENTIAL ALTERATION IN NUTRITION, LESS THAN BODY REQUIREMENTS, related to MUCOSITIS, NAUSEA, ANOREXIA, DIARRHEA, HYPERGLYCEMIA, HYPERTRIGLYCERIDEMIA, BOWEL PERFORATION

Defining Characteristics: In clinical studies, mucositis affected 70% of patients, nausea 43%, diarrhea 27%, and anorexia 40% of patients. Bowel perforation occurs rarely but may be fatal. Presentation includes fever, abdominal pain, metabolic acidosis, bloody stools, diarrhea, and/or acute abdomen. The incidence of hypercholesterolemia is 87%, triglyceridemia 83%, and hyperglycemia was 89%; in terms of grades 3 and 4 toxicities, hyperglycemia occurred in 17% of patients, hypophosphatemia 13%, and hypertriglyceridemia in 6% of patients. mTOR is involved in insulin signaling, which possibly explains the hypertriglyceridemia and hyperglycemia.

Nursing Implications: Assess serum triglycerides, cholesterol, glucose baseline and during treatment with the drug. Teach the patient to report any new or worsening abdominal pain or bloody stools right away and to come to the emergency department for immediate evaluation. Premedicate with antiemetics. Encourage small, frequent meals of cool, bland foods, and increase fluid intake. Assess oral mucosa prior to drug administration and instruct patient to report changes. Teach patient oral hygiene measures and self-assessment. Teach patient to notify physician/nurse if excessive thirst or any increase in volume or frequency of urination. Notify physician of any abnormalities and discuss implications and management.

IV.   ALTERATION IN SKIN INTEGRITY, POTENTIAL, related to RASH

Defining Characteristics: Maculopapular rash is the most common toxicity, affecting 47%; 10% had acne, 14% had a nail disorder, 11% had dry skin, and 19% pruritus.

Nursing Implications: Assess patient skin integrity, including nails baseline and regularly during treatment. Teach patient self-assessment and local comfort measures, including the use of water-based emollients. Teach patient to report skin changes and if self-care ineffective, discuss plan with physician, especially if severe.

V.   ALTERATION IN COMFORT AND ACTIVITY TOLERANCE, POTENTIAL, related to ASTHENIA

Defining Characteristics: Asthenia affects 51% of patients in clinical studies, depression 4%, but at the higher dose of 250 mg q week, 5% had grades 3 and 4 depression.

Nursing Implications: Assess baseline comfort, mental status, and activity tolerance, and reassess during treatment, asking patient to identify what activities now unable to do, sleep habits, and also feeling state. Discuss alternating rest and activity periods and also possibility of other family members or friends assisting with energy-consuming responsibilities to increase energy reserve. Assess baseline alertness, sleep patterns. Assess other drugs taken, especially those with sedating qualities, and alcohol ingestion. Instruct patient to avoid alcohol and to take drug at bedtime. Assess degree of drowsiness and dizziness for safety of patient. If significant, teach measures to ensure safety.

Drug: trametinib (Mekinist)

Class: Kinase inhibitor (MEK kinase inhibitor, first in class).

Mechanism of Action: The mitogen-activated extracellular signal regulated kinase 1 (MEK1) and MEK2 proteins are upstream regulators of the ERK (extracellular signal-related kinase) pathway, which promote cell division. Trametinib is a reversible inhibitor of MEK1 and MEK2 activation, as well as their kinase activity. The BRAF pathway includes MEK1 and MEK2, and if there is a BRAF V600E mutation, this turns on the pathway resulting in a continual signal being sent to the cell nucleus calling for cell proliferation. Trametinib turns this pathway off in tumors with the BRAF V600E mutation, such as certain malignant melanoma tumors, and leads to cell death (apoptosis).

Metabolism: After oral dosing, peak plasma level is reached 1.5 hours after the dose (T_{max}). Mean absolute bioavailability is 72%. Administration with a high-fat, high-calorie meal decreased AUC by 24%, C_{max} by 70%, and delayed T_{max} by about 4 hours, compared to when the drug is taken in a fasting state. Drug is 97.4% bound to plasma proteins. Metabolism occurs by deacetylation alone, or with mono-oxygenation, or in combination with glucuronidation. The elimination half-life of the drug is 3.9–4.8 days. Most (> 80%) of the drug and metabolites are excreted in the feces, with < 20% excreted in the urine. Mild hepatic impairment does not affect drug pharmacokinetics, but the drug was not studied in patients with moderate or severe hepatic impairment. Mild or moderate renal impairment does not affect pharmacokinetics, but the drug was not studied in patients with severe renal dysfunction.

Indications: In combination with dabrafenib, for the treatment of patients with (1) unresectable or metastatic melanoma with *BRAF V600E* or *V600K* mutations as detected by an FDA approved test as a single agent or in combination with dabrafenib; (2) *BRAF V600E or BRAF V600K*-mutation positive melanoma with lymph node involvement after complete resection as adjuvant therapy; (3) metastatic NSCLC with *BRAF V600E* muations as detected by an FDA-approved test; (4) locally advanced or metastatic anaplastic thyroid cancer (ATC) with *BRAF V600E* mutation and without any satisfactory locoregional treatment options.

Limitations of use: Trametinib is not indicated for the treatment of patients with melanoma who have progressed on prior *BRAF*-inhibitor therapy.

Contraindications: None.

Dosage/Range:
- Presence of *BRAF V600 E or V600K* mutation in tumor specimen must be confirmed by a FDA-approved detection test.
- *Unresectable or metastatic melanoma:* Trametinib 2 mg PO once daily, as a single agent or in combination with dabrafenib, until disease progression or unacceptable toxicity. Take at least 1 hour before or at least 2 hours after a meal, at about the same time each day.See dabrafenib drug information.
- *Adjuvant treatment of melanoma:* 2 mg PO daily in combination with dabrafenib, until disease progression or unacceptable toxicity, for up to 1 year. Take at least 1 hour before or at least 2 hours after a meal, at about the same time each day. See dabrafenib drug information.
- *NSCLC:* Trametinib 2 mg PO once daily, as a single agent or in combination with dabrafenib, until disease progression or unacceptable toxicity. Take at least 1 hour before or at least 2 hours after a meal, at about the same time each day. See dabrafenib drug information.
- Anaplastic thyroid cancer (ATC): Trametinib 2 mg PO once daily, as a single agent or in combination with dabrafenib, until disease progression or unacceptable toxicity. Take at least 1 hour before or at least 2 hours after a meal, at about the same time each day. See dabrafenib drug information.

Dose Modifications: When given in combination, trametinib does not receive a dose modification for the following adverse reactions of dabrafenib: noncutaneous malignancies, uveitis; also, there is no dose modification for new primary cutaneous malignancies. See dabrafenib package insert for dabrafenib dose modifications.
- Dose Levels:
  - Trametinib dose reductions: (1) First dose reduction dose is to 1.5 mg orally once daily; (2) second reduction dose is to 1 mg orally once daily; if unable to tolerate 1 mg orally, discontinue trametinib.

- *Venous thromboembolism:*
  - Uncomplicated DVT or PE: hold trametinib for up to 3 weeks; if improved to grades 0–1, resume at a lower dose level; if not, permanently discontinue trametinib.
  - If life-threatening PE, permanently discontinue trametinib.
- *Cardiac:*
  - Asymptomatic, absolute decrease in LVEF of 10% or greater from baseline AND is < institutional LLN from pretreatment value: hold drug up for up to 4 weeks, and if improved to normal LVEF value, resume trametinib dose at a lower dose level; if not improved to normal LVEF, discontinue drug permanently.
  - Symptomatic CHF, or absolute decrease in LVEF > 20% from baseline that is below LLN, permanently discontinue trametinib.
- *Ocular:*
  - Retinal pigment epithelial detachments (RPED): hold drug up to 3 weeks; if improved, resume trametinib at same or a lower dose level; if not improved, permanently discontinue trametinib or resume at a lower dose.
  - Retinal vein occlusion: permanently discontinue trametinib.
- *Pulmonary:*
  - ILD/pneumonitis: permanently discontinue trametinib.
- *Febrile Drug Reaction/Fever:*
  - Fever > 104°F, or fever complicated by rigors, hypotension, dehydration, or renal failure: hold trametinib until fever resolves, then resume trametinib at same or lower dose level.
- *Dermatologic:* Intolerable grade 2 skin toxicity or grade 3 or 4 skin toxicity: Hold trametinib for up to 3 weeks; if improved, resume trametinib at lower dose level; if not improved, discontinue drug permanently.
- *Other Adverse Reactions:*
  - Intolerable grade 2 or any grade 3 adverse reaction: hold trametinib for up to 3 weeks; if improved to grades 0–1, resume each drug at lower dose level; if not improved, permanently discontinue trametinib.
  - First occurrence of grade 4 adverse reaction: hold trametinib until adverse reaction improves to grades 0–1; then resume trametinib at a lower dose level; if no improvement, permanently discontinue drug.
  - Recurrent grade 4 adverse reaction, permanently discontinue trametinib.

Drug Preparation:
- Drug available in 0.5-mg and 2-mg tablets.

Drug Administration:
- Assess LVEF findings (ECHO or MUGA scan prior to initiating drug, then one month after initiation, and then at 2- to 3-month intervals). Hold trametinib for up to 4 weeks if absolute LVEF value decreases by 10% from pretreatment values and is < LLN. See Dose Modifications and package insert. Assess BP baseline and during treatment as HTN may develop.
- Teach patient to (1) take trametinib orally on an empty stomach, at least 1 hour before or at least 2 hours after a meal, at about the same time each day so that the drug dose is separated by 24 hours; (2) DO NOT take a missed dose within 12 hours of the next

trametinib dose, and (3) when given in combination with dabrafenib, to take trametinib with either the morning or evening dose of dabrafenib.

- Teach patient how to contact provider 24/7 and to report or seek emergency medical care for significant changes such as bleeding, difficulty breathing, T> 104°F. See patient teaching pamphlet for patients taking both Taflinar (debrafenib) and Mekinist (trametinib) available at https:// www.tafinlarmekinist.com.

Drug Interactions:
- No formal studies have been conducted.
- Drug is not a substrate of CYP enzymes or efflux transporters P-gp or BCRP in vitro.
- Drug is an inhibitor of CYP2C8 in vitro.
- Drug is an inducer of CYP3A4 in vitro, but administration with the sensitive CYP3A4 substrate everolimus did not clinically affect AUC or C_{max} of everolimus.

Lab Effects/Interference:
- Increased AST (60%), increased ALT (39%), increased alkaline phosphatase (24%).
- Hypoalbuminemia (43%), anemia (38%).
- Hyperglycemia when trametinib is combined with dabrafenib.
- Increased LVEF by ECHO or MUGA.

Special Considerations:
- Warnings and Precautions:
  - *New primary malignancies:* both cutaneous and noncutaneous malignancies can occur when trametinib is administered with dabrafenib.
    - **Cutaneous malignancies:** Incidence of basal cell carcinoma was in patients receiving trametinib with dabrafenib (3.3%). Perform dermatologic evaluations prior to starting combination, every 2 months while on therapy, and for up to 6 months after discontinuance of the combination. No dosage adjustments are recommended for patients who develop primary cutaneous malignancies.
    - **Noncutaenous malignancies**: rare *RAS* mutation-positive cancers (activation of *RAS* through mutation or other mechanisms). Incidence 1–1.4%. Monitor patients closely for signs and symptoms of noncutaneous malignancy, and permanently discontinue drug in patients who develop *RAS* mutation-positive noncutaneous cancers. No dose modification is required for noncutaneous malignancies.
    - *Hemorrhage (*including major symptomatic bleeding in a critical area or organ) can occur. In the COMBI-d study, incidence of hemorrhage in patients receiving dabrafenib and trametinib was 19%. Permanently discontinue trametinib for all grade 4 hemorrhage events, as well as grade 3 events that do not improve. Hold trametinib for up to 3 weeks for grade 3 hemorrhagic events; if improved, resume at the next lower dose level.
    - *Colitis and GI perforation:* can occur, and may be fatal. Incidence is low (colitis 0.6%, GI perforation 0.3%).
    - *Venous thromboembolism:* DVT, PE can occur. Incidence in clinical studies of DVT and PE occurred in 2.8%–4.3% of patients receiving the combination. Teach patients to seek medical care right away if they develop symptoms of DVT or PE (e.g., shortness of breath, chest pain, arm or leg swelling). Discontinue trametinib

if life-threatening PE occurs. Hold trametinib for up to 3 weeks for uncomplicated DVT and PE; if improved, resume trametinib at a lower dose level.

- *Cardiomyopathy* occurred in 3–9% of patients receiving combination, or 11% in receiving trametinib as a single agent in clinical trials. Assess LVEF by ECHO or MUGA scan before trametinib is initiated, one month after drug is started, and then at 2- to 3-month intervals while on treatment. Hold trametinib for up to 4 weeks if absolute LVEF value decreases by 10% from pretreatment values and is < LLN. Permanently discontinue drug for symptomatic cardiomyopathy or persistent asymptomatic LVEF dysfunction of > 20% from baseline that is below LLN that does not resolve within four weeks.
- *Ocular toxicities:*
  - **Retinal vein occlusion** occurred in 0.2% of patients; it may lead to macular edema, decreased visual function, neovascularization, and glaucoma. If patient reports loss of vision or other visual disturbances, patient should have an urgent (within 24 hours) ophthalmological evaluation. Drug should be discontinued if retinal vein occlusion is documented.
  - **Retinal Pigment Epithelial Detachment (RPED, uni or bilateral)** can occur when trametinib is given as a single agent or in combination with dabrafenib. If RPED occurs, it is often bilateral and multifocal in the macular region of the retina. Perform ophthalmological exam baseline, then regularly during therapy and if the patient develops visual symptoms. Hold trametinib if RPED is diagnosed. If within 3 weeks, on repeat ophthalmological evaluation, RPED has resolved, resume trametinib. If no improvement after 3 weeks, reduce the trametinib dose or discontinue drug.
- *ILD* occurred in 2% of patients receiving trametinib as a single-agent, and 2.4% in those receiving the combination. Hold drug in patients presenting with new or progressive pulmonary signs/symptoms, including cough, dyspnea, hypoxia, pleural effusion, or infiltrates, while pulmonary symptoms are worked up. If treatment-related ILD or pneumonitis is found, discontinue trametinib.
- *Serious febrile reactions:* can occur, along with hypotension, rigors or chills, dehydration or renal failure can occur when trametinib is given with dabrafenib; incidence was 17%. Fever (all grades) occurred in 57% of patients with unresectable or metastatic melanoma. Hold trametinnib for fever > 104°F or for serious febrile reactions or fever accompanied by hypotension, rigors/chills, dehydration, renal failure, and evaluate for signs/symptoms of infection. Monitor serum creatinine and renal function tests during and after severe fever. See Dose Modifications and Mekinist package insert. Administer antipyretics as secondary prophylaxis when restarting trametinib if patient had a prior episode of severe febrile reaction or fever with complications. Administer corticosteroids (e.g., prednisone 10 mg qd) for at least 5 days for second or subsequent pyrexia if temperature does not return to baseline within 3 days of onset of fever, or for fever with complications (e.g., dehydration, hypotension, renal failure, severe chills/rigors) and there is no evidence of active infection (Novartis, 2018).
- *Skin toxicity* is common (Trial 1 incidence 87%, 12% severe) and includes rash, dermatitis, acneiform rash, PPES, and erythema. Hold trametinib for intolerable or

severe skin toxicity. If improvement or recovery within 3 weeks, resume trametinib at a reduced dose. See Dose Modifications.

- *Hyperglycemia* may occur when both drugs are administered; patient may require an increase in the dose of insulin or oral hypoglycemic agent, or initiation of insulin, or of an oral hypoglycemic agent, if not already taking it. Monitor serum glucose levels baseline and during therapy, especially in patients with preexisting diabetes or hyperglycemia. Teach patients to report symptoms of hyperglycemia.
- Risks associated with combination treatment: Trametinib is indicated for use in combination with dabrafenib. Review the full pescribeing information on dabrafenib on serious risks of dabrafenib before starting patient on the combination. Teach patient of potential side effects of combination therapy, and events to report right away.
- *Embryo-fetal toxicity.* Counsel women and men of reproductive potential to use highly effective contraception during drug therapy and for 4 months after treatment.
  - If patient is receiving trametinib and dabrafenib, teach patient to use nonhormonal method of contraception, as dabrafenib can make this type of contraceptive ineffective.
  - Teach patient that if pregnancy is suspected, to advise provider right away.
  - Nursing mothers should decide whether to discontinue nursing or discontinue the drug, taking into account the importance of the drug to the mother's health.
  - Drug may impair fertility in female and male patients or reproductive potential.
- Most common side effects: (1) unresectable/metastatic melanoma: pyrexia, nausea, rash, chills, diarrhea, vomiting, HTN, peripheral edema; (2) adjuvant treatment of melanoma: pyrexia, fatigue, nausea, headache, rash, chills, diarrhea, vomiting, arthralgia, and myalgia; (3) NSCLC: pyrexia, fatigue, nausea, vomiting, diarrhea, dry skin, decreased appetite, edema, rash, chills, hemorrhage, cough, dyspnea.

Potential Toxicities/Side Effects and the Nursing Process

I. ALTERATION IN CIRCULATION related to CARDIOMYOPATHY

Defining Characteristics: Cardiomyopathy defined as cardiac failure, LV dysfunction, or decreased LVEF, occurred in 7% of patients in clinical trials. When combined with dabrafenib, incidence was 11%. Median time to onset of cardiomyopathy was 63 days (range 16–156 days). Cardiomyopathy resolved in 71% of patients.

Nursing Implications: Assess baseline cardiac function, including pulse, BP. Review history, and identify patients at risk who have CHF, hypertension, coronary artery disease. Patients should have baseline ECHO or gated blood pool scan to determine left ventricular ejection fraction (LVEF), and this should be monitored at least every 2–3 months during therapy and at the conclusion of therapy. Assess for signs and symptoms at each visit: dyspnea, increased cough, paroxysmal nocturnal dyspnea, peripheral edema, S3 gallop, and decrease in left ventricular function when tested. Teach patient to report cough, weight gain, light-headedness, edema of ankles or feet, difficulty breathing, feeling like the heart is pounding or racing, or need to use more pillows at night. Hold treatment if absolute LVEF value decreases by 10% from pretreatment values and is < LLN. Permanently discontinue drug for symptomatic cardiomyopathy or persistent asymptomatic LVEF dysfunction that does not resolve within four weeks.

II.   ALTERATION IN SENSORY PERCEPTION, POTENTIAL, related to VISUAL CHANGES

Defining Characteristics: Retinal pigment epithelial detachments (RPED) was rare (incidence 0.8%), but may lead to blindness. RPED led to reduced visual acuity that resolved after a median of 11.5 days (range 3–71 days) after drug interruption. Ocular coherence tomography (OCT) abnormalities were present a month after drug interruption in some cases. Retinal vein occlusion can also rarely occur (0.2% of patients), which may lead to macular edema, decreased visual function, neovascularization, and glaucoma.

Nursing Implications: Teach patient that visual changes may occur rarely but must be reported right away to prevent worsening, as rarely blindness may occur. Patient should immediately report blurred vision, loss of vision, other visual changes, seeing color dots, or seeing a halo (blurred outline around objects). Discuss with physician or NP/PA ophthalmologic evaluation baseline. Assess patient for visual changes and ensure patient has an ophthalmological evaluation at any time new or changed visual disturbances are reported. If patient reports loss of vision or other serious visual disturbances, patient should have an urgent (within 24 hours) ophthalmological evaluation. Drug should be discontinued if retinal vein occlusion is found.

III.   ALTERATION IN SKIN INTEGRITY, POTENTIAL, related to RASH, DERMATITIS, ACNEIFORM RASH, PPES, ERYTHEMA

Defining Characteristics: Skin toxicity is common (87%, 12% severe) and includes rash (57% incidence), dermatitis acneiform (19%), dry skin (11%), pruritus (10%), and paronychia (10%). Six percent of patients required hospitalization, commonly for secondary infection. Median time to onset was 15 days (1–221 days), and median time to resolution was 48 days (1–282 days).

Nursing Implications: Assess baseline skin integrity and dryness. Teach patient that these side effects may occur and to report them. Teach self-care measures based on symptoms that arise. For PPES, teach patient to keep skin moisturized, avoid repetitive hand or foot motions such as jogging, avoid hot water, and use tepid bath water. Teach patient to report erythema, edema, desquamation (peeling), or any changes in sensation. Teach patient to keep nails trimmed and clean. If rash itches at night, suggest patient wear cotton gloves to avoid scratching rash and possibly infecting it. Teach patient management of itching, and to avoid scratching, as secondary infections may require IV antibiotics. If paronychia develop, suggest measures to reduce distress, such as steroid tape.

TREATMENT

IV. ALTERATION IN NUTRITION related to DIARRHEA, STOMATITIS

Defining Characteristics: Diarrhea affected 43% of patients (no grades 3–4), and stomatitis 15% (2% grades 3–4).

Nursing Implications: Assess patient for bowel-elimination pattern and status of oral mucosa. Teach patient that these side effects may occur and to report them. Teach patient to self-assess oral mucosa and to use a systematic oral cleansing after meals and at bedtime. Teach patient to report any pain or difficulty eating or drinking. If stomatitis worsens, discuss topical treatment with diphenhydramine or lidocaine plus antacid mixture. See Dose Modifications.

Drug: tretinoin (Vesanoid, ATRA, all-trans-retinoic acid)

Class: Retinoid.

Mechanism of Action: Induces maturation of acute promyelocytic leukemia (APL) cells, thus decreasing proliferation. In patients who achieve a complete response to this therapy, there is an initial maturation of primitive leukemic cells, and then cells in both the bone marrow and peripheral blood are normal, polyclonal blood cells. The exact mechanism is unknown.

Metabolism: This drug is well absorbed orally into the systemic circulation, with peak concentrations in 1–2 hours. Drug is > 95% protein-bound, primarily to albumin. Oxidative metabolism occurs via the cytochrome P450 enzyme system in the liver. Drug is excreted in the urine (63% in 72 hours) and feces (31% in 6 days).

Indication: Indicated for the induction remission of patients with APL (FAB-M3), characterized by the presence of the (15:17) translocation and/or presence of the PML/RAR (alpha) gene.

Dosage/Range:
- 45 mg/m^2 per day.

Drug Preparation:
- None: oral.
- Available as 10-mg capsules.
- Protect from light.

Drug Administration:
- Drug is to be used for induction remission only.
- Administer in evenly divided doses until complete remission (CR) is achieved, then for an additional 30 days, or after 90 days of treatment, whichever comes first.

Drug Interactions:
- Drugs that either inhibit or induce the cytochrome P450 hepatic enzyme system potentially will interact with this drug, but there are no data to suggest that these drugs either increase or decrease tretinoin activity.

- Drugs that induce the enzyme system: rifampin, glucocorticoids, phenobarbital, pentobarbital; drugs that inhibit the enzyme system: ketoconazole, cimetidine, erythromycin, verapamil, diltiazem, cyclosporin.
- Antifibrinolytic agents.

Lab Effects/Interference:
- Increased cholesterol and triglyceride levels (60% of patients).
- Increased LFTs (50–60% of patients).

Special Considerations:
- Absorption is enhanced when taken with food.
- Monitor CBC, platelets, coagulation studies, liver function tests, and triglyceride and cholesterol levels frequently during therapy.

Potential Toxicities/Side Effects and the Nursing Process

I.   ALTERATION IN OXYGENATION, POTENTIAL, related to RETINOIC-ACID-APL SYNDROME

Defining Characteristics: Syndrome occurs in approximately 25% of patients and varies in severity but has resulted in death. Syndrome is characterized by fever, dyspnea, weight gain, pulmonary infiltrates on X-ray, and pleural and/or pericardial effusions. May also be accompanied by impaired myocardial contractility, hypotension, ± leukocytosis, and because of progressive hypoxemia and multisystem organ failure, some patients have died. Usually occurs during first month of treatment, but may follow initial drug dose.

Nursing Implications: Assess VS, pulmonary exam, and weight at each visit. Teach patient to do daily weights and to report any SOB, fever, weight gain. If this occurs, notify physician and discuss obtaining CXR and focused exam. Discuss chest X-ray findings with physician. Be prepared to give high-dose steroids at the first sign of the syndrome (e.g., dexamethasone 10 mg IV q 12 h × 3 days or until symptom resolution (necessary in 60% of patients). Provide pulmonary and hemodynamic support as necessary. Discuss whether drug should be discontinued based on severity and patient's response to high-dose steroids.

II.   ALTERATION IN COMFORT related to VITAMIN A TOXICITY

Defining Characteristics: Almost all patients experience some toxicity, but they do not usually have to discontinue the drug. Toxicity of high-dose vitamin A includes headache (86%) starting the first week of treatment, but fading after that; fever (83%); skin/mucous membrane dryness (77%); bone pain (77%); nausea/vomiting (57%); rash (54%); mucositis (26%); pruritus (20%); increased sweating (20%); visual disturbances (17%); ocular disorders (17%); skin changes (17%); alopecia (14%); changed visual acuity (6%); visual field defects (3%).

Nursing Implications: Teach patient about possible side effects of high-dose vitamin A as above and to report them if they occur. Teach patient symptom management. Assess severity of symptom(s) and discuss with physician symptom management of fever, headache unresponsive to acetaminophen, nausea/vomiting. If headache is severe in a child, have child evaluated for pseudotumor cerebri.

III. POTENTIAL FOR INJURY related to PSEUDOTUMOR CEREBRI

Defining Characteristics: Benign intracranial hypertension has occurred in children treated with retinoids. Early signs and symptoms are papilledema, headache, nausea and vomiting, and visual disturbances.

Nursing Implications: Teach patient/parents to report symptoms. Assess patient for symptomatology on regular basis. If headache is severe, discuss with physician analgesics and therapeutic lumbar puncture.

IV. POTENTIAL DISTURBANCE IN CIRCULATION

Defining Characteristics: The following disturbances may occur: arrhythmia (23%), flushing (23%), hypotension (14%), hypertension (11%), phlebitis (11%), cardiac failure (6%); 3% of patients studied developed cardiac arrest, myocardial infarction, enlarged heart, heart murmur, ischemia, stroke, and other serious disturbances.

Nursing Implications: Assess cardiac status baseline and presence of risk factors (e.g., hypertension). Assess VS at each visit and teach patient in a manner not to induce anxiety to report any symptoms such as chest pain, SOB, heart palpitations, or any changes that occur.

V. ALTERATION IN NUTRITION, LESS THAN BODY REQUIREMENTS, related to GI DYSFUNCTION

Defining Characteristics: Some problems are related to APL, and together with drug may emerge, such as GI bleeding/hemorrhage, which may occur in up to 34% of patients. Other GI problems include abdominal pain (31%), diarrhea (23%), constipation (17%), dyspepsia (14%), abdominal distention (11%), hepatosplenomegaly (9%), hepatitis (3%), and ulcer (3%).

Nursing Implications: Assess GI status and presence of GI dysfunction baseline. Teach patient to report any GI disturbances or changes in bowel status. If these occur, assess severity and need for symptom management, or discussion/intervention with physician. Monitor liver function studies frequently during therapy.

VI. SENSORY/PERCEPTUAL ALTERATIONS related to CHANGES IN EAR SENSATION/HEARING

Defining Characteristics: 23% of patients report earache or fullness in ears. Other ear problems that may occur are reversible hearing loss (5%) and irreversible hearing loss (1%).

Nursing Implications: Teach patient that this may occur and to report it if it occurs. Assess severity and need for intervention.

VII.   POTENTIAL FOR INJURY related to CNS, PERIPHERAL NERVOUS SYSTEM CHANGES, AND AFFECT CHANGES

Defining Characteristics: Changes that may occur include dizziness (20%), paresthesias (17%), anxiety (17%), insomnia (14%), depression (14%), confusion (11%), cerebral hemorrhage (9%), agitation (9%), and hallucinations (6%). Rarely, the following may occur: forgetfulness, gait disturbances, convulsions, coma, facial paralysis, tremor, leg weakness, somnolence, slow speech, aphasia, and other CNS changes.

Nursing Implications: Teach patient in a manner that does not cause anxiety to report any changes in affect, sensorium, or functional ability (e.g., to walk, speak). Assess severity of symptom(s) if they arise and potential for injury. If severe, modify patient's environment to minimize risk of injury and discuss medical intervention with physician.

VIII.   ALTERED URINARY ELIMINATION, POTENTIAL, related to RENAL CHANGES

Defining Characteristics: Uncommonly, renal insufficiency may occur (11%), dysuria (9%), acute renal failure (3%), urinary frequency (3%), renal tubular necrosis (3%), and enlarged prostate (3%).

Nursing Implications: Assess baseline urinary elimination pattern. Teach patient to report any changes. Monitor BUN/creatinine periodically during therapy and discuss any abnormalities with physician.

Drug: vandetanib (Caprelsa)

Class: Kinase inhibitor; multiple TKI.

Mechanism of Action: Vandetanib is a potent, selective inhibitor of multiple tyrosine kinases; it blocks vascular endothelial growth factor receptor (VEGFR-2), as well as the epidermal growth factor receptor (EGFR-1) tyrosine kinases. This inhibits endothelial cell migration, proliferation, survival, and new blood vessel formation during angiogenesis. It inhibits EGFR-dependent cell survival, as well as EGF-stimulated RTK phosphorylation in tumor and endothelial cells, as well as VEGF-stimulated tyrosine kinase phosphorylation in endothelial cells. In mouse tumor models, the drug reduced tumor cell-induced angiogenesis, tumor vessel permeability, and inhibited tumor growth and metastasis. It also blocks RET (rearranged during transfection) kinase, protein tyrosine kinase 6 (BRK), TIE2 (RTK found on endothelial cells and necessary for tumor angiogenesis, as well as normal vascular development), members of the EPH receptors' kinase family (important

TREATMENT

role in cell signaling and cancer development), and members of the SRC family of tyrosine kinases (may contain oncogenic protein), which may be important in certain tumors. There is no relationship between RET mutations and efficacy with vandetanib.

Metabolism: The median plasma half-life is 19 days following daily dosing. The drug is slowly absorbed, with a peak plasma concentration in a median of 6 hours (range 4–10 hours). Food does not affect absorption. Steady state is achieved in about 3 months. Drug is about 90% protein-bound. The drug is metabolized in the liver by enzymes including CYP3A4, forming two major metabolites. Sixty-nine percent of the drug is excreted within 21 days (44% in feces, and 25% in urine), with additional drug being excreted after this time given long half-life.

Indication: Indicated for the treatment of symptomatic or progressive medullary thyroid cancer in patients with unresectable locally advanced or metastatic disease. Use in patients with indolent, asymptomatic, or slowly progressing disease only after careful consideration of the treatment-related risks.

Contraindication: Patients with congenital long QT syndrome. Do not use vandetanib in patients with hypocalcemia, hypokalemia, or hypomagnesemia; moderate or severe hepatic impairment; or patients with a history of hemoptysis of $\geq 1/2$ tsp red blood. Correct hypocalcemia, hypokalemia, and/or hypomagnesemia before administering vandetanib.

Dosage/Range:
- Prescribers and pharmacies distributing vandetanib must be certified through the Vandetanib Risk Evaluation Mitigation Strategy (REMS) program, a restricted distribution program. To enroll in the Vandetanib REMS program, call 1-800-236-9933 or visit www.caprelsarems.com.
- 300 mg once daily, orally with or without food.
- Renal impairment: Starting dose should be reduced to 200 mg once daily in patients with moderate (creatinine clearance 30 to 50 mL/min) to severe (creatinine clearance < 30 mL/min) renal impairment; monitor QTc interval closely.
- Do not start drug in patients whose QTc interval is > 450 ms.

Dosage Modifications:
- For adverse reactions grade 3 or higher, decrease the 300-mg daily dose to 200 mg (two 100-mg tablets), and then if further dose reduction needed, to 100 mg daily. See package insert.
- Interrupt vandetanib for:
  - If QTc (corrected QT interval, see Introduction to *Chapter 3* for how to determine this)> 500 ms, interrupt drug dosing until QTc < 450 ms, then resume at reduced dose. Because of the drug's 19-day half-life, adverse reactions, including prolonged QT interval, may not resolve quickly. Monitor appropriately.
  - CTCAE grade 3 or greater toxicity: once toxicity resolves or improves to CTCAE grade 1, resume at a reduced dose.
- Recurrent toxicities: reduce vandetanib dose to 100 mg after resolution or improvement to CTCAE grade 1, if continued treatment warranted.

- Drug should not be used for/by:
  - Patients with moderate (Child-Pugh Class B) and severe (Child-Pugh Class C) hepatic impairment.
  - Patients with congenital long QT syndrome.
  - Patients with hypocalcemia, hypokalemia, and/or hypomagensemia.
  - Patients with a history of hemoptysis of $\geq$ 1/2 tsp red blood.

Drug Preparation:
- Oral. Available as 100-mg and 300-mg tablets. Do not crush.
- REMS Program: Only prescribers and pharmacies certified with the restricted distribution program are able to prescribe and dispense vandetanib (Caprelsa).

Drug Administration:
- Monitor ECG (QTc interval), electrolytes (serum potassium, calcium, magnesium), TSH baseline, during week 2–4, then again weeks 8–12 after starting vandetanib therapy, then every 3 months. Monitor more frequently if patient develops diarrhea.
- Replete electrolytes so that serum calcium, potassium, and magnesium are WNL before vandetanib administration, as ordered. Monitor periodically during therapy, and correct as needed and ordered. Maintain serum potassium at 4 mEq/L or higher (WNL) and serum magnesium and calcium levels WNL.
- ECG QTc must be < 450 msec for patient to receive vandetanib (AstraZeneca, 2017).
- Teach patient to:
  - Take tablet orally, daily at about the same time, with or without food.
  - If the patient misses a dose, do not take it if less than 12 hours before the next dose.
  - If the patient cannot swallow the tablet whole, disperse the tablet(s) in a glass containing 2 oz. of noncarbonated water, and stir for approximately 10 minutes until well dispersed (will not completely dissolve). To ensure full dose is consumed, add an additional 4 oz. of noncarbonated water swirl to mix the remaining residues and have the patient swallow the solution.
- Dispersed drug can be administered through nasogastric or gastrostomy tubes.
- Avoid direct contact of skin or mucous membranes with crushed drug; if this occurs, wash the area thoroughly.

Drug Interactions:
- Strong CYP3A4 inducers may decrease vandetanib serum concentration (e.g., dexamethasone, phenytoin, carbamazepine, rifampin, rifabutin, rifapentine, phenobarbital), St. John's wort; DO NOT take together.
- Drugs that prolong QT interval [anti-arrhythmic drugs (e.g., amiodarone, disopyramide, procainamide, sotalol, dofetilide); others (chloroquine, clarithromycin, dolasetron, granisetron, haloperidol, methadone, moxifloxacin, pimozide)]: Increase risk of QTc prolongation; avoid concomitant administration.
- Metformin, other drugs transported by the organic cation transporter type 2 (OCT2): increased plasma concentrations of metformin; use together cautiously and monitor for toxicities.
- Digoxin: increased digoxin plasma concentrations: monitor digoxin levels closely, and monitor patients for digoxin toxicity.

Lab Effects/Interference:
- Prolongs QTc interval.
- Decreased serum calcium (57%), decreased serum glucose (24%); increased ALT (51%, 2% grades 3–4).
- Bilirubin increased (13%), creatinine increased (16%).
- Decreased: WBC (19%), Hgb (13%), neutrophils (10%), platelets (9%).
- Proteinuria (10%).
- TSH may be increased if the patient develops hypothyroidism; decreased T_4.

Special Considerations:
- Warnings and Precautions:
  - *QT prolongation and torsades de pointes.*
    - Torsades de pointes (a type of ventricular tachycardia), ventricular tachycardia, and sudden death have occurred in patients receiving the drug.
    - Do not start drug in patients whose QTc interval is > 450 ms.
    - Drug should not be prescribed for patients with a history of torsades de pointes, congenital long QT syndrome, bradyarrhythmias, or uncompensated heart failure.
    - Drug exposure is increased in patients with renal impairment; the starting dose should be reduced to 200 mg in patients with moderate-to-severe renal impairment, and monitor QT interval frequently.
    - Risk of torsades de pointes increased in patients with hypokalemia, hypomagnesemia, and/or hypocalemia.
    - Perform ECG and assess serum potassium, calcium, magnesium, and TSH baseline, at 2–4 weeks, and 8–12 weeks after starting vandetanib, then every 3 months. Monitor electrolytes more frequently if patient develops diarrhea.
    - Maintain serum potassium at 4 mEq/L or higher (within normal range) and maintain serum and calcium levels WNL.
    - Avoid using vandetanib with other drugs that prolong the QT interval, and if medically necessary to coadminister, monitor ECG for QT-interval prolongation more frequently.
    - Following any dose reduction for QT prolongation, or any dose interruption > 2 weeks, assess QT interval as described above.
    - Stop vandetanib in patients who develop a QTc > 500 msec until the QTc returns to < 450 ms. Resume vandetanib at a reduced dose.
    - Drug has not been studied in patients with ventricular arrhythmias or recent myocardial infarction.
  - *Skin reactions and SJS:* severe skin reactions, including SJS and Toxic Epidermal Necrolysis (TEN) have occurred. Photosensitivity reactions can occur during therapy and for 4 months after last dose. Permanently discontinue drug for severe skin reactions and refer patient for urgent medical evaluation. Teach patient to seek urgent medical evaluation and care if a severe skin reaction occurs. Patient may require systemic therapy (e.g., corticosteroids). Photosensitivity reactions can occur during and up to 4 months after vandetanib treatment.
  - *Interstitial lung disease (ILD)*, resulting in death, has been reported; interrupt drug immediately if patient has unexplained dyspnea, cough, and fever. If ILD is confirmed, permanently discontinue drug, and treat ILD.

- *Ischemic cerebrovascular events* occurred in 1.3% of patients. Discontinue vandetanib in patients who experience a severe ischemic cerebrovascular event.
- *Hemorrhagic events* have occurred. Drug should not be prescribed in patients with a recent history of hemoptysis ($\geq$ 1/2 teaspoon of red blood). Discontinue vandetanib if severe hemorrhage occurs.
- *Heart failure* has been observed in patients receiving the drug; it may not be reversible on stopping the drug and may be rarely fatal. Monitor for signs/symptoms of heart failure, and if heart failure develops, drug discontinuance should be considered.
- *Diarrhea*, grade 3 or higher, occurred in 11% of patients. If diarrhea occurs, monitor patient's serum electrolytes and ECGs to reduce risk and enable early detection of QT prolongation resulting from dehydration. Interrupt vandetanib for severe diarrhea; when symptoms improve, resume drug at a reduced dose.
- *Hypothyroidism:* Most patients studied had undergone thyroidectomy. Assess patients for onset of hypothyroidism: assess TSH baseline, then at 2–4 weeks, 8–12 weeks after starting the drug, then every 3 months thereafter. If signs/symptoms of hypothyroidism occur (e.g., fatigue, sluggishness, increased sensitivity to cold, constipation, dry skin, puffy face, hoarse voice, increased serum cholesterol, unexplained weight gain, joint stiffness, muscle weakness, brittle fingernail/hair, depression, heavy menses), assess TSH and discuss with physician or NP/PA, adjustment of thyroid replacement therapy dose as needed.
- *Hypertension* may occur. Monitor all patients for HTN, and discuss vandetanib dose reduction or interruption for uncontrolled HTN. Vandetanib should not be resumed if HTN is not controlled.
- *Reversible posterior leukoencephalopathy syndrome (RPLS)*, a syndrome of subcortical vasogenic edema diagnosed by brain MRI, may occur.
    - If patient presents with seizures, headache, visual disturbances, confusion, or altered mental function, RPLS should be considered in the differential diagnosis.
    - Three out of the four patients who developed RPLS while receiving vandetanib also had HTN.
    - Discontinue vandetanib in patients who develop RPLS.
- *Renal impairment:* vandetanib exposure is increased so starting dose must be reduced to 200 mg in patients with moderate-to-severe renal impairment. Monitor QT interval closely. No information is available for patients with end-stage renal disease who require dialysis.
    - *Hepatic impairment:* Drug is not recommended for patients with moderate (Child-Pugh Class B) or severe (Child-Pugh Class C) hepatic impairment.
    - *Embryo-fetal toxicity:* Drug is fetotoxic. If the drug is used during pregnancy, or if the patient becomes pregnant while receiving the drug, the patient should be apprised of the potential hazard to the fetus. Teach women of childbearing potential to use effective contraception during treatment, and for at least 4 months after the last dose.
    - *Drug interactions:* Avoid coadministration of vandetanib with antiarrhythmic drugs (e.g., amiodarone, disopyramide, procainamide, sotalol, dofetilide) and other drugs which can prolong the QT interval (e.g., chloroquine, clarithromycin, dolasetron, granisetron, haloperidol, methadone, moxifloxacin, pimozide).

- *Caprelsa Risk Evaluation and Mitigation Strategy (REMS) Program:* To minimize the risk of QT prolongation, torsades de pointes, and sudden death, vandetanib is only available through a restricted distribution program. Prescribers and pharmacists must be certified with the program to prescribe and dispense vandetanib.
- Most common adverse drug reactions (≥ 20%, and with a difference between arms of ≥ 5%) were diarrhea/colitis, rash, acneiform dermatitis, nausea, hypertension, headache, URI, decreased appetite, and abdominal pain.
- Most common lab abnormalities (≥ 20%) were decreased serum calcium and glucose, and increased ALT.

Potential Toxicities/Side Effects and the Nursing Process

I. ALTERATION IN CIRCULATION, POTENTIAL, related to QTc PROLONGATION

Defining Characteristics: Patients may develop QT prolongation on EKG. Do NOT administer to patients with prolonged or who may develop prolonged QTc (hypokalemia, hypomagnesemia, hypocalcemia, other drugs that prolong the QTc). Prolonged QTc in the setting of low magnesium and hypokalemia sets the stage for torsades de pointes, with ventricular tachycardia, fibrillation, and sudden cardiac death possible. Incidence of electrolyte disturbances: decreased calcium 57% (6% grades 3–4), decreased magnesium 7% (< 1%), decreased potassium 6% (1%). Fourteen percent had QTc prolonged: 69% had QTc > 450 ms, 7% had QTc > 500 ms. Only physicians certified by the Vandetanib REMS can prescribe, and only certified pharmacies can dispense the drug.

Nursing Implications: Assess patient's drug profile to ensure that the patient is not taking any drugs that may increase the QTc interval. Assess baseline QTc interval. Identify patients at risk for development of prolonged QTc (congenital long QTc) syndrome, prolonged QTc > 450 msec, taking antiarrhythmics or other drugs that can prolong the QTc interval, hypokalemia, hypomagnesemia, concomitant CYP3A4 strong inhibitors. Correct electrolyte abnormalities (e.g., magnesium, calcium, potassium) before starting vandetanib, and monitor periodically during therapy. Hypokalemia, hypocalcemia, and hypomagnesemia in the setting of prolonged QTc may lead to torsades de pointes, ventricular fibrillation, and sudden cardiac death. QTc must be assessed baseline, at 2–4 weeks, and 8–12 weeks after starting vandetanib therapy, then every 3 months thereafter. Following any dose reduction for QT prolongation, or any dose interruptions > 2 weeks, QT assessment should be conducted as previously described. If the patient has diarrhea, serum electrolytes and EKGs will need to be assessed more frequently, and electrolytes repleted. Because of the long half-life of 19 days, a prolonged QT interval may take a few weeks to resolve. Serum potassium level should be maintained at 4 mEq/L or higher (within normal range) and serum magnesium and calcium kept WNL. Teach patient to correctly take vandetanib as prescribed, and to avoid any drugs that may interact with vantedanib, until discussion with the physician, NP, PA, or nurse. Patients with renal impairment should have a dose reduction to avoid increased serum levels of vandetanib. See Introduction to *Chapter 5* for a full discussion of assessing the QT (QTc) interval in patients receiving drugs that may increase the risk of serious complications.

II.   ALTERATION IN CIRCULATION, POTENTIAL, related to BLEEDING AND HYPERTENSION

Defining Characteristics: Like all antiangiogenic agents, vandetanib can cause serious hemorrhagic events and hypertension (HTN).

Nursing Implications: Drug should not be given to patients with a recent history of hemoptysis of ≥ 1/2 tsp. of red blood. Teach patient that bleeding may occur and to come to the emergency department and notify physician or nurse practitioner right away if bleeding (e.g., epistaxis) does not resolve in 15 minutes with local pressure and ice. Ensure that major surgery is planned with adequate time for drug elimination from body (half-life 19 days) and that it is not resumed until after adequate wound healing. Assess patient for hypertension, and if uncontrolled, hypertensive crisis. Assess at each visit, and discuss if needed, medical management of HTN. If not able to be medically controlled, stop drug until HTN well-managed. Drug should be permanently discontinued in patients with severe hemorrhage or uncontrollable hypertension.

III.   POTENTIAL ALTERATION IN SENSORY PERCEPTUAL PATTERNS related to ISCHEMIC CEREBROVASCULAR EVENTS, REVERSIBLE POSTERIOR LEUKOENCEPHALOPATHY SYNDROME (RPLS)

Defining Characteristics: Ischemic cerebrovascular events have occurred and are rarely fatal, with incidence 1.3%. RPLS, a syndrome of subcortical vasogenic edema as shown on brain MRI, may also occur rarely and may be more likely in patients with HTN. Blurred vision affected 9% of patients.

Nursing Implications: Assess baseline neurological status. Teach patient to report any changes in behavior, thinking, visual changes, or any new signs or symptoms. If seizure, headache, visual disturbances, confusion, or altered mental function, discuss patient RPLS evaluation with physician or midlevel practitioner. MRI is used to identify RPLS pathology. Drug should be permanently discontinued in patients who have either ischemic cerebrovascular events or RPLS. If patient complains of blurred vision, discuss with physician or midlevel practitioner, have evaluation by ophthalmologist, and slit lamp examination. Those studied had corneal opacities (vortex keratopathies), which led to halos and decreased visual acuity. If blurred vision, advise patient not to drive or operate machinery.

IV.   POTENTIAL ALTERATION IN SKIN INTEGRITY related to RASH

Defining Characteristics: Rash occurred in 53% of patients, with 5% being grades 3–4. Rash included rash erythematous, generalized, macular, maculopapular, papular, pruritic, exfoliative, dermatitis, dermatitis bullous, generalized erythema, and eczema. Dermatitis acneiform/acne occurred in 35% of patients, while 15% had dry skin, and 11% pruritus. Rash was usually mild to moderate. Photosensitivity reactions are increased (13%). Severe skin reactions, including SJS, have been reported; some have been fatal.

Nursing Implications: Assess skin integrity baseline and periodically during therapy. Teach patient that rash may occur, and give general symptom-management strategies to minimize discomfort. Mild-to-moderate skin reactions (rash, dry skin, dermatitis, pruritus, photosensitivity, PPES) may require topical and systemic corticosteroids, oral antihistamines, and topical and systemic antibiotics. Advise patient to wear sunscreen and protective clothing when exposed to the sun (during drug treatment and for 4 months following discontinuance). If rash is grade 3, then the drug should be stopped until improvement; when resolved or improved, discuss with physician dose reduction or discontinuance. Teach patient to stop drug and notify nurse or physician if rash begins to peel, is severe, or does not resolve with local management. If rash is severe, treatment may require corticosteroids and vandetanib should be permanently discontinued.

V. POTENTIAL ALTERATION IN OXYGENATION related to INTERSTITIAL LUNG DISEASE (ILD)

Defining Characteristics: ILD or pneumonitis may occur rarely and may result in death. EGFR blockade may be responsible for this, as EGF is necessary to repair injury to the lung tissue. Nonspecific respiratory signs and symptoms are hypoxia, pleural effusion, cough, or dyspnea when infectious, malignant, and other causes have been excluded.

Nursing Implications: Assess patient's respiratory patterns baseline and periodically during treatment. Tell patient to report any new or worsening respiratory symptoms right away. Discuss management plan with physician or midlevel practitioner: imaging to identify ILD changes, and rule out other causes. If symptoms are absent or minimal, and radiological changes are suggestive of ILD, physician may continue vandetanib and closely monitor the patient. If symptoms are moderate, vandetanib therapy is often interrupted until symptoms improve, with or without corticosteroids and antibiotics. If symptoms of ILD are severe, vandetanib should be stopped/permanently discontinued, with corticosteroids and antibiotic therapy instituted.

VI. ALTERATION IN NUTRITION, LESS THAN BODY REQUIREMENTS, related to DIARRHEA, NAUSEA, VOMITING, ANOREXIA, INCREASED LIVER FUNCTION TESTS

Defining Characteristics: Diarrhea occurred in 57% of all patients in study, with 11% being grades 3–4; it is usually well managed with routine antidiarrheal agents. Nausea affected 33% (1% grades 3–4) of patients, and vomiting 15% (1% grades 3–4). Twenty-one percent of patients had decreased appetite (4% grades 3–4), and 10% experienced weight loss. ALT was elevated in 51% of patients, 2% grades 3–4.

Nursing Implications: Assess nutritional status, bowel-elimination pattern, and appetite baseline, and repeat at each visit or telephone call during treatment. Assess LFTs baseline, and ALT every 3 months per physician. Inform patient that these side effects may occur. Teach self-administration of antinausea and antidiarrheal medications (e.g., loperamide) and to notify provider if symptoms persist so that dose can be interrupted and more aggressive antidiarrheal strategies implemented. Since electrolytes can be lost with diarrhea, patient will need to recheck serum electrolytes if diarrhea is persistent or severe. If severe, vandetanib should be interrupted until diarrhea is controlled. When controlled, the vandetanib dose should be reduced when drug is resumed. Teach patient dietary modification if nausea and vomiting or diarrhea occur (e.g., for diarrhea, BRAT diet of bananas, rice, applesauce, and toast) and to increase oral fluids to prevent dehydration. Consult a dietitian to see the patient for dietary counseling for anorexia. Discuss any abnormalities with physician or nurse practitioner.

VII. ALTERATION IN COMFORT related to HEADACHE, FATIGUE, ABDOMINAL PAIN

Defining Characteristics: Headache affected 26% of patients (1% grades 3–4), fatigue 24% (6% grades 3–4), abdominal pain 21% (3% grades 3–4), asthenia 15% (3% grades 3–4).

Nursing Implications: Assess patient's baseline comfort, and teach that these symptoms may occur. Teach symptom-management strategies to minimize discomfort. Teach patient to notify physician if fatigue or headache becomes severe and does not respond to local therapy.

Drug: vemurafenib (Zelboraf, PLX4032)

Class: Kinase inhibitor. BRAF-kinase inhibitor; BRAF is a serine-threonine kinase.

Mechanism of Action: 40–60% of patients with malignant melanoma have a mutation in the *BRAF* gene (*BRAF* ^{V600E}), which controls a protein involved in cell signaling. This leads to constitutive activation of downstream signaling via the MAPK pathway (the message for the cell to divide continues to be sent to the cell nucleus via this pathway, even though the cell never received a message to divide from outside the cell). The RAS-RAF pathway is very important in normal cell growth and survival. Mutation of the *BRAF* gene keeps the BRAF protein in an active state causing excessive signaling. Vemurafenib potently inhibits the BRAF protein and turns off the MAPK signaling, so the message no longer is sent to the cell nucleus telling the cell to divide. In addition, blocking the BRAF protein allows cells to undergo apoptosis. However, patients ultimately develop resistance to the drug, so it may require concomitant administration with a MEK or AKT inhibitor. Drug may cross the blood–brain barrier.

Metabolism: After oral administration of 960 mg twice daily for 15 days, the T_{max} was 3 hours, with steady state achieved in 15–22 days. Relationship of dosing with food ingestion has not been studied. Drug is highly protein-bound (> 99%). The drug is excreted in the feces (94%) and urine (1%). The elimination half-life is 57 hours. Drug clearance in

TREATMENT

patients with mild-to-moderate hepatic or renal insufficiency was similar to patients with normal organ function, but clearance in patients with severe dysfunction was not studied. Drug is a substrate of CYP3A4, and both a substrate and inhibitor of the efflux transporter P-glycoprotein (P-gp).

Indication: Drug is indicated for the

- Treatment of patients with unresectable or metastatic melanoma with *BRAF ^{V600E}* mutation as detected by an FDA approved test.
- Treatment of patients with Erdheim-Chester Disease with *BRAF^{V600}* mutation, [Erdheim-Chester is a rare, slow-growing blood cancer involving non-Langerhans cell histiocytosis, where too many histiocytes are produced, which then accumulate in tissues and organs causing dysfunction].
- Not indicated for the treatment of patients with wild-type BRAF melanoma.
- **Contraindications:** None. DO NOT start vemurafenib in patients with uncorrected electrolyte abnormalities, QTc > 500 ms, Long QT syndrome, or in patients taking other medicines known to prolong the QT interval.

Dosage/Range:

- Confirm the presence *of BRAF V600(E)* mutation in tumor specimens prior to initiation of treatment using a FDA-approved diagnostic test.
- 960 mg PO twice daily (four 240-mg tablets), approximately 12 hours apart, with or without a meal. Dose-modify based on toxicity. Doses < 480 mg twice daily are not recommended.

Dose Modifications:

- For new, primary cutaneous malignancies: no dose modifications are necessary.
- For other adverse reactions:
  - Permanently discontinue drug for any of the following:
  - Grade 4 adverse reactions, first appearance (if clinically appropriate), or second appearance.
  - QTc prolongation > 500 msec and increased by > 60 msec from pretreatment values.
  - Withhold vemurafenib for NCI CTCAE (v.4.0) for intolerable grade 2 or higher adverse reactions.
  - Upon recovery to grades 0–1, restart vemurafenib at a reduced dose as follows: (1) 720 mg twice daily for first appearance of intolerable grade 2 or grade 3 adverse reactions; and (2) 480 mg twice daily for the second appearance of intolerable grade 2, or grade 3 adverse reactions, or for the first appearance of grade 4 adverse reaction (if clinically appropriate).
  - Do not dose-reduce to below 480 mg twice daily.
  - Dose Modification for Strong CYP3A4 Inducers:
    - Avoid concurrent use of strong CYP3A4 inducers during vemurafenib therapy, which can lower serum concentration of vemurafenib.
    - If concurrent administration is necessary/unavoidable, increase the dose of vemurafenib by 240 mg (1 tablet) as tolerated.
    - After discontinuation of strong CYP3A4 inducer for 2 weeks, resume vemurafenib dose that was taken before starting the strong CYP3A4 inducer.

Drug Preparation:
- Oral. Available as 240-mg tablet.

Drug Administration:
- Assess baseline labs, including serum creatinine, and LFTs, then periodically during treatment. Discuss with provider baseline ECG documenting QTc interval.
- Teach patient to:
  - Swallow whole with a glass of water, and do not to chew or crush tablet. May take with or without food.
  - If a dose is missed, it can be taken up to 4 hours prior to the next dose. Do not take both doses at the same time. Do not take an additional dose if vomiting occurs, but continue with next scheduled dose.
  - Continue treatment until disease progression or unacceptable toxicity.

Drug Interactions:
- Drug is a substrate of CYP3A4.
  - Strong CYP3A4 inhibitors (ketoconazole, itraconazole, clarithromycin, atazanavir, nefazodone, saquinavir, telithromycin, ritonavir, indinivir, nelfinavir, voriconazole) may increase vemurafenib serum level and increase toxicity. Use alternative drug if possible; if not, use together cautiously if at all, and monitor patient closely for vemurafenib toxicity.
  - Strong inducers (phenytoin, carbamazepine, rifampin, rifabutin, rifapentine, phenobarbital) can decrease vemurafenib concentrations; use alternative drug if possible; if not, use together cautiously if at all, and monitor patient closely for vemurafenib effect.
- Drug is a moderate CYP1A2 inhibitor, a weak CYP2D6 inhibitor, and a CYP3A4 inducer.
- CYP2D6 substrate (dextromethorphan): increased AUC (up to 47%); use together cautiously.
- Midazolam (CYP3A4 substrate): decreased midazolam AUC by 39%.
- Effect of vemurafenib on CYP1A2 substrates: concomitant use of vemurafenib with drugs having a narrow therapeutic window that are predominantly metabolized by CYP1A2 is not recommended.
  - If it cannot be avoided, monitor patient closely for toxicities, and consider a dose reduction of the concomitant CYP1A2 substrate.
  - CYP1A2 substrate (caffeine): increased mean AUC of caffeine by 2.6-fold.
- Warfarin: 18% increase in warfarin AUC (CYP2C9 substrate); use together cautiously and monitor patient's INR closely for warfarin dosing.
- Ipilimumab: increased transaminases and bilirubin in the majority of patients receiving vemurafenib and ipilumumab together.
- Vemurafenib is both a substrate of and an inhibitor of the efflux transporter P-glycoprotein (P-gp). If coadministered with digoxin a sensitive P-gp substrate, digoxin exposure is increased by 1.8-fold.

Lab Effects/Interference:
- Increased LFTs (AST, ALT, alkaline phosphatase, bilirubin).
- Increased QTc interval.

Special Considerations:

- Patients must be BRAF-mutation positive (Cobas 4800 BRAF V600 Mutation test is one test to determine this) to benefit from this drug. It may be possible that the drug, if used in patients with BRAF-wild-type genotype, will cause progression of melanoma (Chapman et al., 2011). In addition, the drug will not work in BRAF-wild-type cancers, and may cause secondary tumors in internal organs in addition to the skin (any organ with squamous epithelium).
- Warnings and Precautions:
  - *New primary malignancies:*
    - Cutaneous squamous cell carcinoma, keratocanthoma, and melanoma occurred at a higher incidence in patients receiving drug, as compared to control arm in Trial 1.
    - Incidence of cutaneous squamous cell carcinomas and keratocanthomas occurred in 24% of patients compared to < 1% in the control.
    - Median time to first appearance of cutaneous squamous cell carcinoma was 7–8 weeks; about 33% of patients who developed this on vemurafenib experienced at least one additional occurrence, with median time between occurrences of 6 weeks.
    - Risk factors included age ≥ 65, prior skin cancer, and chronic sun exposure.
    - Patients should have dermatologic evaluations prior to starting therapy, and every 2 months while on therapy. Manage suspicious skin lesions with excision and dermatopathologic evaluation. Consider dermatologic monitoring for 6 months after last dose of vemurafenib.
  - *Noncutaneous squamous cell carcinoma* (SCC) of the head and neck can occur. Monitor patients closely for this.
    - *Other malignancies:* Vemurafenib may promote malignancies associated with activation of RAS through mutation or other mechanisms. Patients with Erdheim-Chester disease (ECD) may develop myeloid neoplasms; monitor CBC/differential in these patients with co-existing myeloid malignancies. Monitor patients closely for signs or symptoms of other malignancies.
  - *Tumor promotion in BRAF wild-type melanoma:* Paradoxical activation of MAP-kinase signaling and increased proliferation of BRAF wild-type cells exposed to BRAF inhibitors can occur. Ensure drug is only used in patients with tumors having BRAF V600E mutations.
  - *Serious hypersensitivity reactions* may occur, including anaphylaxis, generalized rash and erythema, hypotension, drug reaction with eosinophilia and systemic symptoms (DRESS syndrome) during and upon reinitiation of vemurafenib treatment. Monitor patients closely, permanently discontinue drug, and manage serious hypersensitivity reactions.
  - *Severe dermatologic reactions*, including SJS and toxic epidermal necrolysis (TEN), have occurred. Drug should be permanently discontinued if severe reactions occur.
  - *QT prolongation may occur*, and may lead to increased risk of ventricular arrhythmia, including torsades de pointes.
    - Patients should have an ECG with QTc measurement and serum electrolytes (especially potassium, magnesium, calcium) baseline, then 15 days after treatment

    initiation or dose modification for QTc prolongation, then monthly during the first 3 months, then every 3 months or as clinically indicated.

- DO NOT start vemurafenib in patients with uncorrected electrolyte abnormalities, QTc > 500 ms, or Long QT syndrome, or in patients taking medicines known to prolong the QT interval.
- If QTc > 500 msec (grade 3), withhold drug and assess/correct electrolyte abnormalities; control cardiac risk factors for QT prolongation. Upon recovery to QTc ≤ 500 msec (grade 2 or less), restart vemurafenib at a reduced dose.
- Permanently discontinue vemurafenib if the QTc interval remains > 500 msec and increased > 60 msec from pretreatment values after controlling cardiac risk factors for QT prolongation (e.g., electrolyte abnormalities, CHF, and bradyarrhythmias).
- *Hepatotoxicity:* Abnormal elevations of LFTs may occur, as may liver injury with subsequent coagulopathy. Monitor LFTs (transaminases, alkaline phosphatase, bilirubin) baseline, then monthly during treatment, increasing frequency as needed. Manage laboratory abnormalities by dose interruption, reduction or treatment discontinuation.
  - Concurrent administration with ipilumumab: safety and effectiveness not established; in dose finding study, grade 3 increases in transaminases and bilirubin occurred in a majority of patients.
- *Photosensitivity:* Mild to severe photosensitivity may occur. Teach patient to avoid sun exposure, wear protective clothing, and use a broad-spectrum UVA/UVB sunscreen and lip balm (SPF ≥ 30) when outdoors, as drug can cause photosensitivity.
- *Ophthalmologic reactions* may occur (uveitis, blurry vision, and photophobia), so teach patient to report any visual changes, and discuss ophthalmologic evaluation with physician or midlevel practitioner. Steroid or mydriatic ophthalmic drops may be needed to manage uveitis.
- *Embryo-fetal toxicity:* Drug can cause fetal harm, and fetal drug levels were 5% of maternal levels.
  - Teach women of childbearing age to use effective contraception during therapy and for at least 2 weeks after last dose of vemurafenib.
  - If the drug is used in pregnancy or if the patient becomes pregnant while taking the drug, the patient should be apprised of potential hazard to the fetus.
  - Mothers should make a decision to stop nursing or to stop the drug, taking into account the importance of the drug to the mother's health.
- *Radiation sensitization and radiation recall:* May be severe and involve cutaneous and visceral organs when RT is administered prior to, during, or subsequent to vemurafenib treatment. Monitor patients closely when vemurafenib is administered concurrently or sequentially with RT.
- *Renal failure:* can occur, as can acute interstitial nephritis and acute tubular necrosis. Elevated serum creatinine occurred in 26% of patients receiving vemurafenib compared to 5% in the dacarbazine clinical trial arm. Assess serum creatinine before starting vemurafenib and periodically during treatment.
- *Dupuytren's contracture and plantar fascial fibromatosis:* Usually mild to moderate when these occur, but disabling dupuytren's contracture has been reported. Teach patient to report symptoms.

- Most common adverse events were: (1) melanoma ($\geq$ 30%): arthralgia, rash, alopecia, fatigue, photosensitivity reactions, nausea, pruritus, and skin papilloma; (2) ECD (> 50%): arthralgia, maculo-papular rash, alopecia, prolonged QTc on ECG, and skin papilloma.
- Su et al. (2012) showed that resistance is likely because of reactivation of the RAS/RAF pathway and activation of an alternative pathway. This study supports future studies in which an MEK or AKT inhibitor is added to vemurafenib to combat resistance. Another study comparing combinations of a BRAF inhibitor (GSK436) and an AKT inhibitor (GSK212) showed that the combination was safe with preliminary antitumor activity in patients with advanced melanoma (Infante et al., 2011).
- In trying to understand the increased incidence of squamous cell carcinomas and keratoacanthomas in patients treated with vemurafenib, researchers found that 60% of tumors had an *RAS* mutation, suggesting that perhaps the *BRAF* inhibition activates mutations in RAS. This might be prevented by combining treatment with an MEK inhibitor, as mentioned above.

Potential Toxicities/Side Effects and the Nursing Process

I.   ALTERATION IN COMFORT related to FATIGUE, ARTHALGIA

Defining Characteristics: Fatigue occurred in 38–54%, and arthralgias in 53–67% of patients.

Nursing Implications: Teach patients to report alterations in comfort, especially joint pain and fatigue. Distinguish new onset of symptoms versus those experienced before treatment due to malignancy. Teach patient to manage arthralgias and energy-conserving strategies to manage fatigue.

II.   ALTERATION IN SKIN INTEGRITY, POTENTIAL, related to INCREASED RISK FOR ALOPECIA, KERATOACANTHOMA, SQUAMOUS CELL CARCINOMA, NEW MELANOMA, AND PHOTOSENSITIVITY

Defining Characteristics: Alopecia, photosensitivity, and rarely development of keratocanthoma or squamous cell carcinoma may occur. Keratocanthoma is a common low-grade skin tumor thought to originate from the hair follicle. It is often considered a form of squamous cell carcinoma. It is found in sun-exposed skin (e.g., face, forearms, and hands). It is dome-shaped, symmetrical, and surrounded by inflamed skin. There are often keratin scales and debris. It grows rapidly, and if not treated, will eventually necrose and heal with scarring. New primary melanomas may occur. Rash occurs in up to half of patients. Photosensitivity affects 33–49% of patients, and pruritus up to 30%.

Nursing Implications: Patient should have a baseline dermatologic evaluation prior to beginning therapy, then every 2 months while on therapy, and continuing for 6 months after completion of drug therapy. Any suspicious lesion should be excised and biopsied, then treated as per standard of care. Drug dose is not changed. Assess patient's skin baseline and at each visit. Teach patient to stop taking the drug and call provider right away if the patient develops a severe skin reaction, such as blisters on the skin, in the mouth, fever, peeling of the skin, or redness or swelling of face, hands or soles of feet. Teach patient to self-assess skin regularly, and advise provider if notice a new wart, sore, or bump that bleeds or does not heal, or a mole that changes in color. Teach patient to use strong UVA/UVB sunblock (SPF 30 or higher), lip balm, and protective clothing or to avoid exposing skin to the sun. Teach to wear a hat to protect the scalp, especially if experiencing alopecia, and to cover exposed skin with a shirt or cover. Teach patient to wear sunglasses to protect the eyes when out in the sun if it cannot be avoided. Teach the patient to report any new skin lesions on sun-exposed body parts, especially if it is growing quickly. Discuss with physician referral to dermatology to obtain an excisional biopsy of the lesion.

III.   ALTERATION IN NUTRITION, LESS THAN BODY REQUIREMENTS, related to NAUSEA, DIARRHEA

Defining Characteristics: Nausea occurred in 35–37%, vomiting in 18–26%, diarrhea in 28–29%, and constipation in 12–16% of patients in two clinical trials.

Nursing Implications: Assess weight, bowel-elimination status, and baseline nutritional status, and monitor during therapy. Teach patient that symptoms can occur and ways to minimize this effect, such as self-administration of antinausea and antidiarrheal medications per protocol and to report symptoms that do not resolve with established plan. If patient has constipation, teach diet modifications to increase peristalsis, self-administration of cathartics and hydration as needed. Teach patient to identify nutritionally dense (high calories and protein in the smallest amount) foods and to keep them handy in the refrigerator. Teach patient to eat small, frequent meals and to have a bedtime snack. Teach patient that goal is to drink a glass of fluid every hour while awake. Teach patient to call provider if symptoms do not resolve within 24 hours. Monitor closely patients, such as older persons, who are at risk for dehydration. Discuss any abnormalities with a physician.

IV.   ALTERATION IN CIRCULATION, POTENTIAL, related to QTc PROLONGATION

Defining Characteristics: Patients may develop QT prolongation on ECG. In the setting of low electrolyte levels (potassium, magnesium, calcium), this can set the stage for ventricular arrhythmias, especially torsades de pointes, which may cause sudden death. Drug is not recommended for patients with uncorrectable electrolyte abnormalities, Long QT syndrome, a QTc > 500 ms, or who are taking medications known to prolong the QT interval (e.g., methadone, haloperidol).

Nursing Implications: Assess patients at risk (cardiac history, medications that may prolong QTc including serotonin antagonists, history of cardiac arrhythmias). Assess ECG and serum electrolytes; discuss correction of electrolytes prior to starting drug. Monitor

ECG and electrolytes should be at day 15 after drug initiation, then monthly during first 3 months of therapy, then every 3 months during therapy. If the QTc > 500 msec (grade 3) at any time, stop the drug, correct electrolyte abnormalities, and control cardiac risk factors for QT prolongation (e.g., CHF, bradyarrhythmias). Once the QTc is < 500 msec, restart the drug at a lower dose. Permanently discontinue drug if after correction of risk factors, the QTc increases again both > 500 msec, and > 60 msec change from pretreatment values. See Introduction to *Chapter 5* for a full discussion of assessing the QT (QTc) interval in patients receiving drugs that may increase the risk of serious complications. Teach patient to call provider right away, or go to the emergency room if feeling faint, or have a rapid heartbeat.

Drug: Venetoclax (Venclexta)

Class: BCL-2 inhibitor, first in class.

Mechanism of Action: Drug is a selective, orally bioavailable small-molecule inhibitor of Bcl-2, a protein which halts or prevents apoptosis. *BCL-2* (B-cell lymphoma2) is a gene whose proteins regulate apoptosis (programmed cell death) either by inducing (pro-apoptotic) or inhibiting (antiapoptotic) apoptosis (Yip & Reed, 2008). The Bcl-2 protein is an antiapoptotic protein overexpressed in many cancers, including Chronic Lymphocytic Leukemia (CLL), which leads to tumor cell survival and likely influences chemotherapy resistance (AbbVie, 2016). Blockade of Bcl-2 antiapoptotic protein restores tumor cell apoptosis by binding to the Bcl-2 protein, which displaces the proapoptotic proteins (e.g., BIM). This triggers the outer membrane of the mitochondria to become permeable, and caspases are activated, destroying the tumor cells (see process of apoptosis in chapter introduction).

Metabolism: Taken with food, the maximal plasma concentration of venetoclax is reached in 5–8 hours. Administration with a low-fat meal increases venetoclax exposure by 3.4 times, while administration with a high-fat meal increases exposure by 5.1–5.3 times compared to administration without food. Drug is highly protein-bound, and the terminal elimination half-life is 26 hours. Drug is metabolized by CYP3A4/5 and drug is cleared from the blood by hepatic elimination. Almost all of the drug is excreted in the feces (> 99.9%, with 20.8% as unchanged drug), and < 0.1% excreted in the urine.

Indication(s): Treatment of patients with (1) CLL or small lymphocyte lymphoma (SLL) with or without 17p deletion (adult patients); (2) first line treatment of previously untreated patients with CLL or SLL, in combination with obinutuzumab (Gazyva); (3) acute myeloid leukemia (AML) in combination with azacitidine or decitabine or low-dose cytarabine in newly diagnosed adults aged 75 or older or who have comorbidities that preclude use of intensive induction chemotherapy (accelerated approval).

Contraindications: Concomitant use of venetoclax with strong inhibitors of CYP3A at initiation and during ramp-up phase.

Dosage/Range:
- Assess risk for TLS, discuss with provider and administer prophylactic hydration and antihyperuricemics to patient prior to first dose of venetoclax as ordered.
- Venetoclax dose is ramped up during the first 5 weeks of therapy to gradually reduce tumor burden and decrease risk of TLS. Patient should take venetoclax with a meal and water at about the same time each day. Starting Medication Pack provides the first 4 weeks of venetoclax according to the ramp-up schedule to the recommended daily dose of 400 mg. Use 100-mg tablets (4 tablets) for the 400-mg dose which is supplied in bottles. Drug should be taken PO daily until disease progression or unacceptable toxicity.
- *Ramp-up schedule for patients with CLL/SLL:*
  - Week 1: daily dose is 20 mg PO.
  - Week 2: daily dose is 50 mg PO.
  - Week 3: daily dose is 100 mg PO.
  - Week 4: daily dose is 200 mg PO.
  - Week 5 and beyond: daily dose is 400 mg PO.
- *Venetoclax CLL/SLL starting pack provides the first 4 weeks of venetoclax according to the ramp-up schedule. The 400 mg dose is made up of four 100-mg tablets supplied in the bottle.*
- *Venetoclax in combination with obinutuzumab:*
  - Start obinutuzumab at 100 mg on cycle 1 day 1, followed by 900 mg on cycle 1 day 2. Administer 1000 mg on days 8 and 15 of cycle 1 and on day 1 of each subsequent 28-day cycle, for at total of 6 cycles. See Gayzva package insert for recommended dosing.
  - On cycle 1 day 22, start venetoclax according to the 5-week ramp-up schedule. After completing the ramp-up schedule on cycle 2 day 28, patients should continue on venetoclax 400 mg PO once daily from cycle 3 day 1 until the last day of cycle 12.
- *Venetoclax in combination with rituximab:*
  - Start rituximab administration after the patient has completed the 5-week dose ramp-up schedule, and has received the 400-mg dose for 7 days.
  - Administer rituximab on Day 1 of each 28-day cycle × 6 cycles; Cycle 1 dose of rituximab is 375 mg/m^2 IV, and Cycles 2-6 dose is 500 mg/m^2 IV.
  - Patients should continue venetoclax 400–mg once daily × 24 months from Cycle 1 day1 of rituximab.
- *Venetoclax as monotherapy:* Recommended dose is 400-mg PO once daily after completion of the 5-week ramp-up schedule. Take orally once daily until disease progression or unacceptable toxicity.
- *Venetoclax for acute myeloid leukemia:* Ramp up schedule. Dose depends upon the combination regimen and agent:
  - Venetoclax day1 (100 mg × 1 day), day 2 (200 mg × 1 day), day 3 (400 mg × 1 day).
  - Days 4 and beyond: (1) venetoclax 400 mg when given in combination with azacitidine or decitabine; (2) 600 mg when given with low-dose cytarabine.
  - Continue venetoclax in combination with azacitidine or decitabine, or low-dose cytarabine until disease progression or unacceptable toxicity.
  - All patients should have WBC $< 25 \times 10^9$/L prior to initiation of venetoclax; cytoreduction may be required.

- Before 1st venetoclax dose, give patient prophylactic measures including hydration, anti-hyperuricemic agents and continue ramp-up phase. Assess blood chemistries (potassium, uric acid, phosphorus, calcium, creatinine) and correct pre-existing abnormalities as ordered prior to initiating venetoclax treatment.
- Monitor blood chemistires for TLS at pre-dose, 6–8 hours after each new dose during ramp-up and 24 hours after reaching final dose.
- For patients with TLS risk factors (e, circulating blasts, high burden of leukemic cells in bone marrow, elevated pretreatment LDH, or reduced renal function) consider additional measures to reduce risk of TLS such as increased frequency of lab monitoring and reducing venetoclax dose.
- *Risk assessment for TLS and TLS prophylaxis based on tumor burden in CLL/SLL patients:*
  - If patient at low risk [all LN < 5 cm and absolute lymphocyte count < 25 × 10^9/L]: oral hydration of 1.5-2L (or IV if unable to take PO), allopurinol anti-uric acid, outpatient therapy: For 1st dose of 20 mg and 50 mg: assess serum chemistries predose, at 6-8 hours, and at 24 hours. For subsequent ramp-up doses: pre-dose.
  - Medium risk [any LN 5 cm to < 10 cm or absolute lymphocyte count ≥ 25 × 10^9/L: oral hydration 1,5-2 L and consider additional fluid IV; allopurinol anti hyperuricemic; outpatient; For 1st dose of 20 mg and 50 mg: assess serum chemistries predose, at 6-8 hours, and at 24 hours. For subsequent ramp-up doses: pre-dose. Consider hospitalization for patients with CrCl < 80 mL/min; monitor blood chemistries at 6-8 hours and at 24 hours at each subsequent ramp-up dose.
  - If patient at high risk [e.g., any LN ≥ 10 cm, or absolute lymphocyte count is ≥ 25 × 10^9/L and any LN ≥ 5 cm]: Oral hydration (1.5–2 L) plus IV (150–200 mL/hr as tolerated; allopurinol; consider rasburicase if baseline uric acid is elevated; in hospital, assessment of chemistries: for 1st dose of 20mg and 50 mg dose: predose, at 4, 8, 12, and 24 hours. Outpatient assessment for subsequent ramp up doses: assess predose, 6–8 hours and at 24 hours.

Dose Modifications (see package insert):
- **CLL/SLL:** Interrupt dosing or dose-reduce for toxicities.
- *TLS:* Blood chemistry changes or symptoms suggestive of TLS: Any occurrence. (1) Hold next day's dose; if resolved within 24–48 hours or last dose, resume at same dose. (2) for any blood chemistry changes requiring > 48 hours to resolve, resume at a reduced dose; (3) for any events of clinical TLS, resume at reduced dose following resolution.
- *Non-hematologic toxicities:* Grade 3–4: (1) 1st occurrence: interrupt venetoclax; once toxicity has resolved to grade 1 or baseline level, resume venetoclax at the same dose; (2) 2nd and subsequent occurrences: interrup venetoclax and after resolution, resume following dose reduction guidelines; physician may choose a larger dose reduction.
- *Hematologic toxicities:* Grade 3 neutropenia with infection or fever; or grade 4 hematologic toxicities (except lymphopenia): (1) 1st occurrence: interrupt venetoclax; consider G-CSF to reduce infection risk of neutropenia; once toxicity resolved to grade 1 or baseline level, resume venetoclax at the same dose; (2) 2nd and subsequent occurrences: interrupt venetoclax; consider G-CSF as clinically indicated; after resolution, resume venetoclax following dose reduction guidelines; physician may choose a larger dose reduction.

- *Dose Reduction Guidelines for CLL/SLL:* Dose at interruption, and restart dose (during ramp-up phase, continue the reduced dose for 1 week before increasing the dose): if dose at interruption 400 mg, restart at 300 mg; 300 mg, restart at 200 mg; 200 mg, restart at 100 mg; 100 mg restart at 50 mg; 50 mg, restart at 20 mg; 20 mg, restart at 10 mg. See package insert.
- **Recommended dose modifications for toxicities in AML:**
  - Grade 4 neutropena with/without fever or infection; or grade 4 thrombocytopenia:
    1. occurrence prior to achieving remission: transfuse blood products, administer prophylactic and treatment anti-infectives as clinically appropriate and ordered. In most incidences, azacitidine, decitabine or low-dose cytarabine cycles should not be interrupted due to cytopenias prior to achieving remission (Venclexta, Nov 2018);
    2. first occurrence after achieving remission and lasting at least 7 days: delay subsequent treatment cycle of venetoclax and azacitidine, decitabine, or low-dose cytarabine and monitor blood counts; administer or teach patient to self-administer G-CSF as ordered as ordered for neutropenia. Once the toxicity has resolved to grade 1–2, resume venetoclax therapy at same dose in combination with azacitidine, decitabine or low-dose cytrarabine;
    3. subsequent occurrences in cycles after achieving remission and lasting $\geq$ 7 days: delay subsequent cycles of venetoclax and azacitidine or decitabine or cytarabine and monitor blood counts; administer G-CSF as indicated for neutropenia. Once the toxicity has resolved to grade 1–2, resume venetoclax therapy at the same dose and reduce the cycle duration by 7 dyas for each subsequent cycle.
  - CYP3A and P-gp inhibitors:
    1. CLL/SLL: Coadministration with strong CYP3A inhibitors is CONTRAINDI-CATED at **initiation and during ramp-up phase**. See package insert.
    2. AML; Initiation and ramp up phase: (a) POSACONAZOLE: dose reductions: Day 1–10 mg, day 2–20 mg, day 3–50 mg, day 4–70 mg. After ramp up reduce venetoclax dose to 70 mg as steady daily dose; (b) OTHER STRONG CYP3A INHIBITORS: dose reductions: Day 1–10 mg, day 2–20 mg, day 3–50 mg, day 4–100 mg. After ramp up reduce venetoclax dose to 100 mg as steady daily dose; (c) MODERATE CYP3A INHIBITOR: Reduce the venetoclax dose by at least 50%. (d) P-gp INHIBITOR: Reduce the venetoclax dose by at least 50%. For CLL/SLL, consider alternative medications or reduce the venetoclax dose as above.
    3. Resume the venetoclax dose used prior to concomitant use of a strong or moderate CYP3A inhibitor or P-gp inhibitor 2–3 days after discontinuance of the inhibitor. See package insert.

Drug Preparation:
- Available in 10-mg, 50-mg, and 100-mg tablets.
- Starting pack: provides first 4 weeks of venetoclax according to the ramp-up schedule.
- Once ramp-up completed, the 400 mg dose is made up of 100 mg tablets supplied in bottles.

Drug Administration:
- Assess patient risk factors for developing TLS as drug can cause a rapid tumor cell lysis and release of intracellular and destroyed cell components (e.g., potassium, phosphate)

with changes in blood chemistries within 6–8 hours of the first dose of venetoclax, and at each dose increase.

- Risk is based on tumor burden, and patient comorbidities.
- See package insert for recommended TLS prophylaxis based on tumor burden calculations (1) *low* **tumor burden:** 1.5–2L oral hydration and allopurinol, with blood chemistry monitoring in outpatient predose, and postdose at 6–8 hours, 24 hours with first doses of 20-mg and 50-mg, and also predose at subsequent ramp-up doses; (2) *medium* **risk:** oral hydration 1.5–2 L and consider IV as well, with allopurinol, and blood monitoring predose and postdose at 6–8 hours, 24 hours at first doses of 20-mg and 50-mg, and predose and postdose at subsequent ramp-up doses; discuss hospitalization for patients with **CrCl < 80 mL/min** at first dose of 20-mg and 50-mg with bloods monitored *in hospital* at first dose of 20-mg and 50-mg: predose and postdose at 4, 8, 12, and 24 hours, and *outpatient* at subsequent ramp-up doses predose, postdose at 6, 8, 24 hours; and (3) **high risk:** oral (1.5–2 L) hydration plus IV (150–200 mL/hr as tolerated, with allopurinol (consider rasburicase if baseline uric acid is elevated), and monitor blood chemistries *in hospital* at first doses of 20-mg and 50-mg: predose and postdose at 4, 8, 12, and 24 hours, and *outpatient* at subsequent ramp-up doses predose and postdose at 6, 8, 24 hrs.
- Female patients of reproductive potential should have a pregnancy test before venetoclax is initiated. Teach patient to use effective contraception during therapy and for 30 days after last dose.
- Assess patient ANC, CBC, tumor burden and risk for TLS, and baseline chemistries. If past dose interruption due to grades 3–4 neutropenia, discuss need for G-CSF with physician/NP/PA. Review any recommended dose modifications with physician/NP/PA.
- Teach patient to (1) take venetoclax with a meal and water at about the same time each day, (2) tablets should be swallowed whole, not chewed, crushed or broken prior to swallowing, (3) if a dose is missed within 8 hours of the time it is usually taken, the patient should take the missed dose as soon as possible, and resume the normal daily dosing schedule; if the dose is missed by more than 8 hours, the patient should NOT take the missed dose and should resume the usual dose schedule the next day, (4) if the patient vomits following a dose, no additional dose should be taken that day; take the next prescribed dose at the usual time the next day; and (5) do not drink grapefruit juice, eat grapefruit, Seville oranges (often used in marmalade), or starfruit while taking venetoclax, as any of these will increase the amount of venetoclax in the blood.

Drug Interactions:
- Strong CYP3A inhibitors (ketoconazole, conivaptan, clarithromycin, indinavir, itraconazole, lopinavir, ritonavir, telaprevir, posaconazole, and voriconazole): Contraindicated at initiation of venetoclax and during ramp-up phase due to potential for increased risk of TLS. After ramp-up when patient is on a steady daily dose of venetoclax, reduce the venetoclax dose by at least 75% when used concomitantly with strong CYP3A inhibitors. Resume the venetoclax dose that was used prior to starting the CYP3A inhibitor 2–3 days after discontinuation of the inhibitor.
- Moderate CYP3A inhibitors (erythromycin, ciprofloxacin, diltiazem, dronedarone, fluconazole, verapamil) and P-gp Inhibitors (e.g., amiodarone, azithromycin, captopril,

carvedilol, cyclosporine, felodipine, quercetin, quinidine, ranolazine, rifampin, ticagrelor): Avoid concomitant administration. Consider alternative treatments. If a moderate CYP3A or a P-gp inhibitor myst be used, reduce the venetoclax dose by at least 50%. Monitor the patient closely for signs of venetoclax toxicity. Resume the venetoclax dose used prior to starting the CYP3A or P-gp inhibitor 2–3 days after discontinuation of the inhibitor.

- Strong CYP3A4 inducers (e.g., carbamazepine, phenytoin, rifampin, St. John's wort) or moderate CYP3A inducers (e.g., bosentan, efavirenz, etravirine, modafinil, nafcillin): Avoid concomitant administration and consider alternative treatments with less CYP3A induction.
- Warfarin: venetoclax coadministration increases Cmax and AUC of R-warfarin and S-warfarin. Monitor INR closely in patients receiving venetoclax and warfarin.
- P-gp substrates: Venetoclax may inhibit P-gp substrates in the gut. Avoid coadministration of a P-gp substrate with a narrow therapeutic index (e.g., digoxin, everolimus, sirolimus). If they must be coadministered, the substrate should be taken at least 6 hours before venetoclax.

Lab Effects/Interference:
- Neutropenia, anemia, thrombocytopenia
- TLS abnormalities: hyperkalemia, hyperphosphatemia, hypocalcemia, hyperuricemia.

Special Considerations:
- Most common adverse reactions ($\geq$ 20%): neutropenia, diarrhea, nausea, anemia, URI, thrombocytopenia, fatigue.
- Warnings and Precautions:
  - *TLS:* in patients with high-tumor burden may be fatal, or result in renal failure requiring dialysis. TLS is high for these patients during the initial 5-week ramp-up phase. Changes in blood chemistries from TLS can occur 6–8 hours after the first drug dose, and at each drug increase. See TLS assessment in Drug Administration section and package insert. Monitor patient and blood chemistries carefully and closely, administer TLS prophylaxis (e.g., hydration and antihyperuricemics), manage intensively as risk increases (e.g., IV hydration, hospitalization), interrupt dose if needed.
  - *Neutropenia:* In patients with CLL, grades 3–4 neutropenia occurred in 63–64% of patients, and grade 4 occurred in 31–33% of patients. Febrile neutropenia occurred in 4–6% of patients receiving venetoclax monotherapy or in combination. In patients with AML, baseline neutrophil counts worsened in 97–100% of patients treated with venetoclax in combination with azacitidine or decitabine or low-dose cytarabine. Neutropenia can recur with subsequent cycles of therapy. Monitor CBC/differential throughout treatment and interrupt dose for severe neutropenia. Consider G-CSF. Assess closely for and teach patient to self-assess, for signs and symptoms of infection. If febrile, institute prompt supportive measures as ordered, including antimicrobials.
  - *Infections:* Severe and fatal infections have occurred, such as pneumonia and sepsis. Monitor patients closely for signs/symptoms of infection and administer antimicrobials promptly. Hold venetoclax for grade 3 and higher infections.

- *Immunizations:* Avoid administration of live-attenuated vaccines prior to, during, or after treatment with venetoclax until B-cell recovery occurs as this has not been studied.
- *Embryo-fetal toxicity* may occur. Teach female patients of reproductive potential to use effective contraception to avoid pregnancy during therapy and for at least 30 days after the last dose. These patients should receive a pregnancy test before the drug is initiated. If pregnancy occurs, the patient should be apprised of the potential hazard to the fetus.
  - Mothers should not breast-feed while receiving the drug.
  - Male fertility may be compromised by therapy with venetoclax. Male patients may wish to bank sperm.

Potential Toxicities/Side Effects and the Nursing Process

I.   POTENTIAL FOR INJURY related to TLS

Defining Characteristics: Venetoclax is very effective in rapidly lysing lymphocytes at the beginning of therapy and at each dose increase. Patients at high risk for TLS (e.g., high-tumor burden, other morbidities) who cannot clear the products of destroyed cells may develop renal failure requiring dialysis or life-threatening conditions. Patients must have a calculated TLS risk assessment by the physician, with appropriate TLS prophylaxis, e.g., hydration and antihyperuricemic therapy before receiving venetoclax. TLS occurred in 6% of patients by chemistries, while hypokalemia (20%), hypophosphatemia (15%), hypocalcemia (9%), and hyperuricemia (6%) also occurred.

Nursing Implications: Review patient's risk for developing TLS and aggressive TLS prophylaxis regimen. If patient is at high risk, or has a Crcl < 80 mL/min, therapy for first dose of 20 mg and 50 mg should be administered in the hospital. See Drug Administration and package insert for TLS assessment and hydration/antihyperuricemic regimen. Administer hydration and anti-hyperuricemic regimen as ordered. Monitor serum chemistries and renal function tests closely, and necessary other diagnostics, such as ECG as ordered if laboratory abnormalities occur.

II.   POTENTIAL FOR INFECTION AND BLEEDING related to NEUTROPENIA AND THROMBOCYTOPENIA

Defining Characteristics: In patients with CLL/SLL, neutropenia occurred in 45% of patients, while grades 3–4 neutropenia occurred in 41% of patients. Febrile neutropenia occurred in 5%. Infections in clinical trials were URI (22%) and pneumonia (8%). Anemia occurred in 29% (grades 3–4 in 18%), and thrombocytopenia in 22% (15% grades 3–4).

Nursing Implications: Assess baseline CBC, WBC, differential, and platelet count baseline and monitor closely during the ramp-up phase, then as ordered by physician/NP/PA. Assess for signs/symptoms of infection or bleeding. Teach patient the signs/symptoms of infection or bleeding and to report these immediately, and teach patient self-care measures to minimize risk of infection and bleeding. This includes avoidance of crowds, proximity to people with infections, and OTC aspirin-containing medications. Discuss need for growth factors with physician, PA or NP. Discuss dose reduction based as needed with physician/NP/PA.

III. ALTERATION IN NUTRITION, POTENTIAL related to DIARRHEA, NAUSEA, VOMITING, AND CONSTIPATION

Defining Characteristics: Diarrhea occurred in 25%, nausea in 33%, vomiting in 15%, and constipation in 14% of patients in clinical trials.

Nursing Considerations: Assess nutritional status and bowel-elimination pattern baseline and at each visit. Teach patient to report symptoms, and to manage self-care if symptoms occur: to take OTC antidiarrheal or constipation medication as needed, to take antinausea medicine as prescribed; to modify diet (e.g., increase fiber and fluids if constipated, foods to slow diarrhea and fluids to reverse dehydration; high-calorie, high-protein foods in small amounts if decreased taste, appetite, and weight loss). Teach patient to report any symptoms that do not resolve or improve with the established plan. To increase appetite, encourage patients to use a small plate, take small portions, and not to fill the plate; take antiemetic 30 minutes prior to eating; and to eat small, frequent meals. Arrange dietary consultation if available and needed. Monitor weight at each visit to note trends.

Drug: vismodegib (Erivedge)

Class: Hedgehog pathway inhibitor.

Mechanism of Action: The Hedgehog pathway is vital during embryogenesis, and it is a complicated pathway. A simplified version is described. In the embryo, the Hedgehog pathway is responsible for cell proliferation and differentiation into specialized cells, organ formation, and tissue migration to the correct anatomical position within the developing embryo. That way, the fetus develops with the spinal cord in the right place, with five fingers on each hand, five toes on each foot, and the anatomical part heading in the right direction (tissue polarity). The Hedgehog pathway also plays a role in cell differentiation, stem cell maintenance and wound healing in adults. The Hedgehog gene codes for the sonic hedgehog (SHH) protein, which will bind to a specific cell membrane receptor complex to turn on signal transduction leading to cell proliferation. The receptor complex on the cell membrane is made up of two proteins: patched (PTCH) 1 that binds the ligand SHH, and smoothened (SMO), which turns on the actual signal transduction to activate the target genes controlling cell proliferation. Normally this pathway is almost shut down after the fetus is formed. If the PTCH1 gene becomes mutated, then the PTCH1 protein cannot bind to SMO, releasing SMO to send unlimited messages to the target genes so that unregulated cell proliferation occurs along with angiogenesis. Mutations in PTCH1, PTCH2, SMO, and another gene may be mutated in basal cell carcinoma (BCC). UV exposure mutates PTCH1, and is thought to be responsible for 70% of BCCs (von Gorlin syndrome). Another

10–20% of BCCs appear to be due to mutations in SMO, leading to unregulated signaling to the genes responsible for cell proliferation. Thus, in BCC, the Hedgehog pathway becomes turned on without regulation, resulting in malignant transformation. Hedgehog signaling from the tumor to the stroma (surrounding tissue that stimulates tumor growth) increases tumorigenesis (Gupta et al., 2010). Vismodegib binds to and inhibits SMO, the transmembrane protein that is necessary for activation of signal transduction. By inactivating SMO, the pathway is turned off.

Metabolism: The drug is highly permeable but has low solubility in water. After an oral dose, the absolute bioavailability is 31.8%. The drug binds to plasma proteins > 99%. More than 98% of the total circulating drug components are parent drug. Drug is metabolized by oxidation (CYP2C9, CYP3A4/5), glucuronidation, and pyridine ring cleavage. Drug and metabolites are eliminated via the liver with 82% of administered dose found in the feces, and 4.4% in the urine. Elimination half-life is 4 days after continuous daily dosing, and 12 days after a single dose. Drug has not been studied in patients with hepatic or renal impairment.

Indication: The treatment of adults with (1) metastatic basal cell carcinoma, or with (2) locally advanced basal cell carcinoma that has recurred following surgery or who are not candidates for surgery, and who are not candidates for radiation therapy.

Dosage/Range:
- 150-mg capsule PO daily, with or without food until disease progression or unacceptable toxicity.

Dosage Modifications for Adverse Events
- Hold vismodegib for up to 8 weeks for intolerable adverse reactions until improvement or resolution. Treatment durations < 8 weeks prior to interruption have not been studied.

Drug Preparation:
- None, oral. Available as 150-mg capsules, in a bottle containing 28 capsules. Teach patient to keep bottle at room temperature and out of reach of children and pets.

Drug Administration:
- Verify patient is not pregnant, through testing within 7 days before starting therapy with vismodegib. Teach patient to use effective contraception during therapy and for at least 24 months after the final dose. Teach male patients with female sexual partners with reproductive potential to use condoms to prevent pregnancy during treatment and for at least 3 months after the last drug dose.
- Teach patient to take tablet with or without food and to swallow capsule whole. Do not open or crush capsules. If a dose is missed, do not make it up. Resume drug with next scheduled dose.
- Teach patients not to donate blood or blood products while receiving vismodegib and for 24 months after last drug dose.
- Teach men not to donate semen during therapy and for 3 months after the final drug dose.

Drug Interactions:
- Vismodegib is a substrate of CYP2C9 and CYP3A4; there appear to be no effects from CYP3A4 inducers or inhibitors on vismodegib serum levels.

- Drugs that inhibit the efflux of P-glycoprotein (P-gp) (clarithromycin, erythromycin, azithromycin): since vismodegib is a substrate of P-gp, these drugs may increase vismodegib serum levels and risk for toxicity; avoid concurrent use.
- Drugs that alter gastric pH (PPIs, H_2-receptor antagonists, antacids): may alter vismodegib solubility and reduce bioavailability, thus reducing efficacy; avoid concurrent use.
- Vismodegib is an inhibitor of CYP2C8, CYP2C9, CYP2C19, and the transporter BCRP. The significance is unknown.

Lab Effects/Interference:
- Hyponatremia, hypokalemia, azotemia.

Special Considerations:
- Warnings and Precautions:
  - *Embryo-fetal toxicity:* Drug is teratogenic, embryotoxic, and fetotoxic in rats. It can cause embryo-fetal death and severe birth defects.
    - Verify pregnancy status of females of reproductive potential within 7 days of starting vismodegib to ensure patient is not pregnant before starting vismodegib.
    - Teach women of childbearing potential to use effective contraception during and for 24 months after the last dose of vismodegib.
    - Teach men with female partners of reproductive potential to use condoms, even if they have had a vasectomy, as there is potential risk of drug exposure through semen. Teach males to continue condom use for 3 months after final dose of vismodegib.
    - Teach patients to contact their healthcare provider immediately if they suspect they (or for males, their female partner) may be pregnant.
    - Nursing mothers should make a decision to discontinue nursing or to discontinue the drug, taking into account the importance of the drug to the mother's health.
  - *Blood donation:* Patients should not donate blood or blood products while receiving the drug and for at least 24 months following the last dose of vismodegib.
  - *Semen donation:* Teach males not to donate semen during and for 3 months after the last dose of vismodegib.
  - *Premature fusion of the epiphyses:* has been reported in pediatric patients; in some cases, after drug discontinuation, fusion progressed.
- Most common adverse effects ($\geq 10\%$) are muscle spasms, alopecia, dysgeusia, weight loss, fatigue, nausea, diarrhea, decreased appetite, constipation, arthralgias, vomiting, and ageusia. Drug may cause amenorrhea in women.

Potential Toxicities/Side Effects and the Nursing Process

I.   ALTERATION IN SEXUALITY/REPRODUCTION related to POTENTIAL TERATOGENICITY

Defining Characteristics: Drug is teratogenic and fetotoxic, causing embryo-fetal death and severe birth defects. Drug may be excreted in semen. Amenorrhea has been observed in premenopausal women; it is unknown if it is reversible.

Nursing Implications: Assess reproductive status, sexual activity, and birth control measures used for both men and women. Instruct male patients to use condoms with spermicide, even after a vasectomy, during sexual intercourse with female partners while receiving therapy and for 2 months after the last dose when drug has been stopped. Ensure that women have had a negative pregnancy test within 7 days of starting the drug. Teach women to use highly effective contraception measures that have < 1% risk of failure prior to starting therapy, and to continue using it for 7 months after the last dose of vismodegib has been taken. Teach female patients to tell their providers immediately if pregnant (during therapy or for 7 months posttherapy) or if a male patient's female partner becomes pregnant while the patient is taking vismodegib. Exposure to the drug during pregnancy should be reported to Genentech Adverse Event Line (1-888-835-2555). Encourage the patient to participate in the Erivedge pregnancy pharmaco-vigilance program. Nursing mothers should either discontinue the drug or discontinue nursing. Teach male patients not to donate semen during and for 3 months after therapy (Genentech, 2015).

II. POTENTIAL ALTERATION IN NUTRITION related to NAUSEA, DIARRHEA, CONSTIPATION, VOMITING, DECREASED APPETITE, WEIGHT LOSS, DYSGEUSIA, AGEUSIA

Defining Characteristics: Nausea (incidence 30%), diarrhea (29%), constipation (21%), vomiting (14%), weight loss (45%), decreased appetite (25%), dysgeusia (changes in taste sensation) (55%), and ageusia (inability to taste sweet, sour, bitter, salty) (11%) can occur.

Nursing Implications: Assess nutritional status and bowel-elimination pattern baseline and at each visit. Teach patient self-care measures: to take OTC antidiarrheal or constipation medication as needed, to take antinausea medicine as prescribed; to modify diet (e.g., increase fiber and fluids if constipated, foods to slow diarrhea and fluids to reverse dehydration; high-calorie, high-protein foods in small amounts if decreased taste, appetite, and weight loss); and if taste disturbances, use taste stimulants such as Crazy Jane salt and pepper. Teach patient to report any symptoms that do not resolve or improve with the established plan. To increase appetite, encourage patients to use a small plate, take small portions, and not to fill the plate; take antiemetic 30 minutes prior to eating; and to eat small, frequent meals. Arrange dietary consultation if available and needed. Monitor weight at each visit to note trends.

III. ACTIVITY INTOLERANCE, POTENTIAL, related to FATIGUE, ASTHENIA, HEADACHE

Defining Characteristics: Fatigue occurs commonly in patients with advanced cancer who were studied. Fatigue occurred in 40% of patients.

Nursing Implications: Assess baseline activity and energy level, and teach patient that this symptom may occur. Assess patient's activity patterns, and suggest ways to conserve energy.

IV.   ALTERATION IN BODY IMAGE, POTENTIAL, related to ALOPECIA, SKIN CHANGES

Defining Characteristics: Alopecia occurs in 64% of patients receiving vismodegib.

Nursing Implications: Assess baseline skin integrity, and teach patient that alopecia may occur. Encourage patient to obtain a wig (cranial prosthesis) prior to starting therapy. Assess effect of hair loss on patient's body image, as well as skin changes. Encourage patient to verbalize feelings and provide emotional support. If needed, involve social worker in supportive counseling. Encourage patient to use scarves and hats as appropriate and to attend supportive educational sessions such as ACS Look Good... Feel Better programs if available.

V.   ALTERATION IN COMFORT related to MUSCLE SPASMS, ARTHRALGIAS

Defining Characteristics: Muscle spasms occurred in 72% of patients, and arthralgias, in 16%.

Nursing Implications: Teach patient that these side effects may occur and to report them. Teach patient to use local measures to reduce discomfort, such as use of heat or cold, acetaminophen. Teach patient to report symptoms that do not respond to self-care strategies and discuss with provider muscle relaxants and other measures.

Drug: vorinostat (Zolinza, suberoylanilide hydroxamic acid, SAHA)

Class: Histone deacetylase (HDAC) inhibitor.

Mechanism of Action: Histones are proteins that give structure and support to the DNA helix and DNA coils around the histones. Some tumors have excess HDAC, which causes the DNA to stay tightly packed. The DNA cannot be transcribed, and genes are not expressed and thus are silenced, like important tumor-suppressor genes. Vorinostat inhibits the enzymatic activity of histone deacetylases HDAC1, HDAC2, and HDAC3 (class I) and HDAC6 (class II). This results in increased histone acetylation and uncoiling of DNA so that the DNA is open; genes are expressed and can be transcribed for protein synthesis. These proteins are critical in normal cell-cycle regulation. The drug induces cell-cycle arrest and apoptosis in some transformed cells; the mechanism of action of antineoplastic effect has not been fully characterized.

Metabolism: After oral ingestion, the drug becomes 71% protein-bound. It is metabolized via glucuronidation and hydrolysis followed by α-oxidation, resulting in two inactive metabolites. Drug is eliminated primarily through metabolism, with < 1% of drug recoverable in the urine.

Indication: Indicated for the treatment of cutaneous manifestations of cutaneous T-cell lymphoma (CTCL) in patients who have progressive, persistent, or recurrent disease on or after two systemic therapies.

Dosage/Range:
- 400 mg orally once daily with food until disease progression or unacceptable toxicity.
- If intolerant to therapy, reduce dose to 300 mg orally once daily with food. If necessary, reduce the dose further to 300 mg once daily with food for 5 consecutive days and repeated weekly.
- Reduce dose in patients with mild or moderate hepatic impairment (BR 1–3 × ULN or AST > ULN): 300 mg once daily with food. There are no recommendations for patients with severe hepatic dysfunction (BR > 3 × ULN).
- Dose-reduce for thrombocytopenia, anemia.

Drug Preparation:
- Available in 100-mg gelatin capsules.

Drug Administration:
- Teach patient to:
  - Take vorinostat capsule(s) with food, and not to crush or open capsules.
  - Drink at least 2 L of fluid a day to prevent dehydration and to report vomiting or diarrhea that does not respond to recommended treatment promptly.
  - Verbally repeat signs of DVT, and to report them right away to call their physician/NP/PA.
  - If bleeding occurs, to seek medical attention right away.
  - Avoid direct contact of skin or mucous membranes with the powder and wash the area thoroughly if that occurs. Health care professionals should avoid contact with crushed and/or broken capsules (Merck&Co, Inc., 2018).
  - Teach women of reproductive potential, and men with female sexual partners of reproductive potential, to use effective contraception during drug therapy and for at least 6 months (women) and 3 months (men) after last drug dose.
- Monitor CBC, chemistry tests (electrolytes, glucose, serum creatinine, magnesium) every 2 weeks during first 2 months and then monthly thereafter; ECG with QTc measurement baseline and periodically during treatment.

Drug Interactions:
- Other HDACs (e.g., valproic acid): severe thrombocytopenia, GI bleeding; use together cautiously and monitor platelet count every 2 weeks during first 2 months.
- Coumarin-derivative antigoagulants: prolonged PT and INR. Monitor INR closely and dose accordingly.

Lab Effects/Interference:
- Decreased platelet and red blood cell count.
- Increased serum creatinine (46% of patients) and protein in urine (57% of patients).
- Hyperglycemia, hypokalemia, hyponatremia.
- QT/QTc prolongation, rarely.

Special Considerations:
- Warnings and Precautions:
  - *Pulmonary embolism (PE)* occurred in 5% of patients, and deep vein thrombosis (DVT) has been reported: Monitor for signs and symptoms, especially patients with a

history of thromboembolic events, and teach patient to report SOB, chest pain, other symptoms right away or call 911.

- *Dose-related thrombocytopenia and anemia*; May require dose modification or drug discontinuance. Monitor CBC/differential, platelet count every 2 weeks for the first 2 months, then monthly.
- *Nausea, vomiting, diarrhea:* patients may require antiemetics, antidiarrheals, and fluid and electrolyte replacement to prevent dehydration. Preexisting nausea, vomiting, and diarrhea should be well controlled before starting vorinostat therapy.
- *Hyperglycemia:* Monitor blood glucose every 2 weeks during the first 2 months and then monthly; monitor diabetic patients closely.
- *Clinical chemistry abnormalities:* Measure and correct abnormal electrolytes, creatinine, magnesium, and calcium baseline. Correct hypokalemia and hypomagnesemia before beginning vorinostat therapy. Monitor clinical chemistries as above every 2 weeks for the first 2 months, then at least monthly.
- *Severe thrombocytopenia and GI bleeding* has been reported when HDAC inhibitors are combined (e.g., vorinostat and valproic acid). Monitor platelet counts more frequently.
- *Fetal harm* can occur if administered to a pregnant woman, as drug crosses the placenta and drug is found in fetal animal plasma levels up to 50% of maternal concentrations.
  - Counsel women of reproductive potential to use effective contraception to avoid pregnancy. If drug is used during pregnancy or the patient becomes pregnant while taking the drug, the patient should be apprised of the potential hazard to the fetus.
  - Nursing mothers should decide whether to discontinue nursing or to discontinue vorinostat, taking into consideration the importance of the drug to the mother's health.
- Use in patients with hepatic impairment. Vorinostat AUC increases 50–66% in patients with hepatic impairment, and the incidence of grades 3–4 thrombocytopenia was increased in patients with mild or moderate hepatic impairment. Reduce dose in these patients.
- Most common side effects ($\geq$ 20%):
  - GI: diarrhea, nausea.
  - Constitutional: fatigue.
  - Hematologic: thrombocytopenia.
  - Nutritional disorders: dysgeusia, anorexia.

Potential Toxicities/Side Effects and the Nursing Process

I.   POTENTIAL FOR BLEEDING AND FATIGUE related to THROMBOCYTOPENIA AND ANEMIA

Defining Characteristics: Thrombocytopenia occurs in 25.6% (5.8% grades 3–4) of patients and anemia in 14% (grades 3–4, 2.3%).

Nursing Implications: Monitor CBC, platelet count baseline and periodically during therapy. Assess for signs and symptoms of bleeding, fatigue, and anemia. Teach patient to self-assess for signs and symptoms of bleeding and anemia and to call if they occur. Assess patient medication profile and any OTC medications, such as those containing aspirin or NSAIDs that would increase the risk of bleeding. Instruct patient to avoid these drugs and not to begin any OTC medications without first discussing with nurse or physician. Teach patient to alternate rest and activity periods if feeling fatigued and to organize shopping and chores in a way to minimize energy expenditures.

II. ALTERATION IN NUTRITION, LESS THAN BODY REQUIREMENTS, related to NAUSEA, DIARRHEA, ANOREXIA, DEHYDRATION, VOMITING, DYSGEUSIA, HYPERGLYCEMIA

Defining Characteristics: In clinical trials, these side effects occurred with the following frequency: diarrhea (52%), nausea (41%), dysgeusia (28%), anorexia (24%), dry mouth (16%), vomiting (15%), constipation (15%), and anorexia (14%).

Nursing Implications: Assess weight, bowel-elimination status, baseline nutritional status, and glucose level, and monitor during therapy. Teach patient that symptoms can occur and ways to minimize this effect, such as self-administration of antinausea and antidiarrheal medications and to report symptoms that do not resolve with established plan. Teach patient to identify nutritionally dense (high calories and protein in the smallest amount) foods and to keep them handy in the refrigerator. Teach patient to eat small, frequent meals and to have a bedtime snack. Teach patient that goal is to take in at least 2 quarts of fluid a day and to try to drink a glass of fluid every hour while awake. Monitor those patients at risk for dehydration closely, such as the elderly. Teach patient signs and symptoms of hyperglycemia (excessive thirst, frequent urination) and to report these. Discuss any abnormalities with a physician.

III. POTENTIAL ALTERATION IN CIRCULATION related to PULMONARY EMBOLISM, QTc PROLONGATION, PERIPHERAL EDEMA

Defining Characteristics: Pulmonary embolism occurred in 4.7% of patients, prolongation of the QTc interval occurred but has not been studied definitively, and peripheral edema occurred in 12% of patients.

Nursing Implications: Do baseline assessment of cardiac status, including the presence of peripheral edema, and ensure that baseline EKG with QTc interval has been done and that it is done periodically during treatment. Identify patients at risk for developing QTc prolongation, such as patients on anti-arrhythmic agents and patients with hypomagnesemia or hypokalemia. Check electrolytes and magnesium every 2 weeks during first 2 months of therapy and then monthly after that. Replete magnesium and potassium as ordered, or teach patient about self-administration of medications. Teach patient to report new pain in the back of the leg., a red streak up the leg, or difficulty breathing right away and to come to the emergency department for evaluation.

Chapter *4*
Immunologic Targeted Therapy

Immunologic targeted therapy or immunotherapy has become the single most important advance in cancer treatment (ASCO, 2016) and in 2018, adoptive cell immunotherapy was named the clinical cancer advance of the year (ASCO, 2018). In 2019, American Society of Clinical Oncology (ASCO) identified advances in rare tumors as the major advance so far and that this has been possible through the "successes of immunotherapies and targeted therapies, as well as insights into molecular diagnostics and the microbiome" (ASCO Post, 2019). ASCO notes that 6 years ago (in 2011), ipilimumab (Yervoy®) was recognized as the first drug to improve patient survival from advanced melanoma, while in 2015, combination with nivolumab (Opdivo®), a different immune checkpoint inhibitor targeting the programmed death-1 (PD-1) receptor was more effective than ipilimumab alone (ASCO, 2016). In addition to ipiliumumab, six other immune checkpoint inhibitors have been FDA approved: the programmed death receptor-1 (PD-1) blockers: cimiplimab-rwlc (Libtayo®), nivolumab (Opdivo), pembrolizumab (Keytruda®), and the programmed death-ligand 1 (PD-L1) blockers atezolizumab (Tecentriq®), avelumab (Bavencio®) and durvalumab (Imfinzi™). While all patients do not respond to the immune checkpoint inhibitors, those that do may have long-lasting responses (Ravoon, 2017). Historically, the search for the magic bullet to "turn on" the immune system to identify and kill cancer cells has been continued for decades. One of the limiting factors in cancer therapy has been the tumor's ability to evade the immune system, a hallmark of cancer. As knowledge of the immune system has evolved, efforts to manipulate and strengthen the immune system and direct key parts, such as antigen-presenting T-lymphocytes that can kill and direct other T-cells to kill tumor cells, were documented. However, early efforts such as use of interleukin-2 and lymphokine-activated killer (LAK) cells, as well as tumor infiltrating lymphocyte or TILs adoptive therapy, were only effective in a small percentage of patients. Fortunately, despite many disappointments, experts continued to try to understand the immune system better, and to harness the power of the immune system to target and destroy cancer cells. Tumors are able to take advantage of a number of strategies to circumvent the immune system. For example, the normal immune system uses two key strategies to turn down the immune system to protect normal cells from damage (e.g., autoimmune): (1) CTLA-4 (cytotoxic T-lymphocyte-associated protein), and (2) PD-1 and the ligands for PD-1 called PD-L1 and PD-L2. Currently one FDA-approved therapy blocks CTLA-4, while three block PD-1 and three block PD-L1. This has brought long-term survival to a number of patients with metastatic melanoma, bladder, and NSCLC, among others. In 2019, the first immune checkpoint inhibitor combination with a molecular targeted agent was FDA approved [avelumab (Bavencio) and axitinib for renal cell carcinoma]. The question remains what are the biomarkers that can predict which patients will respond and derive benefit so that clinicians can personalize therapy to the patient's specific tumor. Currently, the only biomarker is the presence of PD-L1 as shown by immunohistochemistry testing. Gajewski (2012) helps us understand this by making the distinction between tumors that are immunologically ignorant and those that are immunologically responsive. The immunologically ignorant tumors are not responsive to immune checkpoint blockade as they are associated with a low mutation load, immune tolerance against self-antigens, and they lack molecules for T-cell homing into tumor sites (e.g., chemokines). In contrast, immunologically responsive tumors are characterized by intrinsic T-cell immune-inhibition and extrinsic tumor-related T-cell immunosuppression (Gajewski, 2012). The intestinal microbiome has been identified as a very important factor in a competent immune system (Belkaid & Hand, 2014) and in the efficacy of immune checkpoint inhibitors (Pinato et al., 2019). Pinato emphasizes that gut microbial diversity strengthens mucosal immunity in the gut, as well as dendritic cell function and antigen presentation, all critical in a successful immune response. Research is underway looking at fecal microbiota and how it enhances the potency of this immune checkpoint inhibitor response (Osman & Luke, 2019). This led investigators to question the effect of antibiotic therapy on patients either before or concurrently during their treatment with an immune checkpoint inhibitor. It is hypothesized that the broad-spectrum antibiotics given prior to immunotherapy adversely changed the gut microbiota. Pinato et al. (2019) found that prior antibiotic therapy reduced overall survival significantly in patients treated for NSCLC, melanoma, and other cancers, compared to similar patients who did not receive antibiotics prior to immunotherapy. However, there was no difference in response or survival if the patient received antibiotic therapy concurrently with immune checkpoint therapy. While antibiotic therapy prior to immune checkpoint inhibitor therapy warrants caution, further research will help to define recommendations. Another variable that appears to affect response to efficacy of PD-(L)1 blockade is the use of baseline steroids. Arbour et al. (2018) studied 640 patients with NSCLC from two international institutions and found that patients who received prednisone $\geq$ 10 mg on day 1 of PD-(L)1 blockade had decreased ORR, PFS, and OS. The findings remained significant after controlling for smoking history, PS, and history of brain metastases. No differences were found when corticosteroids were used during therapy to manage irAEs. While caution is advised when considering corticosteroid use on day 1 of therapy, as more experience is gained with immune checkpoint inhibitor therapy, details that influence response will be identified and validated. The question also remains as what constitutes a genetic "positive" PD-L1 test (e.g., what percentage of staining of tumor cells). As more is learned about the mechanism of action of different immunotherapies, the targets have been refined. Traditionally, drugs are tested in specific cancers, and then if effective, approved to treat those tumors. New thinking, which is individualizing cancer medicine, involves development of drugs that target a specific genetic abnormality or mutation, This is called a *tumor agnostic drug* treatment, and currently there are three drugs with tumor agnostic indications: pembrolizumb (Keytruda), nivolumab (Opdivo), and larotrectinib (Vitrakvi). Pembrolizumab and nivolumab are effective against tumors that have DNA mismatch repair deficiency (dMMR) or microsatellite instability-High (MSI-H). Pembrolizumab is approved for any metastatic or unresectable tumor type with these genetic alterations, and nivolumumab is approved for patients with colorectal cancer with dMMR or MSI-H genetic alterations. Larotrectinib targets the Neurotropic Receptor Tyrosine Kinase (NTRK) fusion gene found in rare tumors that have metastasized and for which there is no alternative therapy: for example, mammary analogue secretory cancer; cellular or mixed congenital mesoblastic nephrome; infantile fibrosarcoma; and some rare forms of NSCLC, papillary thyroid cancer, breast, and sarcoma with the TRK mutation.

Other very promising therapies are defining personalized cancer therapy and include immune manipulation therapies such as chimeric antigen receptor (CAR) T-cell therapy for certain hematologic tumors. For example, tisagenlecleucel-t (Kymriah) is an anti-CD19-CAR retroviral vector-transduced autologous T cell therapy, a precisely targeted therapy against a specific patient's tumor. It is adoptive immunotherapy that uses a patient's own T-cells that have been removed and reprogrammed with a transgene that encodes for a CAR [FDA(a), 2017]. The CAR is made from a mouse single-antibody chain fragment that can recognize the CD-19 antigen. This is fused with parts of genes that control intracellular signaling (CD137 and CD3). This re-engineered CAR when injected into the patient, binds to the CD-19 antigen, and sends an intracellular message to increase proliferation of the new T-cell with the CAR, and also to protect the CAR so it remains in the newly formed T-cells. The CAR identifies and kills CD19-expressing malignant and nonmalignant B-cells bearing the CD-19 antigen. Research studies showed long-lasting remissions in pediatric and young patients with B-cell acute lymphocytic leukemia (ALL) who had relapsed or who were refractory to treatment. While this treatment is ground-breaking, it does come with toxicity; as expected, when the lymphocytes are destroyed, they release cytokines, and the resulting cytokine release syndrome (CRS) can be life-threatening. A second CAR T-cell therapy axicabtagene ciloleucel (Yescarta) is FDA approved for the treatment of adult patients with relapsed or refractory large B-cell lymphoma after 2 or more lines of systemic chemotherapy.

The immune checkpoint inhibitors offer strategies to block cancer's ability to turn down or off the immune system. Monoclonal antibodies (mAbs) have provided a vehicle to launch the immune checkpoint inhibitors. Much work has been and continues to be done to refine the remarkable abilities of mAbs, such as conjugating the mAb to a poison (antibody-drug conjugate [ADC]). Drugs that have been instrumental in demonstrating blockade of immune system features taken advantage of by tumors offer some patients remarkable long-term responses, such as pembrolizumab (Keytruda) and nivolumab (Opdivo). Research to identify biomarkers that will indicate which patients will respond are ongoing. Other FDA-approved agents include the oncolytic viral immunotherapy, talimogene laherparepved (Imlygic® or T-vec), used for intralesional treatment of recurrent melanoma, and the vaccine sipuleucel-t (Provenge) for prostate cancer.

Immune-oncology has been shown to drive more precise cancer treatment. Epitope-based therapy involves taking an epitope, or part of an antigen, and then using it to activate and improve the immune system's response to the patient's specific tumor (Soon-Shiong, 2016). A national conference of key thought leaders, academic and community physicians, and researchers has been held annually at Scripps Oceanographic Institute called the "Future of Genomic Medicine" (FOGM). Since tumor targets are specific, treatments that should be the most effective incubate the patient's tumor antigen and the patient's T-lymphocytes (antigen presenting cells [APCs]), which are then immunologically augmented, then reinjected into the patient to assist the patient's immune system in mounting a powerful response against that specific antigen. Today, these therapies include the autologous vaccine sipuleucel-T (Provenge®), adenoviral vector therapies that are being studied, and chimeric antigen receptor T-lymphocyte (CAR-T cell therapy or CAR-T) therapies, including tisa-genlecleucel (Kymriah), axicabtagene ciloleucel (Yescarta), and others that are also currently under investigation. CAR-T cell therapy is an adoptive cell transfer (ACT), where the patients' immune cells are engineered to attack cells in the patient's tumor. It is called a "living drug" since it uses the patient's own T-lymphocytes, which are removed and then genetically engineered to make special receptors called CARs [NCI, 2014]. These new receptors tell the T-lymphocytes how to recognize the cancer antigen on tumor cells, and billions of copies of these CAR-T cells are made in the laboratory and then injected into the patient. Once in the body, the infused T-cells reproduce and they follow instructions from the engineered receptor to recognize and kill tumor cells with the patient's tumor antigen on their cell surfaces (NCI, 2014). Because billions of T-lymphocytes are used, which also release cytokines, or chemical messengers, all at one time, one of the side effects of CAR-T cell therapy is CRS. This is discussed later in the chapter.

New frontiers are being exploited to try to manipulate the immune system to augment its response against cancer. CRISPR is defined as Clustered Regularly Interspaced Short Palindromic Repeats and is thought to be the "biggest biotechnological discovery of the century" (Martinez-Lage et al., 2018) as it permits precise modification or editing of genes in DNA (Tian et al., 2019). The CRISPR gene-editing tool is being used in clinical trials to genetically alter a patient's T-lymphocytes to identify and attack cancer cells similar to genetically reengineered receptors in CAR T therapy. The engineered T-cell receptors identify and then mount an aggressive attack against the patient's cancer cells, but in addition, the gene for PD-1, which can act as a "brake" for the immune system, is removed. Thus, the patient not only gets the precision aggressive attack on the patient's cancer cells but also PD-1 inhibition. Currently, two patients have received this treatment on a clinical trial—one with sarcoma and one patient with multiple myeloma (NPR, 2019). Other trials are being planned/conducted at other U.S. centers and elsewhere in the world.

Progress can come from many different directions. Platt et al. (2017) were studying a vaccine that produced antibodies against HIV, and unexpectedly found that the C3d immune complement protein was able to block tumor-mediated immune suppression and turn back on the immune system in mice with murine lymphoma and melanoma. The results were an 80–90% reduction in tumor burden, which was long lived. They described tumor escape of immune surveillance by engaging regulators of the T-cell checkpoint, expanding the population of regulatory T-cells, and other mechanisms. The resulting immune response provoked by the C3d protein was independent of B cells, NK cells, and antibodies; the protein increased the number of tumor infiltrating CD8 positive lymphocytes, depleted regulatory T-cells, and by suppressed expression of PD-1 protein by T-cells. Thus, the protein was able to turn off the mechanism that tumors were using to block immune surveillance and turn back on T-cell activation and proliferation (Platt et al., 2017). The authors have a pending patent application for use of the protein as an anticancer agent.

Immunotherapy, the boosting or restoration of the immune system to fight cancer, is now the fifth major cancer treatment modality. Unlike the other four treatments, however, immunotherapy does not directly target the cancer cells; rather, it targets immune processes to block tumors that co-opt the body's normal immune processes or augments the patient's immune system to directly target tumor antigens. See Table 4.1 that compares the

Table 4.1   Comparison of Five Cancer Therapies

Modality	Mechanism of Action	Adverse Events
Immunotherapy	Restores and/or augments normal immune response and killing of tumor cells	Fatigue, immune-related adverse reactions (irAEs), such as rash and pruritis; diarrhea/colitis; hepatitis; endocrinopathies; pneumonitis; hepatitis; dermatologic changes
Molecular-Targeted Therapy	Targets key signaling proteins that are mutated or overexpressed in the tumor, blocking tumor growth and inducing apoptosis	Class-related effects such as bleeding, HTN, impaired wound healing with anti-angiogenic drugs; rash and diarrhea with epidermal growth factor receptor (EGFR) inhibitors; as well as drug-specific toxicities
Chemotherapy	Kills frequently dividing cells	Collateral damage to normal, frequently dividing cells, including the bone marrow with increased risk of infection and bleeding, gonads, GI mucosa, and hair follicles; as well as some organ-specific toxicities.
Radiation	Local treatment to kill tumor cells in RT field	Collateral damage to surrounding normal tissue, although minimized with improved 3D conformal therapy.
Surgery	Local excision of tumor	Postoperative adverse events; risk of tumor seeding if tumor extensive.

five modalities. In this chapter, immunotherapy encompasses biotherapy, biologic therapy, and immune-oncology. This chapter will provide a review of the immune system and an organizing framework to understand cytokines, immune modulating agents, vaccines, and immunologic targeting agents.

THE NORMAL IMMUNE SYSTEM

While the skin and mucous membranes in fact represent the first physical barrier or line of defense against invading micro-organisms, this section will focus on the immune components internally. Theoretically, the immune system should be able to identify and destroy upwards of 100,000 cancer cells (Swann, 2007). The immune system is responsible for identifying invading microorganisms and abnormal cells that might harm the body. It uses immune surveillance to accomplish this, distinguishing self from nonself by markers on the cell surface that match the person's major histocompatibility complex class-1 (MHC-1) proteins, also called human leukocyte antigens (HLA).

The immune system is constantly on the lookout for cells or antigens (proteins) that do not have the MHC nameplate showing that they belong to the body (immune surveillance); once recognized as foreign, the immune elements destroy the cells and remove them from the body. In addition, the immune system destroys and removes abnormal, old, or damaged cells. Because humans live in a biosphere, it is important that the immune system can identify, destroy, and remove invading micro-organisms that do not have self (MHC) proteins. Normally, the immune system is quiet or tolerant as it encounters cells with the correct MHC proteins. However, when a microorganism invades, or a cell without the MHC protein is found, the immune system is turned on to find and destroy it. An antigen can be defined as any substance that can cause an immune response and which then participates in the immune reaction. The distinct, unique surface regions of an antigen that can elicit an immune response are called epitopes, each of which can bind to a specific antibody (Murphy, 2011). Tumor antigens are usually genetically distinct from normal cells and tumor specific (Coulie et al., 2014).

The body has two immune responses that interact to create immunity: (1) the *innate*, a first-line of defense that is immediate, nonantigen specific, and that does not remember the exposure, and (2) the *adaptive*, which is second-line, takes longer to occur, is antigen specific, and has immunologic memory (Murphy, 2011). We are born with innate immunity, while adaptive immunity is acquired.

Our bodies are protected by both the ***innate*** and ***adaptive*** immune responses, which are interconnected. The innate immune response is immediate, as when you get the flu. You may develop fever, malaise, and other symptoms. The innate immune response is the first line of defense, and while immediate, it is not antigen-specific, nor is there immunological memory. Thus, you need to get a flu shot every year to protect against the flu. The key elements in the innate response are phagocytes (e.g., macrophages, monocytes, neutrophils), dendritic cells, and natural killer (NK) cells. NK cells activated by the innate response will kill any potential target it recognizes as "nonself" that does not have an MHC-1 protein. It is not antigen-specific.

In contrast, the adaptive immune response takes longer to evolve initially, is antigen-specific, and your body's immune system remembers the antigen, so the next time the antigen is seen, the adaptive response is much more swift and potent. In the adaptive immune system, the immune cells are able to distinguish self from nonself, to remember the "foreign" antigen(s) to which they have been exposed (memory T and B cells do this), and to mount an immune attack to eliminate the foreign antigen. When the antigen is encountered again, the immune system will mount a rapid and increasingly more potent defense against the antigen. The adaptive immune system has two major parts: (1) humoral immunity, involving antibodies, and complement; and (2) cell-mediated immune system, involving T-lymphocyte cells, called T-cells.

First, the immune system needs to know what the invader looks like so it can mobilize an army of immune cells, seek out the enemy as identified by its antigen, and destroy it. Antigens act as nameplates, and those without MHC do not belong to the body and are identified as foreign. APCs are critical to an effective immune response. When a foreign organism invades the body, macrophages and dendritic cells (a type of B-lymphocyte) will find the organism, engulf and digest it, and then remove a peptide fragment containing the antigen and mount it on their cell surface to show the target to T-lymphocytes and other immune cells. Dendritic cells have great potential in recognizing and orchestrating an immune attack against tumor cell antigens; however, they must mature before they can activate T-lymphocytes. More specifically, after the dendritic cell recognizes the foreign antigen on the surface of the tumor cell, it infiltrates into the tumor, processes intracellular proteins and/or antigens, and matures in a lymph node so that each dendritic cell can express fragments of the antigen on its surface to present to the T-lymphocytes in cell-mediated immunity. The mature dendritic cell uses the MHC to present the foreign antigen; when bound to the T-lymphocyte, a signal is sent to make more T-lymphocytes: the B7 costimulatory molecule on the dendritic cells binds to the CD28 receptor on the T-lymphocyte, which then signals T-lymphocyte replication so that there is rapid proliferation of activated T-lymphocytes to find and kill the invading micro-organism or tumor cell with that antigen. Key warriors in the immune system's army that can be activated by the dendritic cells are cytotoxic T-lymphocytes (CTLs), B-lymphocytes, and NK cells. They can be thought of as "attack dogs" defending the human body. As dendritic cells orchestrate the army's advance against the foreign antigen, they use cytokines as chemical messengers to talk to the different immune cells, and to orchestrate the immune reaction. Thus, the immune cells use cytokines to talk to each other.

Cell-mediated immunity involves activation of specific immune cells such as the thymus-dependent lymphocytes, or T-lymphocytes, often abbreviated T-cells. These cells are involved in the cell-mediated (cytotoxic) immune response and are divided into helper [CD4+ (T4) lymphocytes, which help activated B-lymphocytes make antibody] and cytotoxic T-cells [CD8+ (T8, or effector cells), which kill invading organisms or cancer cells], among others. In order for the CTLs to function, they must be activated, which stimulates them to proliferate and then mature so that they are directed against only the invading antigen (containing cell), which they will kill (Chen & Mellman, 2013). CD8 T-lymphocytes can be *cytotoxic*, killing identified antigen-specific cells or CD8 T-cells can be *regulatory*, which help to turn down the immune response after the invading organism has been neutralized. Because the immune reaction can be so powerful, there has to be a way to turn down the immune system so that the person's organs are not attacked, such as with autoimmune diseases. These are called immune checkpoints. This is one place malignant cells co-opt the immune system and turn down the cytotoxic T-lymphocyte response. Function of any T-cell (helper, cytotoxic, or regulatory) is activated only when the T-lymphocyte binds to its specific antigen when it is presented on an APC (Messerschmidt et al., 2016).

The dendritic cell activates helper T-cells, which produce cytokines that activate appropriate B-lymphocytes and/or T-lymphocytes to seek and destroy the antigen(s) marked for destruction. These helper T-lymphocytes may be activated to differentiate into CTLs, which proliferate rapidly against the specific antigen(s) and kill the cell containing the antigen on its cell surface. See Figure 4.1.

Humoral immunity involves B-lymphocytes, which make antibody and complement. They are derived from the bone marrow cells (Messerschmidt et al., 2016). B-lymphocytes can recognize APCs, and are taught how to recognize the foreign antigen fragment. Once B-cells become activated, including with additional costimulatory signals, they differentiate into plasma cells, which can be thought of as "antibody factories," making an antibody specifically against the invading antigen or protein. The manufactured antibody fits "like a lock and a key" on the epitope of the antigen, and it seeks out and destroys cells with the antigen on its cell surface. See Figure 4.2 for an antibody, where the variable region (top of the Y, F_{ab} portion) is the lock, contoured to fit any microbe or invading antigen epitope (infinite number of shapes so that the antibody will recognize any and all invading antigens encountered in a person's life). The stem of the Y (F_c) is the constant region, which calls members of the immune system to help attack the bound antigen.

The upper Y or variable section of the antibody (F_{ab}) matches the antigen shape exactly, and it binds to the antigen to mark the cell for attack, while the stem of the Y is

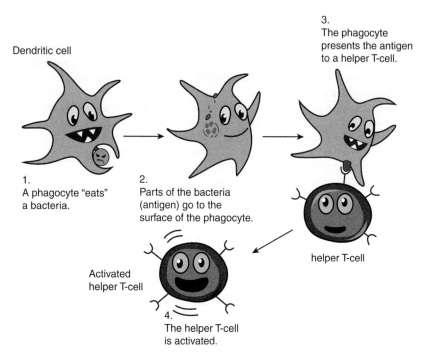

Figure 4.1   Antigen Presentation
Reproduced from "The Immune System—in More Detail." Nobelprize.org. http://www.nobelprize.org /educational/medicine/immunity/immune-detail.html. June 14, 2016. Copyright Nobel Media AB 2014.

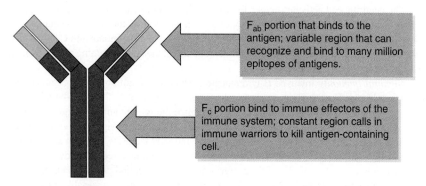

Figure 4.2   Antibody

the constant region (F_c), which calls in the effector cells of the immune system to kill the antigen-containing cell (e.g., NK cells, macrophages).

Antibody is made when the immune system identifies an invading micro-organism, as shown in Figure 4.3.

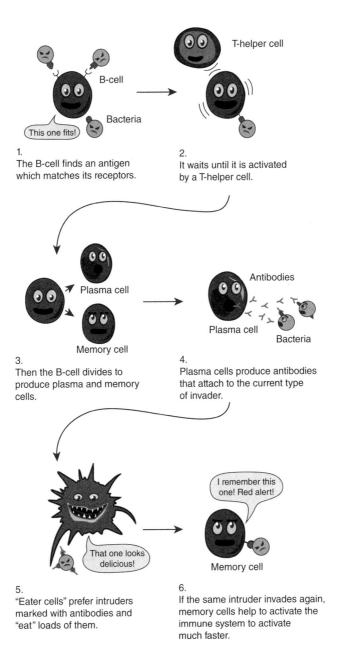

Figure 4.3   Manufacturing Antibodies.

Reproduced from "The Immune System—in More Detail." Nobelprize.org. http://www
.nobelprize.org/educational/medicine/immunity/immune-detail.html. June 14, 2016.
Copyright Nobel Media AB 2014.

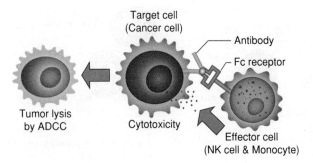

Figure 4.4   Antibody Dependent Cell-mediated Cytotoxicity (ADCC)

Data from Carter P. Improving the efficacy of antibody-based cancer therapies. *Nat Rev Cancer* 2001;1:118-129; Eureka Therapeutics, http://www.eurekainc.com.cn /technology.html. Accessed November 5, 2009.

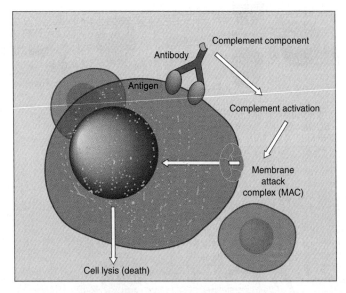

Figure 4.5   Complement-Dependent Cytotoxicity (CDC)

Reproduced from iQ Biosciences. Complement-Dependent Cytotoxicity (CDC) Assay. https://www.iqbiosciences.com/bioservices/in-vitro_bioservices/complement-dependent -cytotoxicity-assays/. 2016.

When an antibody binds to an antigen, the cell is killed in one of two ways: (1) antibody-dependent cell-mediated cytotoxicity (ADCC) or (2) complement-dependent cytotoxicity (CDC). See Figures 4.4 and 4.5. In ADCC, B-lymphocytes become activated and begin manufacturing antibodies against the specific antigen presented by the APCs. See Figures 4.3 and 4.4.

In ADCC, once bound to the antibody/antigen complex, the attracted NK cells release cytotoxic granules, along with cytokines, which kill the cell by digesting the cell membrane and entering the cell, causing apoptosis. In CDC, B lymphocytes bind to the antigen and activate complement, which triggers the complement cascade. The antigen-containing cell is coated with complement, which "punches" holes in the cell membrane, killing the cell (Weinberg, 2014). Complement is a very powerful cell-killing mechanism, and normal cells protect themselves from it by expressing anticomplement proteins on their cell membranes. Unfortunately, some cancer cells have been found to overexpress membrane-bound complement regulatory proteins, which protect them from CDC (Weinberg, 2014).

mAbs are similar to the body's antibodies, but they are a clone of antibodies manufactured to target a single antigen and bind tightly to that antigen like a key in a lock. They are discussed in more detail later in the chapter.

The cancer-immunity cycle was described by Chen and Mellman (2013) as occurring in the following steps as the immune system attempts to recognize and destroy cancer cells:

1. Tumor cell lysis and release of tumor-associated antigens.
2. APCs take up, process, and present fragments of the tumor antigen to the immune system.
3. T-cells are primed and activated, generating effector (cytotoxic) and memory T-cells to the tumor antigen.
4. Activated T-cells seek out and destroy tumor cells with this tumor antigen.
5. Infiltration of T-cells into the tumor.
6. T-cells recognize tumor antigens in cancer cells.
7. T-cells kill tumor antigen-containing cells, leading back to 1, tumor cell lysis and release of tumor-derived antigens.

Cytokines are the messages secreted by immune cells that provide communication between and among the immune system cells. Cytokines regulate the intensity and duration of the immune response to an invading microorganism and are critical to the orchestration of the immune response. Cytokines include interleukins, interferons, and colony-stimulating factors. For example, helper T-cells secrete interferon-γ and interleukin-2 (Messerschmidt et al., 2016).

HOW CANCER EVADES THE IMMUNE SYSTEM

The immune response can be very powerful and potentially can kill the person by attacking and destroying normal tissues if it is not controlled. Immune checkpoints are in place that sense when it is time to turn down or off the immune response, principally by dampening or shutting off the function of activated CTLs. As reviewed in *Chapter 3*, Hanahan and Weinberg (2011) described the strategies tumors use to evade the immune system as a hallmark of cancer, so that the tumor can remain invisible to the body's normal immune defenses.

Cancer cells have learned that if they co-opt or make the patient's immune system develop immune tolerance to the antigen, the cancer antigen is not recognized as foreign and does not ramp up the immune response against it. Cancer cells can evade the immune system by suppressing immune cells locally; in the microenvironment, they can also make the immune system tolerant to the cancer antigens by co-opting the inhibitory immune checkpoints and by using immune editing (Pardoll, 2012; Schreiber et al., 2011).

The knowledge of how cancer evades the immune system is evolving. Zielinski et al. (2013) describe four ways the immune system is circumvented. First, tumors may reduce expression of the class-I MHC molecules so that they are not detected as nonself and an immune response is not activated; thus, the tumor antigen cannot be seen by CTLs. Second, they can turn down (down-regulate) the innate immune system's cancer-fighting NK cells. Third, they can avoid apoptosis by down-regulating the Fas receptor (apoptosis antigen 1) cell surface expression so they are invisible to NK and CTLs, and apoptosis does not occur. Fourth, they can promote an anti-inflammatory state favoring tumor growth through secretion of growth factors that are immunosuppressive to T-lymphocytes and macrophages.

Dunn et al. (2006) describe a theory of immunoediting that spans the time from immune surveillance to tumor escape that occurs in three phases. Initially, in the first phase called "immune surveillance," cancer cells are identified and totally eliminated. The second phase occurs if a cancer cell escapes immune surveillance, is not eliminated, but is held in check by the immune cells, and this is called "immune equilibrium." At this time, there is an occult, dormant tumor whose cells are in a "stand off" with the immune cells fighting them (Messerschmidt et al., 2016). The third phase is called "immune escape," where previously dormant tumor cells have mutated, which allows the cells to evade the immune system. As the mutated cells begin to grow and invade, they are now clinically symptomatic and detectable. The immune system is exhausted, overwhelmed, and metastases occurs.

How do cancer cells co-opt the immune checkpoints? Immune checkpoints are normal pathways that inhibit the immune system, or turn it down or off after the immune system has done its job (self-tolerance). In the human body, the intensity (amplitude) and quality of the immune response is determined by a balance between costimulatory and inhibitory signals (Pardoll, 2012). Otherwise, the uncontrolled immune system could greatly damage organs, peripheral tissues, and could kill the person. The T-cell antigen receptor has been likened to an "ignition switch" turning on the T-cell attack against microinvaders (Johnson, 2017). CD28, a molecule expressed on T-cells gives costimulatory signals that accelerate T-cell activation and survival. In contrast, CTLA-4 acts as the "brakes."

There are probably many immune checkpoints, of which only a few are well known. Unfortunately, tumor cells are known to be able to co-opt immune checkpoints that turn down or turn off the immune system (activation of T-cells). This explains how tumor cells "escape" immune surveillance and control (equilibrium). As the tumor grows, and outgrows its available nutritional supply (oxygen, glucose), the cells without oxygen start to necrose, which leads to inflammation. Now, the immune system gets alerted and responds with an immune response. Tumor cells are able to co-opt: (1) CTLA-4 and (2) PD-1. CTLA-4 can be thought of as an "off" switch for cytotoxic T-cell activation as it controls the amplitude of the T-cell activation (Pardoll, 2012). CTLA-4 is expressed on T-lymphocytes, and its ligand is CD80 (Quezada & Peggs, 2013). The CTLA-4 cell surface protein is a negative regulator of T-lymphocyte function and activation; that is, once activated, it turns down the powerful T-lymphocyte immune response after the immune response is started to protect normal tissues from the ravages of the immune response (Wolchok & Saenger, 2008). Most malignant cells express CTLA-4 (CD152) and use it to escape cytotoxic T-lymphocyte attack (immune resistance). Blockade of CTLA-4 results in antitumor immunity (Wolchok & Saenger, 2008) because it turns back on the switch of T-cell activation (turns off the brakes that would stop T-cell activation), and the tumor cells can no longer escape cytotoxic T-lymphocyte attack. This occurs early in the immune response.

Similarly, the programmed cell death protein-1 (PD-1) or its ligand (PD-L1, PD-L2) modulates T-cell activity in peripheral tissues later in the immune response, limiting T-cell effector functions (Moreno & Ribas, 2015; Pardoll, 2012). The PD-1 receptors are expressed on T-cells and pro-B cells. PD-1 is a receptor that binds the two ligands PD-L1 and PD-L2. PD-1 and its ligand function to prevent activation of T-cells in tissues, which decreases the risk of auto-immunity and injury to normal tissues and also promotes self-tolerance (Moreno & Ribas, 2015). Some tumors increase (upregulate) the production of PD-1 ligands (PD-L1, PD-L2) to try to halt immune surveillance and antitumor responses in the tumor microenvironment (Pardoll, 2012). This allows the cancer cells to circulate invisibly and not be stopped by the immune system.

Other ways the tumor can elude the immune system include the tumor's ability to interfere with dendritic cell maturation, and/or it may block signaling between the costimulatory molecules B7 and CD28, which is required for maturation of activated T-lymphocytes. Without this signaling, cytokines are not produced, such as IL-2, which is necessary for full activation of T-lymphocytes, and the proliferating T-lymphocytes are not fully activated (Scandella & Ludewig, 2005).

CLASSES OF IMMUNOLOGICALLY TARGETED AGENTS

Classes of immunologically targeted agents are discussed separately but may not fall into one simple category. For example, nivolumab (Opdivo) is an immune checkpoint inhibitor that is also a mAb and can be considered an immune-modulating agent (Wilkes, 2017).

CYTOKINES

Cytokines are substances released from activated lymphocytes and include the interferons (IFNs), interleukins (ILs), and colony-stimulating factors (CSFs). Cytokines are responsible for communication between and among immune elements to orchestrate the immune response. Cytokines can either enhance or suppress an immune response. Cytokines can bring other immune cells to an area of infection using chemotaxis (chemotactic cytokines).

Interferons: Interferons occur naturally in the body and were the first cytokine to be studied. The interferons can be divided into two types: type I IFNs bind to cell surface receptors on effector cells, and include IFN-α and IFN-β, which bind to α and β cell surface receptors on effector cells, respectively. Type II IFNs, such as IFN-γ bind to different cell surface receptors. Interferons of both groups help to regulate the immune system, improve resistance to invading microorganisms, and halt cell proliferation. However, each interferon subgroup has specific functions, as will be discussed with each drug.

IFN-α is stimulated by viruses and tumor cells; its antiviral activity is greater than its antiproliferative activity, which is greater than its immunomodulatory effects. There are 20 subtypes of IFN-α. IFN-β is also stimulated by viruses; it has equal antiviral, antiproliferative, and immunomodulatory effects. There are two subtypes of IFN-β. IFN-γ is essential during innate and adaptive immunity responses to infections by viruses, some bacteria, and some protozoa. It is has both proinflammatory actions (e.g., activating macrophages to kill microbes, induction of the Class II MHC), and anti-inflammatory actions. It has been shown to help contain tumor growth and progression by increasing tumor antigen presentation to tumor specific T-cells and increasing the tumor sensitivity to killing by NK cells (Lin and Young, 2013). It is stimulated by the cell-mediated immune response and IL-2; it is released by activated T-lymphocytes and NK cells. It can inhibit viral replication.

Common side effects of interferons include flu-like symptoms, anorexia, and fatigue.

CSFs: CSFs include hematopoietic growth factors. They, too, occur naturally in the body and help immature blood cell elements develop into mature, effective white blood cells, red blood cells, or platelets. Recombinant DNA techniques have permitted the manufacture of large quantities of these substances. An "r" prefix (e.g., r-IL-2) indicates that it was produced using recombinant technology.

Biosimilar cytokines and therapeutic biologicals are being developed and approved by the FDA. The first biosimilar drug, filgrastim sndz (Zarxio®), was FDA approved in 2015. According to the FDA (2017d), a biosimilar product is highly similar to the reference biological product with only minor differences in clinically inactive compounds, and no clinically meaningful differences (e.g., safety, purity, and potency). The FDA (2017e) also states that "bringing new biosimilars to patients" especially in treating costly diseases, "can help spur the competition that can lower health-care costs and increase access to important therapies." In development of a biosimilar, the drug sponsor must not only show "high similarity" to the originator biological, but also biosimilar pharmacokinetics and pharmacodynamics so that the same dose, strength and route of administration can be used (FDA (f) 2017; Isakov et al., 2015). What may not known when the biosimilar is approved, but becomes clear inn post-marketing, is the clinical immunogenicity (e.g., antibody formation and binding, neutralizing, cytokine levels). In addition, there may be immunogenic variation in lot-to-lot drug between manufacturers so it is imperative that any variations in manufacturing are minimized (FDA, 2015a). The FDA recommends parallel study in treatment-naïve patients. A biosimilar drug is named by the FDA by first giving the drug to which the biosimilar is compared, and then adding a 4-letter suffix to the product name, such as filgrastim-sndz, that are randomly generated. Biosimilars have extrapolated indications, that is, while initial research compares the drug used to treat the most sensitive disease, once this is established, the biosimilar indications are extrapolated from the originator biological agent when the mechanism of the drug, PK and PD testing are similar, for example if a rituximab biosimilar is approved for use in treating lymphoma, this could not be extrapolated for use in the treatment of non-malignant rheumatoid arthritis as rituximab is as the mechanism of action, PK and PD findigs are different. Extrapolation, however, is NOT interchangeability, or freely substituting the biosimilar for the originator biological agent through alternation or switching (FDA, 2015b). Additional studies are required for interchangeability involving alternating from the reference (originator) biological to the biosimilar and back to the reference biological. As clinicians and scientists have more experience with use of biosimilars, there is a closer look at differences in antibody dependent cell-mediated cytotoxicity (ADCC) compared to the target product, and also there may be differences within different lots of a biosmiliar drug that are identified in quality assurance studies. Table 4.2 shows biosimilars FDA approved as of June 2019. Biosimilars used for the treatment of rheumatoid arthritis are discussed in the introduction of *Chapter 5*.

Table 4.2   Biosimilars FDA Approved as of June 1, 2019

Biosimilar	Drug Class	Approval Date	Indications (see specific drug sections for full indications)
Bevacizumab-awwb (Mvasi)	VEGF-inhibitor	September 2017	Treatment of patients with metastatic CRC, unresectable non-squamous NSCLC with carboplatin/paclitaxel, glioblastoma, metastatic RCC with interferon alfa, persistent/recurrent/metastatic cervical cancer with paclitaxel and cisplatin or topotecan
Epoetin alfa-epbx (Retacrit™)	rHuEPO; Erythropoiesis-stimulating agent (ESA)	May 2018	Treatment of anemia due to chronic kidney disease, zidovudine in HIV-infected patients, or concomitant myelosuppressive chemotherapy (when at least 2 additional months of chemotherapy is planned); reduction of allogeneic RBC transfusions in patients undergoing elective, noncardiac, non-vascular surgery
Filgrastim-aafi (Nivestym)	rG-CSF	July 2018	Decrease incidence of neutropenic infection in patients receiving myelosuppressive anti-cancer drugs or with nonmyeloid malignancies undergoing BMT; reduce time to neutrophil recovery and duration of fever in AML consolidation treatment; mobilize autologous hematopoietic progenitor cells for leukapheresis collection; reduce incidence and duration of neutropenia in patient siwth congenital neutropenia
Filgrastim-sndz (Zarxio®)	rG-CSF	March 2015	Decrease incidence of neutropenic infection in patients receiving myelosuppressive anti-cancer drugs or with nonmyeloid malignancies undergoing BMT; reduce time to neutrophil recovery and duration of fever in AML consolidation treatment; mobilize autologous hematopoietic progenitor cells for leukapheresis collection; reduce incidence and duration of neutropenia in patient siwth congenital neutropenia
Pegfilgrastim-jmdb (Fulphila™)	rG-CSF	June 2018	Treatment to decrease the incidence of infection (e.g., febrile neutropenia) in patients with non-myeloid malignancy receiving myelosuppressive anti-cancer drugs associated with significant febrile neutropenia
Pegfilgrastim-cbqv (Udenyca®)	rG-CSF	November 2018	Treatment to decrease the incidence of infection (e.g., febrile neutropenia) in patients with nonmyeloid malignancy receiving myelosuppressive anticancer drugs associated with significant febrile neutropenia

(continues)

Table 4.2   (Continued)

Biosimilar	Drug Class	Approval Date	Indications (see specific drug sections for full indications)
Rituximab-abbs (Truxima®)	Anti-CD20	November 2018	Relapsed or refractory low grade or follicular CD20+ NHL, previously untreated follicular NHL, non-progressing low grade NHL as a single agent after 1st line chemo (NOT approved for other Rituxan indications) see package insert
Trastuzumab-dkst (Ogivri®)	HER2/new receptor antagonist	December 2017	Treatment of patients with breast or metastatic gastric or GE junction adenocarcinoma that overexpress the HER2 gene (HER2+)
Traztuzumab-dttb (Ontruzant)	HER2/new receptor antagonist	January 2019	Treatment of HER2 over-expressing breast, gastric or gastroesophageal junction adenocarcinoma
Trastuzumab-qyyp (Trazimera)	HER2/new receptor antagonist	March 2019	
Trastuzumab-pkrb (Herzuma™)	HER2/neu receptor antagonist	December 2018	Treatment of patients with breast cancer that overexpresses the HER2 gene (HER2+) ONLY —not indicated for other Herceptin indications (see package insert)

Key: rG-CSF: recombinant granulocyte-colony stimulation factor; AML: acute myelogenous leukemia; VEGF: vascular endothelian growth factor; HER: human epidermal growth factor receptor; RCC: renal cell carcinoma; NSCLC: non-small cell lung cancer; SQ: subcutaneous.

The use of colony-stimulating, especially myeloid, growth factors, has permitted chemotherapy to be given more safely, and importantly, allowed the maintenance of scheduled dose delivery. Filgrastim (Neupogen®), tbo-filgrastim (Neutroval®, Granix®), and two filgrastim biosimilar agents [filgrastim sndz (Zarxio®), filgrastim-aafi (Nivestym)] are granulocyte-colony-stimulating factors (G-CSFs) approved to prevent infection related to febrile neutropenia following bone marrow suppressive chemotherapy, as well as for other uses. A sustained-duration pegylated formulation requiring less frequent dosing is available (pegfilgrastim or Neulasta®, and pegrastim-jmdb or Fulphila™). This is called primary prophylaxis and begins after the first cycle of chemotherapy. Primary prophylaxis is used to prevent febrile neutropenia in high-risk patients (e.g., age, medical history, disease characteristics, expected chemotherapy myelotoxicity) (Smith et al., 2015). Secondary prophylaxis is when the growth factor is used to prevent the recurrence of febrile neutropenia in a patient who has not used growth factor in the past, and therapeutic use is when the growth factor is used at the time of neutropenia or neutropenic fever in high-risk individuals, such as those with sepsis syndrome, pneumonia, or fungal infection (Hill et al., 2014).

In order to provide guidance and recommendations for evidence-based practice, the American Society of Clinical Oncology (ASCO) published guidelines for the use of colony-stimulating factors in 2015. The guideline emphasizes that the reduction of febrile neutropenia is an important clinical outcome justifying the use of CSFs, regardless of the impact on other factors, when the risk of febrile neutropenia is 20% or more and there is no other equally effective anticancer regimen that does not require CSFs available. An example of a common breast cancer regimen with a 20% or greater incidence of febrile neutropenia is Adriamycin® and Cytoxan® followed by Taxol® (AC→T). Additional regimens can be found in the 2018 Myeloid Growth Factor NCCN Guideline, found at http://www.nccn.org. Patient factors and comorbidities can also increase the risk for febrile neutropenia; these include a history of severe neutropenia with similar chemotherapy, extensive prior chemotherapy, poor performance or nutritional status, age older than 65 years, and bone marrow involvement with tumor (NCCN, 2018). Dose dense regimens that require CSFs should only be used in a clinical trial or if supported by strong evidence to support efficacy (Smith et al., 2015). For example, prophylactic G-CSF permits patients with diffuse aggressive lymphoma, aged 65 or older who are being treated with curative intent, to have reduced risk of febrile neutropenia and infections (Smith et al., 2015). NCCN guidelines (2018) suggest that patients with solid tumors or nonmyeloid malignancies should be evaluated for risk of febrile neutropenia prior to the first cycle of chemotherapy in terms of disease, chemotherapy regimen, patient risk factors (e.g., age 65 or older, prior history of neutropenia), and treatment intent (e.g., cure vs. control vs. palliation). If the risk of febrile neutropenia is high ($> 20\%$), CSF as primary prophylaxis should be used. If the risk is intermediate (10–20%), consider CSF. If it is low, $< 10\%$, CSF should not be prescribed. Following the first cycle of chemotherapy, and with subsequent cycles, if the patient develops febrile neutropenia or a dose-limiting neutropenic event, and G-CSF was used with cycle 1, consider dose reduction or change in treatment regimen. If G-CSF was not used before, consider secondary prophylaxis with CSF. If no febrile or other dose-limiting neutropenic event occurred, reassess after each subsequent treatment cycle. Febrile neutropenia is defined as a single temperature $\geq 38.3°C$ (101°F) orally or $\geq 38°C$ (100.4°F) over 1 hour; neutropenia is defined as < 500 neutrophils/m^3 or $< 1,000$ neutrophils/mm^3 with an anticipated decline to ≤ 500 cells/mm^3 over the next 48 hours. NCCN (2017) recommendations for use of CSF to treat patients who present with febrile neutropenia are as follows: if the patient is currently receiving prophylactic G-CSF (e.g., filgrastim or sargramostim), continue it. If the patient has received prophylactic pegfilgrastim, do not give additional G-CSF. If the patient did not receive prophylactic CSF and has risk factors for an infection-associated complication (e.g., sepsis syndrome, age > 65 years, severe neutropenia with ANC $< 100/mm^3$, neutropenia expected to last more than 10 days in duration, pneumonia, invasive fungal infection, hospitalized at the time of fever, prior episode of febrile neutropenia, and other clinically documented infections), consider giving G-CSF.

Sargramostim, or granulocyte-macrophage colony-stimulating factor (GM-CSF), is approved for myeloid reconstitution after autologous bone marrow transplantation (BMT) and for other uses. It is now being studied in use with dendritic cell vaccines. Both G-CSF and GM-CSF can be used to mobilize stem cells that will be used to rescue the bone marrow after high-dose chemotherapy. However, because it also stimulates the macrophages, fever is a distinct side effect with GM-CSF.

EPO or rHuEPO (erythropoietin) may be given as an adjunct to chemotherapy in certain regimens. Together with the American Society of Hematology Colleagues, ASCO guidelines assert that there is strong evidence to use epoetin as a treatment option for patients with chemotherapy-associated anemia with a hemoglobin concentration below 10 g/dL (Rizzo et al., 2002). However, despite beliefs that increasing the hemoglobin beyond 12 g/dL would improve patient response and quality of life, studies showed the converse; in fact, using erythropoiesis-stimulating agents (ESAs) to target a hemoglobin of 12 g/dL or higher in cancer patients resulted in shortened time to tumor progression in patients with advanced head and neck cancer receiving radiation therapy, shortened overall survival, increased deaths related to disease progression in patients with metastatic breast cancer receiving chemotherapy, and increased risk of death in cancer patients not receiving chemotherapy or radiation therapy (FDA, 2007). Three meta-analyses confirmed these findings in patients with breast, NSCLC, head and neck, lymphoid, and cervical cancers, while two did not (NCCN, 2018). As a result, the FDA issued an alert (on March 9, 2008) that required all ESA package inserts to add to the black-box warning that ESAs be used only on labels (e.g., while patients are receiving on-curative myelosuppressive chemotherapy). ESAs are *not* indicated when the anticipated outcome is cure. In addition, Medicare (CMS) revised their guidelines to tighten reimbursement for ESAs. The target hemoglobin has now been changed to 10 g/dL, with initiation tied to Hgb < 10 g/dL (HCT < 30%) for a maximum of 8 weeks, and the threshold for holding ESAs is the lowest dose necessary to avoid RBC transfusion (NCCN, 2018). In addition, it is imperative to analyze the patient's iron status and replete as necessary. IV iron appears to be superior to oral iron (NCCN, 2018). The NCCN Cancer and Chemotherapy-Induced Anemia Guidelines specify recommendations for administering parenteral iron products (e.g., iron dextran, ferric gluconate, iron sucrose) (NCCN, 2018).

In February 2010, the FDA required that oncologists/hematologists comply with their Risk Evaluation and Mitigation Strategy (REMS), which was later evaluated, leading to a change in this requirement in 2017. As of 2017, no longer is REMS required for erythropoietin stimulating agents. An evaluation of patient treatment during the time of the REMS requirement showed that prescribers were knowledgeable and that the guidelines were followed. However, as the risk of shortened overall survival and/or increased risk of tumor progression or recurrence associated with the drug still exists, along with increased risk of thrombosis of vascual access, the provider must follow the specific drug labelling. For example, the PI for Procrit (epoetin alfa) recommends that patients requiring surgery receiving epoetin alfa receive DVT prophylaxis during the perisurgical period, due to the increased risk of deep venous thrombosis.

In summary, when ESAs are prescribed, based on FDA and NCCN Guidelines (2018):

- Patients with Hgb < 10 g/dL with at least two additional cycles of planned chemotherapy.
  - Review potential risks and benefits with patient.
  - Use the lowest dose to prevent red blood cell transfusion.
  - Use only for treatment of anemia due to concomitant myelosuppressive chemotherapy (noncurative).
  - Use fixed titration.
  - Discontinue ESA therapy following the completion of a chemotherapy course.
- ESAs are not indicated for patients receiving myelosuppressive therapy when the anticipated outcome is cure.

Platelet growth factor, oprelvekin (Neumega), or IL-11 can be used to prevent and treat thrombocytopenia after myelosuppressive chemotherapy and results in a modest increase in platelets. However, it has side effects that have limited its utility. Romiplostim (Nplate®) is a "peptibody," or peptide antibody, that mimics the activity of thrombopoietin to stimulate platelet production. Clinical trials in patients with immune thrombocytopenia purpura (ITP) have shown significant benefit. The drug is FDA approved for the treatment of thrombocytopenia in patients with chronic immune (idiopathic) thrombocytopenia purpura (ITP). An oral agent, eltrombopag (Promacta®), works similarly and is also FDA approved for treatment of ITP. Atatromopag (Doptelet®) is a thrombopoietin receptor agonist indicated for the treatment of thrombocytopenia in adults with chronic liver disease scheduled to undergo surgery. Common side effects of colony-stimulating factors may include bone pain, fatigue, anorexia, and fever.

Interleukins: Interleukin-2 (IL-2) is a naturally occurring cytokine that is made using recombinant technology. IL-2 is thought to amplify the immune response as it possesses the same qualities as IL-2 the body produces. This includes enhanced T-cell proliferation, lymphocyte cytotoxicity, induction of killer cell activity, and induction of interferon-gamma production (Prometheus, 2015). Aldesleukin (Proleukin®, IL-2) is indicated for the treatment of adults with metastatic renal cell carcinoma and adults with metastatic malignant melanoma. Patients require vigilant nursing care, including emergency care if needed. Side effects of interleukins include flu-like symptoms (fever, chills, rigor, malaise, arthralgias, headache, myalgias, and anorexia), and fatigue, as well as substance-specific side effects; for example, IL-2 can cause serious and potentially fatal side effects, depending upon dose, such as capillary leak syndrome (CLS). In CLS, blood vessel leakage of serum into the surrounding interstitial spaces, resulting in potentially severe hypotension, hemo-concentration (concentrated blood due to decreased volume), and hypoalbuminemia. This can lead to multiple-organ failure and shock. Patients must have normal cardiac and pulmonary function, and patients with an ECOG performance status of 0 (zero) when treatment is initiated have a higher response rate and lower toxicity (Prometheus, 2015).

MONOCLONAL ANTIBODIES

Antibodies are immunoglobulins (Ig) made by B-lymphocytes, that recognize antigens. The function of the antibody is twofold: (1) to bind the antigen that elicited the immune response and (2) to call other immune elements and molecules to the antibody to kill the invading micro-organism or abnormal cell. An antibody is shaped like a "Y." The top portion of the Y, shaped like two arms reaching out from a stick, is the variable region (F_{ab}) that is able to bind a specific antigen; it is variable to meet the infinite number of shapes that could be encountered. It is estimated that the B-lymphocytes can recognize more than 10 million or more different antigen fragments (epitopes) and make more than 1 billion different antibodies. B-lymphocytes search the body for specific antigen-containing cells that match the shape of their receptor, and when they find one, they connect to it. Helper T-cells make proteins that will activate the B-lymphocytes so the B-lymphocyte can make many copies of itself (clones) including plasma and memory cells that will remember the intruder with this specific antigen or shape. The plasma cells make antibodies against the identical antigen found on the B-lymphocyte receptor. The F_{ab} (variable) portion is made up of two light chains and two heavy chains. Once it finds the antigen matching the B-lymphocyte receptor shape, it will attach to it like a key in a lock. The F_c region, the bottom or stem of the Y, is the constant region, which is same for all antibodies in a class (e.g., immunoglobulin Gs, IgGs). It calls to it many of the effector immune cells and molecules to kill the antigen-containing cell. See Figure 4.6.

As the body does not know what antigens will be encountered during a person's life, the immune system has evolved to prepare for an infinite number of encounters using the adaptive immune response. The body genetically programs early B-lymphocytes and T-lymphocytes to produce clones of cells with either a B-cell receptor (BCR) or T-cell receptor (TCR) that is unique and three-dimensional. The receptor is complementary in shape to specific antigen epitope(s), so it can fit together like a "key in a lock." The B-cells make a huge number of Igs, with each B-cell making an Ig or antibody for a specific antigen (epitope). The BCR is a membrane-bound Ig that will bind the antigen that is shaped like the BCR. While the BCR can directly bind the antigen epitope encountered, as discussed the TCR must be presented with the epitope or antigen fragment by APCs showing the MHC molecule. In addition to presentation of the antigen fragment by the APC, to complete T-cell activation, the dendritic cell provides a T-cell activator via the costimulatory signals involving a member of the B7 family of costimulatory molecules that bind to their ligand CD28, in the T-cell (Sharman & Allison, 2015). IL-2 is then released and the T-cells are activated. Once the T-cells are activated, since they are so potent, CTLA4 is expressed to down-regulate or turn off T-cell activation by binding to the B7 molecules with much greater avidity than CD28 (Sharman & Allison, 2015). Theoretically, the immune system can bind epitopes of any possible antigen. In malignancy, as the cancer cells mutate, the immune system must adapt to recognize new tumor antigens with TCRs and BCRs matching the newly evolved tumor antigen(s). Tumor antigens are largely cell surface targets that are overexpressed, mutated, or expressed when they should not be, compared to normal tissues but also include antigens located on tumor stromal and vascular cells that are distinct from

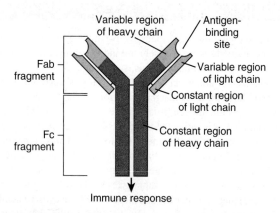

Figure 4.6   **Antibody with Heavy and Light Chains**

normal cells (Scott et al., 2012). T-cells are able to recognize tumor antigens within tumors (Chen & Mellman, 2013). Unfortunately, tumor cells are able to co-opt some of the normal protective immune responses, such as CTLA4, and keep T-cell activation turned down or off (Pardoll, 2012).

A mAb is a copy of a single antibody. Used in immunotherapy, mAbs are a clone of copies of a specific antibody. Initially made by fusing immortal multiple myeloma (MM) cells with mouse spleen containing B-cells (murine hybridoma technique), most mAbs are now made in the laboratory, using recombinant DNA techniques. These antibodies are designed specifically to target or "latch onto" a specific antigen. MAbs made using mice hybridomas are called murine, using mouse antibodies, and are antigenic (capable of causing a hypersensitivity reaction [HSR]) when injected into humans. In an effort to reduce hypersensitivity to the mAbs, human hybridoma techniques are used to make a mixture of mouse and human antibodies called *chimeric* with more than 50% of the antibody being human; *humanized* antibody, which contains > 90% human antibody; and totally *human* antibody (100% human) (Vogel, 2010). See Figure 4.7. The risk of hypersensitivity during mAb administration is highest with murine mAbs, and lowest with human mAbs.

In developing the mAb, the isotype (reflecting the immunoglobulin skeleton of the mAb) of a mAb is a deliberate design element. IgG_1 mAbs stimulate the host immune response and complement activation, and they stimulate ADCC when the mAb attaches to an antigen. ADCC mobilizes immune elements that can destroy cancer cells, such as NK cells and macrophages. Examples of mAbs that are isotype IgG_1 are bevacizumab, trastuzumab, cetuximab, ipilimumab, durvalumab, and ofatumumab. IgG_2 mAbs activate host defenses mildly, if at all; they do activate complement, but they do not activate ADCC. An example of an IgG_2 mAb is panitumumab. Research continues to improve the structural form of mAbs to try to increase effectiveness. While the name of a mAb can sound confusing, there is a syntax that helps to figure out what type of an mAb the drug is as shown in Figure 4.8. Table 4.3 is a list of all mAbs in cancer treatment that the FDA approved in 2017.

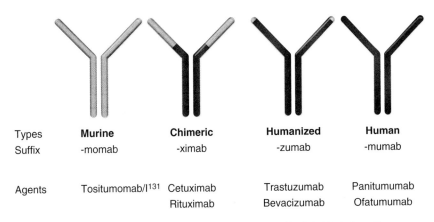

Figure 4.7 **Types of mAbs Depend upon Whether the Antibody is Made from Human, Mouse (murine), or Both Types of Proteins**

1st syllable	Name unique to the product	Tras
2nd syllable	Target, e.g., tumor = tu, li=	tu
3rd syllable	immunomodulating	zu
4th syllable	Composition, where	mab
	o = mouse	Trastuzumab
	xi = chimeric (mouse and human)	
	zu = humanized	
	u = human	
	mab = monoclonal antibody	
	Consonants to link syllables	

Figure 4.8   What's in a Name: Quick Tips on Understanding Monoclonal Antibody Names

January 2017, the FDA (2017) recommended improved naming guidance to provide pharmacovigilance in identifying the correct biological by name. As so many new mAbs were being developed, not only was the FDA running out of names, but many had similar names. The FDA recommendation is the addition of a suffix for the proper naming of an originator biological product, a related biological product or a biosimilar product. This suffix should be unique, have no meaning, be four lowercase letters of which at least 3 are distinct, be non-proprietary, be attached to the core name with a hyphen and be free of legal barriers that would restrict its usage. For example, in 2018, the newly FDA-approved PD-1 blocking agent cemiplimab-rwlc (Libtayo®) uses the new nomenclature, and although it looks at first glance like it is a biosimilar, it is a new, originator biological product NOT a biosimilar.

As mAbs home in on a specific antigen, the mAb can destroy the cell or interrupt malignant cell signaling using (1) antibody direct action such as blockade of a cell receptor and interruption of signaling pathways; (2) immune-mediated (e.g., ADCC, CDC); (3) delivery of a toxic payload that will then kill the cell (e.g., ADC); and (4) lethal effects on tumor stroma and/or vasculature (Scott et al., 2012). For example, trastuzumab inhibits HER2 cell signaling and causes cell death using ADCC, while bevacizumab inhibits VEGF signaling. The antibody can be "naked" or not attached to a toxin, or it can be conjugated and attached to a toxic payload to kill the cell, such as ADCs. Current FDA-approved mAbs for the following tumor antigens are: epidermal growth factor receptor-1 (EGFR; cetuximab and panitumumab), EGFR-2, HER2 or ERBB2 (HER2; trastuzumab, ado-trastuzumab emtansine, and pertuzumab), vascular endothelial growth factor (VEGF; bevacizumab), cytotoxic T-lymphocyte-associated antigen 4 (CTLA4; ipilimumab), programmed death receptor protein and its ligand (PD-1, PD-L1; nivolumab, pembrolizumab), cluster of differentiation (CD) antigens on B-lymphocytes (CD20; rituximab, ofatumumab, obinutuzumab, ibritumomab tiuxetan); CD 30 (brentuximab vedotin), and CD52 (alemtuzumab), and CD19-CD3 bi-specific mAbs (T-cell engager, blinatumomab). In 2017, pembrolizumab was FDA approved for treatment of patients with tumor cells that possessed a genetic flaw: MSI-H. This is the first drug approved for tumors with specific genetic features rather than a specific diagnosis (e.g., site-agnostic) (FDA, 2017b).

Table 4.3   Monoclonal Antibodies and Their Targets and General Indications (see specific-drug detail in chapter for full FDA-indications)

mAb	Target, Type, Composition
ado-trastuzumab emtansine (Kadcyla®)	HER2, ADC with emtansine poison, humanized Indication: HER2+ metastatic breast cancer
Alemtuzumab (Campath®) NOT Lemtrada®	CD-52, naked, humanized Indication: B-cell CLL
Atezolizumab (Tecentriq®)	PD-L1, naked, humanized Indication: (1) Urothelial carcinoma, (2) metastatic NSCLC; (3) triple negative breast cancer with paclitaxel protein bound; (4) SCLC with carboplatin and etoposide .
Avelumab (Bavencio®)	PD-L1, naked, human (IgG1) Indications: (1) Metastatic Merkel cell carcinoma, (2) locally advanced or metastatic urothelial cancer with disease progression after/during platinum-containing chemotherapy, or within 12 months of neoadjuvant or adjuvant treatment with platinum-containing chemotherapy.
Bevacizumab (Avastin®) Bevacizumab-awwb (Mvasi)	Vascular endothelial growth factor (VEGF), naked, humanized Indications: mCRC, NSCLC with carbo/paclitaxel, epithelial ovarian cancer/fallopian tube/primary peritoneal, mRCC, cervical cancer, recurrent GBM
Blinatumomab (Blincyto®)	CD19-CD3 bi-specific T-cell engager (attaches to CD19 on malignant cell) and CD3 on T-cell, engaging T-cell to kill malignant cell Indication: B-cell precursor ALL in 1st or 2nd CR with minimal residual disease; relapsed or refractory B-cell precursor ALL
Brentuximab vedotin (Adcetris®)	CD30, ADC with vedotin poison, chimeric Indication: (1) Hodgkin lymphoma: (a) previously untreated stage III or IV in combination with doxorubicin, vinblastine, and dacarbazine, (b) at high risk of relapse or progression as post-autologous HSCT consolidation, (c) after failure of auto-HSCT or after failure of at least 2 prior multi-agent chemotherapy regimens in patients who are not candidates for auto-HSCT; (2) systemic anaplastic large cell lymphoma (a) previously untreated or other CD-30 expressing peripheral T-cell lymphoma, in combination with systemic cyclophosphamide, doxorubicin, and prednisone, (b) after failure of at least 1 prior multi-agent chemotherapy agent; (3) primary cutaneous anaplastic large cell lymphoma or CD3p expressing mycosis fungoides who have received prior systemic therapy.
Cemiplimab-rwlc (Libtayo®)	PD-1, naked, human (IgG4) Indications: metastatic cutaneous squamous cell carcinoma (CSCC) or locally advanced SCSS who are not candidates for curative surgery or RT.

(continues)

Table 4.3   (Continued)

mAb	Target, Type, Composition
Cetuximab (Erbitux®)	EGFR, naked, chimeric Indication: mCRC (wild-type, EGFR expressing), head and neck cancer
Daratumumab (Darzalex®)	CD38, naked, human Indication: multiple myeloma, in combination or as a single agent
Durvalumab (Imfinzi)	PD-L1, naked, human Indication: locally advanced or metastatic urothelial cancer with disease progression after/during platinum-containing chemotherapy, or within 12 months of neoadjuvant or adjuvant treatment with platinum-containing chemotherapy; Unresectable Stg III NSCLC which has not progressed after concurrent platinum-based chemotherapy and RT.
Elotuzumab (Empliciti®)	SLAMF7 (activates NK cells), naked, humanized Indication: multiple myeloma (with lenalidomide and dexamethasone)
Gemtuzumab ozogamicin (Mylotarg)	CD-33-directed antibody-drug conjugate (ADC), antibody is humanized, conjugated poison is calichaemicin. Indication: (1) newly diagnosed adult patients with CD33 positive AML, (2) relapsed or refractory CD-33 positive AML in adult and pediatric patients 2 years and older
Ibritumomab tiuxetax (Zevalin®)	CD20, radio-immunoconjugate, murine Indication: low-grade or follicular NHL
Inotuzumab ozogamicin (Besponsa)	CD22-directed antibody-drug conjugate (ADC); antibody is humanized; conjugated poison is calichaemicin. Indications: adults with relapsed or refractory B-cell precursor acute lymphoblastic leukemia (ALL).
Ipilimumab (Yervoy)	CTLA4, naked, human Indication: (1) adjuvant melanoma, (2) metastatic or unresectable melanoma; (3) intermediate or poor risk untreated advanced renal cell carcinoma; (4) in combination with nivolumab, patients 12 years or older with MSI-H or dMMR metastatic colorectal cancer that has progressed after treatment with a fluropyrimidine, oxaliplatin, and irinotecan (accelerated approval).
Mogamulizumab-kpke (Poteligeo)	CC chemokine receptor type 4 (CCR4), naked, humanized IgG1 Indication: adult patients with relapsed or refractory mycosis fungoides or Sezary syndrome, after at least 1 prior systemic therapy
Moxetumomab pasudotox-tdfk (Lumoxiti)	CD-22,Immunotoxic composed of recombinant murine IgG variable domain genetically fused to a truncated form of *Psudemomonas* exotoxin (PE38) that inhibits protein synthesis.

Table 4.3　　**(Continued)**

mAb	Target, Type, Composition
	Indication: adult patients with relapsed or refractory hairy cell leukemia who have received at least 2 prior systemic therapies, including treatment with a purine nucleoside analogue (PNA).
Necitumumab (Portrazza®)	EGFR, naked, human Indication: Squamous NSCLC, with gemcitabine and cisplatin.
Nivolumab (Opdivo)	PD-1, naked, human Indications: (1) melanoma: (a) unresectable or metastatic melanoma alone or in combination with ipilimumab, (b) adjuvant treatment of malignant melanoma; (2) metastatic NSCLC, (3) advanced renal cell cancer (a) who have received prior antiangiogenic therapy, (b) intermediate or poor risk previously untreated, with ipilimumab; (4) relapsed or progressive classical Hodgkin lymphoma after (a) HSCT and brentuximab vedotin, or (b) 3 of more lines of systemic therapy including HSCT; (5) recurrent/metastatic squamous cell cancer of the head and neck, (6) locally advanced or metastatic urothelial carcinoma (a) that has progressed during or after platinum-containing therapy, (b) have disease progression within 12 monthso of neoadjuvant or adjuvant platinum-containing chemotherapy; (7) adult and pediatric patients with MSH-H or mismatch repair deficient (dMMR) metastatic CRC that has progressed after treatment with a fluoropyrimidine, oxaliplatin, and irinotecan; (8) hepatocellular carcinoma after treatment with sorafenib; (9) metastatic SCLC with progression after platinum-based chemotherapy and at least 1 other line of therapy (accelerated approval); (10) previously untreated patients with RCC in combination with ipilimumab.
Obinutuzumab (Gazyvz®)	CD20, naked, humanized Indications: relapsed or refractory follicular lymphoma with bendamustine followed by obinutuzumab; previously untreated stage II bulky- IV follicular lymphoma in combination with chemotherapy followed by obinutuzuab after partial response; CLL with chlorambucil
Ofatumumab (Arzerra®)	CD20, naked, human Indication: CLL
Olaratumab (Lartruvo™) Withdrawn from Global Market as Phase III ANNOUNCE trial did not improve survival (4.25.19)	Platelet-derived growth factor receptor alpha (PDGFR-α), naked, human. Indication: Soft tissue sarcoma, with doxorubicin, in adults who are not candidates for curative surgery or radiotherapy available for patients already receiving drug (Lilly, 2019).
Panitumumab (Vectibix®)	EGFR, naked, human Indication: mCRC (wild-type)

(continues)

Table 4.3 *(Continued)*

mAb	Target, Type, Composition
Pembrolizumab (Keytruda)	PD-1, naked, humanized Indication: (1) unresectable or metastatic melanoma; adjuvant therapy for LN+ completely resected melanoma; (2) NSCLC metastatic, as a single agent in PD-L1 expressing tumors (a) high ≥50% or (b) ≥1%); (c) first-line metastatic nonsquamous NSCLC with pemetrexed and carboplatin; (d) first-line treatment of metastatic squamous NSCLC with carboplatin and paclitaxel or nab-paclitaxel; (3) recurrent or metastatic HNSCC; (4) classical Hodgkin disease, refractory or relapsed; (5) locally advanced or metastatic urothelial carcinoma in patients (a) after progression or who are ineligible for cisplatin-containing chemotherapy and whose tumors express PD-L1 (combined positive score ≥10); (b) with disease progression during or after platinum-containing therapy or within 12 months of neoadjuvant or adjuvant therapy with platinum-containing chemotherapy; (6) MSI-H solid tumors which have progressed or CRC that has progressed after treatment with a fluoropyrimidine, oxaliplatin, and irinotecan (adult and pediatric); (7) gastric or GE junction adenocarcinoma expressing PD-L1, progressing on or after 2+ prior therapies; (8) cervical cancer, recurrent or metastatic, expressing PD-L1; (9) adult and pediatric patients with refractory primary mediastinal large B-cell lymphoma, or who have relapsed after 2+ prior therapies; (10) hepatocellular carcinoma; (11) merkel cell carcinoma; (12) renal cell carcinoma, advanced, in combination with axitinib, first line.
Pertuzumab (Perjeta®)	HER2, naked, humanized Indication: HER2+ breast cancer (neoadjuvant, adjuvant, or treatment of metastatic disease)
Polatuzumab vedotin-piiq (Polivy)	CD79b, antibody-drug conjugate (humanized IgG1 mAb for human CD79b, linked to MMAE antimitotic agent) Indication: adults with relapsed or refractory diffuse large B-cell lymphoma, in combination with bendamustine and a rituximab product.
Ramucirumab (Cyramza®)	VEGFR-2, naked, human Indication: metastatic NSCLC, gastric/GE junction, mCRC in combination with other drugs, and HCC as a single agent.
Rituximab (Rituxan®)	CD20, naked, chimeric Indication: NHL: (a) CD20+ low-grade or follicular, relapsed or refractory; (b) previously untreated CD20+ follicular; (c) non-progressing low-grade B-cell after first-line therapy; (d) previously untreated diffuse large B-cell CD20+ with CHOP or other anthracycline-based therapy; CLLCD20+; (e) RA with methotrexate; (f) Wegener's granulomatosis and MPA, together with steroids; moderate to severe Pemphigus Vulgaris in adults.

Table 4.3   *(Continued)*

mAb	Target, Type, Composition
Rituximab-abbs (Truxima®)	BIOSIMILAR to Ritixan; CD20, naked, chimeric Indication: NHL: (a) CD20+ low-grade or follicular, relapsed or refractory; (b) previously untreated CD20+ follicular; (c) non-progressing low-grade B-cell after first-line therapy ONLY not full approval of Rituxan indications.
Rituximab and hyaluronidase human (Rituxan Hycela®)	CD20, naked, chimeric prepared with hyaluronidase human for subcutaneous injection Indication: Follicular lymphoma (relapsed, refractory, previously untreated in combination with first-line chemotherapy; diffuse large B-cell lymphoma, previously untreated, in combination with CHOP or other anthracycline-based regimen; CLL, in combination with fludarabine and cyclophosphamide.
Tagraxofusp-erzs (Elzonr®is™)	CD123; composed of recombinant human IL-3 and truncated diphtheria toxin forming a fusion protein Indication: blastic plasmacytoid dendritic cell neoplasm (BPDCN)
Trastuzumab (Herceptin®) Biosimilars Trastuzumab-dkst (Ogivri®), Trastuzumab-dttb (Ontruzant®), Trastuzumab-qyyp (Trazimera®)	HER2, naked, humanized Indications: HER2+ overexpressing breast cancer; metastatic HER2+ overexpressing gastric or GE junction adenocarcinoma.
Trastuzuab-pkrb (Herzuma®, Biosimilar)	BIOSIMILAR with only Breast Cancer indication (NOT full Herceptin indications: HER2+ breast cancer ONLY), naked, humanized Indication: HER2+ breast cancer
Trastuzumab and hyaluronidase (Herceptin Hylecta™)	HER2; naked, humanized. Indication: HER2 overexpressing breast cancer.

ADC: Antibody-Drug-Conjugate; naked signifies the mAb has no attachment or conjugate; metastatic colorectal cancer (mCRC): metastatic colorectal cancer; CLL: chronic lymphocytic leukemia; NSCLC: nonsmall cell lung cancer; auto-HSCT: autologous hematopoietic stem cell transplantation; mRCC: metastatic renal cell cancer; GBM: glioblastoma multiforme; ALL: acute lymphoblastic leukemia; SLAMF7: Signaling Lymphocytic Activation Molecule Family member 7 (surface glycoprotein) expressed on multiple myeloma cells; NHL: non-Hodgkin's lymphoma; GE junction: esophageal/gastric junction adenocarcinoma; MSI-H: microsatellite instability-high; SCLC: small cell lung cancer.

Figure 4.7 shows mechanisms of mAb therapy. As can be seen, chimeric mAbs contain more mouse than humanized or human mAbs, so premedication is usually required to prevent infusion reactions when administering a chimeric mAb.

IMMUNE CHECKPOINT INHIBITORS

As more research emerges improving the understanding of how the immune system is circumvented by cancer, new drugs are being developed to target these events when the immune system's T-lymphocytes become overwhelmed or tricked by cancer cells. It is important for oncology nurses to be conversant with the elements of the immune system so they can teach patients and their families about them. This is an exploding area of drug development and represents hope to patients who have exhausted chemotherapy treatment options for advanced disease, as demonstrated by the immune checkpoint inhibitors. For example, some patients with recurrent, previously treated NSCLC who received nivolumab had a median OS of 12.2 months, compared to 9.4 months in patients receiving docetaxel chemotherapy, with 51% of patients who received nivolumab alive at 1 year compared to 39% receiving docetaxel (Borghaei et al., 2015). In 2017, a 2-year follow-up of the two randomized controlled trials (Checkmate 017 and 057), showed 23% of squamous cell NSCLC patients receiving nivolumab were alive vs 8% receiving docetaxel, and for non-squamous NSCLC patients, 29% and 16% were alive respectively (Horn et al., 2017). For those patients responding to nivolumab, responses were durable, while no patient receiving docetaxel had a durable response, and treatment related adverse events were less in the nivolumab group (68%, grade 3–4 10%) vs the docetaxel group (88%, grade 3–4, 55%) (Horn et al., 2017).

For decades, different clinical trials explored ways to stimulate and/or augment immune function. The immune response can be very powerful and threaten normal tissues, so there are immune checkpoints that sense when it is time to turn down or off the immune response, principally the activity of activated CTLs. Cancer cells have learned that if they co-opt or make the patient's immune system tolerant of the tumor antigen (immune tolerance), then the cancer antigen is not recognized as foreign and does not ramp up the immune response against it. The six immune checkpoint inhibitors currently FDA approved are ipilimumab (Yervoy), nivolumab (Opdivo), pembrolizumab (Keytruda), atezolizumab (Tecentriq®), durvalumab (Imfinzi™), and avelumab (Bavencio®). Other immune checkpoints being studied along with their inhibitors are LAG and TIM-3. In addition, molecular-targeted agent combinations with immune checkpoint inhibitors are being conducted (Sharman & Allison, 2015).

CTLA-4 is expressed on T-lymphocytes, and its ligand is CD80 (Quezada & Peggs, 2013). The CTLA-4 cell surface protein is a negative regulator of T-lymphocyte function and activation, and it turns down the powerful T-lymphocyte immune response after the pathogen is eliminated to protect normal tissues from the ravages of the immune response (Sharman & Allison, 2015). Most malignant cells express CTLA-4 (CD152) and use it to escape cytotoxic T-lymphocyte attack. Blockade of CTLA-4 should result in immunity against the tumor (Sharman & Allison, 2015).

Ipilimumab (Yervoy) is an immune checkpoint inhibitor that is FDA approved for the treatment of unresectable or metastatic melanoma, as well as the adjuvant treatment of patients with melanoma with lymph node involvement. Ipilimumab is a mAb directed against cytotoxic T-lymphocyte-associated antigen 4 (CTLA-4), designed to augment cytotoxic T-cell function. CTLA-4 acts as the "off" switch to depress T-lymphocyte activation and function as the immune response is winding down. Cancer cells co-opt this process by releasing CTLA-4 and turning off/down activated T-lymphocyte function. Ipilimumab blocks CTLA-4 so no inhibitory protein is sent; T-cell proliferation, activation, and IL-2 production continue so that the CTLs continue to be activated and attack the tumor antigen identified by the APCs (Ribas, 2012).

Another important immune checkpoint is the PD-1 receptor and its ligands PD-L1 and PD-L2, which tumor cells co-opt and use to become invisible to the immune system

(Pardoll, 2012). Many cells express ligands for PD-1; when ligands bind the PD-1 receptor on T-lymphocytes, PD-1 turns down/off activated T-lymphocyte immune response. It does this by interfering with TCR signaling (Sharman & Allison, 2015). The ligands for PD-1 are PD-L1 (expressed on many cells including immune cells), and PD-L2 which is found only on APCs (Sharman & Allison, 2015). PD-1 is also expressed by activated T-lymphocytes when they are exposed to antigens for a long time, which may explain gradual immune tolerance to tumor antigen(s). PD-1's role is to protect the peripheral tissues from autoimmunity. Drugs such as nivolumab and pembrolizumab, which are mAbs, block the PD-1 receptor so that it cannot be stimulated by its ligand, and the activated T-lymphocytes continue their war against the cells with cancer antigens. Both have been FDA approved. The PD-1 inhibiting drugs appear to be most active in tumors that overexpress PD-L1, but more research needs to be done to clarify the best biomarkers (Patel & Kurzrock, 2015). Because the checkpoint inhibitors that block CTLA4 and PD-1 use different pathways, and occur at different times in the immune response, the drugs were combined in the treatment of malignant melanoma in the CheckMate 067 trial (Larkin et al., 2015; Wolchok et al., 2013). Patients receiving the combination showed a higher overall response rate (57.6%) compared to CTLA4 blockade (ipilimumab, 19%) or PD-1 blockade (nivolumab, 43.7%) alone (Wolchok et al., 2016). The combination had the greatest activity compared to either agent alone, and as single agents, nivolumab was superior to ipilimumab. These findings were regardless of PD-L1 or *BRAF* mutation status (Wolchok et al., 2016). In 2017, with a minimum 28-month follow-up, the median PFS was 11.7 months with the combination, versus 6.9 months with nivolumab, and 2.9 months with ipilimumab alone (Larkin et al., 2017). The ORR with the combination was 58.9% (17.2% CR), 44.6% (14.9% CR) with nivolumab alone, and 19% (4.4% CR) for ipilimumab alone. Median duration of response at this writing has not been reached for the combination arm, and is 31.1 months in the nivolumab alone arm, and 18.2 months in the ipilimumab alone arm. The safety profile of the arm was similar to earlier results, and even if patients who discontinued therapy due to toxicity had responses >70% and a significant survival benefit (Larkin et al., 2017).

It has been shown that solid tumors that express MSI-H have strong immune activation (Gatalica et al., 2016), which has led to the FDA approval of pembrolizumab (Keytruda) for the treatment of MSH-I solid tumors, including mCRC. Microsatellites are sections of DNA where short sections containing 2–5 base pairs, are repeated many times (e.g., 5–50 times) throughout the noncoding genome. The number of microsatellites is specific to the species and were used to map the genome. They are very important in the genetic diversity of species, as they are highly prone to mutation. When DNA is inherited, there are a precise number of microsatellites. DNA repair genes help to control the mutations. However, in some cancers, there is a problem with the DNA repair genes, called DNA mismatch repair (MMR) or deficient MMMR (dMMR). This causes instability of the microsatellites. Some tumors are hypermutable, meaning that there are many mutations in the microsatellites; these are called MSI-H. It has been found that tumors that are MSI-H have strong immune activation (Gatalica et al., 2016). Studies have shown that PD-1 blockade is possible in tumors with mismatch-repair deficiency (dMMR) and which are MSI-H (Le et al., 2015). In CRC, MSI-H describes a distinct tumor pathway, made of mutations together with DNA deficient mismatch repair and/or hypermethylation of promoter regions (Gatalica et al., 2016). About 15% of CRCs are MSI-H, where 3% are patients with inherited mutations

(Lynch syndrome) and 12% are those with sporadic mutations (Gatalica et al., 2016). These mutations are believed to encode "nonself" immunogenic antigens in the mutations, and given there are a high number of these mutations due to deficient DNA repair, the result is a tumor capable of strong immune activation (Gatalica et al., 2016). Thus, mismatch repair status predicts clinical benefit from immune checkpoint inhibitors (Le et al., 2015). This helps explain why these tumors are amenable to immune checkpoint inhibition, and pembrolizumab has this indication.

Major side effects of immune checkpoint inhibitors are immune-related (inflammatory), are called irAEs, and may be very serious. These include rash/dermatitis; colitis/diarrhea; endocrinopathies, including adrenal insufficiency, type 1 DM, and thyroid dysfunction; pneumonitis, hepatitis, and a number of less common effects. While the irAE profile is similar between CTLA4 blockers and PD-1 inhibitors, the frequency is higher in anti-CTLA4 therapy (Sharman & Allison, 2015). In 2018, ASCO and NCCN worked together to develop practice guidelines for the management of irAEs in patients treated with immune checkpoint inhibitor therapy (ASCO 2018, NCCN, 2018). These are discussed in detail in the section entitled Nursing Implications.

ADOPTIVE CELL TRANSFER

This immunotherapy technique develops a large population of immune cells that can seek out and destroy cancer cells carrying a tumor-specific antigen, thus restoring immunity against these cancer cells. This technique increases not only the number of immune effector T-cells but also often increases their effectiveness in killing cancer cells. T-lymphocyte-adoptive therapies (called CAR T-cell therapy), use the patient's own genetically engineered or modified T-lymphocytes that are treated so that they proliferate, and seek and attack the patient's specific tumor antigen when reinjected back to the patient. These are truly individualized and personalized cellular cancer therapies, as they are directed toward the patient's own tumor antigen.

The National Comprehensive Cancer Network (NCCN) has developed recommendations for the management of CAR T-cell related toxicities, principally CRS and neurotoxicity (NCCN, 2019). Key points are shown in Table 4.4. The principal nursing concern in caring for patients receiving CAR-T therapy is CRS, which is magnified given the large number of infused T-cells that rapidly release a huge number of cytokines, as well as the numbers of CD19 B-cells killed; patients may develop very high fever, hypotension, and capillary leak/pulmonary edema and CRS may be life-threatening (Smith & Venella, 2017). The higher the disease burden, the higher the risk for more severe CRS. CRS can lead to severe coagulopathy with prolonged PTT (partial thromboplastin time), and low fibrinogen levels, necessitating cryoprecipitate and fresh frozen plasma transfusions. CRS-related inflammation can alter hemodynamics so that patients may develop acute renal injury and dysfunction from decreased renal blood flow (Smith & Venella, 2017). Intervention is aimed at controlling symptoms without interfering with T-cell killing of tumor cells. Supportive therapy includes antipyretics, analgesics, antiemetics, vasopressors, and oxygen. If patients progress to multi-organ failure with worsening pulmonary status, the anti-inflammatory tocilizumab is preferred as it decreases inflammation by blocking IL-6, and does not interfere directly with T-cell efficacy (Smith & Venella, 2017). In contrast, methylprednisolone will directly interfere with CAR T-cell function, so it is only given if other strategies are ineffective. Other side effects of CAR-T cell therapy include neurological symptoms (e.g., seizure, confusion, unresponsiveness), TLS, GVHD, and for CART-19 therapy, B-cell lymphocyte aplasia as the engineered T-cells kill all the CD-19 positive B lymphocytes. These patients will require prophylaxis with levetiracetam at the start of CRS to prevent seizures and for the CART-19 patients, monthly IVIG infusions to prevent infection (Smith & Venella, 2017).

T-cell specificity and the ability to recognize up to a billion (10^9) different antigens is a compelling principle underlying antitumor immunotherapy, but equally important is the

Table 4.4   Key Points in Care of Patients Receiving CAR T-cell Therapy Based on NCCN (2019), Porter et al. (2018), and Lee et al. (2019)

Baseline and during CAR T-cell Infusion	Post CAR T-cell infusion	When to expect toxicities
• Ensure patient has a central venous access device (double or triple lumen) • Cardiac monitoring available for monitoring patients at onset of grade 2 CRS until resolution to ≤ grade 1 • Discuss with provider TLS prophylaxis if patient has large tumor burden and aggressive histology • Discuss with provider seizure prophylaxis if patient at risk with therapy	• Close monitoring (inpatient or outpatient in experienced centers); (a) assess for CRS at least 2×/day or if the patient's status changes during peak period of risk; (b) neuro-toxicity assessment at least 2×/day or when patient status changes; if increased suspicion of neurolotoxicity, assess at least q 8 hours (including cognitive and motor weakness). • Hospitalization recommended for CRS • Monitor CBC, metabolic panel (including magnesium and phosphorus), and coagulation profile. • Baseline CRP and ferritin, with reassessment at least 3 times a week × 2 weeks postinfusion and daily if patient experiences CRS. • Cytopenias may continue for weeks to months after treatment • Long-term B cell aplasia and hypogammaglobulinemia may occur in patients achieving a CR.	1) CRS: onset 2–3 days, duration 7–8 days, signs/symptoms = fever, hypotension, tachycardia, hypoxia, chills; may be associated with cardiac, hepatic, renal impairment. Serious complications may include atrial fibrillation, ventricular tachycardia, cardiac arrest, cardiac failure, renal insufficiency, CLS, hypotension, hypoxia, HLH/MAS. 2) Neurologic toxicity: onset 4–10 days; duration 14–17 days; signs/symptoms = encephalopathy, headache, tremor, dizziness, aphasia, delirium, insomnia, anxiety, auronomic neuropathy, and rarely, agitation, hyperactivity, psychosis; serious events include seizures, cerebral edema. 3) HLH/MAS during CRS: possible if (1) rapidly rising and high ferritin (> 5000 ng/mL) with cytopenias, especially if also 1 or more: (a) grade 3/higher bilirubin, AST, ALT; (b) grade 3/higher oliguria or increase in serum creatinine; (c) grade 3/higher pulmonary edema; (2) hemophagocytosis on bone marrow or organs.

(continues)

Table 4.4 *(Continued)*

Baseline and during CAR T-cell Infusion	Post CAR T-cell infusion	When to expect toxicities
Grading of CRS	Grade 1: fever ≥ 38°C Grade 2: fever with hypotension, not requiring vasopressors +/or hypoxia requiring low-flow nasal cannula Grade 3: fever with hypotension, requiring a vasopressor +/– vasopressin +/or hypoxia requiring high-flow oxygen delivery Grade 4: Fever with hypotension requiring multiple vasopressors +/– hypoxia requiring positive pressure	

Modified from National Comprehensive Cancer Network. Management of Immunotherapy-related Toxicities. Version 2.2019 (April 8, 2019). Porter D, Frey N, Wood P et al. Grading of Cytokine release syndrome associated with CAR T cell therapy tisagenlecleucel. *J Hematology & Oncology.* 2018; 11:35. Available at https://www.ncbi.nlm.nih.gov/pmc/articles/PMC5833070/pdf/13045_2018_Article_571.pdf. Accessed May 12, 2019. Lee DW, Santomasso BD, Locke FL et al. ASTCT consensus grading for cytokine release syndrome and neurologic toxicity associated with immune effector cells. *Biol Blood Marrow Transplant* 2019; 25(4):625-638.

Abbreviations: CLS= capillary leak syndrome; CRS=cytokine release syndrome; HLH/MAS= hemophagocytic lymphohistiocytosis/macrophage activation syndrome; TLS= tumor lysis syndrome

fact that long-term T-cell memory cells are created, and if/when exposed to the tumor antigen again, there is an accelerated immune response (Sharman & Allison, 2015).

Potential neurotoxicity is the second major toxicity of CAR T-cell therapy.

VACCINES
Tumor vaccines stimulate or restore the immune system (NCI, 2015). Vaccines can be *preventative*, such as that for human papilloma virus (HPV), which has been shown to prevent cervical and other HPV-related cancers in young adults, or *therapeutic*, such as sipuleucel-T (Provenge). Therapeutic vaccines involve injection of an antigen to stimulate the immune system, so that cytotoxic T-cells are activated and directed to recognize specific tumor antigen(s) or to manufacture antibodies to bind to the tumor-specific antigen (NCI, 2015). Not only must the vaccine be able to direct an antigen-specific immune response, but it must also be able to overcome the forces that allowed the tumor to evade the immune system in the first place. Sipuleucel-T (Provenge) is an autologous cellular immunotherapy agent that is indicated for the treatment of asymptomatic or minimally symptomatic metastatic, castrate-resistant, prostate cancer. The vaccine is individualized to each patient, and studies showed the vaccine increased median survival by 4.1 months (Kantoff et al., 2010). The vaccine uses prostatic acid phosphatase (PAP, a common antigen found on prostate cancer cells), plus granulocyte-macrophage colony-stimulating factor (sargramostim,

GM-CSF) to stimulate an immune response. Dendritic (APC) cells are removed from the patient by leukaphoresis and sent to the vaccine manufacturer who cultures the cells with PAP plus GM-CSF to stimulate the immune cells and enhance antigen presentation (NCI, 2015). The cultured cells plus GM-CSF are then sent back to the patient's physician, who reinfuses them. This is repeated two more times for a total of three treatments. See Drug Information.

ONCOLYTIC VIRAL THERAPY

Oncolytic virus therapy uses a genetically modified virus, such as herpes virus-1 (HSV-1) to locally kill tumor cells when injected into the lesion, and systemically, to stimulate an immune response much like a vaccine does. Talimogene laherparepved (T-vec, Imlygic®) is FDA approved for the local treatment of unresectable cutaneous, subcutaneous, and nodal melanoma lesions that have recurred after initial surgery. The oncolytic virus destroys tumor cells locally, releasing tumor associated antigens that then can be fragmented and mounted on dendritic APC cells, which can then activate T-cells to kill the tumor antigen-containing cells elsewhere in the body. This therapy theoretically stimulates local and systemic immune responses. Once the tumor is infected by the modified virus, the virus replicates, the tumor cell ruptures, releasing many virons that then infect other tumor cells (Hoffner et al., 2016). The infectious nature of HSV-1 requires adherence to scrupulous biohazard principles, as well as precise and understandable patient and caregiver education. In addition, special care must be given when the drug is injected near the airway as obstructive symptoms may occur (Amgen, 2017). See Drug Information.

BI-SPECIFIC T-CELL ENGAGER

CTLs are highly specific and powerful effector cells, being able to destroy tumor cells. However, they cannot attack free antigens. The CTL has a protein complex on its cell membrane called a TCR, which interacts with APCs. An important protein in the TCR is CD3, which regulates signal transduction to activate T cells, allowing them to recognize and kill this specific (tumor) antigen. Bispecific T-cell Engager (BiTE) technology uses mAbs to bind together CTLs and the malignant antigen. One mAb binds to CTLs via the CD3 receptor, and the other mAb binds to the tumor-specific antigen. Once linked, the CTL produces dissolving substances like perforin and granzymes; when released into the tumor cell, they cause the tumor cell to undergo apoptosis. Blinatumomab (Blincyto®) is the first bispecific CD19-directed CD3 T-cell engager to receive FDA approval; it is indicated for the treatment of Philadelphia-chromosome–negative relapsed or refractory B-cell precursor ALL.

IMMUNOMODULATORY DRUGS

Immunomodulatory drugs modulate the immune system by a variety of not-well understood mechanisms, including antiangiogenic mechanisms, T-cell costimulatory functions, stimulation of NK cells and T-cells. The three generations of immunomodulatory thalidomide analogue drugs are thalidomide (Thalomid®), lenalidomide (Revlimid®), and pomalidomide (Pomalyst®). Lenalidomide and pomalidomide are synergistic with dexamethasone and usually given together. Thalidomide and its analogues are severely embryo-fetal toxic, so pregnancy is an absolute contraindication and strict REMS programs are required for each drug. Venous and arterial thromboembolism are also risks, which with others, are fully described in the drug section.

NURSING IMPLICATIONS

Nurses continue to play a critical role in the teaching and care of patients receiving targeted immunotherapy and their families. This section highlights three important areas: infusion reactions, EGFR inhibitor rash management, and identification and management of immune-mediated toxicity from immune checkpoint inhibitors. ONS recommends that oncology nurses involved in immunotherapy administration have a fundamental knowledge of the immunotherapy classes of drugs and the adverse effects that their patients are receiving (education), and that the nurse uses the same level of care (competence) in the administration of immunotherapy agents as with other antineoplastic agents (ONS, 2016). Further, as patients may receive multimodality therapy, the nurse must use fundamental principles of antineoplastic agents together with immunotherapy, chemotherapy, RT and other treatments. Finally, in terms safe handling, as immunotherapies are a newer modality, there is limited research available, so ONS recommends that each institution has an ongoing process of drug evaluation to determine their policy.

INFUSION REACTIONS

Infusion reactions related to administration of immunotherapy may commonly occur, and each nurse must be prepared to manage them, with emergency medication and equipment as well as a provider who can prescribe emergency medications both readily available. Infusion reactions can be related to an allergic or HSR (IgE mediated), be anaphylactoid (not IgE mediated), or be related to CRS (rapid lysis of lymphocytes releasing active cytokines). These reactions are most likely related to IV administration, but oral drugs can also cause HSRs, including, rarely, anaphylaxis. **mAbs**, especially murine or chimeric mAbs, commonly cause HSRs due to the antigenic murine antibody. CRS risk is increased when the patient tumor burden of lymphocytes is $>25,000/mm^3$.

Allergic or type I HSRs are related to the generation of IgE in the patient's blood on the first exposure to a drug (antigen) in susceptible patients. On the second exposure, the person is sensitized, and IgE is released in large quantities which lyse mast cells and basophils, releasing histamine, inflammatory leukotrienes, prostaglandins, cytokines, and other vasoactive substances. Reactions can vary from mild to severe (anaphylaxis) or can be fatal. Most often, symptoms may be similar to milder infusion reactions, such as fever, chills, or flushing. However, the nurse must be vigilant and precise in patient assessment, as other signs and symptoms may develop. The more quickly the reaction occurs after the initiation of the drug, the more severe the reaction (Kim & Fischer, 2011). HSRs are usually immediate, and often occur within minutes of the patient receiving the drug, but may be delayed up to 10–12 hours (Vogel, 2010). Patient risk factors include history of allergies, and may involve geographical location, such as with cetuximab (Erbitux). Severe anaphylaxis occurs in a small percentage of patients. See Table 4.5, showing Common Toxicity Criteria Adverse Effects (CTCAE) grading of allergic reactions and anaphylaxis.

TREATMENT

Table 4.5   CTCAE v 4.03 Allergic Reaction (Grade 5 is death)

Grade 1	Grade 2	Grade 3	Grade 4
Transient flushing or rash, drug fever <38°C (<100.4°F); intervention not indicated	Intervention or infusion interruption indicated; responds promptly to symptomatic treatment (e.g., NSAIDs, antihistamines, opioids); prophylactic medication indicated for ≤24 h	Prolonged (e.g., not rapidly responsive to symptomatic medication and/or brief interruption of infusion); recurrence of symptoms after initial improvement; hospitalization indicated for clinical sequelae (e.g., renal impairment, pulmonary infiltrates)	Life-threatening consequences; urgent intervention indicated

Modified from National Cancer Institute. Common Terminology Criteria for Adverse Events (CTCAE). Version 4.03 (NIH Publication No. 09-5410). https://evs.nci.nih.gov/ftp1/CTCAE/CTCAE_4.03_2010-06-14_QuickReference_5x7.pdf. June 14, 2010.

Signs and symptoms experienced include the following (Kim & Fischer, 2011; Vogel, 2010):

- Skin: rash, pruritis, flushing, urticaria (hives), erythema, angioedema
- Pulmonary: *Upper airway*: cough, dyspnea, nasal congestion, rhinitis, sneezing, oropharyngeal or laryngeal edema. *Lower airway*: dyspnea, bronchospasm, wheezing, tachypnea, chest tightness
- CNS: throbbing headache, dizziness, confusion, anxiety, sense of impending doom, loss of consciousness (LOC)
- GI: nausea, vomiting, diarrhea, abdominal cramping
- GU: incontinence, uterine cramping or pelvic pain
- Musculoskeletal: arthralgias, myalgias, fatigue, lower back pain
- CV: hypotension, HTN, tachycardia, palpitations, arrhythmia, edema, chest pain, ischemia or infarction, cardiac arrest

As with any drug, the nurse should review the potential for infusion reaction, HSR or CRS before administration. If the nurse's practice, hospital, or clinic has a protocol for management of the reaction, it should be reviewed. The patient's history should be reviewed for past allergic reactions, which increase the risk. If ordered, administer premedications over the recommended time. The goal of nursing management is prevention, which includes anticipation of a potential reaction due to risk factors and patient premedication with acetaminophen, antihistamines, and/or a corticosteroid as ordered. Ensure that emergency equipment and medications are readily available and that a provider who can prescribe is located in the clinical area. In general, patient management follows these steps (Ellis & Dat, 2003; Polovich et al., 2014; Viale et al., 2010; Vogel, 2010):

- Obtain baseline vital signs and note patient's mental status.
- If a reaction develops, stop the infusion, and keep the line open with a plain solution such as normal saline.

- Assess for airway, breathing, and circulation.
- For a *localized allergic response*: Evaluate symptoms; observe for urticaria, wheals, localized erythema.
- Administer diphenhydramine and/or hydrocortisone as per physician's order.
- Monitor vital signs every 15 minutes for 1 hour.
- Discuss patient's response with physician, NP or PA. Often, if the reaction resolves to ≤ grade 1, the infusion is resumed at 50% of the infusion rate when the reaction occurred, as ordered by the provider.
- Document specific observations, intervention, and patient response.

For a *generalized allergic response*, assess for the following signs or symptoms (these usually occur within the first 15 minutes of the start of the infusion or injection). Reaction can be either an *anaphylactoid* (has never been exposed to the drug before) or *anaphylaxis* (severe HSR after having received the drug before). See Table 4.4. However, management is the same for either. Assess for and further evaluate:

- Subjective signs and symptoms: generalized itching, chest tightness, agitation, uneasiness, dizziness, nausea, crampy abdominal pain, anxiety, sense of impending doom, desire to urinate or defecate, chills.
- Objective signs: flushed appearance; localized or generalized urticaria; edema of face, hands, or feet; hoarseness; respiratory distress with or without wheezing; hypotension; cyanosis; difficulty speaking; sense of impending doom. If the patient develops angioedema, the tongue and throat tissues can swell quickly and obstruct the patient's airway. Listen for any hoarseness, which may signal orpharyngeal or laryngeal edema. Once this occurs, it is very difficult to intubate the patient, so the provider should be called immediately, and in some institutions, a code is called.
- Stop the infusion immediately and notify the physician. Change IV bag and tubing to a 0.9% sodium chloride USP to keep a patent IV and so no additional drug is infused from the original bag and tubing. If not contraindicated, ensure maximum rate of infusion if the patient is hypotensive as ordered.
- Position the patient to promote perfusion of the vital organs; the supine position is preferred.
- Monitor vital signs every 2 minutes until stable, then every 5 minutes for 30 minutes, then every 15 minutes as ordered.

Table 4.6   CTCAE v 4.03 Anaphlyaxis (Grade 5 is death)

Grade 1	Grade 2	Grade 3	Grade 4
–	–	Symptomatic broncho-spasm; with or without urticaria; parenteral intervention indicated; allergy-related edema, angioedema; hypotension	Life-threatening consequences; urgent intervention indicated

Modified from National Cancer Institute. Common Terminology Criteria for Adverse Events (CTCAE). Version 4.03 (NIH Publication No. 09-5410). https://evs.nci.nih.gov/ftp1/CTCAE/CTCAE_4.03_2010-06-14_QuickReference_5x7 .pdf. June 14, 2010.

TREATMENT

- Assess LOC and mentation as this reflects level of oxygenation. Oxygen should be administered as needed if patient is hypoxic, or is desaturating based on O_2 sat monitoring, as long as bronchospasm has resolved.
- Reassure the patient and the family.
- Maintain the airway and anticipate the need for cardiopulmonary resuscitation.
- Epinephrine is the drug of choice for anaphylaxis, and should be given immediately if anaphylaxis is suspected, and if the patient is in an ambulatory practice, taken to the hospital right away via ambulance (Kim & Fischer, 2011). Intramuscular injection of epinephrine results in a faster onset of action and higher serum level so is preferred over subcutaneous administration. All medications must be administered with a physician's order (Kim & Fischer, 2011). Recall that the concentration of epinephrine for IM injection is 1:1,000, while that for IV injection is 1:10,000. Accidental injection of 1:1,000 concentration of epinephrine IV can cause tachycardia, HTN, myocardial infarction, and death. Many institutions have substituted epi-pens for vials of 1:1,000 epinephrine on code carts to avoid this error.

Anticipate administering the following medications for the following effects in adults:

a. Vasoconstriction to increase cardiac output and blood pressure, as well as bronchodilation to open the airway: epinephrine (1:1,000, 0.3–0.5 mL **for IM or subcutaneous injection**, repeat every 5–15 minutes).
b. Anti-inflammation/bronchodilation: rapid acting corticosteroid such as hydrocortisone 100-mg IV.
c. Bronchodilation: albuterol inhaler (2 puffs from multidose inhaler).
d. Antihistamines to stop allergic release of histamines:
   1) diphenhydramine: 25–50-mg IVP
   2) ranitidine 50-mg IV or famotidine 20-mg IV
e. Oxygen if bronchospasm is controlled.
f. IV fluids for hypotension.

Document the incident in the medical record according to institution policy and procedures. If severe or anaphylaxis occurs, usually the drug is discontinued. If anaphylaxis occurs, the patient should be admitted for observation as once the half-life of the rescue drugs is reached, anaphylaxis can recur. If not anticipated, the patient might have a fatal outcome if the rescue medications cannot be readministered.

Anaphylactoid reactions occur upon first exposure to an antigen and are not IgE (immune) mediated. The antigen binds to the surface of the mast cells and basophils, causing them to rupture and to release inflammatory mediators (histamine, leukotrienes, prostaglandins), triggering the same signs and symptoms as occur with true anaphylaxis. Management of the patient with an anaphylactoid reaction is identical to that outlined above for the patient with an HSR.

CYTOKINE RELEASE SYNDROME

CRS occurs when administering a mAb and is related to the destruction of cells, which release cytokines. These cytokines cause a systemic inflammatory response, with fever, hypotension, and rigors. If very severe, it is called a cytokine storm, and may involve pulmonary edema. Risk factors include administration of a mAb (e.g., rituximab) and following adoptive T-cell therapies (Lee et al., 2014). Patients with a high white blood cell count $\geq$ 25,000/mm^3 are also at high risk. CRS following adoptive T-cell therapy is discussed separately as it can be more severe and requires more aggressive intervention.

CRS usually occurs on the first treatment, within 30–120 minutes of initiating the drug (Vogel, 2010). The side effects are related to release of cytokines such as IL-2, interferon, and tumor necrosis factor (TNF) (Breslin, 2007) and include fever, chills, nausea, hypotension, tachycardia, headache, rash, dyspnea, and edema of tongue/throat (Breslin, 2007). The CTCAE CRS grading schema is shown in Table 4.7. Nursing priorities are the same as for patients with HSR. Initially, the nurse should stop the infusion and closely monitor the patient until symptoms resolve, usually within 30 minutes. Administer ordered medications, such as diphenhydramine and/or a corticosteroid if the symptoms do not resolve, and resume the infusion at a slower rate as ordered, once the symptoms do resolve (Vogel, 2010).

As investigational agents such as CAR-T cell therapy are studied, the CTCAE v4.0 CRS grading needed revision to reflect the seriousness of immunotherapy-associated CRS. Lee et al. (2014) combined treatment recommendations to correspond to grading assessment. Vigilant supportive care includes empiric treatment of concurrent bacterial infections, maintenance of adequate hydration, and BP for every grade. Immunosuppression (tocilizumab) should be used for grades 3 and 4, and high-risk grade 2. Organ toxicities should be managed by CTCAE v4.0.

- Grade 1: Fever, constitutional symptoms: Vigilant supportive care, assess for infection and treat fever and neutropenia, if present; monitor fluid balance, give antipyretics and analgesics as needed.
- Grade 2: Hypotension which responds to fluids or one low-dose vasopressor; hypoxia responds to < 40% O$_2$; organ toxicity grade 2: if no extensive comorbidities or older age, vigilant supportive care with close monitoring of cardiac and other organ function.

Table 4.7   CTCAE v 4.03 Cytokine Release Syndrome (Grade 5 is death)

Grade 1	Grade 2	Grade 3	Grade 4
Mild reaction; infusion interruption not indicated; intervention not indicated	Therapy or infusion interruption indicated but responds promptly to symptomatic treatment (e.g., antihistamines, NSAIDs, opioids, IV fluid); prophylactic medications indicated for ≤24 h.	Prolonged (e.g., not rapidly responsive to symptomatic medication and/or brief interruption of infusion); recurrence of symptoms after initial improvement; hospitalization indicated for clinical sequelae (e.g., renal impairment, pulmonary infiltrates)	Life-threatening consequences; urgent intervention indicated

Modified from National Cancer Institute. Common Terminology Criteria for Adverse Events (CTCAE). Version 4.03 (NIH Publication No. 09-5410). https://evs.nci.nih.gov/ftp1/CTCAE/CTCAE_4.03_2010-06-14_QuickReference_5x7.pdf. June 14, 2010.

TREATMENT

If extensive comorbidities or older age, give vigilant supportive care, tocilizumab (immunosuppressant) ± corticosteroids.

- Grade 3: Hypotension that requires multiple vasopressors or high dose vasopressors; hypoxia requires ≥ 40% O_2; organ toxicity: grade 3, grade 4 transaminitis: requires vigilant supportive care, tocilizumab (immunosuppressant) ± corticosteroids.
- Grade 4: Mechanical ventilation, organ toxicity grade 4 (excluding transaminitis): requires vigilant supportive care, tocilizumab (immunosuppressant) ± corticosteroids.

EGFR INHIBITOR RASH AND RELATED SKIN PROBLEMS

RASH

With the promise of epidermal growth factor receptor inhibitors (EGFRIs), the dose-limiting toxicities of skin rash and diarrhea are clearly within the domain of nursing practice. Rash is often more severe with mAbs compared to tyrosine kinase inhibitors (TKIs). The degree of rash appears to predict response, with increased likelihood of response in colorectal cancer (CRC), with increased intensity of rash (Saltz et al., 2001). It is also known that patients with mutated *K-RAS/RAS* genes do not respond to EGFRI therapy so that therapy can be tailored to prevent side effects from a drug to which the patient will not respond. As responding patients need to consider this treatment as chronic therapy, the challenge to nurses is to help patients minimize and manage symptoms and to maximize quality of life.

A number of authors have described effective approaches, including Lynch et al. (2007), who reported the results of a consensus group, as have the Multinational Association for Supportive Care in Cancer (MASCC) (Lacouture et al., 2011) and Alberta Health Services in their evidence-based Clinical Practice Guideline (2012). The following describes the pathophysiology of EGFR toxicity. However, there are a few Level I evidence-based interventions.

EGFRs are located in the cells of the epidermis (skin keratinocytes, hair follicles, and sweat and sebaceous glands) and lining of the gastrointestinal tract where EGF is important in stimulating replacement cells and repair of gut mucosal injury. Blockade of EGF pathways in skin results in an inflammatory, sterile rash that then crusts and looks like acne but is pathologically quite distinct. Rash is common in sun-exposed skin with many sebaceous glands (Lacouture et al., 2011). Skin rash is more intense with mAbs, such as cetuximab and panitumumab, whereas the rash with small molecule, oral TKIs (e.g., erlotinib) may last longer, and dark-skinned patients such as African Americans may have fewer rashes than lighter-skinned patients. In addition, rash does not appear in previously irradiated skin, thought to be due to depletion of the EGFRs; however, EGFRIs are radiosensitizers (Lynch et al., 2007).

Normally, when skin epidermis is damaged or aged, it is replaced by underlying keratinocytes that have differentiated and migrated to the skin surface. The skin is the primary protective barrier for the body, preventing UV light damage, and helps to keep in moisture. Lacouture (2006) describes the pathophysiology; thinking of the pathophysiology in phases can help understand the skin toxicity related to EGFRIs.

Phase I: weeks 0–1, erythema and edema like a sunburn. EGFR inhibition in the skin stops the underlying keratinocytes from differentiating and migrating to the skin surface to replace them, and they are arrested. The body senses that these arrested replacement cells should not be there and thus causes them to undergo apoptosis or programmed cell death. The dead keratinocytes cause the release of chemokines, which recruit neutrophils to the area as part of the sterile, inflammatory response. The patient feels a sunburn-like reaction (erythema, tenderness, slight swelling) on the face and areas that have previously been exposed to the sun. The goal is to preserve skin integrity, minimize discomfort, and prevent infection. Key patient teaching includes (1) use perfume-free and hydrophilic moisturing skin cream to keep the skin from drying out; (2) avoid sun exposure, using a sunblock of SPF 25 or higher and protect skin with hat and clothes when out in the sun; (3) wash with lukewarm water and use a mild soap; (4) apply prescribed prophylactic skin creams; (5) report distressing tenderness; (6) keep fingernails clean and trimmed. Some practices begin oral antibiotic prophylaxis with doxycycline or minocycline (Hofheinz et al., 2016) based on a number of studies showing that prophylactic use decreases severity of rash (e.g., Lacouture et al., 2010), although not incidence. A systematic review and meta-analysis of antibiotic prophylaxis for EGFRI-induced skin toxicity showed that, in 12 out of 13 studies, topical and systemic prophylactic measures lowered risk of rash compared to controls, and moderate-to-severe toxicities (grade 2–4) were reduced by nearly 66% in all 13 studies (Petrelli et al., 2016).

Phase II: weeks 1–3, papulopustules appear: This sterile inflammatory process results in death of the keratinocytes (apoptosis) and the formation of debris, which causes a papular rash on the skin. At the same time, the skin is no longer fortified by healthy keratinocytes, and thus, it thins and is unable to preserve water in the body, leading to skin dryness (xerosis) and itching. The rash begins within 7–10 days of starting therapy and peaks in intensity in 2–3 weeks and then gradually gets better. The goal is to prevent infection, promote healing, and maximize comfort and coping during this time. See Drug Information in this chapter, as well as drug package inserts for specific information on holding or discontinuing drug for severe dermatologic adverse effects. Continue teaching and antibiotic prophylaxis if ordered.

Phase III: weeks 3–5, lesions crust. The skin becomes drier (xerosis) with pruritus and the formation of telangiectasias (dilated capillaries in the skin). The skin flakes and itches. For flaking skin, keratolytics such as lactic acid, salicylic acid, or urea-containing topicals such as 12% Lac-Hydrin or other exfoliating lotions can be helpful. Continue reinforcement of teaching, assessment of potential infection, and antibiotic prophylaxis if ordered.

Phase IV: weeks 5–8, persistent dry skin, erythema, other skin/hair changes. While skin rash has usually resolved, EGFR inhibitor blockade of the hair follicles and nail beds results in hair changes (hair thinning or alopecia on scalp but increased hair growth on the eyelids [trichomegaly] or face [hypertrichosis]). The hair texture can change (changes in texture and strength). Paronychia (periungual inflammation) can develop with crusted lesions on nail folds and tenderness. Painful skin fissures on the fingers can develop. It is important to assess eyelashes, and if they are long, they can fold back and irritate the conjunctiva; refer to an ophthalmologist for redirection as needed (Borkar et al., 2013). Teach patient to report skin and hair changes, and suggest patient avoid hot blow-drying of hair (Lacouture et al., 2016).

Management strategies continue to lack strong Level I evidence. Lacouture et al. (2011) studied whether beginning preventive treatment before the rash occurs could decrease severity of panitumumab-related rash. They found that grade 2 or higher rash and other skin changes were significantly reduced in patients who received daily moisturizer, sunscreen, topical hydrocortisone, and oral doxycycline compared to a control group; there was no difference in tumor response. More recently, Melosky et al. (2016) prospectively studied prophylactic skin treatment in the prevention of erlotinib-induced skin rash in a randomized phase III trial and found no difference among arms, as the incidence of rash was 84%. However, interestingly, patients receiving either prophylactic (minocycline) or reactive (after rash developed based on grade) treatment had a longer OS (7.6 and 8 months) compared to those receiving no treatment unless severe (grade 3) rash (survival was 6 months). Rash was not self-limiting (Melosky et al., 2016).

Lacouture et al. (2011) developed clinical practice recommendations. The guideline recommends prophylactic treatment in weeks 1–6 and week 8 of beginning EGFRI therapy. Recommendations are based on Level II evidence for prevention and IV for treatment once it occurs. This includes topical hydrocortisone 1% cream, with moisturizer and sunscreen twice daily, and systemic doxycycline 100 mg PO bid (or minocycline 100 mg daily if in tropical areas as minocycline is not photosensitizing). Lacouture et al. (2016) recommend prophylaxis with doxycycline or minocycline for ≥ 8 weeks. For treatment of rash, Lacouture et al. (2011) recommend topical ointments such as clindamycin 1% cream, and for systemic treatment, doxycycline 100 mg PO bid, or minocycline 100 mg qd. EGFRI dose should be reduced or held based on package insert.

The Alberta Health Services also developed clinical practice guideline (2012), and recommends patients should receive individualized management to permit the patient to receive maximum recommended EGFR inhibitor dose. Treatment based on rash intensity is (1) mild to moderate: topical 2% clindamycin plus hydrocortisone lotion bid until rash resolution; (2) moderate-to-severe: topical 2% clindamycin plus hydrocortisone lotion bid until rash resolution, and oral minocycline 100 mg qd × minimum of 4 weeks, and continuing until rash resolves; (3) persistent: consider EGFR inhibitor dose reduction per label, as well as topical 2% clindamycin plus hydrocortisone lotion bid until rash resolution, and oral minocycline 100 mg qd × minimum of 4 weeks, and continuing until rash resolves; a medrol dose pack may be considered. Recommended supportive and follow-up care include: teaching the patient to (1) use cool or lukewarm water to bathe or wash, not hot, and apply moisturizers immediately following bath to prevent skin drying; (2) avoid alcohol, fragrance or dyed soaps, shampoos, body washes; (3) use alcohol-free emollient creams and hypoallergenic make-up; (4) avoid any skin care products containing alcohol, over-the-counter acne medications such as benzoyl peroxide, and scented laundry detergents; (5) avoid sun exposure by using a sunscreen SPF 30 or higher, when exposed to the sun; and (6) stay hydrated at all times as this will help prevent skin dryness and itching.

In summary, management of rash involves (Alberta Health Services, 2012; Lacouture et al., 2011):

- **Grade 1/mild rash**, which is localized, does not interfere with ADLs and is not infected (Lynch et al., 2007): Maintain current drug dose, observe or give topical hydrocortisone 1% or 2.5% or clindamycin 1% gel (anti-inflammatory benefit); reassess in 2 weeks.
- **Grade 2/moderate**, which is generalized, has mild symptoms, minimal effect on ADLs, and no infection: Continue EGFRI dose; use topicals (hydrocortisone 2.5% or

clindamycin 1% gel). If pustules are present, also add doxycycline 100 mg PO twice daily or minocycline 100 mg PO twice daily (give antimicrobial and anti-inflammatory effect), and reassess after 2 weeks.

- **For a grade 3 or severe rash**, which is generalized, severe, has a significant impact on ADLs, and increased risk of infection: Interrupt dose for up to 21 days or until rash is improved to grade 2. Treat rash with topicals (hydrocortisone 2.5% or clindamycin 1% gel), and patient should receive doxycycline 100 mg PO twice daily or minocycline 100 mg PO twice daily, along with methylprednisolone (Medrol dose pack); reassess after 2 weeks. Restart treatment based on manufacturer's recommendation. Interrupt or discontinue drug if rash worsens (Lynch et al., 2007). If the rash appears infected (exudate, vesicular formation, different appearance), obtain C+S, treat empirically until sensitivity received, and/or obtain dermatology consult.
- **Grade 4**, generally drug is discontinued.

OTHER EGFR INHIBITOR SKIN ISSUES

Pruritis management may be challenging but must be managed to prevent the patient from scratching, especially with unclean fingernails, which may result in serious infection. Lacouture et al. (2011) recommend topical treatment with menthol-pramoxine-doxepin or medium to high potency steroids, along with a systemic antihistamine. If this is unsuccessful, gabapentin/pregabalin or doxepin are possible Class V agents. Xerosis, or excessive drying of the skin, may be prevented by (1) bathing with bath oils or mild moisturizing soap, tepid water and following with regular moisturizing creams; (2) avoidance of extreme temperatures and direct sunlight. Management of mild/moderate xerosis employs (1) emollient creams that are packaged in a jar/tub without irritants; (2) occlusive emollients containing urea, colloidal oatmeal, and petroleum-based creams; (3) exfoliants for scaly areas such as ammonium lactate 12% or lactic acid cream 12%; (4) urea cream (10–40%); (5) salicylic acid 6%; (6) zinc oxide (13–40%); and for severe, (7) medium- to high-potency steroid creams. Fissures may develop on the hands and feet. Prevention involves using protective footwear, avoiding friction with fingertips, toes, and heels; treatment if fissures develop involves (1) application of thick moisturizers or zinc oxide (13–40%) cream, (2) painting the fissure with liquid glue or cyanoacrylate to seal cracks, (3) steroids or steroid tape, hydrocolloid dressings, topical antibiotics, (4) bleach soaks to prevent infection (Level III evidence). Lastly, Lacouture et al. (2011) recommend prevention of paronychia by using diluted bleach soaks and avoiding irritants. Paronychia management involves corticosteroids or calcineurin inhibitors (Level II evidence), and systemic tetracyclines, reserving antimicrobials when culture and sensitivity testing known.

Nursing care of patients receiving EGFR inhibitor therapy focuses on minimizing symptoms and helping patients maximize their quality of life. Patient educational materials are available, such as *Skin Reactions to Targeted Therapies* (March 2015) by the American Society of Clinical Oncology, available at http://www.cancer.net/navigating-cancer-care /side-effects/skin-reactions-targeted-therapies.

Zachariae et al. (2003) found that dermatologic disease-related impairment of quality of life predicted psychological symptoms. Molinari et al. (2005) found that 5 of 13 patients in a study of cetuximab-induced rash felt the rash had significant impact on their quality of life. Wagner et al. (2007) reported that the most commonly distressing aspects of skin toxicity on patients receiving EGFRIs are pain, irritation, pruritus, dryness, hair changes, interference with activities (work or hobbies), and the emotional impact (feeling depressed, frustrated, isolated). Fortunately, in a study by Humblet (2007), patients with CRC who had the most severe rash also tended to have the highest response rate; patients who were most bothered by skin toxicity also had the highest quality-of-life scores and fewest symptoms from cancer. Nurses need to assess the impact of skin changes on patients in terms of function, emotion, social, and physical, such as pain or tenderness.

IMMUNE-MEDIATED ADVERSE EFFECTS OF IMMUNE CHECKPOINT INHIBITORS

The immune checkpoint inhibitors (ICPi's) [ipilimumab (Yervoy), nivolumab (Opdivo), pembrolizumab (Keytruda), atezolizumab (Tecentriq), avelumab (Bavencio), and durvalumab (Imfinzi)] have revolutionized treatment of many cancers today. These drugs work by preventing tumors and the body from turning off activation of the powerful T-lymphocytes at immune checkpoints, and thus continuing a robust immune response. Normally this checkpoint turns down/off T-cell activation so that normal tissue is spared immune activation, and does not develop auto-immune disease(s). However, checkpoint blockade by these agents results in potential toxicities that are related to their immune effect on specific organs called immune-related adverse events or irAEs, and can be fatal. Thus, patients need very focused nursing assessment, patient/family teaching and nursing care. The T-lymphocyte hyperactivated-immune response damages normal organ tissue, such as the skin, GI tract (colitis), liver (hepatitis), lung (pneumonitis), musculoskeletal system, kidneys, bone marrow, cardiovascular system, ocular system or endocrine organs (e.g., thyroid, pituitary, adrenal glands). IrAEs often occur at a predictable time during checkpoint inhibitor drug therapy with rash and mucosal irritation occurring first (after week 3), then diarrhea/colitis occurring after that (Weber et al., 2012).

IrAEs can be severe, and life-threatening. Both ASCO and NCCN have released guidelines for the management of irAEs (ASCO, 2018; NCCN, 2019). Patients require close monitoring during therapy and for 6 months following completion of therapy (Weber et al., 2015).

ASCO (2019) recommendations suggest that if a patients develop symptom(s) while receiving one of these drugs, the nurse and physician should suspect an irAE until it is ruled out. A ICPi is continued with close monitoring if the patient develops a grade 1 toxicity, except for some neurological, hematologic or cardiac toxicities (ASCO, 2018). If a patient develops a grade 2 toxicity, discuss with the physician holding the ICPi until symptoms resolve to ≤ grade 1 with the administration of corticosteroids (initial dose 0.5–1 mg/kg/day of prednisone or equivalent) if warranted (ASCO, 2018). Almost all immune toxicities can be reversed by administration of corticosteroids, which should be used for grade 2 or higher irAEs (see drug package insert as this may vary among drugs, see Table 4.8). If the patient develops a grade 3 toxicity, high dose corticosteroids should be started (1–2 mg/kg/da prednisone or equivalent, or methylprednisolone IV 1–2 mg/kg/day), tapering over 4–6 weeks once a response occurs. If symptoms do not improve with 48–72 hours of high dose corticosteroids, discuss with physician adding another immunsuppressive agent can be added, such as infliximab, a TNF-α inhibitor (Weber et al., 2016; ASCO 2018; NCCN

Table 4.8   Selected Immune Mediated Adverse Effects: Grading and Management, based on ASCO and NCCN guidelines, and Weber (2016). IrAE diagnosis must be confirmed and other possible etiologies excluded. See references for full detail, and consult individual drug package inserts for management of irAEs.

Immune-Related Adverse Effect CTCAE Grading	Management	Follow-Up
Dermatologic toxicity Vitiligo (hair, skin) Skin peeling, blisters Oral ulceration Eosinophilic infiltrates Lichenoid deposits Stevens–Johnson syndrome (SJS) Toxic epidermal necrolysis (TEN)		
Grade 1 (Mild) Sx do not affect QOL or can be controlled with topical regimen and/or oral anti-pyretic	• R/O other causes (e.g., cellulitis, contact dermatitis, other drug reaction, sun exposure, radiation recall) • Continue ICPi • Topical emollients +/or mild-moderate topical corticosteroid cream, anti-itch ointment/cream (e.g., betamethasone 0.1%) • Teach patient to avoid skin irritants, sun exposure	If no improvement within a week, or symptoms worsen, treat as grade ¾ (see below)
Grade 2 Inflammatory reaction affects QOL and requires intervention based on diagnosis. (e.g., intense itching but intermittent; macules/papules/ pustules cover 10–30% of BSA; psychosocial impact limiting instrumental ADLs)	• Consider holding ICPi and monitor weekly for improvement; if it does not resolve, interrupt treatment until skin AE resolves to grade 1 • Consider starting prednisone or equivalent 1 mg/kg tapering over 4 weeks • Topical emollients, oral antihistamines, and medium-to-high potency topical corticosteroid cream, (e.g., moderate=triamcinolone 0.1%, high=betamethasone 0.1%) Oral anti-pyretic agents (e.g., diphenhydramine)	

Table 4.8 *(Continued)*

Immune-Related Adverse Effect

CTCAE Grading	Management	Follow-Up
Grade 3 Same as grade 2 but failure to respond to grade 2 interventions (e.g., intense and constant pruritis; papules/macules associated with local superinfection)	• Hold ICPi (Check package insert) • Dermatology consult and biopsy PRN • Assess for SJS and TEN, and if confirmed, permanently discontinue ICPi • Topical emollients, oral antihistamine, high potency topical corticosteroid • Give oral prednisone (0.5–1 mg/kg/day) or equivalent, tapering over at least 4 weeks Antibiotic therapy for superinfection	If rapid improvement, consider reinitiation of ICP on a case-by-case basis
Grade 4 All severe rashes	• Immediately hold ICPi, urgent dermatology consult, admit patient immediately with direct Oncology involvement • Systemic steroids: IV methylprednisolone (or equivalent (1–2 mg/kg) with slow (at least 4 weeks) taper after toxicity resolves. • Consult derm to see if ICPi can be resumed after toxicity resolves to grade 1 • Refer to package insert.	If no improvement within 48–72 hours, consider adding immunosuppression with infliximab • Monitor closely for progression to Severe Cutaneous Adverse Reaction • Consider alternative antineoplastic therapy over resuming ICPi if irAE does jnot resolve to ≤ grade 1 • If ICPi is patient's only option, consider resuming once toxicity resolves to grade 1
Severe cutaneous adverse reactions (SCAR) including SJS, TEN, AGEP, DRESS, DIHS	• Total body skin exam including mucous membranes • Complete ROS to rule out other etiologies of skin problem (e.g., infection, a drug interaction, or a skin condition linked to another systemic disease).	• Consider serial photography of lesion(s) • Full lab workup; if febrile, include blood cultures • Skin biopsy
Grade 2 (no grade 1) Morbilliform (maculopapular 10–30% BSA with systemic symptoms, lymphadenopathy or facial swelling	• Hold ICPi and monitor closely (q 3 days) for progression • Topical emollients, oral antihistamines, med-high potency ptopical corticosteroids • Consider starting prednisone (0.5–1 mg/kg/da) then taper over at least 4 weeks	

(continues)

Table 4.8   *(Continued)*

Immune-Related Adverse Effect CTCAE Grading	Management	Follow-Up
Grade 3 Skin sloughing <10% BSA with mucosal involvement, associated signs (e.g., erythema, purpura, epidermal detachment and mucous membrane detach-ment	• Hold ICPi and consult dermatology • Topical emollients, petrolatum emollients or dimethicone, oral antihistamines, high strength topical corticosteroids • IV methylprednisolone (or equivalent) 0.5 mg–1 mg/kg, and when responds convert to oral, then taper over at least 4 weeks • Admit to burn/consult wound service, supportive care including fluid and electrolytes, infection prevention	• Consider additional immune suppression if needed (e.g., infliximab) • Consult appropriate services if mucous membrane involvement with SJS, TEN to minimize scarring (e.g., ophthalmology, ENT, urology, GYN) • If DRESS/DIHS occurs, may require prolonged immunosuppression
Grade 4 Skin erythema and blistering/ sloughing (10%–>30% BSA), with associated signs (e.g., erythema, purpura) and/or systemic sx, abnormal labs	• Permanently D/C ICPi. • Admit to burn/consult wound service, supportive care including fluid and electrolytes, infection prevention • Start IV methylprednisolone (or equivalent) 1–2 mg/kg • Consider IVIG or cyclosporine if severe or steroid unresponsive	• Consult appropriate services if mucous membrane involvement with SJS, TEN to minimize scarring (e.g., ophthalmology, ENT, urology, GYN) • Consider pain/palliative consult and admission if presenting with DRESS manifestations
Colitis S/s: abdominal pain, cramping, ↑ in ostomy output, blood or mucus in stool, incontinence. Perforation: peritoneal signs, ileus, sepsis.	Grade 2: Assess CBC, CMP, TSH, ESR, CRP; stool C+S, c.diff, parasite, CMV, other virus, O&P Screening labs: HIV, Hepatitis A+B, blood quantiferon for TB in case needs infliximab Consider CT of abdomen, pelvis, GI endoscopy with biopsy Grade 3/4 as above, repeat endoscopy if unresponsive to steroids or before resuming ICPi	• Begins early by weeks 3–4 with ipilimumab, but occurs later and less commonly with PD-1/PD-L1 blockade, about 6 weeks into treatment • Teach patients to report abdominal pain, nausea, cramping, blood or mucus in stool, change in bowel habits, fever, abdominal distention, obstipation, constipation

Table 4.8 *(Continued)*

Immune-Related Adverse Effect CTCAE Grading	Management	Follow-Up
Grade 1: *Diarrhea:* ↑ of <4 stools/day over baseline; mild ↑ in ostomy output vs. baseline. *Colitis:* asymptomatic, observation only, intervention not indicated	• Distinguish between diarrhea alone and colitis, especially with ipilimumab, which has a 30% incidence • Continue CPIi therapy or temporarily hold and resume; symptomatic treatment • Patient education to ↑ hydration, dietary modification, self-administration of antidiarrheal medications, close telephone contact • If prolonged, GI consult.	R/O infectious cause (e.g., stool for WBC, C&S, *Clostridium difficile*) Diarrhea: increase in number of stools, vs. colitis, characterized by abdominal pain, colon inflammation by endoscopy or imaging Close monitoring for worsening symptoms; teach patient to report these right away.
Grade 2: *Diarrhea:* ↑ of 4–6 stools/day over baseline; moderate ↑ in ostomy output vs baseline. *Colitis:* abdominal pain; mucus or blood in stool; limiting self-care ADL	• **Hold** checkpoint inhibitor until grade 1, consider permanently D/C CTLA-4 agents; administer antidiarrheal therapy once infection ruled out. • Consult GI • Give corticosteroids 1 mg/kg/day prednisone or equivalent • When sx resolve to ≤1, taper corticosteroids over 4–6 weeks before resumingICPi	*If worsens or persists >3–5 days with oral steroids, treat as grade 3/4 *EGD/colonoscopy if grade ≥2 to stratify for early infliximab treatment and safety of resuming CPIi *Stool inflammatory markers (lactoferrin and calprotectin) for grade ≥2 to distinguish functional vs inflammatory diarrhea, monitor calprotectin
Grade 3: *Diarrhea:* ↑ of ≥ 7 stools/day over baseline; incontinence; hospitalization indicated; severe ↑ in ostomy output vs. baseline limiting self-care ADL. *Colitis:* severe abdominal pain; change in bowel habits; medical intervention indicated; peritoneal signs	• Permanently discontinue ipilimumab, may restart PD-1, PD-L1 inhibitors when sx resolve to ≤ grade 1 • Give corticosteroids (initial 1-2 mg prednisone or equivalent), then when improved to grade 1, start taper over at least 1 month • For all, if sx worsen or persist 3–5 days on corticosteroid therapy, or recur after improvement, consider adding noncorticosteroid immunosuppressive medication (e.g., infliximab 5 mg/kg/day if no contraindication)	Hospitalization with IV hydration, corticosteroids, electrolyte replacement Consider endoscopy if diagnosis unclear, rule out bowel perforation Or risk of opportunistic infections (OI) due to immunosuppression (e.g., CMV colitis) Taper corticosteroids over 4 weeks or longer, up to 6–8 weeks if diffuse and severe ulceration or bleeding (O'Kane et al., 2017)

(continues)

Table 4.8   *(Continued)*

Immune-Related Adverse Effect CTCAE Grading	Management	Follow-Up
Grade 4: *Diarrhea:* life-threatening; urgent intervention indicated *Colitis:* life-threatening; urgent intervention indicated	• Permanently discontinue all checkpoint inhibitors. • Admit patient, or closely monitor in ambulatory setting. • Administer methylprednisolone or equivalent 1–2 mg/kg/day until resolve to ≤ grade 1, then start taper over 4–6 weeks. • Lower GI endoscopy if refractory symptoms or possibility of new infecotions.	Consider endoscopy, rule out bowel perforation Add prophylactic antibiotics for opportunistic infections If diarrhea/colitis persists >2–3 days, and no perforation or sepsis exists, add immunosuppressive therapy, e.g., infliximab 5–10 mg/kg/day if no contraindication If refractory to infliximab, consider vedolizumab
Hepatitis	• Diagnostic: (1) Monitor LFTs prior to each infusion +/ or q week if grade 1; (2) Grade ≥2: exclude other causes including viral hepatitis, ETOH history, iron stores, thromboembolic event, liver metastases; (3) if suspect autoimmune cause, assess ANA/ASMA/ANCA; (4) if AlkP alone is elevated, assess GGT; if isolated transaminases elevated, assess creatine kinase	• Incidence <10% ipilimumab, and <5% other checkpoint inhibitors • Onset 8–12 weeks after starting treatment • Teach all patients to report immediately: yellowing of skin, or sclera; severe nausea +/or vomiting; pain on R side abdomen; drowsiness; dark colored urine; easy bruising or bleeding; decreased appetite. • If additional immune-suppression needed, infliximab may not be preferred given potential risk of idiosyncratic liver failure (ASCO, 2018).
Grade 1 Asymptomatic; AST or ALT > ULN to 3.0 × ULN and/or T. bili > ULN to 1.5 × ULN	• Continue CPIi and monitor closely, consider alternate etiologies • Monitor LFTs 1–2 X/week • Symptom control	• If LFTs worsen, treat as grade 2 or 3/4

Table 4.8   *(Continued)*

Immune-Related Adverse Effect

CTCAE Grading	Management	Follow-Up
Grade 2 Asymptomatic; AST or ALT > 3.0 × ULN to ≤ 5 × ULN and/or T. bili > 1.5 ULN to ≤ 3 × ULN	• Hold CPIi, give prednisone ≤ 10 mg/da; resume if recovers to grade ≤1 • For significant symptomatic grade 2 and abnormal LFTs persisting 3–5 days, may give corticosteroid 0.5–1 mg/kg day prednisone or equivalent and monitor LFTs q 3 days. • Assess medication profile and stop unnecessary hepatotoxic drugs	• See ICPi package insert. • Resume ICPi after steroid taper when sx improve to grade 1 or less, and steroid dose ≤10 mg/day; taper over at least 1 month.
Grade 3 AST or ALT > 5–20 × ULN and/or T. bili > 3–10 × ULN; Symptomatic liver dysfunction; fibrosis by biopsy; compensated cirrhosis; reaction of chronic hepatitis	• Permanently discontinue CPIi • Immediately give methylprednisolone or equivalent 1-2 mg/kg • Assess LFTs every 1–2 days • Consider hospitalization if AST/ALT >8 ULN +/or total BR 3 × ULN • If refractory to intervention, consult hepatologist for further definition/pathology of hepatitis	• On corticosteroids, if LFTs do not decrease after 3 days, worsen, or rebound, add mycophenolate mofetil or consider azathioprine (test for thiopurine methyltransferase (TPMT) deficiency first) [ASCO, 2018] • If LFTs resolve to ≤ grade 1, attempt steroid taper at 4–6 weeks, re-escalate if needed; optimal duration not known.
Grade 4 AST or ALT > 20 × ULN and/or T. bili > 10 × ULN; Decompensated liver function (e.g., ascites, encephalopathy, coma)	• Permanently discontinue CPIi • Assess LFTs q day; consider in-hospital monitoring • Give methylprednisolone 2 mg/kg/da or equivalent • Avoid infliximab if immune mediated hepatitis • Add prophylactic antimicrobials for OIs	• If LFTs resolve to ≤ grade 1, attempt steroid taper at 4–6 weeks, re-escalate if needed; optimal duration not known. • Consider transfer to tertiary care facility PRN

(continues)

Table 4.8   (*Continued*)

Immune-Related Adverse Effect CTCAE Grading	Management	Follow-Up
Pneumonitis S/S: dyspnea, chest pain, dry cough, SOB at rest, wheezing; hypoxia, tachypnea, tachycardia	• Diagnostic: focal or diffuse inflammation of lung parenchyma (CT) • Workup: CXR, CT, pulse oximetry • If grade 2+, add nasal swab, sputum C+S, blood C+S, urine C+S	• Uncommon, <10% in CPIi except ipilimumab • For patients on prolonged steroid use (>12 weeks), consider: (1) GI and pneumocystis prophylaxis with PPI and Bactrim; (2) consider calcium and Vitamin D supplements; (3) role of prophylactic fluconazole role is unclear (see institutional guidelines)
Grade 1 Asymptomatic; confined to 1 lobe or the lung or <25% of lung parenchyma; clinical or diagnostic observation only (e.g., CT scan)	• Hold ICPi if XR evidence of pneumonitis progression • Repeat CT in 3–4 weeks; if patient has baseline testing, may offer repeat spirometry/DLCO in 3–4 weeks. • May resume ICPi if improvement on XR • Monitor patient q week with Hx, PE, pulse oximetry; may offer CXR	• If sx worsen, treat as grade 2 or 3/4 • Consider Pulmonary (bronchoscopy and biopsy), and ID consults
Grade 2 Symptomatic (mild to moderate); involves >1 lung lobe or 25–50% of lung parenchyma; medical intervention indicated; sx limit instrumental ADL	• Hold CPIi until resolution to ≤ grade 1 • Prednisone 1–2 mg/kg/day and taper by 5–10 mg/week over 4–6 weeks • Pulmonary and ID consults, consider bronchoscopy with BAL • Consider empiric antibiotics • Monitor q 3 days: Hx, PE, pulse oximetry, consider CXR, Reimage every 1–3 days • Resume checkpoint inhibitor when resolves to grades 0–1 after corticosteroid taper	• If no improvement after 48–72 hours on corticosteroid therapy, or worsens, treat as grade 3/4 • See CPIi package insert.

Table 4.8 *(Continued)*

Immune-Related Adverse Effect

CTCAE Grading	Management	Follow-Up
Grade 3/4 Grade 3: Severe new symptoms; new or worsening hypoxia; hospitalization required; all lung lobes involved or >50% of lung parenchyma; limits self-care ADL; oxygen indicated Grade 4: life-threatening respiratory compromise; urgent intervention indicated (intubation)	• Permanently discontinue CPIi • Administer methylprednisolone IV 1–2 mgkg/daycorticosteroids with taper when improves to grades 0–1, over at least 6 weeks • Pulmonary and ID consults, consider bronchoscopy with BAL +/– transbronchial biopsy (unless clinical picture consistent with pneumonitis) • Add empiric antimicrobials. • Hospitalization for further management	• If no improvement on corticosteroids after 48 hours, or worsening sx, add additional immunosuppressive agent (e.g., infliximab 5 mg/kg or mycophenolate mofetil IV 1 g bid or IVIG × 5 days or mycophenolate mofetil IV 1 g bid), or cyclophosphamide.
Endocrine Adverse Effects	• Teach patients to report: headaches that do not go away or unusual headache pattern; vision changes; rapid heartbeat; increased sweating; extreme tiredness or weakness; muscle aches; weight gain or weight loss; dizziness or fainting; feeling increased hunger or thirst; hair loss; changes in mood or behavior (↓ sex drive, irritability, forgetfulness); feeling cold; constipation; deep voice; urinating more than usual; nausea or vomiting; abdominal pain.	• Although all are uncommon hypophysitis (pituitary inflammation) and hypothyroidism occur most common (incidence up to 10% with ipilimumab) • In hypophysitis, assess for decrease in hormones released by the pituitary (ACTH, TSH, FSH, LH, GH, prolactin)
Adrenal Insufficiency ↑ fatigue, muscle weakness, loss of appetite, nausea, vomiting, diarrhea, hypotension, hypglycemia	• Diagnostic work-up: AM ACTH and cortisol; basic metabolic pattern (Na, K, CO₂, glucose); if indeterminate results, ACTH stimulation test; if primary adrenal insufficiency found (high ACTH, low cortisol): evaluate for precipitating cause of crisis (e.g., infection); adrenal CT to r/o metastasis or hemorrhage (ASCO, 2018),	• Primary adrenal insufficiency: low AM cortisol, high morning ACTH and hyponatremia, hyperkalemia, with orthostasis and volume depletion due to loss of aldosterone (ASCO, 2018) • Teach patients about stress dosing, and need for a medical alert bracelet for adrenal insufficiency so stress dose given if patient has emergency or needs surgery.

(continues)

TREATMENT

Table 4.8 *(Continued)*

Immune-Related Adverse Effect CTCAE Grading	Management	Follow-Up
Grade 1 Asymptomatic or mild sx	• Consider holding ICPi until stabilized on replacement hormone • Endocrine consult • Replacement therapy with prednisone (5–10 mg PO q d) or hydrocortisone (10–20 mg POq am, 5–10 mg PO q 2 PM)	• May require flurocortisone (0.1 mg/da) for mineralocoricoid replacement in primary adrenal insufficiency • Titrate dose up or down as dictated by sx
Grade 2 Moderate sx, able to perform all ADLs	• Consider holding ICPi until stabilized on replacement hormone • Endocrine consult • Start OP treatmentat 2–3 × main-tenance dose (e.g., if prednisone 20 mg qd, or hydrocortisone 20–30 mg on AM, 10–20 mg in afternoon) to manage acute sx	• Taper stress dose corticosteroids down to maintenance doses over 5–10 days • Maintenance therapy as in grade 1
Grades 3/4 Severe sx, medically significant or life-threatening consequences; unable to perform ADL.	• Hold ICPi until patient stabilized on hormone replacement • Endocrine consult • For sx, see in clinic, or ER referral for after hours: 2L+ IV Normal saline, IV stress dose steroids on presentation: hydrocortisone 100 mg or dexamethasone 4 mg (if diagnosis not clear and stimulation testing needed).	• Taper stress dose corticosteroids down to main-tenance doses over 7–14 days after discharge • Maintenance therapy as in grade 1

Table 4.8 *(Continued)*

Immune-Related Adverse Effect

CTCAE Grading	Management	Follow-Up
Hypophysitis Fatigue, lethargy, visual disturbances, confusion, hallucinations, memory loss, emotional lability, dizziness, nausea, vomiting, insomnia, anorexia, diabetes insipidus	• Inflammation of pituitary • Diagnostic: low ACTH with low cortisol; low or normal TSH with low FT4. Hypernatremia and volume depletion with diabetes insipidus (DI); low testosterone or estradiol with low LH and FSH • Assess: ACTH, AM cortisol, TSH, free T4, electrolytes • Consider evaluating LH, FSH, testosterone in males, or estrogen in premenopausal women with fatigue, loss of libido, and mood changes	• Most commonly presenting as central adrenal insufficiency, but may also have central hypothyroidism, DI, and hypogonadism • Consider MRI brain w/wo contrast with pituitarysellar cuts if patient has multiple endocrine abnormalities, +/– new, severe Has, or visual changes (ASCO, 2018) • Corticosteroids must be started first when planning hormone replacement for multiple deficiencies (ASCO, 2018) • Teach patients to take a double dose (stress dosing) and wear medic alert bracelet if has adrenal insufficiency if infection or stress
Grade 1 Asymptomatic or mild sx	• Consider holding ICPi until stabilized on hormone replacement • Hormonal supplementation for primary hypothyroidism and adrenal insufficiency • Testosterone and estrogen therapy if not contraindicated and needed • Endocrine consult.	• Start corticosteroid therapy several days before thyroid hormone replacement to prevent precipitating adrenal crisis • Follow FT4 for thyroid hormone replacement titration as TSH not accurate (ASCO, 2018).
Grade 2 Moderate symptoms, able to do ADLs	• Consider holding ICPi until stabilized on replacement hormone • Endocrine consult • Replacement hormone therapy as in grade 1	Monitor labs

(continues)

Table 4.8 *(Continued)*

Immune-Related Adverse Effect CTCAE Grading	Management	Follow-Up
Grade 3/4 Severe symptoms, medically significant or life threatening, Unable to dp ADLs. hospitalization indicated	• Hold CPIi until stabilized on replacement hormones • Endocrine consult • Hormone replacement as in grade 1 • Consider initial pulse dose corticosteroid with prednisone 1–2 mg/kg oral daily (or equivalent) tapered over at least 1–2 weeks.	Consider pituitary MRI When improvement, taper corticosteroids over at least 1 month once improvement with or without hormones Resume checkpoint inhibitor If adrenal insufficiency, may need to continue steroids with mineralocorticoid component (Weber et al., 2016)
Thyroid Dysfunction *Hyperthyroid (less common)* Weight loss, irritability, palpitations, diarrhea, feeling hot *Hypothyroid (more common)* Fatigue, sluggishness, anorexia, ↓ weight, dry skin, constipation, feeling cold	• Primary hypothyroidism: elevated TSH, normal of low FT4. Assess: TSH and and FT4 q 4–6 weeks as part of routine clinical monitoring or if patient symptomatic • If no risk factors, full replace-ment is estimated on IBW based dose of about 1.6 mcg/kg/day (ASCO, 2018). • For elderly/fragile with multiple co-morbidities, consider titrating up from low dose, starting at 25–50 mcg. • If adrenal insufficiency, ALWAYS replace corticosteroid before thyroid hormone started. (ASCO, 2018).	• Hyperthyroidism: Suppressed TSH and high normal or elevated FT4 and/or T3. Assess TSH, free T4 q 4–6 weeks from start of ICPi therapy or if patient symptomatic; consider TSH receptor antibodies if Graves' disease suspected; closely monitor thyroid function q 2–3 weeks after diagnosis to identify hypothyroidism in patients with thyroiditis and hyperthyroidism
Grade 1 *Hypothyroidism:* TSH < 10 mIU/L and asymptomatic *Hyperthyroidism:* asymptomatic or mild sx	• Continue ICPi with close monitoring of TSH, FT4; if hyperthyroid, monitor q 2–3 weeks until it is definitely hyperthyroidism • Endocrine consult if Graves' disease suspected (e.g., PE findings of ophthalmopathy or thyroid bruit)	• Thyroiditis is transient and resolves in a few weeks to primary hypothyroidism or normal function • Graves' disease is generally persistent and requires anti-thyroid medical therapy

Table 4.8 *(Continued)*

Immune-Related Adverse Effect

CTCAE Grading	Management	Follow-Up
Grade 2 Symptomatic *Hypothyroid*: moderate sx. Able to perform ADLs; TSH persistently > 10 mIU/L *Hyperthyroid*: Moderate sx, able to do ADLs	*Hypothyroid:* • May hold ICPi until sx resolve to baseline; consider endocrine consult • Thyroid hormone replacement (e.g., levothyroxine) as clinically indicated; Monitor TSH q 6–8 weeks while titrating hormone to normal TSH; FT4 can be used short-term (2 weeks) to make sure adequate therapy if FT4 initially low • Resume CPi when symptom-free; monitor TSH q 6 weeks, then when stable, assess annually or based on sx *Hyperthyroid:* • May hold ICPi until sx resolve to baseline; consider endocrine consult • Beta blocker for symptomatic relief • Hydration and supportive care • Consult package insert as most checkpoint inhibitors should be held until clinically stable and symptoms managed.	• Hyperthyroid: corticosteroids are not usually required to shorten duration • For persistent hyperthyroidism (>6 weeks) or if Graves' disease suspected, work up and get endocrine consult.

(continues)

Table 4.8   (Continued)

Immune-Related Adverse Effect CTCAE Grading	Management	Follow-Up
Grade 3/4		
Hypothyroid	*Hypothyroid:*	Work-up:
Severe sx, medically significant or life-threatening; unable to perform ADLs	• Hold ICPi until sx resolve to baseline with supplementation • Endocrine consult • Admit for IV therapy if s/s myxedema (bradycardia, hypothermia)	• Monitor for hyperglycemia or worsening pre-existing DM (baseline, with each treatment cycle during induction × 12 weeks then q 3–6 weeks thereafter • Type I DM: assess ketosis in urine, assess anion gap on metabolic panel; anti-islet cell or anti-insulin antibodies are highly specific for autoimmune DM (ASCO, 2018)
Hyperthyroid		
Severe sx, medically significant or life-threatening; unable to perform ADLs	• Hold ICPi until sx resolve to baseline with appropriate therapy • Endocrine consult • Beta blocker for symptomatic relief • If severe sx or possible thyroid storm, admit patient and start prednisone 1–2 mg/kg/day or equivalent, tapered over 1–2 weeks. Consider use of SSKI or thionamide (methimazole or PTU)	
DM	Type I DM: Autoimmune DM due to islet cell destruction, onset is often acute, with ketosis and requires insulin	
Poly: uria, phagia, dipsia; blurred vision, fatigue; weight loss	Type II DM: Steroid exposure can cause a combination of insulin resistance and insufficiency that may require oral hypoglycemic or insulin • Type I DM insulin: usually lower doses due to preserved sensitivity; need long acting but also prandial coverage • Type II insulin: sliding scale with meals helps to estimate daily requirements	
Grade 1	• Continue ICPi with close follow-up and lab monitoring	
Asymptomatic or mild sx; fasting glucose > ULN-160 mg/dL, no ketosis or lab evidence of Type I DM	• May start oral therapy for new onset Type II DM • Assess for Type I DM if acute onset with prior normal values, or ketosis	

Table 4.8 *(Continued)*

Immune-Related Adverse Effect

CTCAE Grading	Management	Follow-Up
Grade 2 Moderate sx able to do ADLs Fasting glucose value >160–250 mg/dL; ketosis or evidence of T1DM at any glucose level	• May hold ICPi until clinically stable (glucose control); titrate oral hypo-glycemic or add insulin for worsening control of Type II DM • Type I DM requires insulin or is default if not sure of type • Urgent endocrine consult for Type I DM, or internal medicine if no endocrine	• Consider hospitalization if Type I DM if early outpatient evaluation not available or signs of ketoacidosis are present • If ICPi held, resume checkpoint inhibitor when blood glucose well controlled
Grade 3/4 Severe symptoms, medically significant of life threatening consequences. Unable to do ADLS.	• Hold ICPi until blood sugar effectively controlled with antihyperglycemic agents, with resolution of toxicity to grade ≤1 • Urgent endocrine consult for all patients	• If all other potential causes ruled out, forego biopsy, and begin immunosuppressive therapy • Autoimmune cause should be treated swiftly
Grade 3: Glucose >250–500 mg/dL	• Start insulin for all patients (ASCO 2018)	
Grade 4: glucose > 500 mg/dL	• Admit for inpatient management: possible DKA, symptomatic patients regardless of type of DM, new onset Type I DM unable to see endocrine consult. (ASCO 2018)	
Nephritis and Renal Dysfunction	• Exclude other potential causes	
Often asymptomatic; vague nausea +/– vomiting, hematuria, pedal edema, decreased urinary output, cloudy or dark urine	• Monitor serum creatinine prior to each dose • Routine urinalysis not necessary unless to r/o UTI, unless suggested by Renal (Nephrology) consult	
Grade 1 Serum creatinine level increase of >0.3 mg/dL; creatinine 1.5–2.0 × above baseline	• Consider holding ICPi based on other potential causes, e.g., IV contrast, medications, dehydration) • Review medication profile and discuss changing potentially nephrotoxic medications	• R/O hypovolemia, other potential causes • If other cause identified, resume ICPi • If improves to baseline, resume serum creatinine monitoring

(continues)

Table 4.8   *(Continued)*

Immune-Related Adverse Effect

CTCAE Grading	Management	Follow-Up
Grade 2 Serum creatinine 2–3 × above baseline	• Hold ICPi temporarily; cosult Renal service • Monitor serum creatinine every 2–3 days • Rule out other etiologies, and if not found, give prednisone 0.5–1 mg/kg/day (or equivalent) • If renal function worsening or no improvement, increase steroid dose to 1–2 mg/kg/day prednisone equivalents, and permanently discontinue ICPi	• If renal function improves to grade 1 or less, taper corticosteroids over 4–6 weeks • If no recurrence of renal dysfunction, discuss with provider/patient about risks/benefits of resuming ICPi • If elevated serum creatinine persists >7 days or worsens, without any other cause, treat as grade 3
Grade 3 Serum creatinine > 3 × above baseline or > 4.0 mg/dL; hospitalization indicated	• Permanently discontinue ICPi) • Consult Renal (nephrology) • If no other etiology identified, give corticosteroids (initial dose 1–2 mg/kg/day prednisone/equivalent)	• If toxicity improves to grade 1 or less, taper corticosteroids over at least 4 weeks
Grade 4 Life-threatening consequences; dialysis indicated	• If elevated serum creatinine persists >3–5 days (grade 3) or >2–3 days (grade 4) or worsens, consider adding additional immunosuppression (mycophenolate)	
Musculoskeletal Toxicity ***Inflammatory Arthritis***	• Joint pain with joint swelling, and inflammation sx (stiffness after inactivity or in AM lasting > 30 min–1 hr; improves with NSAIDs or corticosteroids but not opioids • Patient with inflammatory RA should have serial rheumatology exams, including inflammatory markers, every 4–6 weeks after starting ICPi therapy (ASCO, 2018)	• Early recognition is very important to prevent erosive joint damage • Corticosteroids can be used initially, but due to need for prolonged treatment, consider starting steroid-sparing therapy.

Table 4.8 *(Continued)*

Immune-Related Adverse Effect CTCAE Grading	Management	Follow-Up
Grade 1 Mild pain with inflammation, erythema, or joint swelling	• Hx and PE: rheumatologic hx, examine all peripheral joints for tenderness, swelling, ROM; spine • Consider plain XR/imaging to rule out metastases, evaluate joint damage (erosions) if appropriate • Consider autoimmune blood panel (ANA, RF, anti-CCP, anti-inflammatory markers ESR and CRP if symptoms persist • Continue ICPi • Start pain analgesia with acetaminophen +/- NSAIDs	• If sx suggestive of reactive arthritis or affect the spine, consider HLA B27 testing (ASCO, 2018)
Grade 2 Moderate pain associated with signs of inflammation, erythema, or joint swelling, limited ability to do instrumental ADLs	• Hold ICPi and resume when sx are controlled and on prednisone ≤ 10 mg/day • Hx and PE, diagnostic labs as in grade 1 • Titrate analgesia (e.g., NSAIDs) as needed; if inadequately controlled, start prednisone or prednisolone 10-20 mg/day or equivalent × 4-6 weeks • If improvement, taper prednisone slowly according to response over 4-6 wees; if no improvement after initial 4-6 weeks, treat as grade 3 • If corticosteroid taper is not possible to <10 mg/day after 3 months, consider adding a disease-modifying anti-rheumatic drug (DMARD) (see *Chapter 5*)	• Consider US +/- MRI of affected joints if persistent arthritis or unresponsive to treatment, to rule out metastases or septic joint • Consider early referral to rheumatologist if there is synovitis (joint swelling) or symptoms persist for >4 weeks • Consider intr-articular steroid injections for pain in large joints

(continues)

Table 4.8 *(Continued)*

Immune-Related Adverse Effect CTCAE Grading	Management	Follow-Up
Grade 3/4 Severe pain associated with signs of inflammation, erythema, or joint swelling; irreversible joint damage; disabling; limited ability to do self-care ADLs	• Hold ICPi and resume in consultation with rheumatology, if sx recover to grade 1 or less • Start oral prednisone 0.5–1 mg/kg; if no improvement after 4 weeks or worsening of sx. Consider synthetic (MTX, leflunomide) or biologic (TNFα receptor inhibitor e.g., infliximab, or IL6 receptor inhibitor DMARD (do not use IL6 receptor inhibitor if patient has colitis as rarely causes perforation)	Test for viral hepatitis B, C, and latent/active TB before starting biological DMARDs Referral to Rheumatology

Modified from Brahmer JR, Lacchetti C, Schneider BJ et al. Management of immune-related adverse events in patients treated with immune checkpoint inhibitor therapy: American Society of Clinical Oncology Clinical Practice Guideline. *J Clin Oncol* 2018; 36:1714-1768; National Comprehensive Cancer Network. Management of immunotherapy-related toxicities (immune checkpoint immune-related toxicities). Version 1.2018 (February 14, 2018). Available at https://www.nccn.org/professionals/physician_gls/pdf/immunotherapy.pdf. Accessed June 18, 2018. Weber JS, Postow M, Lao CD, Schadendorf D. Management of adverse events following treatment with anti-programmed death-1 agents. *Oncologist* 2016; 21:1230–1240. O'Kane GM, Labbe C, Doherty MK et al. Monitoring and management of immune-related adverse effects associated with programmed cell death protein-1 axis inhibitors in lung cancer. *Oncologist* 2017; 22:70–80; Weinstein A, Gordon R-A, Kasler MK, et al. Understanding and managing immune-related adverse events associated with immune checkpoint inhibitors I patients with advanced melanoma. *J Adv Pract Oncol* 2017;8(1):58–72. CTCAE: US Department of Health and Human Services, National Institutes of Health, National Cancer Institute. Common terminology criteria for adverse events (CTCAE). Version 4.03. Available at https://evs.nci.nih.gov/ftp1/CTCAE/CTCAE_4.03_2010-06-14_QuickReference_5x7.pdf. Accessed June 18, 2018.

Abbreviations for Table 4.8:

ACTH: adrenocorticotropic hormone; AE: adverse effects; AGEP: acute generalized exanthematous pustulosis; ALKP: alkaline phosphatase; ALT: alanine aminotransferase; AM: morning; ANA: antinuclear antibodies; ANCA: antineutrophil cytoplasmic antibodies; ASMA: actin smooth muscle antibody; AST: aspartate aminotransferase; CBC: complete blood count; CMP: comprehensive metabolic panel; CRP: C-reactive protein; C+S: culture and sensitivity; CO_2: carbon dioxide; CT: computerized tomography; CTLA-4: cytotoxic T-lymphocyte-associated-4 (CD152); CXR: chest xray; DIHS: drug induced hypersensitivity syndrome; D/C: discontinue; DM: diabetes mellitus; DMARD: disease modifying anti-rheumatoid drug; DRESS: drug reaction with eosinophilia and systemic symptoms; ENT: ears, nose and throat; ESR: erythrocyte sedimentation rate; FSH: follicle stimulating hormone; FT4: free thyroxine (T4); GGT: gamma glutamyl transferase; GH: growth hormone; GI: gastrointestinal; GYN: gynecology; HIV: human immunodeficiency virus; Hx: history; ICPi: immune checkpoint inhibitor; IVIG: Intravenous immune globulin; K: potassium; LFTs: liver function tests; LH: lutenizing hormone; Na: sodium; NSAID: non-steroidal anti-inflammatory drug;

OIs: opportunistic infections (risk increased with administration of corticosteroids); O+P: ova and parasite; PE: physical exam; PD-1: programmed cell death receptor-1; PD-L1: programmed cell death ligand-1; PRN: as needed; QOL: quality of life; RA: rheumatoid arthritis; SCAR: severe cutaneous adverse reactions (changes in struction or function of skin, the appendages, or mucous membranes due to a drug.SJS: Stevens Johnson Syndrome; sx: symptoms; TB: tuberculosis; TEN: toxic epidermal necrolysis; TSH: thyroid stimulating hormone; T. bili: total bilirubin; ULN: upper limit of normal;

2018). Corticosteroid tapering requires at least 4 weeks, starting when toxicity resolves to grade 1. Once improvement occurs, or at the time of taper, change patient from IV corticosteroids to oral equivalent doses. However, recall that bioavailability of oral corticosteroids is lower when calculating equivalent doses (Weber et al., 2016). If unable to taper corticosteroids, see package insert as drug should be discontinued (e.g., pembrolizumab, if unable to wean to corticosteroid dose of 10 mg or less within 12 weeks).

When the patient's symptoms or lab abnormality resolves to ≤grade 1, the patient may be rechallenged with the ICPi; however, if the patient had an early-onset irAE, adjustments are not recommended (ASCO, 2018). If a grade 4 toxicity occurs (except for endocrinopathy that is well controlled with hormone replacement), the ICPi should be permanently discontinued (ASCO, 2018).

Patients receiving PD-1 inhibitors may take a longer time to fully respond than patients receiving ipilimumab a CTLA-4 inhibitor, so they require long-term monitoring (Weber et al., 2015). Also, as cancer does not discriminate, patients often have other chronic illnesses, and often, multiple chronic conditions which require close monitoring while receiving ICPi therapy. If a patient already has an autoimmune disease, the decision to start an ICPi may be a difficult one. The nurse, together with the physician, should help the patient understand the potential risks and benefits to make an informed decision. In general, patients receiving ICPis may experience fevers, chills, and lethargy; maculopapular skin toxicity; diarrhea and colitis; elevated LFTs; and thyroiditis, and less commonly, hypophysitis and adrenal insufficiency. Table 4.8 shows an overview of assessment and management of selected irAEs, based on the literature and recent ASCO and NCCN guidelines (2019). The reader is directed to the primary references for greater detail, and discussion of less common irAEs such as neurological and hematolotic events. In addition, the reader should consult the specific ICPi package insert as some drugs have special requirements to manage toxicity.

Patient and family education is critical as irAEs develop over time, and through close monitoring, early small changes in patient status may reveal an early irAE (ASCO, 2018). Patients should be taught the drug mechanism of action, potential side effects and irAEs, which signs and symptoms to report right away, and how to contact a provider outside of clinic or practice hours.The nurse should pay particular attention to advising the patient who lives far away or has difficulty getting to an emergency department. Patients should tell all their providers about the ICPi they are receiving. The nurse should collaborate with colleagues so that there is consistent assessment and documentation whenever the patient is seen so that changes can be identified over time (ASCO, 2018).

It has been noted that patients receiving ICPi's also receiving the influenza vaccine may have an excessive immune response. Swiss oncologists studied patients receiving PD-1/PD-L1 blockade for lung cancer, from two hospitals, and found that 52.2% experienced immune-related adverse events following the trivalent flu shot (Rothschild et al., 2017). Grades 3–4 events occurred in 26.1% (compared to general rates of IRaEs at these hospitals of 25.5% with 9.8% grades 3–4. While replication of the study in a large patient clinical trial should be performed, in the meanwhile, clinicians should be cautious as they plan influenza vaccination for their patients receiving PD-1/PD-L1 inhibitors.

Ipilimumab (Yervoy), the first immune checkpoint inhibitor, was FDA approved using an REMS program to ensure that providers, patients, and pharmacists were well versed in the potential immune-related adverse effects. The drug enhances and prolongs the activation and proliferation of CTLs so that the immune system can identify and kill the cancer cells. Normally, CTLA-4 slows/stops this immune response after the invading pathogen has been neutralized to protect normal body tissue from the effects of the powerful immune system. Many patients experience adverse effects, which can occur during therapy or be delayed in onset. It is important for the nurse and patient/family to know that adverse reactions, as well as the patient tumor response to ipilimumab, can take months to occur (Rubin, 2012). Skin reactions typically occur after 3–4 weeks (after first or second drug dose), GI tract adverse effects occur 6.5–7 weeks after starting therapy, liver toxicity occurs after 9–10 weeks, and endocrine effects occur after 3–9 weeks (Rubin, 2012; Weber et al., 2015). The safety of administering an immune checkpoint inhibitor to a patient with an underlying autoimmune condition, such as rheumatoid arthritis, or SLE, is unknown (O'Kane et al., 2016). However, it is thought that these drugs will increase risk of autoimmune exacerbation.

Developed as part of a REMS program, which is no longer required, nursing assessment, guide for management, and checklist are available, as well as a patient wallet card from the Yervoy drug-specific website. Early side effects that can occur during the infusion or up to 24–72 hours or more after the infusion are fatigue, nausea, vomiting, diarrhea, fever, headache, dizziness, rash, and pruritus (Fecher et al., 2013). The most common immune-related adverse effects are enterocolitis, hepatitis, dermatitis, and endocrinopathy (Bristol Myers Squibb, 2017). Most reactions begin during treatment, but some may occur weeks to months after the drug has been stopped. Early identification of toxicity is critical so that early intervention can follow and minimize the effect. Most low-grade immune-related adverse effects are managed with supportive care, while moderate or severe toxicity is managed by drug interruption and corticosteroids followed by a taper (Fecher et al., 2013; Yervoy package insert, 2015). Algorithms are available for toxicity management (Fecher et al., 2013). Ipilimumab is discontinued if corticosteroids cannot be tapered to 7.5 mg prednisone/equivalent/day, or failure to complete the full treatment course within 16 weeks from first dose. The other type of ICPi currently used today are inhibitors of the programmed-death receptor-1 (PD-1) and its ligand programmed death receptor ligand-1 (PD-L1). See individual drugs for further discussion. See package inserts or drug information for each specific immune checkpoint inhibitor.

Early identification and intervention are key components to patient safety, and the nurse must be knowledgeable about the potential adverse effects and key points to teach patients and their families. It is important to reassure patients that most side effects are mild to moderate and can be effectively managed (Rubin, 2010, 2012). However, it is critical that the patient/family report any symptoms as they occur as soon as possible, and the nurse should assess the patient in a systematic fashion at each visit. With each potential toxicity, medical management (Fecher et al., 2013) and nursing management (Rubin, 2012) is indicated in Table 4.6.

COST

While it is encouraging to see the possibilities of targeted therapy, the cost is of major concern. Today we are in a healthcare economic crisis. For example, a course (three treatments) of sipuleucel-T (Provenge) costs $93,000 with a resulting median increase in survival of 4.1 months (patients with minimal disease prostate cancer) (Anassi & Ndefo, 2011), while four treatments with ipilimumab (Yervoy) costs $120,000 resulting in a median 3.7-month increase in survival in patients with metastatic melanoma (Fellner, 2012). Larkin et al. (2015) conducted an RCT of patients with untreated melanoma and found a significant survival advantage for patients receiving nivolumab alone or in combination with ipilimumab compared to ipimumab alone, and in patients who had PD-L1 negative tumors, the combination of immune checkpoint inhibitors was significantly superior to either agent alone. However, the combination is expensive at over a million dollars a year ($120,000 for the ipilimumab, plus $12,500 a month for nivolumab) (Winslow, 2015). More and more, studies must look at the cost-effectiveness of these expensive treatments. Kohm et al. (2017) developed a model to estimate lifetime costs and quality-adjusted life years for patients with treatment naïve advanced melanoma expressing wild-type *BRAF.* They studied treatment sequences with first-line nivolumab, ipilimumab, nivolumab plus ipilimumab, pembrolizumab every 2 weeks, and pembrolizumab every 3 weeks. They concluded that pembrolizumab every 3 weeks, followed by second-line ipilimumab was more effective and less expensive than the standard-of-care dacarbazine. The second cost-effective treatment was first line nivolumab followed by second line ipilimumab or ipilimumab followed by nivolumab (Kohn et al., 2017). It is estimated that the out-of-pocket costs for a Medicare patient receiving the combination is $60,000 a year (Andrews, 2015). The American Association of Clinical Oncology *State of Cancer Care in America 2017* reviewed the accomplishments and cost of cancer care in 2016 and found that one in three cancer survivors who were of a working age had accumulated debt for treatment; of these survivors, 55% owed $100,000 or more (ASCO, 2017). Nurses must remain cognizant of costs of therapy, especially the out-of-pocket or copays, which may be in the thousands of dollars. The nurse is an advocate to help patients and their families find the resources, such as pharmacist or social worker, to access indigent programs; nurses must help their physician colleagues discuss cost as well as drug side effects as patients must choose among therapies so that the relative cost vs. benefit risks is understood.

With the success of the two FDA approved chimeric antigen receptor (CAR) T-cell therapies, Medicare and Medicaid Services (CMS) has announced coverage of these procedures, with restrictions and need to collect evidence, but reimbursement rates have been based on stem cell transplant and do not cover the full cost. Recently, CMS has announced an increase in reimbursement as part of the Fiscal Year 2020 Inpatient Prospective Payment System (Silverstein, 2019). However, still in question, is the outpatient management that is practiced in some centers.

Each drug is reviewed and updated based on the current package insert. "Accelerated approval" under Indications refers to the FDA-approval status. Drugs may be approved based on tumor response rate and duration of response. Continued approval for this indication may be contingent upon verification and description of clinical benefit in confirmatory trials (FDA, 2017).

References

Alberta Health Services. (2012). Prevention and treatment of rash in patients treated with EGFR inhibitor therapies. Clinical Practice Guidelines Supp-003. Alberta, CA: Alberta Health Services. Available at http://www.albertahealthservices.ca/assets/info/hp/cancer/if-hp-cancer-guide-supp003 -egfri-rash.pdf. Accessed March 23, 2016.

Alisdawi S, Westin GFM, Al-Kali A, Go RS. Blastic plasmacytoid dendritic cell neoplasm. A population-based analysis for the SEER and NCDB databases. *Blood* 2016; 128:4789-4799.

American Society of Clinical Oncology. ASCO Clinical Cancer Advances 2016. Available at http://cancerprogress.net/sites/cancerprogress.net/files/asco-cca16-web-updated.pdf. Accessed March 16, 2016.

American Society of Clinical Oncology. State of Cancer Care in America 2017. Available at https://www.asco.org/research-progress/reports-studies/state-cancer-care-america-2017. Accessed May 25, 2017.

American Society of Clinical Oncology. Advance of the Year 2017. Available at https://www.asco.org/research-progress/reports-studies/clinical-cancer-advances-2018/advance-year. Accessed September 14, 2018.

American Society of Clinical Oncology. Cancer Clinical Advances of the Year 2019. Available at https://www.ascopost.com/issues/february-10-2019/clinical-cancer-advances-2019. Accessed April 23, 2019.

American Society of Clinical Oncology. Management of immune-related adverse events in patients treated with immune checkpoint inhibitor therapy: American society of clinical oncology clinical practice guidelines. *J Clin Oncol* 2018; 36(17): 1714-1768.

American Society of Health-Systems Pharmacists (ASHP). Discontinued drug bulletin:denileukin diftitox, March 25, 2015. Available at http://www.ashp.org/menu/DrugShortages/DrugsNoLonger Available/bulletin.aspx?id=1009. Accessed September 11, 2016.

Amgen, Inc. Aranesp (darbapoietin alfa) [package insert]. Thousand Oaks, CA. January 2019.

Amgen, Inc. Blincyto (blinatumomab) [package insert]. Thousand Oaks, CA. April 2019.

Amgen, Inc. Epogen (epoetin alfa) [package insert]. Thousand Oaks, CA. July 2018.

Amgen, Inc. Imlygic (talimogene laherparepvec) [package insert]. Thousand Oaks, CA. December 2018.

Amgen, Inc. MVASI (bevacizumab-awwb) [package insert]. Thousand Oaks, CA. September 2017.

Amgen, Inc. Neulasta (pegfilgrastim) [package insert]. Thousand Oaks, CA. April 2019.

Amgen, Inc. Neupogen (filgrastim) [package insert]. Thousand Oaks, CA. June 2018.

Amgen, Inc. Nplate (romiplostim) [package insert]. Thousand Oaks, CA. April 2016.

Amgen, Inc. Kepivance (palifermin) [package insert]. Thousand Oaks, CA. June 2018.

Amgen, Inc. Vectibix (panitumumab) [package insert]. Thousand Oaks, CA. June 2017.

Anassi I, Ndefo UA. Sipuleucel-T (Provenge) Injection. *Pharmacy Therapeutics* 2011; 36(4): 197–202.

Andrews A. Treating with checkpoint inhibitors—Figure $1 million per patient. *Am Health Drug Benefits* 2015; 8 (Special Issue): 9.

Arbour KC, Mezquita L, Long N et al., Impact of baseline steroids on efficacy of programmed cell death-1 and programmed death- ligand 1 blockade in patients with non-small cell lung cancer. *J Clin Oncol* 2018; 36(28):2872-2878.

AstraZeneca Pharmaceuticals LP. Imfinzi (durvalumab) [package insert]. Wilmington, DE. February 2018.

AstraZeneca Pharmaceuticals LP. Lumoxiti (moxetumomab pasudotox-tdfk) [package insert]. Wilmington, DE. September 2018.

Baselga J, Cortes J, Kim SB, et al. Pertuzumab plus Trastuzumab plus Docetaxel for Metastatic Breast Cancer. *N Engl J Med* 2012; 366:109–119.

Beck KE, Blansfield JA, Tran KQ, et al. Enterocololitis in Patients with Cancer after Antibody Blockade of Cytotoxic t-Lymphocyte–associated Antigen 4. *J Clin Oncol* 2006; 24:2283–2289.

Belkaid Y, Hand TW. Role of the microbiota in immunity and inflammation. *Cell* 2014; 157:121–141.

Borghaei H, Paz-Ares L, Horn L, et al. Nivolumab versus Docetaxel in Advanced Nonsquamous Non–Small-Cell Lung Cancer. *N Engl J Med* 2015; 373:1627–1639.

Borkar DS, Lacouture ME, Basti S. Spectrum of Ocular Toxicities from Epidermal Growth Factor Receptor Inhibitors and Their Intermediate-term Follow-up: A Five-year Review. *Support Care Cancer* 2013; 1(4):1167–1174.

Breslin S. Cytokine-Release Syndrome: Overview and Nursing Implications. *Clin J Oncol Nurs* 2007; 11(1 suppl): 37–42.

Bristol-Myers Squibb Co. Empliciti (elotuzumab) [package insert]. Princeton, NJ. November 2018.

Bristol-Myers Squibb Co. Yervoy (ipilimumab) [package insert]. Princeton, NJ. July 2018.

Bristol-Myers Squibb Co. Opdivo (nivolumab) [package insert]. Princeton, NJ. April 2019.

Burstein HJ, Aragon-Ching JB, Baxter NN, et al. Clinical Cancer Advances 2017. Annual Report on Progress Against Cancer from the American Society of Clinical Oncology. *J Clin Oncol* 2017; 35:1341–1367. Available at http://ascopubs.org/doi/abs/10.1200/JCO.2016.71.5292. Accessed May 22, 2017.

Campath® Access Program. Patient access and monitoring form. Available at https://hematologiegron-ingen.nl/protocollen/download/?id=4306. Accessed June 19, 2018.

Cardinale D, Colombo A, Torrisi R, et al. Trastuzumab-induced Cardiotoxicity: Clinical and Prognostic Implications of Troponin I Evaluation. *J Clin Oncol* 2010; 28(25):3910–3916.

Celgene Corp. Pomalyst (pomalidomide) [package insert]. Summit, NJ. May 2018.

Celgene Corp. Thalomid (thalidomide) [package insert]. Summit, NJ. December 2017.

Celgene Corp. Revlimid (lenalidomide) [package insert]. Summit, NJ. May 2019.

Celltrion, Inc. Truxima (rituximab-abbs) [package insert]. Republic of Korea, November 2018.

Centers for Disease Control (CDC). HPV Vaccine information for clinicians. Available at https://www.cdc.gov/hpv/hcp/need-to-know.pdf. Accessed May 8, 2019.

Chen DS, Mellman I. Oncology Meets Immunology: The Cancer-Immunity Cycle. *Immunity* 2013; 39:1–10.

Chu E, DeVita VT. *Physicians Cancer Chemotherapy Drug Manual 2016*. Burlington, MA: Jones and Bartlett Learning, LLC 2016.

Coherus BioSciences Inc. pegfilgrastim-cbqv (Udenyca™) [package insert]. Redwood City, CA. February 2019.

Coulie PG, Van den Eynde BJ, van de Bruggen P, Boon T. Tumor Antigens Recognized by T Lymphocytes: At the Core of Cancer Immunotherapy. *Nature Rev Cancer* 2014; 14:135–146.

Chung CH, Mirakhur B, Chan E, et al. Cetuximab-induced Anaphylaxis and IgE Specific for Galactose-α-1,3-galactose. *N Engl J Med* 2008; 358:1109–1117.

Dendreon Corp, Provenge (sipuleucel-T) [package insert]. Seattle, WA. July 2017.

Dunn GP, Koebel CM, Schreiber RD. Interferons, Immunity, and Cancer Immunoediting. *Nat Rev Immunol* 2006; 6(11):836–848.

Duvic M. Optimizing denileukin diftitox (Ontak) therapy. *Haematologic Rep* 2006; 2(13):57–60.

Eggermont AM, Suciu S, Santinami M, et al. Adjuvant Therapy with Pegylated Interferon alfa-2b versus Observation alone in Resected Stage III Melanoma: Final Results of EORTC 18991, a Randomized Phase III Trial. *Lancet* 2008; 372(9633):117–26.

Eli Lilly and Co. Cyramza (ramucirumab) [package insert]. Indianapolis, IN. May 2019.

Eli Lilly and Co. Lilly to establish an access program for patients as it prepares to withdraw Lartruvo™ (olaratumab) from the global market. Available at https://investor.lilly.com/news-releases/news-release-details/lilly-establish-access-program-patients-it-prepares-withdraw. Accessed May 3, 2019.

Eli Lilly and Co. Portrazza (necitumumab) [package insert]. Indianapolis, IN. November 2015.

Eisai Inc. ONTAK (denileukin diftitox) [package insert]. Woodcliff Lake, NJ. August 2011.

EMD Serona, Inc. Bavencio (avelumab) [package insert]. Rockland, MD. May 2019.

Fakir M. Anti-EGFR Monoclonal Antibody-induced Hypomagnesaemia. *Lancet Oncol* 2007; 8(5): 366–367.

Fecher LA, Agarwala SS, Hodi FS, Weber JS. Ipilimumab and Its Toxicities: A Multidisciplinary Approach. *The Oncologist* 2013; 18(6):733–743.

Fellner C. Ipilimumbab (Yervoy) prolongs survival in advanced melanoma. *P&T* 2012; 37(9): 503–511.

Food and Drug Administration (FDA) (a). Oncologic Drugs Advisory Committee Briefing Document, July 12, 2017. Available at: https://www.fda.gov/downloads/AdvisoryCommittees/CommitteesMeeting Materials/Drugs/OncologicDrugsAdvisoryCommittee/UCM566168.pdf. Accessed July 19, 2017.

Food and Drug Administration (FDA)(b). FDA Grants Accelerated Approval to Pembrolizumab for First Tissue/site Agnostic Indication. Available at https://www.fda.gov/drugs/informationondrugs/approveddrugs/ucm560040.htm. Accessed July 19, 2017.

Food and Drug Administration (FDA) (c). Information on ESAepoetin Alfa., Darbapoietin Alfa. [Issued April 13, 2017]. Available at https://www.fda.gov/Drugs/DrugSafety/ucm109375.htm. Accessed May 12, 2017.

Food and Drug Administration (FDA) (b). Scientific considerations in demonstrating Food and Drug Administration (FDA) (d). Biological product definitions, May 2017. Available at https://www.fda.gov/downloads/Drugs/DevelopmentApprovalProcess/HowDrugsareDevelopedandApproved/ApprovalApplications/TherapeuticBiologicApplications/Biosimilars/UCM581282.pdf. Accessed June 16, 2018.

Food and Drug Administration (FDA) (e). FDA news release (September 14, 2017). Available at https://www.fda.gov/NewsEvents/Newsroom/PressAnnouncements/ucm576112.htm. Accessed June 16, 2018.

Food and Drug Administration (FDA) (f). Considerations in demonstrating interchangeability with a reference product: Guidance for industry. May 2017. Accessed June 16, 2018. Available at https://www.fda.gov/downloads/Drugs/GuidanceComplianceRegulatoryInformation/Guidances/UCM537135.pdf. Accessed June 16, 2018.

Food and Drug Administration (FDA) (a) Nonproprietary naming of biological products: guidance for industry. January 2017. Available at https://www.fda.gov/downloads/drugs/guidances/ucm459987.pdf.

Food and Drug Administration (FDA) (a). Guidance for industry on biosimilars. April 2015. Available at https://www.fda.gov/downloads/Drugs/GuidanceComplianceRegulatoryInformation/Guidances/UCM291128.pdf. Available at https://www.fda.gov/downloads/drugs/guidances/ucm291128.pdf. Accessed June 16, 2018.

Food and Drug Administration (FDA). Keytruda (pembrolizumab) and Tecentriq (atezolizumab): FDA Alerts Health care professionals and investigators – FDA statement-decreased survival in some patients in clinical trials associated with monotherapy. Posted May 18, 2018. Available at:_ https://www.fda.gov/Safety/MedWatch/SafetyInformation/SafetyAlertsforHumanMedicalProducts/ucm608253.htm. Accessed June 30, 2018.

Gajewski TF. Cancer Immunotherapy. *Mol Oncol* 2012; 6(2):242–250.

Gatalica Z, Vranic S, Xiu J, Swensen J. High Microsatellite Instability (MSI-H) Colorectal Carcinoma: A Brief Review of Predictive Biomarkers in the Era of Personalized Medicine. *Familial Cancer* 2016; 15:405–412.

Genentech Inc. Avastin (bevacizumab) [package insert]. South San Francisco, CA. February 2019.

Genentech Inc. Gazyva (obinutuzumab) [package insert]. South San Francisco, CA. November 2017.

Genentech Inc. Herceptin (trastuzumab) [package insert]. South San Francisco, CA. November 2018.

Genentech Inc. Herceptin Hylecta (trastuzumab and hyaluronidase-oysk). [package insert]. South San Francisco, CA. February 2019.

Genentech Inc. Kadcyla (ado-trastuzumab emtansine) [package insert]. South San Francisco, CA. May 2019.

Genentech Inc. Perjeta (pertuzumab) [package insert]. South San Francisco, CA. December 2018.

Genentech Inc. Polivy (polatuzumab vedotin-piiq) [package insert]. South San Francisco, CA. June 2019.

Genentech Inc. Rituxan (rituximab) [package insert]. South San Francisco, CA. January 2019.

Genentech Inc. Rituxan Hylecta injection (rituximab and hyalonuridase human) [package insert]. South San Francisco, CA. April 2018.

Genentech Inc. Tecentriq (atezolizumab) [package insert]. South San Francisco, CA. March 2019.

Genzyme. Thyrogen® (thyrotropin alfa for injection) [package insert]. Cambridge, MA. April 2017.

Genzyme Inc. Campath® (alemtuzumab). [package insert]/ Cambridge, MA. October 2018.

Gill S, June CH. Going viral: Chimeric Antigen Receptor T-cell Therapy for Hematological Malignancies. *Immunol Rev* 2015; 263(1):68–89.

GlaxoSmithKline. Promacta (eltrpombopag) [package insert]. Research Triangle Park, NC. August 2015.

GlaxoSmithKline. Cervarix (human papillomarvairus bivalent vaccine) [package insert]. Research Triangle Park, NC. February 2015.

Hamid O, Robert C, Daud A, et al. Safety and Tumor Responses with Lambrolizumab (Anti-PD-1) in Melanoma. *New Engl J Med* 2013; 369:134–144; doi: 10.1056/NEJMoa1305133.

Hanahan D, Weinberg RA. Hallmarks of Cancer: The Next Generation. *Cell* 2011; 144:646–674.

Hill G, Barron R, Fust K, et al. Primary vs Secondary Prophylaxis with Pegfilgrastim for the Reduction of Febrile Neutropenia Risk in Patients Receiving Chemotherapy for non-Hodgkin's Lymphoma: Cost-effectiveness Analyses. *J Med Econ* 2014; 17(1):32–42.

Hoffner B, Iodice GM, Gasal E. Administration and Handling of Talimogene Laherparepvec: An Intra-lesional Oncolytic Immunotherapy for Melanoma. *Oncologist* 2016; 43(2):219–227.

Hofheinz R-D, Deplanque G, Komatsu Y et al. Recommendations for the prophylactic management of skin reactions induced by epidermal growth factor receptor inhibitors in patients with solid tumors. *The Oncologist* 2016; 21:1483–1491.

Horizon Pharma USA, Inc. Actimmune (interferon gamma-1b) [package insert]. Lake Forest, IL. May 2017.

Horn L, Spigel DR, Vokes EE et al. Nivolumab versus docetaxel in previously treated patients with advanced non-small cell lung cancer: Two-year outcomes from two randomized, open-label, phase III trials (checkmate 017 and checkmate 057).

Housman G, Byler S, Heerboth S, et al. Drug Resistance in Cancer: An Overview. *Cancers (Basel)* 2014; 6(3):1769–1792.

Humblet Y, Peeters M, Siena S. Association of Skin Toxicity (ST) Severity with Clinical Outcomes and Health-related Quality of Life (HRQoL) with Panitumumab. *J Clin Oncol* 2007; 25(18S, June 20 supplement): 4038.

ImClone LLC and Eli Lily. Erbitux (cetuximab) [package insert]. Indianapolis, IN. June 2018.

Isakov L, Jin B, Jacobs IA. Statistical primer on biosimilar clinical development. *Am J Ther* 2016; 23:1075-2765e1903-e1910. Available at https://www.ncbi.nlm.nih.gov/pmc/articles/PMC5102275/pdf/ajt-23-e1903.pdf. Accessed June 17, 2018.

Ismael G, Hegg R, Muehlbauer S, et al. Subcutaneous versus Intravenous Administration of (neo) Adjuvant Trastuzumab in Patients with HER2-positive, Clinical Stage I-III Breast Cancer (HannaH study): A Phase 3, Open-label, Multicenter, Randomized Trial. *Lancet Oncol* 2012; 13(9): 869–78.

Izzedine H, Rixe O, Billemont B, Baumelou A, Deray G. Angiogenesis Inhibitor Therapies: Focus on Kidney Toxicity and Hypertension. *Am J Kidney Dis.* 2007; 50(2):203–218.

Jackisch C, Stroyakovsky D, Pivot X et al. Subcutansous vs intravenous trastuzumab for patients with ERBB2-positive early breast cancer: final analysis of Hannah phase III randomized controlled trial. *JAMA Oncology* 2019; 5(5): e190339; doi: 10.1001/jamaoncol.209.0339.

Jansson Biotech, Inc. Darzalex (daratumumab) [package insert]. Horsham, PA. February 2019.

Jansson Products, LP. Procrit (epoetin alfa) [package insert]. Horsham, PA. April 2017.

Jansson Biotech, Inc. Sylvant (siltuximab) [package insert]. Horsham, PA. May 2018.

Johnson K. Chasing checkpoints: James Allison in *Time* magazine top 100. *Medscape*. May 16, 2017. Available at http://www.medscape.com/viewarticle/880057. Accessed May 22, 2017.

Jonker DJ, O'Callaghan CJ, Karapetis CS, et al. Cetuximab for the Treatment of Colorectal Cancer. *N Engl J Med* 2007; 357:2040–2048.

Kammula US, White D, Rosenberg SA. Trends in the Safety of High-dose Bolus Interleukin-2 Administration in Patients with Metastatic Cancer. *Cancer* 1998; 83(4):797–805.

Kantoff PW, Higano CS, Shore ND, et al. Sipuleucel-T Immunotherapy for Castration-resistant Prostate Cancer. *N Engl J Med* 2010; 363(5):411–422.

Kim H, Fischer D. Anaphlaxis. *Allergy Asthma Clin Immunol* 2011; 7(Suppl 1): S6–12.

Kite Pharma, Inc. Yescarta™ (axicabtagene ciloleucel). [package insert]. Santa Monica, Ca. October 2017.

Kohn CG, Zeichner SB, Chen Q, et al. Cost-effectiveness of Immune Checkpoint Inhibition in BRAF Wild-type Advanced Melanoma *J Clin Oncol* 2017; 35(11):1194–1202.

Kyowa Kirin, Inc. Poteligeo® (mogamulizumab-kpkc). [Package insert.] Bedminster, NJ: August 2018.

Lacouture ME, Anadkat MJ, Bensadoun R-J, et al. Clinical Practice Guidelines for the Prevention and Treatment of EGFR Inhibitor-associated Dermatologic Toxicities. *Support Care Cancer* 2011; 19(8):1079–1095.

Lacouture ME, Mitchell EP, Piperdi B et al. Skin toxicity evaluation protocol with panitumumab (STEPP), a phase II, open-label, randomized trial evaluating the impact of a pre-Emptive Skin treatment regimen on skin toxicities and quality of life in patients with metastatic colorectal cancer. *J Clin Oncol* 2010; 28(8):1351–1357.

Larkin J, Chiarion-Sileni V, Gonzalez R, et al. Combined Nivolumab and Ipilimumab or Monotherapy in Untreated Melanoma. *N Engl J Med* 2015; 373(1):23–34.

Larkin J, Chiarion-Sileni V, Gonzalez R, et al. Overall Survival Results from a Phase III Trial of Nivolumab Combined with Ipilimumab in Treatment-naïve Patients with Advanced Melanoma (CheckMate-067). *Proceedings from the 2017 American Association for Cancer Research Annual MeeTing*. Washington, DC, April 2–5, 2017. Abstract CT075.

Le DT, Uram JN, Wang H, et al. PD-1 Blockade in Tumors with Mismatch-repair Deficiency. *N Engl J Med* 2015; 372(26):2509–2520.

Lee DW, Gardner R, Porter DL, et al. Current concepts in the Diagnosis and Management of Cytokine Release Syndrome. *Blood* 2014; 124(2):188–196. Erratum *Blood* 2014; 124(2):188 (vasopressor doses).

Lin F-C, Young HA. The Talented Interferon-Gamma. *Adv in Biosci Biotechnol* 2013; 4: 6–13.

Lundin J, Kimby E, Bjorkholm M, et al. Phase II Trial of Subcutaneous Anti-CD52 Monoclonal Antibody Alemtuzumab (Campath-1H) as First-line Treatment for Patients with B-cell Chronic Lymphocytic Leukemia (B-CLL). *Blood* 2002; 100:768–773.

Lynch TJ, Kim ES, Eaby B et al. Epidermal Growth Factor Receptor Inhibitor-associated Cutaneous Toxicities: An Evolving Paradigm in Clinical Management. *Oncologist* 2007; 12(5):610–612.

Martinez-Lage M, Puig-Serra P, Menendez P, Torres-Ruiz R, Rodrigues-Perales S. CRISP/Cas9 for cancer therapy: hopes and challenges. Biomedicines 2018; 6:105–113. Available at https://www.ncbi.nlm.nih.gov/pmc/articles/PMC6315587/pdf/biomedicines-06-00105.pdf. Accessed May 8, 2019.

Melosky B, Anderson H, Burkes RL, et al. Pan Canadian Rash Trial: A Randomized Phase III Trial Evaluating the Impact of a Prophylactic Skin Treatment Regimen on Epidermal Growth Factor Receptor-tyrosine Kinase Inhibitor-induced Skin Toxicities in Patients with Metastatic Lung Cancer. *J Clin Oncol* 2016; 34(8):810–815.

Merck & Co. Gardasil 9 (human papillomavirus 9-valent vaccine) [package insert]. Whitehouse Station, NJ. October 2018.

Merck & Co. Sylatron (peginterferon alfa-2b) [package insert]. Whitehouse Station, NJ. September 2015.

Merck & Co. Zostavax (Zoster vaccine live) [package insert]. Whitehouse Station, NJ. June 2019.

Merck & Co. Keytruda (pembrolizumab) [package insert]. Whitehouse Station, NJ. April 2019.

Merck & Co. Ontruzant (trastuzumab-dttb) [package insert]. Whitehouse Station, NJ. January 2019.

Merck, Sharp & Dohme Corp. Intron A (interferon alfa-2b, recombinant) injection [package insert]. Whitehouse Station, NJ. February 2016.

Messerschmidt JL, Prendergast GC, Messerschmidt GL. How Cancers Escape Immune Destruction and Mechanisms of Action for the New Significantly Active Immune therapies: Helping Nonimmunologists. *Oncologist* 2016; 21:233–243.

Molinari E, De Quatrebarbes J, Andre T, Aractingi S. Cetuximab-induced Acne. *Dermatology* 2005; 211:330–333.

Moreno BH, Ribas A. Anti-programmed Cell Death Protein-1/Ligand-1 Therapy in Different Cancers. *Br J Cancer* 2015; 112:1421–1427. doi: 10.1038/bjc.2015.124

Murphy K. *Janeway's Immunobiology*, 8th ed. New York, NY: Garland Science; 2011.

Mylan GmbH. Fulphila (pegfilgrastim-jmdb). [package insert]. Zurich, Switzerland. June 2018.

Mylan GmbH.Ogivri (trastuzumab-dkst). [package insert]. Morgantown. WV. December 2017.

National Cancer Institute. *CAR T-cell Therapy: Engineering Patients' Immune Cells to Treat Their Cancers*. Updated October 16, 2014. Available at http://www.cancer.gov/about-cancer/treatment /research/car-t-cells. Accessed March 14, 2016.

National Cancer Institute. *Cancer vaccines*. Updated December 18, 2015. Available at: http:// www.cancer.gov/about-cancer/causes-prevention/vaccines-fact-sheet#q4. Accessed March 20, 2016.

National Comprehensive Cancer Network. *NCCN Guidelines Version 1.2018* (March 2, 2018). *Myeloid Growth Factors*. Available at https://www.nccn.org/professionals/physician_gls/pdf/myeloid_growth.pdf. Accessed June 16, 2018.

National Comprehensive Cancer Network. *NCCN Guidelines Version 2. 2019* (March 27, 2019) *Cancer- and Chemotherapy-induced Anemia*. Available at https://www.nccn.org/professionals/ physician_gls/pdf/anemia.pdf. Accessed June 16, 2018.

National Comprehensive Cancer Network. *NCCN Guidelines Version 2. 2019* (April 8, 2019) *Management of Immunotherapy-related Toxicities*. Available at https://www.nccn.org/professionals/ physician_gls/pdf/immunotherapy.pdf. Accessed May 3, 2019.

National Immunotherapy Coalition (NIC). *Historical National Coalition Formed to Accelerate Next Generation Immunotherapy in Cancer*. January 11, 2016. Available at http://www.cancermoonshot2020.org/. Accessed March 13, 2016.

National Institutes of Health, National Cancer Institute. Cancer Moonshot Blue Ribbon Panel Report 2016. Available at https://www.cancer.gov/research/key-initiatives/moonshot-cancer-initiative /blue-ribbon-panel/blue-ribbon-panel-report-2016.pdf. Accessed May 25, 2017.

National Public Radio (NPR). First US patients treated with CRISPR at Penn as human gene-editing trials get underway. Available at https://whyy.org/npr_story_post/first-u-s-patients-treated-with -crispr-as-human-gene-editing-trials -get-underway/. Accessed May 9, 2019.

Novartis Pharmaceuticals Corp. Arzerra (ofatumumab) [package insert]. East Hanover, NJ. August 2016.

Novartis Pharmaceuticals Corp. Kymriah™ (tisagenlecleucel). [package insert]. East Hanover, NJ. May 2018.

Novartis Pharmaceuticals Corp. Promacta (eltrombopag) [package insert]. East Hanover, NJ. May 2018.

O'Day, Weber JS, Wolchok JD, et al. Effectiveness of Treatment Guidance on Diarrhea and Colitis across Ipilimumab Studies. *J Clin Oncol* 2011; 29: (suppl; abstr 8554).

O'Kane GM, Labbe C, Doherty MK, et al. Monitoring and Management of Immune-related Adverse Events Associated with Programmed Cell Death Protein-1 Axis Inhibitors in Lung Cancer. *Oncologist* 2017; 22:70–80.

Osman AEG, Luke JJ. The impact of the fecal microbiome on cancer immunotherapy. *BioDrugs* 2019; (331):1–7.

Oncology Nursing Society. Education of the Nurse Who Administers and Cares for the Individual Receiving Chemotherapy and Biotherapy, Revised 2016. Available at https://www.ons.org/sites /default /files/Chemo_Position_Statement.pdf. Accessed May 24, 2017.

Office of the Press Secretary, the White House. *Factsheet: Investing in the National Cancer Moonshot*. Available at https://www.whitehouse.gov/the-press-office/2016/02/01/fact-sheet-investing -national-cancer-moonshot. Accessed August 6, 2016.

Paik S, Bryant J, Tan-Chiu E, et al. Real World Performance of HER2 Testing—National Surgical Adjuvant Breast and Bowel Project Experience. *J Natl Cancer Inst* 2002; 94:852–854.

Pardoll M. The Blockade of Immune Checkpoints in Cancer Immunotherapy. *Nat Rev Cancer* 2012; 12:252–264.

Patel SP, Kurzrock R. PD-L1 Expression as a Predictive Biomarker in Cancer Immunotherapy. *Mol Cancer Ther* 2015; 14(4):847–856.

Petrelli F, Borgonovo K, Cabiddu M et al. Antibiotic prophylaxis for skin toxicity induced by antiepidermal growth factor receptor agents: a systematic review and meta-analysis. *Br J of Dermatology* 2016; 175(6):1166–1174.

Pfizer Injectables. Neumega (oprelvekin) [package insert]. Philadelphia, PA. January 2011.

Pfizer Biosimilars, Manufactured by Hospira. Retacrit™(epoetin alfa-epbx). [package insert]. Lake Forest, IL. May 2018.

Pfizer Biosimilars, Manufactured by Hospira. Nivestym™ filgrastim(filgrastim-aafi). [package insert]. Lake Forest, IL. July 2018.

Pfizer, Inc.Trazimera® (trastuzumab-qyyp). [package insert]. New York, NY. March 2019.

Pinato DJ, Howlett S, Ottaviani D et al. Antibiotic treatment prior to immune checkpoint inhibitor therapy as a tumor-agnostic predictive correlate of response in routine clinical practice. ASCO-SITC Clinical Immuno-Oncology Symposium, San Francisco, CA. February 28–March 2, 2019. Abstract 147, presented March 1, 2019.

Pituskin E, Mackey JR, Koshman S, et al. Prophylactic Beta Blockade Preserves Left Ventricular Ejection Fraction in HER2-Overexpressing Breast Cancer Patients Receiving Trastuzumab: Primary Results of The MANTICORE Randomized, Controlled Trial. 2015 San Antonio Breast Cancer Symposium. Abstract S1-05. Presented December 9, 2015.

Platt JL, Silva I, Balin SJ, et al. C3d Regulates Immune Checkpoint Blockade and Enhances Antitumor Immunity. *JCI Insight* 2017; 2(9):e90201. Available at https:doi.org/10/1172/jci.insight.90201.

Polovich M, Olsen M, LeFebvre KB (eds.). *Chemotherapy and Biotherapy Guidelines and Recommendations for Practice,* 4th ed. Pittsburgh, PA: ONS; 2014: 163–168.

Prometheus Laboratories Therapeutics and Diagnostics. Proleukin (aldesleukin) [package insert]. San Diego, CA. August 2018.

Quezada SA, Peggs KS. Exploiting CTLA-4, PD-1, and PD-L1 to Reactivate the Host Immune Response Against Cancer. *Br J Cancer* 2013; 108:1560–1565.

Ranpura V, Hapani S, Wu S. Treatment-related Mortality with Bevacizumab in Cancer Patients: A Meta-analysis. *JAMA* 2011; 305(5):487–494.

Ravoori S. AACR Annual meeting 2017: Immunotherapy Provides Long-lasting Responses to Certain Cancer Types. Available at http://blog.aacr.org/aacr-annual-meeting-2017-immunotherapy -provides-long-lasting-responses-certain-cancer-types/. Accessed May 22, 2017.

Reidy DL, Chung KY, Timoney JP, et al. Bevacizumab 5 mg/kg can be Infused Safely over 10 minutes. *J Clin Oncol* 2007; 25(19):2691–2695.

Ribas, A. Tumor Immunotherapy Directed at PD-1. *N Engl J Med* 2012; 366(26):2517–2519.

Regeneron Pharmaceuticals, Inc and Sanofi-aventis US LLC. Zaltrap (ziv-aflibercept) [package insert]. Bridgewater, NJ. September 2014.

Regeneron Pharmaceuticals, Inc and Sanofi-aventis US LLC. Libtayo (cemiplimab-rwlc) [package insert]. Bridgewater, NJ. March 2019.

Robert C, Ribas A, Wolchok JD, et al. Anti-programmed-death-receptor-1 Treatment with Pembrolizumab in Ipilimumab-refractory Advanced Melanoma: A Randomised Dose-comparison Cohort of a Phase 1 Trial. *Lancet.* 2014; 384(9948):1109–1117. doi: 10.1016/S0140-6736(14)60958-2.

Rothschild SI, Balmelli C, Kaufmann L, et al. Immune Response and Adverse Events to Influenza Vaccine in Cancer Patients Undergoing PD-1 Blockade. Poster presented at *European Lung Cancer Conference.* Geneva, Switzerland, May 5–8, 2017.

Rubin K. Managing Immune-related Adverse Events to Ipilimumab: A Nurse's Guide. *CJON* 2012; 16(2): E69–E75.

Rubin K. Understanding Immune Checkpoint Inhibitors for Effective Patient Care. *CJON* 2015; 19(6): 709–717.

Saltz L, Hochster H, Tchekmeydian NS, et al. Acne-like Rash Predicts Response in Patients Treated with Cetuximab (IMC-C225) plus Irinotecan (CPT-11) in CPT-11-Refractory Colorectal Cancer (CRC) that expresses Epidermal Growth Factor Receptor (EGFR). *Proc NCI-AACR-EORTC* 2001; 559.

Sandoz Inc. Zarxio (filgrastim-sndz) [package insert]. Princeton, NJ. April 2018.

Sanofi-aventis US LLC. Leukine (sargramostim) [package insert]. Bridgewater, NJ. May 2018.

Sanofi-aventis US LLC. Zaltrap (ziv-aflibercept) [package insert]. Bridgewater, NJ. June 2016.

Scott AM, Wolchok JD, Old LJ. Antibody Therapy of Cancer. *Nature* 2012; 12:278–287.

Scandella E, Ludewig B. Dendridic Cells and Autoimmunity. *Transfusion Med Hemotherapy* 2005; 32(6):363–368.

Schilsky RL. Tumor-agnostic treatment for cancer: an expert perspective. Available at https://www.cancer.net/blog/2018-12/tumor-agnostic-treatment-cancer-expert-perspective. Accessed April 23, 2019.

Schreiber RD, Old LJ, Smyth MJ. Cancer Immunoediting: Integrating Immunity's Roles in Cancer Suppression and Promotion. *Science* 2011; 331:1565–1570.

Seattle Genetics. Adcetris (brentuximab vedotin) [package insert]. Bothell, WA. November 2018.

Sharma P, Allison JP. Immune checkpoint targeting in cancer therapy: Toward combination strategies with curative potential. *Cell* 2015; 161(2):205–214.

Silverstein R. ASH President comments on Medicare proposal for CAR T-cell therapy. *ASCO Post,* April 2019. Available at https://www.ascopost.com/News/59977. Accessed April 29, 2019.

Smith TJ, Bohlke K, Lyman GH, et al. Recommendations for the Use of WBC Growth Factors: American Society of Clinical Oncology Clinical Practice Guideline Update. *J Clin Oncol* 2015; 33(28): 3199–3212.

Smith LT, Venella K. Cytokine Release Syndrome: Inpatient Care for Side Effects of CAR-T Cell Therapy. *Clin J Oncol Nurs* 2017; 21(2):29–34.

Sompayrac L. *How the Immune System Works,* 4th ed. Malden, MA: Blackwell Publishing; 2012.

Soon-Shiong P. Case Study #1 Elisa Long. Presented at the Future of Genomic Medicine (FOGM) IX, Scripps Institution of Oceanography, La Jolla, CA. March 3, 2016.

Spectrum Pharmaceuticals, Inc. Zevalin (90 Y ibritumomab) [package insert]. Irvine, CA. August 2013.

Stemline Therapeutics, Inc. Elzonris™ (tagraxofusp-erzs). [package insert]. New York, NY. December 2018.

Swain SM, Baselga J, Kim SB, et al. Pertuzumab, Trastuzumab, and Docetaxel in HER-2 Positive Metastatic Breast Cancer. *N Engl J Med* 2015; 372(8):724–734.

Swan JT, Zaghloul H, Wagner J, et al. Safety of a rapid, 90-minute Rituximab infusion protocol. *J Clin Oncol* 2011; 29: (suppl; abstr e18551).

Swann JB, Smyth MJ. Immune Survelliance of Tumors. *J Clin Investig* 2007; 117:1137–1146.

Swedish Orphan Biovitrum AB. Kepivance [palifermin] package insert. Stolkholm, Sweden. November 2011.

Teipar S, Piessevaux H, Claes K, et al. Magnesium Wasting Associated with Epidermal-Growth-Factor Receptor Targeting Antibodies in Colorectal Cancer: A Prospective Study. *Lancet Oncol* 2007; 8(5):387–94.

Teva Pharmaceuticals Inc. Granix (tbo-filgrastim) [package insert]. North Wales, PA. March 2019.

Testa U, Pelosi E, Frankel A. CD123 is a membrane biomarker and therapeutic target in hematologic malignancies. *Biomarker Res* 2014: 2:1–11. doi: 10.1186/2050-7771-2-4.

Tian X, Gu T, Patel S, Bode AM et al. CRISP/Cas9—an evolving biological tool kit for cancer biology and oncology. *Nature Partner Journals: Precision Oncology* 2019; 3:8. Available at https://www.nature.com/articles/s41698-019-0080-7. Accessed May 9, 2019.

Topp MS, Gökbuget N, Stein AS, et al. Safety and Activity of Blinatumomab for Adult Patients with Relapsed or Refractory B-Precursor Acute Lymphoblastic Leukaemia: A Multicentre, Single-arm, Phase 2 Study. *Lancet Oncol* 2015; 16:57–66.

United Therapeutics Corp. Unituxin (dinutuximab) [package insert]. Silver Spring, MD. March 2017.

U.S. Department of Health and Human Services. *Common Terminology Criteria for Adverse Events (CTCAE).* Version 4.03. Bethesda, MD: June 14, 2010; 65–67.

Valeant Pharmaceuticals, Inc. Aldara (imiquimod cream) [package insert]. Bridgewater, NJ. April 2018.

Viale PH, Yamamoto DS. Biphasic and Delayed Hypersensitivity Reactions: Implications for Oncology Nursing. *Clin J Oncol Nurs* 2010; 14:347–356.

Vogel W. Infusion Reactions: Diagnosis, Assessment, and Management. *Clin J Oncol Nurs* 2010; 14: E10–E21.

Wagner LI. Psychological Impact and Quality of Life Issues Associated with Therapy-induced Rash. Presentation, 32nd Annual Oncology Nursing Society Congress Ancillary event. Las Vegas, NV: April 25, 2007.

Wang T, Lockhart A. Aflibercept in the Treatment of Metastatic Colorectal Cancer. *Clin Med Insights Oncol* 2012; 6: 19.

Weber J. Review: Anti-CTLA4 antibody ipilumumab: Case Studies of Clinical Response and Immune-related Adverse Events. *Oncologist* 2007; 12(7):864–872.

Weber JS, Yang JC, Atkins MB, Disis ML. Toxicities of Immunotherapy for the Practitioner. *J Clin Oncol* 2015 [Epub ahead of print April 27, 2015]. doi:10.1200/JCO.2014.60.0379

Weber JS, Kahler KC, Hauschild A. Management of Immune-related Events and Kinetics of Response with Ipilimumab. *J Clin Oncol* 2012; 30(21):2691–2697.

Weinberg RA. *The Biology of Cancer,* 2nd ed. New York, NY: Garland Science; 2014.

Wilkes GM. *Immunotherapy in Cancer Treatment.* Available at http://www.inpractice.com/Textbooks/Oncology-Nursing/Cancer-Treatments/Immunotherapy/Chapter-Pages/Page-1. Updated May 2017. Accessed May 22, 2017.

Winslow R. Bristol-Myers Drug Combination Shows Promise Against Melanoma. *The Wall Street Journal,* April 20, 2015.

Wolchok JD, Saenger Y. The Mechanism of Anti-CTL-9.A-4 activity and the Negative Regulation of t-cell Activation. *Oncologist* 2008; 13 (suppl 4): 2–9.

Wolchok JD, Kluger H, Callahan MK, et al. Nivolumab plus Ipilimumab in Advanced Melanoma. *N Engl J Med* 2013; 369:122–133.

Wolchok JD, Chiarion-Sileni V, Gonzalez R, et al. Updated Results from a Phase III Trial of Nivolumab (NIVO) Combined with Ipilimumab (IPI) in Treatment-naïve Patients (pts) with Advanced Melanoma (MEL) (CheckMate 067). *J Clin Oncol* 2016; 34 (suppl; abstract 9505).

Wong RS, et al. A Multicenter, Randomized, Double-Blind, Placebo-Controlled Study of the Efficacy and Safety of Siltuximab, an Anti-interleukin-6 Monoclonal Antibody, in Patients with Multicentric Castleman's Disease. *Blood* 2013; 122:505. (Oral presentation presented at: 55th American Society of Hematology (ASH) Annual Meeting; December 7–11, 2013; New Orleans, LA.)

Wyeth Pharmaceuticals Inc. Mylotarg (gemtuzumab ozogamicin). [package insert]. Philadelphia, PA. April 2018.

Wyeth Pharmaceuticals Inc. Besponsa (inotuzumab ozogamicin). [package insert]. Philadelphia, PA. March 2018.

Zachariae R, Zachariae C, Ibsen HHW. Psychological Symptoms and Quality of Life of Dermatology Outpatients and Hospitalized Dermatology Patients. *Acta Dermatol-Venereol* 2003; 84(3): 205–212.

Zielinski C, Knapp S, Mascaux C, Hirsch F. Rationale for Targeting the Immune System Through Checkpoint Molecule Blockade in the Treatment of Non-Small Cell Lung Cancer. *Ann Oncol* 2013; 24:1170–1179.

Drug: ado-trastuzumab emtansine (Kadcyla)

Class: ADC; HER2-targeted antibody and microtubule inhibitor conjugate.

Mechanism of Action: HER2-targeted mAb (trastuzumab) with microtubule-inhibitor conjugate. The cellular poison DM1 (emtansine), a micro-tubular inhibitor, is linked to trastuzumab. Like a Trojan horse, when the drug attaches to an HER2 receptor, the poison is internalized in the HER2 positive cell, and the poison released intracellularly. Then, MD1 (emtansine) binds to tubulin, preventing cell division, which results in cell cycle arrest and programmed cell death (apoptosis). The drug appears also to inhibit HER2 receptor signaling, mediate ADCC, and prevent shedding of the HER2 extracellular domain in human, HER2 positive, breast cancer cells.

Metabolism: Maximal serum levels occur near the end of the infusion. DM1 is about 93% plasma protein bound, and DM1 is a substrate of P-glycoprotein (P-gp). DM1 is metabolized in the liver by CYP3A4 primarily and by CYP3A5 to a lesser degree but does not inhibit or induce major CYP450 enzymes. The elimination half-life of the drug is about 4 days. Renal impairment (mild or moderate) does not affect clearance.

Indications: Drug is indicated as a single agent for the (1) treatment of patients with HER2 positive, metastatic breast cancer who previously received trastuzumab and a taxane, separately or in combination who have (a) received prior therapy for metastatic disease or (b) developed disease recurrence during or within 6 months of completing adjuvant therapy; or (2) adjuvant treatment of patients with HER2-positive early breast cancer who have residual invasive disease after neoadjuvant taxane and trastuzumab-based treatment. Patients should be selected based on an FDA-approved companion diagnostic for ado-trastuzumab emtansine showing HER2 protein overexpression and/or HER2 gene amplification.

Dosage/Range:
- **Do not substitute trastuzumab for or with Kadcyla (ado-trastuzumab emtansine).**
- Recommended dose is 3.6 mg/kg given as an IV infusion every 3 weeks (21-day cycle), until disease progression or unacceptable toxicity (patients with metastatic breast cancer) or for a total of 14 cycles in patients with early breast cancer unless there is disease recurrence or unmanageable toxicity. Initial dose is 3.6 mg/kg (actual body weight) IV infusion over 90 minutes; subsequent doses are 3.6 mg/kg IV over 30 minutes. DO NOT exceed dose of 3.6 mg/kg. DO NOT substitute drug for or with trastuzumab.
- Drug is not recommended for patients who have previously had trastuzumab permanently discontinued due to infusion-related reactions (IRRs) or HSRs.
- Dose interruption, reduction, or treatment discontinuation for management of increased LFTs, decreased LVEF, thrombocytopenia, ILD, peripheral neuropathy. See full prescribing information.

Dose Modifications Dose Level Reductions
- Dose Level Reductions: Starting dose: 3.6 mg/kg. First dose reduction = dose level 3 mg/kg; second dose reduction = dose level 2.4 mg/kg; if further dose reductions needed, discontinue drug.

Dose Modifications for patients with Metastatic Breast Cancer:
- Do NOT reescalate the drug dose after a dose reduction is made.
- *Increased liver function tests*
  - Increased serum transaminases (AST/ALT): grade 2 (> 2.5 to $\leq 5 \times$ ULN = treat at same dose level); grade 3 (> 5 to $\leq 20 \times$ ULN): hold ado-trastuzumab emtansine until AST/ALT recovers to grade ≤ 2, and then reduce one dose level; grade 4 ($> 20 \times$ ULN): permanently discontinue drug.
  - Hyperbilirubinemia: grade 2 (> 1.5 to $\leq 3 \times$ ULN): hold drug until total bilirubin recovers to $\leq$ grade 1, then treat at same dose level; grade 3 (> 3 to $\leq 10 \times$ ULN): hold drug until total bilirubin recovers to $\leq$ grade 1, then reduce one dose level; grade 4 ($> 10 \times$ ULN): permanently discontinue drug.
- *Drug Induced Liver Injury (DILI):* Permanently discontinue drug in patients with transaminases $> 3 \times$ ULN and concomitant total bilirubin $> 2 \times$ ULN in absence of another likely cause, such as liver metastasis or concomitant medications.
- *Nodular Regenerative Hyperplasia (NRH):* Permanently discontinue drug in patients diagnosed with NRH.
- *Left ventricular dysfunction*
  - Symptomatic CHF: discontinue ado-trastuzumab emtansine.
  - LVEF $< 40\%$: do not administer ado-trastuzumab emtansine; repeat LVEF assessment within 3 weeks. If LVEF $< 40\%$ is confirmed, discontinue drug.
  - LVEF 40% to $\leq 45\%$ and decrease is $\geq 10\%$ points from baseline: hold ado-trastuzumab emtansine. Repeat LVEF assessment within 3 weeks. If LVEF has not recovered to within 10% points from baseline, discontinue drug.
  - LVEF 40% to $\leq 45\%$ and decrease is $< 10\%$ points from baseline, continue treatment with drug; repeat LVEF assessment within 3 weeks.
  - LVEF $> 45\%$: continue treatment with ado-trastuzumab emtansine.
- *Thrombocytopenia*
  - Grade 3 (platelets $25,0000/mm^3$ to $< 50,000/mm^3$): hold drug until platelet count recovers to $\leq$ grade 1 ($\geq 75,000/mm^3$) and then treat at same dose level.

- Grade 4 (platelets $< 25,000/\text{mm}^3$): hold drug until platelet count recovers to $\le$ grade 1 ($\ge 75,000/\text{mm}^3$), then reduce one dose level.
- *Pulmonary Toxicity:* Permanently discontinue drug in patients diagnosed with Interstitial Lung Disease or pneumonitis.
- *Peripheral Neuropathy:* Temporarily discontinue drug in patients experiencing grade 3 or 4 peripheral neuropathy until it resolves to $\le$ grade 2.

Dose Modifications for patients with Early Breast Cancer
- *Increased ALT:* (1) Grades 2–3 (>3.0 to $\le 20 \times$ ULN on day of scheduled treatment: hold ado-trastuzumab emtansine until ALT recovers to grade ≤ 1, and then reduce one dose level; (2) Grade 4 ($>20 \times$ ULN at any time): discontinue ado-trastuzumab emtansine.
- Increased AST: (1) Grade 2 (>3.0 to $\le 5 \times$ ULN on day of scheduled treatment: hold ado-trastuzumab emtansine until AST recovers to grade ≤ 1, and resume at same dose level; (2) Grade 3 (>5 to $\le 20 \times$ ULN on day of scheduled treatment: hold ado-trastuzumab emtansine until AST recovers to grade ≤ 1, and then reduce one dose level; (3) Grade 4 ($>20 \times$ ULN at any time): discontinue ado-trastuzumab emtansine.
- Hyperbilirubinemia: (1) Total Bilirubin (TBILI) >1.0 to $\le 2.0 \times$ ULN on day of treatment: do not administer ado-trastuzumab emtansine until TBILI recovers to $\le 1.0 \times$ ULN and then reduce one dose level; (2) TBILI $>2 \times$ ULN at any time: discontinue ado-trastuzumab emtansine.
- NRH: all grades, discontinue ado-trastuzumab emtansine permanently.
- Thrombocytopenia: (1) Grades 2–3 on day of scheduled treatment (25,000 to $<75,000/\text{mm}^3$): hold ado-trastuzumab emtansine until platelet count recovers to $\le$ grade 1 ($\ge75,000/\text{mm}^3$), then treat at the same dose level. If a patient requires 2 delays due to thrombocytopenia, consider reducing dose by one level; (2) Grade 4 at any time ($<25,000/\text{mm}^3$): hold ado-trastuzumab emtansine until platelet count recovers to $\le$ grade 1 ($\ge75,000/\text{mm}^3$), then reduce one dose level.
- Left Ventricular (LV) Dysfunction: (1) LVEF $<45\%$: Hold ado-trastuzumab emtansine, repeat LVEF assessment within 3 weeks. If LVEF $<45\%$ is confirmed, discontinue ado-trastuzumab; (2) LVEF 45% to $<50\%$ and decrease is $\ge 10\%$ points from baseline prior to starting ado-trastuzumab emtansine: Hold ado-trastuzumab emtansine and repeat LVEF assessment within 3 weeks. If LVEF remains $<50\%$ and has not recovered to $<10\%$ points from baseline, discontinue ado-trastuzumab emtansine; (3) LVEF 45% to $<50\%$ and decrease is $<10\%$ points from baseline; continue ado-trastuzumab emtansine treatment and repeat LVEF assessment within 3 weeks; (4) LVEF $\ge50\%$: continue ado-trastuzumab emtansine treatment.
- Heart Failure: Symptomatic CHF, Grade 3–4 LV systolic dysfunction (LVSD) or Grade 3–4 heart failure or Grade 2 heart failure accompanied by LVEF $<45\%$: discontinue ado-trastuzumab emtansine treatment.
- Peripheral neuropathy: Grades 3–4: hold ado-trastuzumab emtansine until resolution to Grade ≤2.
- Pulmonary toxicity: ILD or pneumonitis: permanently discontinue ado-trastuzumab emtansine.
- Radiotherapy-related Pneumonitis: (1) Grade 2: discontinue ado-trastuzumab emtansine if not resolving with standard therapy; (2) Grades 3–4: discontinue ado-trastuzumab emtansine.

- If a planned dose is delayed or missed, it should be administered as soon as possible; do not wait until the next planned cycle. The treatment schedule should be adjusted to maintain a 3-week interval between doses, at the dose and rate the patient tolerated in most recent infusion.
- Kadcyla Access Solutions available to assist patients in specific access and reimbursement issues, including copay assistance for underinsured patients and free medication for uninsured patients (1-888-249-4918).

Drug Preparation:
- Drug is available in single-use 100- and 160-mg sterile lyophilized powder containing vials. Double-check label to ensure that drug is Kadcyla (ado-trastuzumab emtansine). Do not substitute Herceptin (trastuzumab) for this drug. Double check that drug vial being used is ado-trastuzumab emtansine and NOT trastuzumab.
- Using a sterile syringe, aseptically add 8 mL sterile water for injection into the 160-mg vial, or 5 mL to the 100-mg vial. Vials reconstitute to 20 mg/mL.
- Gently swirl the vial until solution is completely dissolved. Solution should be colorless to pale brown. Do not shake or freeze. Do not use if visible particulate matter or if the solution is cloudy or discolored.
- Aseptically draw up calculated dose volume, and add reconstituted solution to an infusion bag containing 250 mL 0.9% sodium chloride injection. Mix by gentle inversion of infusion bag. DO NOT USE dextrose (5%) solution.
- Do not mix or dilute the drug with any other drugs.
- Reconstituted vials should be used immediately, or may be stored in a refrigerator at 2–8°C (36–46°F) for up to 24 hours prior to use. Do not freeze. Diluted drug infusion bags may be stored in a refrigerator at 2–8°C (36–46°F) for up to 24 hours prior to use. This storage time is additional to the time allowed for the reconstituted vials. Do not freeze or shake.
- Drug contains no preservatives and is for single use only. Discard any unused solution after 4 hours.
- Drug tradename should be recorded in patient's medical record for tracking biological medicinal products.

Drug Administration:
- Prior to administration: Assess LFTs and platelet count baseline and prior to each cycle, LVEF baseline and at least every 3 months during treatment. Verify the pregnancy status of females of reproductive potential prior to starting first dose of drug. Teach women that exposure of the fetus to the drug during or within 7 months prior to conception can result in fetal harm and to use effective contraception during and for at least 7 months following last dose of drug. Assess for signs/symptoms of pulmonary toxicity or peripheral neuropathy, and compare to baseline or prior assessment.
- Administer as an IV infusion only, via a 0.2 or 0.22 micron in-line, nonprotein adsorptive polyethersulfone (PES) filter. Do not use Dextrose (5%) solution; do not administer by IVP or IV bolus.
- Drug dose is 3.6 mg/kg IV infusion every 3 weeks as a 21-day cycle.
- Administer **initial dose** over 90 minutes; subsequent doses over 30 minutes (if prior infusions were well tolerated), at 3-week intervals. Observe patient **during** and following

infusion (at least 90 minutes **following** initial dose, and for at least 30 minutes **following** subsequent doses) for flushing, fever, chills, dyspnea, hypotension, wheezing, bronchospasm, and tachycardia, or other infusion-related reactions.

- The infusion rate should be slowed or interrupted if an infusion reaction occurs. Drug should be permanently discontinued if IRR is life-threatening.
- Incidence in Study 1 was 1.4%, and most reactions resolved over the course of several hours to a day after the infusion was terminated. One patient had severe infusion reaction/anaphylaxis. Emergency equipment and medications should be immediately available.
- If a planned dose is missed or delayed, administer as soon as possible; do not wait until the next planned cycle but adjust the schedule to maintain a 3-week cycle. Administer the infusion at the dose and rate patient tolerated in the most recent infusion (Genentech, 2019).
- Discuss dose modifications for abnormal PE/lab values: increased serum transaminases, hyperbilirubinemia, LV dysfunction, thrombocytopenia, pulmonary toxicity, or peripheral neuropathy.
- Monitor infusion site for possible subcutaneous infiltration during drug administration. Avoid extravasation. Reactions, generally within 24 hours of drug administration, have been reported characterized by erythema, tenderness, skin irritation, pain, and swelling at the infusion site. These were usually mild.

Drug Interactions:
- Incompatible with Dextrose (5%) solutions.
- Strong CYP3A4 inhibitors (e.g., atazanavir, clarithromycin, indinavir, itraconazole, nefazodone, nelfinavir, ritonavir, saquinavir, telithromycin, voriconazole) may increase drug serum level and increase toxicity. Avoid concomitant administration. If concomitant use is unavoidable, consider delaying ado-trastuzumab emtansine until the strong CYP3A4 inhibitor has cleared from the circulation (about three elimination half-lives of the CYP3A4 inhibitor). Assess for signs/symptoms of toxicity.

Lab Effects/Interference:
- Increased LFTs: bilirubin (17%), increased AST (98%), increased ALT (82%).
- Decreased platelet (83%), and neutrophil (39%) counts; decreased hemoglobin (60%).
- Decreased potassium (33%).

Special Considerations:
- Warnings and Precautions:
  - *Hepatotoxicity:* Most commonly in clinical trials, this was manifest as asymptomatic, transient increases in serum transaminases. However, serious hepatotoxicity has rarely been reported, including liver failure and death, in patients with metastatic breast cancer treated with ado-trastuzumab emtansine. This included severe DILI and associated hepatic encephalopathy, and some of the patients had comorbidities and/or concomitant hepatotoxic medications. Assess serum transaminases and bilirubin prior to initiation of ado-trastuzumab emtansine treatment and prior to each dose. Reduce dose or discontinue drug as appropriate in cases of increased serum transaminases or total bilirubin. Nodular regenerative hyperplasia (NRH) may also rarely

occur, but it can be confirmed only by histopathology. Consider NRH in patients with clinical symptoms of portal hypertension and/or cirrhosis-like pattern on CT, but with normal transaminases and no other manifestations of cirrhosis. If NRH is confirmed, drug should be permanently discontinued. Monitor serum transaminases and bilirubin baseline and prior to each ado-trastuzumab emtansine. Dose modify based on AST/ALT and bilirubin values.

- *Left Ventricular (LV) Dysfunction:* ado-trastuzumab emtansine increases risk of LVEF dysfunction. In the EMILIA study, incidence of LVEF dysfunction in patients with metastatic breast cancer (MBC) occurred in 1.8% of patients compared to 3.3% in patients receiving lapatinib plus Capecitabine (Genentech, 2019). In the KATHERINE study of patients with early breast cancer (EBC), LV dysfunction occurred in 0.4% of patients receiving ado-trastuzumab emtansine, compared to 0.6% in the patients receiving trastuzumab (Genentech, 2019). Evaluate LVEF in all patients prior to and during treatment (e.g., every 3 months) with ado-trastuzumab emtansine. The drug has not been studied in patients with a baseline LVEF of <50%.
  - If at routine monitoring of patients with MBC, LVEF is < 40%, or is 40% to 45% with a 10% or greater absolute decrease below the pretreatment value, hold drug and repeat LVEF assessment within approximately 3 weeks. Permanently discontinue ado-trastuzumab emtansine if the LVEF has not improved or has declined further.
  - If at routine monitoring of patients with EBC, LVEF is <45% or is 45% to 49% with a 10% or greater absolute decrease below the pretreatment value, hold ado-trastuzumab emtansine and repeat LVEF assessment within about 3 weeks. Permanently discontinue ado-trastuzumab emtansine if the LVEF has not improved or declined further.
  - The EMILIA and KATHERINE clinical trials excluded patients with a history of symptomatic CHF, serious cardiac arrhythmias, or history of MI or unstable angina within 6 months (Genentech, 2019).
- *Embryo-fetal toxicity:* Embryo-fetal death or birth defects can occur following exposure to ado-trastuzumab emtansine (either during treatment or within 7 months after last dose). *Verify* pregnancy status prior to the initiation of ado-trastuzumab emtansine. Advise female patients and male patients with female sexual partners of reproductive potential of these risks and the need for effective contraception during and for at least 7 months after last treatment. If the drug is administered during pregnancy, if a patient becomes pregnant while receiving the drug, or within 7 months following the last dose of the drug, teach patient about potential hazard to fetus. Report exposure immediately to the Genentech Adverse Event Line (1-888-835-2555). Encourage women who may be exposed during pregnancy to enroll in the MotHER Pregnancy Registry by contacting 1-800-690-6720.
- *Pulmonary Toxicity:* ILD may occur, including pneumonitis (incidence 0.8–1.2% in EMILIA study of patients with MBC), possibly leading to acute respiratory distress syndrome. Incidence was 1.1% in the KATHERINE EBC study of EBC patients. Radiation pneumonitis was reported in 1.8% of patients who received adjuvant

radiotherapy and ado-trastuzumab emtansine. Evaluate symptoms if they arise (e.g., dyspnea, cough, fatigue, and pulmonary infiltrates) and permanently discontinue drug if ILD or pneumonitis is diagnosed. Patients with dyspnea at rest due to complications of advanced cancer and comorbidities may be at increased risk for pulmonary toxicity.

- *IRRs, HSRs:* Drug was not studied in patients with prior hypersensitivity or serious infusion reactions to/from trastuzumab, so drug is not recommended in this group of patients. In clinical studies, incidence of IRRs was 1.4% in patients with MBC, and 1.6% in patients with EBC. IRRs were characterized by one or more of the following: flushing, chills, pyrexia, dyspnea, hypotension, wheezing, bronchospasm, and tachycardia; in most patients, reactions resolved in hours to a day after the infusion. Treatment should be interrupted if a severe IRR occurs. Drug should be permanently discontinued if a life-threatening IRR occurs. Patients should be closely monitored during and after treatment (e.g., monitor patient 90 and 30 minutes after initial and subsequent infusions, respectively). Emergency resuscitation and medication should be immediately available in the infusion area.
- *Thrombocytopenia* occurred in 31% of patients in the EMILIA study of patients with MBC (grade 3 or higher, 15%), and 29% in the KATHERINE study of patients with EBC (6% grade 3 or higher). However, the incidence of thrombocytopenia in Asian patients was higher. In the EMILIA study, the incidence of grade 3 or higher thrombocytopenia was 45%, while in the KATHERINE study, the overall incidence was 50% with incidence of grade 3 or higher was 19% (Genentech, 2019). Nadir occurred by day 8, and generally improved to grades 0–1 by the next scheduled dose. Monitor platelet counts closely especially in Asian patients (baseline and prior to each dose), and teach all patients to self-assess for signs/symptoms of bleeding and self-care measures to minimize bleeding. Discuss dose modification accordingly. Patients with thrombocytopenia ($< 100,000/mm^3$) and patients on anticoagulant treatment should be closely monitored.
- *Hemorrhage:* Fatal hemorrhage has occurred, in patients with and without risk factors. Overall frequency of hemorrhage was 32.2% in clinical trials in the Kadcyla group (1.8% grades 3–4) vs. 16.4% (0.8% grades 3–4) in the lapatinib+capecitabine treated group. Use cautiously in patients with thrombocytopenia or receiving anticoagulation or antiplatelet therapy if drug is medically necessary, and monitor patient very closely.
- *Neurotoxicity:* Peripheral neuropathy occurred primarily as grade 1 and was predominately sensory. In the EMILIA study of patients with MBC, overall incidence was 21% of patients (grade 3 or higher 2.2%) versus 14% in the lapatinib/Capecitabine group (0.2% grade 3 or higher). In the KATHERINE study of patients with EBC, overall incidence was 32% in the Kadcyla group compared to 17% in the trastuzumab group; 30% of patients in the Kadcyla group did not have resolution of motor or sensory neuropathy at the end of the study. Assess for signs/symptoms baseline and before each dose. If the patient develops grade 3 or 4 peripheral neuropathy, the drug should be temporarily discontinued until peripheral neuropathy has resolved to ≤ grade 2.

- *HER2 Testing:* Ensure patient is HER2 positive (overexpression or gene amplification) using an FDA-approved test by laboratories with demonstrated proficiency.
- *Extravasation:* Reactions may occur after extravasation, usually within 24 hours and are usually mild (e.g., erythema, tenderness, skin irritation, or swelling at infusion site). Monitor infusion site closely during administration for possible extravasation.
- Mothers should not breastfeed while receiving the drug.
- Most common side effects (frequency > 25%) are nausea, fatigue, musculoskeletal pain, thrombocytopenia, increased liver transaminases, headache, constipation. Most common grades 3–4 adverse effects in clinical trials were thrombocytopenia, increased transaminases, anemia, hypokalemia, peripheral neuropathy, and fatigue.

Potential Toxicities/Side Effects and the Nursing Process

I.   POTENTIAL FOR BLEEDING, INFECTION, AND FATIGUE related to BONE MARROW SUPPRESSION

Defining Characteristics: Thrombocytopenia occurs in 31.2% (14.5% grades 3–4, while in Asian patients it was 45.1%), anemia in 14.3%, and neutropenia in 6.7%. Fatigue occurs in 36.3%. Epistaxis occurs in 22.5%. Platelet nadir occurs by day 8 and usually returns to grades 0 or 1 by the next scheduled dose. In clinical trials, the incidence of thrombocytopenia was higher in Asian patients.

Nursing Implications: Assess CBC/differential and platelet count baseline and prior to each treatment. Hold drug if platelet count < 75,000 cells/mm^3 and dose-modify per physician/prescribing information. Teach patient to report bleeding, signs/symptoms of bleeding, right away. Teach patient to self-assess for signs/symptoms of infection, bleeding, or severe fatigue. Teach patient to avoid aspirin-containing OTC medications and NSAIDs. Teach patient strategies to manage fatigue and conserve energy, such as alteration of rest and activity and organizing chores.

II.   POTENTIAL FOR SENSORY/PERCEPTUAL ALTERATIONS related to NEUROLOGICAL TOXICITY

Defining Characteristics: Peripheral neuropathy occurs in 21.2% (2.2% grades 3–4), dizziness 10.2%, and headache in 28.2% of patients.

Nursing Implications: Teach patient that these side effects may occur and to report them. Assess sensory/perceptual changes (e.g., numbness, tingling, weakness) baseline and prior to each drug administration. Assess one side versus the other side, and note extent of paresthesias if present (stocking glove distribution), starting at fingertips or tips of toes, and progressing proximally to wrist/ankle like a glove and stocking, and document. Assess patient's ability to do ADLs and impact of neuropathy on functioning. Discuss grade with NP/PA or physician and need to dose-modify or interrupt (hold drug for grades 3–4). Assess for presence of dizziness and risk for falls, and discuss strategies to minimize risk of falling. Assess for headache and discuss self-care strategies to prevent/manage them.

III. ALTERATION IN NUTRITION related to DYSPEPSIA, STOMATITIS, DRY MOUTH, ABDOMINAL PAIN, VOMITING, DIARRHEA, CONSTIPATION, NAUSEA, DYSGEUSIA, INCREASED LFTs

Defining Characteristics: Dyspepsia occurs in 9.2% of patients, stomatitis in 14.1%, dry mouth 16.7%, abdominal pain (18.6%), diarrhea (24.1%), constipation (26.5%), nausea (39.8%), increased transaminases (28.8%), and hypokalemia (10.2%).

Nursing Implications: Assess baseline nutritional status, lab findings, especially LFTs (transaminases, bilirubin), and serum potassium. Discuss abnormalities with physician or NP/PA and understand dose interruption or modification per prescribing information. Teach patient that nutritional impact symptoms may occur and to report them. Discuss with the patient medication and self-care strategies to manage nausea, vomiting, diarrhea, constipation, dyspepsia, and stomatitis if they occur. Discuss dietary modifications as needed. If the patient has persistent diarrhea, discuss lab testing of serum potassium and need for repletion and hydration with physician or NP/PA. If symptoms persist, discuss pharmacologic plan revision with NP/PA or physician.

IV. ALTERATIONS IN COMFORT related to MYALGIAS, ARTHRALGIAS, MUSCULOSKELETAL PAIN

Defining Characteristics: Myalgias occur in 14.1% of patients, arthralgias in 19.2%, and musculoskeletal pain in 36% of patients.

Nursing Implications: Teach patient that these symptoms may occur and to report them. Assess baseline comfort, and teach self-care strategies, such as application of heat or local cooling to manage symptoms. If they persist, discuss pharmacologic management with NP/PA or physician.

Drug: aldesleukin (interleukin-2, Proleukin)

Class: Cytokine.

Mechanism of Action: Interleukin-2 (IL-2), previously called T-cell growth factor, is produced by helper T cells following antibody-antigen reaction (processed antigen is mounted on macrophage) and IL-1. IL-2 amplifies the immune response to an antigen by immunomodulation and immunorestoration. IL-2 stimulates T-lymphocyte proliferation, enhances killer T-cell activity, increases antibody production (secondary to increased B-cell proliferation), helps to increase synthesis of other cytokines (IFNs, IL-1, -3, -4, -5, -6, CSFs), and stimulates production and activation of NK cells and other cytotoxic cells (LAK and TIL).

Metabolism: The half-life of distribution is 13 minutes, whereas the elimination half-life is 85 minutes.

Indication: For the treatment of adults with (1) metastatic renal cell carcinoma (RCC), (2) metastatic melanoma. Patient selection must be careful and exclude patients with significant cardiac, pulmonary, renal, hepatic, or CNS impairment.

Contraindications: In (1) patients with a known history of hypersensitivity to IL-2 or any component of Proleukin; (2) patients with an abnormal thallium stress test or abnormal pulmonary function tests, and those with organ allografts. Retreatment with (3) Proleukin is contraindicated in patients who have experienced the following drug-related toxicities while receiving an earlier course of therapy:

- Sustained ventricular tachycardia ($\geq$ 5 beats), uncontrolled cardiac rhythm disturbances, EKG changes showing angina or MI, cardiac tamponade.
- Intubation > 72 hours.
- Renal failure requiring dialysis > 72 hours.
- Coma or toxic psychosis lasting > 48 hours; difficult to control seizures.
- Bowel ischemia or perforation, GI bleeding requiring surgery.

Delay with resumption of dose after resolution of symptoms and condition resolved or ruled out:
- Persistent atrial fibrillation, supraventricular tachycardia, or bradycardia.
- Hypotension (SBP < 90 mm Hg with need for pressors).
- EKG change showing MI, ischemia, myocarditis.
- O_2 saturation < 90%.
- Mental status changes (confusion, agitation).
- Sepsis.
- Serum creatinine > 4.5 or $\geq$ 4 mg/dL with severe volume overload, acidosis, or hyperkalemia; persistent oliguria, urine output < 10 mL/hour for 16–24 hours with increasing serum creatinine.
- Signs of hepatic failure (encephalopathy, increasing ascites, liver pain, hypoglycemia): stop this course of treatment and reinitiate new course after at least 7 weeks of rest.
- Stool guaiac repeatedly > 3–4+.
- Bullous dermatitis or marked worsening of preexisting skin condition (do not use topical steroid therapy).

Dosage/Range:

Metastatic renal cell carcinoma and metastatic malignant melanoma:
- 600,000 IU/kg (0.037 mg/kg) IVB over 15 minutes every 8 hours for a maximum of 14 doses over 5 days and then a 9-day rest, followed by 14 additional doses, 1 every 8 hours, for a maximum of 28 doses per course as tolerated. Evaluate for response 4 weeks after completion of a course and before the next treatment course. Tumor shrinkage should be seen before retreatment. Seven-week rest period should separate discharge from the hospital and retreatment. Delay and drug holiday should be used rather than drug dose reduction to manage toxicity.
- Dose should be held for atrial fibrillation, supraventricular tachycardia, symptomatic bradycardia; SBP < 90 mmHg; ECG changes consistent with ischemia; O_2 saturation < 90%; mental status changes; sepsis; serum creatinine > 4.0–4.5 mg/dL; persistent

oliguria; hepatic failure; 3–4+ guaiac positive stool; bullous dermatitis. See package insert for resumption of dose after recovery of these signs/symptoms.
- Dose modifications—see package insert (Prometheus, August 2018).

Drug Preparation:
- Vial containing 22 million international units (1.3 mg) should be reconstituted with 1.2 mL of sterile water for injection, USP so each mL contains 18 million international units of drug. DO NOT SHAKE. Further dilute in 50 mL of 5% dextrose injection, USP. If dose is < 1.5 mg, use a smaller volume. Refrigerate and use within 48 hours of preparation. Bring to room temperature before administration.

Drug Administration:
- Baseline and during treatment
  - Assess lab tests (CBC/differential, blood chemistries including electrolytes, renal and hepatic function), and results of CXR baseline and as ordered during treatment. Serum creastinine should be ≤ 1.5 mg/dL before IL-2 treatment started.
  - Review baseline PFTs with arterial blood gases, stress thallium study.
  - Monitor patient daily with T, HR, RR, BP, weight, I/O, and total body balance.
  - If patient hypotensive (SBP < 90 mm Hg), patient should be monitored via cardiac monitor for ectopy. If an abnormal complex or rhythm seen, document it on ECG. If hypotensive, the patient should have hourly vital signs and pulse oximetry.
  - If a patient develops dyspnea or signs of respiratory impairment (tachypnea or rales), discuss with provider arterial blood gases.
  - Cardiac assessment should be done at least daily—if s/s chest pain, murmurs, gallops, irregular rhythm, or palpitations, discuss with provider cardiac enzymes and document status on ECG.
- Final concentration should be between 30 and 70 μg/mL.
- Use plastic IV bags instead of glass bottles, and do not use in-line filters.
- Administer IV over 15 minutes.
  - Concomitant drugs which improve symptom management during administration and continuing for 12 hours after last dose (Prometheus, 2015): (1) antipyretics, including NSAIDs, starting immediately prior to aldesleukin dose (monitor renal function as may be synergistic nephrotoxicity); (2) meperidine to control rigors associated with fever; (3) H_2 antagonists for prophylaxis of GI irritation and bleeding; (4) antiemetics and antidiarrheal agents.
  - Indwelling central lines have an increased risk of gram positive infection and prophylaxis with oxacillin, nafcillin, ciprofloxacin, or vancomycin should be considered.
  - Avoid coadministration of steroids unless life-threatening episode requiring this. Expect that the therapeutic effect of aldesleukin is diminished.

Drug Interactions:
- Potentiation of CNS effects when given in combination with psychotropic drugs.
- The combination with nephrotoxic, myelotoxic, cardiotoxic, or hepatotoxic drugs will increase toxicity of aldesleukin in these organ systems.
- Increased risk of HSR when sequential high-dose aldesleukin combined with dacarbazine, cisplatin, tamoxifen, and IFN-α.

- IFN-α and aldesleukin concurrently: increased risk of myocardial injury (MI, myocarditis, severe rhabdomyolysis).
- Glucocorticoid steroids: decreased antitumor effectiveness. Do not use together.
- β-Blockers, antihypertensives: potentiate hypotension of aldesleukin.
- Iodinated contrast medium: increased risk of atypical adverse reaction (12.6% incidence) characterized by fever, chills, nausea, vomiting, pruritus, rash, diarrhea, hypotension, edema, and oliguria and typically happens when contrast is given within 4 weeks of aldesleukin dosing.

Lab Effects/Interference:
- Anemia, leukopenia, thrombocytopenia
- Elevated LFTs
- Increased serum creatinine
- Acidosis

Special Considerations:
- Patient must have NORMAL cardiac, pulmonary, hepatic, renal (serum creatinine ≤ 1.5 mg/dL), and CNS function before treatment and be free of any known infection.
- Baseline testing includes the following, which should be repeated daily during drug administration:
  - Standard CBC, differential, and platelet counts.
  - Blood chemistries (including electrolytes, renal, and hepatic function tests).
  - Chest x-ray.
  - Baseline PFTs with arterial blood gases (ABGs) with $FEV_1 > 2$ L or ≥ 75% predicted for height and age prior to starting therapy.
  - Baseline stress thallium study with normal ejection fraction and unimpaired wall motion.
  - Daily monitoring during therapy of VS including pulse oximetry, cardiopulmonary exam, weight, and fluid I/O. If the patient has a systolic BP < 90 mm Hg, patient should receive continuous telemetry, EKG documentation of any abnormal rhythm, and hourly VS monitoring. If patient develops dyspnea, assess ABGs. If angina develops, patient should have cardiac enzyme evaluation and further cardiac workup.
- Warnings and Precautions:
  - *Restricted use:* Patients should have normal cardiac and pulmonary function defined by thallium stress testing and formal pulmonary function testing. Extreme caution should be used in patient with a normal thallium stress test, normal PFTs, but a history of cardiac or pulmonary disease.
  - *Hospital setting required under supervision of a qualified physician experienced in the use of anticancer agents:* An ICU and specialists skilled in cardiopulmonary or intensive care medicine must be available.
  - *Capillary Leak Syndrome (CLS):* Proleukin has been associated with CLS (loss of vascular tone and extravasation of plasma proteins and fluid into extracellular space). This may result in hypotension and reduced organ perfusion which can be severe and fatal. CLS may be associated with cardiac arrhythmias (supraventricular and ventricular), angina MI, respiratory insufficiency requiring intubation, GI bleeding or infarction, renal insufficiency, edema, and mental status changes.

- *Impaired neutrophil function* (reduced chemotaxis), with increased risk of disseminated infection (e.g., sepsis, bacterial endocarditis): Preexisting bacterial infections should be fully treated before starting aldesleukin therapy. Patients with indwelling central lines are at high risk for infection with gram-positive microorganisms; antibiotic prophylaxis with oxacillin, nafcillin, ciprofloxacin, or vancomycin has been shown to reduce the incidence of staphylococcal infections.
- *Mental status:* Drug should be withheld in patients developing moderate to severe lethargy or somnolence; continued drug administration may result in coma.
- Drug may worsen symptoms of patients with unknown/untreated CNS metastases. Thorough evaluation and treatment of CNS metastases should precede the treatment.
- Use caution when patient is receiving other drugs that are hepatic or renally toxic.
- Drug may increase rejection in allogeneic transplant patients, exacerbation of autoimmune disease, and inflammatory disorders.
- Drug should be used during pregnancy only if the potential benefit justifies the potential risk to the fetus.
- Nursing mothers should make a decision to discontinue nursing or to discontinue the drug, taking into consideration the importance of the drug to the mother's health.

Potential Toxicities/Side Effects (Dose-1 and Schedule-Dependent) and the Nursing Process

I.   ALTERATION IN COMFORT related to FLU-LIKE SYNDROME

Defining Characteristics: Chills may occur 2–4 hours after dose; rigors are possible; fever to 39–40°C (102–104°F), and headache. Myalgia and arthralgias may occur at high doses because of accumulation of cytokine deposits/lymphocytes in joint spaces. The incidence of chills is 52%, fever 29%, malaise 27%, asthenia 23%, and anorexia 20%.

Nursing Implications: Assess baseline T, VS, neurologic status, and comfort level, and monitor every 4–6 hours if patient is in hospital. Discuss with physician premedication and regular dosing of antipyretic (e.g., acetaminophen ± diphenhydramine, NSAID). If patient is in hospital and experiences rigor, discuss with physician IV meperidine and monitor BP for hypotension.

II.   SENSORY/PERCEPTUAL ALTERATION related to CNS EFFECTS

Defining Characteristics: Confusion, irritability, disorientation, impaired memory, expressive aphasia, sleep disturbances, depression, hallucinations, and psychoses may occur, resolving within 24–48 hours after last drug dose. Mental status abnormalities exaggerated by anxiety and sleep deprivation.

Nursing Implications: Assess baseline mental status and neurologic status before drug administration. Assess patient for changes (impaired memory/attention, disorientation, slow/vague responses to questions, increased lethargy) during treatment. Teach patient to report signs/symptoms. Provide information, emotional support, and interventions to ensure safety if signs/symptoms occur.

III.   ALTERATION IN CARDIAC OUTPUT related to HYPOTENSION (HIGH-DOSE THERAPY)

Defining Characteristics: Increased risk with dose > 100,000 IU/kg. CLS (peripheral edema, CHF, pleural effusions, and pericardial effusions) may occur and is reversible once treatment is stopped. Atrial arrhythmias may occur; occasionally, supraventricular tachycardia, myocarditis, chest pain; and rarely, myocardial infarction. IL-2 causes peripheral vasodilation, decreased systemic vascular resistance, and hypotension that may lead to decreased renal perfusion. A decrease in SBP occurs 2–12 hours after start of therapy and typically will progress to significant hypotension (SBP < 90 or a 20-mm Hg drop from baseline SBP) with hypoperfusion. In addition, protein and fluids will extravasate into the extravascular space, forming edema and new effusions.

Nursing Implications: Assess baseline cardiopulmonary status and patients at risk (the older population, those with preexisting cardiac dysfunction). Monitor VS and pulse oximetry frequently, at least q 4 hours (if hypotensive, q 1 hr), noting rate, rhythm of heartbeat, blood pressure, urinary output, fluid status, I/O q 4 hours or more frequently, and daily weights during therapy. Discuss any abnormalities with physician, and revise plan as needed (e.g., diuretics, plasma expanders). Instruct patient to report signs or symptoms of dyspnea, chest pain, edema, or other abnormalities immediately. Hypotension requires fluid replacement, and patient should be monitored with continuous cardiac monitoring if SBP < 90 mm Hg. Any ectopy should be documented on ECG. Manufacturer states that early administration of dopamine (1–5 mcg/kg/min) to patients with CLS before the onset of hypotension can improve organ perfusion and preserve urinary output. Increased dopamine doses (6–10 mcg/kg/min) or the addition of phenylephrine hydrochloride (1–5 mcg/kg/min) to low-dose dopamine has been described. After blood pressure is stabilized, the use of diuretics is often effective in relieving edema and pulmonary congestion.

IV.   POTENTIAL ALTERATION IN OXYGENATION

Defining Characteristics: Pulmonary symptoms are dose related, such as dyspnea and tachypnea. Pulmonary edema may occur with hypoxia because of fluid shifts.

Nursing Implications: Assess baseline cardiopulmonary status every 4 hours during therapy, noting rate, rhythm, depth of respirations, presence of dyspnea, and breath sounds (presence of wheezes, crackles, rhonchi). Identify patients at risk: those with preexisting cardiac or pulmonary disease, prior treatment with cardio or pulmonary-toxic drugs or radiation, and smoking history. Instruct the patient to report cough, dyspnea, or change in respiratory status. Strictly monitor I/O, total fluid balance, and daily weight. Discuss abnormalities with physician, as well as the need for oxygen, diuretics, or transfer to ICU.

V. POTENTIAL ALTERATION IN NUTRITION, LESS THAN BODY REQUIREMENTS, related to NAUSEA/VOMITING, DIARRHEA, MUCOSITIS, ANOREXIA

Defining Characteristics: Nausea and vomiting are mild and are effectively controlled by antiemetics. Diarrhea is common and can be severe. Stomatitis is common but mild.

Nursing Implications: Assess the patient's baseline nutritional status. Administer antiemetics as ordered. Teach the patient potential side effects and self-care measures, including oral hygiene, and encourage patient to eat favorite high-calorie, high-protein foods. Teach self-administration of prescribed antiemetics and antidiarrheals as needed. Refer to the dietitian as appropriate.

VI. POTENTIAL ALTERATION IN ELIMINATION related to RENAL DYSFUNCTION, HEPATOTOXICITY

Defining Characteristics: IL-2 causes decreased renal blood flow with cumulative doses. Oliguria, proteinuria, increased serum creatinine and BUN, and increased LFTs (bili, AST, ALT, LDH, alk phos) may occur. Anuria occurs in 5% of patients; renal dysfunction is reversible after drug discontinuance. Hepatomegaly and hypoalbuminemia may occur.

Nursing Implications: Assess baseline renal and hepatic functions and monitor during treatment. Assess fluid and electrolyte balance, urine output hourly, and total body balance. Dipstick urine for protein. Discuss abnormalities with physician and revise plan.

VII. POTENTIAL FOR FATIGUE AND BLEEDING related to ANEMIA, THROMBOCYTOPENIA

Defining Characteristics: Anemia occurs in 29% of patients and may require RBC transfusion. Thrombocytopenia occurs commonly but rarely requires transfusion.

Nursing Implications: Assess baseline CBC and platelet count and signs/symptoms of fatigue, severe anemia, bleeding. Instruct the patient to report signs/symptoms immediately and to manage self-care (alternate rest/activity, minimize bleeding by avoidance of OTC aspirin-containing medicines). Transfuse red cells and platelets as ordered.

VIII. POTENTIAL ALTERATION IN SKIN INTEGRITY related to DIFFUSE RASH

Defining Characteristics: Patients may develop diffuse erythematous rash, which may desquamate (soles of feet, palms of hands, between fingers). Pruritus may occur with or without rash.

Nursing Implications: Assess baseline skin integrity. Teach patient to report signs and symptoms. Discuss/teach symptomatic management, including the use of mild soaps and rinsing skin thoroughly after bathing. Encourage the use of alcohol-free, oil-based moisturizers on skin and the protection of desquamated areas.

Drug: alemtuzumab (Campath anti-CD52 monoclonal antibody) NOT Lemtrada

Class: mAb targeting CD52; humanized IgG1 mAb.

Mechanism of Action: Humanized mAb, which targets the CD52 antigen present on the surface of most normal human lymphocyte cells, as well as malignant T-cell and B-cell malignant lymphocytes (lymphomas). Most monocytes, macrophages, NK cells, some granulocytes, and CD4+ cells, also have the CD52 antigen. Once the mAb binds with the CD52 antigen, it initiates ADCC and complement binding, which then lead to apoptosis, or programmed cell death, and activation of normal T-cell cytotoxicity against the malignant cells.

Metabolism: When given subcutaneously or intravenously, pharmacokinetics appear similar, but the absorption is much slower with subcutaneous administration. It takes a higher cumulative dose (an additional 6 weeks) to achieve a therapeutic level. The mean half-life is 11 hours after the first 30-mg dose, 6 hours after the last 30-mg dose, but steady-state plasma levels are not reached until week 6. Levels appear to correlate with the number of circulating CD52-positive cells. Drug clearance decreases with repeated dosing as more leukemic cells are killed. Given subcutaneously, CLL cells were cleared from the blood in 95% of patients in a median time of 21 days (Lundin et al., 2002). Host antibodies may develop 14–21 days after the first dose and theoretically can decrease lymphocyte killing.

Indication: Indicated as a single agent for the treatment of B-cell chronic lymphocytic leukemia (B-CLL).

Dosage/Range:
- Drug is available only through the Campath Access Program (1-877-422-6728) administered by Sanofi Foundation, and is not commercially available.
- Initial dose is 3-mg IV infusion over 2 hours, daily, with dose escalated to 10 mg daily when well tolerated (side effects are grade 2 or less).
- When dose of 10 mg is well tolerated, the dose is increased to 30 mg and becomes the maintenance dose, 30 mg/day, given 3 times a week (e.g., Monday, Wednesday, and Friday) for 12 weeks (maximum weekly dose 90 mg). Total duration of therapy, including dose escalation, is 12 weeks. Dose escalation to 30 mg usually takes 3–7 days.
- Concomitant medications
  - Premedicate with oral antihistamine and acetaminophen 30 minutes prior to first infusion and each dose escalation. Institute appropriate medical management if serious infusion reaction (e.g., steroids, epinephrine, meperidine) as needed and ordered (Sanofi, 2018).

- Administer prophylactic *Pneumocystis jiroveci* pneumonia (PCP) [e.g., trimethoprim/ sulfamethoxazole DS bid three times a week] and herpes virus infection (e.g., famci- clovir 250 mg bid) antimicrobial agents as ordered.
- Continue PCP and herpes viral prophylaxis for a minimum of 2 months after comple- tion of alumtuzimab or until CD4+ count is $\geq$ 200 cells/μL, whichever comes later.
- Withold drug for grade 3–4 infusion reactions.
- Hold drug during serious infection or other serious adverse reactions until resolution.
- Discontinue drug for autoimmune anemia or autoimmune thrombocytopenia.
- Subcutaneous administration is better tolerated and results in similar efficacy (Lundin et al., 2002).

Dose Modification for Neutropenia or Thrombocytopenia:
- ANC $<$ 250/μL and/or platelet count $\leq$ 25,000/μL.
  - First occurrence: hold alemtuzumab; resume alemtuzumab at 30 mg when ANC $\geq$ 500/μL and platelet count $\geq$ 50,000/μL.
  - Second occurrence: hold alemtuzumab; resume alemtuzumab at 10 mg when ANC $\geq$ 500/μL and platelet count $\geq$ 50,000/μL.
  - Third occurrence: discontinue alemtuzumab.
- $\geq$ 50% decrease from baseline in patients initiating therapy with a baseline ANC $\leq$ 250/μL and/or a baseline platelet count $\leq$ 25,000/μL.
  - First occurrence: hold alemtuzumab; resume alemtuzumab at 30 mg upon return to baseline value(s).
  - Second occurrence: hold alemtuzumab; resume alemtuzumab at 10 mg upon return to baseline value(s).
  - Third occurrence: discontinue alemtuzumab.
- If the delay between dosing is $\geq$ 7 days, initiate therapy at alemtuzumab 3 mg and esca- late to 10 mg and then to 30 mg as tolerated.

Drug Preparation:
- Available in **single-use** vials containing 30 mg alemtuzumab in 1 mL of diluent. Inspect for particulate matter and discoloration, and if found, do not use. DO NOT shake vial. Discard vial including any unused portion after dose withdrawal. Contains no preserva- tive and is for single use.
- **Use a syringe calibrated in increments of 0.01 for 3- and 10-mg doses.** Use a syringe calibrated in 0.1 mL increments for the 30-mg dose. Draw up ordered dose:
  - 3-mg dose: withdraw 0.1 mL into a 1-mL syringe calibrated in 0.01 mL increments.
  - 10-mg dose: withdraw 0.33 mL into a 1-mL syringe calibrated in 0.01 mL increments.
  - 30-mg dose: withdraw 1 mL in either a 1- or 3-mL syringe calibrated in 0.1-mL increments.
  - Dilute in 100 mL sterile 0.9% sodium chloride USP or 5% dextrose in water. **Gently invert IV bag to mix.** Use within 8 hours after dilution: store at room temperature (15–30°C) or refrigerated (2–8°C); protect from light.
- Drug is compatible with PVC infusion bags and PVC or polyethylene-lined PVC ad- ministration sets. Do not add or simultaneously infuse other drug substances through the same IV line.

- Drug is available only through the Campath Access Program (Sanofi Foundation), free of charge (1-877-422-6728); it requires healthcare provider documentation and compliance with certain requirements including toxicity reporting (Campath Access Program, 2015).

Drug Administration:
- IV infusion over 2 hours. Initial dose is 3 mg; repeat daily until infusion reactions are less than or equal to grade 2; then administer 10 mg daily until infusion reactions are less than or equal to grade 2; then administer the 30-mg dose as below (subsequent dosing).
- Subsequent dosing: 30-mg IV over 2 hours 3 times/week, for a minimum of 4 weeks, but may continue up to 12 weeks (total duration of therapy is 12 weeks, including dose escalation). Give on Monday, Wednesday, and Friday.
- If dose held more than 7 days, reinstitute gradually with dose escalation as with initial dose.
- Premedicate with acetaminophen 650 mg and diphenhydramine 50 mg 30 minutes prior to beginning each infusion.
- Assess hydration status and need for IV fluids with prescribing physician or NP/PA.
- Assess CBC/differential weekly during alemtuzumab therapy, more frequently if cytopenias.
- Stop drug immediately if a reaction develops during the infusion.
- Severe reactions may require hydrocortisone 200 mg. If drug requires slower infusion, repeat premedications at 4 hours.
- Institute appropriate medical management for infusion reactions as needed (e.g., steroids, epinephrine, meperidine).
- *Anti-infective prophylaxis recommended,* continuing for 2 months after treatment completed/stopped, or CD4+ count ≥ 200 cells/μL, whichever occurs later:
  - PCP prophylaxis with trimethoprim and sulfamethoxazole (Bactrim) DS/twice daily, 3 times a week (or equivalent).
  - Herpes prophylaxis: an antiviral such as famciclovir 250 mg twice daily (or equivalent). Stop the drug immediately if a serious infection occurs.
  - Dose-reduce if ANC < 250/μL and/or platelet count ≤ 25,000/μL. See package insert.
  - Single doses > 30 mg or cumulative doses > 90 mg weekly increase the risk of pancytopenia.
  - Do not give IVP or IVB.

Drug Interactions:
- No formal drug studies have been done.

Lab Effects/Interference:
- An immune response to the drug may interfere with subsequent serum laboratory tests using antibodies.
- Decreased WBC, lymphocyte, red blood cell, and platelet counts.

Special Considerations:
- Most common adverse effects (≥10%) are: cytopenias, infusion reactions, cytomegalovirus (CMV) and other infections, nausea, emesis, diarrhea, and insomnia.

- Warnings and Precautions:
  - *Cytopenias:* severe, including fatal autoimmune anemia and thrombocytopenia; prolonged myelosuppression have been reported. In addition, hemolytic anemia, pure red cell aplasia, bone marrow aplasia, and hypoplasia have been reported after treatment with alemtuzumab at the recommended dose. Escalate dose to 30 mg slowly, and never exceed 90mg in a week.
  - Hold drug for cytopenias (except lymphpenia); discontinue for autoimmune cytopenias or severe hematologic adverse reactions.
  - There is increased risk of serious infection. Administer prophylactic *Pneumocystis jiroveci* pneumonia (PCP) and herpes virus infection antimicrobial agents during alemtuzumab therapy. If a serious infection occurs, stop Campath treatment until infection has resolved.
  - Patients who have received multiple courses of chemotherapy prior to campath-1H are at increased risk for bacterial, viral, and other opportunistic infections.
  - Drug-related immunosuppression results in severe and prolonged lymphopenia, with increased risk of opportunistic infections. Administer PCP and herpes viral prophylaxis during alemtuzumab therapy and for a minimum of 2 months after completion of alemtuzumab therapy or until CD4+ count is $\geq$ 200 cells/ μL, whichever occurs later. Prophylaxis does not eliminate these infections. Drug may reactivate herpes simplex infections.
  - Routinely monitor patients for cytolomegalovirus (CMV) infection during therapy and for 2 months after therapy is completed.
- *Infusion Reactions:*
  - The drug may cause serious infusion reactions during or shortly after drug infusion, characterized by pyrexia, chills/rigors, nausea, hypotension, urticaria, dyspnea, rash, emesis, and bronchospasm. In clinical trials, the highest frequency of infusion reactions was during the first week of treatment.
  - Monitor for signs/symptoms and hold infusion for grades 3–4 reactions. Postmarketing reports have described reactions including syncope, pulmonary infiltrates, ARDS, cardiopulmonary arrest, myocardial infarction, acute cardiac insufficiency, angioedema, and anaphylaxis.
  - The drug dose must be gradually increased at the initiation of therapy or if therapy is interrupted for 7 or more days; in addition, the patient should receive premedication prior to dosing. Institute medical management (e.g., glucocorticoids, epinephrine, meperidine) as needed and ordered.
- *Immunosuppression/Infections:*
  - Hold drug for serious infections and during antiviral treatment for CMV infection or confirmed CMV viremia (PCR positive CMV in $\geq$ 2 consecutive samples obtained 1 week apart).
  - Administer therapeutic ganciclovir or equivalent for CMV infection or confirmed CMV viremia.
- *Laboratory Monitoring:*
  - Assess CBC at weekly intervals during alemtuzumab therapy and more frequently if worsening anemia, neutropenia, or thrombocytopenia occurs.
  - After treatment, assess CD4+ counts until recovery to $\geq$ 200 cells/μL.

- After receiving alemtuzumab for initial CLL therapy, recovery of CD4+ counts to ≥ 200 cells/μL occurred by 6 months' posttreatment (median at 2 months was 183 cells/μL). In previously treated patients, median time to recovery of CD4+ counts to ≥ 200 cells/μL was 2 months; full recovery to baseline CD4+ and CD8+ may take > 12 months.
- *Immunization:* DO NOT administer live viral vaccines to patients who have recently received alemtuzumab as it is unknown if patients will be able to generate an immune response.
- Administer ONLY irradiated blood products to avoid transfusion associated graft versus host disease (TAGVHD), unless emergency.
- Embryo-fetal toxicity:
  - It is not known if alemtuzumab causes fetal harm. Women of reproductive potential should avoid pregnancy by using effective contraception during therapy and for at least 6 months after last drug dose. Drug should be given to a pregnant woman only if clearly needed. Nursing mothers should make a decision whether to discontinue nursing or alemtuzumab, taking into account the elimination half-life of alemtuzumab and the importance of the drug to the mother's health.
- Subcutaneous and intravenous have similar efficacy and effect.
- Following 3-times-a-week therapy, destruction of CLL cells takes about 14 days before being removed from the peripheral blood, with no cells detectable at 5 weeks. Bone marrow clearance takes 6–12 weeks, and bulky lymphadenopathy takes considerably longer. Large, bulky lymph nodes are less responsive to therapy (Chu & DeVita, 2016).
- Lemtrada (alemtuzumab) is FDA indicated for treatment of patients with relapsing multiple sclerosis (MS) and should not be confused with Campath (alemtuzumab).

Potential Toxicities/Side Effects (Dose- and Schedule-Dependent) and the Nursing Process

I.   POTENTIAL FOR INJURY related to INFUSION REACTIONS, HYPERSENSITIVITY REACTION DURING INFUSION

Defining Characteristics: Infusion reactions are common and require premedication to prevent them. Symptoms occur during or shortly after drug infusion (pyrexia, chills/rigors, nausea, hypotension, urticaria, dyspnea, rash, emesis, and bronchospasm) with highest incidence the first week of therapy. Hypotension occurs in 15%, rash in 30%, nausea in 47%, vomiting in 33%, drug-related fever 83%, and rigors in 89% of patients. Infusion reactions usually resolve after 1 week of therapy. Subcutaneous dosing significantly reduces the risk of allergic reactions. Rarely, syncope, pulmonary infiltrates, ARDS, respiratory arrest, cardiac arrhythmias, MI, acute cardiac insufficiency, cardiac arrest, angioedema, and anaphylactoid shock have been described in postmarketing reports.

Nursing Implications: Assess vital signs baseline and frequently during infusion, especially during dose escalation. Teach patient that reactions may occur and to tell nurse or physician immediately. Administer premedication as ordered, usually 500–1,000 mg acetaminophen and 50-mg diphenhydramine 30 minutes prior to infusion. Provide adequate hydration, as this seems to decrease the incidence of infusion reactions (e.g., at least 500 mL before and after dose). Dose is begun low at 3 mg, then gradually increased based on patient tolerance to 10-mg dose, then to a 30-mg dose. If the patient has a treatment break of 7 days or more, then it is necessary to reintroduce drug at the lower dose and gradually escalate dose. Assess skin for integrity and presence of rash. Teach patient to report this, and discuss management with physician. Teach patient that nausea may develop and to report it right away. Discuss antiemetic agent with physician, and administer as ordered. If reaction happens, stop infusion but keep main IV line open, notify physician, and, if rigors, give meperidine and any other medications ordered by physician. Expect reaction to resolve in 20 minutes or so and gradually resume infusion per physician order. Withhold drug for grades 3–4 infusion reactions; give glucocorticoids and/or epinephrine per physician order when needed. Emergency equipment should be available; rarely, reaction can be severe.

II. POTENTIAL FOR INFECTION AND BLEEDING related to BONE MARROW DEPRESSION

Defining Characteristics: Drug kills lymphocytes, plus other infection-fighting cells of the immune system (e.g., monocytes, macrophages, NK cells). Severe lymphopenia and a rapid and sustained decrease in lymphocyte subsets occur after drug is given. In previously untreated patients, CD4+ count was 0 cells at 1 month after treatment (normal is 500–1,500 cells/μL), recovering to 238/μL at 6 months. All patients develop leukopenia, with approximately 99% lymphopenic, and 85% of patients developing neutropenia. The incidence of thrombocytopenia is 71% with platelet recovery weeks 7–12; incidence of anemia is 76%. There is a dramatic fall in WBC during the first week. As both T- and B-cell lymphocytes are killed, patients are at an increased risk for bacterial, viral, and other opportunistic infections. Most patients require prophylactic antimicrobials with/without antiviral therapy, especially heavily pretreated patients. Most common pulmonary infections are opportunistic: *Pneumocystis jiroveci (carinii)* pneumonia (PCP), cytomegalus virus (CMV) pneumonia, and pulmonary aspergillosis. Commonly, there is reactivation of herpes simplex infections and development of oral candidiasis. Rarely, pancytopenia, marrow aplasia, autoimmune anemia, severe autoimmune thrombocytopenia, and prolonged myelosuppression have occurred and may be fatal.

Nursing Implications: Assess baseline leukocyte, platelet, and Hgb/HCT; monitor before each treatment, during therapy at least weekly, and more often as needed. Ensure that a single drug dose does not exceed 30 mg, and that the cumulative weekly drug total does not exceed 90 mg. Hold drug for ANC < 250/μL or platelets ≤ 25,000/μL. See package insert for dose modifications. Teach that patient is at risk for opportunistic infections, to take medications as prescribed, and to report any problems or changes right away. Teach patient about recommended antimicrobials as ordered: trimethoprim/sulfamethoxazole DS twice daily 3 times a week (PCP prophylaxis), and famociclavir 250 mg twice daily as herpetic prophylaxis. Assess risk for infection and integrity of skin and mucous membranes, pulmonary status, and ability to clear secretions, as well as history of past infections, baseline and prior to each treatment. Teach patient to self-administer prophylactic antibiotics, antiviral, and antifungal agents as ordered by physician. Ensure that patient has coverage or can purchase antimicrobial medications. Teach patient to self-administer oral antifungal agent if oral candidiasis develops. Teach patient to self-assess for signs/symptoms of infection and to call provider immediately or come to the emergency room if temperature > 100.5°F, shaking chills, or rash, productive cough, burning on urination, or any signs/symptoms of infection or bleeding. Teach self-care strategies to minimize risk of infection and bleeding, including avoidance of OTC aspirin-containing medications. Following completion of therapy, assess and follow CD4 counts until recovery greater than or equal to 200 cells/μL. If serious infection develops, drug should be interrupted until infection resolves. Patient should NOT receive live vaccines during or recently after Campath treatment. The drug should be permanently discontinued for autoimmune or severe hematologic adverse reactions.

III.   ALTERATION IN OXYGENATION, POTENTIAL, related to HYPOTENSION, HYPERTENSION, TACHYCARDIA

Defining Characteristics: Hypotension is common, affecting 32% of patients in clinical studies, while 11% had hypertension. Eleven percent of patients also had sinus or supraventricular tachycardia.

Nursing Implications: Assess baseline cardiac status, including blood pressure and heart rate, noting rhythm and rate. Assess past medical history for arrhythmia, hypertension. If the heart rate is irregular, document rhythm on EKG, monitor blood pressure for evidence of decompensation, and discuss management with physician. If hypertension noted, discuss management with physician. If hypotension noted, assess patient tolerance and need for intervention; discuss management with physician.

Drug: Atezolizumab (Tecentriq) injection

Class: PD-L1 blocking mAb.

Mechanism of Action: Drug is an Fc-engineered, humanized, mAb (IgG1) that binds to PD-L1 and blocks interaction between PD-1 and B7.1 receptors. PD-L1 may be expressed on tumor cells and tumor-infiltrating immune cells in the microenvironment, which then may help block the body's antitumor immune response. Atezolizumab binds to PD-L1 and blocks its interaction with PD-1 and B7.1 receptors, which releases the blockade PD-L1/PD-1 hold over the patient's immune response. This allows T-lymphocytes to resume doing their job by attacking the invading tumor cells as well as those in the microenvironment. This does not involve antibody-dependent cellular cytotoxicity (ADCC, Genentech, 2016).

Metabolism: Terminal half-life of atezolizumab is 27 days. Steady state is achieved after 6–9 weeks of therapy (2–3 cycles).

Indications: Adult patients with (1) *locally advanced or metastatic urothelial carcinoma* who:

(1a) are ineligible for cisplatin-containing chemotherapy and whose tumors express PD-L1 [PD-L1 stained tumor-infiltrating immune cells [IC] covering $\geq$ 5% of tumor area) as determined by an FDA-approved test, OR (1b) are not eligible for any platinum-containing chemotherapy regardless of level of tumor PD-L1 status;, OR (1c) have disease progression during or following any platinum-containing chemotherapy or within 12 months of neoadjuvant or adjuvant chemotherapy. **Patient selection:** select cisplatin-ineligible patients with previously untreated locally advanced or metastatic urothelial carcinoma for treatment based on the PD-L1 expression on tumor-infiltrating immune cells. [Acelerated approval is based on tumor response and duration of response; continued approval for this indication may be contingent upon verification and description of clinical benefit in confirmatory trials.];

(2) *metastatic NSCLC* who (2a) have non-squamous histology without *EGFR* or *ALK* genomic tumor aberrations, as first-line therapy with bevacizumab, paclitaxel, and carboplatin; (2b) have disease progression during or following platinum-containing chemotherapy. If *EGFR* or *ALK* mutation positive, the patient has disease progression on FDA-approved treatment for the mutation; (3) *unresectable locally advanced or metastatic triple negative breast cancer* (TNBC) whose tumors express PD-L1 as determined by an FDA approved test, together with paclitaxel protein bound (accelerated approval); (4) *extensive stage SCLC* (ES-SCLC) in combination with carboplatin and etoposide (accelerated approval).

Contraindications: None.

Dosing/Range:
- Urothelial carcinoma: 1,200 mg as an IV infusion over 60 minutes every 3 weeks, until disease progression or unacceptable toxicity.
- NSCLC: 1,200 mg as an IV infusion over 60 minutes every 3 weeks; if administered in combination, administer atezolizumab prior to chemotherapy or other antineoplastic drug(s) when administered on the same day.
- Metastatic TNBC: 840 mg IV over 60 minutes followed by 100 mg/m^2 paclitaxel protein-bound. For each 28 day cycle, atezolizumab is administered on days 1 and 15, and paclitaxel protein-bound is administered on days 1, 8 and 15.
- SCLC: 1,200 mg as an IV infusion over 60 minutes every 3 weeks; if administered in combination, administer atezolizumab prior to chemotherapy when administered on the same day.
- If the 1st infusion is well tolerated, give all subsequent infusions over 30 minutes.

Dose Modifications: No dose reductions are recommended. Hold drug until toxicity resolves to grade 0–1, and if corticosteroid are administered, dose is $\leq$ 10 mg prednisone (or equivalent) a day; then resume drug. No dose reductions.
- Hold drug for (1) grade 2 pneumonitis; (2) hepatitis: AST or ALT > 3–8 × ULN or total BR > 1.5–3 × ULN; (3) colitis or diarrhea: grade 2–3; (4) grade 2–4 endocrinopathies or Type I DM; (5) grade 3 irAE involving a major organ, (6) infections grade 3–4: until grade 1 or resolved.

- Permanently discontinue for (1) grades 3–4 pneumonitis; (2) hepatitis: AST or ALT > 8 × ULN or total BR > 3 × ULN; (3) grade 4 colitis or diarrhea: (3) persistent grade 2–3 AEs (except endocrinopathies) that do not receover to grade 0–1 within 12 weeks; (4) inability to taper corticosteroid (to ≤ 10 mg/day or equivalent, within 12 weeks after last drug dose; (5) recurrent grade 3–4 AE.
- Infusion-related reactions: (1) grade 1–2: interrupt or slow infusion rate; (2) grade 3–4: permanently discontinue drug.

Drug Preparation: Drug is available as 840 mg/14 mL (60 mg/mL) and 1,200 mg/20 mL (60 mg/mL) solution in a single-dose vial. Dilute prior to infusion. Solution is colorless to slightly yellow in a single-dose vial.

Prepare solution for infusion:
- Withdraw ordered dose from vial(s).
- Dilute into a 250 mL PVC, polyethylene (PE) or polyolefin (PO) infusion bag containing 0.9% sodium chloride injection USP.
- Dilute with 0.9% sodium chloride injection USP, only.
- Mix diluted solution by gentle inversion; do NOT shake.
- Discard partially used or empty vials of atezolizumab.

Storage of infusion solution:
- Product does not contain a preservative.
- Administer immediately once prepared. If diluted solution is not used immediately, it can be stored either (1) at room temperature for no more than 6 hours from the preparation time (includes room temperature storage of the infusion in the infusion bag and time for drug administration); or (2) under refrigeration at 2–8°C (36–46°F) for no more than 24 hours from time of preparation.
- Do NOT freeze, do not shake.

Drug Administration:
- Infuse the first dose of atezolizumab over 60 minutes through an IV line with or without a sterile, nonpyrogenic, low-protein binding in-line filter (pore size 0.2–0.22 micron).
- If the first infusion is well tolerated, all subsequent infusions can be given over 30 minutes.
- DO NOT administer as IVP or IV bolus. Do not coadminster other drugs thorough the same IV line.

Drug Interactions: Unknown.

Lab Effects/Interference:
- Lymphopenia, anemia
- Increased LFTs (ALT, AST, alkaline phosphatase), serum creatinine, hyperglycemia, hyper- or hypothyroidism (increased or decreased TSH), hyponatremia, hypoalbuminemia
- Increased serum amylase or lipase

Special Considerations:
- FDA (2018) limited the use of atezolizumab and pembrolizumab for patients with locally advanced or metastatic urothelial cancer who are not eligible for cis-platinum containing

therapy. Studies showed decreased survival when either of these drugs was given as a single agent compared to platinum-based chemotherapy in previously untreated patients with locally advanced or metastatic urothelial cancer whose tumors had no or low expression of PD-L1. As of 2018, patients must be ineligible for treatment with a cisplatin containing regimen and have a PD-L1 expression of ($\geq$ 5%) of tumor area (stained tumor-infiltrating immune cells), or be patients who are not eligible for cisplatinum-containing chemotherapy regardless of PD-L1 tumor expression (FDA, 2018).

- Most common adverse reactions ($\geq$ 20%):
- As a single agent: fatigue/asthenia, nausea, cough, dyspnea, and decreased appetite.
- In combination with other antineoplastic drugs in patients with NSCLC and SCLC: fatigue/asthenia, nausea, alopecia, constipation, diarrhea, and decreased appetite.
- In combination with paclitaxel protein-bound in patients with TNBC were: alopecia, peripheral neuropathies, fatigue, nausea, diarrhea, anemia, constipation, cough, headache, neutropenia, vomiting, and decreased appetite.
- Warnings and Precautions:
  - *Immune-related pneumonitis:* Incidence across trials was 2.5%. Median time to onset was 3.6 months, with a median duration of 1.4 months. Monitor patients for signs with radiographic imaging, and assess for symptoms of pneumonitis. Hold drug for grade 2 pneumonitis, and administer corticosteroids at 1–2 mg/kg/day prednisone equivalents for grade 2 or higher pneumonitis, followed by a taper. Permanently discontinue for grades 3–4 pneumonitis.
  - *Immune-related hepatitis:* Across clinical trials, incidence of hepatits was 9% in patients receiving atezolizumab as a single agent. Immune-related hepatitis is defined as requiring corticosteroid therapy. Median time to onset 1.4 months, and median duration was 24 days. Hepatitis resolved in 71% of patients. Monitor for signs and symptoms of hepatitis during drug therapy and after completion. Monitor AST, ALT, and bilirubin baseline and periodically during treatment. Hold drug for grade 2, and administer corticosteroids at 1–2 mg/kg/day prednisone equivalents for grade 2 or higher transaminase elevations with or without concomitant elevation in total bilirubin, followed by a corticosteroid taper. Permanently discontinue for grades 3–4 immune-mediated hepatitis, severe or life-threatening transaminase, or total BR elevation.
  - *Immune-related colitis:* Across clinical trials, incidence of diarrhea and colitis was 20%, with median time to onset 1.5 months. Monitor for signs/symptoms of diarrhea or colitis. Hold drug for grade 2 and higher; if symptoms persist for >5 days, or recur, administer corticosteroids 1–2 mg/kg prednisone or equivalent per day, followed by a taper. Consider IV methylprednisolone 1–2 mg/kg/day and convert to oral steroids once the patient has improved. For both grades 2 and 3 diarrhea or colitis, when symptoms improve to grades 0–1, taper steroids over $\geq$ 1 month. Resume treatment with atezolizumab if the event improves to grades 0–1 within 12 weeks and corticosteroids have been reduced to the equivalent of $\leq$ 10 mg oral prednisone per day. Permanently discontinue for grade 4 diarrhea or colitis.
  - *Immune-related endocrinopathies:* Monitor patients for signs and symptoms of endocrinopathies. See package insert for corticosteroids and hormone replacement recommendations.

- Hypophysitis: incidence of grade <0.1%. For grade 2 or higher, patient should receive prednisone 1–2 mg/kg/day or equivalent followed by taper and hormone replacement as clinically indicated.
- Thyroid disorders: monitor for changes in thyroid function; hold drug for symptomatic thyroid disease.
- Adrenal insufficiency: incidence 0.4%, median time to onset 5.7 months. Monitor for clinical signs and symptoms. For grade 2 or higher, patient should receive prednisone 1–2 mg/kg/day or equivalent followed by taper and hormone replacement as clinically indicated. Drug should be interrupted based on severity.
- Type I diabetes mellitus: incidence <0.1%. Monitor patient for hyperglycemia or other signs/symptoms of diabetes. Patient should receive insulin as ordered and clinically indicated. Drug should be interrupted based on severity.
- *Other immune-related adverse effects:* see package insert for management
  - Neurologic: e.g., *myasthenic syndrome/myasthenia gravis,* Guillain–Barré or meningoencephalitis, motor and sensory neuropathy:
  - ocular inflammatory toxicity (e.g., uveitis iritis)
  - myocarditis
  - dermatologic
  - systemic inflammatory response syndrome
  - hematologic
  - renal dysfunction, nephrotic syndrome, nephritis
  - vasculitis
  - musculoskeletal (e.g., myositis)
  - pancreatitis: Incidence 0.1%.
- *Infection:* Severe infections can occur, and may be fatal. Incidence of infection across clinical trials was 42%. Monitor patient for signs and symptoms of infection and treat with antibacterial(s) for suspected or confirmed bacterial infection. Drug should be held for grade 3 or higher infection, and drug resumed once the patient is clinically stable.
- *Infusion reaction (IRs):* IRs can be severe or life-threatening. Incidence of infusion reactions across all clinical trials was 1.3%. Interrupt or slow the rate of infusion for mild or moderate infusion reactions, and consider pre-medication with subsequent doses. Discontinue for grades 3–4 infusion reactions. Incidence of IRs was similar in patients receiving drug as a single agent or in combination with other antineoplastics.
- *Embryo-fetal toxicity:* Teach women of reproductive potential of the potential risk to the fetus, and use effective contraception to prevent pregnancy during therapy and for at least 5 months after the last drug dose. Mothers should not breastfeed while receiving the drug.

Potential Toxicities/Side Effects and the Nursing Process

I.   ALTERATION IN COMFORT related to FATIGUE, PYREXIA, PERIPHERAL EDEMA, BACK/NECK PAIN, ARTHRALGIA

Defining Characteristics: Fatigue occurred in 52% of patients. Common incidences of pyrexia was 21%, peripheral edema 21%, back/neck pain 15%, and arthralgias 14%.

Nursing Implications: Teach the patient that these events may occur and to report them. Assess baseline comfort and self-care strategies to maintain comfort and energy conservation. Monitor closely during treatment. Develop a plan to assure comfort, depending on the symptoms reported, and assess its efficacy and revise the plan if needed at each visit.

II. ALTERATION IN NUTRITION, POTENTIAL, LESS THAN BODY REQUIREMENTS, related to DECREASED APPETITE, NAUSEA, CONSTIPATION, VOMITING, OR DIARRHEA

Defining Characteristics: Nutritional impact symptoms can occur with the following frequencies across clinical trials: nausea (25%), vomiting (17%), diarrhea (18%), constipation (21%), and decreased appetite (26%).

Nursing Implications: Assess nutritional and bowel-elimination patterns, appetite, and presence of nausea and/or vomiting at baseline and at each visit. Teach that diarrhea, constipation, nausea, vomiting, and decreased appetite may occur and to report them. Assess nutrition impact symptoms and discuss their management with the physician. Teach the patient to self-administer antidiarrheal or antiemetic medication, if needed, and to report symptoms that do not improve. In addition, teach patients to report immediately any diarrhea, blood in stool or black stools, and severe stomach pain or tenderness so that the potential for colitis may be further evaluated.

III. ALTERATION IN SKIN INTEGRITY, POTENTIAL, related to RASH, PRURITUS, OR EDEMA

Defining Characteristics: Skin integrity can be affected by rash, edema, and pruritis.

Nursing Implications: Teach the patient that rash, pruritus, and peripheral edema may occur and to report them. Assess the patient's skin integrity and determine the presence of edema, both at baseline and regularly during therapy. Teach patient self-care measures to reduce pruritis.

IV. POTENTIAL ALTERATION IN OXYGENATION related to PNEUMONITIS

Defining Characteristics: In all clinical trials, pneumonitis incidence was 2.6% with median time to onset of 2.6 months in urothelial cancer patients and 3.3 months with median duration of 1.4 months for patients with NSCLC.

Nursing Implications: Teach the patient to report new or worsening cough, chest pain, or shortness of breath. Monitor the patient for signs and symptoms of pneumonitis. Discuss findings with the physician/NP/PA. Expect that after exclusion of other diagnoses, the patient will be evaluated with imaging and pulmonary and infectious disease consultation if respiratory status changes occur. See Special Considerations.

V.   POTENTIAL ALTERATION IN ELIMINATION related to COLITIS

Defining Characteristics: Incidence of diarrhea or colitis was 18.7% in patients with urothelial carcinoma and 19.3% in NSCLC patients. Grade 3–4 diarrhea occurred in 1.9% of patients. Incidence of immune-mediated colitis or diarrhea was 0.8%, with median time to onset of 1.7 months.

Nursing Implications: Monitor patients for immune-mediated colitis. Teach the patient to report signs and symptoms of colitis right away (diarrhea, blood in stools or tarry stools, severe abdominal pain). Ensure patient remains well hydrated. Monitor the patient for immune-mediated colitis, and administer corticosteroids as ordered. See Special Considerations.

VI.   POTENTIAL ALTERATION IN NUTRTION related to HEPATITIS

Defining Characteristics: Immune-mediated hepatitis (defined as requiring use of corticosteroids and no clear alternate etiology) and abnormal LFTs may occur. Incidence of immune-mediated hepatitis was 1.3% of urothelial cancer patients and 0.9% in NSCLC patients. Median time to onset was 1.1 months (urothelial) and 28 days (NSCLC). No patient developed recurrence of hepatitis once therapy resumed after temporary interruption. Signs and symptoms of hepatitis include elevated transaminases and total bilirubin, icterus, severe nausea and vomiting, right-sided abdominal pain, drowsiness, dark urine, increased bruisability or bleeding, and anorexia.

Nursing Implications: Assess LFTs at baseline and monitor regularly during therapy. Evaluate the patient for right-sided abdominal pain, drowsiness, dark urine, increased bruising or bleeding, and loss of appetite. Teach the patient to report any yellowing of the skin or whites of the eyes, as well as severe nausea or vomiting. See Special Considerations.

VIII.   POTENTIAL ALTERATION IN ENDOCRINE FUNCTION related to HYPOTHYROIDISM, HYPERTHYROIDISM, HYPERGLYCEMIA, OR ADRENAL CRISIS

Defining Characteristics: Incidence in all urothelial cancer clinical trials for hypothyroidism was 2.5% and for NSCLC patients was 4.2%. Type 1 diabetes mellitus may occur (incidence 0.2–0.3%).

Nursing Implications: Monitor thyroid function at baseline and periodically during therapy. Monitor for hyperglycemia. Teach the patient to report signs and symptoms of hyper- and hypothyroidism, such as headaches that do not go away, extreme tiredness, weight gain or loss, changes in mood or behavior, dizziness or fainting, hair loss, feeling cold, constipation, and deep and/or hoarse voice. Discuss and teach the patient about ordered hormone replacement therapy for hypothyroidism, or medical management of hyperthyroidism. If hypothyroidism occurs, the patient should receive hormone replacement therapy. If hyperthyroidism occurs, discuss medical management with the physician/NP/PA. Teach patient to self-assess for and report signs/symptoms of hypo- and hyperglycemia. See package insert for further assessment and management (Genentech, 2019).

Drug: Avelumab (Bavencio)

Classification: PD-L1 blocking human IgG1 lambda mAb.

Mechanism of Action: Tumor cells and tumor-infiltrating immune cells express PD-L1, which turns-off the antitumor immune response in the tumor microenvironment. The PD-L1 receptors on these cells bind to PD-1 and B7.1 receptors on the patient's T-cells and APCs, which then turns off cytotoxic T-cell activity, T-cell proliferation, and cytokine production (EMD Serano, Inc. 2017). Avelumab binds to PD-L1, thus preventing PD-L1 from binding to its receptors PD-1 and B7.1. By blocking this interaction, PD-L1 no longer suppresses the immune response so antitumor cytotoxity is restored.

Metabolism: Steady-state is reached after approximately 4–6 weeks (2–3 cycles of drug) with repeated dosing. Avelumab is eliminated from the body by proteolytic degradation, with a terminal half-life of 6.1 days at a dose of 10 mg/kg.

Indications: Treatment of patients with (1) *metastatic Merkel cell carcinoma* (MCC) (adults and pediatric patients aged 12 years and older); (2) *locally advanced or metastatic urothelial carcinoma* (UC) who (a) have disease progression during or after platinum-containing chemotherapy, or (b) have disease progression within 12 months of neoadjuvant or adjuvant treatment with a cisplatinum-containing chemotherapy; (3) advanced renal cell cancer, as first line in combination with axitinib. Indications (1–2) are accelerated approvals based on tumor response and response duration. Continued approval may be contingent upon verification and description of clinical benefit.

Contraindication: None.

Dosage Range:
- 800 mg IV infusion over 60 minutes every 2 weeks until progression or unacceptable toxicity. For RCC, drug is given in combination with axitinib 5 mg PO bid (12 hours apart) with or without food. Dose escalation of axitinib above initial 5 mg dose may be considered at intervals of 2 weeks or longer. See axitinib prescribing guidelines.
- Patients should be premedicated with an antihistamine and acetaminophen *prior to the first 4 infusions*, then as needed prior to subsequent cycles of therapy.

Dose Modifications:
- Pneumonitis: *Grade 2*, hold avelumab; resume in patients with complete or partial resolution (grades 0–1) after corticosteroid taper. *Grades 3–4, or recurrent grade 2 pneumonitis*: permanently discontinue avelumab.
- Hepatitis:
  - Monotherapy:
    - *AST/ALT >3 to 5 × ULN or total bilirubin > 1.5 and up to 3 × ULN:* Hold avelumab, and resume in patients with complete or partial resolution (grades 0–1) of hepatitis after corticosteroid taper.

- *AST/ALT > 5 × ULN or total bilirubin > 3 × ULN:* permanently discontinue avelumab.
- In combination with axitinib for first line treatment of RCC:
  - If *AST/ALT >3 to 5 × ULN or total bilirubin ≥ 1.5 and up to 3 × ULN:* Hold avelumab and axitinib until recovery to grades 0-1. If persistent (>5 days), consider corticosteroid therapy [initial dose 0.5–1 mg/kg/day] prednisone/equivalent followed by taper. Consider rechallenge with a single drug or sequential rechallenge with both drugs after recovery. Dose reduce per axitinib package insert if rechallenging with axitinib.
  - If *AST/ALT ≥ 5 × ULN or total bilirubin > 3 × ULN with total bilirubin ≥ 2 × ULN or total bilirubin ≥ 3 × ULN,* permanently discontinue avelumab and axtinib and consider corticosteroid therapy [initial dose 1–2 mg/kg/day prednisone/equivalent followed by a taper].
- Colitis: *Grades 2–3 diarrhea or colitis:* hold avelumab; resume in patients with complete or partial resolution (grades 0–1) of colitis or diarrhea after corticosteroid taper. *Grade 4 diarrhea or colitis, or recurrent grade 3 diarrhea or colitis:* permanently discontinue avelumab.
- Endocrinopathies (e.g., hypothyroidism, hyperthyroidism, adrenal insufficiency, hyperglycemia): *Grades 3–4:* hold avelumab; resume in patients with complete or partial resolution (grades 0–1) of endocrinopathies after corticosteroid taper.
- Nephritis and Renal Dysfunction: *Serum creatinine > 1.5 and up to 6 × ULN:* hold avelumab; resume in patients with complete or partial resolution (grades 0–1) of nephritis and renal dysfunction after corticosteroid taper. *Serum creatinine > 6 × ULN:* permanently discontinue avelumab.
- Other immune-related adverse reactions (see package insert): *Moderate or severe clinical signs or symptoms, or grades 3–4 endocrinopathies:* hold avelumab pending clinical evaluation; resume in patients with complete or partial resolution (grades 0–1) of other immune-mediated adverse reactions after corticosteroid taper.
  - For moderate or severe clinical signs or symptoms of an immune-mediated adverse reaction not described in package insert or grade 3-4 endocrinopathies: hold avelumab pending clinical evaluation. Resume avelumab in patients with complete or partial resolution (grade 0–1) or other immune-mediated adverse reactions after corticosteroid taper.
  - Stevens Johnson Syndrome (SJS), toxic epidermal necrolysis (TEN), rhabdomyolysis, myasthenia gravis, histiocytic necrotizing lymphadenitis, demyelination vasculitis, hemolytic anemia, hypophysitis, iritis, and encephalopathy: Permanently discontinue avelumab for (1) life-threatening adverse reaction excluding endocrinopathies, (2) recurrent severe immune-mediated adverse reaction, (3) requirement for 10 mg per day or more prednisone/equivalent for >12 weeks or longer.
- Infusion-related: *Grades 1–2:* interrupt or slow rate of infusion. *Grades 3–4:* permanently discontinue avelumab. Grades 3–4, permanently discontinue avelumab.

Drug Preparation:
- Preparation:
  - Available as 200 mg/10 mL (20 mg/mL) in a single dose vial.

- Visually inspect for particulate matter and discoloration (should be clear, colorless to slightly yellow) and discard vial if cloudy, discolored or contains particulate matter.
- Asceptically withdraw calculated volume required from avelumab vial, and inject into a 250 mL infusion bag containing either 0.9% Sodium Chloride Injection or 0.45% Sodium Chloride Injection. Gently invert bag to mix and avoid foaming or excessive shearing.
- Inspect solution (should be clear, colorless, and free of visible particles).
- Discard any partially used or empty vials.
- Storage:
  - At room temperature (up to 77°F [25°C]) for no more than 4 hours from time of dilution, OR.
  - Refrigerated (36–46°F [2–8°C]) for no more than 24 hours from time of dilution; allow to come up to room temperature prior to administration.
  - Do not freeze or shake diluted solution.

Drug Administration:
- Assess for signs/symptoms of immune mediated adverse effects (e.g., pneumonitis, hepatitis, colitis, hyperglycemia/type 1 DM, nephritis/renal dysfunction, and other immune-mediated effects [see package insert]).
- Assess laboratory parameters baseline and prior to each cycle, then periodically: CBC, metabolic profile including LFTs, serum glucose; monitor thyroid function tests (TFTs) and serum creatinine baseline and then periodically.
- Administer premedication as ordered (antihistamine, acetaminophen) for first 4 cycles and then if needed for subsequent cycles.
- Administer diluted solution over 60 minutes through patent IV containing a sterile, nonpyrogenic, low-protein binding in-line filter (pore size 0.2 micron).
- Monitor for infusion reaction and manage per guidelines.
- Do not coadminister other drugs through the same IV line.

Drug Interactions: None known.

Laboratory Effects/Interference:
- Increased AST, ALT; serum lipase, amylase, bilirubin, glucose, creatinine, potassium, bilirubin.
- Decreased serum sodium.
- Anemia, lymphopenia, thrombocytopenia, neutropenia.

Special Considerations:
- Most common adverse reactions (≥20%): fatigue, musculoskeletal pain, diarrhea, nausea, IRRs, rash, decreased appetite, peripheral edema.
- Warnings and Precautions:
  - *Immune-related (IR) pneumonitis:* hold avelumab for moderate pneumonitis; permanently discontinue for severe, life-threatening, or recurrent moderate pneumonitis.
  - *IR hepatitis:* Monitor for changes in liver function. Hold avelumab for moderate hepatitis. Permanently discontinue for severe or life-threatening hepatitis. Incidence of hepatotoxicity (grade 3–4 ALT and AST elevation) is higher when avelumab is

combined with axitinib. Consider more frequent monitoring of LFTs when the combination is given. Hold avelumab and axitinib for moderate (grade 2) hepatotoxicity, and permanently discontinue the combination for severe or life-threatening (grade 3–4) hepatotoxicity. Administer corticosteroids as needed and ordered.

- *IR colitis:* hold avelumab for moderate or severe colitis. Permanently discontinue for life-threatening or recurrent severe colitis.
- *IR endocrinopathies:* Hold drug for severe (grade 3) or life-threatening (grade 4) endocrinopathies.
- Monitor for signs and symptoms of adrenal insufficiency (e.g., extreme fatigue, weight loss, decreased appetitie, hyperpigmentation, hypotension, salt craving, hypoglycemia, nausea, vomiting, diarrhea) during and after treatment. Administer corticosteroids as ordered.
- Assess for hypothyroidism and hyperthyroidism, which can occur at any time during treatment.
- Assess for Type I diabetes mellitus.
- *IR nephritis and renal dysfunction:* hold avelumab for moderate or severe nephritis or renal dysfunction. Permanently discontinue for life-threatening nephritis or renal dysfunction.
- *Other IR advaerse events:* may involve any organ system, most occurring during treatment with avelumab, but some may appear after last drug dose. See package insert.
- *IRRs:* Premedicate with an antihistamine and acetaminophen as ordered. Monitor for signs/symptoms of IRRs including pyrexia, chills, flushing, hypotension, dyspnea, wheezing, back pain, abdominal pain, and urticaria. Interrupt or slow the infusion rate for mild or moderate IRRs. Stop the infusion and permanently discontinue for severe or life-threatening IRRs.
- *Major adverse cardiovascular events (MACE):* Avelumab in combination with axitinib may cause severe and fatal cardiovascular events. Consider baseline LVEF determination and periodic evaluation during therapy. Reduce risk by controlling HTN, DM, or dyslipidemia. Discontinue avelumab and axitinib for grade 3–4 cardiovascular events. Incidence of MACE was 7% compared to 3.4% in the sunitinib-treated group. Events included death due to cardiovascular events (1.4%), grade 3–4 MI (2.8%), grade 3–4 CHF (1.8%). Mean time to onset was 4.2 months.
- *Embryo-fetal toxicity:* Avelumab can cause fetal harm. Teach female patients of reproductive potential to use effective contraception during treatment and for 1 month after last drug treatment to avoid pregnancy.
- Mothers should not breastfeed while receiving avelumab or for 1 month after last dose.

Potential Toxicities/Side Effects and the Nursing Process

I.   ALTERATION IN COMFORT related to FATIGUE, ASTHENIA, MUSCULOSKELETAL PAIN, ARTHRALGIA, RASH, PRURITIS, PERIPHERAL EDEMA

Defining Characteristics: In clinical trials, symptoms occurred in the following frequencies: fatigue and asthenia occurred in 50% of patients; musculoskeletal pain occurred in

32%, arthralgia in 16%, and peripheral edema in 20%; rash occurred in 22%, and pruritus in 10%.

Nursing Implications: Teach the patient that these events may occur and to report them. Assess baseline comfort and self-care strategies to maintain comfort and energy conservation. Assess the patient's skin integrity and determine the presence of edema, both at baseline and regularly during therapy. Monitor closely during treatment. Develop a plan to assure comfort, depending on the symptoms reported, and assess its efficacy and revise the plan if needed at each visit.

II. ALTERATION IN NUTRITION, POTENTIAL, LESS THAN BODY REQUIREMENTS, related to DECREASED APPETITE, NAUSEA, CONSTIPATION, DIARRHEA, VOMITING, IR HEPATITIS

Defining Characteristics: Nutritional impact symptoms of nausea, vomiting, diarrhea, constipation, and decreased appetite can occur as demonstrated in clinical trials. Diarrhea occurred in 23%, nausea in 22%, decreased appetite in 20%, constipation in 17%, and vomiting in 13%. IR hepatitis occurred in 0.9% of patients. When given in combination with axitinib, grades 3 and 4 increased ALT and AST occurred in 9% and 7% respectively. Median time to onset was 2.8 months, and median duration of hepatitis was 15 days.

Nursing Implications: Assess nutritional and bowel-elimination patterns, appetite, and presence of nausea and/or vomiting, and weight at baseline and at each visit. Assess LFTs baseline and periodically during treatment, identifying any abnormalities and discussing possibility of hepatitis for any abnormalities. Assess for signs/symptoms of hepatitis. Teach patient that diarrhea, constipation, nausea, vomiting, and decreased appetite may occur and to report them. Assess nutrition impact symptoms and discuss their management with the physician. Teach the patient to self-administer antidiarrheal stool softeners if constipation is present, or antiemetic medication, if needed, and to report symptoms that do not improve. In addition, teach patients to report immediately any diarrhea, blood in stool or black stools, and severe stomach pain or tenderness so that the potential for colitis may be further evaluated. See Problem IV.

III. POTENTIAL ALTERATION IN OXYGENATION related to PNEUMONITIS

Defining Characteristics: In all clinical trials, incidence was 1.2%, including 0.5% with grades 3–5. Median time to onset was 2.5 months (range 3 days to 11 months), and median duration was 7 weeks.

Nursing Implications: Teach the patient to report new or worsening cough, chest pain, or shortness of breath. Monitor the patient for signs and symptoms of pneumonitis. Discuss findings with the physician/NP/PA. Expect that after exclusion of other diagnoses, the patient will be evaluated with imaging and expect drug to be interrupted for grade 2 and higher, permanently stopped for grades 3–4 or recurrent grade 2; patient should be treated with corticosteroids with a taper, and drug may be resumed in patients with complete or partial resolution to grades 0–1.

IV. POTENTIAL ALTERATION IN ELIMINATION related to COLITIS

Defining Characteristics: Incidence of diarrhea or colitis was 1.5% with 0.4% of patients having grade 3. Median time to onset was 2.1 months, and median duration was 6 weeks.

Nursing Implications: Teach the patient to report signs and symptoms of colitis (diarrhea, blood in stools or tarry stools, severe abdominal pain). Drug should be held for grade 2 and higher (permanently discontinued for grade 4 or recurrent grade 3 diarrhea or colitis). Patients should receive a corticosteroid taper, and if complete or partial resolution (grades 0–1) those with grade 2 or 3 diarrhea or colitis may be restarted on the drug.

V. POTENTIAL ALTERATION IN NUTRTION related to HEPATITIS

Defining Characteristics: Immune-mediated hepatitis (defined as requiring use of corticosteroids and no clear alternate etiology) and abnormal LFTs may occur. Incidence in clinical trials was 0.9%. Signs and symptoms of hepatitis include elevated transaminases and total bilirubin, icterus, severe nausea and vomiting, right-sided abdominal pain, drowsiness, dark urine, increased bruisability or bleeding, and anorexia.

Nursing Implications: Assess LFTs at baseline and periodically as ordered during therapy. Evaluate the patient for right-sided abdominal pain, drowsiness, dark urine, increased bruising or bleeding, and loss of appetite. Teach the patient to report any yellowing of the skin or whites of the eyes, as well as severe nausea or vomiting. See dose modification section for management based on abnormal LFTs.

VI. POTENTIAL ALTERATION IN URINE ELIMINATION related to IMMUNE-MEDIATED NEPHRITIS AND RENAL DYSFUNCTION

Defining Characteristics: IR nephritis occurred in 0.1% of patients in clinical studies.

Nursing Implications: Assess the patient's baseline renal function and periodically during therapy. Teach the patient to report signs and symptoms such as a decrease in the amount of urine, blood in urine, ankle swelling, loss of appetite. Drug should be held for grade 2 (serum creatinine > 1.5–6 × ULN), and permanently discontinued for grades 3–4 (serum creatinine >6 × ULN). Patients with grade 2 nephritis can resume treatment once complete or partial resolution (grades 0–1) after corticosteroid therapy with taper.

VII. POTENTIAL ALTERATION IN ENDOCRINE FUNCTION related to HYPOTHYROIDISM, HYPERTHYROIDISM, HYPERGLYCEMIA, OR ADRENAL CRISIS

Defining Characteristics: Incidence in clinical trials for hypothyroidism was 5%, and for hyperthyroidism, 0.4%. Type 1 diabetes mellitus may occur (in clinical trials 0.1%). Adrenal insufficiency was uncommon (0.5%).

Nursing Implications: Monitor thyroid function at baseline and periodically during therapy. Monitor for hyperglycemia. Teach the patient to report signs and symptoms of hyper and hypothyroidism, such as headaches that do not go away, extreme tiredness, weight gain or loss, changes in mood or behavior, dizziness or fainting, hair loss, feeling cold, constipation, and deep and/or hoarse voice. Discuss and teach the patient about ordered hormone replacement therapy for hypothyroidism, or medical management of hyperthyroidism. If patient is hyperglycemic administer insulin as ordered, teach patient self-management. Monitor for signs/symptoms of adrenal insufficiency (chronic fatigue, muscle weakness, weight loss, nausea, vomiting, hypotension, hyperpigmentation of skin), hypophysitis/hypopituitarism (fatigue, lethargy, loss of libido, amenorrhea, dizziness, nausea, vomiting, diabetes insipidus). Drug should be held for grades 3–4, and can be when resolved to grades 0–1 after a corticosteroid taper.

Drug: axicabtagene ciloleucel (Yescarta™) suspension for IV infusion

Class: CD-19 directed genetically modified autologous T cell immunotherapy (CAR-T, Chimeric Antigen Receptor–T cell therapy)

Mechanism of Action: CD-19 directed genetically modified autologous T cell immunotherapy binds to CD-19 expressing malignant cells and normal B cells; the engagement of the of the anti-CD-19 chimeric antigen receptor T cells and the CD-19 expressing target cells turns on CD28, CD3-zeta costimulatory domains which then activate signaling to activate T-cells, and other processes (e.g., T-cell proliferation, acquisition of effector functions, and secretion of inflammatory cytokines and chemokines) that lead to killing the CD-19 expressing cells.

Metabolism: After drug infusion, peak elevation of cytokines (IL-6,8,10,15; TNF-α, IFN-γ, others),occurred within the first 14 days, returning to baseline within 28 days usually. B cell aplasia occurred as a result of killing of normal CD19 B-cells. After the drug infusion, the anti-CD-19 CAR T cells peaked around the first 7–14 days, and showed a rapid expansion followed by return to baseline by 3 months. The number of anti-CD19 CAR Tcells in the blood was positively associated with CR or PR. The median anti-CD19 cell Cmax in responders were 205% higher than non-responders, with median AUC of responders days 0–28 was 251% higher than non-responders. Patients that required immunosuppression for cytokine release syndrome (CRS) either tocilizumab or corticosteroids, had significantly higher anti-CD19 CAR T cells. The drug was not studied in patients with renal or hepatic impairment.

Indication: Treatment of adult patients with relapsed or refractory large B-cell lymphoma after 2+ lines of systemic therapy, including diffuse large B-cell lymphoma (DLBCL) not otherwise specified, primary mediastinal large B-cell lymphoma, high-grade B-cell lymphoma, and DLBCL arising from follicular lymphoma.

Limitations of Use: Axicabtagene ciloleucel in not indicated for treatment of patients with primary CNS lymphoma.

Dosage Range: Drug is available only through a restricted program under a Risk Evaluation and Mitigation Strategy (REMS) called Yescarta REMS. Axicabtagene ciloleucel is for autologous use only (patient's T-cells are removed, re-engineered to make a chimeric receptor that increases efficacy against the CD19 receptor on the B-lymphocytes, and increases proliferation of identical T-cells once reinfused into the patient's body to attack the malignant cells..

- Each single infusion bag contains a suspension of chimeric antigen receptor (CAR)-positive T cells in about 68 mL. The patient's target dose is 2×10^6 CAR-positive viable T-cells per kg body weight (maximum 2×10^8 CAR-positive viable T-cells) (Kite Pharma, 2017).

Drug Preparation:

Drug Administration: Drug is for autologous use only.
- Patient's identity must match patient identifiers on axicabtagene ciloleucel cassette and infusion bag. DO NOT administer if they do not match.
- Preparing patient for infusion: confirm availability of prepared axicabtagene ciloleucel prior to starting lymphodepletion regimen.

Pre-treatment: Administer lymphodepleting chemotherapy regimen (Cyclophophosphamide 500 mg/m^2 IV and fludarabine 30 mg/m^2 IV in the fifth, fourth, and third day before the planned infusion.

Premedication:
- Give acetaminophen 650 mg PO, diphenhydramine 12.5 mg IV or PO approximately 1 hr before axicabtagene ciloleucel infusion.
- Avoid prophylactic use of systemic corticosteroids as this may interfere with drug activity.
- Confirm availability of tocilizumab prior to infusion.

Preaparation of axicabtagene ciloleucel *for infusion:* Coordinate the timing of axicabtagene ciloleucel thaw and infusion. Confirm the infusion time in advance, and adjust the start time of thaw such that it will be ready for infusion when the patient is.
- Confirm patient identify with the patient identifiers on the axicabtagene ciloleucel cassette. DO NOT remove the drug bag from the cassette UNLESS the patient identifiers match. Once a match is confirmed, remove the axicabtagene ciloleucel product bag from the cassette and make sure it matches the drug bag label.
- Inspect the product bag for any loss of integrity (e.g., breaks, cracks) before thawing. If the bag is compromised, follow guidelines or call Kite Pharma at 1-844-454-KITE.
- Place the infusion bag inside a second sterile bag.
- Thaw axicabtagene ciloleucel at 37°C using a water bath or dry thaw method until no visible ice in infusion bag. Gently mix bag contents to disperse clumps of cells. Small clumps of cellular material should disperse with gentle maual mixing. DO NOT wash, spin down, or re-suspend bag contents.
- Once thawed, axicabtagene ciloleucel can remain at room temperature (20°C–25°C) for up to 3 hours.

Administration of axicabtagene ciloleucel (autologous use ONLY)
- Assess laboratory parameters. In women of reproductive potential, who are sexually active, pregnancy status should be verified as drug is not recommended during pregnancy.

- Ensure that tocilizumab and emergency equipment available prior to infusion and during patient recovery period.
- Do NOT use a leukodepleting filter; Central venous access is recommended for the infusion.
- Confirm patient's identity matches the patient identifiers on the axicabtagene ciloleucel product bag.
- Prime tubing with normal saline prior to infusion.
- Infuse entire contents of axicabtagene ciloleucel infusion bag withint 30 minutes by gravity or a peristaltic pump.
  - Gently agitate product bag during axicabtagene ciloleucel infusion to prevent cell clumping
  - Remember axicabtagene ciloleucel is stable at room temperature for up to 3 hours after thaw.
- After all infusion bag contents have been infused, infuse any remaining cells in the tubing by rinsing the tubing contents with normal saline at the same rate, to ensure all drug is infused.
- Use Universal Precautions and biosafety guidelines for handling and disposal of tubing, bags, and during administration, as axicabtagene ciloleucel contains human blood cells genetically altered with replication incompetent retroviral vector, and it is imperative to prevent potential transmission of infectious diseases.

Monitoring:
- Drug can only be administered at a certified healthcare facility.
- Monitor patients at least daily for 7 days at the certified healthcare facility after infusion for signs/symptoms of cytokine release syndrome (CRS) and neurologic toxicity. Ensure patients understand that they must remain within proximity of the certified healthcare facility for at least 4 weeks after the infusion.
  - CRS Grading and Management:
    - If CRS suspected, manage as below (Kite, 2017). Patients with grade 2 or greater symptoms should be monitored by continuous cardiac telemetry and pulse oximetry. If CRS is severe, assess ECHO to assess cardiac function. For severe, or life threatening CRS, consider ICU supportive therapy.
    - *Grade 1* (requires symptomatic treatment only, e.g., fever, nausea, fatigue, headache, malaise, myalgia); *Grade 2* (requires moderate intervention (e.g., oxygen requirement is <40% FiO$_2$; hypotension responsive to IV fluids or low dose vasopressor (1 only); grade 2 organ toxicity; *treatment:* administer tocilizumab 8 mg/kg IV over 1 hour (max dose 800 mg); repeat q 8 hrs $\times$ 3 so maximum 4 doses in 24 hr if not responsive to IV fluids or increasing need for supplemental oxygen; add corticosteroids as with grade 3 if no improvement within 24 hr on tocilizumab; *Grade 3* (requires aggressive intervention, O$_2$ > 40% FiO$_2$ or hypotension requiring high dose or multiple vasopressors or grade 3 organ toxicity or grade 4 transaminitis; *treatment:* tocilizumab per grade 2 plus methylprednisolong 1 mg/kg IV bid or equivalent dexamethasone (e.g., 10 mg IV q 6 h); continue corticosteroids until event is grade 1 or less, then taper over 3 days; *Grade 4* life threatening, requires ventilator, continuous veno-venous hemodialysis (CVVHD) or grade 4 organ toxicity (excluding transaminitis); *treatment:*

Tocilizumab same as grade 2, methylprednisolone 1,000 mg IV q d × 3 days; if improves, manage as above.
- Neurologic toxicity:
  - If toxicity grade 2 or higher, monitor with contiuous cardiac telemetry and pulse oximetry. Provide intensive care supportive therapy for severe or life-threatening toxicity. Consider non-sedating, anti-seizure medications (e.g., levetiracetam) for seizure prophylaxis for any grade 2 or higher nurologic toxicity.
  - Grade 2: (a) if concurrent CRS: administer tocilizumab for management of grade 2 CRS; if no improvement within 24 hours, give dexamethasone 10 mg IV q 6 hr if not already on a corticosteroid; continue dexamethasone until event is grade 1 or less, then taper over 3 days; (b) if no concurrent CRS: give dexamethasone 10 mg IV q 6 hr until event ≤grade 1, then taper over 3 days.
  - Grade 3: (a) if concurrent CRS, administer tocilizumab as in CRS grade 2 administer dexamethasone 10 mg IV with first dose of tocilizumab then q 6 hr; continue dexamethasone until event is grade 1 or less, then taper over 3 days; (b) If no concurrent CRS, give dexamethasone 10 mg IV q 6 hr, and continue until event is grade 1 or less, then taper over 3 days.
  - Grade 4: (a) if concurrent CRS, administer tocilizumab as in CRS grade 2; give methylprednisolone 1,000 mg IV per day with 1st dose of tocilizumab and continue methylprednisolone 1,000 mg IV per day for 2 more days; if improves, then manage as above; (b) if no concurrent CRS: Administeer methylprednisolone 1,000 mg IV per day for × 3 days; if improves, then manage as above
- During infusion assess for HSRs, CRS, and neurotoxicity during and after drug infusion.
- Teach patient they must remain near the certified healthcare facility for at least 4 weeks after infusion. Patient must have daily assessment for CRS and neurotoxicity, as well as other adverse effects × 7 days at the certified healthcare facility. In addition, the patient must be monitored closely for an additional 4 weeks.

Drug Interactions: Unknown.

Lab Effects/Interference:
- Lymphopenia, leukopenia, neutropenia, anemia, thrombocytopenia.
- Hypophosphatemia, hyponatremia, hypokalemia.
- Increased uric acid, direct bilirubin, alanine aminotransferase.
- Hypogammaglubulinemia.
- Anti-product antibodies: drug may induce these but no evidence they alter effect.

Special Considerations:
- Drug is likely fetotoxic as are cyclophosphamide and fludarabine; assess pregnancy status of women with reproductive potential before starting therapy, and teach patient to use effective contraception during therapy. This has not been studied.
- Warnings and Precautions:
  - *CRS:* incidence is about 94%, and may be fatal. Median time to onset was 2 days, and median duration 7 days. CRS is manifested by fever (78%), hypotension (41%), tachycardia (28%), hypoxia (22%), chills (20%); may be associated with cardiac arrhythmias (including atrial fibrillation and ventricular tachycardia), cardiac arrest,

cardiac failure, renal insufficiency, capillary leak syndrome (CLS), hypotension, hypoxia, hemophagocytic lymphohistiocytosis/macrophage activation syndrome (HLH/MAS). **Two doses of tociliziumab** MUST be available prior to starting infusion of axicabtagene ciloleucel. Monitor patient at least daily × 7 days at the certified healthcare facility after infusion for signs/symptoms of CRS. Patient should be monitored for signs/symptoms of CRS × 4 weeks after infusion. Teach patient to seek emergency care immediately if signs/symptoms of CRS occur at any time. Implement supportive care, tocilizumab or tociliost common were encephalopathy (57%) which may be prolonged, headache (44%), tremor (31%), dizziness (21%), aphasia (18%), delirium (17%), insomnia (9%), and anxiety (9%). Other serious events were leukoencephalopathy, seizures, and rarely cerebral edema which may be fatal. Monitor patient daily for at least 7 days at the certified healthcare facility after the infusion of axicabtagene ciloleucel, then continue monitoring patient for 4 weeks after the infusion. Intervene promptly if signs/symptoms identified.

- *Yescarta REMS:* because of risk of CRS and neurologic toxicity, drug is available only through a restricted program under a Risk Evaluation and Mitigation Strategy (REMS) called Yescarta REMS. This requires: 1) healthcare facility that dispenses and administers axicabtagene ciloleucel must be enrolled and comply with the REMS requirements (be certified, have on-site, immediate access to tocilizumab, and ensure a minimum of 2 doses of tocilizumab are available for each patient for infusion withint 2 hours after the axicabtagene ciloleucel infusion if needed for treatment of CRS; 2) certified healthcare facilities must ensure that healthcare providers who prescribe, dispense, or administer axicabtagene ciloleucel are trained about the management of CRS and neurological toxicities.
- *HSRs:* Allergic reactions may occur, including anaphylaxis, due to dimethyl sulfoxide (DMSO) or residual gentamicin in the axicabtagene ciloleucel infusate.
- *Serious infections:* Severe or life-threatening infections may occur. All grade infections occurred in 38% of patients, and were grade 3 or higher in 23% of patients. Febrile neutropenia occurred in 36% of patients, and may be concurrent with CRS. Drug should not be given to a patient with active systemic infection. Monitor closely for signs/symptoms of infection, and teach patient to self-assess and report them right away. Administer prophylactic anti-microbials per local guidelines. Manage with broad spectrum antibiotics, other microbials per culture, IV fluids, and other supportive care as indicated. Screen for HBV, HCV, HIVbefore collecting cells for manufacturing as treatment may reactivate HBV which may result in fulminant hepatitis, hepatic failure and death.
- *Prolonged cytopenias:* Cytopenia may be prolonged for several weeks after lymphodepleting chemotherapy and axicabtagene ciloleucel infusion. In a clinical trial 28% of patients had grade 3 or higher cytopenia that lasted 30 days or longer, including thrombocytopenia (18%), neutropenia (15%), and anemia (3%). Monitor blood counts after axicabtagene ciloleucel infusion.
- *Hypogammaglobulinemia:* B-cell aplasia and hypogammaglobulinemia can occur (incidence about 15%); monitor immunoglobulin levels after treatment and manage using infection precautions, antibiotic prophylaxis, and immunoglobulin replacement. Vaccination with live viral vaccines has not been studied; it is not recommended for

at least 6 weeks prior to the start of lymphodepleting chemotherapy, during axicabtagene ciloleucel therapy, and until immune recovery after treatment.

- *Secondary Malignancies:* may develop after treatment with axicabtagene ciloleucel and require life-long monitoring.
- *Efects on ability to drive and use machines:* Because of the potential neurotoxicity, including altered mental status and seizures, patients are at risk for decreased consciousness and coordination for up to 8 weeks after the axicabtagene ciloleucel infusion. Teach patients not to drive or use hazardous equipment during this intial period.

Potential Toxicities/Side Effects and the Nursing Process

I.   ALTERATION IN HOMEOSTASIS, POTENTIAL, related to CYTOKINE RELEASE SYNDROME

Defining Characteristics: CRS is a systemic inflammatory response that occurs when cytokines are released into the systemic circulation by the activation and proliferation of modified T cells and the subsequent killing of normal and malignant B-lymphocytes (FDA(a), 2017). Incidence is 94% all grades, with 13% grade 3/4. Onset occurred after a median of 2 days after infusion and lasted a median of 7 days. ICU care may be necessary. Symptom constellation includes high fevers, rigors, fatigue, anorexia, nausea, vomiting, diarrhea, diaphoresis, headache, encephalopathy, myalgia/arthralgia, rash, hypotension (which may require vasopressors), CLS, tachypnea, and hypoxia (which may require ventilator support). DIC and macrophage activation syndrome (MAS) may occur. CRS may be life-threatening or fatal. Rarely, hemophagocytic lymphohistiocytosis/macrophage activation syndrome (HLH/MAS) may complicate CRS. CLS, if it occurs, is characterized by loss of vascular tone and extravasation of plasma proteins and fluid into the extravascular space. This results in hypotension and decreased organ perfusion. CLS may be associated with cardiac arrhythmias, angina, MI, respiratory insufficiency requiring intubation, GI bleeding, edema, and mental status changes.

Nursing Implications: Assess baseline temperature, vital signs, pulmonary, cardiac, and neurologic status, and comfort level, baseline, and monitor closely at least daily after infusion × 7 days in the certified healthcare facility; continue to monitor closely for 4 more weeks. Ensure that at least 2 doses of tocilizumab are available prior to the dose administration, as well as emergency medical equipment. Assess LFTs and other laboratory tests as ordered. Teach the patient to report any difficulty breathing, or other signs and symptoms of CRS and to seek emergency medical assistance right away. Be prepared to institute emergency medical orders, and transfer to ICU if needed. Provide supportive care as ordered per CRS algorithm (see Nursing Administration section), including IL-6 blockade (e.g., tocilizumab) and corticosteroid administration for immunosuppression.

II.   SENSORY/PERCEPTUAL ALTERATIONS related to NEUROLOGIC TOXICITY

Defining Characteristics: Neurotoxicity occurred in 87% of patients. Most (98%) occurred within the first 8 weeks following the axicabtagene ciloleucel infusion. Although the

TREATMENT

mechanism is not well understood, noninfectious encephalopathy/delirium has occurred with T-cell therapy, characterized by aphasia, tremor, seizures, confusion, and encephalopathy (FDA(a), 2017). Encephalopathy occurred in 57% of patients and occurred during or immediately after CRS; it was self-limiting and resolved with the treatment of CRS. Most common other neurotoxicities were tremor (31%), dizziness (21%), aphasia (18%), delirium (17%), incomnia (9%), anxiety (9%), but other serious events were leukoencephalopathy, seizures and rare cerebral edema which may be fatal.

Nursing Implications: Assess baseline mental status, neurologic status, and consciousness before drug administration. Monitor closely daily post infusion × 7 days in the certified healthcare facility, and continue close monitoring for 4 weeks following that. If CRS develops, as well as neurotoxicity, administer tocilizumab and corticosteroids as ordered (see Nursing Administration section), and monitor the patient closely. Teach the patient to report any changes in mental or neurologic status right away and to seek medical care.

III.   POTENTIAL FOR INJURY related to INFECTION

Defining Characteristics: Febrile neutropenia occurred in 36% of patients within the 8-week postinfusion period. It was related to both the disease process and lymphodepleting chemotherapy. Grade 3/4 occurred in 23% of patients who had both neutropenia and fever. Infections occurred in 38% of patients and were grade 3 in 23% (Kite, 2017). Patients may have hypogammaglobulinemia (15%), lymphopenia (100%), neutropenia (93%), anemia (66%), and thrombocytopenia (58%).

Nursing Implications: Assess baseline CBC, ANC, and platelet count and monitor closely during therapy and follow-up daily × 7 days, then an additional 4 weeks. Discuss prophylactic antibiotics with physician/provider. Evaluate for infection, including assessment of central line and blood cultures, and administer broad-spectrum antibiotics as ordered. Teach the patient to self-assess and to report any fever or other signs and symptoms of infection, and to avoid potential sources of infection.

Drug: bevacizumab (Avastin); Biosimilar bevacizumab-awwb (Mvasi) [These are NOT interchangeable medications. Avastin is indicated for treatment of recurrent ovarian cancer but this was not included in the initial MVASI label.]

Class: Recombinant humanized mAb targeted against VEGF; angiogenesis inhibitor.

Mechanism of Action: VEGF binds to receptors on endothelial cells, turning on the cell surface receptors KDR and Flt-1, which then function as tyrosine kinases sending the message to the cells to proliferate and migrate. This leads to the establishment of new blood vessels (neovascularization) in tumors. Studies show that tumors that express VEGF tend to be more aggressive, more invasive, and more likely to metastasize. Bevacizumab binds to all human forms of VEGF-A, thus preventing it from binding to its receptors on the endothelial cells. This theoretically prevents one step in the process of angiogenesis from occurring. In addition, it appears that VEGF is necessary to maintain existing tumor blood vessels, and when blocked by bevacizumab, these blood vessels normalize, have less permeability, which reduces tumor interstitial pressure, and allows normal blood flow throughout the tumor. When given with chemotherapy, this theoretically results in increased flow of chemotherapy within the tumor and increased cell kill. Bevacizumab may augment the body's antitumor immune response by helping dendritic cells function more effectively. Finally, bevacizumab is an IgG_1 mAb that theoretically recruits immune effector cells such as NK cells and macrophages, which attack tumor cells (antibody-dependent cellular cytotoxicity), as well as stimulating complement-mediated killing of tumor cells. Chu and DeVita (2016) describe avenues leading to bevacizumab resistance: (1) increased expression of pro-angiogenic factor ligands, such as hepatocyte growth factor, (2) circumventing angiogenic signaling by recruitment of bone marrow derived cells which restores neovascularization and tumor angiogenesis, (3) increased pericyte coverage of tumor blood vessels reducing need for VEGF-mediated survival signaling, and (4) activation and enhancement of invasion and metastasis, which allows access to normal tissue blood vessels.

Metabolism: Humanized via recombinant technologies resulting in a 93% human mAb. It is widely distributed throughout the body and has a terminal half-life of approximately 20 days (range 11–50 days). It appears to reach steady state in 100 days. Drug clearance varies by body weight, gender, and tumor burden: men and patients with a large tumor burden have higher clearances than females, but this does not appear to decrease drug efficiency. Drug clearance has not been studied in patients with either renal or hepatic impairment, but it appears that there is minimal drug clearance by these organs. Concurrent administration of 5-fluourouracil, carboplatin, doxorubicin, cisplatin, or paclitaxel does not affect pharmacokinetics of the drug.

Indication: FDA-approved for the treatment of (1) metastatic CRC, first- or second-line, in combination with IV fluorouracil-based regimen; (2) metastatic CRC, that has progressed on first line bevacizumab, as second-line, in combination with fluoropyrimidine-irinotecan- or fluoropyrimidine-oxaliplatin-based chemotherapy; (3) unresectable, locally advanced, recurrent or metastatic nonsquamous NSCLC, as first-line, in combination with carboplatin and paclitaxel; (4) glioblastoma, recurrent, in adults; (5) metastatic renal cell carcinoma in combination with interferon alfa; (6) cervical cancer that is persistent, recurrent, or metastatic, in combination with paclitaxel and cisplatin or paclitaxel and topotecan;

Avastin indication (not MVASI) also includes (7) recurrent epithelial ovarian, fallopian tube, or primary peritoneal cancer (a) in combination with carboplatin and paclitaxel, followed by bevacizumab as a single agent, for stage III-IV disease after initial surgical resection; (b) in combination with paclitaxel, pegylated liposomal doxorubicin, or topotecan for platinum-resistant recurrent disease who received no more than 2 prior chemotherapy regimens; (c) in combination with carboplatin and paclitaxel, or carboplatin and gemcitabine, followed by bevacizumab as a single agent, for platinum-sensitive recurrent disease.

Dosage/Range:
- DO NOT administer bevacizumab until at least 28 days following surgery and the wound is fully healed (Genentech, 2019).
- Metastatic CRC (mCRC)

- Metastatic CRC: 5 mg/kg IV every 2 weeks with bolus-IFL.
- Metastatic CRC: 10 mg/kg IV every 2 weeks with FOLFOX4.
- Metastatic CRC: 5 mg/kg every 2 weeks or 7.5 mg/kg every 3 weeks when used in combination with a fluoropyrimidine-irinotecan or fluoropyrimidine-oxaliplatin based chemotherapy regimen in patients who have progressed on a first-line Avastin containing regimen.
- *First line Nonsquamous NSCLC:* 15 mg/kg every 3 weeks when combined with carboplatin and paclitaxel.
- *Recurrent glioblastoma:* 10 mg/kg IV every 2 weeks.
- *Metastatic renal cell cancer (mRCC):* 10 mg/kg IV every 2 weeks with interferon-alfa.
- *Persistent, recurrent, or metastatic cervical cancer:* 15 mg/kg every 3 weeks with paclitaxel/cisplatin or paclitaxel/topotecan.
- *Stage III or IV epithelial ovarian cancer*, fallopian tube cancer, orprimary peritoneal cancer following initial surgical resection: 15 mg/kg IV every 3 weeks in combination with carboplatin/paclitaxel for up to 6 cycles, followed by 15 mg/kg IV every 3 weeks as a single agent, for a total of up to 22 cycles;
- *Platinum-resistant recurrent epithelial* ovarian, fallopian tube, or primary peritoneal cancer: (a) 10 mg/kg IV every 2 weeks with paclitaxel, pegylated liposomal doxorubicin, or weekly topotecan; (b) 15 mg/kg IV every 3 weeks with topotecan given every 3 weeks.
- *Platinum-sensitive recurrent epithelial ovarian*, fallopian tube, or primary peritoneal cancer: (a) 15 mg/kg IV every 3 weeks in combination with carboplatin/paclitaxel for 6–8 cycles, followed by 15 mg/kg IV every 3 weeks as a single agent; (b) 15 mg/kg IV every 3 weeks in combination with carboplatin/gemcitabine for 6–10 cycles, followed by 15 mg/kg every 3 weeks as a single agent.
- Drug is NOT indicated for the adjuvant treatment of colon cancer.
- Discontinue bevacizumab for:
  - GI perforation, fistula formation involving an internal organ or GI tract, non-GI fistula.
  - Wound dehiscence and wound-healing complications requiring medical intervention.
  - Serious (grade 3 or 4) hemorrhage requiring medical intervention.
  - Severe arterial thromboembolic events (ATEs).
  - Venous thromboembolism, grade 4.
  - Hypertensive crisis or hypertensive encephalopathy.
  - Posterior reversible encephalopathy syndrome (PRES).
  - Nephrotic syndrome.
  - CHF (any).
  - Severe infusion reactions.
- Temporarily suspend bevacizumab for:
  - At least 4 weeks (28 days) prior to elective surgery; do not reinitiate for at least 28 days after surgery and until the surgical wound is fully healed.
  - Recent history of hemoptysis of 1/2 tsp (2.5 mL) or more.
  - Severe hypertension not controlled with medical management; resume once controlled.
  - Moderate to severe proteinuria pending further evaluation (e.g., $\geq$ 2 g of proteinuria/24 hours in absence of nephrotic syndrome).

- Severe clinically significant infusion reactions: interrupt infusion, resume at a decreased rate after symptoms resolve.
- Mild, clinically insignificant infusion reactions: decrease infusion rate.

Drug Preparation:
- Available in single dose vials: 100 mg/4 mL (25 mg/mL) and 400 mg/16 mL (25 mg/mL). Solution is colorless to pale brown.
- Visually inspect solution for particulate matter or discoloration.
- Aseptically withdraw ordered amount of bevacizuab and dilute in a total volume of 100 mL of 0.9% sodium chloride injection USP. DO NOT administer with or mix with dextrose solution.
- Discard unused portions of the vial as drug does not contain preservatives.
- Store diluted bevacizumab at 2–8°C (36–46°F) for up to 8 hours. Protect from light. Do not freeze or shake.

Drug Administration:
- Do not administer as an IV push or bolus.
- Do not initiate bevacizumab for 28 days following major surgery and until surgical wound is fully healed.
- Patients with active hemoptysis ($\geq$ 1/2 tsp of red blood) should not receive the drug.
- Administer IV over 90 minutes for the first infusion.
  - Subsequent infusions. If first infusion tolerated well (e.g., without fever and/or chills), administer second dose over 60 minutes; if this is well-tolerated, administer all subsequent doses as a 30-minute infusion.
  - Bevacizumab 5 mg/kg has been shown to be safely infused over 10 minutes (Reidy et al., 2007).

Drug Interactions:
- Paclitaxel/carboplatin combination: may decrease paclitaxel exposure after 4 cycles of treatment (day 63).
- Incompatible with dextrose solutions.

Lab Effects/Interference:
- Thrombocytopenia
- Proteinuria
- Leukopenia and neutropenia
- Hypokalemia
- Bilirubinemia

Special Considerations:
- Bevacizumab is **not** indicated for adjuvant treatment of colon cancer.
- Black box warnings discuss risk of (1) gastrointestinal perforations (incidence in patients with CRC was 2.4%, NSCLC 0.9%, 3.2% in cervical cancer patients with prior pelvic irradiation), sometimes associated with intra-abdominal abscesses, and fistula formation; (2) complications of surgery and wound healing; and (3) hemorrhage (fatal hemoptysis occurred in five patients with NSCLC—incidence was 31% in patients with squamous cell and 2.3% in patients with adenocarcinoma histology).

- Warnings and Precautions:
  - *Gastrointestinal perforation and Fistulae* (GI perforation, intra-abdominal abscesses, and/or fistula formation) occurs in up to 3.2% of patients, and highest incidence was in patients with cervical cancer and who had received prior pelvic radiation.
  - Presentation may include abdominal pain, nausea, emesis, constipation, and fever; generally occurs within the first 50 days of bevacizumab therapy.
  - Perforation can be complicated by intra-abdominal abscess, fistula formation, and the need for diverting ostomies. Avoid drug in ovarian cancer patients with evidence of recto-sigmoid involvement.
  - GI fistula can occur; in patients with cervical cancer, the incidence of GI-vaginal fistulae was 8.2% in the bevacizumab treated group, compared to 0.9% in the control patients, all patients had had prior pelvic radiation.
  - Permanently discontinue drug if GI perforation, tracheoesophageal fistula, or any grade 4 fistula occurs.
  - *Non-GI fistula formation* (tracheoesophageal, bronchopleural, biliary, vaginal, renal, bladder sites). Most events occurred within the first 6 months of therapy. Permanently discontinue drug if patient develops a tracheoesophageal (TE) fistula, any grade-4 fistula, or if a fistula forms involving an internal organ.
  - *Surgical and wound-healing complications:* Incidence of patients with mCRC who underwent surgery during bevacizumab therapy was 15 vs. 4% in those who did not. Suspend drug at least 28 days before elective surgery, and do not initiate drug for at least 28 days after surgery and until the surgical wound is fully healed. Discontinue drug for wound healing complications requiring medical intervention. Necrotizing fasciitis, most commonly related to wound healing complications, GI perforation or fistula formation have occurred and some cases have been fatal. Discontinue drug in patients who develop necrotizing fasciitis.
  - *Hemorrhage:* There are two patterns of bleeding: (a) minor hemorrhage, most commonly grade 1 epistaxis, and (b) serious hemorrhagic events (e.g., hemorrhage, hemoptysis, GI bleeding, hematamesis, CNS hemorrhage, epistaxis, vaginal hemorrhage), which in some cases were fatal. The incidence of grade 3 or higher hemorrhage in bevacizumab patients was 1.2–6.9%.
    - Drug is not indicated in NSCLC patients with squamous histology, as the incidence of serious or fatal pulmonary hemorrhage was 31% in these patients. In NSCLC patients with CNS metastases who had completed RT and surgery > 4 weeks prior to the start of bevacizumab, the incidence of grade 2 CNS hemorrhage was documented in 1.2% of patients. Intracranial hemorrhage in patients with previously treated glioblastoma was 8/163 patients.
    - Do NOT give bevacizumab to patients with recent hemoptysis of ≥ 1/2 teaspoon of red blood; discontinue bevacizumab in patients with hemorrhage.
  - *Arterial Thrombotic Events (ATEs)* with increased risk of cerebral infarction, myocardial infarction, transient ischemic attacks, and angina have occurred compared to control patients (grade ≥ 3 2.6%, vs. 0.8% in control). Highest incidence of grade 3-5 ATE was in patients with GBM.
    - The risk of developing ATE increased in patients with a history of arterial thrombo-embolism, diabetes, age > 65 years.

- Permanently discontinue drug if a severe ATE occurs. Safety of resuming bevaci-zumab after resolution of an ATE has not been studied.
- *Venous thromboembolic events (VTEs):* increased risk of VTEs (11% vs 5% without bevacizumab); discontinue drug if grade 4 VTE including pulmonary embolism.
- *Hypertension (HTN):* Monitor BP and treat HTN. The incidence of grades 3–4 HTN was 5–18% in bevacizumab patients. Continue to monitor BP regularly in patients with bevacizumab-induced or exacerbated HTN after bevacizumab is discontinued. Tempo-rarily suspend bevacizumab if HTN not medically controlled. Permanently discontinue drug if hypertensive crisis or encephalopathy occurs.
- *Posterior reversible encephalopathy syndrome (PRES)* has an incidence of < 0.5%, with signs and symptoms of headache, seizure, lethargy, confusion, blindness, and other vi-sual changes occurring from 16 hours to 1 year after bevacizumab was begun. It may be associated with mild-moderately severe HTN. Confirm diagnosis of PRES with MRI. Discontinue drug in patients developing PRES. Symptoms likely resolve or improve within days, although some patients have ongoing neurological sequelae.
- *Renal injury and proteinuria, rare nephrotic syndrome:* Monitor urine protein by urine dipstick/urinalysis baseline and serially during bevacizumab therapy; if the urine dipstick is 2+ or greater, perform a 24-hour urine sample for protein.
  - Suspend drug for moderate proteinuria (≥ 2 g of protein/24 hours in a 24-hour urine) and resume when 24-hour urine for protein is < 2 g/24 hr. Discontinue drug if ne-phrotic syndrome develops.
  - There is a poor correlation between urine protein/creatinine ratio (UPCR) and the 24-hour urine protein, so a 24-hour urine collection is necessary.
  - Median time to onset of proteinuria was 5.6 months (15 days to 37 months) after starting bevacizumab.
- *Infusion reactions* may occur rarely (< 3%, with 0.2% severe) manifested by hyper-tension, hypertensive crisis associated with neurologic signs and symptoms, wheezing, oxygen desaturation, grade-3 hypersensitivity, chest pain, headaches, rigors, and diapho-resis. Stop infusion if a severe infusion reaction occurs and treat as medically appropriate and ordered.
- *Ovarian failure:* Teach patients of childbearing age that this may occur (incidence in one study of premenopausal women was 34% compared to 2% in control arm). After discon-tinuance of bevicizumab, recovery of ovarian function occurred in 22% of these patients.
- *Embryo-fetal toxicity:* Drug is teratogenic. Women of childbearing age should use highly effective contraceptive measures during treatment to avoid pregnancy, and for 6 months after the drug is stopped. Bevacizumab use during pregnancy is only if the potential ben-efit to the pregnant woman justifies the potential risk to the fetus. Nursing mothers should decide whether to discontinue nursing, or to discontinue the drug, taking into account the half-life of bevacizumab (approximately 20 days, range 11–50 days) and the importance of the drug to the mother's health.
- *Congestive Heart Failure (CHF):* Bevacizumab is not indicated in combination with anthracycline-based chemotherapy.
- Incidence of grade 3 or higher decline in LVEF was 1% in patients receiving bevacizumab vs 0.6% in patients receiving chemotherapy alone; in patients with prior anthracycline treatment, the incidence was 4% vs 0.6% for patients receiving chemotherapy alone.

- Time to onset of LV dysfunction or CHF was 1–6 months after the first dose of bevacizumab in at least 85% of patients and was resolved in 62% of patients who developed CHF.
- The incidence of neutropenia and febrile neutropenia are increased in patients receiving bevacizumab plus chemotherapy compared to patients receiving chemotherapy alone.
- The incidence of grade ≥ 3 left ventricular dysfunction was 1% in bevacizumab patients compared to the control arm across indications.
- Most common toxicities (> 10%, twice control group incidence): epistaxis, headache, hypertension, rhinitis, proteinuria, taste alterations, dry skin, rectal hemorrhage, lacrimation disorder, back pain, exfoliative dermatitis.
- Drug toxicities that occur more commonly in the elderly (≥ 2%) were asthenia, sepsis, deep thrombophlebitis, hypertension, hypotension, myocardial infarction, congestive heart failure, diarrhea, constipation, anorexia, leukopenia, anemia, dehydration, hypokalemia, and hyponatremia. In those aged 75 or older, in addition, dyspepsia, gastrointestinal hemorrhage, edema, epistaxis, increased cough, and voice alteration occurred more commonly than those under age 65.
- Ranpura et al. (2011) performed a meta-analysis of RCTs and found that bevacizumab, in combination with chemotherapy or biological therapy compared to chemotherapy alone, was associated with increased mortality.

Potential Toxicities/Side Effects and the Nursing Process

I. ALTERATION IN INTESTINAL AND SKIN INTEGRITY related to GASTROINTESTINAL PERFORATION, FISTULAE, AND WOUND DEHISCENCE

Defining Characteristics: Rarely, patients may develop gastrointestinal perforation, sometimes fatal. It may be associated with intra-abdominal abscesses, or fistula, and occur at variable times during the treatment. Incidence across all studies was 3.2%, and for patients with cervical cancer the highest incidence was in patients who had received prior pelvic radiation. Presenting symptoms were abdominal pain associated with nausea and constipation. Colonoscopy has a similar risk of GI perforation, so drug should be stopped 28 days before a planned colonoscopy.

It is unknown how long the interval between surgery and treatment with bevacizumab should be, but it may be greater than 2 months, and the surgical incision should be completely healed; similarly, it is not known how long the interval should be between treatment with bevacizumab and elective surgery, but it certainly should be longer than the elimination time of the drug (half-life 20 days).

The incidence of GI-vaginal fistulae in the cervical cancer trial was 8.2% in the bevacizumab arm, compared to 0.9% in the control group. All patients who developed vaginal-GI fistulae had had prior pelvic RT.

The incidence of non-GI fistulae is increased but is uncommon, and generally occurs within the first 6 months of treatment.

Exfoliative dermatitis occurred in 19% of patients receiving 5-FU/LV plus bevacizumab. GI perforation has occurred in patients with NSCLC and advanced breast cancer receiving bevacizumab.

Nursing Implications: Assess baseline bowel, skin integrity, and healing of any wounds or incisions; assess for dehiscence and integrity of skin or wound at each visit. Teach patient that very rarely GI perforation or wound dehiscence may occur and to report or come to the emergency room for severe abdominal pain associated with nausea, vomiting, constipation, or other symptoms or problems with wound healing right away for immediate evaluation. Bevacizumab should be discontinued if perforation or wound dehiscence occurs. Bevacizumab should be held prior to elective surgery based on the drug half-life of 20 days (range, 10–50 days) and not started until at least 28 days after major surgery; the surgical incision must be fully healed. For patients who are undergoing metastectomy, the drug may be stopped 2 months before and not resumed for at least 60 days after hepatectomy. Teach patient to self-assess changes in skin or wound integrity and to report it right away. Bevacizumab should be discontinued if the patient develops GI perforation, tracheoesophageal fistula, grade-4 fistula, or fistula formation involving an internal organ.

II.   ALTERATION IN HEMOSTASIS related to BLEEDING AND THROMBOSIS

Defining Characteristics: Two patterns of bleeding may rarely occur: minor hemorrhage such as mild (grade 1) epistaxis, and serious hemorrhage. The incidence of epistaxis is 35% compared to 10% in the chemotherapy-only mCRC group. Epistaxis is easily controlled with pressure application. Of note, hemorrhage (pulmonary) occurred when drug was being studied in patients with lung cancer, with a higher incidence (31% in a small study) in patients with squamous cell histology; thus the drug is contraindicated in patients with squamous cell histology or those with hemoptysis. Many of these patients bled from a cavitation or area of necrosis in the pulmonary tumor. Rare severe hemorrhage includes hemoptysis, gastrointestinal (GI) bleeding, hematemesis, CNS hemorrhage, epistaxis, and vaginal bleeding occurred 5 times more frequently in the group receiving bevacizumab than the group receiving only chemotherapy. The incidence of severe (grade 3 and higher) hemorrhage was 1.2–4.6%. The incidence of grade 2 CNS hemorrhage in NSCLC patients with CNS metastasis was 1.2% in the bevacizumab arm, while intracranial hemorrhage occurred in 4.9% of patients with previously treated glioblastoma, with 1.2% grades 3–4.

Thrombocytopenia may occur in 5% of patients. Deep vein thrombosis may occur in 6–9% of patients. Patients on low-dose Coumadin for implanted port patency had no increased risk of bleeding. There was an increased incidence of venous thromboembolism in patients with cervical cancer receiving bevacizumab with chemotherapy (10.6 vs. 5.4% in patients receiving chemotherapy alone).

Nursing Implications: Assess baseline hematologic parameters and monitor during therapy. Teach patient that bleeding may occur and is most commonly epistaxis but may also rarely occur as bleeding in the gastrointestinal tract, vagina in women, or elsewhere, and to report signs/symptoms of bleeding, changes in mental status, mobility, vision, weakness, or any new sign or symptom right away. Teach patient to assess for and report right away signs/symptoms of thrombosis: new swelling, pain, skin warmth, and/or change in color (e.g., erythema, mottling) on the legs or thighs; new onset pain in the abdomen; dyspnea or shortness of breath, rapid heartbeat, chest pain, or pressure that may signal a pulmonary embolism; and any changes in vision, new onset of severe headache, lightheadedness, or dizziness. Assess baseline mental status and neurologic signs, and monitor during therapy, especially in patients with brain metastasis. Teach patients to apply pressure if epistaxis occurs. Discuss any abnormalities with physician. Bevacizumab should be discontinued if the patient develops serious hemorrhage, and it should not be given to patients with recent hemoptysis ($\geq$ 1/2 tsp bright red blood). Drug should be discontinued in patients who develop a severe arterial thrombotic event or a life-threatening (grade 4) venous thrombotic event including pulmonary embolism.

III. POTENTIAL ALTERATION IN CIRCULATION related to HYPERTENSION AND CONGESTIVE HEART FAILURE

Defining Characteristics: Bevacizumab increases the incidence and severity of hypertension, a class effect of all angiogenesis inhibitors believed caused by inhibition of VEGF, which decreases nitric oxide and prevents blood vessel dilation. Across clinical studies, incidence of grades 3–4 HTN ranged from 5 to 18%.

Nursing Implications: Assess baseline BP prior to and during treatment, at least for the first treatment, then prior to each drug administration. BP should be monitored every 2–3 weeks during treatment. If the patient has a history of hypertension, monitor BP more closely, although hypertension develops over time rather than during the drug infusion. Blood pressure should continue to be monitored after patient has stopped the drug. Teach patient drug administration, potential side effects, and self-care measures if prescribed antihypertensive medication, such as angiotensin-converting enzyme inhibitors, beta-blockers, diuretics, and calcium channel blockers. Drug should be temporarily suspended in patients with severe hypertension until BP can be controlled with medical management. Drug should be permanently discontinued if the patient develops hypertensive crisis (diastolic blood pressure >120 mm Hg) or hypertensive encephalopathy.

IV. ALTERATION IN RENAL FUNCTION related to NEPHROTIC SYNDROME

Defining Characteristics: Nephrotic syndrome and proteinuria may occur. Thirty-six percent of mCRC patients receiving bevacizumab developed grades 1–4 proteinuria; and 20% of patients with renal cell cancer receiving bevacizumab and IFN-α; grades 3–4 proteinuria ranged from 0.7–7.4% across studies. Median time to onset of proteinuria was 5.6 months after starting drug, and median time to resolution was 6.1 months. Proteinuria did not resolve in 40% of patients.

Nursing Implications: Assess baseline renal function and presence of protein in urine (1+ or greater by dipstick), and monitor prior to each treatment. Discuss any abnormalities with the physician. Patients with 2+ or higher proteinuria by urine dipstick should be asked to collect a 24-hour urine sample for protein. Drug should be held for proteinuria $\geq$ 2 g/ 24 hr, and resume when proteinuria < 2 g/24 hr. Monitor patients closely if moderate to severe proteinuria until improved or resolved. Drug should be discontinued if the patient develops nephrotic syndrome.

Drug: blinatumomab (Blincyto)

Class: Bispecific CD19-directed CD3 T-cell engager, first in class.

Mechanism of Action: Agent is made up of two mAbs that bind and link together (1) CD19-expressed cells on the surface of B-lineage cells (the antigen), and (2) CD3 expressed on the surface of T-lymphocytes, which in turn activates T-lymphocytes. CD3 is located in the TCR. When it complexes with CD19 on benign and malignant cells, it activates the T-lymphocytes, making them cytotoxic. The cytotoxic T-cells produce and release cytolytic proteins and inflammatory cytokines, and stimulate the proliferation of more T-cells, which then attack and lyse the CD19+ cells.

Metabolism: When blinatumomab was given as a 4-week continuous infusion (CI), T-cell activation occurred, with a resulting decrease in peripheral B-cells and a transient increase in cytokine levels. The metabolic pathway of the agent is unknown. Clearance is reduced in patients with moderate renal impairment.

Indication: For the treatment of adults and children with: (1) B-cell precursor acute lymphoblastic leukemia (ALL) in first or second CR with minimal residual disease (MRD) > 0.1% (accelerated approval); (2) relapsed or refractory B-cell precursor acute lymphoblastic leukemia (ALL).

Contraindications: Patients with known hypersensitivity to blinatumomab or to any component of the product formulation.

Dosage/Range (see package insert April 2019):

I. MRD-positive B-cell precursor ALL
- Treatment course is 1 cycle of blinatumomab for induction followed by up to 3 additional cycles for consolidation.
- A single cycle of treatment for induction or consolidation consists of 28 days of continuous IV infusion followed by a 14-day treatment free interval (total 42 days). If in the hospital, drug can be mixed in 24 or 48 hour infusion bags, and at home, 7 day infusion bags can be prepared. See package insert.
- Induction (cycle 1) and consolidation (cycles 2–4) doses for patients with weight ≥ 45 kg, dose is 28 mcg/day (fixed dose) days 1–28, while that for patients weighing <45 kg is 15 mcg/m^2/day (BSA based, not to exceed 28 mcg/day) days 1–28. Days 29–42 are treatment-free (14 days).
- Hospitalization recommended for the first 3 days of cycle 1, and first 2 days of second cycle. For all subsequent cycle starts and re-initiations (e.g., if treatment interrupted for 4+ hours), supervision by a healthcare professional or hospitalization is recommended.
- Premedicate with prednisone or equivalent: *adults:* prednisone 100 mg IV or equivalent (e.g., dexamethasone 16 mg) 1 hour prior to first dose of blinatumomab in each cycle. *Pediatrics:* 5 mg/m^2 dexamethasone to a maximum dose of 20 mg prior to the first dose of blinatumomab in cycle 1 and when restarting an infusion after an interruption of 4+ hours in cycle 1.

II. Relapsed or refractory B-cell precuror ALL

- Treatment course consists of up to 2 cycles of blinatumomab for induction, followed by 3 cycles for consolidation treatment and up to 4 additional cycles of continued therapy. Cycle 1 (induction) is a step increase dose.
- A single cycle of treatment of blinatumomab INDUCTION or CONSOLIDATION consists of 28 days of continuous IV infusion followed by a 14-day treatment-free interval (total 42 days).
- A single cycle of blinatumomab CONTINUED THERAPY consists of 28 days of continuous IV infusion blinatumomab, followed by a 56-day treatment-free interval (total 84 days).
- Patients who weight at least 45 kg receive a fixed dose:
  - Cycle 1: 9 mcg/day continuous infusion for days 1–7, and 28 mcg/day continuous infusion on days 8–28, followed by a 14-day rest (days 29–42).
  - Subsequent cycles (2–5): 28 mcg/day continuous infusion on days 1–28 of each 6-week cycle for Induction cycle 2, and consolidation cycles 3–5.
  - Continued therapy cycles 6–9: 28 mcg/day days 1–28, with a 56-day treatment-free interval days 29–84.
- Patient weight < 45 kg (BSA-based dosing):
  - Induction Cycle 1: 5 mcg/m^2/day (not to exceed 9 mcg/day) days 1–7, and 15 mcg/m^2/day (not to exceed 28 mcg/day) days 8–28, followed by a 14-day treatment-free interval (days 29-42.
  - Induction cycle 2, and consolidation cycles 3–5: 15 mcg/m^2/day (not to exceed 28 mcg/day) days 1–28, followed by a 14-day treatment-free interval (days 29–42).
  - Continued therapy cycles 6–9: 15 mcg/m^2 (not to exceed 28 mcg/day) days 1–28, followed by 56-day treatment-free interval (days 29–84).
  - Hospitalization is recommended for the first 9 days of cycle 1, and the first 2 days of cycle 2. For all subsequent starts and re-initiation (e.g., if treatment is interrupted for 4+ hours), supervision by a healthcare professional or hospitalization is recommended.
  - Premedicate with dexamethasone: *adult* patients: dexamethasone 20 mg 1 hour prior to first dose of blinatumomab of each cycle, prior to a step dose (e.g., cycle 1 d8) and when restarting an infusion after an interruption of 4+ hours. *Pediatrics:* dexamethasone 5 mg/m^2 (maximum dose 20 mg) prior to first dose cycle 1, prior to a step dose (e.g., cycle 1 d8) and when restarting an infusion after an interruption of 4+ hours.

Dose Modifications

- ***Dose Interruption:*** If the interruption after an adverse event is not > 7 days, continue the same cycle to a total of 28-days of infusion inclusive of days before and after the interruption in that cycle. If an interruption due to an adverse event is >7 days, start a new cycle.
- CRS: *Grade 3*: Interrupt blinatumomab. Administer dexamethasone: *patients 45 kg or more*: 8 mg every 8 hours IV/PO for up to 3 days and taper thereafter over 4 days; patients <45 kg: 5 mg/m^2 (maximum 8 mg) every 8 hours PO/IV for up to 3 days and taper thereafter over 4 days. When CRS resolved restart at (1) Weight $\geq$45 kg: 9 mcg/day;

escalate to 28 mcg/day after 7 days if CRS does not recur; (2) Patients <45 kg: 5 mcg/m^2/day; escalate to 15 mcg/m^2 after 7 days if toxicity does not recur. *Grade 4*: Permanently discontinue blinatumomab. Administer dexamethasone as instructed for grade 3 CRS.

- Neurological toxicity: (1) Seizure: Permanently discontinue blinatumomab if more than 1 seizure occurs. (2) *Grade 3*: Withhold blinatumomab until no more than grade 1 (mild) and for at least 3 days, then restart at (1) Weight ≥45 kg: 9 mcg/day; escalate to 28 mcg/day after 7 days if the toxicity does not recur. If the toxicity occurred at 9 mcg/day, or if the toxicity takes >7 days to resolve, permanently discontinue blinatumomab; (2) Patient <45 kg: 5 mcg/m^2/day; escalate to 15 mcg/m^2/day after 7 days if toxicity does not recur; if the toxicity occurred at 5 mcg/m^2/day, or if the toxicity takes >7 days to resolve, permanently discontinue blinatumab. *Grade 4:* Permanently discontinue blinatumomab.

- Other clinically relevant adverse reactions: *Grade 3 (severe)*: Withhold blinatumomab until no more than grade 1 (mild), then restart at (1) Weight ≥45 kg: 9 mcg/day; escalate to 28 mcg/day after 7 days if the toxicity does not recur. If the toxicity takes more than 14 days to resolve, permanently discontinue blinatumomab; (2) Patient <45 kg: 5 mcg/m^2/day; escalate to 15 mcg/m^2/day after 7 days if the toxicity does not recur. If the toxicity takes more than 14 days to resolve, permanently discontinue blinatumomab. *Grade 4 (life-threatening)*: Consider discontinuing blinatumomab permanently.

Drug Preparation (See package insert for specific instructions)
- FDA-required updated REMS safety information: Preparation and administration errors. Review package insert for preparation, infusion rates, and administration. See www.blincytorems.com.
- Key points:
  - The instructions for preparation/admixing and administration MUST BE strictly followed to minimize the risk of medication errors.
  - Blinatumab can be infused over 24 hours (preservative-free) or 48 hours (preservative-free) or 7 days (with preservative). The prescribing physician should consider the frequency of bag changes, and the weight of the patient as the 7-day infusion is NOT recommended for patients weighing <22 kg. Call AMGEN for questions about reconstitution or preparation of drug: 1-800-77-AMGEN (May 2018).
- **See package insert for aseptic preparation requirements,** e.g., USP compliant facility using a ISO Class 5 laminar airflow hood (minimum) by personnel trained in aseptic manipulation and admixture of oncology drugs. PPE should be worn, and gloves and surfaces should be disinfected (Angen, 2018).
- **Incompatibility:** drug is incompatible with di-ethylhexylphthalate (DEHP) due to possible particle formation and cloudy solution. **Must use** polyolefin, PVC DHEP-free or ethyl vinyl acetate (EVA) infusion bags/pump cassettes, and polyolefin, PVC DHEP-free or EVA IV tubing sets.
- Available as 35 mcg lyophilized powder in a single-use vial for reconstitution with one vial of IV solution stabilizer.
- Use IV solution stabilizer provided to coat the prefilled IV bag prior to the addition of reconstituted blinatumomab. **DO NOT use the IV solution stabilizer for reconstitution!**

- **Follow instructions exactly.** See package insert for specific information and for preparation of drug. *Use specific volumes described in admixture instructions*, as dosage errors may occur.

Drug Administration:
- FDA-required updated REMS safety information: Preparation and administration errors. Review package insert for preparation, infusion rates, and administration. See www.blincytorems.com.
- Verify pregnancy status of females of reproductive potential before initiating blinatumomab.
- See package insert for preparation. **See package insert for specific infusion rates** based on infusion duration and dose for patients weighing <45 kg. Tubing should be primed with prepared solution for infusion.
- Perform independent double check of infusion device (24-hour, 48-hour, or 7-day) as well as drug infusion bag.
- Administer blinatumomab as a continuous IV infusion at a constant flow rate using an infusion pump that is programmable, lockable, nonelastomeric, and has an alarm.
  - Must use polyolefin, PVC DHEP-free or ethyl vinyl acetate (EVA) infusion bags/pump cassettes, and polyolefin, PVC DHEP-free, or EVA IV tubing sets.
  - **Incompatibility:** drug is incompatible with di-ethylhexylphthalate (DEHP) due to possible particle formation and cloudy solution.
  - Administer using IV tubing that contains a sterile nonpyrogenic, low-protein-binding, 0.2-micron in-line filter for bags infused over 24 or 48 hours. An in-line filter is not required if drug is administered over 7 days (patients weighing >45 lbs).
  - The IV bag should be infused over 24 or 48 hours (preservative free) or 7 days (with preservative, not recommended for patients weighing < 22 kg). See package insert for specific infusion rates based on infusion duration as well as dose of patients weighing <45 kg.
- Use a dedicated IV lumen.
- *Do not* **flush the blinatumomab infusion line, especially when changing infusion bags, as this may cause overdose with increased complications.**
- Hospitalization:
- *MRD-positive B-cell precursor **ALL**:*
  - Hospitalization is recommended for first 3 days of first cycle and first 2 days of second cycle. For all subsequent cycle starts, and drug re-initiation (if treatment interrupted for 4+ hours), infusion should be supervised by a healthcare professional in the hospital.
  - Premedicate with prednisone or equivalent: (1) adults: prednisone 100 mg IV (equivalent dexamethasone is 16 mg) 1 hr prior to first dose of each cycle; (2) pediatrics: premedicate with 5 mg/m^2 dexamethasone (max dose 20 mg) prior to first drug dose in first cycle, and when restarting an infusion after a 4+ hour interruption.
- *Relapsed or refractory B-cell precursor ALL:*
  - Hospitalization is recommended for the first 9 days of cycle 1 and first 2 days of cycle 2. All subsequent cycle starts, and reinitiaiton if treatment interrupted for 4+ hours, should be supervised by a healthcare professional or hospitalization is recommended.

- Premedicate with dexamethasone 1 hour prior to first dose of each cycle, prior to a step dose (e.g., cycle 1 day 8), and when an infusion is restarted after a 4 hour or longer interruption.
  - Adults: 20 mg
  - Pediatric: 5 mg/m^2 (max 20-mg dose)
- **Strictly follow instructions** for administration in package insert (e.g., no flushing of line), as this may result in an dosing errors with increased toxicity.
- Assess for toxicity: CNS toxicity (e.g., confusion) and CRS are major toxicities that occur during the infusion.
- At the end of the infusion, discard any unused the blinatumomab solution in the IV bag, along with the IV lines. The starting volume is greater than the volume infused to the patient.
- Monitor the patient closely for signs and symptoms of infection and ensure prompt treatment.
- Assess the patient's ability to drive or use machines; teach the patient to avoid driving or using hazardous machinery while blinatumomab is being administered.
- Assess patients aged > 65 years old closely for cognitive disorder, confusion, other neurological toxicities.
- Assess pediatric patients for serious adverse reactions to benzyl alcohol preservative (e.g., gasping syndrome of CNS depression, metabolic acidosis, gasping respirations). Thus 7-day infusion bags containing benzyl alcohol are not recommended for patients weighing <45 kg.
- Monitor LFTs baseline and during treatment; treatment should be held if transaminases increase to > 5 × ULN or bilirubin increases to > 3 × ULN.
- When the treatment is interrupted for an adverse event, if it is NO LONGER than 7 days, continue the same cycle to a total of 28 days of the infusion inclusive of days before and after the interruption in that cycle. If an interruption is > 7 days, start a new cycle.

Drug Interactions: CYP450 enzymes may be suppressed by transient cytokine elevation.

Lab Effects/Interference:
- Neutropenia, anemia, thrombocytopenia
- Decreased serum potassium, phosphate, and magnesium
- Increased serum ALT, AST, total bilirubin, and glucose

Special Considerations:
- Warnings and Precautions: Interrupt or discontinue as needed for the following events:
  - *CRS*, which may be fatal; closely monitor during infusion for headache, fever, nausea, asthenia, hypotension, ↑ AST, ↑ total bilirubin, DIC; interrupt or discontinue as ordered. Incidence was 15% in patients with relapsed/refractory ALL, and 7% in patients with MRD-positive ALL. Median time to onset of CRS was 2 days after start of infusion with resolution if it occurred in 5 days (Amgen, 2019). There is overlap of symptoms of infusion reactions, capillary leak syndrome, and hemophagocytic histiocytosis/macrophage activation syndrome (MAS). Monitor patient closely in the hospital or clinic, and teach patients to self-assess and contact their provider right away if signs/symptoms develop and seek emergency medical care as

directed. If severe CRS develops, interrupt blinatumomab until CRS resolves. Discontinue drug permanently if life threatening. Administer corticosteroids for severe or life-threatening CRS.

- *Neurologic toxicity*, which may be severe, life-threatening, and fatal; incidence is approximately 65%, with a median time to onset of first 2 weeks. Monitor patients for headache, tremor, dizziness, and altered LOC. Grade 3 occurred after drug initiation in 13% (encephalopathy, convulsions, speech disorder, disturbance of consciousness, confusion, disorientation, and coordination and balance disorders. Most symptoms/signs resolved with drug interruption, but some persisted after drug discontinuation (Amgen, 2018). Teach patients receiving outpatient therapy to self-monitor and report right away any signs or symptoms.

- *Serious infections* occur in about 25% of patients. Discuss with provider prophylactic antibiotics and surveillance testing during blinatumomab therapy.Monitor patient closely during therapy for bacterial and opportunistic infections, as well as catheter-related infections.

- *Tumor lysis syndrome* (TLS) may occur and be life-threatening.
  - Use prophylactic measures, including pretreatment nontoxic cytoreduction and on-treatment hydration to prevent TLS.
  - Monitor for signs and symptoms of TLS, including laboratory assessment, and manage TLS with medication management, as well as with temporary interruption or discontinuation of blinatumomab.

- *Neutropenia and febrile neutropenia.* Monitor laboratory parameters (e.g., ANC) during infusion. Interrupt drug if prolonged neutropenia occurs.

- *Effects on ability to drive or use machines:* Patients are at risk for LOC related to the potential neurologic events, including seizures, which may occur with blinatumomab administration. Advise patients *not* to drive or engage in hazardous occupations or activities such as operating heavy or potentially dangerous equipment while blinatumomab is being administered.

- *Elevated liver enzymes (transient) may occur*, with a median time to onset of 3 days when associated with CRS. If outside of CRS, the median time of onset is 19 days. Monitor LFTs closely (AST, ALT, GGT, total bilirubin) baseline and during treatment. Interrupt blinatumomab therapy if transaminases rise to more than 5 × ULN, or if bilirubin rises to more than 3 × ULN.

- *Pancreatitis:* has been reported in patients receiving blinatumomab combined with dexamethasone; monitor for signs and symptoms. Discuss temporary interruption vs. discontinuation of blinatumomab and dexamethasone with physician if pancreatitis occurs.

- *Leukoencephalopathy* has occurred in patients receiving blinatumomab, especially if they have received prior treatment with cranial irradiation and antileukemic chemotherapy, including systemic high-dose methotrexate or intrathecal cytarabine.

- *Preparation and administration errors* have occurred; instructions for preparation and administration should be followed exactly to minimize medication errors

- *Immunizations:* safety of immunization with live viral vaccines has not been studied, and is not recommended for at least 2 weeks prior to the start of blinatumomab treatment, during treatment, and until immune recovery following last cycle of blinatumumab.

- *Risk of serious adverse reactions in pediatric patients due to benzyl alcohol preservative.* Gasping syndrome may occur in neonates and infants receiving benzyl alcohol-preserved drugs. See package insert. Infusion of 7-days should only be used for patients weighing 22 kg or more.
- Most common adverse reactions (incidence ≥ 20%): pyrexia, headache, peripheral edema, febrile neutropenia, nausea, hypokalemia, tremor, rash, and constipation.
- Infusion reactions may occur and may be clinically indistinguishable from CRS manifestations.
- *Embryo-fetal toxicity:* Blinatumomab may cause fetal toxicity. Verify pregnancy status of female patients of reproductive potential before initiating the drug. Teach patients to use effective contraception while receiving the drug to prevent pregnancy. The drug should be used during pregnancy only if the potential benefit justifies the potential risk to the fetus. Mothers should not breastfeed while receiving the drug, and should decide whether to discontinue the drug or nursing, taking into account the importance of the drug to the mother.

Potential Toxicities/Side Effects and the Nursing Process

I.   ALTERATION IN COMFORT AND HOMEOSTASIS, POTENTIAL, related to CYTOKINE RELEASE SYNDROME

Defining Characteristics: Incidence is 11%. Symptom constellation may include pyrexia (62%), headache (36%), asthenia (17%), hypotension (11%), increased ALT and AST (11–12%), and increased total bilirubin. Other signs and symptoms are fever, fatigue, dizziness, nausea, vomiting, chills, face swelling, wheezing or trouble breathing, and skin rash. CRS may be rarely life threatening or fatal. Rarely, disseminated intravascular coagulation (DIC), CLS, and hemophagocytic lymphohistiocytosis/macrophage activation syndrome (HLH/MAS) may complicate CRS. CLS, if it occurs, is characterized by loss of vascular tone and extravasation of plasma proteins and fluid into the extravascular space. This results in hypotension and decreased organ perfusion. CLS may be associated with cardiac arrhythmias, angina, MI, respiratory insufficiency requiring intubation, GI bleeding, edema, and mental status changes. Infusion reactions may also occur and be clinically indistinguishable from CRS signs and symptoms. HSRs occur in 1% of patients. Peripheral edema occurs in 25% of patients, dyspnea in 15%, and hypotension in 11%.

Nursing Implications: Assess baseline temperature, vital signs, pulmonary and neurologic status, and comfort level, and monitor every 4–6 hours when the patient is hospitalized. Assess LFTs and other laboratory tests as ordered. Teach the patient to report any difficulty breathing, or other signs and symptoms of CRS. Be prepared to institute medical orders to manage signs and symptoms and expect that the drug may be temporarily interrupted or discontinued depending on their severity. Teach outpatients to self-assess for CRS signs/symptoms and to notify healthcare provider right away and seek emergency medical care as directed.

II.   SENSORY/PERCEPTUAL ALTERATIONS related to NEUROLOGIC TOXICITY

Defining Characteristics: Approximately 50% of patients experience neurologic toxicity, with 15% having grade 3 or higher reactions (severe, life-threatening, or fatal). Mean time to development is 7 days. Toxicity may include encephalopathy, seizures, speech disorders, disturbances in consciousness, confusion, disorientation, and disorders of balance and coordination. Most events resolve with drug interruption, but some require permanent discontinuation of the drug.

Nursing Implications: Assess baseline mental status, neurologic status, and consciousness before drug administration. Assess for changes during the infusion, such as decreased consciousness, confusion, disorientation, loss of balance or coordination, changes in speech, or seizures; if identified, discuss with physician regarding management and interruption of drug. Teach the patient to report any changes in mental or neurologic status or seizure occurrence.

III.   POTENTIAL FOR INJURY related to INFECTION

Defining Characteristics: Febrile neutropenia occurs in 25% of patients, with 23% having grade 3 or higher. The incidence of neutropenia is 16%, thrombocytopenia 11%, and anemia 18%. Serious infections occur in 25% of patients, including sepsis (7%), pneumonia (9%), bacteremia, opportunistic infections, and catheter-site infections. Bacterial infections account for 19% of all infections, fungal 15%, and viral 13%. Fifteen percent of patients have chills.

Nursing Implications: Assess baseline CBC, ANC, and platelet count and monitor during therapy. Assess patients for signs and symptoms of infections. Teach the patient to self-assess and to report any fever, or other signs and symptoms of infection. Teach self-care measures to minimize risk of infection and bleeding, including avoidance of OTC aspirin-containing medications. Discuss with physician/NP/PA prophylactic antibiotics and any surveillance testing as appropriate. Discuss possible signs and symptoms of infection with physician/NP/PA, and implement antimicrobial medication(s) as ordered. Discuss drug interruption with physician/NP/PA for prolonged neutropenia.

IV.   POTENTIAL FOR ALTERATION IN NUTRITION, LESS THAN BODY REQUIREMENTS, related to NAUSEA, CONSTIPATION, DIARRHEA, VOMITING

Defining Characteristics: Nausea occurs in 25% of patients, constipation 20%, diarrhea 20%, and vomiting 13%. Eleven percent of patients had increased weight, but 25% had peripheral edema.

Nursing Implications: Assess the patient's baseline nutritional status and weight, and monitor it during therapy. If the patient experiences weight gain, assess for peripheral edema. Teach the patient to report nausea, vomiting, or change in bowel status that does not resolve. Discuss management strategies with physician/NP/PA. Teach the patient self-care strategies to manage diet and symptoms.

Drug: brentuximab vedotin (Adcetris®)

Class: CD-30 directed antibody-drug conjugate (ADC) made up of (1) Chimeric (mouse/human) IgG_1 antibody cAC10, specific for human CD30, (2) microtubule disrupting agent MMAE (monomethyl auristatin E), and (3) protease-cleavable linker covalently attaching MMAE to cAC10 (Seattle Genetics, 2018).

Mechanism of Action: CD30, a member of the TNF factor family, is expressed on Hodgkin Reed-Sternberg cells in classical Hodgkin Lymphoma (cHL) as well as on the surface of systemic anaplastic large cell lymphoma (sALCL) cells. The ADC binds to CD-30 expressed cells, is internalized into the malignant cells, MMAE is released which disrupts the microtubule network necessary for cell division, causing cell cycle arrest and cell death (apoptosis). There also appears to be antibody-dependent cellular phagocytosis (Seattle Genetics, 2018).

Metabolism: Maximum ADC concentration occurs at the end of the infusion and dose-proportional. Steady state is reached at 21 days with 3-week dosing. Maximal concentration for MMAE occurred 1–3 days after dose, with steady state at 21 days. The MMAE exposure decreased 50–80% of the first dose with subsequent dosing. Only a small amount of released MMAE is metabolized, primarily by oxidation (CYP3A4/5), with about 24% of MMAE recovered in urine and feces (72%, unchanged) over 1 week. In patients with severe renal failure, the AUC of MMAE is 2-fold higher and 2.3-fold higher in patients with moderate and severe hepatic impairment.

Indications: Treatment of adult patients with: (1) *classical Hodgkin lymphoma (cHL):* (a) previously untreated Stage III or IV cHD in combination with doxorubicin, vinblastine, dacaarbazine; (b) cHD at high risk of relapse or progression as post-autologous hematopoietic stem cell transplantation (auto-HSCT) consolidation; (c) cHD after failure of auto-HSCT or after failure of at least 2 prior multi-agent chemotherapeutic regimens in patients who are not candidates for auto-HSCT; (2) *Anaplastic large cell lymphoma (sALCL):* (a) Previously untreated sALCL or other CD30-expressing peripheral T-cell lymphomas (PTCL), including angioblastic T-cell lymphoma and PTCL not otherwise specified, in combination with cyclophosphamide, doxorubicin, and prednisone; (b) sALCL after failure of at least 1 prior multi-agent chemotherapeutic regimen; (3) *primary cutaneous anaplastic large cell lymphoma (pcALCL)* or CD-30 expressing mycoses fungoides (MF) who have received prior systemic therapy.

Contraindications: Concomitant use with bleomycin due to pulmonary toxicity.

Dosage(s):
• Administer only as an IV infusion over 30 minutes.

Malignancy:
- **Previously untreated stage III or IV cHL**: 1.2 mg/kg (max 120 mg) together with chemotherapy. Administer q 2 weeks until a maximum of 12 doses, disease progression or unacceptable toxicity. If concurrently receiving AVD chemotherapy, administer G-CSF beginning with cycle 1.
- **cHL consolidation**: 1.8 mg/kg (maximum 180 mg). Start therapy within 4–6 weeks post-auto-HSCT or upon recovery from auto-HSCT. Administer every 3 weeks until a maximum of 16 cycles, disease progression or unacceptable toxicity.
- **Relapsed cHL**: 1.8 mg/kg (maximum 180 mg). Administer every 3 weeks until disease progression or unacceptable toxicity.
- **Previously untreated sALCL or other CD30-expressing Peripheral T-cell Lymphoma (PTCL):** 1.8 mg/kg (maximum 180 mg) in combination with chemotherapy. Administer every 3 weeks with each cycle of chemotherapy for 6–8 doses. Patients with PTCL who are receiving brentuximab vedotin with cyclophosphamide, doxorubicin, and prednisone (CHP) chemotherapy, give G-CSF beginning with cycle 1.
- **Relapsed sALCL:** 1.8 mg/kg (maximum 180 mg). Administer every 3 weeks until disease progression or unacceptable toxicity.
- **Relapsed primary Cutaneous ALCL or CD-30 expressing mycosis fungoides**: 1.8 mg/kg (maximum 180 mg). Administer every 3 weeks until a maximum of 16 cycles, disease progression or unacceptable toxicity.

Dose Modifications for Organ Impairment [if patient weighs > 100 kg, calculate based on 100 kg]

Renal impairment.
(1) **For recommended dose 1.2 mg/kg (max 120mg) q 2 weeks:** (a) Normal or mild (CrCL > 50–80 mL/min) or moderate (CrCL 30–50 mL/min): 1.2 mg/kg (maximum 120 mg q 2 weeks; (b) Severe (CrCL < 30 mL/min): avoid use.
(2) **For recommended dose 1.8 mg/kg (max 180 mg) q 3 weeks):** (a) Normal or mild (CrCL > 50–80 mL/min) or moderate (CrCL 30–50 mL/min): 1.8 mg/kg (maximum 180 mg q 3 weeks; (b) Severe (CrCL < 30 mL/min): avoid use.

Hepatic impairment.
(1) **For recommended dose 1.2 mg/kg (max 120 mg) q 2 weeks:** (a) Normal: 1.2 mg/kg (Max 120 mg q 2 weeks; (b) Mild (Child-Pugh A): 0.9 mg/kg (max 90 mg) q 2 weeks; (c) Moderate or Severe (Child-Pugh B, C): Avoid use.
(2) **For recommended dose 1.8 mg/kg (max 180 mg) q 3 weeks:** (a) Normal: 1.8 mg/ kg (max 180 mg) q 3 weeks; (b) Mild (Child-Pugh A): 1.2 mg/kg (max 180 mg) q 3 weeks; (c) Moderate or severe (Child-Pugh B, C): avoid use.

Dose Modification for Toxicity [if patient weighs > 100 kg, calculate based on 100 kg]:

Peripheral Neuropathy
(1) **For recommended dose 1.2 mg/kg (max 120 mg) q 2 weeks, in combination with chemotherapy:** (A) Grade 2: Reduce dose to 0.9 mg/kg (max 90 mg) q 2 weeks; (B) Grade 3: Hold brentuximab until improvement to grade 2 or lower; restart at 0.9 mg/kg

(max 90 mg) q 2 weeks, consider modifying dose of other neurotoxic chemotherapy; (C) Grade 4: discontinue drug.

(2) **For recommended dose 1.8 mg/kg (max 180 mg) q 3 weeks:**
   a. **MONOTHERAPY:** (A) New or worsening grade 2 or 3: Hold brentuximab until improvement to baseline or grade 1; restart at 1.2 mg/kg (max 120 mg) q 3 weeks; (B) Grade 4: discontinue drug.
   b. **IN COMBINATION WITH CHEMOTHERAPY:** (A) Grade 2: Sensory neuropathy: continue treatment at same dose; Motor neuropathy: reduce dose to 1.2 mg/kg up to a maximum of 120 mg every 3 weeks; (B) Grade 3: sensory neuropathy: reduce dose to 1.2 mg/kg up to a maximum of 120 mg every 3 weeks; motor neuropathy: discontinue drug; (C) Grade 4: discontinue drug.

Neutropenia

In combination with chemotherapy:
(1) **For recommended dose 1.2 mg/kg (max 120mg) q 2 weeks:** Grades 3 or 4: Administer G-CSF prophylaxis for subsequent cycles if patient did not receive primary G-CSF prophylaxis.
(2) **For recommended dose 1.8 mg/kg (max 180 mg) q 3 weeks:** Grades 3 or 4: Administer G-CSF prophylaxis for subsequent cycles if patient did not receive primary G-CSF prophylaxis.

As monotherapy:
(1) **For recommended dose 1.8 mg/kg (max 180 mg) q 3 weeks:** (A) Hold dosing until improvement to baseline or grade 2 or lower, consider G-CSF prophylaxis for subsequent cycles; (B) Recurrent grade 4 despite G-CSF prophylaxis: Consider drug discontinuation or dose reduction to 1.2 mg/kg up to a maximum of 120 mg q 3 weeks.

Dose for patients weighing >100 kg should be calculated based ona weight of 100 kg.

Drug Preparation:
Available as 50 mg of brentuximab vedotin as a sterile, white to off-white lyophilized preservative-free cake or powder in a single dose vial for reconstitution.
- Use safe handling precautions, including PPE, when preparing and disposing of drug and equipment.
- Determine the number of 50-mg vials needed based on patient weight and prescribed dose.
- Asceptically, reconstitute each 50-mg vial with 10.5 mL Sterile Water for Injection USP to yield a single dose solution of 5 mg/mL concentration of brentuximab vedotin.
- Direct the stream of diluent toward the vial wall rather than directly into the cake or powder. Gently swirl vial contents but Do Not Shake.
- Inspect reconstituted solution: it should be clear to slightly opalescent, colorless, and free of visible particles.
- Following reconstitution, dilute immediatey into an infusion bag. If not diluted immediatedly, store the solution at 2–8°C (36–46°F) and use within 24 hours of reconstitution. Do Not Freeze.
- Discard any unused portion of drug left in vial.

- To dilute into an infusion bag, calculate the required volume of reconstituted brentuximab vedotin (5 mg/mL), aseptically withdraw from vial, and add it to an infusion bag containing a minimum of 100 mL solution (0.9% Sodium Chloride, 5% Dextrose Injection, or Lactated Ringer's Injection) to achieve a final concentration of 0.4 mg/mL–1.8 mg/mL brentuximab vedotin.
- Gently invert bag to mix the solution.
- Administer the diluted drug immediately, or may store the solution at at 2–8°C (36–46°F) and use within 24 hours. Do Not Freeze.

Drug Administration:
- Administer G-CSF beginning with cycle 1 to patients with: (a) previously untreated stage III or IV cHL receiving brentuximab vedotin with doxorubicin, vinblastine, and dacarbazine (AVD), and (b) previously untreaeted PTCL who are treated with brentuximab vedotin and cyclophosphamide, doxorubicin and prednisone (CHP).
- Assess patient for signs/symptoms of (a) neuropathy, and compare to baseline unless first dose, and if so, document baseline for serial comparisons; (b) CBC absolute neutrophil count, platelet count, presence of signs/symptoms of infections, risk of developing TLS, renal and hepatic function, skin integrity, pulmonary and GI status.
- Teach patient potential side effects, self-care measures, and what and how to report any significant side effects right away.
- Verify pregnancy status of female patients of reproductive potential. Teach women of reproductive potential the drug is fetotoxic and and to avoid pregnancy during and after treatment by using effective contraception during and for at least 6 months after last drug dose.
- Teach male patients with female partners of reproductive potential to use effective contraception during and for at least 6 months after last drug dose. Teach male patients that their fertility may be compromised by brentuximab vedotin therapy and provide sperm banking information/resources as requested and appropriate.
- Administer brentuximab vedotin only as an IV infusion over 30 minutes.
- Assess for infusion reactions and anaphylaxis during the infusion, and stop the infusion if they occur. If a patient has experienced an infusion reaction in prior doses, discuss premedication with acetaminophen, an antihistamine, and a corticosteroid with the NP, PA, or physician.

Lab Interactions/Effects:
- Neutropenia, thrombocytopenia, anemia.
- Elevated liver enzymes, bilirubin.

Drug Interactions:
- CYP3A4 inhibitors/inducers: MMAE is a substrate of CYP3A4/5, and primarily metabolized by CYP3A4.
  - Inhibitor: Coadministration with ketoconazole (potent CYP3A4 inhibitor) increased AUC by about 34%.
  - Coadministration with potent inducer rifampin decreases AUC by about 46%
- P-glycoprotein (P-gp) inhibitors: MMAE is a substrate of efflux transporter P-gp; coadministration may increase exposure to MMAE.

- ABVD: Bleomycin should NOT be given as additive pulmonary toxicity; patient should receive AVD (doxorubicin, vinblastine, dacarbazine) when ordered in combination with brentuximab vedotin.

Special Considerations:
- Most common adverse reactions were neutropenia, anemia, peripheral sensoty neuropathy, nausea, fatigue, constipation, diarrhea, vomiting, pyrexia.
- Warnings and Precautions:
  - *Progressive multifocal leukoencephalopathy (PML):* JC virus infection may occur resulting in PML and death. Assess for and discuss any new-onset CNS neurological changes with physician or NP/PA right away (e.g., worsening general weakness, clumsiness, balance issues, sensory loss, personality changes). Hold drug if PML suspected, and drug should be discontinued if PML diagnosis is confirmed. Patients at risk include those who have received prior therapies or underlying disease that is immunsuppressive.
  - *Peripheral neuropathy (PN):* 62% incidence, primarily sensory, but motor neuropathy can occur with monotherapy. When given with AVD, the incidence is 67% (all grades PN), and was 52% in patients receiving brentuximab vedotin and CHP. Monitor for symptoms of PN such as hypoesthesia, hyperesthesia, paresthesia, discomfort, burning sensation, neuropathic pain or weakness. If a patient experiences new onset or worsening PN, discuss treatment delay with provider, change in dose, or drug discontinuation as appropriate.
  - *Anaphylaxis and infusion reactions:* Monitor patient closely during infusion. Interrupt infusion if a reaction occurs, discuss management with provider. If anaphylaxis occurs, drug should be permantly discontinued, and medical intervention instituted immediately.
  - *Hematologic Toxicities:* Febrile neutropenia can be prolonged and severe ($\geq$1 week), and grade 3 or 4 thrombocytopenia and anemia can occur. When drug is combined with chemotherapy, G-CSF prophylaxis should begin with Cycle 1 (e.g., previously untreated stage III/IV cHL or previously untreated PTCL) receiving chemotherapy. Assess CBC/differential prior to each dose, and more frequently if low or grade 3 or 4 neutropenia develops. Monitor for fever, and teach patient self-care strategies, and to report fever right away. Consider dose delay, reduction, drug discontinuation or G-CSF prophylaxis with next dose (if not used previously) for grade 3 or 4 neutropenia and monitor for fever and infection closely.
  - *Serious infection and opportunistic infections:* Pneumonia, bacteremia, and sepsis/septic shock has occurred. Monitor patients closely for bacterial, fungal, or viral infections and treat promptly.
  - *Tumor Lysis Syndrome (TLS):* Patients with high tumor burden and rapidly proliferating tumors are at increased risk for TLS; anticipate and discuss prophylaxis with physician or NP/PA.
  - *Increased toxicity in patients with severe renal impairment.* Drug should not be given to patients with severe renal impairment (CrCL < 30 mL/min).
  - *Increased toxicity in patients with moderate or severe hepatic impairment.* Do not administer drug to patients with moderate (Child-Pugh B) or severe (Child-Pugh C) hepatic impairment.

- *Hepatotoxicity:* Hepatocellular injury can occur, characterized by elevated serum transaminases and/or bilirubin. Risk may be higher in patients with preexisting liver disease, elevated baseline transaminases and bilirubin. Hold, change dose, or discontinue drug in patients with worsening or recurrent hepatotoxicity.
- *Pulmonary toxicity:* Non-infectious pulmonary toxicity (e.g., pneumonia, interstitial lung disease, ARDS) has occurred. Assess patients for cough and dyspnea, and other signs/symptoms of pulmonary toxicity. If new or worsening symptoms develop, discuss with provider holding drug until evaluation and symptomatic improvement.
- *Serious dermatologic reactions:* Stevens Johnson Syndrome (SJS) and toxic epidermal necrolysis (TEN) have occurred; if either is suspected or occurs, hold or discontinue drug and give appropriate ordered therapy.
- *Gastrointestinal (GI) complications:* Acute pancreatitis has been reported, as well as serious and potentially fatal GI complications such as perforation, hemorrhage, ulcer, obstruction, enterocolitis, neutropenic colitis, and ileus. Patients with lymphoma having GI involvement may have increased risk of perforation. Hold drug and discuss with provider prompt evaluation of any new or worsening GI symptoms.
- *Embryo-fetal toxicity:* Drug can cause fetal harm. Confirm pregnancy status of women of reproductive potential prior to starting drug. Teach these women of reproductive potential should to avoid pregnancy by using effective contraception during and for at least 6 months after last drug dose. Brentuximab vedotin may damage spermatozoa and testicular tissue with resulting genetic abnormalities so men with female sexual partners of reproductive potential should use effective contraception during therapy and for at least 6 months after final dose of brentuximab vedotin.
- Teach new mothers not to breastfeed while receiving the drug.

Potential Toxicities/Side Effects and the Nursing Process

I.   POTENTIAL FOR INJURY related to HYPERSENSITIVITY/ANAPHYLAXIS and INFUSION REACTION

Defining Characteristics: Infusion reactions across 4 studies with brentuximab vedotin given as monotherapy showed an incidence of 13% (grade 3 in 10% of these), most commonly characterized by chills, nausea, dyspnea, pruritis, pyrexia, and cough. The incidence decreased to 9% when combined with chemotherapy. Rarely, anaphylaxis has been reported.

Nursing Implications: Assess baseline mental status and vital signs/oxygenation prior to drug administration, and periodically during infusion, as needed. If infusion reaction occurs, interrupt infusion and discuss rate decrease or medical intervention with provider. Discuss premedication and administer this for patients who have had a prior infusion reaction. If anaphylaxis occurs, stop and discontinue the drug immediately, assess patient vital signs, and implement physician or NP/PA medical orders. Recall signs/symptoms of anaphylaxis: subjective symptoms include generalized itching, nausea, chest tightness, crampy abdominal pain, difficulty speaking, anxiety, agitation, sense of impending doom, uneasiness, desire to urinate/defecate, dizziness, and chills. Objective signs are flushed appearance; angioedema of face, neck, eyelids, hands, and feet; localized or generalized urticaria; respiratory distress with or without wheezing; hypotension; and cyanosis. Review standing physician orders or nursing procedures for patient management of anaphylaxis, and be prepared to stop drug immediately and change IV to a plain NS solution to keep vein patent, notify physician, keep patent airway, monitor VS, and administer ordered medications, which may include epinephrine 1:1,000 IM in the thigh, IV hydrocortisone sodium succinate, and IV diphenhydramine. Teach patient to report any unusual symptoms. Patient should be observed after each treatment, and longer periods may be required if the patient experiences an infusion reaction. Discuss management with provider: e.g., for mild-to-moderate infusion reactions (grades 1–2), decrease infusion rate permanently by 50%, and drug should be discontinued in patients who experience severe infusion reactions (grades 3–4).

II.   POTENTIAL FOR INFECTION AND BLEEDING related to BONE MARROW DEPRESSION

Defining Characteristics: Neutropenia is common, with an incidence of 54%-981 across studies. Febrile neutropenia occurs in 19% of patients receiving brentuximab vedotin and AVD chemotherapy. Febrile neutropenia may be severe and prolonged (≥ 1 week). Anemia incidence is 27%–98%, and thrombocytopenia 15%–28%. Grade 3 and 4 thrombocytopenia or anemia may occur.

Nursing Implications: Assess baseline CBC/absolute neutrophil count baseline and monitor before each treatment, and more often as needed. See dose modification for grade 3 and 4 neutropenia. Assess for signs/symptoms of viral, bacterial and fungal infection. Ensure patients receiving brentuximab vedotin and AVD chemotherapy also receive prophylactic G-CSF starting with Cycle 1. Assess risk for infection and integrity of skin and mucous membranes, pulmonary status, and ability to clear secretions, as well as history of past infections, baseline and prior to each treatment. Teach patient to self-assess for signs/symptoms of infection and to call provider immediately or come to the emergency room if temperature > 100.5°F, shaking chills, or rash, productive cough, burning on urination, or any signs/symptoms of infection or bleeding. Teach self-care strategies to minimize risk of infection and bleeding, including avoidance of OTC aspirin-containing medications. If a patient develops neutropenia and is not receiving prophylactic G-CSF discuss with provider starting this. See dose reductions for patients with renal or hepatic dysfunction. Drug should not be given to patients with severe renal impairment or moderate or severe hepatic impairment.

Drug: cemiplimab-rwlc (Libtayo®)

Class: Programmed death receptor-1 (PD-1) blocking antibody.

Mechanism of Action: The body protects itself from uncontrolled immune response by turning the response down or off, by binding the PD-1 ligands PD-L1 and PD-L2 to the PD-1 receptor found on T cells, inhibiting T-cell and cytokine production. Some tumor cells are able to turn up (upregulare) the action of PD-1 ligands turning the immune response off so the T-cells cannot seek the tumor cells and kill them. Cemiplimab-rwlc binds to PD-1, thus preventing PD-L1 and PD-l2 ligands from binding to the T-cell receptor, the pathway is not inhibited or turned off, and the immune response is kept in the ON position, so tumor cell immune surveillance and tumor cell killing continues.

Metabolism: With continued every 3 week IV dosing, steady-state is reaching in 4 months, with an elimination half-life of 19 days.

Indications: Treatment of patients with metastatic cutaneous squamous cell carcinoma (CSCC) or locally advanced CSCC who are not candidates for curative surgery or RT.

Contraindications: None.

Dosage/Range: 350 mg IV infusion over 30 minutes every 3 weeks until disease progression or unacceptable toxicity.

Dose Modification

Severe and potentially fatal immune-related adverse effects (irAEs):
- Pneumonitis: Grade 2: hold cemiplimab-rwlc; grades 3–4: permanently discontinue drug.
- Colitis: Grades 2–3: hold cemiplimab-rwlc; grade 4: permanently discontinue drug.
- Hepatitis: (1) AST or ALT ↑ to >3 and up to 10 times ULN or if total bilirubin ↑ up to 3 × ULN: hold cemiplimab-rwlc; (2) AST or ALT ↑ to > 10 times ULN or if total bilirubin ↑ > 3 × ULN: permanently discontinue drug.
- Endocrinopathies: Grades 2,3,4: hold cemiplimab-rwlc if clinically necessary.
- Other immune reactions involving a major organ: Grade 3: hold cemiplimab-rwlc; grade 4: permanently discontinue drug.
- Recurrent or persistent IRAEs: Permanently discontinue drug for (1) recurrent Grade 3,4; (2) Grade 2–3 persistent for 12 weeks or longer after last cemiplimab-rwlc dose, or (3) requirement of 10 mg/day or greater prednisone or equivalent lasting 12 weeks or longer after last cemiplimab-rwlc dose.

Other AEs: Infusion-related reactions:
- Grade 1–2: interrupt or slow the rate of infusion.
- Grade 3–4: permanently discontinue cemiplimab-rwlc.

Drug Preparation:
- Cemiplimab-rwlc is available as 350 mg/7 mL (50 mg/mL) solution in a single-dose vial.
- Visually inspect vial; vial contents should be clear to slightly opalescent, colorless to pale yellow solution but may contain trace amounts of translucent to white particles. Discard vial if cloudy, discolored, or has extraneous particulate matter other than described.
- Preparation: Do not shake. Withdraw 7 mL from vial and dilute with 0.9% Sodium Chloride Injection USP or 5% Dextrose Injection USP to a final concentration between

1 mg/mL–20 mg/mL. Mix diluted solution by gentle inversion; do not shake. Discard any unused product.

- Storage of Infusion Solution: Store at room temperature up to 25°C (77°F) for no more than 8 hours from preparation time to the end of the infusion, or at 2°C–8°C (36°F–46°F) for no more than 24 hours from time of preparation to the end of the infusion.

Drug Administration:
- Teach patient about potential irAEs, and infusion reaction.
- Teach patient to self-assess and to report right away (1) new or worsening cough with SOB, chest pain; (2) diarrhea, black stools or with blood or mucous, severe stomach pain; (3) skin, severe nausea, vomiting, pain on right side of stomach; (4) dark urine, bleeding or bruising; (5) changes in how you feel, rapid heart beat, weight gain or loss, deep voice, changes in mood; (6) blood in urine, or decrease in volume of urine; (7) rash or itching of skin; (8) any other changes.
- Assss patient for signs/symptoms of irAEs baseline and prior to each treatment. Assess serum chemistries, LFTs, thyroid function tests, glucose baseline, and as ordered during therapy. Discuss any abnormalities with provider.
- Verify negative pregnancy test of female patients of reproductive potential.
- Administer cemiplimab-rwlc 350 mg IV infusion over 30 min, through an IV line containing a sterile, in-line or add-on 0.2 micron to 5-micron filter.
- Monitor patient for signs/symptoms of infusion reaction, and teach patient to report asap chills, itching/rash, SOB, dizziness, fever, feeling like passing out, back or neck pain, facial swelling.
- Teach female patients of reproductive potential to use effective contraception during and for at least 4 months after the last cemiplimab-rwlc dose.

Drug Interactions:
- None known. Corticosteroids ≥ 10 mg equivalency of prednisone given baseline (with or before the PD-1 and PD-L1 inhibitors) has been associated with decreased drug efficacy in treatment of NSCLC (Arbour et al., 2018).

Lab Effects/Interference:
- Increased AST, INR, serum calcium.
- Decreased serum albumin, phosphate, sodium

Special Considerations:
- Most common side effects (≥20%), in clinical trials were: fatigue, rash, diarrhea.
- Women should not breast feed while receiving the drug and for at least 4 months after last cemiplimab-rwlc dose.
- Warnings and Precautions:
  - *Severe and fatal immune-mediated adverse reactions (irAEs):* irAEs can occur in any organ system or tissue, usually during but can also occur after receiving PD-1 inhibitors. Early identification and intervention are critical.
    - Monitor patient for signs/symptoms of irAEs. Monitor serum chemistries, including LFTs and thyroid function tests, baseline and periodically during treatment. Intervene promptly to manage irAEs, and discuss specialty consults as needed with MD/NP/PA.

- Expect that in general, hold cemiplimab-rwlc for grade 3–4, and certain grade 2 irAEs. Drug should be permanently discontinued for grade 4 and certain grade 3 irAEs.
- Expect to administer ordered corticosteroids (1–2 mg/kg/da) or equivalent for grade 3–4 and certain grade 2 irAEs until improvement to grade 0–1 followed by a corticosteroid taper over 1 month. If toxicity uncontrolled with this, expect order for other systemic immunosuppressant.
- Expect hormone replacement therapy for endocrinopathies as indicated.
- Immune related pneumonitis: incidence 2.4% and was grade 5 in 0.2%, grade 3 (0.7%), and grade 2 (1.3%).Corticosteroids were necessary in all patients with pneumonitis and 85% received doses ≥ 40 mg/day or equivalent. Pneumonitis resolved in 62% of patients.
- Immune-related colitis: Incidence 0,9% of patients (grade 3 in 0.4%, grade 2 in 0.6%). All patients received corticosteroids, and 60% received doses ≥40 mg/day or equivalent, resulting in resolution in 80% of patients.
- Immune-mediated colitis: Incidence 0.9% (Grade 5 in 0.2%, grade 4 in 0.2%, grade 3, 1.7%). All patients received corticosteroids, and 91% received doses ≥40 mg/day or equivalent, resulting in resolution in 64% of patients.
- Immune-mediated endocrinopathies included adrenal insufficiency, hypophysitis, hypothyroidism, hyperthyroidis, and Type 1 diabetes mellitus (DM).
- Immune-related nephritis with renal dysfunction: Incidence was 0.6% (grade 3, 0.4%, grade 2, 0.2%. All patients received corticosteroids, and 67% received doses ≥40 mg/day or equivalent, resulting in resolution in 100% of patients.
- Immune-related dermatologic AEs included erythema multiforme and pemphigoid: Incidence 1.7% (grade 3 in 1.1%, grade 2 in 0.6%. Stevens Johnson syndrome (SJS) and toxic epidermal necrolysis (TEN) has lso occurred. All patients received corticosteroids, and 89% received doses ≥40 mg/day or equivalent, resulting in resolution in 33% of patients. About 22% of patients experienced recurrence after reinstitution of cemiplimab-rwlc.
- Other irAEs occurring in <1% of patients included: neurological (e.g., meningitis, myelitis, encephalitis, myasthenia gravis, demyelination), cardiovascular (e.g., myocarditis, pericarditis, vascultitides), ocular (e.g., uveitis, iritis, retinal detachment, visual impairment, blindness), GI (e.g., pancreatitis), musculoskeletal/connective tissue (e.g., arthritis, myositis, rhabdomyolysis), and hematologic/immunologic changes (e.g., hemolytic anemia, aplastic aneia, systemic inflammatory response syndrome). If uveitis occurs in combination with other irAEs, discuss possible Vogt-Koyanagi-Harada like syndrome which may require systemic corticosteroids to prevent blindness.
- *Infusion-related reactions (IRRs):* Severe IRRs (grade 3) occurred in 0.2% of patients. Monitor patients during infusion for signs/symptoms of IRRs. Grade 1–2 IRRs: interrupt or slow infusion rate as ordered; grade 3–4, permanently discontinue cemiplimab-rwlc as ordered by provider.
- *Embryo-fetal toxicity:* Drug is feto-toxic. Teach female patients of reproductive potential to use effective contraception during cemiplimab-rwlc and for at least 4 months after last dose.

Potential Toxicities/Side Effects and the Nursing Process

I.   ALTERATION IN COMFORT related to FATIGUE, MUSCULOSKELETAL PAIN

Defining Characteristics: Fatigue occurred in 29% of patients. Musculoskeletal pain occurred in 17% of patients..

Nursing Implications: Teach the patient that these events may occur and to report them. Assess baseline comfort and self-care strategies to maintain comfort and energy conservation. Monitor closely during treatment. Develop a plan to assure comfort, depending on the symptoms reported, and assess its efficacy and revise the plan if needed at each visit.

II.   ALTERATION IN NUTRITION, POTENTIAL, LESS THAN BODY REQUIREMENTS, related to DECREASED APPETITE, NAUSEA, CONSTIPATION, VOMITING, OR DIARRHEA

Defining Characteristics: Nutritional impact symptoms of nausea, vomiting, diarrhea, constipation, and decreased appetite can occur: diarrhea (22%), nausea (19%), constipation (12%), and decreased appetite (10%).

Nursing Implications: Assess nutritional and bowel-elimination patterns, appetite, and presence of nausea and/or vomiting at baseline and at each visit. Teach that diarrhea, constipation, nausea, vomiting, and decreased appetite may occur and to report them. Assess nutrition impact symptoms and discuss their management with the patient, including dietary modification. Teach the patient to self-administer antidiarrheal or antiemetic medication, if needed, and to report symptoms that do not improve. In addition, teach patients to report immediately any diarrhea, blood or mucus in the stool or black, tarry stools, or severe stomach pain or tenderness so that the potential for colitis may be promptly further evaluated.

III.   ALTERATION IN SKIN INTEGRITY, POTENTIAL, related to RASH, PRURITUS

Defining Characteristics: Skin integrity can be affected by rash, and pruritis, especially if the patient itches the skin. Rash occurred in 25% of patients, and pruritis 15%.

Nursing Implications: Teach the patient that rash, and pruritus may occur and to report them. Assess the patient's skin integrity both at baseline and regularly during therapy. Teach patient self-care measures to reduce pruritis and maintain intact skin (e.g., if very itchy, wear thin white gloves at night when sleeping).

IV.   POTENTIAL ALTERATION IN OXYGENATION related to PNEUMONITIS

Defining Characteristics: In clinical trials, incidence was 2.4%. See Warnings and Precautions.

Nursing Implications: Teach the patient to report new or worsening cough, chest pain, or shortness of breath. Monitor the patient for signs and symptoms of pneumonitis. Discuss findings with the physician/NP/PA. Expect that after exclusion of other diagnoses, the patient will be evaluated with imaging and pulmonary and infectious disease consultation if respiratory status changes occur. If pneumonitis confirmed, expect the drug to be held until resolution, and corticosteroids administered. Administer ordered corticosteroids followed by a 1-month taper. Monitor daily.

V. POTENTIAL ALTERATION IN ELIMINATION related to COLITIS

Defining Characteristics: Incidence of immune-related colitis was 0.9%. Expect corticostoids to be ordered for all patients with a confirmed diagnosis of ir-colitis. Monitor patients for immune-mediated colitis.

Nursing Implications: Teach the patient to report signs and symptoms of colitis (diarrhea, blood in stools or tarry stools, severe abdominal pain). Monitor the patient for immune-mediated colitis, and administer corticosteroids as ordered.

VI. POTENTIAL ALTERATION IN NUTRTION related to HEPATITIS

Defining Characteristics: Immune-mediated hepatitis (defined as requiring use of corticosteroids and no clear alternate etiology) and abnormal LFTs may occur. Incidence in clinical trials was 2.1%. Signs and symptoms of hepatitis include elevated transaminases and total bilirubin, icterus, severe nausea and vomiting, right-sided abdominal pain, drowsiness, dark urine, increased bruisability or bleeding, and anorexia.

Nursing Implications: Assess LFTs at baseline and monitor regularly during therapy. Evaluate the patient for right-sided abdominal pain, drowsiness, dark urine, increased bruising or bleeding, and loss of appetite. Teach the patient to report any yellowing of the skin or whites of the eyes, as well as severe nausea or vomiting. Expect corticosteroids to be ordered for all patients with ir-hepatitis. Monitor patient closely.

VII. POTENTIAL ALTERATION IN URINE ELIMINATION related to IMMUNE-MEDIATED NEPHRITIS AND RENAL DYSFUNCTION

Defining Characteristics: Immune-related nephritis defined as renal dysfunction or grade 2 or higher increased creatinine, requirement for corticosteroids, and no clear alternate etiology, can occur. Incidence with cemiplimab-rwlc was 0.6%.

Nursing Implications: Assess the patient's baseline renal function, and monitor closely during therapy. Teach the patient to report signs and symptoms such as a decrease in the amount of urine, blood in urine, ankle swelling, loss of appetite. Hold drug and administer ordered corticosteroids to all patients with ir-nephritis, and once resolved, taper over 1 month as ordered.

Drug: cetuximab (Erbitux)

Class: Chimeric (mouse/human) monoclonal IgG_1 antibody targeted against epidermal growth factor receptor (EGFR1).

Mechanism of Action: Epidermal growth factor receptor (EGFR, HER1) is a transmembrane glycoprotein receptor tyrosine kinase (RTK) that is turned on (constitutively expressed) in many normal epithelial tissues, such as the skin and hair follicles. Activation of this RTK is also seen in cancers in the head and neck, colon, and rectum, as well as others. Cetuximab binds specifically to EGFR in normal and tumor cells, has a 10 times greater binding affinity to EGFR than the EGF ligand. It competitively inhibits the binding of its ligand EGF and others, such as transforming growth factor-α (TGF-α). This prevents dimerization and initiation of cell signaling via RTK phosphorylation; thus, the message telling the cell to divide does not occur and is not sent down the cell's communication pathway. In addition to cell growth inhibition, there is induction of apoptosis and decreased matrix metalloproteinase and VEGF production so invasion and metastasis is blocked. As an IgG1 mAb, it may also recruit immune effector cells via ADCC, as well as complement activation. Drug is synergistic with chemotherapy and radiotherapy, as it appears to prevent the malignant cell from repairing DNA damage. Drug is effective only if *KRAS* and *NRAS* genes are normal (called wild-type). If *KRAS* gene is mutated, it turns itself on and sets up an independent signaling cascade, bringing a message to the nucleus that tells the cell to divide regardless of whether or not EGFR is blocked by cetuximab. *KRAS* gene is mutated in about 30% of patients with mCRC, but rarely in patients with SCCHN. Resistance to cetuximab appears related to EGFR mutations causing decreased binding affinity, decreased EGFR expression, increased expression of TGF-α ligand, *KRAS* mutation in codons 12 and 13, *BRAF* mutations, *NRAS* mutations, increased HER-2 expression through gene amplification, and increased HER-3 expression (Chu & DeVita, 2016).

Metabolism: Drug is an IgG_1 chimerized antibody, and it is postulated that clearance is via binding of the antibody to EGFR of hepatocytes with internalization of the cetuximab-EGFR complex. Mean elimination half-life is approximately 97 hours (range, 41–213 hours). Steady state reached by third weekly infusion. Mean half-life is 112 hours. Females have a 25% lower clearance of drug than males, but there was no difference in efficacy. No differences were found related to race, age, and hepatic and renal functional impairment.

Indication: Treatment of patients with
- *Head and neck cancer* (1) locally or regionally advanced squamous cell carcinoma in combination with radiation therapy; (2) recurrent locoregional disease or metastatic squamous cell carcinoma in combination with platinum-based therapy with 5-FU; (3) recurrent or metastatic squamous cell carcinoma progressing after platinum-based therapy.
- *CRC,* **K-Ras** *mutation-negative (wild-type),* EGFR-expressing metastatic (mCRC), as determined by FDA-approved tests (1) in combination with FOLFIRI (irinotecan, 5-Fluorouracil, leucovorin) for first-line treatment; (2) in combination with irinotecan in patients refractory to irinotecan-based chemotherapy; and (3) as a single agent in patients

who have failed oxaliplatin- and irinotecan-based chemotherapy, or who are intolerant to irinotecan.
- **Indicated only in mCRC patients with *RAS* wild-type tumors**, as determined by an FDA-approved test. Patients with *KRAS* gene mutation in codon 12 or 13 (exon 2) or mutation in *NRAS* have not shown a treatment benefit and in fact may do worse so drug is not recommended in these patients. Signal transduction through the EGFR results in activation of wild-type *KRAS* or *NRAS* protein. However, in cells with activating *KRAS* or *NRAS* (somatic) mutations, the mutant KRAS or NRAS protein is continually active and appears independent of EGFR regulation.

Dosage/Range:
- Premedicate with an H_1 antagonist 30–60 minutes before cetuximab.

SCCHN
- Monotherapy: Administer 400 mg/m^2 initial dose as a 120-minute IV infusion followed by 250 mg/m^2 weekly infused over 60 minutes.
- In combination with RT or platinum-based therapy and fluorouracil
  - Initiate cetuximab initial dose 400 mg/m^2 IV one week prior to initiation of RT or on the first day of platinum-based therapy/fluorouracil, as a 120-minute infusion.
  - Complete cetuximab administration 1 hour prior to platinum-based therapy with 5-FU and FOLFIRI.
  - Subsequent doses for all other infusions are 250 mg/m^2 weekly as a 60-minute infusion for the duration of RT (6–7 weeks) or until disease progression or unacceptable toxicity when administered in combination with platinum-based therapy with fluorouracil.

CRC
- Monotherapy or in combination with irinotecan or FOLFIRI (irinotecan, fluorouracil, leucovorin):
  - Administer 400 mg/m^2 initial dose as a 120-minute IV infusion
  - Then 250 mg/m^2 weekly infused over 60 minutes until disease progression or unacceptable toxicity
  - *Complete cetuximab 1 hour before irinotecan or FOLFIRI.*
- Reduce the infusion rate by 50% for NCI CTC grade 1 or 2 infusion reactions.
- Permanently discontinue for grade 3 or 4 infusion reactions.
- Dermatologic toxicities and infectious sequelae: grade 3 or 4.
- First occurrence: delay infusion 1–2 weeks; if improvement, continue at 250 mg/m^2; if no improvement, discontinue cetuximab.
- Second occurrence: delay infusion 1–2 weeks; if improvement, decrease dose to 200 mg/m^2; if no improvement, discontinue cetuximab.
- Third occurrence: delay infusion 1–2 weeks; if improvement, decrease dose to 150 mg/m^2; if no improvement, discontinue cetuximab.
- Fourth occurrence: discontinue cetuximab.
- Pulmonary toxicity: Acute onset or worsening pulmonary symptoms: delay infusion 1–2 weeks; if improvement, continue at dose administered at time of occurrence. If no improvement in 2 weeks or if interstitial lung disease (ILD) is confirmed, discontinue cetuximab.

Drug Preparation:
- Available in 100 mg/50 mL and 200 mg/100 mL single-use vials, with concentration of 2 mg/mL, as a sterile, injectable liquid without preservatives.
  - Do not shake or dilute. Solution should be clear and colorless, and may contain small, white particles of cetuximab that are easily visible.
  - Inspect vial, and do not use if discolored or particulate matter present.
- Store vials under refrigeration at 2–8°C (36–46°F). Do not freeze. Increased particulate formation may occur at temperatures at or below 0°C. Drug contains no preservatives.
- Drug prepared in infusion containers are chemically and physically stable for 12 hours at 2–8°C (36–46°F), and for 8 hours at controlled room temperature (20–25°C or 68–77°F). Discard any remaining solution in the infusion container after 8 hours at room temperature, or 12 hours at 2–8°C (36–46°F). Discard any unused portion of the vial.

Drug Administration:
- Assess baseline labs and before each treatment, including serum magnesium and potassium. Ensure electrolyte values are WNL before treatment.
- Drug must be filtered using a low protein-binding 0.22-μm in-line filter prior to infusion.
- Administer as an IV infusion over 2 hours for a loading dose, and 1 hour for a maintenance dose, using an infusion pump or syringe pump. Do not exceed infusion rate of 10 mg/min.
- Premedicate with an antihistamine before administration, and administer at a maximum of 10 mg/min. Observe patient for 1 hour following infusion, or longer (as needed) if an infusion reaction develops.
- Flush with 0.9% saline solution at the end of the infusion.

Drug Interactions:
- Synergy with cytotoxic chemotherapy (e.g., irinotecan) or radiotherapy
- Radiation sensitizer

Lab Effects/Interference:
- Hypomagnesemia; also related hypocalcemia, hypokalemia.

Special Considerations:
- Most common adverse reactions in cetuximab clinical trials (incidence ≥25%) include cutaneous adverse reactions (e.g., rash, pruritis, nail changes), headache, diarrhea, and infection.
- Warnings and Precautions
  - *Infusion reactions:* Incidence of severe (grades 3–4) infusion reactions low (2–5%), but may be fatal (1/1,000). Risk of anaphylaxis may be increased in patients with a history of tick bites, red meat allergy, or in the presence of IgE antibodies directed against galactose-α-1,3-galactose (alpha-gal). Ninety percent of severe reactions occur during first infusion despite premedication and are characterized by rapid onset of airway obstruction (stridor, hoarseness, bronchospasm), hypotension, shock, LOC, myocardial infarction, and/or cardiac arrest. Treat with epinephrine, corticosteroids, antihistamines, bronchodilators, oxygen as needed, and keep available. Drug

should be discontinued if severe reaction occurs. Mild-to-moderate reactions require infusion-rate reduction and prophylactic diphenhydramine.

- Premedicate with antihistamine.
- Monitor patients for 1 hour after drug infusion in a setting with resuscitation equipment and medications to treat anaphylaxis (e.g., epinephrine, corticosteroids, IV antihistamines, bronchodilators, and oxygen).
- Monitor patients longer (>1 hour) to confirm resolution if the patient requires treatment for an infusion reaction. Resume infusion at a slower rate if reaction resolves, as ordered.
- Immediately and permanently discontinue cetuximab if patient has a serious infusion reaction.

- *Cardiopulmonary arrest:* cardiopulmonary arrest/sudden death occurred in 2% of patients treated with RT and cetuximab vs none in the patients receiving RT alone, in one clinical trial. Carefully consider cetuximab use in combination with RT or platinum-based therapy with 5-FU in head and neck cancer patients with history of coronary artery disease, CHF, or arrhythmia. In addition, electrolytes including magnesium, calcium, and potassium should be closely monitored during and after cetuximab therapy, as low serum magnesium, calcium, and potassium increase risk of development of torsades de pointes, with subsequent ventricular tachycardia and sudden death.
- *Pulmonary toxicity:* Very rarely (< 0.5%), ILD may occur. Hold drug and evaluate patients who develop acute or worsening pulmonary symptoms. Permanently discontinue the drug if ILD is found.
- *Dermatologic toxicity:* Skin toxicity (including acneiform rash, skin drying and fissuring, paronychial inflammation, infectious sequelae, cellulitis, blepharitis, conjunctivitis, keratitis/ulcerative keratitis with decreased visual acuity, chelitis) and hypertrichosis (long eyelashes) occurs. Rash occurred in 76–88% and was severe in 1–17% of patients in clinical trials.
  - Rash usually develops within the first 2 weeks of therapy and resolves after treatment cessation, but in >50%, continued >28 days. Life-threatening and fatal bullous mucocutaneous disease with blisters, erosions, skin sloughing has been observed, but it is unclear if directly related to cetuximab.
  - Monitor patients for skin toxicity and infection of the rash.
  - Teach patients to wear sunscreen and hats, as well as to limit sun exposure. Rash is not acne but a sterile, inflammatory rash (see introduction to this chapter for a complete discussion).
- *Use of cetuximab in combination with RT and cisplatin:* patients develop an increased incidence of grade 3/4 mucositis, radiation recall syndrome, acneiform rash, cardiac events, and electrolyte disturbances compared to patients receiving RT and cisplatin alone. The addition of cetuximab to RT and cisplatin did not improve PFS (Eli Lily, 2016).
- *Hypomagnsemia and electrolyte abnormalities:* Hypomagnesemia occurred in 55% of patients during clinical trials, and was severe in 6–17%. Onset of hypomagnesemia and other electrolyte disturbances occurred days to months after beginning cetuximab. Monitor serum electrolytes baseline and periodically during treatment for hypomagnesemia,

hypocalcemia, and hypokalemia during and for at least 8 weeks after last dose of cetuximab. Repeat as necessary.

- *Increased tumor progression*, increased mortality, or lack of benefit inpatients with *Ras*-mutant mCRC (somatic mutations in exon 2 (codons 12,13), exon 3 (codons 59,61), and exon 4 (codons 117,146) of either *K-Ras* or *N-Ras*).
- *EGFR expression and response:* almost all patients with SCCHN have EGFR positive tumors. In clinical studies of patients with mCRC, response rate did not correlate with either the percentage of positive cells or intensity of EGFR expression (Eli Lily, 2016).
- *Ebryo-fetal toxicity:* Women of childbearing age should use effective contraception, during therapy and extending for 2 months from the last dose of cetuximab. If cetuximab is administered to a pregnant woman, it should be done only if the benefit outweighs the potential risk. Nursing mothers should discontinue nursing during cetuximab therapy and for 2 months from the last dose of the drug.
- Cetuximab improved overall survival when compared with best supportive care (BSC), which led to its second indication in treatment of patients with advanced CRC: patients receiving cetuximab had a 23% improvement in OS and a 32% reduction in risk of disease progression. OS was 6 months in the cetuximab arm compared with 4.5 months in the BSC arm (Jonker et al., 2007).

Potential Toxicities/Side Effects and the Nursing Process

I.   POTENTIAL FOR INJURY related to HYPERSENSITIVITY/ANAPHYLAXIS and INFUSION REACTION

Defining Characteristics: Across all studies, some patients (15–21%) experienced an infusion reaction, largely (90%) with the first infusion, as evidenced by pyrexia, chills, rigors, dyspnea, bronchospasm, angioedema, urticaria, hypertension, and hypotension. Grades 3–4 reactions occurred in 2–5% of patients and were fatal in one patient. Severe infusion reactions can be characterized by rapid onset of airway obstruction (bronchospasm, stridor, hoarseness), hypotension, shock, LOC, myocardial infarction, and/or cardiac arrest. Treat with epinephrine, corticosteroids, antihistamines, bronchodilators, oxygen as ordered, and keep these medications close by and available. The incidence of anaphylaxis is geographically predicted, with an incidence of 20% in Tennessee to Missouri, about 11% in California, and 0.6% in Boston (Chung et al., 2008).

Nursing Implications: Ensure patient receives premedication with diphenhydramine as ordered. Assess baseline VS and mental status prior to drug administration, at 15 minutes, and periodically during infusion, as needed. Remain with patient during first 15 minutes of first infusions. Recall signs/symptoms of anaphylaxis, and if these occur, stop drug immediately, notify physician, and assess patient's vital signs. Subjective symptoms are generalized itching, nausea, chest tightness, crampy abdominal pain, difficulty speaking, anxiety, agitation, sense of impending doom, uneasiness, desire to urinate/defecate, dizziness, and chills. Objective signs are flushed appearance; angioedema of face, neck, eyelids, hands, and feet; localized or generalized urticaria; respiratory distress with or without wheezing; hypotension; and cyanosis. Review standing physician orders or nursing procedures for patient management of anaphylaxis, and be prepared to stop drug immediately and change IV to a plain NS solution to keep vein patent, notify physician, keep patent airway, monitor VS, and administer ordered medications, which may include epinephrine 1:1,000 IM in the thigh, IV hydrocortisone sodium succinate, and IV diphenhydramine. Teach patient to report any unusual symptoms. Patient should be observed for 1 hour after each treatment, and longer periods may be required if the patient experiences an infusion reaction. For mild-to-moderate infusion reactions (grades 1–2), decrease infusion rate permanently by 50%, and continue prophylactic diphenhydramine. Drug should be discontinued in patients who experience severe infusion reactions (grades 3–4).

II. POTENTIAL ALTERATION IN BODY IMAGE, SKIN INTEGRITY, COMFORT, related to SKIN RASH, CHANGES IN EYES AND HAIR FOLLICLES

Defining Characteristics: Drug inhibits epidermal growth factor receptor, so major toxicity is manifested in the skin. Most patients (88–90%) develop a mild-to-moderate acne-like rash that is self-limiting. Grades 3–4 rash across all studies occurred in 9–18% of patients. Rash is a sterile, suppurative rash with multiple follicular or pustular lesions that appear during the first 2 weeks of therapy in areas of sun exposure: face, upper chest, and back, but in some cases, it is extended to the arms. Rash maximizes within 4 weeks, and then improves. Rash also resolves when treatment is stopped. However, in 50% of patients, it takes longer than 28 days to resolve. Dry skin and itching often occur. Scratching with dirty hands or nails can lead to fissures and infection. Nail changes occur, as well as paronychia. Eye changes are related to EGFR blockade and inflammation, and include blepharitis (inflammation of eyelid), conjunctivitis, keratitis/ulcerative keratitis with decreased visual acuity, and hypertrichosis (excessive hair). Infection can be treated with topical clindamycin or oral antibiotics. It appears that patients who have significant rash also have a tumor response.

Nursing Implications: Teach patient that rash most likely will occur due to mechanism of drug action. Assess baseline skin integrity on areas of face, neck, and trunk; assess baseline comfort and satisfaction with body image, and monitor at each treatment. Teach patient to report any distress and assess extent of rash. For severe rash, first occurrence, hold drug for 1–2 weeks, and if improvement, continue drug at usual dose. For second occurrence, hold for 1–2 weeks, and then if improved, reduce dose to 200 mg/m^2. If third occurrence of severe rash, hold drug for 1–2 weeks, and if improvement, dose-reduce to 150 mg/m^2. For the fourth occurrence or if there is no improvement after holding drug for 2 weeks in prior occurrences, drug is stopped. If skin appears to be infected (exudate, vesicle formation, abnormal appearance), obtain C+S and discuss empiric treatment with physician. *For rash management, refer to introduction in this chapter.* Teach all patients to (1) use a water-based emollient frequently during the day to prevent dryness, (2) stay hydrated, (3) avoid sun exposure and wear SPF 30 (zinc-based). Do not use antiacne medications. Tetracycline analogues provide anti-inflammatory benefit. Grade 1/mild rash (localized, does not interfere with ADLs, and is not infected): Goal is to preserve skin integrity, minimize discomfort, and prevent infection. Key patient teaching includes (1) use a mild soap with active ingredients that reduce skin drying, such as pyrithione zinc (Head & Shoulders),

(2) consider applying aloe gel to red, tender areas, (3) report distressing tenderness, as pramoxine (lidocaine topical anesthetic) may help, (4) keep fingernails clean and trimmed, and (5) apply zinc ointment to rectal mucosa after washing. Management: maintain current drug dose, observe or give topical hydrocortisone 1 or 2.5% or clindamycin 1% gel (anti-inflammatory benefit), reassess in 2 weeks. For grade 2/moderate, which is generalized, mild symptoms, has minimal effect on ADLs, and no infection: Goal is to prevent infection and promote comfort. Continue EGFRI dose; use topicals (hydrocortisone 2.5% or clindamycin 1% gel) and consider adding doxycycline 100 mg PO twice daily or minocycline 100 mg PO twice daily (give antimicrobial and anti-inflammatory effect) and reassess after 2 weeks. For grades 3–4 or severe rash (generalized, severe, has a significant impact on ADLs, and increased risk of infection): The goal is to prevent infection or identify it early to minimize complications and to promote effective coping. Interrupt drug. Treat rash with topicals (hydrocortisone 2.5%, or clindamycin 1% gel), doxycycline 100 mg PO twice daily or minocycline 100 mg PO twice daily, and methylprednisolone (Medrol dose pack); reassess after 2 weeks. Resume drug when rash improved to grade 2, at full or reduced dose (Lynch et al., 2007; Lacouture et al., 2011). If rash appears infected (exudate, vesicular formation, different appearance), obtain C+S, treat empirically until sensitivity received, and/or obtain dermatology consult.

III.   ALTERATION IN ELECTROLYTE BALANCE related to HYPOMAGNESEMIA, POTENTIAL

Defining Characteristics: Magnesium wasting appears related to EGFR inhibition in the renal tubular epithelial cells so that excreted magnesium is not resorbed in the distal convoluted tubules. This leads to initial magnesium wasting, followed by losses of calcium and potassium. Hypomagnesemia occurs in about 55% of patients receiving the drug and is severe in 6–17% of patients. It begins within days to months of receiving the drug, and there is much interpatient variability. There appears to be a direct relationship between the duration of cetuximab treatment and severe hypomagnesemia (Fakih, 2007). Symptoms of grades 3–4 hypomagnesemia include fatigue, cramps, and somnolence.

Nursing Implications: Assess baseline electrolyte balance before initial treatment and before each successive weekly treatment. Grade 1 is a serum level of 1.0 mg/dL LLN, grade 2 is 0.9–1.0 mg/dL, grade 3 is 0.7–0.8 mg/dL, and grade 4 is ≤ 0.6 mg/dL. Replete magnesium, calcium, and potassium as needed. Oral magnesium may be ineffective and result in diarrhea (Tejpar et al., 2007). Magnesium repletion regimens include weekly IV replacement of 4-g magnesium sulfate for grade 2. For grades 3–4, patients may be symptomatic, and magnesium replacement may involve once to twice weekly IV infusions of 6–10 g. Provide support for patients, as magnesium replacement infusions require lengthy time in clinic, as an 8-g infusion requires 4 hours. Post-IV replacement with every other day serum magnesium monitoring is important until the patient develops a steady state (Fakih, 2007). Continue to monitor after drug has been discontinued (half-life of the drug and time drug persists, e.g., 8 weeks). Magnesium replacement in IV hydration, beginning when a patient has grade-1 hypomagnesemia, may be effective in preventing worsening hypomagnesemia.

For patients who have refractory grade-4 hypomagnesemia, a stop-and-go approach has been effective where cetuximab is held for 4–8 weeks until the magnesium corrects; it is reported that grade-4 hypomagnesemia does not recur when cetuximab is then reintroduced (Fakih, 2007).

IV. ALTERATION IN NUTRITION, LESS THAN BODY REQUIREMENTS, related to NAUSEA, VOMITING, DIARRHEA, STOMATITIS/MUCOUS MEMBRANE DISORDER, CONSTIPATION, WEIGHT LOSS

Defining Characteristics: Incidence of mild-to-moderate digestive symptoms includes nausea (64% for patients across all trials, 19–64%, diarrhea (19–66%), vomiting (0–40%), stomatitis/mucous membrane disorder (MMD) (0–32%), weight loss (0–15%), anorexia (0–30%), and constipation (0–53%). Seven percent of patients develop MMD; 86% of patients with squamous cell cancer of the head and neck receiving concurrent RT experienced mucositis.

Nursing Implications: Assess baseline weight and nutritional status. Teach patient that these symptoms may occur and to report them. Administer antiemetic and other symptom management medications as ordered. Teach patient self-administration of these medications at home. Monitor serum electrolytes (magnesium, calcium) prior to each dose, and replete magnesium as needed. Teach patient dietary modifications to address symptoms such as anorexia (small, frequent high-calorie, high-protein foods, stimulants as permitted by protocol); constipation (high-fiber, high-fluid, high-roughage foods, stool softeners); diarrhea (BRAT diet: bananas, rice, applesauce, and toast); nausea (avoid food preparation odors by cooking in zipped plastic bag, or having someone else cook; choose cool, soft, nonspicy, or fatty foods); mucositis (blenderized high-calorie, protein-dense foods, cold or cool soft foods, avoidance of spicy or acidic foods; or percutaneous endoscopically placed gastrostomy [PEG] tube feedings when unable to swallow, local anesthetics to reduce oral and esophageal discomfort/pain). Assess efficacy of intervention and revise plan as needed.

V. POTENTIAL FOR INFECTION AND FATIGUE related to LEUKOPENIA AND ANEMIA

Defining Characteristics: Leukopenia occurs in about 25% of patients (combination vs. 1% monotherapy) with 17% grades 3–4 (combination) and anemia in 16% (combination vs. 10% monotherapy) with 4–5% grades 3–4.

Nursing Implications: Assess baseline WBC, hematocrit, and hemoglobin, and monitor prior to each treatment, especially if drug is given in combination with irinotecan. Teach patient to monitor temperature and report temperature > 100.5°F. Assess level of fatigue and teach energy baseline and prior to each treatment. Teach patient that fatigue may occur due to anemia, and teach energy-conserving strategies such as alternating rest and activity periods.

Drug: Daratumumab (Darzalex)

Class: Monoclonal IgG1 antibody, targeting the CD38 protein on hematopoietic cells

Mechanism of Action: CD38 is a transmembrane protein that is expressed on the cell surface of hematopoietic cells, including MM cells; its functions include receptor-mediated adhesion, cell signaling, and modulation of cyclase and hydrolase activity (Janssen Biotech, Inc, 2015). Daratumumab binds to CD38 and inhibits tumor growth, and leads to apoptosis directly via Fc mediated cross linking as well as immune-mediated tumor cell lysis (CDC, ADCC, and antibody dependent cellular phagocytosis [ADCP]). As myeloid derived suppressor cells, NK cells, and a subset of regulatory T cells also express CD38, lysis of these cells represents collateral damage (Janssen, 2015).

Metabolism: Steady state is reached about 5 months into the every 4-week dosing period. The estimated terminal half-life of the drug is about 18 days. Renal impairment did not influence drug level or concentration. Mild hepatic impairment did not make a clinical difference, but drug was not studied in patients with moderate or severe hepatic impairment.

Indications: Treatment of patients with MM (1) in combination with bortezomib, melphanan and prednisone for the treatment of patients with newly diagnosed MM who are ineligible for a autologous stem cell transplant; (2) in combination with lenalidomide and dexamethasone, or bortezomib and dexamethasone for patients who have received at least 1 prior therapy; (3) in combination with pomalidomide in patients who have received at least 2 prior therapies including a lenalidomide and a proteasome inhibitor; and (4)) as monotherapy, in patients who have received at least 3 prior lines of therapy including a proteasome inhibitor (PI), an immunomodulatory agent (I), or who are double-refractory to a PI and I.

Contraindications: Patients with a history of hypersensitivity to daratumumab of any of the components of the forumulation.

Dosage/Range: 16 mg/kg actual body weight as an IV infusion. Administer pre- and postinfusion medications. Administer only as an IV infusion after dilution with 0.9% Sodium Chloride Injection, USP.

(1) Newly diagnosed MM: In combination with bortezomib, melphalan, prednisone (VMP)-6-week cycle dosing regimen in patients ineligible for autologous stem cell transplant.
   a. Weeks 1–6 = weekly doses × 6
   b. Weeks 7–54 = every 3 week dosing schedule (total of 16 doses)
   c. Weeks 55 onward until disease progression = every 4-week dosing schedule
(2) Relapsed/refractory MM: Monotherapy combination therapy with lenalidomide or pomalidomide and low-dose dexamethasone (4-week cycle dosing regimen)
   a. Weeks 1–8 = weekly × 8 (total of 8 doses)
   b. Weeks 9–24 = every 2 week dosing (total of 8 doses)
   c. Week 25 onwards until disease progression = every 4 week dosing

(3) Relapsed/refractory MM:
   a. Monotherapy and combination therapy with bortezomib and dexamethasone (4-week cycle regimen)
      i. Weeks 1–8 = weekly (total of 9 doses)
      ii. Weeks 9–24 = every 3 weeks (total of 5 doses)
      iii. Week 25 onward until disease progression = every 4 weeks
(4) b. Combination therapy with bortezomib and dexamethasone (3-week cycle regimen)
      i. Weeks 1–9= weekly × 9
      ii. Weeks 10–24= every 3 weeks (total 5 doses)
      iii. Week 25 onward until disease progression = every 4 weeks
(5) Missed daratumumab doses: administer missed dose as soon as possible and adjust dosing schedule accordingly to keep the treatment interval.
(6) To facilitate administration, the first prescribed 16 mg/kg dose at week 1 may be split over 2 consecutive days (e.g., 8 mg/kg on day 1 and 8 mg/kg on day 2).

- **Use infusion rate shown in Drug Administration.**
- Daratumumab does not contain a preservative so must be given immediately at room temperature (15–25°C [59–77°F]) and in room light. Diluted solution can be kept at room temperature for a maximum of 15 hours (including infusion time).
- If not used immediately, the diluted solution can be stored prior to administration for up to 24 hours at refrigerated conditions (2–8°C [36–46°F]) and protected from light.

Dose Modifications:
- No dose adjustments; dose delay may be necessary to permit bone marrow recovery. Interrupt for infections and treat with antimicrobial therapy.
- Discontinue drug for severe, life-threatening infusion reactions.

Drug Preparation: Available in 100 mg/5 mL and 400 mg/20 mL solutions in a single-dose vial.
- Prepare the infusion solution using aseptic technique
  - Calculate the dose (mg), total volume (mL) of drug required and the number of daratumumab vials needed based on ordered dose and patient's actual body weight.
  - Inspect daratumumab solution: it should be colorless to pale yellow. Do not use if opaque particles, discoloration, or other foreign particles present.
  - Aseptically remove a volume of 0.9% sodium chloride injection USP from infusion bag/container equal to the required volume of daratumumab solution.
  - Withdraw necessary amount of daratumumab solution and dilute to appropriate volume (1,000 mL first infusion, 500 mL infusion 2 and subsequent unless patient had a reaction) by adding to a 0.9% Sodium Chloride Injection USP infusion bag/container. Infusion bag or container must be made of PVC, polypropylene (PP), polyethylene (PE), or polyolefin blend (PP+PE). Use aseptic technique.
  - Gently invert bag/container to mix; do not shake.
  - Following dilution, diluted infusion bag should be administered immediately at room temperature as infusion does not contain a preservative. Otherwise, infusion bag/container may be stored for up to 24 hours in a refrigerator at 2–8°C (36–46°F), protected from light. Do not freeze. After allowing bag/container to come to room temperature use immediately since prepared drug contains no preservative.

- Inspect drug product for particulate matter and discoloration before administration. Very small, translucent to white proteinaceous particles may be visible as drug is a protein. Do not use if visibly opaque particles, discoloration, or other foreign particles are observed.
- Do not administer daratumumab concomitantly in the same IV line with other agents.

Drug Administration:
- Ensure a type and screen has been sent to the blood bank prior to starting treatment. Inform blood bank that patient will be receiving daratumumab.
- Ensure immediate access to emergency equipment and appropriate medical support to manage infusion reactions if they occur. **Drug should be interrupted** for any grade/severity of infusion reaction.
- If infusion bag refrigerated, allow to come to room temperature.
- Assess vital signs, baseline and monitor patient closely during infusion for reactions. Stop drug and discuss/implement medical intervention as ordered.
- Adminster preinfusion and postinfusion medications as ordered.
- **Preinfusion medications** to all patients 1–3 hours before every daratumumab infusion: (1) corticosteroid, long or medium acting [(*Monotherapy*: methylprednisolone 100 mg or equivalent IV before infusions 1 and 2, then after the second infusion, the dose may be reduced (IV or oral 60 mg); *Combination therapy*: dexamethasone 20 mg or equivalent prior to each infusion (first infusion should be IV, then can consider oral for subsequent infusions); Additional background regimen-specific corticosteroids (e.g., prednisone) should not be taken on daratumumab infusion days when patient receives dexamethasone (or equivalent) as premedication.(2) antipyretic (oral acetaminophen 650–1,000 mg); (3) antihistamine (PO or IV diphenhydramine 25–50 mg or equivalent).
- Administer diluted solution as an IV infusion using an infusion set fitted with a flow regulator and an in-line, sterile, nonpyrogenic, low-protein-binding polyethersulfone (PES) filter (pore size 0.22 or 0.2 micrometer). Polyurethane (PU), polybutadiene (PDB), PVD, PP, or PE administration sets must be used.
- Infusion line should be a dedicated line without other agents infusing concomitantly.
- **Infusion should be completed within 15 hours** as there is no preservative.
- Infusion rate (Maximum rate 200 mL/hr) [see package insert, table 4, 2019):
  - **First infusion**: 1,000 mL at 50 mL/hr initial rate, increase 50 mL/hr every hour, to maximum rate 200 mL/hr; increase infusion rate only in absence of infusion reactions.
  - **Second infusion**: 500 mL at 50 mL/hr initial rate, increase 50 mL/hr every hour, to maximum rate 200 mL/hr; increase infusion rate only in absence of infusion reactions. Use a dilution volume of 500 mL only if there were NO grade 1 (mild), or greater infusion reactions **during the first 3 hours of the FIRST infusion**. Otherwise continue to use the dilution volume of 1,000 mL and instructions for first infusion.
  - **Subsequent infusions** (third infusion onward): 500 mL at 100 mL/hr initial rate, increase 50 mL/hr every hour, to maximum rate 200 mL/hr. **Use the modified initial rate ONLY if there were no grade 1 (mild) or greater infusion reactions during a final infusion rate of ≥ 100 mL/hr in the first two infusions.** Otherwise follow instructions for the second infusion.

- **Postinfusion medication:** to reduce the risk of delayed infusion reaction for all patients.
  - *Monotherapy:* Oral corticosteroid (intermediate or long-acting) [20 mg methylprednisolone or equivalent]on each of 2 days (1, 2) following all infusions; start day after the infusion
  - *Combination therapy:* Consider giving low-dose oral methylprednisolone (≤20 mg) or equivalent on the day after the daratumumab infusion. If the background regimen-specific corticosteroid (e.g., dexamethasone) is administered the day after the daratumumab infusion, it may not be necessary to give additional postinfusion medications.
  - Patients with a history of COPD, consider short- and long-acting bronchodilators, and inhaled corticosteroids. If the patient tolerates the first 4 infusions without major infusion reactions, these additional inhaled medications can be discontinued.
- **Prophylaxis for herpes zoster reactivation:** Start antiviral prophylaxis within 1 week of starting daratumumab and continue for 3 months following end of treatment.
- If a dose is missed, administer the dose as soon as possible and adjust the dose schedule accordingly.
- *Infusion reactions of any severity:* interrupt daratumumab immediately and manage the symptom(s), such as further reduction in infusion rate; if life-threatening, discontinue drug. See above.
  - Grades 1–2 (mild-moderate): once symptoms resolve, resume infusion at no more than half the rate at which the reaction occurred. If patient does not experience further symptoms, rate can be escalated at appropriate increments and intervals (e.g., 50 mg/hr) to the maximum rate of 200 mL/hr.
  - Grade 3 (severe): Once reaction symptoms have resolved, consider restarting infusion at no more than half the rate at which the reaction occurred. If the patient does not experience additional symptoms, resume infusion rate escalation at prescribed increments and intervals. If there is a recurrence of grade 3 symptoms, stop drug, manage symptoms, then consider resumption at no more than half the infusion rate at which the symptoms recurred once resolved, and consider reescalation at appropriate increment and interval if no further reaction occurs. If a third episode of grade 3 or greater infusion reaction occurs, permanently discontinue drug.
  - Grade 4 (life threatening): permanently discontinue drug.

Drug Interactions: None known.

Lab Effects/Interference:
- Interference with indirect antiglobulin tests (Coombs Test): drug binds to CD38 on red blood cells, and results in a positive Indirect Antiglobulin Test (indirect Coombs test); this may persist for up to 6 months after last infusion. Daratumab bound to RBCs masks detection of antibodies to minor antigens in the serum but this does not interfere with determining the patient's ABO, Rh blood type (Janssen Biotech, 2016).
- Anemia, thrombocytopenia, neutropenia, lymphopenia.
- Increase in CD4+ and CD8+ T-cells.
- Decrease in myeloid derived suppressor cells, NK cells, and certain regulatory T-cells.

Special Considerations:
- Type and screen patients prior to starting treatment. Inform blood banks that the patient is receiving daratumumab and that type and screen blood bank specimens drawn after first treatment will be inaccurate.
- Most common side effects were infusion reactions, neutropenia, thrombocytopenia, fatigue, nausea,diarrhea, constipation, vomiting, muscle spasms, arthralgia, back pain, pyrexia, chills, dizziness, insomnia, cough, dyspnea, peripheral edema, peripheral sensory neuropathy, and URI.
- Warnings and Precautions:
  - *Infusion reactions:* Daratumumab can cause severe infusion reactions. Forty-six percent of patients have an infusion reaction, most during the first infusion and were grade 1–2; however, reactions can occur with subsequent infusions. Almost all infusion reactions during or occur within 4 hours of completing the infusion.
  - With postinfusion medication(s), incidence of subsequent or postinfusion reactions is significantly less. Most occur during the infusion or within 4 hours of completing the infusion. Before postinfusion medications were administered, reactions occurred up to 48 hours after the infusion.
  - Severe reactions have occurred, including bronchospasm, hypoxia, dyspnea, HTN, laryngeal edema, and pulmonary edema.
  - Assess for signs and symptoms of infusion reaction including respiratory symptoms (cough, nasal congestion, throat irritation), chills, vomiting, and nausea. Less common symptoms were wheezing, allergic rhinitis, pyrexia, chest discomfort, pruritis, and hypotension.
  - Adhere to premedication and postmedication administration guidelines (including an oral corticosteroid to all patients after the infusion) to decrease risk of infusion reactions. Monitor patient closely during the entire infusion. Interrupt infusion for any reaction and manage symptoms as ordered. Infusion rate should be reduced for all grade 1–3 reactions, and drug should be permanently discontinued for grade 4 reactions. If a patient has a grade 1–3 reaction, ensure infusion rate is reduced when restarting the infusion.
  - If a patient has COPD, consider adding to postinfusion medications: short- and long-acting bronchodilators and inhaled steroids (2019).
- *Interference with serological testing:* Patient should have a **type and screen performed prior to starting therapy**, and the blood bank should be notified that the patient is receiving this drug. See Lab Interference section.
- *Neutropenia:* Daratumumab may increase the neutropenia caused by the other drugs when used in combination. Monitor CBC/differential baseline and periodically during treatment as ordered. Monitor patients for signs/symptoms of infection, and teach to report them right away. Drug may need to be delayed until neutrophil recovery, but daratumumab dose is not reduced. Consider growth factor support.
- *Thrombocytopenia:* Daratumumab may increase thrombocytopenia caused by the other drugs when used in combination. Monitor CBC/differential baseline and periodically during treatment as ordered. Monitor patients for signs/symptoms of bleeding, and teach to report them right away. Daratumab may need to be delayed until platelet recovery, but daratumab dose is not reduced.

- *Interference with determination of complete response:* Drug is an IgG kappa mAb that can be detected on both serum protein electrophoresis (SPE) and immunofixation (IFE) assays used in monitoring endogenous M-protein; this interference may interfere with determining whether the patient with IgG kappa myeloma has had a CR or disease progression (Janssen Biotech, 2016).
- Teach women and men of reproduction potential to use effective contraception during and for 3 months after the last daratumumab dose.
  - IgG$_1$ mAbs cross the human placenta and theoretically may cause fetal myeloid or lymphoid-cell depletion, and increased bone density.
  - Do not administer live vaccines to neonates or infants exposed to daratumumab in utero until a hematology evaluation is completed.
- Published data suggest breast milk antibodies do not enter the neonatal or infant circulation during breastfeeding. If breastfeeding desired, risks and benefits should be weighed.

Potential Toxicities/Side Effects and the Nursing Process

I.   POTENTIAL FOR INJURY related to INFUSION-RELATED REACTIONS

Defining Characteristics: IRRs are common, with 46% occurring during the first infusion, 5% with the second infusion, and 4% with subsequent infusions. Second and subsequent infusion reactions were all < grade 3. Median time to onset was 1.5 hours and 37% of infusions were interrupted due to a reaction. Median duration of infusions were 7.0 hours for first infusion, 4.6 hours for second infusion, and 3.4 hours for subsequent infusions. Severe reactions can occur, characterized by bronchospasm, dyspnea, hypoxia, and hypertension.

Nursing Implications: Ensure that premedications and postinfusion medications are administered. If patient has obstructive pulmonary disease, discuss with provider use of inhalers (see administration). Ensure that medications necessary for the management of severe infusion reactions are readily available (e.g., epinephrine, antihistamines, corticosteroids) and that provider is locally available to assess patient and prescribe orders. Assess baseline VS and monitor frequently during the infusion. Follow infusion rate guidelines (see Drug Administration section) for first, second, and subsequent infusions. Escalate dose as ordered only if there were no grade 1 or greater infusion reactions during the first 3 hours of first infusion, or for the first two infusions, no grade 1 or higher infusion reactions during a final infusion rate of ≥ 100 mL/hr. Stop the infusion for ANY infusion reaction and discuss symptom management with provider. For grades 1–2, once symptoms resolve, resume infusion at no more than half the rate at which the reaction occurred, and if no further reactions, resume incremental infusion rate increases at prescribed interval as ordered. If grade 3, when reaction symptom(s) decrease to grade 2 or less, discuss with provider resumption of the infusion at no greater than half the infusion rate when the symptoms occurred; if no additional symptoms occur, resume infusion rate escalation at increments and intervals as outlined in administration. Monitor VS, and notify physician of changes, especially during/ after rate escalation. Be prepared to provide emergency support as necessary (including IV saline, epinephrine, antihistamines, bronchodilators).

II.   ALTERATION IN COMFORT related to FATIGUE, PYREXIA, COUGH, BACK PAIN, ARTHRALGIA

Defining Characteristics: Fatigue occurred in 39%, pyrexia 21%, cough 21%, back pain 23%, arthralgia 17%. Anemia occurred in 45% (19% grade 3).

Nursing Implications: Assess baseline comfort prior to each infusion, and tolerance of past infusion. Discuss strategies to manage symptoms. Teach patient strategies to conserve energy. If symptoms are severe, discuss management with physician.

III.   POTENTIAL FOR INJURY related to INFECTION and BLEEDING

Defining Characteristics: URI occurred in 20%, nasopharyngitis 15%, pneumonia 11%. Neutropenia occurred in 60% (17% grade 3, 3% grade 4), lymphopenia 72% (30% grade 3, 10% grade 4). Thrombocytopenia occurred in 48% (10% grade 3, 8% grade 4).

Nursing Implications: Monitor CBC, platelets baseline and regularly during treatment. If the patient develops cytopenia, monitor more frequently. Assess for signs/symptoms of infection, bleeding, fatigue, and chest pain prior to each treatment. Teach patient to self-assess for these, including taking temperature, and instruct to report them immediately. Transfuse red cells and platelets as ordered.

IV.   ALTERATION IN NUTRITION, POTENTIAL, related to NAUSEA, DIARRHEA, CONSTIPATION, VOMITING, DECREASED APPETITE

Defining Characteristics: Nausea affected 27% patients in clinical trials, diarrhea 16%, constipation 15%, and vomiting 14%. Decreased appetite affected 15%.

Nursing Implications: Assess baseline nutritional status, and presence of nutritional impact symptoms. Teach patient these side effects may occur and to report them. Assess patient each day of treatment and discuss self-care strategies including over-the-counter management of constipation and diarrhea; if these strategies are not effective, discuss prescription pharmacological management with provider.

Drug: darbepoetin alfa (Aranesp)

Class: Cytokine, CSF.

Mechanism of Action: Recombinant DNA protein that is an erythropoiesis-stimulating protein, closely resembling erythropoietin. Drug is produced in the Chinese hamster ovary. Drug stimulates erythropoiesis in the same way that endogenous erythropoietin does in response to hypoxia. Darbepoetin alfa interacts with progenitor stem cells to stimulate red blood cell production.

Metabolism: Following subcutaneous administration of Aranesp to patients with chronic kidney disease (CKD) (receiving or not receiving dialysis), absorption was slow and C_{max} occurred at 48 hours (range: 12–72 hours). In patients with CKD receiving dialysis, the average $t_{1/2}$ was 46 hours (range: 12–89 hours), and in patients with CKD not receiving dialysis, the average $t_{1/2}$ was 70 hours (range: 35–139 hours). Aranesp apparent clearance was approximately 1.4 times faster on average in patients receiving dialysis compared to patients not receiving dialysis. The bioavailability of Aranesp in patients with CKD receiving dialysis after subcutaneous administration was 37% (range: 30–50%).

Indication: For the treatment of anemia due to (1) effects of concomitant myelosuppressive chemotherapy, and upon initiation, there is a minimum of 2 additional months of planned chemotherapy; (2) CKD in patients on dialysis and patients not on dialysis. Drug has not been shown to improve quality of life, fatigue, or patient well-being.

Not Indicated: For use (1) in patients with cancer receiving hormonal agents, biologic products, or RT, unless also receiving concomitant myelosuppressive chemotherapy; (2) in patients with cancer receiving myelosuppressive chemotherapy when the anticipated outcome is cure; (3) in patients with cancer receiving myelosuppressive chemotherapy in whom the anemia can be managed by transfusion; (4) as a substitute for RBC transfusions in patients who require immediate correction of anemia.

Contraindications: Patients with (1) uncontrolled hypertension; (2) pure red cell aplasia that begins after treatment with darbapoietin or other erythropoietin protein drugs; (3) serious allergic reactions to darbapoietin.

Limitations of Use: darbopoietin has not been shown to improve quality of life, fatigue, or patient well-being. Aranesp is not indicated for: (1) patients with cancer receiving hormonal agents, biological products, or RT, unless also receiving concomitant myelosuppressive chemotherapy; (2) patients with cancer receiving myelosuppressive chemotherapy when the anticipated outcome is cure; (3) patients with cancer receiving myelosuppressive chemotherapy in whom the anemia can be managed by transfusion; (4) as a substitute for RBC transfusions in patients requiring immediate correction of anemia.

Dosage/Range:
- Use the *lowest dose* of darbepoetin alfa necessary to avoid RBC transfusion. Should not be used if goal is cure.
- Cancer patients receiving chemotherapy: initiate only if Hgb < 10 g/dL and there is a minimum of 2 additional months of planned chemotherapy:
  - 2.25 mcg/kg subcutaneously q week until completion of a chemotherapy course, OR
  - 500 mcg every 3 weeks subcutaneously until completion of a chemotherapy course.

Dose Modifications:
- If Hgb increases by > 1.0 g/dL in 2-week period or when Hgb reaches level to avoid RBC transfusion, reduce dose by 40% of the prior dose when using weekly or every 3-week schedule.
- If Hgb > level to avoid RBC transfusion, hold dose until Hgb falls to point where transfusion may be needed and restart at 40% below previous dose, when using weekly or every 3-week schedule.

- If Hgb increases by < 1 g/dL and remains < 10 g/dL after 6 weeks of therapy, increase dose to 4.5 micrograms/kg/week when given weekly, but not when given every 3 weeks.
- If there is no response as measured by Hgb levels or if RBC transfusions are still required after 8 weeks of therapy, or following completion of a chemotherapy course, discontinue Aranesp whether weekly or every 3-week schedule is being used.
- Dose increases should not occur more frequently than once a month.
- Goal is to prevent or treat deficit of oxygen-carrying capacity (NCCN, 2014): (1) if asymptomatic, in hemodynamically stable chronic anemia without acute coronary syndrome (ACS), goal is Hgb 7–9 g/dL; (2) symptomatic anemia: (a) acute hemorrhage with evidence of hemodynamic instability or inadequate oxygen delivery: transfuse to correct; (b) Hgb < 10 g/dL with tachycardia, postural hypotension, goal is maintain Hgb 8–10 g/dL; (c) anemia with ACS or acute MI: transfusion goal to maintain Hgb ≥ 10 g/dL.
- CKD on dialysis: start darbapoietin therapy when Hgb level is <10 g/dL; if Hgb approaches or exceeds 11 g/dL, reduce or interrupt darbapoietin dose. Recommended starting dose is 0.45 mcg/kg IV or SQ as a weekly dose or 0.75 mcg/kg once every 2 weeks. Use IV route for patients receiving hemodialysis.
- Chronic renal failure patients not on dialysis: Consider starting darbapoietin therapy when Hgb level is < 10 g/dL AND rate of Hgb decline indicates need of RBC transfusion, or to reduce risk of alloimmunization or other RBC transfusion risks. Dose is 0.45 micrograms/kg IV or SC q weekly, OR 0.75 mcg/kg IV, or SQ every 2 weeks. See package insert for pediatric patients with CKD.
  - If increase in Hgb is < 1.0 g/dL over 4 weeks and iron stores are adequate, increase dose by 25% of the previous dose; dose may be increased at 4-week intervals until Hgb is 10–12 g/dL; dose increase no more frequently than once a month.
  - If Hgb rises rapidly (>1 g/dL in any 2-week period), reduce the dose by 25%; if the Hgb continues to increase, hold the dose until Hgb starts to decline, and reinstitute drug at 25% less than prior dose.
  - If Hgb increases by > 1 g/dL in 2-week period, decrease dose by 25% to maintain the lowest hemoglobin to avoid red blood cell transfusion, not to exceed 12 g/dL.
  - Convert from epoetin alfa to darbepoetin alfa (see Special Considerations).
- NCCN alternative regimens (NCCN, 2014).
  - Darbepoetin 100 mcg/week fixed dosing—titrate up to 150–200 micrograms fixed dose weekly subcutaneously.
  - Darbepoetin 200 mcg every 2 weeks fixed dosing—titrate up to 300 mcg fixed dose every 2 weeks subcutaneously.
  - Darbepoetin 300 mcg every 3 weeks fixed dosing—titrate up to 500 mcg fixed dose every 3 weeks subcutaneously.
- Contraindicated in uncontrolled HTN, pure red cell aplasia, or if patient has serious allergic reactions to Aranesp.

Drug Preparation:
- Drug available in single-dose vials containing: 25, 40, 60, 100, 200, 300, and 500 mcg/mL and 150 mcg/0.75 mL, and contains polysorbate.
- Single-dose prefilled syringes containing: 25 mcg/0.42 mL, 40 mcg/0.4 mL, 60 mcg/0.3 mL, 100 mcg/0.5 mL, 150 mcg/0.3 mL, 200 mcg/0.4 mL, 300 mcg/0.6 mL, or 500 mcg/1 mL.

- Do not shake drug, as it may denature it; keep out of bright light; do not dilute; visually inspect drug for discoloration or particulate matter prior to parenteral administration, and discard if found.
- Store at 2–8°C (36–46°F). Do not freeze or shake, and protect from light.

Drug Administration:
- Administer weekly to start, subcutaneously or intravenously, and may be able to give every 2 weeks, depending upon response to drug.

Drug Interactions:
- No studies have been performed.

Lab Effects/Interference:
- Increased hemoglobin and hematocrit.
- Rare pure red-cell aplasia, severe anemia related to neutralizing antibodies.

Special Considerations:
- Warnings and Precautions:
  - *Increased mortality, myocardial infarction, stroke, and thromboembolism:* ESAs increased the risk for death, myocardial infarction, stroke, venous thromboembolism, thrombosis of vascular access when using ESAs to target an Hgb > 11 g/dL.
  - *Increased mortality and/or increased risk of tumor progression or recurrence in cancer patients.*
  - Shortened overall survival and/or increased the risk of tumor progression or recurrence in clinical studies of patients with breast, NSCLC, head and neck cancer, lymphoid, and cervical cancers.
  - Decreased locoregional control also occurred.
  - Decreased progression-free survival and overall survival in metastatic breast cancer trials.
  - Darbopoietin alfa did not demonstrate superiority to placebo for OS or PFS in a double-bind, placebo-controlled trial of patients with advanced NSCLC (Amgen, 2019).
- *Hypertension (HTN):* control HTN prior to initiating and during drug therapy. Patients who have controlled hypertension should have regular assessment of blood pressure. Patients should be encouraged to be compliant with their antihypertensive medication regimen.
- *Seizures:* drug increases the risk for seizures in patients with CKD.
- *Lack or loss of hemoglobin response to Epogen:* rule out other causes such as iron deficiency, infection, inflammation, bleeding, and if it appears related to drug, follow dosing recommendations.
  - *Pure red cell aplasia (PRCA):* if severe anemia and low reticulocyte count develop, hold drug and evaluate patient for neutralizing antibodies to erythropoietin. Permanently discontinue drug if pure red-cell aplasia is diagnosed.
  - *Serious allergic reactions* can occur, including anaphylactic reactions, angioedema, bronchospasm, skin rash, and urticarial. Immediately and permanently discontinue drug and administer supportive care as ordered if serious reactions occur.

- *Severe cutaneous reactions:* Blistering and skin exfoliation have occurred, including erythema multiforme and Steven Johnson Syndrome (SJS). Discontinue drug if severe skin reactions occur.
- *Dialysis management:* After starting darbopoietin alfa, patients may need adjustments to their dialysis prescriptions (e.g., patient may require increased anticoagulation with heparin).
- *Laboratory monitoring:* Evaluate transferrin saturation and serum ferritin before and during epoietin alfa therapy. Give supplemental iron therapy as ordered when ferritin is < 100 mcg/L or when serum transferrin saturation is <20%. Monitor Hgb after starting therapy and after each dose adjustment, weekly until the Hgb is stable and sufficient to minimize the need for RBC transfusion.
- Rarely, patients may develop antibodies that neutralize the effect, which can lead to red-cell aplasia. If a patient loses response to darbepoetin alfa, evaluation should be done to find cause, including presence of binding and neutralizing antibodies to darbepoetin alfa, native erythropoietin, and any other recombinant erythropoietin administered to the patient.
- The possibility that darbepoetin alfa can stimulate tumor growth, especially as a growth factor of myeloid malignancies, has not been studied.
- No studies have been performed on use of the drug in pregnant women. Drug should be used only if potential benefit outweighs risk to the fetus; it is unknown whether the drug is excreted in human milk, so caution should be used if given to a nursing mother.
- See package insert for conversion from epoietin alfa to darbapoietin.

Potential Toxicities/Side Effects and the Nursing Process

I.   ACTIVITY INTOLERANCE related to FATIGUE

Nursing Implications: Assess baseline activity and energy levels. Assess baseline fluid.

II.   ALTERATION IN SKIN INTEGRITY, POTENTIAL, related to PERIPHERAL EDEMA, RASH

Nursing Implications: Perform baseline skin assessment, assess baseline weight and presence of edema. Teach patient to report development of peripheral edema. Teach patient self-assessment of skin, weight, and peripheral edema and to report rash right away. Assess degree of peripheral edema if it develops, and discuss significant edema with physician to determine etiology and management. Teach patient local skin care, including avoidance of tight clothing and shoes, keeping skin moisturized to prevent cracking, and local comfort measures. If rash develops, assess extent, presence of urticaria, and implications regarding allergic reaction and drug discontinuance.

III. ALTERATION IN COMFORT related to HEADACHE, DIZZINESS, FEVER, MYALGIA, ARTHRALGIA

Nursing Implications: Teach patient that bone pain may occur and discuss use of non-steroidal anti-inflammatory drugs with patient and physician for symptom management. Teach patient to remain seated or lying down if feeling dizzy, and when dizziness has resolved, to change position gradually. Monitor hemoglobin weekly during dose determination period, and weekly for at least 4 weeks after each dose adjustment. Teach patient that headache, fever, dizziness, myalgia, and arthralgia may occur and to report them if they do not respond to usual management strategies.

IV. ALTERATION IN ELIMINATION related to DIARRHEA

Nursing Implications: Assess baseline patient bowel elimination pattern. Teach patient to report these side effects so that they can be evaluated. Teach patient self-care measures, including dietary modification, local comfort measures, and OTC antidiarrheal medication. Teach patient to report symptoms that persist, and discuss with physician possible other etiologies and management plan.

V. KNOWLEDGE DEFICIT related to SELF-ADMINISTRATION TECHNIQUE

Defining Characteristics: Drug is administered once weekly, or if response is adequate, may be given once every 2 weeks.

Nursing Implications: Assess baseline psychomotor ability, knowledge, and willingness to learn technique of self-injection. Teach how to refrigerate drug, self-administer using prefilled syringes, activate needle guard, and safely collect used syringes for proper disposal. Drug insert has "Information for Patients and Caregivers." Use written and video supplements to teach process and have patient correctly demonstrate technique prior to performing at home. Make referral to visiting-nurse agency to reinforce teaching if needed. Teach patient telephone number and whom to call if questions or problems arise, and ensure that patient can correctly repeat information.

Drug: dinutuximab (Unituxin)

Class: mAb; binds GD2.

Mechanism of Action: Dinutuximab binds to the glycolipid GD2, which is expressed on neuroblastoma cells and normal cells derived from the neuroectoderm. Through binding, the drug induces cell lysis of GD2-expressing cells through ADCC and CDC.

Metabolism: Drug terminal half-life is 10 days.

Indication: In combination with GM-CSF, interleukin-2 (IL-2), and 13-*cis*-retinoic acid (RA) for the treatment of pediatric patients with high-risk neuroblastoma who achieve at least a partial response to prior first-line multiagent, multimodality therapy.

Contraindications: Patients who have had anaphylaxis to dinutuximab.

Dosage/Range:
- 17.5 mg/m²/day as a diluted IV infusion over 10–20 hours for 4 consecutive days for up to 5 cycles. Infusion is started at 0.875 mg/m²/hr for 30 minutes; infusion rate can be gradually increased as tolerated to a maximum rate of 1.75 mg/m²/hr. Dose modify according to package insert.
- Cycles 1, 3, and 5 are 24 days in duration, and are given in combination with GM-CSF.
- Cycles 2 and 4 are 32 days in duration, and are given in combination with IL-2.
- Required pretreatment with hydration, opioid analgesia, antihistamine, and antipuretic.

Dose Modifications:
- Permanently discontinue drug for grades 3 or 4 anaphylaxis; grades 3 or 4 serum sickness; grade 3 pain, unresponsive to maximal supportive measures; grade 4 sensory neuropathy or grade 3 sensory neuropathy that interferes with daily activities for more than 2 weeks; grade 2 or greater peripheral motor neuropathy; grade 4 hyponatremia despite appropriate fluid management; subtotal or total vision loss, urinary retention that persists following discontinuation of opioids, transverse myelitis, and RPLS.
- Mild to moderate symptoms (e.g., transient rash, fever, rigors, localized urticaria that responds promptly to symptomatic treatment):
  - Onset of reaction: Reduce dinutuximab rate to 50% of previous rate, and monitor closely.
  - After resolution, gradually increase rate up to a maximum rate of 1.75 mg/m²/hr.
- Prolonged or severe adverse reactions (e.g., mild bronchospasm without other symptoms, angioedema that does not affect the airway):
  - Onset: Immediately interrupt dinutuximab infusion.
  - After resolution, if signs and symptoms resolve rapidly, resume dinutuximab at 50% of the previous rate and monitor closely.
  - First recurrence: Discontinue dinutuximab until the following day. If symptoms resolve and continued treatment is warranted, premedicate with hydrocortisone 1 mg/kg (maximum 50 mg) IV and administer dinutuximab at a rate of 0.875 mg/m²/hr in an ICU.
  - Second recurrence: Permanently discontinue dinutuximab.
- Capillary leak syndrome:
  - Moderate to severe but not life-threatening CLS:
    - Onset: Immediately interrupt dinutuximab.
    - After resolution: Resume dinutuximab at 50% of the previous rate.
  - *Life-threatening CLS:*
    - Onset: Discontinue dinutuximab for the current cycle.
    - After resolution: In subsequent cycles, administer dinutuximab at 50% of the previous rate.
  - First recurrence: Permanently discontinue dinutuximab.

- Hypotension (symptomatic, systolic BP [SBP] < lower limit of normal for age, or SBP decreased by more than 15% compared to baseline) requiring medical intervention:
  - Onset: Interrupt dinutuximab infusion.
  - After resolution: Resume dinutuximab infusion at 50% of previous rate. If BP remains stable for ≥ 2 hours, increase the infusion rate as tolerated up to a maximum rate of 1.75 mg/m^2/hr.
- Severe infection or sepsis: At onset of reaction, discontinue dinutuximab until resolution of infection; then proceed with subsequent cycles of therapy.
- Neurologic disorders of the eye (e.g., blurred vision, photophobia, mydriasis, fixed or unequal pupils, optic nerve disorder, eyelid ptosis, papilledema):
  - Onset of reaction: Discontinue dinutuximab until resolution.
  - After resolution: Reduce dinutuximab dose by 50%.
  - First recurrence or if accompanied by visual impairment: Permanently discontinue dinutuximab.

Drug Preparation: Available as injection solution of 17.5 mg/5 mL (3.5 mg/mL) in a single-use vial.

- Store vials in a refrigerator at 2–8°C (36–46°F). Protect from light by storing in the outer carton. *Do not freeze or shake vials.*
- Visually inspect for particulate matter and discoloration, and do not use the vial if the solution is cloudy or discolored, or contains particulate matter.
- Aseptically withdraw the required volume of dinutuximab from the single-use vial and inject into a 100-mL bag of 0.9% sodium chloride injection USP. Mix by gentle inversion. Do not shake. Discard any unused drug in the vial.
- Store the diluted dinutuximab solution under refrigeration (2–8°C [36–46°F]). Initiate infusion within 4 hours of preparation.
- Discard diluted dinutuximab solution 24 hours after preparation.

Drug Administration:
- Cycles 1, 3, and 5 are 24 days in duration; cycles 2 and 4 are 32 days in duration.
- Assess serum electrolytes daily and monitor CBC/differential closely during dinutuximab therapy.
- Assess temperature, blood pressure, respirations, neurologic vital signs (including pupil size, reactivity to light, and bilateral strengths); ask if patient has experienced any visual changes, numbness/tingling, motor weakness, or changes in ability to do ADLs. Assess for signs and symptoms of infection. Assess level of comfort and presence of pain.
- Pretreatment:
  - *IV hydration* of 10 mL/kg of 0.9% sodium chloride injection USP IV over 1 hour just prior to starting each dinutuximab infusion.
  - *Analgesics:*
    - Morphine sulfate 50-mcg/kg IV immediately prior to initiation of dinutuximab, then continue as a morphine drip at an infusion rate of 20–50 mcg/kg/hr during and for 2 hours after the completion of dinutuximab.
    - Administer additional 25-mcg/kg to 50-mg/kg IV doses of morphine sulfate as needed for pain up to once every 2 hours, followed by an increase in the morphine sulfate infusion rate in clinically stable patients.

- Consider fentanyl or hydromorphone if morphine sulfate is poorly tolerated.
  - If pain is inadequately managed with opioids, consider gabapentin or lidocaine in conjunction with IV morphine.
- *Antihistamines and antipyretics:*
  - Administer an antihistamine such as diphenhydramine (0.5–1 mg/kg; maximum dose of 50 mg) IV over 10–15 minutes starting 20 minutes prior to the start of dinutuximab, and as tolerated every 4–6 hours during dinutuximab infusion.
  - Administer acetaminophen (10–15 mg/kg; maximum dose of 650 mg) 20 minutes prior to each dinutuximab infusion, and every 4–6 hours as needed for fever or pain. Administer ibuprofen (5–10 mg/kg) every 6 hours as needed for control of persistent fever or pain.
- Initiate infusion at a rate of dinutuximab 0.875 $mg/m^2/hr$ for 30 minutes. Gradually increase the rate as tolerated to a maximum rate of 1.75 $mg/m^2/hr$.
- Monitor patient closely for signs and symptoms of an infusion reaction during and for 4 hours after the end of the infusion. Immediately interrupt the dinutuximab infusion for severe infusion reactions, and permanently discontinue it if anaphylaxis occurs.

Drug Interactions: No drug–drug studies have been conducted.

Lab Effects/Interference:
- Hyponatremia, hypokalemia, hypocalcemia, hypoalbuminemia, hypophosphatemia, and hypomagnesemia: Immediately interrupt therapy
- Thrombocytopenia, lymphopenia, anemia, and neutropenia
- Hyperglycemia and hypertriglyceridemia
- Increased ALT, AST, and serum creatinine
- Proteinuria

Special Considerations:
- Black box warnings:
  - Serious and potentially life-threatening infusion reactions occurred in 26% of patients; administer prehydration and premedication (including antihistamines) prior to each dinutuximab infusion. Monitor patients closely for signs and symptoms of an infusion reaction during and for 4 hours after the end of each dinutuximab infusion. Interrupt the drug for severe reactions, and permanently discontinue it if anaphylaxis occurs.
  - Severe neuropathic pain occurs in most patients during the infusion. Administer IV opioids prior to, during, and for 2 hours after the end of each infusion. Grade 3 peripheral sensory neuropathy occurred in 2–9% of patients. Severe motor neuropathy was observed in adults receiving dinutuximab, and may not resolve in all cases. The drug should be permanently discontinued for severe unresponsive pain, severe sensory neuropathy, or moderate to severe peripheral motor neuropathy.
- Warnings and Precautions:
  - *Serious infusion reactions*
  - *Neurotoxicity*
  - *Neurological disorders of eye:* Interrupt dinutuximab for dilated pupil with sluggish light reflex or other visual disturbances and permanently discontinue drug for recurrent eye disorders or loss of vision.

- *Prolonged urinary retention and transverse myelitis:* Permanently discontinue drug and institute supportive care.
- *RPLS:* Permanently discontinue drug and institute supportive care for signs and symptoms (e.g., severe headache, HTN, visual changes, lethargy, and seizures).
- *CLS:* Administer required prehydration and monitor patients closely during treatment. Incidence of grades 3–5 was 23% in study 1. If patients have symptomatic or severe CLS, immediately interrupt or discontinue dinutuximab, and institute supportive measures.
- *Hypotension* may occur. Incidence of severe (grade 3/4) hypotension was 16% in study 1 vs. 0% in control. Ensure prehydration is given and monitor BP closely during drug infusion. If patient develops symptomatic hypotension, SBP < LLN for age, or SBP that has decreased >15% compared to baseline, immediately interrupt or discontinue drug.
- *Infection (systemic):* Incidence of grades 3–4 bacteremia requiring IV antibiotics or other urgent intervention occurred in 13% in study 1, while sepsis occurred in 18%. Monitor patients closely for signs/symptoms of systemic infection, and temporarily discontinue dinutuximab in patients with systemic infection until infection resolves.
- *Bone marrow suppression:* Severe (grades 3–4) thrombocytopenia occurred in 39%, anemia in 34%, neutropenia in 34%, and febrile neutropenia in 4% in study 1. Monitor peripheral blood counts closely during therapy.
- *Electrolyte disturbances:* Incidence is at least 25% (hyponatremia, hypokalemia, hypocalcemia). Severe hypokalemia occurred in 37% of patients, and severe hyponatremia occurred in 23%. Monitor serum electrolytes daily during therapy.
- *Atypical hemolytic uremic syndrome (HUS):* Permanently discontinue dinutuximab and provide supportive management for signs of HUS.
- *Embryo-fetal toxicity:* Drug may cause fetal harm. Teach female patients of reproductive potential to use effective contraception during treatment and for 2 months after last dose.
- Nausea and vomiting: Incidence rates are 46% (6% grades 3–4) and 19% (2% grades 3–4) of patients, respectively. Incidence of diarrhea is 43% (13% grades 3–4).
- Most common adverse reactions (≥25%) are pain, pyrexia, thrombocytopenia, lymphopenia, infusion reactions, hypotension, hyponatremia, increased ALT, anemia, vomiting, diarrhea, hypokalemia, CLS, neutropenia, urticarial, hypoalbuminemia, increased AST, and hypocalcemia.
- Most common serious reactions (≥5%) are infections, infusion reactions, hypokalemia, hypotension, pain, fever, and CLS.

Potential Toxicities/Side Effects and the Nursing Process

I. POTENTIAL FOR INJURY related to INFUSION-RELATED REACTIONS

Defining Characteristics: Infusion reactions usually occurred during or within 24 hours of dinutuximab infusion. Serious infusion reactions (grades 3 or 4) occurred in 26% of patients receiving dinutuximab with RA compared to 1% receiving RA alone. Urgent intervention was required for facial and upper airway edema, dyspnea, bronchospasm, stridor, urticaria, and hypotension. Signs and symptoms may overlap with HSRs. One patient had multiple cardiac arrests and died within 24 hours after dinutuximab infusion.

Nursing Implications: Ensure that premedications are administered prior to dinutuximab infusion. Monitor the patient closely during the infusion and for 4 hours after the infusion is completed. The clinical setting should have resources for cardiopulmonary resuscitation (medications, equipment, qualified responders) if needed. For mild-to-moderate infusion reactions (e.g., rash, fever, rigors, and localized urticaria) that respond promptly to antihistamines or antipyretics, reduce the infusion rate and monitor the patient closely. If severe or prolonged infusion reactions occur, immediately interrupt or permanently discontinue dinutuximab, and provide supportive management. If life-threatening effects occur, dinutuximab should be permanently discontinued. Urgent interventions for severe infusion reactions include interruption of dinutuximab, BP support, bronchodilator therapy, and corticosteroids.

II.   ALTERATION IN COMFORT related to PAIN

Defining Characteristics: Up to 85% of patients experience pain despite opioid analgesic pretreatment, and it is severe (grade 3) in 51%. Pain occurs during the infusion and is characterized as abdominal, generalized, extremity, back musculoskeletal chest pain, neuralgia, or arthralgia.

Nursing Implications: Document baseline comfort level and any analgesics used. Premedicate with analgesics (including opioids) prior to each dinutuximab dose; continue analgesics as a continuous infusion during the dinutuximab infusion, and for 2 hours after the dose is completed. If pain is severe, decrease the dinutuximab infusion rate to 0.875 mg/m^2/hr. If pain persists despite opioids, other analgesics, and infusion rate reduction, dinutuximab should be discontinued.

III.   ALTERATION IN ACTIVITY, POTENTIAL, related to NEUROPATHY

Defining Characteristics: Peripheral neuropathy occurred in 13% of patients, and 3% experienced grade 3 (severe) effects. Peripheral sensory neuropathy affected 9% of patients, with a median duration of 9 days. Peripheral motor neuropathy is more common in adult patients compared to pediatric patients.

Nursing Implications: Assess patient for signs and symptoms of peripheral sensory (e.g., paresthesias, dysesthesias) and motor neuropathy (e.g., weakness). Discuss any findings with physician/NP/PA. Dinutuximab should be permanently discontinued in patients with grade 2 peripheral motor neuropathy, grade 3 sensory neuropathy (interferes with ADLs for more than 2 weeks), or grade 4 sensory neuropathy.

IV.   ALTERATION IN SENSORY PERCEPTION, VISUAL, related to NEUROLOGIC DISORDERS OF THE EYE

Defining Characteristics: Incidence is 2–15% and includes blurred vision, photophobia, mydriasis, fixed or unequal pupils, optic nerve disorder, eyelid ptosis, and papilledema. Median duration is 4 days.

Nursing Implications: Assess the patient for pupil equality in size and reaction to light; assess for ptosis. Ask if patient has experienced any changes in vision, and discuss findings with physician/NP/PA. Teach the patient to report any changes in vision immediately. Dinutuximab should be interrupted if the patient experiences dilated pupils with sluggish light reflex or other visual disturbances that do not cause visual loss. Once this reaction is resolved, dinutuximab dose should be reduced by 50% if further therapy is warranted. The drug should be permanently discontinued if the patient has recurrent signs and symptoms following dose reduction, or if the patient experiences loss of vision.

V.   INCREASED RISK OF INFECTION, BLEEDING related to BONE MARROW DEPRESSION

Defining Characteristics: Incidence in clinical trials was 66% for thrombocytopenia (39% grades 3–4), 62% for lymphopenia (51% grades 3–4), 51% for anemia (34% grades 3–4), and 39% for neutropenia (34% grades 3–4). Infections included sepsis (incidence 18%; 16% grades 3–4) and device-related infection (16%; 16% grades 3–4). Hemorrhage occurred in 17% of patients (6% grades 3–4).

Nursing Implications: Assess CBC/differential. Assess the patient for signs and symptoms of systemic infection and bleeding, and discuss with physician/NP/PA the possibility of drug interruption until the infection resolves. Teach the patient self-care strategies to minimize the risks of infection and bleeding, and to report any signs and symptoms of infection or bleeding right away.

VI.   ALTERATION IN HOMEOSTASIS related to CAPILLARY LEAK SYNDROME

Defining Characteristics: CLS occurred in 40% of patients and was severe (grades 3–4) in 23%. Hypotension occurred in 60% (16% grades 3–4). Hypoxia was reported by 24% of patients (12% grades 3–4). CLS is characterized by loss of vascular tone and extravasation of plasma proteins and fluid into the extravascular space. This results in hypotension and decreased organ perfusion. CLS may be associated with cardiac arrhythmias, angina, MI, respiratory insufficiency requiring intubation, GI bleeding, edema, and mental status changes.

Nursing Implications: Assess the patient at baseline and during the infusion for signs and symptoms of CLS, including hypotension. Ensure prehydration is administered. If signs and symptoms are identified, discuss interventions immediately with physician/NP/PA *as infusion should be immediately interrupted.* If the patient has mild or moderate signs and symptoms, expect that when the patient's symptoms return to baseline, the infusion will be resumed at 50% of the previous rate. If life-threatening reaction occurs, discontinue the drug for the current cycle. In addition, be prepared to implement orders for emergency, supportive management. For subsequent cycles, after life-threatening CLS has resolved, the patient should receive the dinutuximab infusion at 50% of the previous rate. If signs and symptoms of CLS recur, the drug should be permanently discontinued.

Drug: Durvalumab (Imfinzi)

Classification: PD-L1 blocking antibody.

Mechanism of Action: Drug is an IgG Mab that blocks the interaction of programmed cell death ligand 1 (PD-L1) with PD-1 and CD80 (B7.1) molecules. Blockade of PD-L1/PD-1 and PD-L1/CD80 releases the inhibition of the immune response so that the body's T cells can hunt and kill tumor cells; it does this without inducing antibody dependent cell-mediated cytotoxicity (ADCC). Expression of PD-L1 can be turned on by inflammatory signals, such as IFN-gamma, and may be expressed on tumor cells and tumor-associated immune cells in the tumor microenvironment (AstraZeneca, 2017). PD-L1 is meant to limit possible damage by the immune system on normal organs and tissues. PD-L1 blocks T-cell function and activation through by binding to PD-1 and CD80 (B7.1). Cytotoxic T-cell activity is turned off, as is T-cell proliferation and cytokine production. PD-L1 blockade by durvalumab increased T-cell activation and decreased tumor size in animal models.

Metabolism: Mean terminal half-life is approximately 17 days. It is unknown if severe renal impairment or moderate or severe hepatic impairment alter the pharmacokinetics (AstraZeneca, 2017).

Indication: Treatment of patients with (1) locally advanced or metastatic urothelial cancer who have disease progression during or following platinum-containing chemotherapy, or disease progression within 12 months of neoadjuvant or adjuvant treatment with platinum-containing chemotherapy; and (2) unresectable stage III NSCLC whose disease has progressed following concurrent platinum-based chemotherapy and RT..

Indication (1) is an accelerated approval based on tumor response rate and duration of response. Continued approval for this indication may be contingent upon verification and description of clinical benefit in confirmatory trials (AstraZeneca, 2017).

Contraindication: None

Dosage Range:
- Urothelial cancer: 10 mg/kg IV infusion over 60 minutes every 2 weeks until disease progression or unacceptable toxicity. Drug should be diluted prior to infusion.
- NSCLC: 10 mg/kg IV infusion over 60 minutes every 2 weeks until disease progression, unacceptable toxicity, or a maximum of 12 months. Drug should be diluted prior to infusion.
- Dosage Modifications (No dose reductions; hold or discontinue drug):
  - Pneumonitis: *grade 2*: hold dose, give initial dose of 1–2 mg/kg/day prednisone or equivalent, followed by taper; *grades 3–4*: permanently discontinue, give initial dose of 1–4 mg/kg/day prednisone or equivalent, followed by taper.
  - Hepatitis: *grade 2–3* AST/ALT to ≤8 × ULN or total bilirubin ≤ 5 × ULN: hold dose while for *grade 3* or concurrent ALT or AST > 3 × ULN AND total bilirubin >

2 × ULN with no other cause, permanently discontinue. For all, give initial dose of 1–2 mg/kg/day prednisone or equivalent, followed by taper.

- Colitis or diarrhea: *grade 2* hold dose, while *grades 3–4,* permanently discontinue; for all, give initial dose of 1–2 mg/kg/day prednisone or equivalent, followed by taper.
- Hypothyroidism: *grades 2–4*: initiate thyroid hormone replacement as clinically indicated.
- Hyperthyroidism: *grades 2–4;* hold dose until clinically stable, then symptomatic management.
- Adrenal insufficiency, hypophysitis/hypopituitarism: *grades 2–4;* hold dose until clinically stable, then give initial dose of 1–2 mg/kg/day prednisone or equivalent, followed by taper and hormone replacement as clinically indicated.
- Type I diabetes mellitus: *grades 2–4;* hold dose until clinically stable, then initiate insulin therapy as clinically indicated.
- Nephritis: *grade 2 (creatinine >1.5–3 × ULN)*: hold dose, while for *grades 3–4,* permanently discontinue drug, then for both, give initial dose of 1–2 mg/kg/day prednisone or equivalent, followed by taper.
- Rash or dermatitis: *grade 2 for >1 week, or grade 3,* hold dose, while for *grade 4,* permanently discontinue, then for both, give initial dose of 1–2 mg/kg/day prednisone or equivalent, followed by taper.
- Infection: *grades 3–4,* hold dose, manage symptomatically with anti-infectives for suspected or confirmed infections.
- IRRs: *grades 1–2,* interrupt or slow the infusion rate and consider premedication with subsequent doses*; grades 3–4,* permanently discontinue drug.
- Other: *grade 3,* hold dose, and manage symptomatically; *grade 4,* permanently discontinue and consider give initial dose of 1–4 mg/kg/day prednisone or equivalent, followed by taper.

Drug Preparation:

- Preparation (available in 120 mg/2.4 mL (50 mg/mL) and 500 mg/10 mL single-dose vials):
  - Visually inspect drug for particulate matter and discoloration, and do not used if seen. Drug should be clear to opalescent, colorless to slightly yellow solution without visible particules.
  - Do not shake the vial.
  - Withdraw the required volume from the vial(s) of darvalumab and transfer into a 0.9% Sodium Chloride Injection, USP or 5% Dextrose Injection, USP, IV bag. Mix solution by gentle inversion. Do not shake solution. The final concentration of the diluted solution should be between 1 and 15 mg/mL.
  - Discard partially used or empty vials of darvalumab.
- Storage:
  - 24 hours in a refrigerator at 2–8°C (36–46°F)
  - 4 hours at room temperature (up to 25°C [77°F])
  - Do not freeze; do not shake.

Drug Administration:
- Assess patient for signs/symptoms of immune-related adverse effects.
- Administer IV infusion over 60 min through an IV line containing a sterile, low-protein binding 0.2 or 0.22 micron in-line filter. Monitor closely for infusion reactions.
  - Interrupt or slow infusion rate if patient develops mild or moderate infusion reactions (IRs)
  - Permanently discontinue drug in patients with grade 3 or 4 infusion reactions (bronochospasm, anaphylaxis)
- Do not coadminister other drugs through the same infusion line.
- Teach patient to report right away: new or worsening cough, SOB, chest pain; yellowing of skin, severe nausea or vomiting, right-sided abdominal pain, dark (tea) colored urine, increased bruising; increased frequency of bowel movements, black stools; decreased urination, blood in urine, ankle swelling; signs/symptoms of infection; chills or shaking, wheezing, dizziness, swelling of face; any new signs/symptoms or changes.

Drug Interactions: None known.

Laboratory Effects/Interference:
- Lymphopenia, anemia, neutropenia.
- Decreased serum sodium, potassium, albumin.
- Increased alkaline phosphatase, AST, ALT, hyperbilirubinemia; serum calcium, magnesium, glucose, creatinine, potassium.

Special Considerations:
- Most common adverse reactions ($\geq$15%): fatigue, musculoskeletal pain, constipation, decreased appetite, nausea, peripheral edema, UTI. Grade 3–4 adverse events were reported in 43% of patients.
- In clinical trials, infection, and immune related adverse events (e.g., pneumonitis, hepatitis, colitis, thyroid disease, diabetes and adrenal insufficiency) were seen.
- Warnings and Precautions:
  - *Immune-mediated pneumonitis:* uncommon but may be fatal. Incidence is 5%, with median time to onset was 1.8 months. Evaluate patients closely, and if pneumonitis is suspected, patient should receive radiological imaging, corticosteroid therapy and treatment modification. Moderate grade 2: prednisone 1–2 mg mg/kg/day (or equivalent; if more severe prednisone 1–4 mg/kg/day for (grades 3–4), followed by taper over at least 4 weeks. Drug should be interrupted or discontinued depending upon severity.
  - *Immune-related hepatitis:* uncommon but may be fatal. Incidence 12%, with median time to onset was 1.2 months. Monitor LFTs each cycle during treatment and manage with treatment modification and corticosteroids: See package insert.
  - *Immune-related colitis:* incidence across studies was 18%, with median time to onset was 1.4 months. Manage with treatment modifications, antidiarrheal agents, and corticosteroids. If needed, patient may require nonsteroidal immunosuppressants. See package insert.
  - *Immune related endocrinopathies* (see package insert): monitor thyroid function and blood glucose baseline and periodically during treatment. Assess for signs/symptoms of hypo/hyperthyroidism, adrenal insufficiency, type 1 DM, and hypophysitis.

Manage by hormonal replacement, as indicated, treatment modification. See package insert.

- *Immune-related nephritis:* Monitor patients for renal dysfunction prior to and periodically during treatment. Interrupt treatment and treat with prednisone (or equivalent) followed by taper (see package insert). Discontinue drug if severe.
- *Immune-related dermatologic issues: RASH:* bullous dermatitis, SJS, TEN have been described. Monitor for signs/symptoms of rash. Interrupt treatment and treat with prednisone (or equivalent) followed by taper (see package insert). Discontinue drug if severe.
- *Other immune-mediated adverse reactions:* rash, asceptic meningitis, hemolytic anemia, immune thrombocytopenic purpura, myocarditis, myositis, and ocular inflammatory toxicity (e.g., uveitis, keratitis) may occur rarely ($\leq 1\%$). Assess renal function baseline and each cycle during treatment. Monitor for signs/symptoms. Manage with treatment modification, and corticosteroid therapy as indicated followed by taper. See package insert.
- *Infection:* In study 1, infections occurred in 29.7% of patients, and was grade 3 or 4 in 6%. Incidence of infections in the combined safety database was 37.6% of patients. Most common grade 3–4 infection was UTI. Monitor patients for signs/symptoms of infection, and discuss anti-infective treatment with provider. Severe infections included sepsis, necrotizing fasciitis, and osteomyelitis.
- *Infusion related reactions:* In study 1, incidence was 1.6%. A few patients developed urticarial within 48 hours of the drug dose. Assess for signs/symptoms of IRR and interrupt infusion if it occurs. If mild-moderate, interrupt or slow infusion rate; if grade 3 or higher, permanently discontinue.
- *Embryo-fetal toxicity:* Teach patients of reproductive potential that drug can cause fetal harm and to use effective contraception to prevent pregnancy during treatment and for at least 3 months after last dose.
- Teach patients not to breastfeed while receiving the drug and for at least 3 months after last dose.

Potential Toxicities/Side Effects and the Nursing Process

I. **ALTERATION IN COMFORT related to FATIGUE, ASTHENIA, MUSCULOSKELETAL PAIN, OR ARTHRALGIA, PERIPHERAL EDEMA, PYREXIA**

Defining Characteristics: Fatigue, and asthenia occurred in 39% of patients. Musculoskeletal pain also occurred. Peripheral edema and pyrexia/tumor associated fever occurred in 15% and 14% respectively.

Nursing Implications: Teach the patient that these events may occur and to report them. Assess baseline comfort and self-care strategies to maintain comfort and energy conservation. Monitor closely during treatment. Develop a plan to assure comfort, depending on the symptoms reported, and assess its efficacy and revise the plan if needed at each visit.

II.   ALTERATION IN NUTRITION, POTENTIAL, LESS THAN BODY REQUIREMENTS, related to DECREASED APPETITE, NAUSEA, CONSTIPATION, DIARRHEA, OR CONSTIPATION

Defining Characteristics: Nutritional impact symptoms of nausea, vomiting, diarrhea, constipation, and decreased appetite can occur. Constipation occurred in 21% of patients, nausea in 16%, and diarrhea/colitis in 13%.

Nursing Implications: Assess nutritional and bowel-elimination patterns, appetite, and presence of nausea and/or vomiting, and weight at baseline and at each visit. Assess LFTs baseline and with each cycle, identifying any abnormalities and discussing possibility of hepatitis for any abnormalities. Teach that diarrhea, constipation, nausea, vomiting, and decreased appetite may occur and to report them. Assess nutrition impact symptoms and discuss their management with the physician. Teach the patient to self-administer antidiarrheal, stool softeners if constipation is present, or antiemetic medication, if needed, and to report symptoms that do not improve. In addition, teach patients to report immediately any diarrhea, blood in stool or black stools, and severe stomach pain or tenderness so that the potential for colitis may be further evaluated.

III.   ALTERATION IN SKIN INTEGRITY, POTENTIAL, related to RASH, PRURITUS, OR EDEMA

Defining Characteristics: Skin integrity can be affected by rash, edema, and pruritis.

Nursing Implications: Teach the patient that rash, pruritus, and peripheral edema may occur and to report them. Assess the patient's skin integrity and determine the presence of edema, both at baseline and regularly during therapy. Teach patient self-care measures to reduce pruritis.

IV.   POTENTIAL ALTERATION IN OXYGENATION related to PNEUMONITIS

Defining Characteristics: In all clinical trials, incidence was 2.3% with median time to onset of 55 days.

Nursing Implications: Teach the patient to report new or worsening cough, chest pain, or shortness of breath. Monitor the patient for signs and symptoms of pneumonitis. Discuss findings with the physician/NP/PA. Expect that after exclusion of other diagnoses, the patient will be evaluated with imaging and pulmonary and/or infectious disease consultation if signs/symptoms of pneumonitis occur. Expect drug to be interrupted for grade 2, and permanently stopped for grades 3–4; patient should be treated with prednisone as above in dose modifications.

V.   POTENTIAL ALTERATION IN ELIMINATION related to COLITIS

Defining Characteristics: Incidence of diarrhea or colitis was 12.6% (study 1) with 1.1% of patients having grade 3–4.

Nursing Implications: Teach the patient to report signs and symptoms of colitis (diarrhea, blood in stools or tarry stools, severe abdominal pain). Monitor the patient for immune-mediated colitis, and administer corticosteroids as ordered. Drug should be held for grade 2, and permanently discontinued for grade 3–4.

VI. POTENTIAL ALTERATION IN NUTRTION related to HEPATITIS

Defining Characteristics: Immune-mediated hepatitis (defined as requiring use of corticosteroids and no clear alternate etiology) and abnormal LFTs may occur. Incidence in clinical trials was 1.1%. Signs and symptoms of hepatitis include elevated transaminases and total bilirubin, icterus, severe nausea and vomiting, right-sided abdominal pain, drowsiness, dark urine, increased bruisability or bleeding, and anorexia.

Nursing Implications: Assess LFTs at baseline and at each cycle of therapy. Evaluate the patient for right-sided abdominal pain, drowsiness, dark urine, increased bruising or bleeding, and loss of appetite. Teach the patient to report any yellowing of the skin or whites of the eyes, as well as severe nausea or vomiting. Expect the following orders if abnormal LFTs occur: see dose modifications. Drug should be held for grade 2 and higher, and permanently discontinued for grade 3+ (ALT or AST $> 8\times$ ULN or total bilirubin $> 5 \times$ ULN) or grade 4. Corticosteroid therapy should be given for grade 2 or higher.

VII. POTENTIAL ALTERATION IN URINE ELIMINATION related to IMMUNE-MEDIATED NEPHRITIS AND RENAL DYSFUNCTION

Defining Characteristics: Immune-related nephritis defined as renal dysfunction or grade 2 or higher increased creatinine, requirement for corticosteroids, and no clear alternate etiology, can occur.

Nursing Implications: Assess the patient's baseline renal function, and monitor at each cycle during therapy. Teach the patient to report signs and symptoms such as a decrease in the amount of urine, blood in urine, ankle swelling, loss of appetite. Drug should be held for grade 2 (serum creatinine > 1.5–$3 \times$ ULN), and permanently discontinued for grades 3–4; all patients should receive corticosteroid therapy with taper.

VIII. POTENTIAL ALTERATION IN ENDOCRINE FUNCTION related to HYPOTHYROIDISM, HYPERTHYROIDISM, HYPERGLYCEMIA, OR ADRENAL CRISIS

Defining Characteristics: Incidence in clinical trials for hypothyroidism was 5.5%, and for hyperthyroidism, 4.9%. Type 1 diabetes mellitus may occur (in clinical trials $<0.1\%$). Adrenal insufficiency was uncommon (0.9%).

Nursing Implications: Monitor thyroid function at baseline and periodically during therapy. Monitor for hyperglycemia. Teach the patient to report signs and symptoms of hyper- and hypothyroidism, such as headaches that do not go away, extreme tiredness, weight gain or loss, changes in mood or behavior, dizziness or fainting, hair loss, feeling cold, constipation, and deep and/or hoarse voice. Discuss and teach the patient about ordered hormone replacement therapy for hypothyroidism, or medical management of hyperthyroidism. If the patient is hyperthyroid, drug should be held until clinically stable. If patient is hyperglycemic, administer insulin as ordered, teach patient self-management, and hold drug for grades 2–4 until clinically stable. Monitor for signs/symptoms of adrenal insufficiency (chronic fatigue, muscle weakness, weight loss, nausea, vomiting, hypotension, hyperpigmentation of skin), hypophysitis/hypopituitarism (fatigue, lethargy, loss of libido, amenorrhea, dizziness, nausea, vomiting, diabetes insipidus); drug should be held for grades 2–4 until patient is clinically stable, and patient should receive corticosteroids followed by a taper.

Drug: Elotuzumab (Empliciti)

Class: mAb, targets SLAMF7 (Signaling Lymphocytic Activation Molecule Family member 7) protein, which is expressed on myeloma cells.

Mechanism of Action: SLAMF7 is expressed on myeloma cells (independent of cytogenetic abnormalities) and NK cells. Drug facilitates NK killing of myeloma cells through ADCC. When combined with lenalidomide, NK activation is enhanced with greater myeloma cell kill (greater than either elotuzumab or lenalidomide alone).

Metabolism: When given with lenalidomide and dexamethasone, 97% of maximum steady-state concentration is predicted to be eliminated in 82.4 days. Clearance increases with increasing body weight, supporting a weight-based dosing.

Indications: Treatment of adult patients with MM (1) in combination with lenalidomide and dexamethasone who have received 1–3 prior therapies; (2) in combination with pomalidomide and dexamethasone who have received at least 2 prior therapies including lenalidomide and a proteasome inhibitor.

Dosage/Range:
- With lenalidomide and dexamethasone: 10-mg/kg IV every week for the first 2 cycles (28-day cycle), then every 2 weeks thereafter until disease progression or unacceptable toxicity (see administration schema in Table 1, package insert (2018).
- With pomalidomideand dexamethasone: 10-mg/kg IV every week for the first 2 cycles and 20 mg/kg every 4 weeks thereafter until disease progression or unacceptable toxicity.
  - See administration schema in Table 2, package insert (2018).
  - Administer dexamethasone dose as follows:
    (1) On days that elotuzumab is administered, (a) age 75 years old or younger, dose is 28 mg PO between 3–24 hours before elotuzumab dose plus dexamethasone 8 mg IV between 45–60 minutes before elotuzumab as premedication; (b) if age >75 years, dexamethasone 8 mg PO between 3–24 hours before elotuzumab dose plus dexamethasone 8 mg IV between 45–60 minutes before elotuzumab as premedication.

(2) On days that elotuzumab is not given, but a dose of dexamethasone is scheduled (days 8, 15, 22 of cycle 3 and all subsequent cycles), give dexamethasone 40 mg PO to patients aged 75 or younger, and 20 mg PO to patients older than 75 years.

- Premedicate with 8 mg IV, diphenhydramine 25–50 mg PO/IV or equivalent, ranitidine 50 mg IV or equivalent, and acetaminophen 650–1000 mg PO, 45–90 minutes before each elotuzumab dose.

Dose Modifications:
- If dose of one drug in regimen is delayed, interrupted, or discontinued, other drugs may continue to be given as scheduled. If dexamethasone is delayed or discontinued, decide about administration of elotuzumab based on risk of hypersensitivity.
- Interrupt infusion for grade 2 or higher infusion reactions, and institute appropriate medical and supportive measures.
  - When resolved to grade 1 or lower, restart drug at 0.5 mL/minute and gradually increase at the rate of 0.5 mL/min every 30 minutes as tolerated to the rate at which the infusion reaction occurred. Resume the escalation regiment if there is no recurrence of infusion reaction.
  - If a patient experiences an infusion reaction, monitor VS every 30 minutes × 2 hours after the end of the elotuzumab infusion. If the infusion reaction recurs, stop the elotuzumab infusion and do not restart on that day. If reaction severe, permanently discontinue elotuzumab.
  - Dose delays and modifications for dexamethasone, pomalidomide, and lenalidomide per prescribing information for each drug.

Drug Preparation:
- Available as 300 or 400 mg lyophilized powder in a single-dose vial for reconstitution
- Calculate dose (mg) and determine the number of vials needed for 10 mg/kg dose. Aseptically add the following volume of sterile water for injection USP:
  - 300 mg vial: add 13 mL, deliverable volume in vial is 12 mL, with concentration of 25 mg/mL.
  - 400 mg vial: add 17 mL, deliverable volume in vial is 16 mL, with concentration of 25 mg/mL.
- Once added, hold the vial upright and swirl the solution by rotating the vial to dissolve the lyophilized cake. Invert the vial a few times to dissolve any powder that may be on the inside top of the vial. DO NOT SHAKE. Lyophilized powder should dissolve in <10 minutes.
- Once dissolved, allow to stand 5–10 minutes. Solution should be colorless to slightly yellow, clear to slightly opalescent. Inspect visually for particulate matter and discoloration prior to administration, and discard if found.
- Aseptically withdraw calculated volume for ordered dose up to a maximum of 16 mL from the 400-mg vial, and 12 mL from the 300-mg vial. Further dilute with 230 mL of either 0.9% sodium chloride injection USP or 5% dextrose injection USP into an infusion bag made of polyvinyl chloride or polyolefin.
- Adjust volume of 0.9% sodium chloride injection USP or 5% dextrose injection USP so not as to exceed 5 mL/kg of patient weight at any given dose of elotuzumab.

- Complete elotuzumab infusion within 24 hours of reconstitution. If not used immediately, the infusion solution may be stored under refrigerated conditions (2–8°C [36–46°F]) and protected from light for up to 24 hours (maximum 8 hours of the total 24 hours can be at room temperature, 20–25°C [68–77°F] and room light).

Drug Administration:
- Assess patient for infection (e.g., fever), treat promptly, and hold drug.
- Three drug regimen is feto-toxic, so ensure female patient of reproductive potential has a negative pregnancy test, and that restrictions and REMS governing lenalidomide use are followed.
- Administer elotuzumab ONLY after premedications given [H1 blocker diphenhydramine 25–50 mg PO or IV, H2 blocker ranitidine 50-mg IV, acetaminophen 650–1,000 mg PO. When given with lenalidomide, divide dexamethasone dose into an oral and IV dose (e.g., 28 mg PO and 8 mg IV, see package insert); give the 8 mg dexamethasone IV dose as part of the premedication plan.
- Schedule Elotuzumab in combination with lenalidomide and dexamethasone:
  - Cycles are 28 days. See Table 1 in package insert for full schema (2018).
  - Administer **dexamethasone**: (1) on days that elotuzumab is administered, give dexamethasone 28 mg PO between 3 and 24 hours before elotuzumab dose plus 8-mg IV between 45 and 90 minutes before elotuzumab dose; (2) on days that elotuzumab is not administered, but a dose of dexamethasone is scheduled (days 8, 22 of cycle 3 and all subsequent cycles), give 40 mg PO.
  - Lenalidomide: Days 1–21.
- Elotuzumab in combination with pomalidomide and dexamethasone:
  - Cycles are 28 days. See Table 2 in package insert for full schema (2018).
  - Administer dexamethasone dose as follows:
  - (1) On days that elotuzumab is administered, (a) age 75 years old or younger, dose is 28 mg PO between 3-24 hours before elotuzumab dose plus dexamethasone 8 mg IV between 45–60 minutes before elotuzumab as premedication; (b) if age >75 years, dexamethasone 8 mg PO between 3–24 hours before elotuzumab dose plus dexamethasone 8 mg IV between 45–60 minutes before elotuzumab as premedication.
  - (2) On days that elotuzumab is not given, but a dose of dexamethasone is scheduled (days 8, 15, 22 of cycle 3 and all subsequent cycles), give dexamethasone 40 mg PO to patients aged 75 or younger and 20 mg PO to patients older than 75 years.
  - Pomalidomide: Days 1–21 for each cycle.
- Interrupt for grade 2 or higher infusion reactions, and permanently discontinue for severe reactions. Institute appropriate medical and supportive measures. When resolved to grade 1 or lower, restart drug at 0.5 mL/min and gradually increase at the rate of 0.5 mL/min every 30 minutes as tolerated to the rate at which the infusion reaction occurred. Resume the escalation regiment if there is no recurrence of infusion reaction.
- If an infusion reaction, monitor VS every 30 minutes × 2 hours after the end of the elotuzumab infusion. If infusion reaction recurs, stop infusion and do not restart on that day. Severe infusion reactions may require drug discontinuation.
- If dose of one drug in regimen is delayed, interrupted or discontinued, other drugs may continue to be given as scheduled. If dexamethasone is delayed or discontinued, decide about administration of elotuzumab based on risk of hypersensitivity.

Drug Administration:

- Use infusion set and sterile, nonpyrogenic, low-protein-binding filter (pore size 0.2–1.2 micrometer) using an automated infusion pump.
- Administer premedication (dexamethasone [see regimen bullet], diphenhydramine 25–50 mg PO/IV), ranitidine (50 mg IV or 150 mg PO), and acetaminophen (650–1,000 mg) so administration is completed 45–90 minutes before elotuzumab is administered.
- Regimen is Elotuzumab 10 mg/kg administered IV every week for the first 2 cycles (28-day, drug given on days 1, 8, 15, 22 with lenalidomide and dexamethasone. Starting cycle 3, drug is given every 2 weeks (28 day cycle) on days 1 and 15. Dexamethasone is given IV (8 mg) and PO (40 mg) on concurrent days with elotuzumab cycles 1–2, and on days 1 and 15 of cycles 3 and subsequent cycles. See package insert.
- Infusion rate elotuzumab 10 mg/kg:
- Start infusion at 0.5 mL/min; increase rate if no infusion reaction as follows:
  - Cycle 1, dose 1: at 0–30 minutes: rate 0.5 mL/min; at 30–60 minutes: rate 1 mL/min; at 60 minutes+: rate 2 mL/min.
  - Cycle 1, dose 2: at 0–30 minutes: rate 3 mL/min; at 30 minutes+: rate 4 mL/min.
  - Cycle 1, doses 3 and 4 and all subsequent cycles: infusion rate 5 mL/min.
- Infusion rate elotuzumab 20 mg/kg: Start infusion rate at 3 mL/min. Infusion rate is increased in a stepwise fashion. If no infusion reactions, maximum infusion rate is 5 mL/min.
  - Dose 1: time 0–30 min, rate is 3 mL/min; time 30 min or more, rate is 4 mL/min.
  - Dose 2 and all subsequent doses: rate is 5 mL/min.
  - Adjust infusion rate if patient has a grade 2 or higher infusion reaction.
  - Do not mix any other drugs with, or administer as an infusion with, other medications.

Drug Interactions:

- Synergy with lenalidomide, pomalidomide.
- No formal drug–drug interactions have been performed.

Lab Effects/Interference:

- Elotuzumab: Interference with assays used to monitor M-protein, impacting the determination of complete response (CR) vs. relapse.
- Three drug regimen: Leukopenia, lymphopenia, thrombocytopenia; increased LFTs; hyperkalemia, hypocalcemia, decreased serum bicarbonate, hyperkalemia, hyperglycemia, hypoalbuminemia, elevated alkaline phosphatase.

Special Considerations:

- Most common adverse reactions (20% or higher): fatigue, diarrhea, pyrexia, constipation, cough, peripheral neuropathy, nasopharyngitis, URI, decreased appetite, pneumonia.
- Warnings and Precautions:
  - *Infusion reactions:* Occurred in 10% of patients in one clinical trial, and 3.3% in another, Grade 3 occured in 1% of patients. Symptoms included fever, chills, hypertension, as well as bradycardia, hypotension, or chest disomfort in some patients during infusions. Most reactions (70%) occur during the first dose. Ensure all patients receive premedications as ordered. Interrupt infusion for grade 2 or higher and medically manage. See Drug Administration.

- *Infections:* Occurred in 65–81% (7–28% grade 3, 5–24% grade 4) across clinical trials. Infections were fatal in 2.2–5% of patients. Opportunistic infections occurred in 9–22% of patients. Infections included fungal (5–10%) and herpes zoster (1.8–14%). Assess patients for signs/symptoms of infection and institute appropriate antimicrobial therapy promptly.
- *Second primary malignancy:* higher incidence (9.1%) compared to control (5.7%) in one trial. Monitor patients for development of a second primary malignancy (hematologic, solid, or skin).
- *Hepatotoxicity* occurred in 2.5% of patients: monitor LFTs and stop drug if hepatotoxicity grade 3 or higher suspected (e.g., AST/ALT > 5× ULN, total bilirubin > 3× ULN, alkaline phosphatase > 5× ULN). Monitor baseline and during therapy.
- *Interference with determination of CR:* elotuzumab can confuse response evaluation for CR, and possibly relapse from CR in patients with IgG kappa myeloma protein (Bristol-Myers Squibb, 2015).
- *Abnormalities in VS that occurred during infusion:* SBP ≥ 160 mm Hg 33.3%; DBO ≥100 mm Hg 17.3%; SBP < 90 mm Hg 28.9%; HR ≥100 bpm 47.8%; HR < 60 bpm 66%.

Potential Toxicities/Side Effects and the Nursing Process

I.   POTENTIAL FOR INJURY related to INFUSION-RELATED REACTIONS

Defining Characteristics: IRRs occurred in 10% of patients, with 70% occurring during the first infusion. All were grade 3 or lower. Reactions were characterized by fever, chills, and hypertension; bradycardia and hypotension also occurred during infusions. In the trial, 5% of patients had an infusion interruption, for a median of 25 minutes, and 1% discontinued the drug due to the reaction. Incidence of pyrexia was 37.4% in all patients.

Nursing Implications: Ensure that premedications are administered. Ensure that medications necessary for the management of severe infusion reactions are readily available (e.g., epinephrine, antihistamines, corticosteroids) and that provider is locally available to assess patient and prescribe orders. Assess baseline VS and monitor frequently during the infusion. Follow infusion rate guidelines (see Drug Administration section) for first, second, and subsequent infusions. Interrupt infusion for grade 2 or higher infusion reactions, and provide medical interventions as ordered.

II.   POTENTIAL FOR INJURY related to INFECTION

Defining Characteristics: URI occurred in 22.6%, nasopharyngitis 24.5%, pneumonia 20.1%. Infections were reported in 81.4% (28% grades 3/4) of patients compared to 74.4% (24.3% grades 3/4) in patients receiving only lenalidomide and dexamethasone. Opportunistic infections were reported in 22% of patients (9.7% fungal, 13.5% herpes zoster).

Nursing Implications: Assess for signs/symptoms of infection prior to each treatment. Teach patient to self-assess for these, including taking temperature, and instruct to report them immediately. If patient has signs/symptoms, have the patient assessed by provider, and implement treatment plan as ordered.

III. ALTERATION IN COMFORT related to FATIGUE, PYREXIA, COUGH, PAIN IN EXTREMITIES, HEADACHE, OROPHARYNGEAL PAIN

Defining Characteristics: Fatigue occurred in 61.6%, pyrexia 37.4%, cough 34.3%, pain in extremities 16.4%, headache 15.4%, and oropharyngeal pain 10.1%.

Nursing Implications: Assess baseline comfort prior to each infusion, and tolerance of past infusion. Discuss strategies to manage symptoms. Teach patient strategies to conserve energy. If symptoms are severe, discuss management with physician.

IV. POTENTIAL SENSORY/PERCEPTUAL ALTERATIONS related to PERIPHERAL NEUROPATHY

Defining Characteristics: Peripheral neuropathy occurs in 26.7% (3.8% grades 3–4).

Nursing Implications: Teach patient that these side effects may occur and to report them. Assess sensory/perceptual changes (e.g., numbness, tingling, weakness) baseline and prior to each drug administration. Assess one side versus the other side, and note extent of paresthesias if present (stocking glove distribution), starting at fingertips or tips of toes, and progressing proximally to wrist/ankle like a glove and stocking, and document. Assess patient's ability to do ADLs, and impact of neuropathy on functioning. Discuss new onset and worsening of existing peripheral neuropathy with NP/PA or physician for further evaluation and need to dose-modify or interrupt therapy. Assess risk for falls, and discuss strategies to minimize risk of falling.

V. ALTERATION IN NUTRITION, POTENTIAL, related to DIARRHEA, CONSTIPATION, VOMITING, DECREASED WEIGHT

Defining Characteristics: Diarrhea affected 46.9% patients in clinical trials, constipation 35.5%, decreased appetite 20.8%, and vomiting 14.5%. Decreased weight affected 13.8%.

Nursing Implications: Assess baseline nutritional status, weight, and presence of nutritional impact symptoms. Teach patient these side effects may occur and to report them. Assess patient each day of treatment, and discuss self-care strategies including over-the-counter management of constipation and diarrhea; if these strategies are not effective, discuss prescription pharmacological management with provider. Discuss significant weight changes with provider and how this may impact plan of care.

Drug: epoetin alfa (Epogen®, erythropoietin, Procrit®); epoetin alfa-epbx (Retacrit)

Class: Cytokine, CSF.

Mechanism of Action: Stimulates the division and differentiation of erythrocyte stem cells in the bone marrow and is a hormone produced by recombinant DNA techniques. Has a naturally occurring counterpart, erythropoietin. Results in the release of reticulocytes into the bloodstream in 7–10 days, where they mature into erythrocytes, taking 2–6 weeks to increase hemoglobin.

Metabolism: Following SC injection, 21–31% of drug is bioavailable, with rapid distribution to tissues. Drug is taken up in the liver, kidneys, and bone marrow. Onset of action in a few days to 2 weeks; peak effect in 2–3 weeks. Half-life is 4–13 hours. Eliminated via the liver and urine (10% unchanged drug).

Indication: (A) Treatment of anemia due to (1) CKD in patients on or not on dialysis; (2) zidovudine in HIV-infected patients; (3) the effects of concomitant myelosuppressive chemotherapy and upon initiation, there is a minimum of 2 additional months of planned chemotherapy; and (B) reduction of allogeneic RBC transfusions in patients undergoing elective, noncardiac, nonvascular surgery.

Limitations of Use: Procrit has not been shown to improve quality of life, fatigue, or patient well-being. Drug is not indicated in (1) patients with cancer receiving hormonal agents, biologic products, or RT, unless also receiving concomitant myelosuppressive chemotherapy; (2) patients with cancer myelosuppressive chemotherapy when the anticipated outcome is cure; (3) in patients with cancer receiving myelosuppressive chemotherapy in whom the anemia can be managed by transfusion; (4) patients scheduled for surgery willing to donate autologous blood; (5) patients undergoing cardiac or vascular surgery; (6) as a substitute for RBC transfusions in patients requiring immediate correction of anemia.

Contraindications: Patients with (1) uncontrolled hypertension; (2) pure red-cell aplasia that begins after treatment with erythropoietin-stimulating drugs; (3) serious allergic reaction to the drug; (4) use of multidose vials in neonates, infants, pregnant women, and nursing mothers that contain benzyl alcohol (Epogen, Procrit and not available for Retacrit).

Dosage/Range:
- Use the *lowest dose* of epoetin alfa that will gradually increase the hemoglobin concentration to the lowest level sufficient to avoid the need for red blood cell transfusion.
- Cancer patients receiving chemotherapy (nonmyeloid, noncurative) with Hgb < 10 g/dL, and at least 2 additional months of chemotherapy are planned:
  - Initial adult dose is 150 U/kg subcutaneous three times a week or 40,000 U subcutaneously weekly, until completion of a chemotherapy course.
  - Age 5–18 years old: Initial pediatric dose 600 units/kg IV weekly until completion of a chemotherapy course.
  - Reduce dose by 25% if (1) Hgb approaches a level sufficient to avoid RBC transfusion or (2) Hgb increases > 1 g/dL in any 2-week period.

- Hold dose if Hgb > level needed to avoid RBC transfusion and resume at 25% below previous dose.
- Increase dose if after 4 weeks of epoietin alfa Hgb increases by < 1 g/dL AND remains < 10 g/dL:
  - Three times weekly: increase dose to 300 U/kg 3 times a week in adults.
  - Weekly: increase to 60,000 U weekly in adults.
- Weekly (children): 900 units/kg (maximum 60,000 units).
- After 8 weeks of therapy, if there is no response by Hgb or RBC transfusions are required, discontinue drug.
- Discontinue epoietin alfa after the completion of a chemotherapy course.
- Goal is to prevent or treat deficit of oxygen-carrying capacity (NCCN, 2019): (1) if asymptomatic, in hemodynamically stable chronic anemia without ACS, goal is Hgb 7–9 g/dL; (2) symptomatic anemia: (a) acute hemorrhage with evidence of hemodynamic instability or inadequate oxygen delivery: transfuse to correct; (b) Hgb < 10 g/dL with tachycardia, postural hypotension, goal is maintain Hgb 8–10 g/dL; (c) anemia with ACS or acute MI: transfusion goal to maintain Hgb ≥ 10 g/dL.
- Surgery patients (preoperative use for reduction of allogeneic red blood cell transfusion):
  - Assess Hgb: must be > 10–13 g/dL. Patients should also receive venous thrombosis prophylaxis during epoietin alfa therapy (Amgen, 2018).
  - Dose is 300 U/kg/day subcutaneously × 15 days (10 days before surgery, on the day of surgery, and for 4 days after surgery) or 600 units/kg subcutaneously in 4 doses administered 21, 14, and 7 days before surgery, and on the day of surgery.
  - All patients should receive adequate iron supplementation to start at least by the beginning of epoietin alfa therapy.
  - Patients should also receive prophylactic anticoagulation to prevent DVT.
- Chronic renal failure: See package insert.
  - Ensure adequate patient iron stores (transferrin saturation at least 20%, ferritin at least 100 ng/mL).
  - 50–100 U/kg tiw (adult) or 50 U/kg tiw (pediatric) to maintain Hgb between 10 and 12 g/dL.
  - Initiate in pediatrics only when hgb is < 10 mg/dL; if the hgb level rises to 12g/dL, interrupt or reduce the dose; recommended starting dose for children 1 month or over: 50 mg/kg three times a week IV or SQ.
  - Reduce dose by 25% if Hgb approaches 12 g/dL; if Hgb continues to increase, hold dose until Hgb begins to decline, and then reinstitute drug at dose 25% less than previous dose.
  - Reduce dose by 25% if Hgb increases by > 1 g/dL in a 2-week period.
  - Increase dose by 25% if Hgb does not increase by 2 g/dL after 8 weeks of therapy, or Hgb rise is > 1 g/dL over 4 weeks, and iron stores are adequate (transferrin saturation > 20%); do not increase dose more frequently than once a month; monitor Hgb twice weekly for 2–6 weeks after dose increase.
  - Maintain lowest dose to avoid red blood cell transfusion but not to exceed 12 g/dL.
- Zidovudine-treated HIV-infected adult patients (see package insert):
  - Adult starting dose is 100 units/kg IV or SQ 3 times per week.

- Increase dose if Hgb does not increase after 8 weeks of therapy, by 50–100 U/kg 3 times weekly subcutaneously, or IV and evaluate response every 4–8 weeks thereafter, and adjust dose in 50–100 U/kg increments 3 times a week SQ, or IV to a dose that reaches a level to avoid RBC transfusions or 300 U/kg.
- Hold drug if Hgb > 12 g/dL until Hgb < 11 g/dL, and then resume drug with a 25% dose reduction of previous dose.
- Surgery patients: 300 Units/kg qd × 15 days or 600 units/kg weekly.
- Discontinue erythropoietin if an increase in Hgb does not occur at a dose of 300 U/kg for 8 weeks.

Drug Preparation:
- DO NOT SHAKE vial, as it may denature the glycoprotein.
- Available as preservative-free, single-dose vials for injection in 2,000, 3,000, 4,000, and 10,000 U/mL. Soulution is clear and colorless. Vials must be refrigerated, and unused portions should be discarded.
- Multidose injection vials, preserved with benzyl alcohol: available as 10,000 U/mL (20,000 U/2 mL) and 20,000 U/mL (1 mL); discard 21 days after initial entry. This formulation contraindicated in neonates, infants, pregnant, or lactating women due to benzyl alcohol component.
- Store at 2–8°C (36–46°F).
- Do not dilute or administer with other drugs.
- Subcutaneous administration: At the time of injection, may admix in the syringe, bacteriostatic 0.9% sodium chloride injection USP with benzyl alcohol 0.9% (bacteriostatic saline) to the preservative-free epoetin from single-use vial to reduce injection-site discomfort.

Drug Administration:
- Evaluate iron status before and during treatment and maintain iron repletion. Correct or exclude other causes of anemia before initiating treatment.
- Subcutaneous or IV (chronic renal failure on dialysis at end of dialysis) injection.
- See package insert for patient education diagram.

Drug Interactions:
- None reported.

Lab Effects/Interference:
- Expect increase in Hgb/HCT in 2–6 weeks.

Special Considerations:
- Warnings and Precautions:
  - *Increased mortality, myocardial infarction, stroke, and thromboembolism:* ESAs increased the risk for death, myocardial infarction, stroke, venous thromboembolism, thrombosis of vascular access when using ESAs to target a Hgb > 11 g/dL.
  - *Increased mortality and/or increased risk of tumor progression or recurrence in cancer patients.*
    - Decreased progression-free survival and OS: Shortened overall survival and/or increased the risk of tumor progression or recurrence in clinical studies of patients with breast, NSCLC, head and neck cancer, lymphoid, and cervical cancers.

- Decreased locoregional control also occurred.
- *Hypertension (HTN):* control HTN prior to initiating and during drug therapy.
- *Seizures:* drug increases the risk for seizures in patients with CKD.
- *Lack or loss of hemoglobin response to Epogen:* rule out other causes such as iron deficiency, infection, inflammation, bleeding, and if it appears related to drug, follow dosing recommendations.
- *Pure red cell aplasia:* if severe anemia and low reticulocyte count develop, hold drug and evaluate patient for neutralizing antibodies to erythropoietin. Permanently discontinue drug if pure red-cell aplasia is diagnosed.
- *Serious allergic reactions* can occur, including anaphylactic reactions, angioedema, bronchospasm, skin rash, and urticarial. Immediately and permanently discontinue drug and administer supportive care as ordered if serious reactions occur.
- *Severe cutaneous reactions:* Blistering and skin exfoliation reactions including erythema multiforme and Stevens-Johnson Syndrome (SJS). Toxic epidermal necrolysis (TEN) has been reported in patients receiving ESAs including Epogen. Discontinue drug immediately.
- *Risk of serious adverse reactions due to benzyl alcohol preservative:* This formulation contraindicated in neonates, infants, pregnant, or lactating women due to benzyl alcohol component. Do not mix epoetin alfa with bacteriostatic saline, which also contains benzyl alcohol.
  - *Albumin (human)* is contained in the drug and carries a remote risk of viral disease (e.g., transmission [Creutzfeld–Jakob disease]).
  - *Dialysis management:* Dialysis prescriptions may need to be adjusted after the drug is started, such as increased anticoagulation with heparin to prevent clotting of the extracorporeal circuit during hemodialysis.
  - *Laboratory monitoring:* Evaluate transferrin saturation and serum ferritin before and during epoietin alfa therapy. Give supplemental iron therapy as ordered when ferritin is < 100 mcg/L or when serum transferrin saturation is <20%. Monitor Hgb after starting therapy and after each dose adjustment, weekly until the Hgb is stable and sufficient to minimize the need for RBC transfusion.
  - Use the lowest dose to avoid RBC transfusions.
  - Use ESAs only for anemia from noncurative, myelosuppressive chemotherapy.
  - Discontinue following the completion of a chemotherapy course.
- Patients receiving ESAs preoperatively to reduce the need for allogeneic blood cell transfusions had a higher incidence of deep venous thrombosis if not also receiving prophylactic anticoagulation. DVT prophylaxis is recommended.
- Iron stores need to be assessed and replaced to maximize response to therapy.

Potential Toxicities/Side Effects (Dose- and Schedule-Dependent) and the Nursing Process

I.   ALTERATION IN COMFORT related to PYREXIA, FATIGUE, HEADACHE

Defining Characteristics: May be due to HIV disease, rather than drug, and occurs in 20–25% of patients. Allergic reactions including urticaria may occur. Anaphylaxis has not been reported.

Nursing Implications: Assess baseline T and energy level. Instruct patient to report signs/ symptoms, and discuss measures to increase comfort.

II.   POTENTIAL ALTERATION IN OXYGENATION related to POLYCYTHEMIA

Defining Characteristics: Polycythemia may result if target range is exceeded with consequent complications (Hgb > 12 g/dL).

Nursing Implications: Monitor weekly Hgb until stable dose is achieved. Dose should be interrupted if Hgb approaches 12 g/dL and then resumed at 75% dose once HCT is < 11 g/dL. When Hgb has stabilized, discuss monitoring Hgb with physician (e.g., testing).

III.   KNOWLEDGE DEFICIT related to SELF-ADMINISTRATION TECHNIQUE

Defining Characteristics: Most often drug is administered subcutaneously 3 times/week or weekly.

Nursing Implications: Assess baseline psychomotor ability, knowledge, and willingness to learn technique of self-injection. Teach how to prepare drug, self-administer, and safely collect used syringes for proper disposal. Use written and video materials as supplements to teaching process and have patient correctly demonstrate technique prior to performing at home. Make referral to visiting-nurse agency to reinforce teaching.

Drug: filgrastim (Neupogen, G-CSF); Biosimilar dilgrastim-sndz (Zarxio), filgrastim-aafi (Nivestym) [These are NOT interchangeable medications.]

Class: Cytokine, CSF.

Mechanism of Action: Recombinant DNA protein (G-CSF) that regulates the production of neutrophils in the bone marrow (proliferation, differentiation, activation of mature neutrophils). Drug is produced by the insertion of the human G-CSF gene into *Escherichia coli* bacteria.

Metabolism: Elimination half-life is 3.5 hours.

Indication: (1) To decrease the incidence of infection (febrile neutropenia) in patients with nonmyeloid malignancies receiving myelosuppressive anticancer drugs associated with a significant incidence of severe neutropenia with fever; (2) reducing time to neutrophil recovery and duration of fever, following induction or consolidation chemotherapy in adults with acute myeloid leukemia (AML); (3) to reduce the duration of neutropenia and neutropenia-related clinical sequelae (e.g., febrile neutropenia) in patients with nonmyeloid malignancies undergoing myeloablative chemotherapy followed by marrow transplantation; (4) mobilization of hematopoietic progenitor cells into the peripheral blood for collection by leukapheresis, as this increases the numbers of progenitor cells capable of engraftment; (5) to reduce the incidence and duration of sequelae of neutropenia (e.g., fever, infections, oropharyngeal ulcers); and (6) Neupogen: to increase survival in patients acutely exposed to myelosuppressive doses of radiation (hematopoietic syndrome of acute radiation syndrome).

Contraindications: Patients with known hypersensitivity to *E. coli*–derived proteins, filgrastim, or any component of the product.

Dosage/Range:
- Starting dose 5 µg/kg/day subcutaneous or IV; dose increase by 5 µg/kg for each chemotherapy cycle, based on duration and severity of neutropenia at nadir.
- BMT: After BMT, 10 µg/kg/day as IV infusion of 4 or 24 hours, or as a continuous subcutaneous, 24-hour infusion, and then titrated based on ANC.
- Mobilization of peripheral blood progenitor cells (PBPC) is 10 µg/kg/day subcutaneous at least 4 days until the first leukapheresis procedure, and continued until the last leukapheresis. Modify dose if WBC > 100,000/mm^3.
- Patients with AML receiving induction or consolidation: 5 µg/kg/day subcutaneous beginning 24 hours after last dose of chemotherapy until ANC > 1,000/mm^3 for 3 consecutive days.
- Acute

Exposure to myelosuppressive RT doses (Neupogen): 10 mcg/kg daily SQ starting as soon as possible after suspected or confirmed exposure to RT dose > 2 gray (Gy). Patient's absorbed radiation dose should be estimated (e.g., biodosimetry if available, information from public health, or clinical time to onset of vomiting or lymphocyte depletion kinetics). Obtain baseline CBC and then serial CBC's every third day until ANC remains > 1,000/mm^3 for 3 consecutive CBCs. Do not delay dose if a CBC is not readily available. Continue administration until the ANC > 1,000/mm^3 for 3 consecutive CBCs or > 10,000/mm^3.

Drug Preparation:
- Drug available in refrigerated single-dose vials or prefilled syringes.
- **Vials** of 300 mcg/mL or 480 mcg/1.6 mL in single dose dispensing packs of 10. Teach patient to discard unused portions.
- **Prefilled** syringe (SingleJect) with 27-gauge, 1/2-inch needle with an UltraSafe Needle Guard available in 300 mcg/0.5 mL (600 mcg/mL) or 480 mcg/0.8 mL (600 mcg/mL) syringes, in dispensing packs of 1 or 10.
- Needle cover of prefilled syringes contains dry natural rubber, a derivative of latex. Patients with a latex allergy should use drug available in the single dose vial.
- Filgrastim should be stored in the refrigerator at 2–8°C (36–46°F).
- Avoid shaking.
- Remove from refrigerator 30 minutes prior to injection. Discard if left out > 6 hours.

Drug Administration:
- Subcutaneous or intravenously daily, beginning at least 24 hours post-administration of chemotherapy, continuing up to 2 weeks or until ANC > 10,000/mm^3. Prior to use, remove vial or prefilled syringe from refrigerator and allow to reach room temperature for a minimum 30 minutes and maximum 24 hours. Discard any vial or syringe left at room

temperature >24 hours. Visually inspect solution for clarity and absence of color, and do not administer if particulate matter or discoloration seen.

- Teach patient/caregiver to prepare and self-administer filgrastim. See patient education material in package insert. Administer in outer area of upper arms, abdomen, thighs, or upper outer areas of buttock.
- Assess CBC/differential/platelet count baseline, then 2×/week during filgrastim therapy; discontinue filgrastim when ANC ≥ 10,000/mm³ after the expected chemotherapy-induced nadir.
- BMT: assess CBC/platelet counts at a minimum 3×/week following marrow infusion to monitor the recovery of marrow reconstitution.

Drug Interactions:
- None significant.

Lab Effects/Interference:
- Increased WBC and neutrophil counts.
- Increased LDH, uric acid, alkaline phosphatase.

Special Considerations:
- Warnings and Precautions:
  - *Splenic rupture:* has been reported following Neupogen injection. Immediately evaluate patients who report LUQ and/or shoulder tip pain for an enlarged spleen or splenic rupture.
  - *ARDS* has been reported, probably as a result of an influx of neutrophils to the site of lung inflammation. If patient develops fever, lung infiltrates, or respiratory distress, immediately evaluate for ARDS; if diagnosed, hold drug until resolution or discontinue and give appropriate medical management of ARDS.
  - *Serious allergic reactions,* including anaphylaxis, may occur on initial or subsequent treatment. Most often occur within 30 minutes of administration, especially if given IV but can occur within days after discontinuation of initial antiallergy treatment. Provide symptomatic treatment as ordered. Administration of corticosteroids, antihistamines, bronchodilators and/or epinephrine brings rapid resolution of symptoms. Permanently discontinue drug if a serious reaction occurs. Drug is contraindicated in patients with a history of serious allergic reactions to human G-CSF such as filgrastim or pegfilgrastim.
  - *Sickle cell disorders:* severe sickle cell crisis has occurred, sometimes fatal. Drug should be administered to these patients only after careful consideration of risks and benefits by a sickle cell expert physician.
  - *Glomerulonephritis:* has occurred in patients receiving the drug, characterized by azotemia, hematuria, proteinuria, and renal biopsy. Most reactions resolve after drug is discontinued. If glomerulonephritis occurs, rule out other possible causes, and if appears related, consider dose-reduction or dose interruption,
  - *Alveolar hemorrhage and hemoptysis* have been reported in patients undergoing PBPC mobilization, which is not an approved indication of the drug.

- *Patients with severe chronic neutropenia (SCN):* may develop myelodysplastic syndrome (MDS) or AML during Neupogen therapy. If a patient with SCN develops abnormal cytogenetics or myelodyspasia, risks and benefits of continuing Neupogen should be carefully considered.
- *CLS* has been reported after G-CSF administration, characterized by hypotension, hypoalbuminemia, edema, and hemoconcentration. If CLS suspected, monitor the patient closely and implement physician orders. Patient may require ICU monitoring and care.
- *Thrombocytopenia* has been reported in patients receiving Neupogen. Monitor platelet counts baseline and during therapy.
- *Leukocytosis:* Discontinue Neupogen if the ANC exceeds 10,000/mm^3 after the chemotherapy-induced nadir has occurred. Monitor CBCs at least twice weekly during therapy. Once Neupogen is discontinued, ANC usually is reduced by 50% in 1–2 days, with return to pretreatment levels in 1–7 days. If Neupogen is used for PBPC collection and therapy, discontinue Neupogen if the leukocyte count rises to >100,000/mm^3.
- *Cutaneous vasculitis:* has been reported in patients receiving Neupogen and was moderate to severe. Hold filgrastim in patients with cutaneous vasculitis; when symptoms resolve, and ANC has decreased, Filgrastim may be started at a reduced dose.
- *Potential effect on malignant cells:* Filgrastim is a growth factor for neutrophils, but it is unknown if also can act as a growth factor for tumor cells.
- *Simultaneous use with chemotherapy and RT* not recommended. The safety of administration during concurrent therapy has not been established.
- *Nuclear imaging:* Transient positive bone-imaging studies may occur due to increased bone marrow activity due to growth factor stimulation.
- *Aortitis:* Manifested by fever, abdominal pain, kalaise, back pain, and increased inflammatory markers (e.g., CRP, wbc). May occur as early as first week of treatment. If aortitis cannot be excluded, discontinue filgrastim.
- **Do not administer drug** within 24 hours of chemotherapy administration (within 24 hours before and 24 hours after).
- Patients with SCN should have a confirmed diagnosis before starting filgrastim therapy. MDS and AML have been reported as part of the natural history of congenital neutropenia without cytokine therapy but have also occurred in patients treated for SCN with filgrastim.

Potential Toxicities/Side Effects (Dose- and Schedule-Dependent) and the Nursing Process

I.   ALTERATION IN COMFORT related to SKELETAL PAIN

Defining Characteristics: Patients (22%) may report transient skeletal pain, believed due to the expansion of cells in the bone marrow in response to G-CSF.

Nursing Implications: Teach patient that this may occur, and discuss use of NSAIDs with patient and physician for symptom management. Monitor WBC and ANC twice weekly during 10,000/mm^3.

II.   KNOWLEDGE DEFICIT related to SELF-ADMINISTRATION TECHNIQUE

Defining Characteristics: Drug is administered daily for up to 2 weeks by subcutaneous injection (outpatients).

Nursing Implications: Assess baseline psychomotor ability, knowledge, and willingness to learn technique of self-injection. Teach how to prepare drug, self-administer, and safely collect used syringes for proper disposal. Use written and video supplements to teaching process, and have patient correctly demonstrate technique prior to performing at home. Make referral to visiting-nurse agency to reinforce teaching. Patient instructions in English are on package insert. Video and more detailed patient education are available from Amgen (Thousand Oaks, CA) representative.

Drug: Gemtuzumab ozogamicin (Mylotarg)

Class: Antibody-drug conjugate (ADC); CD-33 directed ADC.

Mechanism of Action: CD-33 directed ADC where the antibody recognizes and binds to CD-33, bringing with it an attached (via linker) cytotoxic agent calicheamicin; once it binds to the CD-33 receptor on the leukemic blast cells (tumor), the ADC-CD33 complex is internalized, releasing the poison into the tumor cell. This causes double stranded DNA breaks, cell cycle arrest, and apoptosis (programmed cell death).

Metabolism: Calichaemicin portion is 97% protein bound to human plasma proteins. It is extensively metabolized via nonenzymatic reduction. Terminal plasma half-life after first dose was 62 hours, and 90 hours after second dose.

Indications: (1) newly diagnosed CD33-positive AML in adults; (2) relapsed or refractory CD33-positive AML in adults and pediatric patients aged 2 years and older.

Contraindications: Hypersensitivity to MYLOTARG or any of its components.

Dosage/Range:
- Newly diagnosed, de novo AML (combination regimen):
  - *Induction:* 3 mg/m^2 (up to one 4.5 mg vial) on Days 1, 4, and 7 in combination with daunorubicin and cytarabine.
  - *Consolidation:* 3 mg/m^2 (up to one 4.5 mg vial) on Day 1 in combination with daunorubicin and cytarabine.
- Newly diagnosed AML (single agent regimen):
  - *Induction:* 6mg/m^2 (NOT limited to one 4.5 mg vial) on Day 1, and 3mg/m^2 (NOT limited to one 4.5 mg vial) on Day 8.
  - *Continuation:* For patients without evidence of disease progression after induction, up to 8 continuous courses of gemtuzumab ozogamicin 2mg/m^2 (NOT limited to one 4.5 mg vial) on Day 1 every 4 weeks.
- Relapsed/refractory AML (single agent regimen): 3mg/m^2 (up to one 4.5 mg vial) on Days 1, 4, and 7.

- Premedicates with a corticosteroid, antihistamine, and acetaminophen 1 hour before drug administration.
- Monitor cbc/ANC count frequently at least 3X/week through recovery from treatment related toxicities.
- *Dose Modifications:*
  - Combination therapy:
    - Persistent thrombocytopenia: if platelet count does not recover to ≥ 100K within 14 days after the planned start date of consolidation cycle (14 days after hematologic recovery after previous cycle), discontinue drug (NO consolidation cycles)
    - Persistent neutropenia: if neutrophil count does not recover to ≥ 500 cells/mm^3 within 14 days after the planned start date of consolidation cycle (14 days after hematologic recovery after previous cycle), discontinue drug (NO consolidation cycles)
  - Monotherapy or combination therapy
    - Veno-occusive disease (VOD): discontinue drug
    - Total bilirubin > 2 × ULN or AST and/or ALT > 2.5 × ULN: delay drug until recovery of total bilirubin to ≤ 2 × ULN, and AST and ALT to ≤ 2.5 × ULN prior to each dose. Omit scheduled dose if delayed > 2 days between sequential infusions.
    - Infusion related reactions: (1) Interrupt infusion and institute appropriate management; (2) administer acetaminophen, diphenhydramind and/or methylprednisolone, PRN; (3) provide supportive care measures; (4) for mild, moderate or severe infusion reactions, once symptoms resolve, consider resuming infusion at NO MORE than half the rate at which the reaction occurred; if symptoms recur, repeat; (5) permanently discontinue drug if a severe infusion reaction or any life-threatening reaction occurs.
    - Other severe or life-threatening non-hematologic toxicities: (1) Delay treatment with gemtuzumab ozogamicin until recovery to a severity of ≤ mild; (2) omit scheduled dose if delayed >2days between sequential infusions.dfadsfs

Drug Preparation:
- Available as 4.5 mg in a lyophilized cake or powder in a single-dose vial for reconstitution and dilution.
- *Reconstitution:* (1) Use safe handling precautions for cytotoxic drugs; (2) Calculate dose (mg) and number of vials needed; (3) Allow drug vial(s) to reach ambient temperature for 5 minutes; (4) Reconsitute each vial with 5 mL Sterile Water for Injection USP resulting in a concentration of 1 mg/mL which delivers 4.5 mL (4.5 mg) of Mylotarg; (5) Gently swirl vial but do not shake to dissolve; (6) Inspect solution for particulate matter and discoloration; solution may contain small white, opaque to translucent fiber like particles; (7) contains NO bacteriostatic preservatives; (8) use reconstituted solution immediately or after being refrigerated at 2°–8°C (36°–46°F) for up to 1 hour. PROTECT FROM LIGHT.
- *Dilution:* (1) Calculate required volume of diluted drug to obtain the prescribed dose based on BSA, and aseptically withdraw from vial using a syringe. (2) PROTECT FROM LIGHT; discard any unused reconstituted solution left in vial.

- Doses: MUST BE MIXED TO A CONCENTRATION BETWEEN 0.075 mg/mL and 0.234 mg/mL as follows:
  - Doses < 3.9 mg must be prepared for administration by syringe. Add the reconstituted MYLOTARG solution to a syringe with 0.9% Sodium Chloride Injection to a final concentration of 0.075–0.234 mg/mL PROTECT FROM LIGHT.
  - Doses ≥ 3.9 mg must be diluted in a syringe or an IV bag in an appropriate volume of 0.9% Sodium Chloride Injection to a final concentration of 0.075–0.234 mg/mL PROTECT FROM LIGHT.
  - Gently invert the infusion container to mix the diluted solution; do not shake.
- Following dilution with 0.9% Sodium Chloride Injection MYLOTARG solution should be infused immediately. If not used immediately, store at room temperature at 15°–25°C (59°–77°F) for up to 6 hours which includes the 2 hour infusion time and 1 hour if needed to allow the refrigerated diluted solution to equilibrate to room temperature. The diluted solution can be refrigerated at 2°–8°C (36°–46°F) for up to 12 hours which includes the 1 hour in the vial post-reconstituion. PROTECT FROM LIGHT and DO NOT FREEZE.

Drug Administration:
- Assess CBC/ANC and LFTs.
- Assess patient, toxicity from prior treatment if appropriate.
- Administer pre-medications.
- Use an in-line 0.2 micron polyethersulfone)PES) filter for MYLOTARG infusion.
- Protect the IV bag from light using a light-blocking cover; IV tubing does not require protection from light.
- Infuse drug over 2 hours.
- Do not mix MYLOTARG with, or administer as an infusion with, other medicinal products.

Drug Interactions: None known.

Lab Effects/Interference:
- Decreased platelets, neutrophils, which may be prolonged.
- Decreased serum phosphate, sodium, potassium.
- Increased aljaline phosphatase, aspartate aminotransferase, alanine aminotransferase, blood bilirubin.

Special Considerations:
- Most common adverse reactions (>15%) were hemorrhage, infection, fever, nausea, vomiting, constipation, headache, increased AST, increased ALT, rash, mucositis.
- Warnings and Precautions:
  - *Hepatotoxicity including veno-occlusive liver disease (VOD):* hepatotoxicity can be life-threatening and VOD may be fatal. Incidence of VOD was 5% during or after treatment, or following HSCT. Median time from dose to onset of VOD was 9 days, but may occur up to 28 days or more after last dose. Risk appears higher in patients who recive higher doses of MYLOTARG as monotherapy, and in patients with moderate or severe hepatic impairment prior to receiving MYLOTARG where the risk was 8.7 times higher. Assess ALT, ALT, total bilirubin (BR), alkaline phosphatase

prior to each dose of MYLOTARG, and after treatment, monitor patient closely for signs/symptoms of VOD (e.g., elevated AST, ALT, total BR, hepatomegaly which may be painful, rapid weight gain, and ascites. Discuss dose modification or discontinuation for any abnormalities. If VOD is diagnosed, discontinue MYLOTARG and implement ordered therapy.

- *Infusion-related reactions (IRs) including anaphylaxis:* IRs can occur, and may be life-threatening or fatal, during or within 24 hours of infusion of MYLOTARG. Signs and symptoms include fever, chills, hypotension, tachycardia, hypoxia, and respiratory failure. Ensure premedication is administered prior to drug administration. Interrupt infusion immediately if patient develops an IR, especially dyspnea, bronchospasm, or hypotension. Monitor patient closely during and for at least 1 hour after the end of the infusion, or until signs/symptoms completely resolve. Drug should be discontinued if patient develops anaphylaxis, including severe respiratory symptoms or clinically significant hypotension (Wyeth, 2018).

- *Hemorrhage:* Bleeding occurred in 90% (all grades) and 20% (grades 3/4) in one clinical trial of patients receiving combined MYLOTARG and chemotherapy, related to prolonged thrombocytopenia. Assess CBC prior to each MULOTARG dose and monitor CBC frequently after treatment. Monitor for, and teach patients to report, signs/symptoms of bleeding during treatment. If severe bleeding occurs, drug should be delayed or discontinued with appropriate supportive care.

- *QT Interval Prolongation:* Calicheamicin may cause QTc prolongation. Patients at risk have a history of or predisposition for QTc prolongation, are taking other drugs which prolong the QTc interval, or patients with electrolyte disturbances. If patient is at risk, ensure electrolytes are monitored, abnormalities corrected (expecially serum magnesium, calcium, potassium) prior to treatment and PRN during treatment.

- *Use in AML with Adverse-Risk Cytogenetics:* The addition of MYLOTARG does not confer added benefit when added to chemotherapy.

- *Embryo-fetal toxicity:* Drug is fetotoxic. Teach women of reproductive potential to use effective contraception during treatment with MYLOTARG and for 6 months after last dose. If a patient does become pregnant or it is suspected while receiving the drug, the patient should advise the provider right away. Men with female partners of reproductive potential receiving the drug should use effective contraception during treatment with MYLOTARG and for 3 months after last dose. Nursing mothers should not breastfeed while receiving the drug.

Potential Toxicities/Side Effects and the Nursing Process

I.   POTENTIAL FOR INJURY related to ACUTE INFUSION-RELATED EVENTS

Defining Characteristics: Patients often experience an infusion reaction during or after the infusion, characterized by chills, fever, nausea, vomiting, headache, hypotension, hypertension, hypoxia, and/or dyspnea. The incidence is decreased when premedication is administered. Rarely, life-threatening or fatal reactions may occur during or within 24 hours of the infusion. Incidence is greatest with first treatment, and less with second treatment.

Nursing Implications: Premedicate with corticosteroid, acetaminophen and diphenhydr-amine as ordered 1 hour before gemtuzumab ozogamicin administration. If TLS is possible/suspected, discuss with provider hydration and allopurinol to reduce risk. Monitor VS/O$_2$ saturation (O$_2$ sat) baseline and every 15–30 minutes during the infusion and for at least 1 hour after the infusion. Interrupt infusion immediately for signs/symptoms of infusion reaction and discuss management with provider. Monitor patient's VS/O$_2$ saturation closely until signs and symptoms completely resolve. Discuss resuming infusion at ≤50% of the rate at which the reaction occurred with provider. Discontinue drug for a severe infusion or life-threatening reaction. If patient develops signs/symptoms of anaphylaxis, including severe respiratory symptoms or clinically significant hypotension, gemtuzumab ozogami-cin should be discontinued. Ensure that medications are necessary for the management of hypersensitivity/anaphylaxis are readily available (e.g., epinephrine, antihistamines, corti-costeroids). Be prepared to provide emergency support as necessary Iincluding changing IV line to IV saline so no further drug is infused, epinephrine, antihistamines, bronchodilators).

II.   POTENTIAL FOR INFECTION, BLEEDING, AND FATIGUE, related to BONE MARROW DEPRESSION

Defining Characteristics: Gemtuzumab ozogamicin is myelosuppressive causing throm-bocytopenia and neutropenia that may be persistent, especially when administered with chemotherapy. Grade 3/4 infection and hemorrhage incidence in combination therapy was 47%/18% respectively in induction, 55%/5% in consolidation 1 and 50%/6% consolida-tion 2. These incidences compared with 39%/9% after induction, 42%/0, and 50%/0 after consolidation 1 and 2 in patients receiving daunorubicin and cytarabine only. In patients receiving gemtuzumab ozogamicin monotherapy, the incidence of Grade 3 sepsis was 32%, fever 16%, pneumonia 7%, bleeding 7%; there was no grade 4 toxicity (Wyeth, 2018).

Nursing Implications: Monitor CBC/platelets baseline and regularly during and before each treatment. Dose modify for persistent thrombocytopenia or neutropenia. Assess for signs/symptoms of infection, bleeding and fatigue baseline, between treatment, and prior to each treatment. Teach patients to self-assess for these, including taking temperature, and instruct to report abnormal results immediately. Teach patient measures to minimize these side effects by avoiding crowds, not takin gOTC medicines containing aspirin or NSAIDs. Teach patient strategies to minimize energy expenditure and to conserve energy. Transfuse red blood cells and platelets as ordered.

Drug: human papillomavirus 9-valent vaccine, recombinant suspension for intramuscular injection (Gardasil 9) [The only HPV vaccine recommended in the US by the CDC since 2017]

Class: Vaccine.

Mechanism of Action: Drug is prepared by using recombinant techniques. Animal studies suggest that the efficacy of L1 VLP vaccines is related to the development of the humoral immune response, and this is postulated as the mechanism of action in humans (Merck, 2018). The exact mechanism of protection is unknown.

Indication: Indicated in

(1) girls and women 9 through 45 years of age for the prevention of the following diseases caused by HPV: types included in the vaccine:
- Cervical, vulvar, vaginal, and anal cancer caused by HPV types 16, 18, 31, 33, 45, 52, 58
- Genital warts (condyloma acuminata) caused by HPV types 6, 11
- Precancerous or dysplastic lesions caused by HPV types 6, 11, 16, 18, 31, 33, 45, 52, 58 (cervical intraepithelial neoplasia (CIN) grades 2–3 and cervical adenocarcinoma in situ; CIN grade 1; vulvar intraepithelial neoplasia (VIN) grades 2 and 3; vaginal intraepithelial neoplasia (VaIN) grades 2 and 3; anal intraepithelial neoplasia (AIN) grades 1, 2, and 3).

(2) Indicated in boys and men 9 through 45 years of age for the prevention of the following diseases caused by HPV types included in the vaccine:
- Anal cancer caused by HPV types 16, 18, 31, 33, 45, 52, 58
- Genital warts (condyloma acuminata) caused by HPV types 6, 11
- Precancerous or dysplastic lesions caused by HPV types 6, 11, 16, 18, 31, 33, 45, 52, 58:
- Anal intraepithelial neoplasia (AIN) grades 1, 2, and 3.

Limitations of Use and Effectiveness:
- Does not eliminate necessity for women to undergo recommended cervical cancer screening.
- Recipients of vaccine should not discontinue recommended anal cancer screening.
- Vaccine has not been shown to provide protection against disease from HPV types to which a person has been exposed previously through sexual activity.
- Vaccine only protects against HPV 6, 11,16, 18, 31, 33, 45, 52, 58 and does not protect against other HPV types.
- Vaccine is not a treatment for external genital lesions; cervical, vulvar, vaginal, and anal cancers; CIN, VIN, VaIN, or AIN.
- Not all vulvar, vaginal, and anal cancers are caused by HPV, and vaccine only protects against those vulvar, vaginal, and anal cancers caused by HPV 16, 18, 31, 45, 52, and 58.
- Vaccine does not protect against genital diseases not caused by HPV.
- Vaccination with Gardasil 9 vaccine may not result in protection in all vaccine recipients.

(3) Contraindicated if hypersensitivity including severe allergic reactions to yeast or after a previous dose of Gardasil 9 or Gardasil.

Dosage/Range: Dose is Gardasil 9 (0.5 mL) as an IM injection
- Age 9–15 years: (a) 2 dose regimen: administer a dose at 0, 6, to 12 months (if the second dose is administered earlier than 5 months after the first dose, administer a third dose at least 4 months after the second dose (Merck, 2018); (b) 3-dose regimen with a dose at 0, 2, and 6 months.
- Age 15 through 45 years: 3-dose regimen administered at 0, 2, and 6 months.

- Patients who have previously received vaccinations with Gardasil and now plan to receive Gardasil 9 have not been studied.

Drug Preparation: Available as a 0.5 mL suspension for injection as a single-dose vial and pre-filled syringe.

Drug Administration:
- For IM use only.
- Shake well before use. Thoroughly agitate immediately before use to maintain vaccine suspension. Do not dilute or mix with other vaccines. After thorough agitation, vaccine is a white, cloudy liquid. Visually inspect the solution for particulate matter or discoloration, and discard if either is found.
- *Single dose vial:* aseptically withdraw the 0.5-mL dose using a sterile needle and syringe and use promptly.
- *Prefilled syringe:* shake well before use; attach a sterile needle by twisting in a clockwise direction until needle fits securely on the syringe.
- Prepare site with alcohol swab, and administer IM in the deltoid region of the upper arm or in the higher anterolateral area of the thigh.
- Observe the patient for 15 minutes after administration; patient should be sitting down, as syncope may occur.
- Vaccine may cause syncope, which can result in the patient falling and becoming injured.
- Patient should be observed for 15 minutes postinjection.
- Syncope has been associated with tonic–clonic movement and other seizure-like activity.
  - If this occurs, place the patient in a supine or Trendelenburg position to restore cerebral perfusion.
  - Seizure-like activity is usually transient and resolves with supine positioning.

Drug Interactions:
- Immunosuppressive medications may reduce immune response to vaccines

Lab Effects/Interference:
- Unknown.

Special Considerations:
- Vaccine is FDA-approved for use in females and males aged 9 through 45 years.
- *Limitations of use:* see Indications.
- Most common adverse reactions ($\geq$10%): (a) *Girls and women aged 16 through 26 years old*: injection-site pain (89.9%), injection site swelling (40%), injection site erythema (34%), headache (14.6%); (b) *Girls aged 9 through 15*: injection-site pain (89.3%), injection site swelling (47.8%), injection site erythema (34.1%), headache (11.4%); (c) *boys and men aged 16 through 26*: injection-site pain (63.4%), injection site swelling (20.2%), injection site erythema (20.7%); (d) *boys aged 9 through 15*: injection-site pain (71.5%), injection site swelling (26.9%), injection site erythema (24.9%).

Warnings/Precautions:
- *Syncope:* Vaccine may cause syncope, which can result in the patient falling and becoming injured.
  - Patient should be observed for 15 minutes postinjection.
  - Syncope has been associated with tonic–clonic movement and other seizure-like activity. If this occurs, place the patient in a supine or Trendelenburg position to restore cerebral perfusion. Seizure-like activity is usually transient and resolves with supine positioning.
- *Allergic Reaction:* If the patient has an allergic reaction, institute appropriate medical treatment as ordered. Supervision must be readily available in case of anaphylaxis, which has been reported following Gardasil 9 administration.
- Safety has not been established in pregnant women. Register women who receive the vaccine while pregnant in the pregnancy registry by calling 1-800-986-8999. Safety has not been established in children below the age of 9 years.
- Immunocompromised individuals may have a diminished response to the vaccine.

Potential Toxicities/Side Effects and the Nursing Process

I. ALTERATION IN COMFORT related to INJECTION-SITE DISCOMFORT, HEADACHE

Defining Characteristics: Injection site pain, swelling and redness can occur. Headache also occurred.

Nursing Implications: Teach patient that these may occur, and teach local strategies to minimize discomfort, such as warm compresses for injection-site discomfort. Teach patients to report discomfort that does not resolve. Observe patient for at least 15 minutes after injection in case of syncope.

Drug: ^{90}Y ibritumomab tiuxetan, Ibritumomab (Zevalin)

Class: mAb chelated to radioisotope ^{90}Y yttrium.

Mechanism of Action: Ibritumomab tiuxetan is a mAb that targets the cell surface antigen CD20, which is found on the surface of normal and malignant B-cell lymphocytes. The CD20 antigen is also present (expressed) on more than 90% of B-cell non-Hodgkin's lymphoma (NHL) cells, but fortunately is not found on normal bone marrow stem cells, pre-B cells, or other normal tissues. The complex is made up of a murine anti-CD20 mAb conjugated to the linker chelator tiuxetan, which then securely chelates the radioisotope ^{90}Y yttrium. The complex attaches to the CD20 receptor, and then the radioisotope delivers high beta energy waves to the malignant cell, causing cell death. The isotope delivers high energy with a short half-life of 64 hours. It appears that if the malignant cells are pretreated with an anti-CD20 antibody (e.g., rituximab), this clears malignant and normal B lympho-cytes from the blood, and ^{90}Y ibritumomab tiuxetan is better able to target the lymphoma B-lymphocytes.

Metabolism: ^{90}Y yttrium has a half-life of 64 hours, and effective half-life in the blood of 28 hours, median biologic half-life of 47 hours, and median area under the curve (AUC) of 25 hours (Wiseman et al., 1996).

Indication: CD20 directed radiotherapeutic antibody administered as part of the Zevalin therapeutic regimen indicated for treatment of patients with
- Relapsed and/or refractory, low-grade, follicular or transformed B-cell NHL, including patients refractory to rituximab therapy.
- Previously untreated follicular NHL who achieve a partial or complete response to first-line chemotherapy.

Dosage/Range:
- Biodistribution is determined prior to dosing determination and administration.
- Day 1: administer rituximab 250 mg/m^2 intravenously.
- Days 7, 8, or 9: administer rituximab 250 mg/m^2 IV infusion.
  - If platelets $\geq$ 150,000/mm^3: within 4 hours after rituximab infusion, administer 0.4 mCi/kg (14.8 MBq/kg) Y-90 Zevalin, intravenously.
  - If platelets $\geq$ 100,000 but $\leq$ 149,000/mm^3 in relapsed or refractory patients: within 4 hours after rituximab infusion, administer 0.3 mCi/kg (11.1 MBq/kg) Y-90 Zevalin, intravenously.
  - Maximum ibritumomab dose is 32 mCi.
- Initiate Zevalin therapeutic regimen following recovery of platelet counts to $\geq$ 150,000/mm^3 at least 6 weeks and no more than 12 weeks, following the last dose of first-line chemotherapy.
- Do not treat patients with platelet counts < 100,000/mm^3.
- No contraindications, but drug should not be given to patients with altered biodistribu-tion of Y-90 ^{Zevalin}, and patients with $\geq$ 25% lymphoma marrow involvement or impaired bone marrow reserve.
- Administer rituximab/Zevalin only in facilities where immediate access to resuscitative measures is available.

Drug preparation/procedure for determining radiochemical purity and radiation dosimetry:
- Zevalin available as 3.2 mg/2 mL in a single-use vial.
- See package insert.

Drug Administration:
- Assess CBC/differential and platelet count. Assess medication profile for drug(s) that interfere with platelet function or coagulation. Assess platelet count more frequently in these patients.
- Day 1: administer rituximab 250 mg/m^2 intravenously.
  - Premedicate with oral acetaminophen 650 mg and diphenhyramine 50 mg before rituximab infusion.

- Administer rituximab at an initial rate of 50 mg/hr, and if no infusion reaction, escalate the infusion rate in 50-mg/hr increments every 30 minutes to a maximum of 400 mg/hr. Do not mix or dilute rituximab with other drugs.
- Immediately stop the rituxmab for serious infusion reactions, and discontinue Zevalin therapeutic regimen.
- Temporarily slow or interrupt the rituximab infusion for less severed infusion reactions; if symptoms improve, continue the infusion at one-half the previous rate.
- Days 7, 8, or 9:
  - Premedicate with oral acetaminophen 650 mg and diphenhyramine 50 mg before rituximab infusion.
  - Administer rituximab at initial rate of 50 mg/hr; and if no infusion reaction, escalate the infusion rate in 50 mg/hr increments every 30 minutes to a maximum of 400 mg/hr. Do not mix or dilute rituximab with other drugs.
  - Administer Y-90 Zevalin injection through a free-flowing IV line within 4 hours after rituximab infusion finishes. Use a 0.22 micron low-protein-binding in-line filter between the syringe and the infusion port. After infusion, flush the line with at least 10 mL of normal saline.
    - **If platelet count $\geq$ 150,000/mm^3,** administer Y-90 Zevalin over 10 minutes as an IV injection at a dose of 0.4 mCi/kg (14.8 MBq/kg) actual body weight.
    - **If platelet count $\geq$ 100,000/mm^3 but < 149,000/mm^3,** in relapsed or refractory patients, Y-90 Zevalin over 10 minutes as an IV injection at a dose of 0.3 mCi/kg (11.1 MBq/kg) actual body weight.
    - Do NOT administer more than 32 mCi/kg (1,184 MBq) Y-90 Zevalin dose regardless of the patient's body weight.
  - Monitor patient closely for extravasation during Y-90 injection. Immediately stop infusion and restart in another limb if signs/symptoms of extravasation occur.

Drug Interactions:
- Increased bone marrow suppression if combined with other myelosuppressive drugs or drugs interfering with blood clotting.
- Monitor patients receiving medications that interfere with platelet function or coagulation more frequently for thrombocytopenia.

Lab Effects/Interference:
- Decreased WBC and neutrophil, platelet count, and Hgb/HCT.

Special Considerations:
- Warnings and Precautions:
  - *Infusion reactions:* Rituximab, alone or with Y-90 Zevalin, can cause severe, including fatal, infusion reactions. Typically, these are seen during the first rituximab infusion (onset 30–120 minutes).
    - Signs and symptoms of a severe reaction can include urticaria, hypotension, angioedema, hypoxia, bronchospasm, pulmonary infiltrates, ARDS, MI, ventricular fibrillation, and cardiogenic shock. Immediately discontinue rituximab and Y-90 Zevalin for severe infusion reactions.

- Less severe reactions: temporarily slow or interrupt the rituximab infusion. Ensure resuscitation resources are immediately available in infusion area.
- *Prolonged and severe cytopenias* are most common severe adverse reactions. Onset is delayed and duration prolonged, sometimes > 12 weeks after infusion. May be complicated by hemorrhage and severe infection.
  - Incidence of severe thrombocytopenia and neutropenia greater in patients with baseline mildly thrombocytopenic counts (e.g., $\geq$ 100,000/mm^3 but $\leq$ 149,000/mm^3).
  - Do NOT administer Zevalin therapeutic regimen to patients with $\geq$ 25% lymphoma marrow involvement and impaired bone marrow reserve.
  - Monitor CBC/differential and platelet counts weekly until levels recur, or as clinically indicated. Monitor patients for cytopenias and their complications (e.g., febrile neutropenia, hemorrhage) for up to 3 months after Zevalin therapeutic regimen is given. Avoid using drugs that interfere with platelet function or coagulation after Zevalin therapeutic regimen.
- *Severe cutaneous and mucocutaneous reactions:* Erythema multiforme, Stevens–Johnson syndrome (SJS), toxic epidermal necrolysis (TEN), bullous dermatitis, and exfoliative dermatitis, sometimes fatal, have been reported. May occur a few days to 4 months after administration of the Zevalin therapeutic regimen. Discontinue Zevalin therapeutic regimen in patients experiencing a severe cutaneous or mucocutaneous reaction.
- *Altered biodistribution:* 1.3% of patients recorded in a postmarketing registry had altered biodistribution.
- *Risk of secondary malignancy:* MDS and/or AML were reported in 5.2% of patients with relapsed or refractory NHL enrolled in clinical studies. Median time to diagnosis was 1.9 years after Zevalin therapeutic regimen administration. Incidence in patients who received Zevalin therapeutic regimen after first line chemotherapy was 12.7% compared to 6.8% in the control arm.
- *Vaccines:* Do not administer live viral vaccines after Zevalin therapeutic regimen is given.
- *Use radionucleotide precautions* during and after radiolabeling Zevalin with Y-90.
- *Embryo-fetal toxicity:* Y-90 Zevalin can cause fetal harm. Teach women of reproductive potential to use effective contraception to avoid pregnancy for a minimum of 12 months. If Zevalin therapeutic regimen is administered during pregnancy, the patient should be apprised of the potential hazard to the fetus.
- Because IgG is excreted in human milk, nursing mothers should make a decision whether to discontinue nursing or not receive the Zevalin therapeutic regimen, taking into account the importance of the drug to the mother's health.
- After treatment, there is rapid reduction in malignant and normal B-cell lymphocytes, with circulating B cells undetectable for the first 12 weeks, followed by recovery of normal B cells starting in the sixth month after therapy.
- Common adverse events ($\geq$ 10%): cytopenias, fatigue, nasopharyngitis, nausea, abdominal pain, asthenia, cough, diarrhea, and pyrexia.

Potential Toxicities/Side Effects and the Nursing Process

I. POTENTIAL FOR INJURY related to ANAPHYLAXIS

Defining Characteristics: Rare but potentially life-threatening reaction may occur. Mouse antibodies are used that are foreign and may stimulate anaphylaxis. Rare, fatal anaphylactic reactions have occurred within 24 hours of rituximab dose. Of the reactions, 80% occur during the first rituximab infusion, and within 30–120 minutes of the infusion. Severe infusion reactions include pulmonary infiltrates, acute respiratory distress syndrome, myocardial infarction, ventricular fibrillation, and cardiogenic shock.

Nursing Implications: Assess baseline T, VS. Administer premedications prior to rituximab as ordered, usually acetaminophen and diphenhydramine. Initiate infusion at 50 mg/hour, and increase in 50 mg/hour increments q 30 minutes to a maximum of 400 mg/hour. If patient develops discomfort, slow infusion; stop infusion if reaction is severe. Once symptoms have improved, resume rate at 50% of previous rate. Have emergency equipment and medications nearby, including epinephrine and corticosteroids. Assess patient for signs/symptoms, including generalized flushing and urticaria leading to pallor, cyanosis, bronchospasm, hypotension, unconsciousness. Teach patient to report signs/symptoms, including sense of doom, tickle in throat. If signs/symptoms occur, stop infusion immediately, assess VS, notify physician. Physician may prescribe epinephrine 0.3 mL (1:1,000) subcutaneous if hypotensive. Oxygen, antihistamines, corticosteroids may also be used.

II. POTENTIAL FOR INFECTION, BLEEDING, AND FATIGUE, related to BONE MARROW SUPPRESSION

Defining Characteristics: Neutropenia common, with 77% incidence, and 25–32% of patients experiencing grade-4 neutropenia, with a median nadir of 900–1,100/mm^3; thrombocytopenia incidence 95% with median platelet nadir of 49,500/mm^3; anemia incidence 61% with median nadir for red blood cells 9.9 g/dL hemoglobin. Nadir occurred around 7–9 weeks after treatment, and duration of cytopenias was 22–35 days. Chills and fever were common, affecting 27.5 and 21.6% of patients in one study. There appears to be increased hematologic toxicity in patients with bone marrow involvement by tumor, as expected. Rare fatal cerebral hemorrhage, severe infections.

Nursing Implications: Drug contraindicated in patients with > 25% bone marrow hypocellular bone marrow, or history of failed stem cell collection. Assess baseline CBC, platelet count, and monitor closely during and after therapy at least weekly for the first 12 weeks after treatment. Assess risk for increased hematologic toxicity, for example, whether bone marrow involvement by tumor. Teach patient that blood counts will fall and potential signs/symptoms of infection, bleeding, and fatigue. Teach patient self-care measures, including self-assessment for signs/symptoms of infection, bleeding, and anemia; self-care strategies to minimize risk for infection (e.g., avoiding crowds and proximity to people with colds), bleeding (e.g., avoid aspirin-containing OTC medicines), and fatigue (e.g., alternating rest and activity periods), and what/where to report fever, bleeding, signs/symptoms of infection. Most studies show that few patients developed severe infections, and there were few if any deaths from treatment-related infections. Transfuse red blood cells and platelets as ordered.

III.   ALTERATION IN COMFORT related to ASTHENIA, NAUSEA, ABDOMINAL PAIN, HEADACHE

Defining Characteristics: Asthenia commonly affects 21.6%, nausea (grades 1 or 2) 21.6%, and abdominal pain and headache 9.8%. Nausea, vomiting, diarrhea, increased cough, dizziness, arthralgia, anxiety may occur.

Nursing Implications: Assess baseline comfort and energy level. Teach patient that these side effects may occur, and strategies to manage them. If the symptom persists or is unresolved, teach patient to report it, and discuss with physician other management strategies.

IV.   POTENTIAL FOR INJURY related to RADIATION EXPOSURE

Defining Characteristics: ^{90}Y Zevalin is a beta-emitter so that patients should protect others from exposure to their body secretions (saliva, stool, blood, urine).

Nursing Implications: Teach patient importance of specific radiation precautions, beginning at the start of treatment, and continuing for 1 week after treatment is completed: use condom during sexual intercourse, refrain from deep kissing; avoid transfer of body fluids; wash hands thoroughly after using the toilet; and continue effective contraception for 12 months following completion of treatment.

Drug: imiquimod 5% topical cream (Aldara®)

Class: Immune response modifier.

Mechanism of Action: Stimulates the immune system to release cytokines, including interferon, which stimulate Langerhans cells to kill skin cancer cells. Has been shown to reduce the expression of Bcl-2 (a protein that causes the cell to avoid apoptosis, or programmed cell death, by preventing the activation of the proapoptotic proteins called capases) and increase apoptosis of basal skin cancer cells.

Metabolism: Unknown.

Indications: For the topical treatment of patients with (1) actinic keratosis, (2) superficial basal cell carcinoma (sBCC), (3) external genital warts.

Dosage/Range: Imiquimod 5% topical cream is applied to the sBCC lesion (must be 2 cm or less in diameter), including a 1-cm margin around the lesion, as shown in the table below.

Drug Preparation: Wash hands before and after application of cream, and wear gloves. Wash skin area(s) with mild soap and water, then dry thoroughly before application, and again, after 8 hours application. Apply cream to lesion with an additional 1 cm surrounding the lesion(s), at bedtime leaving the cream on at least 8 hours, 5 nights a week, for 6 weeks.

Drug Interactions: Unknown.

Lab Effects/Interference: None known.

Special Considerations:
- Indicated for the treatment of sBCC on the body, neck, arms, or legs (not the face, hands, or feet) when surgical removal is not an option.
- Drug is also used for the treatment of external genital and nongenital warts, molluscum contagiosum, solar keratoses.

Potential Toxicities/Side Effects (More Severe with Higher Dosing) and the Nursing Process

I. POTENTIAL ALTERATION IN SKIN INTEGRITY AND COMFORT related to SKIN IRRITATION

Defining Characteristics: Redness, swelling, development of a sore or blister, peeling, itching, and burning are common application-site reactions. Response to therapy cannot be determined until the skin reaction resolves, sometimes up to 12 weeks.

Nursing Implications: Explain to the patient that these side effects may occur. Teach patient to wash skin prior to application, and again after 8 hours. Teach patient to assess skin reactions, and to report any symptoms that interfere with activities of daily living, as a rest period of a few days may be necessary if symptoms are severe. In addition, instruct patient to stop cream and report infection in the application area right away.

II. KNOWLEDGE DEFICIT related to SELF-ADMINISTRATION OF CREAM

Defining Characteristics: Treatment is for 6 weeks and must be applied properly for adequate tumor exposure.

Nursing Implications: Teach patient self-administration of the cream and to keep a diary to keep track of the application schedule. Teach patient to wash hands before and after application. Teach patient verbally and through demonstration to wash treatment area with mild soap and water, then to dry prior to application. Cream should be applied to extend 1 cm beyond the lesion borders, and rubbed into the treatment area until no longer visible. Keep cream away from eyes. Cream should be on for at least 8 hours, and then removed using mild soap and water.

Drug: Inotuzumab ozogamicin (Besponsa)

Class: Antibody-Drug Conjugaate (ADC); CD22- directed ADC.

Mechanism of Action: Mab recognizes CD22 and binds to it on tumor cells; the ADC is internalized, releasing calicheamicin which induces double-strand DNA breaks, leading to cell cycle arrest and apoptosis.

Metabolism: Calicheamicin compound is 97% protein bound to human plasma proteins. It is primarily metabolized by nonenzymatic reduction. Terminal half-life of the ADC is 12.3 days.

Indications: Adult patients with relapsed or refractory B-cell precursor acute lymphoblastic leukemia (ALL).

Contraindications: None.

Dosage/Range:
- Premedicate with a corticosteroid, antipyretic, and antihistamine.
- If patient has circulating lymphoblasts, cytoreduction is recommended with a combination of hydroxyurea, steroids and/or vincristine to a peripheral blast count of $\leq 10,000/$ mm^3 prior to first inotuzumab ozogamicin dose.
- **All patients Cycle 1**: Dose is 1.8 mg/m^2 in 3 divided doses: Day 1 = 0.8 mg/m^2; Day 8 = 0.5 mg/m^2; Day 15 = 0.5 mg/m^2. Cycle is 21 days (but may be extended to 28 days if recovering from toxicity).
- **Subsequent cycles:**
  - **Patients who have achieved a CR or CRi** (CR with incomplete hematologic recovery): Dose is 1.5 mg/m^2 divided in 3 doses: Day 1 = 0.5 mg/m^2; Day 8 = 0.5 mg/m^2; Day 15 = 0.5 mg/m^2. Cycle 28 days.
  - **Patients who HAVE NOT achieved a CR or Cri:** Dose is 1.8 mg/m^2 in 3 divided doses: Day 1 = 0.8 mg/m^2; Day 8 = 0.5 mg/m^2; Day 15 = 0.5 mg/m^2. Cycle 28 days. If patient does not achieve a CR or CRi within 3 cycles, the drug should be discontinued.
- If a patient is going on to HSCT, 2 cycles only are recommended. If the patient does not achieve a CR or CRi, and MRD (minimal residual disease) after 2 cycles, then a third cycle can be considered.
- **Dose Modifications**: If the dose is reduced, then it should not be re-escalated.
  - *Hemataologic toxicities:*
    - If prior to treatment, ANC was $\geq 1 \times 10^9$/L: If ANC decreases, then interrupt the next cycle until recovery of ANC to $\geq 1 \times 10^9$/L; discontinue inotuzumab ozogamicin if low ANC persists for >28 dyas and is suspected related to inotuzumab ozogamicin.
    - If prior to treatment, platelet count was $\geq 50 \times 10^9$/L: If platelet count decreases, then interrupt the next cycle until recovery of platelets to $\geq 50 \times 10^9$/L; discontinue inotuzumab ozogamicin if low platelets persists for >28 days and is suspected related to inotuzumab ozogamicin.

- If prior to treatment, ANC was $< 1 \times 10^9$/L and/or platelet count was $< 50 \times 10^9$/L: If ANC or platelet count decreases, then interrupt the next cycle until at least 1 of the following occurs: (1) ANC and platelet counts recover to at least baseline levels for the prior cycle, OR (2) ANC recovers to $\geq 1 \times 10^9$/L and platelet count recovers to $\geq 1 \times 10^9$/L independent of transfusion(s); OR (3) Stable or improved disease (based on most recent bone marrow assessment) and the ANC and platelet count decrease is considered to be due to the underlying disease (not considered to be due to inotuzumab ozogamicin-related toxicity).
- Non-hematologic toxicities:
  - Veno Occlusive Disease (VOD) or other severe liver toxicity: permanently discontinue drug.
  - Total bilirubin $> 1.5 \times$ ULN and AST/ALT > 2.5 ULN: Interrupt dosing until recovery of total bilirubin to $\leq 1.5 \times$ ULN and AST/ALT to $\leq 2.5 \times$ ULN prior to each dose unless due to Gilbert's syndrome or hemodialysis. Permanently discontinue treatment if total bilirubin does not recover to $\leq 1.5 \times$ ULN or AST/ALT does not recover to $\leq 2.5 \times$ ULN.
  - Infusion-related (IR) reaction: Interrupt the infusion and institute ordered medical management. Depending upon severity, consider discontinuation of the infusionor administration of steroids and antihistamines. For severe or life-threatening IRs, permanently discontinue drug.
  - Non-hematologic toxicity $\geq$ grade 2: Interrupt treatment until recovery to grade 1 or pre-treatment grade levels prior to each dose.
- Dose modifications depending upon duration of dosing interruption due to non-hematologic toxicities:
  - Less than 7 days: Interrupt the next dose (maintain a minimum of 6 days between doses).
  - ≥ 7 days: Omit the next dose within the cycle.
  - ≥ 14 days: Once adequately recovered, decrease the total dose by 25% for the subsequent cycle. If further dose modification is required, then reduce the number of doses to 2 per cycle for subsequent cycles. If a 25% decrease in the total dose is followed by a decrease to 2 doses per cycle is not tolerated, then permanently discontinue treatment.
  - >28 days: Consider permanent discontinuance of drug.

Drug Preparation: is available as 0.9 mg as a white to off-white lyophylized powder in a single- dose vial for reconstitution and further dilution. PROTECT the reconstituted and diluted solutions from light. Do NOT freeze either solution. The maximum time from reconstitution through the end of administration should be ≤ 8 hours, with **4 hours or less between reconstitution and dilution**.

Reconstitution:
- Use PPE; calculate dose (mg) and number of vials needed. Aseptically add 4 mL Sterile Water for Injection USP to obtain a concentration of 0.25 mg/mL; vial delivers 3.6 mL (0.9 mg).

- Gently swirl contents of vial to dissolve, DO NOT SHAKE. Inspect solution for particulates and discoloration—should be clear to opalescent, colorless to slightly yellow, without visible foreign matter.
- Storage: (a) Reconstituted solution should be used immediately or after being refrigerated for up to 4 hours at 2°C–8°C; 36°F–46°F; (b) after start of dilution, use diluted solution immediately or after storage at room temperature (20°–25°C, 68°–77°F) for up to 4 hours, or refrigerated (2°C–8°C; 36°F–46°F) for up to 3 hours. PROTECT FROM LIGHT AND DO NOT FREEZE.
- There should ONLY be ≤ 4 hours between reconstitution and dilution.

Dilution:
- Calculate the required volume of reconstituted solution for the dose (recheck BSA and dose); withdraw this amount from vial(s) using a syringe, and discard any unused drug.
- Add reconstituted solution to an IV container of 0.9% Sodium Chloride USP to make a total volume of 50mL. Use an infusion container of polyvinyl chloride (DEHP or non-DEHP containing), poyolefin, or ethylene vinyl acetate (EVA).
- Gently invert the infusion container to mix; DO NOT SHAKE.

Drug Administration:
- Assess cbc/ANC, LFTs, electrolytes prior to each treatment, and ECG prior to initial treatment. Assess patient for signs/symptoms of adverse reactions prior to next cycle.
- Assess pregnancy status of female patients of reproductive potential prior to first dose.
- If diluted solution is refrigerated, allow to equilibrate at room temperature for approximately 1 hour prior to administration. Administer diluted solution WITHIN 8 HOURS of reconstitution
- Premedicate with a corticosteroid, antipyretic, and antihistamine.
- Infuse diluted drug over 1 hour at a rate of 50 mL/h at room temperature (20°C–25°C; 68°F–77°F). PROTECT FROM LIGHT.
  - [Drug does not require filtration. If a filter is used, ensure filter is made of polyethersulfone (PES)-, polyvinylidene fluoride (PVDF)–,or hydrophilic polysulfone (HPS).
  - Do not use filters made of nylon or mixed cellulose ester (MCE)].
- Use IV tubing made of PVC (DEHP- or non-DEHP-containing), polyolefin (polypropylene and/or polyethylene), or polybutadiene.
- Observe patient during treatment and for at least 1 hour after the end of the infusion for signs/symptoms of IRs.

Drug Interactions: Low potential for drug interactions.

Lab Effects/Interference:
- Decreased neutrophils, lymphocytes, platelets, and red blood cells.
- Increased serum bilirubin, AST, ALT, GGT, alkaline phosphatase, lipase, uric acid, amylase
- QTc prolongation

Special Considerations:
- Most common adverse reactions (≥20%): thrombocytopenia, neutropenia, infection, anemia, leukopenia, fatigue, hemorrhage, pyrexia, nausea, headache, febrile neutropenia,

increased serum transaminases, abdominal pain, gamma-glutamyltransferase increased, hyperbilirubinemia.
- Mothers should not breast feed while receiving the drug.
- Warnings and Precautions:
  - Hepatotoxicity, including fatal and life-threatening Veno-Occlusive Disease (VOD, sinusoidal obstruction syndrome) have occurred in patients receiving inotuzumab ozogamicin. Incidence was 14% during or after treatment or after HSCT completion. VOD occurred up to 56 days after the last drug dose, and median time to onset of VOD after inotuzumab ozogamicin and subsequent HSCT was 15 days. Patients at risk are those who undergo HSCT after inotuzumab ozogamicin treatment, who are exposed to conditioning regimens of 2 alkylating agents, and whose last total bilirubin was ≥ ULN before HSCT. Other risk factors for other patients are current or prior liver disease, prior HSCT, increased age, later salvage treatment lines, and a greater number of cycles of inotuzumab ozogamicin therapy (Wyeth, 2018). Patients with serious liver disease, or who have experienced prior VOD are also at risk for VOD as well as worsening liver disease. Patients should be monitored closely for signs/ symptoms of VOD (elevated total bilirubin, hepatomegaly, rapid weight gain, ascites). Patients for whom HSCT is planned after treatment should only receive 2 cycles of inotuzumab ozogamicin, unless a third cycle is necessary if patient did not achieve CR or CRi and MRD after 2 cycles. If a patient proceeds to HSCT after inotuzumab ozogamicin therapy, monitor LFTs closely during the first month post transplant. For all patients, monitor LFTs closely baseline, and prior to, and after each dose. See Dose Modifications.
  - *A higher post-HSCT non-relapse mortality* rate occurred in patients receiving inotuzumab ozogamicin.Post-HSCT non-relapse mortality was 39% for the patient arm receiving inotuzumab ozogamicin vs 23% in the investigator's chemotherapy of choice arm. In those patients receiving inotuzumab ozogamicin, the most common causes of death were VOD and infection. Monitor patients closely post-HSCT for signs/ symptoms of infection and VOD.
  - *Myelosuppression:* Occurs frequently, with thrombocytopenia in 51% (grade 3/4, 14/28%) and neutropenia 49% (grade 3/4, 20/27%) of patients. Febrile neutropenia occurred in 26% of patients. Platelet recovery (to > 50,000/mm$^{3)}$ in patients who achieved a CR or CRi was later than 45 days in 9% of patients. Infections (bacterial, viral, fungal) occurred in 48%, and were fatal in 5%. Hemorrhage occurred in 33% with grade 3/4 events in 5% of patients. The most common event was epistaxis, although fatal intra-abdominal hemorrhage occurred in 1% of patients. Monitor CBC/ ANC prior to each dose and monitor patient closely for signs/symptoms of infection and bleeding. Discuss prophylactic anti-infectives with provider and perform surveillance testing during and after treatment with inotuzumab ozogamicin as ordered. Manage adverse reactions with appropriate medical interventions as ordered and if severe, with dose modification or permanent discontinuation of drug.
  - *Infusion related reactions (IRRs):* All IRRs were grade 2 in 2% of patients with most occurring during Cycle 1 shortly after the end of the inotuzumab ozogamicin infusion, resolving spontaneously or with medical management. Administer premedication with a corticosteroid, antipyretic, and antihistamine. Monitor patients closely

during and for 1 hour after the infusion for IRRs (e.g., fever, chills, rash, dyspnea). In an IRR occurs, stop the infusion, and administer medical intervention as ordered (e.g., hold, administer steroids and antihistamines and resume, or if severe, permanently discontinue drug).

- *QTc prolongation:* occurred in 3% of patients (QTcF ≥ 60 msec from baseline), 2% grade 2. No grade 3 or torsades de pointes has been reported. Use drug cautiously in patients (1) with a history or predisposition for QTc prolongation, (2) who are taking drugs which prolong the QTc, or (3) have electrolyte disturbances. Assess ECG and electrolytes prior to start of inotuzumab ozogamicin treatment, after initiation of any drug which can prolong the QTc, and as indicated during treatment. Correct any electrolyte imbalance as ordered.

- *Embryo-fetal toxicity:* Drug is feto-toxic. Verify pregnancy status of female patient of reproductive potention, prior to starting drug Teach women of reproductive potential to use effective contraception during and for at least 8 months after last drug dose. Teach male patients with female partners of reproductive potential to use effective contraception during treatment and for 5 months following last dose.

Potential Toxicities/Side Effects (More Severe with Higher Dosing) and the Nursing Process

I.   POTENTIAL FOR INFECTION, BLEEDING, AND FATIGUE, related to BONE MARROW DEPRESSION

Defining Characteristics: Inotuzumab ozogamicin is myelosuppressive causing thrombocytopenia in 51% of patients (42% grade 3/4), and neutropenia in 49% of patients (48% grade 3/4). Hemorrhage occurred in 33% (5% grade 3/4) and febrile neutropenia in 26% (26% grade 3/4).Anemia occurred in 36% (grade 3/4 in 24%) Fatigue affected 35% of patients. [Wyeth, 2018].

Nursing Implications: Monitor cbc/ANC baseline, before each treatment, and as indicated. Assess for signs/symptoms of infection, bleeding and fatigue baseline, between treatment, and prior to each treatment. Teach patients to self-assess for these, including taking temperature, and instruct to report abnormal results immediately or to go to the ED. Teach patient measures to minimize these side effects by avoiding crowds, not taking OTC medicines containing aspirin or NSAIDs. Teach patient strategies to minimize energy expenditure and to conserve energy. Transfuse red blood cells and platelets as ordered.

II.   ALTERATION IN NUTRITION, POTENTIAL related to NAUSEA, VOMITING, ABDOMINAL PAIN, HEPATOTOXICITY

Defining Characteristics: Nausea occurred in 31% of patients, vomiting 15%, abdominal pain 23%, diarrhea 17%, constipation 16%, and stomatitis 13%. Serum transaminases (GGT, AST, ALT) were elevated in 57–71% of patients, alkaline phosphatase elevated in 49%, and increased bilirubin in 36%. VOD occurred in 14% (during, after, or after HSCT).

TREATMENT

Nursing Implications: Assess need for antiemetic and administer as ordered prior to drug administration as has received a corticosteroid as premedication. Ensure patient has a prescription for antiemetic for home use, and instruct to call if nausea/vomiting occur, and are refractory to the medication.assess bowel elimination status and need for counseling to prevent diarrhea or constipation while receiving the drug. Assess oral mucosa and teach oral hygiene care after meals and at bedtime, and instruct to call if the patient develops pain or ulcers. Teach patient importance to promote intact oral mucosa to prevent infection. Assess LFTs baseline, and before each treatment. Discuss abnormalities with provider. Teach patients dietary strategies to minimize nausea, vomiting, diarrhea, constipation and stomatitis as appropriate. Asess for VOD, especially in patients with hepatic dysfunction or prior HSCT: elevated total bilirubin, hepatomegaly, rapid weight gain, ascites, and discuss urgently with provider. Treatment with inotuzumab ozogamicin should be interrupted if hepatotoxicity occurs and the drug discontinued if VOD occurs.

Drug: interferon alfa (2') (alpha interferon, IFN, interferon alpha-2a, rIFN-A, Roferon A)

Class: Cytokine (interferon).

Mechanism of Action: Antiviral, antiproliferative, and immunomodulatory effects. Activates prenatural killer cells, increases cytotoxicity of NK cells, and enhances immune response.

Metabolism: Well absorbed following subcutaneous or IM injection with 90% bioavailability after subcutaneous injection. Drug peaks at 6–8 hours and has an elimination half-life of 2 hours (IM/IV) and 3 hours (subcutaneous). Renal filtration and tubular reabsorption as catabolites; minor hepatic metabolism and biliary excretion.

Indications: For the treatment of patients with (1) chronic hepatitis C, (2) hairy-cell leukemia in adults age 18 and over; (3) chronic phase, Philadelphia chromosome (Ph) positive chronic myelogenous leukemia (CML) who are minimally pretreated (within 1 year of diagnosis).

Contraindications: Patients with (1) hypersensitivityto Roferon-A or any of its components; (2) autoimmune hepatitis; (3) hepatic decompensation (Child-Pugh class B and C) before or during treatment; also contraindicated in neonates and infants, as it contains benzyl alcohol.

Target Tumor Diameter	Size of Cream Droplet to Be Used (diameter) (mm)	Amount of Imiquimod Cream Used (mg)
0.5 to 1.0 cm	4	10
≥1.0 to 1.5 cm	5	25
≥1.5 to 2.0 cm	7	40

Available in single-use packets, supplied 12 per box.

Dosage/Range:
- Hepatitis C: 3 million international units 3X (tiw) a week SQ for 12 months (48–52 weeks) OR induction dose of 6 million international units tiw for the first 3 months (12 weeks) followed by 3 million international units tiw for 9 months (36 weeks).
  - Normalization of serum ALT usually occurs within a few weeks of initial dose; about 90% of patients who respond to Roferon A do so within the first 3 months of treatment.
  - If the patient has no response in the first 3 months, drug discontinuation should be considered.
- CML: 9 million international units daily subcutaneous for up to 18 months.
  - Short-term tolerance is improved by gradually increasing the dose over the first week from 3 million international units daily for 3 days, to 6 million international units daily for 3 days, then to the target dose of 9 million international units for the rest of the treatment period.
  - Median time to a complete hematologic response was 5 months in one study but may take up to 18 months. Treatment should be continued until disease progression.
  - If severe side effects occur, interrupt treatment or reduce dose or frequency of injections to achieve the individual maximally tolerated dose.
- Hairy-cell leukemia: Induction 3 million international units daily for 16–24 weeks SQ; maintenance 3 million international units 3 times/week for 6–24 months.
  - If dose reductions needed for severe adverse reactions, reduce dose by one-half or hold individual doses. Do not exceed doses higher than 3 million international units.
  - Patient should be evaluated for response to therapy by assessment of peripheral blood and bone marrow for hairy cells monthly. If patient does not respond within 6 months, treatment should be discontinued.

Drug Preparation:
- Available for subcutaneous administration as prefilled syringes:
  - 3 million international units/0.5 mL/syringe, in boxes of 1 or 6.
  - 6 million international units/0.5 mL/syringe in boxes of 1 or 6.
  - 9 million international units/0.5 mL/syringe in boxes of 1 or 6.
  - Store in refrigerator at 2–8°C (36–46°F). Do not shake or freeze. Store in refrigerator and protect from light during storage.

Drug Administration: Intramuscular, subcutaneous, or intravenous.
- Assess CBC/platelet counts and clinical chemistry tests baseline then periodically during therapy. Carefully monitor any patients with ANC $< 1,500/mm^3$, platelet count $< 75,000/mm^3$, Hgb < 10 g/dL, and creatinine > 1.5 mg/dL. Also, monitor patients with leukemia closely during the initial phase of treatment for severe BMD.
- Assess ECG baseline and during therapy in patients with preexisting cardiac abnormalities and/or in advanced stages of cancer.
- Assess LFTs in patients with chronic hepatitis C: serum ALT baseline, then at week 2 and monthly thereafter.
- Assess thyroid stimulating hormone (TSH) baseline and every 3 months in patients with preexisting thyroid abnormalities, as they can be treated with the drug as long as TSH is normal.

• Assess triglycerides baseline and during therapy and manage medically as needed. If patient has consistently elevated triglycerides (e.g., >1,000 mg/dL) associated with symptoms of pancreatitis (abdominal pain, nausea, or vomiting), drug should be discontinued.

Drug Interactions:
• May decrease elimination of aminophylline by 33–81% via inhibition of cytochrome P450 enzyme system.
• Increased effects of CNS depressants.
• Increased bone marrow suppressant effects with zidovudine (AZT).
• Drug may affect P450 oxidative metabolic process.
• Drug may increase neurotoxic, hematotoxic, or cardiotoxic effects of prior or concomitant drugs.
• IL-2 given concomitantly with Roferon-A, potentiation of risk for developing renal failure.
• Hyperglycemia.

Lab Effects/Interference:
• Dose-dependent; leukopenia, thrombocytopenia, anemia; elevated liver serum transaminases.
• Elevated triglycerides.

Special Considerations:
• Warnings and Precautions:
  • Neuropsychiatric disorders: Depression and suicidal behavior have been reported, including suicide attempts.
    • Use drug with extreme caution in patients with a history of depression and follow patient closely if used. Teach patient to report depression or suicidal thoughts immediately.
    • Psychiatric intervention and/or drug cessation should be considered for depressed patients, but suicides have occurred after the drug was stopped.
    • CNS adverse reactions have been reported: Decreased mental status, dizziness, impaired memory, agitation, manic behavior, psychotic reactions, and rarely coma. Most were reversible with dose reduction or drug cessation within a few days–3 weeks. Use drug cautiously in patients with a seizure disorder or compromised CNS function.
• Cardiovascular disorders: Use drug cautiously in patients with cardiac disease, as drug may exacerbate preexisting cardiac disease; rarely, MI and cardiomyopathy have occurred.
• Cerebrovascular disorders: Ischemic and hemorrhagic cerebrovascular events have occurred.
• Hypersensitivity: May rarely occur (e.g., urticaria, angioedema, bronchoconstriction, anaphylaxis) as well as skin rashes. If a serious reaction occurs, drug must be discontinued and appropriate emergency medical care instituted. Transient rash does not necessitate drug interruption.

- Hepatic disorders: Transient liver abnormalities have been reported in patients with hepatitis C; if the patient has poorly compensated liver disease, results in ascites, hepatic failure, or death.
- GI disorders: Ulcerative and hemorrhagic/ischemic colitis have been reported within 12 weeks of starting therapy (characterized by abdominal pain, bloody diarrhea, fever); drug should be immediately discontinued if this occurs, and colitis usually resolves within 1–3 weeks of drug discontinuance.
- Infections: Must distinguish between fever as part of flu-like symptomatology versus fever and infection, especially if patient has neutropenia. Serious bacterial, viral, fungal infections have occurred; if this happens, appropriate antimicrobial therapy should be instituted and interferon therapy discontinued.
- Bone marrow toxicity: Drug suppresses bone marrow function, resulting in cytopenias and anemia, which may be severe. Assess CBC baseline and routinely during therapy. Discontinue drug if ANC < 500 cells/mm^3 or platelets < 25,000 cells/mm^3.
- Endocrine disorders: Drug causes or exacerbates hypothyroidism and hyperthyroidism. Hyperglycemia has occurred. Diabetic patients may require adjustment of their antidiabetic medications. Assess baseline glucose and monitor during therapy, especially in diabetic patients.
- Pulmonary disorders may be induced or exacerbated; monitor for dyspnea, pulmonary infiltrates, pneumonia, bronchiolitis obliterans, interstitial pneumonitis, and sarcoidosis; evaluate promptly. If patient develops persistent or unexplained pulmonary infiltrates or impaired pulmonary function, interferon should be discontinued.
- Ophthalmologic disorders: Patients should have baseline eye exam; if patient has preexisting ophthalmologic disorders (e.g., diabetic or hypertensive retinopathy), they should receive ongoing periodic exams during interferon therapy. If patient develops symptoms, this should prompt a complete eye exam, and drug should be discontinued if new or worsening ophthalmologic disorders occur.
- Pancreatitis: Marked triglyceride elevation is a risk factor. Drug should be interrupted if symptoms arise, and drug discontinued if the diagnosis of pancreatitis is confirmed.
- Most common adverse effects were: (1) in patients with chronic hepatitis C (3 million international unit dose): flu-like symptoms (fatigue, myalgia/arthralgia, fever, chills, asthenia, sweating, leg cramps, malaise), headache, nausea, vomiting, diarrhea, injection-site reaction; (6 million international unit dose): higher incidence of severe psychiatric events. Fewer adverse events occur in the second 6 months of treatment than in the first 6 months; (2) patients with CML: fever, asthenia, or fatigue, myalgia, chills, arthalgia/bone pain, headache, anorexia, nausea/vomiting, diarrhea, headache, depression; (3) patients with hairy-cell leukemia: fever, fatigue, headache, chills, weight loss, skin rash, myalgia, anorexia, nausea/vomiting, diarrhea, dizziness.
- Roferon-A should be used in pregnant women only if the potential benefit justifies the potential risk to the fetus. Teach females of reproductive potential and men to use effective contraception during interferon therapy.
- Nursing mothers should make a decision whether to discontinue nursing or discontinue the drug, taking into account the importance of the drug to the mother's health.

Potential Toxicities/Side Effects (More Severe with Higher Dosing) and the Nursing Process

I.   ALTERATION IN COMFORT related to FLU-LIKE SYNDROME

Defining Characteristics: Chills 3–6 hours after dose in 40–60% of patients; fever (74–98% of patients) with onset 30–90 minutes after chill, lasting up to 24 hours. Temperature 39–40°C (102–104°F), tachyphylaxis (decrease in severity/occurrence after successive treatments) common. Fatigue (89–95% of patients) and malaise are cumulative and dose-limiting. Headache, myalgias occur in 60–70% of patients, as well as arthralgias (5–24% of patients).

Nursing Implications: Assess baseline T, VS, neurologic status, and comfort level; monitor every 4–6 hours if patient is in hospital. Discuss with physician premedication and regular dosing of antipyretic (e.g., acetaminophen ± diphenhydramine, NSAID). Teach patient self-care measures, including monitoring T, comfort level, self-administration of prescribed medications prior to dose and regularly postdose, as well as the use of heat or cold for myalgias, arthralgias. Encourage patient to increase oral fluids and alternate rest and activity periods. If patient is in hospital and experiences rigor, discuss with physician IV meperidine (25 mg IV q 15 min to maximum 100 mg in 1 hour) and monitor BP for hypotension. Teach patient to alternate rest and activity periods.

II.   POTENTIAL FOR INFECTION AND BLEEDING related to NEUTROPENIA AND THROMBOCYTOPENIA

Defining Characteristics: Although uncommon, increased risk with increased dose; dose-limiting thrombocytopenia; reversible. Onset usually in 7–10 days, nadir at day 14, but may be delayed in hairy-cell leukemia (20–40 days); recovery in 21 days.

Nursing Implications: Assess baseline CBC, WBC, differential, and platelet count, and signs/symptoms of infection or bleeding. Discuss any abnormalities with physician before drug administration. Teach patient signs/symptoms of infection and bleeding and to report them immediately. Teach patient self-care measures to minimize infection and bleeding, including avoidance of OTC aspirin-containing medications and oral hygiene regimen.

III.   ALTERATION IN NUTRITION, LESS THAN BODY REQUIREMENTS, related to NAUSEA, DIARRHEA, ANOREXIA

Defining Characteristics: Anorexia occurs (46–65% of patients) and is cumulative and dose-limiting. Nausea (32–51% of patients) is mild with tachyphylaxis after 1 week. Diarrhea (29–42% of patients) is mild, and vomiting is rare (10–17% of patients). Taste alterations and xerostomia may occur.

Nursing Implications: Assess baseline nutritional status. Teach patient potential side effects and self-care measures, including oral hygiene. Encourage patient to prepare favorite high-calorie, high-protein foods ahead of time so able to snack when hungry. Teach self-administration of prescribed antiemetics and antidiarrheals as needed. Refer to dietitian as appropriate.

IV.   SENSORY/PERCEPTUAL ALTERATION related to CNS EFFECTS

Defining Characteristics: Dizziness (21–41% of patients), confusion (8–10% of patients), decreased mental status (17% of patients), and depression (16% of patients). Somnolence, irritability, poor concentration, seizures, paranoia, hallucinations, psychoses may occur in 70% of patients but are reversible. Use drug cautiously in patients with history of seizures or CNS dysfunction.

Nursing Implications: Assess baseline mental status and neurologic status prior to drug administration. Assess patient for changes (impaired memory/attention, disorientation, slow/vague responses to questions, increased lethargy) during treatment. Instruct patient to report signs/symptoms; provide information and emotional support, as well as interventions to ensure safety if signs/symptoms occur.

V.   POTENTIAL ALTERATION IN CARDIAC OUTPUT related to TACHYCARDIA, CHEST PAIN, DYSRHYTHMIAS

Defining Characteristics: Uncommon but dose-related with increased risk in elderly and patients with preexisting cardiac dysfunction: tachycardia, pallor, cyanosis, chest pain, orthostatic hypotension or hypertension arrhythmias, CHF, syncope.

Nursing Implications: Assess baseline cardiopulmonary status and risk (elderly, preexisting cardiac dysfunction). EKG testing is done baseline and during treatment for high-risk individuals. Monitor VS and I/O, every 4 hours while receiving drug in hospital. Teach patient to report signs/symptoms of dyspnea, chest pain, edema, or other abnormalities immediately.

VI.   POTENTIAL ALTERATION IN ELIMINATION related to RENAL AND HEPATIC DYSFUNCTION

Defining Characteristics: Dose-related increased BUN, creatinine, LFTs (increased AST 42–46%) may occur, as well as proteinuria. Patient may develop interstitial nephritis.

Nursing Implications: Assess baseline renal and hepatic function studies and urinalysis prior to drug initiation, and periodically during therapy. Discuss abnormalities with physician.

VII.   POTENTIAL FOR SEXUAL DYSFUNCTION related to IMPOTENCE, MENSTRUAL IRREGULARITIES

Defining Characteristics: Impotence and decreased libido, menstrual irregularities, and increased spontaneous abortions have occurred. Drug is excreted in breastmilk.

Nursing Implications: Assess patient's baseline sexual patterns and discuss potential alterations. Provide information, emotional support, and referral as appropriate and needed. Encourage patient to use contraceptive measures; mothers receiving the drug should not breastfeed.

VIII. POTENTIAL ALTERATION IN SKIN INTEGRITY related to RASH, PARTIAL ALOPECIA, DRYNESS

Defining Characteristics: Partial alopecia (8–22% of patients), rash (11–18% of patients), throat dryness (15% of patients), as well as skin dryness, flushing, pruritus, and irritation at injection site may occur.

Nursing Implications: Assess baseline skin integrity. Instruct patient to report signs/symptoms. Discuss/teach symptomatic management, including the use of mild soaps and rinsing skin thoroughly after bathing. Encourage patient to use alcohol-free, oil-based moisturizers on skin.

IX. KNOWLEDGE DEFICIT related to SELF-ADMINISTRATION TECHNIQUE

Defining Characteristics: Often patients must receive daily dosing or thrice weekly dosing in the home setting by subcutaneous injection, and they are unfamiliar with technique.

Nursing Implications: Assess baseline psychomotor ability, knowledge, and willingness to learn technique of self-injection. Teach how to prepare drug, self-administer, and safely collect used syringes for proper disposal. Use written and video materials as supplements to teaching process and have patient correctly demonstrate technique prior to performing at home. Make referral to visiting-nurse agency to reinforce teaching.

Drug: interferon alfa-2b (Intron A, IFN-alpha-2b recombinant, α-2-interferon, rIFN-α-2)

Class: Cytokine (interferon).

Mechanism of Action: Antiviral, antiproliferative, and immunomodulatory effects. Activates prenatural killer cells, increases cytotoxicity of NK cells, and enhances immune response.

Metabolism: Well absorbed following subcutaneous or IM injection with 90% bioavailability after subcutaneous injection. Drug peaks at 6–8 hours, and has an elimination half-life of 2 hours (IM/IV) and 3 hours (subcutaneous). Renal filtration and tubular reabsorption as catabolites; minor hepatic metabolism and biliary excretion.

Indications: For the treatment of (1) adults 18 years or older with hairy-cell leukemia; (2) adults age 18 years or older with malignant melanoma, who are free of disease but at high risk for systemic recurrence, within 56 days of surgery; (3) adults age 18 years or older with clinically aggressive follicular NHL in conjunction with anthracycline-containing combination chemotherapy (efficacy in patients with low-grade, low-tumor burden follicular NHL has not been demonstrated); (4) selected adults age 18 years or older with condylomata acuminata involving external surfaces of the genital and perianal areas; (5) selected adults age 18 years or older with AIDS-related Kaposi's sarcoma (response is more likely in patients without systemic symptoms, limited lymphadenopathy, and relatively intact immune system, as indicated by total CD4 count); (6) adults age 18 years or older with chronic hepatitis C with compensated liver disease who have a history of blood or blood-product exposure and/or are HCV antibody positive (studies show clinically meaningful effects [e.g., normalization of ALT and reduction in liver necrosis and degeneration]; compensated liver disease is defined as (i) absence of history of decompensation [e.g., hepatic encephalopathy, variceal bleeding, ascites], (ii) bilirubin stable and WNL, (iii) PT $<$ 3 seconds prolonged, (iv) WBC $\geq$ 3,000/mm^3, and platelets $\geq$ 70,000/mm^3); (7) patients 1 year of age or older with chronic hepatitis B with compensated liver disease (serum HBsAg positive for at least 6 months and have evidence of HBV replication [serum HBeAg positive] with elevated serum ALT).

Contraindications: Patients with (1) hypersensitivity to interferon alpha or any product component, (2) autoimmune hepatitis, (3) decompensated liver disease. Intron A and Rebetol® combination therapy is contraindicated in (1) patients with hypersensitivity to ribavirin or any other product component, (2) pregnant women, (3) men whose female partners are pregnant, (4) patients with hemoglobinopathies (e.g., thalassemia major, sickle cell anemia), (5) patients with creatinine clearance $<$ 50 mL/min.

Dosage/Range:
- Hairy-cell leukemia: IFN-α: 2 million international units (MIU)/m^2 IM or subcutaneous 3 times/week for 2–6 months.
  - If platelet count is $<$ 50,000/mm^3, drug should be administered SQ not IM.
  - Dosage forms: powder: 10 million international units/mL; solution 18 million international units multidose; solution 25 million international units multidose.
  - If severe reactions, dose-reduce 50% or temporarily interrupt therapy until resolve, then resume at 50% dose (e.g., 1 million international unit/m^2 tiw).
  - If severe reactions recur, discontinue drug.
  - Discontinue drug if progressive disease or failure to respond after 6 months of treatment.
- Malignant melanoma: Induction: 20 million international units/m^2 IV infusion over 20 minutes, on days 1–5 weekly for 4 weeks.
  - Use powder ONLY: 10 million international units (10 million international units/mL), 18 million international units/mL, 50 million international units/mL. Reconstituted drug is preservative-free and single-use only.
  - Dose modifications: Hold drug for severe adverse reactions, including ANC $>$ 250/mm^3 but $<$ 500/mm^3 or ALT/AST $>$ 5–10 $\times$ ULN, until adverse effects abate, then resume at 50% of the previous dose.
  - Permanently discontinue drug for persistent toxicity, severe adverse effects that recur on a reduced dose, or if ANC is $<$ 250/mm^3 or ALT/AST $>$ 10 $\times$ ULN.

- Maintenance: 10 million international units/m^2 subcutaneous 3 times/week for 48 weeks.
- Use powder ONLY: 10 million international units (10 million international units/mL), 18 million international units/mL single dose, 18 million international units multidose (6 million international units/mL), or 25 million international units/mL (10 million international units/mL). Reconstituted drug is preservative-free and single-use only.
- Dose modifications: Hold drug for severe adverse reactions, including ANC > 250/mm^3 but < 500/mm^3 or ALT/AST > 5–10 × ULN, until adverse effects abate, then resume at 50% of the previous dose.
- Permanently discontinue drug for persistent toxicity, severe adverse effects that recur on a reduced dose, or if ANC is < 250/mm^3 or ALT/AST > 10 × ULN.
- Follicular NHL: 5 million international units SQ 3 times a week (tiw) for up to 18 months in conjunction with an anthracycline-containing regimen and following completion of chemotherapy.
  - Powder: 10 million international units single dose; solution: 18 million international unit multidose (6 million international unit/mL), 25 million international units (10 million international unit/mL).
  - Dose adjustment: CHOP chemotherapy doses were reduced 25% and cycle length increased by 33% from full dose when alpha-interferon was added to the regime. Delay chemotherapy cycle if ANC < 1,500/mm^3 or platelet count < 75,000/mm^3.
  - Permanently discontinue Intron A if AST > 5 × ULN or serum creatinine is > 2.0 mg/dL.
  - Hold Intron A for ANC < 1,000/mm^3 or platelet count < 50,000/mm^3.
  - Reduce Intron A dose by 50% (2.5 million international units tiw) for ANC > 1,000/mm^3 but < 1,500/mm^3; dose may be reescalated to starting dose of 5 million international units tiw after resolution and ANC > 1,500/mm^3.
- Condylomata Acuminata: 1 million international unit per lesion in a maximum of 5 lesions in a single course. The lesions should be injected 3 times weekly on alternate days for 3 weeks. An additional course may be administered at 12–16 weeks.
  - DO NOT use the 18 million international units or 50 million international unit powder or the 18 million international unit multidose solution for this indication.
  - Use powder 10 million international units (single-dose), or solution 25 million international units multidose (10 million international units/mL).
  - See package insert for injection technique.
- AIDS-related Kaposi's sarcoma: IFN-α2b: 30 million international units/m^2/dose subcutaneous or IM 3 times/week, until disease progression or maximal response achieved after 16 weeks of treatment. Dose reduction is frequently needed.
  - Use powder 50 million international units (50 million international units/mL). DO NOT use solution for injection. Reconstituted powder does not contain preservatives and is a single-use vial.
  - Dose adjustment: Reduce dose 50% for severe adverse reactions; resume at this lower dose after reactions abate with dosing interruption. Drug should be permanently discontinued if severe reactions persist or recur at the reduced dose.

- Chronic Hepatitis C: 3 million international units 3 times a week (tiw) SQ or IM. Patients tolerating therapy with normalization of ALT at 16 weeks of treatment can have treatment extended to 18–24 months, same dose, to improve the response rate.
  - If patient does not normalize ALT or have persistently high HCV RNA levels after 16 weeks, it is unlikely that he or she will get a sustained response with continued treatment; consider drug discontinuance.
  - Intron A combined with Rebetol: see package insert.
  - Dose adjustment: Dose-reduce 50% for severe adverse reactions, or therapy should be temporarily discontinued.
- Chronic Hepatitis B: Adults: 30–35 million international units per week SQ or IM, either as 5 million international units daily (QD) or as 10 million international units 3 times a week (tiw) for 16 weeks. Pediatrics: see package insert.
  - Use dosage forms: Powder 10 million international units (single-dose) or solution 25 million international units multidose (10 million international units/mL). Reconstituted powder is preservative-free, so is a single-use vial.
  - Dose adjustment: Severe adverse effects or laboratory abnormalities: 50% dose reduction, or discontinue drug as appropriate. If WBC $<$ 1,500/mm^3, ANC $<$ 750/mm^3, OR platelet count $<$ 50,000/mm^3: reduce dose 50%. If WBC $<$ 1,000/mm^3, ANC $<$ 500/mm^3, or platelet count $<$ 25,000/mm^3, permanently discontinue drug. Intron A therapy was resumed at up to 100% of the initial dose when WBC, ANC, and platelet counts returned to normal or baseline values. See package insert.

Drug Preparation:
- IFN-α2b (Intron A): Available in (1) powder for injection/reconstitution and (2) solution for injection vials. Not all dosage forms and strengths are appropriate for some indications.
- Powder for injection is preservative-free, so vial must be discarded after reconstitution and withdrawal of a single dose.
- See package insert.
- Allow solution to come to room temperature before using.

Drug Administration:
- Administer in the evening to enhance tolerability. Acetaminophen may also be administered at the same time.
- Intramuscular, subcutaneous, or IVB, intermittent or continuous infusion.
- Ensure patient has adequate hydration, especially during treatment for malignant melanoma; this may require IV hydration.
- Assess baseline CBC/differential/platelet count, blood chemistries including LFTs and TSH, electrolytes, and results of periodic assessment during therapy.
- Assess ECG of patients with preexisting cardiac abnormalities or advanced cancer baseline and periodically during therapy.
- Malignant melanoma induction: Assess differential WBC count, LFTs weekly, and then monthly during maintenance.

Drug Interactions:
- May decrease elimination of aminophylline by 33–81% via inhibition of cytochrome P450 enzyme system.

- Increased effects of CNS depressants.
- Increased bone marrow suppressant effects with zidovudine (AZT).
- Increased risk of peripheral neuropathy when combined with vinblastine.

Lab Effects/Interference:
- Dose-dependent; leukopenia; elevated liver serum transaminases.

Special Considerations:
- Warnings and Precautions:
  - Alpha interferons, including Intron A, can cause or aggravate fatal or life-threatening neuropsychiatric, autoimmune, ischemic, and infectious disorders. **Monitor patients closely using clinical exam and laboratory evaluations. If patient has persistently severe or worsening signs or symptoms of these conditions, Intron A therapy should be withdrawn.**
  - Flu-like symptoms can be severe and should be used cautiously in patients with debilitating medical conditons (e.g., COPD, or DM prone to acidosis) or patients with coagulation disorders (thrombophlebitis, PE) or severe myelosuppression.
  - Cardiovascular disorders: Use cautiously in patients with a history of MI or arrhythmia disorders who should be monitored closely, as drug can cause HTN, hypotension, arrhythmia, tachycardia $\geq$ 150 beats/min, and rarely, cardiomyopathy.
  - Cerebrovascular disorders: Ischemic and hemorrhagic cerebrovascular events have occurred.
  - Neuropsychiatric disorders: Depression and suicidal behavior, including suicidal ideation, have occurred.
    - If the patient develops psychiatric problems, including clinical depression, patient should be carefully monitored during treatment and in the 6-month follow-up period.
    - Drug should be used cautiously in patients with a history of psychiatric disorders and should be discontinued in any patient developing a severe psychiatric disorder during treatment. These effects usually reverse promptly after drug discontinuance, but full resolution may take up to 3 weeks.
    - If psychiatric symptoms persist or worsen, or suicidal ideation or aggressive behavior toward others occurs, drug should be discontinued and patient followed with psychiatric intervention until resolved.
    - Preexisting symptoms of psychiatric disorders may be exacerbated; if patient has a history of substance abuse, consider need for drug screening and periodic health evaluation, including psychiatric symptom-monitoring.
  - Bone marrow toxicity: Drug suppresses bone marrow function and may cause cytopenias, including aplastic anemia. Monitor CBC baseline and routinely during treatment. Discontinue drug if ANC < 500 cells/mm³ or platelet count < 25,000/mm³.
  - Ophthalmologic disorders: May be induced or aggravated; patients should have a comprehensive eye exam baseline, and if preexisting disorders (e.g., diabetic or hypertensive retinopathy), should receive periodic ophthalmologic exams. If a patient presents with ocular symptoms, a prompt and complete eye exam should be done. If the patient develops a new or worsening ophthalmologic disorder, interferon alfa-2b treatment should be discontinued.

- Endocrine disorders: Infrequently, patients may develop hypo- or hyperthyroidism. Assess baseline TSH, and repeat if patients develop symptoms of thyroid dysfunction. If the patient has a preexisting thyroid abnormality and normal thyroid function cannot be managed, Intron A should not be administered. Diabetes may occur; if it is unable to be controlled, drug should be stopped.
- GI disorders: Hepatotoxicity may occur. Monitor patients with liver function abnormalities closely, and discontinue drug if needed.
- Pulmonary disorders: May be induced or worsened (e.g., dyspnea, pulmonary infiltrates, pneumonia, bronchiolitis obliterans, interstitial pneumonitis, pulmonary hypertension, sarcoidosis). If a patient presents with fever, cough, dyspnea, or other respiratory symptoms, a CXR should be assessed. If there are pulmonary infiltrates, or evidence of pulmonary function impairment, monitor the patient closely and discontinue drug as appropriate.
- Autoimmune disorders: May occur (e.g., thrombocytopenia, vasculitis, RA, lupus erythematosius, rhabdomyolysis). If a patient develops an autoimmune disorder during therapy, monitor the patient closely and discontinue drug if appropriate.
- Human albumin is used in the drug manufacture and carries a theoretical, remote risk of Creutzfeldt–Jakob disease (CJD).
- AIDS-related Kaposi's sarcoma: Drug should not be used if patient has rapidly progressive visceral disease. Patients receiving zidovudine and Intron A may have synergistic effect, with a higher incidence of neutropenia. Monitor the WBC closely.
- Chronic hepatitis C and chronic hepatitis B: Drug should not be used in patients with decompensated liver disease, autoimmune hepatitis, a history of autoimmune disease, or patients who are immunosuppressed transplant recipients.
- Peripheral neuropathy: Has been reported when drug is administered with telbivudine.
- Use with ribavirin (Rebetol) may cause birth defects and/or death of unborn child. Confirm a negative pregnancy test immediately before planned initiation of therapy. Teach female patients to use at least 2 forms of contraception and have monthly pregnancy tests. Combination with ribavirin may also cause hemolytic anemia, with anemia occurring within 1–2 weeks of starting ribavirin.
- Acute serious HSRs (e.g., urticaria, angioedema, bronchoconstriction, anaphylaxis) may rarely occur. Provide appropriate medical care as ordered, and drug should be discontinued for acute reactions.
- Elevated triglycerides may occur and may result in pancreatitis. If patient has persistently elevated triglycerides > 1,000 mg/dL, drug should be discontinued.

Potential Toxicities/Side Effects (More Severe with Higher Dosing) and the Nursing Process

I.   ALTERATION IN COMFORT related to FLU-LIKE SYNDROME

Defining Characteristics: Chills 3–6 hours after dose in 40–60% of patients; fever (74–98% of patients) with onset 30–90 minutes after chill, lasting up to 24 hours. Temperature 39–40°C (102–104°F); tachyphylaxis (decrease in severity/occurrence after successive treatments) common. Fatigue (89–95% of patients) and malaise are cumulative and dose-limiting. Headache, myalgias occur in 60–70% of patients, as well as arthralgias (5–24% of patients).

Nursing Implications: Assess baseline T, VS, neurologic status, and comfort level; monitor every 4–6 hours if patient is in hospital. Discuss with physician premedication and regular dosing of antipyretic (e.g., acetaminophen ± diphenhydramine, NSAID). Teach patient self-care measures, including monitoring T, comfort level, self-administration of prescribed medications prior to dose and regularly postdose, as well as the use of heat or cold for myalgias, arthralgias. Encourage patient to increase oral fluids and alternate rest and activity periods. If patient is in hospital and experiences rigor, discuss with physician IV meperidine (25 mg IV q 15 min to maximum 100 mg in 1 hour) and monitor blood pressure for hypotension. Teach patient to alternate rest and activity.

II. POTENTIAL FOR INFECTION AND BLEEDING related to NEUTROPENIA AND THROMBOCYTOPENIA

Defining Characteristics: Although uncommon, increased risk with increased dose; dose-limiting thrombocytopenia, reversible. Onset in 7–10 days, nadir in 14 days (may be delayed 20–40 days in patients with hairy-cell leukemia) and recovery at day 21.

Nursing Implications: Assess baseline CBC, white blood count, differential, and platelet count, and signs/symptoms of infection or bleeding. Discuss any abnormalities with physician before drug administration. Teach patient signs/symptoms of infection and bleeding, and to report them immediately. Teach patient self-care measures to minimize infection and bleeding, including avoidance of OTC aspirin-containing medications, and oral hygiene regimen.

III. ALTERATION IN NUTRITION, LESS THAN BODY REQUIREMENTS, related to NAUSEA, DIARRHEA, ANOREXIA

Defining Characteristics: Anorexia occurs (46–65% of patients) and is cumulative and dose-limiting. Nausea (32–51% of patients) is mild with tachyphylaxis after 1 week. Diarrhea (29–42% of patients) is mild, and vomiting is rare (10–17% of patients). Taste alterations and xerostomia may occur.

Nursing Implications: Assess baseline nutritional status. Teach patient potential side effects and self-care measures including oral hygiene. Encourage patient to prepare favorite high-calorie, high-protein foods ahead of time so able to snack when hungry. Teach self-administration of prescribed antiemetics and antidiarrheals as needed. Refer to dietitian as appropriate.

IV. SENSORY/PERCEPTUAL ALTERATION related to CNS EFFECTS

Defining Characteristics: Dizziness (21–41% of patients), confusion (8–10% of patients), decreased mental status (17% of patients), and depression (16% of patients). Somnolence, irritability, poor concentration, seizures, paranoia, hallucinations, psychoses may occur in 70% of patients but are reversible. Use drug cautiously in patients with history of seizures or CNS dysfunction.

Nursing Implications: Assess baseline mental status and neurologic status prior to drug administration. Assess patient for changes (impaired memory/attention, disorientation, slow/vague responses to questions, increased lethargy) during treatment. Instruct patient to report signs/symptoms; provide information and emotional support, as well as interventions to ensure safety if signs/symptoms occur.

V. POTENTIAL ALTERATION IN CARDIAC OUTPUT related to TACHYCARDIA, CHEST PAIN, DYSRHYTHMIAS

Defining Characteristics: Uncommon but dose-related with increased risk in elderly and patients with preexisting cardiac dysfunction: tachycardia, pallor, cyanosis, chest pain, orthostatic hypotension or hypertension arrhythmias, CHF, syncope.

Nursing Implications: Assess baseline cardiopulmonary status and risk (elderly, preexisting cardiac dysfunction). ECG testing is done baseline and during treatment for high-risk individuals. Monitor VS and I/O every 4 hours while receiving drug in hospital. Teach patient to report signs/symptoms of dyspnea, chest pain, edema, or other abnormalities immediately.

VI. POTENTIAL ALTERATION IN ELIMINATION related to RENAL AND HEPATIC DYSFUNCTION

Defining Characteristics: Dose-related increased BUN, creatinine, LFTs (increased AST in 42–46%) may occur, as well as proteinuria. Patient may develop interstitial nephritis.

Nursing Implications: Assess baseline renal and hepatic function studies and urinalysis prior to drug initiation, and periodically during therapy. Discuss abnormalities with physician.

VII. POTENTIAL FOR SEXUAL DYSFUNCTION related to IMPOTENCE, MENSTRUAL IRREGULARITIES

Defining Characteristics: Impotence and decreased libido, menstrual irregularities, and increased spontaneous abortions have occurred. Drug is excreted in breastmilk.

Nursing Implications: Assess patient's baseline sexual patterns and discuss potential alterations. Provide information, emotional support, and referral as appropriate and needed. Encourage patient to use contraceptive measures; mothers receiving the drug should not breastfeed.

VIII. POTENTIAL ALTERATION IN SKIN INTEGRITY related to RASH, PARTIAL ALOPECIA, DRYNESS

Defining Characteristics: Partial alopecia (8–22% of patients), rash (11–18% of patients), throat dryness (15% of patients), as well as skin dryness, flushing, pruritus, and irritation at injection site may occur.

Nursing Implications: Assess baseline skin integrity. Instruct patient to report signs/ symptoms. Discuss/teach symptomatic management, including the use of mild soaps and rinsing skin thoroughly after bathing. Encourage patient to use alcohol-free, oil-based moisturizers on skin.

IX. KNOWLEDGE DEFICIT related to SELF-ADMINISTRATION TECHNIQUE

Defining Characteristics: Often patients must receive daily dosing or thrice weekly dosing in the home setting by subcutaneous injection, and they are unfamiliar with technique.

Nursing Implications: Assess baseline psychomotor ability, knowledge, and willingness to learn technique of self-injection. Teach how to prepare drug, self-administer, and safely collect used syringes for proper disposal. Use written and video materials as supplements to teaching process and have patient correctly demonstrate technique prior to performing at home. Make referral to visiting-nurse agency to reinforce teaching.

Drug: interferon gamma-1b (Actimmune®, IFN-gamma [γ], rIFN-gamma)

Class: Cytokine (Interferon).

Mechanism of Action: Actimmune is interferon gamma-1b. It has antiviral, antiprolifera-tive, and immunomodulatory effects. Activates phagocytes and appears to generate toxic oxidative metabolites in phagocytes; interacts with interleukins to orchestrate immune effect, and enhances antibody-dependent cellular cytotoxicity, NK activity, and mounting of antigen on monocytes (Fc expression).

Metabolism: Slowly absorbed following subcutaneous or IM injection, with 89% bioavailability. Peaks in 4–13 hours following IM injection, and 6–7 hours after subcutaneous injection. Elimination half-lives for IV injection are 30–60 minutes, and 2–8 hours for IM or subcutaneous injection. Renal filtration and tubular reabsorption as catabolites; minor hepatic metabolism and biliary excretion.

Indication: (1) For reducing the frequency and severity of serious infections associated with Chronic Granulomatous Disease (CGD), and (2) delaying time to disease progression in patients with severe, malignant osteopetrosis (SMO).

Contraindications: Patients with known or developed hypersensitivity to interferon-gamma, *E. coli*–derived products, or any product components.

Dosage/Range:
- CGD and SMO:
  - BSA > 0.5 m^2: 50 mcg/m^2 (1 million international units/m^2) SQ 3 times a week (e.g., M, W, F).
  - BSA ≤ 0.5 m^2: 1.5 mcg/kg/dose SQ 3 times a week.
  - Dose modification: dose-reduce 50% for severe adverse reactions, or interrupt dose until reaction abates.

- Safety and efficacy of doses higher or lower than those recommended (50 mcg/m^2) have not been studied.

Drug Preparation:
- May use either sterilized glass or plastic disposable syringes.
- Drug is clear, colorless in a single-use vial for subcutaneous injection. Each 0.5 mL of Actimmune contains 100 mcg (2 million international units). It is available as a single vial or in cartons of 12.
- Vials should be stored in a refrigerator at 2–8°C (36–46°F) immediately upon receipt. DO NOT FREEZE. Avoid vigorous shaking. An unentered vial of Actimmune should not be left at room temperature for a total time > 12 hours prior to use; if it is left out for > 12 hours, it should be discarded.

Drug Administration:
- Prior to the beginning of therapy, in addition to indicated tests for each diagnosis, the following tests should be assessed baseline and every 3 months while on therapy:
  - CBC/differential/platelet count
  - Blood chemistries (including renal, LFTs); in patients < 1 year of age, LFTs should be assessed monthly
  - Urinalysis
- Available as 100 mcg (2 million International Units) per 0.5 mL solution in a single-use vial. Solution is sterile and should be clear and colorless. Inspect before drawing up.
- Administer SQ in the right or left deltoid or anterior thigh. Can be administered using either sterilized glass or plastic disposable syringes. Do not mix other drugs in the same syringe.
- As appropriate, teach patient or caregiver SQ technique and drawing up medication, aseptic technique, safe handling, and disposal of hazardous waste. Set up home delivery of medication, syringes, and alcohol wipes as well as hazardous waste needle disposal container.

Drug Interactions:
- Concomitant use of drugs with neurotoxic, hematotoxic, or cardiotoxic effects may increase the toxicity of interferons.
- Avoid simultaneous administration of interferon gamma with other heterologous serum proteins or immunological preparations (e.g., vaccines).
- May decrease elimination of aminophylline by 33–81% via inhibition of cytochrome P450 enzyme system.
- Increased effects of CNS depressants.
- Increased bone marrow suppressant effects with zidovudine (AZT), other bone marrow suppressive agents.

Lab Effects/Interference:
- Dose-dependent, leukopenia; elevated liver serum transaminases.
- Increased serum creatinine, BUN, proteinuria.

Special Considerations:
- Most common adverse reactions (≥2%) include fever, headache, rash, chills, injection site erythema or tenderness, fatigue, and diarrhea.

- Warnings and Precautions:
  - *Cardiovascular disorders:* Acute and transient flu-like syndrome (fever, chills) may exacerbate preexisting cardiac problems. Use drug cautiously in patients with ischemia, CHF, or arrhythmia.
  - *Neurologic disorders:* Abnormal neurological symptoms may occur but are reversible soon after drug discontinuation. Most are mild and include decreased mental status, gait disturbance, dizziness. Use drug cautiously in patients with a history of seizures.
  - *Bone marrow toxicity:* Reversible neutropenia and thrombocytopenia may occur and be severe, especially when given in combination with other potentially myelosuppressive agents. Monitor patient blood counts closely.
  - *Hepatic toxicity:* May occur with elevations of AST and/or ALT (up to 25-fold). This occurs more often in children younger than 1 year, compared to older children; these children should have monthly LFT assessment. Elevated values are reversible with dose reduction or drug interruption. If hepatic toxicity occurs, reduce dose or discontinue to reverse severe AST and ALT elevations; monitor LFTs monthly in patients <1 year old. Patients with advanced hepatic disease receiving repeated dosing may accumulate drug; frequent monitoring of LFTs is recommended.
  - *Renal toxicity:* monitor renal function regularly when giving interferon gamma, in patients with severe renal insufficiency as drug accumulation may occur.
  - *HSTs:* Acute serious HSRs may occur; if so, discontinue the drug immediately and provide appropriate medical intervention as ordered. Transient cutaneous rash has occurred requiring treatment interruption.
  - *Allergic reactions to natural rubber:* vial stopper contains natural rubber, a derivative of latex. Use caution if patient has a latex allergy.
  - Drug should be used during pregnancy only if the potential benefit justifies the potential risk to the fetus.
  - Nursing mothers should make a decision to discontinue nursing or to discontinue the drug, taking into consideration the importance of the drug to the mother's health.

Potential Toxicities/Side Effects (More Severe with Higher Dosing) and the Nursing Process

I.   ALTERATION IN COMFORT related to FLU-LIKE SYNDROME

Defining Characteristics: Chills 3–6 hours after dose in 14% of patients; fever (52% of patients), with onset 30–90 minutes after chill. Tachyphylaxis (decrease in severity/occurrence after successive treatments) common. Fatigue (14% of patients) and myalgia (6%) can occur. Headache occurs in 33% of patients.

Nursing Implications: Assess baseline T, VS, neurologic status, and comfort level; monitor every 4–6 hours if patient is in hospital. Discuss with physician premedication and regular dosing of antipyretic (e.g., acetaminophen ± diphenhydramine, NSAID). Teach patient self-care measures, including monitoring temperature, comfort level, self-administration of prescribed medications prior to dose and regularly postdose, as well as the use of heat or cold for myalgias, arthralgias. Encourage patient to increase oral fluids and alternate rest and activity periods. If patient is in hospital and experiences rigor, discuss with physician

IV meperidine (25 mg IV q 15 min to maximum 100 mg in 1 hour) and monitor blood pressure for hypotension. Teach patient to alternate rest and activity.

II.   POTENTIAL FOR INFECTION AND BLEEDING related to NEUTROPENIA AND THROMBOCYTOPENIA

Defining Characteristics: Although uncommon, increased risk with increased dose; dose-limiting thrombocytopenia; reversible.

Nursing Implications: Assess baseline CBC, white blood count, differential, and platelet count, and signs/symptoms of infection or bleeding. Discuss any abnormalities with physician before drug administration. Teach patient signs/symptoms of infection and bleeding, and to report them immediately. Teach patient self-care measures to minimize infection and bleeding, including avoidance of OTC aspirin-containing medications, and oral hygiene regimen.

III.   ALTERATION IN NUTRITION, LESS THAN BODY REQUIREMENTS, related to NAUSEA, DIARRHEA

Defining Characteristics: Nausea (10% of patients) is mild with tachyphylaxis after 1 week. Diarrhea (14% of patients) is mild, and vomiting is rare (13% of patients).

Nursing Implications: Assess baseline nutritional status. Teach patient potential side effects and self-care measures, including oral hygiene. Encourage patient to prepare favorite high-calorie, high-protein foods ahead of time so able to snack when hungry. Teach self-administration of prescribed antiemetics and antidiarrheals as needed. Refer to dietitian as appropriate.

IV.   KNOWLEDGE DEFICIT related to SELF-ADMINISTRATION TECHNIQUE

Defining Characteristics: Often patients must receive daily dosing or thrice weekly dosing in the home setting by subcutaneous injection, and they are unfamiliar with technique.

Nursing Implications: Assess baseline psychomotor ability, knowledge, and willingness to learn technique of self-injection. Teach how to prepare drug, self-administer, and safely collect used syringes for proper disposal. Use written and video materials as supplements to teaching process, and have patient correctly demonstrate technique prior to performing at home. Make referral to visiting-nurse agency to reinforce teaching.

Drug: ipilimumab (Yervoy)

Class: Immune checkpoint inhibitor. Human cytotoxic T-lymphocyte antigen-4 (CTLA-4) blocking antibody; IgG1 human mAb.

Mechanism of Action: Ipilimumab is a negative regulator of T-cell activation. CTLA-4 is an antigen that is expressed on human activated T-lymphocytes that is important in regulating the body's immune response; it has an affinity for B7 costimulatory molecules, which determine how the T-lymphocyte will interact with APCs. T-lymphocytes are important in immune surveillance to distinguish between self and nonself-antigens. CTLA-4 down-regulates (turns off) T-lymphocytes after the invading antigen has been removed so that the immune system does not injure normal tissue. Ipilimumab is a fully human mAb that binds to CTLA-4 and blocks its interaction with ligands CD80/CD86. This augments T-cell activation and proliferation. Ipilimumab's effect on malignant melanoma cells is indirect, probably via T-cell mediated antitumor activity.

Metabolism: When given IV every 3 weeks, steady state is achieved after the third dose. The terminal half-life is 14.7 days. Systemic clearance was increased with increasing body weight, but this did not require dose adjustments. Patients with renal or hepatic impairment did not require dose adjustments. Lab testing of pregnant animals showed that there was a higher incidence of abortion, stillbirth, premature delivery, and infant mortality when given in the third trimester.

Indication: Treatment of patients with (1) malignant melanoma: (a) unresectable or meta-static melanoma, in adults and pediatric (aged 12 years or older); (b) adjuvant treatment of cutaneous melanoma with pathologic involvement of regional lymph nodes of > 1 mm who have undergone complete resection, including total lymphadenectomy; (2) advanced renal cell carcinoma (RCC) with intermediate or poor risk, previously untreated advanced renal cell carcinoma (RCC), in combination with nivolumab; (3) microsatellite instability-hgh (MSI-H) or mismatch repair deficient (dMMR) metastatic CRC (mCRC) in adult and pediatric (aged 12 years or older) patients which has progressed after treatment with a fluoropyrimidine, oxaliplatin, and irinotecan, in combination with nivolumab (accelerated approval).

Contraindications: none.

Dosage/Range:
- *Unresectable or Metastatic Melanoma:* 3 mg/kg IV infusion over 90 minutes, every 3 weeks × 4 doses. Treatment delays may occur, but all treatment must be administered within 16 weeks of the first dose.
- *Adjuvant Treatment Melanoma:* 10 mg/kg IV over 90 minutes every 3 weeks for 4 doses, followed by 10 mg/kg every 12 weeks for up to 3 years. In the event of toxicity, doses are omitted not delayed.
- *Advanced RCC:* Nivolumab 3 mg/kg IV over 30 minutes, followed by ipilimumab 1 mg/kg IV over 30 minutes on the same day, every 3 weeks for a maximum of 4 doses. Then after completing the combination for 4 doses, give nivolumab as a single agent, either 240 mg every 2 weeks or 480 mg every 4 weeks, administered IV over 30 minutes until disease progression or unacceptable toxicity. Use separate infusion bags and filters for each infusion when given in combination.
- *mCRC:* Ipilimumab 1 mg/kg IV infusion over 30 minutes, immediately following nivolumab administered on the same day, every 3 weeks for up to × 4 doses or until unacceptable toxicity or disease progression. See nivolumab prescribing information.
- Permanently discontinue for severe adverse reactions.

Dose Modifications for Immune Mediated Adverse Reactions:
- Endocrine: (1) symptomatic endocrinopathy: hold ipilimumab; resume in patients with complete or partial resolution of adverse reaction (grades 0–1) and who are receiving < 7.5 mg prednisone or equivalent per day; (2) symptomatic reactions lasting 6 weeks or longer, inability to reduce corticosteroid dose to 7.5 mg prednisone or equivalent per day: permanently discontinue ipilimumab.
- Ophthalmologic: Grades 2 through 4 reactions not improving to grade 1 within 2 weeks while receiving topical therapy or requiring systemic therapy: permanently discontinue ipilimumab.
- All other: (1) Grade 2: hold ipilimumab, resume in patients with complete or partial resolution of adverse reactions (grades 0–1) and who are receiving < 7.5 mg prednisone or equivalent per day. (2) Grade 2 reactions lasting > 6 weeks or longer, inability to reduce corticosteroid dose to < 7.5 mg prednisone or equivalent per day, or grades 3–4: permanently discontinue ipilimumab.
- Drug should be permanently discontinued for any of the following:
  - Persistent moderate adverse reactions or inability to reduce corticosteroid to 7.5 mg prednisone or equivalent per day.
  - Failure to complete full treatment in 16 weeks from administration of first dose of patients with metastatic melanoma
  - Severe adverse reactions or life-threatening adverse reactions, including any of the following:
  - Colitis with abdominal pain, fever, ileus, peritoneal signs, 7 or more stools per day over baseline, stool incontinence, need for IV hydration > 24 hours, GI hemorrhage, or GI perforation.
  - Significantly abnormal LFTs: AST or ALT > 5 times ULN, or total bilirubin > 3 times ULN.
  - SJS, TEN, or rash complicated by full thickness dermal ulceration, or necrotic bullous or hemorrhagic manifestations.
  - Severe motor or sensory neuropathy, Guillain–Barré syndrome, or myasthenia gravis.
  - Severe immune-mediated reactions involving any organ system (e.g., nephritis, pneumonitis, pancreatitis, noninfectious myocarditis); institute systemic high-dose corticosteroid therapy.
  - Immune-mediated ocular disease that is unresponsive to topical immunosuppressive therapy.

Drug Preparation:
- Available in 50-mg/10-mL (5-mg/mL) and 200-mg/40-mL (5-mg/mL) vials.
- Allow drug vial to come to room temperature over 5 minutes prior to mixing. Inspect and discard if any particulate matter or discoloration is found.
- Withdraw the ordered amount and aseptically add to either 0.9% sodium chloride injection USP or 5% dextrose injection, USP to create a final concentration of 1–2 mg/mL.
- Mix solution by gently inverting bag. Do not shake.
- Drug may be stored under refrigeration (2–8°C, 36–46°F) or at room temperature (20–25°C, 68–77°F) for ≤ 24 hours.

Drug Administration:
- Assess LFTs, TFTs, and clinical chemistries prior to each dose. Assess for immune-related AEs (irAEs) from prior dosing.
- Administer IV over 90 minutes via sterile, nonpyrogenic, low-protein binding in-line filter (e.g., 0.22 micron). Flush IV line with 0.9% sodium chloride injection USP or 5% dextrose injection, USP after administration to ensure all drug is administered. Do not mix ipilimumab with any other medicines (with or as an infusion with).
- IV infusion may be associated with infusion reactions, such as chest pain, flushed/red face, and back pain. Stop infusion and assess response. Administer ordered antihistamines (H1 and H2) and corticosteroid.
- When given in combination with nivolumab,, infuse nivolumab first, followed by ipilimumab on the same day, each over 30 minutes IV. Use separate infusion bags and filters for each drug. See specific information for nivolumab (Opdivo) for toxicity and administration.

Drug Interactions:
- Vemurafenib: concurrent administration has resulted in increased grade 3 rise in transaminases, with or without increased bilirubin.

Lab Effects/Interference:
- Elevated LFTs (must distinguish between liver metastases and immune hepatitis).
- Alterations in cortisol, ACTH, testosterone, TSH, free T4 levels.

Special Considerations:
- Increased T-lymphocyte activation, proliferation and resulting inflammation are responsible for the major immune-related toxicities: dermatitis, enterocolitis, and hypophysitis (rare). Rarely, inflammation of the eyes (uveitis), pituitary, thyroid, kidneys (nephritis), lungs (alveolitis), adrenal glands can occur, as can aseptic meningitis and arthritis. Grades 3–4 events are largely reversible with high-dose steroids therapy (Weber, 2007).
- Warnings and Precautions:
  - *Severe irAEs:* Permanently discontinue drug.
  - *Moderate IRs:* Hold dose for moderate immune-mediated adverse effects until return to baseline, improvement to mild severity, or complete resolution, and patient is receiving < 7.5 mg prednisone or equivalent per day. Administer high-dose corticosteroids for severe, persistent, or recurring immune-mediated reactions.
  - *Assess patient at each visit for signs and symptoms of toxicity.*
    - **Immune-mediated enterocolitis:** Incidence in patients receiving ipilimumab alone was 32%, while in combination with nivolumab was 7–10%. Median time to onset in combination patients was 1.7–2.4 months. Monitor patient for signs/symptoms of enterocolitis (e.g., diarrhea, abdominal pain, mucus or blood in stool, fever) as well as of bowel perforation (e.g., peritoneal signs, ileus). Rule out other possible causes and consider endoscopy for persistent or severe problems. Hold drug for moderate enterocolitis, administer antidiarrheal medications, and if persistent for >1 week, start systemic corticosteroids. Permanently discontinue drug for severe enterocolitis and start systemic corticosteroids; upon improvement

to grades 0–1, begin taper over at least 1 month. If enterocolitis is unresponsive to corticosteroids within 3–5 days, or recurring after symptom improvement, discuss with physician adding anti-TNF or other immunosuppressant agent. When combined with nivolumab for the treatment of RCC, incidence was 10%. Most patients responded to corticosteroids but some required further immunosuppression with infliximab. See Nursing Implications.

- **Immune-mediated hepatitis:** Evaluate LFTs and assess patient for signs/symptoms of hepatitis, before each dose of ipilimumab. If hepatitis occurs, rule out infectious or malignant causes, and increase frequency of LFTs monitoring until resolution. Hold ipilimumab for grade 2 hepatotoxicity. Permanently discontinue ipilimumab if grades 3–4 hepatotoxicity occurs, and administer corticosteroids; when LFTs improve to baseline, start corticosteroid taper over 1 month. If hepatitis persists despite high-dose corticosteroids, discuss with physician administering mycophenolate treatment. When combined with nivolumab, incidence was 7%.

- **Immune-mediated dermatitis:** Monitor for signs/symptoms of dermatitis (e.g., rash, pruritis), and consider immune-related unless other cause found. Permanently discontinue in patients with SJS, TEN, or rash complicated by full thickness dermal ulceration, or necrotic, bullous, or hemorrhagic manifestations. Give systemic corticosteroids as ordered, and when dermatitis is controlled, taper over at least 1 month. Hold ipilimumab in patients with moderate or severe signs and symptoms.

- **Immune-mediated neuropathies:** Monitor for signs/symptoms of motor or sensory neuropathy (e.g., unilateral or bilateral weakness, sensory alterations, or paresthesias). Hold ipilimumab for moderate neuropathy (not interfering with daily activities). Permanently discontinue ipilimumab if severe neuropathy develops (interferes with ADLs). Implement ordered medical management for severe neuropathy; discuss administration of systemic corticosteroids.

- **Immune-mediated endocrinopathies:** Monitor TFT, adrenocorticotropic hormone (ACTH) level, and clinical chemistries baseline, prior to each dose, and as clinically indicated. Evaluate at each visit for signs/symptoms of endocrinopathy (e.g., hypophysitis, adrenal insufficiency/adrenal crisis, hyper- or hypothyroidism); be alert for signs/symptoms: fatigue, headache, changes in mental status, abdominal pain, unusual bowel habits, hypotension) and discuss need for replacement hormone(s) as needed with physician or midlevel practitioner. Hold ipilimumab if patient is symptomatic, consider endocrine consult, and start systemic corticosteroids as ordered.

- **Infusion reactions (IRs):** Incidence 4.2-5.1% of patients. Severe reactions can occur with nivolumab and ipilimumab. Interrupt or slow the rate of infusion in patients with mild or moderate IRs. Permanently discontinue ipilimumab in patients with severe or life-threatening IRs.

- **Other immune-mediated adverse reactions (irAEs) including ocular:** Ocular toxicity may include blurred vision and reduced visual acuity, and may be associated with retinal detachment or permanent visual loss. Rarely, in combination trials, patients developed myocarditis, rhabdomyolysis, myositis, pericarditis and other reactions. Permanently discontinue ipilimumab for clinically significant or severe irAEs; administer ordered systemic corticosteroids, tapering over at least 1 month when toxicity resolves to grade 1 or less. Administer and teach patient self-administration of corticosteroid eye drops for uveitis, iritis, or episcleritis; if unresponsive to local immunosuppressive treatment, ipilimumab should be permanently discontinued.

- **Embryo-fetal toxicity**: Toxic effect greatest in second and third trimester of pregnancy. Teach female patients of reproductive potential to use effective contraception during treatment and for 3 months after last dose.

- Patient education medication guide is available at http://packageinserts.bms.com/ medguide /medguide_yervoy.pdf.

- May take up to 3 months after drug is stopped to see a response. Patients may have short-term progression followed by delayed regression with a prolonged duration of clinical response or stable disease (Weber, 2007; Weber et al., 2015).

- Nursing mothers should decide whether to discontinue nursing or to discontinue the drug, taking into account the importance of the drug to the mother's health. IgG1 is known to cross the placental barrier, and it is not known if the drug is excreted in human milk.

- Patients should be given a wallet card stating the patient is receiving ipilimumab so that if the patient needs to go to the emergency room, physicians there will know that the patient may be experiencing immune-mediated side effects.

Potential Toxicities/Side Effects and the Nursing Process (see chapter introduction for additional information)

I.   ALTERATION IN ELIMINATION, POTENTIAL, related to DIARRHEA, ENTEROCOLITIS

Defining Characteristics: In initial clinical trials for patients with metastatic melanoma: Incidence of diarrhea is 32% with 7% grades 3–5; colitis affected 8% of patients, with 5% being grades 3–5. Uncontrolled diarrhea may progress to enterocolitis. Rarely, enterocolitis can result in bowel perforation. In the drug studies ($n = 511$), 1% developed intestinal perforation, 0.8% died as a result of complications, and 5% of patients were hospitalized for severe enterocolitis. The median time to onset of grade 2 enterocolitis was 6.3 weeks (range 0.3–18.9 weeks), and to grades 3–5 severe enterocolitis was 7.4 weeks (range 1.6–13.4 weeks). Eighty-five percent of patients with grades 3–5 enterocolitis were treated with high-dose corticosteroids ($\geq$ 40 mg prednisone equivalent per day), with a median dose of 80 mg/day for a median duration of treatment of 2.3 weeks (ranging up to 13.9 weeks), followed by a corticosteroid taper. For patients studied who had moderate grade 2 enterocolitis, 46% were not treated with high-dose corticosteroids, 29% were treated with < 40 mg prednisone/equivalent/day for a median duration of 5.1 weeks. Twenty-five percent were treated with high-dose corticosteroids for a median duration of 10 days prior to taper. Infliximab was administered to 8% of patients with moderate, severe, or life-threatening immune-mediated enterocolitis if the patient did not have an adequate response to high-dose corticosteroids. In most patients, symptoms resolved. O'Day et al. (2011) tested a GI management protocol and found that if followed, there was resolution of diarrhea/colitis during ipilimumab treatment: Grade 1 diarrhea: Treat symptomatically without immunosuppressives, unless diarrhea continued for more than 5 days; grade 2: Treat symptomatically, and if persists for 3–5 days or worsens, treat with corticosteroids; grade 3 or higher: Treat with systemic high-dose corticosteroids. Median time to resolution to a lower grade was 1 week, and median time to resolution was 2 weeks.

For patients receiving ipilimumab for **adjuvant treatment**, 16% of patients developed grades 3–5 immune-related enterocolitis, and grade 2 enterocolitis occurred in 14%. Intestinal perforation occurred in 1.5% and 0.6% patients died from complications. Median time to onset for grades 3–4 enterocolitis was 1.1 months (range 1 day–20.6 months). Ninety-five percent of patients with grades 3–4 enterocolitis were treated with systemic corticosteroids (median duration of treatment was 4.7 months). Most patients with moderate enterocolitis (75%) were treated with systemic corticosteroids, median duration of treatment 3.5 months. Noncorticosteroid immunosuppression (infliximab) was used to treat 36% of patients with grades 3–4 and 15% of patients with a grade 2 event. Most patients with grades 3–4 (86%) experienced complete resolution to grade 1, and 11% did not improve. Complete resolution in patients with grade 2 enterocolitis occurred in 94% of patients, 3% improvement to grade 1, and 3% no improvement.

Nursing Interventions: Assess patient's baseline bowel elimination status, and history of bowel dysfunction, such as colitis. Ask about any changes in normal bowel habits or changes from baseline, or last visit: diarrhea, abdominal pain, blood or mucus in stool with/without fever, peritoneal signs consistent with bowel perforation, ileus. In symptomatic patients, rule out infectious etiologies and consider endoscopic evaluation for persistent or severe symptoms. Teach patient that diarrhea may occur, to report diarrhea > 4 stools over baseline/day, loose stools, and blood or mucus in the stool. Review the patient's medication profile to identify any bowel medications, and to teach patient to avoid stool softeners and laxatives. Teach patient to take loperamide (or recommended antidiarrheal medication) after the first loose stool if it occurs, and to report right away if diarrhea does not resolve in 24 hours, or if the patient has nausea and/or vomiting and cannot take fluids. MODERATE diarrhea or enterocolitis is defined as diarrhea up to 4–6 stools over baseline/24 hours, abdominal pain, mucus, or blood in stool (grade 1 is < 4 stools over baseline, grade 2 is 4–6 stools over baseline ± abdominal pain, mucus or blood in stool). Ipilipimab should be withheld for moderate enterocolitis. Antidiarrheals such as loperamide are used, and the stool tested to ensure another cause is not ignored. Ipilimumab is resumed if symptoms have improved to mild (< 4 stools/day) or resolved completely. If symptoms continue for more than 1 week, expect systemic corticosteroids (e.g., 0.5 mg/kg/day prednisone/equivalent) to be started and continued until improvement or resolution. The corticosteroids should be tapered. Ipilimumab can be resumed when symptoms have improved to at least mild severity and the steroid dose is 7.5 mg prednisone or equivalent, or less. SEVERE, life-threatening, or fatal immune-mediated enterocolitis (grades 3–5) is defined as having diarrhea (7 or more stools over baseline/24 hours), fever, ileus, peritoneal signs. Bowel perforation must be ruled out, and if present, corticosteroids are not started. Expect endoscopy and colonoscopy to be performed, with biopsies, for a definitive diagnosis. If enterocolitis is found, high-dose IV corticosteroids (1–2 mg/kg/day of prednisone or equivalent) are initiated. Once symptoms have resolved, patient should resume nutrition with a progressive low-fat, low-fiber diet. IV corticosteroids can be converted to oral, and the patient discharged home on an oral steroid. The corticosteroid taper should be done over at least 1 month (Weber, 2007). If symptoms do not resolve, the patient should be continually evaluated for evidence of gastrointestinal perforation or peritonitis. Repeat endoscopy should be considered, as should alternative immunosuppressive therapy. If the patient is refractory to high-dose parenteral steroids (e.g., unresponsive within 3–5 days, or recurring after symptom improvement), consider adding an anti-TNF or other immunosuppressant agents (e.g., infliximab [Remicade], a chimeric MAb targeting TNF-a, as a single dose may be prescribed [Beck et al., 2006]). This requires TB testing, as it can reactivate dormant TB. Teach patient to go to the ED or call 911 if severe abdominal pain, with or without vomiting and constipation, occurs, as the patient needs to be evaluated for bowel perforation right away, although this is a rare event. If bowel perforation occurs, anticipate and prepare patient for immediate surgical intervention. Teach patient not to take any OTC medications or dietary supplements until discussing it first with nurse or physician.

II.   ALTERATION IN SKIN INTEGRITY, POTENTIAL, related to DERMATITIS

Defining Characteristics: Dermatitis is a common side effect, often associated with pruritus. Biopsy may show T-lymphocyte infiltrates. In clinical studies, pruritus occurred in 31% of patients, and rash in 29% of patients (2% severe grades 3–5). Severe (grades 3–5) dermatitis appeared in 2.5% of all study patients (e.g., as SJS, TEN, or rash complicated by full thickness dermal ulceration, or necrotic, bullous, or hemorrhagic manifestations). One patient died of TEN. Twelve percent of patients had moderate (grade 2) dermatitis. Median time to onset of moderate, severe, or life-threatening dermatitis was 3.1 weeks (range up to 17.3 weeks from initiation of ipilimumab). Fifty-four percent of patients with severe dermatitis received high-dose corticosteroids (median dose 60 mg of prednisone/equivalent) for a median of 14.9 weeks followed by steroid taper. Time to resolution ranged up to 15.6 weeks. Less than half of the patients with moderate dermatitis received high-dose corticosteroids (median dose 60 mg/day prednisone/equivalent), for a median of 2.1 weeks. Eleven percent were treated with topical corticosteroids only, while 49% had neither topic nor systemic steroids. Seventy percent of patients had complete resolution of symptoms, 11% improved to grade 1, and 19% had no improvement.

Patients receiving adjuvant ipilimumab had an incidence of 4% immune-related dermatitis. Median time for onset of grades 3–4 was 14 days, and for grade 2 was 11 days. Eighty-four percent of patients with grades 3–4 dermatitis received systemic corticosteroids for a median of 21 days, resulting in complete resolution in a median time of 4.3 months. However, of the 16% of patients not treated with systemic or topical corticosteroids, 11% had complete resolution and 1 had improvement to grade 1.

Nursing Interventions: Assess baseline skin integrity and presence of abnormalities, and monitor during therapy. Teach patient that dermatitis may occur. Moderate dermatitis is defined as diffuse, covering 50% or less of skin surface. If this occurs, ipilimumab dose is held, and topical or systemic corticosteroids administered if there is no improvement of symptoms within 1 week. If symptoms resolve or improve to mild (localized) symptoms, and systemic steroid dose is 7.5 mg prednisone equivalent or less, ipilimumab can be resumed. Severe or life threatening dermatitis is defined as SJS, TEN, or rash complicated by full thickness dermal ulceration, or necrotic, bullous, or hemorrhagic manifestations. Ipilimumab must be permanently discontinued, and high-dose corticosteroids (1–2 mg/kg/day) started immediately. When the dermatitis is controlled, the corticosteroid should be tapered over at least 1 month. Other symptom management agents that may be used are antipruritic medications such as diphenhydramine and hydroxyzine.

III.   ALTERATION IN NUTRITION related to IMMUNE HEPATITIS

Defining Characteristics: Uncommon, but may occur characterized by increasing LFTs. Rarely, severe, and fatal liver inflammation can occur. In patients receiving adjuvant ipilimumab, grades 3–4 hepatitis occurred in 11% and moderate grade 2 occurred in 5%. Liver biopsy performed in 6 patients with grades 3–4 showed toxic or autoimmune hepatitis. Median time to onset for grades 3–4 was 2 months (range 1 day to 4.2 months), and for grade 2 hepatitis was 1.4 months Most (94%) of patients with grades 3–4 experienced complete resolution, 4% improvement to grade 1, and 2% no improvement. Resolution in patients with grade 2 occurred in 91% patients, while 9% did not improve. Most (90%) of patients with grades 3–4 hepatitis were treated with systemic corticosteroids for a median duration of 4.4 months. Three-quarters (73%) of patients with moderate hepatitis were treated with systemic corticosteroids for a median duration of 2.6 months. If vemurafenib was given concurrently, grade 3 increases in transaminases with or without increases in bilirubin, occurred in 60% of patients.

Nursing Interventions: Assess LFTs and signs and symptoms of hepatitis baseline and prior to each drug dose. If increasing LFTs (AST, ALT, total bilirubin), check labs every 3 days until stable or decreasing and then weekly per physician's order. Hold drug if moderate elevation in LFTs (AST or ALT > 2.5 times but 1.5 times but 5 times ULN, total bilirubin > 3 times ULN), or failure to complete full treatment course within 16 weeks from administration of first dose. Anticipate that the physician will rule out any infectious or malignant cause. If LFTs continue to rise and immune hepatitis suspected, systemic high-dose corticosteroids (1–2 mg/kg/day prednisone equivalent) should be started, with increased frequency of LFT monitoring until resolution. Once LFTs show sustained improvement or resolve to baseline, the corticosteroid dose should be tapered over at least 1 month. If symptoms do not resolve, consider alternative immunosuppressive therapy, such as mycophenolate mofetil, tacrolimus, or infliximab (Weber, 2007).

IV.   POTENTIAL FOR SENSORY/PERCEPTUAL ALTERATIONS related to NEUROPATHY, GUILLAIN–BARRE SYNDROME, MYASTHENIA GRAVIS

Defining Characteristics: Neurological side effects are rare. A number of cases of Guillain–Barré, one fatal, one case of severe (grade 3) peripheral motor neuropathy, and a case of myasthenia gravis have been reported. In the adjuvant trial, 2% of patients experienced grades 3–5 immune-related neuropathy, and moderate grade 2 neuropathy occurred in 0.2%. Time to onset ranged from 1.4–27.4 months. Patients with grades 3–4 neuropathy were treated with systemic corticosteroids (range 3 days–38.3 months) and 3 patients also received tacrolimus.

Nursing Interventions: Assess baseline neurological status, and symptoms of motor or sensory neuropathy, such as unilateral or bilateral weakness, sensory alterations, or paresthesias, and monitor for these, as well as patient's ability to perform ADLs prior to each dose. Teach patient to report any changes in sensation, perception, or in ability to perform ADLs. Ipilimumab should be held for moderate neuropathy (not interfering with ADLs) but must be permanently discontinued when peripheral neuropathy becomes severe (patient cannot perform ADLs). The drug should also be discontinued if new onset or worsening of severe motor or sensory neuropathy, Guillain–Barré syndrome or myasthenia gravis or failure to complete the full treatment course within 16 weeks from date of first dose. Anticipate that medications appropriate to the type of neurological condition will be instituted; high-dose corticosteroid therapy (1–2 mg/kg/day prednisone/equivalent) should also be considered.

V. ALTERATION IN BODY FUNCTION AND METABOLISM related to IMMUNE-MEDIATED ENDOCRINOPATHIES, e.g., HYPOPHYSITIS (inflammation leading to hypopituitarism)

Defining Characteristics: Uncommon but significant because symptoms are vague initially (e.g., fatigue, headaches, low TSH, and serum cortisol levels), and if untreated, dysfunction of the hypophysis (such as pituitary enlargement) is far-reaching (e.g., severe headaches, severe fatigue, memory loss, loss of libido) (Weber et al., 2015). In clinical studies, 1.8% of patients developed grades 3–4 immune-mediated endocrinopathy (requiring hospitalization, urgent medical interventions, or interfering with patient's ability to perform ADLs). Patients all had hypopituitarism; in addition, some had adrenal insufficiency, hypogonadism, and hypothyroidism; 2.3% of patients had moderate endocrinopathy requiring hormone replacement or medical intervention (grade 2), and conditions included hypothyroidism, adrenal insufficiency, hypopituitarism; one patient had hyperthyroidism, and one had Cushing's syndrome. Median time to onset for moderate to severe immune-mediated endocrinopathy was 11 weeks, with a range up to 19.3 weeks after the first ipilimumab dose.

In the adjuvant trial, grades 3–4 immune-related endocrinopathies occurred in 8% of patients, most commonly hypopituitarism, and 20% had grade 2 endocrinopathies. Median time to onset for grades 3–4 was 2.2 months, while median time to grade 2 was 2.1 months.

Nursing Interventions: Monitor TST and clinical chemistries baseline and prior to each ipilimumab dose. Assess baseline activity and comfort levels and at each visit. Teach patient to report onset of worsening fatigue, headaches, changes in mental status, abdominal pain, unusual bowel habits, dizziness (hypotension), or new onset nonspecific symptoms. If hypophysitis is suspected, discuss evaluation with physician or NP/PA: MRI to compare size of pituitary baseline, cortisol, ACTH, TSH, and free T4 levels. If the diagnosis of hypophysitis is confirmed, teach patient about and administer ordered high-dose steroids and hormonal replacement as needed (e.g., thyroid hormone, testosterone for male patients). Expect that most patients will continue on low-dose hydrocortisone to protect the pituitary gland (Blansfield et al., 2005). Ipilimumab should be held for moderate immune-mediated reactions or any symptomatic endocrinopathy until complete resolution or the patient is stable on hormone replacement therapy. Some patients require systemic corticosteroids (1–2 mg/kg/day prednisone/equivalent, as well as hormone-replacement therapy. Ipilimumab should be permanently discontinued if unable to reduce corticosteroid dose to 7.5 mg prednisone/equivalent/day, or failure to complete full treatment course in 16 weeks from first ipilimumab dose.

Drug: lenalidomide (Revlimid)

Class: Immunomodulator with antiangiogenic and antineoplastic properties; thalidomide analogue.

Mechanism of Action: Drug is an analogue of thalidomide with immunomodulatory, antiangiogenic, and antineoplastic properties. Drug inhibits proliferation and induces apoptosis of some hematopoietic tumor cells, including MM, MCL, and del (5q) MDS cells. Drug modulates the immune system (is immunomodulatory) by activating T-lymphocytes and NK cells, increasing the numbers of NK T-cells, and inhibiting pro-inflammatory cytokines (e.g., TNF-α and IL-6). Lenalidomide is synergistic with dexamethasone in inhibiting cell proliferation and inducing apoptosis in multiple myeloma (MM) cells.

Metabolism: Rapidly absorbed after oral administration, with maximal plasma concentrations occurring 0.5–6 hours after dose in patients with MM or MDS. Taking the drug with a high-fat meal decreased the AUC about 20% and decreased C_{max} 50% in healthy subjects. However, the studies establishing efficacy and safety did not specify, so the drug can be taken without regard to food intake. Drug exposure (AUC) in MM and MDS patients with normal or mildly impaired renal function (CrCl $\geq$ 60 mL/min) was about 60% higher than in young, healthy male subjects. Drug has approximately 30% protein binding. Drug is primarily excreted by the kidneys, with 90% of a radioactive dose excreted in the urine within 10 days; 4% is excreted in the feces. About 82% of the drug is excreted in the urine as lenalidomide within 24 hours. The mean half-life of the drug is 3 hours in healthy subjects and 3–5 hours in patients with MM, MCL, and MDS.

Indications: Drug is indicated for the treatment of adult patients with (1a) MM in combination with dexamethasone; (1b) MM as maintenance therapy after autologous hematopoietic stem cell transplantation (auto-HSCT); (2) transfusion-dependent anemia due to low- or intermediate-1-risk MDS associated with a deletion 5q abnormality with or without additional cytogenetic abnormalities; (3) mantle cell lymphoma (MCL) whose disease has relapsed or progressed after two prior therapies, one of which included bortezomib; (4) follicular lymphoma (FL), previously treated in combination with a rituximab product; (5) marginal zone lymphoma (MZL), previously treated in combination with a rituximab product.

Limitations of use: NOT indicated and not recommended for the treatment of patients with CLL outside a controlled clinical trial. Toxicity and mortality were higher in CLL patients.

Contraindications: (1) Pregnancy as drug can cause fetal harm (ABSOLUTE CONTRA-INDICATION); (2) severe allergic (hypersensitivity) reaction (e.g., angioedema, SJS, TEN) to lenalidomide.

Dosage/Range:
Multiple Myeloma
- **MM Combination therapy**: Recommended starting dose is 25 mg once daily orally with or without food, days 1–21 of repeated 28-day cycles, together with dexamethasone. See package insert 14.1 for dexamethasone doses. Dexamethasone dose can be reduced in patients older than 75 years.
- **MM maintenance following autologous HSCT** (if ANC ≥ 1,000/mcL, platelets ≥75,000/mcL): 10 mg PO once daily continuously on days 1–28 of repeated 28-day cycles. If revlimid well tolerated after 3 cycles of maintenance therapy, dose can be increased to 15 mg PO qd.
- Starting dose for renal impairment shown below. Starting dose for patients >75 years old may be reduced. Treatment is continued or modified based upon clinical and laboratory findings. See package insert for dose modification guidelines.
- An alternative regimen for dexamethasone is 40 mg PO on days 1, 8, 15, 22 of a 28-day cycle (Chu and DeVita, 2016).
- In patients *eligible for auto-HSCT*, stem cell mobilization should occur within 4 cycles of lenalidomide containing therapy. In patients ineligible for auto-HSCT, treatment should continue until disease progression or unacceptable toxicity.
- **MDS**: 10 mg once daily orally. Starting dose for renal impairment shown below. Treatment is continued or modified based upon clinical and laboratory findings. **See package insert for dose modification guidelines**.
- **MCL**: 25 mg once daily orally on days 1–21 of repeated 28-day cycles. Starting dose for renal impairment shown below. Treatment is continued until disease progression or unacceptable toxicity. See package insert for dose modification guidelines.
- **FL or MZL:** 20 mg PO once daily on days 1–21 of repeated 28-day cycles for up to 12 cycles.

Dose Modifications for renal impairment:
- After initiation of lenalidomide, subsequent dose modification is based on individual patient treatment tolerance, as shown in package insert.
- Renal impairment: Adjust starting dose based on Creatinine Clearance (CrCl) patients with moderate or severe renal impairment and on dialysis.
  - Moderate renal impairment (CrCl 30–60 mL/min): MM, MCL, FL, MZL = 10 mg once daily; Maintenance after Auto-HSCT, MDS = 5 mg every 24 hours
  - Severe renal impairment (CrCl < 30 mL/min, not requiring dialysis): MM, MCL = 15 mg every other day; FL, MZL = 5 mg once daily; Maintenance after Auto-HSCT, MDS = 2.5 mg once daily.
  - End-stage renal disease (CrCl < 30 mL/min, requiring dialysis): On dialysis days, administer after dialysis; MM, MCL, FL, MZL = 5 mg once daily; MDS = 2.5 mg once daily; administer after dialysis on dialysis days.

- Lenalidomide combination therapy for MM: CrCl 30–60 mL/min: consider escalating dose to 15 mg after 2 cycles if the patient tolerates the 10-mg dose.
- Lenalidomide maintenance therapy after Auto-HSCT for MM, and for MCL and MDS: base subsequent dose increase or decrease on individual patient treatment tolerance.
- Lenalidomide combination therapy for FL and MZL: CrCl 30–60 mL/min: after 2 cycles, consider increasing the lenaidomide dose to 15 mg PO if patient has tolerated therapy.

Dose Modifications for Neutropenia, Thrombocytopenia, other adverse effects: see package insert for each disease category.

Drug Preparation:
- Oral available in 2.5-, 5-, 10-, 15-, 20-, and 25-mg capsules. Available only under a restricted distribution program called REVLIMID REMS program. Prescribers and pharmacists must be registered with the program.
- Patients must meet all the conditions of the REVLIMID REMS program and read, agree, and comply with all of the REMS requirements. Previously this was known as the RevAssist Program.
- Pregnancy test results must be verified by the prescriber and the pharmacist prior to dispensing the prescription, as drug cannot be given to a pregnant woman.
- See prescribing guidelines for Revlimid for dose modifications.

Drug Administration:
- Oral, at the same time each day, with or without food. Capsules should be swallowed whole with water, and they should not be opened, broken, or chewed.
- Check to make sure that pregnancy tests are negative 10–14 days and 24 hours prior to therapy, monthly, and for 4 weeks after drug is stopped.
- Assess that the patient is using an effective method of contraception. See Nursing Problem IV.
- Assess CBC/ANC weekly for cycles 1 and 2, days 1 and 15 of cycle 3, then every 28 days (4 weeks) for MM patients taking drug with dexamethasone or on lenalidomide maintenance therapy. If patient has MDS, assess cbc/ANC weekly × first 8 weeks, then at leasat monthly. If the patient has MCL, assess cbc/ANC weekly × 1 month, then every 2 weeks during cycles 2–4, then monthly thereafter.
- Assess CBC/ANC in patients with FL and MZL weekly for the first 3 weeks of cycle 1 (28 days), then every 2 weeks during cycles 2–4, and then monthly thereafter.
- Discuss dose modifications with provider based on laboratory findings.

Drug Interactions:
- Digoxin: lenalidomide may increase C_{max} and AUC of digoxin; closely monitor digoxin plasma levels.
- Erythropoietin-stimulating agents or estrogen-containing therapies: may increase risk of venous thromboembolism. Use together cautiously in MM patients taking lenalidomide and dexamethasone.
- Additive antitumor effect when combined with dexamethasone in the treatment of MM.

Lab Effects/Interference:
- Decreased neutrophil, lymphocyte, platelet, and red blood cell counts.
- Decreased potassium, magnesium, sodium, phosphate, and calcium.
- Increased alanine aminotransferase.

Special Considerations:
- Warnings and Precautions:
  - *Embryo-fetal toxicity:* Lenalidomide may cause birth defects or embryo-fetal death. Revlimid is available only through a restricted distribution program called the Revlimid REMS program. For females of reproductive potential: must avoid pregnancy for at least 4 weeks before beginning lenalidomide therapy, during therapy, during dose interruptions, and for at least 4 weeks after completing therapy; (2) must commit to prevention of pregnancy during treatment by the use of two reliable methods of contraception, or commit to continuous abstinence from heterosexual sex, beginning 4 weeks before beginning lenalidomide therapy, during therapy, during dose interruptions, and for at least 4 weeks after completing therapy; (3) have two negative pregnancy tests prior to beginning therapy, one within 10–14 days and the second within 24 hours before prescribing lenalidomide, then weekly during the first month, then monthly thereafter in women with regular menstrual cycles, or every 2 weeks in women with irregular menstrual cycles. As the drug is found in sperm, men receiving lenalidomide must always use a latex or synthetic condom during any sexual contact with females of reproductive potential and for up to 4 weeks after discontinuing lenalidomide, even if they have had a successful vasectomy; men receiving the drug must not donate sperm. Nursing mothers should discontinue nursing or discontinue use of the drug. See Nursing Problem IV. (3) Patients must not donate blood when receiving lenalidomide, and for 4 weeks after last dose as blood may be given to a pregnant patient.
  - *REVLIMID REMS Program:* Required components include: (a) Prescribers must be certified with the Revlimid REMS program by enrolling and complying with the REMS requirements; (b) patients must sign a Patient–Physician agreement form and comply with the REMS requirements; female patients of reproductive potential who are not pregnant must comply with the pregnancy testing and contraception requirements, and males must comply with contraception requirements; (c) pharmacies must be certified with the Revlimid REMS program, must only dispense to patients who are authorized to receive Revlimid, and comply with REMS requirements.
  - *Hematologic events:* Drug is associated with significant neutropenia and thrombocytopenia. Monitor patients with neutropenia for signs of infection; teach patients to assess for infection and bleeding and to report them right away Monitor CBC/differential for (1) MM patients taking lenalidomide and dexamethasone, or lenalidomide (alone) as maintenance therapy, every 7 days for the first 2 cycles, on days 1 and 15 of cycle 3, and every 28 days (4 weeks) thereafter; (2) MDS patients: weekly for the first 8 weeks, and then at least monthly. If the patient has MCL, assess CBC/ANC weekly $\times$ 1 month, then every 2 weeks during cycles 2–4, then monthly thereafter. Assess CBC/ANC in patients with FL and MZL weekly for the first 3 weeks of cycle 1 (28 days), then every 2 weeks during cycles 2–4, and then monthly thereafter.

Based on testing results, discuss dose modification recommended in package insert (Celgene, 2019).

- *Venous and arterial thromboembolism:* Risk is increased in MM patients taking lenalidomide and dexamethasone, as is risk for MI and stroke (CVA). Help patient modify modifiable risk factors, and discuss interventions with physician (e.g., hyperlipidemia, HTN, smoking). Thromboprophylaxis is recommended, based on patient's underlying risk. ESA and estrogen may each increase risk further. Teach patient to report signs/symptoms of thrombotic events right away.
- *Second primary cancers* occurred at a greater frequency in controlled trials of newly diagnosed MM patients receiving lenalidomide compared to controls (e.g., acute myelogenous leukemia and MDS).
- *Increased mortality in patients with CLL* treated with Revlimid—drug is not indicated for CLL.
- *TLS:* Drug may cause TLS in patients with large tumor burdens prior to treatment that lyse quickly when lenalidomide is given, and it may be fatal. Discuss TLS prophylaxis with physician and closely monitor patients.
- *Tumor flare reaction*, characterized by lymph node swelling, low-grade fever, pain, and rash, have occurred when the drug was studied in patients with CLL (for which the drug is NOT indicated) or lymphoma. In MCL studies, the incidence was 10%, and was grades 1–2, generally occurring during the first cycle. Tumor flare reactions may mimic tumor progression. If needed, corticosteroids, NSAIDs, and/or narcotic analgesics may be considered. If a patient has a grades 3 or 4 reaction, hold lenalidomide until it resolves to ≤ grade 1. Monitor patients with MCL for tumor flare reactions.
- *Impaired stem cell mobilization* may occur, with a decreased number of CD34+ cells collected after > 4 cycles. If autologous stem cell transplant is planned, referral to a transplant center should occur early in treatment.
- *Hepatotoxicity*, including hepatic failure, has occurred and some cases have been fatal. Monitor LFTs and stop drug upon elevation of liver enzymes; drug can be resumed after liver enzymes return to baseline, and consider dose reduction.
- *Increased mortality in patients with MM when pembrolizumab is added to a thalidomide analogue and dexamethasone:* Combination with a PD-1 or PD-LI blocker is not advised outside of a clinical trial.
- *Thyroid disorders:* Both hypo- and hyperthyroidism have been reported. Assess TFTs baseline and during therapy.
- *Severe cutaneous reactions including hypersensitivity reactions* can occur, including angioedema, SJS, and TEN, and they can be fatal. Discontinue drug immediately if reactions are suspected, or if rash is grade 4. DO NOT resume lenalidomide if these reactions are verified. Drug is contraindicated in these patients. Consider lenalidomide interruption or discontinuation for grades 2–3 skin rash.
- *Early mortality in patients with MCL:* higher risk for death in patients with high tumor burden, high wbc at baseline ($\geq 10 \times 10^9$/L), and MIPI (Mantle cell prognosis score) score at diagnosis.

- Drug is largely excreted unchanged by the kidneys; use cautiously in patients with renal impairment, and dose-reduce per package insert (see Dose Modifications).

- Elderly MM patients receiving lenalidomide and dexamethasone have a higher risk of developing DVT, PE, atrial fibrillation, and renal failure following use of lenalidomide.
- Patients must not donate blood during lenalidomide treatment and for 1 month following last drug dose, as the blood may be given to a pregnant female whose fetus would then be exposed to lenalidomide. Men taking thalidomide must not donate sperm.
- Most common side effects in patients with MM: fatigue, neutropenia, constipation, diarrhea, muscle cramp, anemia, pyrexia, peripheral edema, nausea, back pain, URI, dyspnea, dizziness, thrombocytopenia, tremor, rash.
- Most common side effects in patients with MDS: thrombocytopenia, neutropenia, diarrhea, pruritus, rash, fatigue, constipation, nausea, nasopharyngitis, arthralgia, pyrexia, back pain, peripheral edema, cough, dizziness, headache, muscle cramp, dyspnea, pharyngitis, epistaxis.
- Most common side effects in patients with MCL: neutropenia, thrombocytopenia, fatigue, diarrhea, anemia, nausea, cough, pyrexia, rash, dyspnea, pruritus, constipation, peripheral edema, leukopenia.

Potential Toxicities/Side Effects and the Nursing Process

I.   POTENTIAL FOR INFECTION AND BLEEDING related to BONE MARROW SUPPRESSION

Defining Characteristics: Significant neutropenia and thrombocytopenia may occur, requiring dose adjustments. In MDS patients, neutropenia occurred in 61.5% of patients, thrombocytopenia in 61.5%, and anemia in 11.5%. Grade 3 or 4 hematologic toxicity was seen in 80% of patients enrolled in the MDS study, and 48% developed grades 3–4 neutropenia. In this study, the median time to onset of neutropenia was 42 days, and median time to recovery was 17 days. In this study, 54% of patients developed grades 3–4 thrombocytopenia, with a median time to onset of 28 days, and median time to recovery was 22 days. In MM patient clinical trials (taking lenalidomide and dexamethasone), incidence of neutropenia was 42.2% (grades 3–4 in 33.4% of patients), thrombocytopenia 21.5% (with 12.2% grades 3–4), and anemia 31.4% (with 9.9% grades 3–4). The incidence in MCL patients was: neutropenia, 49%, thrombocytopenia 36%, and anemia 31%.

Nursing Implications: Assess baseline CBC, WBC, differential, and platelet count prior to lenalidomide, then (1) for MDS patients: weekly for the first 8 weeks of treatment, then monthly; (2) for MM patients: every 2 weeks for first 12 weeks, then monthly; (3) for MCL patients: weekly for first cycle (28 days), every 2 weeks during cycles 2–4, then monthly. Based on CBC/differential, discuss dose modifications as indicated in Revlimid package insert, with physician. Assess for signs/symptoms of infection or bleeding. Teach patient the signs/symptoms of infection or bleeding, and to report these immediately, and teach patient self-care measures to minimize risk of infection and bleeding. This includes avoidance of crowds, proximity to people with infections, and OTC aspirin-containing medications (except if used for thromboprophylaxis). Discuss need for blood product support with physician or NP/PA. Drug should be used in combination with another agent that does not cause bone marrow suppression, like bortezomib (Velcade), rather than chemotherapy.

II.   ALTERATION IN COMFORT related to ITCHING, RASH, FATIGUE, LIGHT-HEADEDNESS, AND LEG CRAMPS

Defining Characteristics: Patients may develop itching (7.6% MM/dexamethasone patients, 41.9% MDS patients, 17% MCL patients); rash (21.2% MM/dexamethasone patients, 35.8% MDS patients, 22% MCL patients); and dry skin (9.3% MM/dexamethasone patients and 14.2% MDS patients). In addition, 31.1–43.9% of patients experience fatigue; 16–26.3% peripheral edema, 8–21.6% arthralgias; 13–25.8% back pain; and 18.2–33.4% muscle cramps or 13% muscle spasms. About 19.6–23.2% of patients reported dizziness or headache.

Nursing Implications: Assess patient's baseline comfort, and teach patient that these symptoms may occur. Assess skin integrity baseline and during therapy. Teach symptom management strategies to minimize discomfort. Teach patient to notify nurse or physician if fatigue, rash, itching, or leg cramps are severe, or do not resolve with local management. Teach patient to change position slowly and to report severe dizziness. Teach patient to report leg cramps or new onset of shortness of breath or chest pain right away, and evaluate for DVT or PE.

III.   ALTERATION IN NUTRITION, LESS THAN BODY REQUIREMENTS, related to DIARRHEA, CONSTIPATION, OR NAUSEA, ELECTROLYTE DISTURBANCE

Defining Characteristics: In clinical studies, diarrhea occurred in 38.5% of MM/dexamethasone patients, 48.6% of MDS patients, and 31% of MCL patients. Constipation occurred in 40.5%, 23.6%, and 16% of patients respectively. Nausea affected 26.1%, 23.6%, and 30% of patients, while vomiting affected 12.2%, 10.1%, and 12%, respectively. Around 15.3% of MM patients receiving lenalidomide/dexamethasone had dysgeusia.

Nursing Implications: Assess baseline nutrition, electrolytes, and bowel elimination pattern. Teach patient that diarrhea, constipation, nausea, and less commonly vomiting, may occur. Teach patient self-care strategies to minimize symptoms and to report them if they do not resolve. Teach patient self-administration of antiemetics or antidiarrheals as prescribed, and to notify provider if diarrhea persists. Teach patient dietary modification if diarrhea, constipation, nausea, or vomiting occur (e.g., the BRAT diet for diarrhea: bananas, rice, applesauce, and toast), and to increase oral fluids to prevent dehydration. Assess electrolytes baseline, as needed if patient develops diarrhea or vomiting, and periodically during treatment. Assess patient taste changes, and suggest dietary modifications if dysgeusia occurs.

IV.   KNOWLEDGE DEFICIT, POTENTIAL, related to PATIENT INSTRUCTIONS (Revlimid REMS), CONTRACEPTION, AND PREGNANCY TESTING   .

Defining Characteristics: Drug is fetotoxic. Patients must be able to understand the risk to the fetus, comply with REMS requirements, and be able to safeguard the drug in the home.

Nursing Implications: Assess patient's ability to understand rationale, importance of pregnancy testing in women of childbearing age, and to avoid pregnancy 4 weeks prior to drug prescription, and during treatment, treatment holidays, and for 4 weeks following drug discontinuance. Assess the understanding and ability of patients with childbearing potential to comply with contraception requirement and other self-care strategies and agree to the following:

- Female patients: (1) avoiding pregnancy for at least 4 weeks before beginning lenalidomide therapy, during therapy, during dose interruptions, and for at least 4 weeks after completing therapy; (2) committing to either continuous abstinence from heterosexual intercourse or to use two methods of reliable birth control beginning 4 weeks prior to starting lenalidomide therapy, during therapy, during dose interruptions, and continuing for 4 weeks following discontinuance of lenalidomide; (3) complying with pregnancy testing 10–14 days and within 24 hours prior to starting lenalidomide; then weekly during first month and monthly thereafter in women with regular menstrual cycles, or every 2 weeks in women with irregular menstrual cycles; and (4) having two negative pregnancy tests before the drug is prescribed.
- Male patients: (1) must always use a latex condom during any sexual contact with females of childbearing potential, as drug is present in the semen; (2) must continue contraception for 28 days after stopping the drug, even if the man has had a successful vasectomy; (3) must not donate sperm.
- Teach patient to notify the physician immediately under the following conditions:
  - Female patient becomes pregnant, thinks she might be pregnant, thinks birth control has failed, stops birth control, misses her menses, or has unusual menstrual bleeding. If so, she must stop taking the drug and notify the physician immediately;
  - Male patient has unprotected sex with a woman who can become pregnant, or if he thinks his sexual partner may be pregnant.
- Patients must not donate blood during treatment with lenalidomide and for 1 month following drug discontinuation.
- Assess ability of patient to keep drug/drug supply out of the reach of children and pets, and NEVER to share drug with anyone else, even if they have similar symptoms. Discuss any concerns with the physician.

Drug: Mogamulizumab-kpkc (Poteligeo)

Class: Human IgG1 monoclonal antibody, recombinant; binds to CCR4, receptor for CC chemokines involved in lymphocyte trafficking.

Mechanism of Action: Mogamulizumab-kpkc targets CC chemokine receptor 4 (CCR4)-expressing cells. CCR4 is expressed on surface of some T-cell tumor cells, and is expressed on regulatory T-cells (Treg) and a subset of helper (Th2) T-cells (Kyowa Kirin, 2018). Once CCR4 binding occurs, the tumor cell is targeted for antibody-dependent cellular cytotoxicity (ADCC) and cell death.

Metabolism: Steady state is reached after 8 doses (12 weeks). Terminal half-life is 17≈days (66%).

Indications: Treatment of adult patients with relapsed or refractory mycosis fungoides (MF) or Sezary syndrome, after at least 1 prior systemic therapy. Mycosis fungoides and Sezary syndrome are types of cutaneous T-cell lymphoma with proliferation of helper T cells.

Contraindications: None.

Dosage/Range:
- Premedicate with diphenhydramine and acetaminophen for the first mogamulizumab-kpkc dose.
- Dose is 1 mg/kg IV infusion over at least 60 minutes on days 1, 8, 15, and 22 of the first 28-day cycle; then on days 1 and 15 of each subsequent 28-day cycle until disease progression or unacceptable toxicity.
- Administer mogamulizumab-kpkc within 2 days of scheduled dose; if a dose is missed, give the next dose as soon as possible and resume dosing schedule.
- DO NOT administer SQ or by rapid IV administration.
- Dose Modifications:
  - *Dermatologic toxicity* (1) permanently discontinue for life-threatening (grade 4) rash or Stevens Johnson syndrome (SJS) or toxic epidermal necrolysis (TEN); (2) if either SJS or TEN is suspected, stop drug and do not resume until these diagnoses have been excluded and cutaneous reaction has resolved to grade ≤1; (3) if moderate or severe (grades 2 or 3) rash occurs, interrupt drug and administer at least 2 weeks of topical corticosteroids; if rash improves to grade 1 or less, resume mogamulizumab-kpkc; (4) if mild (grade 1) rash, consider topical corticosteroids.
  - *Infusion reactions* (1) permanently discontinue mogamulizumab-kpkc for life-threatening (grade 4) infusion reaction; (2) temporarily interrupt the infusion of mogamulizumab-kpkc for mild to severe (grades 1–3) infusion reactions and treat symptoms; (3) reduce infusion rate by at least 50% when restarting the infusion after symptoms resolve; (4) if reaction recurs and is unmanageable, discontinue infusion; (5) if an infusion reaction occurs, administer premedications for subsequent mogamulizumab-kpkc infusions.

Drug Preparation:
- Available as 20 mg/5 mL (4 mg/mL) in a single-dose vial.
- Visually inspect drug product solution for particulate matter and discoloration prior to administration (should be clear to slightly opalescent colorless); if cloudiness, discoloration or particulates are observed, discard solution.
- Calculate the dose (mg/kg) and number of vials of mogamulizumab-kpkc needed to prepare the dose.
- Aseptically withdraw the reqired volume of mogamulizumab-kpkc into the syringe, and transfer into an IV bag containing 0.9% Sodium Chloride Injection, USP. The final concentration of the diluted solution should be between 0.1 mg/mL to 3.0 mg/mL. Diluted solution is compatible with polyvinyl chloride (PVC) or polyolefin (PO) infusion bags.
- Mix diluted solution by gentle inversion; do not shake.

TREATMENT

- Discard any unused portion left in vial.
- Storage of diluted solution: after preparation, infuse mogamulizumab-kpkc solution immediately, or store under refrigeration at 2°C–8°C (36°F–46°F) for no more than 4 hours from the time of infusion preparation. Do not freeze or shake.

Drug Administration:
- If patient a female of reproductive potential, verify patient is not pregnant prior to starting mogamulizumab-kpkc.
- Premedicate for first dose, and if patient has an infusion reaction, premedicate prior to subsequent mogamulizumab-kpkc doses.
- Administer mogamulizumab-kpkc solution over at least 60 minutes through an IV line with a sterile, low protein binding, 0.22 micron (or equivalent) in-line filter.
- Do not mix mogamulizumab-kpkc with other drugs; do not co-administer with other drugs through same IV line.

Drug Interactions: Unknown.

Lab Effects/Interference:
- Decreased CD4 (helper) lymphocytes, WBC, platelets, neutrophils, RBC
- Decreased serum albumin, calcium, phosphate, magnesium, glucose
- Increased serum calcium, uric acid, glucose, AST, ALT, alkaline phosphatase

Special Considerations:
- Most common adverse reactions (≥ 20%): rash, infusion related reactions, fatigue, diarrhea, musculoskeletal pain, URI.
- Drug is not recommended in pregnant women. Female patients of reproductive potential should have a negative pregnancy test before starting mogamulizumab-kpkc, and should be taught to use effective contraception during treatment and for at least 3 months after last dose of mogamulizumab-kpkc.
- Warnings and Precautions:
  - *Dermatologic toxicity:* Stevens-Johnson syndrome (SJS) and toxic epidermal necrolysis (TEN), which may be life-threatening or fatal, have occurred. In Trial 1, incidence of dermatologic toxicity was 25%, with 18% grade 3, while in all clinical trials incidence of grade 3 skin toxicity was 3.6%. Onset of drug eruption is variable, with median time to onset 15 weeks in Trial 1, and 25% of cases occurring after 31 weeks. Most commonly reported were papular or maculopapular rash, lichenoid, spongiotic or granulomatous dermatis; mobilliform rash; scaly plaques, pustular eruption, folliculitis, non-specific dermatitis, and psoriasiform dermatitis. Monitor patients closely throughout treatment for rash. Management includes topical corticosteroids and interruption or permanent discontinuation of mogamulizumab-kpkc (see Dosage Modifications). Discuss skin biopsy with provider to distinguish drug eruption from disease progression. For any life-threatening (grade 4) reaction, SJS or TEN, permanently discontinue mogamulizumab-kpkc. If SJS or TEN is suspected, interrupt mogamulizumab-kpkc and do not resume until diagnosis is ruled out, and cutaneous reaction has resolved to ≤grade 1.
  - *Infusion reactions:* Incidence in Trial 1 was 35% (8% grade 3), most occurring during or shortly after first infusion although they can occur with subsequent infusions as

well. Most common signs included chills, nausea, fever, tachycardia, rigors, headache, vomiting. Consider premedicating all patients for first infusion: incidence in Trial was 42% without premedication and 32% with premedication. Monitor patients closely during infusion and interrupt infusion for signs/symptoms of infusion reaction (any grade), and manage promptly.

- *Infections:* In Trial 1, incidence of grade 3 or higher infection was 18%, including sepsis, pneumonia, and skin infection. Monitor patients closely for infection and discuss prompt management with provider.
- *Autoimmune complications:* Discuss with provider risk and benefit ration in patients with a history of autoimmune disease. Fatal and life-threatening immune-mediated complications have been reported in patient sreceiving mogamulizumab-kpkc such as grade 3 or higher myocarditis, polymyositis, hepatitis, pneumonitis, and a variant of Guillain-Barre syndrome. Mogamulizumab-kpkc use should be interrupted or permanently discontinued in patients with a history of autoimmune disease if immune-mediated adverse reactions are suspected based on risk and benefit analysis.
- *Complications of allogeneic hematopoiectic stem cell transplantation (HSCT) after mogamulizumab-kpkc administration:* There are increased risks of transplant complications in patients who received HSCT after mogamulizumab-kpkc. These include severe (grade 3–4) GVHD, steroid refractory GVHD, and transplant related death. There appears to be increased risk if mogamulizumab-kpk is given within 50 days before the HSCT. Patients should be followed closely for early signs/symptoms of transplant related complications (Kyowa Kirin, 2018).

Potential Toxicities/Side Effects and the Nursing Process

I.   POTENTIAL ALTERATION IN BODY IMAGE, SKIN INTEGRITY, COMFORT, related to DERMATOLOGIC TOXICITY

Defining Characteristics: Rash is common, with an incidence of 25% in Trial 1, called drug eruption, and occurring as grade 3 in 18% of patients. Rarely, SJS and TEN can occur. Onset is variable, and in Trial 1 median time to onset was 15 weeks, where 25% occurred later than 31 weeks (Kyowa Kirin, 2018).

Nursing Implications: Assess patient skin integrity, comfort, and body image baseline, and periodically during therapy. Teach patient that skin eruption may occur and to report this. Discuss management with provider, including topical corticosteroids, dose interruption, drug discontinuance, and skin biopsy if difficult to distinguish drug interruption from disease progression. If SJS or TEN is suspected, drug should be stopped, and not restarted until either diagnosis is ruled out, and cutaneous reaction has resolved to ≤ grade 1 reaction.

II.   POTENTIAL FOR INJURY related to ACUTE INFUSION-RELATED EVENTS

Defining Characteristics: About 1/3 (35%) of patients experience an infusion reaction during or after the infusion, characterized by chills, fever, nausea, vomiting, headache, hypotension, hypertension, hypoxia, and/or dyspnea. Most (90%) occur during or shortly after the first infusion but may occur with subsequent infusions. Rarely, life-threatening or fatal reactions may occur during or within 24 hours of the infusion. Premedication reduces incidence of reactions from 42% to 32% in Trial 1.

Nursing Implications: Premedicate with acetaminophen and diphenhydramine as ordered 1 hour before mogamulizumab-kpkc administration, at least prior to initial treatment and if patient has an infusion reaction, premedicate for subsequent infusions. Monitor patient and VS/O_2 saturation (O_2 sat) closely, baseline and during the infusion. Permanently discontinue mogamulizumab-kpkc if patient has a grade 4 (life-threatening) infusion reaction. Temporarily interrupt infusion immediately for signs/symptoms of grade 1–3 infusion reaction and discuss management with provider to manage symptoms. Monitor patient's VS/O_2 saturation closely until signs and symptoms completely resolve. If patient develops signs/symptoms of anaphylaxis, including severe respiratory symptoms or clinically significant hypotension, mogamulizumab-kpkc should be permanently discontinued. Ensure that medications necessary for the management of hypersensitivity/anaphylaxis are readily available (e.g., epinephrine, antihistamines, corticosteroids). Be prepared to provide emergency support as necessary Iincluding changing IV line to IV saline so no further drug is infused, epinephrine, antihistamines, bronchodilators).

Drug: Moxetumomab pasudotox-tdfk (Lumoxiti)

Class: Immunotoxin (first in class) using a monoclonal antibody and toxin; CD22- directed immunoglobulin (variable domain, recombinant murine Ig genetically fused to a truncated form of *Pseudomonas* exotoxin PE 38.

Mechanism of Action: Moxetumomab pasudotox-tdfx is a CD22-directed cytotoxin which binds to CD22 on the cell surface of B-cells and is then internalized resulting in inhibition of protein synthesis and apoptosis. Specifically the internalization causes ADP-ribosylation of elongation factor 2 which then inhibits protein synthesis.

Metabolism: In studies, as CD22 B-cell counts are difficult, CD19+B cells were used as a surrogate. Drug was effective in reducing circulating CD19+B cells on day 8 by 89% from baseline and after the first 3 infusions. Mean elimination half-life of moxetumomab pasudotox-tdfk was 1.4 hours. The metabolism of the drug is unknown but proteolytic degradation into small peptides and amino acids via catabolic pathways is suspected (AstraZeneca, 2018). If the patient develops anti-drug antibodies (ADA), presence of ADA post-baseline was associated with lower cmax at later cycles (Cycle 3 and beyond).

Indications: Adult patients with relapsed or refractory hairy-cell leukemia who have received at least 2 prior systemic therapies, including treatment with a purine nucleoside analog (PNA). Not indicated for patients with severe renal impairment (CrCl ≤ 29 mL/min).

Contraindications: None. Not recommended in patients with severe renal impairment (CrCl ≤ 29 mL/min). Not recommended in patients with a PMH of hemolytic uremic syndrome (HUS) or severe thrombotic microangiopathy (TMA).

Dosage/Range:
- 0.04 mg/kg as an IV infusion over 30 min on days 1, 3, and 5 of each 28-day cycle. Continue moxetumomab pasudotox-tdfx treatment for a maximum of 6 cycles, or until disease progression or unacceptable toxicity.
- Premedicate, hydrate, and consider low-dose aspirin aministration days 1–8 of each cycle. See administration.

Drug Preparation (See package insert for detailed instructions):
- *Dose:* Available as 1 mg lyophilized cake or powder in a single-dose vial for reconstitution and further dilution. Use asenptic technique; calculate dose and number of vials needed (1 mg/vial) to be reconstituted. The final concentration of the reconstituted solution is 1 mg/mL do NOT round down for partial vials. Use patient's actual body weight prior to first dose of the first treatment cycle. A CHANGE in dose should only be made between cycles when a change in weight is >10% from weight used to calculate first dose. No change in dose should be made during a particular cycle.
- *Reconstitution:* Use only Sterile Water for Injection USP.
  - Reconstitute each vial with 1.1 ml Sterile Water for Injection USP resulting in 1 mg/mL solution and withdrawal of 1 mL of drug.
    - Direct diluent along walls of vial, not directly into the lyophilized cake or powder
    - Gentliy swirl vial until completely dissolved. Invert the vial to ensure all cake or powder in the vial is dissolved; DO NOT shake.
  - Visually inspect reconstituted solution for any discoloration or particles—solution should be clear to slightly opalescent, colorless to slightly yellow, and free from visible particles.
  - Use reconstituted solution immediately. DO NOT store reconstituted vials as there is no preservative.
- *Dilution:* Add IV Solution Stabilizer (packaged separately) to the infusion bag prior to adding the moxetumomab pasudotox-tdfx.
  - Add 1 mL IV Solution Stabilizer to the 50 mL bag of 0.9% Sodium Chloride Injection USP. **Use only 1 vial of stabilizer** for each administration of moxetumomab pasudotox-tdfx; gently invert the bag to mix the solution; do not shake.
  - Withdraw the required volume of reconstituted moxetumomab pasudotox-tdfx solution as calculated, and inject into the 50 mL infusion bag of .9% Sodium Chloride Injection USP and 1 mL IV Solution Stabilizer; gently invert the bag to mix the solution; do not shake.
  - Discard any partially used or empty vials of moxetumomab pasudotox-tdfx.
- Storage Times:
  - Reconstituted solution cannot be stored as it contains no preservative.
  - Diluted solution: use immediately or after storage at room temperature (20°C–25°C; 68°F–77°F) for up to 4 hours or store refrigerated at 2°C–8°C (36°F–46°F) for up to 24 hours. Protect from light. Do NOT freeze. DO NOT shake.
  - Administration: if the diluted solution is refrigerated (at 2°C–8°C (36°F–46°F) , allow to equilibrate at room temperature (20°C–25°C; 68°F–77°F) for no more than 4 hours prior to administration. Administer diluted solution within 24 hours of reconstitution as a 30- minute infusion. Protect from light.

Drug Administration:
- Patient Assessment for Capillary Leak Sydrome (CLS) and hemolytic uremic syndrome (HS):
  a. CBC/ANC, blood chemistries before each dose, and on day 8 of each cycle.
  b. Before each infusion **assess for CLS**: weight and BP;
     i. if weight has increased by 5.5 lbs (2.5 kg) or 5% greater from day 1 of the cycle, and the patient is hypotensive, promptly check for peripheral edema, hypoalbuminemia and respiratory symptoms, including SOB and cough;
     ii. if CLS is suspected, assess for a decrease in oxygen saturation and evidence of pulmonary edema +/or serosal effusions.
     iii. If patient develops grade 2 or higher CLS should receive appropriate supportive measures including treatment with oral or IV corticosteroids, with monitoring of weight, albumin levels, and BP until resolution.
     iv. CLS Grading and Management Guidelines:
         1. Grade 2: symptomatic, medical intervention indicated: delay moxetumomab pasudotox-tdfx dosing until symptoms resolve.
         2. Grade 3: severe symptoms, medical intervention indicated, grade 4: life-threatening consequences, urgent intervention indicated: discontinue moxetumomab pasudotox-tdfx.
  c. Before each infusion **assess for HUS**: assess hemoglobin level, platelet count, serum creatinine.
     i. If HUS is suspected, promptly check blood LDH, indirect bilirubin, and blood smear schistocytes for evidence of hemolysis.
     ii. Discontinue moxetumomab pasudotox-tdfx in patients with HUS; administer ordered supportive measures and fluid replacement, and monitor blood chemistries, cbc, and renal function closely.
     iii. If patient has a normal baseline serum creatinine, and serum creatinine is increasing:
         1. delay dosing if grade 2 or higher ($>$1.5 × baseline or the ULN); resume drug upon recovery to grade 1 (1–1.5 × baseline or between ULN and 1.5 ULN)
         2. If baseline serum creatinine is grade 1 or 2, delay dosing for creatinine increases to grade 3 or higher ($>$3 × baseline or ULN); resume drug upon recovery to baseline grade or lower.
- *Hydration:*
  a. Administer 1 L isotonic solution (e.g., 5% Dextrose Injectin USP or 0.45% or 0.9% Sodium Chloride Injectin USP) over 2–4 hours prior to and after each moxetumomab pasudotox-tdfx infusion. If patient weighs $<$50 kg, administer 0.5L
  b. Teach patient to hydrate with up to 3 L [(12) 8-oz glasses] of oral fluids (e.g., water, milk, juice) every 24 hours on days 1 through 8 of each 28-day cycle. If patient weighs $<$50 kg, increase oral fluids to 2 L [(8) 8-oz glasses] per 24 hours.
  c. Monitor fluid balance and serum electrolytes to prevent fluid overload and/or electrolyte abnormalities.
- *Thromboprophylaxis:*
  a. Consider low-dose aspirin on days 1 through day 8 of each 28-day cycle.
  b. Monitor for signs/symptoms of thrombosis.

- *Premedication:*
  a. Premedicate 30–90 minutes before each dose with (1) antihistamine (e.g., diphenhydramine), (2) acetaminophen, and (3) histamine-2 receptor antagonist (e.g., ranitidine, famotidine, or cimetidine).
  b. If a severe infusion-related (IR) reaction occurs, interrupt drug and administer ordered medical interventins. Once reaction resolves, and as ordered, administer oral or IV corticosteroid approximately 30 minutes before resuming infusion and before each subsequent dose of the drug thereafter.
- Drug Administration: Administer moxetumomab pasudotox-tdfx as an IV infusion over 30 minutes on days 1, 3, and 5 of a 28-day cycle for a maximum of 6 cycles.
- *Post-infusion medication:*
  a. Consider oral antihistamines and antipyretics for up to 24 hours after moxetumomab pasudotox-tdfx infusion.
  b. Administer oral corticosteroid (e.g., 4 mg dexamethasone) as ordered to decrease nausea and vomiting.
  c. Maintain adequate oral fluid intake.
- Monitor for infusion related (IR) reactions.

Drug Interactions: None known.

Lab Effects/Interference:
- Anemia
- Increased creatinine, ALT, AST
- Decreased serum albumin, calcium, phosphate

Special Considerations:
- Most common toxicities ($\geq$ 20%): IR reactions, edema, nausea, fatigue, headache, pyrexia, constipation, anemia, diarrhea.
- Teach female patients of reproductive potential to use effective contraception during and for at least 30 days after last dose. Advise women not to breastfeed.
- Warnings and Precautions:
  - *Capillary Leak Syndrome (CLS):* Occurs in 34% of patients, including grade 2 in 23%, grade, 3 1.6%, and grade 4, 2%. Assess for 1) weight gain (increase in 5.5 lbs or 2.5 kg) or $\geq$ 5% from day 1 of current cycle; 2) hypotension; 3) peripheral edema; 4) SOB or cough; 5) pulmonary edema and/or serosal effusions; 6) hypoalbuminemia, elevated HCT, leukocytosis, thrombocytosis. Teach patient that urgent care is required if patient develops symptoms of CLS, and to go to ER or seek immediate care. If patient develops CLS, patient should be hospitalized as medically indicated, and receive concomitant oral or IV corticosteroids. Moxetumomab pasudotox-tdfx should be held for grade 2 CLS until resolution, and permanently discontinued for grades 3–4. may be life-threatening, and occurs in approximately 34% of patients. Most episodes occurred within first 8 days of a treatment cycle; median time to resolution of CLS was 12 days. Monitor patient weight and BP prior to each drug dose, and as clinically indicated during treatment.
  - *Hemolytic Uremic Syndrome (HUS):* HUS is characterized by triad of microangiopathic hemolytic anemia, thrombocytopenia, and progressive renal failure. Incidence

with moxetumomab pasudotox-tdfx is 7% (including grade 3 of 3%; grade 4 of 0.8%). Most cases occurred within the first 9 days of a treatment cycle. Median time to resolution was 11.5 days, and all cases resolved. Drug should be avoided inpatients with a prior history of severe thrombotic microangiopathy (TMA) or HUS. Monitor blood chemistry and CBC prior to each dose and on Day 8 of each treatment cycle, as well as mid-cycle. Consider HUS if patient develops hemolytic anemia, worsening or sudden onset thrombocytopenia, increase in serum creatinine levels, elevation of bilirubin and/or LDH, and have evidence of hemolysis (based on peripheral blood smear schistocytes). If HUS is suspected, prompt medical therapy should be instituted to prevent progressive renal failure requiring dialysis, with fluid repletion, hemodynamic monitoring, and hospitalization as clinically indicated. Moxetumomab pasudotox-tdfx should be discontinued.

- *Renal Toxicity:* Occurs in about 26% of patients, including acute kidney injury, renal failure, renal impairment, increased serum creatinine, and proteinuria. Most cases are mild to moderate. In patients who develop HUS, those ≥ 65 years old, or those with baseline renal impairment may be at increased risk for worsening renal function after treatment with moxetumomab pasudotox-tdfx. Monitor renal function prior to each drug dose, and as clinically indicated. Delay moxetumomab pasudotox-tdfx dose in patients with grade 3 or higher elevations in serum creastinine, or upon worsening from baseline by ≥ 2 grades.
- *IR reactions:* Were characterized by chills, cough, dizziness, dyspnea, feeling hot, flushing, headache, HTN, hypotension, myalgia, nausea, pyrexia, sinus tachycardia, vomiting, or wheezing, occurred in 50% of patients in 1 study, with 11% grade 3. Most common IR reactions were nausea, pyrexia, chills, vomiting, headache, and infusion related reaction. IR reactions may occur during any treatment cycle, and patient should receive premedication. If a severe infusion reaction occurs, interrupt moxetumomab pasudotox-tdfx infusion and implement ordered medical intervention. As ordered administer oral or IV corticosteroid therapy about 30 minutes before resuming the infusion once the reaction has resolved.
- *Electrolyte abnormalities:* More than 50% of patients experience electrolyte abnormalities, most commonly hypocalcemia (25%). Monitor serum electrolytes prior to each dose and on day 8 of each treatment cycle, and mid-cycle as ordered.

Potential Toxicities/Side Effects and the Nursing Process

I.   ALTERATION IN CARDIAC OUTPUT, POTENTIAL related to CLS

Defining Characteristics: CLS is a leakage of proteins and fluid out of the capillaries into surrounding tissues, resulting in hypotension, hypoalbuminemia, hemoconcentration (low HCT), and symptoms of fluid overload. CLS incidence is 34% of patients receiving moxetumomab pasudotox-tdfx, including grade 2 in 23%, grade 3, 1.6%, and grade 4, 2%. Most patients develop symptoms in the first 8 days of a treatment cycle, and median time to resolution was 12 days (AstraZeneca, 2018). If not treated promptly and effectively, CLS can cause organ failure and death.

Nursing Implications: Assess cardiopulmonary status and weight baseline, before each treatment and between treatments as indicated. Assess cbc, albumin, electrolytes and serial weights before treatment. During the infusion, monitor VS and pulse oximetry, urinary output, and fluid status., Assess for 1) weight gain (increase of 5.5 lbs or 2.5 kg, or $\geq$ 5% from Day 1 of current cycle; 2) hypotension; 3) peripheral edema; 4) SOB or cough; 5) signs/ symptoms of pulmonary edema and/or serosal effusions; 6) hypoalbuminemia, elevated HCT, leukocytosis, thrombocytosis. Teach patient that urgent care is required if patient develops symptoms of CLS (egm dyspnea, chest pain, edema), and to go to ER or seek immediate care. If patient develops CLS, patient should be hospitalized as medically indicated, and receive concomitant oral or IV corticosteroids. Moxetumomab pasudotox-tdfx should be held for grade 2 CLS until resolution, and permanently discontinued for grades 3–4. may be life-threatening, and occurs in approximately 34% of patients. Discuss any abnormalities with physician, and revise plan as needed (e.g., corticosteroids, diuretics, plasma expanders).

II. POTENTIAL ALTERATION IN ELIMINATION related to Hemolytic Uremic Syndrome (HUS)

Defining Characteristics: HUS is a thrombotic microangiopathy which occurs rarely and is characterized by the triad of 1) abnormal destruction of red blood cells (microangiopathic hemolytic anemia), and 2) platelets (thrombocytopenia) which then results in the blockage of the renal capillaries causing 3) acute renal injury (progressive renal failure). The incidence in moxetumomab pasudotox-tdfx clinical trials was 7%; grade 3 occurred in 3% , and grade 4 in 0.8% of patients. Most patients develop HUS in the first 9 days of a treatment cycle, but it can happen at other times as well. Drug should not be given to patients with a PMH of severe thrombotic microangiopathy (TMA) or HUS.

Nursing Implications: Assess patient hyedration status, CBC, renal and liver function, and serum electrolytes baseline and before each treatment. Discuss any abnormalities with provider to see if treatment will proceed. Ensure that patient understands pretreatment hydration schedule [drink up to 3 L [(12) 8-oz glasses] of oral fluids (e.g., water, milk, juice) every 24 hours on Days 1 through 8 of each 28-day cycle. If patient weighs <50 kg, increase oral fluids to 2 L [(8) 8-oz glasses) per 24 hours]. Administer pre-and post-treatment IV hydration, and monitor I+O closely. Discuss prophylactic administration of low dose aspirin to prevent patient thrombosis, with provider. If patient develops grade 3 or higher elevation in serum creatinine, or worsening from baseline by 2 or more grades, moxetumomab pasudotox-tdfx should be delayed. HUS should be suspected in patient with: hemolytic anemia, worsening or sudden onset of thrombocytopenia, increase in serum creatinine, elevation of bilirubin and/or LDH, or evidence of hemolysis on peripheral blood smear (schistocytes). If HUS is suspected, LDH, indirect bilirubin and blood smean schistocytes should be assessed right away. If HUS is confirmed, drug should be discontinued, and patient treated with supportive measures, including fluid replacement, and monitoring of blood chemistry, CBC, and renal function until HUS resolves.

III.   POTENTIAL FOR INJURY related to ACUTE INFUSION-RELATED (IR) EVENTS

Defining Characteristics: About half of patients experience an infusion reaction during or after the moxetumomab pasudotox-tdfx infusion, characterized by chills, cough, dizziness, dyspnea, feeling hot, flushing, headache, HTN, infusion related reaction, myalgia, nausea, pyrexia, sinus tachycardia, vomiting, or wheezing (AstraZeneca, 2018). Grade 3 IRs occurred in 11% of patients in one study. Most common IRs are nausea, pyrexia, chills, vomiting, and headache, IRs can occur during any treatment cycle.

Nursing Implications: Premedicate with acetaminophen, diphenhydramine and a H2 receptor antagonist as ordered 30–90 minutes before moxetumomab pasudotox-tdfx administration. If a patient develops a severe IR, interrupt the infusion and administer ordered oral or IV corticosteroid 30 minutes before resuming the infusion once symptoms have resolved, or before the next infusion as ordered. Monitor patient and VS/O_2 saturation (O_2 sat) closely, baseline and during the infusion. Administer post-infusion medication as ordered (e.g., oral antihistamine, antipyretic for up to 24 hours post), oral corticosteroid (e.g., 4 mg dexamethasone to decrease risk of nausea/vomiting), and teach patient to maintain oral fluid intake.

Drug: necitumumab (Portrazza)

Class: mAb targeted against EGFR, Humanized IgG1 mAb.

Mechanism of Action: Binds to the ligand (EGF) binding site, thus preventing expression and activation of EGFR, which is associated with malignant progression, induction of angiogenesis, and inhibition of apoptosis. Binding of mAb to EGFR binding site results in internalization and degradation of EGFR, and binding also leads to ADCC in EGFR-expressing cells.

Metabolism: Necitumumab is genetically engineered in mammalian NSO cells. Elimination half-life is approximately 14 days. Time to reach steady state is about 100 days.

Indications: Treatment of patients with metastatic squamous NSCLC, in first line setting, in combination with gemcitabine and cisplatin. Drug is NOT indicated for the treatment of nonsquamous NSC LC patients.

Dosage/Range: 800 mg (absolute dose) IV infusion over 60 minutes on days 1 and 8 of each 3-week cycle.

Dose Modifications:
- IRRs: (1) Grade 1: reduce infusion rate by 50%; (2) Grade 2: stop the infusion until signs/ symptoms have resolved to grades 0–1, then resume infusion at 50% reduced rate for all subsequent infusions; (3) permanently discontinue drug for grades 3–4 infusion reaction.
- Dermatologic toxicity: (1) Grade 3 rash or acneiform rash: hold drug until symptoms resolve to grade 2 or less, then resume dose at reduced dose of 400 mg for at least 1 treatment cycle. If symptoms do not worsen, may increase dose to 600 and 800 mg in

subsequent cycles; (2) permanently discontinue drug if (a) grade 3 rash or acneiform rash does not resolve to grade ≤2 within 6 weeks; (b) reactions worsen or become intolerable at a dose of 400 mg; (c) patient experiences grade 3 skin induration/fibrosis; (d) grade 4 dermatologic toxicity.

Drug Preparation: Drug available in a single dose vial of 800 mg/50 mL (16 mg/mL).
- Inspect vial contents for particulate matter and discoloration before dilution, and discard if found.
- Store vials in a refrigerator at 2–8°C (36–46°F) until time of use. Keep vial in outer carton to protect from light.
- Dilute the required volume of necitumumab with 0.9% sodium chloride injection, USP in an IV infusion container to a final volume of 250 mL. Do NOT use solutions containing dextrose.
- Gently invert container to mix. DO NOT FREEZE or SHAKE the infusion solution. DO NOT dilute with other solutions or coinfuse with other electrolytes or medication.
- Discard vial with any unused portion of necitumumab.

Drug Administration:
- Visually inspect diluted solution for particulate matter and discoloration prior to administration, and discard solution if found.
- Administer diluted necitumumab infusion via infusion pump over 60 min through a separate infusion line. Flush the line with 0.9% sodium chloride injection USP at the end of the infusion.
- If a patient experiences a grade 1 infusion reaction, reduce infusion rate by 50%. Stop the infusion for grade 2 until signs/symptoms have resolved to grade 0/1; resume at 50% reduced infusion rate for all subsequent infusions. Permanently discontinue necitumumab for grades 3 or 4 infusion reactions.
- If a patient experienced a previous grade 1 or 2 infusion reaction, premedicate with diphenhydramine or equivalent prior to all subsequent infusions. If a patient experiences a second grade 1 or 2 infusion reaction, premedicate for all subsequent infusions with diphenhydramine or equivalent, acetaminophen and dexamethasone (or equivalent) prior to each necitumumab infusion.

Drug Interactions: Necitumumab, gemcitabine and cisplatin: AUC of gemcitabine increased by 22% and C_{max} increased by 63%; cisplatin exposure unchanged.

Lab Effects/Interference:
- Hypomagnesemia
- Hypokalemia, hypocalcemia, hypophosphatemia

Special Considerations:
- Warnings and Precautions:
  - Cardiopulmonary arrest/sudden death occurred in 3% of patients receiving combination therapy. Patients had comorbid conditions including coronary artery disease, hypomagnesemia, COPD, and HTN. Closely monitor serum electrolytes, including serum magnesium, potassium and calcium during therapy, and aggressively replace during and after necitumumab administration.

- Hypomagnesemia occurred in 83% of patients receiving the combination therapy, and was severe in 20%: Monitor patient for hypomagnesemia, hypocalcemia, and hypokalemia prior to each necitumumab infusion and for at least 8 weeks following the completion of necitumumab therapy. Hold drug for grades 3–4 electrolyte abnormalities; subsequent cycles of necitumumab may be administered once abnormalities are corrected to ≤grade 2. Replete electrolytes as ordered.
- Venous and thromboembolic events (VTE and ATE). Incidence of VTE was 9%, vs. 5% in the control group, and most common VTEs were PE (5%) and DVT (2%). Incidence of ATEs was 5% vs. 4% in control, while grade 3 or higher was 4% vs. 2% in control. Most common ATEs were cerebral stroke and ischemia (2%) and MI (1%). Discontinue necitumumab for severe VTE or ATE.
- Dermatologic toxicities (rash, dermatitis acneiform, dry skin, pruritis, generalized rash, skin fissures, maculo-papular rash, erythema) occurred in 79% of patients and was severe in 8%. Onset of skin toxicity was within first 2 weeks of therapy, and resolved within 17 weeks after onset. Monitor for toxicities. Dose modify for grade 3 skin reactions, and discontinue necitumumab for grade 4 (severe) toxicity or grade 3 skin induration/fibrosis. Teach patient to limit and protect self from sun exposure.
- IRRs occurred in 1.5% of patients, with 0.4% grade 3. Patients were not premedicated prior to the first dose, and most IRRs occurred after the first or second administration. Monitor during and following infusion for signs/symptoms of infusion reaction. Discontinue necitumumab for serious or life-threatening reactions.
- Increased toxicity in nonsquamous cell NSCLC, with increased morbidity and mortality. Drug is NOT indicated for treatment of patients with nonsquamous NSCLC.
- Embryo-fetal toxicity: can cause fetal harm and death. Teach women of reproductive potential to use effective contraception during therapy and for 3 months after last dose. Mothers should not breastfeed while receiving the drug and for 3 months after last dose.
- Most common adverse reactions (all grades) occurring ≥ 30 and ≥2% higher than gemcitabine/cisplatin alone: rash and hypomagnesemia.

Potential Toxicities/Side Effects and the Nursing Process

I. POTENTIAL FOR INJURY related to INFUSION REACTION

Defining Characteristics: IRRs occurred in 1.5% of patients, with 0.4% grade 3. Patients were not premedicated prior to the first dose, and most IRRs occurred after the first or second administration.

Nursing Implications: Monitor during and following infusion for signs/symptoms of infusion reaction. Assess baseline VS and mental status prior to drug administration, and periodically during infusion, as needed. Recall signs/symptoms of anaphylaxis, and if these occur, stop drug immediately, notify physician, and assess patient's vital signs. Subjective symptoms are generalized itching, nausea, chest tightness, crampy abdominal pain, difficulty speaking, anxiety, agitation, sense of impending doom, uneasiness, desire to urinate/defecate, dizziness, and chills. Objective signs are flushed appearance; angioedema of face, neck, eyelids, hands, and feet; localized or generalized urticaria; respiratory distress with or without wheezing; hypotension; and cyanosis.

If a patient experiences a grade 1 infusion reaction, reduce infusion rate by 50%. Stop the infusion for grade 2 until signs/symptoms have resolved to grade 0/1; resume at 50% reduced infusion rate for all subsequent infusions. Permanently discontinue necitumumab for grade 3 or 4 infusion reactions.

If a patient experienced a previous grade 1 or 2 infusion reaction, premedicate with diphenhydramine or equivalent prior to all subsequent infusions. If a patient experiences a second grade 1 or 2 infusion reaction, premedicate for all subsequent infusions with diphenhydramine or equivalent, acetaminophen, and dexamethasone (or equivalent) prior to each necitumumab infusion.

II. POTENTIAL ALTERATION IN BODY IMAGE, SKIN INTEGRITY, COMFORT related to SKIN RASH, CHANGES IN EYES AND HAIR FOLLICLES

Defining Characteristics: Drug inhibits epidermal growth factor receptor, so major toxicity is manifested in the skin. Most patients (87%) develop a mild-to-moderate acne-like rash that is self-limiting. Skin toxicity was severe in 8% of patients. Rash is a sterile, suppurative rash with multiple follicular or pustular lesions that appear during the first 2 weeks of therapy in areas of sun exposure: face, upper chest, and back, but in some cases, it is extended to the arms. Rash resolves within 17 weeks. Dry skin and itching occur in 7% of patients. Scratching with dirty hands or nails can lead to fissures and infection. Nail changes occur, as well as paronychia in 7% of patients. Eye lid changes are related to EGFR blockade and inflammation, and include blepharitis (inflammation of eyelid), conjunctivitis, and visual impairment. It appears that patients who have significant rash also have a tumor response.

Nursing Implications: Teach patient that rash most likely will occur due to mechanism of drug action. Assess baseline skin integrity on areas of face, neck, and trunk; assess baseline comfort and satisfaction with body image, and monitor at each treatment. Teach patient to report any distress and assess extent of rash. Teach patient to report any eye or vision changes.

Hold drug for grade 3 rash or acneiform rash until symptoms resolve to grade ≤2, then resume necitumumab at a reduced dose of 400 mg for at least 1 treatment cycle. If symptoms do not worsen, may increase dose to 600 mg and then to 800 mg in subsequent cycles.

Permanently discontinue necitumumab for (1) grade 3 rash or acneiform rash does not resolve to grade ≤2 within 6 weeks; (2) reactions worsen or become intolerable at a dose of 400 mg; (3) patient experiences grade 3 skin induration/fibrosis; and (4) grade 4 dermatologic toxicity.

If skin appears to be infected (exudate, vesicle formation, abnormal appearance), obtain C+S and discuss empiric treatment with physician. *For rash management, refer to introduction in this chapter.* Teach all patients to (1) use a water-based emollient frequently during the day to prevent dryness, (2) stay hydrated, (3) avoid sun exposure and wear SPF 30 (zinc-based). Do not use antiacne medications. Tetracycline analogues provide anti-inflammatory benefit. Grade 1/mild rash (localized, does not interfere with ADLs, and is not infected): Goal is to preserve skin integrity, minimize discomfort, and prevent infection. Key patient teaching includes (1) use a mild soap with active ingredients that reduce skin drying, such as pyrithione zinc (Head & Shoulders), (2) consider applying aloe gel to red, tender areas, (3) report distressing tenderness, as pramoxine (lidocaine topical anesthetic) may help, (4) keep fingernails clean and trimmed, and (5) apply zinc ointment to rectal mucosa after washing. Management: maintain current drug dose, observe or give topical hydrocortisone 1% or 2.5% or clindamycin 1% gel (anti-inflammatory benefit), reassess in 2 weeks. For grade 2/moderate, which is generalized, mild symptoms, has minimal effect on ADLs, and no infection: Goal is to prevent infection and promote comfort. Continue EGFRI dose; use topicals (hydrocortisone 2.5% or clindamycin 1% gel) and consider adding doxycycline 100 mg PO twice daily or minocycline 100 mg PO twice daily (give antimicrobial and anti-inflammatory effect) and reassess after 2 weeks. For grades 3–4 or severe rash (generalized, severe, has a significant impact on ADLs, and increased risk of infection): The goal is to prevent infection or identify it early to minimize complications and to promote effective coping. Interrupt drug. Treat rash with topicals (hydrocortisone 2.5%, or clindamycin 1% gel), doxycycline 100 mg PO twice daily or minocycline 100 mg PO twice daily, and methylprednisolone (Medrol dose pack); reassess after 2 weeks. Resume drug when rash improved to grade 2, at full or reduced dose (Lacouture et al., 2011; Lynch et al., 2007). If rash appears infected (exudate, vesicular formation, different appearance), obtain C+S, treat empirically until sensitivity received, and/or obtain dermatology consult.

III. ALTERATION IN ELECTROLYTE BALANCE related to HYPOMAGNESEMIA, POTENTIAL

Defining Characteristics: Magnesium wasting appears related to EGFR inhibition in the renal tubular epithelial cells so that excreted magnesium is not resorbed in the distal convoluted tubules. This leads to initial magnesium wasting, followed by losses of calcium and potassium. Cisplatin also causes proximal and distal renal tubular damage in the kidneys, resulting in hypomagnesemia, hypocalcemia, and hypokalemia. Hypomagnesemia occurs in about 83% (incidence 13% more than that of patients receiving cisplatin and gemcitabine alone), and is severe in 20% (grades 3 and 4). Median time to hypomagnesemia and electrolyte abnormalities is 6 weeks after starting necitumumab therapy. Symptoms of grades 3–4 hypomagnesemia include fatigue, cramps, and somnolence. Incidence of hypokalemia is 28% (5% grades 3 or 4); hypocalcemia 45% (6% grades 3 or 4); hypophosphatemia 31% (8% grades 3 or 4).

Nursing Implications: Assess baseline electrolyte balance before initial treatment and before each successive weekly treatment. Grade 1 is a serum level of 1.0 mg/dL LLN, grade 2 is 0.9–1.0 mg/dL, grade 3 is 0.7–0.8 mg/dL, and grade 4 is ≤ 0.6 mg/dL. Replete magnesium, calcium, and potassium as needed and ordered. Oral magnesium may be ineffective and result in diarrhea (Tejpar et al., 2007). Magnesium repletion regimens include weekly IV replacement of 4-g magnesium sulfate for grade 2. For grades 3–4, patients may be symptomatic, and magnesium replacement may involve once to twice weekly IV infusions of 6–10 g. Provide support for patients, as magnesium replacement infusions require lengthy time in clinic, as an 8-g infusion requires 4 hours. Post-IV replacement with every other day serum magnesium monitoring is important until the patient develops a steady state (Fakih, 2007). Continue to monitor after drug has been discontinued (half-life of the drug and time drug persists, e.g., 8 weeks). Magnesium replacement in IV hydration, beginning when a patient has grade 1 hypomagnesemia, may be effective in preventing worsening hypomagnesemia.

IV.   ALTERATION IN NUTRITION, LESS THAN BODY REQUIREMENTS, related to NAUSEA, VOMITING, DIARRHEA, STOMATITIS/MUCOUS MEMBRANE DISORDER, CONSTIPATION, WEIGHT LOSS

Defining Characteristics: Incidence of mild-to-moderate digestive symptoms includes vomiting (29%), diarrhea (16%), stomatitis (11%), and decreased weight (13%).

Nursing Implications: Assess baseline weight and nutritional status. Teach patient that these symptoms may occur and to report them. Administer antiemetic and other symptom management medications as ordered. Teach patient self-administration of these medications at home. Monitor serum electrolytes (magnesium, calcium) prior to each dose, and replete magnesium as needed. Teach patient dietary modifications to address symptoms such as diarrhea (BRAT diet: bananas, rice, applesauce, and toast) and mucositis (blenderized high-calorie, protein-dense foods, cold or cool soft foods, avoidance of spicy or acidic foods). Assess efficacy of intervention, and revise plan as needed.

Drug: nivolumab (Opdivo) injection

Class: Immune checkpoint inhibitor mAb. Human PD-1–blocking antibody; IgG_4 humanized mAb against PD-1.

Mechanism of Action: One of the ways cancer evades the immune system is by taking advantage of the body's process to turn down activated T-lymphocytes after an immune response, which is intended to protect the body's organs from autoimmune injury. The programmed cell death receptor-1 (PD-1) is found on T-lymphocytes, especially if they have been exposed to an antigen for a long time. The PD-1 receptor is activated by its ligand, PD-L1 (also known as B7-H1 or CD274), which is often found in the tumor microenvironment (Hamid et al., 2013). PD-1 also has another ligand, PD-L2 (also known as B7-DC or CD273), which is preferentially expressed on APCs. When the ligands PD-L1 and PD-L2 bind to the PD-1 receptor on T-lymphocytes, T-cell proliferation and cytokine production are turned off (Bristol-Myers Squibb Co., 2015). Some tumors upregulate PD-1 ligands—a phenomenon that contributes to loss of immune surveillance. mAb drugs that block the ligand PD-L1 from binding to its receptor PD-1 prevent activated T-lymphocytes from being turned down/off so that these cells can continue to attack cancer cells. See the chapter introduction for *Immunotherapy*. Because it blocks this immune checkpoint inhibitor, nivolumab has less immune toxicity than ipilimumab, which blocks the inhibitory receptor cytotoxic T-lymphocyte–associated antigen 4 (CTLA-4) and occurs earlier in the immune response. However, immune-related toxicity may occur, although it is less common. When nivolumab (anti-PD-1) and ipilimumab (anti-CTLA4) are combined, T-cell function is enhanced to a degree greater than either one of the drugs alone, with increased anti-tumor effect.

Metabolism: Steady-state drug concentrations are reached by week 12 when nivolumab is administered at 3 mg/kg every 2 weeks; its elimination half-life is 26.7 days. Clearance increases as body weight increases, so the dose is weight based. Renal impairment and mild hepatic impairment do not affect clearance, but the drug was not studied in patients with moderate or severe hepatic impairment.

Indications: Treatment of patients with:
(1) Melanoma
   • Unresectable or metastatic melanoma, as a single agent or in combination with ipilimumab.
   • Adjuvant treatment of melanoma: for patients with lymph node involvement or metatatic disease who have undergone complete resection.
(2) Metastatic NSCLC with progression on or after platinum-based chemotherapy. Patients with EGFR or ALK genomic tumor aberrations should have disease progression on FDA-approved therapy for these aberrations prior to receiving nivolumab.
(3) Small cell lung cancer (SCLC): metastatic SCLC with progression after platinum-based chemotherapy and at least one other line of therapy. Accelerated approval.
(4) Advanced renal cell carcinoma (RCC):
   • Single agent in patients with advanced RCC who have received prior antiangiogenic therapy.
   • In combination with ipilimumab, in patients with intermediate or poor risk, previously untreated advanced RCC.
(5) Classical Hodgkin lymphoma in adults that has relapsed or progressed after (a) autologous hematopoietic stem cell transplantation (HSCT) and brentuximab vedotin, or (b) 3 or more lines of systemic therapy that includes autologous HSCT. Accelerated FDA approval based on response rate.
(6) Squamous cell carcinoma of the head and neck: Recurrent or metastatic squamous cell carcinoma of the head and neck (SCCHN) with disease progression on or after a platinum-based therapy.
(7) Locally advanced or metastatic urothelial carcinoma in patients who (a) have disease progression during or following platinum-containing chemotherapy, or (b) have disease progression within 12 months of neoadjuvant or adjuvant treatment with platinum-containing chemotherapy. Accelerated FDA approval based on tumor response rate and duration of response.
(8) Microsatellite instability-high (MSI-H) or Mismatch Repair Deficient (dMMR) metastatic colorectal cancer: Treatment of adult and pediatric patients (12 years and older) with MSH-H or mismatch repair deficient (dMMR) metastatic CRC that has progressed following treatment with a fluoropyrimidine, oxaliplatin, and irinotecan (a) as a single agent; or (b) in combination with ipilimumab after progression on fluoropyrimidine, oxaliplatin, and irinotecan. [accelerated approval].
(9) Hepatocellular carcinoma (HCC) previously treated with sorafenib. Accelerated approval.

Dosage/Range:
- Nivolumab is administered IV over 30 minutes.
- *Unresectable or metastatic melanoma*
  - Single agent: 240 mg IV infusion over 60 minutes every 2 weeks, or 480 mg IV infusion every 4 weeks, until disease progression or unacceptable toxicity.
  - with ipilimumab: nivolumab 1 mg/kg IV over 30 minutes followed by ipilimumab 3 mg/kg IV over 90 min, on the same day, every 3 weeks for a maximum of 4 doses or until unacceptable toxicity, After completing 4 doses of the combination, administer nivolumab as a single agent either 240 mg IV infusion every 2 weeks, or nivolumab 480 mg every 4 weeks until disease progression or unacceptable toxicity.
- *Adjuvant treatment of melanoma:* Nivolumab 240 mg every 2 weeks or 480 mg q 4 weeks IV until disease progression or unacceptable toxicity for up to 1 year.
- *Metastatic NSCLC:* nivolumab 240 mg IV every 2 weeks or 480 mg IV every 4 weeks until disease progression or unacceptable toxicity.
- *Metastatic SCLC:* 240 mg IV over 30 minutes every 2 weeks until disease progression or unacceptable toxicity.
- *Advanced RCC:* (a) single agent, nivolumab 240 mg IV infusion every 2 weeks or 480 mg IV every 4 weeks until disease progression or unacceptable toxicity; (b) combination with ipilimumab: nivolumab 3 mg/kg IV infusion over 30 minutes, followed by ipilimumab 1 mg/kg IV over 30 minutes on the same day, every 3 weeks × 4 doses. After completing the 4 ipilimumab doses, give nivolumab as a single agent 240 mg IV infusion every 2 weeks or 480 mg IV every 4 weeks until disease progression or unacceptable toxicity.
- *Classical Hodgkin's lymphoma:* nivolumab 240 mg IV infusion every 2 weeks or 480 mg IV every 4 weeks until disease progression or unacceptable toxicity.
- *Recurrent or metastatic SCCHN:* nivolumab 240 mg IV every 2 weeks or 480 mg q 4 weeks until disease progression or unacceptable toxicity.
- *Locally advanced or metastatic urothelial carcinoma:* nivolumab 240 mg IV infusion every 2 weeks or 480 mg q 4 weeks until disease progression or unacceptable toxicity.
- *MSI-H or mMMR metastatic CRC:* (a) Single agent: (1) adults and children aged 12 years or older and weighing 40 kg or more: nivolumab 240 mg IV infusion every 2 weeks or 480 mg IV infusion every 4 weeks, until disease progression or unacceptable toxicity; (2) children ≥12 years old weighing <40 kg: nivolumab 3 mg/kg every 2 weeks IV infusion over 30 minutes until disease progression or unacceptable toxicity; b) combination with ipilimumab (1) for adults and children aged 12 and above weighing >40 kg: nivolumab 3 mg/kg IV infusion over 30 minutes, followed by ipilimumab 1 mg/kg IV over 30 minutes on the same day, every 3 weeks × 4 doses. After completing the 4 ipilimumab doses, give nivolumab as a single agent 240 mg IV infusion every 2 weeks or 480 mg IV every 4 weeks until disease progression or unacceptable toxicity; for children aged 12 and above, weighing <40 kg: nivolumab 3 mg/kg IV infusion over 30 min, followed by ipilimumab 1 mg/kg IV infusion after the nivolumab, every 3 weeks × 4 weeks; after completing 4 doses of ipilimumab, give nivolumab 3 mg/kg as a single agent every 2 weeks IV over 30 minutes until disease progression or unacceptable toxicity.
- *Hepatocellular carcinoma (HCC):* nivolumab 240 mg IV every 2 weeks, or 480 mg q 4 weeks until disease progression or unacceptable toxicity.

TREATMENT

Dose Modifications:
* Interrupt or slow the infusion rate in patients with mild or moderate infusion reactions based on grade; discontinue nivolumab if reaction is severe or life-threatening.
* If nivolumab is held, ipilimumab should be held as well in patients receiving the combination.
* No recommended dose modification for hypo- or hyperthyroidism.
* Recommended Dose Modifications for nivolumab:
  (1) Colitis: (a) grade 2 diarrhea or colitis: hold dose and resume when adverse reaction returns to grade 0/1; (b) grade 3 diarrhea or colitis as a single agent: hold dose and resume when adverse reaction returns to grade 0/1; (c) grade 3 diarrhea or colitis when given with ipilimumab: permanently discontinue; grade 4: permanently discontinue.
  (2) Pneumonitis: (a) grade 2: hold dose and resume when adverse reaction returns to grade 0/1; (b) grades 3 or 4: permanently discontinue.
  (3a) Hepatitis/ non HCC: (a) AST/or ALT $>$ 3–5 $\times$ ULN or total bilirubin $>$ 1.5–3 $\times$ ULN: hold dose and resume when adverse reaction returns to grade 0/1; (b) AST or ALT $>$5 $\times$ ULN or total bilirubin $>$ 3 $\times$ ULN, permanently discontinue.
  (3b) Hepatitis/HCC: (a) Hold dose and resume when AST/ALT return to baseline if (1) AST/ALT WNL at baseline and inceases to $>$3X and up to 5 $\times$ ULN: (2) if AST/ALT is $>$1 and up to 3 $\times$ ULN at baseline and increases to to $>$5 $\times$ and up to 10 $\times$ ULN; or if AST/ALT is $>$3 and up to 5 $\times$ ULN at baseline and increases to $>$8 and up to 10 $\times$ ULN. (b) Permanently discontinue drug if AST/ALT increase to $>$10 $\times$ ULN or total bilirubin increases to $>$3 $\times$ ULN.
  (4) Hypophysitis: (a) grades 2–3: hold dose and resume when adverse reaction returns to grade 0/1; (b) grade 4: permanently discontinue.
  (5) Adrenal insufficiency: (a) grade 2: hold dose and resume when adverse reaction returns to grade 0/1; (b) grades 3–4: permanently discontinue.
  (6) Type 1 Diabetes Mellitus: (a) grade 3 hyperglycemia: hold dose and resume when adverse reaction returns to grade 0/1; (b) grade 4: permanently discontinue.
  (7) Nephritis and renal dysfunction: (a) serum creatinine $>$1.5 to 6 $\times$ ULN, hold dose and resume when adverse reaction returns to grade 0/1; (b) serum creatinine $>$ 6 $\times$ ULN: permanently discontinue.
  (8) Skin rash: (a) grade 3 rash or suspected SJS or TEN, hold dose and resume when adverse reaction returns to grade 0/1; (b) grade 4 or confirmed SJS or TEN: permanently discontinue.
  (9) Encephalitis: (a) new-onset moderate or severe neurologic signs or symptoms, hold dose and resume when adverse reaction returns to grade 0/1; (b) immune-mediated: permanently discontinue.
  (10) Other: (a) Other grade 3 adverse reaction: first occurrence, hold dose and resume when adverse reaction returns to grade 0/1; recurrence of same grade 3 reaction, permanently discontinue; (b) life-threatening or grade 4 adverse reaction: permanently discontinue; (c) grade 3 myocarditis: permanently discontinue; (d) requirement for 10 mg/day or greater prednisone or equivalent for $>$12 weeks, permanently discontinue; (e) persistent grade 2 or 3 adverse reactions lasting $>$ 12 weeks, permanently discontinue.

Drug Preparation: Available as 10 mg/mL conentrations: 40 mg/4 mL,100 mg/10 mL, and 240 mg/24 mL solutions in single-use vials.

- Visually inspect drug for particulate matter or discoloration (should be opalescent, colorless to pale yellow) and discard if any is found.
- *Preparation:* Withdraw the required drug volume and transfer it to an IV container; dilute with either 0.9% sodium chloride USP or 5% dextrose injection USP, to prepare an infusion with a final concentration 1–10 mg/mL. The total volume of infusion must not exceed 160 mL. For adult and pediatric patients weighing <40 kg, the total infusion volume must not exceed 4 mL/kg of body weight. Mix diluted solution by inversion, and *do not shake*. Discard any partially used or empty vials.
- *Storage:* As the drug does not contain a preservative, store at room temperature for no more than 8 hours from the time of preparation (includes room-temperature storage of infusion in the IV container **and time for administration of the infusion**). Or, store under refrigeration (2–8°C [36–46°F]), and nivolumab infusion is stable for up to 24 hours from time of infusion preparation. *Do not freeze.*

Drug Administration:
- Administer as an infusion over 30 minutes through an IV line containing a sterile, nonpyrogenic, low-protein-binding in-line filter (pore size, 0.2–1.2 micrometer).
- When administered in combination with ipilimumab, **infuse nivolumab first** followed by ipilimumab on the same day. Use separate infusion bags and filters for each infusion.
- Do not administer other drugs through the same line.
- Flush the IV line at the end of the infusion.
- Interrupt or slow the infusion rate in patients with mild or moderate infusion reactions; discontinue nivolumab if reaction is severe or life-threatening. Assess and monitor patient closely. Provide supportive medical intervention as ordered.

Drug Interactions: Studies have not been conducted.

Lab Effects/Interference:
- Decreased serum sodium, potassium, magnesium, and calcium.
- Decreased lymphocyte, red cell, and platelet counts.
- Increased creatinine, calcium, potassium, AST, ALT, alkaline phosphatase, glucose, triglycerides, cholesterol.

Special Considerations:
- Most common adverse effects (≥20% of patients) treating patients with: (1) as a single agent, fatigue,r ash, musculoskeletal pain, pruritus, diarrhea, nausea, asthenia, cough,dyspnea, constipation: fatigue, rash, pyrexia, diarrhea, nausea, vomiting, dyspnea; in combination with ipilimumab: fatigue, rash, diarrhea, nausea, pyrexia, vomiting, dyspnea; (2) melanoma with combined nivolumab and ipilimumab; (3) renal cell carcinoma with ipilimumab and nivolumab: fatigue, rash, diarrhea, musculoskeletal pain, pruritus, nausea, cough, pyrexia, arthralgia, decreased appetite.
- Severe infusion reactions have been reported in < 1.0% of patients. Incidence of all infusion reactions ranged from 2.7 to 6%. Interrupt or slow the infusion rate in patients

with mild or moderate infusion reactions. Discontinue drug if patient has a severe or life-threatening reaction.

- Immune-mediated adverse reactions (irAEs) are possible. If suspected, exclude other causes.
  - Based on the severity of the reaction, withhold nivolumab and administer high-dose corticosteroid, and as appropriate, administer hormone-replacement therapy.
  - Upon improvement to grades 0–1, begin corticosteroid taper and continue for at least 1 month. Consider restarting nivolumab after the taper is completed if reasonable, but recognize that the drug may require permanent discontinuation.
- Warnings and Precautions:
  - irAEs (see Opdivo package insert):
    - *Pneumonitis:* Definition of pneumonitis is requiring use of corticosteroids without alternate etiology. In single agent clinical trials, incidence was 3.1% (increasing to 6% with ipilimumab). Most patients (84%) required high-dose corticosteroids for a median duration of 30 days. Monitor patients for signs and symptoms of pneumonitis with imaging and history. Administer corticosteroids 1–2 mg/kg/day prednisone as ordered or equivalent for moderate (grade 2) or more severe (grade 3–4) pneumonitis, followed by taper. Grade 2: hold nivolumab and resume when signs/symptoms and imaging resolved. Permanently discontinue for severe (grade 3) or life-threatening (grade 4). See "Potential Toxicities/Side Effects and the Nursing Process."
    - *Colitis:* Incidence of diarrhea or colitis was 2.9% of patients as a single agent, with median time to onset for immune colitis of 5.3 months (increased to 26% with ipilimumab with median onset at 1.6 months). Monitor patients for signs/symptoms of colitis. If diagnosed, (a) hold drug for grade 2 and grade 3 colitis, and permanently discontinue for grade 4 or recurrent colitis; (b) grade 2 (moderate) lasting >5 days: administer 0.5–1 mg/kg/da prednisone equivalents followed by taper; and if worsening or no improvement, increase to 1–2 mg/kg/day prednisone; grade 3 (severe) or grade 4 (life-threatening): Administer 1–2 mg/kg/day prednisone equivalents, followed by taper over at least 4 weeks. Some patients will need additional immune suppression with infliximab. See "Potential Toxicities/Side Effects and the Nursing Process."
    - *Hepatitis:* Monitor LFTs baseline and during treatment. Non HCC patients; hold the drug for grade 2 hepatotoxicity and permanently discontinue for severe (grade 3) or life-threatening (grade 4). HCC patients: Hold, discontinue, or continue based on severity (see package insert); if drug is held or discontinued, give corticosteroids for prednisone 1–2 mg/kg/day or equivalent followed by a taper.
    - *Hypophysitis:* Incidence ranges from 0.6% (9% with ipilimumab). Monitor for signs and symptoms. Replace hormone(s) as ordered based on labs. Hold drug and administer corticosteroids for moderate (grade 2) or grade 3. Permanently discontinue drug for severe (grade 4).
    - *Adrenal insufficiency:* incidence ranged from 1% (5% with ipilimumab). Assess for signs and symptoms during therapy and after treatment. Hold drug for grade

2 or higher, administer corticosteroids for grade 3 or higher, and discontinue drug for grade 3 or higher. Taper corticosteroids over at least 1 month.

- *Type I Diabetes Mellitus* can occur. Monitor for hyperglycemia. Administer insulin, and hold drug for grade 3 hyperglycemia until metabolic control achieved. Permanently discontinue drug for grade 4 hyperglycemia.
- *Nephritis and renal dysfunction:* Monitor serum creatinine baseline and periodically during treatment. Hold drug for grade 2 or 3 and permanently discontinue for grade 4. Administer corticosteroids with taper for grade 2 or higher.
- *Hypothyroidism and hyperthyroidism:* Incidence in clinical trials for hypothyroidism ranged from 9% (22% with ipilimumab), and for hyperthyroidism, 2.7% (8% with ipilimumab). Monitor thyroid function at baseline and periodically during therapy. If hypothyroidism occurs, the patient should receive hormone replacement therapy. If hyperthyroidism occurs, discuss medical management with the physician/NP/PA. The drug dose does not require modification.
- *Immune-related rash:* Incidence ranged from 9% (22.6% in ipilimumab combination). Monitor for rash as severe rash may occur (e.g., TEN). Hold drug if SJS or TEN is suspected, and obtain dermatology consult/biopsy. Permanently discontinue if SJS or TEN diagnosis is confirmed. Hold drug and administer corticosteroids with taper for grade 3 or higher rash, and permanently discontinue for grade 4 (severe, life-threatening) rash.
- *Immune-related encephalitis* is rare (0.2%); hold drug in patients with new-onset moderate to severe neurologic signs/symptoms and further evaluate to rule out infectious or other causes of neurological deterioration. This may include neurology consult, brain MRI, LP. If all other possible etiologies ruled out, corticosteroids with taper should be administered.
- *Other immune-mediated adverse reactions* (irAEs) may occur, including after the drug is discontinued. These reactions are uncommon, but include uveitis, iritis, pancreatitis, autoimmune neuropathy, systemic inflammatory response syndrome (SIRS) and vasculitis. Consider corticosteroid therapy based on the severity of the reaction, and taper over a month once resolved (grades 0–1).
- *Infusion Reactions:* Rare (<1%); Interrupt or slow infusion rate for mild to moderate infusion reactions, and discontinue drug if severe or life-threatening. Rarely, signs/symptoms may occur within 48 hours of infusion. Teach patient to self-assess and report right away.
- *Complications of allogeneic HSCT after nivolumab.* Follow patients closely for early evidence of transplant-related complications (e.g., hyperacute GVHD, severe (grades 3–4) GVHD, steroid-requiring febrile syndrome, hepatic veno-oclusive disease (VOD) and other possible reactions.
- *Embryo-fetal toxicity:* Nivolumab can cause fetal harm. Teach women of reproductive age to use effective contraception to avoid pregnancy during treatment and for 5 months following the last dose. Women should not breastfeed while receiving the drug.
- *Increased mortality in patients with multiple myeloma when nivolumab is added to a thalidomide analogue and dexamethasone:* Do not administer PD-1 or PD-L1 blocking antibody to multiple myeloma patients in combination with a thalidomide analogue plus dexamethasone.

Potential Toxicities/Side Effects and the Nursing Process

I. ALTERATION IN COMFORT related to FATIGUE, ASTHENIA, MUSCULOSKELETAL PAIN, OR ARTHRALGIA

Defining Characteristics: Asthenia and fatigue were common. Arthralgia, back pain, and musculoskeletal pain can also occur.

Nursing Implications: Teach the patient that these events may occur and to report them. Assess baseline comfort and self-care strategies to maintain comfort and energy conservation. Monitor closely during treatment. Develop a plan to assure comfort, depending on the symptoms reported, and assess its efficacy and revise the plan if needed at each visit.

II. ALTERATION IN NUTRITION, POTENTIAL, LESS THAN BODY REQUIREMENTS, related to DECREASED APPETITE, NAUSEA, CONSTIPATION, VOMITING, OR DIARRHEA

Defining Characteristics: Nutritional impact symptoms of nausea, vomiting, diarrhea, constipation, and decreased appetite can occur.

Nursing Implications: Assess nutritional and bowel-elimination patterns, appetite, and presence of nausea and/or vomiting at baseline and at each visit. Teach that diarrhea, constipation, nausea, vomiting, and decreased appetite may occur and to report them. Assess nutrition impact symptoms and discuss their management with the physician. Teach the patient to self-administer antidiarrheal or antiemetic medication, if needed, and to report symptoms that do not improve. In addition, teach patients to report immediately any diarrhea, blood in stool or black stools, and severe stomach pain or tenderness so that the potential for colitis may be further evaluated.

III. ALTERATION IN SKIN INTEGRITY, POTENTIAL, related to RASH, PRURITUS, OR EDEMA

Defining Characteristics: Skin integrity can be affected by rash, edema, and pruritis.

Nursing Implications: Teach the patient that rash, pruritus, and peripheral edema may occur and report them. Assess the patient's skin integrity and determine the presence of edema, both at baseline and regularly during therapy. Teach patient self-care measures to reduce pruritis.

IV. POTENTIAL ALTERATION IN OXYGENATION related to PNEUMONITIS

Defining Characteristics: In all clinical trials, incidence was 3.1–6% (increasing to 6% with ipilimumab), with median time to onset of 1.6 (with combination) to 3.5 months (single agent).

Nursing Implications: Teach the patient to report new or worsening cough, chest pain, or shortness of breath. Monitor the patient for signs and symptoms of pneumonitis. Discuss findings with the physician/NP/PA. Expect that after exclusion of other diagnoses, the patient will be evaluated with imaging and pulmonary and infectious disease consultation if respiratory status changes occur.

- Grade 1 (x-ray changes only): Discuss management with provider, e.g., holding nivolumab, and monitor every 2–3 days. Reassess at least every 3 weeks, and if improved, resume nivolumab. If the patient's condition worsens, treat as it as grade 2 or 3/4.
- Grade 2 or higher: Withhold the drug until resolution for moderate (grade 2) or higher severity, and permanently discontinue it for severe (grade 3) or life-threatening (grade 4) pneumonitis. Administer corticosteroids at a dose of 1–2 mg/kg/day (prednisone or equivalent) for grade $\geq$ 2, followed by a taper. Monitor daily. Consult pulmonary and infectious disease specialists, and consider bronchoscopy and lung biopsy. If the patient improves and returns to baseline, taper steroids over at least 1 month. For grade 2 pneumonitis which has resolved, after the taper is completed, consider resuming nivolumab.

V.   POTENTIAL ALTERATION IN ELIMINATION related to COLITIS

Defining Characteristics: Incidence of diarrhea or colitis was 25–31% (increased to 56% with ipilimumab), but incidence of immune-mediated colitis (requiring corticosteroids without alternate etiology) was 2.4–4.1% (26% with nivolumab and ipilimumab combination). Time to onset was 1.6–6.7 months. Monitor patients for immune-mediated colitis.

Nursing Implications: Teach the patient to report signs and symptoms of colitis (diarrhea, blood in stools or tarry stools, severe abdominal pain). Monitor the patient for immune-mediated colitis, and administer corticosteroids as ordered.

- *Grade 1:* Continue nivolumab.
- *Grade 2:* Hold nivolumab as ordered. If colitis symptoms persist for more than 5 days, or recur, expect a corticosteroid to be ordered at a dose of 0.5–1 mg/kg/day (prednisone or equivalent). Once the patient is improved, and after corticosteroid taper over at least 1 month if used, nivolumab can be resumed. If symptoms worsen or persist for longer than 3–5 days with oral steroids, treat as grade 3/4.
- *Grade 3/4:* Hold drug and administer prescribed corticosteroids 1–2 mg/kg/day (prednisone or equivalent), followed by a taper.
- *Grade 3:* Hold nivolumab until the patient is at grades 0–1, then taper the steroids over at least 1 month. If symptoms persist or worsen or are grade 4, permanently discontinue nivolumab. If the patient's condition is improved from persistent grade 3 or 4, continue steroids until the patient is at grade 1, then taper over at least 1 month. Lower GI endoscopy should be considered if needed.
- When administered with ipilimumab, hold nivolumab for moderate (grade 2) colitis. Permanently discontinue nivolumab for severe or life-threatening colitis (grades 3–4) or for recurrent colitis upon restarting nivolumab.

VI.   POTENTIAL ALTERATION IN NUTRTION related to HEPATITIS

Defining Characteristics: Immune-mediated hepatitis (defined as requiring use of corticosteroids and no clear alternate etiology) and abnormal LFTs may occur. Incidence in clinical trials was 0.3–2.3% (13% with nivolumab/ipilimumab combination).

  Signs and symptoms of hepatitis include elevated transaminases and total bilirubin, icterus, severe nausea and vomiting, right-sided abdominal pain, drowsiness, dark urine, increased bruisability or bleeding, and anorexia.

Nursing Implications: Assess LFTs at baseline and monitor regularly during therapy. Evaluate the patient for right-sided abdominal pain, drowsiness, dark urine, increased bruising or bleeding, and loss of appetite. Teach the patient to report any yellowing of the skin or whites of the eyes, as well as severe nausea or vomiting. Expect the following orders if abnormal LFTs occur:

- *Grade 1:* AST or AST > ULN to 3.0 × ULN and/or total bilirubin > ULN to 1.5 × ULN: Continue nivolumab and closely monitor LFTs.
- *Grade 2:* AST or ALT > 3.0 to < 5 × ULN and/or total bilirubin > 1.5 to ≤ 3 × ULN: Hold nivolumab and assess LFTs every 3 days; administer 0.5–1 mg/kg/day prednisone equivalents. If LFTs improve to grade 1 or baseline, resume nivolumab; if steroids were administered, taper them over at least 1 month before resuming nivolumab. Monitor baseline and LFTs routinely.
- *Grade 3/4:* AST or ALT > 5 × ULN and/or total bilirubin > 3 × ULN: Permanently discontinue nivolumab, and increase LFT monitoring to every 1–2 days. Consult GI specialist and administer corticosteroids 1–2 mg/kg/day (prednisone or equivalent). When the patient has improved to grade 0–1, taper steroids over at least 1 month. If lab abnormalities persist for more than 3–5 days, worsen, or rebound, add noncorticosteroid immunosuppressive medication. Discontinue drug for grades 3 or 4 transaminase elevations with or without concomitant total bilirubin elevation.

VII.   POTENTIAL ALTERATION IN URINE ELIMINATION related to IMMUNE-MEDIATED NEPHRITIS AND RENAL DYSFUNCTION

Defining Characteristics: Immune-related nephritis defined as renal dysfunction or grade 2 or higher increased creatinine, requirement for corticosteroids, and no clear alternate etiology, can occur.

Nursing Implications: Assess the patient's baseline renal function, and monitor closely during therapy. Teach the patient to report signs and symptoms such as a decrease in the amount of urine, blood in urine, ankle swelling, loss of appetite.

- *Grades 2 (moderate) to 3 (severe):* Expect the following: hold nivolumab and administer corticosteroids (prednisone or equivalent of 0.5–1 mg/kg/day, then taper over at least 1 month). If patient worsens or there is no improvement, increase dose to 1–2 mg/kg/day and permanently discontinue nivolumab.
- *Grade 4:* Permanently discontinue nivolumab. Give corticosteroids 1–2 mg/kg/day (prednisone or equivalent), then taper over 1 month.

VIII. POTENTIAL ALTERATION IN ENDOCRINE FUNCTION related to HYPOTHYROIDISM, HYPERTHYROIDISM, HYPERGLYCEMIA, OR ADRENAL CRISIS

Defining Characteristics: Incidence in clinical trials for hypothyroidism ranged from 7 to 9% (22% with ipilimumab), and for hyperthyroidism, 1.4–4.4% (8% with ipilimumab). Type 1 diabetes mellitus may occur.

Nursing Implications: Monitor thyroid function at baseline and periodically during therapy. Monitor for hyperglycemia. Teach the patient to report signs and symptoms of hyper and hypothyroidism, such as headaches that do not go away, extreme tiredness, weight gain or loss, changes in mood or behavior, dizziness or fainting, hair loss, feeling cold, constipation, and deep and/or hoarse voice. Discuss and teach the patient about ordered hormone replacement therapy for hypothyroidism, or medical management of hyperthyroidism. Monitor thyroid function at baseline and periodically during therapy. If hypothyroidism occurs, the patient should receive hormone replacement therapy. If hyperthyroidism occurs, discuss medical management with the physician/NP/PA. The drug dose does not require modification. If patient is hyperglycemic administer insulin as ordered, and hold drug for grade 3 hyperglycemia until control achieved. Discontinue drug for grade 4 hyperglycemia.

Expect the following medical management:
- *Asymptomatic endocrinopathy* (TSH < 0.5 × LLN or TSH > 2 × ULN, or consistently out of range in 2 subsequent assessments; include free T_4 at subsequent cycles as clinically indicated): Continue nivolumab; consider endocrine consult.
- *Symptomatic endocrinopathy:* Continue nivolumab for hypothyroidism or hyperthyroidism, but hold drug for other endocrinopathies with abnormal lab/pituitary scan. Monitor endocrine function, and consider pituitary scan if not already done; repeat lab tests in 1–3 weeks, and MRI in 1 month if symptoms persist but lab tests and pituitary scan are within normal limits. Consider endocrine consult, and start hormone replacement if the patient is symptomatic with abnormal lab tests and pituitary scan.
- *Suspicion of adrenal crisis:* Hold nivolumab, rule out sepsis, obtain an endocrine consult, administer stress-dose of IV steroids with mineralocorticoid activity, and give IV hydration.

Drug: obinutuzumab injection (Gazyva®)

Class: IgG_1 mAb (humanized) targeted at the CD_{20} molecule on B-cell lymphocyte membranes.

Mechanism of Action: Mab binds to the CD_{20} antigen on pre B- and mature B-lymphocytes, and lyses the B-lymphocytes directly through activation of intracellular death pathways, activation of the complement cascade, and indirectly through engagement of immune effector cells (e.g., antibody-dependent cellular cytotoxicity and ADCP).

Metabolism: Half-life approximately 28.4 days.

Indications: Obinutuzumab (Gazyva) is indicated (1) in combination with chlorambucil for the treatment of patients with previously untreated CLL; (2) in combination with bendamustine followed by obinutuzumab monotherapy in patients with follicular lymphoma (FL) who relapsed after or who are refractory to a rituximab-containing regimen; (3) in combination with chemotherapy followed by obinutuzumab monotherapy in patients achieving at least a PR, for the treatment of adult patients with previously untreated stage II bulky, III or IV FL.

Contraindications: patients with known hypersensitivity reactions (e.g., anaphylaxis) to obinutuzumab or any of the excipients, including serum sickness with prior obinutuzumab use.

Dosage/Range:
- Premedicate with a glucocorticoid (e.g., IV 20 mg dexamethasone or 80 mg methylprednisolone), acetaminophen (650–1,000 mg), and antihistamine (e.g., diphenhydramine 50 mg) before each infusion. Hydrocortisone is not used, as it is not effective in reducing the rate of infusion reactions.
- Administer prophylactic hydration and anti-hyperuricemics to patients at high risk for TLS as ordered.
- Doses:
  - CLL (six 28-day treatment cycles):
    - Cycle 1: 100 mg day 1 infused at 25 mg/hr over 4 hours. Do NOT increase the infusion rate. Day 2: 900 mg at 50 mg/hr if no previous infusion reaction; infusion rate can be escalated in increments of 50 mg/hr every 30 min to a maximum rate of 400 mg/hr.
    - Cycle 1, days 8, 15 and cycles 2–6, day 1; 1,000 mg; if no previous infusion reaction and the final infusion rate was 100 mg/hr or faster, infusions can be started at 100 mg/hr and increased by 100 mg/hr every 30 minutes to a maxium of 400 mg/hr. If an infusion reaction occurred during prior infusion, administer at 50 mg/hr. Rate can be excalated in increments of 50 mg/hr every 30 minutes to a maximum rate of 400 mg/hr.
    - If a planned dose of obinutuzumab is missed, administer the missed dose as soon as possible and adjust dosing schedule to maintain the time interval between doses. If appropriate, patients who do not complete the day 1 cycle 1 dose may proceed to the day 2 cycle 1 dose.
  - FL: 28-day cycle; 1,000 mg IV each dose. Six to eight treatment cycles, followed by monotherapy.
    - Cycle 1 (loading doses) day 1: administer at 50 mg/hr; infusion rate can be escalated in 50 mg/hr increments every 30 min to a maximum of 400 mg/hr On Cycle 1, Day 8 and 15: if no IR or a grade 1 IR, and the last infusion rate was 100 mg/hr, infusion can be started at 100 mg/hr. For cycles 2–6 or 2–8, Day 1 only, then every 2 months for up to 2 years: if no previous infusion reaction and the final infusion rate was 100 mg/hr or faster, infusions can be started at 100 mg/hr and increased by 100 mg/hr every 30 minutes to a maxium of 400 mg/hr. If an infusion reaction of grade 2 or higher occurred in prior infusion, start infusion at 50 mg/hr; escalate infusion rate in increments of 50 mg/hr every 30 minutes to a maximal dose of 400 mg/hr.

- Patients with relapsed or refractory FL: administer obinutuzumab in combination with bendamustine in six 28-day cycles. If patient achieves stable disease, CR or PR to the initial 6 cycles, continue obinutuzumab 1000 as monotherapy for up to 2 years.
- For patients with previously untreated FL, administer obinutuzumab with one of the following chemotherapy regimes: (a) six 28-day cycles in combination with bendamustine; (b) six 28-day cycles in combination with CHP followed by 2 additional 21-day cycles of obinutuzumab alone; (c) eight 21-day cycles in combination with CVP.
- Patients with previously untreated FL who achieve a CR or PR after initial 6 or 8 cycles should continue on obinutuzumab 1,000 mg as monotherapy for up to 2 years.
- If a planned dose of obinutuzumab is missed, administer the missed dose as soon as possible and adjust dosing schedule to maintain the time interval between doses. During monotherapy, maintain original dosing schedule for subsequent doses. Monotherapy should start approximately 2 months after the last dose of obinutuzumab administered during the induction phase.
- Premedication for microbial prophylaxis: Neutropenic patients should receive antiviral and antifungal prophylaxis.
- Consider treatment interruption for infection, grades 3–4 cytopenia, or ≥ grade 2 non-hematologic toxicity.

Drug Preparation:
- Available in 1,000 mg/40 mL (25 mg/mL) single-use vials.
- Inspect vial for any particulate matter, discoloration; do not use if found.
- Aseptically dilute into a 0.9% sodium chloride PVC or non-PVC polyolefin infusion bag. **Do not use** other diluents (e.g., dextrose 5%).
- CLL:
  - Cycle 1, day 1 (100 mg) and day 2 (900 mg): withdraw 40 mL Gazyva from vial. Dilute 4 mL (100 mg) into a 100-mL 0.9% sodium chloride infusion bag for immediate administration. Dilute the remaining 36 mL (900 mg) into a 250-mL 0.9% sodium chloride infusion bag at the same time for use on day 2 and store at 2–8°C (36–46°F) for up to 24 hours. After allowing the diluted bag to come to room temperature, use immediately. CLEARLY label each infusion bag.
  - Cycle 1, days 8 and 15, and day 1, cycles 2–6: withdraw 40 mL of Gazyva solution (1,000 mg) from the vial and dilute in 250-mL 0.9% sodium chloride infusion bag.
  - FL: withdraw 40 mL of Gazyva solution (1,000 mg) from the vial and dilute in 250-mL 0.9% sodium chloride infusion bag.
    - Gently rotate bag to mix, but do not shake or freeze.
    - Use diluted infusion immediately, or within 24 hours when refrigerated at 2–8°C (36–46°F).
- Administer at a final concentration of 0.4–4 mg/mL.

Drug Administration:
- Ensure all patients have had HBV screening before drug is initiated. If patient is HBV-positive, monitor them during and after treatment closely. If HBV is reactivated, discontinue obinutuzumab.
- Administer IV infusion only, never IVP or IVB through a *dedicated line*. Do not mix with other drugs.

- Premedicate before each infusion.
- Provide prophylactic hydration and antihyperuricemics as ordered for patients at high risk for TLS.
- Monitor CBC/differential baseline and regularly during therapy as ordered.
- Appropriate medical support and emergency equipment must be readily available to manage infusion reactions if they occur (and may be fatal).

Administer Premedication:
- Cycle 1: (a) CLL Day 1,2; (b) FL: Day 1: (1) IV glucocorticoid (e.g., 20 mg dexamethasone or 80 mg methylprednisolone) completed at least 1 hour prior to obinutuzumab infusion; (2) PO acetaminophen (650–1,000 mg) and antihistamine (e.g., 50 mg diphenylhydramine) given at least 30 minutes prior to obinutuzumab infusion.
- All subsequent infusions (CLL, FL): (1) all patients: PO acetaminophen 650–1,000 mg at least 30 minutes prior to obinutuzumab infusion; (2) patients with an infusion reaction grades 1–2 in previous infusion: acetaminophen and antihistamine at least 30 minutes before obinutuzumab infusion; (3) patients with a grade 3 infusion reaction with previous infusion OR lymphocyte count $>25 \times 10^9$/L prior to next treatment: IV glucocorticoid (dexamethasone 20 mg or 80 mg methylprednisolone) completed at least 1 hour prior, acetaminophen, and antihistamine given at least 30 minutes prior to obinutuzumab infusion (Genentech, 2017).
- TLS Prophylaxis: If the patient has a high tumor burden, and/or high number of circulating lymphocytes ($> 25 \times 10^9$/L) or renal impairment, premedicate with antihyperuricemics (e.g., allopurinol) as ordered, starting 12–24 hours before initiating obinutuzumab (Gazyva) therapy, and continue prophylaxis prior to each obinutuzumab infusion as needed. Also, ensure adequate hydration to prevent TLS.
  - **Antimicrobial Prophylaxis:** Patients with grades 3–4 neutropenia lasting >1 week should receive antimicrobial prophylaxis until resolution of neutropenia to grades 1–2. Consider antiviral and antifungal prophylaxis.
  - **Treatment interruption for toxicity:** Consider treatment interruption for grades 3–4 cytopenias, or $\geq$ nonhematologic toxicity.
- Ensure emergency medications, equipment, and support personnel are available in the even that severe infusion reaction(s) occur.
- Monitor CBC/differential baseline and at regular intervals.
- Infusion Administration
- CLL (six 28-day treatment cycles):
  - Cycle 1: 100 mg day 1 infused at 25 mg/hr over 4 hours. Do NOT increase the infusion rate. Day 2: 900 mg at 50 mg/hr if no previous infusion reaction; infusion rate can be escalated in increments of 50 mg/hr every 30 min to a maximum rate of 400 mg/hr.
  - Cycle 1, days 8, 15, and cycles 2–6, day 1; 1,000 mg; if no previous infusion reaction and the final infusion rate was 100 mg/hr or faster, infusions can be started at 100 mg/hr and increased by 100 mg/hr every 30 minutes to a maxium of 400 mg/hr. If an infusion reaction occurred during prior infusion, administer at 50 mg/hr. Rate can be excalated in increments of 50 mg/hr every 30 minutes to a maximum rate of 400 mg/hr.
  - If a planned dose of obinutuzumab is missed, administer the missed dose as soon as possible and adjust dosing schedule to maintain the time interval between doses. If

appropriate, patients who do not complete the day 1 cycle 1 dose may proceed to the day 2 cycle 1 dose.

- FL: 28-day cycle; 1,000 mg IV each dose. Six to eight treatment cyces, followed by monotherapy.
  - Cycle 1 (loading doses) day 1: administer at 50 mg/hr; infusion rate can be escalated in 50 mg/hr increments every 30 min to a maximum of 400 mg/hr Days 8, 15, cycles 2–6 or day 1, cycles 2–8 only, then every 2 months for up to 2 years: if no previous infusion reaction and the final infusion rate was 100 mg/hr or faster, infusions can be started at 100 mg/hr and increased by 100 mg/hr every 30 minutes to a maxium of 400 mg/hr. If an infusion reaction of grade 2 or higher occurred in prior infusion, start infusion at 50 mg/hr; escalate infusion rate in increments of 50 mg/hr every 30 minutes to a maximal dose of 400 mg/hr.
  - Patients with relapsed or refractory FL: administer obinutuzumab in combination with bendamustine in six 28-day cycles. If patient achieves stable disease, CR or PR to the initial 6 cycles, continue obinutuzumab 1000 as monotherapy for up to 2 years.
  - For patients with previously untreated FL, administer obinutuzumab with one of the following chemotherapy regimes: (a) six 28-day cycles in combination with bendamustine; (b) six 28-day cycles in combination with CHP followed by 2 additional 21-day cycles of obinutuzumab alone; (c) eight 21-day cycles in combination with CVP.
  - Patients with previously untreated FL who achieve a CR or PR after initial 6 or 8 cycles should continue on obinutuzumab 1,000 mg as monotherapy for up to 2 years.
  - If a planned dose of obinutuzumab is missed, administer the missed dose as soon as possible and adjust dosing schedule to maintain the time interval between doses. During monotherapy, maintain original dosing schedule for subsequent doses. Monotherapy should start approximately 2 months after the last dose of obinutuzumab administered during the induction phase.
- **Infusion Reactions:**
  - Grade 4 (life-threatening): Stop infusion, manage symptoms per provider, and permanently discontinue obinutuzumab.
  - Grade 3 (severe): Interrupt and manage symptoms. When resolved, consider resuming obinutuzumab at no more than half the previous infusion rate. If the patient does not have further infusion reactions, escalate the infusion rate per cycle day as above. If the patient again has a grade 3 infusion reaction when rechallenged, stop infusion and permanently discontinue. FOR CLL patients only, the day 1 infusion rate may be increased back up to 25 mg/hr after 1 hour but NOT increased further.
  - Grade 1–2 (mild-moderate): reduce infusion rate or interrupt infusion, and manage symptoms. When symptoms resolve, continue or resume infusion. If the patient has no further infusion reaction, escalate infusion rate per treatment cycle as above. FOR CLL patients only, the day 1 infusion rate may be increased back up to 25 mg/hr after 1 hour but NOT increased further.
  - Hypotension may occur during obinutuzumab infusion; consider having patients taking antihypertensive medications hold their medication 12 hours prior to and throughout each obinutuzumab infusion and for the first hour after obinutuzumab administration.

Drug Interactions:
- No formal studies have been done.

Lab Effects/Interference:
- Neutropenia, lymphopenia, leukopenia, thrombocytopenia, anemia.
- Increased AST, ALT
- Decreased serum calcium, sodium, albumin, potassium.

Special Considerations:
- Warnings and Precautions:
  - *Hepatitis B reactivation:* may occur, which rarely may result in fulminant hepatitis, hepatic failure, and death. All patients should be screened for HBV infection (measuring HBsAg and anti-HBc) before starting obinutuzumab therapy. If patient shows evidence of hepatitis B infection, consult with a hepatitis expert about monitoring and consideration for HBV antiviral therapy. Monitor all patients with current or prior HBV infection closely (clinical and laboratory) for signs of hepatitis and HBV reactivation (e.g., increased transaminase levels, bilirubin) during and after completion of treatment. If a patient does experience HBV reactivation, discontinue obinutuzumab and concomitant chemotherapy.
  - *JC (John Cunningham) virus infection* called PML, may rarely occur. The infection occurs in the brain white matter, damaging cells that make myelin (neuronal insulation). While many people carry the JC virus, it is only virulent if immunosuppressed, and then can be fatal. Consider JC in the differential of any patient with new onset or changes in neurological status. Consider evaluation by a neurologist, brain MRI, and LP. Discontinue obinutuzumab, and consider cessation of chlorambucil if the patient develops PML. Teach patients to report any new neurologic symptoms such as confusion, dizziness, loss of balance, difficulty talking or walking, or vision problems right away.
  - *Infusion reactions* occurred in 65% of CLL patients during the infusion of the first 1,000 mg of drug infused, but reactions can also occur with later infusions within 24 hours of the infusion. In CLL clinical trials, when premedication was administered and the initial dose divided into 2 days, the incidence of infusion reactions decreased to 47%. Thirty-eight percent of the patients with relapsed or refractory NHL patients experienced an infusion reaction on Day 1. Premedicate patients with acetaminophen, antihistamine, and glucocorticoid agents, and divide CLL first dose (see Drug Administration). Slowly escalate dose as ordered (see Drug Administration). Monitor patients closely during infusions, and stop the drug if a reaction occurs. Most frequent symptoms are nausea, fatigue, dizziness, vomiting, diarrhea, HTN, flushing, headache, fever, chills. However, more severe symptoms including hypotension, tachycardia, dyspnea, respiratory symptoms (e.g., bronchospasm, laryngeal and throat irritation, wheezing, laryngeal edema) can occur. Manage severe reactions as needed with glucocorticoids, epinephrine, bronchodilators, and/or oxygen and administer medications as ordered. Stop the drug and permanently discontinue if patient develops anaphylaxis, or any other life-threatening symptoms. For grade 3 reactions, interrupt drug until symptoms resolve. For grades 1–2, interrupt or slow infusion rate (see Drug Administration).

- *Hypersensitivity reactions (HSRs) including serum sickness:* Hypersensitivity has been reported with immediate-onset signs of dyspnea, bronchospasm, hypotension, urticaria, and tachycardia. Late-onset sign/symptoms of hypersensitivity (serum sickness) includes chest pain, diffuse arthralgias, and fever. It may be difficult to distinguish from IRRs. However, HSRs rarely occur on first dose, rather they occur after sensitization in subsequent cycles. If HSR suspected, stop infusion if during, and permanently discontinue. Do not rechallenge. Reaction may occur after the end of the infusion. Teach patient signs/symptoms to report right away and how to get emergency medical care.
- *TLS*: Rapid lymphocyte lysis can cause TLS within 12–24 hours of initial drug infusion, characterized by acute renal failure, hyperkalemia, hyperuricemia, and/or hyperphosphatemia. Patients with high tumor burden and/or high circulating lymphocyte counts ($> 25 \times 10^9$/L) are at high risk and should receive TLS prophylaxis prior to receiving first drug infusion (e.g., antihyperurecemic agent, allopurinol, or rasburicase) beginning 12–24 hours before dose. Monitor laboratory tests during initial treatment if patient at risk for TLS. If TLS occurs, correct electrolyte abnormalities, monitor renal function, ensure hydration and fluid balance, and provide supportive care as needed.
- *Infections:* Drug is *immunosuppressive, especially in combination with chlorambucil or bendamustine,* and may result in serious bacterial, fungal, and new/reactivated viral infections during or after therapy with obinutuzumab. Grade 3–5 infections occurred in 29% of patients receiving both obinutuzumab and bendamustine (3% fatal), and incidence was 15% in patients receiving obinutuzumab plus CHOP or CVP. Do not give drug to patients with an active infection, and closely monitor patients with a history of recurring or chronic infections.
- *Neutropenia:* Neutropenia can occur, or be of late onset (>28 days after completion of treatment and/or be prolonged (lasting >28 days). Consider dose delays for grade 3 or 4 nuetropenia, and give antimicrobial prophylaxis until neutropenia resulves to grade 1–2.
  - Thrombocytopenia: can occur in patients receiving both obinutuzumab and chemotherapy, and it may be severe and life-threatening. It can begin in cycle 1. Monitor platelet count, and patient for thrombocytopenia and hemorrhage. Consider dose delays based on platelet count, and consider holding concomitant medications that can increase the risk of bleeding (platelet inhibitors, anticoagulants) especially during cycle 1.
- *Immunization:* Do not immunize patients with live or attenuated viral vaccines during treatment until B-lymphocytes have recovered.
- Drug may cause worsening of preexisting cardiac conditions.
- Drug may lead to progressive multifocal leukoencephalopathy (PML), which may be fatal.
- The most common side effects were (1) CLL: infusion reactions, neutropenia, thrombocytopenia, and diarrhea; (2) relapsed or refractory NHL: infusion reaction, neutropenia, constipation, cough, pyrexia, URI, arthralgia, sinusitis, asthenia, UTI; constipation, fever, thrombocytopenia, vomiting, URI, decreased appetite, arthralgia, sinusitis, (3) previously untreaeted NHL: infusion reactions, neutropenia, URI, cough, constipation, diarrhea,

headache, herpesvirus infection, arthralgia, insomnia, pneumonia, thrombocytopenia, decreaed appetite, alopecia, pruritis.

* Administration of drug to a pregnant woman is likely to cause fetal B-cell lymphocyte depletion.

Potential Toxicities/Side Effects and the Nursing Process

I.   POTENTIAL FOR INFECTION related to NEUTROPENIA, IMMUNOSUPPRESSION, AND THROMBOCYTOPENIA

Defining Characteristics: Obinutuzumab in combination with chlorambucil resulted in 40% incidence of neutropenia in clinical trials, 34% grades 3–4; this increases risk for infections. The incidence of infections was 38%, 9% grades 3–4. Cough occurs in 10% of patients, as does pyrexia. Thrombocytopenia occurred in 15% of patients, 11% grades 3–4. Anemia occurred in 12% of patients; Incidence of neutropenia in CLL patients with chlorambucil across trials was 38–76% (33–39% grades 3–4) and in patients with indolent NHL with bendamustine followed by monotherapy was 35% (33% grades 3–4). Incidence of thrombocytopenia in CLL patients was 14–48% (10–13% grades 3–4). Rarely, acute thrombocytopenia can occur within 24 hours of the infusion. Drug is immunosuppressive, especially in combination with chlorambucil or bendamustine, and may result in serious bacterial, fungal, and new/reactivated viral infections during or after therapy with obinutuzumab. Do not give drug to patients with an active infection, and closely monitor patients with a history of recurring or chronic infections.

Nursing Implications: Assess baseline WBC, lymphocyte, and neutrophil counts, platelet count, and hemoglobin, and monitor frequently during therapy, especially if the patient develops neutropenia or thrombocytopenia. Assess skin integrity, potential for infection, and teach patient measures to prevent infection (e.g., keeping skin intact, avoiding sources of infection, good hand-washing), bleeding, or worsening fatigue. Teach patient to report any signs/symptoms of infection (e.g., redness, heat, exudate on skin, temperature ≥ 100.4°F, cough, sputum production, dysuria), or bleeding. Assess for signs/symptoms of infection during therapy and at each visit, as well as for bleeding and fatigue. If a patient develops an infection, discuss with physician or midlevel practitioner interrupting or discontinuing drug and beginning appropriate antimicrobial treatment. Neutropenic patients should receive antimicrobial prophylaxis throughout treatment, and antiviral and antifungal prophylaxis should be considered. All patients should be screened for HBV infection (measuring HBsAg and anti-HBc) before starting obinutuzumab therapy. Closely monitor all patients with current or prior HBV infection (clinical and laboratory) for signs of hepatitis and HBV reactivation (e.g., increased transaminase levels, bilirubin) during and after completion of treatment.

II.   POTENTIAL FOR INJURY related to INFUSION REACTION

Defining Characteristics: Obinutuzumab can cause infusion reactions, so premedication is required. Incidence in CLL with chlorambucil was 60%, and 69% for indolent NHL given with bendamustine or as monotherapy was 69%. Most frequent symptoms are nausea, fatigue, dizziness, vomiting, diarrhea, HTN, flushing, headache, fever, chills. More severe reaction is characterized by hypotension, tachycardia, dyspnea, bronchospasm, laryngeal edema, and wheezing. The risk for severe infusion reaction may be increased in patients with preexisting cardiac or pulmonary conditions.

Nursing Implications: Ensure patient receives premedication with acetaminophen, diphenhydramine or equivalent, and glucocorticoid (dexamethasone or prednisolone). See Drug Administration. Begin infusion using slow infusion rate as in Administration section. Assess for signs/symptoms of infusion reaction, and be prepared to stop infusion. Recall signs/symptoms of an infusion reaction, as well as anaphylaxis; if these occur, stop drug immediately, notify physician, and assess patient's vital signs. Subjective symptoms of anaphylaxis are generalized itching, nausea, chest tightness, crampy abdominal pain, difficulty speaking, anxiety, agitation, sense of impending doom, uneasiness, desire to urinate/defecate, dizziness, and chills. Objective signs are flushed appearance; angioedema of face, neck, eyelids, hands, and feet; localized or generalized urticaria; respiratory distress with or without wheezing; hypotension; and cyanosis. Review standing orders or nursing procedures for patient management of anaphylaxis and be prepared to stop drug immediately, notify physician, monitor VS, and administer ordered medications, which may include epinephrine 1:1,000 glucocorticoids, bronchodilator, oxygen, and diphenhydramine. Teach patient to report any unusual symptoms. STOP the infusion for ALL infusion reactions. For severe reactions, institute medical management urgently, such as for angina or other signs/symptoms of myocardial insufficiency. Drug is permanently discontinued for anaphylaxis. If initial reaction is grade 3, interrupt infusion until reaction resolves. For grades 1, 2, interrupt infusion or slow infusion rate, and manage symptoms per physician or mid-level practitioner. Teach patient to report any signs and symptoms of infusion reaction within 24 hours of the infusion (e.g., fever, chills, rash, breathing problems). Closely monitor patients with preexisting cardiac or pulmonary conditions during drug infusion and postinfusion period, as these patients may have more severe reactions. Discuss with physician/mid-level practitioner withholding antihypertensive treatment 12 hours prior to the infusion, during the infusion, and for 1 hour after administration to reduce the risk of hypotension.

Drug: ofatumumab (Arzerra)

Class: IgG_1 mAb (fully human) targeted at the CD_{20} molecule on B-cell lymphocyte membranes.

Mechanism of Action: Drug is a CD_{20}-directed cytolytic mAb. Drug binds specifically to both the small and large extracellular loop epitope on the CD_{20} molecule and is released very slowly from the site. An epitope is a location on the antigen that can elicit an immune response. The CD_{20} molecule is expressed on normal B lymphocytes (B-lymphocyte lineage from pre-B to mature B-lymphocyte) and on B-cells in CLL patients. The Fab portion of ofatumumab binds to the CD_{20}, and the Fc portion calls in immune effector cells to kill the B-lymphocytes. Drug has stronger CDC than rituximab, is more effective in killing tumor cells with lower expression of CD_{20} cells, and is able to kill CD_{20} cells resistant to rituximab.

Metabolism: Ofatumumab is eliminated via target-independent and B-cell–mediated routes. As the B-lymphocytes are killed, the clearance of the drug is slower, so the infusions are scheduled every 4 weeks following 8 weekly infusions. The mean $t_{1/2}$ between infusion 4 and 12 was approximately 14 days (range 2.3–61.5 days). Although volume of distribution and clearance increase with increased body weight, this is not clinically significant.

Indications: For the treatment of
1. In combination with chlorambucil, previously untreated patients with CLL for whom fludarabine-based therapy is considered inappropriate.
2. Patients with relapsed CLL in combination with fludarabine and cyclophosphamide.
3. Extended treatment of patients who are in CR or PR after at least 2 lines of therapy for recurrent or progressive CLL.
4. Patients with CLL refractory to fludarabine and alemtuzumab.

Dosage/Range:
- Premedicate 30 minutes to 2 hours prior to each dose of ofatumumab with oral acetaminophen 1,000 mg (or equivalent), oral or IV antihistamine (cetirizine 10 mg or equivalent), and IV corticosteroid (prednisolone 100 mg or equivalent).
- Ofatumumab doses (IV infusion), in a setting prepared to monitor for, and to manage infusion reactions. Dose should be prepared in 1,000 mL of 0.9% sodium chloride injection USP.
  1. *CLL previously untreated, in combination with chlorambucil:* (a) 300 mg on cycle 1, day 1, followed by (b) 1,000 mg on cycle 1, day 8, by IV infusion. (3) 1,000-mg IV infusion on day 1 of subsequent 28-day cycles for a minimum of 3 cycles until best response or a maximum of 12.
  2. *CLL refractory to fludarabine and alemtuzumab:* 12 doses as follows: (a) Dose 1: 300-mg initial dose infused at 12 mL/hr (3.6 mg/hr), followed 1 week later by (b) doses 2–8: 2,000 mg weekly for 7 doses, followed 4 weeks later by (c) doses 9–12: 2,000 mg every 4 weeks for 4 doses.
  3. *Extended treatment in CLL:* Single agent (a) 300 mg on day 1, followed by (b) 1,000 mg 1 week later on day 8, followed by (c) 1,000 mg 7 weeks later, and every 8 weeks thereafter for up to a maximum of 2 years.
  4. *Relapsed CLL* relapsed, in combination with fludarabine and cyclophosphamide: (a) 300 mg on day 1, followed by (b) 1,000 mg on day 8 (cycle 1), then (c) 1,000 mg on day 1 of each subsequent 28-day cycle for a maximum of 6 cycles.

Drug Preparation:
- Available as 100-mg/5-mL and 1,000-mg/50-mL single-use vials. Do not shake product. Inspect parenteral drug products for particulate matter and discoloration before administration. Drug should be a clear to opalescent, colorless solution. If discolored or cloudy, or if there are foreign particulates, do not use.

- For the 300-mg dose:
  - Withdraw and discard 15 mL from a 1,000-mL polyolefin bag of 0.9% sodium chloride injection, USP.
  - Withdraw 5 mL from each of three 100-mg vials of ofatumumab and add to the IV bag. Mix diluted solution by gentle inversion.
- For the 1,000-mg dose:
  - Withdraw and discard 50 mL from a 1,000-mL polyolefin bag of 0.9% sodium chloride injection, USP.
  - Withdraw 50 mL from 1 single-use 1,000-mg vial of ofatumumab and add to the IV bag. Mix diluted solution by gentle inversion.
- For the 2,000-mg dose:
  - Withdraw and discard 100 mL from a 1,000-mL polyolefin bag of 0.9% sodium chloride injection, USP.
  - Withdraw 50 mL from 2 single-use 1,000-mg vials of ofatumumab and add to the IV bag. Mix diluted solution by gentle inversion.
- Store diluted solution at 2–8°C (36–46°F). No incompatibilities between ofatumumab and polyvinylchloride or polyolefin bags and administration sets have been seen.
- START infusion within 12 hours of drug preparation, and discard the prepared solution after 24 hours.

Drug Administration:
- Dilute and administer as an IV infusion; do not administer as an IV push or bolus, or as a subcutaneous injection. All doses should be mixed in 1,000 mL of 0.9% sodium chloride injection USP.
- Premedicate before each infusion. The infusion environment should permit adequate patient monitoring and treatment of infusion reactions.
- **Premedications and Ofatumumab:**

Previously Untreated CLL, Relapsed CLL or Extended Treatment CLL:
- *Premedications:* (a) Infusion numbers 1 and 2: IV corticosteroid (prednisolone 50 mg or equivalent), oral acetaminophen 1,000 mg, PO/IV diphenhydramine 50 mg or cetirizine 10 mg (or equivalent); (b) infusions 3 and beyond: IV corticosteroid 0–50 mg (may be reduced or omitted if no grade 3 or higher infusion reaction with prior infusion), acetaminophen and diphenhydramine or cetirizine.
- *Ofatumumab:*
  - For initial 300 mg dose: begin infusion at a rate of 3.6 mg/hr (12 mL/hr).
  - For subsequent infusions of 1,000 mg: initiate infusion at a rate of 25 mg/hr (25 mL/hr); if patient had a grade 3 or higher infusion related adverse event in previous infusion, start infusion at 12 mg/hr.
  - If no infusion-related adverse event, may increase infusion rate every 30 minutes. Do not exceed an infusion of 400 mL/hr. See Tables 4.7 and 4.8 in drug package insert.

Refractory CLL:
- *Premedications:* (a) Infusions 1, 2, 9: IV corticosteroid 100 mg, acetaminophen 1,000 mg PO, diphenhydramine 50 mg or cetirizine 10 mg PO/IV; Infusions 3–8: IV corticosteroid 0–100 mg (may be reduced or omitted if no grade 3 or higher infusion reaction with prior infusion), acetaminophen, diphenhydramine, or cetirizine;

Table 4.9   Infusion Rates for Arzerra in Previously Untreated CLL, Relapsed CLL, and Extended Treatment in CLL

Interval after Start of Infusion (min)	Initial 300-mg Dose (mL/hr) [Median Duration of Infusions = 4.8–5.2 hr]	Subsequent Infusions 1,000 mg (mL/hr) [Median Duration of Infusions 4.2–4.4 hrs]
0–30	12	25
31–60	25	50
61–90	50	100
91–120	100	200
121–150	200	400
151–180	300	400
>180	400	400

Reproduced from Novartis Pharmaceuticals Corp. Arzerra (ofatumumab) package insert. East Hanover, NJ, August 2016.

Table 4.10   Infusion Rates for Arzerra in Refractory CLL

Interval after Start of Infusion (min)	Infusions 1 and 2 (mL/hr) 300 and 2,000-mg Doses: [Median Duration of Infusions = 6.8 hr] (mL/h)	Subsequent Infusions 3–12 Dose 2,000 mg: [Median Durations of Infusions = 4.2–4.4 hours] (mL/h)
0–30	12	25
31–60	25	50
61–90	50	100
91–120	100	200
>120	200	400

Reproduced from Novartis Pharmaceuticals Corp. Arzerra (ofatumumab) package insert. East Hanover, NJ, August 2016.

infusions 10–12: IV corticosteroid 50–100 mg (if no grade 3 or higher infusion reaction with infusion 9, prednisolone dose may be reduced to 50–100 mg), acetaminophen, and diphenhydramine or cetirizine.

- *Ofatumumab:*
  - Infusion 1 (300-mg dose): Initiate infusion at a rate of 3.6 mg/hr (12 mL/hr)
  - Infusion 2 (2,000-mg dose): initiate infusion at a rate of 24 mg/hr (12 mL/hr)
  - Infusion 3–12 (2,000-mg doses): initiate infusion at a rate of 50 mg/hr (25 mL/hr)
  - If no infusion-related event, the infusion rate may be increased every 30 minutes as shown in the following table; do not exceed 400 mL/hr.
- Do not mix drug with, or administer as an infusion with, other medicines.
- Administer using an infusion pump and an administration set.

- Flush the IV line with 0.9% sodium chloride injection USP before and after each dose.
- Start infusion within 12 hours of preparation. Discard prepared solution after 24 hours.
- The following infusion rates should be used after the patient has received premedication:

Infusion Rate Dose Modification for Infusion Reaction
- Interrupt infusion for any infusion reactions. Infusion may be resumed at the discretion of the treating physician. As a guide,
  - If the infusion reaction resolves or remains ≤grade 2, resume infusion with modifications according to grade
    - Grades 1–2: infuse at one-half of the previous infusion rate
    - Grades 3–4: infuse at a rate of 12 mL/hr
- After resuming the infusion, rate may be increased according to above tables based on patient tolerance.
- Consider permanently discontinuing ofatumumab if severity of infusion reaction does not decrease to ≤ grade 2 despite adequate intervention.
- Permanently discontinue ofatumumab if patient develops anaphylaxis.

Drug Interactions:
- Coadministration of ARZERRA did not result in clinically relevant effects on the pharmacokinetics of fludarabine, cyclophosphamide, chlorambucil, or its active metabolite, phenylacetic acid mustard.

Lab Effects/Interference:
- Decreased neutrophil, platelet, red blood cell count.

Special Considerations:
- Warnings and Precautions:
  - *Infusion Reactions:* Ofatumumab can cause infusion reactions; when given with chlorambucil, 56% occurred during the initial infusion, 23% on the second-day infusion, and less frequently during subsequent infusions. The infusion reaction may be characterized by bronchospasm, dyspnea, laryngeal edema, pulmonary edema, flushing, hypertension, hypotension, syncope, cardiac ischemia/infarction, back pain, abdominal pain, pyrexia, rash, urticaria, and angioedema. STOP the infusion with all infusion reactions. For severe reactions, institute emergency medical management urgently, such as for angina or other signs/symptoms of myocardial insufficiency. All patients should receive premedication with acetaminophen, antihistamine, and corticosteroid. If an anaphylactic reaction occurs, immediately and permanently discontinue ofatumumab.
  - *Cytopenias:* Neutropenia and thrombocytopenia are side effects and can be prolonged (> 1 week) and severe. In clinical trials, the incidence of grades 3–4 neutropenia was 42% (18% grade 4) and sometimes lasted for > 2 weeks. CBC/platelets should be assessed baseline and regularly during therapy, with more frequent blood tests in patients who have grades 3–4 cytopenias. Cytopenias can have late-onset.
  - *PML* can occur, so any patient with a new onset of, or changes in preexisting, neurologic signs or symptoms should be evaluated for PML, including a neurology consult, brain MRI, and LP exam. Ofatumumab should be discontinued if PML is suspected.

Teach patients to report any new neurologic symptoms such as confusion, dizziness, loss of balance, difficulty talking or walking, or vision problems right away.

- *Reactivation of hepatitis B* can occur with mAb therapy against CD20, including fulminant hepatitis and death. Screen ALL patients for HBV infection prior to starting the drug (hepatitis B surface antigen (HBsAg) and hepatitis B core antibody positive (anti-HBc). Carriers of hepatitis B should be monitored closely for signs/symptoms of active HBV infection during ofatumumab therapy and for 6–12 months following the last dose of therapy. Ofatumumab must be discontinued in patients who develop viral hepatitis or reactivation of HBV and should then be treated with appropriate antiviral therapy. The reintroduction of ofatumumab after HBV therapy has not been studied. Teach patients at risk for HBV to report increasing fatigue and yellow discoloration of skin or eyes.
- *TLS:* Rapid lymphocyte lysis can cause TLS within 12–24 hours of initial drug infusion, characterized by acute renal failure, hyperkalemia, hyperuricemia, and/or hyperphosphatemia. Patients with high tumor burden and/or high circulating lymphocyte counts ($> 25 \times 10^9$/L) are at high risk and should receive TLS prophylaxis prior to receiving first drug infusion (e.g., antihyperuricemic agent such as allopurinol, hydration beginning 12–24 hours before dose). If TLS occurs, correct electrolyte abnormalities, monitor renal function and ensure hydration and fluid balance, and provide supportive care as needed.
- *Hepatitis B virus (HBV) infection.*
- *Immunizations:* Do not give patient live viral vaccines during or following administration of ofatumumab as the ability to generate an immune response has not been studied.
- Obstruction of the small intestines can occur, and patients should have a diagnostic workup to rule this out if symptoms (e.g., abdominal pain, nausea) develop.
- Immunizations: Live vaccines should NOT be administered to patients receiving ofatumumab, and the ability of the patient to generate an immune response to any vaccine is unknown following administration of ofatumumab.
- Drug has not been studied in patients with renal or hepatic impairment; use cautiously in these patients.
- Drug may cause fetal harm. Teach women of childbearing age to use effective contraception to avoid pregnancy. Caution should be used if a mother nurses her baby. Published data suggest that neonatal and infant consumption of breastmilk does not result in substantial absorption of maternal antibodies into circulation. However, the local GI and limited systemic exposure of ofatumumab effects are not known.
- Most common side effects (10% or greater incidence) were (1) previously untreated CLL: infusion reactions, neutropenia; (2) refractory CLL: neutropenia, followed by pneumonia, pyrexia, cough, diarrhea, anemia, fatigue, dyspnea, rash, nausea, bronchitis, URI; and (3) Extended treatment in CLL: infusion reactions, neutropenia, URI. The most common serious adverse reactions in patients who received 2,000 mg of ofatumumab were infections (pneumonia and sepsis), neutropenia, and pyrexia. Infections were bacterial, viral, and fungal, affecting 70% of patients. Twenty-nine percent had grade 3 or higher infections, and 12% were fatal. This was less than the incidence (17%) of fatal infections in the group of patients receiving fludarabine and alemtuzumab.

Potential Toxicities/Side Effects and the Nursing Process

I.   POTENTIAL FOR INJURY related to HYPERSENSITIVITY and INFUSION REACTION

Defining Characteristics: Ofatumumab can cause infusion reactions, so premedication is required. Incidence of infusion reactions is highest with first 2 infusions. In clinical trial with chlorambucil plus Arzerra, the incidence was 67% (10% grade 3 of higher), and as a single agent 46% (4% grade 3 or higher). The infusion reaction is characterized by bronchospasm, dyspnea, laryngeal edema, pulmonary edema, flushing, hypertension, hypotension, syncope, cardiac ischemia/infarction, back pain, abdominal pain, pyrexia, rash, urticaria, and angioedema. The risk for infusion reaction may be increased in patients with moderate to severe COPD.

Nursing Implications: Ensure patient receives premedication with acetaminophen, diphenhydramine or equivalent, and IV corticosteroid (prednisolone or equivalent). See Drug Administration. Begin infusion using slow infusion rate table. Recall signs/symptoms of anaphylaxis, and if these occur, stop drug immediately, notify physician, and assess patient's vital signs. Subjective symptoms are generalized itching, nausea, chest tightness, crampy abdominal pain, difficulty speaking, anxiety, agitation, sense of impending doom, uneasiness, desire to urinate/defecate, dizziness, and chills. Objective signs are flushed appearance; angioedema of face, neck, eyelids, hands, and feet; localized or generalized urticaria; respiratory distress with or without wheezing; hypotension; and cyanosis. Review standing orders or nursing procedures for patient management of anaphylaxis and be prepared to stop drug immediately if an infusion reaction occurs. Notify physician or NP/PA, monitor VS, and administer ordered emergency medications, if needed which may include epinephrine 1:1,000, hydrocortisone sodium succinate, oxygen, and diphenhydramine. Teach patient to report any unusual symptoms. STOP the infusion for ALL infusion reactions. For severe reactions, institute medical management urgently, such as for angina or other signs/symptoms of myocardial insufficiency. If initial reaction is grades 1, 2, or 3, after resolution or if reaction remains ≤ grade 2, resume at one-half the previous infusion rate (for grades 1–2) or at 12 mL/hr (grade 3). After resuming the infusion, the infusion rate may be increased according to the infusion rate table (every 30 minutes as long as asymptomatic). Teach patient to report any signs and symptoms of infusion reaction within 24 hours of the infusion (e.g., fever, chills, rash, breathing problems).

II.   POTENTIAL FOR INFECTION AND BLEEDING related to NEUTROPENIA AND THROMBOCYTOPENIA

Defining Characteristics: Neutropenia, thrombocytopenia, and anemia are side effects. Neutropenia can have late onset (grades 3–4, onset at least 42 days after treatment dose) and/or be prolonged (not resolved in 24–42 days after last treatment dose) and be severe. In clinical trials, the incidence of grades 3–4 neutropenia was 42% (18% grade 4), and sometimes lasted for > 2 weeks. The incidence of neutropenia in patients taking chlorambucil in combination with ofatumumab was 27–66% (26–29% grade 3 and higher), while that in patients taking ofatumumab alone was 24% (22% grade 3 or higher). The incidence of infection is 80% (bacterial, viral, and fungal), primarily pneumonia and sepsis. Twelve percent of patients die from their infections. Pyrexia occurs in 20% of patients. Drug may also reactivate HBV infection, so carriers must be monitored closely. In patients who took chlorambucil in combination with Azerra, pancytopenia, agranulocytosis, and fatal neutropenic sepsis have occurred.

Nursing Implications: Assess CBC and differential/platelets baseline and regularly during therapy, with more frequent blood testing in patients who have grades 3–4 cytopenias. Assess hepatitis B viral screening findings for high-risk individuals and ensure the results are negative before starting drug. Teach patient to report fever and signs/symptoms of infection or bleeding right away. Assess medication profile and OTC medications taken. Teach patient to avoid OTC medications containing NSAIDs or aspirin. Teach patient to talk to nurse or physician before beginning any OTC medications. Monitor before each treatment, during therapy, and more often as needed. Assess risk for infection and integrity of skin and mucous membranes, pulmonary status, and ability to clear secretions, as well as history of past infections, baseline and prior to each treatment. Teach patient to self-administer prophylactic antibiotics, antiviral, and antifungal agents as ordered by physician. Ensure that patient has coverage or can purchase antimicrobial medications if ordered. Teach patient to self-administer oral antifungal agent if ordered for oral candidiasis if it develops. Teach patient to self-assess for signs/symptoms of infection and to call provider immediately or come to the emergency room if temperature > 100.4°F, shaking, chills, rash, productive cough, burning on urination, or any signs/symptoms of infection or bleeding. Teach self-care strategies to minimize risk of infection and bleeding, including avoidance of OTC aspirin-containing medications. Closely monitor hepatitis B carriers for clinical and laboratory signs of active HBV during therapy and for 6–12 months after the last infusion of ofatumumab. Discontinue the drug in patients who develop viral hepatitis or reactivation of viral hepatitis and implement antiviral therapy. Do not administer live viral vaccines to patients who have recently received the drug.

Drug: oprelvekin (Neumega®)

Class: Biologic (interleukin).

Mechanism of Action: IL-11 is a thrombopoietin growth factor that directly stimulates the bone marrow stem cells and megakaryocyte progenitor cells so that the production of platelets is increased. Produced by recombinant DNA technology. Results in higher platelet nadir and accelerates time to platelet recovery postchemotherapy.

Metabolism: Peak serum concentrations reached in approximately 3 ± 2 hours, with a terminal half-life of approximately 7 ± 1 hours. Bioavailability is < 80%. Clearance decreases with age, and drug is rapidly cleared from the serum, distributed to organs with high perfusion, metabolized, and excreted by the kidneys. Little intact drug is found in the urine.

Indications: For the prevention of severe thrombocytopenia and the reduction in the need for platelet transfusions after myelosuppressive chemotherapy in adult patients with non-myeloid malignancies who are at high risk of severe thrombocytopenia.

Contraindication: Patients with a history of hypersensitivity to Neumega or any component of the product. Drug is NOT indicated following myeloablative chemotherapy, as there is increased toxicity.

Dosage/Range:
• Adults: 50 µg/kg subcutaneous daily.

Drug Preparation:
• Available as single-use vial containing 5 mg of oprelvekin as a lyophilized, preservative-free powder. This is reconstituted with 1 mL sterile water for injection, USP, gently swirled to mix, and results in a concentration of 5 mg/1 mL in a single-use vial. NOTE: 5 mL of diluent is supplied, but only 1 mL should be withdrawn to reconstitute drug. Drug should be used within 3 hours of reconstitution. If not used immediately, store reconstituted solution in refrigerator or at room temperature, but DO NOT FREEZE OR SHAKE.

Drug Administration:
• The drug should be administered subcutaneously every day (abdomen, thigh or hip, or upper arm). Begin daily administration 6–24 hours after the completion of chemotherapy, and continue until the postnadir platelet count is equal to or greater than 50,000 cells/mL.
  • Do not give for more than 21 days, and stop at least 2 days before starting the next planned cycle of chemotherapy.
  • Drug has *not* been evaluated in patients receiving chemotherapy regimens longer than 5 days, nor has it been shown to cause delayed myelosuppression (e.g., mitomycin C, nitrosoureas).
• Assess for allergic reactions (e.g., edema of face, tongue, larynx); SOB, wheezing, chest pain, hypotension including shock; dysarthria, LOC; mental status changes; rash; urticaria; flushing and fever. Drug should be discontinued if patient develops an allergic or HSR.

Drug Interactions:
• Unknown.

Lab Effects/Interference:
• Increase in platelet count.
• Anemia associated with increased circulating plasma volume.

Special Considerations:
• Allergic reactions including anaphylaxis have occurred.
• Increased toxicity following myeloablative therapy for which the drug is not indicated.
• Causes fluid retention, so must be used with caution in patients with CHF or in patients receiving chronic diuretic therapy.
• Monitor platelet count frequently during oprelvekin therapy, and at the time of the expected nadir to identify when recovery will begin.
• Drug should not be used during pregnancy or by nursing mothers.

TREATMENT

Potential Toxicities/Side Effects and the Nursing Process

I. ALTERATIONS IN FLUID AND ELECTROLYTE BALANCE related to FLUID RETENTION

Defining Characteristics: Most patients develop mild to moderate fluid retention (peripheral edema, dyspnea on exertion) but without weight gain. Fluid retention is reversible in a few days after drug is stopped. Patients with preexisting pleural effusions, pericardial effusions, or ascites may develop increased fluid, and may require drainage. Patients receiving chronic administration of potassium-excreting diuretics should be monitored extremely closely, as there are reports of sudden death due to severe hypokalemia in patients receiving ifosfamide and chronic diuretic therapy. CLS has *not* been reported. Dilutional anemia has occurred.

Nursing Implications: Assess baseline fluid and electrolyte balance, and weight prior to beginning drug. Assess presence of history of cardiac problems, or CHF, and risk of developing fluid volume overload. If diuretic therapy is ordered, monitor fluid and electrolyte balance very carefully, and replete electrolytes as indicated and ordered. Teach patients that mild-to-moderate peripheral edema and shortness of breath on exertion are likely to occur during the first week of treatment and will disappear after treatment ends. If the patient has CHF or pleural effusions, instruct to report worsening dyspnea to their nurse or physician.

II. ALTERATION IN CIRCULATION related to ATRIAL FIBRILLATION

Defining Characteristics: Some patients (10%) experience transient arrhythmias, including atrial fibrillation or flutter, after treatment with oprelvekin; it is believed to be caused by increased plasma volume rather than the drug itself. Arrhythmias may be symptomatic, are usually brief in duration, and are not clinically significant. Some patients have spontaneous conversion to a normal sinus rhythm, while others require rate-controlling drug therapy. Most patients can receive drug without recurrence of the atrial arrhythmia. Risk factors for developing atrial arrhythmias are (1) advancing age, (2) use of cardiac medications, (3) history of doxorubicin exposure, and (4) history of atrial arrhythmia. Other cardiovascular events include tachycardia, vasodilatation, palpitations, and syncope.

Nursing Implications: Assess baseline risk. If patient has history or presence of atrial arrhythmias, discuss with the physician potential benefit versus risk, and monitor very closely. Monitor baseline heart rate and other vital signs at each visit. Instruct patient to report immediately palpitations, lightheadedness, dizziness, or any other change in condition, especially if patient has any risk factors.

III. ALTERATION IN SENSORY PERCEPTION related to VISUAL BLURRING

Defining Characteristics: Transient, mild visual blurring has been reported, as has papilledema in 1.5% of patients. Dizziness (38%), insomnia (33%), and infection of conjunctiva (19%) may also occur.

Nursing Implications: Assess risk for papilledema (existing papilledema, CNS tumors); assess for changes in pupillary response in these patients. Teach patients that dizziness and insomnia may occur; tell them to change positions slowly and to hold onto supportive structures. If insomnia is severe, discuss sleep medications with physician.

IV.   ALTERATION IN NUTRITION, LESS THAN FULL BODY REQUIREMENTS, related to GI SYMPTOMS

Defining Characteristics: Nausea, vomiting, mucositis, and diarrhea may occur, although percentage was not significantly greater than placebo control. Oral candidiasis occurred in 14% of patients, and this was significantly greater than control.

Nursing Implications: Instruct patient to report changes, and assess impact on nutrition. Inspect oral mucosa and teach patient how to inspect it. Because patient is receiving myelosuppressive chemotherapy, teaching should include oral hygiene regimen and frequent self-assessment by patient.

V.   ALTERATIONS IN BREATHING PATTERN, INEFFECTIVE, POTENTIAL, related to DYSPNEA, COUGH

Defining Characteristics: Dyspnea (48% of patients), rhinitis (42%), increased cough (29%), pharyngitis (25%), and pleural effusions (10%) may occur.

Nursing Implications: Assess baseline pulmonary status and presence of pleural effusions. Instruct patient to report dyspnea and any other changes. Discuss significant changes with physician.

Drug: palifermin (Kepivance)

Class: Mucocutaneous epithelial (Keratinocyte) growth factor.

Mechanism of Action: Palifermin is a keratinocyte growth factor (KGF) produced by recombinant DNA technology, similar to the naturally occurring, endogenous KGF. Once EGF binds to its receptor found on epithelial cells—including those of the tongue, buccal mucosa, mammary gland, skin (hair follicles and sebaceous gland), lung, liver, and the lens of the eye—it stimulates proliferation, differentiation, and migration of epithelial cells. KGF decreases the incidence and duration of severe stomatitis in patients with hematologic malignancies who undergo high-dose chemotherapy and radiation therapy with stem cell rescue.

Metabolism: Palifermin has an elimination half-life of 4.5 hours (average).

Indication: To decrease the incidence and duration of severe oral mucositis in patients with hematologic malignancies receiving myelotoxic therapy requiring hematopoietic stem cell

(HSC) support; indicated as supportive care for preparative regimens predicted to result in ≥ WHO grade 3 mucositis in the majority of patients.

Safety and efficacy of drug have not been established in patients with nonhematologic malignancies. Drug is not recommended for use with melphalan 200 mg/m² as a conditioning regimen.

Dosage/Range:
- 60 mcg/kg/day IV bolus for 3 consecutive days before and 3 consecutive days after myelotoxic therapy, for a total of 6 doses.
  - The first 3 doses prior to chemotherapy, with the third dose 24–48 hours before myelotoxic therapy.
  - Administer the last 3 doses after myelotoxic therapy with the first of the doses on the day of HSC infusion after the infusion is completed, and more than 4 days after the most recent administration of palifermin.

Drug Preparation:
- Available as 6.25-mg lyophilized powder in a single-use vial.
- Reconstitute Kepivance lyophilized powder with sterile water for injection USP, aseptically, by slowly injecting 1.2 mL sterile water for injection USP to yield final volume of 5 mg/mL. Do not shake or agitate the vial.
- Protect from light.
- Drug should be used immediately. If not, reconstituted solution may be refrigerated in its carton for up to 24 hours at 2–8°C (36–46°F); prior to injection, may leave at room temperature for up to 1 hour protected from light. Inspect for discoloration or particulates; if found, do not use. The drug contains no preservatives, so any unused portion should be discarded.
- Do not filter drug during reconstitution or administration.
- Prior to administration, allow palifermin to reach room temperature for a maximum of 1 hour protected from light. Discard drug if left at room temperature > 1 hour.

Drug Administration:
- Administer IV bolus; if heparin used to maintain an IV line, rinse the line with saline prior to and after palifermin administration.
- Premyelotoxic therapy: The third dose should be 24–48 hours before myelotoxic chemotherapy is administered.
- Postmyelotoxic therapy: The first of the three doses should be given after, but on the same day of the HSC infusion, and at least 4 days after the most recent administration of palifermin.

Drug Interactions:
- Heparin: Palifermin binds to heparin, so drugs should not be used concomitantly; flush central line well with saline prior to administration of palifermin.
- Myelotoxic chemotherapy: If given with chemotherapy, KGF increases the severity and duration of oral mucositis. Palifermin should NOT be administered within 24 hours before, during infusion of, or after the administration of myelotoxic chemotherapy.

Lab Effects/Interference:
- Increase in serum amylase and lipase.

Special Considerations:
- Potential for stimulation of tumor growth may exist in nonhematologic malignancies.
- Drug is embryotoxic to lab animals when given in higher doses; drug should be used in pregnant women only when the potential benefit to the mother exceeds the risk to the fetus.
- Nursing mothers should make a decision to discontinue nursing or to discontinue the drug, taking into account the importance of the drug to the patient's health.
- Most common adverse reactions are skin toxicities (rash, erythema, edema, pruritis), oral toxicities (dysesthesia, tongue discoloration, tongue thickening, alteration of taste), pain, arthralgias, and dysesthesia (usually localized to the perioral area).

Potential Toxicities/Side Effects and the Nursing Process

I.   POTENTIAL ALTERATION IN SKIN INTEGRITY related to SKIN RASH

Defining Characteristics: Skin rash was the most common serious adverse reaction and occurred in 62% of patients in clinical studies. Skin toxicity was manifested by rash, erythema (32%), edema (28%), and pruritus (35%). Median time to onset was 6 days after the first of 3 doses, and lasted a median of 5 days.

Nursing Implications: Teach patient that skin cha nges may occur and to report them. Teach patient self-care strategies to promote comfort and reduce the risk of infection.

II.   ALTERATION IN NUTRITION AND COMFORT related to ORAL TOXICITIES

Defining Characteristics: Dysesthesia, tongue discoloration, tongue thickening, alterations in taste occur related to the increased keratin layer on the lining of the oral cavity.

Nursing Implications: Inform patient that these side effects may occur. Teach patient systematic oral cleansing after meals and at bedtime. Inform patient to report discomfort or inability to chew or swallow, and develop plan with measures to promote comfort and nutrition. Many patients are already receiving TPN. If taste alterations are bothersome, suggest dietitian referral for measures to stimulate taste.

III.   ALTERATION IN COMFORT related to PAIN, ARTHRALGIAS, AND DYSESTHESIAS

Defining Characteristics: Dysesthesia, pain, and arthralgias may occur and affect about 12% of patients.

Nursing Implications: Assess baseline comfort, as well as existing arthralgias and dysesthesias. Perform a basic neurologic assessment. Inform patient these side effects may occur and to report them if they occur. Develop a plan of care that includes self-care activities to promote comfort, such as the use of heat or cold for arthralgias. If pain related to stomatitis is severe, then patient-controlled analgesia may be necessary. Teach patient to report any dysesthesias, hyperesthesias, hypoesthesias, or paresthesias that occur. Develop a plan to minimize discomfort, such as keeping sheets off feet if patient has hyperesthesias.

Drug: panitumumab (Vectibix)

Class: IgG_2 human mAb targeted against EGFR.

Mechanism of Action: Drug is a human IgG_2 mAb. It blocks growth factor (ligand, such as epidermal growth factor and TGF-α) from binding to EGFR, thus preventing dimerization and initiation of cell signaling via RTK phosphorylation; thus, the message telling the cell to divide does not occur. The drug competes with natural ligands but has a higher affinity for the EGFR than the ligands. In addition to cell growth inhibition, there is induction of apoptosis, and decreased matrix metalloproteinase and VEGF production. This decreases angiogenesis. Drug is effective only if *KRAS/RAS* genes are normal (called wild-type, WT). If *KRAS/RAS* genes are mutated, the gene turns itself on and sets up an independent signaling cascade bringing a message to the nucleus telling the cell to divide regardless of whether EGFR is blocked by panitumumab.

Metabolism: Steady-state reached by third infusion. Elimination half-life is approximately 7.5 days.

Indication: Treatment of patients with wild-type *KRAS* (defined as wild-type in both *KRAS* and *NRAS* as determined by an FDA-approved test for this use in metastatic CRC (mCRC).
- In combination with FOLFOX for first-line treatment.
- As monotherapy following disease progression after prior treatment with fluoropyrimidine, oxaliplatin, and irinotecan chemotherapy-containing regimens.
- Not indicated for the treatment of patients with *RAS* mutant mCRC or for whom *RAS* mutation status is unknown.
- Before first treatment, assess *RAS* mutational ststus, and confirm the absence of a RAS mutation in exon 2 (codons 12,13), exon 3 (codons 59.61), and exon 4 (codons 117, 146) of both *KRAS* and *NRAS*.

Dosage/Range:
- 6 mg/kg IV infusion every 14 days over 1 hour for doses ≤1,000 mg, or 90 minutes for doses >1,000 mg. If first infusion is well-tolerated, subsequent infusions can be given over 30–60 minutes.
- Infusion reactions: reduce infusion rate by 50% for mild reactions; terminate infusion for severe reactions. Depending upon the severity and/or persistence of the reaction, permanently discontinue panitumumab. Medical resources for the treatment of severe infusion reactions should be in the infusion area.
- Dermatologic toxicities[hold or discontinue for severe or intolerable dermatologic toxicity; reduce dose for recurrent grade 3 toxicity):
  - Upon first occurrence of a grade 3 dermatologic reaction, withhold 1–2 doses of panitumumab. If the reaction improves to < grade 3, reinitiate panitumumab at the original dose.

- Upon second occurrence of a grade 3 dermatologic reaction, withhold 1–2 doses of panitumumab. If the reaction improves to < grade 3, reinitiate panitumumab at 80% of the original dose.
- Upon third occurrence of a grade 3 dermatologic reaction, withhold 1–2 doses of panitumumab. If the reaction improves to < grade 3, reinitiate panitumumab at 60% of the original dose.
- Upon the fourth occurrence of a grade 3 dermatologic reaction, permanently discontinue panitumumab.
- Permanently discontinue panitumumab after the occurrence of a grade 4 dermatologic reaction or for a grade 3 dermatologic reaction that does not recover after withholding 1–2 doses.

Drug Preparation:
- Available as single-use (20-mg/mL vials): 100 mg/5 mL, and 400 mg/20 mL.
- Inspect drug (should be colorless; do not administer if solution is discolored).
- Do not shake.
- Use a 21-gauge or smaller needle to withdraw ordered dose (e.g., 6 mg/kg unless dose reduced); DO NOT use needle-free devices (e.g., vial adapters) to withdraw vial contents.
- Dilute to a total volume of 100 mL with 0.9% sodium chloride injection, USP; doses > 1,000 mg should be diluted to 150 mL 0.9% sodium chloride injection, USP. Final concentration should be ≤ 10 mg/mL. Mix diluted solution by gentle inversion.
- Use the diluted infusion solution within 6 hours of preparation if stored at room temperature, or within 24 hours of dilution if stored at 2–8°C (36–46°F). DO NOT FREEZE. Discard any unused portion remaining in the vial.

Drug Administration:
- Administer IV infusion using low-protein binding 0.2 or 0.22-μm in-line filter using infusion pump over 60 minutes (90 minutes for dose > 1,000 mg). DO NOT administer as an IV push or bolus.
- Infuse doses of ≤ 1,000 mg over 60 minutes though a peripheral IV line or indwelling IV catheter. If infusion tolerated, administer subsequent infusions over 30–60 minutes. Administer doses > 1,000 mg over 90 minutes.
- Do NOT administer panitumumab by IV push or bolus.
- Flush line before and after panitumumab infusion with 0.9% sodium chloride injection, USP. Do not mix with other drug products or IV solutions.
- Reduce the infusion rate by 50% if patient experiences a mild or moderate (grades 1–2) infusion reaction for the remainder of the infusion.
- Stop and discontinue drug for severe reactions, or persistent reactions, for example, grades 3–4 infusion reactions (symptomatic bronchospasm or anaphylaxis).
- Postmarketing reports indicate that severe infusion reactions occur in 1% of patients and may be fatal.
- Hold drug for severe or intolerable skin toxicity; may resume at 50% dose if toxicity improves.

Drug Interactions:
- IFL: Severe diarrhea (1 fatality). DO NOT COADMINISTER.

Lab Effects/Interference:

• Decreased magnesium 6 weeks after beginning therapy.
• Decreased calcium in some patients.

Special Considerations:

• Panitumumab is not indicated for use in patients with *KRAS* mutation or if mutational status is unknown. Patients with *KRAS* gene mutation in codon 12 or 13 have not shown a treatment benefit, so drug is not recommended in these patients. In fact, increased tumor progression, increased mortality, or lack of benefit was seen in *K-RAS* mutant mCRC (Amgen, 2015). Signal transduction through the EGFR results in activation of wild-type KRAS protein. However, in cells with activating *KRAS* (somatic) mutations, the mutant KRAS protein is continually active and appears independent of EGFR regulation. *K-RAS* tumor status must be determined before using the drug.
• Warnings and Precautions:
  • *Dermatologic toxicities* were reported in 90% of patients and were severe in 15% of patients receiving monotherapy in Study 1. Clinical manifestations included dermatitis cuneiform, pruritus, erythema, rash, skin exfoliation, paronychia, dry skin, and skin fissures. Teach patient to avoid sun exposure, and to use SPF and hat protection if going outside. Closely monitor the patient with rash for the development of inflammatory or infectious sequelae. Life-threatening and fatal infections, including necrotizing fasciitis, abcesses, bullous mucocutaneous skin disease, and sepsis have occurred. Rare cases of SJS and TEN have been reported postmarketing. Follow dose modifications for grades 3 and 4. Hold drug or discontinue drug for dermatologic or soft-tissue toxicity, associated with severe or life-threatening inflammatory or infectious complications.
  • *Increased tumor progression, increased mortality, or lack of benefit* in patients with RAS-mutant mCRC
  • *Electrolyte Depletion/Monitoring:* Drug may cause grades 3–4 hypomagnesemia in 7% of patients. Hypomagnesemia occurred ≥ 6 weeks after starting panitumumab. Some patients had both hypomagnesemia and hypocalcemia. Assess electrolytes baseline and periodically during and for 8 weeks after the completion of panitumumab therapy. Replete electrolytes as needed.
  • *Severe infusion reactions* occurred in 1% of patients (NCI grades 3–4), and 4% experienced infusion reactions in Study 1. Infusion reactions characterized by fever, chills, dyspnea, bronchospasm, and hypotension. Reactions may appear to be anaphylactoid reaction without prior drug exposure for sensitization. Fatal infusion reactions have occurred post-marketing. Terminate the infusion for severe infusion reactions and provide emergency medical care.
  • *Acute renal failure in combination with chemotherapy:* Severe diarrhea and dehydration, leading to acute renal failure and other complications, have occurred when panitumumab is administered with chemotherapy.
  • *ILD*, a class effect, may occur in 1% of patients, but caution should be used when treating patients with a history of interstitial pneumonitis, pulmonary fibrosis, as after the first fatality, these patients were excluded from clinical trials. Permanently discontinue panitumumab if ILD is confirmed. If the patient has a history of interstitial

pneumonitis or pulmonary fibrosis, or evidence of interstitial pneumonitis or pulmonary fibrosis, risk versus benefit must be carefully considered.

- *Photosensitivity:* sunlight exposure can exacerbate dermatolotic toxicity; teach patients to wear sunscreen, hats, and limit sun exposure while receiving panitumumab.
- *Ocular toxicities:* keratitis and ulcerative keratitis which are known risk factors for corneal perforation have been reported. Monitor for signs/symptoms of keratitis, and interrupt or discontinue therapy for worsening or acute keratitis. Consult ophthalmologist as needed.
- *Increased mortality and toxicity* with panitumumab when added to bevacizumab and chemotherapy so this combination should NOT be used:
- *Embryo-fetal toxicity:* Drug is fetotoxic. Women of reproductive potential should use effective birth control measures to avoid pregnancy during and for at least 2 months after last dose.. Physicians are encouraged to enroll pregnant patients in Amgen's Pregnancy Surveillance Program (1-800-772-6436). Mothers should not breastfeed while receiving the drug; a decision should be made to discontinue nursing or discontinue the drug, taking into account the importance of the drug to the mother's health.
- Compared with BSC, panitumumab significantly improved PFS, but there was no significant difference in overall survival (OS) between groups.
- Most common adverse reactions ($\geq$ 20%) were (1) as monotherapy, skin rash, paronychia, fatigue, nausea, diarrhea; (2) in combination with FOLFOX, diarrhea, stomatitis, mucosal inflammation, asthenia, paronychia, anorexia, hypomagnesemia, hypokalemia, rash, acneiform dermatitis, pruritis, and dry skin.

Potential Toxicities/Side Effects and the Nursing Process

I.   POTENTIAL ALTERATION IN BODY IMAGE, SKIN INTEGRITY, COMFORT related to SKIN RASH, PARONYCHIA, SKIN FISSURES, PRURITUS

Defining Characteristics: Drug inhibits epidermal growth factor receptor, so major toxicity is manifested in the skin with 90% of patients experiencing some type of skin toxicity. Most patients develop a mild-to-moderate acne-like rash that is self-limiting. Sixteen percent report a grade 3–4 rash. Rash is a sterile, suppurative rash with multiple follicular or pustular lesions that appear during the first 2 weeks of therapy on the face, upper chest, and back, but in some cases, extended to the arms. Rash resolves when treatment is stopped, without scar formation. Pruritus affects 57%, dry skin 10%, acneform dermatitis 57%, skin desquamation 25%, erythema 65%, paronychia 25%, macular rash 22%, skin fissures 20%, stomatitis 7%, and oral mucositis 6%. Fissures can become infected; infection can be treated with topical clindamycin, or oral antibiotics. However, severe dermatologic toxicities can result in infectious complications including sepsis, death, and abscesses requiring incision and drainage. Eye-related toxicities occurred in 15% of patients (conjunctivitis 4%, hyperemia 3%, lacrimation 2%, eyelid irritation 1%), median time to most severe toxicity 15 days from starting drug; median time to solution was 84 days. Exposure to UV light exacerbates intensity and severity of rash.

Nursing Implications: Teach patient that rash most likely will occur due to mechanism of drug action. Assess baseline skin integrity on areas of face, neck, and trunk; assess baseline comfort and satisfaction with body image, and monitor at each treatment. Teach patient to report any distress and assess extent of rash. For severe rash (grades 3–4 or intolerable), hold drug for up to one month until it resolves to grade 2 or less; if it does not, discontinue drug. When rash resolves to grade 2 and the patient is symptomatically improved and no more than two doses have been held, resume drug at 50% of the original dose. If skin toxicity recurs, discontinue drug. If skin appears to be infected (exudate, vesicle formation, abnormal appearance), obtain C+S and discuss empiric treatment with physician. For rash, fissure, and paronychia management refer to the introduction to *Chapter 5*. Teach all patients to (1) use a water-based emollient frequently during the day to prevent dryness, (2) stay hydrated, (3) avoid sun exposure and wear SPF 30 (zinc-based). Do not use anti-acne medications. Tetracycline analogues provide anti-inflammatory benefit. **Grade 1 or mild rash (localized, does not interfere with ADLs, and is not infected):** The goal is to preserve skin integrity, minimize discomfort, and prevent infection. Key patient teaching includes (1) use a mild soap with active ingredients that reduce skin drying such as pyrithione zinc (Head & Shoulders), (2) consider aloe gel for red, tender areas, (3) report distressing tenderness, as pramoxine (lidocaine topical anesthetic) may help, (4) keep fingernails clean and trimmed, and (5) apply zinc ointment to rectal mucosa after washing. Management: maintain current drug dose, observe or give topical hydrocortisone 1 or 2.5% or clindamycin 1% gel (anti-inflammatory benefit) with or without oral doxycycline or minocycline 100 mg BID; reassess in 2 weeks. **For grade 2 or moderate rash that is generalized, mild symptoms, and has minimal effect on ADLs, and no infection:** The goal is to prevent infection and promote comfort. Continue EGFRI dose; use topicals (hydrocortisone 2.5% or clindamycin 1% gel) and add doxycycline or minocycline 100 mg PO twice daily (give antimicrobial and anti-inflammatory effect) and reassess after 2 weeks. **For grades 3–4 or severe rash (generalized, severe, has a significant impact on ADLs, and increased risk of infection):** The goal is to prevent infection or to identify it early to minimize complications and to promote effective coping. Dose-reduce EGFRI drug based on manufacturer's recommendation, and treat rash with topicals (hydrocortisone 2.5% or clindamycin 1% gel), doxycycline 100 mg PO twice daily or minocycline 100 mg PO twice daily, and consider systemic hydrocorticosteroids; reassess after 2 weeks, and interrupt or discontinue drug if rash worsens (Lynch et al., 2007). If rash appears infected (exudate, vesicular formation, different appearance), obtain C+S, treat empirically until sensitivity received, and/or obtain dermatology consult. The STEPP study (Lacouture, 2010) showed that preventive therapy in patients receiving panitumumab, of daily moisturizer, sunscreen, topical hydrocortisone and oral doxycycline 100 mg bid (or minocycline 100 mg daily), reduced the incidence of grade 2 or higher rash compared to patients who received only moisturizer and sunblock, when starting panitumumab therapy.

II.   ALTERATION IN NUTRITION, LESS THAN BODY REQUIREMENTS, related to NAUSEA, VOMITING, DIARRHEA, STOMATITIS, CONSTIPATION, ANOREXIA, ABDOMINAL PAIN

Defining Characteristics: Incidence of mild-to-moderate digestive symptoms include nausea (23%), diarrhea (21%), abdominal pain (25%), vomiting (19%), constipation (21%), stomatitis (7%), hypomagnesia (39%), and oral mucositis (6%) in patients in clinical trials.

Nursing Implications: Assess baseline weight and nutritional status. Inform patient that these symptoms may occur, and to report them. Administer antiemetic and other symptom management medications as ordered. Teach patient self-administration of these medications at home. Monitor serum electrolytes (magnesium, calcium) prior to each dose, and replete magnesium as needed. Teach patient dietary modifications to address symptoms such as anorexia (small, frequent high-calorie, high-protein foods, stimulants as permitted by protocol); constipation (high-fiber, high-fluid, high-roughage foods, stool softeners); diarrhea (bananas, rice, applesauce, and toast); nausea (avoid food preparation odors by cooking in zipped plastic bag, or having someone else cook; choose cool, soft, nonspicy, or fatty foods). Teach patient to report any symptoms that do not resolve or improve on the plan. Assess efficacy of intervention, and revise plan as needed. Dehydration is a worrisome complication of diarrhea; teach patient to call right away if diarrhea persists, and/or is unable to drink fluids (e.g., 8 oz every hour while awake).

III.   POTENTIAL FOR ALTERATION IN COMFORT related to FATIGUE, DYSPNEA, PERIPHERAL EDEMA, PYREXIA, ARTHRALGIA

Defining Characteristics: In clinical trials, the following symptoms were reported in patients with advanced CRC: fatigue (51%), cough (18%), dyspnea (14%), peripheral edema (14%), pyrexia (14%), arthralgia (14%), back pain (12%), headache (12%), dizziness (11%), insomnia (11%).

Nursing Implications: Assess patient comfort level, self-care measures baseline and periodically during therapy. Teach patient that these symptoms may arise, either from the drug and/or the treatment. Develop a plan for symptom management, assess efficacy, and revise as needed. Assess level of fatigue and teach energy-conserving strategies, baseline and prior to each treatment. Inform patient that fatigue may occur due to anemia, and teach energy-conserving strategies such as alternating rest and activity periods.

IV.   ALTERATION IN ELECTROLYTE BALANCE related to HYPOMAGNESEMIA, POTENTIAL

Defining Characteristics: Magnesium wasting appears related to EGFR inhibition in the renal tubular epithelial cells so that excreted magnesium is not resorbed in the distal convoluted tubules. This leads to initial magnesium wasting, followed by losses of calcium and potassium. Hypomagnesemia occurs in about 38% of patients receiving the drug and is severe in 2–4% of patients. It begins within days to months of receiving the drug, and there is much interpatient variability. There appears to be a direct relationship between duration of EGFRI MAb treatment and severe hypomagnesemia (Fakih, 2007). Symptoms of grade 3–4 hypomagnesemia include fatigue, cramps, and somnolence.

Nursing Implications: Assess baseline electrolyte balance prior to initial treatment and prior to each successive weekly treatment. Grade of hypomagnesemia: Grade 1 is a serum level of < LLN–1.2 mg/dL, grade 2 is 0.9–1.2 mg/dL, grade 3 is 0.7–0.9 mg/dL, and grade 4 is ≤ 0.7 mg/dL. Replete magnesium, calcium, and potassium as needed. Oral magnesium may be ineffective and may result in diarrhea (Tejpar et al., 2007). Magnesium repletion regimens include weekly IV replacement of 4 g magnesium sulfate for grade 2. For grades 3–4, patients may be symptomatic and magnesium replacement may involve once- to twice-weekly IV infusions of 6–10 g. Provide support for patients as magnesium replacement infusions require lengthy time in clinic, as an 8-g infusion requires 4 hours. Post-IV replacement with every other day serum magnesium monitoring is important until the patient develops a steady state (Fakih, 2007). Continue to monitor after drug has been discontinued (half-life of the drug and time drug persists [e.g., 8 weeks]). Magnesium replacement in IV hydration starting when a patient has grade 1 hypomagnesemia may be effective in preventing worsening hypomagnesemia. For patients who have refractory grade 4 hypomagnesemia, a stop-and-go approach has been effective where EGFRI MAb is held for 4–8 weeks until the magnesium corrects; it is reported that grade 4 hypomagnesemia does not recur when cetuximab is then reintroduced (Fakih, 2007).

Drug: pegfilgrastim (Neulasta); Biosimilar pegfilgrastim-jmdb (Fulphila™), pegfilgrastim-cbqv (Udenyca™)—NOT interchangeable

Class: Cytokine, CSF, Leukocyte growth factor.

Mechanism of Action: Recombinant DNA protein (G-CSF) that regulates the production of neutrophils in the bone marrow (proliferation, differentiation, activation of mature neutrophils). Drug is produced by the insertion of the human G-CSF gene into *E. coli* bacteria. Drug has longer half-life and different excretion pattern as compared to the parent drug, filgrastim.

Metabolism: Clearance of drug decreases with increased dose and body weight, and is directly related to the number of neutrophils so that as neutrophil recovery begins after myelosuppressive chemotherapy, serum concentration of pegfilgrastim declines rapidly. In patients with increased body weight, systemic exposure to the drug was higher, despite dose normalized for body weight. Pharmacokinetics are variable, with a half-life of 15–80 hours after subcutaneous injection. Pharmacokinetics did not vary with age (elderly) or gender.

Indications: To (1) decrease the incidence of infection, as manifested by febrile neutropenia, in patients with nonmyeloid malignancies receiving myelosuppressive anticancer drugs associated with a clinically significant incidence of febrile neutropenia; (2) Neulasta only: increase survival in patients acutely exposed to myelosuppressive doses of radiation (Hematopoietic Subsyndrome of Acute Radiation Syndrome). Peg-filgrastim is not indicated for the mobilization of PBPC for HSCT.

Contraindication: Patients with a history of serious allergic reactions to human G-CSFs such as pegfilgrastim or filgrastim products.

Dosage/Range:
- Patients with cancer receiving myelosuppressive chemotherapy: 6 mg subcutaneous (SQ) once per chemotherapy cycle. Do not administer between 14 days before and 24 hours

after administration of cytotoxic chemotherapy. Use weight-based dosing for pediatric patients weighting < 45 kg. See package insert.

- Patients acutely exposed to myelosuppressive doses of radiation (>2 gray [Gy]): 2 doses, 6 mg each, SQ, 1 week apart. Administer the first dose as soon as possible after suspected or confirmed exposure to myelosuppressive doses of radiation, and a second dose a week later. Use weight based dosing for pediatric patients weighting < 45 kg. See package insert. Obtain a baseline CBC. Do not delay if CBC not readily available. Estimate patient's absorbed radiation dose (e.g., level of radiation exposure) based on dosimetry, public health information, or clinical findings such as time to onset of vomiting or lymphocyte depletion kinetics.

Drug Preparation:

- Drug available in (1) 6-mg/0.6-mL prefilled syringes for manual use, and (2) Neulasta only: 6 mg/0.6 mL solution in a single-use prefilled syringe co-packaged with the On-body Injector for Neulasta.
- Needle cap on prefilled syringes contains dry natural rubber; if the patient has a latex allergy, the syringe should not administer these products.
- A healthcare provider must fill the On-body Injector with Neulasta using the prefilled syringe, and then apply the On-body Injector to the patient's skin (abdomen or back of arm). The back of the arm may only be used if there is a caregiver available to monitor the status of the injector. Approximately 27 hours after the injector is applied, Neulasta will be delivered over approximately 45 minutes. A healthcare provider may initiate administration with the On-body Injector for Neulasta on the same day as chemtotherapy administration, as long as the injector delivers Neulasta no less than 24 hours after cytotoxic chemotherapy administration.
  - The prefilled syringe co-packaged in Neulasta Onpro™ kit must only be used with the On-body Injector for Neulasta, and it contains additional solution to compensate for lost liquid during delivery. If the syringe is used for manual SQ injection, the patient will receive an overdose, while if the manual prefilles syringe is used with the On-body Injector, the patient may receive an underdose.

Drug Administration:

- Subcutaneous × 1 *at least 14 days prior to or more than 24 hours after* chemotherapy administration.
  - Pegfilgrastim is administered as a subcutaneous injection as a single prefilled syringe either (1) via manual injection or (2) via the On-Body Injector for Neulasta, which is copackaged with a single prefilled syringe.
  - Ensure patient instructions from package insert are reviewed with patient and caregiver, and all questions answered.
- Do not use the On-body Injector for Neulasta to deliver any other drug; use only to administer the copackaged Neulasta prefilled syringe.
  - Apply On-body Neulasta Injector only on intact, nonirritated skin on arm or abdomen.
  - A missed dose may occur due to failure or leakage of the On-body Injector for Neulasta; if this occurs a new dose should be administered by single prefilled syringe for manual use, as soon as possible after detection.

Drug: pegfilgrastim **1161**

TREATMENT

- See Healthcare Provider Instructions for Use for the On-body Injector for Neulasta for full administration information; see patient information section attached to package insert and review with patient and caregiver.
- If a patient receives administration via the On-body Injector for Neulasta, teach patients (1) to avoid activities such as traveling, driving or operating heavy machinery during hours 26–29 following application (this includes the 45-minute delivery period plus an hour postdelivery). Patients should have a caregiver nearby when using for the first time; (2) give patient dose delivery information written on the Patient Instructions for Use; (3) ensure that the patient understands when the dose delivery will begin and how to monitor the On-body Injector for Neulasta for completed delivery; (4) ensure the patient understands how to identify signs of malfunction of the injector.
- The On-body Injector for Neulasta uses acrylic adhesive. For patients who have reactions to acrylic adhesives, use may result in a significant reaction.

Drug Interactions:
- Lithium: may potentiate the release of neutrophils from the bone marrow; monitor neutrophil count more frequently.

Lab Effects/Interference:
- Increased white blood cell count and neutrophil count.

Special Considerations:
- Most common adverse effects ($\geq 5\%$ difference compared to placebo): bone pain an pain in extremity.
- Contraindicated in patients with known hypersensitivity to *E. coli*–derived proteins, pegfilgrastim, filgrastim, or any product component.
- Warnings and Precautions:
  - *Fatal splenic rupture* has been reported in patients receiving the parent drug, filgrastim, for PBPC. If a patient receiving pegfilgrastim complains of left upper abdominal or shoulder tip pain, patient should be evaluated immediately for an enlarged spleen or splenic rupture.
  - *Adult respiratory distress syndrome* has been reported in neutropenic patients with sepsis receiving the parent drug filgrastim, probably related to the influx of neutrophils to inflamed pulmonary sites. Neutropenic patients receiving pegfilgrastim who develop fever, lung infiltrates, or respiratory distress should be immediately evaluated for ARDS. If ARDS is suspected, pegfilgrastim should be stopped until ARDS resolves with appropriate medical care.
  - *Serious allergic reactions,* including anaphylaxis; permanently discontinue drug if this occurs.
  - *On-body injector contains uses acrylic adhesive:* if patient who have reactions to acrylic adhesives, using this produce may result in a significant reaction.
  - *Use in sickle cell disorders:* Severe sickle cell crisis, rarely fatal, has been reported in patients with sickle cell disease (homozygous sickle cell anemia, sickle/hemoglobin C disease, sickle/α-thalassemia) who received filgrastim, the parent drug. Pegfilgrastim should be used in this population only when the potential benefit outweighs the

risk, and patients should be well hydrated and closely monitored for sickle cell crisis, with immediate intervention.

- *Glomerulonephritis:* characterized by azotemia, hematuria, proteinuria, and confirmed by renal biopsy. If glomerulonephritis is suspected, rule out other possible causes, and if appears due to pegfilgrastim, discuss drug interruption or dose reduction.
- *Leukocytosis:* Monitor CBC during use of pegfilgrastim as WBC of $\geq 100 \times 10^9$ may occur
- Neulasta only: *Potential device failure*: teach patients to notify their provider if they believe the on-body injector is not functioning as expected.

- *Capillary Leak Syndrome (CLS)* has been reported, characterized by hypoalbuminemia, edema, and hemoconcentration. Monitor patients intensively if signs/symptoms develop and treat emergently.
- *Potential for tumor growth stimulatory effect on malignant cells:* G-CSF receptor to which drug binds is also found in tumor cell lines (some myeloid, T-lymphoid, lung, head and neck, and bladder cancer), and the potential for the drug to be a tumor growth factor exists.
- Aoritis has been described in patients receiving Neulasta (e.g., fever, abdominal pain, malaise, back pain, increased inflammatory markers).
- *Nuclear imaging*: Increased hematopoietic bone marrow activity driven by growth factor may be associated with positive bone imaging changes; radiologist should consider this when interpreting bone imaging studies.
- *(Neulasta only)-Body Injector:* A healthcare provider must fill the injector with Neulasta using the prefilled syringe, then apply the injector to the patient's skin (abdomen or back of arm). The back of the arm can be used only if a caregiver will monitor the status of the injector. Approximately 27 hours after the On-Body Injector is applied to intact, nonirritated skin, Neulasta will be administered over 45 minutes. See patient education material attached to package insert.
  - A healthcare provider may apply the injector to the patient's skin on the same day as chemotherapy is administered as long as the injector delivers Neulasta no less than 24 hours after the chemotherapy is administered.
  - The copackaged prefilled syringe contains additional solution to compensate for loss during delivery, so the syringe can be used *only with the injector*. If the syringe is used for manual administration, the patient will receive an overdose of Neulasta. If a manual prefilled syringe is used for the injector, the patient will be underdosed.
  - If a dose is missed due to failure or leakage of the injector, a new dose should be administered as soon as possible once detected.
- Pegfilgrastim should not be administered within *14 days prior to* and *for 24 hours after chemotherapy administration* because of the potential for an increase in sensitivity of rapidly dividing myeloid cells to the chemotherapy.
- Allergic reactions to pegfilgrastim, including anaphylaxis, skin rash, and urticaria, have been reported, most often on initial exposure to the drug but in some instances after the drug was stopped. If a serious allergic reaction occurs, the drug should be discontinued and the patient closely monitored for several days.
- Drug may exacerbate preexisting psoriasis, Sweet's syndrome (neutrophilic dermatitis), and cutaneous vasculitis.

• Drug should not be used for PBPC mobilization.
• Drug should be used in pregnant women only when the potential benefit outweighs risk of fetal harm, as there are no adequate controlled studies in pregnant women, and laboratory animals had increased number of abortions and wavy ribs in fetuses.

Potential Toxicities/Side Effects (Dose- and Schedule-Dependent) and the Nursing Process

I. ALTERATION IN COMFORT related to SKELETAL PAIN, HEADACHE, MYALGIA, ABDOMINAL PAIN, ARTHRALGIA

Defining Characteristics: Patients (26%) may report transient mild-to-moderate skeletal pain believed due to the expansion of cells in the bone marrow in response to G-CSF. About 12% used nonopioid analgesics, and less than 6% required opioid analgesics. Leukocytosis of more than $100-10^9/L$ occurred in $< 1\%$ of patients. Other pain related to headache, myalgia and arthralgia, and abdominal pain may occur less commonly, but is easily managed.

Nursing Implications: Teach patient that bone pain may occur, and discuss use of nonsteroidal anti-inflammatory drugs with patient and physician for symptom management. Monitor WBC, hematocrit, and platelet count as appropriate prior to each cycle of chemotherapy. Teach patient that headache, myalgia, arthralgia, abdominal pain may occur and to report them if they do not respond to usual management strategies.

II. ALTERATION IN NUTRITION, POTENTIAL, related to NAUSEA, VOMITING, CONSTIPATION, DIARRHEA, ANOREXIA, STOMATITIS, MUCOSITIS

Defining Characteristics: Nutritional symptoms are rarely reported and may be related to the underlying malignancy.

Nursing Implications: Perform baseline patient nutritional assessment, history of nausea and vomiting, bowel elimination pattern, oral assessment, and usual appetite. Teach patient to report these side effects so that they can be evaluated. Teach patient self-care measures, including dietary modification and local comfort measures, as well as pharmacologic management as determined by the nurse/physician team. Teach patient to report symptoms that persist and do not respond to the planned therapy.

III. ALTERATION IN SKIN INTEGRITY, POTENTIAL, related to PERIPHERAL EDEMA, ALOPECIA

Defining Characteristics: Peripheral edema and alopecia are rarely reported, and may be related to other factors, such as the chemotherapy agents administered.

Nursing Implications: Perform baseline skin and scalp assessment. Teach patient to report development of peripheral edema, hair loss. If hair loss occurs, discuss acceptable management strategies with patient, depending upon impact of hair loss. Assess degree of peripheral edema if it develops, and discuss significant edema with physician to determine etiology and management. Teach patient local skin care, including avoidance of tight clothing and shoes, keeping skin moisturized to prevent cracking, and local comfort measures.

IV.   KNOWLEDGE DEFICIT related to SELF-ADMINISTRATION TECHNIQUE

Defining Characteristics: Drug is administered once per chemotherapy cycle, more than 14 days prior to chemotherapy administration or more than 24 hours after chemotherapy is given.

Nursing Implications: Assess baseline psychomotor ability, knowledge, and willingness to learn technique of self-injection. Assess which administration technique patient will use. (1) If On-body Injector for Neulasta, See the healthcare provider instructions for use of the On-Body Injector for Neulasta for complete information. Teach patient the following: (1) avoid traveling, driving, or operating heavy machinery during hours 26–29 following application of the injector (including the 45-minute delivery period plus an hour postdelivery); (2) have a caregiver nearby for first use of the injector; (3) review the patient instructions for use of the Neulasta On-Body Injector with the patient and caregiver and ensure understanding of when the dose delivery of Neulasta will begin, how to monitor the On-Body Injector for completed delivery, and how to identify signs of malfunction of the injector. (2) If manual injection, teach how to self-administer using manual prefilled syringes, activate needle guard, and safely collect used syringes for proper disposal. Drug insert has "Information for Patients and Caregivers." Use written and video supplements in teaching process, and have patient correctly demonstrate technique prior to performing at home. Make referral to visiting-nurse agency to reinforce teaching if needed. Teach patient telephone number and whom to call if questions or problems arise, and ensure that patient can correctly repeat information.

Drug: peginterferon alfa-2b (Sylatron)

Class: Interferon, cytokine

Mechanism of Action: Drug is a pleiotropic cytokine. The exact mechanism of antimelanoma effect is unknown, but it relates to immune effects. Interferon alfa-2b has antiviral, antiproliferative, and immunomodulatory effects. In addition, it activates pre-NK cells, increases cytotoxicity of NK cells, and enhances immune response.

Metabolism: After subcutaneous injection, the mean terminal half-life was about 51 hours in clinical study. The mean terminal half-life is about 43 hours. Drug is metabolized by cytochrome P-450 enzymes (CYP2C9 and CYP2D6). In patients with renal dysfunction, the AUC increased by 1.3-, 1.7-, and 1.9-fold in mild, moderate, and severe renal impairment.

Indication: For the adjuvant treatment of melanoma with microscopic or gross nodal involvement within 84 days of definitive surgical resection, including complete lymphadenectomy.

Contraindication: Patients with (1) history of anaphlyaxis to peginterferon alfa-2b or interferon alfa-2b; (2) autoimmune hepatitis; (3) hepatic decompensation (Child-Pugh score > 6 [class B and C]).

Dosage/Range:
- 6 mcg/kg/week subcutaneously for 8 doses, followed by 3 mcg/kg/week subcutaneously for up to 5 years. Premedicate with acetaminophen 500–1,000 mg orally 30 minutes prior to first dose, and as needed for subsequent injections.
  - Dose reduce in patients with moderate or severe renal impairment and end-stage renal disease.
  - Moderate (CrCl 30–50 mL/min): initial 4.5 mcg/kg/week × 8 weeks, then 2.25 mcg/kg/wk × 5 yr
  - Severe (CrCl < 30 mL/min): initial 3 mcg/kg/week × 8 weeks, then 1.5 mcg/ kg/week × 5 yr
  - End-stage renal disease (on dialysis): initial 3 mcg/kg/week × 8 weeks, then 1.5 mcg/kg/week × 5 yr

Dose Modifications:
- Permanently discontinue drug for:
  - Persistent or worsening severe neuropsychiatric disorders
  - Grade 4 nonhematologic toxicity
  - Inability to tolerate a dose of 1 mcg/kg/wk
  - New or worsening retinopathy
- Withhold drug dose for any of the following:
  - ANC < 0.5×10^9/L
  - Platelet count < 50×10^9/L
  - ECOG performance status (PS) > 2 (see below)
  - Nonhematologic toxicity > grade 3
- Resume dosing at a reduced dose when ANC > 0.5×10^9/L, platelet count > 50×10^9/L, ECOG PS 0–1, nonhematologic toxicity has completely resolved or improved to grade 1. SYLATRON

Dose Modifications:

Starting Dose (mcg/kg/week)	Dose Modifications for Doses 1–8
6	1st dose modification: 3 mcg/kg/week
	2nd dose modification: 2 mcg/kg/week
	3rd dose modification: 1 mcg/kg/week
	If unable to tolerate 1 mcg/kg/week, permanently discontinue drug
3	1st dose modification: 2 mcg/kg/week
	2nd dose modification: 1 mcg/kg/week
	If unable to tolerate 1 mcg/kg/week, permanently discontinue drug

Drug Preparation:
- Drug is available in 200, 300, and 600 mcg of deliverable lyophilized powder per single-use vial. Reconstitute vial with 0.7 mL of sterile water for injection USP. Upon reconstitution, the final concentration of the drug will be:
  - 200 mcg in 0.5 mL (final concentration 40 mcg per each 0.1 mL) of peginterferon alfa-2b (Sylatron)
  - 300 mcg in 0.5 mL (final concentration 60 mcg/each 0.1 mL) of peginterferon alfa-2b (Sylatron)
  - 600 mcg in 0.5 mL (final concentration 120 mcg/each 0.1 mL) of peginterferon alfa-2b (Sylatron)
- Swirl gently to dissolve the lyophilized powder. DO NOT SHAKE. Visually inspect the solution for particulate matter, cloudiness, or discoloration, and discard if present.
- Do not withdraw > 0.5 mL of reconstituted solution from each vial. If reconstituted solution is not used immediately, store at 2–8°C (36–46°F) for no more than 24 hours. Discard remaining solution after 24 hours. DO NOT FREEZE. For single-use only. Discard any unused portion.

Drug Administration:
- Administer subcutaneously. Rotate injection sites.
- Teach patient/caregiver self-administration, drug preparation, safe handling, and waste disposal of hazardous drug.
- Assess labs including CBC/differential/platelets; monitor hepatic function with serum bilirubin, ALT, AST, alkaline phosphatase, and LDH at 2 and 8 weeks, and 2 and 3 months following initiation of drug, then every 6 months while receiving the drug.
- Assess baseline TSH, chemistries.
- Teach patient and caregiver to immediately report any symptoms of depression or suicidal ideation to their provider. Monitor and evaluate patients for signs and symptoms of depression and other psychiatric symptoms every 3 weeks during the first 8 weeks of treatment, and every 6 months thereafter. Monitor patient during treatment and for at least 6 months after the last dose; permanently discontinue peginterferon-alfa-2b for suicidal or homicidal ideation, aggressive behavior toward others, or any other severe or persistent psychiatric symptoms. Institute psychiatric intervention and follow-up as needed.

Drug Interactions:
- Drugs metabolized by CYP2C9 (e.g., glyburide, glipizide, indocin, phenobarbital, phenytoin) or CYP2D6 (e.g., SSRIs, TCAs, beta-blockers, Type 1A antiarrythmics); therapeutic effect of these drugs may be altered.
- Caffeine (CYP1A2 substrate) or desipramine (CYP2D6 substrate) increased the exposure to caffeine 36% and to desipramine 30%, with potential increased toxicity from caffeine and desipramine.

Lab Effects/Interference:
- Increased: ALT or AST, alkaline phosphatase, GGT, serum triglycerides.
- Proteinuria, anemia

Special Considerations:

- Warnings and Precautions:
  - Depression and other serious neuropsychiatric adverse reactions may occur, including suicide, suicidal ideation, homicidal ideation, depression, and an increased risk of relapse of recovering drug addicts.
    - Teach patient/caregivers to report immediately symptoms of depression or suicidal thoughts.
    - Assess for signs and symptoms of depression and other psychiatric problems every 3 weeks for the first 8 weeks of treatment, then at least every 6 months.
    - Monitor patients during treatment and for at least 6 months after therapy ends, and discuss concerns with physician, NP/PA.
    - Drug should be permanently discontinued if persistent or worsening psychiatric symptoms or behaviors occur; refer for psychiatric evaluation.
  - Cardiovascular adverse reactions: MI, bundle branch block, tachycardia, and supraventricular arrhythmias occurred in 4% of patients. Drug should be permanently discontinued for new onset of ventricular arrhythmias or cardiovascular decompensation.
  - Drug can cause a decrease in visual acuity or blindness due to retinopathy.
    - Retinal and ocular changes include macular edema, retinal artery or vein thrombosis, retinal hemorrhages and cotton wool spots, optic neuritis, papilledema, and serous retinal detachment; they can be induced or aggravated by treatment with peginterferon alfa-2b.
    - Although rare, patients should receive an eye examination that includes assessment of visual acuity and indirect ophthalmoscopy or fundus photography at baseline in patients with preexisting retinopathy, and at any time during treatment.
    - Teach patients to report any changes in vision IMMEDIATELY. Permanently discontinue drug in patients who develop new or worsening retinopathy.
  - Hepatic failure: Drug increases the risk of hepatic decompensation and death in patients with cirrhosis.
    - Monitor hepatic function with serum bilirubin, ALT, AST, alkaline phosphatase, and LDH at 2 and 8 weeks, and 2 and 3 months following initiation of drug, then every 6 months while receiving the drug.
    - Permanently discontinue the drug if evidence of severe (grade 3) hepatic injury or hepatic decompensation (Child-Pugh score $>$ 6 [class B and C]).
  - Drug can cause new onset or worsening of hypothyroidism, hyperthyroidism, and diabetes mellitus. Overall incidence of endocrinopathies was 2% compared to $<$ 1% in the observation group. Obtain TSH level 4 weeks prior to the start of peginterferon alfa-2b, at 3 and 6 months following initiation, and every 6 months thereafter. The drug should be permanently discontinued in patients who develop hypothyroidism, hyperthyroidism, or diabetes mellitus that cannot be effectively managed.
  - Drug should be used during pregnancy only when the potential benefit justifies the potential hazard to the fetus.
  - Nursing mothers should decide to discontinue nursing or to discontinue the drug, taking into consideration the importance of the drug to the mother's health.

- FDA-approval based on an open-label, multicentered randomized trial evaluating the safety and efficacy of peginterferon alfa-2b in 1,256 patients with surgically resected stage III melanoma within 84 days of lymph node dissection (Eggermont et al., 2008). The primary endpoint was RFS. Median RFS for the peginterferon alfa-2b group was 34.8 months compared to 25.5 months in the observation group. Secondary endpoint was OS. There was no statistically significant difference in survival between the treatment and observation arms. Some patients (16%) did not continue on the 3 mcg/kg/week regimen. Patients (52%) had dose reductions, and 70% required dose delays (average delay 2.2 weeks). Some patients (33%) discontinued treatment due to adverse reactions.

ECOG status assesses a patient's level of functioning (e.g., self care, physical ability), and ranges from 0, where the patient is fully active, able to carry on all activities as the patient had prior to illness, to 5, which is dead. The grading 1 is used for ambulatory patients with slight restriction on strenuous activity but patient able to work a light job. Grade 2 indicates the patient is up at least 50% of the time, but cannot do work. Grade 3 indicates the patient is confined to bed or chair >50% of waking hours, while Grade 4 indicates completely disabled, unable to do any self-care, and totally confined to bed or chair.

The ECOG Performance Status is in the public domain, therefore available for public use. To duplicate the scale, please cite the reference above and credit the Eastern Cooperative Oncology Group, Robert Comis.

Potential Toxicities/Side Effects and the Nursing Process

I.   ALTERATION IN COMFORT related to FLU-LIKE SYNDROME

Defining Characteristics: Most commonly patients experienced fatigue (94%), pyrexia (75%), headache (70%), myalgia (68%), nausea (64%), and chills (63%). Joint pain also occurred. Fatigue was severe in 7%, pyrexia in 3%.

Nursing Implications: Assess baseline T, VS, neurologic status, and comfort level and teach patient/caregiver to report severe symptoms. Teach patient to premedicate with acetaminophen 30 minutes prior to the first dose, and as needed prior to subsequent doses. Teach patient to take dose at bedtime. Teach patient self-care measures, including hydration of one 8-oz. glass of fluid every hour while awake to minimize risk of dehydration, self-assessment and monitoring of temperature, comfort level, self-administration of prescribed medications prior to dose, as well as the use of heat or cold for myalgias, arthralgias. Encourage patient to increase oral fluids and alternate rest and activity periods, medications, and oral hygiene regimen.

II.   ALTERATION IN NUTRITION, LESS THAN BODY REQUIREMENTS, related to NAUSEA, VOMITING, DIARRHEA, ANOREXIA

Defining Characteristics: Anorexia (69%) occurs and is cumulative. Nausea (64%) is mild with tachyphylaxis after 1 week. Diarrhea (37%) is mild, and vomiting (26%) may occur. Aphthous stomatitis, pancreatitis, and colitis were reported post-marketing.

Nursing Implications: Assess baseline nutritional status. Teach patient potential side effects and self-care measures, including oral hygiene. Encourage patient to prepare favorite high-calorie, high-protein foods ahead of time to be able to snack when hungry. Teach self-administration of prescribed antiemetics and antidiarrheals as needed. Refer to dietitian as appropriate.

III. SENSORY/PERCEPTUAL ALTERATION related to CNS EFFECTS, DEPRESSION, SUICIDAL IDEATION

Defining Characteristics: Depression occurred in 59% of patients compared to 24% in the observation group. It was severe or life-threatening in 7% of patients receiving peginterferon alfa-2b, compared to < 1% in observation group. These effects are reported up to 6 months after discontinuation of the drug. Drug can also result in aggressive behavior, psychoses, hallucinations, bipolar disorders, mania, and encephalopathy. Patients also reported headache (70%), dysgeusia (38%), dizziness (35%), olfactory nerve disorder (23%), and paresthesias (21%).

Nursing Implications: Assess baseline mental status and neurologic status prior to drug administration. Assess patient for changes (depression, impaired memory/attention, change in behavior, disorientation, slow/vague responses to questions, increased lethargy) during treatment. Instruct patient to report signs/symptoms, provide information and emotional support, as well as interventions to ensure safety if signs/symptoms occur. Teach patients and their caregivers to report immediately any symptoms of depression or suicidal ideation to their healthcare provider. Monitor and evaluate patients for signs and symptoms of depression and other psychiatric symptoms every 3 weeks during the first 8 weeks of treatment, and every 6 months thereafter. Monitor patients during treatment and for at least 6 months after the last dose of peginterferon alfa-2b. Permanently discontinue drug for persistent severe or worsening psychiatric symptoms or behaviors and refer for psychiatric evaluation.

IV. POTENTIAL ALTERATION IN CARDIAC OUTPUT related to TACHYCARDIA, CHEST PAIN, DYSRHYTHMIAS

Defining Characteristics: In the clinical trial, cardiac adverse reactions, including MI, bundle-branch block, ventricular tachycardia, and supraventricular tachycardia occurred in 4% of patients compared with 2% in the observation group. In post-marketing, patients reported hypotension, cardiomyopathy, and angina pectoris.

Nursing Implications: Assess baseline cardiopulmonary status and risk (elderly, preexisting cardiac dysfunction). Discuss EKG testing, baseline and during treatment, for high-risk individuals. Monitor vital signs at each visit. Teach patient to report signs/symptoms of palpitations, dyspnea, chest pain, edema, or other abnormalities immediately. Drug should be permanently discontinued for new onset of ventricular arrhythmias or cardiovascular decompensation.

V.   POTENTIAL ALTERATION IN ELIMINATION related to RENAL AND HEPATIC DYSFUNCTION

Defining Characteristics: Dose-related increased ALT or AST occurred in 77% of patients, GGT in 8%, and increased alkaline phosphatase in 23% of patients. Drug increases the risk of hepatic decompensation and death in patients with cirrhosis. Proteinuria may occur.

Nursing Implications: Monitor hepatic function with serum bilirubin, ALT, AST, alkaline phosphatase, and LDH baseline, at 2 and 8 weeks, and 2 and 3 months following initiation of drug, then every 6 months while receiving the drug. The drug should be permanently discontinued if evidence of severe (grade 3) hepatic injury or hepatic decompensation (Child-Pugh score > 6 [class B and C]).

VI.   POTENTIAL ALTERATION IN SKIN INTEGRITY related to RASH, PARTIAL ALOPECIA, DRYNESS

Defining Characteristics: Injection-site reaction occurs in 62% of patients. Exfoliative rash occurred in 36% of patients and alopecia in 34%.

Nursing Implications: Assess baseline skin integrity. Instruct patient to report signs/symptoms. If skin site is painful, try applying ice to the site 5–10 minutes prior to the injection. Discuss/teach symptomatic management, including the use of mild soaps and rinsing skin thoroughly after bathing. Encourage patient to use alcohol-free, oil-based moisturizers on skin. Teach patient to report any severe symptoms, and discuss management with physician/midlevel.

VII.   KNOWLEDGE DEFICIT related to SELF-ADMINISTRATION TECHNIQUE

Defining Characteristics: Patient or caregiver must administer drug weekly in the home setting by subcutaneous injection and is unfamiliar with technique.

Nursing Implications: Assess baseline psychomotor ability, knowledge, and willingness to learn technique of self-injection. Teach how to prepare drug, self-administer, and safely collect used syringes for proper disposal. Use written and video materials as supplements to teaching process and have patient correctly demonstrate technique prior to performing at home. Make referral to visiting-nurse agency to reinforce teaching if needed.

Drug: pembrolizumab (Keytruda)

Class: Immune checkpoint inhibitor. Human programmed death-1 (PD-1)-blocking antibody; humanized mAb against PD-1.

Mechanism of Action: One of the ways cancer evades the immune system is by taking advantage of the body's process to turn down activated T-lymphocytes after an immune response to protect the body's organs from autoimmune injury. The programmed cell death 1 (PD-1) receptor is found on T-lymphocytes, especially if they have been exposed to an antigen for a long time. It is activated by its ligand, PD-L1 (also known as B7-H1 or CD274), which is often found in the tumor microenvironment (Hamid et al., 2013). PD-1 also has another ligand, PD-L2 (also known as B7-DC or CD273), which is preferentially expressed by APCs. When the ligands PD-L1 and PD-L2 bind to the PD-1 receptor on T-lymphocytes, they turn off T-cell proliferation and cytokine production (Merck & Co., 2017). Some tumors upregulate PD-1 ligands. mAb drugs that block the ligand PD-L1 from binding to its receptor PD-1 prevent activated T-lymphocytes from being turned down/off so they can continue to attack cancer cells. See chapter introduction on *Immunotherapy*. By blocking this immune checkpoint inhibitor, pembrolizumab has less immune toxicity than others, such as ipilimumab, which blocks the inhibitory receptor cytotoxic T-lymphocyte-associated antigen 4 (CTLA-4). However, immune-related adverse effects may occur. In mice, this decreases tumor growth (Merck & Co., 2017). Solid tumors that have MSI-H are responsive to checkpoint inhibitors. About 15% of CRC tumors are MSI-H, due to a mutation in the mismatch (DNA) repair pathway (MMR). Microsatellites are repeating tandem sections of DNA that have insertion and deletion mutations, as well as nucleotide substitutions throughout the length of the DNA (Gatalica et al., 2016). MSI-H tumors have strong immune activation (Gatalica et al., 2016), which may explain why these tumors are sensitive to checkpoint inhibitors.

Indication: Treatment of patients with

(1) **Melanoma:** (a) unresectable or metastatic melanoma; (b) adjuvant treatment of patients with lymph node involvement, following complete resection.

(2) **Metastatic NSCLC**: (a) in combination with pemetrexed and platinum chemotherapy, as first-line treatment of non-squamous NSCLC without EGFR or ALK genomic tumor aberrations; (b) in combination with carboplatin and either paclitaxel or nab-paclitaxel as first-line treatment of squamous NSCLC; (c) as a single agent of patients whose tumors express PD-L1 (Tumor Proportion Score, TPS ≥1%) as determined by an FDA-approved test, with disease progression on or after platinum-containing chemotherapy, or if EGFR or ALK-mutation positive, patient has disease progression on FDA-approved treatments for these mutations.

(3) **Stage III not surgical or definitive chemoradiation candidates or metastatic NSCLC:** as a single agent for first line treatment expressing PD-LI (Tumor Proportion Score, TPS ≥1%) as determined by an FDA-approved test without EGFR or ALK genomic tumor aberrations.

(4) **Head and Neck Squamous Cell Cancer (HNSCC)**: (a) as a single agent in patients with recurrent or metastatic HNSCC with disease progression on or after platinum-containing chemotherapy; (b) in combination with platinum and fluorouracil (FU) for first line treatment of patients with metastatic or with unresectable, recurrent HNSCC; (c) as a single agent for the first line treatment of patients with metastatic or with unresectable, recurrent HNSCC whose tumors express PD-L1 (Combined Positive Score (CPS) ≥1 as determined by a FDA-approved test).

(5) **Classical Hodgkin Lymphoma** (cHL): adult and pediatric patients with refractory cHL or who have relapsed after 3 or more prior lines of therapy (accelerated approval);

(6) **Primary mediastinal large B-cell lymphoma (PMBCL)**: adult and pediatric patients with refractory PMBCL, or who have relapsed after 2 or more prior therapy; pembrolizumab is not recommended for treatment of PMBCL patients who need urgent cytoreductive treatment. (accelerated approval);

(7) **Urothelial carcinoma,** locally advanced or metastatic, patients:
   (a) who are NOT eligible for cisplatin-containing chemotherapy and whose tumors express PD-L1 (combined positive score (CPS) $\geq$ 10 as determined by an FDA-approved test, or in patients who are not eligible for any platinum-containing chemotherapy regardless of PD-L1 status (accelerated approval);
   (b) who have locally advanced or metastatic urothelial carcinoma who have disease progression during or following platinum-containing chemotherapy or within 12 months of neoadjuvant or adjuvant treatment with platinum-containing chemotherapy;

(8) **Microsatellite High (MSI-H) or mismatch-repair deficient (dMMR) cancers**: adult and pediatric patients with unresectable or metastatic MSI-H or dMMR; (a) solid tumors that have progressed following prior treatment and who have no satisfactory alternative treatment options, or (b) CRC that has progressed following treatment with a fluoropyrimidine, oxaliplatin, and irinotecan (accelerated approval). Limitation of use: safety and efficacy not established in pediatric patients with MSI-H CNS cancers.

(9) **Gastric cancer that is recurrent locally advanced or metastasized or gastroesophageal (GEJ) adenocarcinoma** that express PD-L1 (combined positive score (CPS) $\geq$1) as determined by an FDA-approved test, with disease progression on or after 2+ lines of therapy including fluoropyrimidine- and platinum-containing chemotherapy and if appropriate, HER2/neu-targeted therapy; acelerated approval.

(10) **cervical cancer** that is recurrent or metastatic with disease progression on or after chemotherapy whose tumors express PD-L1 (CPS $\geq$ 1) as determined by an FDA-approved test (accelerated approval).

(11) Hepatocellular carcinoma (HCC): who have previously been treated with sorafenib. Accelerated approval.

(12) Merkel cell carcinoma (MCC): in adult and pediatric patients with recurrent locally advanced or metastatic Merkel cell carcinoma. Accelerated approval.

(13) **renal cell carcinoma (RCC),** advanced, in combination with axitinib for first-line treatment.

Indications that are approved under accelerated approval are based on tumor response rate and durability of response. Continued approval may be contingent upon verification and description of clinical benefit in confirmatory trials.

Dosaage: Patients requiring positive PD-L1 expression: stage III NSCLC who are not candidates for surgery or definitive chemoradiation, metastatic NSCLC, first-line treatment of metastatic or unresectable, recurrent HNSCC, metatatic urothelial carcinoma, metastatic gastric cancer, recurrent or metatatic cervical cancer.

Dosage/Range: (IV infusion over 30 minutes)
- All doses administered as an IV infusion over 30 minutes every 3 weeks until disease progression or unacceptable toxicity; or in patients with melanoma receiving adjuvant therapy up to 12 months if no recurrence; or in patients with cHL, PMBCL, NSCLC, HNSCC, urothelial carcinoma, gastric cancer, cervical cancer, HCC, MSI-H, or renal cell carcinoma up to 24 months in patients without disease progression.

Melanoma: 200-mg every 3 weeks (until disease progression, unacceptable toxicity, or in adjuvant patients, for up to 12 months if no disease recurrence).
- *NSCLC:* 200-mg every 3 weeks until disease progression, unacceptable toxicity, or up to 24 months in patients without disease progression. If administering pembrolizumab in combination with chemotherapy, administer pembrolizumab prior to chemotherapy when given on the same day.
- *HNSCC:* 200-mg every 3 weeks until disease progression, unacceptable toxicity, or up to 24 months in patients without disease progression. If administering pembrolizumab in combination with chemotherapy, administer pembrolizumab **prior to** chemotherapy when given on the same day.
- *cHL or PMBCL:* 200-mg every 3 weeks for adults; for pediatric patients, 2-mg/kg (up to 200 mg) every 3 weeks, until disease progression, unacceptable toxicity, or up to 24 months in patients without disease progression.
- *Urothelial carcinoma:* 200-mg every 3 weeks, until disease progression, unacceptable toxicity, or up to 24 months in patients without disease progression.
- *MSI-H cancers:* 200-mg every 3 weeks for adults; for pediatric patients, 2-mg/kg (up to 200 mg) every 3 weeks, until disease progression, unacceptable toxicity, or up to 24 months in patients without disease progression.
- *Gastric cancer:* **200-mg every 3 weeks,** until disease progression, unacceptable toxicity, or up to 24 months in patients without disease progression.
- *Cervical cancer:* 200-mg every 3 weeks, until disease progression, unacceptable toxicity, or up to 24 months in patients without disease progression.
- *HCC:* 200-mg every 3 weeks, until disease progression, unacceptable toxicity, or up to 24 months in patients without disease progression.
- *MCC:* 200-mg every 3 weeks; for pediatric patients, 2-mg/kg (up to 200 mg) every 3 weeks, until disease progression, unacceptable toxicity, or up to 24 months in patients without disease progression.
- *RCC:* 200-mg every 3 weeks in combination with axitinib 5 mg PO bid; consider dose escalation of axitinib at intervals of 6 weeks or longer as appropriate (Merck, 2019). Treatment can continue for up to 24 months if no disease progression.

Dose Modifications: Do not reduce dose of pembrolizumab, rather, withhold or discontinue drug as follows (see package insert for more detail):
- **Hold pembrolizumab for**:
  (1) grade 2 pneumonitis, (2) grades 2–3 colitis, (3) hepatitis AST/ALT >3x–<5× ULN, (4) grades 3–4 endocrinopathies, (4) grade 4 hematological toxicity cHL and PMBCL; (5) grade 2 nephritis, (6) grade 3 severe skin reactions or suspected Stevens-Johnson syndrome (SJS) or toxic epidermal necrolysis (TEN); (7) AST or ALT > 3 and up to 5 × ULN or total bilirubin > 1.5–3 × ULN (patient without HCC); (8) RCC patients

receiving axitinib plus pembrolizumab: if ALT or AST $\geq$ 3 $\times$ ULN but <10 $\times$ ULN without concurrent total bilirubin $\geq$ 2 $\times$ ULN. Consider corticosteroid therapy. Consider rechallenge with a single drug or sequential rechallenge with both drugs after recovery. If rechallenging with axitinib, consider dose reduction as per axitinib prescribing information; (9) any other grade 2 or grade 3 toxicity based on severity and type of reaction; (9) resume pembrolizumab when patient recovers to grade 0–1.

- **Permanently discontinue pembrolizumab** for (1) any life-threatening adverse reaction (excluding endocrinopathies controlled with hormone-replacement therapy or hematologic toxicity in patients with cHL or PMBCL); (2) grades 3–4 pneumonitis or recurrent pneumonitis of grade 2 severity; (3) grades 3–4 nephritis; (4) grade 4 severe skin reactions or confirmed SJS or TEN; (5) AST or ALT > 5 $\times$ ULN or total bilirubin > 3 $\times$ ULN [for patients with liver metastasis who begin treatment with grade 2 AST or ALT, if AST or ALT increases by $\geq$50% relative to baseline and lasts for at least 1 week]; (6) grade 3 or 4 myocarditis, encephalitis, or Guillain-Barre syndrome; (7) grades 3–4 Infusion-related reactions (IIIRs); (8) inability to reduce corticosteroids dose to 10 mg or less of prednisone or equivalent per day within 12 weeks; (9) persistent grades 2–3 adverse reactions (excluding endocrinopathies controlled with hormone replacement therapy) that do not recover to grade 0–1 within 12 weeks after last dose of pembrolizumab; (10) severe grade 3 treatment-related adverse reaction based on severity and type or grade 4; (11) recurrent grades 3 or 4 adverse effects; (12) RCC patients without liver metastases, AST or ALT >5 $\times$ ULN, or total bilirubin >3 $\times$ ULN; if patient has liver metastases and grade 2 AST or ALT at baseline with an increase in AST or ALT of 50% or more relative to baseline that persists for at least 1 week; (13) RCC in patients receiving axitinib with pembrolizumab, if ALT or AST $\geq$ 10 $\times$ ULN or >3 $\times$ ULN with concurrent total bilirubin $\geq$ 2 $\times$ ULN, discontinue both drugs permanently and consider corticosteroid therapy.

Drug Preparation:
- Pembrolizumab is available as a 50-mg *lyophilized powder* for injection in a single-use vial for reconstitution, and as a 100 mg/4 mL (25 mg/mL) *solution* in a single-use vial.
- To reconstitute 50-mg lyophilized powder:
  - Add 2.3 mL sterile water for injection, USP by injecting the water along the walls of the vial (not directly into the lyophilized powder), resulting in a concentration of 25 mg/mL.
  - Swirl the vial contents slowly and gently. Allow up to 5 minutes for the bubbles to clear.
  - *Do not shake the vial.*
- To prepare IV solution:
  - Visually inspect the solution for particulate matter or discoloration. The solution should be clear to slightly opalescent, colorless to slightly yellow. If visible particles or discoloration are seen, discard the vial.
  - Dilute pembrolizumab injection (solution) or reconstituted lyophilized powder prior to IV administration.
  - Aseptically withdraw the ordered volume from the vial(s) and transfer to an IV bag containing 0.9% sodium chloride injection, USP or 5% dextrose injection USP. The final concentration of the diluted solution should be between 1 and 10 mg/mL

- Mix the diluted solution by gentle inversion. Discard any unused drug left in the vial.
- Storage of reconstituted and diluted solutions:
  - Store reconstituted and diluted solution from the pembrolizumab 50-mg vial either
  - At room temperature for no more than 6 hours from time of reconstitution until time the infusion finishes (including room-temperature storage of reconstituted vials, storage of infusion solution in the IV bag, and duration of infusion) **or**
  - Under refrigeration at 2–8°C (36–46°F) for no more than 24 hours from the time of reconstitution. If refrigerated, allow the diluted solution to come to room temperature prior to administration.
  - Store the diluted solution from the pembrolizumab 100 mg/4 mL vial either
    - At room temperature $\leq$ 6 hours from the time of dilution (including room-temperature storage of the infusion solution in the IV bag and duration of infusion), **or**
    - Under refrigeration at 2–8°C (36–46°F) for no more than 24 hours from the time of dilution. If refrigerated, allow the diluted solution to come to room temperature prior to administration.
  - Do not freeze.

Drug Administration:
- When pembrolizumab is given in combination with chemotherapy, administer pembrolizumab prior to chemotherapy when given on the same day.
- Assess for any immune-related adverse effects (irAEs) such as signs/symptoms of pneumonitis, colitis, or others from prior treatment doses; assess cbc/differential and metabolic panel, endocrine function tests, as ordered and discuss any abnormalities with provider prior to treatment.
- Administer infusion solution IV over 30 minutes through an IV line containing a sterile, nonpyrogenic, low-protein-binding 0.2 to 0.5 micron in-line or add-on filter.
- Do not coadminister with other drug(s) through the same line.

Drug Interactions:
- Unknown. No formal studies have been conducted.

Lab Effects/Interference:
- Anemia, hypocalcemia, hyponatremia, hypoalbuminemia, decreased bicarbonate
- Hyperglycemia, hypertriglyceridemia, increased AST and ALT, increased alkaline phosphatase.

Special Considerations:
- In a study of 173 patients with advanced melanoma refractory to ipilimumab, Robert et al. (2014) found a response rate of 26% lasting 1.4–8.5 months or longer. Hamid et al. (2013) found the response rate did not differ significantly between patients who had received prior ipilimumab treatment and those who had not. Most responses seen within the first 12 weeks of treatment.
- **Most common adverse events** ($\geq$ 20% of patients) (1) melanoma: included fatigue, nausea, pruritus, rash, decreased appetite, constipation; (2) NSCLC: included fatigue, decreased appetite, dyspnea, and cough.

- FDA (2018) limited the use of atezolizumab and pembrolizumab for patients with locally advanced or metastatic urothelial cancer who are not eligible for cis-platinum containing therapy. Studies showed decreased survival when either of these drugs was given as a single agent compared to platinum-based chemotherapy in previously untreated patients with locally advanced or metastatic urothelial cancer whose tumors had low expression of PD-L1. For pembrolizumab, as of 2018, patients must be **ineligible** for treatment with a cisplatin containing regimen and express PD-L1 (have a combined positive score (CPS) ≥10), or be patients who are not eligible for cisplatinum-containing chemotherapy regardless of CPS score (FDA, 2018).
- Warnings and Precautions:
  - *Immune-related pneumonitis*: occurred in 3.4% of patients studied receiving pembrolizumab; median time to onset 3.3 months. with 0.8% grade 2 and 0.4% grade 3; median time to onset was 4.3 months with a median duration of 2.6 months. Incidence in patients with NSCLC receiving pembrolizumab as first line therapy for advanced disease was 8.2% (including grade 3–4 in 3.2% of patients). If the patient had a history of prior thoracic RT, incidence was 17%. Pneumonitis resolved in 51% of the patients. Monitor patients for signs and symptoms of pneumonitis, evaluate any suspicious symptoms promptly with imaging and discuss management with provider. For grade 2 or higher, expect to hold drug and administer corticosteroids (1–2 mg/kg/day prednisone equivalent) followed by a taper over 4 weeks or more. Permanently discontinue pembrolizumab in patients with grades 3 or 4 pneumonitis, or recurrent moderate grade 2 pneumonitis.
  - *Immune-related colitis*: occurred in 1.7 % of patients; median time to onset was 1.3 months Monitor patients for signs and symptoms of colitis. Hold drug for grade 2 or higher and administer corticosteroids (1–2 mg/kg/day prednisone equivalents/taper over at least 4 weeks; permanently discontinue drug for grade 4 colitis.
  - *Immune-related hepatitis*: Incidence in melanoma patients was 10.7% with median time to onset was 1.3 months. Risk of grades 3–4 hepatotoxicity is higher in patients receiving axitinib with pembrolizumab (RCC). Increased incidences of grades 3–4 ALT (20%) and AST (13%) hepatotoxicity were seen, with a median time to onset for ALT of 2.3 months. Monitor LFT baseline and regularly during therapy, with more frequent monitoring of patients when another drug is given with pembrolizumab (e.g., axitinib). For patients rechallenged, with either pembrolizumab or axitinib monotherapy or with both, 55% had no recurrence of ALT > 3 × ULN. Manage hepatotoxicity in most patients with corticosteroids, followed by a corticosteroid taper. Hold or discontinue drug based on severity of changes in liver enzymes.
  - *Immune-related endocrinopathies (see package insert)*
    - **Hypophysitis:** occurred in 0.6% of patients. Median time to onset was 3.3 months with median duration 3.7 months. Monitor for signs and symptoms of hypophysitis (including hypopituitarism and adrenal insufficiency). Hold drug and give corticosteroids/taper and replacement as clinically indicated. Hold drug for moderate (grade 2) and hold or discontinue drug for grades 3–4.
    - **Thyroid disorders:** Immune-mediated hyperthyroidism and hypothyroidism: occurred in 3.4% and 8.5% of patients respectively; , median time to onset was 1.4–3.5 months respectively. Monitor thyroid function studies baseline, during

treatment, and monitor for signs and symptoms of hyper- and hypothyroidism. Administer replacement hormones for hypothyroidism, and manage hyperthyroidism with thionamides and beta-blockers as needed. Hold or discontinue drug for severe (grade 3) or life threatening (grade 4) hyperthyroidism.

- **Type 1 diabetes mellitus:** Incidence 0.2%. Monitor for hyperglycemia and signs/ symptoms of diabetes. Administer insulin for immune Type1 DM; hold pembrolizumab and give antihyperglycemics to patients with *severe* hyperglycemia.
- *Immune-mediated nephritis:* in 0.3% of patients when pembrolizumab was given as a single agent; median time to onset was 5.1 months and median duration was 3.3 months. When administered with pemetrexed and platinum, the incidence was 1.7%; median time to onset was 3.2 months, and duration 1.6–16.8+ months. Monitor renal function. Hold drug and give corticosteroids/taper for grade 2 or higher nephritis. Permanently discontinue drug for grade 3 and 4 nephritis.
- *Immune-mediated skin adverse reactions:* Monitor skin integrity and teach patient to report any changes. If SJS, TEN, bullous phemphigoid or exfoliative dermatitis is suspected, exclude other causes. If severe, hold or permanently discontinue drug and administer corticosteroids/taper as ordered. Discuss with provider or get a dermatitis consult.
- *Other immune-mediated adverse reactions occurred* during or after pembrolizumab was discontinued. Incidence was < 1% of patients and included exfoliative dermatitis, uveitis, arthritis, myositis, pancreatitis, hemolytic anemia, partial seizures, myasthenic syndrome, optic neuritis, rhabdomyolysis, and adrenal insufficiency. Evaluate; if severe, interrupt drug and give corticosteroids. When resolved to grade 1 or less, start corticosteroid taper and continue for > 1 month. Permanently discontinue drug for any severe or grade 3 immune-mediated adverse reaction. If uncontrolled with corticosteroids consider other systemic immunosuppressant therapy. Solid organ transplant rejection has been reported in post-marketing reports; pembrolizumab may increase the risk of rejection so the risk vs benefit must be carefully discussed with the transplant patient.Myelitis and myocarditis were reported during clinical trials, and in post-marketing reports.
- *Infusion-related reactions:* Incidence of severe and life-threatening reactions 0.1%. Monitor patients for signs/symptoms of infusion related reactions (e.g., rigors, chills, wheezing, pruritis, flushing, rash, hypotension, hypoxemia, fever). Stop infusion and permanently discontinue pembrolizumab for severe or life-threatening infusion reactions.
- *Complications of allogeneic hSCT* have occurred.Risk vs benefit discussion must occur before patient decides on pembrolizumab therapy as patient may be at increased risk of GVHD. (a) *Allogeneic HSCT after treatment with pembrolizumab*: in one trial of patients with cHL26% developed GVHD and 9% developed veno-occlusive disease (VOD); (b) *Allogeneic HSCT prior to treatment with pembrolizumab*: if patient experienced GVHD after transplant, there is a possible increased risk for GVHD after treatment with pembrolizumab Follow patients closely for signs/symptoms of transplant-related comlications (e.g., hyperacute GVHD, severe acute GVHD, febrile syndrome requiring steroids, hepatic VOD) and discuss plan to intervene promptly.

- **Increased mortality in patients with multiple myeloma when pembrolizumab is added to a thalidomide analogue and dexamethasone**: In 2 RCTs of patients with multiple myeloma, the addition of pembrolizumab to thalidomide analogue and dexamethasone increased mortality. No PD-1 or PD-L1 blocking antibody is indicated in combination with thalidomide analogue and dexamethasone for multiple myeloma. Treatment of patients with multiple myeloma should receive PD-1 or PD-L1 inhibitor therapy ONLY in a controlled clinical trial (Merck, 2019).
- *Drug causes embryo-fetal toxicity* as PD-1/PDL-1 signaling pathways maintain maternal immune tolerance to fetal tissue. Teach women of reproductive potential to use highly effective contraception to avoid pregnancy during treatment and for 4 months after treatment has ended. Mothers should not nurse while receiving pembrolizumab.

Potential Toxicities/Side Effects and the Nursing Process

I.   POTENTIAL FOR INJURY related to IMMUNE related ADVERSE EFFECTS (see Special Considerations, and package insert Table 2.14)

II.   ALTERATION IN NUTRITION, POTENTIAL, LESS THAN BODY REQUIREMENTS, related to DIARRHEA, NAUSEA, DECREASED APPETITE

Defining Characteristics: Symptom incidence by disease is indicated as melanoma/NSCLC patients. Diarrhea affected 20%/15%, nausea 0%/18%, vomiting 0%/12%, decreased appetite 16%/25%, and constipation 22%/15%. Hyperglycemia, hypertriglyceridemia, hypoalbuminemia, and increased AST/ALT occurred.

Nursing Implications: Assess nutritional and bowel-elimination patterns, appetite, and presence of nausea and/or vomiting baseline and at each visit. Teach that diarrhea, constipation, nausea, vomiting, and decreased appetite may occur, and to report them. Assess control of nutrition impact symptoms and discuss management with physician. Teach patient to self-administer antidiarrheal or antiemetic medication, if needed, and to report symptoms that do not improve. Monitor LFTs, glucose, albumin, triglycerides baseline and periodically during therapy as ordered.

III.   ALTERATION IN COMFORT related to FATIGUE, ASTHENIA, MYALGIA, HEADACHE, PYREXIA, CHILLS, AND ABDOMINAL PAIN

Defining Characteristics: Fatigue was common, affecting 28%/44%; arthralgia occurred in 14%/15%; headache in 14%/0%, pyrexia in 14%/12%, abdominal pain 13/0%, and anemia.

Nursing Implications: Teach patient that these events may occur and to report them. Assess comfort and hemoglobin/hematocrit baseline, and monitor closely during treatment. Develop a plan to assure comfort, depending on symptoms reported, teach patient self-care strategies, and assess efficacy and revise plan if needed at each visit.

IV. ALTERATION IN SKIN INTEGRITY, POTENTIAL, related to RASH, PRURITUS, AND VITILIGO

Defining Characteristics: Incidence is expressed as percentage melanoma/NSCL patients. Pruritis affected 28%/12%, rash affected 24%/18%, and vitiligo 13%/0%. Peripheral edema also occurred.

Nursing Implications: Teach patient that rash, pruritus, vitiligo, and peripheral edema may occur and to report these signs and symptoms. Assess patient skin integrity and presence of edema, baseline and regularly, during treatment. Teach strategies to patient to maintain skin integrity, reduce itching, and evaluate response.

Drug: pertuzumab (Perjeta)

Class: HER-2/neu receptor dimerization inhibitor (HDI). Specifically, it is a recombinant humanized (IgG1) that inhibits human epidermal growth factor receptor dimerization, the first of its class. It is a HER-2 receptor antagonist.

Mechanism of Action: In order for a growth signal to be sent to the cell nucleus, a growth factor (ligand) attaches to the human epidermal growth factor receptor, or HER. The growth factor receptor now needs to dimerize or pair with another growth factor receptor to activate the RTK; for example, HER-2 receptor needs to dimerize or pair with another HER receptor, such as HER-1 (EGFR), HER-3, or HER-4. Pertuzumab is an IgG_1 mAb that binds to the dimerization domain of HER (subdomain II) so the binding of the antibody directly inhibits the ability of HER-2 to dimerize with other HER proteins and no other proteins can bind to it to activate the receptor. Without activation, the signal is not sent to downstream effectors such as mitogen-activated protein kinase (MAP kinase) and phosphoinositide 3-kinase (P13K) pathways, which control cell growth and survival. This leads to cell growth arrest and apoptosis (programmed cell death). In addition, pertuzumab mediates ADCC. Drug blocks a different HER-2 receptor location from that of trastuzumab so drugs can be given together to maximize blockade of HER signaling. This leads to greater antitumor activity than either agent alone (Baselga et al., 2012). Drug is a recombinant, humanized mAb.

Metabolism: Steady state concentration of pertuzumab is reached after the first maintenance dose following loading dose. Median drug half-life is 18 days. Pertuzumab exposure in patients with mild and moderate renal impairment was similar to patients with normal renal function.

Indication: Treatment of patients with HER2-positive breast cancer:
(1) Metastatic Breast Cancer (mBC), who have not received prior anti-HER2 therapy or chemotherapy for metastic disease, in combination with trastuzumab and docetaxel;
(2) Early breast cancer (EBC), in combination with trastuzumab and chemotherapy for
  • Neoadjuvant treatment of patients with HER2-positive, locally advanced, inflammatory, or EBC (either > 2 cm in diameter or node-positive) as part of a complete treatment regimen for early breast cancer.

- Adjuvant treatment of patients with HER2-positive early breast cancer at high risk of recurrence.
(3) Patients should be selected based on HER2 protein overexpression or HER2 gene amplification in tumor specimens using FDA-approved tests specific for breast cancer by laboratories with demonstrated proficiency.

Dosage/Range:

Initial loading dose:
- 840-mg IV infusion as a 60-minute infusion, followed every 3 weeks thereafter by a 420-mg IV infusion over 30–60 minutes.
- When administered with pertuzumab, trastuzumab dose is 8 mg/kg as a 90-minute infusion initially, followed q 3 weeks by 6 mg/kg administered IV infusion over 30–90 minutes.
- Pertuzumab, trastuzumab, and taxane should be administered sequentially. Pertuzumab and trastuzumab can be given in any order, but taxane should be administered AFTER pertuzumab and trastuzumab. A 30–60 min observation period after the pertuzumab infusion is completed is recommended and before starting trastuzumab or taxane infusion (Genentech, 2018).
- If the patient is receiving an anthracycline-based regimen, pertuzumab and trastuzumab should be administered AFTER completion of the anthracycline (Genentech, 2018).
- *HER-2 positive metastatic breast cancer (MBC):* pertuzumab IV infusion every 3 weeks, in combination with trastuzumab and docetaxel. Docetaxel dose is 75 mg/m^2 IV infusion, and mag be escalated to 100 mg/m^2 q 3 weeks if initial dose is well tolerated.
- *Neoadjuvant treatment of breast cancer in HER2-positive patients with locally advanced, inflammatory, or early stage breast cancer:* pertuzumab IV infusion preoperatively every 3 weeks for 3–6 cycles, as part of one of the following treatment regimes for early breast cancer:
  - Four preoperative cycles of pertuzumab in combination with trastuzumab and docetaxel, followed by 3 post-operative cycles of fluorouracil, epirubicin, and cyclophosphamide (FEC), as given in NeoSphere (see package insert).
  - Three or four preoperative cycles of FEC alone, followed by 3 or 4 preoperative cycles of pertuzumab in combination with docetaxel and trastuzumab, as given in TRYPHAENA and BERENICE, respectively (see package insert).
  - Six preoperative cycles of pertuzumab in combination with docetaxel, carboplatin, and trastuzumab (TCH) (escalation of docetaxel above 75 mg/m^2 is not recommended), as given in TRYPHAENA (see package insert).
  - Four preoperative cycles of dose-dense doxorubicin and cyclophosphamide (ddAC) alone followed by 4 preoperative cycles of pertuzumab in combination with paclitaxel and trastuzumab as given in BERENICE study (see package insert).
  - FOLLOWING SURGERY, patients should continue to receive pertuzumab with trastuzumab every 3 weeks for a total of 1 year of treatment (up to 18 cycles),
- When pertuzumab, trastuzumab, and docetaxel are given, drugs should be given sequentially, with docetaxel administered **after** pertuzumab and trastuzumab. An observation period of 30–60 minutes is recommended after each pertuzumab infusion and before starting the subsequent infusion of trastuzumab or docetaxel.

- *Adjuvant treatment of breast cancer:*
  - Pertuzumab should be administered in combination with trastuzumab q 3 weeks for a total of 1 year (up to 18 cycles) or until disease recurrence or unmanageable toxicity, whichever occurs first;
  - This is as part of a complete regimen for early breast cancer, including standard anthracycline and/or taxane-based chemotherapy as given in APHINITY (see package insert).
  - Pertuzumab and trastuzumab should start on Day 1 of the first taxane-containing cycle.

Dose Modification:

- For delayed or missed doses, if the time between two sequential infusions is < 6 weeks, administer the 420-mg dose of pertuzumab; do not wait for the next planned dose. If the time between two sequential infusions is 6 weeks or more, the initial dose of pertuzumab 840 mg should be readministered as a 60-minute IV infusion, followed every 3 weeks thereafter by a dose of 420-mg IV infusion over 30–60 minutes.
- Pertuzumab should be discontinued if trastuzumab is discontinued. Dose reductions of pertuzumab are not recommended. See docetaxel prescribing information for docetaxel dose modifications.
- LVEF: Assess LVEJ baseline before pertuzumab and regularly during treatment
  - MBC: If pretreatment ≥50%, repeat LVEF q 12 weeks; (a) hold pertuzumab and trastuzumab for at least 3 weeks for a LVEF < 40% or 40–45% with a fall of ≥10% points < pretreatment value; (b) resume pertuzumab and trastuzumab after 3 weeks if LVEF has recovered to either >45% or 40–45% with a fall of <10% points below pretreatment value
  - Early breast cancer: When pretreatment LVEF is ≥ 55%, monitor LVEF every 12 weeks (once during neoadjuvant therapy). (a) If the patient is receiving anthracycline-based chemotherapy, a LVEF of ≥ 50% is required after completion of the anthracyclines before starting pertuzumab and trastuzumab, (b) Hold pertuzumab and trastuzumab dosing for at least 3 weeks if LVEF is <50% with a fall of ≥10% points below pretreatment value; (c) Resume pertuzumab and trastuzumab when either LVEF is ≥50%, or <10% points below pretreatment value.
- If after a repeat assessment within approximately 3 weeks, the LVEF has not improved or has declined further, discontinuation of pertuzumab and trastuzumab should be considered, unless the benefits for the individual patient are deemed to outweigh the risks.
- IRRs: slow or interrupt infusion if patient develops an IRR.
- HSRs/anaphylaxis: discontinue infusion immediately, provide medical intervention immediately as ordered, and pertuzumab should be discontinued as pertuzumab is contraindicated in patients with known hypersensitivity to pertuzumab or to any of its excipients.

Drug Preparation:

- Available as a single-use vial of 420 mg/14 mL (30 mg/mL). Use 0.9% sodium chloride injection bags ONLY. Do not use D5W.
- After inspecting vial to ensure no particulates or discoloration, aseptically withdraw appropriate volume of drug and dilute in 250 mL 0.9% sodium chloride injection PVC or

non-PVC polyolefin infusion bag. Mix solution by gentle inversion, but do not shake. Administer immediately after preparation.
- Use immediately once prepared. If drug containing infusion bag is not used immediately, it can be stored at 2–8°C (36–46°F) for up to 24 hours.
- Dilute with 0.9% sodium chloride injection only. DO NOT use dextrose (5%) solution.

Drug Administration:
- When pertuzumab is administered with trastuzumab and a taxane, they should be administered sequentially: taxane should be given AFTER pertuzumab and trastuzumab, After pertuzumab administration, there should be a 30–60 minute observation period before giving the trastuzumab or taxane. If the patient is receiving an anthracycline, pertuzumab and trastuzumab should be administered after the completion of the anthracycline (Genentech, 2017).
- Assess pregnancy status prior to first dose, as drug is embryo-fetotoxic. Teach patient to use effective contraception during and for 7 months following last dose of pertuzumab.
- Assess findings of ECHO or MUGA scan for LVEF, baseline and at least every 3 months during treatment.
- Initial: IV infusion over 60 minutes (loading dose) then subsequent: IV infusion over 30–60 min (maintenance doses) every 3 weeks. Do NOT give IVB or IVP. Reduce infusion rate or interrupt if infusion reaction occurs. Permanently discontinue for severe reactions.
- Observe patients closely for 60 minutes after the first infusion, and 30 minutes after subsequent infusions, and before administering trastuzumab or docetaxel. If a significant infusion reaction occurs, stop the infusion and administer HSR medications as ordered. Monitor patient closely until complete resolution of signs and symptoms. Consider permanent drug discontinuance in patients with severe infusion reactions.

Drug Interactions:
- No drug-drug interactions observed between pertuzumab and trastuzumab, or between pertuzumab and docetaxel.

Lab Effects/Interference:
- Neutropenia, anemia when given with docetaxel and trastuzumab.

Special Considerations:
- FDA approval based on results of the Clinical Evaluation of Pertuzumab and Trastuzumab (CLEOPATRA) clinical trial demonstrating that the addition of pertuzumab significantly increased PFS compared to trastuzumab and docetaxel alone (18.5 vs. 12.4 months, $p < 0.001$). Superior overall survival was confirmed at 56.4 months with this first-line regimen, demonstrating a 15.7-month advantage compared to patients receiving placebo/trastuzumab/docetaxel (Swain et al., 2015). Addition of pertuzumab did not increase toxicity: febrile neutropenia (48.9 vs. 45.8% in control), grade 3 or higher diarrhea (7.9 vs. 5%), but no increase in left ventricular systolic dysfunction (1.2 vs. 2.8%) (Baselga et al., 2012).
- Warnings and Precautions:
  - *Left Ventricular Dysfunction:* pertuzumab can result in subclinical and clinical heart failure, manifesting as CHF, and decreased LVEF. Evaluate cardiac function prior to and during treatment. Discontinue pertuzumab treatment for a confirmed clinically

significant decrease in LVEF. Drug has not been studied in patients with a pretreatment LVEF value of ≤50%, history of CHF, decreases in LVEF to <50% during prior trastuzumab therapy, or in patient with a prior cumulative anthracycline exposure of >360 mg/m² of doxorubicin or its equivalent.

* *Drug is embryo-fetal toxic.* Women of childbearing age should use effective contraception to prevent pregnancy during treatment and for 7 months after the last dose. Teach patient to contact provider immediately if pregnancy is suspected while receiving the drug or within 7 months of last dose. If drug is administered during pregnancy, provider should contact Genentech Adverse Event Line (1-888-835-2555), and pregnant women should enroll in MotHER Pregnancy Registry (1-800-690-6720).

* *Infusion related-reactions (IRRs):* Monitor for IRRs closely for 60 minutes after the first infusion and for 30 minutes after subsequent infusions. Interrupt infusion for IRR, give ordered medical therapy, monitoring patient until signs/symptoms resolve. If reaction is severe, discuss drug discontinuation with provider.

* *HSRs:* Monitor patient closely during drug infusion. Stop drug and administer rescue medications as ordered, and have emergency equipment and medication close by.

* *HER2 testing* should be performed using FDA approved tests by laboratories with demonstrated proficiency.

* Overall, the most common toxicities when pertuzumab was given with trastuzumab and docetaxel were diarrhea, alopecia, neutropenia, nausea, fatigue, rash, and peripheral neuropathy.

Potential Toxicities/Side Effects and the Nursing Process

I.   POTENTIAL FOR INJURY related to HYPERSENSITIVITY/ANAPHYLAXIS AND INFUSION REACTION

Defining Characteristics: When pertuzumab was administered alone on a separate day in Study 1, the incidence of infusion reactions was 13% (compared to 9.8% in the placebo group) with < 1% grade 3 or 4. Most commonly, infusion reaction was characterized by pyrexia, chills, fatigue, headache, asthenia, hypersensitivity, and vomiting. In the second cycle, when all drugs were given on the same day, the most common infusion reactions were fatigue, dysgeusia, hypersensitivity, myalgia, and vomiting.

Incidence of hypersensitivity/anaphylaxis was 10.8% in pertuzumab group compared to 9.1% in control group, with grades 3–4 HSR 2% in the pertuzumab group and 2.5% in the placebo group. In Study 3, overall frequency of hypersensitivity/anaphylaxis was highest in the pertuzumab + TCH group (13.2%), of which 2.6% were grades 3–4.

Nursing Implications: Assess baseline VS and mental status prior to drug administration and periodically during infusion, as needed. Remain with patient during first 15 minutes of first infusions, and observe patient for 30–60 minutes depending upon cycle after drug has finished infusing. Recall signs/symptoms of anaphylaxis; if these occur, stop drug immediately, notify physician, and assess patient's vital signs. Subjective symptoms are generalized itching, nausea, chest tightness, crampy abdominal pain, difficulty speaking, anxiety, agitation, sense of impending doom, uneasiness, desire to urinate/defecate, dizziness, and chills. Objective signs are flushed appearance; angioedema of face, neck, eyelids, hands, and feet; localized or generalized urticaria; respiratory distress with or without wheezing; hypotension; and cyanosis. Review standing physician orders or nursing procedures for patient management of anaphylaxis, and be prepared to stop drug immediately and change IV to a plain NS solution to keep vein patent, notify physician, keep airway patent, monitor VS, and administer ordered medications, which may include epinephrine 1:1,000 IM in the thigh, IV hydrocortisone sodium succinate, and IV diphenhydramine. Teach patient to report any unusual symptoms. Patient should be observed for 1 hour after the initial treatment, 30 minutes after subsequent treatments, and before trastuzumab and docetaxel are administered. Slow infusion or interrupt the drug if patient develops an infusion reaction, and administer ordered medications. Discontinue the drug if the patient has a serious HSR, and provide emergency intervention and medications as ordered.

II.   POTENTIAL FOR INFECTION related to NEUTROPENIA

Defining Characteristics: Neutropenia occurred in 53% of patients compared to 50% in the control group without pertuzumab. Grades 3–4: 49 vs. 46%. Febrile neutropenia occurred in 13.8% compared to 7.6% in controls. Pyrexia occurred in 18.7% of patients, similar to controls.

Nursing Implications: Assess baseline blood counts, WBC, and differential. Teach patient to report fever and signs/symptoms of infection right away (e.g., $T \geq 100.4°F$, dysuria, productive cough). Assess medication profile and OTC medications taken. Teach patient to avoid OTC medications containing NSAIDs or aspirin. Teach patient to talk to nurse or physician before starting any OTC medications.

III.   POTENTIAL ALTERATION IN NUTRITION related to DIARRHEA, NAUSEA, VOMITING, CONSTIPATION, STOMATITIS, DECREASED APPETITE, DYSGEUSIA

Defining Characteristics: In Study 1 of patients with MBC, diarrhea was most common, affecting 66.7% of patients (grades 3–4 7.9%); compared to 46% in control group without pertuzumab (5% grades 3–4), and ranging in severity from grades 1–3. Nausea and vomiting affected 42 and 24% patients respectively, similar to the control group. Constipation affected 15%, significantly less than the control (25%). Stomatitis occurred in 19% compared to 15% in control group. Decreased appetite affected 29 vs. 26% in control, and dysgeusia occurred in 18% of patients (16% in control group).

Nursing Implications: Assess bowel elimination patterns and nutritional status, baseline and prior to each treatment. Teach patient self-care strategies depending upon symptom: to take antidiarrheal medications if diarrhea, to take antiemetic medication as ordered if nausea/vomiting; if constipation, to take fiber supplements or laxatives as needed. To decrease symptoms, teach patient dietary modifications, which might include high fiber, high fluids for constipation, BRAT diet for diarrhea unless it is persistent, and then modify with more protein; avoid fatty and spicy foods if nausea/vomiting. Teach patient to report any symptoms that do not resolve or improve with the established plan. Teach patient strategies to increase appetite (use small plate with small portions of food; take antiemetic pill prior to eating if needed; use small frequent feedings of high-protein, high-calorie foods, including bedtime snack if tolerated; if dysgeusia, based on sensory change, use plastic utensils if metallic taste, and use spices such as Crazy Jane salt).

IV.   ACTIVITY INTOLERANCE, POTENTIAL, related to FATIGUE, ASTHENIA, HEADACHE

Defining Characteristics: Fatigue occurs commonly in patients with advanced cancer who were studied. Fatigue occurred in 38% of patients similar to control group. Asthenia occurred in 26%, less than the control group of 30%. Headache occurred in 21% of patients, and anemia 23% compared to 19% in control group.

Nursing Implications: Assess baseline activity and energy level, and teach patient that this symptom may occur. Assess patient's activity patterns and suggest ways to conserve energy. Teach patient that headache may occur and to use self-care measures, such as taking acetaminophen, finding a quiet place without bright light to rest until the headache resolves. Monitor HGB/HCT.

V.   ALTERATION IN BODY IMAGE, POTENTIAL, related to ALOPECIA, SKIN CHANGES

Defining Characteristics: Alopecia occurs in 61% of patients receiving docetaxel, trastuzumab, and pertuzumab, same as the control group without pertuzumab. Skin changes included rash (33.7 vs. 24% in control), nail disorder (same as control, 23%), pruritus (14 vs. 10%), and dry skin (10.6 vs. 4.3%).

Nursing Implications: Assess baseline skin integrity and skin moisture. Teach patient that skin changes, including alopecia, may occur. Encourage patient to obtain a wig (cranial prosthesis) prior to starting therapy. Assess effect of hair loss on patient's body image, as well as skin changes. Encourage patient to verbalize feelings and provide emotional support. If needed, involve social worker in supportive counseling. Encourage patient to use scarves or hats as appropriate and to attend supportive educational sessions such as ACS Look Good . . . Feel Better program. Teach patient to assess for skin and nail changes, use skin emollients, and report nail changes. Discuss management of nail changes with nurse practitioner or physician.

Drug: polatuzumab (Polivy)

Class: Antibody-drug conjugate (ADC); CD79b-directed ADC.

Mechanism of Action: Drug is an ADC composed of (a) humanized IgG1 mAb specific for humanCD79b; (b) small molecule antimitotic agent MMAE (monomethyl auristatin E);

and (c) cleavable linker that covalently attaches MAE to the polatuzumab antibody. Like a Trojan horse, when the drug attaches to the CD79b cell membrane receptor, the poison is internalized in the CD79b- positive cell, intracellular lysosomal proteases cleave the linker, and the poison MMAE is released into the cell. It then binds to the microtubules (cell division mitotic apparatus), and kills dividing cells (inhibits cell division and induces apoptosis) (Genentech, 2019).

Metabolism: Antibody-conjugated MMAE terminal half-life is about 12 days by cycle 6, while the unconjugated MMAE terminal half-life is about 4 days after the first drug dose. While the metabolism has not been studied, it is believed to undergo catabolism to small peptides, amino acids, unconjugated MMAE and catabolites of unconjugated MMAE. MMAE is a substrate for CYP3A4. In patients studied with mild hepatic impairment there was a clinically insignificant 40% increase in MMAE exposure. The effect on MMAE pharmactokinetics of severe renal impairment, ESRD, moderate to severe hepatic impairment (AST or ALT$>$2.5 $\times$ ULN or total bilirubin $>$1.5 $\times$ ULN), or liver transplantation is unknown.

Indication: Treatment of adult patients with relapsed or refractory diffuse large B-cell lymphoma (DLBCL) after at least two prior therapies, in combination with bendamustine and rituximab product.

Contraindication: None. Avoid administration to patients with moderate or severe hepatic impairment (bilirubin $>$1.5 $\times$ ULN).

Drug Dosage/Range:
- Polatuzumab vedotin-piiq dose is 1.8 mg/kg IV infusion over 90 minutes on day 1 every 21 days for 6 cycles in combination with bendamustine and a rituximab product. Subsequent infusions can be administered over 30 minutes if previous infusion well tolerated. Monitor patient during and for at least 30 minutes after the 30-minute infusion.
  - Recommended dose of bendamustine is 90 mg/m^2/day on days 1 and 2 of each cycle;
  - Recommended dose of rituximab product is 375 mg/m^2 on day 1 of each cycle.
- Premedicate with an antihistamine and antipyretic at least 30 minutes before administering polatuzumab vedotin-piiq (unless previously premedicated).
- Consider prophylactic G-CSF.
- If a planned dose of polatuzumab vedotin-piiq is missed, administer as soon as possible and re-adjust the schedule to maintain 21 days between polatuzumab vedotin-piiq doses of each cycle.

Dose Modifications:
- *Peripheral neuropathy:* (a) **grade 2–3**: hold polatuzumab vedotin-piiq until improvement to $\leq$ grade 1; if recovered to $\leq$ grade 1 on or before day 14, restart polatuzumab vedotin-piiq with the next cycle at a permanently reduced dose of 1.4 mg/kg; if patient's dose has been previously reduced to 1.4 mg/kg, discontinue drug. If not recovered to $\leq$ grade 1 on or before day 14, discontinue drug; (b) **grade 4:** discontinue hold polatuzumab vedotin-piiq.
- *Infusion-related reaction (IRR):* (a) **grade 1–3 IRR**: interrupt polatuzumab vedotin-piiq and give ordered supportive treatment; for first instance of grade 3 wheezing,

bronchospasm, or generalized urticarial, permanently discontinue drug. For recurrent grade 2 wheezing or urticaria or for recurrence of any grade 3 symptom, permanently discontinue polatuzumab vedotin-piiq. Otherwise, upon complete resolution of symptoms, resume infusion at 50% of the prior rate before interruption; if no infusion related symptoms, infusion rate can be escalated in increments of 50 mg/hr every 30 minutes. For the next cycle, infuse polatuzumab vedotin-piiq over 90 minutes; if no IRRs, subsequent infusions can be administered over 30 minutes. Ensure premedications are always given for all cycles; (b) **grade 4:** stop infusion immediately and provide ordered supportive treatment; permanently discontinue polatuzumab vedotin-piiq.

* *Myelosuppression:* Severity on day 1 of any cycle; if primary cause is lymphoma, may not need dose delay or reduction. (a) **grade 3–4 neutropenia:** (1) Hold all treatments until ANC recovers to >1,000/mL. if recovery to >1,000/mL occurs on or before day 7, resume all treatments without any additional dose reductions; consider adding G-CSF for subsequent cycles if not previously given; (2) If ANC recovers to >1,000/mL after day 7, restart all treatment once recovered, consider G-CSF for subsequent cycles if not already given; if G-CSF prophylaxis given, consider dose reduction of bendamustine. If bendamustine already dose reduced, consider decreasing polatuzumab vedotin-piiq dose to 1.4 mg/kg. (b) **grade 3–4 thrombocytopenia:** (1) Hold all treatment until platelets recover to >75,000/mL. If recovery is on or before day 7, resume all treatment without any additional dose reductions; (2) if recovery to >75,000/mL is after day 7, restart all treatment, with dose reduction of bendamustine. If bendamustine already dose reduced, consider dose reduction of polatuzumab vedotin-piiq dose to 1.4 mg/kg.

Drug Preparation:

* Available as 140 mg polatuzumab vedotin-piiq as a lyophylized powder in a single-dose vial.

Reconstitution:

* Reconstitute vial immediately before dilution. Calculate the dose required, total volume of reconstituted drug needed, and number of vials needed.
* Aseptically add 7.2 mL of Sterile Water for Injection USP to each 140 mg vial by injecting stream toward the inside wall of the vial; concentration is 20 mg/mL.
* Swirl solution slowly but do not shake, until completely dissolved. Inspect for discoloration and particulate matter, and if found, do not use. Should be colorless to slightly brown, clear to slightly opalescent, and free of visible particulates. Do not freeze or expose to direct sunlight.
* If needed, can store unused reconstituted polatuzumab vedotin-piiq solution refrigerated at 2–8°C (36–46°F) for up to 48 hours or at room temperature (9–25°C, 47–77°F) for a maximum of 8 hours prior to dilution. Discard vial when cumulative storage time prior to dilution >48 hours.

Dilution:

* Dilute polatuzumab vedotin-piiq to a final concentration of 0.72–2.7 mg/mL in an IV infusion bag with a minimum volume of 50 mL containing 0.9% sodium chloride injection USP, 0.45% sodium chloride injection USP, or 5% dextrose injection USP.

- Recalculate ordered dose to double check math, then determine volume of 20 mg/mL required to deliver the ordered dose.
- Asceptically withdraw the required volume of reconstituted drug using a sterile syringe and dilute into the IV infusion bag. Discard any unused drug left in the vial. Gently mix by slowly inverting bag but do not shake. Inspect solution for particulates and discard if present.
- If not used immediately, store the diluted polatuzumab vedotin-piiq as follows but do not freeze or expose to direct sunlight:
  - 0.9% sodium chloride injection USP: Up to 24 hours at 2–8°C (36–46°F) or up to 4 hours at room temperature (9–25°C, 47–77°F).
  - 0.45% sodium chloride injection USP: Up to 18 hours at 2–8°C (36–46°F) or up to 4 hours at room temperature (9–25°C, 47–77°F).
  - 5% dextrose injection USP: Up to 36 hours at 2–8°C (36–46°F) or up to 6 hours at room temperature (9–25°C, 47–77°F).
- LIMIT transportation to 30 minutes at 9–25°C or 12 hours at 2–8°C (36–46°F). Total storage plus transportation times of diluted product should not exceed storage time in bullet above (storage).
- Limit agitation stress that can result in aggregation during preparation and transportation to administration site. Do not transport diluted product through automated pneumatic tube or automated cart. If the prepared solution will be transported to a different facility, remove air from infusion bag to prevent aggregation, and use a vented spike infusion set to ensure accurate dosing during the infusion (see package insert).

Drug Administration:
- Ensure that female patients of reproductive potential have a negative pregnancy test before starting therapy. Teach patients to use effective contraception during treatment and for 3 months after the last dose. Patients should not breastfeed while receiving the drug. Teach male patients with female sexual partners to use effective contraception during therapy and for at least 5 months after the last dose.
- Drug may impair male fertility. Assess patient's interest in sperm banking before starting therapy.
- Review prescription for or administer *Pneumocystis jiroveci* pneumonia and herpesvirus prophylaxis throughout treatment with polatuzumab vedotin-piiq.
- Discuss with provider prophylactic G-CSF for cycle 1, or if prior grade 3–4 neutropenia, ensure patient receives prophylactic G-CSF for subsequent cycles. See package insert.
- Discuss with provider patient risk for developing TLS and administer prophylaxis as ordered (or teach patient about home hydration, antiurecimic therapy before cycle 1).
- If not already premedicated for rituximab product, administer an antihistamine and anytipyretic at least 30–60 minutes before polatuzumab vedotin-piiq to prevent IRRs.
- Administer as an IV infusion only, using a dedicated IV and infusion line; use a sterile, nonpyrogenic, low-protein-binding in-line or add-on filter (0.2 or 0.22 micron pore size).
- Do NOT mix drug with or administer as an infusion with other drugs.
- Administer first dose over 90 minutes, and monitor for IRRs. If the first infusion is well tolerated, next infusion can be infused over 30 minutes, again monitoring patient closely for IRRs during, and for 30 minutes after the infusion is completed.

TREATMENT

- Managing IRRs:
  - **grade 1–3 IRR:** interrupt polatuzumab vedotin-piiq and give ordered supportive treatment; for first instance of grade 3 wheezing, bronchospasm, or generalized urticaria, permanently discontinue drug.
  - For recurrent grade 2 wheezing or urticaria, or for recurrence of any grade 3 symptom, permanently discontinue polatuzumab vedotin-piiq.
  - Otherwise, upon complete resolution of symptoms, resume infusion at 50% of the prior rate before interruption; if no infusion related symptoms, infusion rate can be escalated in increments of 50 mg/hr every 30 minutes. For the next cycle, infuse polatuzumab vedotin-piiq over 90 minutes; if no IRRs, subsequent infusions can be administered over 30 minutes.
  - Ensure premedications are always given for all cycles;
  - **grade 4:** Stop infusion immediately and provide ordered supportive treatment; permanently discontinue polatuzumab vedotin-piiq.

Drug Interactions (physiologically based modeling, see package insert):
- Strong CYP3A4 inhibitors (e.g., ketoconazole): concomitant use should increase unconjugated MMAE AUC by 45%.
- Strong CYP3A4 inducer (e.g., rifampin): concomitant use should decrease AUC of unconjugated MMAE by 63% and reduce drug efficacy.
- Sensitive CYP3A4 substrate (e.g., midazolam): concomitant use should not affect exposure to substrate.
- MMAE is a P-gp substrate but it does not inhibit P-gp.

Lab Effects/Interference:
- Decreased lymphocyte, neutrophil, platelet counts, decreased Hgb.
- Decreased serum calcium, phosphorus, potassium, albumin.
- Increased serum creatinine, SGPT/ALT, SGOT/AST, lipase, amylase.

Special Considerations:
- Most common adverse reactions ($\geq$20%): neutropenia, thrombocytopenia, anemia, peripheral neuropathy, fatigue, iarrhea, pyrexia, decreased appetite, pneumonia.
- Concomitant use of strong CYP3A inhibitors or inducers has the potential to affect the exposure to unconjugated MMAE and influence incidence of adverse effects or efficacy.
- Hepatic dysfunction has the potential to increase exposure to MMAE and increase toxicity; monitor patient closely for adverse effects.
- Warnings and Precautions:
  - *Peripheral Neuropathy:* Overall incidence in combination with bendamustine and rituximab product is 40%, and in one study, median time to onset was 2.1 months. Incidence was grade 1 in 26% of patients, grade 2 in 12%, and grade 3 in 2.3%. Most patients (65%) had improvement or resolution after a median of 1 month, and 48% had complete resolution. While primarily sensory, motor and sensorimotor periphera neuropathy may occur. Monitor patient for symptoms such as hypoesthesia, hyperesthesia, paresthesias, dysesthesia, neurpathic pain, burning sensation, weakness, gait disturbance. If symptoms are new or worsening existing symptoms, discuss grade

and implications for holding drug, reducing dose, or discontinuing drug (see dose modifications).

- *IRRs:* While most reactions occur during or soon after the infusion, delayed reactions occurring up to 24 hours after the infusion have occurred. Incidence in clinical studies was 18%, but with premedication, incidence is 7% (grade 1 in 67%, grade 2 in 25%, and grade 3 in 8%). Monitor patient during infusion and after (for 30 minutes after the 30 min infusion) for fever, chills, flushing, dyspnea, hypotension, and urticarial. If an IRR occurs, stop infusion, implement ordered interventions, and if mild, anticipate the drug will be resumed at a 50% reduced infusion rate. If recurrent grade 3 or new instance of a grade 4 (e.g., bronchospasm, anaphylaxis), stop drug immediately, institute emergency management as ordered, and permanently discontinue. See Dose Modifications.

- *Myelosuppression:* Incidence of neutropenia 49% (42% grade 3 or higher), thrombocytopenia 49% (40% grade 3 or higher), anemia 47% (24% grade 3 or higher), febrile neutropenia 13% (13% grade 3 or higher). Pyrexia occurred in 30%, pneumonia in 13–22% and sepsis in 6% (all grade 3 or higher). Fatalities occurred in patients with pneumonia and sepsis. Monitor cbc/ANC baseline, day 1 of each cycle, and as needed. See Dose Modifications for dose delay, reduction, or drug discontinuance. Consider prophylactic G-CSF administration.

- *Serious and opportunistic infections (OIs):* Serious, and sometimes fatal, infections can occur including OIs such as sepsis, pneumonia (including *P. jiroveci* and other fungal pneumonia), herpesvirus infection, and cytomegalovirus infection have occurred. Grade 3 or higher infections occurred in 32% of patients, and infection-related deaths were reported in 2.9% of patients within 90 days of lst treatment. Discuss with provider recommended prophylaxis for *P. jiroveci* snf herpesvirus. Monitor patients closely for signs/symptoms of infection during therapy and teach patient signs/symptoms to report right away.

- *Progressive multifocal leukoencephalopathy (PML):* Rarely PML can occur (0.6% incidence). Monitor patient for signs/symptoms of new or worsening neurological, cognitive, or behavioral changes. Hold drug and concomitant chemotherapy if PML suspected, and if confirmed, permanently discontinue drug.

- *TLS:* Discuss risk and prophylaxis with provider: high tumor burden, rapidly proliferating tumor. If at risk, teach patient recommended/ordered regimen: hydration, uricemic agent as ordered. Monitor patient closely.

- *Hepatotoxicity:* Hepatocellular injury may occur, including elevation of transaminases and/or bilirubin. Grade 3 and 4 transaminase elevations occurred in 1.9% of patients respectively. Preexisting liver disease, elevated baseline liver enzymes and concomitant medications that are hepatotoxic may increase risk. Monitor serum transaminases and bilirubin baseline and before each cycle.

- *Embryo-fetal toxicity:* Drug is fetotoxic. Assess pregnancy test for female patients of reproductive potential before beginning therapy, and teach patients to use effective contraception during and for 3 months after last dose. Teach male patients with female sexual partners of reproductive potential to use effective contraception during and for at least 5 months after last dose.

Potential Toxicities/Side Effects and the Nursing Process

I.   POTENTIAL FOR INJURY related to INFUSION REACTIONS

Defining Characteristics: Infusion reactions may occur despite premedication with an antihistamine and antipyretic but the incidence is decreased (from 18% to 7%) and may occur as late as 24 hours after the drug dose. Most commonly characterized by fever, chills, flushing, dyspnea, hypotension, and urticarial.

Nursing Implications: Ensure patient receives premedications. Assess baseline mental status and vital signs including oxygenation prior to drug administration and periodically during infusion, as needed. If infusion reaction occurs, interrupt infusion and discuss rate decrease or medical intervention with provider. If anaphylaxis occurs, stop and discontinue the drug immediately, assess patient vital signs, and implement physician or NP/PA emergency medical orders. Recall signs/symptoms of anaphylaxis: subjective symptoms include generalized itching, nausea, chest tightness, crampy abdominal pain, difficulty speaking, anxiety, agitation, sense of impending doom, uneasiness, desire to urinate/defecate, dizziness, and chills. Objective signs are flushed appearance; angioedema of face, neck, eyelids, hands, and feet; localized or generalized urticaria; respiratory distress with or without wheezing; hypotension; and cyanosis. Review standing physician orders or nursing procedures for patient management of anaphylaxis, and be prepared to stop drug immediately and change IV to a plain NS solution to keep vein patent, notify physician, keep patent airway, monitor VS, and administer ordered medications, which may include epinephrine 1:1,000 IM in the thigh, IV hydrocortisone sodium succinate, and IV diphenhydramine. Teach patient to report any unusual symptoms. Patient should be observed after each treatment, and longer periods may be required if the patient experiences an infusion reaction. Initial infusion is administered over 90 minutes and if well tolerated, infusion time can be decreased to 30 minutes, with a 30-minute observation period following drug infusion completion. Discuss management with provider: see Dose Modification section.

II.   POTENTIAL FOR INFECTION AND BLEEDING related to BONE MARROW DEPRESSION and IMMUNE SUPPRESSION

Defining Characteristics: Serious or severe myelosuppression can occur. Neutropenia is common, with an incidence of 49% (42% grade 3 or higher). Lymphopenia occurred in 13% and was grade 3-4. Febrile neutropenia occurs in 13% of patients receiving polatuzumab vedotin-piiq and chemotherapy. Anemia incidence is 28–47%, and thrombocytopenia 31–49%. Grade 3 and 4 thrombocytopenia or anemia may occur. Risk for pneumonia and sepsis should be assessed as these may be fatal infections. Incidence of pneumonia is 22% and sepsis 6%. Opportunistic infections (OIs) can occur. Patients should receive prophylaxis for *Pneumocystis jiroveci* and herpesvirus.

Nursing Implications: Assess baseline cbc/absolute neutrophil count baseline and monitor before each treatment, and more often as needed. Patients at risk should receive G-CSF prophylaxis. See dose modification for grade 3 and 4 neutropenia. Assess for signs/symptoms of viral, bacterial, and fungal infection. Assess risk for infection and integrity of skin and mucous membranes, pulmonary status, and ability to clear secretions, as well as history of past infections, baseline and prior to each treatment. Teach patient to self-assess for signs/symptoms of infection and to call provider immediately or come to the emergency room if temperature > 100.5°F, shaking chills, or rash; productive cough; burning on urination; or any signs/symptoms of infection or bleeding. Teach self-care strategies to minimize risk of infection and bleeding, including avoidance of OTC aspirin-containing medications. If a patient develops neutropenia and is not receiving prophylactic G-CSF discuss with provider starting this for subsequent cycles.

III.   POTENTIAL FOR SENSORY/PERCEPTUAL ALTERATIONS related to PERIPHERAL NEUROPATHY

Defining Characteristics: Peripheral neuropathy (PN) occurs in 40% (2.3% grades 3–4), and dizziness, in 13% of patients. PN is primarily sensory but motor or sensorimotor PN may occur. Median time to onset of PN was 2.1 months in clinical studies and was grade 1 in 26% of patients, grade 2 in 12%, and grade 3 in 2.3%. Peripheral neuropathy was largely reversible (65% of patients reported improvement/resolution after a median of 1 month, and 48% reported complete resolution (Genetech, 2019).

Nursing Implications: Teach patient that these side effects may occur and to report them. Assess sensory/perceptual changes (e.g., numbness, tingling (paresthesias), weakness, sensory changes (such as hypoesthesia, hyperesthesia, dysesthesia), neuropathic pain, burning sensations, gait disturbance baseline and prior to each drug administration. Assess one side versus the other side, and note extent of paresthesias if present (stocking glove distribution), starting at fingertips or tips of toes, and progressing proximally to wrist/ankle like a glove and stocking, and document. Assess patient's ability to do ADLs and impact of neuropathy on functioning. Discuss grade with NP/PA or physician and need to dose-modify or interrupt (hold drug for grades 3–4). Assess for presence of dizziness and risk for falls, and discuss strategies to minimize risk of falling. Assess for headache and discuss self-care strategies to prevent/manage them.

IV.   ALTERATION IN NUTRITION related to DIARRHEA, VOMITING, DECREASED APPETITE, HEPATIC INJURY

Defining Characteristics: Patients received combination therapy with increased incidence of symptoms from bendamustine. Diarrhea occurred in 38–45% of patients, vomiting in 18–27% of patients, decreased appetite in 29%, increased transaminases (36–38%), and hypokalemia (24%).

Nursing Implications: Assess baseline nutritional status, lab findings, especially LFTs (transaminases, bilirubin), and serum potassium and prior to each cycle of therapy. Discuss abnormalities with physician or NP/PA, and discuss management and dose modification (see section on Dose Modification). Teach patient that nutritional impact symptoms may occur and to report them. Discuss with the patient medication and self-care strategies to manage nausea, vomiting, diarrhea, and decreased appetite if they occur. Discuss dietary modifications as needed. If the patient has persistent diarrhea, discuss lab testing of serum potassium and need for potassium repletion and hydration with physician or NP/PA. If symptoms persist, discuss pharmacologic plan revision with NP/PA or physician.

Drug: pomalidomide (Pomalyst)

Class: Immunomodulator with antiangiogic and antineoplastic properties; thalidomide analogue.

Mechanism of Action: Third-generation thalidomide analogue that is an immunomodulatory agent with antineoplastic activity. Drug has been shown to inhibit proliferation and cause apoptosis of hematopoietic tumor cells, and to have activity in lenalidomide-resistant MM cell lines. It is synergistic with dexamethasone to bring about tumor cell apoptosis. Pomalidomide enhances T-cell and NK cell-mediated immunity and inhibits production of pro-inflammatory cytokines (TNF-α and IL-6). Drug also has antiangiogenic activity.

Metabolism: After oral administration, C_{max} occurs at 2 and 3 hours after dosing. Drug is distributed in the semen at a concentration of 67% of plasma level 4 hours post dose. In healthy subjects, drug binds to plasma proteins 12–44%. Drug is primarily metabolized in the liver by CYP1A2 and CYP3A4, and to a lesser degree by CYP2C19 and CYP2D6. Median plasma half-life is 9.5 hours in healthy subjects, and 7.5 hours in patients with MM. Drug is excreted primarily in the urine (73%, 2% unchanged), and feces (15%, 8% unchanged drug). Drug is a substrate for P-glycoprotein (P-gp).

Indication: In combination with dexamethasone, the treatment of patients with MM who have received at least two prior therapies, including lenalidomide and a proteasome inhibitor , and have disease progression on or within 60 days of completing last therapy. Clinical benefit has not been verified.

Contraindications: Pregnant females, as pomalidomide can cause fetal harm.

Dosage/Range:
- Females of reproductive potential must have negative pregnancy testing and use contraception methods before initiating pomalidomide.
- 4 mg orally, daily on days 1–21 of repeated 28-day cycles until disease progression, in combination with dexamethasone. See package insert for doses of dexamethasone (Section 14.1).
- Dosage adjustment for:
  - Concurrent strong CYP1A2 inhibitors: avoid; if must use, reduce pomalidomide dose by 50%
  - Severe renal impairment on hemodialysis: recommended starting dose is 3 mg PO daily (25% dose reduction), taken after completion of dialysis procedure on hemodialysis days.

- Hepatic impairment: Mild or moderate (Child-Pugh classes A+B)=3 mg PO daily (25% dose reduction); severe (Child-Pugh C)=2 mg PO qd (50% dose reduction)
- To initiate a new cycle of pomalidomide, the neutrophil count must be at least 500 per mcL and the platelet count at least 50,000 per mcL. If toxicities occur after dose reductions to 1 mg, then discontinue pomalidomide.
- Permanently discontinue pomalidomide for angioedema, skin exfoliation, bullae, or other severe dermatologic reactions.
- For other grade 3–4 toxicities, hold treatment and restart treatment at 1 mg less than the previous dose when toxicity has resolved to ≤ grade 2 at the physician's discretion.

Dose Modifications:
- Neutropenia (ANC < 500 per mcL, or febrile neutropenia [fever ≥ 38.5°C and ANC < 1,000 per mcL]): interrupt pomalidomide; follow CBC weekly and resume drug at 3 mg daily when ANC ≥ 500 per mcL; for each subsequent decrease to ANC < 500 per mcL, interrupt drug then resume at a reduced dose 1 mg less than previous dose, once ANC returns to ANC ≥ 500 per mcL.
- Thrombocytopenia (platelets < 25,000 per mcL): interrupt pomalidomide, follow CBC weekly, resume drug at 3 mg daily once platelets return to > 50,000 per mcL; for each subsequent drop in platelets < 25,000 per mcL, interrupt drug then resume at a reduced dose 1 mg less than previous dose, once platelet count returns to > 50,000 per mcL.
- Other grade 3 or 4 toxicities: interrupt drug, then restart treatment at 1 mg less than the previous dose when toxicity has resolved to ≤ grade 2 at physician's discretion.
- If toxicities occur after dose reductions to 1 mg daily, discontinue pomalidomide.

Drug Preparation:
- Drug is available only through a restricted distribution program called POMALYST REMS. Prescribers and pharmacists must be certified with the program and patients must sign an agreement and comply with requirements.
- Drug is available as capsules in 1-, 2-, 3-, and 4-mg strengths.

Drug Administration:
- Ensure females of reproductive potential are not pregnant: (1) patient must commit to either abstain continuously from heterosexual sexual intercourse or to use two methods of reliable birth control, beginning 4 weeks prior to initiating treatment with pomalidomide, during therapy, during dose interruption, and continuing for 4 weeks after last dose of pomalidomide; (2) two negative pregnancy tests must be obtained before patient starts therapy, test 1 within 10–14 days and then the second test within 24 hours prior to prescribing, then weekly during the first month, then monthly thereafter in women with regular menses, or every 2 weeks in women with irregular menses.
- Ensure male patients understand that pomalidomide is present in semen, so patient must always use a latex or synthetic condom during any sexual contact with females of reproductive potential while receiving pomalidomide, and for 28 days after last dose, even if the patient has undergone a successful vasectomy. Patient should NOT donate sperm.
- Assess CBC/ANC baseline and weekly for first 8 weeks of treatment, then monthly thereafter. Monitor serum chemistries and LFTs baseline and monitor LFTs at least monthly.

- Assess for signs/symptoms of neuropathy, skin changes baseline and during therapy.
- Teach patient NOT to donate blood during pomalidomide treatment or for 1 month after last dose as blood might be given to a pregnant female patient whose fetus then is exposed to the drug. Fetus should NOT be exposed to pomalidomide.
- Teach patient to take pomalidomide and water, with or without food. Drug capsule should be taken with water and should not be broken, chewed, or opened.
- Pomalidomide is excreted primarily in the urine. Do not administer to patients with serum creatinine > 3.0 mg/dL.
- Pomalidomide is metabolized in the liver. Avoid pomalidomide in patients with serum bilirubin > 2.0 mg/dL.
- Discuss VTE prophylaxis based on individual patient's underlying risk factors with provider prior to starting therapy. Teach patient to report signs/symptoms of VTE right away for evaluation.

Drug Interactions:
- Pomalidomide is primarily metabolized by CYP1A2 and CYP3A; pomalidomide is also a substrate for P-glycoprotein (P-gp).
- Drugs that may increase pomalidomide plasma concentrations:
  - CYP1A2 inhibitors (strong): pomalidomide plasma concentrations may be increased when drug is coadministered with a strong CYP1A2 inhibitor (e.g., fluvoxamine) in the presence of a strong CYP3A4/5 and P-gp inhibitor (e.g., ketoconazole). Ketoconazole in the absence of a CYP1A2 inhibitor does not increase pomalidomide serum levels.
  - Thus, AVOID coadministration of strong CYP1A2 inhibitors (e.g., ciprofloxacin and fluvoxamine) unless medically necessary; and if necessary to coadminister, pomalidomide dose must be reduced.
  - If a CYP1A2 inhibitor without coadministration of a CYP3A4 and P-gp inhibitor is given, monitor patient closely for toxicity, and reduce pomalidomide dose as needed.
- Drugs/substances that may reduce pomalidomide plasma concentrations:
  - Smoking: may reduce pomalidomide serum level due to CYP1A2 induction and reduce efficacy; teach patients that smoking may reduce drug's effectiveness.
  - CYP1A2 inducers: have not been studied, and may reduce pomalidomide serum level. Dexamethasone, a weak CYP3A4 inducer, in combination with pomalidomide, did not change the pharmacokinetics of pomalidomide.

Lab Effects/Interference:
- Neutropenia, thrombocytopenia, anemia.
- Hyperglycemia, hypercalcemia.
- Hyponatremia, hypocalcemia, hypokalemia.
- Increased serum creatinine.

Special Considerations:
- Warnings and precautions:
  - *Embryo-fetal toxicity:* Pomalyst is contraindicated in pregnancy. Drug is a thalidomide analogue which is known to cause severe life-threatening birth defects.

Pregnancy must be excluded in females of reproductive potential before start of treatment (2 negative pregnancy tests, one 10–14 days and the second within 24 hours prior to prescribing pomalidomide therapy), then weekly during the first month, then monthly thereafter in females with regular menstrual cycles, or q 2 weeks in women with irregular menstrual cycles. Patient must prevent pregnancy by using two reliable methods of contraception starting 4 weeks prior to therapy initiation, during therapy and dose interruptions, and continuing for 4 weeks after last pomalidomide dose. Men receiving the drug will have drug in their semen; they must always use a latex or synthetic condom during any sexual contact with females of reproductive potential; this should continue for 4 weeks after last pomalidomide drug dose.Drug is only available through a restricted program called Pomalyst REMS.

- *Pomalyst REMS Program:* Required components of the program include (a) Prescribers must be certified with the Pomalyst REMS program by enrolling and complying with the REMS requirements; (b) Patients must sign a Patient–Physician Agreement Form and comply with the REMS requirements (e.g., female patients of reproductive potential who are not pregnant must comply with the pregnancy testing and contraception requirements, and males must comply with contraception requirements); (c) Pharmacies must be certified with the Pomalyst REMS program, must only dispense to patients who are authorized to receive Pomalyst and comply with REMS requirements.

- *Venous and ATEs:* VTE, deep vein thrombosis (DVT), and pulmonary embolism (PE) may occur; as may arterial thrombotic events (MI, stroke). When anticoagulant therapies were mandated in clinical trials, the incidence of thromboembolic events was 8.0% in patients receiving pomalidomide plus low-dose dexamethasone, and 3.3% in patients receiving pomalidomide plus high-dose dexamethasone. Efforts to reduce modifiable risk factors should occur, such as effective control of hyperlipidemia, HTN, smoking. Thromboprophylaxis is recommended, with selection of regimen based on patient's underlying risk factors.

- *Increased mortality in patients with muldiple myeloma when pembrolizumab is added to thalidomide analogue and dexamethasone* found in 2 randomized clinical trials. PD- and PD-L1 blocking antibody is not indicated in this setting, and should not be combined with thalidomide analogues/dexamethasone unless part of a controlled clinical trial.

- *Hematologic Toxicity:* Neutropenia occurs in 51% of patients with an incidence of 46% grades 3–4; anemia and thrombocytopenia also occur. Patients should have CBC/differential and platelet counts monitored weekly for the first 8 weeks, then monthly. Dose interruption and modification are used to manage toxicity.

- *Hepatotoxicity:* hepatic failure has occurred. Monitor LFTs monthly. Stop pomalidomide if elevation of LFTs and evaluate. Consider resuming at a lower dose once LFTs have returned to baseline.

- *Severe cutaneous reactions including HSRs:* HSRs may occur, including angioedema and severe dermatologic reactions. Permanently discontinue pomalidomide for angioedema, skin exfoliation, bullae, or any other severe dermatologic reactions. DO NOT resume therapy.

- *TLS* may occur. Patients at risk are those with a high tumor burden before initial treatment; discuss TLS prophylaxis with physician, and monitor patient closely.
- *Dizziness and confusional state:* Drug can cause dizziness (14%) and confusion (7%). Teach patient to avoid driving and operating heavy machinery until the patient knows the drug's effects, and to avoid any other concurrent medications that can cause dizziness or a confusional state.
- *Neuropathy:* In Trials 1 and 2 (Pomalyst and low-dose dexamethasone), neuropathy occurred in 18% of patients, with 12% having peripheral neuropathy. No grade 4 neuropathy was reported.
- *Risk of second primary tumor:* AML has been reported in patients receiving pomalidomide in clincal trials outside of MM.
- Most common adverse reactions were fatigue, asthenia, neutropenia, anemia, constipation, nausea, diarrhea, dyspnea, URIs, back pain, pyrexia.
- Patients must not donate blood during treatment with pomalidomide or for one month after discontinuing the drug, as the blood may be given to a pregnant patient whose fetus must not be exposed to the drug.
- Men should be counseled not to donate sperm, as drug is distributed in semen.
- Nursing mothers should discontinue the drug or stop nursing.

Potential Toxicities/Side Effects and the Nursing Process

I. POTENTIAL FOR INFECTION, BLEEDING, FATIGUE, related to BONE MARROW SUPPRESSION

Defining Characteristics: In Trial 1, neutropenia occurred in 57% of patients receiving pomalist only, while 55% of those also receiving low-dose dexamethasone had neutropenia. In trial 2, 51.3% patients receiving pomalidomide plus low-dose dex had neutropenia, while only 20.7% of those receiving pomalidomide plus high-dose dexamethasone did Thrombocytopenia in 29.7–29.3% of patients receiving pomalidomide plus either low or high dose dexamethasone. Fever, chills, pneumonia and URI were also reported, as was rare neutropenic sepsis. In trial 2, fatigue and asthenia occurred in 42.7–46.7% of patients.

Nursing Implications: Assess baseline CBC, WBC, differential, and platelet count baseline and weekly for the first 8 weeks, then monthly. Hold drug if ANC < 500 cells/mm^3 or platelets < 50,000 cells/mm^3 and dose-modify when ANC and/or platelet count recovers (see dosing section). Assess for signs/symptoms of infection or bleeding. Teach patient the signs/symptoms of infection (e.g., T > 100.4°F, productive cough, dysuria, dyspnea) or bleeding (e.g., epistaxis, pink urine, after brushing teeth), and to report these immediately. Teach patient self-care measures to minimize risk of infection and bleeding. This includes avoidance of crowds, proximity to people with infections, and OTC aspirin-containing medications (except 325 mg PO aspirin daily as DVT prophylaxis), and NSAIDs. Discuss any abnormalities with physician or NP/PA. Teach patient strategies to manage fatigue, and conserve energy, such as altering rest and activity, organizing chores, engaging in gentle exercise.

II.   ALTERATION IN NUTRITION, LESS THAN BODY REQUIREMENTS, related to DIARRHEA, CONSTIPATION, NAUSEA, VOMITING, DECREASED APPETITE, WEIGHT LOSS

Defining Characteristics: Nutrition impact symptoms may occur. In trial 2, the following incidences were reported in patients receiving pomalidomide with low-dose dex/high dose dex: diarrhea in 22%/18.7%; constipation in 21.7%/14.7%; nausea in 15%/11.3%; and vomiting in 7.3%/4%.; and decreased appetite 12.7%/8%. Hypokalemia and hypocalcemia occurred in <10% of patients.

Nursing Implications: Assess baseline nutritional status, including weight and serum lab values (e.g., electrolytes and glucose). Assess bowel elimination pattern, energy level/activity, and appetite. Teach patient that symptoms may occur and to report them. Teach patient self-care management strategies for diarrhea, constipation, nausea, vomiting, and to report if symptom(s) do not resolve. Teach dietary modifications based on symptoms, such as the BRAT diet for diarrhea (bananas, rice, applesauce, and toast), and to increase oral fluids to prevent dehydration. Involve dietitian as needed and available.

III.   ALTERATION IN COMFORT related to BACK PAIN, MUSCULOSKELETAL CHEST PAIN, MUSCLE SPASMS, ARTHRALGIA, EDEMA

Defining Characteristics: In Trial 2, symptoms occurred with the following incidences (pomalidomide with low dose dex/high dose dex): back pain (19.7%/16%%), bone pain (18%/14%), muscle spasms (15.3%/7.3%), arthralgia (18.7%/4.7%), and peripheral edema (17.3%/11.3%).

Nursing Implications: Assess patient's baseline comfort, as bone involvement by MM may increase discomfort. Teach patient that these symptoms may occur, and to report them. Teach patient self-management strategies and to report them if ineffective, including use of warmth/heat and cold, as tolerated and preferred. Discuss analgesics with physician/NP/PA, recommendations for the patient, and need for prescription analgesics. Teach patient to report rash, and to have it evaluated to rule out allergic reaction.

IV.   POTENTIAL FOR KNOWLEDGE DEFICIT, POTENTIAL, related to PATIENT INSTRUCTIONS (Pomalyst REMS), CONTRACEPTION, AND PREGNANCY TESTING

Defining Characteristics: Drug is fetotoxic. Patients must be able to understand the risk to the fetus, comply with REMS requirements, and be able to safeguard the drug in the home.

Nursing Implications: Assess patient's ability to understand rationale, importance of pregnancy testing in women with reproductive potential, and to avoid pregnancy starting 4 weeks prior to drug prescription, during treatment, treatment holidays, and for 4 weeks following drug discontinuance. Assess the understanding and ability of patients with childbearing potential to comply with contraception requirement and other self-care strategies and agree to the following:

- Pregnancy testing to verify that females of reproductive potential are not pregnant: (1) patient must commit to either abstain continuously from heterosexual sexual intercourse or to use two methods of reliable birth control, beginning 4 weeks prior to initiating treatment with pomalidomide, during therapy, during dose interruption, and continuing for 4 weeks after last dose of pomalidomide; (2) two negative pregnancy tests must be obtained before patient starts therapy, test #1 within 10–14 days and then the second test within 24 hours prior to the drug being prescribed, then weekly during the first month, then monthly thereafter in women with regular menses, or every 2 weeks in women with irregular menses.
- Male patients must understand that pomalidomide is present in semen, so patient must always use a latex or synthetic condom during any sexual contact with females of reproductive potential while receiving pomalidomide, and for 28 days after last dose, even if the patient has undergone a successful vasectomy. Patient should NOT donate sperm.
- Teach patient to notify the physician immediately under the following conditions:
  - Female patient becomes pregnant, thinks she might be pregnant, thinks birth control has failed, stops birth control, misses her menses, or has unusual menstrual bleeding. If so, she must stop taking the drug and notify the physician immediately;
  - Male patient has unprotected sex with a woman who can become pregnant, or if he thinks his sexual partner may be pregnant.
- Patients must not donate blood during treatment with pomalidomide and for 1 month following drug discontinuation.
- Assess ability of patient to keep drug/drug supply out of the reach of children and pets, and NEVER to share drug with anyone else, even if they have similar symptoms. Discuss any concerns with the physician.

Drug: ramucirumab injection (Cyramza)

Class: Recombinant human, IgG_1 mAb targeted against vascular endothelial growth factor receptor 2 (VEGFR2); angiogenesis inhibitor.

Mechanism of Action: Binds to the VEGF receptor 2 (VEGFR2), as opposed to bevacizumab, which targets the ligand VEGF. Thus, it prevents binding of the ligand VEGF to the receptor, prevents VEGF receptor activation, and subsequent proliferation and migration of endothelial cells to form tumor blood vessels (angiogenesis).

Metabolism: Unknown.

Indication: Ramucirumab is indicated for the treatment of patients with (1) advanced gastric or gastro-esophageal junction (G-E) adenocarcinoma with disease progression on or after prior fluoropyrimidine- or platinum-containing chemotherapy, as a single agent or in combination with paclitaxel; (2) metastatic NSCLC with disease progression on or after platinum-based chemotherapy, in combination with docetaxel, if tumor has EGFR or ALK genomic tumor aberrations the patient should have disease progression on FDA-approved therapies for these specific aberrations prior to receiving ramucirumab; (3) metastatic CRC with disease progression on or after prior therapy with bevacizumab, oxaliplatin, and a fluoropyrimidine, in combination with FOLFIRI (folinic acid, irinotecan, 5-FU; (4) hepatocellular cancer (HCC) with an alpha fetoprotein of $\geq$ 400 ng/mL who have previously been treated with sorafenib, as a single agent.

Dosage/Range:
- *Gastric cancer:* as a single agent or in combination with weekly paclitaxel: 8 mg/kg IV every 2 weeks, as an IV infusion over 60 minutes. Continue drug until disease progression or unacceptable toxicity.
- *NSCLC:* 10-mg/kg IV on Day 1 of a 21-day cycle, as an IV infusion over 60 minutes prior to docetaxel infusion. Continue drug until disease progression or unacceptable toxicity.
- CRC: 8-mg/kg IV every 2 weeks, as an IV infusion over 60 minutes, prior to FOLFIRI administration. Continue drug until disease progression or unacceptable toxicity.
- HCC: 8-mg/kg every 2 weeks IV infusion over 30 minutes; continue drug until disease progression or unacceptable toxicity.
- Premedication: (1) Prior to each ramucirumab dose, administer IV histamine H1 antagonist (e.g., diphenhydramine HCl); (2) if patient has experienced a grade 1or 2 infusion reaction, also premedicate with dexamethasone (or equivalent) and acetaminophen prior to each ramucirumab infusion.

Dose Modifications:
- Infusion reactions: Grades 1–2: reduce infusion rate by 50%; grades 3–4: permanently discontinue drug.
- Hypertension (HTN): Interrupt drug for severe HTN until controlled with antihypertensive therapy. Permanently discontinue drug for severe HTN that cannot be controlled with antihypertensive therapy.
- Proteinuria: Assess dipstick/urinalysis before each treatment and if 2+ or greater protein, assess 24-hour urine protein.
  - Interrupt drug for urine protein level $\geq$ 2 g/24 hr. When urine protein < 2 g/24 hr, reinitiate drug at a reduced dose (if initial dose was 8 mg/kg, first dose reduction to 6 mg/kg, and if initial dose was 10 mg/kg, first dose reduction to 8 mg/kg). If protein level $\geq$ 2 g/24 hr happens again, interrupt drug, and when urine protein is < 2 g/24 hr, reinitiate drug at a further reduced dose (second dose reduction) of 5 mg/kg for gastric and CRC patients (6 mg/kg for NSCLC patients) every 2 weeks. Thus for initial dose of ramucirumab 8 mg IV, 1st dose reduction is to 5 mg/kg, and second dose reduction to 5 mg/kg. If initial dose was 10 mg/kg, 1st dose reduction is to 8 mg/kg, and second dose reduction to 6 mg/kg (Eli Lilly, 2017).
  - Permanently discontinue drug if urine protein level > 3 g/24 hr or if patient develops nephrotic syndrome.
- Wound healing complications: Interrupt drug prior to scheduled surgery and until the surgical wound is fully healed.
- Arterial thrombotic events, GI perforation, or grades 3–4 bleeding: Permanently discontinue drug.
- For toxicities related to paclitaxel docetaxel, or FOLFIRI drugs, see current prescribing information.

Drug Preparation:
- Available in 100-mg/10 mL or 500-mg/50 mL in a concentration of 10-mg/m, as single-dose vials.
- Inspect vials and ensure no particulate matter or discoloration prior to use, and discard if found. Store vials in refrigerator at 2–8°C (36–46°F) until use. Keep the vial in the outer carton in order to protect from light.
- Calculate dose and aseptically withdraw ordered amount. Further dilute in 0.9% sodium chloride in an IV infusion container to make a final volume of 250 mL. Do not use dextrose solutions. Gently invert to mix, and do not shake or freeze. Do not dilute with other solutions or add anything or coinfuse with electrolytes or medications.
- Store diluted infusion bag at 2–8°C (36–46°F) for up to 24 hours, or 4 hours at room temperature (below 25°C [77°F]).
- Discard any unused drug in the vial.

Drug Administration:
- Assess BP and urine for protein (1+ or greater by dipstick/urinalysis), and monitor prior to each treatment. Discuss any abnormalities with the physician. Patients with 2+ or higher proteinuria by urine dipstick/urinalysis should be asked to collect a 24-hour urine sample for protein. Drug should be held for proteinuria $\geq$ 2 g/24 hr, and resume when proteinuria $<$ 2 g/24 hr at a reduced rate. Monitor patients closely if moderate to severe proteinuria until improved or resolved. Drug should be discontinued if the patient develops nephrotic syndrome or urine protein $>$ 3 g/24 hr.
- Visually inspect infusion bag for particulate matter and discoloration; if found, discard solution.
- Premedicate with an IV histamine H1 antagonist (e.g., diphenhydramine). If the patient has had a prior grades 1–2 infusion reaction, add dexamethasone and acetaminophen to the premedications given.
- Infuse drug over 60 minutes via an infusion pump, through a separate line. Do not give IVP or IVB.
- Use of a protein-sparing 0.22 micron filter is recommended.
- Flush with sterile 0.9% sodium chloride for injection at the end of the infusion.

Drug Interactions:
- No studies have been done. Ramucirumab is incompatible with dextrose solutions.

Lab Effects/Interference:
- Serum hyponatremia; urine proteinemia.
- Anemia.

Special Considerations:
- Warnings and Precautions:
  - *Hemorrhage:* Increased risk of hemorrhage and GI hemorrhage, which may be severe and fatal. In study 1, incidence was 3.4% for ramucirumab vs. 2.6% for placebo, and in study 2, incidence of severe bleeding was 4.3% for ramucirumab vs. 2.4% for placebo; in study 3 the incidence of ramucirumab plus docetaxel was 2.4% and that of placebo was 2.3%; and in study 4, incidence of severe bleeding was 2.5% for

ramucirumab plus FOLFIRI vs. 1.7% for placebo plus FOLFIRI (Eli Lilly, 2017). The drug should be permanently discontinued if severe bleeding occurs.

- *Arterial thrombotic events (ATE):* Serious ATEs including MI, cardiac arrest and CVA have occurred. Incidence in gastric patients receiving ramucirumab alone was 1.7% in study 1.
- *Hypertension (HTN):* Increased incidence of severe HTN in patients receiving ramucirumab. Control HTN prior to starting therapy with ramucirumab. Monitor BP at least every 2 weeks during treatment. Temporarily suspend ramucirumab for severe HTN until it can be medically controlled. Permanently discontinue drug in patients with hypertensive crisis or hypertensive encephalopathy.
  - *Infusion related reactions:* Most occur during first or second infusion. Symptoms included rigors/tremors, back pain/spasm, chest pain and/or bronchospasm, SVT, hypotension. Administer premedications and monitor patient during infusion. Emergency equipment, medications and personnel should be available in the infusion unit. Immediately and permanently discontinue ramucirumab for grades 3–4 infusion reactions.
  - *GI perforations:* although rare, GI perforation can occur. Drug should be permanently discontinued in patients with GI perforation.
  - *Impaired wound healing:* Hold the drug for 28 days prior to elective surgery, and do not administer ramucirumab for at least 28 days following a major surgical procedure and until the wound is fully healed. Discontinue ramucirumab if the patient develops wound healing complications requiring medical intervention.
- Worsening of preexisting hepatic impairment: Clinical deterioration in patients with Child-Pugh Class B or C cirrhosis has occurred including new or worsening encephalopathy, ascites, or hepatorenal syndromes. Risk versus potential benefit should be discussed with the patient, and ramucirumab given only if potential benefits outweigh risks in these patients. In patients with Child-Pugh A liver cirrhosis, the incidence of hepatic encephalopathy and hepatorenal syndrome was higher (6%) than in patients receiving placebo (0%) (Lilly, 2019).
- *RPLS:* rarely reported. If patient has symptom(s), evaluate and confirm the diagnosis by MRI and discontinue ramucirumab in patients with RPLS.
- *Proteinuria including nephrotic syndrome:* Occurred in patients recieving ramucirumab plus FOLFIRI, and was severe in 3% compared to 0.2% in patients receiving placebo and ramucirumab. Monitor urine for proteinuria prior to drug administration. Patients with 2+ or higher proteinuria by urine dipstick/urinalysis should be asked to collect a 24-hour urine sample for protein. Drug should be held for proteinuria $\geq$ 2 g/24 hr, and resume when proteinuria $<$ 2 g/24 hr at a reduced dose. Monitor patients closely if moderate to severe proteinuria until improved or resolved. Drug should be discontinued if the patient develops nephrotic syndrome or urine protein $>$ 3 g/24 hr.
- *Thyroid dysfunction:* Monitor during treatment with ramucirumab. In study 4, the incidence of hypothyroidism was 2.6% in the ramucirumab plus FOLFIRI arm, compared to 0.9% in the placebo/ramucirumab arm.
- *Embryofetal toxicity:* based on mechanism of action, drug can cause fetal harm. Teach women of reproductive potential to use effective contraception during and for at least 3 months after the last dose of ramucirumab. Mothers should not breastfeed.

- Single agent ramucirumab (≥ 2% more than placebo): HTN, diarrhea.
  - Together with paclitaxel (≥ 30% incidence and 2% > placebo): fatigue, neutropenia, diarrhea, epistaxis.
  - Together with docetaxel (≥ 30% incidence and 2% > placebo): neutropenia, fatigue/ asthenia, stomatitis/mucosal inflammation.
  - Together with FOLFIRI (≥ 30% incidence and 2% > placebo): diarrhea, neutropenia, decreased appetite, epistaxis, stomatitis.

Potential Toxicities/Side Effects and the Nursing Process

I. POTENTIAL FOR INJURY related to INFUSION REACTION

Defining Characteristics: Incidence in clinical trials occurred prior to standardly prescribing premedications, and was 16%, including 2 severe events. Most infusion reactions occur during or after first or second drug infusion.

Nursing Implications: Ensure patient receives premedication with diphenhydramine as ordered, and if prior grades 1–2 infusion reactions, also administer dexamethasone and acetaminophen as ordered. Assess baseline VS and mental status prior to drug administration, at 15 minutes and periodically during infusion, as needed. Remain with patient during first 15 minutes of infusions. Signs and symptoms included rigors/tremors, back pain/spasms, chest pain/tightness, chills, flushing, dyspnea, wheezing, hypoxia, paresthesia. Rarely, in severe cases, bronchospasm, supraventricular tachycardia, and hypotension occurred. Recall signs/symptoms of infusion reactions; if these occur, stop drug immediately, notify physician, and assess patient's vital signs. If the infusion reaction is grade 1 or 2, infusion rate should be reduced by 50%. Drug should be permanently discontinued for grades 3–4. Review standing physician orders or nursing procedures for patient management of infusion reaction, and be prepared to stop drug immediately and change IV to a plain NS solution to keep vein patent; notify physician. Ensure oxygen and resuscitation equipment is nearby in infusion area. If severe, keep patent airway, monitor VS, and administer ordered medications, which may include epinephrine 1:1,000 IM in the thigh, IV hydrocortisone sodium succinate, and IV diphenhydramine. Teach patient to report any unusual symptoms.

II. POTENTIAL ALTERATION IN CIRCULATION related to HYPERTENSION

Defining Characteristics: Hypertension occurred in 8–16% of patients (8% grades 3–4) in clinical trials.

Nursing Implications: Assess baseline BP prior to administering first dose of ramucirumab, and at least every 2 weeks during treatment. If the patient has a history of hypertension, monitor BP more closely, although hypertension develops over time rather than during the drug infusion. Blood pressure should continue to be monitored after patient has stopped the drug. Teach patient drug administration, potential side effects, and self-care measures if prescribed antihypertensive medication, such as angiotensin-converting enzyme inhibitors, beta-blockers, diuretics, and calcium channel blockers. Ramucirumab should be temporarily suspended in patients with severe hypertension until BP can be controlled with medical management. Drug should be permanently discontinued if HTN cannot be controlled with antihypertensive therapy, the patient develops hypertensive crisis (diastolic blood pressure > 120 mm Hg), or develops hypertensive encephalopathy.

III. ALTERATION IN NUTRITION, POTENTIAL, related to DIARRHEA, RARE RISK GI PERFORATION

Defining Characteristics: Diarrhea occurs in 14% of patients and was grades 3–4 in 1% of patients.

Nursing Implications: Assess baseline nutritional status and bowel elimination status. Teach patient that diarrhea may occur, and much more rarely, bowel perforation. Discuss with patient self-care strategies to manage diarrhea if it occurs. Teach patient that GI perforation may rarely occur, and to report and go to the emergency room right away if severe diarrhea, vomiting, and/or severe pain in the abdomen occurs.

Drug: rituximab (Rituxan); Biosimilar rituximab-abbs (Truxima): indicated for treatment of NHL (1-3) ONLY

Class: mAb (anti-CD20 antibody).

Mechanism of Action: Anti-CD20 antibody that is genetically engineered (chimeric mAb, or part mouse/part human) directed against the CD20 antigen found on the surface of normal and malignant B-cell lymphocytes. The CD20 antigen is also present (expressed) on more than 90% of B-cell NHL cells, but fortunately is not found on normal bone marrow stem cells, pre-B cells, normal plasma cells, or other normal tissues. A section of the rituximab (Fab domain), CD20 binds to the CD20 antigen on B lymphocytes; another section of the rituximab (Fc domain) calls together other immune effectors, resulting in lysis of the B lymphocyte.

Metabolism: Serum and half-life of drug vary with dose and sequence, and at 375 mg/m^2, the median serum half-life was 76.3 hours after the first infusion, as compared to 205 hours after the fourth infusion. Drug was detected in patient serum up to 3–6 months after completion of treatment.

Indications: The treatment of patients with:
Rituxan, Truxima:
- **NHL:** (1) relapsed or refractory, low-grade or follicular, CD-20 positive, B-cell NHL as a single agent; (2) previously untreated follicular, CD-20 positive, B-cell NHL in combination with first-line chemotherapy and, in patients achieving a CR or PR response to rituximab in combination with chemotherapy, as single-agent maintenance therapy; (3) nonprogressing (including stable disease), low-grade, CD-20 positive B-cell NHL as a single agent after first-line CVP chemotherapy;

Rituxan ONLY:

- **NHL:** (4) previously untreated diffuse large B-cell, CD-20 positive NHL, in combination with CHOP or other anthracycline-based chemotherapy regimens.
- **CLL** in combination with fludarabine and cyclophosphamide (FC) for the treatment of patients with previously untreated or treated CD20-positive CLL.
- **RA,** in combination with methotrexate, in adult patients with moderately-to-severely active rheumatoid arthritis (RA) who have had an inadequate response to one or more TNF antagonist therapies.
- **Granulomatosis with Polyangiitis (GPA) (Wegener's Granulomatosis [WG]), and microscopic polyangiitis (MPA)** in adult patients in combination with glucocorticoids for the treatment of active GPA (WG) and (MPA).
- Moderate to severe Pemphigus Vulgaris (PV) in adult patients.
- **Rituximab** is not recommended for use in patients with severe, active infections.

Dosage/Range:

- **Premedications:**
  - Premedicate before each infusion with acetaminophen and an antihistamine. For patients receiving rituximab infusion over 90 minutes, administer glucocorticoid prior to infusion.
  - For RA (rheumatoid arthritis) patients, methylprednisolone 100-mg IV or its equivalent is recommended 30 minutes prior to each infusion.
  - *Pneumocystis jiroveci* pneumonia (PCP) and antiherpetic viral prophylaxis is recommended for patients with CLL during treatment and for up to 12 months following treatment, as appropriate.
  - PCP prophylaxis is recommended for patients with GPA and MPA during treatment and for 6 months following last rituximab infusion.

Rituximab doses
NHL: 375 mg/m² IV infusion:

- **Relapsed or refractory, low-grade or follicular, CD20-positive, B-cell NHL.**
  - 375 mg/m² given as IV infusion weekly for 4 or 8 doses.
  - Retreatment for relapsed or refractory, low-grade or follicular, CD-20 positive B-cell NHL: Administer once weekly for 4 doses.
- **Previously untreated, follicular, CD20-positive, B-cell NHL.**
  - 375 mg/m² IV infusion day 1 of each cycle of chemotherapy for up to 8 doses.
  - If CR or PR, start rituximab maintenance therapy 8 weeks following completion of rituximab in combination with chemotherapy. Administer rituximab as a single agent every 8 weeks for 12 doses.
- **Nonprogressing, low-grade, CD20-positive, B-cell NHL after first-line CVP chemotherapy.**
  - Following completion of 6–8 cycles of CVP chemotherapy, administer rituximab 375 mg/m² IV infusion, once weekly for 4 doses every 6 months for up to 16 doses.
- **Diffuse large B-cell NHL (DLBCL)**
  - 375 mg/m² IV infusion day 1 of each cycle of chemotherapy for up to 8 infusions.

Chronic lymphocytic leukemia (CLL):
- 375 mg/m² initially on the day prior to the start of FC chemotherapy, then 500 mg/m² IV on day 1 of cycles 2–6 administered every 28 days.
- PCP and antiherpetic viral prophylaxis is recommended during treatment and for up to 12 months following treatment as needed.

As a component of Zevalin (ibritumomab tiuxetan) therapeutic regimen:
- Rituximab 250-mg/m² IV within 4 hours prior to the administration of Indium-111-(In-111-) Zevalin, and within 4 hours prior to the administration of Yttrium-90-(Y-90-) Zevalin.
- Administer rituximab and In-111-Zevalin 7–9 days prior to rituximab and Y-90-Zevalin. Refer to Zevalin package insert for full prescribing information regarding Zevalin therapeutic regimen.

Rheumatoid arthritis: Administer rituximab as two 1,000-mg **(NOT per meter squared)** *IV infusions separated by 2 weeks (one course);*
- Administer glucocorticoids (methylprednisolone 100 mg IV or equivalent) 30 minutes prior to each infusion to reduce incidence and severity of infusion reactions.
- Subsequent courses should be administered every 24 weeks or based on clinical evaluation, but not sooner than every 16 weeks.
- Rituximab is given in combination with methotrexate.

Granulomatosis with polyangiitis (GPA, Wegener's granulomatosis or WG) and Microscopic Polyangiitis (MPA):
- 375 mg/m² IV once weekly for 4 weeks, together with glucocorticoid.
- Methylprednisolone 1,000 mg IV per day for 1–3 days, followed by oral prednisone 1 mg/kg/day (not to exceed 80 mg/day and tapered per clinical need) are recommended to treat severe vasculitis symptoms; this regimen should begin within 14 days prior to or with the initiation of rituximab and may continue during and after the 4-week course of rituximab treatment.
- PCP and antiherpetic viral prophylaxis is recommended during treatment and for at least 6 months following the last rituximab treatment.
- There is limited data on the safety and efficacy of subsequent courses of rituximab in patients with GPA and MPA.

Pemphigus Vulgaris (PV)
- Two 1,000 mg IV infusions separated by 2 weeks in combination with a tapering of glucocorticoids.
- Maintenance treatment: 500 mg IV infusion at month 12 and every 6 months thereafter or based on clinical evaluation.
- Relapse treatment: 1,000mg IV infusion upon relapse and consider resuming or increasing the glucocorticoid dose based on clinical evaluation.

Drug Preparation:
- Do not mix with or dilute with other drugs.
- Store at 2–8°C (36–46°F) and protect vials from direct sunlight.
- Available as 100-mg (10-mL) and 500-mg (50-mL) single-use preservative-free vials.
- Inspect for particulate matter and discoloration prior to administration. Do not use vial if particulates or discoloration is present.

TREATMENT

- Aseptically withdraw the ordered dose and dilute to a final concentration of 1–4 mg/mL in an infusion bag of either 0.9% sodium chloride USP or 5% dextrose in water. Gently invert to mix, and inspect for presence of any particulate matter or discoloration. Discard any unused drug left in the vial.
- Drug is stable in infusion solution at 2–8°C (36–46°F) for 24 hours. While studies have shown stability at room temperature for another 24 hours, since rituximab infusions do not contain a preservative, refrigeration is recommended.

Drug Administration:
- DO NOT GIVE AS AN INTRAVENOUS PUSH OR BOLUS.

Laboratory monitoring:
- **Malignancies:**
  - Patients receiving monotherapy should have a CBC and platelet count prior to each rituximab infusion.
  - During treatment with rituximab and chemotherapy, CBC and platelets should be monitored with weekly to monthly intervals or more frequently if cytopenias develop.
- **RA, WG, or MPA:** Patients should have a CBC and platelet count at 2- to 4-month intervals during rituximab therapy.
- **Premedicate** before each infusion with acetaminophen and an antihistamine and other medications as needed for diagnosis or prior infusion reaction.
- Infusion area should have emergency equipment, medications, and personnel available.
- **First infusion:** Initiate infusion at a rate of 50 mg/hr; if no infusion-related problems occur, increase the infusion rate in 50-mg/hr increments every 30 minutes to a maximum of 400 mg/hr. If infusion reaction occurs, slow or stop the infusion depending on severity. If not severe, may continue the infusion at half the previous rate (minimum 50% rate reduction) once symptoms resolve. Discontinue drug if infusion reaction is severe.
- **Subsequent infusions:**
  - *Standard infusion:* If the first infusion is well tolerated, administer at initial rate of 100 mg/hr, and increase by 100-mg/hr increments every 30 minutes, to a maximum of 400 mg/hr as tolerated.
  - For *previously untreated follicular NHL and DLBCL patients:* If patient did not experience a grade 3–4 IRR during cycle 1, a 90-minute infusion can be administered in cycle 2 with a glucocorticoid-containing chemotherapy regimen. Most of the CD20 lymphocytes have been lysed in the first treatment, so the risk of CRS is minimal (Swan et al., 2011).
  - Initiate at a rate of 20% of the total dose given in the first 30 minutes, with the remaining 80% of the total dose given over the next 60 minutes.
  - If the 90-minute infusion is well tolerated in cycle 2, the same rate can be used when giving the remainder of the treatment regimen (through cycle 6 or 8).
  - **Do not use the 90-min** infusion for patients who have clinically significant cardiovascular disease or who have circulating lymphocyte counts $\geq$5,000/mm^3 before cycle 2.
- Administer glucocorticoid component of chemotherapy prior to rituximab infusion.
- Interrupt the infusion or slow the rate if an infusion reaction occurs. Continue the infusion at one-half the previous rate upon symptom improvement.

- Fatal infusion reactions have rarely occurred within 24 hours of rituximab dose, characterized by hypoxemia, pulmonary infiltrates, ARDS, MI, VF, and shock. Eighty percent of the fatal reactions occurred with the first infusion.

Drug Interactions:
- Renal toxicity when rituximab used in combination with cisplatin. Combination not indicated.

Lab Effects/Interference:
- Decreased lymphocyte count (B cells); decreased IgM and IgG serum levels.
- Hypophosphatemia and hyperuricemia.

Special Considerations:
- Warnings and Precautions:
  - *Infusion reactions:* Although infusion reactions are common (fever, chills) during the first infusion, severe infusion reactions can also occur and some cases are fatal. Appropriate emergency medical support to manage severe infusion reactions must be available.
    - Severe reactions typically occurred during the first infusion with onset 30–120 minutes, but they can occur within 24 hours.
    - Signs/symptoms include involving urticaria, hypotension, angioedema, bronchospasm, hypoxia, pulmonary infiltrates, acute respiratory distress syndrome, myocardial infarction, ventricular fibrillation, cardiogenic shock, anaphylactoid events, and death.
    - Patients should be premedicated with an antihistamine and acetaminophen prior to drug administration (RA patients should receive methylprednisolone 100 mg IV or equivalent 30 minutes prior to dose).
    - STOP infusion for severe reactions and institute emergency medical management (e.g., glucocorticoids, epinephrine, oxygen, bronchodilators, saline) for infusion reactions as needed.
    - Depending upon severity of reaction and required interventions, temporarily or permanently discontinue rituximab.
    - For mild-to-moderate infusion reactions, once symptoms have resolved, rituximab may be resumed at 50% of the previous rate. Closely monitor patients who have preexisting cardiac or pulmonary conditions, those who have had prior cardiopulmonary side effects, and those with high numbers ($\geq 25,000/m^3$) of circulating tumor cells. Infusion reaction is a cytokine release reaction related to the cytokines released when the tumor cells are rapidly lysed by rituximab. The higher the number of circulating tumor cells, the higher the risk of an infusion reaction or CRS.
    - Emergency medications should be readily available: epinephrine, antihistamines, and corticosteroids.
  - *Severe mucocutaneous reactions* may occur, some resulting in death.
    - Reactions include paraneoplastic pemphigus, SJS, lichenoid dermatitis, vesiculobullous dermatitis, and TEN.
    - Onset can be as early as the first day of therapy to 13 weeks following rituximab dose.

- Drug should be stopped if a reaction develops; a skin biopsy should be performed.
- If the patient has a severe mucocutaneous reaction, the drug should be discontinued.
- *Hepatitis B (HPV) reactivation* can occur in hematologic patients treated with rituximab, usually about 4 months after the first rituximab dose, and about 1 month after the last dose.
  - Reactivation can result in fulminant hepatitis, hepatic failure, or death.
  - All patients at high risk for HPV should be screened for HPV prior to starting rituximab therapy.
  - Carriers of hepatitis B should be closely monitored for clinical and laboratory signs of active HPV infection for several months following rituximab therapy.
  - Patients who develop viral hepatitis should have rituximab discontinued, along with any concomitant chemotherapy, and start appropriate treatment, including antiviral therapy.
  - It is unknown whether rituximab can be safely resumed in these patients.
- *PML* can occur following rituximab therapy, usually within 12 months of the last rituximab infusion, and can be fatal.
  - PML is caused by the JC virus, and the disease occurs in patients who have been immunosuppressed, such as patients with hematologic malignancies who received chemotherapy along with rituximab or as part of a stem cell transplant, or with autoimmune disease in patients who had prior or concurrent immunosuppressive therapy.
  - Most cases of PML were diagnosed within 12 months of their last rituximab dose. If a patient receiving rituximab has a new-onset neurologic problem, consider PML in the differential, with evaluation by a neurologist, along with brain MRI and lumbar puncture.
  - Rituximab should be discontinued, and the discontinuation or reduction of any concomitant chemotherapy or immunosuppressive therapy in the patient who develops PML should be considered.
- *TLS* may occur within 12–24 hours after the first infusion of rituximab for NHL, with acute renal failure, hyperkalemia, hypocalcemia, hyperuricemia, or hyperphosphatemia.
  - Patients at risk for TLS are those with a high number of circulating tumor cells ($\geq$ 25,000/mm^3), high tumor burden, and high LDH.
  - Prepare patients at risk prior to rituximab with aggressive IV hydration and anti-hyperuricemic therapy, correct electrolyte abnormalities, monitor renal function and fluid balance, and administer supportive care, including dialysis, if needed.
- *Serious infections* can occur during and up to 1 year after the last rituximab-based therapy, including potentially fatal bacterial, fungal, and new or reactivated viral infections (e.g., CMV, herpes simplex, parvovirus B19, varicella zoster, West Nile, hepatitis B and C).
  - If a patient develops a severe infection, discontinue rituximab and begin appropriate antimicrobial therapy.
  - Drug should NOT be administered to patients with severe active infections.

- *Cardiovascular adverse reactions:* Cardiac arrhythmias and angina can occur and be life-threatening.
  - Patients who develop clinically significant arrhythmias should receive cardiac monitoring during and after all subsequent infusions of the drug.
  - Patients with a history of arrhythmias and angina should be cardiac monitored during infusion and immediately postinfusion for evidence of recurrence of these problems.
  - Rituximab should be discontinued if serious or life-threatening cardiac arrhythmias occur.
- *Severe renal toxicity* can occur in patients with NHL after rituximab therapy, including renal toxicity in patients who develop TLS.
  - Patients should be monitored closely for signs of renal failure.
  - Discontinue rituximab in patients with a rising serum creatinine or oliguria.
- *Bowel obstruction and perforation* can occur rarely in NHL patients receiving rituximab and chemotherapy and sometimes result in death.
  - Typically, abdominal pain, bowel obstruction, and perforation occurred 6 days (range 1–77) after rituximab dosing.
  - Patients with abdominal pain should have a thorough diagnostic evaluation to rule out obstruction or perforation.
  - *Immuniation:* Do not administer live viral vaccines as it has not been studied. For patients with RA, follow current immunization guidelines and give nonlive vaccines at least 4 weeks prior to a course of rituximab. The effect of rituximab on immune response to pneumococcal vaccinations (T-cell independent antigen) was lower in RA patients receiving rituximab and MTX, while response to tetanus toxoid vaccine (T-cell dependent antigen with existing immunity) was positive (Genentech, 2016).
  - *Embryo-fetal toxicity:* Drug can cause fetal harm due to B-cell lymphocyteopenia. Teach women of reproductive potential to use effective contraception during therapy and for 12 months after last rituximab dose.
  - *Laboratory monitoring:* Monitor CBC, platelet count regularly during therapy.
  - *Concomitant use of biologic agents and DMARDS* other than Methotrexate: limited safety data in RA patients with peripheral B-cell depletion following treatment with rituximab; observe patients closely for signs of infection. Concomitant immunosuppressants other than corticosteroids have not been studied in WG or MPA patients exhibiting peripheral B-cell depletion following treatment with rituximab.
  - *Use in RA patients who have not had prior inadequate response to TNF antagonists:* use of rituximab is not recommended.
  - *Retreatment in patients with granulomatosis with polyangiitis (GPA) (Wegener's Granulomatosis) and microscopinc polyangiitis (MPA): safety and efficacy has not been established for retreatment.*
- Cytopenias that develop during rituximab therapy can last months beyond the treatment period.
- Retreatment in patients with GPA, WG, and MPA: there are limited data; safety and efficacy have not been established.

- Nursing mothers: caution should be used when administering rituximab to a nursing mother.
- Most common adverse reactions:
  - NHL ($\geq 25\%$): Infusion reactions, fever, lymphopenia, chills, infection, and asthenia;
  - CLL: infusion reactions, neutropenia.
  - RA ($\geq 10\%$): URI, nasopharyngitis, UTI, bronchitis; other less-frequent reactions: infusion reactions, serious infections, cardiovascular events.
  - GPA and MPA ($\geq 15\%$): infections, nausea, diarrhea, headache, muscle spasms, anemia, peripheral edema; other less frequent: infusion reactions.

Potential Toxicities/Side Effects and the Nursing Process

I.   POTENTIAL FOR INJURY related to INFUSION-RELATED REACTIONS

Defining Characteristics: IRRs occurred within 30 minutes to 2 hours of the beginning of the first infusion. Fever and chills/rigors affect most patients during the initial infusion. Other infusion-related symptoms include: nausea; urticaria; fatigue; headache; pruritus; bronchospasm; dyspnea; sensation of swelling of tongue, throat; hypotension; flushing; and pain at disease site. Infusion-related reactions generally resolve with slowing or interrupting the drug infusion, and/or symptomatic treatment (IV saline, acetaminophen, diphenhydramine). Premedications often reduce the severity and/or occurrence of these reactions. In patients who receive retreatment after having completed at least one course of drug therapy, reactions that were reported include: fever, chills, asthenia, pruritus, and infusion-related events (fever, chills, pain, and throat irritation). The incidence of abdominal pain, anemia, dyspnea, hypotension, and neutropenia is higher in patients with bulky tumors > 10 cm. Infusion reaction is more likely during or after initial treatment, as it is related to the release of cytokines from the lysed CD20-positive cells. In successive treatments, fewer CD20 cells remain to be lysed, so there is significantly less cytokine release.

Nursing Implications: Discuss with physician or NP/PA the use of premedications, such as acetaminophen and an antihistamine before drug therapy. Ensure that medications necessary for the management of severe infusion reactions are readily available (e.g., epinephrine, antihistamines, corticosteroids). Assess baseline VS and monitor frequently during the infusion. Follow infusion rate guide (see Drug Administration section) for first and subsequent infusions. Slow or stop the infusion if severe IRRs occur. Monitor VS, and notify physician. Be prepared to provide emergency support as necessary (including IV saline, epinephrine, antihistamines, bronchodilators). If/when symptoms resolve, resume the infusion at 50% of the rate of the previous infusion, as directed by the physician.

II.   ALTERATION IN ELIMINATION, RENAL, related to TUMOR LYSIS SYNDROME

Defining Characteristics: Patients with high tumor burden receiving rituximab for the first time are at risk for rapid tumor lysis. TLS occurs as a result of rapid release of intracellular contents into the bloodstream. The risk of TLS appears higher in patients with a high num- ber of circulating lymphocytes, for example, $> 25{,}000/mm^3$.

Nursing Implications: For first infusion, expect patient orders to include: Hydration at 150 mL/hr with or without alkalinization, oral allopurinol, strict monitoring of I/O, daily weight, and body balance determination. Monitor baseline and daily BUN, creatinine, po- tassium, phosphorus, uric acid, and calcium. Monitor for renal, cardiac, neuromuscular signs/symptoms, hyperkalemia, hyperphosphatemia, hypomagnesemia, hypocalcemia, and elevated uric acid.

III.   POTENTIAL FOR INFECTION related to LYMPHOPENIA AND BONE MARROW DEPRESSION

Defining Characteristics: B-cell lymphocytes are reduced in some patients, together with a decrease in immunoglobulins in some patients. Bacterial infections that occurred in these patients were not associated with neutropenia, and some were severe, involving sepsis due to *Listeria, Staphylococcus*, and polymicrobials; posttreatment infections included rare sepsis, and viral infections (herpes simplex and herpes zoster). Leukopenia occurs in some patients, thrombocytopenia in some, and neutropenia in some others. Serious bone marrow suppression was uncommon and may occur up to 30 days following treatment. These in- clude severe neutropenia, thrombocytopenia, and severe anemia. Rarely, transient aplastic anemia or hemolytic anemia may occur. Incidence of neutropenia, anemia, and abdominal pain was higher, as was the severity, in patients with bulky tumors > 10 cm. Limited data is available about safety of biologic agents and DMARDS (other than methotrexate) in RA, as rituximab will deplete peripheral B-cells. Post-marketing reports have noted prolonged rare pancytopenia, marrow hypoplasia, grades 3–4 prolonged or late onset neutropenia.

Nursing Implications: Monitor CBC, platelets baseline and regularly during treatment. If the patient develops cytopenia, monitor more frequently. Assess for signs/symptoms of infection, bleeding, fatigue, and chest pain prior to each treatment. Teach patient to self-assess for these, including taking temperature, and instruct to report them immediately. Transfuse red cells and platelets as ordered. Observe patients with RA who are also taking DMARDS (other than methotrexate) closely for signs of infection.

IV.   LOSS OF SKIN INTEGRITY, POTENTIAL, related to SEVERE MUCOCUTANEOUS REACTIONS

Defining Characteristics: Severe skin reactions have occurred rarely and, in some cases, ended in death of patient. Skin abnormalities include paraneoplastic pemphigus (uncom- mon autoimmune disorder, may be related to underlying malignancy), SJS (may be caused by HSV or other infectious disorder), lichenoid dermatitis, vesiculobullous dermatitis, and TEN. Onset is 1–13 weeks following rituximab exposure.

Nursing Implications: Assess baseline skin and mucous membrane integrity. Teach pa- tient that rarely skin and mucous membrane reactions may occur, and to report any changes right away. Manufacturer recommends stopping rituximab therapy and obtaining skin biopsy to determine cause. Discuss with physician. Teach the patient local care strategies depending upon symptoms.

V.   ALTERATION IN COMFORT related to ASTHENIA, HEADACHE, NAUSEA, VOMITING, PRURITUS, MYALGIA, AND DIZZINESS

Defining Characteristics: From single-agent Rituxan studies for relapsed or refractory, low-grade or follicular NHL, there was some incidence of asthenia. Headache, nausea, pruritus, vomiting, myalgia, and dizziness may also occur.

Nursing Implications: Assess baseline comfort prior to each infusion, and tolerance of past infusion. Discuss strategies to manage symptoms. If symptoms are severe, discuss management with physician.

Drug: Rituximab and hyaluronidase human injection (Rituxan Hycela injection)

Class: mAb with agent to increase subcutaneous absorption.

Mechanism of Action: Rituximab is an mAb that targets the CD20 antigen on the surface of pre-B and mature B-lymphocytes. When the drug binds to the CD20 antigen, it causes B-lymphocyte lysis (death) probably by CDC and antibody-dependent cell-medicated cytotoxicity (ADCC). Hyaluronase is a polysaccharide found in the subcutaneous tissue extracellular matrix; it is depolymerized by the enzyme hyaluronidase, which increases the subcutaneous permeability for the subcutaneous injection of rituximab. Hyanuronidase increases the absorption of the drug systemically. The hyaluronidase effects are temporary, and normal skin permeability is restored within 24–48 hours.

Indications: Treatment of adult patients with (1) *follicular lymphoma (FC)* (a) relapsed or refractory, follicular lymphoma as a single agent, (b) previously untreated follicular lymphoma in combination with first-line chemotherapy and, in patients who achieve a CR or PR to rituximab in combination with chemotherapy, as single-agent maintenance therapy, (c) nonprogressing (including SD) follicular lymphoma as a single agent after first-line cyclophosphamide, vincristine, and prednisone (CVP) chemotherapy; (2) *diffuse large B-cell lymphoma (DLBCL)* previously untreated in combination with cyclophosphamide, doxorubicin, vincristine, prednisone (CHP), or other anthracycline-based chemotherapy regimen; (3) *chronic lymphocytic leukemia (CLL),* untreated or previously treated, in combination with fludarabine and cyclophosphamide (FC).

Limitations of Use: (1) Rituximab hyaluronidase injection should be used ONLY after patients have received at least one full dose of a rituximab product by IV infusion; (2) drug is NOT indicated for treatment of nonmalignant conditions.

Contraindications: None.

Dosage Range: Drug is for SUBCUTANEOUS INJECTION ONLY.

- Rituximab hyaluronidase injection should only be administered by a healthcare professional with available medical support to manage severe reactions if they occur because they can be fatal.
- Rituximab hyaluronidase injection should be used ONLY after patients have received at least one full dose of a rituximab product by IV infusion WITHOUT experiencing a severe adverse reaction. If the patient has a severe reaction while receiving rituximab IV infusion, then the patient should continue receiving IV rituximab until a full IV dose is successfully administered (Genentech, 2017).
- Recommended premedication:
  - Acetaminophen and an antihistamine before each dose of rituximab hyaluronidase injection; consider also administering a glucocorticoid drug.
  - Patients with CLL: Prophylaxis for PCP and herpes virus during treatment and for up to 12 months after treatment as appropriate.
- Doses are fixed, NOT BSA.
  - FL: Rituximab 1,400 mg/23,400 hyaluronidase human units SQ. Premedicate before each dose.
    - *Relapsed or refractory FL:* once weekly × 3 or 7 weeks following a full dose of a rituximab product by IV infusion at week 1 (i.e., 4 or 8 weeks total).
    - *Retreatment for relapsed or refractory, FL:* once weekly × 3 weeks following a full dose of a rituximab product by IV infusion at week 1 (i.e., 4 weeks total).
    - *Previously untreated FL:* administer on day 1 of cycles 2–8 chemotherapy (every 21 days) for up to 7 cycles following a full dose of a rituximab product by IV infusion on day 1 cycle 1 of chemotherapy (i.e., up to 8 cycles in total). If CR or PR, patient should receive rituximab/hyaluronidase maintenance treatment 8 weeks after completion of rituximab/hyaluronidase in combination with chemotherapy. Administer rituximab/hyaluronidase as a single-agent every 8 weeks × 12 doses.
      - *Nonprogressing FL after first-line CVP chemotherapy:* Following completion of 6–8 cycles of CVP chemotherapy and a full dose of a rituximab product by IV infusion at week 1, administer once weekly for 3 weeks (e.g., 4 weeks in total) at 6-month intervals to a maximum of 16 doses.
  - DLBCL: Rituximab 1,400 mg/23,400 hyaluronidase human units SQ. Patient should receive one full dose of a rituximab product by IV infusion in combination with CHOP chemotherapy before starting the subcutaneous drug. Premedicate before each dose. Administer Rituximab 1,400 mg/23,400 hyaluronidase human units SQ on day 1 of cycles 2–8 of CHOP chemotherapy for up to 7 cycles (up to 6–8 cycles total).
  - CLL: Rituximab 1,600 mg/26,800 hyaluronidase human units SQ. Patient should receive one full dose of a rituximab product by IV infusion in combination with FC chemotherapy before starting the subcutaneous drug. Premedicate before each dose. Administer rituximab 1,600 mg/26,800 hyaluronidase human units SQ on day 1 of cycles 2–6 (every 28 days) for a total of 5 cycles.

Drug Preparations:
- Drug is ready to use. Available as (1) Injection: 1,400 mg rituximab and 23,400 units hyaluronidase human per 11.7 mL (120 mg/2,000 units/mL) in a single-dose vial; and

(2) Injection: 1,600 mg rituximab and 26,800 units hyaluronidase human per 13.4 mL (120 mg/2,000 units/mL) in a single-dose vial.

- Attach hypodermic injection needle to the syringe immediately before administration to avoid needle clogging. Drug is compatible with polypropylene and polycarbonate syringe material and stainless steel transfer and injection needles.
- Inspect drug product for any particulate matter or discoloration, and do not use if found.
- Storage: Once rituximab/hyaluronidase injection is withdrawn from the vial, it should be labeled with the peel-off sticker and used immediately. If not used immediately, prepare in controlled and validated aseptic conditions. Once transferred from vial to syringe, store the solution in refrigerator at 2°–8°C (36–46°F) up to 48 hours and subsequently for 8 hours at room temperature up to 30°C (86°F) in diffuse light.

Drug Administration:
- Inject rituximab/hyaluronidase human injection into the SQ tissue of the abdomen over 5–7 minutes and AVOID injection into skin that is red, bruised, tender, or hard, or areas with moles or scars. No data are available about injection to other subcutaneous areas.
- Rituximab 1,400 mg/hyaluronidase 23,400 units dose is a volume of 11.7 mL; inject SQ into abdomen over 5 minutes.
- Rituximab 1,600 mg/hyaluronidase 26,800 units dose is a volume of 13.4 mL; inject SQ into abdomen over 7 minutes.
- If interrupted during administration, continue administering at the same or a different site but only in the abdomen.
- Observe patient for at least 15 minutes following Rituximab/hyaluronidase SQ injection.
- DO NOT administer other medications for SQ use at the same sites used for rituximab/hyaluronidase injection.

Drug Interactions: cisplatin: increased risk of renal toxicity.

Lab Effects/Interference:
- When given with chemotherapy, neutropenia, thrombocytopenia
- Increased risk of TLS: hyperuricemia, hyperkalemia, renal dysfunction

Special Considerations:
- Most common adverse reactions (incidence ≥ 20%):
  - FL: infections, neutropenia, nausea, constipation, cough, fatigue
  - DLBCL: infections, neutropenia, alopecia, nausea, anemia
  - CLL: infections, neutropenia, nausea, thrombocytopenia, pyrexia, vomiting, injection site erythema
- Warnings and Precautions:
  - *Severe mucocutaneous reactions:* Rarely, potentially fatal mucocutaneous reactions may occur such as paraneoplastic pemphigus, SJS, lichenoid dermatitis, vesiculobullous dermatitis, and TEN. If this occurs, discontinue the drug.
  - *Hepatitis B virus reactivation:* Characterized by an abrupt increase in HBV replication (rapid increase in serum HBV DNA levels or detection of HBsAg in a person who was previously negative, and anti-HBc positive, can occur. HBV reactivation is often followed by hepatitis as evidenced by increased serum transaminases. In some cases, fulminant hepatitis, hepatic failure, and death have occurred.

- Screen all patients for HBV infection (e.g., measure HBsAg and anti-HBc) before starting a rituximab-containing product. Monitor patients with evidence of current or prior HBV infection for signs/symptoms of hepatitis or HBV reactivation for several months following last dose of rituximab-containing product. HBV reactivation has been reported up to 24 months after completion of rituximab therapy (Genentech, 2017).
- If patient does develop HBV reactivation, immediately discontinue rituximab/hyaluronidase human and any concomitant chemotherapy, and follow physician orders to implement appropriate treatment.
- *PML:* JC virus infection resulting in PML and death has occurred in patients receiving rituximab-containing products. Monitor for new-onset neurologic manifestations, and expect thorough evaluation of PML including neurology consult, brain MRI, and LP. Drug should be discontinued if PML is diagnosed, and chemotherapy or immunosuppressive therapy should be discontinued or dose reduced (Genentech, 2017).
- *Hypersensitivity and other administration reactions:* Patients must receive one full dose of rituximab product by IV infusion before being able to receive SQ rituximab/hyaluronidase human injection as the risk of infusion reactions is highest during the first infusion. These reactions are believed to be related to CRS and/or release of other chemical mediators and are managed by slowing or stopping the infusion.
  - CRS is often indistinguishable from acute HSRs, except that a true HSR typically occurs within minutes after starting the infusion, whereas CRS occurs later.
  - IRRs: IV administration of rituximab-containing product has been associated with severe, fatal IRRs characterized by pulmonary events, fever, chills, rigors, hypotension, urticarial, angioedema, and other symptoms, occurring within 30 minutes to 2 hours after starting the first IV infusion. Anaphylaxis and other HSRs may also occur.
  - Severe CRS is characterized by severe dyspnea, often associated with bronchospasm and hypoxia, fever, chills, rigors, urticarial, and angioedema, occurring 1–2 hours after starting the infusion. ARDS and death may occur rarely. There is increased risk of poor outcome in patients with a history of pulmonary insufficiency or with lymphoma infiltrating the lung.
  - Interrupt the rituximab product *immediately* if a severe reaction occurs, and treat symptoms aggressively as ordered. Closely monitor patients with (a) preexisting cardiac or pulmonary conditions, (b) those who have experienced prior cardiopulmonary adverse reactions, and (c) those with a high number of circulating tumor cells ($\geq 25,000/mm^3$).
  - Give ordered premedication (e.g., antihistamine and acetaminophen) before administering the SQ injection and discuss with provider the addition of a glucocorticoid as appropriate.
  - Observe patient for at least 15 minutes after the SQ injection and for longer periods if patient is at increased risk for HSRs.
  - Local cutaneous reactions including injection-site reactions may occur (e.g., pain, swelling, induration, hemorrhage, erythema, pruritus, and rash) and may be delayed for more than 24 hours. The incidence in clinical studies was 16% and was

mild or moderate, resolving without treatment. Most reactions occurred during cycle 2 with the first of the SQ injections, and incidence decreased with subsequent injections.

- *TLS:* This can occur 12–24 hours after rituximab-containing product administration, especially in patients with a high circulating tumor volume (e.g., $\geq 25,000/mm^3$). Discuss with provider aggressive IV hydration and anti-hyperuricemic therapy if patient is at high risk. Monitor and correct electrolyte abnormalities and monitor renal function and intake/output (fluid balance); if needed, hemodialysis can be used to reverse renal compromise.
- *Infections:* Serious bacterial, fungal, and new or reactivated viral (e.g., CMV, herpes simplex, varicella zoster) infections can occur during and after rituximab-containing product therapy ends. Patients with CLL was 56% in those receiving IV rituximab versus 49% in those receiving SQ injection. In patients with FL or DLBCL, the incidence is 46 and 41%, respectively. Drug should be discontinued for serious infections and patient treated with appropriate anti-infective agents.
- *Cardiovascular adverse reactions:* Ventricular fibrillation, MI, and cardiogenic shock have occurred with rituximab-containing product administration. Discontinue drug for serious or life-threatening arrhythmia or angina.
- *Renal toxicity:* Severe, potentially fatal, renal toxicity occurred after administration of rituximab-product-containing drug, especially in patients who developed TLS, or in patients receiving concomitant cisplatin therapy, during clinical trials. The combination of rituximab/hyaluronidase human and cisplatin is not an approved treatment regimen. Monitor patient for signs of renal failure, and discontinue drug if serum creatinine is rising or if the patient develops oliguria.
- *Bowel obstruction and perforation:* Abdominal pain, bowel obstruction, and perforation have been described in patients receiving rituximab, including patients receiving SQ rituximab/hyaluronidase human in combination with chemotherapy. Time to GI perforation was 6 (range 1–77) days. If patient develops symptoms of GI obstruction (e.g., abdominal pain or repeated vomiting), patients should be evaluated promptly.
- *Immunization:* Do not vaccinate patient with live vaccines during treatment with rituximab/hyaluronidase human.
- *Embryo–fetal toxicity:* Drug can cause B-cell lymphocytopenia in the infants exposed to rituximab in utero. Teach patients of childbearing potential to use effective contraception to prevent pregnancy during treatment and for 12 months after last dose of rituximab-hyaluronidase human.
- Counsel nursing mothers not to breastfeed while receiving the drug.

Potential Toxicities/Side Effects and the Nursing Process

I. POTENTIAL FOR INJURY related to INFUSION-RELATED REACTIONS

Defining Characteristics: IRRs occurred within 30 minutes to 2 hours of the beginning of the first infusion. Fever and chills/rigors affect most patients during the initial infusion. Other infusion-related symptoms include nausea, urticaria, fatigue, headache, pruritus, bronchospasm, dyspnea, sensation of swelling of tongue and throat, hypotension, flushing, and pain at disease site. Infusion-related reactions generally resolve with slowing or interrupting the drug infusion, and/or symptomatic treatment (IV saline, acetaminophen, diphenhydramine). Premedications often reduce the severity and/or occurrence of these reactions. In patients who receive retreatment after having completed at least one course of drug therapy, reactions that were reported include fever, chills, asthenia, pruritus, and infusion-related events (fever, chills, pain, and throat irritation). The incidence of abdominal pain, anemia, dyspnea, hypotension, and neutropenia is higher in patients with bulky tumors >10 cm. Infusion reaction is more likely during or after initial treatment, as it is related to the release of cytokines from the lysed CD20-positive cells. In successive treatments, fewer CD20 cells remain to be lysed, so there is significantly less cytokine release.

Nursing Implications: Administer ordered premedications (e.g., diphenhydramine, acetaminophen) and discuss with physician or NP/PA the need for/use of corticosteroid premedications. Ensure that medications necessary for the management of severe infusion reactions are readily available (e.g., epinephrine, antihistamines, corticosteroids). Assess baseline VS and observe the patient for 15 minutes after the SQ injection. If a severe reaction occurs while administering the drug, stop the injection. Monitor VS and notify physician right away. Be prepared to provide emergency support as necessary (including IV saline, epinephrine, antihistamines, bronchodilators).

II.   ALTERATION IN ELIMINATION, RENAL, related to TUMOR LYSIS SYNDROME

Defining Characteristics: Patients with high tumor burden receiving rituximab for the first time are at risk for rapid tumor lysis. TLS occurs as a result of rapid release of intracellular contents into the bloodstream. The risk of TLS appears higher in patients with a high number of circulating lymphocytes (e.g., >25,000/mm^3). Although the occurrence of TLS is most likely during the first cycle given as an IV infusion, it is possible that TLS can occur after SQ injection if the circulating tumor volume is still >25,000/mm^3.

Nursing Implications: If the patient is at high risk for TLS (e.g., high circulating tumor volume), expect patient orders to include hydration at 150 mL/hour with or without alkalinization, oral allopurinol, strict monitoring of I/O, daily weight, and body balance determination. Monitor baseline and daily BUN, creatinine, potassium, phosphorus, uric acid, and calcium. Monitor for renal, cardiac, neuromuscular signs/symptoms, hyperkalemia, hyperphosphatemia, hypomagnesemia, hypocalcemia, and elevated uric acid.

III.   POTENTIAL FOR INFECTION related to LYMPHOPENIA AND BONE MARROW DEPRESSION

Defining Characteristics: B-cell lymphocytes are reduced in some patients, together with a decrease in immunoglobulins in some patients. Bacterial infections that occurred in these patients were not associated with neutropenia, and some were severe, involving sepsis due to *Listeria, Staphylococcus*, and polymicrobials; posttreatment infections included rare sepsis and viral infections (herpes simplex and herpes zoster). Leukopenia occurs in some patients, thrombocytopenia in some, and neutropenia in some others. Serious bone marrow suppression was uncommon and may occur up to 30 days following treatment. These include severe neutropenia, thrombocytopenia, and severe anemia.

Nursing Implications: Monitor CBC, platelets baseline and regularly during treatment. If the patient develops cytopenia, monitor more frequently. Assess for signs/symptoms of infection, bleeding, fatigue, and chest pain before each treatment. Teach patient to self-assess for these, including taking temperature, and instruct to report them immediately.

IV.   LOSS OF SKIN INTEGRITY, POTENTIAL, related to SEVERE MUCOCUTANEOUS REACTIONS, INJECTION-SITE REACTIONS

Defining Characteristics: Severe skin reactions have occurred rarely and, in some cases, were fatal. Skin abnormalities include paraneoplastic pemphigus (uncommon autoimmune disorder, which may be related to underlying malignancy), SJS (may be caused by HSV or other infectious disorder), lichenoid dermatitis, vesiculobullous dermatitis, and TEN. Onset is 1–13 weeks following rituximab exposure. Patients receiving SQ rituximab/hyaluronidase human may develop local cutaneous reactions such as pain, swelling, induration, hemorrhage, erythema, pruritus, and rash. Incidence is about 16%, and reactions were mild or moderate in clinical trials and did not require treatment.

Nursing Implications: Assess baseline skin and mucous membrane integrity. Teach patient that rarely skin and mucous membrane reactions may occur, and ask them to report any changes right away. Manufacturer recommends stopping rituximab therapy and obtaining skin biopsy to determine cause. Discuss with physician. Teach the patient local care strategies depending on symptoms. Assess for site reactions before administering SQ rituximab/hyaluronidase human, and avoid areas on the abdomen that are red, bruised, tender, or hard, or areas where there are moles or scars. Document where the drug was administered in the medical record so that an assessment can be made of any skin reaction before the next SQ injection.

V.   ALTERATION IN COMFORT related to NAUSEA, VOMITING, PYREXIA, COUGH, FATIGUE

Defining Characteristics: Incidence was ≥20% in patients with FL (nausea, constipation, cough, fatigue), DLBCL (nausea), and CLL (nausea, pyrexia, vomiting).

Nursing Implications: Assess baseline comfort before each infusion and tolerance of past infusion. Discuss strategies to manage symptoms. If symptoms are severe, discuss management with physician.

Drug: sargramostim (Leukine, GM-CSF)

Class: Cytokine (GM-CSF, granulocyte macrophage growth factor).

Mechanism of Action: GM-CSF that regulates growth of all levels of granulocytes and stimulates production of monocytes and macrophages; GM-CSF induces synthesis of other cytokines and enhances cytotoxic action. Manufactured using recombinant DNA technology.

Metabolism: Peak serum levels 2–3 hours after injection. Initial half-life 12–17 minutes, with a terminal half-life of 1.6–2.6 hours.

Indication: Patients with/undergoing (1) AML following induction chemotherapy in adults aged 55 years and older to shorten time to neutrophil recovery and to reduce incidence of severe and life-threatening infection, and infections resulting in death; (2) autologous peripheral blood progenitor cell mobilization and collection; (3) autologous peripheral blood progenitor cell bone marrow transplantation for acceleration of myeloid recovery in patients with NHL, acute lymphoblastic leukemia (ALL), and Hodgkin's disease; (4) acceleration of myeloid recovery in adult and pediatric patients aged 2 years and older undergoing allogeneic BMT from HLA-matched related donors (myeloid reconstitution after allogeneic BMT); (5) delayed neutrophil recovery or graft failure after allogeneic or autologous bone marrow transplantation in adult and pediatric patients 2 years and older; (6) acute exposure to myelosuppressive doses of radiation [Hematopoietic Syndrome of Acute Radiation Syndrome (H-ARS)].

Contraindication: In patients with (1) known hypersensitivity to GM-CSF, yeast-derived products, or any product component; (2) use cautiously, if at all, in patient with excessive leukemic myeloid blasts in the bone marrow or peripheral blood ($\geq$ 10%); (3) do not administer concomitantly with chemotherapy and/or radiotherapy.

Dosage/Range:
- *Neutrophil recovery following chemotherapy in AML:* 250 mcg/m^2/day as a 4-hour infusion, beginning approximately on day 11 or 4 days after the completion of induction chemotherapy, if the day 10 bone marrow is hypoplastic with < 5% blasts.
  - Continue therapy until ANC > 1,500 cells/mm^3 for 3 consecutive days or a maximum of 42 days.
  - Discontinue drug immediately if leukemic regrowth occurs.
  - If a severe reaction occurs, dose can be reduced by 50% or interrupted until the reaction abates.
  - To prevent excessive leukocytosis (WBC > 50,000 cells/mm^3 or ANC > 20,000 cells/mm^3) assess CBC/differential twice weekly during therapy. Drug should be interrupted or dose-reduced by half if the ANC > 20,000 cells/mm^3.
- *Mobilization of PBPC:* 250 g/m^2/day IV over 24 hours or SQ once daily. Continue same dose through the period of PBPC collection. Saragramostim dose should be reduced by 50% if WBC > 50,000 cells/mm^3.
- *PBPC transplantation:* 250 g/m^2/day IV over 24 hours or SQ once daily, beginning immediately following infusion of progenitor cells and continuing until an ANC > 1,500 cells/m^3 is attained for 3 consecutive days.

- *Myeloid reconstitution after autologous or allogeneic BMT:* 250 g/m²/day IV over 2 hours beginning 2–4 hours after bone marrow infusion, and not less than 24 hours after the last dose of chemotherapy or radiotherapy.
  - Do not give until the postmarrow infusion ANC is < 500 cells/mm³; continue sargramostim until an ANC > 1,500 cells/mm³ for 3 consecutive days occurs.
  - If a severe adverse reaction occurs, sargramostim dose can be 50% dose-reduced or interrupted until reaction abates. Discontinue the drug immediately if blast cells appear or disease progression occurs.
  - To prevent excessive leukocytosis (WBC > 50,000 cells/mm³ or ANC > 20,000 cells/mm³), assess CBC/differential twice weekly during therapy. Drug should be interrupted or dose-reduced by half if the ANC > 20,000 cells/mm³.
- *BMT or engraftment delay:* 250 g/m²/day IV over 2 hours for 14 days; dose can be repeated after 7 days off therapy if engraftment has not occurred.
  - If engraftment still has not occurred, a third course of 500 mcg/m²/day IV for 14 days may be tried after 7 days off therapy.
  - If there is still no improvement, it is unlikely that an increased dose will be successful.
  - If a severe adverse reaction occurs, sargramostim dose can be 50% dose-reduced or interrupted until reaction abates. Discontinue the drug immediately if blast cells appear or disease progression occurs.
  - To prevent excessive leukocytosis (WBC > 50,000 cells/mm³ or ANC > 20,000 cells/mm³), assess CBC/differential twice weekly during therapy. Drug should be interrupted or dose-reduced by half if the ANC > 20,000 cells/mm³.
- Acute exposure to myelosuppressive doses of radiation (H-ARS) daily subcutaneous injection:
  - 7 mcg/kg in adult and pediatric patients weighing >40 kg.
  - 10 mcg/kg in pediatric patients weighing 16–40 kg.
  - 12 mcg/kg in pediatric patients weighing <15 kg.
  - Administer sargramostim as soon as possible after suspected or confirmed exposure to radiation doses >2 gray (Gy).
  - Estimate a patient's absorbed radiation dose (i.e., level of radiation exposure) based on information from public health authorities, biodosimetry, if available, or clinical findings such as time to onset of vomiting or lymphocyte depletion kinetics (Sanofi-aventis, 2018).
  - Assess baseline cbc with differential and then serial cbcs every third day until the ANC remains >1,000/mm³ for 3 consecutive cbcs. Do not delay administration of sargramostim if a cbc is not available.
  - Continue administration of sargramostim until the ANC remains >1,000/mm³ for 3 consecutive cbcs or exceeds 10,000/mm³ after a radiation-induced nadir.

Drug Preparation:
- Sargramostim must not be administered with or within 24 hours preceeding cytotoxic chemotherapy or radiotherapy or within 24 hours following chemotherapy.
- Dosage forms and strengths:
  - For injection (lyophylized powder): 250 mcg of sargramostim in single-dose vial for reconstitutions;
  - Injection (solution): 500 mcg/mL in a multiple-dose vial.

- *Leukine injection* is preserved with benzyl alcohol as an injectable solution (500 mcg/mL) in a vial. Once entered, the vial can be stored up to 20 days at 2–8°C. Discard any remaining solution after 20 days.
- *Lyophilized Leukine* is preservative-free (250 mcg) that requires reconstitution with 1 mL sterile water for injection, USP, or 1 mL Bacteriostatic Water for Injection, USP. Do not mix the the contents of vials reconstituted with different diluents together. Use preservative-free reconstituted sargramostim for injection within 6 hours following reconstitution and/or dilution for injection. Do not reenter or reuse the vial. Neonates and infants MUST receive lyophylized solution reconstituted with Sterile Water for Injection without preservatives to avoid benzyl alcohol exposure. Bacteriostatic water containing solutions should not be used for neonates. For sargramostim that is has preservatives (benzyl alcohol), diluted drug can be stored for up to 20 days at 2–8°C once the vial has been entered; discard any remaining solution after 20 days. See package insert for reconstitution directions.
- SQ administration: do not further dilute.
- IV administration requires further dilution in 0.9% sodium chloride. If final concentration is < 10 g/mL, human albumin at a final concentration of 0.1% should be added to the saline prior to adding Leukine to prevent absorption of drug in IV container and tubing. (To obtain a final concentration of 0.1% albumin [human], add 1 mg albumin per 1 mL 0.9% sodium chloride injection USP [e.g., use 1 mL 5% albumin (human) in 50 mL 0.9% sodium chloride injection USP].)
- Do *not* use an in-line membrane filter when administering drug IV.
- Store liquid and reconstituted lyophilized Leukine under refrigeration at 2–8°C (36–46°F); do not freeze.

Drug Administration:
- Administer SQ or IV per Dosage/Range section.
- CBC twice a week during therapy; monitor renal and hepatic function in patients with baseline impairment in either system biweekly during therapy. Monitor body weight and hydration status closely during therapy.
- DO NOT administer sargramostim simultaneously with cytotoxic chemotherapy or radiotherapy, or within 24 hours preceding or following chemotherapy or radiotherapy.

Drug Interactions:
- Corticosteroids, lithium: may increase myeloproliferation.

Lab Effects/Interference:
- Increased stem cell, granulocyte, macrophage production.
- Serum glucose, BUN, cholesterol, bili, creatinine, ALT, alk phos; ↓ serum albumin, Ca.
- Leukocytosis, eosinophilia.

Special Considerations:
- Produces fever more commonly than G-CSF.
- Warnings and Precautions:
  - *HSRs:* serious HSRs including anaphylaxis have been reported. When sargramostim is administered IV, appropriate trained personnel and emergency equipment should

be close by. If a serious allergic or anaphylactic reaction occurs, immediately discontinue the drug and institute emergency medical intervention as ordered, as well as ABCs of resuscitation. Discontinue drug permanently in these patients.

- *IRRs:* may occur, characterized by respiratory distress, hypoxia, flushing, hypotension, syncope, and/or tachycardia after first dose of sargramostim in a particular cycle. These symptoms usually resolve, and do not recur in subsequent doses in the same cycle of treatment. Monitor patient closely for symptoms, especially patients with preexisting lung disease. If patients have dyspnea or other acute symptoms, reduce the rate of infusion by 50% as ordered. If symptoms persist or worsen despite rate reduction, discontinue infusion as ordered.

- *Risk of severe myelosuppression when sargramostim administered within 24 hours of chemotherapy or radiotherapy.* Do not administer sargramostim simultaneously with or within 24 hours preceding cytotoxic chemotherapy or radiotherapy or within 24 hours after chemotherapy. See package insert.

- *Effusions and Capillary Leak Syndrome (CLS):* Edema, CLS, pleural and/or pericardial effusion have been described. Usually these are reversible after drug interruption or dose reduction with or without diuretic therapy. Use drug cautiously in patients with preexisting fluid retention, pulmonary infiltrates, or CHF, and monitor patient closely. Assess patient closely during and immediately after infusions, especially in patients with preexisting lung disease. Monitor and document body weight and hydration status carefully during sargramostim administration.

- *Supraventricular arrhythmias:* may occur, especially in patients with previous history of cardiac arrhythmias. These are reversible when sargramostim is discontinued. Use drug cautiously in patients with preexisting cardiac disease.

- *Leukocytosis:* wbc $\geq$ 50,000/mm^3 may occur. Monitor CBC/ANC twice a week; base decision whether to dose reduce or interrupt treatment as ordered based on patient's clinical condition. Once sargramostim discontinued, excessive blood counts returned to normal within 3–7 days.

- *Potential effect on malignant cells:* It is possible that drug can act as a growth factor for any tumor type, particularly myeloid malignancies. Use drug cautiously in patients with myeloid malignant characteristics. Discontinue sargramostim if disease progression occurs during sargramostim administration.

- *Immunogenicity:* Sargramostim treatment may result in neutralizing antidrug antibody formation. In a study of patients receiving the drug for 12 months, 82.9% developed antisargramostim neutralizing antibodies with loss of efficacy of drug. Use sargramostim for the shortest time possible.

- *Risk of serious adverse reactions in infants due to benzyl alcohol preservative:* Use only preservative free solution for neonates and low birth-weight infants. Gasping syndrome is a potentially serious and fatal reaction, characterized by CNS depression, metabolic acidosis and gasping respirations.

- *Respiratory symptoms:* Sequestration of granulocytes in pulmonary circulation has occurred, resulting in dyspnea. If patient develops dyspnea during the infusion, slow infusion rate by 50%; if respiratory symptoms worsen despite slowing infusion, discontinue drug. Subsequent infusions can be given per standard dose schedule with careful monitoring. Use cautiously and monitor closely hypoxic patients.

- *Cardiovascular symptoms:* Occasional supraventricular arrhythmia has occurred, especially in patients with a history of arrhythmias. This is reversible after drug discontinuation.
- *Renal and hepatic dysfunction:* Monitor lab values baseline and during treatment.
- Stop drug when WBC > 50,000 cells/mm^3, ANC > 20,000 cells/mm^3, or platelets > 500,000 cells/mm^3.
- Administer > 24 hours after last chemotherapy (usually 4 days following completion of induction chemotherapy).
- Drug should be administered to pregnant women or nursing mothers only if clearly needed.

Potential Toxicities/Side Effects (Dose- and Schedule-Dependent) and the Nursing Process

I.   ALTERATION IN COMFORT related to FLU-LIKE SYNDROME

Defining Characteristics: Fever, myalgias, chills, rigors, fatigue, and headache may occur.

Nursing Implications: Assess baseline T, VS, neurologic status, and comfort level, and monitor q 4–6 hours if patient in hospital. Discuss with physician premedication and regular dosing of antipyretic (e.g., acetaminophen ± diphenhydramine, NSAID). Teach patient self-care measures, including monitoring temperature, comfort level, self-administration of prescribed medications prior to dose and regularly postdose, as well as the use of heat or cold for myalgias, arthralgias. Encourage patient to increase oral fluids and alternate rest and activity periods. If patient is in hospital and experiences rigor, discuss with physician IV meperidine (25 mg IV every 15 minutes to maximum 100 mg in 1 hour) and monitor blood pressure for hypotension.

II.   ALTERATION IN COMFORT related to SKELETAL PAIN

Defining Characteristics: Transient skeletal pain may occur and is believed to be due to bone marrow expansion in response to GM-CSF.

Nursing Implications: Teach patient this may occur and discuss use of NSAIDs with patient and physician for symptom management. Monitor WBC, absolute neutrophil count (ANC) twice weekly during therapy; dose reduction or discontinuation depends on purpose of drug.

III.   POTENTIAL ALTERATION IN SKIN INTEGRITY related to RASH, FLUSHING, INJECTION-SITE REACTION

Defining Characteristics: Facial flushing, generalized rash, and inflammation at injection site may occur.

Nursing Implications: Teach patient that these may occur, and instruct to report rash, inflammation. Teach patient to rotate injection sites. Assess rash, and teach symptomatic management.

IV. POTENTIAL ALTERATION IN OXYGENATION related to DYSPNEA AND FLUID RETENTION

Defining Characteristics: Some patients developed dyspnea during initial 2–6 hours of continuous infusion GM-CSF, thought to be due to migration of neutrophils in the lung. Fluid retention may also occur.

Nursing Implications: Assess baseline pulmonary and fluid status. Teach patient to monitor weight daily and instruct to report any changes in weight, breathing (e.g., dyspnea).

Drug: siltuximab (Sylvant®)

Class: Interleukin-6 (IL-6) antagonist, chimeric mAb.

Mechanism of Action: Drug is a chimeric mAb that binds human Interleukin-6 (IL-6), thus preventing IL-6 from binding to its IL-6 receptors. IL-6 is a cytokine produced by various cells (e.g., T- and B-lymphocytes, monocytes, fibroblasts, endothelial cells). IL-6 normally induces immunoglobulin secretion. A dysregulated, overproduction of IL-6 from activated B-lymphocytes in affected lymph nodes is believed to cause multicentric Castleman's disease (MCD) with its systemic manifestations (e.g., enlarged lymph nodes, fever, weakness, fatigue, night sweats, weight loss, nausea, vomiting, loss of appetite, nerve damage, and increased risk of infection). Treatment with siltuximab in a clinical trial resulted in significant tumor and symptomatic responses (Wong et al., 2013).

Metabolism: Following IV administration, C_{max} occurred near the end of the infusion. With every 3-week dosing, steady state is reached by the 6th infusion. Mean terminal half-life ($t_{1/2}$) after the first infusion is 20.6 days (range 14.2–29.7 days). There was no difference in clearance in patients with preexisting mild, moderate, and severe renal impairment compared to normal patients, nor any difference in patients with mild or moderate hepatic impairment compared to patients with normal hepatic function. Patients with end-stage renal disease or severe hepatic dysfunction (Child-Pugh Class C) were not studied.

Indication: Drug approved for the treatment of patients with multicentric Castleman's disease (MCD) who are human deficiency virus- (HIV-) negative and human herpes virus-8- (HHV-8-) negative.

- MCD, a rare blood disorder similar to lymphoma, affects about 1,100–1,300 Americans. It is a serious, chronic disease characterized by an abnormal overgrowth of lymphocytes in lymph nodes and in lymphoid tissue such as the liver and spleen, which become enlarged. The cause is unknown, but it is associated with an overproduction of IL-6. Disease symptoms include fever, night sweats, weight loss, weakness, fatigue, and a weakened immune system leading to infection. Infection, multi-organ system failure, and malignancies, including malignant lymphoma, are common causes of death in MCD.
- Drug has not been studied in patients who are HIV-positive or HHV-8 positive because drug does not bind to virally produced IL-6 in a nonclinical study.

- MCD2001 was the clinical trial leading to FDA priority review and approval, which showed that of 79 patients with symptomatic MCD randomized to BSC alone or the combination BSC/siltuximab, 34% of patients receiving the combination had a durable tumor and symptomatic response persisting for a minimum of 18 weeks without treatment failure, compared to zero in the BSC arm ($p = 0.0012$). Sixty-one percent of anemic patients had an increase in hemoglobin of 1.5 g/dL in the combination group vs zero in the BSC group ($p < 0.05$).
- **Contraindication:** patients having a severe HSR to the drug or its excipients.

Dosage/Range:
- 11 mg/kg administered as a 1 hr IV infusion every 3 weeks, until treatment failure.
- Assess CBC/differential, platelet count prior to each dose for the first 12 months, then every 3 cycles theraefter.
- Prior to first siltuximab dose, labs must be: ANC $\geq 1.0 \times 10^9$/L, platelet count $\geq 75 \times 10^9$/L, Hgb < 17 g/dL.
- Prior to subsequent siltuximab doses, labs must be: ANC $\geq 1.0 \times 10^9$/L, platelet count $\geq 50 \times 10^9$/L, Hgb < 17 g/dL.
- DO NOT administer drug to patients with severe infections until the infection resolves.
- Discontinue drug in patients with severe infusion-related reactions, anaphylaxis, severe allergic reactions, or CRSs. Do not reinstitute treatment in patients who have had a severe HSR to siltuximab or any of its excipients.

Drug Preparation:
- Available in 100 and 400 mg of lyophilized powder in single-use vials. Obtain 250-mL infusion bags of 5% dextrose in water, made of PVC with Di (2-ethylhexyl), phthalate (DEHP), or Polyolefin (PO), as well as IV administration sets lined with PVC with DEHP or polyurethane (PU), containing a 0.2 micron in-line polyethersulfone (PES) filter.
- Calculate dosage required, total volume or reconstituted drug needed, and number of vials.
- Using a 21-gauge 1-1/2 inch needle, aseptically add 5.2 mL sterile water for injection, USP, to the 100-mg vial, or 20 mL of sterile water for injection, USP, to the 400-mg vial. Each vial will have a concentration of 20 mg/mL. Gently swirl the reconstituted vials until completely dissolved; DO NOT shake or swirl vigorously. Dissolving the lyophilized powder should take < 60 minutes.
- Once reconstituted and prior to further dilution, inspect for particulate matter and discoloration, and do not use if found or if visibly opaque. Further dilute into the infusion bag within 2 hours.
- Aseptically remove the calculated dose volume (that will be added) from a 250-mL bag of sterile dextrose 5% in water that is made of PVC with DEHP or PO; then slowly add the total calculated volume for the ordered dose of reconstituted siltuximab to the 5% dextrose in water infusion bag. Gently invert to mix.
- Drug will be administered by IV infusion over 1 hour, completed within 4 hours of dilution of the reconstituted solution to the infusion bag.
- Reconstituted drug does not contain preservatives, so any unused portion should be disposed of as hazardous waste.

Drug Administration:
- Assess CBC/ANC prior to each treatment for the first 12 months, then every 3 dosing cycles.
  - Prior to initial drug dose: ANC must be $\geq 1.0 \times 10^9/L$, platelet count $\geq 75 \times 10^9/L$, and Hgb < 17 g/dL.
  - Prior to subsequent doses: ANC must be $\geq 1.0 \times 10^9/L$, platelet count $\geq 50 \times 10^9/L$, and Hgb < 17 g/dL.
  - If lab parameters are not met, delay dose but do not reduce dose.
- Assess for signs/symptoms of infection; drug should not be given if patient has had a severe IRR, anaphylaxis, severe allergic reactions or CRS previously.
- Drug must be diluted in 250-mL infusion bags of 5% dextrose in water made of PVC with Di2-ethylhexyl phthalate (DEHP) or Polyolefin (PO), and administered by IV administration sets lined with PVC with DEHP or polyurethane (PU), containing a 0.2 micron in-line polyethersulfone (PES) filter.
- Administer by IV infusion over 1 hour; infusion must be completed within 4 hours of the time the reconstituted solution was placed into the infusion bag.
- Do not infuse concomitantly with other drugs in the same IV line.
- Stop the infusion if the patient has an infusion reaction. Ensure that the infusion setting has resuscitation equipment, emergency medications, and personnel trained in emergency resuscitation.
  - Mild to moderate reaction: if the reaction resolves, may restart drug at a lower infusion rate per MD or NP/PA; consider premedication with antihistamines, acetaminophen, and corticosteroids. Discontinue drug if the patient does not tolerate the infusion with these interventions.
  - Anaphylaxis: stop the infusion, provide immediate medical intervention, and discontinue siltuximab.

Drug Interactions:
- Cytochrome P450 substrates: infection and inflammation, and cytokines (e.g., IL-6) down regulate cytochrome P450 enzymes in the liver. When IL-6 is inhibited, this may restore CYP450 enzyme activity to higher levels leading to increased metabolism of CYP450 substrates (drugs that are metabolized by CYP450 enzymes). When starting or stopping siltuximab for patients being treated with CYP450 substrates with a narrow therapeutic index, perform therapeutic monitoring of effect (e.g., warfarin or drug concentration such as cyclosporine or theophylline), and adjust dose as needed. The effect of siltuximab on CYP450 enzyme activity can persist for several weeks after stopping siltuximab.
- CYP3A4 substrates (e.g., oral contraceptives, lovastatin, atorvastatin): exercise caution when coadministering, as a decrease in effectiveness may occur and is undesirable.

Lab Effects/Interference:
- Decreased C-reactive protein (CRP), platelet count.
- Hypertriglyceridemia, hypercholesteremia, hyperuricemia.

Special Considerations:
- The most common adverse effects ($> 10\%$) were pruritus, increased weight, rash, hyperuricemia, URI.

- Warnings and Precautions:
  - *Concurrent acute severe infections: Do not administer drug to patients with severe infections* until the infection has resolved. Drug may mask signs and symptoms of acute inflammation including suppression of fever, and acute phase reactants such as CRP. Monitor patients receiving siltuximab closely for infections, stop drug, and promptly treat with anti-infective therapy.
  - *Vaccinations: Do not administer live vaccines* because inhibition of IL-6 may interfere with the normal immune response to new antigens.
  - *Infusion related reactions (IRRs) or HSRs:* While uncommon, anaphylaxis has occurred. Incidence of IRRs is 5.1–6.3%, with 1.3% severe reactions; none were fatal. Symptoms included back pain, chest pain, or discomfort, nausea, vomiting, flushing, erythema, and palpitations. Clinical area where drug is administered must have emergency resuscitation equipment and trained personel.
    - Anaphylaxis: stop infusion immediately, change to plain IV solution so remaining drug in tubing does not infuse; manage ABCs and implement ordered emergency plan as ordered. Drug should be permanently discontinued.
    - Mild to moderate IRR: Stop infusion, and if reaction resolves, restart at a lower infusion rate as ordered; discuss premedication with antihistamines, acetaminophen, and corticosteroids. Discontinue drug if patient does not tolerate the infusion despite these changes.
  - *GI perforation:* reported in clinical trials, though not MCD trials. Use drug cautiously in patients at risk for GI perforation. Patients presenting with symptoms suggestive of GI perforation should be evaluated immediately.
- Infants born to pregnant women treated with siltuximab may be at increased risk of infection; caution is advised in the administration of live vaccines to these infants. Drug should be used during pregnancy only if the potential benefit justifies the potential risk to the fetus. Advise patients of childbearing potential to avoid pregnancy, using contraception during and for 3 months after treatment ends.
- Nursing mothers: a decision should be made whether to discontinue nursing or to discontinue the drug, taking into account the importance of the drug to the mother's health.

Potential Toxicities/Side Effects and the Nursing Process

I.   POTENTIAL FOR INJURY related to HYPERSENSITIVITY/ANAPHYLAXIS and INFUSION REACTION

Defining Characteristics: Infusion reactions were reported in 4.8% of patients; symptoms were back pain, chest pain or discomfort, nausea, vomiting, flushing, erythema, and palpitations. Anaphylaxis occurred in one patient of the approximately 750 patients treated with siltuximab.

Nursing Implications: Ensure resuscitation equipment, emergency medicines, and oxygen are located in the infusion area. Assess baseline VS and mental status prior to drug administration, at 15 minutes, and periodically during infusion, as needed. Remain with patient during first 15 minutes of first infusions. Recall signs/symptoms of anaphylaxis; if these occur, stop drug immediately, notify physician, and assess patient's vital signs. Subjective symptoms are generalized itching, nausea, chest tightness, crampy abdominal pain, difficulty speaking, anxiety, agitation, sense of impending doom, uneasiness, desire to urinate/defecate, dizziness, and chills. Objective signs are flushed appearance; angioedema of face, neck, eyelids, hands, and feet; localized or generalized urticaria; respiratory distress with or without wheezing; hypotension; and cyanosis. Review standing physician orders or nursing procedures for patient management of anaphylaxis, and be prepared to stop drug immediately and change IV to a plain NS solution to keep vein patent, notify physician or NP/PA, keep airway patent, monitor VS, and administer ordered medications, which may include epinephrine 1:1,000 IM in the thigh, IV hydrocortisone sodium succinate, and IV diphenhydramine. Teach patient to report any unusual symptoms. Stop infusion if a reaction occurs. For mild-to-moderate infusion reactions (grades 1–2), the drug maybe resumed at a decreased infusion rate per MD or NP/PA; also, consider premedication with an antihistamine, acetaminophen, and a corticosteroid for subsequent treatments. Drug should be discontinued in patients who experience anaphylaxis.

II. POTENTIAL ALTERATION IN SKIN INTEGRITY related to RASH, PRURITUS, EDEMA

Defining Characteristics: Rash and pruritus each affected 28% of patients during the initial 8 infusions. Edema was reported in 26%.

Nursing Implications: Assess baseline skin integrity, and teach patient that rash, pruritus, and edema may occur, and to report it. If it occurs, assess need for intervention and discuss with MD or NP/PA if it persists or worsens.

Drug: sipuleucel-T (Provenge)

Class: Autologous cellular immunotherapy agent.

Mechanism of Action: Sipuleucel-T induces an immune response in the patient directed against PAP, an antigen expressed in most prostate cancers. In the laboratory, the patient's APCs are cultured with PSP-GM-CSF so that the APCs can take up and process the recombinant target antigen into small peptides that are then displayed on the APC surface. These pieces of the tumor antigen can then be recognized by the patient's immune system by T-lymphocytes and NK cells, which will then seek and destroy the prostate cancer cells.

Metabolism: Unknown. Neutralizing antibodies to GM-CSF were transient.

Indication: Drug is FDA-approved for the treatment of asymptomatic or minimally symptomatic metastatic castrate-resistant (hormone refractory) prostate cancer.

Dosage/Range: Recommended course is 3 complete doses at 2-week intervals.
• Each dose of sipuleucel-T contains a minimum of 50 million autologous CD54+ (APCs that carry a piece of the patient's prostate cancer [antigen] to present to the immune system

to stimulate it to attack the patient's prostate cancer cells), activated with PAP-GM-CSF, suspended in 250 mL of lactated Ringer's injection, USP, in a sealed, patient-specific infusion bag. The bag may also contain other immune cells that have been leukophoresed.
- Each infusion is preceded by a leukapheresis procedure approximately 3 days prior.

Drug Preparation:
- Drug is shipped directly to the patient's physician, who will infuse the drug.
- Sipuleucel-T will arrive in a cardboard shipping box with the drug inside a special insulated polyurethane container. Verify the product and patient-specific label on the top of the insulated container. Do NOT remove the container from the box or open the lid until the patient is ready to receive the infusion.
- Do NOT infuse the drug until confirmation of product release has been received from Dendreon, the manufacturer. They will send a Cell Product Disposition Form containing patient identifiers, expiration date and time, and the disposition status (approved for infusion or rejected) to the infusion site.
- Infusion must begin prior to the expiration date and time indicated on the Cell Product Disposition Form and product label. DO NOT initiate infusion of expired drug. Once the infusion bag is removed from the insulated container, it should remain at room temperature for no more than 3 hours. DO NOT return the infusion bag to the shipping container.
- Once the patient is prepared for infusion, and the Cell Product Disposition Form and product label have been received, remove the sipuleucel-T infusion bag from the insulated container and inspect for signs of leakage. Contents will be clear to opaque, with a white to red color, including shades of off-white, cream, light yellow, and orange. Gently mix and resuspend the contents of the bag, inspecting for clumps and clots, which can be gently dispersed by manual mixing. DO NOT administer if the bag leaks or if clumps remain in the bag.
- Prior to the infusion, match the patient's identity with the patient identifiers on the Cell Product Disposition Form and the infusion bag.
- Sipuleucel-T is to be used for autologous use only.
- Sipuleucel-T should be used with caution in patients with risk factors for thromboembolic events.
- Sipuleucel-T is not routinely tested for transmission of infectious diseases and may transmit disease to healthcare professionals. Use universal precautions.

Drug Administration:
- Confirm patient identity (must be same patient leukophoresed that is receiving the drug).
- Inspect the infusion bag; do not administer if there are leaks or clumps that cannot be dissolved.
- Check that the infusion time is prior to the expiration date and time on the Cell Product Disposition Form and product label. Do not use expired sipuleucel-T.
- Administer premedication (acetaminophen and antihistamine such as diphenhydramine).
- Do NOT use a cell filter, and infuse over 60 minutes.
- If the patient has an acute infusion reaction, interrupt or slow the infusion depending upon severity, and discuss further management with physician/NP/PA. If the infusion is interrupted, and then is reinitiated, make sure that the infusion bag has not been standing at room temperature for more than 3 hours. Syncope and hypotension have also been

observed. Closely monitor patient, especially those patients with cardiac or pulmonary conditions.
- Observe the patient for 30 minutes after completion of the infusion.

Drug Interactions:
- Unknown, as no studies have been performed.
- Concomitant use of chemotherapy and immunosuppressive medications with sipuleucel-T has not been studied.

Lab Effects/Interference:
- Anemia.

Special Considerations:
- Drug is indicated solely for AUTOLOGOUS use.
- Warnings and Precautions:
  - *Acute infusion reactions* have been observed (within 1 day of infusion). Symptom constellation may include nausea, vomiting, fatigue, fever, rigors, chills, respiratory events (dyspnea, hypoxia, bronchospasm), syncope, hypotension, HTN and tachycardia. In contolled clinical trials, 71.2% of patients had an acute IRR, most often characterized by chills, fever, and fatigue; 95% had mild or moderate reaction. This may require stopping the infusion or slowing it down, depending upon the severity of the reaction. Closely monitor patients with preexisting cardiac or pulmonary problems.
  - *Thromboembolic events:* including DVT and PE, may occur. Use drug cautiously in patients with risk factors for thromboembolic events.
  - *Vascular disorders:* CVA and TIA have been observed rarely following drug administration MI was also seen, although it is not clear if related to drug infusion; (a) cerebrovascular disease: incidence was 3.5% in the Provenge group compared to 2.6% in the control group. Monitor patients closely who have risk factors; (b) cardiovascular disorders: incidence of MI was 0.8% in the Provenge group versus 0.3% in the control group. In postmarketing reports, postinfusion MI has occurred; monitor patients with risk factors closely during and after the infusion.
  - *Potential transmission of infectious diseases:* Use universal precautions when handling the drug. Sipuleucel-T is not routinely tested for transmissible infectious diseases and may transmit disease to healthcare providers handling the product.
  - *Concomitant use of chemotherapy and immunosuppressive medications* with sipuleucel-T have not been studied and is not recommended.
  - *Product safety testing:* The drug is released once testing for microbial and sterility has been successful. The final 7-day incubation sterility tests are not available when the infusion occurs. If the results become positive after the drug has been approved for administration, Dendreon will contact the treating physician.
- In two clinical studies, patients receiving sipuleucel-T had significantly longer overall survival (25.8/25.9 months vs. 21.7/21.4 months, $p = 0.032, p = 0.010$).
- The most common side effects are chills, fatigue, fever, back pain, nausea, joint ache, and headache. Suspected adverse reactions can be reported to the FDA at www.fda.gov /medwatch.

- Severe adverse events were reported in 24% of patients, compared to 25% in the control group. These included infusion reactions, cerebrovascular events, and single-case reports of eosinophilia, rhabdomyolysis, myasthenia gravis, myositis, and tumor flare.
- Side effects of leukophoresis 3 days prior to the therapy included citrate toxicity (14%), oral paresthesia (12%), paresthesia (11%), and fatigue (8%).

Potential Toxicities/Side Effects and the Nursing Process

I.   POTENTIAL FOR INJURY related to HYPERSENSITIVITY AND INFUSION REACTION

Defining Characteristics: Sipuleucel-T can cause acute infusion reactions within 1 day of infusion. In clinical trials, the incidence was 71%, and of these, 95% were mild or moderate, characterized by chills, fever, and fatigue that resolved within 2 days. Severe or grade 3 reactions occurred in 3.5% of patients and included chills, fever, fatigue, asthenia, dyspnea, hypoxia, bronchospasm, dizziness, headache, HTN, muscle ache, nausea, and vomiting. The incidence of severe reactions was greatest after the second infusion (2.1%) compared to infusion 1 (0.8%). Rarely patients were admitted for management of acute infusion reactions. There were no grade 4 or 5 reactions.

Nursing Implications: Ensure patient identifiers are closely checked. Ensure patient receives premedication with acetaminophen, diphenhydramine, or equivalent. Begin infusion slowly; then speed up to complete within 1 hour. Closely monitor patients with cardiac or pulmonary conditions. Have physician or NP nearby in case of reaction. Recall signs/symptoms of anaphylaxis/infusion reaction, and if these occur, stop drug immediately, notify physician, and assess patient's vital signs. Subjective symptoms are generalized itching, nausea, chest tightness, crampy abdominal pain, difficulty speaking, anxiety, agitation, sense of impending doom, uneasiness, desire to urinate/defecate, dizziness, and chills. Objective signs are flushed appearance; angioedema of face, neck, eyelids, hands, and feet; localized or generalized urticaria; respiratory distress with or without wheezing; hypotension; and cyanosis. Review standing orders or nursing procedures for patient management of anaphylaxis and be prepared to stop drug immediately, notify physician, monitor VS, and administer ordered medications, which may include epinephrine 1:1,000, hydrocortisone sodium succinate, oxygen, and diphenhydramine. Teach patient to report any unusual symptoms. If the patient develops an acute infusion reaction, if severe, stop the reaction; if mild or moderate, discuss with physician or nurse practitioner whether the infusion should be slowed down or interrupted. If severe, institute medical management urgently, such as for angina or other signs/symptoms of myocardial insufficiency. Teach patient to report any signs and symptoms of infusion reaction within 24 hours of the infusion (e.g., fever, chills, rash, breathing problems).

II.   ALTERATION IN COMFORT related to CHILLS, FATIGUE, FEVER, BACK PAIN, NAUSEA, JOINT ACHE, HEADACHE

Defining Characteristics: In clinical trials there were chills (53%), fatigue (41%), fever (31%), back pain (29%), nausea (21%), joint ache (19%), headache (18%). Most patients have one or more of these side effects, and in 67% of patients, they are mild or moderate. Back pain and chills were severe in about 2% of patients.

Nursing Implications: Assess baseline comfort level and teach patient that these side effects may occur. Teach self-management for comfort and teach patient to call if symptomatic treatment does not resolve issue in 1–2 days. Discuss with physician or nurse practitioner prescription medication to improve comfort for symptoms that do not respond to conservative management.

Drug: tagraxofusp-erzs (Elzonris™)

Class: C123 –directed cytotoxin composed of recombinant human interleukin-3 (IL-3) and truncated diphtheria toxic (DT) fusion protein.

Mechanism of Action: The cytotoxin is directed by the attached IL-3 to cells containing CD123 on the membrane, and brings the fusion protein DT into the cell, where it causes cell death. Blastic plasmacytoid dendritic cell neoplasm (BPDCN) has CD123 overexpressed on its cell membrane, although it is a rare malignancy with an incidence of 1% or less of the U.S. population. It is highly lethal, unless HSCT is performed. The bone marrow is the primary site of involvement, followed by skin, heart, mediastinum and pleura (Alsidawi et al., 2016). While CD123 appears on the cell membranes of hematopoietic progenitor cells, is overexpressed on the cell membranes of other hematologic malignancies including AML, B-ALL, and Hairy cell leukemia (Testa et al., 2014).

Indication: Treatment of BPDCN in adults and pediatric patients 2 years and older.

Contraindication: None.

Dosage/Range: 12 mcg/kg IV over 15 minutes once daily on days 1–5 of a 21-day cycle. Dosing period may be extended for dose delays up to day 10 of the cycle. Continue treatment until disease progression or unacceptable toxicity. Requires premedication (see Drug Administration). Cycle 1 should be administered in the inpatient setting with at least 24 hours of observation after drug administration, in a setting skilled in treatment of leukemic patients. Subsequent cycles can be administered in inpatient or outpatient settings that are equipped with appropriate monitoring for leukemic patients receiving treatment. Patients should be observed for at least 4 hours after ever infusion. Drug can cause capillary leak syndrome (CLS) which can be fatal if not properly managed.

Dose Modification (prior to preparing each drug dose):
- Serum albumin:
  - Prior to 1st dose of tagraxofusp-erzs in Cycle 1: if serum albumin < 3.2 g/dL, administer tagraxofusp-erzs when serum albumin is ≥3.2 g/dL.
  - During tagraxofusp-erzs therapy:
    - (1) if serum albumin is < 3.5 g/dL or is reduced ≥ 0.5 g/dL from the serum albumin value measured prior to initiation of the current cycle: (a) interrupt tagraxofusp-erzs; (b) administer 25 g IV albumin (q 12 hours or more frequently

as practical, until serum albumin is ≥3.5 g/dL AND not more than 0.5 g/dL lower than the value measured prior to dosing initiation of the current cycle.

- (2) a predose body weight is increased by ≥ 1.5 kg over the previous day's predose weight (a) interrupt tagraxofusp-erzs; (b) administer 25 g IV albumin (q 12 hours or more frequently as practical, (b) manage fluid status as clinically indicated (e.g., IV fluids and vasopressors if hypotensive and with diuretics if normotensive or hypertensive) until body weight increase has resolved (e.g., increase is no longer ≥ 1.5 kg > previous day's predose weight).
- (3) Edema,fluid overload and/or hypotension: (a) interrupt tagraxofusp-erzs; (b) administer 25 g IV albumin (q 12 hours or more frequently as practical, until serum albumin is ≥3.5 g/dL; (b) Administer methylprednisolone 1 mg/kg (or equivalent) per day until resolution of CLS signs/symptoms or as clinically indicated; (c) aggressive management of fluid status and hypotension if present (e.g., including IV fluids, diuretics or other blood pressure management) until resolution of CLS signs/symptoms or as clinically indicated.
- Elevated AST or ALT > 5 × ULN: Hold tagraxofusp-erzs until transaminases are ≤ 2.5 × ULN.
- Serum creatinine > 1.8 mg/dL (159 micromol/L) or ceatinine clearance ≤ 60 mL/min: Hold tagraxofusp-erzs until serum creatinine resolves to ≤ 1.8 mg/dL or creatinine clearance ≥ 560 mg/mL.
- SBP ≥ 160 mm Hg or ≤ 80 mm Hg: Hold tagraxofusp-erzs until SBP <160 mm Hg or >80 mm Hg.
- HR ≥ 130 bpm or ≤ 40 bpmL: Hold tagraxofusp-erzs until HR is < 130 bpm, or >40 bpm.
- Body temperature ≥ 38°C: Hold tagraxofusp-erzs until body temperature is <38°C.
- HSR: (a) mild or moderate: Hold tagraxofusp-erzs until resolution of mild/moderate signs/symptom; resume at the same infusion rate; (b) severe or life-threatening: Permanently discontinue tagraxofusp-erzs.

Drug Preparation:

- Available as an injection of 1000 mcg in 1 mL clear colorless solution in a single-dose vial. Drug vial is stored in the freezer between –25°C and –15°C (–13°F to 5°F). Protect drug vial from light by storing in original package until time of use. Thaw vials at room termperature between 15°C and 25°C (59°F and 77°F) prior to preparation.
- See Elzonris package insert for preparation for administration
- Administer tagraxofusp-erzs within 4 hours of preparation. Prepared drug should remain at room temperature for up to 4 hours after preparation..

Drug Administration:

- Assess patient laboratory results: CBC/differential, serum albumin, creatinine, glucose, LFTs and electrolytes. Assess patient baseline weight and on each treatment day; auscultate breath sounds, heart rate, O_2 saturation, and BP baseline and vital signs during treatment. Verify negative pregnancy test within 7 days of treatment date in females of reproductive potential.

- Drug may cause capillary leak syndrome (SLS). Assesses patient tolerance of prior therapy, and signs/symptoms of CLS: weight gain, hypotension and presence of edema. Monitor this through subsequent treatment cycles. See Dose Modifications.
- Before first dose of tagraxofusp-erzs, ensure that serum albumin is ≥ 3.2 g/dL before administering the drug.
- Establish venous access and maintain IV with 9% Sodium Chloride Injection USP.
- Administer cycle 1 infusion in an inpatient setting skilled in the care of leukemic patients, undergoing treatment, and the patient should receive 24 hours monitoring after the infusion; subsequent cycles can be administered inpatient or as an outpatient equipeed with appropriate monitoring for patients with hematopoietic malignancies, and be monitored for at least 4 hours after each dose.
- Premedicate approximately 1 hour before each tagraxofusp-erzs infusion, with an H1-histamine antagonist (e.g., diphenhydramine HCl), H-2 histamine antagonist (e.g., ranitidine), corticosteroid (e.g., 50 mg IV methylprednisolone or equivalent), acetaminophen or equivalent.
- Administer tagraxofusp-erzs and a saline flush by an infusion syringe pump over 15 minutes (see package insert).
- During and after infusion, assess for signs/symptoms of CLS, infusion reaction and hypersensitivity to drureaction; see Dosage Modifications.
- Teach patients that neutropenia, anemia, and thrombocytopenia may occur. Teach patient to self-assess for infection and bleeding, and to report this ASAP. Teach patients measures to reduce the risk of infection and bleeding, and systematic oral cleansing of the mouth to minimize infection if stomatitis develops.
- Teach female patients drug is feto-toxic, and that the patient should use effective contraception during therapy and for at least 1 week after the last drug dose. Women should not breastfeed while receiving the drug and for at least 1 week after the last dose.

Drug Interactions: Unknown.

Lab Effects/Interference:
- Decreased platelets, hemoglobin, neutrophils.
- Increased serum glucose, ALT, AST, creatinine, alkaline phosphatase, potassium, bilirubin, magnesium, sodium.
- Decreased serum albumin, calcium, sodium, potassium, phosphate, magnesium, glucose.

Special Considerations:
- Most common adverse effects (≥30%) in clinical trials were: CLS, nausea, fatigue, peripheral edema, pyrexia, weight increase. Most common laboratory abnormalities (incidence ≥50%) were decreases in serum albumin, platelets, Hgb, calcium, sodium, and increases in glucose, ALT, and AST.
- Patient at risk for bleeding, infection and fatigue. Platelets were decreased in 67% of patients (grade 3–4, 53%), decreased Hgb (60%, grade 3–4, 35%), and neutrophils decreased in 37% (grade 3–4, 31%). Febrile neutropenia occurred in 20% of patients, pyrexia 43%. Monitor CBC/differential, and teach patients self-assessment and to report any signs/symptoms of infection or bleeding.

- Antibodies to the drug may occur (see package insert).
- Warnings and Precautions:
  - *CLS:* CLS can be life-threatening and fatal, so patient requires careful and ongoing assessment to identify early risk factors and intervene promptly. Incidence in clinical trials was 55% (grade 1–2 in 46% of patients and grade 3 in 6% and grade 4 in 1% and grade 5, 2% (2 patients died). Common signs and symptoms occurring ≥20% were hypoalbuminemia, edema, weight gain, and hypotension. Before starting tagraxofusp-erzs, (1) ensure patient has a serum albumin of ≥ 3.2 g/dL and adequate cardiac function; (2) during treatment monitor serum albumin levels prior to starting each subsequent dose, and as clinically indicated; (3) assess patients before each treatment and afterwards for signs or symptoms of CLS, including weight gain, new onset or worsening edema, including pulmonary edema, or hymodynamic instability.
- *Hypersensitivity (HSR):* Incidence of HSRs in clinical trials was 46%, with 10% grade 3. Reported signs/symptoms (≥5% incidence were rash, pruritis, stomatitis, and wheezing. Monitor patients for HSE during the infusion. Interrupt infusion and provide supportive care as ordered, including maintaining an IV with plain solution (e.g., 0.9% Sodium Chloride USP), monitoring VS/oxygen saturation frequently, and discussing management with provider promptly.
- *Hepatotoxicity:* In clinical trials, 88% of patients had increases in LFTs, including grade 1–2 in 48% of patients, grade 3 in 36%, and grade 4 in 4%. Monitor ALT and AST baseline and prior to each drug infusion. Temporarily hold tagraxofusp-erzs if transaminases rise to >5 × ULN and resume treatment when transaminases normalize or abnormality resolves.

Potential Toxicities/Side Effects and the Nursing Process

I. POTENTIAL FOR INJURY related to HYPERSENSITIVITY AND INFUSION REACTION

Defining Characteristics: HSR occurred in 46% of patients in clinical trials, and were grade 3 or higher in 10%.,

Nursing Implications: Ensure patient identifiers are closely checked. Ensure patient receives premedication with acetaminophen, diphenhydramine, or equivalent, and ranitidine or equivalent. Keep IV patent with 0.9% Sodium Chloride USP. Infuse drug over 15 minutes, then follow with saline flush. Closely monitor patients, especially those with cardiac or pulmonary conditions. Have physician or NP nearby in case of reaction. If patient has signs/symptoms of a reaction (e.g., rash, pruritis, stomatitis, or wheezing) stop drug immediately and replace IV line with 0.9% Sodium Chloride USP (so no further drug infuses in IV tubing). with Recall signs/symptoms of anaphylaxis/infusion reaction, and if these occur, stop drug immediately, notify physician, and assess patient's vital signs. Subjective symptoms are generalized itching, nausea, chest tightness, crampy abdominal pain, difficulty speaking, anxiety, agitation, sense of impending doom, uneasiness, desire to urinate/defecate, dizziness, and chills. Objective signs are flushed appearance; angioedema of face, neck, eyelids, hands, and feet; localized or generalized urticaria; respiratory distress with or without wheezing; hypotension; and cyanosis. Review standing orders or nursing procedures for patient management of anaphylaxis. ug immediately, notify physician, monitor VS, and administer ordered medications, which may include epinephrine, hydrocortisone sodium succinate, oxygen, and diphenhydramine. Teach patient to report any unusual symptoms. If the patient develops an acute infusion reaction, if severe, stop the reaction; if mild or moderate, discuss with physician or nurse practitioner whether the infusion should be slowed down or interrupted. Teach patient to report any signs and symptoms of infusion reaction within 24 hours of the infusion (e.g., fever, chills, rash, breathing problems).

POTENTIAL ALTERATION IN OXYGENATION related to CLS

Defining Characteristics: Incidence of CLS is 55%, hypotension 29%, and hypertension 15%. Peripheral edema occurred in 43% and weight increase in 31%. Pyrexia occurred in 43% of patients. Pulmonary symptoms are dose related, such as dyspnea and tachypnea. Pulmonary edema may occur with hypoxia because of fluid shifts.

Nursing Implications: Asess baseline risk of CLS based on serum albumin level,serum creatinine level, presence of peripheral edema, and weight gain. Assess baseline cardiopulmonary status at least every 1 hours during therapy and observation period after infusion, noting rate, rhythm, depth of respirations, presence of dyspnea, and breath sounds (presence of wheezes, crackles, rhonchi). Identify patients at risk: those with preexisting cardiac or pulmonary disease, prior treatment with cardio or pulmonary-toxic drugs or radiation, and smoking history. Instruct the patient to report cough, dyspnea, or change in respiratory status. Strictly monitor serum albumin, serum creatinine, peripheral edema, I/O, total fluid balance, and daily weight before each infusion. See Dosage Modifications for management if serum albumin is low, weight increases, development of peripheral edema, or serum creatinine increases. Discuss abnormalities with physician, as well as the need for IV albumin infusion, oxygen, diuretics, vasopressors, or transfer to ICU.

III. POTENTIAL ALTERATION IN NUTRITION, LESS THAN BODY REQUIREMENTS, related to NAUSEA/VOMITING, DIARRHEA, ANOREXIA, DECREASED APPETITE, AND HEPATOTOXICITY

Defining Characteristics: Nausea and vomiting are mild and are effectively controlled by antiemetics. Nausea occurred in 49%, constipation in 23%, vomiting in 21%, and diarrhea in 20%. ALT and AST were elevated in 82% and 79% of patients, and glucose was elevated in 87% of patients but decreased in 11% of patients.

Nursing Implications: Assess the patient's baseline nutritional status. Assess serum glucose, AST and ALT values, as well as chemistries baseline and prior to each infusion. Administer antiemetics as indicated and ordered. Teach the patient potential side effects and self-care measures, including oral hygiene, and encourage patient to eat favorite high-calorie, high-protein foods. Teach self-administration of prescribed antiemetics and antidiarrheals as needed. Analyze whether weight gain is fluid, as development of peripheral edema suggests CLS.

Discuss abnormalities with physician and revise plan.

Drug: Talimogene laherparepvec (Imygic®, T-vec)

Class: Oncolytic viral therapy; genetically modified oncolytic viral therapy

Mechanism of Action: Talimogene laherparepvec is an attenuated herpes simplex virus (HSV) genetically manipulated to be less virulent and made more immunogenic by encoding human granulocyte-macrophage CSF (GM-CSF) into the viral genome. Once injected into a tumor, the virus is thought to (1) preferentially replicate in the tumor cells and directly kill the tumor cells; and (2) release newly made virons, which then infect and kill neighboring cells, releasing tumor associated antigens, and (3) send signals that help stimulate an immune response against tumor cells with displaying tumor-associated antigens.

Metabolism: Imlygic DNA was found in the tumor, blood, spleen, lymph nodes, liver, heart and kidneys of mice in laboratory testing. Imlygic DNA was found in the injected tumor for 84 days and for 14 days in the blood following first administration of Imlygic.

Indications: Local treatment of unresectable cutaneous, subcutaneous, and/or nodal lesions in patients with melanoma recurrent after initial surgery. Talimogene laherparepvec has not been shown to improve overall survival or have an effect on visceral metastases.

Contraindications: Immunocompromised patients, pregnant patients.

Dosage/Range:
- *Recommended starting dose* is up to a maximum of 4 mL talimogene laherparepvec at a concentration of 10^6 (1 million) plaque-forming units (PFU) per mL. Prioritize lesions to be injected as follows: (1) inject largest lesion(s) first, (2) prioritize injection of remaining lesion(s) based on size until maximum injection volume is reached or until all injectable lesion(s) have been treated.
- *Subsequent doses* (3 weeks after initial treatment): should be administered up to 4 mL of talimogene laherparepvec at a concentration of 10^8 (100 million) PFU per mL. Prioritize lesions to be injected as follows: (1) inject any new lesion(s) that have developed since initial treatment first; (2) remaining lesion(s) should be prioritized by size with the largest being injected first and so forth until maximum injection volume is reached or until all injectable lesion(s) have been injected.
- Recommended dose and schedule: total injection volume for each treatment is a maximum of 4 mL for all injected lesions combined. Because of this, it may not be possible to inject all lesions at each treatment or over the full course of treatment.
  - Initial treatment: (4 mL); Dose is 10^6; inject largest legion(s) first, then prioritize injection based on lesion size (as previous and next bullet below).
  - Second treatment: (4 mL); 3 weeks after initial treatment, dose is now 10^8 PFU/mL. Inject any new lesions since the last treatment first, then prioritize as above.

- All subsequent treatments including reinitiation: (4 mL); 10^8 PFU; inject any new lesions since the last treatment first, then prioritize as above.
- *Dose volume determination* based on lesion size:
  - Size > 5 cm = injection volume up to 4 mL
  - Size > 2.5 to 5 cm = injection volume up to 2 mL
  - Size > 1.5 to 2.5 cm = injection volume up to 1 mL
  - Size > 0.5 to 1.5 cm = injection volume up to 0.5 mL
  - Size $\leq$ 0.5 cm = injection volume up to 0.1 mL
  - If lesions are clustered together, inject them as a single lesion as above.
- *Continue* intralesional treatment for at least 6 months unless other treatment is required or until there are no injectable lesions to treat.
- *Reinitiate* talimogene laherparepvec if new, unresectable cutaneous, subcutaneous, or nodal lesions appear after a CR.

Drug Preparation:
- Healthcare providers who are immunocompromised or pregnant should not prepare or administer talimogene laherparepvec and should NOT come into direct contact with the talimogene laherparepvec injection sites, dressings, or body fluids of treated patients.
- Avoid accidental exposure to talimogene laherparepvec (especially skin, eyes, mucous membranes): wear PPE (safety glasses or face shield along with gloves and protective gown) while preparing or administering talimogene laherparepvec.
  - Cover any exposed wounds before handling.
  - For an accidental occupational exposure, flush with clean water for at least 15 minutes.
  - For broken skin or needle stick, clean the affected area thoroughly with soap and water, and/or disinfectant.
  - Clean all surfaces that may have come into contact with talimogene laherparepvec, and treat any spills with a virucidal agent such as 1% hypochlorite or 70% isopropyl alcohol and blot using absorbent materials.
  - Dispose of all materials that may have come into contact with talimogene laherparepvec as biohazardous waste (e.g., vial, syringe, needle, cotton gauze, gloves, mask, dressings).
  - Teach patients to place used dressings and cleaning materials into a ziploc or sealed plastic bag and dispose in household waste (Amgen, 2018).
- Available as injection 10^6 (1 million) PFU per mL, and 10^8 (100 million) PFU per mL in single use vials.
- Thawing talimogene laherparepvec vials: determine the total volume required, up to 4 mL. Thaw frozen vial(s) at room temperature [20–25°C (68°–77°F)] until talimogene laherparepvec is liquid (approximately 30 minutes). Do not expose the vial to higher temperatures. Keep vial in original carton during thawing. Swirl gently but DO NOT shake.
- After thawing, administer talimogene laherparepvec immediately.
- If not used immediately, store in its original vial and carton protected from light (a) in a refrigerator [2–8°C (36–46°F)] 10^6 (1 million) PFU per mL = 24 hours, 10^8 (100 million) PFU per mL= 1 week (7 days); (b) at up to 25°C (36–46°F):10^6 (1 million) PFU per mL= 12 hours, 10^8 (100 million) PFU per mL= 24 hours.

- Prepare sterile syringes and needles based on number of lesions. Use a detachable 18–26-gauge needle to withdraw the drug, and a 22–26-gauge detachable needle for injection. Small unit syringes, e.g., 0.5 mL insulin syringes, are recommended for better injection control.
- Use a biological safety cabinet (BSC). Be careful not to generate aerosols when loading syringes.

Drug Administration:
- FOR intralesional injection only. DO NOT administer IV.
- Wear PPE and use a BSC if available. Using aseptic technique, remove vial cap and withdraw talimogene laherparepvec from the vial ensuring that the correct volume is drawn up. Avoid generating aerosols when loading syringes.
- **Pre-injection:** (1) clean the lesion and surrounding areas with alcohol swab and let dry; (2) treat the injection site with a topical or local anesthetic agent, if needed. Do not inject anesthetic agent directly into lesion, but inject around the periphery of the lesion.
- **Injection:** (1) inject talimogene laherparepvec intralesionally into cutaneous, subcutaneous, and/or nodal lesions that are visible, palpable, or detectable by ultrasound guidance. (2) using a single insertion point, inject talimogene laherparepvec along multiple tracks as far as the radial reach of the needle permits within the lesion to obtain even and complete dispersion; (3) multiple insertion points may be used if the lesion is larger than the radial reach of the lesion; (4) inject talimogene laherparepvec evenly and completely within the lesion by pulling the needle back without exiting the lesion. Redirect the needle as many times as necessary while injecting the remainder of the dose. Continue until the full dose is evenly and completely dispersed; (5) when removing the needle, withdraw it from the lesion slowly to avoid leakage of talimogene laherparepvec at the insertion point; (6) repeat steps 1–2 under pre-injection and steps 1–5 under injection for other lesions to be injected; (7) use a new needle any time the needle is completely removed from a lesion and each time a different lesion is injected.
- **Postinjection:** (1) apply pressure to the injection site(s) with sterile gauze for at least 30 seconds; (2) swab the injection site(s) and surrounding area with alcohol; (3) change gloves and cover the injected lesion(s) with an absorbent pad and dry occlusive dressing; (4) wipe exterior of occlusive dressing with alcohol; (5) teach patients to (a) keep the injection site(s) covered at least for the 1st week after each treatment visit or longer if the injection site is weeping or oozing; (b) replace the dressing if it falls off.
- Assess for injection site complications such as persistent infection or delayed healing, and if either develops, discuss the risks and benefits with physician and patient before continuing therapy. Risk for developing complications is increased in patients with prior RT or lesions in poorly vascularized areas.
- Teach patients they may develop herpetic infections, including cold sores and herpetic keratitis. Teach them not to scratch the injection sites or their occlusive dressings to try to avoid transfer of the virus. Teach patient to report any suspicious herpes-like lesions to report them right away to be evaluated. In addition, if close contacts develop suspected herpetic infections, they should contact their healthcare provider for care. While talimogene laherparepvec is sensitive to acyclovir, it or other antiviral agents may decrease the effectiveness of talimogene laherparepvec.

- Teach patients that close contacts (e.g., household members, caregivers, sex partners, or persons sharing the same bed), pregnant women, and newborns should NOT have direct contact with the injected lesions, dressings, or body fluids of treated patients.
- Accidental exposure to talimogene laherparepvec may lead to transmission of talimogene laherparepvec and herpetic infection. Avoid direct contact with injected lesions, dressings, or body fluids of treated patients. Teach patient to use gloves when handling dressing and to place the used dressing in a sealed plastic bag, avoiding touching any other surface.
- If healthcare provider is immunocompromised or pregnant, the healthcare provider should NOT prepare or administer the drug. If accidental exposure occurs, clean the affected area immediately.
- AVOID accidental exposure and follow universal biohazard precautions for preparation, administration, and handling of talimogene laherparepvec, especially exposure to skin, eyes, and mucous membranes:
  - Cover any exposed wounds before handling.
  - In the event of an accidental occupational exposure (e.g., through a splash to the eye or mucous membranes), flush with clean water for at least 15 minutes. For other areas, wash the area thoroughly with soap and water and/or a disinfectant,
  - In the event of exposure to broken skin or needle stick, clean the affected area thoroughly with soap and water and/or a disinfectant.
- Treat spills of talimogene laherparepvec with a virucidal agent such as 1% sodium hypochlorite and blot using absorbent materials.
- Dispose of all materials that may have come into contact with talimogene laherparepvec (e.g., vial, syringe, needle, cotton gauze, gloves, masks or dressings) in accordance with universal biohazard precautions.
- Teach patients to place used dressings and cleaning materials into a sealed plastic bag and dispose in household waste.
- Teach patients who develop herpetic infection(s) to follow standard hygienic practices to prevent viral transmission.
- Drug is a live, attenuated replicating virus. Dedicated exam room and biological safety cabinet should be washed with 10% bleach, and terminally cleaned after use with talimogene laherparepvec (T-vec). Any staff participating in the care of a patient receiving talimogene laherparepvec should receive special inservices about drug preparation, preventing exposure and managing spills.

Drug Interactions:
- Talimogene laherparepvec (Imlygic) is sensitive to acyclovir so acyclovir or other antiherpteic viral agents may interfere with talimogene laherparepvec's effectiveness.
- No drug interaction studies have been conducted.

Lab Effects/Interference: None known.

Special Considerations:
- Most common reported adverse drug reactions (≥25%) were fatigue, chills, pyrexia, nausea, influenza-like illness, injection site pain.
- Warnings and Precautions:

- *Accidental exposure:* see Administration. Healthcare providers should avoid direct contact with injected lesions, dressings, or body fluids of treated patients. As patients in the clinic or infusion area waiting room may be immunocompromised, ask patients receiving talimogene laherparepvecto wait in a private area or exam room.
- *Herpetic infection:* Patients may develop herpetic infection; if so, they should be taught to follow standard hygienic practices to prevent viral transmission. Teach patients not to scratch or itch injection sites or occlusive dressings. Suspected herpetic infections should be reported to Amgen (1-855-465-9442).
- *Injection site complications:* assess for persistent infection or delayed healing, and if either develops, discuss the risks and benefits with physician and patient before continuing therapy. Factors which impair healing include prior RT to the injection site or lesions in poorly vascularized areas. Use careful wound care and infection precautions. One patient had a lower extremity amputation 6 months after a Talimogene laherparepvec injection due to a wound infection and inability to heal; area had previously received surgery and RT (Amgen, 2018).
- *Immune-mediated events* may occur. In clinical studies, these included glomerulonephritis, vasculitis, pneumonitis, worsening psoriasis, and vitiligo. Physician should discuss the potential risks and benefits of starting therapy in patients with an underlying autoimmune disease, or before continuing treatment in patients who develop an immune-mediated event.
- *Plasmocytoma at injection site* may occur (in one patient with smoldering myeloma); physician should discuss the risks and benefits in patients with MM or in whom plasmocytoma develops during treatment.
- *Obstructive airway disorder:* Has been reported following talimogene laherparepvec therapy. Use caution when injecting lesions close to major airways.
- Pregnancy is a contraindication. Teach women of reproductive potential to use effective contraception. Mothers should not breastfeed and either discontinue nursing or the drug.

Potential Toxicities/Side Effects and the Nursing Process

I.   ALTERATION IN COMFORT, POTENTIAL, related to FATIGUE, CHILLS, PYREXIA, INFLUENZA-LIKE ILLNESS, MYALGIA, ARTHRALGIA, PAIN IN EXTREMITY, HEADACHE, AND INJECTION SITE PAIN

Defining Characteristics: In clinical trials, fatigue occurred in 50.3% of patients, chills 48.6%, pyrexia 42.8%, influenza-like illness (30.5%), injection site pain 27.7%, myalgia 17.5%, arthralgia 17.1%, pain in extremity 16.4%, and headache 18.8%.

Nursing Implications: Assess comfort level before each treatment. Teach patient that these side effects may occur. Teach self-care strategies to relieve discomfort, and teach patient to notify the nurse/provider if symptoms persist.

II.   ALTERATION IN NUTRITION, POTENTIAL, related to NAUSEA, VOMITING, DIARRHEA, AND CONSTIPATION

Defining Characteristics: Nausea occurred in 35.6% of patients in clinical trials, vomiting in 21.2%, diarrhea 18.8%, and constipation 11.6%.

Nursing Implications: Assess baseline nutritional status, and presence of nutritional impact symptoms. Teach patient these side effects may occur and to report them. Assess patient each day of treatment, and discuss self-care strategies including over-the-counter management of constipation and diarrhea; if these strategies are not effective, discuss prescription pharmacological management with provider.

Drug: tbo-filgrastim (Granix, Neutroval)

Class: G-CSF.

Mechanism of Action: Tbo-filgrastim binds to G-CSF receptors and stimulates neutrophil proliferation, differentiation commitment, and other actions that increase neutrophil number and activity.

Metabolism: After subcutaneous dosing, bioavailability is 33%, median time to maximal concentration is 4–6 hours, and median elimination half-life is 3.2–3.8 hours. Peak serum levels (C_{max}) are reached between days 3 and 5, returning to baseline at day 21.

Indication: In adult and pediatric patients 1 month and older to reduce the duration of severe neutropenia in patients with nonmyeloid malignancies receiving myelosuppressive anticancer drugs associated with a clinically significant incidence of febrile neutropenia.

Contraindications: Patients with a history of serious allergic reactions to filgrastim or pegfilgrastim products.

Dosage/Range:
- 5 mcg/kg/day administered subcutaneously.
- Administer first dose no earlier than **24 hours after** myelosuppressive chemotherapy;
  - Continue with daily dosing until the expected neutrophil nadir has passed, and neutrophil count has recovered to the normal range.
  - Do not administer within 24 hours prior to chemotherapy.
- Monitor CBC/differential prior to chemotherapy and twice per week until recovery.

Drug Preparation:
- Tbo-filgrastim is available in single-dose prefilled syringe or vial:
- Prefilled syringe:
  - 300 microgram/0.5 mL (600 mcg/mL) in single-use prefilled syringe.
  - 480 microgram/0.8 mL (600 mcg/mL) in single-use prefilled syringe.

- Vial:
  - 300 microgram (mcg)/1 mL solution in single-dose vial
  - 480 mcg/1.6 mL (300 mcg/mL)
- Dispense only the prefilled syring without a safety needle guard to patient or caregiver.

Drug Administration (see package insert for health professional administration and patient education sheet at the end of the package insert):
- Drug can be administered by a patient, caregiver, or healthcare professional.
  - If the patient or caregiver wishes to administer the drug, ensure patient is a an appropriate candidate for self-administration or administration by a caregiver.
  - Patient/caregiver must be taught and understand storage, preparation, and administration technique and demonstrate competence through return demonstration of these concepts.
  - Teach patients to use the Instructions for Use provided with the GRANIX prefilled syringe to correctly administer the drug after prior teaching by a healthcare professional.
- Visually inspect parenteral drug products for particulate matter and discoloration prior to administration; do not use if found.
- Ensure correct volume for prescribed dose. Prefilled syringe and vial are for single-dose use only so unused portions should be discarded. No natural rubber latex is used.
- Administer a single-use, prefilled syringe subcutaneously; recommended sites are abdomen (> 2 inches from navel), front of the middle thigh, upper outer area of buttock, and upper back portion of upper arms. Rotate sites daily.
- Avoid areas that are tender, red, bruised, hard, or have scars or stretch marks.

Drug Interactions:
- Drugs that may potentiate release of neutrophils (e.g., lithium); use with caution.

Lab Effects/Interference:
- Increased neutrophil count.

Special Considerations:
- Drug should not be used during pregnancy unless the risk to the fetus is outweighed by benefit for the mother. Caution should be used if drug is used in nursing mothers, as it is not known if drug is secreted in human milk.
- Most common adverse reaction is bone pain.
- Drug should be used during pregnancy only if the potential benefit justifies the potential risk to the fetus.
- Warnings and Precautions:
  - *Splenic rupture* can occur after administration of G-CSFs and be fatal. Evaluate patients who have upper abdominal or shoulder pain after receiving tbo-filgrastim for enlarged spleen and discuss emergency management. If splenic rupture is suspected or confirmed, discontinue drug.
  - *Acute respiratory distress syndrome (ARDS)* can occur in patients receiving G-CSFs. Evaluate any patient receiving tbo-filgrastim who develops fever and lung infiltrates or respiratory distress for ARDS, discuss emergency management with provider. Drug should be discontinued for ARDS.

- *Serious allergic reactions* (e.g., from anaphylaxis and angioneurotic edema to allergic dermatitis rash, pruritic rash, urticaria) may occur. Do not administer tbo-filgrastim to patients who have a history of serious allergic reactions to filgrastim or pegfilgrastim.
- Reactions can occur with first dose. If a serious allergic reaction occurs, manage per ordered antihistamines, steroids, bronchodilators, or epinephrine to reduce reaction severity; if anaphylaxis occurs, patient should be admitted for close observation as symptoms may recur when the half-life of rescue drugs has passed.
- If a serious allergic reaction occurs, permanently discontinue drug.
- *Use in patients with sickle cell disease:* Sickle cell crisis can be precipitated by G-CSF, which may be fatal. Patients with sickle cell disease should weigh the risks and benefits. Do not administer to patients in sickle cell crisis, and discontinue the drug if sickle cell crisis occurs.
- *Glomerulonephritis:* can occur in patients receiving filgrastim products, characterized by azotemia, hematuria, proteinuria, and confirmed by renal biopsy. Most often, glomerulonephritis resolves after dose reduction or drug discontinuation. If no other cause can be found, and glomerulonephritis is likely caused by tbo-filgrastim, discuss with physician dose reduction or drug interruption.
- *Capillary Leak Syndrome (CLS):* can occur in patients receiving filgrastim products, characterized by hypotension, hypoalbuminemia, edema, and hemoconcentration. Treatment must be instituted immediately and may require ICU care. Monitor patients closely.
- *Potential for tumor growth stimulatory effects on malignant cells:* G-CSF receptors have been found on tumor cells, raising the possibility that tbo-filgrastim can act as a growth factor for any tumor type. The drug is not approved for use in myeloid malignancies or myelodysplasia.
- *Leukocytosis:* Rarely, WBC of $\geq$ 100,000/mm^3 have occurred in 2% of patients. Monitor ANC and discontinue tbo-filgrastim if the ANC surpasses 10,000/mm^3 after the expected chemotherapy nadir has occurred. Monitor CBC/ANC at least twice weekly during therapy. ANC values >10,000/mm^3 may not increase clinical benefit. For patients receiving myelosuppressive chemotherapy, discontinuation of filgrastim usually results in a 50% decrease in circulating neutrophils within 1–2 days, and return to pretreatment levels in 1–7 days.
- *Simultaneous use with chemotherapy and radiation therapy not recommended:* Due to potential sensitivity of rapidly dividing myeloid cells to chemotherapy and death of stimulated neutrophils. Patients receiving concurrent RT with filgrastim have not been studied. Do not use tbo-filgrastim in the period 24 hours before through 24 hours after the administration of cytotoxic chemotherapy.
- *Nuclear imaging:* Filgrastim stimulated bone marrow activity may be seen as a transient positive bone-imaging change and should be considered when the imaging is interpreted.
- *Aortitis:* has been reported rarely with another filgrastim product, possibly occurring as early as the first week after starting filgrastim (fever, abdominal pain, malaise, back pain, increased inflammatory markers (e.g., CRP and wbc count)). If aortitis is suspected, discontinue tbo-filgrastim.

- *Alveolar hemorrhage:* has been reported related to another filgrastim product, manifested as pulmonary infiltrates and hemoptysis requiring hospitalization in the mobilization of periperhal blood progenitor cells in healthy donots. The use of tbo-filgrastim for stem cell mobilization is not an approved indication.

Potential Toxicities/Side Effects (Dose- and Schedule-Dependent) and the Nursing Process

I.   ALTERATION IN COMFORT related to BONE PAIN

Defining Characteristics: Patients may report bone pain, believed to be due to the expansion of cells in the bone marrow in response to G-CSF. The incidence in cycle 1 during clinical trials was 3.4%.

Nursing Implications: Teach patient that this may occur, and discuss use of NSAIDs with patient and physician for symptom management. Monitor WBC and ANC twice weekly during therapy; dose should be discontinued when ANC has recovered to the normal range.

Drug: thalidomide (Thalomid)

Class: Immunomodulatory and antiangiogenic agent.

Mechanism of Action: While the mechanism of action is not fully understood, drug has immunomodulatory, anti-inflammatory, and antiangiogenic properties. Drug probably suppresses excessive TNF-α production and modulates some cell surface adhesion molecules involved in leukocyte migration. In MM, drug treatment is accompanied by an increase in the number of circulating NK and T-cell derived cytokines associated with cytotoxic activity. Thalidomide inhibits angiogenesis, possibly by blocking the proliferation of endothelial cells.

Metabolism: Slow absorption after oral administration. Mean peak serum level reached at 2–5 hours after drug administration. Drug is not a substrate of the P450 hepatic enzyme system. The mean elimination half-life was 5.5–7.3 hours. The majority of a radioactive dose is excreted within 48 hours, primarily in the urine as hydrolic metabolites (91.9%), with minor fecal excretion ($<$ 2% of drug). There is a linear relationship between body weight and estimated thalidomide clearance.

Indication: Drug is indicated for the treatment of patients with:
- Newly diagnosed MM in combination with dexamethasone.
- Acute treatment of cutaneous manifestations of moderate to severe ENL and maintenance therapy for the prevention and suppression of the cutaneous manifestations of ENL recurrence.
- Drug is not indicated as monotherapy for ENL treatment if the patient has moderate-severe neuritis.

Dosage/Range:
- Drug is only available through a restricted distribution program, the THALOMID REMS program. This requires that:
  - Prescribers must be certified with THALOMID REMS program by enrolling and complying with the REMS requirements.
  - Patients must sign a patient–provider agreement form and comply with the REMS requirements (e.g., pregnancy testing for females of reproductive potential, and contraception for females and males, see Drug Preparation/Administration).
  - Pharmacies must be certified with THALOMID REMS program, must dispense only to patients who are authorized to receive thalidomide, and comply with REMS requirements.
- *Females of reproductive potential: prescription is contingent upon initial and continued confirmation of negative pregnancy testing.*
- *Consider dose reduction, delay, or discontinuation in patients who develop NCI CTC grade 304 adverse reactions and/or based on clinical judgment.*

Multiple myeloma (MM):
- In combination with dexamethasone in 28-day treatment cycles: Thalidomide 200 mg orally once daily with water, preferably at bedtime, at least 1 hour after the evening meal. Give dexamethasone 40 mg orally daily on days 1–4, 9–12, 17–20, every 28 days.
- Patients who develop constipation, somnolence, or peripheral neuropathy or other adverse events, may benefit by either temporarily discontinuing the drug or continuing at a lower dose.
- With abatement of these adverse reactions, the drug may be started at a lower dose or at the previous dose based on clinical judgment.
- Consider thromboprohylaxis based on individual patient's underlying risk factors.

Cutaneous erythema nodosum leprosum:
- For an episode of ENL: 100–300 mg/day, administered once daily with water, preferably at bedtime, at least 1 hour after the evening meal. Patients weighing < 50 kg should be started at the low end of the dose range.
- Patients with severe ENL reaction, or those who required higher doses to control the reaction: Start at higher doses up to 400 mg/day once daily at bedtime, or in divided doses with water, at least 1 hour after meals.
- Patients with moderate to severe neuritis associated with a severe ENL reaction: corticosteroids may be started concomitant with thalidomide. Steroid usage can be tapered and discontinued when neuritis has improved.
- Thalidomide is not indicated as monotherapy for acute treatment in the presence of moderate-severe neuritis.
- Thalidomide is usually continued until signs and symptoms of active reaction have subsided, usually a period of at least 2 weeks. Patients may be tapered off thalidomide in 50-mg decrements every 2–4 weeks.
- Patients with a documented history of requiring prolonged maintenance treatment to prevent the recurrence of cutaneous ENL, or who flare during tapering, should be maintained on the minimum dose necessary to control the reaction. Tapering off medication should be attempted every 3–6 months, in decrements of 50 mg every 2–4 weeks.

Drug Preparation/Administration:
- Drug is contraindicated in a pregnant woman or in patients with demonstrated hypersensitivity to the drug or its components.
- Available as 50-, 100-, 150-, and 200-mg capsules.
- Pregnancy must be excluded prior to starting therapy, and female patients with reproductive potential must use two reliable methods of contraception.
  - Females of reproductive potential must avoid pregnancy for at least 4 weeks before beginning thalidomide, during therapy, during dose interruptions, and for at least 4 weeks after completing therapy.
  - Females must commit either to abstain continuously from heterosexual intercourse, or to use two reliable methods of birth control, beginning at least 4 weeks before beginning thalidomide, during therapy, during dose interruptions, and for at least 4 weeks after discontinuance of thalidomide therapy.
  - Two negative pregnancy tests must be obtained prior to initiating therapy. First test should be performed within 10–14 days, and the second test within 24 hours prior to prescribing thalidomide therapy, then weekly during the first month, then monthly thereafter in women with regular menstrual cycles or every 2 weeks in women with irregular menstrual cycles.
- Men must always use a latex or synthetic condom during any sexual contact with females of reproductive potential when taking thalidomide and for up to 28 days after thalidomide discontinuance, even if the man has undergone a successful vasectomy. Drug is present in semen.
- Initiate thalidomide treatment only if ANC is $\geq$ 750 cells/mm^3.
  - CBC/differential should be monitored on an ongoing basis, especially in patients prone to neutropenia, such as HIV-seropositive patients.
  - If ANC $<$ 750 cells/mm^3 while on treatment, reevaluate the patient's medication regimen, and if neutropenia persists, consider withholding thalidomide if clinically appropriate.
- Oral, give at bedtime if possible, at least 1 hour after the evening meal.
  - Females of reproductive potential should avoid contact with thalidomide capsules, and capsules should be stored in blister packs until ingestion. If there is skin contact with nonintact capsules or the powder contents, exposed area should be washed with soap and water.
  - Healthcare providers should wear gloves if handling drug capsules to prevent potential cutaneous exposure. If exposed to body fluids from patients receiving thalidomide, exposed area should be washed with soap and water.
- Teach patient that if a dose is missed and it has been $<$ 12 hours since the regular time to take the dose, to take the dose as soon as it is remembered. If it has been $>$ 12 hours, the missed dose should be skipped. The patient should not take 2 doses at the same time.

Drug Interactions:
- Opioids, antihistamines, antipsychotics, antianxiety agents, other CNS depressants including alcohol: increased sedation; avoid coadministration.
- Drugs that cause bradycardia (e.g., calcium channel blockers, beta blockers, alpha/beta-adrenergic blockers, digoxin, cimetidine, famotidine, lithium, tricyclic antidepressants, succinylcholine): possible additive bradycardic effect; use together cautiously.

- Drugs that cause peripheral neuropathy (e.g., bortezomib, amiodarone, cisplatin, docetaxel, paclitaxel, vincristine, disulfiram, phenytoin, metronidazole, alcohol): possible additive effect; use together with caution.
- Hormonal contraceptives increase the risk of thromboembolism. It is unknown if concomitant use of hormonal contraceptives further increases risks for thromboembolism when given with thalidomide.
- Drugs that interfere with hormonal contraceptives (e.g., HIV-protease inhibitors, griseofulvin, modafinil, penicillins, rifampin, rifabutin, phenytoin, carbamazepine, or certain herbal supplements like St. John's wort) when used concomitantly with hormonal contraceptive agents may reduce the effectiveness of contraception up to one month after discontinuation of these concomitant therapies. Women requiring treatment with one or more of these drugs must use 2 OTHER effective or highly effective methods of contraception while taking thalidomide.
- Erythropoietic agents may increase the risk of thromboembolism, as may estrogen containing therapies; use cautiously if at all in patients with MM receiving thalidomide with dexamethasone.
- PD-1 and PD_L1 inhibitors in combiniation with thalidomide analogue and dexamethasone not recommended as increased mortality.

Lab Effects/Interference:
- Decreased leukocytes, neutrophils.
- Hyperglycemia.
- Hypocalcemia.
- Increased serum bilirubin.
- HIV RNA levels may be increased in HIV-seropositive patients.

Special Considerations:
- Warnings and Precautions:
  - *Embryo-fetal toxicity:* Thalidomide is a powerful teratogen that induces a high frequency of severe and life-threatening birth defects, even after a single dose. Thalidomide is ABSOLUTELY CONTRAINDICATED IN PREGNANCY.
  - Women of reproductive potential should not handle thalidomide capsules, and capsules should be stored in blister packs until ingestion. Healthcare providers should use gloves when handling drug, and if any cutaneous exposure occurs, wash the area thoroughly with soap and water. Females of reproductive potential must avoid pregnancy for at least 4 weeks before starting thalidomide, during therapy, during dose interruption, and for at least 4 weeks after completing therapy. Females must commit either to abstain continuously from heterosexual intercourse or to use two methods of reliable birth control, beginning 4 weeks prior to starting thalidomide therapy, during therapy, during dose interruptions, and continuing for 4 weeks after drug discontinuation. Two negative pregnancy tests must be obtained before starting therapy, the first 10–14 days and the second within 24 hours prior to prescribing thalidomide therapy, then weekly during the first month, then monthly thereafter in women with regular menstrual cycles, or every 2 weeks in women with irregular menstrual cycles. Women taking hormonal contraception concomitantly with drugs that may reduce effectiveness of contraception MUST use two other effective or

highly effective methods of contraception when on thalidomide therapy. See Drug Interactions.

- Men must always use a latex or synthetic condom during any sexual contact with females of reproductive potential while taking thalidomide, and for up to 4 weeks after discontinuing the drug even if they have had a successful vasectomy. The drug is present in semen. Men must not donate sperm.
- Patients must not donate blood during thalidomide treatment and for 4 weeks after drug is discontinued.
- *Thalomid REMS program:* Required components of the program include (a) Prescribers must be certified with the Thalomid REMS program by enrolling and complying with the REMS requirements; (b) patients must sign a Patient-Physician Agreement Form and comply with the REMS requirements, e.g., female patients of reproductive potential who are not pregnant must comply with the pregnancy testing and contraception requirements, and males must comply with contraception requirements; (c) pharmacies must be certified with the Thalomid REMS program, must only dispense to patients who are authorized to receive Pomalyst, and comply with REMS requirements.

- *Venous and arterial thromboembolism:* Thalidomide when used to treat MM increases risk of VTE, such as DVT and pulmonary embolism (PE). This risk is significantly increased when combined with dexamethasone. In one controlled trial, the incidence was 22.5% in patients receiving thalidomide plus dexamethasone, compared to 4.9% in patients receiving dexamethasone alone ($p = 0.002$). Consider thromboprophylaxis based on assessment of individual patient's risk factors. Assess patients for signs/symptoms of VTE, and teach patient to call healthcare provider/get medical care right away for SOB, chest pain, arm or leg swelling.
  - *Drowsiness and somnolence:* Teach patients to avoid situations where drowsiness may be a problem and not to take other drowsiness-inducing medicines. Teach patients that their ability to perform hazardous tasks, such as driving a car, or operating complex or dangerous machinery, may be impaired (mentally and/or physically) and to avoid these activities. Thalidomide dosage may need to be reduced.
  - *Increased mortality in patients with muldiple myeloma when pembrolizumab is added to thalidomide analogue and dexamethasone* found in 2 randomized clinical trials. PD- and PD-L1 blocking antibody is not indicated in this setting, and should not be combined with thalidomide analogues/dexamethasone unless part of a controlled clinical trial.
- *Peripheral neuropathy* is common, affecting ≥ 10% of patients, and may be irreversible.
  - Peripheral neuropathy generally occurs with chronic use over a period of months but occurrence after relatively short-term use has been reported. Symptoms may occur after thalidomide treatment has been stopped, and resolve slowly if at all.
  - Assess patients for signs/symptoms of peripheral neuropathy (e.g., numbness, tingling or pain in the hands and feet) baseline, at least monthly for the first 3 months, then periodically during thalidomide therapy.
  - Consider electrophysiological testing (measurement of sensory nerve action potential [SNAP] amplitudes) baseline, and every 6 months to identify asymptomatic neuropathy.

- If symptoms of drug-induced neuropathy develop, discontinue thalidomide immediately to limit further nerve damage, if clinically appropriate. Usually, thalidomide is reinitiated only if neuropathy returns to baseline status.
  - Use medications known to be associated with neuropathy cautiously in patients receiving thalidomide.
- *Dizziness and orthostatic hypotension* may occur. Teach patients to sit upright for a few minutes before standing up from a recumbent position.
- *Neutropenia:* Thalidomide should be initiated only if ANC is $\geq$ 750 cells/mm^3, and CBC/differential should be monitored on an ongoing basis, especially in patients who are prone to neutropenia (e.g., HIV-seropositive patients). Reevaluate patient's medication regimen if ANC falls to < 750 cells/mm^3 while on treatment. If neutropenia persists, consider withholding thalidomide if clinically appropriate. Patients may require dose reduction.
- *Thrombocytopenia:* may occur, including grades 3–4. Monitor CBC/ANC and platelet count. Monitor for signs and symptoms of bleeding (e.g., petechiae, epistaxis, GI bleeding) especially if taking concomitant medication that may increase bleeding risk.
- *Increased plasma HIV viral load* may occur in HIV seropositive patients. Measure viral load baseline, after the first and third months of treatment, and then every 3 months thereafter.
- *Bradycardia* in patients receiving thalidomide has been reported. Monitor patients for bradycardia and syncope. Dose reduction or discontinuance may be required. Medications known to decrease heart rate should be used cautiously in patients receiving thalidomide.
- *SJS and TEN:* Severe dermatological reactions, including SJS and TEN have been reported, and may be fatal. Stop thalidomide if rash occurs, and resume thalidomide only after appropriate clinical evaluation. If rash is exfoliative, purpuric, or bullous, or if SJS or TEN is suspected, do not resume thalidomide.
- *Seizures,* including grand-mal seizures, have been reported post-approval. If a patient has a history of seizures, or other risk factors for developing seizures, monitor the patient closely for clinical changes that could precipitate acute seizure activity.
- *TLS* may occur in patients with a high tumor burden before treatment. Identify these patients, and discuss with physician, NP, or PA TLS prophylaxis.
- *Hypersensitivity to thalidomide* has been reported, characterized by erythematous macular rash, possibly associated with fever, tachycardia, and hypotension; if severe, interrupt thalidomide therapy. If the reaction occurs again after drug is resumed, discontinue thalidomide.
- *Contraceptive risks:* Because some patients receiving thalidomide may develop sudden, severe neutropenia and/or thrombocytopenia, use of an intrauterine device (IUD) or implantable contraceptive may increase the risk of infection or bleeding either at insertion, removal, or during use. Thalidomide treatment in the presence of an underlying malignancy and/or use of an estrogen-containing contraceptive can each increase the risk of VTE. While it is not known if the risks of VTE are additive, the risks should be considered when the patient is selecting contraceptive methods.
- Patients receiving thalidomide should not donate blood during treatment or for one month after the drug has been discontinued, as the blood might be given to a pregnant woman, putting the fetus at risk of exposure to thalidomide.

- Most common side effects when thalidomide is used to treat MM are fatigue, hypocalcemia, edema, constipation, sensory neuropathy, dyspnea, muscle weakness, leukopenia, neutropenia, rash/desquamation, confusion, anorexia, nausea, anxiety/agitation, asthenia, tremor, fever, weight loss, thrombosis/embolism, motor neuropathy, weight gain, dizziness, dry skin.
- Most common side effects when thalidomide is used to treat ENL: somnolence, rash, headache.
- Safety and effectiveness in pediatric patients < 12 years old have not been established.
- In study 2 of MM patients receiving thalidomine with dexamethasone, patients 65 years of age or older had higher incidences of atrial fibrillation, constipation, fatigue, nausea, hypokalemia, DVT, hyperglycemia, PE, and asthenia compared to patients < 65.

Potential Toxicities/Side Effects and the Nursing Process

I.   ALTERATION IN SEXUALITY/REPRODUCTION related to POTENTIAL TERATOGENICITY

Defining Characteristics: Drug is teratogenic and a single dose can cause birth defects. Drug is distributed in semen.

Nursing Implications: Assess reproductive status, sexual activity, and birth control measures used for both men and women. The THALOMID REMS program requires that prescribers be certified with the program (enrolling and complying with REMS), patients must sign a patient–prescriber agreement form and comply with the REMS requirements, and pharmacies must be certified with the THALOMID REMS program, must only dispense to authorized patients, and must comply with REMS requirements. Women of reproductive potential must commit to using two forms of reliable contraception (or abstain continuously from heterosexual sexual intercourse) to avoid pregnancy for 4 weeks before starting thalidomide, during therapy, during dose interruptions, and for at least 4 weeks after drug has been discontinued. Two negative pregnancy tests must be verified prior to starting therapy, one 10–14 days before, and one within 24 hours of prescribing thalidomide therapy, then weekly for the first month, then monthly if regular menses, or every 2 weeks in women with irregular menstrual cycles.

Male patients must commit to always using a latex or synthetic condom during any sexual contact with females of reproductive potential while taking thalidomide, and for up to 28 days after discontinuing the drug. This is regardless of whether the man has had a successful vasectomy. Men should be told not to donate sperm.

Teach women to tell their healthcare provider right away if they have unprotected sex or think that their birth control has failed. If the patient thinks she has become pregnant, she should stop taking thalidomide right away and call her healthcare provider. Teach men to tell their healthcare provider if they have unprotected sexual contact with a female who is or could become pregnant; if their female partner becomes pregnant, they should tell their healthcare provider right away. If the healthcare provider is not available, the patient can call 1-800-332-1088 for medical information. Healthcare providers and patients should report all pregnancies to FDA MedWatch at 1-800-332-1088, and Celgene Corporation at 1-888-423-5436.

II. ALTERATION IN OXYGENATION, POTENTIAL, related to VENOUS THROMBO EMBOLISM

Defining Characteristics: In MM patients, VTE risk is significantly increased when thalidomide is combined with dexamethasone. In one controlled trial, the incidence was 22.5% in patients receiving thalidomide plus dexamethasone, compared to 4.9% in patients receiving dexamethasone alone ($p = 0.002$). In the safety study, DVT occurred in 13% of patients compared to 2% in placebo/dexamethasone group. Risk is further increased in patients receiving concomitant erythropoietic agent or estrogen containing therapy.

Nursing Implications: Assess for signs/symptoms of VTE at each visit. Discuss with physician or NP/PA need for thromboprophylaxis given the individual patient's underlying risk for developing VTE. Teach MM patients taking thalidomide and dexamethsone that there may be an increased risk of blood clots in the veins of the legs and lungs; and the patient should call the healthcare provider or get medical help right away if the patient experiences SOB, chest pain, or arm or leg swelling. Discuss risks and benefits of concomitant erythropoietin or estrogen containing therapy as risk for VTE is increased.

III. ALTERATION IN SENSORY/PERCEPTUAL PATTERNS related to PERIPHERAL NEUROPATHY, DIZZINESS, SEIZURE

Defining Characteristics: Sensory neuropathy occurs commonly ($\geq$ 10%) and in the safety study in combination with dexamethasone, the incidence was 54% (4% grades 3–4). Motor neuropathy occurred in 22% (8% grades 3–4). Neuropathy is potentially severe and may be irreversible. Neuropathy generally occurs after chronic use over a period of months, but reports after short-term use have been made. Symptoms may occur after thalidomide has been stopped, and may resolve slowly or not at all. Confusion was reported in 28% of MM patients receiving thalidomide and dexamethasone in the safety study 1. Dizziness/light-headedness occurred in 20% of MM patients. Orthostatic hypotension may occur. Seizures, including grand mal, have been described in post-marketing reports.

Nursing Implications: Assess baseline neurologic status, especially presence of neuropathy. Teach patient to stop drug and report immediately numbness, tingling, pain, or a burning sensation in hands, legs, or feet. Perform assessment for neuropathy at every visit. Patient should have a monthly examination for the first 3 months of therapy, and regularly after that for signs/symptoms of neuropathy. Manufacturer recommends consideration of electrophysiological testing (measurement of sensory nerve action potential or SNAP amplitudes) baseline and every 6 months to detect asymptomatic neuropathy. Teach patient to avoid any situation where dizziness might be unsafe, and to avoid taking other medicines that increase dizziness or light-headedness. Teach patient to change position slowly, sitting for a few minutes after moving from a lying position, before standing up. Monitor patients with a history of seizures, or who are at risk of a lowered seizure threshold (e.g., other medications) closely for any changes that could precipitate seizure activity. Teach patient to report any changes.

IV.   ALTERATION IN SENSORY/PERCEPTUAL PATTERNS related to DROWSINESS

Defining Characteristics: Drug has sedative qualities, and drowsiness is a frequent side effect. Tolerance to daytime drowsiness occurs over several weeks of use.

Nursing Implications: Assess baseline alertness, sleep patterns. Assess other drugs taken, especially those with sedating qualities, and alcohol ingestion. Instruct patient to avoid alcohol and to take drug at bedtime. Assess degree of drowsiness and dizziness and safety of patient. If significant, teach measures to ensure safety. Advise patients to avoid driving a car or operating machinery.

V.   ALTERATION IN SKIN INTEGRITY, POTENTIAL, related to RASH, PRURITUS

Defining Characteristics: Pruritic, erythematous macular rash may occur. Incidence was 30% in MM patients (rash/desquamation) and 20.8% in ENL patients. Hypersensitivity has been reported with signs/symptoms of erythematous macular rash, possibly associated with fever, tachycardia, and hypotension. Drug rechallenge often results in immediate reaction of rash, tachycardia, and fever. Rash resolves with drug discontinuation. Serious dermatological reactions can occur, including SJS and TEN, which can be fatal.

Nursing Implications: Assess patient for rash/desquamation at each visit. Teach patient to self-assess for rash; if rash occurs, patient should stop thalidomide and to call provider for evaluation. If rash is exfoliative, purpuric, or bullous, or if SJS or TEN is suspected, drug should not be resumed. Teach patient that an allergic reaction may occur and if the patient develops a red, itchy rash, fever, a fast heartbeat, or if the patient feels dizzy or faint, to call the healthcare provider or get medical help right away.

VI.   ALTERATION IN ELIMINATION related to CONSTIPATION

Defining Characteristics: Mild constipation occurs commonly, with an incidence of 55% in MM patients (Safety Study 1).

Nursing Implications: Instruct patient to prevent constipation by using stool softeners, mild laxatives if needed (e.g., Milk of Magnesia), and to use bulk (e.g., psyllium). In addition, teach dietary interventions (e.g., increased fiber, fluids of 3 quarts/day), and mild exercise. Instruct patient to report constipation unresponsive to these interventions.

VII.   POTENTIAL FOR INFECTION related to NEUTROPENIA

Defining Characteristics: Neutrophils are decreased in 31% of MM patients (20% grade 3–4) (Safety Study 1).

Nursing Implications: Determine baseline WBC and ANC. Do not initiate therapy if ANC $< 750/mm^3$. If on treatment, ANC $< 750/mm^3$, the patient's medication regimen should be reevaluated, and if neutropenia persists, consideration should be given to withholding the drug. Drug may be reinstituted after neutrophil recovery. WBC and ANC should be monitored in an ongoing fashion in all patients, especially in patients prone to neutropenia, such as HIV-seropositive patients.

Drug: thyrotropin alfa for injection (Thyrogen®)

Class: Recombinant hormone (human TSH) for tumor remnant ablation.

Mechanism of Action: Patients with thyroid cancer normally have surgery (subtotal or total thyroidectomy) followed by radioactive iodine to remove remaining normal tissue and any malignant cells. In order to stimulate the thyroid to take up the iodine, the TSH level has to be elevated. This drug binds to TSH receptors on remaining normal thyroid epithelial cells and differentiated thyroid cancer cells, stimulating the uptake of iodine and organification, as well as synthesis and secretion of thyroglobulin (T_g), triiodothyronine (T_3), and thyroxine (T_4). An alternative to increasing the TSH level to destroy tumor remnant is to stop taking thyroid hormone replacement therapy, but this has significant side effects. Thyrotropin alfa for injection allows patients to continue to take their hormone replacement therapy with significantly higher quality of life (Genzyme, 2008). This drug is also used as a diagnostic tool in assessment of well-differentiated thyroid cancer recurrence.

Metabolism: After a single 0.9-mg IM dose, mean peak concentrations were reached in 3–24 hours (median 10 hours). The mean elimination half-life is 25 ± 10 hours. The drug appears to be metabolized and excreted by the liver and kidneys.

Indication: (1) Diagnostic: adjunctive tool for serum thyroglobin testing with or without radioiodine imaging in the follow-up of patients with well-differentiated thyroid cancer who have undergone thyroidectomy; (2) use as adjunctive treatment for radioiodine ablation of thyroid tissue remnants in patients who have undergone a near-total or total thyroidectomy for well-differentiated thyroid cancer and who do not have evidence of distance metastases.

Limitations of Use: (a) Thyrogen stimulated serum thyroglobulin (Tg) levels are lower than those after thyroid hormone withdrawal; (b) anti-Tg antibodies may confound the Tg assay; (c) the effect on long-term thyroid cancer outcomes has not been determined.

Dosage/Range:
- 2-injection regimen: 0.9 mg IM followed by a second 0.9 mg injection 24 hours later. If remnant ablation is performed, radioiodine will be administered 24 hours after the second injection of THYROGEN.
- In dialysis-dependent patients with ESRD, drug elimination is slower, resulting in prolonged TSH level elevation; expect that these patients may have an increased risk for headache and nausea.

Drug Preparation:
- Reconstitute with provided 1.2-mL sterile water for injection, resulting in a 0.9-mg thyrotropin alfa in 1.0-mL solution immediately prior to administration.

- If necessary, reconstituted solution can be stored for 24 hours, protected from light, at 2–8°C (36–46°F).

Drug Administration:
- Administer IM ONLY, in the buttock.
- Give 0.9 mg thyrotropin alfa for injection IM daily × 2 doses 24 hours apart.
- Consider pretreatment with glucocorticosteroids in patients who may develop local tumor extension or swelling that could compromise vital structures (trachea, CNS brain, or spinal metastases, extensive macroscopic lung metastases).
- Use cautiously and closely monitor older patients with functional thyroid tumors, as they may experience palpitations or cardiac rhythm disturbances (atrial).
- Consider hospitalization for administration and monitoring postdrug dose for patients with known heart disease, extensive metastases, or known serious underlying disease.
- For radioiodine imaging or remnant ablation, give radioiodine 24 hours after the second (final) thyrotropin alfa injection. Diagnostic scanning should be done 48 hours after the radioiodine administration; post-therapy scanning can be delayed additional days (to allow background activity to decline).
- For serum T_g testing, obtain a sample 72 hours after the second (final) injection.

Drug Interactions:
- None known.
- When used for radioiodine imaging in euthyroid patients, clearance of radioiodine is increased 50% compared with hypothyroid patients and should guide selection of the radioiodine used.

Lab Effects/Interference:
- Euthyroid patients for whom the drug is used for diagnostic imaging will have a significant, transient rise in TSH.
- No patients developed antibodies to thyrotropin alfa.

Special Considerations:
- Drug is indicated as an adjunctive.
- Use cautiously in patients who have previously received bovine TSH and those patients who have had HSRs to TSH administration in the past.
- It is unknown whether the drug is toxic to a fetus and thus should be given to a pregnant woman only when clearly needed; mothers should not breastfeed when receiving the drug.
- Successful ablation can be inferred when thyrogen-stimulated serum T_g level is < 2 ng/mL.
- Rarely, patient may develop hypersensitivity to the injection, characterized by urticaria, rash, pruritus, flushing, and respiratory symptoms; treat symptomatically.
- Warnings and Precautions:
  - Drug causes *a transient but significant rise in serum thyroid hormone* when given to patients who still have substantial remaining thyroid tissue; use cautiously, and monitor closely those patients with heart disease.

- *Stroke* has occurred within 72 hours of drug administration in patients with known CNS metastases.
- *Sudden rapid tumor enlargement or pain at distant metastases* can occur after treatment with the drug with symptoms dependent upon the anatomical location of the tissue: acute hemiplegia, hemiparesis, and loss of vision 1–3 days after drug administration.
  - Laryngeal edema, pain at metastatic tumor site, and respiratory distress requiring tracheostomy have also occurred.
  - Pretreatment with glucocorticoids should be considered for patients at risk for tumor expansion that may compromise vital anatomic structures.

Potential Toxicities/Side Effects (Dose- and Schedule-Dependent) and the Nursing Process

I. ALTERATION IN COMFORT related to FLU-LIKE SYMPTOMS

Defining Characteristics: Transient flu-like symptoms can occur lasting < 48 hours, characterized by fever, chills, myalgia, arthralgia, fatigue, asthenia, malaise, headache, and chills.

Nursing Implications: Assess baseline T, VS, and comfort level, and teach patient that this may occur and how to manage uncomfortable side effects (e.g., acetaminophen). Teach patient self-care measures, including monitoring temperature, comfort level, the use of heat or cold for myalgias, arthralgias. Encourage patient to increase oral fluids and alternate rest and activity periods.

II. POTENTIAL ALTERATION IN NUTRITION, LESS THAN BODY REQUIREMENTS, related to NAUSEA, VOMITING

Defining Characteristics: Nausea is mild and occurs in 11.9%, with vomiting in 2.3% of patients. Nausea and vomiting were severe when the dose was inadvertently given intravenously.

Nursing Implications: Assess baseline nutritional status. Teach patient that nausea may occur and that vomiting is rare; self-care measures, including oral hygiene and preparing favorite high-calorie, high-protein foods ahead of time so that the patient can snack when hungry. Teach the patient to report unrelieved nausea and vomiting if it occurs.

III. ALTERATION IN COMFORT related to HEADACHE

Defining Characteristics: Headache occurs in 7.3%.

Nursing Implications: Assess baseline comfort and teach patient that these side effects may occur. Teach local comfort measures to minimize local injection reactions.

Drug: tisagenlecleucel (Kymriah)

Class: Chimeric Antigen Receptor T cell (CAR-T) therapy that is manufactured for each individual patient; Anti-CD19-CAR retroviral vector-transduced autologous T-cells; genetically modified antigen-specific immunotherapy. First in class.

Mechanism of Action: T-lymphocytes are removed from a patient's blood, then genetically reengineered to give them a specific CAR on the T Cell Receptor (TCR) that will recognize and bind to the tumor antigen, in this case CD19. CD19 is found on B-cells, both malignant B-cell acute lymphoblastic leukemia cells and normal B-lymphocytes. More specifically, the patient's T cells are given a genetically engineered receptor that allows the new supercharged T-cells to seek the specific tumor antigen when reinjected into the patient's body and also to create exponentially more of the same T-cells with the same CAR receptor in the body to continue to locate and eliminate the tumor cells with that antigen. This is accomplished by the outside of the CAR protein having a murine single-chain antibody fragment (scFv) that will recognize the CD19 target antigen. Once the CAR protein binds to the target antigen (e.g., CD19) on the cell surface, it turns on the domains within the receptor. Inside the CAR protein, the T-cell signaling domain (CD3) and costimulatory domains (CD28) coordinate T-cell activation (so that the T-cell population can expand) and T-cell persistence (so they remain in the body to locate and kill the tumor cells with the target antigen) (FDA(a), 2017). Of note, in order to get the CAR inserted into the T-cell, a retroviral-based gene therapy vector (in this case, a lentiviral vector), the vector is integrated into the chromosomes of the T cells and then directs the transcription of the tisagenlecleucel CAR (FDA(a), 2017). This ensures the CAR T-cell will keep an intact modified receptor for the life of the T cell, even if it divides, and ensures a long-term "living drug." The laboratory manufacturing the reengineered T cells must have stringent quality control standards because this affects both patient safety and the biologic activity of the CAR-T cells (FDA(a), 2017):

Indication: treatment of patients: (a) patients up to 25 years old with B-cell precursor acute lymphoblastic leukemia (ALL) that is refractory or in second or later relapse; (b) adult patients with relapsed or refractory large B-cell lymphoma after 2+ lines of systemic therapy, including diffuse large B-cell lymphoma (DLBCL) not otherwise specified, high grade B-cell lymphoma and DLBCL arising from follicular lymphoma.

Limitations of use: tisagenlecleucel is not indicated for treaetment of patients with primary CNS lymphoma.

Dosage/Range: For AUTOLOGOUS use only
- Pediatric and young adult B-cell ALL: a single dose of tisagenlecleucel contains 0.2-5.0 $\times$ 10^6 CAR-positive viable T cells per kg of body weight (patients 50 kg or less), or 0.1 $- 2.5 \times 10^8$ CAR-positive viable T cells for patients weighing > 50 kg, suspended in a patient-specific infusion bag for IV infusion.
- Adult relapsed or refractory diffuse large B-cell lymphoma: a single dose of tisagenlecleucel contains 0.6–6.0 $\times$ 10^8 CAR-positive viable T cells suspended in one or more patient-specific infusion bag for IV infusion.

Drug Administration: .
Preparing patient for tisagenlecleucel administration:
- Confirm availability of tisagenlecleucel prior to starting lymphodepletion regimen
- Lymphodepletion regimen
  - Pediatric to 25 years old relapsed or refractory B-cell ALL
    - Fludarabine 30 mg/m^2 IV daily $\times$ 4 days, and cyclophosphamide 500 mg/m^2 IV daily $\times$ 2 days starting with first dose of fludarabine.
    - Infuse tisagenlecleucel 2–14 days after completion of the lymphodepletion regimen.
  - Adult relaps ed or refractory DLBCL
    - Fludarabine 25 mg/m^2 IV daily $\times$ 3 days, and cyclophosphamide 250 mg/m^2 IV daily $\times$ 3 days starting with first dose of fludarabine.
    - Alternative lymphodepleting chemotherapy: bendamustine 90 mg/m^2 IV daily $\times$ 2 days if a patient had prior grade 4 hemorrhagic cystitis with cyclophosphamide, or demonstrates resistance to a previous cyclophosphamide containing regimen.
    - Infuse tisagenlecleucel 2–11 days after completion of the lymphodepletion regimen.
    - Lymphodepletion chemotherapy may be omitted if a patients wbc is $\leq 1 \times 10^9$/L within 1 week prior to tisagenlecleucel infusion.

Preparation of tisagenlecleucel for infusion and administration
- Delay the tisagenlecleucel infusion if a patient has unresolved serious adverse reactions from preceeding chemotherapies (e.g., pulmonary, cardiac, or hypotension), active uncontrolled infection, active GVHD, or worsening leukemia burden following lymphodepleting chemotherapy.
- Tisagenlecleucel dose may be contained in up to 3 cyropreserved patient specific infusion bags.
  - Verify the number of bags received for the dose with the Certificate of Conformance (CoC) and Certificate of Analysis (CoA).
  - Coordinate the timing of thaw of tisagenlecleucel and infusion: (1) confirm infusion time in advance and make adjust the start time of the thaw so the drug is available for infusion when the patient is ready; (2) if >1 bag has been received for the treatment dose, thaw 1 bag at a time; (3) wait to thaw/infuse the next bag until it is determined the prior bag has been safely administered.

Preparation of tisagenlecleucel for infusion
- Verify tocilizumab and emergency equipment is available prior to infusion and during recovery period.
- Premedicate patient with acetaminophen and diphenhydramine or another H1-antihistamine approximately 30–60 minutes before tisagenlecleucel infusion planned. Do Not use systemic corticosteroids as this may interfere with the drug activity.
- Confirm patient identity: Before tisagenlecleucel preparation, match the patient's identity with the patient identifiers on each tisagenlecleucel infusion bag(s). Tisagenlecleucel is for autologous use ONLY. Use universal precautions in handling drug to avoid potential transmission of infectious diseases (viral vector used in making drug). The patient identifier number may be preceded by the letters DIN or Aph ID (Novartis, 2018).

- Inspect the infusion bag(s) for any breaks or cracks prior to thawing. If a bag is compromised, do not infuse the contents and contact Novartis at 1-844-4KYMRIAH.
- Place the infusion bag inside a second sterile bag in case of a leak and to protect ports from contamination.
- Thaw each infusion bag one at a time at 37°C using either a water bath or dry thaw method until there is no visible ice in the infusion bag. Remove bag from thawing device immediately; **do not** store product bag at 37°C. Once infusion bag has thawed, and is at room temperature (20–25°C), it should be infused within 30 minutes. **Do not** wash, spin down, and/or resuspend tisagenlecleucel in new media prior to infusion.
- Inspect thawed infusion bag contents for any visible cell clumps, and if found, gently mix the contents of the bag by gentle manual mixing of small clumps of cellular material which should disperse. Do not infuse tisagenlecleucel if clumps are not dispersed, the infusion bag is leaking or damaged, orotherwise appears compromised. Call Novartis.

Administration
- Confirm patient's identify with patient identifiers on the infusion bag and have a second independent check.
- Administer tisagenlecleucel as an IV infusion at 10 mL–20 mL/min, adjusted as appropriate for smaller children and volumes. The volume in the infusion bag ranges from 10–50 mL.
  - Do NOT use a leukocyte-depleting filter
  - If >1 bag is being infused for the treatment dose, wait to thaw/infuse the next bag until it is determined that the previous bag is safely administered.
  - Prime tubing prior to infusion with normal saline.
  - Infuse all contents of infusion bag.
  - Rinse the infusion bag with 10 mL–30 mL of sterile normal saline while maintaining a closed tubing system to assure all cells in the bag and tubing are infused into the patient for the full dose..
- Use biosafety guidelines (universal precautions, PPE) inhandling and disposing of bag, tubing, etc. as drug contains human cells genetically modified with a lentivirus.

Monitoring
- Administer drug only at a certified healthcare facility.
- Monitor patient 2–3 times during first 7 days after tisagenlecleucel infusion at the certified healthcare facility for signs/symptoms of cyctokine release syndrome (CRS) and neurotoxicity.
- Teach patient to remain within the proximity of the certified healthcare facility for at least 4 weeks after the tisagenlecleucel infusion. Teach patient to come to call/come to certified healthcare facility right away if signs/symptoms or CRS or neurotoxicity appear.
- CRS: Identify based on clinical presentation, and evaluate for and treat other causes of fever, hypoxia, hypotension. If CRS suspected manage based on severity as follows (and ordered):
  - ***Prodromal syndrome***: low-grade fever, fatigue,anorexia: Observe patient and exclude infection; administer antibiotics per local guidelines if neutropenic; give symptomatic support.

- **CRS requiring mild intervention (with 1+ of the following):** high fever, hypoxia, mild hypotension. Administer antipyretics, oxygen, IV fluids and/or low dose vasopressors as needed.
- **CRS requiring moderate to aggressive intervention (with 1+ of the following):** *(1)* hemodynamic instability despite IV fluids and vasopressor support; (2) worsening respiratory distress including pulmonary infiltrates, increasing oxygen requirement including high flow O_2 and/or need for mechanical ventilation; (3) rapid clinical deterioration. Management: (a) Administer high dose or multiple vasopressors, O_2, mechanical ventilation and/or other supportive care as needed; (b) administer tocilizumab (12 mg/kg IV if <30 kg, 8 mg/kg weight ≥30 kg (max 800 mg), IV over IV; repeat tocilizumab PRN q 8 hr if no clinical improvement; if no response to second dose of tocilizumab, consider a third dose or seek alternative measures to treat CRS (limit maximum 4 tocilizumab doses). If no clinical improvement within 12–18 hr of the first tocilizumab dose, or worsening at any time, administer methylprednisolone 2 mg/kg as an initial dose, then 2 mg/kg per day until vasopressors and high flow O_2 are no longer needed, then taper.

Drug Interactions: Unknown.

Lab Effects/Interference:
- Increased proliferation of T-lymphocytes, including CD4 helper and CD8 cytotoxic T cells.
- Neutropenia, thrombocytopenia, increased C-reactive protein; prolonged B-cell aplasia resulting in hypogammaglobulinemia (continues for as long as modified T cells persist in the patient).
- Hypokalemia, hypophosphatemia.
- Increased AST, ALT, bilirubin.
- False positive HIV test.
- Reactivated HBV, HCV, HIV.

Special Considerations:
- Patient identify must be verified at every step of the process. Manufacturing quality control must be efficient for ensuring identity, safety, purity, and potency of CAR-T cells. Tisagenlecleucel is made using a self-inactivating lentiviral vector that contains extensively modified sequences from HIV-1 (FDA(a), 2017).
- Mild infusion reactions may occur and are reduced by premedication with acetaminophen and antihistamines. If a febrile reaction occurs, infection must be ruled out.
- Most common (>20%): (a) Pediatric and young adult B-cell ALL: CRS, hypogammaglobulinemia, infections-pathogens unspecified, pyrexia, decreased appetite, headache, encephalopathy, hypotension, bleeding episodes, tachycardia, nausea, diarrhea, vomiting, viral infectious disorders, hypoxia, fatigue, acute kidney injury, edema, cough and delirium; (b) adult relapsed/refractory DBLCL: CRS, infections-pathogens unspecified, pyrexia, diarrhea, nausea, fatigue, hypotension, edema, headache.
- The incidence of grade 3/4 CRS was 47%, with a median duration of 8 days. Other significant toxicities were grade 3 neurotoxicity (15%) and grade 3/4 infections within 8 days of the infusion.

- Drug is available only through a restricted program under a Risk Evaluation and Mitigation Strategy (REMS) called the Kymriah REMS.
- Warnings and Precautions:
  - *CRS:* may belief-threatening or fatal. Ensure that 2 doses of tocilizumab are available prior to drug infusion. Monitor patient for at least 4 weeks after treatment to identify CRS early and institute aggressive symptom and support. See problem I.
  - *Neurological toxicities:* Occurred frequently, and included severe or life-threatening reactions. Monitor patients closely for neurological toxicity and exclude other causes. Provide supportive care as needed. See problem II.
  - *Kymriah REMS to mitigate CRS, Nneurological toxicities:* Drug is available only through a restricted program under a Risk Evalation and Mitigation Strategy (REMS) called the Kymriah REMS. Required components are (a) healthcare facilities that dispense and administer tisagenlecleucel must be enrolled and comply with the REMS requirements, and have on-site, immediate access to tocilizumab and ensure that a minimum of 2 doses are available for each patient for administration within 2 hours after tisagenlecleucel infusion if needed for treatment of CRS; (b) certified healthcare facilities must ensure that healthcare providers who prescribe, dispense, or administer tisagenlecleucel are trained about the management of CRS and neurological toxicity.
  - *HSRs:* may occur, including anaphylaxis, due to dimethyl sulfoxide (DMSO) or dextran 40 in tisagenlecleucel.
  - *Serious infections:* may occur, including life-threatening and fatal infections. Incidence was 55% with 33% being grade 3 or higher. Febrile neutropenia occurred in 37% of ALL patients, and 17% of patients with DCBCL, and was grade 3 or higher in these patients. Prolonged cytopenias may occur, including neutropenia (40% of patients). Prior to tisagenlecleucel infusion, institute infection prophylaxis following ordered local guidelines. Do not administer tisagenlecleucel treatment if the patient has an active infection; give drug only when infection has resolved. Patient should be screened for HBV, HCV, and HIV as infection may be reactivated after drug infusion, leading to fulminant hepatitis, hepatic failure and death if HBV reactivation occurs. Monitor patients closely for signs/symptoms of infection after drug infusion, and treat promptly.
  - *Prolonged cytopenias:* may follow lymphodepleting chemotherapy and tisagenlecleucel infusion and last for several weeks. Grade 3 or higher cytopenias (neutropenia and thrombocytopenia) may not resolve by day 28, and some may persist at day 56 after tisagenlecleucel. Prolonged neutropenia is associated with increased risk of infection, but myeloid growth factors, especially GM-CSF, are not recommended during the first 3 weeks after tisagenlecleucel dose, or until CRS resolves (Novartis, 2018).
  - *Hypogammaglobulinemia* and agammaglobulinemia (IgG) related to B-cell aplasia can occur inpatients with CR after tisagenlecleucel infusion. Monitor immunoglobulin levels after treatment with tisagenlecleucel and manage with infection precautions, prophylactic antibiotics, and immunoglobulin replacement. Use of live viral vaccines during or after tisagenlecleucel therapy has not been studied. Vaccination with live viral vaccines is not recommended for at least 6 weeks before the start of lymphodepleting chemotherapy, during tisagenlecleucel therapy, and until immune recovery after tisagenlecleucel. A pregnant woman who has received tisagenlecleucel

may have hypogammaglobulinemia; newborns of these mothers should have immunoglobulin levels assessed (Novartis, 2018).

- *Secondary malignancies:* may occur, or the patient's cancer may recur. Monitor the patient life-long for secondary malignancies. Contact Novartis Pharmaceuticals Corporation to get information about patient samples to collect, at 1-844-4KYMRIAH.
- *Effects on ability to drive and use machines:* Patients should not drive for 8 weeks after tisagenlecleucel infusion as the potential for neurological events, e.g., altered mental status, seizures, decreased coordination may occur. Teach patients not to drive or operate hazardous machinery during this period.

Potential Toxicities/Side Effe cts and the Nursing Process

I.   ALTERATION IN HOMEOSTASIS, POTENTIAL, related to CYTOKINE RELEASE SYNDROME

Defining Characteristics: CRS is a systemic inflammatory response that occurs when cytokines are released into the systemic circulation by the activation and proliferation of modified T cells and the subsequent killing of normal and malignant B-lymphocytes (FDA(a), 2017). Incidence is 74–79% all grades (DLBCL and ALL patients respectively), with 23–49% grade 3/4 (DLBCL and ALL patients respectively). Onset occurred after a median of 3 days after infusion and lasted a median of 8 days. ICU care was necessary for 44% of patients, and median duration in ICU was 8 days. Symptom constellation includes high fevers, rigors, fatigue, anorexia, nausea, vomiting, diarrhea, diaphoresis, headache, encephalopathy, myalgia/arthralgia, rash, hypotension (which may require vasopressors), CLS, tachypnea, and hypoxia (which may require ventilator support). DIC and macrophage activation syndrome (MAS) may occur. CRS may be life threatening or fatal. Rarely, disseminated intravascular coagulation (DIC), CLS, and hemophagocytic lymphohistiocytosis/macrophage activation syndrome (HLH/MAS) may complicate CRS. CLS, if it occurs, is characterized by loss of vascular tone and extravasation of plasma proteins and fluid into the extravascular space. This results in hypotension and decreased organ perfusion. CLS may be associated with cardiac arrhythmias, angina, MI, respiratory insufficiency requiring intubation, GI bleeding, edema, and mental status changes. Risk factors for severe CRS in pALL patients are high pre-infusion tumor burden (>50% blasts in bone marrow), uncontrolled or accelerating tumor burden following lymphodepleting chemotherapy, active infections, and/or inflammatory processed; risk factors in patients with DLBCL are unknown.

Nursing Implications: Ensure 2 doses of tocilizumab are available on site before infusing drug. Assess baseline temperature, vital signs, pulmonary and neurologic status, and comfort level, and monitor closely for signs/symptoms of CRS for at least 4 weeks after treatment, the first week at the certified healthcare facility. Assess LFTs and other laboratory tests as ordered. Teach the patient to report and seek immediate medical attention for any difficulty breathing, fever (100.4°F/38°C or higher), chills/shaking chills, confusion, severe nausea, vomiting, diarrhea, severe muscle or joint pain, feeling dizzy or lightheaded, or other signs and symptoms of CRS. Be prepared to institute emergency medical orders, and transfer to ICU if needed. Provide supportive care via CRS algorithm and IL-6 blockade (e.g., tocilizumab).

II.   SENSORY/PERCEPTUAL ALTERATIONS related to NEUROLOGIC TOXICITY

Defining Characteristics: Incidence of severe or life-threatening neurotoxicity was 72% in ALL patients (21% grade 3 or higher), and 58% in patients with DLBCL (18% grade 3 or higher), and most (88%) occurred within 8 weeks after drug infusion. Median time to first event was 6 days, and median duration was 6 days (ALL) and 14 days (DLBCL). The onset of neurotoxicity can be concurrent with CRS, after CRS resolves, or without CRS. Most common were headache, encephalopathy, sleep disorders, dizziness, tremor, and peripheral neuropathy. Although the mechanism is not well understood, noninfectious encephalopathy/delirium has occurred with T-cell therapy, characterized by aphasia, tremor, seizures, confusion, and encephalopathy (Novartis 2018). Encephalopathy occurred in 34% of ALL patients, and 16% of DLBCL patients. If it occurred during or immediately after CRS, it was self-limiting and resolved with the treatment of CRS.

Nursing Implications: Assess baseline mental status, neurologic status, and consciousness before drug administration. Monitor closely if CRS develops to identify early neurotoxocity. Teach the patient to report any changes in mental or neurologic status, right away and to seek medical attention right away.

III.   POTENTIAL FOR INJURY related to INFECTION

Defining Characteristics: Incidence of infection was 55% after tisagenlecleucel infusion, with. 33% of infections grade 3 or higher. Febrile neutropenia occurred in 37% of ALL patients and 17% of patients with DLBCL within the 8-week postinfusion period, and may be concurrent with CRS. Prolonged cytopenias have occurred, with grade 3 or higher neutropenia which have not resolved by day 56 after tisagenlecleucel infusion, which increase the risk of infection. Risk of infection is related to both the disease process and lymphodepleting chemotherapy. HBV or other viral illness may be reactivated by tisagenlecleucel therapy; HBV reactivation has resulted in fulminating hepatitis, liver failure, and death. .

Nursing Implications: Assess patient for signs/symptoms of active infection; if found, patient should not receive tisagenlecleucel infusion until the infection has resolved. Ensure patient has had screening tests for HBV, HCV, and HIV, and that results are negative, prior to T-cell collection and manufacturing. Assess baseline CBC, ANC, and platelet count and monitor during therapy and follow-up. Evaluate for infection, including assessment of central line and blood cultures, and administer broad-spectrum antibiotics as ordered, along with IV fluids and other supportive care. Teach the patient to self-assess and to report any fever or other signs and symptoms of infection right away.

Drug: trastuzumab (Herceptin®); Biosimilars: (1) ALL indications of Herceptin (a) trastuzumab-dkst (Ogivri), (b) trastuzumab-dttb (Ontruzant), (c) trastuzumab-qyyp (Trazimera); (2) only 1 indication of Herceptin: trastuzumab-pkrb (Herzuma) with indication ONLY for treatment of HER2-overexpressing breast cancer [These biosimilar drugs are NOT interchangeable.]

Class: mAb, unconjugated, targeted against HER-2; humanized anti-HER-2 antibody; HER2/neu receptor antagonist.

Mechanism of Action: Recombinant humanized mAb targeted against the human epidermal growth factor receptor 2 (*HER-2*). *HER-2* is an oncogene that is overexpressed in a number of cancers, including 13–15% of breast cancers. The drug binds to HER-2 tightly, thus inhibiting cell signaling and cell proliferation. This mAb is believed to act through 3 different mechanisms: (1) the antagonizing function of the growth-signaling properties of *HER-2*, (2) signaling immune cells to attack and kill malignant cells with this receptor (ADCC), and (3) synergistic and/or additive effects seen with many chemotherapeutic agents. Herceptin-mediated ADCC preferentially attacks HER2 overexpressing cancer cells compared to non-HER2 expressing cells. HER-2 signaling appears necessary for repair of cardiac damage; this explains why cardiotoxicity develops when administered following a cardiotoxic agent, such as doxorubicin. Mechanisms of resistance include: (1) mutations in HER-2 receptor leading to decreased binding affinity with trastuzumab; (2) decreased expression of HER-2 receptors; (3) increased expression of HER-3; (4) activation/induction of alternative signaling pathways in the cell (Chu & DeVita, 2016).

Metabolism: Initial studies using a loading dose of 4 mg/kg followed by a weekly maintenance dose of 2 mg/kg, a mean half-life of 6 days, with a range of 1–32 days was seen. The mean half-life is 16 days (range, 11–23 days) when a loading dose of 8 mg/kg followed by a 3-weekly 6 mg/kg dose is used. Steady state is reached between weeks 6 and 37.

Indications:
Herceptin (trastuzumab), Ogivri (trastuzumab-dkst), Herzuma (trastuzumab-pkrb), Ontruzant (trastuzumab-dttb), Trazimera (trastuzumab-qyyp):
(1) *HER-2 overexpressing breast cancer*
• Adjuvant treatment of HER-2 overexpressing node-positive or node-negative (ER/PR negative or with one high-risk feature) breast cancer: breast cancer.
  • As part of a treatment regimen consisting of doxorubicin, cyclophosphamide, and either paclitaxel or docetaxel.
  • As part of a treatment regimen with docetaxel and carboplatin.
  • As a single agent following multimodality anthracycline-based therapy.
• Metastatic breast cancer.
  • In combination with paclitaxel for first-line treatment.
  • As a single agent in patients who have received one or more chemotherapy regimens for metastatic disease.

Herceptin (trastuzumab), Ogivri (trastuzumab-dkst), Ontruzant (trastuzumab-dttb), Trazimera (trastuzumab-qyyp):
(2) HER-2 overexpressing metastatic gastric cancer or gastroesophageal junction adenocarcinoma, in combination with cisplatin and capecitabine or 5-fluorouracil, in patients who have not received prior treatment for metastatic disease.

Dosage/Range:
- Assessment of HER2 protein overexpression and *HER2* gene amplification should be performed using FDA-approved tests **specific for breast or gastric cancer** by labs with demonstrated expertise.
- **DO NOT substitute Herceptin (trastuzumab) for or with ado-trastuzumab emtansine, or Herceptin-Hylecta.**
- Do not administer as an IV push or bolus. Do not mix trastuzumab with other drugs.

(1) HER-2 overexpressing breast cancer
*Adjuvant Doses and Schedule Options (for a total of 52 weeks)***:**
- When given **during and following** paclitaxel, docetaxel, or docetaxel/carboplatin:
  - Initial dose of 4 mg/kg IV infusion over 90 minutes week 1, then at 2 mg/kg as an IV infusion over 30 minutes weekly during chemotherapy for the first 12 weeks (paclitaxel or docetaxel) or 18 weeks (docetaxel/carboplatin).
  - One week following the last weekly dose of trastuzumab, administer trastuzumab at 6 mg/kg as an IV infusion over 30–90 minutes every 3 weeks.
- As a single agent within 3 weeks following completion of multimodality, anthracycline-based chemotherapy regimens:
  - Initial dose at 8 mg/kg as an IV infusion over 90 minutes.
  - Subsequent doses at 6 mg/kg as an IV infusion over 30–90 minutes every 3 weeks.
  - Extending adjuvant therapy beyond 1 year is not recommended.

*Metastatic Treatment for Breast Cancer***:**
- Administer trastuzumab, alone or in combination with paclitaxel, at an initial dose of 4 mg/kg as a 90-minute infusion, followed by subsequent once-weekly doses of 2 mg/kg as a 30-minute IV infusion, until disease progression.

(2) Metastatic Gastric Cancer:
- Administer trastuzumab at an initial dose of 8 mg/kg as a 90-minute IV infusion, followed by subsequent doses of 6 mg/kg IV infusion over 30–90 minutes every 3 weeks, until disease progression.
- **Dosing Considerations:** (1) if the patient has missed a dose of trastuzumab by ≤ 1 week, then administer the usual maintenance dose (weekly schedule 2 mg/kg; 3-weekly schedule 6 mg/kg) as soon as possible. Do not wait until next planned cycle. Subsequent trastuzumab maintenance doses should be administered 7 or 21 days later according to the weekly or 3-weekly scheduled; (2) if the patient missed a dose by >1 week, a reloading dose should be administered over approximately 90 minutes (weekly schedule 4 mg/kg; 3-weekly schedule 8 mg/kg) as soon as possible. Subsequent trastuzuab doses should be administered 7 days (2 mg/kg weekly) or 21 days (6 mg/kg every 3 weeks) later based on a weekly or 3-weekly schedule.

- *If infusion reaction occurs,* (1) decrease the rate of infusion for mild or moderate reaction; (2) interrupt the infusion in patients with dyspnea or clinically significant hypotension; (3) discontinue trastuzumab for severe or life-threatening infusion reactions.
- *Cardiomyopathy: Assess LVEF baseline* prior to starting trastuzumab therapy, and at regular intervals during treatment.
  - Hold trastuzumbab dose for at least 4 weeks for either (1) ≥ 16% absolute decrease in LVEF from pretreatment value, or (2) LVEF below institutional limits of normal and ≥ 10% absolute decrease in LVEF from pretreatment values.
  - Resume trastuzumab if, within 4–8 weeks, the LVEF returns to normal limits and the absolute decrease from baseline is ≤ 15%.
  - Permanently discontinue trastuzumab for a persistent (> 8 weeks) LVEF decline or for suspension of trastuzumab dosing on > 3 occasions for cardiomyopathy.

Drug Preparation:
- Check drug label to make sure drug being prepared is trastuzumab (Herceptin) or trastuzumab-dkst (Ogivri) and NOT ado-trastuzumab emtansine.
- Herceptin is available as a lyophilized sterile powder of 420 mg per multi-dose vial or as a single dose (150 mg) dose for parenteral administration, and Ogivri contains 420 mg of drug in the multi-dose vial. Single dose (150mg) is available with Herceptin. Requires refrigeration at 2–8°C (36–46°F). DO NOT FREEZE.
- *Multi-dose vial:* Reconstitute multi-dose vial with 20 mL of bacteriostatic water for injection, USP, containing 1.1% benzyl alcohol, to make a multidose solution containing 21 mg/mL of drug. If the patient is allergic to benzyl alcohol, reconstitute with 20 mL sterile water for injection without preservative to yield a single-use solution and use immediately after preparation. DO NOT SHAKE. *For Herceptin single-dose vial (150 mg),* add 7.4 mL sterile water for injection, to make a solution of 21 mg/mL. This single dose must be used immediately upon preparation as it contains no preservative.
- Using a sterile syringe, aseptically and slowly inject the 20 mL diluent into the vial, directing the stream into the lyophilized cake.
- Swirl the vial gently to mix; DO NOT SHAKE.
- Slight foaming may occur; allow vial to stand undisturbed for about 5 minutes.
- Inspect for particulate matter or discoloration, and if found, do not use. Solution should be clear to slightly opalescent, colorless to pale yellow, without particles.
- Store reconstituted trastuzumab at 2–8°C (36–46°F); discard unused trastuzumab after 28 days. If reconstituted with sterile water for injection without preservatives, use immediately and discard any unused portion.
- Determine the dose in mg ordered. Calculate the volume needed (reconstituted solution contains 21 mg/mL). Further dilute ordered dose in 250 mL of 0.9% sodium chloride injection, USP. DO NOT use dextrose (5%) solution. Gently invert to mix.
- Further dilute in a 250-mL infusion bag containing 0.9% Sodium Chloride Injection USP (PVC or polyethylene). Gently invert bag to mix. DO NOT USE 5% DEXTROSE SOLUTIONS.
- IV infusion bag can be stored at 2–8°C (36–46°F) for 24 hours or less prior to use. DO NOT FREEZE.

- Vial is designed for multiple use and is stable for 28 days following reconstitution at 2–8°C (36–46°F). If patient is hypersensitive to this bacteriostatic diluent, use 20 mL sterile water for injection without preservatives as a single solution (not multidose).

Drug Administration:
- Administered IV infusion; initial loading dose is administered over 90 minutes, and initial maintenance dose (week 2 or dose 2) is administered over 30–60 minutes. Never give as IV push or bolus.
- Observe patient for 1 hour following completion of initial loading dose, and if well tolerated, observe patient for 30 minutes following completion of initial maintenance dose (week or dose 2). If well tolerated, no further postinfusion observation is needed in subsequent weekly infusions.
- Subsequent maintenance doses are administered over 30 minutes if prior administration was well tolerated without fever or chills.
- Continue to administer over 90 minutes if fever, chills experienced in prior administrations.
- Assess results of ECHO or MUGA for LVEF, baseline then every 3 months and upon completion of trastuzumab therapy.
- If trastuzumab is held for significant LV dysfunction, assess LVEF findings at 4-week intervals.
- Subcutaneous administration offers comparable efficacy and safety as shown in 6-year follow-up of the HannaH trial (Jackisch et al., 2019).

Drug Interactions:
- Increased risk of cardiotoxicity when trastuzumab used in conjunction with anthracyclines and/or taxanes (Chu & DeVita, 2016).
- Doxorubicin, anthracyclines: additive cardiotoxicity; DO NOT GIVE CONCURRENTLY.
- Possible increased risk of cardiac dysfunction in patients who receive an anthracycline after stopping trastuzumab. Ideally should wait up to 7 months after stopping trastuzumab before starting anthracycline-based therapy. If anthracyclines are used before 7 months, the patient's cardiac function should be carefully monitored.
- Myelosuppressive chemotherapy: increased neutropenia and febrile neutropenia.

Lab Effects/Interference:
- Decreased LVEF; monitor baseline and throughout treatment.
- Decreased ANC when given with chemotherapy.

Special Considerations:
- HER-2 protein overexpression must be determined prior to treatment. Use FDA-approved tests for the specific tumor type (e.g., breast or gastric/GE junction adenocarcinoma) to assess HER-2 protein overexpression and HER-2 gene amplification. Use laboratories with demonstrated proficiency. FISH (tests for HER-2 gene amplification) are more accurate in identifying HER-2 overexpression; in some centers, patient tumors are tested with IHC (measures HER-2 protein overexpression), and if 2+, sent for FISH testing. IHC 3+ demonstrates definite HER-2 overexpression. Discordant lab values (false negatives or positives) occur more commonly in labs doing less than 100 tests per month (24%) compared with a lab doing 100 or more a month (3%) (Paik et al., 2002).

- Warnings and Precautions:
  - *Cardiomyopathy:* Trastuzumab can cause left ventricular (LV) cardiac dysfunction, arrhythmias, HTN, disabling cardiac failure, and cardiac death. Drug can also cause asymptomatic decline in LV ejection fraction (LVEF). Highest absolute incidence occurs when trastuzumab is administered with an anthracycline so they should not be administered concurrently. Perform a thorough cardiac assessment including LVEF by ECHO or MUGA scan baseline immediately before first dose, every 3 months during and upon completion of trastuzumab. If drug is held for significant LVEF dysfunction, repeat LVEF every 4 weeks. Once trastuzumab therapy is completed, LVEF should be assessed every 6 months for at least 2 years. See package insert for incidence of CHF in adjuvant breast cancer studies and incidence of cardiac dysfunction in metatatic breast cancer studies.
  - *Infusion reactions:* characterized by fever, chills, and possibly nausea, vomiting, pain, headache, dizziness, dyspnea, hypotension, rash and asthenia. Rarely reaction is serious and fatal and occurred during or immediately after the initial infusion. Interrupt trastuzumab infusion in all patients experiencing dyspnea, clinically significant hypotension, and intervention of medical therapy (e.g., epinephrine, corticosteroids, diphenhydramine, bronchodilators, oxygen). Continue to monitor patient closely until all signs/symptoms have resolved. If reaction is severe, consider drug discontinuation. Most reactions occur during or immediately after the drug infusion. In postmarketing reports, some patients showed improvement followed by rapid clinical deterioration, and in some instances, death occurred within hours to days following a serious infusion reaction. No data exists identifying patients that can safely be retreated after severe infusion reaction (Genetech, 2019). However, patients who had treatment resumed, after a serious IRR, received premedication with antihistamines and/or corticosteroids.
  - *Embryo-fetal toxicity:* drug can cause fetal harm. Verify pregnancy status of females of reproductive potential before beginning trastuzumab, and teach patients that exposure to the drug during pregnancy or within 7 months prior to conception can result in fetal harm. Teach females of reproductive potential to use effective contraception during trastuzumab therapy and for 7 months after last dose.
  - *Pulmonary toxicity:* Trastuzumab use can cause serious and fatal pulmonary toxicity (e.g., dyspnea, interstitial pneumonitis, pulmonary infiltrates, pleural effusions, noncardiogenic pulmonary edema, pulmonary insufficiency, hypoxia, ARDS and pulmonary fibrosis. Patients with preexisting symptomatic intrinsic lung disease or with extensive tumor in the lungs, resulting in dyspnea at rest, are at increased risk.
  - *Exacerbation of chemotherapy-induced neutropenia:* Higher incidences of grade 3–4 neutropenia and febrile neutropenia occurs in patients receiving trastuzumab with myelosuppressive chemotherapy compared to patients receiving chemotherapy alone. However, mortality was the same in both groups.
- Trastuzumab is generally very well-tolerated; given that it is a humanized antibody, no premedication is recommended
  - Severe infusion reactions and pulmonary toxicity can occur within 24 hours of the drug dose. Interrupt treatment for dyspnea or significant hypotension. Discontinue drug if patient develops anaphylaxis, angioedema, interstitial pneumonitis, or ARDS.

- Phase III clinical trials studied coadministration together with doxorubicin/cyclophosphamide (AC) showed an increased risk of subclinical and clinical cardiomyopathy (CHF and decreased LVEF). DO NOT give trastuzumab concurrently with anthracycline chemotherapy. Left ventricular function should be evaluated prior to and during treatment with trastuzumab therapy.
- Evaluate LVEF in all patients prior to and during treatment with trastuzumab. If clinically significant decrease in LVEF, discontinue trastuzumab in patients receiving adjuvant therapy and withhold in patients with metastatic disease.
- Withhold trastuzumab for $\geq$ 16% absolute decrease in LVEF from pretreatment values or an LVEF value < institutional limits of normal and $\geq$ 10% absolute decrease in LVEF from pretreatment values.
- Cardiac monitoring: Patient should have a thorough cardiac assessment, including history, physical exam, and LVEF determination (by ECHO of MUGA scan) at the recommended schedule:
  - Baseline LVEF immediately prior to beginning trastuzumab.
  - LVEF measurements every 3 months during and upon completion of trastuzumab.
  - Repeat LVEF measurements at 4-week intervals if trastuzumab is withheld for significant left ventricular cardiac dysfunction.
  - LVEF measurements every 6 months for at least 2 years following trastuzumab when used in the adjuvant setting.
- Planned assessment of LVEF is intended to prevent the development of clinical cardiomyopathy. In an Italian study, Troponin I was an independent predictor of trastuzumab-induced cardiotoxicity (able to identify patients early who would be at risk for developing trastuzumab-induced cardiotoxicity), as well as those for whom cardiotoxicity would be irreversible (Cardinale et al., 2010).
- Prophylactic beta blockade using bisoprolol prevented trastuzumab-related decreases in LVEF in a randomized, double blind adjuvant clinical trial (Pituskin, 2016).
- Resistance to trastuzumab develops with the loss of the tumor suppressor protein PTEN and hyperactivation of the P13K/AKT pathway. PTEN is a tumor suppressor that helps to ensure that the cell cycle is controlled and that uncontrolled cell division does not occur. To do this, it suppresses activation of the P13K/AKT/mTOR pathway. Thus, when PTEN is silenced, P13K/AKT is hyperactivated, which can lead to inhibition of apoptosis and resistance to drugs like trastuzumab and cisplatin (Housman et al., 2014). More recently, microRNA-21 (or miRNA-21) has been identified as the culprit in trastuzumab resistance by turning off the PTEN gene. miRNA are pieces of a gene that control cell behavior by turning certain genes on and off (Rehman et al., 2010). HER-2+ tumor cells with high levels of miRNA became resistant to trastuzumab by turning off the PTEN gene, which led to increased cell proliferation.
- Subcutaneous injection over 5 minutes of a subcutaneous formulation of trastuzumab was noninferior in terms of pharmakokinetic, efficacy, and safety, when compared to IV administration (Ismael et al., 2012). Results of the HannaH phase III RCT showed at 6 years comparable efficacy and safety of subcutaneous trastuzumab compared to IV trastuzumab (Jackisch et al., 2019).

Potential Toxicities/Side Effects and the Nursing Process

I. ALTERATION IN CIRCULATION related to CARDIOMYOPATHY

Defining Characteristics: Trastuzumab administration may result in ventricular dysfunction and congestive heart failure. The risk is significantly greater when given with doxorubicin (28% compared with 7% with AC alone), and thus, trastuzumab should NOT be given with doxorubicin and cyclophosphamide. It should begin after the completion of AC in the adjuvant setting. In addition, there is a theoretical slight increase when given together with paclitaxel, but clinical studies have shown a similar incidence of 2% when trastuzumab is given as monotherapy after adjuvant AC to that of AC followed by paclitaxel. Thus, the two drugs can be given concurrently. The 52-week incidence of trastuzumab-related cardiotoxicity, when given to follow AC concurrent with paclitaxel for 12 weeks and then as a single agent, is about 4%. If allowed to progress, failure may be severe, and the following have been reported: severe cardiac failure, death, and mural thrombosis leading to stroke. Thus, during adjuvant therapy, it is critical that cardiac function be monitored baseline and at least every 3 months. Rare events described following treatment with trastuzumab were vascular thrombosis, pericardial effusion, heart arrest, hypotension, syncope, hemorrhage, shock, and arrhythmia. Risk factors in the NSABP B-31 clinical trial were declining LVEF after completion of AC chemotherapy and increasing age.

Nursing Implications: Assess baseline cardiac function, including apical pulse, BP. Review history, and identify patients at risk who have CHF, hypertension, coronary artery disease. Patients should have baseline ECHO or gated blood pool scan to determine left ventricular ejection fraction (LVEF), and this should be monitored at least every 3 months during adjuvant trastuzumab therapy and at the conclusion of therapy. Repeat LVEF test every 4 weeks if trastuzumab is held for significant changes in LVEF. After completion of adjuvant therapy, assess LVEF every 6 months for at least 2 years. Assess for signs and symptoms at each visit: dyspnea, increased cough, paroxysmal nocturnal dyspnea, peripheral edema, S3 gallop, and decrease in left ventricular function when tested. Teach patient to report cough, weight gain, edema of ankles, difficulty breathing, or need to use more pillows at night. If patient develops a significant decrease in LVEF, the drug should be held for at least 4 weeks and LVEF repeated every 4 weeks for either of the following: (1) $\geq$ 16% absolute decrease in LVEF from pretreatment values below institutional LLN and (2) $\geq$ 10% absolute decrease in LVEF from pretreatment values and below LLN. Resume drug if within 4–8 weeks, the LVEF returns to normal limits, and the absolute decrease from baseline is 15% or less. Discontinue drug for a persistent ($>$ 8 weeks) LVEF decline or for suspension of trastuzumab dosing on more than three occasions for cardiomyopathy. LVEF should continue to be monitored every 6 months for at least 2 years following completion of trastuzumab adjuvant therapy.

Research is with ultra sensitive troponin and other biomarkers to identify early cardiotoxicity.

II.   POTENTIAL FOR INJURY related to HYPERSENSITIVITY, INFUSION RATE

Defining Characteristics: IRRs (e.g., fever and/or chills) were reported in about 40% of patients with their first treatment, and 10% with subsequent infusions. Infusion reactions are characterized by a symptom complex of fever and chills, with or without nausea, vomiting, pain (may be at tumor site), headache, dizziness, dyspnea, hypotension, rash, and asthenia. Severe HSRs are rare but have been reported, including postmarketing serious and fatal infusion reactions. Bronchospasm, anaphylaxis, angioedema, hypoxia, and severe hypotension can occur during or immediately after the infusion but may have an initial improvement followed by rapid clinical deterioration. Severe deterioration may be delayed by hours to days after a serious infusion reaction.

Nursing Implications: Assess VS baseline and frequently during infusion, especially during initial loading dose, and subsequent maintenance infusions. Observe patient for 1 hour following completion of loading dose, and 30 minutes after initial maintenance dose if loading dose was well tolerated. If not well tolerated, continue to monitor for 60 minutes until well tolerated. Notify physician if fever or chills develop and assess need for acetaminophen and slowing of infusion. Although severe allergic reactions are uncommon, have emergency equipment available and nearby, and be prepared to provide emergency support if necessary. **Stop drug if patient develops dyspnea,** severe bronchospasm, hypoxia, or severe hypotension. Notify physician/midlevel and be prepared to administer epinephrine, corticosteroids, diphenhydramine, bronchodilators, and oxygen. Discuss permanent discontinuation of drug for severe infusion reactions. A reaction can occur within 24 hours of the drug dose, and thus, if the patient is symptomatic, consider admitting patient for observation. Discontinue drug for severe and life-threatening infusion reactions. If the patient is to receive the drug again after an infusion reaction during the prior administration, discuss with the physician, and ensure that the patient is premedicated with antihistamines and corticosteroids. Monitor the patient very carefully during the infusion, as despite the premedications, severe infusion reactions can still occur.

III.   ALTERATION IN OXYGENATION, POTENTIAL, related to DYSPNEA, PULMONARY COMPLICATIONS

Defining Characteristics: After trastuzumab, patients have rarely developed serious and fatal pulmonary toxicity. Pulmonary events that have been described include dyspnea, interstitial pneumonitis, pulmonary infiltrates, pleural effusions, noncardiogenic pulmonary edema, pulmonary insufficiency, hypoxia, ARDS, and pulmonary fibrosis. These may be complications of infusion reactions.

Nursing Implications: Assess patient's baseline pulmonary status, including history of pulmonary disease, breath sounds, and respiratory rate. Patients at risk for developing pulmonary complications are (1) those with symptomatic intrinsic lung disease, and (2) those patients with extensive tumor involvement of the lungs so that they are dyspneic at rest. Monitor patients closely during the infusion, and teach patient to report any changes in respiratory function or dyspnea right away. If dyspnea or other symptoms are severe, the patient should come to the emergency room right away for evaluation.

IV. ALTERATION IN COMFORT related to PAIN, ASTHENIA

Defining Characteristics: Generalized pain may affect 11% of patients, and asthenia 5%. Abdominal pain may specifically affect 3% of patients.

Nursing Implications: Teach patients to report alterations in comfort, especially pain and dyspnea. Distinguish new onset of symptoms versus those experienced prior to treatment due to malignancy. Discuss intensity of symptoms and need for pharmacologic and non-pharmacologic interventions. Monitor response to intervention between weekly treatments, and need for alternative strategies.

V. POTENTIAL FOR INFECTION related to EXACERBATION OF CHEMOTHERAPY-INDUCED NEUTROPENIA

Defining Characteristics: In patients with metastatic breast cancer, the incidences of grades 3 and 4 neutropenia, and febrile neutropenia were higher in patients receiving trastuzumab in combination with myelosuppressive chemotherapy.

Nursing Implications: For patients with metastatic breast cancer receiving chemotherapy and trastuzumab, monitor CBC, platelet count baseline and prior to each treatment. Assess for signs and symptoms of infection (e.g., $T \geq 100.4°F$, dysuria, productive cough). Teach patient self-care measures to prevent or minimize the risk of infection. Teach patient self-assessment for signs and symptoms of infection and to call the provider immediately if they occur.

Drug: trastuzumab and hyaluronidase-oysk (Herceptin Hylecta™)

Class: HER2/neu receptor antagonist combined with hyaluronidase an endoglycosidase to permit subcutaneous (SQ) dosing.

Mechanism of Action: Recombinant humanized mAb targeted against the human epidermal growth factor receptor 2 (*HER-2*). *HER-2* is an oncogene that is overexpressed in a number of cancers, including 13–15% of breast cancers. The drug binds to HER-2 tightly, thus inhibiting cell signaling and cell proliferation. This mAb is believed to act through 3 different mechanisms: (1) the antagonizing function of the growth-signaling properties of *HER*-2, (2) signaling immune cells to attack and kill malignant cells with this receptor (ADCC), and (3) synergistic and/or additive effects seen with many chemotherapeutic agents. Herceptin-mediated ADCC preferentially attacks HER2 overexpressing cancer cells compared to non-HER2 expressing cells. HER-2 signaling appears necessary for repair of cardiac damage; this explains why cardiotoxicity develops when administered following a cardiotoxic agent, such as doxorubicin. Mechanisms of resistance include: (1) mutations in HER-2 receptor leading to decreased binding affinity with trastuzumab; (2) decreased expression of HER-2 receptors; (3) increased expression of HER-3; (4) activation/induction of alternative signaling pathways in the cell (Chu & DeVita, 2016). Hyaluronase is a polysaccharide found in the subcutaneous tissue extracellular matrix; it is depolymerized by the enzyme hyaluronidase, which increases the subcutaneous permeability for the subcutaneous injection of rituximab. Hyanuronidase increases the absorption of the drug systemically. The hyaluronidase effects are temporary, and normal skin permeability is restored within 24–48 hours.

Metabolism: Initial studies using a loading dose of 4 mg/kg followed by a weekly maintenance dose of 2 mg/kg, a mean half-life of 6 days, with a range of 1–32 days was seen. The mean half-life is 16 days (range, 11–23 days) when a loading dose of 8 mg/kg followed by a 3-weekly 6 mg/kg dose is used. Steady state is reached between weeks 6 and 37.

Indications: HER2-overexpressing breast cancer (as determined by a FDA-approved companion diagnostic for trastuzumab in laboratories with demonstrated proficiency): (1) Adjuvant treatment (node positive or node negative (ER/PR negative or with one high risk feature) (a) as part of a treatment regimen consisting of doxorubicin, cyclophosphamide, and either paclitaxel or docetaxel; (b) as part of a treatment regimen with docetaxel and carboplatin; (c) as a single agent following multi-modality anthracycline based therapy; (2) metastatic breast cancer in adults (a) in combination with paclitaxel for first-line treatment, or (b) as a single agent in patients who have received one or more chemotherapy regimens for metastatic disease.

Contraindications: None. For subcutaneous administration ONLY.

Dosage/Range:
- DO NOT SUBSTITUTE HERCEPTIN HYLECTA for or with ado-trastuzumab emtansine, or instead of any other Herceptin preparation.
- 600 mg/10,000 units (trastuzumab 600 mg/hyaluronidase 10,000 units) q 3 weeks.
- No loading dose required; no dose adjustments for patient body weight or for different concomitant chemotherapy regimens.
- Treatment duration: (a) *adjuvant*: 52 weeks (1 year) or until disease recurrence if it occurs. Do not administer for >1 year (Genentech, 2019); (b) metastatic breast cancer: continue therapy until disease progression.
- If a dose is missed, it is recommended to administer the next 600 mg/10,000 units (e.g., the missed dose) as soon as possible. Interval between subsequent Herceptin Hylecta doses should not be < 3 weeks.

Dose Modification:
- Cardiomyopathy: assess LVEF prior to starting drug, and at regular intervals during treatment. Herceptin Hylecta dosing should be held for at least 4 weeks for (a) ≥ 16% absolute decrease in LVEF from pre-treatment values, or (b) LVEF < institutional limits of normal and ≥ 10% absolute decrease in LVEF from pretreatment values.
- Drug may be resumed if, withint 4–8 weeks, the LVEF returns to normal limits and the absolute decrease from baseline is ≤15%.
- Drug should be permanently discontinued for a persistent (>8 week) LVEF decline or for suspension of Herceptin Hylecta dosing on >3 occasions for cardiomyopathy.

TREATMENT

Drug Preparation:
- Drug should be refrigerated (2°C–8°C) in the original carton and protected from light. Do not shake or freeze. Once removed from the refrigerator, the drug must be administered within 4 hours and temperature not allowed to exceed 30°C (86°F).
- Available as a 600 mg trastuzumab/10,000 units hyaluronidase (600 mg/10,000 units) single use, ready-to-use solution and does not require dilution. Inspect solution for particulate matter in solution, or discoloration prior to administration, and do not use if found. Solution should be colorless to yellowish, clear to opalescent.
- Independent double check that drug label identifies that the drug being prepared and administered is Herceptin Hylecta and NOT ado-trasntuzumab emtansine or IV trastuzumab or IV Herceptin.
- Under aseptic conditions, withdraw Herceptin/Hylecta from the vial into the syringe, replace the transfer needle with a syringe closing cap. Label the syringe with the peel-off sticker and patient name and date.
- Attach the hypodermic injection needle to the syringe immediately prior to administration followed by volume adjustment to 5 mL. Drug is compatible with polypropylene and polycarbonate syringe materials, stainless steel transfer and injection needles.
- If not used immediately, syringe can be stored in the refrigerator (2°C–8°C) for up to 24 hours, and subsequently at room temperature (20°C–25°C) °for up to 4 hours. Protect from light. Do not shake or freeze.

Drug Administration:
- Administer drug subcutaneously in left or right thigh muscle, and rotate sites.
- Administer new injections at least 2.5 cm from previous site on healthy skin and avoid areas of redness, bruising, tenderness, moles or scars, or areas that are hard. Administer the dose over 2–5 minutes.

Drug Interactions:
- Anthracyclines: potential increased risk for cardiotoxicity due to long wash-out period of Herceptin Hylecta; it is recommended to wait at least 7 months after Herceptin Hylecta treatment to begin anthracycline therapy. Continue close monitoring of cardiac function if anthracyclines are given.

Lab Effects/Interference:
- Decreased LVEF; monitor baseline and throughout treatment.
- Decreased ANC when given with chemotherapy.

Special Considerations:
- Most common adverse effects (≥10%): fatigue, arthralgia, diarrhea, injection site reaction, URI, rash, myalgia, nausea, headache, edema, flushing, pyrexia, cough, pain in extremity.
- Warnings and Precautions:
  - *Cardiomyopathy:*
    - Herceptin Hylecta can cause ventricular cardiac dysfunction, arrhythmias, HTN, cardiac failure (can be disabling), cardiomyopathy, and cardiac death.
    - Compared to patients who do not receive trastuzumab, there is a 4–6 times increase in the incidence of symptomatic myocardial dysfunction in those who receive trastuzumab either as a single agent or in combination therapy.

- The highest incidence occurs in patients when trastuzumab is administered with an anthracycline.
- The cardiac dysfunction was similar between IV and SQ administered trastuzumab.
- Cardiac Monitoring:
  - Patients should receive a thorough cardiac assessment (e.g., history, PE, study of LVEF by echocardiogram or MUGA scan).
    - Schedule:
      - Baseline LVEF immediately prior to starting Herceptin Hylecta
      - Every 3 months during and upon completion of drug therapy
      - Repeat LVEF measurement at 4 week intervals if drug is **withheld for significant LVEF dysfunction** ($\geq$ 16% absolute decrease in LVEF from pretreatment values or LVEF value below institutional limits of normal and $\geq$ 10% absolute decrease in LVEF from pretreatment values.
      - LVEF measurements every 6 months for at least 2 years after completion of Herceptin Hylecta as a component of adjuvant therapy.
  - Management: Hold drug if significant LVEF dysfunction (see bullet above).
- *Embryo-fetal toxicity:* Drug can cause fetal harm when given during pregnancy.
  - Verify the pregnancy status of female patients of reproductive potential before starting the drug.
  - Teach patients to use effective contraception during and for 7 months following treatment with Herceptin Hylecta.
- *Pulmonary Toxicity:* Pulmonary toxicity may occur and be serious or fatal.
  - Highest risk is in patients with symptomatic intrinsic lung disease, or extensive tumor involvement in the lungs resulting in dyspnea at rest.
  - Characterized by dyspnea, interstitial pneumonitis, pulmonary infiltrates, pleural effusions, non-cardiogenic pulmonary edema, pulmonary insufficiency, hypoxia, ARDS, or pulmonary fibrosis.
  - Assess patients closely, especially those patients with dyspnea at rest.
- *Exacerbation of chemotherapy-induced neutropenia:*
  - Incidence of grade 3–4 neutropenia and febrile neutropenia when given with combination myelosuppressive chemotherapy is higher when trastuzumab is.
  - Monitor patients CBC/differential (ANC) closely, and teach patient self care measures to avoid infection, and to report signs/symptoms of infection right away.
- *Hypersensitivity and administration-related reactions:*
  - Severe administrative reactions including HSR and anaphylaxis my occur, with patients having dyspnea at rest due to advanced malignancy and comorbidities at highest risk
  - Incidence of grade 1–4 HSRs was 9% and anaphylaxis 4.2%. Incidence of grades 3–4 HSR was 1%, and anaphylactic reactions was <1%.
  - Monitor patients closely especially during/after first administration.
  - Drug should be permanently discontinued in patients experiencing anaphylaxis or severe HSR.
  - Ensure emergency equipment and medications are available for immediate use if needed.

- If a patient has a grade 1–2 HSR, discuss with provider premedication with analgesic, antipyretic, and/or antihistamine prior to readministration of trastuzumab/hyaluronidase-oysk, and before subsequent doses.

Potential Toxicities/Side Effects and the Nursing Process

I. ALTERATION IN CIRCULATION related to CARDIOMYOPATHY

Defining Characteristics: Trastuzumab (in combination with hyaluronidase-oysk) administration may result in ventricular dysfunction and congestive heart failure. The risk is significantly greater when trastuzumab is given with doxorubicin (28% compared with 7% with AC alone), and thus, trastuzumab should NOT be given with doxorubicin and cyclophosphamide. It should begin after the completion of AC in the adjuvant setting. In addition, there is a theoretical slight increase when given together with paclitaxel, but clinical studies have shown a similar incidence of 2% when trastuzumab is given as monotherapy after adjuvant AC to that of AC followed by paclitaxel. Thus, the two drugs can be given concurrently. The 52-week incidence of trastuzumab-related cardiotoxicity, when given to follow AC concurrent with paclitaxel for 12 weeks and then as a single agent, is about 4%. If allowed to progress, failure may be severe, and the following have been reported: severe cardiac failure, death, and mural thrombosis leading to stroke. Thus, during adjuvant therapy, it is critical that cardiac function be monitored baseline and at least every 3 months. Rare events described following treatment with trastuzumab were vascular thrombosis, pericardial effusion, heart arrest, hypotension, syncope, hemorrhage, shock, and arrhythmia. Risk factors in the NSABP B-31 clinical trial were declining LVEF after completion of AC chemotherapy and increasing age.

Nursing Implications: Assess baseline cardiac function, including apical pulse, BP. Review history, and identify patients at risk who have CHF, hypertension, coronary artery disease. Patients should have baseline ECHO or gated blood pool scan to determine left ventricular ejection fraction (LVEF), and this should be monitored at least every 3 months during adjuvant trastuzumab therapy and at the conclusion of therapy. Repeat LVEF test every 4 weeks if trastuzumab is held for significant changes in LVEF. After completion of adjuvant therapy, assess LVEF every 6 months for at least 2 years. Assess for signs and symptoms at each visit: dyspnea, increased cough, paroxysmal nocturnal dyspnea, peripheral edema, S3 gallop, and decrease in left ventricular function when tested. Teach patient to report cough, weight gain, edema of ankles, difficulty breathing, or need to use more pillows at night. If patient develops a significant decrease in LVEF, the drug should be held for at least 4 weeks and LVEF repeated every 4 weeks for either of the following: (1) $\geq$ 16% absolute decrease in LVEF from pretreatment values below institutional LLN and (2) $\geq$ 10% absolute decrease in LVEF from pretreatment values and below LLN. Resume drug if within 4–8 weeks, the LVEF returns to normal limits, and the absolute decrease from baseline is 15% or less. Discontinue drug for a persistent (> 8 weeks) LVEF decline or for suspension of trastuzumab dosing on more than three occasions for cardiomyopathy. Research is ongoing in an effort to find sensitive biomarkers to identify early cardiotoxicity, e.g., troponin.

II.   POTENTIAL FOR INJURY related to HYPERSENSITIVITY, INFUSION RATE

Defining Characteristics: Patients receiving trastuzumab (in combination with hyaluronidase-oysk) may experience severe administration related reactions. Grade 1–4 HSRs occurred in 9% of patients, while 4.2% experienced anaphylaxis in studies (HannaH, SafeHER, Genetech, 2019). Grade 3–4 HSR occurred in 1%, and anaphylactic reactions occurred in <1%. Patients experiencing dyspnea at rest due to advanced breast cancer or comorbidities may be at increased risk (Genetech, 2019).

Nursing Implications: Closely monitor patients for systemic HSRs especially during, after first treatment. Assess VS baseline and after injection. Have emergency equipment and emergency drugs available and nearby, and be prepared to provide emergency support if necessary. **Stop drug injection if patient develops dyspnea,** severe bronchospasm, hypoxia, or severe hypotension. Notify physician/midlevel and be prepared to administer epinephrine, corticosteroids, diphenhydramine, bronchodilators, and oxygen. Discuss permanent discontinuation of drug for severe infusion reactions. If the patient has a grade 1–2 HSR, discuss premedication with an analgesic, antipyretic and/or antihistamine prior to readministration and before subsequent treatments.

III.   ALTERATION IN OXYGENATION, POTENTIAL, related to DYSPNEA, PULMONARY COMPLICATIONS

Defining Characteristics: After trastuzumab (in combination with hyaluronidase-oysk), patients have rarely developed serious and fatal pulmonary toxicity. Pulmonary events that have been described include dyspnea, interstitial pneumonitis, pulmonary infiltrates, pleural effusions, noncardiogenic pulmonary edema, pulmonary insufficiency, hypoxia, ARDS, and pulmonary fibrosis. Patients with symptomatic intrinsic lung disease or with extensive pulmonary tumor involvement with dyspnea at rest may be at increased risk for severe toxicity.

Nursing Implications: Assess patient's baseline pulmonary status, including history of pulmonary disease, breath sounds, and respiratory rate, and prior to each injection. Monitor patients closely between treatments, and teach patient to report any changes in respiratory function or dyspnea right away. If dyspnea or other symptoms are severe, the patient should come to the emergency room or seen by their oncology provider right away for evaluation.

IV.   POTENTIAL FOR INFECTION related to EXACERBATION OF CHEMOTHERAPY-INDUCED NEUTROPENIA

Defining Characteristics: The incidences of grades 3 and 4 neutropenia, and febrile neutropenia were higher in patients receiving trastuzumab in combination with myelosuppressive chemotherapy than patients receiving chemotherapy alone. However, the incidence of septic death was similar between both groups (Genetech, 2019).

Nursing Implications: Monitor CBC/differential (ANC), platelet count baseline and prior to each treatment. Assess for signs and symptoms of infection (e.g., $T \geq 100.4°F$, dysuria, productive cough). Teach patient self-care measures to prevent or minimize the risk of infection. Teach patient self-assessment for signs and symptoms of infection and to call the provider immediately if they occur.

Drug: ziv-aflibercept (Zaltrap®)

Class: Angiogenesis inhibitor: VEGF trap, recombinant fusion protein.

Mechanism of Action: Drug is a soluble decoy receptor that binds to VEGF-A, VEGF-B, and placental growth factor (PIGF) so that the VEGF growth factors cannot bind to their receptors on the endothelial cells. It is made up of portions of the external receptors (extracellular domains of VEGF Receptor 1 and 2) for the VEGF ligands, that are fused to the Fc (constant region) of a human IgG1 antibody. The fusion protein attracts VEGFs (VEGF-A, B, PIGF) more strongly than do the tumor VEGF receptors so that VEGF binds to the trap and not to the tumor VEGF receptors. This theoretically inhibits tumor angiogenesis and causes the tumor to regress (shrink). VEGFs have an 800 times stronger affinity to aflibercept than to bevacizumab.

Metabolism: Terminal elimination half-life is 4–7 days. Steady state is reached by the second dose. Patients weighing $\geq$ 100 kg had a 29% increase in systemic exposure compared to patients weighing 50–100 kg. There are no changes in pharmacokinetics in patients with mild or moderate hepatic dysfunction, or mild, moderate, or severe renal impairment. The drug was not studied in patients with severe liver impairment.

Indication: Drug is indicated for the treatment of patients with mCRC that is resistant to or has progressed following an oxaliplatin-containing regimen, in combination with 5-fluorouracil, leucovorin, irinotecan (FOLFIRI).

Dosage/Range: 4 mg/kg IV infusion every 2 weeks in combination with 5-fluorouracil, leucovorin, irinotecan (FOLFIRI).

Dose Modifications:
- Temporarily suspend drug for (1) at least 4 weeks before elective surgery; (2) recurrent or severe hypertension until controlled; upon resumption of drug, permanently dose-reduce to 2 mg/kg; (3) proteinuria $\geq$ 2 g/24 hr and resume drug when urine protein $<$ 2 g/24 hr. For recurrent proteinuria, suspend drug until proteinuria is $<$ 2 g/24 hr, and then permanently reduce aflibercept dose to 2 mg/kg.
- Discontinue drug for (1) severe hemorrhage, (2) GI perforation, (3) compromised wound healing, (4) fistula formation, (5) hypertensive crisis or hypertensive encephalopathy, (6) arterial thrombotic events (ATE), (7) nephrotic syndrome or thrombotic microangiopathy (TMA), (8) RPLS.

Drug Preparation:
- Available in single-use vials: 100 mg/4 mL (25 mg/mL), and as 200 mg/8 mL (25 mg/mL). Inspect vial before use: drug is clear, colorless to pale yellow solution. Do not reenter the vial after initial puncture. Withdraw ordered dose and dilute in 0.9% sodium chloride or

5% dextrose solution for injection USP to achieve a final concentration of 0.6–8 mg/mL. Use PVC infusion bags containing bis-(2-ethylhexyl) phthalate (DEHP) or polyolefin infusion bags.
- Store diluted drug at 2–8°C (36–46°F) for up to 24 hours. Discard any unused portion left in the infusion bag.

Administration:
- Assess CBC/differential baseline and before each cycle. Ensure that ANC ≥ 1.5×10^9/L. Assess urine dipstick/urinalysis for protein.
- Administer as an IV infusion over 1 hour, through a 0.2 micron polyethersulfone filter (do not use polyvinylidene fluoride (PVDF) or nylon filters), every 2 weeks. *Do not administer IV push or bolus.* Administer prior to any component of FOLFIRI regimen on the day of treatment. Do not combine aflibercept with other drugs in the same infusion bag or IV line. Administer using an infusion set made of (1) PVC containing DEHP, (2) DEHP-free PVC containing trioctyl-trimellitate (TOTM), (3) polypropylene, (4) polyethylene-lined PVC, or (5) polyurethane.

Drug Interactions:
- None known, but specific studies not done.

Lab Effects/Interference:
- Proteinuria (62% of patients in the VELOUR study).
- Leukopenia, thrombocytopenia, neutropenia.
- Increased serum creatinine.
- Increased AST, ALT.

Special Considerations:
- Drug has angiogenesis inhibitor class (side) effects: hypertension, proteinuria (although the incidence is higher with aflibercept compared to bevacizumab), GI, hemorrhage, and compromised wound healing.
- Warnings and Precautions:
  - *Hemorrhage:* drug increases risk of hemorrhage. Monitor patients for signs/symptoms of bleeding. Discontinue drug if hemorrhage is severe.
  - *GI perforation:* Monitor for signs/symptoms of GI perforation, and discontinue drug if it develops.
  - *Compromised wound healing:* Suspend drug at least 4 weeks prior to elective surgery, and do not resume for at least 4 weeks following major surgery and until the surgical wound is fully healed. Grade 3 impaired wound healing occurred in 0.3% of patients compared to 0 in the placebo/FOLFIRI arm. Minor surgery such as port placement, biopsy, or tooth extraction; drug may be resumed after the surgical wound has fully healed.
  - *Fistula formation:* Higher incidence of GI and non-GI fistula compared to patients receiving chemotherapy alone. In patients with mCRC, sites of fistulae were anal, enterovesical, enterocutaneous, colovaginal, and intestinal sites. Discontinue drug if fistuala develops.
  - *HTN:* monitor BP and treat hypertension. Monitor BP every 2 weeks or more frequently as clinically indicated during therapy. Treat with appropriate antihypertensive

agent(s) and continue monitoring BP regularly. Temporarily suspend drug if hypertension is uncontrolled. Discontinue drug if hypertensive crisis or hypertensive encephalopathy develops.

- *Arterial thrombotic events (ATE):* e.g., TIAs, CVA, angina pectoris, may develop. Drug should be discontinued if ATE occur.
- *Proteinuria:* Severe proteinuria, nephrotic syndrome and thrombotic microangiopathy (TMA) occurred more frequently in patients treated with ziv-aflibercept. Monitor urine protein and/or urinary protein/creatinine ratio (UPCR) for the development or, or worsening of proteinuria during therapy. If patients have a dipstick of ≥2+ for protein, or a UPCR >1, obtain a 24-hour urine collection for protein. Hold drug for proteinuria ≥2 g/24 hours, and resume when proteinuria is < 2 g/24 hr. If it recurs, hold drug until proteinuria is < 2 g/24 hr, and then permanently dose reduce ziv-alflibercept. Discontinue drug if patient develops nephrotic syndrome or TMA.
- *Neutropenia and neutropenic complications:* The incidence of febrile neutropenia and neutropenic infection was higher in group receiving ziv-alflibercept. Monitor CBC, differential baseline prior to starting drug, and before starting each cycle. Delay ziv-alflibercept/FOLFIRI until ANC is 1,500/mm^3 or higher.
- *RPLS:* Patients with suspected RPLS should have an MRI, and if diagnosis confirmed, ziv-alflibercept should be discontinued. Symptoms usually resolve or improve within days after drug discontinuance.
- *Diarrhea and dehydration* may be severe and the incidence of severe diarrhea is increased in patients receiving aflibercept/FOLFIRI (grades 3–4 in 19% vs. 8% receiving FOLFIRI alone); ensure that patients are monitored closely, taught to report symptoms and to remain hydrated. Incidence of diarrhea is increased in patients age 65 or older, compared to those < 65 years old; monitor elderly patients with diarrhea more closely.
- *Embryo-fetal toxicity:* Drug may cause fetal harm. Females and males of reproductive potential should use highly effective contraception to prevent pregnancy

- Most common side effects (incidence ≥ 20%) were leukopenia, diarrhea, neutropenia, proteinuria, increased AST, stomatitis, fatigue, thrombocytopenia, increased ALT, hypertension, decreased weight, anorexia, epistaxis, abdominal pain, dysphonia, increased serum creatinine, and headache.
- Grades 3–4 drug side effects of aflibercept plus FOLFIRI were diarrhea, asthenia, fatigue, stomatitis, infection, hypertension, GI or abdominal pain, neutropenia or neutropenic complications, and proteinuria.

Potential Toxicities/Side Effects and the Nursing Process

I. **POTENTIAL ALTERATION IN CIRCULATION related to HYPERTENSION, ARTERIAL THROMBOTIC EVENTS (ATE), HEMORRHAGE**

Defining Characteristics: Hypertension is a class effect of angiogenesis inhibitors, and it may occur. In general, hypertension was more common (41% of patients) with 20% grade 3 or higher, than with bevacizumab combined with FOLFIRI in the 1st line setting of mCRC (AVIRI study, 28% overall, 10% grade 3 or higher). ATE occurred in 2.6% (grades 3–4, 1.8%) of patients compared to 1.7% (0.7%) in patients receiving placebo plus FOLFIRI.

The incidence of bleeding/hemorrhage in study patients was 38% (3% grades 3–4) compared to 19% (1% grades 3–4) in patients receiving placebo/FOLFIRI.

Nursing Implications: Assess baseline BP prior to and during treatment, at least for the first treatment, then prior to each drug infusion. If the patient has a history of hypertension, monitor BP more closely, although hypertension develops over time rather than during the drug infusion. BP monitoring should continue after the patient has stopped the drug. Teach patient potential drug side effects and self-care measures. Discuss prescription of antihypertensive medications as needed. Angiotensin-converting enzyme (ACE) inhibitors or angiotensin II receptor blockers are preferred as they have low interaction potential with angiogenesis inhibitors, help reduce proteinuria, and prevent the expression of plasminogen-activator inhibitor-1 (may be stimulated by angiogenesis inhibitors and increasing risk of thrombosis) (Izzedine et al., 2007; Wang & Lockhart, 2012). Review patient medical history for history of bleeding, hemorrhage, or ATEs. Assess patient for signs/symptoms of bleeding, or arterial thrombotic events, and teach patient to report/seek emergency care immediately if any bleeding or ATE events occur.

II.   POTENTIAL FOR FLUID VOLUME DEFICIT related to DIARRHEA, DEHYDRATION

Defining Characteristics: The incidence of diarrhea and dehydration is increased when aflibercept is added to FOLFIRI. Diarrhea in the combination occurred in 69% of patients (19% grades 3–4) compared to 57% (8% grades 3–4) in patients receiving placebo/FOLFIRI. Dehydration was similarly increased: combination: 9% (4% grades 3–4) versus 3% (1% grades 3–4) in the placebo/FOLFIRI group. Incidence of diarrhea is increased in patients age 65 or older, compared to those < 65 years old.

Nursing Implications: Assess baseline bowel elimination and hydration status. Teach patient that these side effects may occur and to report uncontrolled diarrhea (persisting > 24 hours despite antidiarrheal medication) or inability to drink 2–3 L of fluid in 24 hours. Involve caregiver in the discussion and emphasize need to drink fluids, 8 oz an hour while awake, to maintain hydration status, especially fluids that contain salt or electrolytes. Teach patient to take immodium per irinotecan recommendations (4 mg at first instance of diarrhea, then 2 mg every 2 hours until 12 hours without diarrhea) to prevent uncontrolled diarrhea and to report severe (persistent, bloody, or with mucus). If the patient is elderly, telephone the patient a day or two following treatment to assess tolerance and status and to report any difficulties early. Teach patient to self-assess temperature, as (FOLFIRI) nadir may occur while the patient is experiencing diarrhea, leading to sepsis.

III.   POTENTIAL FOR INFECTION AND BLEEDING related to NEUTROPENIA, THROMBOCYTOPENIA

Defining Characteristics: Neutropenia and neutropenic complications are more common when aflibercept is added to FOLFIRI than FOLFIRI alone. The incidence of neutropenia was 67% (37% grades 3–4) in the combination group compared to 57% (30% grades 3–4) in the placebo/FOLFIRI group. Febrile neutropenia occurred in 4% of patients receiving the combination, compared to 2% of patients receiving placebo/FOLFIRI. Neutropenic infection/sepsis occurred in 1.5% of patients compared to 1.2% treated with placebo/FOLFIRI. Thrombocytopenia occurred more frequently in the combination arm (48% [3% grades 3–4]) versus 35% (2% grades 3–4) in the placebo/FOLFIRI arm. Epistaxis occurred in 28% patients (0.2% grades 3–4) in the combination arm, compared to 7% in the placebo/FOLFIRI arm.

Nursing Implications: Assess patient baseline and prior to each treatment for risk of infection as well as signs and symptoms of infection and bleeding. Ensure that ANC $\geq$ 1.5×10^9/L. Teach patient self-care measures to avoid infection (e.g., avoid crowds, avoid close proximity to people with colds, wash hands frequently, but especially after touching anything that may be unclean), and to self-assess for signs/symptoms of infection (e.g., temperature $\geq$ 100.4°F, productive cough, pain on urination) and to report these right away. Teach patient and caregiver that diarrhea will increase the risk for infection if the ANC is low and to contact the nurse or physician immediately with a fever and uncontrolled diarrhea. Teach patient to avoid injury and increased risk for bleeding. Review medication profile and ensure the patient is not taking aspirin or NSAIDs. Teach patient to report signs/symptoms of bleeding right away. Teach patient to apply pressure to the bridge of the nose if epistaxis occurs, and to report a nosebleed that does not resolve in 15–20 minutes.

Drug: zoster vaccine live (Zostavax®)

Class: Vaccine.

Mechanism of Action: Initially, varicella zoster virus (VZV) produces chickenpox (varicella). The virus remains dormant in dorsal root or sensory ganglia until reactivation, when zoster occurs. In the body, as the VZV-specific immunity decreases, the virus can become reactivated. The person develops painful, vesicular lesions along a dermatome distribution of the body (on one side). Pain can occur during the prodrome, acute eruptive phase, and the postherpetic phase, which is called post-herpetic neuralgia. Serious complications of herpes zoster, besides pain, include cranial and motor palsies, encephalitis, visual impairment, hearing loss, and death. The vaccine appears to boost varicella-zoster virus immunity to protect against zoster and its complications (Merck, 2019).

Metabolism: Vaccine is a live attenuated virus vaccine.
• Unknown.

Indication: For the prevention of herpes zoster (shingles) in individuals 50 years of age and older. It is not indicated for the treatment of zoster or postherpetic neuralgia or prevention of primary varicella infection (chickenpox).

Contraindication: Patients (1) with a history of anaphylactic/anaphylactoid reaction to gelatin, neomycin, or any other component of the vaccine; (2) with immunosuppression or immunodeficiency; (3) who are pregnant.

Dosage/Range:
- Entire contents (0.65 mL) of reconstituted vaccine lyophilized vial containing at least 19,400 PFU (plaque-forming units) of OKA/Merck strain VZV.

Drug Preparation:
- Remove the lyophilized vaccine powder from the freezer, and immediately and aseptically reconstitute using the provided diluent (stored at room temperature), using a sterile syringe and needle. Inject the entire volume of diluent, and gently agitate the vial to mix thoroughly but not to cause foaming.
- When reconstituted, solution is a semi-hazy to translucent, off-white to pale yellow liquid.
- Use within 30 minutes of reconstitution, but ideally drug should be given immediately after reconstitution to minimize loss of potency.
- Draw up entire contents of vial, and inject subcutaneously into subcutaneous tissue of upper arm (preferable).
- Vaccine lyophilized powder should be stored in the freezer at 15°C (+5°F) or colder, and protect from light. Diluent can be stored at room temperature or in the refrigerator.

Drug Admiinistration:
- Use within 30 minutes of reconstitution, but ideally drug should be given immediately after reconstitution to minimize loss of potency. Draw up entire contents of vial, and inject subcutaneously into subcutaneous tissue of upper arm (preferable).
- Teach women of reproductive potential to use effective contraception to avoid pregnancy for 3 months after the vaccination.

Drug Interactions:
- Pneumovax23 given concurrently: reduced immune response to zoster vaccine live was observed in patients receiving both pneumovax and zoster vaccine live. At least 4-week separation between administration of each drug recommended.

Lab Effects/Interference:
- None known.

Special Considerations:
- Drug is a live, attenuated virus, which may cause more extensive vaccine-associated rash in patients who are immunosuppressed; the drug's efficacy in patients receiving immunosuppressive drugs, inhaled, oral low-dose, or topical corticosteroids, has not been studied. Drug is contra-indicated in patients who are immunosuppressed.
- Warnings and Precautions:
  - *HSRs*, including anaphylaxis: have occurred. Have emergency medications (e.g., epinephrine 1,000 for IM injection) available for use if anaphylactic/anaphylactoid reactions occur, as ordered.
  - *Transmission of vaccine virus* may occur between vaccines and susceptible contacts. Use protective biohazard precautions when preparing the drug.
  - *Concurrent illness:* If acute illness (e.g., fever) or in patients with active untreated TB, defer vaccination.

- *Limitations of vaccine effectiveness:* Protection is not conferred for all vaccine recipients. The duration of protection beyond 4 years after vaccination is unknown, as is the need for revaccination (Merck, 2019).
- Avoid pregnancy for 3 months following vaccination.
- Most common adverse effects (occurring in ≥1% of patients) were injection-site reactions and headache.
- Overall vaccine efficacy is 51% (64% in those aged 60–69; 41% in those aged 70–79; and 18% for those patients aged ≥ 80).
- Drug is NOT a substitute for the vaccine VARIVAX (Varicella Virus Live Vaccine).
- Patients should be taught there is a theoretical risk of transmitting the live vaccine to varicella-susceptible individuals.

Potential Toxicities/Side Effects (Dose- and Schedule-Dependent) and the Nursing Process

I. ALTERATION IN COMFORT related to INJECTION-SITE REACTIONS, RASH, AND HEADACHE

Defining Characteristics: Injection-site reactions included erythema (34%), pain/tenderness (34%), swelling (24%), and pruritus (7%). Headache occurred in 1.4% of patients. Rarely, patients can develop varicella rash.

Nursing Implications: Assess baseline comfort, and teach patient that these side effects may occur. Teach local comfort measures to minimize local injection reactions. Teach patient to report rash right away, and to avoid contact with varicella-sensitive individuals, especially pregnant women.

Chapter 5
Chemobiotherapy for Noncancer Diseases

Today, a number of autoimmune diseases, such as rheumatoid arthritis (RA), are being treated with chemotherapy or biotherapy (here defined by the general term *chemotherapy*), using drugs that in many cases have traditionally been used to treat cancer. This chapter will focus on treatment of RA. Drug administration and care of the patient receiving the drug often become the responsibility of the oncology infusion nurse, or the generalist nurse on a medical–surgical unit. Although oncology nurses usually have resources to learn about such drugs, generalist nurses lack these resources. It is important to understand the rationale for using these drugs, as well as the drug mechanism of action, potential side effects, and nursing implications to administer the drugs safely, as they are considered hazardous. The Oncology Nursing Society (ONS, 2017) has issued a position statement on the education of the RN who administers and cares for individuals receiving chemotherapy and biotherapy, and this includes the following, which the RN will find in the 2020 ONDH:

- Principles, types, classifications, and pharmacology of chemotherapy and biotherapy.
- Pertinent biomarkers.
- Chemotherapy and radiotherapy protectants.
- Principles of safe preparation, storage, labeling, transportation, and disposal of chemotherapeutic and biologic agents.
- Administration procedures.
- Appropriate use and disposal of personal protective equipment (PPE).
- Assessment, monitoring, and management of patients receiving therapy in the care setting.
- Patient and family education for these agents, specific to side effects and related symptom management and processes for urgent and ongoing follow-up.
- Assessment of education on and management of posttreatment care, including follow-up care procedures, late or long-term side effects and physical and psychosocial aspects of survivorship.

Following discussion of why these agents are used to treat RA, this chapter presents selected drugs FDA-indicated for its treatment. Please see *Chapter 1 Introduction* for nursing assessment of the patient prior to chemotherapy administration, and standardized nursing care plan for the management of hypersensitivity reactions (HSRs)/infusion reactions. Please also see *Chapter 1* for a discussion of methotrexate (MTX), and *Chapter 4* for a discussion of rituximab and monoclonal antibodies.

Autoimmune diseases represent the third-largest major illness group in the United States, and it includes more than 100 distinct diseases (AARDA, 2013). One of the most common autoimmune diseases is RA. While the side effect profile of many of the drugs used to treat autoimmune diseases is similar to those used to treat patients with cancer, the doses are usually lower so the side effects are less frequent or severe. However, certain side effects remain the same: HSRs and secondary infections (Zack, 2012).

The cause of RA is not known, but hormones, environmental factors such as smoking and genetic factors may all play a role (RA Fact Sheet, 2008). The disease affects more than a million people and tends to affect women more than men; the peak incidence is between ages 35 and 50 years (Dewing et al., 2012). The average age of the person with RA is 66.8 years (Helmick et al., 2008). RA is characterized by chronic inflammation of the joint lining with subsequent destruction of the underlying cartilage and bone, orchestrated by a flawed immune system. This leads to disability and increased morbidity.

Normally, the immune system is very powerful in identifying and removing invading microorganisms from the body, and also identifying and removing abnormal or damaged cells like cancer cells. The body is able to identify antigens that are "self" (by recognizing HLA or human leukocyte antigen) and distinguish the antigen from "nonself" (i.e., foreign). Foreign antigens are targeted and neutralized. The immune system does this by directly attacking the invading organism or foreign antigen by macrophages, dendritic cells, and killer T-lymphocytes, and also calling in other immune cells to kill cells elsewhere in the body with the same antigen. Once the foreign antigen is located, white blood cells migrate to the area and begin an inflammatory response. Macrophages and dendritic cells can mount fragments of the antigen on the cell surface and become antigen-presenting cells (APCs). They travel to a lymph node to become activated, and then signal more immune cell elements to attack any cell that has this antigen. It also uses inflammatory cytokines such as tumor necrosis factor (TNF-α), a proinflammatory cytokine, and by making an antibody that coats the foreign antigen, it attracts more immune cells. Complement proteins work with antibodies to punch holes in the cell membrane of the invading cell with the foreign antigen, killing it. Once the war against the invader is won, the body needs to turn off the immune fight so that normal cells and tissues are not harmed. Because the immune system is so powerful, specialized regulatory T-lymphocytes usually turn off the immune attack once the invading microorganism (e.g., antigen) is neutralized.

However, in RA, the immune system does not recognize antigens on cells lining the joint that belong to self (the body); the immune system makes autoantibodies against the normal cells in the lining of the synovium (joint lining). Once activated, the T-lymphocytes and macrophages invade the synovial lining and cause the proinflammatory cytokine TNF-α and interleukins (IL-1, 2, 6, 8, 10, 17) to be released. This results in inflammation and proliferation of the synovial tissue and cartilage, along with bone destruction. Interleukin (IL) is also a proinflammatory cytokine and is very important in communicating and orchestrating inflammatory responses. IL-6 is also produced in the joint by synovial and endothelial cells when the joint becomes inflamed. Sarilumab (Kevzara) is an IL-6 receptor antagonist indicated for the treatment of adult patients with moderate to severe RA. In addition, B-lymphocytes infiltrate the synovium, produce immunoglobulins, and activate synovial fibroblasts that destroy the matrix and tissue of the joint. Unfortunately, the regulatory T-lymphocytes do not shut off the immune response. The inflammation is chronic and leads to a thickened synovium and swollen joints. Over time, the immune elements in the inflamed synovium invade and destroy the underlying joint cartilage and bone, as discussed above. RA usually affects symmetric joints, often the wrist and finger joints, which become warm, edematous, and tender. RA symptoms include morning stiffness, which improves with movement, and it may also include systemic symptoms of anorexia, weakness, low-grade fever, and fatigue (Dewing et al., 2012).

The goal of treatment is medical remission or low disease activity (Singh et al., 2016), using NSAIDs and disease-modifying anti-rheumatic drugs (DMARDs). It has been found that joint damage from RA occurs early, often within the first 2 years following diagnosis (El-Miedany, 2002). While DMARDs should be started upon diagnosis, they are often delayed. In 2015, the American College of Rheumatology (ACR) guidelines were updated to guide rheumatologists in the management of RA. Recommendations are based on how long the person has had RA, how severe the RA is, and what prior treatments the patient has received. The 2015 American College of Rheumatology Guideline for the Treatment of Rheumatoid Arthritis outlines treatment strategies (see reference citation to access online).

NSAIDs, including selective COX-2 inhibitors, help to promote comfort by reducing the production of proinflammatory and pain-producing prostaglandins, and salicylates, which are used together with DMARDs (Dewing et al., 2012). In order to reduce the occurrence of adverse effects, medications to protect the stomach should be taken along with, or combined with the NSAID (e.g., proton pump inhibitor, or combination ibuprofen+famotidine, or naproxen+lansoprazole). Low-dose oral glucocorticoids, low-dose delayed-release prednisone, or glucocorticoid injections are sometimes used short-term to help control pain until a DMARD is effective (Dewing et al., 2012).

DMARDs are categorized as nonbiologic or biologic. Nonbiologic therapies are used first and include hydroxychloroquine, leflunomide, MTX, minocycline, and sulfasalazine. MTX is a well-known chemotherapeutic agent that is a folic acid antagonist and is used first line (Wilkie, 2010). Patients receiving MTX should have their LFTs assessed baseline, at 1 month, and then every 8–12 weeks to identify any potential liver toxicity. Folic acid 1–2 mg daily should be prescribed with MTX to minimize the occurrence of side effects (e.g., stomatitis, nausea, hepatic toxicity, alopecia [Wilkie, 2010]).

Biologic DMARDs target either receptors on the B-lymphocytes that help orchestrate inflammation, or proinflammatory cytokines that cause inflammation and joint damage. They are classified as non-TNF or anti-TNF. TNF-α is a proinflammatory cytokine. Non-TNF biologics are abatacept (Orencia, a fully human monoclonal antibody that binds to CD80/86 on the lymphocyte, blocking activation of T-lymphocytes), rituximab (Rituxan, a monoclonal antibody that depletes circulating B lymphocytes with CD20 on their cell surface), and tocilizumab (Actemra, which binds to IL-6 receptors, blocking proinflammatory changes). Anti-TNF biologics are used second line, and include adalimumab (Humira), certolizumab pegol (Cimzia), etanercept (Enbrel), golimumab (Simponi), and infliximab (Remicade). When used, infliximab should be combined with MTX to prevent neutralizing antibodies to infliximab (Wilkie, 2010). The anti-TNF agents are significantly immunosuppressive. All patients should be screened for TB before starting anti-TNF therapy. TNF is critical for the formation of granulomas, so when blocking TNF, TB may complicate therapy (Wilkie, 2010). Because of the immunosuppressive action of anti-TNF agents, infections can progress quickly and become severe; patients need to be taught self-assessment of signs/symptoms of infection and to report them right away. The drug should be interrupted as the patient receives anti-infective therapy. Anti-TNF agents may also increase the risk of CHF, malignancy, and very rarely, demyelinating disease (e.g., multiple sclerosis).

The severity of the patient's RA, symptom duration, risks vs. benefits, and comorbidities help the rheumatologist determine which agents should be used. As a better understanding of the specific immune elements involved in RA emerges, new biological agents will emerge. Tofacitinib (Xeljanz), a Janus kinase inhibitor, is an oral small molecule kinase inhibitor that is FDA-approved, as is baricitinib (Olumiant). It blocks transmission of the message to the white blood cells to turn on inflammation (blocking signaling proteins, which transmit the message). Because all of the biologic DMARDs interfere with the inflammatory and immune processes that are amplified in RA, the most important and dangerous side effect is infection. Nurses play a key role in teaching patients and their families self-care strategies to avoid/reduce the risk of infection and to self-assess and tell providers right away if they develop signs/symptoms of infection for prompt intervention. Other recommendations for patient care are to encourage patients to do regular aerobic exercise and strengthening exercises to improve and maintain function.

Biological DMARDs can be expensive and a company may control access to a single drug. In an effort to help stimulate competition and, hopefully, reduce cost, biosimilars have emerged. According to the FDA (2015), a biosimilar product is highly similar to the reference biological product with only minor differences in clinically inactive compounds and no clinically meaningful differences (e.g., safety, purity, and potency). The FDA also states that "bringing new biosimilars to patients" especially in treating costly diseases, "can help spur the competition that can lower health-care costs and increase access to important therapies." In development of a biosimilar, the drug sponsor must not only show "high similarity" to the originator biological but also biosimilar pharmacokinetics and pharmacodynamics so that the same dose, strength, and route of administration can be used (FDA 2015). However, biosimilar drugs are **not interchangeable** with the reference drug, unless they have undergone specific studies showing that the biosimilar will work the same in every patient as does the reference drug and that switching back and forth from the reference drug to the biosimilar does not cause changes in safety or efficacy; study results must be reviewed by the FDA and interchangeability status granted by the FDA.

Table 5.1 lists a number of biologic DMARDs that are FDA approved for the treatment of RA but not necessarily all other indications. For example, rituximab (Rituxan) has a biosimilar that is FDA approved for cancer treatment, but as no studies were done with RA patients, it does not have this RA indication. Biosimilars are named with the reference drug generic name followed by a randomly generated four-letter suffix.

Table 5.1 Selected common agents used in the management of RA.

Drug NSAIDs			
Diclofenac sodium	Voltaren	Ibuprofen	Motrin, Advil

Drug Glucorticosteroids			
Betamethasone	Celestone (injectable)	Prednisone	Rayos
DMARDs	**Brand Name**	**Drug**	**Brand Name**
methotrexate	Rheumaatrex. Trexall	Leflunomide	Arava

Biologic DMARDs	Trade Name	Mechanism of Action
abatacept	Orencia	Selective T cell co-stimulation modulator
adalimumab adalimumab-adaz adalimumab-adbm adalimumab-atto	Humira Hyrimoz (biosimilar) Cyltezo (biosimilar) Amjevita (biosimilar)	TNF-blocker, mAb
Anakinra	Kineret	IL-1 receptor antagonist
Baricitinib	Olumiant	JAK inhibitor, small molecule
certolizumab pegol	Cimzia	TNF-blocker, mAb
etanercept, etanercept-szzs etanercept-ykro	Enbrel Ereizi (biosimilar) Eticova (biosimilar)	TNF-blocker, mAb
Goliimumab	Simponi	TNF blocker, mAb
infliximab infliximab-dyyb infliximab-abda	Remicade Inflectra (biosimilar) Renflexis (biosimilar)	TNF-blocker, mAb
Sarilumab	Kevzara	IL-6 receptor antagonist, mAb
Tocilizumab	Actemra	IL6 receptor antagonist
Tofacitinib	Xeljanz	JAK inhibitor, small molecule

Abbreviations: DMARDs: disease modifying anti-rheumatic drugs; Biological DMARDs: affect biological process that interferes with inflammatory processes causing rheumatic injury; mAb: monoclonal antibody that is administered parenterally; small molecule: targeted agent that is small and administered orally; JAK: Janus kinase: tyrosine kinase that transduces cytokine-mediated signaling via the JAK-STAT signaling pathway in cells; cytokine: chemical messenger among the immune system elements, which orchestrate inflammation amonth other processes; interleukin (IL): a type of cytokine released by white blood cells to help regulate the immune response; IL-1: cytokines that help regulate the immune and inflammation responses; IL-6: pro-inflammatory cytokine, central in acute phase reactions, and plays an essential role in B-cell maturation; TNF- tumor necrosis factor, alpha, is a pro-inflammatory cytokine produced mainly by macrophages and is involved in acute inflammation; NSAIDs: nonsteroidal anti-inflammatory drugs.

Table 5.2   Biosimilar drugs FDA approved as of June 1, 2019

Reference Drug	Biosimilar Drug	Approval Date
Adalimumab (Humira)	adalimumab-adaz (Hyrimoz)	9/2016 but will not be launched in United States until 2023
	adalimumab-adbm (Cyltezo)	8/2017
	adalimumab-atto (Amjevita)	10/2018
Etanercept (Enbrel)	etanercept-szzs (Erelzi)	8/2016
	etanercept-ykro (Eticovo)	4/2019
Infliximab (Remicade)	infliximab-abda (Renflexis)	12/2016
	infliximab-dyyb (Inflectra)	3/2019

References

AbbVie Inc. Humira (adalimumab) [package insert]. North Chicago, IL. January 2019.

AARDA (American Autoimmune-Related Diseases Association). Available at https://www.aarda.org/mission_statement.php. Accessed May 22, 2019.

Amgen. Enbrel (etanercept) [package insert]. Thousand Oaks, CA. November 2017.

Amgen. Amjevita (adalimumab-atto) [package insert]. Thousand Oaks, CA. September 2016.

Arthritis Foundation. *Rheumatoid Arthritis Fact Sheet.* Available at http://www.arthritis.org/files/images/advocacy/ambassador-kit/RAFactSheet.pdf. Accessed May 22, 2019.

Boehringer Ingelheim Pharmaceuticals, Inc. Cyltezo (adalimumab-adbm) [package insert]. Ridgefield, CT. August 2017.

Bristol Myers Squibb, Orencia (abatacept) [package insert]. Princeton, NJ. March 2019.

Dewing KA, Setter SM, Slusher BA. *Osteoarthritis and rheumatoid arthritis 2–12: Pathophysiology, diagnosis, and treatment.* Available at https://www.nphealthcarefoundation.org/media/filer_public/c0/d1/c0d118bc-16a4-4114-a5cc-69901adfb298/osteoarthritis_and_ra_2012.pdf. Accessed August 7, 2016.

El-Meidany Y. The Evolving Therapy of Rheumatic Diseases, the Future is Now. *Curr Drug Targets Immune Endocr Metabol Disord* 2002; 2(1): 1–11.

Food and Drug Administration (FDA) Guidance for industry on biosimilars. April 2015. Available at https://www.fda.gov/drugs/biosimilars/biosimilar-and-interchangeable-products. Accessed May 22, 2019.

Genentech Inc. Actemra (tocilizumab) [package insert]. South San Francisco, CA. April 2019.

Helmick C, Felson D, Lawrence R, Gabriel S, et al. Estimates of the Prevalence of Arthritis and Other Rheumatic Conditions in the United States. *Arthritis Rheumatism* 2008; 58(1): 15–25.

Janssen Biotech, Inc. Simponi Aria (golimumab IV) [package insert]. Horsham, PA. May 2018.

Janssen Biotech, Inc. Simponi (golimumab SQ) [package insert]. Horsham, PA. May 2018.

Janssen Biotech, Inc. Remicade (infliximab) [package insert]. Horsham, PA. October 2017.

Merck Sharpe & Dohme Corp. Renflexis (infliximab-abda) [package insert]. Whitehouse Station, NJ. March 2019.

Oncology Nursing Society. *Oncology Nursing Society position on education of the RN who administers and cares for the individual receiving chemotherapy, targeted therapy, and immunotherapy.* Available at https://www.ons.org/sites/default/files/2019-04/Chemo_Administrators_Position_statement_April2019.pdf. Reviewed October 2017. Accessed May 22, 2019.

Pfizer Labs. Xeljanz (tofacitinib) [package insert]. New York, NY. October 2018.

Pfizer Labs, (Pfizer Biosimilars). Inflectra (Infliximab-dyyb) [package insert]. New York, NY. April 2019.

Samsung Bioepis Co, Ltd. Eticovo (etanercept-ykro) [package insert]. Incheon, Republic of Korea. April 2019.

Sandoz Inc. Erelzi (etanercept-szzs) [package insert]. Princeton NJ. August 2016.

Sanofi-aventis and Regeneron Pharmaceuticals Inc. Kevzara (sarilumab) [package insert]. Bridgewater NJ and Tarrytown NY, April 2018.

Singh JA, Saag KG, Bridges L, et al. American College of Rheumatology Guideline for the Treatment of Rheumatoid Arthritis. *Arthritis Care Res.* Available at https://www.rheumatology.org /Portals/0 /Files/ACR%202015%20RA%20Guideline.pdf. Accessed August 7, 2016.

Singh JA, Saag KG, Bridges L, et al. American College of Rheumatology Guideline for the Treatment of Rheumatoid Arthritis. *Arthritis Rheumatol* 2016; 68(1): 1–26.

Swedish Orphan Biovitrum AB (publ) [SOBI]. Kineret (anakinra) [package insert]. Stockhom, Sweden. June 2018.

UCB Inc. Cimzia [package insert]. Smyrna GA. April 2019.

Wilkie WS. (2012). Rheumatoid Arthritis. *Cleveland Clinic Center for Medical Education.* Available at http://www.clevelandclinicmeded.com/medicalpubs/diseasemanagement/rheumatology/ rheumatoid-arthritis/. Accessed May 31, 2016.

Zack E. Chemotherapy and Biotherapeutic Agents for Autoimmune Diseases. *Clin J Oncol Nurs* 2012; 16(4): E125–E132.

Drug: abatacept (Orencia)

Class: Selective T-cell costimulation modulator.

Mechanism of Action: Abatacept is a soluble fusion protein made up of the extracellular domain of the human cytotoxic T-lymphocyte associated antigen4 (CTLA-4) linked to a modified Fc (constant antibody domain) of the immunoglobulin IgG1. The drug is made using recombinant DNA technology. The drug inhibits T-lymphocyte activation by binding to CD80 and CD86, which blocks interaction with CD28. Blocking this interaction stops the full T-lymphocyte activation, which otherwise causes inflammation and damage to the joint synovium in RA. In addition, the drug decreases T-lymphocyte proliferation, and inhibits the production of TNF-α, interferon gamma and interleukin-2, all proinflammatory cytokines. This results in suppressed inflammation and decreased antibody production.

Metabolism: Bioavailability following subcutaneous administration is 78.6%. Pharmacokinetics of IV and subcutaneous administration are similar. Terminal half-life is 13–16 days.

Indication: (1) Adult RA that is moderately to severely active, as monotherapy or concomitantly with DMARDs other than TNF antagonists; (2) Juvenile idiopathic arthritis (JIA) that is moderately to severely active in patients 2 years of age or older, as monotherapy or concomitantly with methotrexate; (3) Adult psoriatic arthritis autoinjec (PsA).

Important Limitations: Drug should NOT be given concomitantly with TNF antagonists.

Contraindications: None.

Dosage/Range:
- Drug can be administered IV or SQ.
- **IV Dose Adult RA and Adult PsA:** (a) weight $<$ 60 kg = 500 mg (2 vials); (b) 60–100 kg = 750 mg (3 vials); (c) $>$100 kg = 1000 mg (4 vials). After initial IV dose, next dose is given at 2 and 4 weeks after first infusion, then every 4 weeks.
- **SQ dose Adult RA and Adult PsA:** 125 mg every week via prefilled syringes or in ORENCIA ClickJect™ autoinjector.

Adult RA SQ administration:
- Subcutaneous for adult RA: Administer SQ once weekly with or without an IV loading dose. If patient starts therapy with an IV loading dose, administer a single IV dose (per weight above) followed by the first 125 mg subcutaneously given within a day of the IV infusion.
  - If a loading dose is given, abatacept should be initiated with a single IV loading dose (as above), followed within a day by the first 125-mg subcutaneous injection.
  - Patients transitioning from abatacept IV therapy to subcutaneous administration should administer the first subcutaneous dose instead of the next scheduled IV dose.

Juvenile idiopathic arthritis (JIA):
- May be given IV or SQ; IV infusion only in children 6 years or older, and SQ in patients 2 years of age and older. May be given as monotherapy or concomitantly with methotrexate.
- IV infusion: 30-minute infusion based on body weight (patients aged 6 and above): (a) $<$75 kg = 10 mg/kg; (b) 75 kg or higher = follow adult IV dosing regimen not to exceed 1000 mg. After the initial IV dose, abatacept should be given at 2 and 4 weeks after first dose, then every 4 weeks.
- Subcutaneous administration for JIA based on body weight and given **once weekly**: (a) 0 to $<$25 kg = 50 mg; (b) 25 to $<$50 kg = 87.5 mg; (c) 50 kg or more = 125 mg.
- The safety and efficacy of ORENCIA ClickJect autoinjector for subcutaneous injection has not been studied in patients $<$18 years old.

Adult PsA:
- IV: see above for Adult RA and PsA patients.
- Administer by subcutaneous injection once weekly without the need of an IV loading dose (see doses above).
- Patients transitioning from abatacept IV to SQ administration should administer the first SQ dose instead of the next scheduled IV dose.

Drug Preparation:
- Drug is available in a 250-mg lyophilized powder in single-use vials for IV infusion, or 125-mg/mL solution in a single-dose prefilled syringe (PFS) for subcutaneous injection, or as a 125-mg filled autoinjector for SQ use.
- For IV infusion: Aseptically add 10 mL of sterile water for injection USP using only the **silicone-free disposable syringe** provided with each vial, and an 18- to 21-gauge needle. Silicone syringes may cause development of translucent particles and cannot be used. Direct the stream to the glass wall of the vial. Rotate with gentle swirling motion until completely dissolved. Do not shake or agitate. Vent with a needle to dissipate any foam

that may be present. The reconstituted solution contains 25 mg/mL. Solution should be clear and colorless to pale yellow.

- Inspect prepared solution for opacity, discoloration, or particulate matter; do not use if found.
- Further dilute reconstituted drug to 100 mL. From a 100-mL infusion bag or bottle, withdraw a volume of 0.9% sodium chloride USP equal to the volume of the reconstituted drug solution required for the dose. Slowly add the reconstituted solution to the infusion bag, using the same silicone-free disposable syringe provided with the vial. Do not shake the bag or bottle. The final concentration depends on the amount of added drug but will not be more than 10 mg/mL.
- Administer using a filter (sterile, nonpyrogenic, low-protein binding filter with pore size 0.2 μm to 1.2μm) over 30 min. Infusion must be completed within 24 hours of reconstitution of ORENCIA vials. The fully diluted drug solution may be stored at room temperature or refrigerated at 2–8°C (36–46°F) before use. Discard the fully diluted solution if not administered within 24 hours.
- Inspect again for color and presence of particulate matter.

Drug Administration:
- Ensure patient has had a latent TB test, and if positive, patient has begun anti-TB therapy before starting abatacept; patients should also be screened for hepatitis B (HBV).
- Juvenile idiopathic arthritis (JIA) patients should have all necessary immunizations prior to starting abatacept, as drug may blunt effectiveness of immunizations.
- Adult patients: abatacept may be administered either by IV or SQ route.
- *Intravenous Infusion:*
  - Administer as a 30-minute IV infusion via a sterile, nonpyrogenic low-protein binding filter (pore size 0.2–1.2 μm). Use a separate IV line and do not mix with other agents.
  - Drug infusion must be completed within 24 hours of reconstitution of abatacept vials. If needed, store the fully diluted solution at room temperature or refrigerated at 2–8°C (36°–46°F).
  - Following initial dose, give at 2 and 4 weeks, then every 4 weeks.
- *Subcutaneous Injection:*
  - 125-mg syringe is not intended for IV infusion. Patient may have an initial IV loading dose, with the first SQ dose within a day of the IV loading dose.
  - Patient may be taught self-administration if appropriate. Drug available as 50 mg/0.4 mL, 87.5 mg/0.7 mL, and 125 mg/mL in a single-dose prefilled glass syringe. The autoinjector single dose prefilled ClickJect is 125 mg/mL. Solution is clear to slightly opalescent, colorless to pale yellow in color.
  - Syringe contents should be visually inspected for color or particulate matter and not used if present. Color should be clear, colorless to pale yellow.
  - Teach patient to aseptically inject the entire 1 mL (125 mg) and to rotate sites, avoiding sites if the skin is tender, bruised, red, or hard.

Drug Interaction:
- TNF antagonists: do not coadminister, as there is an INCREASED RISK OF SERIOUS INFECTION.
- Other biologic DMARDs: do not give concurrently.
- Live vaccines: do not give concurrently or for 3 months after last dose.

Lab Effects/Interference:
- Falsely elevated blood glucose readings on the day of infusion.

Special Considerations:
- Warnings and Precautions:
  - *Concomitant administration with TNF antagonist* increases risk of infection significantly and does not improve efficacy. Do **not** coadminister.
  - *Hypersensitivity, anaphylaxis, and anaphylactoid reactions* may occur. Very rarely, patients may have a HSR, characterized by hives, facial edema, dyspnea. Emergency equipment and medications should be available where IV infusions are administered. Patients receiving subcutaneous medications should be taught to seek emergency care if this occurs. In postmarketing experience, one case of fatal anaphylaxis after the first dose has been reported.
  - *Infections:* Serious infections including sepsis have been reported.
  - Patients with history of recurrent or underlying conditions predisposing to infections may develop more infections.
  - If a patient develops a new infection while being treated with abatacept, monitor patient closely.
  - Discontinue abatacept if a serious infection develops.
  - Screen for latent TB infection prior to initiating therapy. Patients testing positive should be treated before starting abatacept.
  - Live vaccines should not be given concurrently or for 3 months after last dose.
  - Patients with JIA should be brought up to date on all immunizations prior to starting abatacept. Abatacept may blunt some immunizations, based on its mechanism of action.
  - Patients with COPD may develop more frequent respiratory adverse events.
  - *Immunizations:* Do not give live vaccines during or within 3 months of treatment with abatacept. Abatacept may blunt effectiveness of some immunizations.
  - *Use in patients with COPD:* In clinical trials, patients with COPD had more frequent adverse events compared to those treated with placebo, including COPD exacerbations, cough, rhonchi, and dyspnea. Abatacept treatment for patients with adult RA and COPD should be undertaken cautiously.
  - *Immunosuppression:* Drugs such as abatacept that inhibit T cell activation may decrease host defenses against infection and cancer and increase incidence of infection and malignancy.
- Most common side effects are headache, URI, nasopharyngitis, and nausea.
- Pregnancy category C: Women of childbearing potential should be counseled that the drug should be used during pregnancy only if the potential benefit to the mother outweighs the risk.
- Nursing mothers should make a decision to discontinue nursing or discontinue the drug, taking into consideration the importance of the drug to the mother's health.

Potential Toxicities/Side Effects and the Nursing Process

I.   POTENTIAL FOR INFECTION related to IMMUNOSUPPRESSION

Defining Characteristics: Patients receiving abatacept are at increased risk for developing infections. Nasopharyngitis occurred in 12% of patients during clinical trials, and UTIs in 6% of patients.

Nursing Implications: Assess results of patient's latent TB test and HBV testing and discuss any abnormalities with physician/NP/PA. If TB is positive, patient should begin anti-TB therapy before beginning abatacept therapy. Assess baseline patient risk for infection (e.g., comorbidities, preexisting infections, any concomitant immunosuppressive drugs). Patient should not receive this drug together with any other biologic DMARD, including anti-TNF agents. Teach patient to self-assess for signs/symptoms of infection (e.g., $T > 100.4°F$, cough, chest pain, sputum production, dysuria), and to report them right away. Closely monitor patient for signs/symptoms of infection during and after treatment with abatacept, including TB reactivation, even if latent TB test is negative, and teach patient to report any changes (e.g., fever, sweats, chills, cough, SOB, blood in sputum, weight loss). Drug should be discontinued if patient develops a serious infection or sepsis, and appropriate antimicrobial therapy should be instituted right away.

II.   KNOWLEDGE DEFICIT related to SUBCUTANEOUS INJECTION TECHNIQUE

Defining Characteristics: Selected patients may choose to self-inject their abatacept doses.

Nursing Implications: Assess patient or caregiver readiness to learn, and assess learning style and limitations. Review with patient drug administration schedule, and to not administer, and notify physician/nurse if patient develops an infection. Provide Medication Guide and Instructions for Use available from Bristol Myers Squibb, the drug manufacturer. Teach patient how to care for drug (PFSs) should be stored in refrigerator at 2–8°C (36–46°F) in the original container until used, and protected from light. Patient should inspect syringe for cloudiness or particles and not use it if these are found. Patient should be careful and protect glass syringe, as it may break. Drug should be kept out of reach of children and pets. Teach patient hand-washing, aseptic technique, subcutaneous injection technique, and how to dispose of syringe/needle. Teach patient to rotate sites and to apply local measures if injection-site reactions occur. Validate patient understanding by having patient describe measures taught, and ideally, by repeating the demonstration of subcutaneous injection technique. Teach patient to develop documentation tool to record site rotation and any site irritation or reaction.

Drug: adalimumab (Humira); Biosimilars adalimumab-atto (Amjevita) and adalimumab-adbm (Cyltezo) for indications RA, JIA, PsA, AS, CD, UC, Ps only

Class: TNF inhibitor, human monoclonal antibody.

Mechanism of Action: Adalimumab binds to TNF-α and blocks its ability to bind to TNF cell surface receptors (p55, p75), thus decreasing the proinflammatory and immune action of TNF-α. The drug also lyses surface TNF expressing cells when complement is present, further decreasing TNF effect. This decreases levels of acute phase reactants of inflammation (C-reactive protein [CRP]) and the proinflammatory cytokine IL-6. Drug decreases leukocyte migration immune response. Elevated TNF levels are found in synovial joint fluid of patients with RA, JIA, psoriatic arthritis (PsA), and ankylosing spondylitis (AS), and they contribute to inflammation and joint destruction.

Metabolism: Following subcutaneous injection, the absolute bioavailability of adalimumab is 64%. Maximum serum concentration is reached in 131 ± 56 hours, and the mean terminal half-life of the drug is approximately 2 weeks (10- to 20-day range). Adalimumab concentrations in the synovial fluid ranged from 31 to 96%. MTX reduces adalimumab clearance by 29% after single dosing, and 44% after multiple doses.

Indications:
(1) Rheumatoid arthritis (RA): to reduce signs and symptoms, induce major clinical response, inhibit progression of structural damage, and improve physical functioning in adults with moderately to severely active RA.
(2) Juvenile idiopathic arthritis (JIA): to reduce signs and symptoms of moderately to severely active polyarticular JIA in children 4 years and older.
(3) Psoriatic arthritis (PsA): to reduce signs and symptoms, inhibit progression of structural damage, and improve physical functioning in adults with active PsA.
(4) Ankylosing spondylitis (AS): to reduce signs/symptoms in adult patients with active AS.
(5) Adult Crohn's disease (CD): to reduce signs/symptoms and induce and maintain clinical remission in adults with moderately to severely active Crohn's disease who have had an inadequate response to conventional therapy, who have lost the response, or who are intolerant to infliximab.
(6) Pediatric Crohn's disease (CD): to reduce signs/symptoms and induce and maintain clinical remission in children aged 6 years of age and older with moderately to severely active Crohn's disease who have had an inadequate response to corticosteroids or immunomodulators such as azathioprine, 6-mercaptopurine (6-MP), or MTX.
(7) Ulcerative colitis (UC): to induce and sustain clinical remission in adults with moderately to severely active UC who have had an inadequate response to immunosuppressants (e.g., corticosteroids, azathioprine, or 6-MP). The effectiveness of adalimumab has not been established in patients who have lost a response to or were intolerant of TNF blockers.
(8) Plaque psoriasis (Ps): to treat adults with moderate to severe chronic Ps who are candidates for systemic therapy or phototherapy, and when other systemic therapies are medically less appropriate.

(9) Hidradenitis Suppurativa (HS): the treatment of moderate to severe HS in patients 12 years of age and older.
(10) Uveitis (UV): noninfectious intermediate, posterior, and panuveitis in adults and pediatric patients aged 2 years and older.

Dosage/Range: Administered as a subcutaneous injection.

- RA, PsA, AS: 40 mg every other week; some RA patients not receiving MTX may benefit from increasing the frequency to 40 mg weekly. Patients may continue taking MTX, other nonbiologic DMARDs, glucocorticoids, NSAIDs, and/or analgesics concurrently.
- JIA (aged 2 or older) or pediatric uveitis: (a) 10 kg (22 lbs) to < 15 kg = 10 mg every other week; (b) 15 kg (33 lbs) to < 30 kg (66 lbs) = 20 mg every other week; (c) weight ≥ 30 kg (66 lbs) = 40 mg every other week (40 mg pen or prefilled syringe). Patients may continue glucocorticoids, NSAIDs, and/or analgesics concurrently.
- Adult Crohn's Disease and UC: initial dose (day 1): 160 mg (four 40-mg injections in 1 day or two 40-mg injections per day on 2 consecutive days); second dose 2 weeks later (day 15): 80 mg; third dose 2 weeks later (day 29): begin maintenance dose of 40 mg every other week. Patients with UC only: continue adalimumab only in patients who have shown evidence of clinical remission by 8 weeks (day 57) of therapy.
- Pediatric Crohn's disease:
  1. 17 kg (37 lbs) to < 40 kg (88 lbs): initial dose (day 1) = 80 mg on day 1 and 40 mg 2 weeks later (day 15; then 2 weeks later (day 29) = begin maintenance dose of 20 mg every other week.
  2. > 40 kg (88 lbs): initial dose (day 1) = 160 mg (two 80-mg injections in 1 day or split over 2 consecutive day (e.g., one 80-mg injection per day for 2 consecutive days); second dose 2 weeks later (day 15) = 80 mg (one 80-mg injection in 1 day); 2 weeks later (day 29) = begin maintenance dose of 40 mg every other week.
- Ps or adult uveitis: 80-mg initial dose, followed by 40 mg every other week, starting 1 week after initial dose.
- HS:
  - Adults: Initial dose (day 1): 160 mg (four 40-mg injections in 1 day or two 40-mg injections per day on days 1 and 2); second dose 2 weeks later (day 15) = 80 mg (two 40-mg injections in 1 day); third dose (day 29), and subsequent doses = 40 mg every week.
  - Adolescents (12 years and older) ≥ 60 kg (132 lbs): Initial dose (day 1) = 160 mg (given in 1 day or split over 2 consecutive days); second dose 2 weeks later (day 15) = 80 mg; third dose (day 29) and subsequent doses = **40 mg every week**.
  - Adolescents (12 years and older) 30 kg (66 lbs) to <60 kg (132 lbs): Initial dose (day 1) = 80 mg; second dose (day 8) and subsequent doses = 40 mg **every other week**.

Drug Preparation:
- Prefilled HUMIRA pen (single dose): available in 80 mg/0.8 mL, 40 mg/0.8 mL, and 40 mg/0.4 mL.
- Prefilled glass syringe (single dose): available in 80 mg/0.8 mL, 40 mg/0.8 mL, 40 mg/0.4 mL, 20 mg/0.4 mL, 20 mg/0.2 mL, 10 mg/0.3 mL, 10 mg/0.1 mL.
- Institutional use: 40 mg/0.8 mL in a single glass vial.

Drug Administration:

- Ensure patient has had TB test and that it is negative for latent infection and that patient is tested periodically during therapy.
- For subcutaneous injection, rotate sites on thigh or abdomen. Do not inject drug into areas that are tender, red, hard, or bruised.
- Do not start drug during an active infection.
- Anaphylaxis or serious allergy can rarely occur. Monitor patient closely and teach patient signs and symptoms to prompt seeking emergency medical care.
- As appropriate, teach patient or caregiver subcutaneous administration of drug using prefilled glass syringe or pen, as well as disposal of syringe/pen.
- May leave PFS or pen at room temperature for 15–30 minutes prior to injection (make sure cap remains on the device). Inspect solution for discoloration or particles, and do not use if found. Teach patients with latex allergies NOT to touch the latex needle cover as it contains latex.
- Teach patient or caregiver to inject the entire contents of the syringe. Provide patient or caregiver instructions in package insert, including images for self-injection.
- As the healthcare provider in a physician's office or institution, aseptically withdraw ordered amount from institutional vial (1 dose per vial) using a sterile needle and syringe, and administer promptly.

Drug Interactions:

- Abatacept (Orencia) or anakinra (Kineret) in combination with adalimumab: increased risk of serious infection; do not give concomitantly.
- Live vaccines: do not administer while patient is receiving adalimumab.
- CYP450 enzyme formation may be suppressed by increased levels of cytokines, and once inflammation is suppressed, may change the enzyme formation. Monitor patients taking CYP450 substrate drug with a narrow therapeutic window (e.g., warfarin) closely, or monitor drug concentrations (e.g., cyclosporine or theophylline) closely and adjust dose as needed.

Lab Effects/Interference:

- Rare cytopenias, pancytopenia.
- Rare increases in cholesterol, lipids, and alkaline phosphatase.
- Rare increases in LFTs.

Special Considerations:

- Warnings and Precautions:
  - *Serious infections* may occur.
    - Adalimumab increases the risk for serious infections requiring hospitalization, including TB, bacterial sepsis, invasive fungal infections (e.g., histoplasmosis), and other opportunistic infections.
    - Most patients who developed serious infections were also taking concomitant immunosuppressants, such as MTX or corticosteroids.
    - If an infection develops, monitor patient carefully and stop drug if infection becomes serious. Drug should be discontinued if patient develops a serious infection or sepsis.

- Risk benefit evaluation should be done prior to starting drug in patients with chronic or recurrent infections.
- Monitor patients closely for signs/symptoms of infection during and after adalimumab therapy, including the possible development of TB in patients who tested negative for latent TB prior to starting therapy.
- *Malignancies*:
  - Lymphoma and leukemia in patients receiving TNF blockers: Postmarketing reports document cases of hepatosplenic T-cell lymphoma, a rare, aggressive, fatal, T-cell lymphoma in young adults with inflammatory bowel disease.
    - Most patients had Crohn's disease or UC, were adolescent or young adults, and had received prior treatment with immunosuppressants azathioprine or 6-MP concomitantly with a TNF-blocker.
    - The combination of adalimumab with either azathioprine or 6-MP should be used with caution.
- *HSRs*: Anaphylaxis and angioneurotic edema have occurred after adalimumab administration.
  - If anaphylaxis occurs, immediately discontinue the drug and provide emergency interventions as ordered.
  - Reactions reported in clinical trials in adults include allergic rash, anaphylactoid reaction, fixed drug reaction, nonspecific drug reaction, and urticaria.
- *HBV reactivation can occur.* Monitor HBV carriers during and for several months after therapy. If reactivation occurs, stop drug and begin antiviral therapy.
- *Neurological reactions*: Demyelinating disease can be exacerbated; rarely, there may be new onset such as Guillain–Barré syndrome. Use cautiously in patients with pre-existing or recent onset central or peripheral nervous system demyelinating disorders.
- *Hematologic reactions*: Cytopenias and pancytopenias may rarely occur; patient should be evaluated and should consider discontinuing drug. Teach patients to report persistent fever, bruising, bleeding, or pallor right away.
- *Combination of adalimumab and anakinra (interleukin-1 antagonist)* increase risk of infection and neutropenia; **do not use together.**
- *Heart failure* may worsen, or there may be new onset of CHF with adalimumab. Monitor patients with preexisting heart failure closely.
- *Autoimmunity:* patients may rarely develop auto-antibodies and develop a lupus-like syndrome. If this occurs the drug should be discontinued.
- *Immunizations:* Pediatric patients should complete their immunizations prior to starting therapy with adalimumab.
- *Use with Abatacept:* **combination with abatacept resulted in increased incidence of serious infections without increased efficacy; do not use together**.
- If the patient develops a systemic illness, consider empiric antifungal therapy for those who reside in or travel to regions where mycoses are endemic.
- All patients should have test for latent TB; if positive, anti-TB treatment should start before beginning adalimumab. Consider anti-TB therapy in patients with a past history of latent or active TB and in whom an adequate course of treatment cannot be confirmed.
  - Cases of TB reactivation and new onset of TB infection have occurred in patients receiving adalimumab who previously received treatment for latent or active TB (e.g., pulmonary and extrapulmonary [disseminated]).

- Consider anti-TB therapy prior to starting adalimumab in patients who have had latent or active TB but for whom it cannot be confirmed whether they completed an adequate course of TB therapy.
- All patients should be monitored for TB during treatment, even if their latent TB test was negative.
- Pregnancy category B: Teach women of reproductive potential that the drug should be used in pregnancy only if the potential benefit to the mother outweighs the potential risk to the fetus, as there are no well-controlled studies. If pregnancy occurs, patient should be encouraged to register with the Pregnancy Registry at 1-877-311-8972.
- Most common adverse effects were infections (e.g., URI, sinusitis), injection-site reactions, headache, and rash.

Potential Toxicities/Side Effects and the Nursing Process

I. POTENTIAL FOR INFECTION related to IMMUNOSUPPRESSION

Defining Characteristics: Patients receiving adalimumab are at increased risk for developing serious infections requiring hospitalization. Although uncommon and occurring in patients receiving multiple immunosuppressant medications (e.g., MTX and corticosteroids), opportunistic infections may be disseminated on presentation, such as fulminating fungal infections. In clinical trials, most common infections were URI (17%), sinusitis (14%), pharyngitis (11%), and UTI (8%).

Nursing Implications: Assess results of patient's latent TB and HBV testing and discuss any abnormalities with physician, NP, or PA. If TB test is positive, patient should begin anti-TB therapy before beginning adalimumab therapy. Assess baseline risk for infection (e.g., comorbidities, preexisting infections, concomitant immunosuppressants like MTX or corticosteroids). Teach patient to self-assess for signs/symptoms of infection (e.g., $T > 100.4°F$, cough, chest pain, sputum production, dysuria), and to report them right away. Closely monitor patient for signs/symptoms of infection during and after treatment with adalimumab, including TB reactivation even if latent TB test is negative, and teach patient to report any changes (e.g., fever, sweats, chills; cough; SOB; blood in sputum; weight loss; warm, red, or painful skin or sores on body; diarrhea or stomach pain; burning when urinating; urinating more often than usual; feeling very tired). Drug should be discontinued if patient develops a serious infection or sepsis, and appropriate antimicrobial therapy instituted right away. If the patient is at risk for fungal infection and develops severe systemic illness, discuss with physician, NP, or PA empiric antifungal therapy.

II. KNOWLEDGE DEFICIT related to SUBCUTANEOUS INJECTION TECHNIQUE

Defining Characteristics: Drug is administered subcutaneously, and appropriate patients (or caregivers) can be taught to administer the drug.

Nursing Implications: Assess patient or caregiver readiness to learn, learning style, and limitations. Review with patient drug administration schedule; tell patient not to administer, and to notify physician/nurse, if patient develops an infection. Provide Medication Guide and Instructions for Use available from AbbVie Inc, the drug manufacturer. Teach patient how to care for drug (should be stored in refrigerator at 2–8°C [36°–46°F] in the original container until used, and it should be protected from light). Patient should inspect syringe for cloudiness or particles and should not use if these are found. Patient should be careful to protect glass syringe, as it may break. Drug should be kept out of reach of children and pets. Teach patient hand-washing, aseptic technique, subcutaneous injection technique, and how to dispose of syringe/needle. Teach patient to rotate sites and to apply local measures if injection-site reactions occur. Validate patient understanding by having patient describe measures taught, and ideally, by returning the demonstration of subcutaneous injection technique. Teach patient to develop documentation tool to record site rotation and any site irritation or reaction.

Drug: anakinra (Kineret)

Class: Interleukin-1 (IL-1) receptor antagonist.

Mechanism of Action: Inflammation results in the production of IL-1, and IL-1 mediates inflammatory and immunological responses. L-1 is involved in cartilage degradation and stimulation of bone resorption (breakdown). IL-1 (α and β) blockade reduces inflammation, joint destruction, and other symptoms of autoinflammation (SOBI, 2018).

Metabolism: Absolute bioavailability after SQ injection is 95%, with maximal plasma concentrations in RA patients at 3–7 hours after dosing. Drug's terminal half-life is 4–6 hours. Mean plasma clearance was reduced in patients with renal dysfunction, by 16% in mild renal (CrCl 50–80 mL/min) and 50% in moderate (CrCl 30–49 mL/min) renal impairment. In patients with severe and end stage renal disease had reduction of 70% and 75% respectively in mean plasma clearance of drug that requires a dose adjustment. No studies in patients with hepatic impairment were conducted.

Indication: Treatment of (1) patients 18 years of age or older with moderately to severely active RA who have failed 1 or more DMARDs to reduce signs/symptoms and to slow the progression of structural damage of RA; (2) infants with cryopyrin-associated periodic syndrome (CAPS) who have neonatal-onset multisystem inflammatory disease (NOMID).

Contraindication: Known hypersensitivity to *E. coli*–derived proteins, anakinra (Kineret), or to any component of the product. Do not start drug in patients with active infection, and do not continue its administration in patients with a serious infection. The safety of the drug in patients with immunosuppression or with chronic infections has not been studied.

Dosage/Range:
RA:
- 100 mg/day SQ at about the same time every day.
- Severe renal insufficiency or end stage renal disease (ESRD) (CrCl, 30 mL/min) 100 mg SQ **every other day.**

- CAPS: 1–2 mg/kg daily starting dose, individually adjusted (in 0.5–1.0 mg/kg increments) to a maximum of 8 mg/kg/day. In NOMID patients with renal insufficiency or ESRD, administer dose every other day.

Drug Preparation:
- Available as an injection form 100 mg/0.67 mL solution in a single-use prefilled syringe.
- Graduated syringe allows for doses between 20–100 mg.
- Check package expiration date, and do not use if passed. Visually inspect solution (should be translucent to white amorphous particles of protein in the solution); do not use if cloudy or discolored, if foreign particles are present or if number of amorphous particles is excessive (see package insert).

Drug Administration:
- As appropriate, teach patient and/or caregiver SQ injection technique (see Information for Patients insert (package insert). Teach patient to (1) wash hands; (2) select site avoiding moles, scars, areas of tenderness, bruises, and red, hard, or open (not intact) skin areas; (3) aseptically prepare SQ site with alcohol swab; (4) inject drug; (5) dispose of syringe (and any unused drug); and (6) rotate sites. Supervise patient's or caregiver's return demonstration, and if successful, empower patient or caregiver to (self-administer at home). Drug available in single-use glass syringe delivering 100 mg of anakinra in 0.67 mL.

Drug Interaction:
Lab Effects/Interference:
Special Considerations:
- Fetal risk unknown. Teach female patients of reproductive potential to use effective contraception during treatment.
- Most common adverse events in (a) RA patients ($\geq$5%) were: injection site reaction, worsening of RA, URI, headache, nausea, diarrhea, sinusitis, arthralgia, flu like-symptoms, and abdominal pain; (b) NOMID patients (>10%) during the first 6 months of treatment were injection site reaction, headache, vomiting, arthralgia, pyrexia, and nasopharyngitis.
- The elderly may be at higher risk to develop infection.
- Warnings and Precautions:
  - *Serious infections*: Patients had an increased risk of infection (2%) compared to control group (<1%). Discontinue drug if patient develops a serious infection, and do not start anakinra in patients with an active infection.
    - The safety of the drug in patients with immunosuppression or with chronic infections has not been studied.
    - Patient may be at increased risk for TB or other atypical or opportunistic infections (OI). Patient should be tested for latent TB before starting drug, and if positive, patient started on antimycobacterial treatment for TB before starting therapy with anakinra.
      - *Use with TNF Blocking Agents*: Do not use concurrently as risk of infection increased without evidence of benefit.

- *HSRs*: may occur, including anaphylaxis and angioedema. If a severe HSR occurs, anakinra should be discontinued permanently and emergency medical intervention instituted.
- *Immunosuppression*: The impact of anakinra immunosuppression on active/ chronic infections and the development of malignancy is unknown.
- *Immunizations*: Do not administer live vaccines concurrently with anakinra.
- *Neutrophil count*: May be decreased. Assess ANC baseline and while receiving anakinra monthly for 3 months, and then quarterly for a period of up to 1 year.

Potential Toxicities/Side Effects and the Nursing Process

I.   POTENTIAL FOR INFECTION related to IMMUNOSUPPRESSION

Defining Characteristics: Patients receiving anakinra are at increased risk of developing infections: incidence was 39% compared to 37% in the placebo group, and of serious infections, 3% in the anakinra group compared to 2% in the placebo group. Most common infections were bacterial manifesting as pneumonia, cellulitis, and bone and joint infections. No serious OIs were reported, but in postmarketing experience, OIs included fungal, mycobacterial, and bacterial pathogens.

Nursing Implications: Review patient history; drug should not be given to a patient with active infection. Assess results of patient's latent TB testing and discuss any abnormalities with physician, NP, or PA. If TB test is positive, patient should take anti-TB therapy before beginning anakinra therapy. Anti-TB therapy should also be considered for patients with a history of latent or active TB, and an adequate course of therapy cannot be confirmed. Monitor all patients for active TB during treatment, even if initial latent TB test is negative. Physician should discuss risks vs. benefits of anakinra in patients with chronic or recurrent infections, exposed to TB, with a history of a serious OI, who have resided or traveled to an area of endemic TB or mycoses, or with underlying conditions besides RA that may predispose them to infection.

Assess CBC/differential baseline labs and at then monthly $\times$ 3 months, then every 3 months for 1 year. Assess baseline risk for infection (e.g., comorbidities, history of infections). Teach patient to self-assess for signs/symptoms of infection (e.g., $T > 100.4°F$, cough, chest pain, sputum production, dysuria), stop drug, and report any signs/symptoms of infection immediately. Closely monitor patient for signs/symptoms of infection, including TB, during and after treatment with anakinra, and teach patient to report any changes (e.g., fever, sweats, rigors, weight loss, blood in sputum). Drug should be interrupted if patient develops a serious infection. If a patient develops a new infection while receiving anakinra therapy, prompt and comprehensive evaluation of an immunocompromised patient should be done, and antimicrobial therapy should be given promptly.

II.   ALTERATION IN COMFORT related to INJECTION SITE REACTIONS

Defining Characteristics: The most common adverse event was injection site reactions, which occurred in 71% of patients during the first month of therapy. Most were mild

(72.6%) or moderate (24.1%), while 3.2% were considered severe. Infection site reaction typically lasted 14–28 days and were characterized by erythema, ecchymosis, inflammation, and pain.

Nursing Implications: Teach patient that injection site reactions may occur and to treat symptomatically. If the reaction does not resolve, the patient should report this to the nurse or physician. Teach patient symptomatic management, such as application of warm or cold to the site, and administration of analgesics, such as acetaminophen. If the area is painful with ecchymosis, then review with patient injection technique to avoid bruising. Revise plan as needed.

Drug: baricitinib (Olumiant)

Class: Janus Kinase (JAK) inhibitor; small molecule kinase inhibitor.

Mechanism of Action: JAKs are enzymes within the cell that carry messages from receptors on the cell surface, which have been activated by cytokine or growth factors, to the cell nucleus. JAKs tell the immune system to turn on and to activate other blood cells using phosphorylation, which activates signal transducers and transcription (STATs), which in turn regulate cell activities, as well as turning on genes in the cell's DNA. JAK inhibitors modulate the signaling pathway, thus stopping this message from being sent so that STATs are not activated and the immune system (inflammation) is not turned on. After treatment with baricitinib there is a rapid decrease in serum CRP within a week and is maintained throughout dosing.

Metabolism: After oral administration, peak plasma levels reached in 1 hour, with steady state reached in 2–3 days with daily dosing. Absolute bioavailability is 80%, and a high fat meal decreased the mean AUC and C_{max} by 11% and 18%, respectively. Drug is 50% bound to plasma proteins, and 45% bound to serum proteins. Baricitinib is a substrate of the Pgp, BCRP, OAT3, and MATE2-K transporters (drug distribution). Elimination half-life in patients with RA is about 12 hours. Drug is primarily metabolized by CYP3A4 microenzyme system, with only 6% of the administered dose appearing as metabolites in the urine and feces. Drug is principally excreted in the urine (75%, almost all (69%) unchanged drug), and about 20% (15% unchanged drug) in the feces.

Indications: For the treatment of adult patients with moderately to severely active RA who has had an inadequate response or intolerance to one or more TNF antagonist therapies.

Limitations of use: Use of baricitinib in combination with other JAK inhibitors, biologic DMARDs, or with potent immunosuppressants (e.g., azathioprine and cyclosporine) is not recommended.

Contraindication: None. Do not administer drug unless patient's absolute lymphocyte count (ALC) $\geq$ 500 cells/mm^3, ANC $\geq$ 1000 cells/mm^3, and Hgb $\geq$8 g/dL. Do not give baricitinib if the patient has active TB. Do not administer baricitinib to patients with active, serious infection, including localized infection. Drug not recommended in patients with moderate or severe renal impairment (GFR < 60 mL/min/1.73 m^2—see package insert

8.7 and 12.3) or in patients with severe hepatic impairment. Do not administer baricitinib to patients also taking probenecid or other strong OAT3 inhibitors.

Dosage/Range:
- 2 mg PO once daily, with or without food; may be used as monotherapy or concurrently with MTX or other DMARDs.
- Patients must have an absolute lymphocyte count (ALC) $\geq$ 500 cells/mm^3, ANC $\geq$ 1000 cells/mm^3, and Hgb $\geq$8 g/dL and be without serious infection, including localized infection.
- Test patient for latent TB; if positive, patient should receive TB treatment before starting baricitinib therapy.

Dose Modifications
- *Serious infections:* If a patient develops a serious infection, hold baricitinib therapy until infection is controlled.
- *Lymphopenia:* (1) ALC $\geq$ 500 cells/mm^3 = maintain dose; (2) ALC <500 cells/mm^3 = interrupt baricitinib until ALC $\geq$ 500 cells/mm^3.
- *Neutropenia:* **(1)** ANC $\geq$ 1000 cells/mm^3 = maintain dose; (2) ALC <1000 cells/mm^3 = interrupt baricitinib until ANC $\geq$ 1000 cells/mm^3.
- *Anemia:* (1) Hgb $\geq$8 g/dL = maintain dose; (2) Hgb <8 g/dL = interrupt baricitinib until Hgb > 8 g/dL.
- *Renal or Hepatic Impairment:* (1) Assess GFR: if < 60 mL/min/1.73 m^2 drug is not recommended; (2) if patient has severe hepatic impairment, drug is not recommended.
- *In combination with strong Organic Anion Transporter 3 (OAT3) inhibitors:* Do not give concurrently (e.g., probenecid).

Drug Preparation: None. Available in 2-mg tablets.

Drug Administration:
- Ensure patient has had a TB test and that it is negative. If positive, talk with physician about holding drug until anti-TB therapy has begun.
- Review medication profile: If patient is taking probenecid, or other OAT3 inhibitor, talk with provider/pharmacist about alternative drugs to replace OAT3 inhibitors.
- Assess patient's CBC/differential, LFTs, renal GFR, lipids, and assess patient for any signs/symptoms of infection. Discuss any abnormalities or positive findings with physician.
- Assess serum lipids 12 weeks after patient starts baricitinib.
- Teach patient to take tablet around the same time every day, with or without meals. Teach signs/symptoms of infection and to stop drug and call provider right away if fever, productive cough, or painful urination or other signs/symptoms of infection.

Drug Interactions:
- **OAT3 inhibitors:** probenecid, cimetidine, etc; decreases renal excretion of baricitinib, increases baricitinib serum concentration and toxicity.

Lab Effects/Interference:
- Decreased ALC, ANC, Hgb.
- Increased liver enzymes (AST, ALT), lipids (total cholesterol, LDL, cholesterol, HDL).

Special Considerations:
- Most common adverse effects (≤1%) include URI, nausea, herpes simplex, and herpes zoster.
- Warnings and Precautions:
  - *Serious infections:* Serious and sometimes fatal infections may occur. Opportunistic infections (OIs) by bacterial, mycobacterial, invasive fungal, viral, and other pathogens can occur. Some patients may present with disseminated rather than localized infection, especially if taking other concomitant immunosuppressants such as methotrexate or corticosteroids. Closely monitor patients for signs/symptoms of infection.
    - Avoid use of drug in patients with active, serious infection, including localized infections. Use drug cautiously in patients with chronic or recurrent infection, who have been exposed to TB, have a history of a serious or an OI, who have lived or traveled in areas of endemic TB or mycoses or with underlying conditions that may predispose them to infections. If an infection is suspected, patient should promptly undergo complete diagnostic evaluation for an immunocompromised patient. If infection identified, antimicrobials should be started promptly and patient closely monitored. Baricitinib should be interrupted if patient does not respond to therapy and not resumed until the infection is controlled.
    - TB: All patients should be tested for latent TB before starting baricitinib therapy, and if TB identified, patient should receive standard antimycobacterial therapy before starting baricitinib. Baricitinib should NOT be administered to a patient with active B. See package insert. Monitor patients for signs/symptoms of TB during baricitinib therapy even if latent TB tests have been negative.
    - Viral reactivation: Monitor patients with history of exposure to viral infection closely such as herpes zoster, hepatitis B or C exposure [(e.g., monitor HBV DNA if positive hepatitis B surface antibody and core antibody without surface antigen (see package insert)].
  - *Malignancy and lymphoproliferative disorders:* Consider risk carefully in patients who have a known cancer (not including a successfully treated nonmelanoma skin cancer). Also, nonmelanoma skin cancers have been reported in patients receiving baricitinib therapy. Assess skin baseline and then periodically during therapy for patients who are at risk for skin cancer.
  - *Thrombosis:* Patients receiving baricitinib therapy are at increased risk for venous and arterial thromboses, including DVT, PE, and arterial thrombosis of the extremities. The cause is unknown. Use drug cautiously in patients at risk for thrombosis. Teach patients to call provider for signs/symptoms suggestive of PE or DVT and to seek medical care right away. Patient should be promptly evaluated and managed.
  - *GI perforation:* Use drug cautiously in patients at risk for GI perforation (e.g., have history of diverticulitis). If a patient presents with new onset abdominal symptoms, patient should be promptly evaluated and GI perforation ruled out.
  - *Laboratory abnormalities:* (a) neutropenia; (b) lymphopenia; (c) anemia; (d) elevated liver enzymes; (e) lipid elevations. Assess labs baseline and periodically during treatment or more frequently if abnormal. Assess serum lipids 12 weeks after starting baricitinib.

- *Vaccinations:* Do not use live vaccines while patient is receiving baricitinib. Update all immunizations per guidelines prior to starting baricitinib.

Potential Toxicities/Side Effects and the Nursing Process

I. POTENTIAL FOR INFECTION related to IMMUNOSUPPRESSION

Defining Characteristics: Patients receiving baricitinib are at increased risk of developing serious infections (e.g., bacterial, mycobacterial, viral, fungal, protzoan). Lymphopenia and neutropenia may occur with lymphocyte counts < 500 cells/mm^3 and ANC $< 1,000$ cells/mm^3. Latent TB may become reactivated TB (pulmonary or extrapulmonary). Opportunistic infections (OIs) may occur, including invasive fungal infections that may be disseminated on presentation (especially if patients were also taking concomitant immunomodulating agents such as MTX or corticosteroids). Most common OIs were TB, esophageal candidiasis, pneuomocystosis, cryptococcosis, BK virus, and cytomegalovirus. Most common infections are pneumonia, herpes zoster, and UTIs. Baricitinib can cause viral reactivation; patients who tested positive for hepatitis B or C were excluded from studies.

Nursing Implications: Review patient history; drug should not be given to a patient with active infection, including localized infections. Assess results of patient's latent TB testing and discuss any abnormalities with physician, NP, or PA. If TB test is positive, patient should take anti-TB therapy before beginning baricitinib therapy. Anti-TB therapy should also be considered for patients with a history of latent or active TB, and an adequate course of therapy cannot be confirmed. Monitor all patients for active TB during treatment, even if initial latent TB test is negative. Physician should discuss risks vs. benefits of baricitinib in patients with chronic or recurrent infections, exposed to TB, with a history of a serious OI, who have resided or traveled to an area of endemic TB or mycoses, or with underlying conditions besides RA that may predispose them to infection.

If the patient screened positive for hepatitis B or C, discuss with physician whether patient is a candidate for the drug, as baricitinib may react with hepatitis virus. If the patient is treated with baricitinib, teach the patient to report immediately increased fatigue, yellow conjunctiva (eyes looking yellow), anorexia, vomiting, clay-colored bowel movements, fever, chills, stomach discomfort, muscle aches, dark urine, or skin rash.

Assess CBC/differential baseline labs and at each visit prior to drug administration, and verify that lymphocyte count is > 500 cells/mm^3 and ANC $> 1,000$ cells/mm^3. Assess baseline risk for infection (e.g., comorbidities, history of infections). Teach patient to self-assess for signs/symptoms of infection (e.g., $T > 100.4°$F, cough, chest pain, sputum production, dysuria), stop drug, and report any signs/symptoms immediately. Closely monitor patient for signs/symptoms of infection, including TB, during and after treatment with baricitinib, and teach patient to report any changes (e.g., fever, sweats, rigors, weight loss, blood in sputum). Drug should be interrupted if patient develops a serious infection, opportunistic infection, or sepsis. If a patient develops a new infection while receiving baricitinib therapy, prompt and comprehensive evaluation of an immunocompromised patient should be done, and antimicrobial therapy should be given.

Teach patient strategies to manage fatigue and conserve energy, such as alteration of rest and activity and organizing chores.

Drug: certolizumab pegol (Cimzia)

Class: TNF blocker (antagonist).

Mechanism of Action: Drug binds to human TNF-α, a key proinflammatory cytokine. By neutralizing TNF-α effect, none of the immune inflammatory molecules are activated, so inflammation is suppressed. The drug does not have an Fc (fragment crystallizable of the antibody) region, so it cannot fix complement, cause antibody-dependent cell-mediated cytotoxicity (ADCC), or cause apoptosis (programmed cell death). Elevated levels of TNF-α are found in Crohn's disease (bowel wall) and RA patients (synovial fluid), and TNF-α plays a central role in disease and progression.

Metabolism: After subcutaneous administration, peak plasma concentrations are found 54–171 hours after injection. Bioavailability is 80%. Terminal half-life is about 14 days. The antibody (Fab portion) is cleaved and excreted primarily in the urine.

Indication: For (1) reducing signs and symptoms of Crohn's disease (CD) and maintaining clinical response in adult patients with moderately to severely active disease who have had an inadequate response to conventional therapy; (2) treatment of adult patients with moderately to severely active RA; (3) treatment of adult patients with active psoriatic arthritis (PsA); (4) treatment of adults with active ankylosing spondylitis (AS); (5) treatment of adults with nonradiographic axial spondyloarthritis with objective signs of inflammation; (6) treatment of adults with moderate to severe plaque psoriasis who are candidates for systemic therapy or phototheapy.

Contraindications: Serious HSRs to certolizumab pegol or to any of the excipients.

Dosage/Range:
The initial dose is 400 mg initially (two subcutaneous injections of 200 mg each).
- **CD:** 400 mg initially (two subcutaneous injections of 200 mg each), and again at weeks 2 and 4; if response occurs, follow with 400 mg subcutaneously every 4 weeks.
- **RA:** 400 mg initially (two subcutaneous injections of 200 mg each), and at weeks 2 and 4, followed by 200 mg every other week; for maintenance dosing, 400 mg subcutaneously every 4 weeks can be considered.
- **PsA:** 400 mg initially and at weeks 2 and 4, followed by 200 mg every other week for maintenance dosing; 400 mg every 4 weeks can be considered.
- **AS:** 400 mg (given as two subcutaneous injections of 200 mg each) initially, and at weeks 2 and 4, followed by 200 mg every other week, or 400 mg every 4 weeks.
- **Nonradiolographic axial spondyloarthritis**: 400 mg initially (two subcutaneous injections of 200 mg each), and at weeks 2 and 4, followed by 200 mg every other week or 400 mg subcutaneously every 4 weeks.
- **Plaque Psoriasis**: 400 mg (two subcutaneous injections of 200 mg each) every other week. If body weight is $\leq$ 90 kg consider administering certolizumab pegol 400 mg

(given as 2 subcutaneous injections of 200 mg each) initially, at week 2 and week 4, followed by 200 mg every other week.

Drug Preparation:

- Remove vials from refrigerator 30 minutes before reconstitution; do not warm the vials in any other manner. Use aseptic technique in reconstituting and administering drug.
- Drug available as lyophilized powder or prefilled syringe:
- 200-mg lyophilized powder for reconstitution, in a single-use glass vial, to be reconstituted with 1 mL of sterile water for injection, USP; use 20-gauge needle included with vial.
  - Direct stream of diluent to the inside wall of the vial, not directly on the lyophilized drug. Gently swirl each vial for 1 minute but do not shake so that all the drug powder is dissolved. Continue gentle swirling every 5 minutes of undissolved drug particles remain, and it may take 30 minutes.
  - The final solution should be clear to opalescent, colorless to pale yellow liquid free of particles.
  - Allow filled reconstituted solution to remain at room temperature for up to 2 hours prior to administration.
  - Use a new syringe to aspirate the contents of each vial (1 mL = 200 mg certolizumab pegol) so that each syringe contains 1 mL. Replace 20-gauge needle with a 23-gauge needle for administration.
  - 200-mg/mL solution in a single-use prefilled glass syringe. The needle shield inside the removable cap of the prefilled syringe contains a derivative of natural rubber latex that may cause an allergic reaction; handle with caution by latex-sensitive individuals.
- Inspect solution carefully for particulate matter, discoloration prior to administration, and do not use if cloudy or particulate matter found.

Drug Administration:

- Ensure patient has been screened for both active and latent TB (e.g., tuberculin skin test and CXR). A finding of skin induration $\geq$ 5 mm is considered positive. If results are positive, ensure that the patient has begun anti-TB therapy prior to starting therapy with certolizumab pegol. Discuss with physician/NP/PA anti-TB therapy in patients with a past history of latent or active TB and in whom an adequate course of treatment cannot be confirmed; as well as patients with risk factors for TB despite having a negative latent TB test.
- For subcutaneous injection, rotate injection sites and avoid areas where skin is tender, bruised, red, or hard.
- When administering a 400-mg dose, two injections of 200 mg should be given at separate sites in the thigh or abdomen. Ensure that entire contents of syringes are injected.
- Teach patient or caregiver to administer certolizumab pegol using PFS, when appropriate.
- Assess for HSR as patients have had reactions including angioedema, anaphylaxis, serum sickness, and uricaria. Teach patient who is self-administering drug and caregiver, to seek emergency medical care right away if this happens.

Lab Effects/Interference:

- Certolizumab pegol may interfere with APTT tests.

Drug Interactions:
- Biological DMARDs: increased risk of infection; do not use concomitantly.
- Live vaccines: do not give with certolizumab pegol.

Special Considerations:
- Most common side effects are URI (18%), rash (9%), and UTI (8%).
- Warnings and Precautions:
  - *Serious infections:* Drug increases risk of serious infections leading to hospitalization or death, with highest risk in patients receiving another concomitant immunosuppressive drug like MTX or corticosteroids. Other patients at risk and for whom risks and benefits should be reviewed: those with chronic or recurrent infection who have been exposed to TB with a history of opportunistic infection (OI); those who have resided or traveled in areas of endemic TB or mycoses (e.g., histoplasmosis, coccidioidomycosis or blastomycosis); and those with underlying conditions that may predispose them to infection.
    - Opportunistic infections (OI) include TB and invasive fungal infections where the patient may present with disseminated disease.
    - Consider empiric antifungal therapy in patients who reside in or travel to regions where mycoses are endemic.
  - Do not start drug if patient has an active infection, and discontinue drug if a serious infection develops.
  - Invasive fungal infections: if a patient develops a systemic illness on certolizumab pegol, consider empiric antifungal treatment for those who reside/travel to regions where mycoses are endemic.
- Patients should be closely monitored for signs/symptoms of infection during and after treatment, including the development of TB in patients who tested negatively for latent TB.
- Prior to initial therapy, patients should be evaluated for active TB and tested for latent infection.
- If initial TB test is positive, patients should begin anti-TB therapy prior to beginning certolizumab pegol.
- Monitor all patients for active TB during and after treatment, even if initial latent TB test is negative.
  - *Malignancy:* Cases of lymphoma and other malignancies have been observed in patients receiving TNF blockers.
    - These have been reported in children, adolescents, and young adults. Drug is not indicated for the treatment of pediatric patients.
    - Half of cases were lymphomas (HD and NHL).
    - Most patients were receiving immunosuppressants as well; diagnosis occurred after a median of 30 months of therapy.
    - Hepatosplenic T-cell lymphoma (aggressive, often fatal) has been reported in patients treated with TNF blockers, in adult males with Crohn's disease or UC.
    - Most had drug in combination with immunosuppressants.

- Melanoma and Merkel cell carcinoma have been reported. Periodic skin examinations are recommended for all patients, especially those with risk factors for skin cancer.
- *Heart failure* may occur either as worsening preexisting HF or new onset.
- *HSR:* Rarely, serious allergic reactions, including anaphylaxis, may occur.
  - Assess for angioedema, dyspnea, hypotension, rash, serum sickness, and urticaria during infusion.
  - If reaction occurs, discontinue drug and institute appropriate medical interventions as ordered.
  - Patients with latex sensitivity should use the prefilled syringe removable cap very carefully as the needle shield inside contains a derivative of natural rubber latex.
- *HBV reactivation.* Test for HBV prior to starting certolizumab pegol.
  - If the test is positive for HBV surface antigen, discuss whether to proceed with a physician specializing in the treatment of patients with HBV.
  - If the patient is an HBV carrier, closely monitor for signs/symptoms of disease activation during and for several months following last dose of certolizumab pegol.
  - If reactivation occurs, stop certolizumab pegol and begin antiviral therapy.
- *Neurologic Reactions:* CNS demyelinating disease, both new onset and progression of existing disease, has rarely occurred in patients receiving certolizumab pegol. Carefully consider risks versus benefit in using drug in patients with demyelinating disease.
- *Hematologic Reactions:* TNF blockers have been associated rarely with pancytopenia, including aplastic anemia. Cytopenias and pancytopenia have occurred rarely. Monitor patients with preexisting blood abnormalities closely. Teach patients to seek immediate medical attention if they develop symptoms suggestive of blood dyscrasias or infection (e.g., persistent fever, bruising, bleeding, pallor) [UCB, 2019].
- *Use with Biological DMARDs:* Serious infections occurred with concurrent use of anakinra, an IL-1 antagonist, and another TNF blocker etanercept without added benefit compared to etanercept alone. Do not use other biological DMARDs with certolizumab pegol.
- *Autoimmunity:* Patients may develop autoantibodies, and rarely, the development of a Lupus-like syndrome may rarely occur; if it does occur, discontinue certolizumab pegol.
- *Immunizations:* Do not administer live or live attenuated vaccines while the patient is receiving certolizumab pegol.
- *Immunosuppression:* TNF mediates inflammation and modulates the cellular immune responses, and theoretically, TNF blockade reduces host defenses against infections and the development of malignancy.
- Pregnancy category B: Counsel women of reproductive potential that the drug should be used during pregnancy only if the benefit exceeds the potential risk, as there are no well-controlled studies in pregnancy. If pregnancy develops, encourage the patient to register in the Pregnancy Surveillance Program (1-877-311-8972). Nursing mothers should decide whether to stop nursing or stop using the drug.

Potential Toxicities/Side Effects and the Nursing Process

I.   POTENTIAL FOR INFECTION related to IMMUNOSUPPRESSION

Defining Characteristics: Patients receiving certolizumab pegol are at increased risk of developing serious infections requiring hospitalization. Although uncommon and occurring in patients receiving combination immunosuppressant medications (e.g., MTX and corticosteroids), opportunistic infections may be disseminated on presentation, such as fulminating fungal infections. In clinical trials, most common infections were URI and UTI.

Nursing Implications: Assess results of patient's latent TB and HBV testing and discuss any abnormalities with physician, NP, or PA. If TB test is positive, patient should begin anti-TB therapy before beginning certolizumab pegol therapy. If HBV is positive, discuss if patient should receive therapy (see above). Assess baseline risk for infection (e.g., comorbidities, preexisting infections, concomitant immunosuppressants like MTX or corticosteroids). Teach patient to self-assess for signs/symptoms of infection (e.g., $T > 100.4°F$, cough, chest pain, sputum production, dysuria), and to report them right away. Closely monitor patient for signs/symptoms of infection during and after treatment with certolizumab pegol, including TB reactivation even if latent TB test is negative; teach patient to report any changes (e.g., fever, sweats, chills, cough, SOB, blood in sputum, weight loss). Drug should be discontinued if patient develops a serious infection or sepsis, and appropriate antimicrobial therapy instituted right away. If the patient is at risk for fungal infection and develops severe systemic illness, discuss with physician, NP, or PA empiric antifungal therapy.

II.   KNOWLEDGE DEFICIT related to SUBCUTANEOUS INJECTION TECHNIQUE

Defining Characteristics: Drug is administered subcutaneously, and appropriate patients (or caregivers) can be taught to administer the drug.

Nursing Implications: Assess patient or caregiver readiness to learn, and assess learning style and limitations. Review with patient drug administration schedule; teach patient not to administer and to notify physician or nurse if patient develops an infection. Provide Medication Guide and Instructions for Use from the drug manufacturer UCB, Inc. Teach patient how to care for drug; it should be stored in refrigerator at 2–8°C (36°–46°F) in the original container until used, and it should be protected from light. Drug must not be frozen. Patient should inspect syringe for cloudiness or particles, and should not use if these are found. Patient should be careful to protect glass syringe, as it may break. Drug should be kept out of reach of children and pets. Teach patient hand-washing, aseptic technique, subcutaneous injection technique, and how to dispose of syringe/needle. Teach patient to rotate sites and to apply local measures if injection-site reactions occur. Validate patient understanding by having patient describe measures taught, and ideally, by returning the demonstration of subcutaneous injection technique. Teach patient that allergic reactions are rare, but to call provider right away or seek emergency care if signs/symptoms of allergic reaction occur (e.g., hives, swollen face, trouble breathing, chest pain). Teach patient to develop documentation tool to record site rotation and any site irritation or reaction.

Drug: etanercept (Enbrel); biosimilars etanercept-szzs (Erelzi), and etanercept-ykro (Eticovo)

Class: TNF blocker (antagonist).

Mechanism of Action: TNF is a proinflammatory cytokine and plays a central role in the inflammatory processes of RA, PJIA, PsA, AS, and psoriasis (PsO). Elevated levels of TNF are found in the joints and tissues of these patients. Etanercept prevents TNF from binding to its two TNF receptors (α and β) so TNF is unable to stimulate the proinflammatory response. The drug also modulates other immune and biological responses regulated by TNF.

Metabolism: Maximal peak serum level is reached in 69 $\pm$ 34 hours after a single dose, and mean drug half-life is 102 $\pm$ 30 hours.

Indication: Treatment of patients with (1) RA; (2) Polyarticular Juvenile Idiopathic Arthritis (JIA) in patients ages 2 and older; (3) psoriatic arthritis (PsA); (4) ankylosing spondylitis (AS); (5) plaque psoriasis (PsO) who are 4 years or older.

Contraindication: sepsis.

Dosage/Range: By subcutaneous injection:
- Adult RA and PsA: 50 mg once weekly with or without MTX.
- AS: 50 mg once weekly.
- Adult PsO: starting dose 50 mg twice weekly for 3 months, followed by maintenance dose of 50 mg once weekly.
- Pediatric PsO or JIA:
  - weight $<$ 63 kg (138 lbs): 0.8 mg/kg weekly (max 50 mg weekly); weight 63 kg (138 lbs) or more: 50 mg weekly.
  - To achieve pediatric doses other than 25 mg or 50 mg, use reconstituted lyophilized powder (Enbrel).
- Adult RA, AS, PsA: MTX, glucocorticoids, salicylates, NSAIDs, or analgesics can be continued with etanercept treatment.

Drug Preparation:
Enbrel:
- Injection: 25 mg/0.5 mL and 50 mg/mL solution in a single-dose prefilled syringe;
- Injection 50 mg/mL solution in single-dose prefilled SureClick autoinjector;
- For injection: 25 mg lyophilized powder in a multiple-dose vial for reconstitution;
- Injection: 50 mg/mL solution in Enbrel Mini single-dose prefilled cartridge for use with the AutoTouch reusable autoinjector only.
- Allow PFS or SureClick Autoinjector to reach room temperature (15–30 and 30 minutes, respectively); do not remove needle cover. Check to see if the amount of liquid falls between the two purple fill-level indicator lines on the PFS. If there is too little liquid, do not use that syringe. Inspect for discoloration and particulate matter in the syringe and do not use if found. There may be small white proteinaceous particles, which is acceptable.

- 25-mg multiuse vial (25 mg etanercept):
  - Use 1 mL of the supplied sterile bacteriostatic water for injection USP (0.9% benzyl alcohol), giving a solution of 25 mg etanercept/1.0 mL.
  - Use the supplied vial adapter to aseptically reconstitute the lyophilized powder, unless multiple doses will be withdrawn; in that case, use a 25-gauge needle to reconstitute and withdraw dose. Label multidose vial (must be used within 14 days).
  - If using the vial adapter, twist the adapter onto the diluent syringe. Then place the vial adapter over the Enbrel vial and insert the vial adapter into the vial stopper. Push down on the plunger to inject the diluent into the Enbrel vial.
  - If the vial will be used as a multidose vial, use a 25-gauge needle, and attach the sticker indicating the date and time of reconstitution. Reconstituted solution must be refrigerated at 36–46°F (2–8°C) and used within 14 days. DO NOT leave reconstituted solution at room temperature.
  - If using a 25-gauge needle to reconstitute and withdraw the Enbrel dose, inject the diluent very slowly into the Enbrel vial. Normally, some foaming occurs.
  - Keep the diluent syringe in place and gently swirl the contents of the vial; do not shake or vigorously agitate.
  - Drug should dissolve in 10 minutes. Inspect for cloudiness or particulate matter, and if found, do not use. Withdraw the correct dose of reconstituted drug into the syringe. Some foam or bubbles may be present.
  - Remove the syringe from vial adapter or remove the 25-gauge needle from syringe. Place 27-gauge needle to inject drug. Do not filter at any time.

Eticovo
- Injection: 25 mg/0.5 mL, and 50 mg/mL solution in a single-dose prefilled syringe.

Erelzi
- Injection: 25 mg/0.5 mL and 50 mg/mL solution in a single-dose prefilled syringe with BD UltraSafe Passive Needle Guard.
- Injection: 50 mg/mL solution in single-dose prefilled Sensoready pen.

Drug Administration:
- Drug should be given subcutaneously.
- Teach patient or caregiver to inject patient when appropriate and if certain that they will comply with medical follow-up as necessary.
- Children should have recommended immunizations given before starting etanercept.

Drug Interactions:
- Live vaccines: do not give with etanercept.
- Immune-modulating biological products (e.g., anakinra): increased immunosuppression; do not give concomitantly.
- Cyclophosphamide: do not use with etanercept.

Lab Effects/Interference:
- Hypoglycemia in diabetic patients (rare).
- Rare cytopenias.

Special Considerations:

- Most common are infections and injection-site reactions.
- Warnings and Precautions:
  - *Serious infections*: Etanercept increases risk of serious infections leading to hospitalization or death, with risk highest in individuals aged 65 or greater, having comorbid conditions, and/or receiving another concomitant immunosuppressive drug like MTX or corticosteroids.
    - Opportunistic infections include TB and invasive fungal infections where the patient may present with disseminated disease.
    - Consider empiric antifungal therapy in patients at risk for invasive fungal disease who develop severe systemic illness.
    - Do not administer etanercept to patients with active infection including important localized infections. Discontinue drug if a serious infection develops. Drug is contraindicated in sepsis.
    - Risk benefit evaluation should be discussed in patients with chronic or recurrent infections, have been exposed to TB, with a history of opportunistic infection, or who have traveled/lived in areas of endemic TB or mycoses (e.g., histoplasmosis), or with underlying conditions that may predispose the patient to infection, such as advanced or poorly controlled diabetes.
    - Fungal infections: see package insert for empiric antifungal therapy in high-risk individuals with systemic illness.
    - Monitor patient closely for signs/symptoms of infection during and after treatment with etanercept.
  - Patients should be closely monitored for signs/symptoms of infection during and after treatment, including the development of TB in patients who tested negatively for latent TB.
    - Prior to initial therapy, patients should be evaluated for active TB and tested for latent TB infection.
    - If initial latent TB test is positive, begin anti-TB therapy prior to beginning etanercept.
    - Monitor all patients for active TB during and after treatment, even if initial latent TB test is negative.
  - Drug may lead to reactivation of HBV.
    - Patients should be tested for HBV infection before starting etanercept. If the test is positive for HBV surface antigen, discuss whether to proceed with a physician specializing in the treatment of patients with HBV.
    - If the patient is a HBV carrier, close monitoring for signs/symptoms of disease activation should occur during and following treatment.
    - Etanercept should be stopped if HBV is reactivated, and antiviral therapy should be started.
  - *Neurological:* Demyelinating disease, both new onset and progression of existing disease, has rarely occurred to patients receiving etanercept. New onset of seizures has been described in patients receiving etanercept. Carefully consider risk versus benefit in using drug in patients with demyelinating disease.

- *Malignancies:* Lymphoma, leukemia, melanoma and nonmelanoma skin cancer, and other malignancies have been reported. Patients at risk for skin cancer should have regular skin screening examinations.
- *Heart failure* has been reported; monitor patients with heart failure closely while receiving etanercept.
- *Hematologic events:* rare pancytopenia, aplastic anemia. Patients should be taught to seek immediate medical treatment if they develop signs/symptoms such as bleeding, persistent fever, bruising, or pallor.
- *Hepatitis B virus reactivation:* Monitor patients previously infected with HBV for reactivation during and several months after therapy ends. If reactivation occurs, physician should consider stopping etanercept and beginning antiviral therapy.
- *Allergic reactions* have occurred in < 2% of patients, and anaphylaxis has been reported. Drug should be discontinued if anaphylaxis occurs and patient given emergency medical care.
- *Immunizations:* Live vaccines should not be given concurrently with the drug. Pediatric patients should receive what immunizations they need to be brought up to date before starting etanercept.
- *Autoimmunity:* Stop drug if patient develops lupus-like syndrome or autoimmune hepatitis.
- *Immunosuppression:* unclear impact on host defenses.
- Use in Wegener's Granulomatosis patients is not recommended.
- Use with anakinra or abatacept is not recommended.
- Use in patients with moderate to severe alcoholic hepatitis: mortality equal to placebo at 1 month of treatment, but was significantly higher at 6 months. Use drug cautiously in patients with moderate to severe alcoholic hepatitis.
- Pregnancy category B: Counsel women of reproductive potential that drug should be used in pregnancy only if benefit outweighs potential risk.

Potential Toxicities/Side Effects and the Nursing Process

I.   POTENTIAL FOR INFECTION related to IMMUNOSUPPRESSION

Defining Characteristics: Patients receiving etanercept are at increased risk of developing serious infections requiring hospitalization. Although uncommon and occurring in patients receiving multiple immunosuppressant medications (e.g., MTX and corticosteroids), opportunistic infections may be disseminated on presentation, such as fulminating fungal infections. In clinical trials, 50–81% of RA patients developed infections. The most common infections were URI (38–65%), while non-URI infections were 21–54%.

Nursing Implications: Assess results of patient's latent TB test and HBV testing and discuss any abnormalities with physician, NP, or PA. If TB test is positive, patient should begin anti-TB therapy before beginning etanercept therapy. Assess baseline patient risk for infection (e.g., comorbidities, preexisting infections, any concomitant immunosuppressive drugs). Teach patient to self-assess for signs/symptoms of infection (e.g., $T > 100.4°F$, cough, chest pain, sputum production, dysuria), and to report them right away. Closely monitor patient for signs/symptoms of infection during and after treatment with etaner-cept, including TB reactivation even if latent TB test is negative, and teach patient to report any changes (e.g., fever, sweats, chills, cough, SOB, blood in sputum, weight loss). Drug should be discontinued if patient develops a serious infection or sepsis, and appropriate antimicrobial therapy should be instituted right away. If the patient is at risk for fungal infection and develops severe systemic illness, discuss with physician empiric antifungal therapy.

II. KNOWLEDGE DEFICIT related to SUBCUTANEOUS INJECTION TECHNIQUE

Defining Characteristics: Drug is administered subcutaneously, and appropriate patients (or caregivers) can be taught to administer the drug.

Nursing Implications: Assess patient or caregiver readiness to learn, and assess learning style and limitations. Review with patient drug administration schedule, and teach patient not to administer and to notify physician/nurse if patient develops an infection. Provide Medication Guide and Instructions for Use from the drug distributor, Amgen. Teach patient how to care for drug; it should be stored in refrigerator at 2–8°C (36°–46°F) in the original container until used, and it should be protected from light. Drug must not be frozen. Patient should inspect syringe for cloudiness or particles and should not use if these are found. Patient should be careful to protect glass syringe, as it may break. Drug should be kept out of reach of children and pets. Teach patient hand-washing, aseptic technique, subcutaneous injection technique, and how to dispose of syringe/needle. Teach patient to rotate sites, and to apply local measures if injection-site reactions occur. Validate patient understanding by having patient describe measures taught, and ideally, by demonstrating the subcutaneous injection technique. Teach patient that allergic reactions are rare, but to call provider right away or seek emergency care if signs/symptoms of allergic reaction occur (hives, swollen face, trouble breathing, chest pain). Teach patient to develop documentation tool to record site rotation and any site irritation or reaction.

Drug: golimumab (Simponi, Simponi Aria)

Class: TNF blocker (antagonist).

Mechanism of Action: Golimumab is a human monoclonal antibody that binds to soluble and transmembrane forms of TNF-α, a proinflammatory cytokine that plays a central role in inflammation of arthritic joints. High levels of TNF-α are found in blood, synovium, and joints of patients with RA, PsA, and AS. Thus, golimumab blocks TNF-α so it is unable to bind to its receptors, suppressing joint inflammation and destruction.

Metabolism: Following subcutaneous injection, the absolute bioavailability of golimumab is 53%. Time to maximum serum concentration is 2–6 days, and steady state is reached by week 12. There is limited extravascular distribution. Median terminal half-life is about 2 weeks. MTX combined with golimumab reduces the formation of antigolimumab antibodies, so the combination should be used in patients with RA. In the PsA and AS trials, concomitant MTX did not appear to influence clinical efficacy or safety. Combinations of NSAIDs, oral corticosteroids, or sulfasalazine with golimumab does not affect golimumab clearance.

Indications: Simponi: (1) RA: adult patients with moderately to severely active RA in combination with MTX; (2) PsA: adult patients alone or in combination with MTX; (3) AS: adult patients with active AS; (4) UC: adult patients with moderately to severely active UC who have demonstrated corticosteroid dependence or who have had an inadequate response to or failed to tolerate oral aminosalicylates, oral corticosteroids, azathioprine, or 6-MP for (a) inducing and maintaining clinical response; (b) improving endoscopic appearance of the mucosa during induction; (c) inducing clinical remission; (d) achieving and sustaining clinical remission in induction responders.

Simponi Aria: Treatment of adult patients with (1) moderately or severely active RA, in combination with MTX; (2) active psoriatic arthritis (PsA); (3) active ankylosing spondylitis (AK).

Contraindications: None.

Dosage/Range:
Simponi (subcutaneous):
- RA: 50-mg subcutaneous injection once a month.
- RA patients should receive MTX in combination with golimumab; for patients with PsA or AS, golimumab may be given with or without MTX or other nonbiologic DMARDs.
- RA, PsA, AS patients: corticosteroids, nonbiologic DMARDs, and/or NSAIDs can be continued during golimumab therapy.
- UC: 200 mg initially administered by subcutaneous injection at week 0, followed by 100 mg at week 2, and then maintenance dose of 100 mg every 4 weeks.

Simponi Aria (intravenous):
- 2 mg/kg IV infusion over 30 minutes at weeks 0, 4, then every 8 weeks.
- All patients: Prior to beginning golimumab and periodically during therapy, patients should be evaluated for active TB and tested for latent infection. In addition, prior to starting drug, patients should be tested for HBV viral infections.

Drug Preparation:
- Simponi is available in 50- and 100-mg strengths for SQ injection:
- Smartject® autoinjector:
    - Each 50-mg single-dose SmartJect® autoinjector contains a prefilled glass syringe (27-gauge 1/2-inch) providing 50 mg of golimumab per 0.5-mL solution.
    - Each 100-mg single-dose SmartJect® autoinjector contains a prefilled glass syringe (27-gauge 1/2-inch) providing 100 mg of golimumab per 1.0-mL solution.
- Prefilled Syringe (PFS):
    - Each 50-mg single-dose prefilled glass syringe (27-gauge 1/2-inch) contains 50 mg of golimumab per 0.5 mL of solution. Each 100-mg single-dose prefilled glass syringe (27-gauge 1/2-inch) contains 100 mg of golimumab per 1.0-mL solution.

- Simponi Aria is available in 50-mg golimumab per 4 mL of solution (12.5 mg of golimumab per mL) in a single-use vial.
  - Ensure vial solution is colorless to yellow and without particulate matter (a few translucent particles of protein are acceptable).
  - Calculate dose (2 mg/kg) and each 4 mL of solution contains 50 mg of golimumab.
  - Dilute the total volume with 0.9% sodium chloride Injection USP to a final volume of 100 mL (e.g., withdrawing a volume of the 0.9% sodium chloride injection USP from the 100-mL infusion bag or bottle equal to the total volume of Simponi Aria. Slowly add the total volume of Simponi Aria solution to the 100-mL infusion bag or bottle). Gently mix and discard any unused drug. Alternatively, 0.45% w/v sodium chloride for infusion can be used.
  - Once diluted, the infusion solution can be stored for 4 hours at room temperature.

Drug Administration:

Simponi subcutaneous:

- Teach patient or caregiver proper aseptic SQ injection technique if/when appropriate.
- Allow the PFS or autoinjector to sit at room temperature for 30 minutes outside the carton prior to SQ administration. Do not warm in any other way.
- Inspect syringe for particles or discoloration, and do not use if present; solution should be clear to slightly opalescent or light yellow.
- Do not use any leftover product in the PFS or autoinjector.
- The needle cover contains dry natural rubber (latex derivative) on PFS and PFS with autoinjector cap, and should not be handled by people with a latex sensitivity.
- When multiple injections are given, give in different sites. Rotate injection sites, avoiding where skin is tender, bruised, red, or hard.

Simponi Aria intravenous:

- Use an infusion set with an inline, sterile, nonpyrogenic, low-protein binding filter (pore size 0.22 micrometer or less).
- The line must be dedicated for the infusion, and no other drugs can be given concomitantly.
- Infuse the diluted drug over 30 minutes.

Drug Interactions:

- MTX: increased response with golimumab in RA patients.
- Biologic DMARDs (e.g., abatacept, anakinra): increased risk of serious infection; DO NOT administer concomitantly.
- Live vaccines: do not administer while patient is receiving golimumab.
- CYP450 enzyme formation may be suppressed by increased levels of cytokines (e.g., TNF) during chronic inflammation, and thus may be normalized with golimumab when TNF levels are reduced. Assess INR frequently in patients receiving warfarin, or closely monitor patient receiving other CYP450 substrates with a narrow therapeutic window.

Lab Effects/Interference:

- Increased ALT, AST.
- Rare pancytopenia, leukopenia, neutropenia, thrombocytopenia; very rare aplastic anemia.

Special Considerations:
- Most common adverse reactions: *IV*: URI, viral infection, bronchitis, HTN, rash; *Subcutaneous*: URI, injection-site reaction, and viral infections. Rarely, psoriasis may occur or worsen in patients with the disease who receive subcutaneous golimumab therapy.
- Warnings and Precautions:
  - *Serious infections*: Drug increases risk of serious infections leading to hospitalization or death.
    - Patients at greatest risk are those > 65 years old, those with comorbid conditions, and/or those taking concomitant immunosuppressants, such as corticosteroids or MTX.
    - Opportunistic infections include TB, HBV infection, and invasive fungal infections where the patient may present with disseminated disease.
    - Consider empiric antifungal therapy in patients with systemic infection who reside in or travel to regions where mycoses are endemic. Other serious infections include sepsis.
    - Do not start the drug if patient has an active infection, and monitor patient closely for signs/symptoms of infection during and after therapy, including TB infection in patients who initially tested negative for latent TB. If an infection develops, stop drug if the infection becomes serious.
  - TB: Prior to initial therapy, patients should be evaluated for active TB (CXR) and tested for latent infection (e.g., induration $\geq$ 5 mm is a positive TB skin test, even if previously vaccinated with BCG). If initial latent TB test is positive, patient should begin anti-TB therapy prior to beginning golimumab.
    - Test for active and latent TB during and after golimumab therapy, even if initial latent TB test is negative.
    - Treatment of latent TB prior to TNF-blocker therapy has been shown to reduce the risk of TB reactivation during therapy.
    - Consider anti-TB therapy prior to golimumab therapy in patients with a past history of latent or active TB, when it cannot be confirmed that an adequate course of therapy has been completed.
    - Cases of active TB have occurred in patients treated with golimumab during and after treatment for latent TB.
    - Monitor patients for signs and symptoms of TB during golimumab therapy even if the patients tested negative for latent TB infection prior to starting therapy, patients were on treatment for latent TB, or patients were previously treated for TB.
  - Invasive fungal infections:
    - Consider empiric antifungal therapy in patients who develop systemic disease and who reside in or travel to regions where mycoses are endemic.
    - Antigen/antibody testing for histoplasmosis may be negative in some patients with active infection. Consult with an expert in treatment of fungal infections.
  - HBV reactivation: Drug may lead to reactivation of HBV.
    - Patients should be tested for HBV infection before starting golimumab. If the test is positive for HBV surface antigen, discuss whether to proceed with a physician specializing in the treatment of patients with HBV.

- If the patient is an HBV carrier, closely monitor the patient for signs/symptoms of disease activation during and following treatment.
- Golimumab should be stopped if HBV is reactivated, and antiviral therapy should be begun.
- *Malignancies:* Lymphoma and other malignancies have been reported in children, adolescent, and young adult patients receiving TNF-blockers who started therapy at or younger than 18 years of age.
  - Median onset was 30 months after starting TNF-blocker therapy, and most patients were receiving concomitant immunosuppressants.
  - Rare postmarketing reports of hepatosplenic T-cell lymphoma in patients receiving TNF-blockers, a rare and aggressive lymphoma, primarily in patients with Crohn's disease who had previously received azathioprine or 6-MP.
  - Melanoma has been reported, and Merkel cell cancer in patients receiving TNF blockers. Patients at risk for skin cancer should have regular screenings for skin cancer.
- *CHF:* CHF, new onset or worsening of existing disease, has occurred rarely.
- *Demyelinating disorder:* TNF-blockers have rarely been associated with new onset or worsening of CNS demyelinating disorders, such as MS. Use drug cautiously in patients with existing demyelinating disorders and monitor closely. Drug should be discontinued if this occurs.
- *Autoimmunity:* Treatment with TNF-blockers may result in the production of antinuclear antibodies (ANA), as well as lupus-like syndrome. If a patient develops a lupus-like syndrome the drug should be discontinued and patient further evaluated.
- *HSR:* Serious HSRs, including anaphylaxis, have rarely occurred with both subcutaneous and IV formulations. Reactions include hives, pruritus, dyspnea, and nausea during IV infusion, and generally after 1 hour of the infusion. If a serious HSR reaction occurs, immediately stop the drug, and implement ordered emergency medical care.
- *Do not administer with other TNF-blockers* (e.g., abatacept) or IL-1 antagonist (anakinra) as there is increased risk of serious infections with potentially no increase in benefit.
- *Switching between Biological DMARDs:* Switching biologicals should only be done carefully as overlapping toxicity increases risk of serious infections.
- *Cytopenias and pancytopenia* have rarely occurred. Drug should be given cautiously in patients who have or have had existing cyptopenias.
- *Vaccinations and therapeutic infectious agents:* Do not administer live vaccines as this may initiate an infection that may become disseminated; live attenuated bacteria (e.g., BCG in bladder cancer also should not be given concurrently).
- Pregnancy category B: Counsel women of reproductive potential that drug should be used during pregnancy only if benefit exceeds potential risk to the fetus, as there have been no controlled trials.
  - Infants who were exposed to the drug in utero should not receive live vaccinations for 6 months following the mother's last dose of golimumab.
  - Nursing mothers should decide whether to stop nursing or discontinue the drug.

Potential Toxicities/Side Effects and the Nursing Process

I.   POTENTIAL FOR INFECTION related to IMMUNOSUPPRESSION

Defining Characteristics: Patients receiving golimumab are at increased risk for developing serious infections (e.g., bacterial, viral, fungal) requiring hospitalization. Although uncommon and occurring in patients receiving multiple immunosuppressant medications (e.g., MTX and corticosteroids), opportunistic infections may be disseminated on presentation, such as fulminating fungal infections (e.g., histoplasmosis, coccidiodomycosis, candidiasis, aspergillosis, pneumocystosis) or extrapulmonary TB. In clinical trials, most common infections were URI (17%), sinusitis (14%), pharyngitis (11%), and UTI (8%).

Nursing Implications: Assess results of patient's latent TB and HBV testing and discuss any abnormalities with physician, NP, or PA. If TB test is positive (e.g., induration of 5 mm or greater on skin tuberculin test), patient should begin anti-TB therapy before beginning golimumab therapy. Assess baseline risk of infection (e.g., comorbidities, preexisting infections, concomitant immunosuppressants like MTX or corticosteroids). Teach patient to self-assess for signs/symptoms of infection (e.g., $T > 100.4°F$, cough, chest pain, sputum production, dysuria), and to report them right away. Closely monitor patient for signs/symptoms of infection during and after treatment with golimumab, including TB reactivation even if latent TB test is negative, and teach patient to report any changes (e.g., fever, sweats, chills, cough, SOB, blood in sputum, weight loss). Drug should be discontinued if patient develops a serious infection or sepsis, and appropriate antimicrobial therapy instituted right away. If the patient is at risk for fungal infection and develops severe systemic illness, discuss empiric antifungal therapy with physician, NP, or PA.

II.   KNOWLEDGE DEFICIT related to SUBCUTANEOUS INJECTION TECHNIQUE

Defining Characteristics: Drug is administered subcutaneously, and appropriate patients (or caregivers) can be taught to administer the drug.

Nursing Implications: Assess patient or caregiver readiness to learn, and assess learning style and limitations. Review with patient drug administration schedule, and teach not to administer and to notify physician/nurse if patient develops an infection. Provide Patient Instructions for Use available from Janssen Biotech (patient package insert). Teach patient how to care for drug; it should be stored in refrigerator at 2–8°C (36–46°F) in the original container until used, and protected from light. Patient should inspect syringe for cloudiness or particles, and not use if these are found. Patient should be careful to protect glass syringe, as it may break. Teach patient not to use any leftover product remaining in the PFS/autoinjector. Teach patients with a latex sensitivity not to handle the needle cover on the PFS/autoinjector, as it contains dry natural rubber (derivative of latex), and to use gloves. Drug should be kept out of reach of children and pets. Teach patient hand-washing, aseptic technique, subcutaneous injection technique, and how to dispose of syringe/needle. Teach patient to rotate sites and to apply local measures if injection-site reactions occur. If multiple injections are needed, teach patient to use separate injection sites. Validate patient understanding by having patient describe measures taught, and ideally, by demonstrating the subcutaneous injection technique. Teach patient to develop documentation tool to record site rotation and any site irritation or reaction.

Drug: infliximab (Remicade); Biosimilars (1) infliximab-dyyb (Inflectra), (2) infliximab-abda (Renflexis)

Class: TNF blocker (antagonist).

Mechanism of Action: Chimeric monoclonal antibody targeting TNF. TNF-α is important in initiating the acute phase reaction in systemic inflammation. TNF-α functions to induce proinflammatory cytokines (e.g., IL1 and IL6), enhances leukocyte migration, activates neutInflrophil and eosinophilic functional activity, induces acute phase reactants and other liver proteins, as well as tissue-degrading enzymes produced by cells in the joints (synoviocytes and/or chronrocytes). Infliximab is a chimeric monoclonal antibody, made up of 25% mouse and 75% human protein, that binds to soluble and transmembrane TNF-α so that TNF-α cannot bind to its receptors. This neutralizes TNF-α effect and reduces inflammation. TNF-α concentrations are elevated in tissues/fluids of patients with RA, Crohn's disease, UC, AS, PsA, and Ps. The drug reduces inflammatory cell infiltration into tissue, levels of IL-6, and CRP.

Metabolism: After IV infusion, median terminal half-life of infliximab is 7.7–9.5 days. Development of antibodies to infliximab increases its clearance. Coadministration with MTX decreases formation of antibodies to infliximab.

Indication: For the treatment of patients with (1a) Crohn's disease (CD) to reduce the signs and symptoms, and induce and maintain clinical remission in adult patients with moderately to severely active disease who have had an inadequate response to conventional therapy; as well as (1b) to reduce the number of draining enterocutaneous and rectovaginal fistulae, and to maintain fistula closure in adult patients with fistulizing disease; (2) pediatric Crohn's disease (Pediatric CD), to reduce the signs and symptoms, and induce and maintain clinical remission in children aged 6 years old and older, with moderately to severely active disease who have had an inadequate response to conventional therapy; (3) Ulcerative Colitis (UC), to reduce signs and symptoms, to induce and maintain clinical remission and mucosal healing, and to eliminate corticosteroid use in adult patients with moderately to severely active disease who have had an inadequate response to conventional therapy; (4) pediatric UC, to reduce signs and symptoms, and to induce and maintain clinical remission in children, aged 6 years and older, with moderately to severely active disease who have had an inadequate response to conventional therapy; (5) RA in combination with MTX, to reduce signs and symptoms, to inhibit the progression of structural damage, and to improve physical function in patients with moderately to severely active disease; (6) Ankylosing Spondylitis (AK) to reduce signs and symptoms in patients with active disease; (7) Psoriatic arthritis (PsA) to reduce signs and symptoms of active arthritis and to prevent the progression of structural damage and improve physical functioning; (8)

Plaque psoriasis (Ps), in adult patients with chronic severe (extensive or disabling) disease who are candidates for systemic therapy and when other systemic therapies are medically less appropriate.

Contraindication: (1) DO NOT administer doses > 5 mg/kg to patients with moderate-to-severe heart failure; (2) drug is contraindicated in patients who have a severe HSR to the drug or to murine proteins.

Dosage/Range:
- Crohn's disease: 5 mg/kg at 0, 2, and 6 weeks, then every 8 weeks as maintenance therapy. Some adults who respond may benefit from increasing the dose to 10 mg/kg if responsiveness is lost. Patients who do not respond by week 14 are unlikely to respond, and drug should be discontinued.
- Pediatric Crohn's disease: 5 mg/kg at 0, 2, and 6 weeks, then every 8 weeks as maintenance therapy.
- UC: 5 mg/kg at 0, 2, and 6 weeks, then every 8 weeks as maintenance therapy.
- Pediatric UC: 5 mg/kg at 0, 2, and 6 weeks, then every 8 weeks as maintenance therapy.
- RA in conjunction with MTX, 3 mg/kg at 0, 2, and 6 weeks, then every 8 weeks as maintenance therapy. Some patients may benefit from increasing the dose up to 10 mg/kg or treating as often as every 4 weeks. However, incidence of infection is higher with higher doses.
- AS: 5 mg/kg at 0, 2, and 6 weeks, then every 6 weeks as maintenance therapy.
- PsA and Ps: 5 mg/kg at 0, 2, and 6 weeks, then every 8 weeks as maintenance therapy.
- DO NOT administer doses > 5 mg/kg to patients with moderate-to-severe heart failure.
- Drug is contraindicated in patients who have a severe HSR to the drug or to murine proteins.
- Prior to starting infliximab therapy, and during therapy, patient should be evaluated for active TB and tested for latent infection.

Drug Preparation:
- Available as 100 mg of lyophilized infliximab in a 20-mg vial for IV use for infliximab and biosimilars.
- IV:
  - Calculate the dose, the total volume of reconstituted infliximab solution required, and the number of vials needed. Each vial will contain 100 mg of the infliximab antibody.
  - Reconstitute each vial with 10 mL sterile water for injection USP, using a syringe with a 21-gauge or smaller needle as follows: Remove the flip top from the vial and wipe the top with an alcohol swab. Insert the needle aseptically into the vial through the center of the rubber stopper and direct the stream of sterile water to the glass wall of the vial. Gently swirl the solution by rotating the vial to dissolve the lyophilized powder, but do not shake or use vigorous agitation. Foaming of the solution may occur; allow the reconstituted solution to stand for 5 minutes.
  - Inspect the solution; it should be colorless to light yellow and opalescent, and it may contain a few translucent particles of infliximab, as it is a protein. Do not use if lyophilized cake has not fully dissolved or if opaque particles, discoloration, or other foreign particles are seen.

- Dilute the total volume of the reconstituted infliximab dose to 250 mL with sterile 0.9% sodium chloride injection, USP by withdrawing a volume equal to the volume of reconstituted drug from the 250 mL bag of 0.9% sodium chloride injection, USP. Slowly add the entire volume of reconstituted drug to the bag or infusion bottle, then gently mix. The resulting infusion concentration should range from 0.4 to 4 mg/mL.
- Begin the infliximab infusion within 3 hours of reconstituting and diluting the drug.

Drug Administration:
- Infusion reactions: 20% of patients experienced an infusion reaction in clinical trials; monitor patient closely during the infusion, as anaphylaxis may occur at any time. Discuss with physician, NP, or PA premedications (e.g., antihistamines, acetaminophen, corticosteroid) to reduce the risk.
- Administer IV over a minimum of 2 hours, using an infusion set with a low-protein-binding, nonpyrogenic, low-binding filter (pore size 1.2 micrometer or less).
  - Mild–moderate infusion reactions: slow or stop infusion; once it resolves, resume at lower infusion rate; and/or administer antihistamines, acetaminophen, and/or corticosteroids.
  - If patient cannot tolerate infusion with these interventions, discontinue drug.
  - If patient has a severe infusion reaction during or after the infusion, drug should be discontinued.
  - Severe infusion reactions: manage signs and symptoms as ordered and have emergency equipment and personnel readily available.
- Assess baseline TB and HBV screening results. Anti-TB therapy should be started before starting infliximab. Retest for latent TB during therapy as ordered as initial negative testing can become positive during therapy.
- Drug should be discontinued if patient has a severe infusion-related HSR.
- Do not give the drug if patient has an active infection, including a clinically important localized infection, or if patient develops lupus-like syndrome.
- Live vaccines should not be given with infliximab. Bring pediatric patients up to date with all vaccinations prior to initiating infliximab.
- Use caution when switching between biological DMARDs, as there may be overlapping biological activity with further increased risk of infection.
- Common adverse effects during administration are flulike symptoms, headache, dyspnea, hypotension, transient fever, chills, GI symptoms, skin rash.

Drug Interactions:
- Anakinra (Kineret), abatacept (Orencia), tocilizumab (Actemra), etanercept (Enbrel), or other biological therapies: concurrent use increases risk of neutropenia and serious infections; DO NOT GIVE CONCOMITANTLY.
- MTX and other concomitant medications (e.g., NSAIDs, folic acid, corticosteroids): may decrease the incidence of anti-infliximab antibody production, and increase infliximab concentrations and potential efficacy.
- Immunosuppressants: reduce number of infusion reactions in patients with Crohn's disease; when used baseline, drugs such as corticosteroids, antibiotics (metronidazole or ciprofloxacin) and aminosalicylates do not appear to affect serum infliximab concentrations.

- Cytochrome (CYP) P450 substrates: formation of CYP450 enzymes may be suppressed by increased cytokine levels (TNF-α, IL-1, IL-6, IL-10, IFN) during chronic inflammation; thus, when infliximab is administered, it is likely that CYP450 enzyme levels will normalize; monitor for increased drug interactions.
- Live vaccines: may result in clinical infection; do not give concurrently.
- BCG, other therapeutic infectious agents: can result in clinical infection and dissemination; do not give concurrently.

Lab Effects/Interference:
- Decreased leucocyte, platelet, and red blood cell counts.
- Rare elevation of LFTs.

Special Considerations:
- Most common adverse effects: infections (URI, sinusitis, pharyngitis), infusion-related reactions, headache, and abdominal pain.
- Warnings and Precautions:
  - *Serious infections*: Due to severe immunosuppression, patients are at increased risk for developing serious infections that require hospitalization and that may be fatal. Patients at risk are those taking concomitant immunosuppressants like MTX or corticosteroids. Drug should be discontinued if a serious infection or sepsis develops, and patient should be given appropriate antimicrobial therapy immediately.
    - Patients should be tested for latent TB prior to infliximab use; if needed, patients should begin anti-TB medications prior to starting infliximab therapy in patients at risk for invasive fungal disease who develop severe systemic illness. Patients have had reactivated TB or new TB infections develop while receiving infliximab. Patients should be tested for latent TB prior to therapy, and then periodically during infliximab therapy. When skin testing, induration of 5 mm or greater is considered positive for latent TB.
    - Infliximab should be discontinued if a patient develops a serious infection or sepsis and antimicrobials and medical care given.
    - Patients should be closely monitored for signs/symptoms of infection during and after treatment, including TB, even if the patient tested negatively for latent TB.
    - Invasive fungal infections: If a patient who lives/travels to a region with endemic mycoses then develops systemic infection, a fungal infection should be suspected. Empiric antifungal therapy should be considered while awaiting confirmation of the diagnosis.
  - *Lymphoma and other malignancies,*
  - Especially in children and adolescents with Crohn's disease or UC. Patients at risk received prior treatment with azathioprine or 6-MP concomitantly with infliximab. Melanoma and Merkel cell carcinoma have occurred in some patients. All patients should receive baseline and periodic skin examinations, especially those with increased risk factors for skin cancer.
  - *Drug may lead to reactivation of HBV*. Patients should be tested for HBV infection before starting infliximab. If the test is positive for HBV surface antigen, discuss whether to proceed with a physician specializing in the treatment of patients with

HBV. If the patient is an HBV carrier, closely monitor the patient for signs/symptoms of disease activation during and following treatment. Infliximab should be stopped if HBV is reactivated, and antiviral therapy should be begun.

- *Severe hepatotoxicity* may occur, beginning 2 weeks to > 1 year after starting infliximab. Evaluate all patients with signs/symptoms of liver dysfunction; if jaundice or marked elevation in liver enzymes occur ($\geq 5 \times$ ULN), discontinue infliximab and evaluate patient thoroughly.
- *Heart failure:* Infliximab has been shown to worsen heart failure. Patients should be advised of the potential risk versus benefit, and if drug is given, patient should be closely monitored during therapy. Drug should be discontinued if new or worsened symptoms occur.
- *Cytopenias:* Drug may cause leukopenia, neutropenia, thrombocytopenia, and pancytopenia. Infliximab should be discontinued if significant hematology abnormalities occur.
- *HSRs* can occur during or within 2 hours of drug infusion (e.g., urticaria, dyspnea, hypotension) and may be serious, including anaphylaxis and serum-like sickness.
  - Rarely, serum sickness-like reaction can occur and is associated with development of anti-infliximab antibodies (e.g., fever, rash, headache, sore throat, myalgias, polyarthralgias, hand and facial edema, dysphagia).
  - Discontinue drug for severe HSRs and have emergency medications and equipment in the infusion room; treat with acetaminophen, antihistamines, corticosteroids, and/or epinephrine per physician.
  - In RA, Crohn's disease, and psoriasis clinical trials, there was a higher incidence of reactions when the drug was readministered after a long treatment break. See Prescribing Information.
- *Cardiovascular and cerebrovascular reactions:* CVA, MI, and arrhythmias have been reported during and within 24 hours of infliximab infusion. Monitor patients closely during infusion, and if a serious reaction occurs, discontinue the infusion.
- *Demyelinating disease*: Rarely, CNS reactions have occurred (e.g., systemic vasculitis, seizures, and CNS demyelinating disorders such as multiple sclerosis). Exacerbation of existing disease or onset of new disease may occur. Caution should be used when deciding to use infliximab in patients with preexisting neurological disorders.
- *Lupus-like syndrome:* stop infliximab if this develops.
  - *Live vaccines:*
  - Do not give live vaccines to patients receiving infliximab, as it has resulted in clinical infections. Caution is advised when giving live vaccines born to women treated with infliximab during pregnancy, as drug crosses the placental barrier and can persist in the serum of infants born to mothers treated with infliximab during pregnancy for up to 6 months. At least a 6-month waiting period following birth is recommended before the administration of live vaccines to infants exposed *in utero* to infliximab.
  - All pediatric patients should be brought up to date with all vaccinations prior to starting infliximab.
  - Care should be taken when switching from one biological DMARD to another, as overlapping biological activity may increase risk of infection.

Potential Toxicities/Side Effects and the Nursing Process

I.   POTENTIAL FOR INJURY related to INFUSION-RELATED REACTIONS

Defining Characteristics: Infliximab is a chimeric monoclonal antibody with at least 25% murine protein, which increases the risk of HSRs. About 20% of patients in clinical trials had infusion reactions (e.g., flu-like symptoms, headache, dyspnea, hypotension, transient fever, chills, GI symptoms, and skin rashes). Although rare, anaphylaxis may occur at any time during the infusion (incidence < 1%). Patients who developed antibodies to infliximab were more likely to have an infusion reaction.

Nursing Implications: Discuss with physician premedications (e.g., acetaminophen plus antihistamine or corticosteroid) prior to drug infusion. Ensure that emergency medications (e.g., epinephrine, antihistamines, corticosteroids) and equipment are readily available if needed for a severe infusion reaction. Assess baseline vital signs and monitor frequently during infusion (see http://www.janssenaccessone.com/pages/remicade/pubs/infusion/infusion.jsp for a template for documentation of infliximab monitoring and infusion). Stop infusion for infusion reactions, assess patient, and discuss next steps with physician, NP, or PA. If severe, in addition, keep vein open with 0.9% normal saline or other IV solution via new tubing (without infliximab in it) and prepare to give emergency support (see *Chapter 1*). Mild-to-moderate infusion reactions may improve after slowing or interrupting the infusion. Once the reaction has been treated and resolves, resume the infusion at a slower rate per physician, NP, or PA. If the patient does not tolerate the infusion after these steps, or if the infusion reaction is severe, infliximab should be discontinued.

II.   POTENTIAL FOR INFECTION related to IMMUNOSUPPRESSION

Defining Characteristics: Patients receiving infliximab are at increased risk of developing serious infections (e.g., bacterial, viral, fungal) requiring hospitalization. Although uncommon and occurring in patients receiving multiple immunosuppressant medications (e.g., MTX and corticosteroids), opportunistic infections may be disseminated on presentation, such as fulminating fungal infections. In clinical trials, most common infections were URI, which occurred in 32% of patients with RA receiving four or more infliximab infusions, sinusitis (14%), pharyngitis (12%), bronchitis (10%), and UTI (8%).

Nursing Implications: Assess results of patient's latent TB and HBV testing and discuss any abnormalities with physician, NP, or PA. If TB test is positive, patient should begin anti-TB therapy before beginning infliximab therapy. Assess baseline risk of infection (e.g., comorbidities, preexisting infections, concomitant immunosuppressants like MTX or corticosteroids). Teach patient to self-assess for signs/symptoms of infection (e.g., *T* > 100.4°F, cough, chest pain, sputum production, dysuria), and to report them right away. Closely monitor patient for signs/symptoms of infection during and after treatment with infliximab, including TB reactivation, even if latent TB test is negative, and teach patient to report any changes (e.g., fever, sweats, chills, cough, SOB, blood in sputum, weight loss). Drug should be discontinued if patient develops a serious infection or sepsis, and appropriate antimicrobial therapy should be instituted right away. If the patient is at risk for fungal infection and develops severe systemic illness, discuss empiric antifungal therapy with physician, NP, or PA.

Drug: sarilumab (Kevzara)

Class: Interleukin-6 (IL-6) receptor antagonist

Mechanism of Action: Drug binds to soluble and membrane-bound IL-6 receptors and inhibits IL-6-mediated signaling to the receptors, thus stopping messages to the cell that drive inflammation. IL-6 is a proinflammatory cytokine produced by a number of immune cells, including T and B lymphocytes, monocytes, and fibroblasts. IL-6 participates in T-lymphocyte activation, immunoglobulin secretion, and initiation of hepatic acute phase protein synthesis, and it is produced by synovial and endothelial cells (Sanofi-aventis, 2018). In RA, IL-6 helps produce joint inflammation. Blockade of IL-6 turns off inflammation.

Metabolism: After a single SQ dose, inflammation markers rapidly fell (e.g., CRP) with return to normal in 2 weeks after treatment started. Neutrophil nadir days 3–4, and then recovered to baseline. Tmax reached in 2–4 days, with steady state reached in 14–16 weeks. As the drug is a mAb, metabolism is likely catabolic degradation into small peptides and amino acids. Drug elimination at high doses is a linear, proteolytic pathway, while at lower doses, it is eliminated by a nonlinear pathway (Sanofi-aventis, 2018). Drug half-life is concentration dependent so that at 200 mg every 2 weeks, half-life is 10 days at steady state, while at a dose of 150 mg every 2 weeks, the half-life was up to 8 days. Elimination is nonrenal and nonhepatic.

Indication: Treatment of adult patients with moderately to severely active RA who have had an inadequate response or intolerance to one or more DMARDs.

Contraindication: Known hypersensitivity to sarilumab or any of its inactive ingredients. Drug is not recommended for patients with an ANC $<2000/mm^3$, platelet count $<150,000/mm^3$, or who have ALT or AST $> 1.5 \times$ ULN. Do not give other biologic DMARDs because of increased risk of infection. Do not give drug to patients with active infections. Drug not recommended for patients with active hepatic disease or hepatic impairment (Sanofi-aventis, 2018).

Dosage/Range:
- Sarilumab may be given as monotherapy or in combination with MTX or other conventional DMARDs.
- Recommended dose is 200-mg SQ every 2 weeks.
- Reduce dose to 150-mg SQ every 2 weeks for management of neutropenia, thrombocytopenia, elevated liver enzymes.

Dose Modifications:
- Neutropenia: (a) ANC > 1000 cells/mm^3, maintain current dose; (b) if ANC 500–1000 cells/mm^3, hold treatment until ANC >1000 cells/mm^3, then resume at a decreased dose

of 150 mg every 2 weeks. Dose can be increased back to 200 mg every 2 weeks as clinically appropriate and ordered; (c) ANC <500 cells/mm^3, discontinue drug. Use ANC results at the end of the dosing interval based on pharmacodynamics.

- Thrombocytopenia: (a) 50–100,000 cells/mm^3, hold treatment until platelet count $>100,000$ cells/mm^3, then drug can be resumed at a reduced dose of 150 mg every 2 weeks. Dose can be increased back to 200 mg every 2 weeks as clinically appropriate and ordered; (b) $<50,000$ cells/mm^3, repeat test and if verified, discontinue drug.
- Elevated transaminases: (a) ALT $>$ ULN to 3 $\times$ ULN = consider dosage modification of concomitant DMARDs as clinically appropriate; (b) ALT $>$ 3 $\times$ ULN to 5 $\times$ ULN or less = hold Sarilumab until ALT $<$ 3 $\times$ ULN; resume drug at a 150 mg every 2 weeks, and may increase back to 200 mg every 2 weeks as clinically appropriate; (c) ALT $>$ 5 $\times$ ULN = discontinue drug. When clinically indicated further evaluation hepatic function by assessing bilirubin.

Drug Preparation:
- Available as 150 mg/1.14 mL or 200 mg/1.14 mL solution in a single prefilled syringe.
- Available as 150 mg/1.14 mL or 200 mg/1.14 mL solution in a single prefilled pen.

Drug Administration:
- Assess baseline labs, and do not treat if ANC <2000 cells/mm^3, platelet count $<150,000$ cells/mm^3, or those who have ALT or AST $>$ 1.5 $\times$ ULN.
- Monitor ANC, platelet count, AST/ALT, and serum lipids at 4–8 weeks after beginning of therapy, then every 3 months for all except lipids, which should be reassessed at 6-month intervals.
- Ensure patient has had TB test for latent TB, and that it is negative. If it is positive, hold treatment and discuss with provider starting anti-TB medications.
- Assess patient for signs/symptoms of infection, and do not treat if patient has an active infection.
- Administer drug SQ or teach patient/caregiver if appropriate to administer drug.
  - Teach patient to wash hands, and prepare a clean work area. Allow prefilled syringe or pen to sit at room temperature for 30 min and 60 min respectively. Keep cap on, and do not heat syringe any other way.
  - Inspect syringe contents for clear and colorless to pale yellow color; do not use if cloudy discolored or contains particles.
  - Teach patient to select site, prep with an alcohol wipe, and inject full amount in the syringe or pen.
  - Teach patient to rotate sites and to avoid areas that are tender, damaged, bruised, or have a scar.
- Teach patient self-assessment for signs/symptoms of infection and to notify provider right away and hold dose if identified (e.g., fever, productive cough, burning on urination).

Drug Interactions:
- IL-6 inhibition may alter CYP microenzyme function. When drug is started or discontinuation of sarilumab, if a patient is also receiving a CYP substrate drug such as warfarin or theophylline with a narrow therapeutic window, monitor closely and adjust dose of substrate.

TREATMENT

- Use cautiously when a giving IL-6 inhibitor with CYP3A4 substrate where a decrease in effectiveness of the substrate is not desireable (e.g., loss of effectiveness of oral contraceptives, decrease effect of statins [e.g., lovastatin, atorvastatin]).
- Live vaccines: Do not give concurrently as infection and dissemination may occur.

Lab Effects/Interference:
- Increased Hgb, serum albumin, serum lipids, ALT, AST.
- Decreases in fibrinogen, serum amyloid A, ANC, platelet count.

Special Considerations:
- Most common adverse effects
  - Effects of sarilumab on fetus during pregnancy are unknown. Drug is transported via the placenta to the fetus in the third trimester, which may affect the immune response of the *in utero* exposed infant. If a patient is pregnant while receiving sarilumab, physicians are encouraged to register patients, and pregnant women can also register themselves at 1-877-311-8972.
- Warnings and Precautions
  - *Serious infections*: occur, and may be fatal. Opportunistic infections (OI) are caused by bacterial, mycobacteria, invasive fungal, viral, or other OI pathogen. Most common infections are pneumonia and cellulitis.
    - Presentation may be disseminated rather than localized disease, especially in patients also taking MTX or corticosteroids, which are immunosuppressive.
    - Do not give sarilumab to patients with active infections, including localized infections. Use cautiously, if at all, in patients with chronic or recurrent infection, a history of serious or OI, underlying conditions besides RA that may increase risk of infection, been exposed to TB, or lived in or traveled to areas of endemic TB or mycoses.
    - Closely monitor patients for signs/symptoms of infection during treatment as signs/symptoms may be lessened due to suppression of acute phase reactants by IL-6 blockade. Hold treatment if patient develops a serious infection or OI; ensure patient has a comprehensive evaluation/diagnostics for possible infection, appropriate for an immune-compromised patient. If an infection is identified, treat promptly with antimicrobials and closely monitor the patient.
    - TB: All patients should be tested for latent TB before starting therapy; if positive, patient should receive antimycobacterial therapy before starting sarilumab. Consider anti-TB treatment in patients with a PMH or latent or active TB in whom an adequate course of treatment cannot be confirmed, and for patients with a negative latent TB test but who have risk factors for TB. Closely monitor patients for signs/ symptoms of TB even if patient tested negative for latent TB.
    - Viral reactivation: may occur, such as herpes zoster. Patients with hepatitis B were not studied.
  - *Laboratory abnormalities:* Neutropenia, thrombocytopenia, increased transaminase levels, and increased serum lipid levels may occur. See Dose Modification section. See Drug Administration for frequency of laboratory monitoring.
  - *GI perforation:* may occur, as a complication of diverticulitis, or in patients taking concomitant NSAIDs or corticosteroids. Patients presenting with new onset abdominal symptoms should be promptly evaluated.

- *Immunosuppression:* may result in increased risk for the development of malignancy. Patients should be monitored over time.
- *HSRs:* have been reported and require drug discontinuation in 0.2–0.3% of patients. Injection site rash, rash, and urticaria were most common signs. Teach patients to seek immediate medical attention if they experience an HSR. If anaphylaxis or other serious HSR occurs, stop drug administration immediately.
- *Active hepatic disease or disease impairment:* Treatment with sarilumab not recommended.
- *Live vaccines:* Do not administer to patients receiving sarilumab due to potentially increased risk of infection from a live vaccine.
- Review with patient Medication Guide in package insert.

Potential Toxicities/Side Effects and the Nursing Process

I.   POTENTIAL FOR INFECTION related to IMMUNOSUPPRESSION

Defining Characteristics: Patients receiving sarilumab are at increased risk of developing serious infections (e.g., bacterial, mycobacterial, viral, fungal, protozoan) leading to hospitalization or death. Although uncommon and often occurring in patients receiving other immunosuppressant medications (e.g., MTX, corticosteroids), opportunistic infections may be disseminated on presentation, which in addition to RA predispose the patient to infection. Patients with latent TB may develop activated TB. Viral infections can be reactivated, such as herpes zoster. Signs and symptoms of acute inflammation may be reduced due to suppression of acute phase reactants. Neutrophils and platelets may be decreased.

Nursing Implications: Review patient history; drug should not be given to a patient with active infection, including localized infections. Physician should review the risks and benefits of using sarilumab therapy in patients with chronic or recurrent infections, as well as those who have been exposed to TB, have a history of serious or opportunistic infection, have lived or traveled in areas of endemic TB or other mycoses, or with underlying conditions that may predispose them to infection. Assess results of patient's latent TB testing and discuss any abnormalities with physician, NP, or PA. If TB test is positive, patient should begin anti-TB therapy before beginning sarilumab therapy. Anti-TB therapy should also be considered, based on input from a TB specialist, for those patients with a history of latent or active TB where an adequate course of therapy cannot be confirmed, or if the patient tested negative for latent TB but has risk factors.

Assess baseline labs, and verify that ANC > 2,000 cells/mm^3 and platelet count is > 100,000 cells/mm^3. ANC and platelet count should be monitored baseline, then at 4–8 weeks after drug is started, then at 3 months and as needed. Assess baseline risk for infection (e.g., comorbidities, preexisting infections, concomitant immunosuppressants like MTX or corticosteroids). Teach patient to self-assess for signs/symptoms of infection (e.g., $T >$ 100.4°F, cough, chest pain, sputum production, dysuria) and to report them right away. Closely monitor patient for signs/symptoms of infection during and after treatment with sarilumab, and teach patient to report any changes. Drug should be interrupted if patient develops a serious infection, opportunistic infection, or sepsis. If a patient develops a new infection while receiving sarilumab therapy, prompt and comprehensive evaluation of an immunocompromised patient should be done.

II.   POTENTIAL FOR INJURY related to HYPERSENSITVITY

Defining Characteristics: Patients can develop a hypersensitivity reaction after sarilumab administration. The percentage of patients who discontinued the drug due to HSR in clinical trials was 0.2–0.3%, and over time was the same as the placebo-controlled group. Signs included injection site rash, rash, and urticarial.

Nursing Implications: If administering the SQ injection, assess patient baseline, during and after the injection. If teaching patient or caregiver to self-administer the drug, teach patients to seek immediate medical attention if they experience an HSR. If anaphylaxis or other serious HSR occurs, stop drug administration immediately.

Drug: tocilizumab (Actemra)

Class: Interleukin-6 (IL-6) receptor antagonist.

Mechanism of Action: Drug binds to soluble and membrane-bound IL-6 receptors to inhibit IL-6-mediated signaling to the receptors, thus stopping messages to the cell that drive inflammation. IL-6 is a proinflammatory cytokine produced by a number of immune cells, including T and B lymphocytes, monocytes, and fibroblasts. IL-6 participates in T-lymphocyte activation, immunoglobulin secretion, and initiation of hepatic acute phase protein synthesis, and it is produced by synovial and endothelial cells. In RA, IL-6 helps produce joint inflammation. Blockade of IL-6 turns off inflammation.

Metabolism: Steady state is reached after the first infusion. The terminal half-life of the drug is concentration-dependent and is 11–13 days for adults with RA, and 16–23 days in children. Doses > 800 mg per infusion are not recommended.

Indication: For the treatment of (1) adults with moderately to severely active RA who have had an inadequate response to one or more DMARDs; (2) patients 2 years of age and older with active polyarticular juvenile idiopathic arthritis (PJIA); (3) patients with active systemic juvenile idiopathic arthritis (SJIA) 2 years of age and older; (4) adults with giant cell arteritis; (5) adults and pediatric patients aged 2 and older with chimeric antigen receptor (CAR) T cell-induced or life-threatening cytokine release syndrome (CRS).

   Drug is not recommended for patients with active hepatic disease or hepatic impairment.

   Contraindication: Known hypersensitivity to drug. Drug is not recommended for patients with active hepatic disease or hepatic impairment.

Dosage/Range:
* RA, PJIA, and SJIA: Drug may be used as monotherapy or concomitantly with MTX; RA, other DMARDs may be combined (nonbiologic). Given as an IV infusion or as a subcutaneous injection.

- Drug should not be started in patients (EXCEPT those with CRS) with an ANC < 2,000 cells/mm^3, platelet count < 100,000 cells/mm^3, or who have ALT or AST ≥ 1.5 × ULN. If ANC < 500 cells/mm^3, drug should be discontinued.
- When transitioning from IV to SQ administration, administer the first SQ dose instead of the next scheduled IV dose.
- RA, CRS: IV doses > 800 mg per IV infusion should not be given.
- Monitor CBC, LFTs, lipids baseline and at 4–8 weeks after start of therapy, then every 3 months.
- **RA:**
- IV infusion:
  - 4 mg/kg IV infusion over 60 minutes every 4 weeks, followed by an increase to 8 mg/kg every 4 weeks based on clinical response. Doses should not exceed 800 mg per infusion.
  - Interrupt drug, and when toxicity resolved, dose-reduce from 8 to 4 mg/kg if for neutropenia (ANC < 1,000 cells/mm^3), thrombocytopenia (< 100,000 cells/mm^3), elevated LFTs (see package insert).
- SQ injection:
  - Patients < 100 kg weight: 162 mg SQ every other week, followed by an increase to every week based on clinical response;
  - Patients ≥ 100 kg weight: 162 mg SQ every week.
  - Interrupt dose or reduce frequency of SQ administration from every week to every other week to manage elevated ALT/AST, neutropenia, and thrombocytopenia.

Giant Cell Arteritis (GCA):
- 162 mg SQ once every week, in combination with a tapering dose of glucocorticoids. If special considerations necessary, dose can be given every other week in combination with a tapering dose of glucocorticoids. Tocilizumab can be used as monotherapy after discontinuation of glucocorticoids. IV administration not approved for GCA.
- Interrupt if low neutrophil or platelet count, increased LFTs. See dose modifications.

PJIA: Alone or in combination with MTX. Do not change dose based solely on a single visit weight as body weight may fluctuate. Give IV or SQ.
- IV: over 60 minutes, every 4 weeks.
  - Patients weighing < 30 kg = 10 mg/kg;
  - Patients weighing ≥ 30 kg = 8 mg/kg.
- SQ:
  - Patients weighing < 30 kg = 162 mg once every 3 weeks;
  - Patients weighing ≥ 30 kg = 162 mg once every 2 weeks.
- Interrupt if low neutrophil or platelet counts, increased LFTs; consider dose modification if MTX also given; see package insert.

SJIA: Give IV or SQ alone or in combination with MTX; do not change dose based solely on a single visit weight as weight may fluctuate.
- IV: over 60 minutes once every 2 weeks.
  - Patients < 30 kg weight: 12 mg/kg.
  - Patients > 30 kg weight: 8 mg/kg.

- SQ:
  - Patients < 30 kg weight: 162 mg every 2 weeks.
  - Patients ≥ 30 kg weight: 162 mg every week.
  - Interrupt if low neutrophil or platelet counts, increased LFTs; consider dose modification if MTX also given; see package insert.

Cytokine Release Syndrome (CRS):
- Administer IV over a 60-minute infusion as need rapid onset of action. Give alone or in combination with corticosteroids.
  - Patients < 30 kg = 12 mg/kg.
  - Patients ≥ 30 kg = 8 mg/kg.
- If no clinical improvement in signs/symptoms of CRS after the first infusion, can give up to 3 additional doses with at least an 8-hour interval between consecutive doses.
- Do not exceed 800 mg per infusion; SQ administration is not approved for CRS.

Dose Modifications:
- *Serious infections:* Hold tocilizumab until the infection is controlled.
- *RA and GCA:*
  - Liver enzyme abnormalities: (a) >**1 to 3 × ULN**: dose modify concomitant DMARDs (RA) or immunomodulatory agents (GCA) if appropriate. If persistent increases in this range: IV tocilizumab: reduce dose to 4 mg/kg or hold until AST and ALT have normalized; SQ tocilizumab: decrease injection frequency to every other week or hold dosing until ALT or AST have normalized; resume tocilizumab at every other week and increase frequency to every week once clinically appropriate. (b) >**3 to 5 × ULN** (confirmed by repeat testing): Hold tocilizumab until < 3 × ULN, and follow recommendations for persistent increases > 3 × ULN, discontinue tocilizumab; (c) >5 × ULN: discontinue tocilizumab.
  - Neutropenia: (a) ANC > 1000 cells/mm^3, maintain dose; (b) ANC 500–1000 cells/mm^3, hold tocilizumab until ANC > 1000 cells/mm^3, resume IV: at 4 mg/kg and increase to 8 mg/kg when clinically appropriate, or resume SQ: at every other week interval, and increase frequency to every week as clinically appropriate; (c) ANC <500 cells/mm^3, discontinue tocilizumab.
  - Thrombocytopenia: (a) 50,000-100,000 cells/mm^3 = hold tocilizumab until platelet count >100,000 cells/mm^3 then resume IV: at 4 mg/kg and increase to 8 mg/kg when clinically appropriate, or resume SQ: at every other week interval, and increase frequency to every week as clinically appropriate.
- *Polyarticular and Systemic Juvenile Idiopathic Arthritis:* Dose modifications have not been studied but recommendations for RA and GCA above should be followed. If appropriate, dose modify or stop concomitant MTX and/or other medications and hold ocilizumab dosing until clinically evaluated. The physician should make a decision to discontinue tocilizumab based on individual medical assessment (Genetech, 2019).

Drug Preparation:
- IV: Available in single-use vials (20 mg/mL): 80 mg/4 mL, 200 mg/10 mL, and 400 mg/20 mL (clear, colorless to pale yellow solution).

- Subcutaneous: Single-use prefilled glass syringe providing 162 mg of tocilizumab in 0.9 mL or autoinjector (0.9 mL).

IV:
- Aseptically prepare IV infusion bag.
  - Patients weighing > 30 kg: use a 100-mL infusion bag or bottle of 0.9% or 0.45% sodium chloride injection USP.
  - Patients weighing < 30 kg: use a 50-mL infusion bag or bottle of 0.9% or 0.45% sodium chloride injection USP.
- Preparation:
  - Withdraw volume equal to the volume of tocilizumab required for the patient dose from the IV bag or bo ttle. [4 mg/kg = 0.2 mL/kg (adult RA); 8 mg/kg (adult RA, SJIA, PJIA and CRS ≥ 30 kg body weight) = 0.4 mL/kg; 10 mg/kg (PJIA < 30 kg of body weight) = 0.5 mL/kg; 12 mg/kg (SJIA (< 30 kg of body weight) = 0.6 mL/kg]
  - Withdraw the ordered amount of tocilizumab for IV infusion from the vial(s). Slowly add tocilizumab for IV infusion to the infusion bag or bottle; gently invert bag to mix.
  - Fully diluted drug can be stored at 2–8°C (36–46°F) or room temperature for up to 24 hours; protect from light. If using 0.45% sodium chloride injection USP, refrigerated solution is stable for up to 24 hours, but at room temperature, it is stable only for 4 hours. Allow refrigerated drug to come to room temperature prior to infusion.
- Inspect for particulate matter and discoloration; if found, do not use.

SQ: Do not use for IV administration.
- If appropriate, patient (adult) /caregiver (for adult or pediatric patients) can be taught to prepare and administer the drug. Use Instructions for Use in package insert for teaching tool. Teach patient to (1) wash hands; (2) select site avoiding moles, scars, areas of tenderness, bruises, and red, hard or open (not intact) skin areas; (3) aseptically prepare SQ site; (4) inject drug; (5) dispose of syringe; and (6) rotate sites. Supervise patient's or caregiver's return demonstration, and if successful, empower patient or caregiver to (self-) administer at home. Drug available in single-use glass syringe delivering 162 mg of tocilizumab in 0.9 mL or in an autoinjector (0.9 mL).

Drug Administration:
- Monitor CBC, LFTs, lipids baseline, then 4–8 weeks after start of therapy, then every 3 months.
- ANC must be > 2,000 cells/mm³, platelet count > 100,000 cells/mm³, and ALT/AST ≤ 1.5 × ULN (EXCEPT for patients with CRS) to begin therapy.
- Assess results of latent TB test, and if positive, patient must begin anti-TB therapy prior to starting tocilizumab therapy.
- Patients with PJIA and SJIA should have their immunizations brought up to date before starting drug.
- IV: Administer by IV infusion **over 60 minutes** with an infusion set. DO NOT administer IVP or bolus; do not infuse concomitantly in the same IV line with other drugs. Monitor for infusion reactions.
- SQ: If appropriate, patient (adult) /caregiver (for adult or pediatric patients) can be taught to prepare and administer the drug. Use Instructions for Use in package insert

for teaching tool. Teach patient to (1) wash hands; (2) select site avoiding moles, scars, areas of tenderness, bruises, and red, hard, or open (not intact) skin areas; (3) aseptically prepare SQ site; (4) inject drug; (5) dispose of syringe; and (6) rotate sites. Supervise patient's or caregiver's return demonstration, and if successful, empower patient or caregiver to (self-) administer at home. Drug available in single-use glass syringe delivering 162 mg of tocilizumab in 0.9 mL or in an autoinjector (0.9 mL).

- Inspect for particulate matter, cloudiness, and discoloration; if found, do not use prefilled syringe. Drug should be clear and colorless to pale yellow.
- Teach patient to call healthcare professional before giving the next dose if patient has an allergic reaction to the injection. If patient has a **serious** reaction, patient should seek immediate medical attention.

Drug Interactions:
- Biologic DMARDs: increased immunosuppression, increased risk for infection; DO NOT give concomitantly.
- Live vaccines: do not give during tocilizumab therapy.
- Simvastatin (a CYP3A4 and OATP1B1 substrate): simvastatin effect may be reduced.
- Omeprazole (CYP2C19 and CYP3A4 substrate): omeprazole effect may be reduced.
- Dextromethorphan (CYP2D6 and CYP3A4 substrate): dextromethorphan effect may be increased after drug infusion.
- Monitor patients receiving drugs that are CYP substrates closely to determine effect (e.g., patients on warfarin) and monitor INR.

Lab Effects/Interference:
- Neutropenia, thrombocytopenia.
- Increased LFTs.
- Increased total cholesterol, triglycerides, LDL, and HDL cholesterol.

Special Considerations:
- Warnings and Precautions:
  - *Serious infections:*
    - Serious infections may occur, and patients receiving other concomitant immunosuppressant medications are at greatest risk (e.g., MTX, corticosteroids); opportunistic infections include invasive fungal infections that may present as disseminated rather than localized disease. Do not administer drug during an active infection, including localized infections. Interrupt drug if a serious infection develops. Risk benefit ratio should be assessed in patients (a) with chronic or recurrent infections; (b) have been exposed to TB; (c) with a history of serious or opportunistic infection; (d) who have lived/traveled in areas of endemic TB or mycoses; (e) with underlying conditions predisposing the patient to infection.
    - TB: All patients should be tested for latent TB, and if positive, anti-TB therapy should be started prior to beginning tocilizumab therapy. Closely monitor patient during tocilizumab therapy for signs/symptoms of infection, including TB, even if the patients had a negative latent TB test.
    - Viral reactivation can occur.

- *GI perforation:* Use drug cautiously in patients at risk for GI perforation, as this has rarely occurred. Any patient, especially those with a PMH of diverticulitis, should be promptly evaluated for new onset abdominal symptoms to identify any GI perforation early.
- *Laboratory parameters:* RA patients: monitor Absolute Neutrophil Count (ANC), platelet count, serum lipids, and LFTs: baseline. Monitor ANC, platelet count, and ALT and AST levels 4–8 weeks after start of therapy, then every 3 months thereafter. Risk of hepatotoxicity (increased LFTs) is greater in patients also receiving MTX. Patients with PJIA should have baseline and repeat testing at the time of the second infusion, then every 4–8 weeks; SJIA patients should have these labs tested every 2–4 weeks. Lipids should be monitored every 4–8 weeks.
- *Immunosuppression:* Treatment with immunosuppressants may result in an increased risk of malignancy, which has occurred with tocilizumab.
- *HSRs,* including anaphylaxis: Rarely, HSRs have occurred (incidence 0.1–0.7%), including anaphylaxis, which may be fatal. IV tocilizumab should only be administered in a setting equipped to manage anaphylaxis. Teach patients receiving SQ tocilizumab to seek immediate emergency assistance if HSR occurs. If severe HSR occurs, drug should be permanently discontinued and emergency measures instituted.
- *Demyelinating disorders:* Rarely, demyelinating disorders have been reported in RA patients. Use drug cautiously in patients with preexisting or recent onset demyelinating disorders.
- *Active hepatic disease and hepatic impairment:* Tocilizumab is not recommended in patients with active liver disease or impairment.
- *Vaccinations:* Live vaccines should not be given to patients receiving tocilizumab.
- Tocilizumab can cause infusion reactions. Patients did not receive premedication in clinical studies, and during 24 hours surrounding drug administration between 4 and 20% developed infusion reactions (e.g., rash, nausea, hypotension, dizziness, urticaria, diarrhea, epigastric distress, arthralgia, headache), but only 0.1–0.2% involved anaphylaxis or HSRs requiring treatment discontinuation; these occurred despite premedication.
- Most common side effects are URI, nasopharyngitis, headache, HTN, and increased ALT.
- Drug may cause fetal harm. Counsel women of reproductive potential to use effective contraception while receiving tocilizumab and that drug should be used in pregnancy only if benefit exceeds potential risks, as there are no well-controlled studies. If drug is used in pregnancy, either the patient or provider can register the patient on the Pregnancy Exposure Registry at 1-877-311-8972. Nursing mothers should stop nursing or discontinue the drug.

Potential Toxicities/Side Effects and the Nursing Process

I.   POTENTIAL FOR INFECTION related to IMMUNOSUPPRESSION

Defining Characteristics: Patients receiving tocilizumab are at increased risk of developing serious infections (e.g., bacterial, mycobacterial, viral, fungal, protozoan) leading to hospitalization or death. Although uncommon and often occurring in patients receiving other immunosuppressant medications (e.g., MTX, corticosteroids), opportunistic infections may be disseminated on presentation, which in addition to RA predispose the patient to infection. In clinical trials, most common infections were URI (6–8%), nasopharyngitis (4–7%), and bronchitis (3–4%), while serious infections were pneumonia, UTI, cellulitis, herpes zoster, gastroenteritis, diverticulitis, sepsis, and bacterial arthritis. Patients with latent TB may develop activated TB. Viral infections can be reactivated, such as herpes zoster. Signs and symptoms of acute inflammation may be reduced due to suppression of acute phase reactants.

Neutrophils (17% over 12 weeks) and platelets (4% over 12 weeks) may be decreased.

Nursing Implications: Review patient history; drug should not be given to a patient with active infection, including localized infections. Physician should review the risks and benefits of using tocilizumab therapy in patients with chronic or recurrent infections, as well as those who have been exposed to TB, have a history of serious or opportunistic infection, have lived or traveled in areas of endemic TB or other mycoses, or with underlying conditions that may predispose them to infection.

Assess results of patient's latent TB testing and discuss any abnormalities with physician, NP, or PA. If TB test is positive, patient should begin anti-TB therapy before beginning tocilizumab therapy. Anti-TB therapy should also be considered, based on input from a TB specialist, for those patients with a history of latent or active TB where an adequate course of therapy cannot be confirmed, or if the patient tested negative for latent TB but has risk factors.

Assess baseline labs, and verify that ANC > 2,000 cells/mm^3, and platelet count is > 100,000 cells/mm^3. ANC and platelet count should be monitored baseline and every 4–8 weeks. Assess baseline risk for infection (e.g., comorbidities, preexisting infections, concomitant immunosuppressants like MTX or corticosteroids). Teach patient to self-assess for signs/symptoms of infection (e.g., T > 100.4°F, cough, chest pain, sputum production, dysuria), and to report them right away. Closely monitor patient for signs/symptoms of infection during and after treatment with tocilizumab, and teach patient to report any changes. Drug should be interrupted if patient develops a serious infection, opportunistic infection, or sepsis. If a patient develops a new infection while receiving tocilizumab therapy, prompt and comprehensive evaluation of an immunocompromised patient should be done.

II.   POTENTIAL FOR INJURY related to INFUSION-RELATED REACTIONS

Defining Characteristics: Patients can develop infusion reactions during or within 24 hours of tocilizumab administration. Incidence of reactions during the infusion ranged from 4 to 6%. Reactions within 24 hours after the infusion occurred in 16–20%. Anaphylaxis was reported in < 1% of patients. Symptoms that occurred during the infusion included headache, nausea, and hypotension; reactions occurring during the 24 hours following infusion were rash, urticaria, diarrhea, epigastric discomfort, arthalgia, dizziness, and hypotension. Incidence of HSRs requiring drug discontinuation were < 0.2%.

Nursing Implications: Discuss with physician premedications (e.g., acetaminophen plus antihistamine or corticosteroid) prior to drug infusion. While anaphylaxis is rare, ensure that emergency medications (e.g., epinephrine, antihistamines, corticosteroids) and equipment are readily available if needed. Assess baseline vital signs before and after the infusion, as well as during the infusion if needed. Stop infusion for infusion reactions, assess patient, and discuss next steps with physician, NP, or PA. If severe, in addition, keep vein open with 0.9% Normal Saline or other IV solution via new tubing (without tocilizumab in it) and prepare to give emergency support (see *Chapter 1*).

Drug: tofacitinib citrate (Xeljanz, Xeljanz XR)

Class: Janus kinase inhibitor (JAK inhibitor); small molecule kinase inhibitor.

Mechanism of Action: JAKs are enzymes within the cell that carry messages from receptors on the cell surface, which have been activated by cytokine or growth factors, to the cell nucleus. JAKs tell the immune system to turn on and to activate other blood cells using phosphorylation, which activates signal transducers and transcription (STATs), which in turn regulate cell activities, as well as turning on genes in the cell's DNA. JAK inhibitors modulate the signaling pathway, thus stopping this message from being sent so that STATs are not activated and the immune system (inflammation) is not turned on. Drug causes dose-dependent decreases in circulating Natural Killer lymphocytes (NK, CD16/56+ cells) with maximal effect in 8–10 weeks after therapy has started. Changes resolve in 2–6 weeks after the drug is discontinued. After treatment with tofacitinib, there is a rapid decrease in serum CRP that takes longer than the drug's half-life to reverse.

Indications: For the treatment of adult patients with (1) moderately to severely active RA who has had an inadequate response or intolerance to MTX. It may be used as monotherapy or in combination with MTX or other nonbiologic DMARDs; (2) psoriatic arthritis who have had an inadequate response or intolerance to MTX or other DMARDs; (3) moderately to severely active ulcerative colitis.

Limitations of use: Use of tofacitinib citrate with biologic DMARDs or with potent immunosuppressants (e.g., azathioprine and cyclosporine) is not recommended.

Contraindication: None.

Dosage/Range:
- Do not start tofacitinib citrate therapy if absolute lymphocyte count <500 cells/mm^3, ANC <1000 cells/mm^3, or Hgb < 9 g/dL. Do not use Xeljanz XR in patients with severe hepatic impairment.
- RA:
  - Tofacitinib (Xeljanz) 5 mg orally twice daily without regard to meals or Xeljanz XR 11 mg once daily.
  - Moderate and severe renal impairment or moderate hepatic impairment doses: recommended dose is tofacitinib citrate 5 mg once daily.
  - As monotherapy or in combination with MTX or other nonbiologic DMARD.
  - Do not use drug if patient develops a serious infection until the infection is controlled.

- Dose interruption for management of lymphopenia, neutropenia, and anemia.
- Switching from tofacitinib citrate tablets to Xeljanz XR tablets: start the XR tablets the day following the last dose of tofacitinib citrate tablets.
- Dose modifications:
  - Lymphocyte count < 500 cells/mm^3 (confirm by repeat testing): discontinue drug.
  - ANC 500–1,000 cells/mm^3: interrupt drug until ANC > 1,000 cells/mm^3 and then resume at usual dose (5 mg bid or Xeljanz XR 11 mg); if ANC < 500 cells/mm^3 (repeat testing confirmation), discontinue drug.
  - Hgb: < 8 g/dL or a decrease of > 2 g/dL: interrupt drug until hemoglobin values have normalized.
- If given with strong CYP3A4 inhibitor (e.g., ketoconazole): reduce dose to 5 mg orally once daily.
- If given with a moderate CYP3A4 inhibitor **and** a potent inhibitor of CYP2C19 (e.g., fluconazole): decrease dose to 5 mg orally once daily. If taking Xeljanz XR, switch to tofacitinib citrate 5 mg tablet once daily.
- If given with potent CYP3A4 inducers (e.g., rifampin, St. John's wort): may reduce or nullify clinical response. Do not coadminister. Teach patient not to take St. John's wort.
- Patients with moderate or severe renal impairment or moderate hepatic impairment: 5 mg once daily. If undergoing hemodialysis: administer dose after dialysis on dialysis days. If dose was taken before dialysis, do not give supplemental dose after dialysis (Pfizer, 2018). Do not give Xeljanz XR to these patients: they should be prescribed immediate release tofacitinib citrate 5 mg tablet once daily.
- See package insert for doses, dose modification for psoriatic arthritis and ulcerative colitis.

Drug Preparation:
- Available as tofacitinib immediate release 5-mg and 10-mg tablets and 11-mg tofacitinib extended release (XR).

Drug Administration:
- Assess results of tests for active and latent TB and viral hepatitis screens.
- Assess lymphocyte and neutrophil count, hemoglobin, LFTs, and lipids baseline and frequently during therapy. Lymphocyte count must be ≥ 500 cells/mm^3, and ANC ≥ 1,000 cells/mm^3 for drug to be given. Hgb should be ≥ 9.0 g/dL.
- Stop drug during active infection, including localized infections.
- Interrupt tocilizumab if a serious infection develops, and do not resume until the infection is controlled.
- Do not give drug to patients with severe hepatic impairment.
- Monitor ANC and Hgb baseline, then after 4–8 weeks of treatment, then every 3 months; lymphocyte counts baseline and every 3 months; monitor LFTs, lipids baseline, then lipids after 4–8 weeks.

Drug Interactions:
- Strong CYP 3A4 inhibitors (e.g., ketoconazole): increased tofacitinib serum level (because drug metabolism is reduced); reduce tocilizumab dose if coadministered (see *Chapter 4 Introduction* for a review of CYP3A4).

- Moderate CYP3A4 inhibitors (e.g., fluconazole) and potent CYP2C19 inhibitors: increased tofacitinib serum levels; reduce tocilizumab dose if coadministered.
- Potent CYP3A4 inducers (e.g., St. John's wort): decreased tofacitinib serum level with decreased tofacitinib activity. Do not take concurrently.
- Immunosuppressive drugs (e.g., azathioprine, tacrolimus, cyclosporine), or other DMARDs: increased risk of infection; DO NOT give concomitantly.

Lab Effects/Interference:
- Initial lymphocytosis at 1 month, followed by a decrease in mean absolute lymphocyte counts below baseline of 10% during 12 months of therapy. Lymphocyte counts < 500 cells/mm^3 were associated with increased risk of serious infection.
- Decreased lymphocyte and neutrophil counts (rare).
- Increased LDL and HDL cholesterol, total cholesterol, triglycerides.
- Increased LFTs.
- Anemia.

Special Considerations:
- Warnings and Precautions:
  - *Serious Infections:* Serious infections requiring hospitalization, sometimes fatal, including TB and bacterial, invasive fungal, and viral opportunistic infections may occur; monitor patient closely.
    - Most common serious infections included pneumonia, cellulitis, herpes zoster, and UTI.
    - Opportunistic infections included mycobacterial infections, cryptococcosis, esophageal candidiasis, pneumocystosis, multidermatomal herpes zoster, cytomegalovirus, and BK virus. Some patients presented with disseminated disease and were often taking concomitant immunomodulating agents, such as MTX or corticosteroids.
    - Tofacitinib should not be given to patients with (1) active, serious infections, including localized infections. Risk versus benefit should be carefully assessed before starting drug in patients (1) with chronic or recurrent infections; (2) who have been exposed to TB; (3) a history of a serious infection or opportunistic infection; (4) Who have traveled to areas of endemic TB or endemic mycoses or who have an underlying condition predisposing them to infection.
    - Viral reactivation, including herpes have occurred. Patients should be screened for viral hepatitis prior to starting drug.
    - Prior to beginning therapy, patient should be tested for latent TB; if positive, delay tofacitinib until anti-TB treatment is started. Monitor all patients closely for active TB during treatment, even if latent TB test is negative. See package insert.
    - Risk of infection may be higher in patients with (1) a history of chronic lung disease or those who develop interstitial lung disease; (2) increasing degrees of lymphopenia—monitor lymphocyte counts.
    - Interrupt drug if patient develops a serious infection, an opportunistic infection, or sepsis, until infection is controlled. Appropriate antimicrobial intervention should occur promptly.

- *Malignancy and Lymphoproliferative Disorders:* Lymphoma and other opportunistic malignancies have occurred in patients treated with tofacitinib. An increased incidence of Epstein–Barr virus associated posttransplant lymphoproliferative disorder has been observed in renal transplant patients treated with tofacitinib and concomitant immunosuppressive medications.
- *GI perforation* has occurred; use cautiously in patients at increased risk, such as those taking NSAIDs, MTX, or corticosteroids.
- *Hypersensitivity reactions (HSRs):* Angioedema and urticarial have been observed. If serious HSRs occur, promptly discontinue tofacitinib while further evaluation for cause of the reaction. Implement ordered emergency interventions.
- Laboratory Monitoring: Assess and monitor
  - Lymphocyte counts baseline and every 3 months thereafter; do not start treatment with tofacitinib if lymphocyte count is < 500 cells/mm³. If a patient has a confirmed absolute lymphocyte count < 500 cells/mm³, patient should not be treated with tofacitinib.
  - Neutrophil count baseline and after 4–8 weeks of treatment, then every 3 months thereafter. Do not start tofacitinib therapy if ANC < 1,000 cells/ mm³, and if patient has a persistent ANC 500–1,000 cells/ mm³, interrupt tofacitinib until ANC ≥ 1,000 cells/ mm³. If patient develops an ANC <500 cells/mm³, tofacitinib treatment is not recommended.
  - Hgb baseline and after 4–8 weeks of treatment, then every 3 months thereafter. Tofacitinib should not be started if Hgb < 9 g/dL. Treatment should be interrupted if Hgb < 8 g/dL during treatment or if a patient's Hgb drops > 2 g/dL on treatment.
  - LFTs: monitor liver enzymes baseline and regularly during therapy. If abnormalities develop, evaluate cause and if drug-induced hepatic injury is suspected, interrupt tofacitinib until this is excluded. If it appears increased serum transaminases are related to drug-induced liver injury, drug should be interrupted until this has been excluded.
  - Lipids (total cholesterol, HDL, LDL): baseline and 4–8 weeks after starting therapy. Elevations usually noted within 6 weeks. Manage elevated lipids according to clinical guidelines per physician/NP/PA.
- *Vaccinations:* Do not give live immunizations (vaccines) while patient is receiving tofacitinib. Patient should receive updated immunizations per guidelines prior to starting tofacitinib therapy.
- *Risk of GI obstruction with a nondeformable extended-release formulation such as Xeljanz XR.* Use caution when administering tofacitinib XR tablets to patients with preexisting severe GI narrowing (pathologic or iatrogenic strictures) as rare reports of obstruction have been made.
- Nonmelanoma skin cancer has been reported in patients; perform periodic skin assessment in patients at risk for skin cancer.
- Pregnancy category C: Counsel women of reproductive potential that drug should be used in pregnancy only if benefit outweighs potential risk, as there are no well-controlled

studies. In laboratory studies, at very high doses, tocilizumab may be fetocidal and tera-togenic. Nursing mothers should discontinue nursing or stop using tocilizumab.

* Most common side effects during first three months of therapy are URI (4.5%), headache (4.3%), diarrhea (4%), and nasopharyngitis (3.8%).

Potential Toxicities/Side Effects and the Nursing Process

I.   POTENTIAL FOR INFECTION related to IMMUNOSUPPRESSION

Defining Characteristics: Patients receiving tofacitinib are at increased risk of developing serious infections (e.g., bacterial, mycobacterial, viral, fungal, protzoan). Lymphopenia and neutropenia may occur rarely with lymphocyte counts < 500 cells/mm^3 occurring in 0.04% of patients and ANC $< 1,000$ cells/mm^3 occurring in 0.07% of patients. There was no association between neutropenia and infection. Latent TB may become reactivated TB (pulmonary or extrapulmonary). Opportunistic infections (OIs) may occur, including inva-sive fungal infections (e.g., cryptococcus and pneumocystosis) that may be disseminated on presentation (patients were usually taking tofacitinib with concomitant immunomodu-lating agents such as MTX or corticosteroids). Most common OIs were TB, mycobacterial infections, cryptococcus, esophageal candidiasis, pneuomocystosis, and cytomegalovirus. Most common infections are pneumonia, cellulitis, herpes zoster, and UTIs. Tofacitinib can cause viral reactivation; patients who screen tested positive for hepatitis B or C were excluded from studies.

Nursing Implications: Review patient history; drug should not be given to a patient with active infection, including localized infections. Assess results of patient's latent TB test-ing and discuss any abnormalities with physician, NP, or PA. If TB test is positive, patient should begin anti-TB therapy before beginning tofacitinib therapy. Anti-TB therapy should also be considered for patients with a history of latent or active TB, and an adequate course of therapy cannot be confirmed. Monitor all patients for active TB during treatment, even if initial latent TB test is negative. Physician should discuss risks vs. benefits of tofacitinib in patients with chronic or recurrent infections, exposed to TB, with a history of a serious OI, who have resided or traveled to an area of endemic TB or mycoses, or with underlying conditions besides RA that may predispose them to infection.

If the patient screened positive for hepatitis B or C, discuss with physician whether pa-tient is a candidate for the drug, as tofacitinib may react with hepatitis virus. If the patient is treated with tofacitinib, teach the patient to report immediately increased fatigue, yellow conjunctiva (eyes looking yellow), anorexia, vomiting, clay-colored bowel movements, fe-ver, chills, stomach discomfort, muscle aches, dark urine, or skin rash.

Assess CBC/differential baseline labs and at each visit prior to drug administration, and verify that lymphocyte count is > 500 cells/mm^3 and ANC $> 1,000$ cells/mm^3. As-sess baseline risk for infection (e.g., comorbidities, history of infections). Teach patient to self-assess for signs/symptoms of infection (e.g., $T > 100.4°F$, cough, chest pain, sputum production, dysuria), stop drug, and report any signs/symptoms immediately. Closely mon-itor patient for signs/symptoms of infection, including TB, during and after treatment with tofacitinib, and teach patient to report any changes (e.g., fever, sweats, rigors, weight loss, blood in sputum). Drug should be interrupted if patient develops a serious infection, opportunistic infection, or sepsis. If a patient develops a new infection while receiving tofacitinib therapy, prompt and comprehensive evaluation of an immunocompromised patient should be done, and antimicrobial therapy should be given.

Teach patient strategies to manage fatigue and conserve energy, such as alteration of rest and activity, and organizing chores.

Section 2
Symptom Management

Chapter *6*
Pain

Pain in the patient with cancer may result from a variety of stimuli. A careful assessment is critical in order to identify the physical causes and psychosocial factors that modulate pain intensity and perception. Pain can be acute or chronic. Acute pain results from stimuli such as surgical procedures, pathologic fractures, and obstruction of a hollow viscous where the stimulus can be removed (e.g., healing, radiation to the bone metastatic site, or resection of obstructing tumor), while chronic pain reflects the more common cancer pain where the stimulus cannot be removed, such as pain resulting from tissue inflammation caused by tumor. Patients often have both acute and chronic components of pain. Acute pain lasts from minutes to months and ceases when the cause of pain is removed (e.g., pain caused by spinal cord compression is removed when the patient undergoes laminectomy or radiotherapy to relieve the compression). This type of pain is often associated with anxiety, and one sees symptoms of sympathetic nervous system arousal (increased heart rate, increased/decreased BP) as well. In contrast, chronic pain lasts from months to years; the cause cannot be removed, and this type of pain is often associated with depression. The long duration of chronic pain dampens sympathetic response, so the patient does not manifest changes in heart rate or BP. Many patients with cancer pain have persistent pain that requires around-the-clock (ATC) analgesia to prevent pain. In addition, patients can develop breakthrough pain (BTP), which may be precipitated by an anticipated event, such as movement, or it just may occur. It is estimated that 64–89% of patients with chronic cancer pain have BTP, with most episodes lasting 120 minutes or less, and a single patient having four to seven episodes a day (Zeppetella et al., 2000). Less commonly, pain can be intermittent, and this is characteristic of acute pain. Here, short-acting analgesia is given intermittently.

Symptoms often accompanying unrelieved pain are sleeplessness, anorexia (loss of appetite), fatigue, irritability, and fear. In fact, as early as the first century AD, it was recognized that fear of pain was significant. Epictetus (AD 55–135) is reported to have said "It is not death or pain that is to be dreaded, but the fear of pain or death" (Crossley, 2006). Nurses play a critical role in advocating for effective cancer pain management and alleviation of other accompanying symptoms. Fortunately, there are a variety of available analgesic medications, including nonopioid and opioid, adjuvant agents such as antidepressants, as well as nonpharmacologic techniques such as relaxation exercises.

Opioid agents are available in immediate-onset formulations for acute pain, and long-duration agents that allow superior control for chronic pain by avoiding the peaks and valleys of serum drug levels associated with immediate preparations. While analgesics do not remove the source or stimulus for the pain, they decrease or modulate the impulse so that the pain impulse perceived by the patient is reduced or absent, thus decreasing the distress and discomfort perceived by the patient. *Nonopioid* medications are helpful for mild-to-moderate pain, and some, such as acetaminophen, provide added analgesia as well. *Adjuvant* medications include acetaminophen, antidepressants, and bisphosphonates.

As the "opioid crisis" became a national public health emergency, states attempted to regulate the prescription of opioids limiting and controlling dispensation of opioids. In 2015, with the significant increase in opioid overdose deaths in the United States, in an effort to prevent misuse and abuse, the Centers for Disease Control (CDC) issued restrictive guidelines for the prescribing of opioids. Unfortunately, it was not clear that these restrictions were intended only for primary care providers, and nationally, there were unintended consequences with difficulties for patients with cancer pain and sickle cell pain to gain access to effective opioid analgesia. The CDC guidelines were also applied by some insurers to determine reimbursement for opioid analgesics. In an effort to clarify the CDC guidelines vis à vis cancer pain and sickle cell disease pain, key members of the National Comprehensive Cancer Network (NCCN), American Society for Clinical Oncology (ASCO), and American Society of Hematology (ASH) met with the CDC, and in February 2019, the CDC issued a clarification stating that the CDC guideline was intended to provide recommendations for primary care clinicians who prescribe opioids for patients with chronic pain outside of active cancer treatment, palliative care, and end-of-life care. The intent was to ensure that physicians and patients consider all safe and effective treatment options for pain management to reduce inappropriate use (ASCO, 2019). The CDC further stated that oncology specialty pain guidelines (NCCN, ASCO) are updated more frequently than the CDC and provide guidance to control cancer pain in cancer patients and survivors without worsening the current opioid crisis (ASCO, 2019). ONS has also reaffirmed its position on cancer pain management (ONS, 2019). While Narcan (naloxone HCl) nasal spray has been available since 2017, the Food and Drug Administration, in an effort to increase availability of the opioid rescue and reduce the significant number of deaths in the United States from opioid drug overdose, approved the first generic naloxone nasal spray to make the antidote more available and accessible (FDA, 2019). It is available without a prescription from any pharmacy, and it is estimated a pack of two Narcan nasal sprays cost between $130–150 (Adapt Pharma, 2017), and it is hoped the generic version will be cheaper and thus more accessible.

Most nonopioid analgesics work peripherally to decrease prostaglandin synthesis (e.g., NSAIDs), but some agents may have a central action as well, such as acetaminophen. Pain receptors appear to be sensitized to mechanical and chemical stimulation by prostaglandins, so interruption of prostaglandin synthesis diminishes the painful impulse. For example, bone destruction and pain from metastasis appear to be mediated by prostaglandins, so NSAIDs that inhibit prostaglandin synthesis are first-line analgesics, together with opioid analgesics. Also bisphosphonates have shown to reduce pain from bony metastases. A Cochrane meta-analysis (2002) of randomized controlled trials showed that "bisphosphonates provided some pain relief for bone metastases," but there was insufficient evidence to recommend this as a first line analgesic. However, the recommendation was that they can be added to opioid analgesia and RT, as needed to enhance analgesia. Other studies have shown more effect but were not randomized controlled trials. In addition, the anti-inflammatory action of NSAIDs contributes to analgesia. Principal side effects of this class are alteration in hemostasis (aspirin inhibits platelet aggregation, while other salicylates may alter hepatic synthesis of blood coagulation factors); alteration in GI mucosal integrity (aspirin and other NSAIDs can erode GI mucosal surface, causing bleeding or ulceration); and altered renal elimination due to inhibition of renal prostaglandins responsible for renal blood flow and function.

NSAIDs achieve their anti-inflammatory effect by inhibiting the enzyme cyclooxygenase (COX), which is necessary for synthesis of prostaglandins and thromboxanes. There are two isoforms of the enzyme: COX-1, which appears to protect the gastric mucosa and is found in most tissues, including platelets, and COX-2, which is found in brain and kidney tissue, as well as other body tissues at the site of inflammation. NSAIDs traditionally inhibit both COX-1 and COX-2 isoforms, resulting in a high risk of gastric ulceration and perforation. As many patients with cancer, and cancer pain, are elderly and at risk for GI complications and renal insufficiency, it is possible to provide prophylaxis against peptic ulceration by concomitantly giving misoprostol or proton pump inhibitors (PPI) concurrently (NCCN, v2.2017). Patients should have their renal function assessed periodically (e.g., baseline and every 3 months).

Acetaminophen is thought to exert central analgesic effects. As there is a maximal daily dosage of 4 g of acetaminophen in patients without renal compromise, it is important to caution patients receiving combination drugs, such as oxycodone–acetaminophen (Percocet), not to take additional acetaminophen. If the patient is receiving the opioid–acetaminophen combination chronically, the NCCN recommends a maximum daily dose of acetaminophen (including with opioid) of 4 g a day for patients with normal hepatic function, or 3 g a day with chronic administration and/or concern about hepatic function (NCCN, 2.2017). Thus, when a NSAID and acetaminophen are combined, they provide both central (acetaminophen) and peripheral (NSAID) analgesic effects.

Adjuvant analgesics play a vital role in cancer pain management. These drugs are indicated for purposes other than analgesia but can be combined with primary analgesics to increase analgesia and/or manage symptoms related to pain or the adverse effects of the opioids. There may be wide variations in patient responses. The major classes used as adjuvant drugs are antidepressant (*Chapter 9*), corticosteroid (*Chapter 1*), anticonvulsant, and specialty drugs for bony metastasis (*Chapter 10*).

The *antidepressants* enhance pain-modulating pathways that are mediated by serotonin and norepinephrine. Not only can these agents help reduce the depression associated with chronic pain, but they can also relieve sleep problems, and often offer significant benefit in the management of neuropathic pain (McDonald & Portenoy, 2006). Antidepressant groups that offer benefit include the tricyclic antidepressants (TCAs), the serotonin-reuptake inhibitors, as well as others such as venlafaxine, bupropion, and duloxetine. Duloxetine (Cymbalta) has been shown to significantly reduce painful chemotherapy-induced peripheral neuropathy, and also improved function and quality of life (Smith et al., 2013). In dosing antidepressants, the starting dosage should be low and given at bedtime. The dose should be titrated up slowly to the usually effective range. It is important to allow 1 week between dose titrations to evaluate the benefit of a given dose. Side effects include sedation, orthostatic hypotension, constipation, dry mouth, dizziness and, less commonly, precipitation of acute angle-closure glaucoma, urinary retention, and arrhythmia.

Corticosteroids are useful in both acute and chronic pain management, such as that associated with metastatic bone pain, neuropathic pain, lymphedema, hepatic capsular distension, and brain metastasis. The dosing is individualized to the etiology of the pain and patient requirements, from low doses to high doses for patients with brain metastasis. It is important to identify patients at risk for peptic ulceration, and then to use corticosteroids cautiously if at all. In addition, patients need to be cautioned not to take concomitant aspirin.

Anticonvulsants may provide analgesia for lancinating, neuropathic pain. Second-generation drugs (gabapentin, pregabalin, and lamotrigine) have largely replaced first-generation drugs (carbamazepine, phenytoin, clonazepam, and valproate).

Specialty drugs for the management of bony metastasis are bisphosphonate pamidronate disodium (Aredia) and zoledronate (Zometa), indicated for use in managing bony metastases. Pamidronate and zoledronate have been shown to inhibit osteoclast activity and reduce pain from bony metastasis. Treatment is given IV every 4 weeks. Radiopharmaceuticals such as strontium-89 are taken up in bone mineral preferentially, in sites of metastasis. However, the subsequent development of acute leukemia has limited interest in radiopharmaceutical management of pain.

CANCER PAIN MANAGEMENT

According to McCaffery (1982), pain is "whatever the patient says it is, occurring where the patient says it is." Use of quantifiable measurement tools is helpful to identify pain intensity (see Figure 6.1) and pain *relief* in response to intervention. The World Health Organization recommends a two-step approach to cancer pain management, beginning with non-opioids for slight-to-mild pain and adding an opioid as the pain intensity increases. Opioids have different potencies, and when a patient is changed from one opioid to another, it is imperative that equianalgesic dosages be used. Equianalgesic dose tables are based on comparative potencies to morphine (see Table 6.1). Opioids and nonopioids can be combined for additive analgesia. Opioid agonist-antagonists, such as pentazocine (e.g., Talwin), should be used with caution, if at all, since they may cause withdrawal syndrome.

Opioid analgesics are the cornerstone of management of moderate-to-severe cancer pain. These drugs, opiate agonists, attach to specific opiate receptors in the limbic system, thalamus, hypothalamus, spinal cord, and organs such as intestines. This leads to altered pain perception at the spinal cord and higher CNS levels. Because of this action, side effects that may occur include suppressed cough reflex; alterations in consciousness and mood (drowsiness, sedation, euphoria, dysphoria, mental clouding); respiratory depression; nausea/vomiting; constipation; and dependence. A recent study compared sustained-release oral morphine to transdermal fentanyl and oral methadone in cancer pain management (Mercadante et al., 2008). No differences in pain or symptom intensity were found or in adverse effects during titration or chronic treatment. Methadone was significantly less expensive. However, oral methadone requires skill in dosing and management (NCCN, v2.2016) due to the drug's biphasic half-life when used for chronic pain.

Unfortunately, some patients with cancer pain suffer needlessly because healthcare providers (physicians) underprescribe and (nurses) undermedicate (Marks & Sacher, 1973). Chronic cancer pain requires the patient to self-administer opioids "ATC" rather than "as needed (PRN)" to prevent moderate-to-severe pain. As improper prescription of opioids for noncancer pain has led to addiction, overdose, and death, the Centers for Disease Control

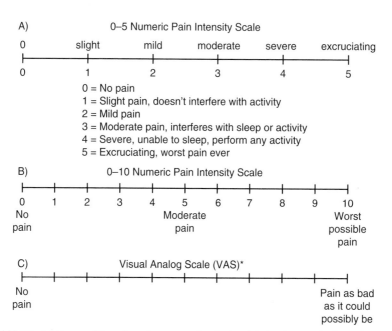

Figure 6.1   Examples of Measure Tools of Pain Intensity

Data from Agency for Healthcare Research and Quality. Acute Pain Management: Operative or medical procedures and trauma. *Clinical Practice Guideline No. 1 (AHCPR Publication No 92-0032)*. Rockville, MD: Agency for Healthcare Research and Quality; 1992; 116–117.

published guidelines to help primary care providers (Dowell et al., 2016). It is important for patients to understand that this is to address a problem in pain management of noncancer patients and their prescribers, NOT patients with cancer and the restrictions do not apply. Too often patients with cancer pain fear "addiction" and remain in pain. It is important to clarify for patients that addiction is a "psychological dependence" where the patient takes the drug for a perceived "high" or sensation, NOT to relieve pain. When the patient with cancer takes a prescribed opiate for pain, addiction is very unlikely. The NCCN Cancer Pain Guidelines (2019) provide an excellent resource for cancer professionals to provide a comprehensive patient pain assessment, including consideration of a patient's cultural and linguistic ability so that patient and family education can be tailored to the patient, and reassessment can be accurate. Key concepts in cancer pain management are tolerance, physical and psychological dependence. Tolerance is the ability to receive larger amounts of a drug without ill effect and to show decreased effect (i.e., pain relief) with continued use of the same drug dose. Tolerance occurs over time, depending on the drug and the route of administration. In addition, tolerance to the respiratory depressant effects of opiates

Table 6.1   Equianalgesic Dose Table

Drug Opioid Agonist	Approximate Equianalgesic Oral Dose	Approximate Equianalgesic Parenteral Dose	Recommended Starting Dose (Adults > 50 kg Body Weight)	
			Oral	Parenteral
Morphine IV to PO = 3	30 mg q 3–4 h (around-the-clock dosing) 60 mg q 3–4 h (single dose or intermittent dosing)	10 mg q 3–4 h	30 mg q 3–4 h	10 mg q 3–4 h
Codeine	200 mg q 3–4 h	75 mg q 3–4 h	60 mg q 3–4 h	60 mg q 2 h (IM, SQ)
Fentanyl	—	0.1 (100 mcg)	—	
Hydromorphone (Dilaudid) IV to PO = 5	7.5 mg q 3–4 h	1.5 mg q 3–4 h	6 mg q 3–4 h	1.5 mg q 3–4 h
Hydrocodone (in Lorcet, Lortab, Vicodin, others)	30 mg q 3–4 h	Not available	10 mg q 3–4 h	Not applicable
Methadone (Dolophine, others)	20 mg q 6–8 h	10 mg q 6–8 h	20 mg q 6–8 h	10 mg q 6–8 h
Oxycodone (Roxicodone, also in Percocet, Percodan, Tylox, others)	15–20 mg q 3–4 h	Not available	10 mg q 3–4 h	Not applicable
Oxymorphone (Numorphan)	10 mg	1 mg q 3–6 h	10 mg q 3–6	1 mg q 3–6 h

Modified from Agency for Healthcare Research and Quality. Acute Pain Management: Operative or medical procedures and trauma. *Clinical Practice Guideline No. 1 (AHCPR Publication No 92-0032)*. Rockville, MD: Agency for Healthcare Research and Quality; 1992; 116–117; National Comprehensive Cancer Network. NCCN Clinical Practice Guidelines in Oncology (NCCN Guidelines®): Adult Cancer Pain (v.2.2016). Available at http://www.nccn.org/professionals/physician_gls/pdf/pain.pdf. Accessed May 29, 2016; Kishner S et al. Opioid Equivalents and Conversion. Medscape News, April 10, 2016. Available at http://emedicine.medscape.com/article/2138678-overview. Accessed May 29, 2016.

develops over time with chronic usage for prevention of cancer pain. For instance, a patient with severe cancer pain who has been receiving escalating doses over a period of time may require very high doses to finally eliminate or reduce the pain to acceptable levels, as in the case of a patient with head and neck cancer who required 1,200 mg/h of morphine yet was still ambulatory and able to interact with family and friends. Opiate agonists may cause physical dependence (causing physical signs and symptoms of withdrawal if drug is stopped abruptly after chronic usage) and addiction (psychological dependence). However, addiction is VERY RARE in cancer patients, occurring in less than 0.1% of patients (Marks & Sacher, 1973). This is important for healthcare professionals, as under-medication of patients with cancer pain causes the patient to have to "watch the clock" and request pain medication whenever it is due, giving the uninformed healthcare professional the impression the patient is "drug seeking" when, in fact, the patient is not receiving adequate analgesics.

BTP management continues to be a significant challenge for healthcare professionals. Recognizing the different needs of different patients has led to a variety of formulations, especially of fentanyl, for the treatment of BTP in opioid-tolerant patients. Fentanyl is available as a transdermal patch delivery of fentanyl (20 times more potent than morphine) and as an immediate-release oral lozenge with mucosal absorption system (Actiq and generic equivalents). Other formulations available are fentanyl buccal tablet, sublingual tablet, sublingual spray, and as a nasal spray.

Recently suppliers of street drugs have found it easier and more lucrative to manufacture fentanyl tablets (National Institute on Drug Abuse [NIDA], 2016). It has been found by drug abusers that adding fentanyl to street-sold heroin or cocaine significantly increases their potency and, of course, risk of overdose and death (NIDA, 2016). Because of an increase in deaths from overdose, scientists are working on a vaccine to prevent addiction and the deaths from overdose from fentanyl and heroin (NIDA, 2016). The unfortunate effect for patients with cancer is that the news media paints a picture of persons using fentanyl as drug abusers or addicts, when in fact this excellent drug has been very effective in treating cancer pain. It is important for oncology nurses to help clarify this information for patients so that they understand the difference between using fentanyl to treat cancer pain and those who abuse the drug.

In addition, in an effort to avoid the pitfalls of the individuals who abuse drugs, Oxy-Contin was reformulated to discourage abuse. In the past, abusers were able to use the controlled-release product to release a large quantity of oxycodone all at once. The reformulated OxyContin has tamper-resistant properties, although unfortunately it can still be abused. In 2006, more than 4 million people aged 12 and over reported using Oxy-Contin for nonmedical uses at least once in their lifetime, and more than 500,000 were new, nonmedical users (U.S. Substance Abuse and Mental Health Services Administration, 2007, 2008). All long-acting and extended-release opioid analgesics now require an accompanying Risk Evaluation and Mitigation Strategy (REMS) program. Similar to that for ESAs, the REMS includes a patient medication guide and provider educational programs and materials (which include appropriate patient selection and dosing) so that prescribers, pharmacists, and patients will understand their responsibilities for the safe prescription, dispensing, and self-administration of the drug. Some drugs, such as the new fentanyl formulations, require a signed patient educational review.

MANAGEMENT

A REMS for transmucosal immediate release fentanyl (TIRF) is required by the FDA to assure standardization between/among products and to ensure informed risk-benefit decisions before starting and during treatment. TIRF medications are indicated only for the management of BTP in adult cancer patients age 18 and over (age 16 and over for Actiq and generic equivalents) who are already receiving and are tolerant to ATC opioid therapy for cancer-related persistent pain. Opioid-tolerant is defined as taking at least: 60 mg of oral morphine/day, 25 mcg transdermal fentanyl/hour, 30 mg oral oxycodone/day, 8 mg oral hydromorphone/day, 25 mg oral oxymorphone/day, or an equianalgesic dose of another opioid/day for a week or longer. Patients receiving TIRF medications should be screened for, and taught about avoidance of, drugs that are CYP3A4 inhibitors, as the drug interaction may result in an increased fentanyl plasma serum level and increased toxicity (e.g., possibly fatal respiratory depression).

All opioids now require a Risk Evaluation and Mitigation Strategy (REMS). Healthcare providers must review REMS-compliant education. In addition, healthcare providers must:

a. Complete a REMS-compliant education program offered by an accredited CE provider or another education program that includes all the elements of the FDA Education Blueprint for Health Care Providers Involved in the Management or Support of Patients with Pain. The blueprint can be found at www.fda.gov/OpioidAnalgesicREMSBlueprint.
b. Discuss the safe use, serious risks, and proper storage and disposal of opioid analgesics with patients and/or their caregivers every time these medicines are prescribed. The Patient Counseling Guide can be obtained at www.fda.gov/OpioidAnalgesicREMSPCG.
c. Emphasize to patients and their caregivers the importance of reading the Medication Guide that they will receive from their pharmacist every time an opioid analgesic is dispensed to them.

Consider using other tools to improve patient, household, and community safety, such as patient–prescriber agreements that reinforce patient–prescriber responsibilities. When trying to evaluate an opioid intervention, it is important to recall that this is the century of genomics. It is now clear that there is considerable genetic polymorphism in the cytochrome P450 family of enzymes (Bernard & Bruera, 2000), and that this can influence analgesic effect. For example, Payne (1998) states that 15% of Caucasians lack the enzyme CYP2D6 that is required to metabolize codeine to morphine, so this group will require higher doses to achieve the same effect. As genotyping becomes more a part of designing a plan of care, it is important to remember this. In addition, as nurses have always done, when one opioid is ineffective, care planning with physician colleagues is necessary to make sure that another opioid from a different class is tried.

Nonopioids: To meet the increasing needs of alternative administration formulations, ketorolac and acetaminophen are available as *parenteral* formulations.

Numerous practice guidelines are available, led by the National Comprehensive Cancer Network (NCCN, v2.2016). The guidelines give titration recommendations for patients who are either opioid-naïve or opioid-tolerant. Key points include the need for rapid titration of short-acting opioids to manage severe pain, before then determining the optimal analgesic regimen to control the patient's pain. For opioid-tolerant patients with a pain rating of > 4 (on a score of 0–10), calculate the previous 24-hour opioid requirement, convert to IV equivalent, and give 10–20% of the total dose. Other key points in the NCCN guidelines are (1) supplemental doses of analgesics should be administered when a pain from a procedure is anticipated, (2) if a patient is receiving a continuous IV PCA and it must be stopped due to a procedure/transport, administer the prescribed IV bolus dose immediately before the procedure/transport and give a subcutaneous dose equivalent to a 2-hour basal infusion rate, (3) anxiolytics should be given preemptively when feasible, and (4) titrate an opioid with caution in patients with risk factors, such as decreased renal/hepatic function, sleep apnea, or poor performance status.

References

Adapt Pharma Inc. Narcan (naloxone HCl) [package insert]. Radnor, PA. February 2017.

American Society of Clinical Oncology. CDC issues key clarification on guidelines for prescribing opioids for chronic pain in patients with cancer and sickle cell disease. Available at https://www.asco.org/advocacy-policy/asco-in-action/cdc-issues-key-clarification-guideline-prescribing-opioids-chronic. Accessed May 29, 2019.

Centers for Disease Control. CDC Guidelines for Prescribing Opioids for Chronic Pain. *Recommendations and Reports* [March 18, 2016]; 65(1):1–49. Available at http://www.cdc.gov/drugoverdose/prescribing/guideline.html. Accessed May 29, 2016.

Dowell D, Haegench TM, Chou R. CDC Guideline for Prescribing Opioids for Chronic Pain-United States, 2016. *J Am Med Assoc* 2016; 315(15):1624–1645.

Endo Pharmaceuticals, Inc. Opana ER (oxymorphone HCl tablet extended release) [package insert]. Malvern, PA. September 2018.

Endo Pharmaceuticals Inc. Opana (oxymorphone HCL tablets) [package insert]. Malvern, PA. September 2018.

Epictetus, arranged and translated by Hastings Crossley as part of the Gutenberg Project (released 2006). *The Golden Sayings of Epictetus. The Project Gutenberg E Book*. Available online at http://www.gutenberg.org/files/871/871-h/871-h.htm. Accessed July 2, 2011.

Ferrell BR, Rivera LM. Cancer Pain Education for Patients. *Semin Oncol Nurs* 1997; 13: 42–48.

Food and Drug Administration. Opioid analgesic REMS. Available at www.opioidanalgesicrems.com. Accessed May 29, 2019.

Food and Drug Administration. Opioid analgesic REMS Blueprint. Available at www.fda.gov/OpioidAnalgesicREMSBlueprint. Accessed May 29, 2019.

Food and Drug Administration 2012. *Transmucosal Immediate Release Fentanyl Risk Evaluation Mitigation Strategy Access Program.* Available at http://www.tirfremaccess.com. Accessed June 22, 2012.

Food and Drug Administration (FDA). FDA requests removal of Opana ER for risks related to abuse. June 8, 2017. Available at https://www.fda.gov/NewsEvents/Newsroom/PressAnnouncements/ucm562401.htm. Accessed July 23, 2017.

Food and Drug Administration (FDA). FDA approves first generic naloxone nasal spray to treat opioid overdose. April 19, 2019. Available at https://www.fda.gov/news-events/press-announcements/fda-approves-first-generic-naloxone-nasal-spray-treat-opioid-overdose. Accessed May 30, 2019.

Galena Biopharma. Abstral (fentanyl sublingual tablets) [package insert]. Portland, OR. July 2014.

Horizon Pharma USA Inc. *Duexis Prescribing Information*. Northbrook, IL. June 2017.

Hospira Inc. Ketorolac Tromethamine [package insert]. Lake Forest. IL. July 2015.

Impax Generics. Oxymorphone HCl. [package insert]. Hayward, CA. April 2016.

Insys Therapeutics. Subsys (fentanyl sublingual spray) [package insert]. Chandler, AZ. December 2016.

Jacox A, Carr DB, Payne R. Management of Cancer Pain. *Clinical Practice Guideline No 9 (AHCPR Pub No 94–0592)*. Rockville, MD: Agency for Health Care Policy & Research USDHHS; 1994.

Janssen Pharmaceuticals. Duragesic (fentanyl transdermal system) [package insert]. Titusville, NJ. September 2018.

Kishner S, Schraga ED. Opioid Equivalents and Conversions. Updated April 10, 2016. Available at http://emedicine.medscape.com/article/2138678-overview. Accessed May 29, 2016.

Mallinckrodt Pharmaceuticals. Exalgo (hydromorphone HCl) extended release tablets [package insert]. Hazelwood, MO. December 2016.

Mallinckrodt Pharmaceuticals. Ofirmev (acetaminophen) injection [package insert]. Hazelwood, MO. March 2018.

Mallinckrodt Pharmaceuticals. Oral transmucosal fentanyl citrate [package insert]. Hazelwood, MO. March 2017.Marks RM, Sacher EJ. Undertreatment of Medical Inpatients with Opioid Analgesics. *Ann Intern Med* 1973; 78:173–181.

McCaffery M. *Nursing. Management of the Patient with Pain.* Philadelphia, PA: JB Lippincott Co.; 198

McDonald AA, Portenoy RK. How to Use Antidepressants and Anticonvulsants as Adjuvant Analgesics in the Treatment of Neuropathic Cancer Pain. *Supportive Oncol* 2006; 4(1):43–52.

Mercadante S, Porzio G, Ferrera P, et al. Sustained-Release Oral Morphine Versus Transdermal Fentanyl and Oral Methadone in Cancer Pain Management. *Eur J Pain* published online at doi: 10.1016/j.ejpain.2008.01.013. Accessed June 24, 2008.

Mylan Pharmaceuticals Inc. Fentanyl transdermal system [package insert]. Morgantown, WV. May 2014.

National Comprehensive Cancer Network (NCCN). *Adult Cancer Pain.* v.2. 2019. Rockville, MD. Available at https://www.nccn.org/professionals/physician_gls/pdf/pain.pdf. Accessed May 30, 2019.

National Comprehensive Cancer Network. New effort launched to bridge differences in clinical practice guidelines for treatment of cancer pain. Available at https://www.nccn.org/about/news/member_ebulletin/ebulletindetail.aspx?ebulletinid=1552. Accessed May 29, 2019.

National Institute on Drug Abuse (NIDA). Fentanyl. Available at https://www.drugabuse.gov/drugs-abuse/fentanyl. Accessed May 30, 2019.

Oncology Nursing Society. Cancer Pain Management: ONS Position Statement. March 2019. Available at https://www.ons.org/advocacy-policy/positions/practice/pain-management. Accessed May 29, 2019.

Parke-Davis. Neurontin (gabapentin) [package insert]. New York, NY. September 2015.

Parke-Davis. Lyrica (pregabalin) [package insert]. New York, NY. March 2016.

Payne R. *Pharmacologic Management of Pain, Section IA3. Berger A, Portenoy RK, Weissman DE, Principles and Practice of Supportive Oncology.* Philadelphia, PA: Lippincott-Raven Publishers; 1998.

Purdue Pharma. Oxycontin Prescribing Information. Stamford, CT: Purdue Pharma LP. September 2018.

Rades D, Schild SE, Abrahm JL. Treatment of Painful Bone Metastases. *Nat Rev Clin Oncol* 2010; 7(4): 220–229.

Roxane Laboratories. Dear Doctor Letter: Important Safety Information Regarding Morphine Sulfate Oral Solution 100 mg per 5 mL (20 mg/mL). December 2010.

Sentynl Therapeutics, Inc. Abstral (fentanyl sublingual tablets) [prescribing information]. Solana Beach, CA. December 2016.

Smith EM, Pang H, Cirrincione C, et al. Effect of Duloxetine on Pain, Function, and Quality of Life among Patients with Chemotherapy-induced Painful Peripheral Neuropathy: A Randomized Clinical Trial. *J Am Med Assoc* 2013; 309(13):1359–1367.

Teva Pharmaceuticals USA Inc. Fentora (fentanyl buccal tablets) [package insert]. North Wales, PA. December 2016.

Teva Pharmaceuticals USA Inc. Actiq (fentanyl citrate oral transmucosal lozenge) [package insert]. North Wales, PA. December 2016.

U.S. Substance Abuse and Mental Health Services Administration, Office of Applied Studies. *Results from the 2006 National Survey on Drug Use and Health: National Findings.* 1007; NSDUH Series H-32, DHHS Publication No (SMA) 07–4293. Rockville, MD; 2007.

U.S. Substance Abuse and Mental Health Services Administration. Oxycontin Prescription Drug Abuse: 2008 Revision. *Substance Abuse Treatment Advisory* 2008; 7(1):1–8.

Wilkie D. Neural Mechanisms of Pain: A Foundation for Cancer Pain Assessment and Management. Maguire DB, Yarbro CH, Ferrell BR, *Cancer Pain Management,* 2nd ed. Sudbury, MA: Jones and Bartlett Publishers; 1995: 61–87.

West Therapeutic Development LLC. Lazanda (Fentanyl nasal spray CII) [package insert]. Northbrook, IL. August 2018.

Wong RKS, Wiffen PJ. Bisphosphonates for the relief of pain secondary to bone metastases. Cochrane Database Systematic Reviews 2002, Issue 2. Art. No. CD002068. DOI: 10.2002/14651858. CD002068

Zeppetella G, O'Doherty CA, Collins S. Prevalence and Characteristics of Breakthrough Pain in Cancer Patients Admitted to a Hospice. *J Pain Symptom Manage* 2000; 20:87–92.

NON-OPIOID ANALGESICS

Drug: acetaminophen (Acephen, Actamin, Anacin-3, Apacet, Anesin, Dapa, Datril, Genapap, Genebs, Gentabs, Halenol, Liquiprin, Meda Cap, Panadol, Panex, Suppap, Tempra, Tenol, Ty Caps, Tylenol)

MANAGEMENT

Class: Miscellaneous analgesic/antipyretic.

Mechanism of Action: Appears to inhibit prostaglandin synthesis centrally, thus preventing sensitization of pain receptors to chemical or mechanical stimulation. Mechanism is similar to salicylates but is not uricosuric. May have weak anti-inflammatory effects in nonrheumatoid conditions (e.g., after oral surgery). Reduces fever by direct effect on hypothalamus; heat is lost through vasodilation and increased peripheral blood flow. Analgesic and antipyretic action similar to aspirin.

Metabolism: Rapidly absorbed from GI tract; 25% serum protein-binding. Elimination half-life is 1–3 hours. Metabolized by the liver and excreted in the urine.

Indication: For the relief of pain and discomfort, and to reduce fever.

Dosage/Range:
- 325–650 mg every 4–6 hours PRN for pain, discomfort. Some individuals may need increased single doses of 1 g.
- Maximum dose in 24 hours: Adults: 10 tablets (3,250 mg) and in children 5 tablets (1,625 mg).

Drug Preparation:
- Ensure seals on tamper-resistant package are intact when opening new package.

Drug Administration:
- Oral, rectal, elixir.

Drug Interactions:
- Hopanaepatotoxicity of acetaminophen may be increased by chronic use of high doses of drugs using hepatic microsomal enzyme system: barbiturates, carbamazepine, rifampin, phenytoin, sulfinpyrazone.

- Alcohol: increased risk of hepatic damage with chronic, excessive use.
- Diflunisal: increased acetaminophen serum level; avoid concurrent use.
- Phenothiazines: possible severe hypothermia may occur when used concomitantly.

Lab Effects/Interference:
- None known.

Special Considerations:
- Elixirs contain alcohol (Tylenol, Valadol).
- Contraindicated in patients with known hypersensitivity; use cautiously, if at all, in patients with hepatic or renal dysfunction.
- Chronic ingestion of large doses of acetaminophen may slightly potentiate effects of coumarin and other anticoagulants.

Potential Toxicities/Side Effects and the Nursing Process

I.   KNOWLEDGE DEFICIT related to SELF-ADMINISTRATION

Defining Characteristics: Fever curve or excessive fever can be masked by self-dosing with acetaminophen.

Nursing Implications: Instruct patient to report temperature over 38.3°C (101°F) or persistent or recurrent fever. Assess other over-the-counter (OTC) medicines the patient may be taking.

II.   POTENTIAL INJURY related to HEPATOTOXICITY

Defining Characteristics: Excessive alcoholic intake and other drugs can increase risk for hepatotoxicity.

Nursing Implications: Assess total acetaminophen dosage/24 hours, taking into account OTC medications. Assess baseline LFTs, especially if the patient has primary hepatoma or liver metastasis. Teach patient to avoid excessive alcohol intake and/or excessive acetaminophen intake.

Drug: acetaminophen injection (Ofirmev)

Class: Miscellaneous analgesic/antipyretic.

Mechanism of Action: Appears to inhibit prostaglandin synthesis centrally, thus preventing sensitization of pain receptors to chemical or mechanical stimulation. Mechanism is similar to salicylates but is not uricosuric. May have weak anti-inflammatory effects in nonrheumatoid conditions (e.g., after oral surgery). Reduces fever by direct effect on hypothalamus; heat is lost through vasodilation and increased peripheral blood flow. Analgesic and antipyretic action similar to aspirin.

Metabolism: C_{max} (maximum concentration) reached at end of 15-minute IV infusion, and is about 70% higher than that achieved with oral administration of the same dose. However, the AUC is similar following oral and IV administration of the same dose. Low binding (10–25%) to plasma proteins. Metabolized by the liver (primarily CYP2E1 micro-enzyme) and metabolites excreted in the urine (< 5% intact drug). Elimination half-life is 1–3 hours, with > 90% of the administered dose excreted within 24 hours.

Indications: FDA-indicated for the management of adults and pediatric patients aged 2 and older with (1) mild-to-moderate pain; (2) moderate-to-severe pain with adjunctive opioid analgesics; and in adults and pediatric patients for (3) reduction of fever.

Contraindications: Patients with (1) severe liver impairment, (2) severe active liver disease, or (3) hypersensitivity to drug or its components.

Dosage/Range:
- Adults and adolescents weighing > 50 kg: 1,000 mg every 6 hours or 650 mg every 4 hours to a maximum of 4,000 mg/day. Minimum dosing interval is 4 hours.
- Adults and adolescents weighing < 50 kg: 15 mg/kg every 6 hours or 12.5 mg/kg every 4 hours to a maximum of 75 mg/kg/day. Minimum dosing interval is 4 hours. Maximum dose in 24 hr = up to 3,750 mg.
- Children > 2 to 12 years old: 15 mg/kg every 6 hours or 12.5 mg/kg every 4 hours to a maximum of 75 mg/kg/day. Minimum dosing interval is 4 hours. Maximum dose in 24 hr = up to 3,750 mg.
- Neonates: including premature neonates born at ≥ 32 weeks, gestational age to 28 days chronological age: 12.5 mg/kg q 6 hr to a maximum of 50 mg/kg/day. Minimal dosing interval is 6 hr.
- Infants (29 days to 2 years of age): 15 mg/kg q 6 hr to a maximum of 60 mg/kg/day. Minimum dosing interval is 6 hr.
- Use cautiously in patients with liver impairment or active hepatic disease, alcoholism, chronic malnutrition, severe hypovolemia, or severe renal impairment.

Drug Preparation: Injection for IV infusion: each 100-mL glass vial contains 1,000-mg acetaminophen (10 mg/mL). Inspect the vial for any particulate matter or discoloration, and discard if found. Aseptically, attach a vented intravenous (IV) set into the septum of the 100-mL vial for patients ordered for 1,000-mg dose. Drug can be administered without further dilution. Do not add any other medications to the vial or infusion device.

For doses < 1,000 mg, aseptically withdraw the ordered amount from an intact sealed vial and place in a separate, empty sterile container (e.g., glass bottle, plastic IV container, or syringe) for IV infusion.
- Available in carton of 24 vials. Store at 20–25°C (68–77°F).
- Vial is a single-use, preservative-free vial, and any unused portion must be discarded. Put small-volume pediatric doses up to 60 mL in a syringe and administer over 15 minutes.
- Once vacuum seal of the glass vial has been penetrated, or the contents transferred to another container, administer the dose within 6 hours.
- DO NOT add other medications to IV tubing; for example, diazepam and chlorpromazine HCl are physically incompatible.

MANAGEMENT

Drug Administration:
- Administer acetaminophen dose IV via vented IV set over 15 minutes, ensuring that at the completion of the infusion, the tubing is shut off to prevent inadvertent air embolism.
- Administer as a single or repeated dose.

Drug Interactions:
- Incompatible with diazepam and chlorpromazine HCl.
- Ethanol: Increased risk of hepatotoxicity.
- Substances that induce or regulate hepatic cytochrome enzyme may alter the metabolism of acetaminophen and increase its hepatotoxicity.
- CYP2E1 may alter the metabolism of acetaminophen and increase its hepatotoxic potential (substrates are acetaminophen, alcohol; inhibitors are disulfiram [Antabuse]; inducers are ethanol and isoniazid [Laniazid]). Ethanol has a complex relationship with acetaminophen: Excess ethanol intake can induce hepatic cytochromes, but it also acts as a competitive inhibitor of acetaminophen metabolism.
- Anticoagulants: Increased INR when administered with chronic administration of oral acetaminophen at 4,000 mg/day; data shows INR increases in some patients who have been stabilized on sodium warfarin; assess INR more frequently and dose warfarin accordingly.

Lab Effects/Interference: May increase LFTs.

Special Considerations:
- Warnings and Precautions:
  - *Hepatic Injury:* Do not exceed recommended doses as it may result in liver failure and death in some instances. Use caution when administering acetaminophen to patients with hepatic impairment or active hepatic disease, alcoholism, chronic malnutrition, severe hypovolemia (due to dehydration or blood loss) or severe renal impairment.
  - *Serious Skin Reactions:* Rarely, severe skin reactions can occur such as acute generalized exanthematous pustuloisis (AGEP), Stevens-Johnson Syndrome (SJS), and toxic epidermal necrolysis (TEN). Teach patients to report rash right away. If AGEP, SJS, or TEN is confirmed, discontinue the drug immediately.
  - *Risk of Medication Errors:* Ensure that dose in milligrams (mg) and milliliters (mL) is not confused, dosing is based on weight for patients weighing <50 kg, infusion pumps are properly programmed, and the total daily dose of acetaminophen from all sources does not exceed maximum daily limits. Use scrupulous technique and double checks to avoid medication dosing errors.
- *Allergy and Hypersensitivity:* Hypersensitivity and anaphylaxis have occurred, characterized by swelling of the face and throat, respiratory distress, urticaria, rash, and pruritus. Discontinue drug immediately if allergic or hypersensitivity reactions occur. DO NOT administer to patients with an allergy to acetaminophen.
- Most common adverse reactions were nausea, vomiting, headache, and insomnia in adult patients; in children, nausea, vomiting, constipation, pruritus, agitation, and atelectasis are most common.
- Overdosage: acute overdosage is dose-dependent and potentially fatal. Sequelae are hepatic necrosis (90% hepatic damage in patients with acetaminophen level > 300 mcg/mL

at 4 hours after ingestion; minimal damage if plasma level < 150 mcg/mL at 4 hours or < 37.5 mcg/mL at 12 hours), renal tubular necrosis, hypoglycemic coma, and thrombocytopenia. Early symptoms of potentially hepatotoxic overdose: nausea, vomiting, diaphoresis, general malaise. Laboratory evidence of hepatotoxicity may not be apparent until 48–72 hours, postingestion. Antidote is *N*-acetylcysteine (NAC, e.g., Mucomyst), which should be administered emergently. Poison Control Center 1-800-222-1222.

- Use in special populations:
  - Drug is pregnancy class C: Use drug only if clearly needed (no studies have been done with IV formulation).
  - Nursing mothers: Studies show infant receives about 1–2% of the mother's dose; use drug cautiously, if at all, in nursing mothers.
  - Pediatrics < 2 years old: Has not been studied, and is not recommended.
  - Severe renal impairment (creatinine clearance < 30 mL/min): Consider reduced daily dose given with longer dosing intervals.

Potential Toxicities/Side Effects and the Nursing Process

I.   KNOWLEDGE DEFICIT related to SELF-ADMINISTRATION

Defining Characteristics: Fever curve or excessive fever can be masked by self-dosing with acetaminophen.

Nursing Implications: Instruct patient to report temperature over 38.3°C (101°F) or persistent or recurrent fever. Assess other OTC medicines the patient may be taking.

II.   POTENTIAL INJURY related to HEPATOTOXICITY

Defining Characteristics: Excessive alcoholic intake and other drugs can increase risk for hepatotoxicity.

Nursing Implications: Assess total acetaminophen dosage/24 hours, taking into account OTC medications. Assess baseline LFTs, especially if the patient has primary hepatoma or liver metastasis. Teach patient to avoid excessive alcohol intake and/or excessive acetaminophen intake.

Drug: aspirin, acetylsalicylic acid (ASA, Aspergum, Bayer Aspirin, Easprin, Ecotrin, Empirin)

Class: Salicylate.

Mechanism of Action: Inhibits prostaglandin synthesis, peripherally preventing sensitization of pain receptors by mechanical and chemical stimuli. Also has anti-inflammatory effect, producing analgesic and antipyretic effects. Central action via hypothalamus unclear.

MANAGEMENT

Metabolism: Rapidly and well absorbed from GI tract, and distributed throughout the body with high concentrations in liver and kidney. Drug is bound to serum proteins, especially albumin. Metabolized by liver and excreted in urine.

Indication: For the relief of pain and the reduction of fever.

Dosage/Range:
- 325–650 mg PO or PR every 4 hours PRN for pain or fever (maximum 3.9 g/day).

Drug Preparation:
- Keep in closed container, away from heat, to prevent drug decomposition.
- Do not use if strong, vinegar-like odor is present. Do not crush enteric-coated aspirin.

Drug Administration:
- Oral or rectal suppositories. Give oral dose with 240-mL water or milk to decrease gastric irritation.
- Oral solution may be made from effervescent aspirin powders (e.g., Alka-Seltzer); Alka-Seltzer chewable aspirin tablets available.

Drug Interactions:
- Ammonium chloride, ascorbic acid, or methionine (urine acidifiers): Decrease ASA excretion, so increase risk of ASA toxicity.
- Antacids, urinary alkalizers: May increase ASA excretion, so may decrease the ASA effect. Alcohol increases the risk of GI ulceration, bleeding.
- Decreased effect of angiotensin-converting enzyme (ACE) inhibitors. When used together, the effect of anticoagulants may be enhanced (additive hypothrombinemic effect), leading to prolonged bleeding time. DO NOT USE TOGETHER.
- Beta-adrenergic blockers (e.g., propranolol): Possible decrease in antihypertensive effect.
- Corticosteroids: Increase in aspirin excretion with decrease in aspirin effect.
- Methotrexate: Increase in methotrexate serum levels with increased toxicity. DO NOT USE CONCURRENTLY.
- NSAIDs: Decrease in NSAID serum concentration; may have increased incidence of GI side effects. Not recommended to be used together.
- Probenecid, sulfinpyrazone: aspirin (doses $\geq$ 3 g/day) antagonizes uricosuric drug effect.
- Spirolactone: Aspirin may inhibit diuretic effect.
- Sulfonylureas, exogenous insulin: Aspirin may have hypoglycemic effect and may potentiate these drug actions. Monitor for hypoglycemia.
- Valproic acid: Aspirin displaces drug and decreases its excretion, resulting in increased serum levels and possible valproic acid toxicity.

Lab Effects/Interference:
- Prolonged bleeding time, leukopenia, thrombocytopenia.

Special Considerations:
- Patients receiving myelosuppressive chemotherapy should be cautioned not to take aspirin due to increased risk of bleeding.
- Patients should be instructed to take drug with food or milk.

- Use cautiously in patients with asthma, rhinitis, or nasal polyps (can cause severe bronchospasm).
- Drug is contraindicated in patients with GI ulcer, GI bleeding, hypersensitivity to aspirin, increased bleeding tendencies.
- Use cautiously in patients with liver damage, hypoprothrombinemia, or with vitamin K deficiency.
- Aspirin administration in patients with breast cancer may reduce recurrence and death, as aspirin appears to inhibit metastases. A study showed that women who were alive for at least 1 year after being diagnosed with breast cancer, who took aspirin (1–7 days of aspirin use per week), had a decreased risk of recurrence and death compared to those who did not take aspirin (Holmes et al., 2010).

Potential Toxicities/Side Effects and the Nursing Process

I. ALTERATION IN NUTRITION, LESS THAN BODY REQUIREMENTS, related to GI TOXICITY

Defining Characteristics: Nausea, dyspepsia (5–25% of patients), heartburn, epigastric discomfort, anorexia, and acute, reversible hepatotoxicity may occur. Risk increases with dose. May potentiate peptic ulcer disease.

Nursing Implications: Teach patient self-administration with 8-oz (240-mL) water or milk. If GI distress develops, discuss use of enteric-coated aspirin (e.g., Ecotrin). If patient receiving high doses of aspirin, monitor LFTs. Drug contraindicated in patients with peptic ulcer disease.

II. POTENTIAL FOR BLEEDING related to INHIBITION OF PLATELET AGGREGATION

Defining Characteristics: Aspirin may cause prolongation of bleeding time, leukopenia, thrombocytopenia, purpura, shortened erythrocyte survival time.

Nursing Implications: Teach patient to avoid aspirin and aspirin-containing drugs if receiving myelosuppressive chemotherapy. Review concurrent medications to identify risk for drug interactions. Monitor Hgb, HCT over time; teach patient signs/symptoms of anemia, and instruct to report them (headache, fatigue, chest pain, irritability). Monitor stool guaiacs.

III. INJURY related to MILD SALICYLISM

Defining Characteristics: Administration of large doses of salicylates may cause salicylism, characterized by dizziness, tinnitus, diminished hearing, nausea, vomiting, diarrhea, mental confusion, CNS depression, headache, sweating, and hyperventilation at serum salicylate concentration 150–300 μg/mL (use in cancer patients usually 100 μg/mL).

Nursing Implications: Teach patient to reduce dose, interrupt dose if signs/symptoms occur. Assess concurrent medications for possible drug interactions.

MANAGEMENT

Drug: choline magnesium trisalicylate (Trilisate)

Class: Choline and magnesium salicylate combination.

Mechanism of Action: Analgesic effect through peripheral and central pathways, decreasing pain perception. Prostaglandin inhibition probably involved in peripheral mechanism. Antipyretic effect via hypothalamic heat regulation center. Does not interfere with platelet aggregation.

Metabolism: Rapidly absorbed from GI tract. Metabolized by the liver and excreted in the urine.

Indication: For the relief of pain, including pain related to osteoarthritis, RA.

Dosage/Range:
• Trilisate 750 mg bid or dose-increase to maximum 3,200 mg/day.

Drug Preparation:
• Trilisate liquid 5 mL or Trilisate 500-mg tablet contains ASA equivalent of 650 mg.
• Trilisate 750-mg tablet contains 975 mg ASA.
• Trilisate 1,000-mg tablet contains 1,300 mg ASA.

Drug Administration:
• Oral.

Drug Interactions:
• Antacids, urine alkalinizers: Increase salicylate excretion and decrease drug effect. Do not administer with antacids.
• Ammonium chloride, ascorbic acid, methionine (urine acidifiers): Decrease salicylate excretion, so increased risk of salicylate toxicity.
• Concomitant administration with alcohol, steroids, other NSAIDs may increase GI side effects.
• Corticosteroids: May increase salicylate excretion and decrease trilisate effect.
• Warfarin: May have increased warfarin levels and increased PT; monitor patient closely, and reduce warfarin dosage as needed.

Lab Effects/Interference:
• Free T_4 may be increased with a concurrent decrease in total plasma T_4 (does not affect thyroid function).

Special Considerations:
• Drug does not interfere with platelet aggregation.
• Use cautiously in patients with chronic renal failure, gastritis.
• Contraindicated if known hypersensitivity to salicylates.
• Drug contains magnesium, so periodic evaluation of serum magnesium should be performed.

Potential Toxicities/Side Effects and the Nursing Process

I.   ALTERATION IN NUTRITION, LESS THAN BODY REQUIREMENTS, related to GI TOXICITY

Defining Characteristics: Fewer GI side effects than aspirin. Nausea, dyspepsia (5–25% of patients), heartburn, epigastric discomfort, anorexia, and acute reversible hepatotoxicity may occur. Risk increases with dose. May potentiate peptic ulcer disease.

Nursing Implications: Teach patient self-administration with food, or 8-oz (240-mL) water or milk. If patient is receiving antacid, administer antacid 2 hours after meals and Trilisate before meals. Assess baseline liver and renal function and monitor if patient is receiving high doses on ongoing basis. Guaiac stool to assess occult blood, as gastric ulceration may occur.

II.   INJURY related to MILD SALICYLISM

Defining Characteristics: Administration of large doses of salicylates may cause salicylism, characterized by dizziness, tinnitus, diminished hearing, nausea, vomiting, diarrhea, mental confusion, CNS depression, headache, sweating, and hyperventilation at serum salicylate concentration 150–300 µg/mL (use in cancer patients usually 100 µg/mL).

Nursing Implications: Teach patient to reduce dose, interrupt dose if signs/symptoms occur. Assess concurrent medications for possible drug interactions.

III.   POTENTIAL ALTERATION IN URINARY ELIMINATION related to RENAL PROSTAGLANDIN INHIBITION

Defining Characteristics: Rarely, elevated serum BUN and creatinine may occur.

Nursing Implications: Assess baseline serum BUN, creatinine, and monitor during therapy.

Drug: clonidine hydrochloride (Duraclon)

Class: Antiadrenergic agent.

Mechanism of Action: Acts centrally to stimulate alpha-2-adrenergic receptors in the CNS, thus inhibiting sympathetic vasomotor centers. When given epidurally, the drug is believed to mimic norepinephrine activity at presynaptic and postjunctional alpha-2-adrenoceptors in the dorsal horn of the spinal cord. Is administered together with opioids for severe cancer pain to maximize analgesia. Clonidine HCl shows best efficacy against neuropathic pain.

MANAGEMENT

Metabolism: Drug is highly lipid-soluble and rapidly distributes into extravascular sites and into the CNS; enters the plasma via the epidural veins, leading to hypotensive effect. Drug is metabolized and excreted in the urine (72% of the administered dose in 96 hours, and 40–50% of that is unchanged drug).

Indication: In combination with opiates for the treatment of severe pain in cancer patients that is not adequately relieved by opioid analgesics alone. Drug may be more effective in patients with neuropathic pain than somatic or visceral pain.

Contraindicated in patients sensitive or allergic to clonidine HCl; epidural administration contraindicated if (1) injection-site infection occurs, (2) patient is receiving anticoagulation, (3) patient has bleeding diathesis, (4) administered above the C4 dermatome, (5) patient has severe cardiac disease or is hemodynamically unstable, or (6) used in obstetrical or postoperative analgesia.

Dosage/Range:

To be administered in combination with opioids via epidural route:
• Initial: Starting dose is 30 µg/hr.
• May be titrated up to 40 µg/hr or down, based on degree of pain relief and extent of side effects.

Drug Preparation:
• Preservative-free preparation.
• Given epidurally in combination with opioid via continuous epidural infusion device.

Drug Interactions:
• CNS depressants (e.g., alcohol, barbiturates): Potentiation of CNS depression.
• Opioid analgesics: May potentiate hypotension due to clonidine.
• TCAs: May antagonize hypotensive effect of clonidine.
• Beta-blockers: May exacerbate hypertensive symptoms of clonidine withdrawal.
• Epidural local anesthetics: Clonidine may prolong pharmacologic effects of local anesthetic; both motor and sensory blockade.

Lab Effects/Interference:
• None known.

Special Considerations:
• Use cautiously in patients receiving digitalis, calcium channel blockers, and beta-blockers, as there may be additive effects of bradycardia and AV block.
• Severe hypotension may occur during first 2 days of clonidine therapy, especially when drug is infused into the upper thoracic spinal segments—monitor vital signs frequently.
• Do not suddenly withdraw drug, as this may result in nervousness, agitation, headache, tremor, rapid increase in blood pressure; scrupulously maintain drug administration equipment to prevent accidental interruption of drug. Drug dose should be gradually decreased over 2–4 days. If patient is receiving a beta-blocker, the beta-blocker should be discontinued several days before the gradual discontinuation of epidural clonidine. Teach patient NOT to discontinue drug on own.

Potential Toxicities/Side Effects and the Nursing Process

I.   ALTERED TISSUE PERFUSION related to HYPOTENSION

Defining Characteristics: Hypotension usually occurs within the first 4 days after beginning epidural clonidine but may also occur throughout treatment. Increased risk in patients receiving infusion into upper-thoracic spinal segments, in women, and in patients who have low body weight. Hypotension may be accentuated by concurrent opiate administration. Clonidine decreases sympathetic CNS outflow, decreasing peripheral resistance, decreasing renal vascular resistance, and decreasing heart rate and BP.

Nursing Implications: Monitor T, BP, HR frequently, especially during first few days of therapy. Notify physician of significant changes. Expect IV fluids to be given to correct hypotension, and if needed, IV ephedrine. Symptomatic bradycardia can be treated with atropine.

II.   ALTERED TISSUE PERFUSION related to REBOUND HYPERTENSION

Defining Characteristics: Withdrawal symptoms can occur if drug is interrupted or stopped abruptly; characterized by nervousness, agitation, headache, tremor, rapid increase in BP. Increased risk in patients receiving high drug doses, patients receiving beta-blockers, or patients with a history of hypertension. Rarely, this may result in CVA, hypertensive encephalopathy, or death.

Nursing Implications: Scrupulously manage/maintain catheter and pump to prevent interruption in flow; teach patient catheter and pump care and use; instruct patient never to abruptly discontinue medicine; anticipate physician will discontinue beta-blockers prior to gradual taper of drug over 2–4 days when drug is being discontinued.

III.   POTENTIAL FOR INFECTION related to IMPLANTED DEVICE

Defining Characteristics: Implanted epidural catheter may become infected, leading to epidural abscess or meningitis.

Nursing Implications: Scrupulously maintain catheter, using sterile technique; teach patient catheter care and management; monitor for signs/symptoms of infection and teach patient this assessment. If in the hospital, monitor for fever and pain and notify the physician immediately if either occurs. Instruct patient to report fever, pain to the physician immediately if at home.

Drug: gabapentin (Neurontin)

Class: Anticonvulsant.

Mechanism of Action: Not clearly understood. Drug is structurally related to neurotransmitter GABA (gamma-amino-butyric acid), but drug does not bind to GABA receptor

MANAGEMENT

sites. It is unclear whether drug has activity at NMDA receptor sites. Drug has been shown to bind to receptor sites in neocortex and hippocampus.

Metabolism: Bioavailability of drug decreases as dose increases, and drug absorption unaffected by food. Drug half-life is 5–7 hours, and drug excreted unchanged in the urine. Plasma clearance may be reduced in elderly and is reduced in renal insufficiency.

Indication: For the management of patients with (1) postherpetic neuralgia in adults; and (2) adjunctive therapy in the treatment of partial-onset seizures in adults and children aged 3 and older with epilepsy.

Contraindication: Hypersensitivity to the drug or any of its ingredients.

Dosage/Range:
Postherpetic neuralgia (see package insert for epilepsy dosing).
- Initial titration: 300 mg on day 1, 300 mg bid on day 2, and 300 mg tid on day 3.
- As needed, dose may be titrated up to 400 mg tid, in increments, to a maximum dose of 600 mg tid (1,800 mg total dose per day).
- Dose-reduce in renal insufficiency:

Creatinine Clearance (mL/min)	Drug Dose
30–60	300 mg bid
15–30	300 mg/day
< 15	300 mg every other day

Drug Preparation:
- Available as 100-, 300-, and 400-mg capsules; 600- and 800-mg tablets; 250 mg/mL oral solution.

Drug Administration:
- Oral, take without regard to food intake.
- Take 1 hour before, or 2 hours after, antacid.
- Take initial dose at bedtime to enhance somnolence and minimize dizziness, fatigue, and ataxia.
- Doses should not be separated by > 12 hours (must be tid, e.g., every 8 hours).
- If drug is discontinued or changed to another anticonvulsant, gradually discontinue drug over 1 week.

Drug Interactions:
- Antacids: decrease bioavailability of drug.
- Cimetidine: decreases renal excretion of drug with potential for excess toxicity; monitor patient closely and dose-reduce if both drugs must be given concomitantly.

Lab Effects/Interference:
- Urinary protein test using Ames N-Multistix may be falsely positive.
- Drug may cause leukopenia, anemia, thrombocytopenia.

Special Considerations:
- Most common side effects when used for postherpetic neuralgia: dizziness, somnolence, peripheral edema.
- Warnings and Precautions:
  - Drug reaction with eosinophilia and systemic symptoms (multi-organ hypersensitivity): discontinue drug if an alternate explanation cannot be found.
  - Anaphylaxis and angioedema: discontinue drug and implement medical orders.
  - Driving impairment: Drug may cause dizziness, fatigue, somnolence, sedation, drowsiness, ataxia, so patient should be taught to avoid activities requiring mental acuity, such as driving, until after full effect of drug is known.
  - Increased seizure incidence/frequency in patients with seizure disorder if gabapentin abruptly discontinued.
  - Suicidal ideation and behavior: monitor for suicidal thoughts and behavior.
  - Neuropsychiatric adverse effects in children 3–12 years of age: monitor patient closely.
- Dose-reduce in patients with renal insufficiency, and consider dose reduction in the elderly.
- Drug helpful in the management of painful peripheral neuropathies.

Potential Toxicities/Side Effects and the Nursing Process

I.   SENSORY/PERCEPTUAL ALTERATIONS related to CNS CHANGES

Defining Characteristics: The most common side effects are somnolence, ataxia, dizziness, and fatigue. Less commonly, nystagmus, tremor, nervousness, dysarthria, amnesia, depression, abnormal thought processes, incoordination, headache, confusion, emotional lability, paresthesia, areflexia, anxiety, hostility, syncope, hypesthesia may occur. Seizures have been reported, as have suicidal tendencies. Other sensory side effects that rarely occur are diplopia, abnormal vision, dry eyes, photophobia, ptosis, and hearing loss.

Nursing Implications: Assess baseline neurologic status and document. Instruct patient of general side effects that may occur, and to report them. Assess for suicidal ideation. If significant CNS changes occur, discuss dose reduction or change to an alternative drug with physician. Instruct patient not to drive a car or to do activities that require mental acuity until full effect of drug is known.

II.   ALTERATION IN NUTRITION related to GI TOXICITY

Defining Characteristics: Nausea and vomiting may occur. Less commonly, dyspepsia, dry mouth, constipation, increased or decreased appetite, thirst, stomatitis, taste changes, increased salivation, fecal incontinence may occur.

Nursing Implications: Assess patient tolerance of GI side effects. Instruct patient to report side effects. If nausea and vomiting occur, discuss changing to another medication or adding antiemetic agent to regimen if relief of peripheral neuropathy is achieved.

MANAGEMENT

III.   ALTERATION IN SKIN INTEGRITY related to RASH

Defining Characteristics: Rash may occur, as may pruritus, acne, alopecia, hirsutism, herpes simplex, dry skin, and increased sweating.

Nursing Implications: Perform baseline skin assessment, and note any areas that are not intact. Teach patient to self-assess for rash, other changes, and to report them. If rash develops, instruct patient to notify provider immediately. If itch occurs, discuss symptomatic management.

IV.   ALTERATION IN RESPIRATORY PATTERN related to RHINITIS, COUGH

Defining Characteristics: Rhinitis, pharyngitis, coughing, pneumonia, dyspnea may occur. Rarely, epistaxis and apnea have been reported.

Nursing Implications: Assess baseline respiratory pattern, and instruct patient to report any changes. Discuss any significant changes with physician, and discuss management versus change of drug.

V.   ALTERATION IN URINARY ELIMINATION related to URINARY CHANGES

Defining Characteristics: Hematuria, dysuria, frequency, urinary incontinence, cystitis, urinary retention may occur.

Nursing Implications: Assess baseline urinary elimination pattern, and instruct patient of possible side effects and to report them. Discuss symptomatic management, or discuss drug change with physician if changes are significant.

VI.   POTENTIAL FOR SEXUAL DYSFUNCTION related to VAGINAL CHANGES AND IMPOTENCE

Defining Characteristics: Vaginal hemorrhage, amenorrhea, dysmenorrhea, menorrhagia, inability to climax, abnormal ejaculation, and impotence have been reported.

Nursing Implications: Assess baseline sexuality, and instruct patient to report any changes. If changes occur, discuss impact and distress caused, and together with physician and patient, discuss drug alternatives.

VII.   POTENTIAL ALTERATION IN OXYGENATION related to TACHYCARDIA, HYPOTENSION

Defining Characteristics: Rarely, hypertension, vasodilatation, hypotension, angina pectoris, peripheral vascular disease, palpitation, tachycardia, and appearance of a murmur may occur.

Nursing Implications: Assess baseline cardiovascular status, and instruct patient to notify provider if any changes occur. Instruct patient to report palpitations, fast heartbeat, dizziness, or chest pain immediately. If significant changes occur, discuss alternative drug therapy with physician.

Drug: ibuprofen (Advil, Genpril, Haltran, Ibuprin, Midol 200, Nuprin, Rufen; parenteral Caldolor injection)

Class: NSAID.

Mechanism of Action: Peripherally acting analgesic, anti-inflammatory, and antipyretic agent; anti-inflammatory action probably due to prostaglandin synthetase inhibition, but is not well understood.

Metabolism: 80% of oral dose absorbed from GI tract, and absorption rate is slowed by administration with food. Peak serum concentrations with tablet occur in 2 hours; suspension in 1 hour. Highly protein-bound (90–99%) and has a plasma half-life of 2–4 hours. Excreted in urine. The parenteral form has an elimination half-life of 2.22–2.44 hours.

Indications: (1) PO: relief of mild-to-moderate pain, pain from RA and osteoarthritis, treatment of primary dysmenorrhea; (2) IV formulation indicated for the short-term management of mild-to-moderate pain, for management of moderate-to-severe pain as an adjunct to opioid analgesia, and for the reduction of fever. Use lowest dosage for shortest duration to achieve desired effect. Drug may cause serious and potentially fatal cardiovascular thrombotic events, as well as serious and potentially fatal GI reactions.

Dosage/Range:
- Oral: 200–800 mg every 4–8 hours PRN to maximum of 3,200 mg/24 hours.
- IV: Pain: 400–800 mg IV over 30 minutes every 6 hours as needed; fever: 400-mg IV over 30 minutes, followed by 400 mg every 4–6 hours or 100–200 mg every 4 hours as needed.

Drug Preparation:
- Tablets: 200, 300, 400, 600, 800 mg.
- Caplets: 200 mg.
- Oral suspension: 100 mg/5 mL.
- IV: Available as 400 mg/4 mL and 800 mg/8 mL (100 mg/mL). Aseptically add ordered dose to 200 mL (for 800-mg dose) or 100 mL (for 400-mg dose) 0.9% sodium chloride, 5% dextrose injection USP, or lactated Ringer's solution, so final concentration is 4 mg/mL or less. Stable for up to 24 hours at ambient temperature (20–25°C) and room lighting.

Drug Administration:
- Oral.
- IV: Administer over at least 30 minutes. Patients must be well-hydrated before drug is given.

MANAGEMENT

Drug Interactions:
- Oral anticoagulants, thrombolytic agents: Possible increase in PT with increased bleeding; use with caution and monitor patient closely.
- Other NSAIDs, aspirin: Possible increase in GI toxicity; do not administer concomitantly.
- Furosemide, thiazide diuretics: Decreased diuretic effect when administered concomitantly.
- ACE inhibitors: NSAIDs may diminish the antihypertensive effect of ACE inhibitors.

Lab Effects/Interference:
- Slight decrease in Hgb not exceeding 1 g/dL without signs of bleeding; decrease in Hgb > 1 g/dL may be associated with signs of bleeding.
- IV formulation: Elevated hepatic transaminases, which may progress to liver failure.

Special Considerations:
- Contraindicated in patients with known hypersensitivity, asthmatic patients with nasal polyps and other patients who develop bronchospasm or angioedema with aspirin or other NSAIDs, and patients with peptic or duodenal ulcer. IV formulation also contraindicated during the perioperative period in the setting of coronary artery bypass graft (CABG) surgery.
- Use cautiously in patients with cardiac or renal dysfunction.
- NSAIDs may increase the risk of serious cardiovascular thrombotic events, myocardial infarction, and stroke, which can be fatal; risk appears to increase with duration of use.
- Discontinue IV formulation if abnormal LFTs persist or worsen.
- Long-term administration of NSAIDs can lead to papillary necrosis and other renal injury. Use cautiously in patients at risk (e.g., elderly; patients with renal impairment, heart failure, hepatic dysfunction, taking diuretics or ACE inhibitors).
- Fluid retention, edema, CHF can occur with NSAIDs; use cautiously in patients with edema or heart failure.
- Hypertension can occur with NSAIDs; monitor BP during therapy.
- Anaphylactoid reactions can occur with patients receiving NSAIDs. Discontinue drug if this occurs.
- Rarely, drug can cause serious skin reactions, such as epidermal necrolysis, which can be fatal. Discontinue drug if rash or other allergic signs or symptoms occur.

Potential Toxicities/Side Effects and the Nursing Process

I.   ALTERATION IN NUTRITION, LESS THAN BODY REQUIREMENTS, related to GI SIDE EFFECTS

Defining Characteristics: Dyspepsia, heartburn, nausea, vomiting, anorexia, diarrhea, constipation, stomatitis, bloating, epigastric and abdominal pain may occur.

Nursing Implications: Assess history of GI symptoms and history of ulcer disease. Teach patient to take NSAID with meals or milk. Teach patient potential side effects, and instruct to report them. If symptoms are severe, discuss alternative NSAIDs with physician.

II.   POTENTIAL FOR BLEEDING related to INHIBITION OF PLATELET AGGREGATION

Defining Characteristics: Drug can prolong bleeding time and inhibit platelet aggregation. Peptic ulceration and occult GI bleeding can occur and be life-threatening. Increased risk factors: smoking, alcoholism.

Nursing Implications: Assess risk, history of peptic ulcer disease or GI bleeding. Assess baseline Hgb, HCT, and presence/absence of occult bleeding by guaiac of stools. Instruct patient to report signs/symptoms of abdominal pain, black stools, blood per rectum, epistaxis, menorrhagia. If patient is at risk for bleeding, discuss with physician use of misoprostol to protect GI mucosa. Teach patient to avoid concurrent use of aspirin, other NSAIDs.

III.   POTENTIAL SENSORY/PERCEPTUAL ALTERATIONS related to CNS CHANGES

Defining Characteristics: Dizziness, headache, nervousness, fatigue, drowsiness, malaise/light-headedness, anxiety, confusion, mental depression, and emotional lability may occur. Decreased hearing, visual acuity, changes in color vision, conjunctivitis, diplopia, and cataracts have been reported. In addition, though rare, aseptic meningitis has occurred.

Nursing Implications: Assess baseline neurologic and mental status. Instruct patient to report changes in sensory/perceptual pattern, especially VISUAL CHANGES. If visual changes occur, discuss with physician referral to ophthalmologist as soon as possible. Assess for rare occurrence of aseptic meningitis (fever, coma). Discuss drug continuance with physician for significant symptoms.

IV.   ALTERATION IN NUTRITION, LESS THAN BODY REQUIREMENTS, related to HEPATIC TOXICITY

Defining Characteristics: Severe and sometimes fatal hepatotoxicity has occurred. Jaundice and hepatitis occur rarely. Borderline increase in LFTs occurs in 15% of patients, while values increase by 3 times in 1%.

Nursing Implications: Assess baseline LFTs and monitor periodically during long-term therapy. Instruct patient to report jaundice, abdominal pain. Discuss discontinuance of drug with physician for significant toxicity.

V.   ALTERATION IN RENAL ELIMINATION related to INHIBITION OF RENAL PROSTAGLANDINS

Defining Characteristics: Acute renal failure may occur rarely within first few days of treatment in patients with preexisting renal dysfunction. Other signs/symptoms of renal dysfunction that may occur rarely are azotemia, cystitis, hematuria, increased serum BUN and creatinine, and decreased creatinine clearance. Peripheral edema has also been described.

Nursing Implications: Assess baseline renal function. Instruct patient to report any changes in urinary function. Monitor periodic serum BUN, creatinine during chronic therapy.

VI.   ALTERATION IN SKIN INTEGRITY related to RASH

Defining Characteristics: Rash (urticaria, vesicles, or erythematous macular) may occur, as may Stevens–Johnson syndrome, flushes, alopecia, rectal itching, and acne.

Nursing Implications: Assess baseline skin integrity and presence of lesions. Teach patient to report abnormalities. Provide symptomatic relief for rashes, pruritus.

VII.   POTENTIAL FOR FATIGUE, THROMBOCYTOPENIA, AND INFECTION related to BONE MARROW INJURY

Defining Characteristics: Neutropenia, agranulocytosis, aplastic anemia, hemolytic anemia, and thrombocytopenia may occur *rarely*.

Nursing Implications: Assess baseline CBC, WBC, differential, and platelet count. Discuss abnormalities with physician. Instruct patient to report severe fatigue, infection, bleeding. Monitor lab values periodically during treatment.

Drug: ibuprofen/famotidine (Duexis)

Class: Combination NSAID and histamine H_2-receptor antagonist.

Mechanism of Action: Ibuprofen appears to provide analgesic and antipyretic actions via prostaglandin synthetase inhibition, which can increase the risk of gastrointestinal (GI) ulceration, especially in the setting of gastric acid. Famotidine is a competitive inhibitor of histamine H_2-receptor antagonist, which inhibits gastric secretion, resulting in suppression of both acid concentration and volume of gastric secretion.

Metabolism: Both ibuprofen and famotidine are rapidly absorbed, resulting in maximal ibuprofen serum concentration (C_{max}) in 1.9 hours after oral administration. C_{max} for famotidine is reached about 2 hours after dosing. Ibuprofen is extensively bound to plasma proteins, while 15–20% of famotidine is protein bound. Ibuprofen is eliminated from systemic circulation 2 hours after administration; it is rapidly metabolized and excreted in the urine so that ibuprofen is totally excreted in 24 hours after the last dose. Famotidine has a half-life of 4 hours, and is excreted by renal (65–70%) and metabolic routes.

Indication: (1) Relief of signs and symptoms of RA and osteoarthritis, and (2) reduction in the risk of developing upper GI ulcers (e.g., gastric and/or duodenal ulcers) in patients taking ibuprofen for those indications.

Contraindications: (1) Known hypersensitivity to drug or its components; (2) history of asthma, urticaria, or allergic-type reactions after taking aspirin or other NSAIDs; (3) in the setting of CABG surgery; (4) known hypersensitivity to other H_2-receptor antagonists.

Dosage/Range: Drug tablet contains fixed-dose combination of ibuprofen 800 mg and famotidine 26.6 mg. One tablet orally, 3 times/day.

Drug Preparation: None. Tablet contains ibuprofen 800 mg and famotidine 26.6 mg.

Drug Administration:
- Oral: Teach patient to swallow drug whole, and not to cut to supply a lower dose. Do not chew, divide, or crush tablet. If a dose is missed, it should be taken as soon as possible. If the next scheduled dose is due, do not take the missed dose but take the next dose on time. Do not take 2 doses at one time to make up for a missed dose.
- Drug is not recommended in patients with renal creatinine clearance < 50 mL/min as the elimination half-life of famotidine is increased and may exceed 20 hours.

Drug Interactions:
- Warfarin-type anticoagulants: Increased risk of serious GI bleeding.
- Aspirin: Increased risk of GI bleeding, other adverse events.
- Corticosteroids, antiplatelet drugs: Increased risk of GI bleeding.
- ACE-inhibitors and diuretics: Ibuprofen may reduce the effectiveness of these drugs.
- Lithium: Increased lithium levels (by ibuprofen interaction).
- Methotrexate: NSAIDs may decrease tubular secretion of methotrexate in the kidney; also displaces methotrexate from plasma proteins, increasing risk of methotrexate toxicity; use together cautiously. Selective serotonin reuptake inhibitors (SSRIs): Increased risk of GI bleeding.
- Cholestyramine: Delayed absorption of ibuprofen.

Lab Effects/Interference: Increased LFTs, anemia, abnormal serum creatinine.

Special Considerations:
- Most common adverse effects (> 1% than ibuprofen alone): nausea, diarrhea, constipation, upper abdominal pain, headache.
- Warnings and Precautions:
  - Cardiovascular thrombotic events: Increased risk of cardiovascular thrombotic events, MI and stroke has been demonstrated in selective COX-2 inhibitors and nonselective NSAIDs. Drug should not be used in patients with a recent MI unless benefits exceed risk or recurrent thrombotic events.
  - GI bleeding, ulceration and perforation: Reduce risk by using lowest effective dosage, do not take more than one type of NSAIDs at a time, avoid use of drug in patients at high risk, assess for signs/symptoms so that prompt evaluation occurs, and if the patient takes low dose aspirin for cardiac prophylaxis, monitor the patient closely for bleeding.
  - Active bleeding: if the patient's baseline Hgb is ≤ 10 g/dL, and the patient is receiving long-term therapy, monitor the Hgb regularly.
  - Hepatotoxicity: Assess LFTs and if abnormal results persist or worsen, or if clinical signs and symptoms of hepatotoxicity develop, drug should be discontinued. Teach

MANAGEMENT

patient to report signs/symptoms of nausea, fatigue, lethargy, diarrhea, pruritus, jaundice, RUQ tenderness, "flu-like" symptoms.

- HTN: new onset or worsening of existing HTN can occur. Patient response to antihypertensives such as ACE inhibitors, thiazide diuretics, or loop diuretics may have an impaired response when taking NSAIDs. Monitor BP.
- Heart failure and edema may occur. Avoid use of the drug in patients with severe heart failure unless benefit outweighs the risk.
- Renal toxicity and hyperkalemia: Long-term use of NSAIDs may result in renal injury (e.g., renal papillary necrosis). Avoid use of drug in patients with advanced renal impairment. Monitor renal function in patients with renal or hepatic impairment, heart failure, dehydration, or hypovolemia.
- Anaphylaxis has occurred. Teach patient to seek emergency care if signs/symptoms occur.
- Seizures may occur related to famotidine in patients with moderate or severe renal impairment (CrCl < 50 mL/min). Drug is not recommended for patients with a CrCl < 50 mL/min.
- Exacerbation of asthma related to aspirin sensitivity. If patient has preexisting asthma, monitor for signs/symptoms of worsening asthma.
- Serious skin reaction: exfoliative dermatitis, Stevens–Johnson syndrome, and toxic epidermal necrolysis has occurred. Teach patient to stop drug and report skin changes suggesting of these severe reactions right away.
- Premature closure of the ductus arteriosus in the fetus may occur in pregnant women of 30 weeks gestation or later. Drug should not be used in pregnant women starting at 30 weeks.
- Hematologic toxicity: Monitor for signs/symptoms of bleeding.
- Masking of inflammation and fever occurs.
- Laboratory monitoring: when used long-term, monitor CBC, chemistries regularly.
- Concomitant NSAID use: other NSAIDs should not be used by patients taking this drug.
- Aseptic meningitis: may occur rarely with ibuprofen use. If signs and symptoms develop, consider ibuprofen as etiology.
- Ophthalmological effects: Rarely, blurred vision, scotomata, or changes in color vision have occurred. If patient has changes in vision, drug should be immediately discontinued and patient evaluated by an ophthalmologist, which includes central visual fields and color vision testing.
- The elderly are at greatest risk for toxicity. Monitor patients closely.
- Nursing mothers: Use drug with caution, as it is unknown if drug is excreted in human milk.

Potential Toxicities/Side Effects and the Nursing Process

I.   ALTERATION IN NUTRITION, LESS THAN BODY REQUIREMENTS, related to GI SIDE EFFECTS

Defining Characteristics: Dyspepsia, heartburn, nausea, vomiting, anorexia, diarrhea, constipation, stomatitis, bloating, epigastric, and abdominal pain may occur.

Nursing Implications: Assess history of GI symptoms and history of ulcer disease. Teach patient to take NSAID with meals or milk. Teach patient potential side effects, and instruct to report them. If symptoms are severe, discuss alternative NSAIDs with physician.

II. POTENTIAL FOR BLEEDING related to INHIBITION OF PLATELET AGGREGATION

Defining Characteristics: Drug can prolong bleeding time and inhibit platelet aggregation. Peptic ulceration and occult GI bleeding can occur and be life-threatening. Increased risk factors: smoking, alcoholism.

Nursing Implications: Assess risk, history of peptic ulcer disease or GI bleeding. Assess baseline Hgb, HCT, and presence/absence of occult bleeding by guaiac of stools. Instruct patient to report signs/symptoms of abdominal pain, black stools, blood per rectum, epistaxis, menorrhagia. If patient is at risk for bleeding, discuss with physician use of misoprostol to protect GI mucosa. Teach patient to avoid concurrent use of aspirin, other NSAIDs.

III. POTENTIAL SENSORY/PERCEPTUAL ALTERATIONS related to CNS CHANGES

Defining Characteristics: Dizziness, headache, nervousness, fatigue, drowsiness, malaise/light-headedness, anxiety, confusion, mental depression, and emotional lability may occur. Decreased hearing, visual acuity, changes in color vision, conjunctivitis, diplopia, and cataracts have been reported. In addition, though rare, aseptic meningitis has occurred.

Nursing Implications: Assess baseline neurologic and mental status. Instruct patient to report changes in sensory/perceptual pattern, especially VISUAL CHANGES. If visual changes occur, discuss with physician referral to ophthalmologist as soon as possible. Assess for rare occurrence of aseptic meningitis (fever, coma). Discuss drug continuance with physician for significant symptoms.

IV. ALTERATION IN NUTRITION, LESS THAN BODY REQUIREMENTS, related to HEPATIC TOXICITY

Defining Characteristics: Severe and sometimes fatal hepatotoxicity has occurred. Jaundice and hepatitis occur rarely. Borderline increase in LFTs occurs in 15% of patients receiving NSAIDs, while values increase by three times in 1%.

Nursing Implications: Assess baseline LFTs and monitor periodically during long-term therapy. Instruct patient to report jaundice, abdominal pain. Discuss discontinuance of drug with physician for significant toxicity.

MANAGEMENT

V.   ALTERATION IN RENAL ELIMINATION related to INHIBITION OF RENAL PROSTAGLANDINS

Defining Characteristics: Acute renal failure may occur rarely within first few days of treatment with NSAIDs in patients with preexisting renal dysfunction. Other signs/symptoms of renal dysfunction that may occur rarely are azotemia, cystitis, hematuria, increased serum BUN and creatinine, and decreased creatinine clearance. Peripheral edema has also been described. Drug should not be used in patients with creatinine clearance < 50 mL/min.

Nursing Implications: Assess baseline renal function. Instruct patient to report any changes in urinary function. Monitor periodic serum BUN, creatinine during chronic therapy.

VI.   ALTERATION IN SKIN INTEGRITY related to RASH

Defining Characteristics: Rash (urticaria, vesicles, or erythematous macular) may occur, as may Stevens–Johnson syndrome, flushes, alopecia, rectal itching, and acne.

Nursing Implications: Assess baseline skin integrity and presence of lesions. Teach patient to report abnormalities. Provide symptomatic relief for rashes, pruritus. Discuss drug discontinuance with physician/midlevel if rash develops.

VII.   POTENTIAL FOR FATIGUE, THROMBOCYTOPENIA, AND INFECTION, related to BONE MARROW INJURY

Defining Characteristics: Neutropenia, agranulocytosis, aplastic anemia, hemolytic anemia, and thrombocytopenia may occur rarely in patients taking NSAIDs.

Nursing Implications: Assess baseline CBC, WBC, differential, and platelet count. Discuss abnormalities with physician. Instruct patient to report severe fatigue, infection, bleeding. Monitor lab reports periodically during treatment.

Drug: indomethacin (Indocin, Indocin SR, Indotech)

Class: NSAID, structurally related to sulindac.

Mechanism of Action: Actions similar to other NSAIDs: anti-inflammatory action, probably by inhibition of prostaglandin synthesis, as well as by inhibiting migration of leukocytes to infection site and stabilization of neutrophils so lysosomal enzymes cannot be released; may also interfere with the production of autoantibodies (mediated by prostaglandins). Analgesic and antipyretic effects appear to result from inhibition of prostaglandin synthesis. Probably reduces tumor-associated fever by inhibition of synthesis of prostaglandin (PGE_1) in hypothalamus. However, drug has serious side effects, so should not be used routinely as an antipyretic.

Metabolism: Rapidly and completely absorbed from GI tract. When administered with food or antacid (aluminum and magnesium hydroxide), peak plasma drug concentrations may be slightly decreased or delayed. Drug is 99% bound to plasma proteins. Crosses BBB slightly, and placenta freely. Metabolized by liver, undergoes enterohepatic circulation, and is excreted in urine.

Indication: Effective for the treatment in active stages of (1) moderate to severe RA including acute flares; (2) moderate-to-severe anklylosing spondylitis; (3) moderate-to-severe osteoarthritis; (4) acute painful shoulder (bursitis and/or tendinitis); and (5) acute gouty arthritis.

Dosage/Range:
- Capsules: 10, 25, 50, 75 mg, given in 2–4 divided doses.
- Sustained release: 75 mg, given once or bid.
- Oral suspension: 25 mg/5 mL, given in 2–4 divided doses.
- Suppositories: 50 mg, given in 2–4 divided doses.

Drug Preparation:
- Drug is sensitive to light. Store capsules in well-closed containers at temperatures < 40°C (104°F).
- Oral suspension should be stored in tight, light-resistant containers at 30°C (86°F).
- Suppositories should be stored at temperatures < 30°C (86°F).

Drug Administration:
- Give with food or antacid to protect GI mucosa.
- Rectal suppository must remain in rectum for at least 1 hour for maximum absorption.
- Consider reduced dose in patients with renal dysfunction.
- Indocin suspension contains 1% alcohol.

Drug Interactions:
- Indomethacin can displace or be displaced by other protein-bound drugs: oral anticoagulants, hydantoins (e.g., phenytoin), salicylates, sulfonamides, sulfonylureas. Therefore, if taking any of these medications with indomethacin, the patient must be assessed for increased toxicity of each drug.
- Antihypertensive effect of hydralazine, captopril, furosemide, beta-adrenergic blockers, or thiazide diuretics may be decreased.
- NSAIDs: concurrent administration with salicylates does not improve drug effects but increases toxicity (GI, aplastic anemia) so should NOT be given concurrently. Diflunisal may decrease renal excretion of indomethacin and increase risk of GI hemorrhage; AVOID concurrent use.
- Triamterene: may precipitate renal failure. DO NOT USE CONCURRENTLY.
- Digoxin: serum levels may be increased and prolonged, so digoxin levels should be monitored closely.
- Methotrexate, especially HIGH DOSE: increased, prolonged serum methotrexate levels can be fatal; AVOID concurrent use.
- Potassium (K+) supplements, K+ sparing diuretics: indomethacin may increase serum K+ concentrations, especially in the elderly or patients with renal dysfunction. Use with caution and monitor K+ serum levels.

MANAGEMENT

- Lithium: may increase plasma lithium levels; assess patient for lithium toxicity.
- Cyclosporine: possible increased nephrotoxicity; use with caution and monitor renal function.
- Probenecid: increased plasma level and therapeutic effects of indomethacin; decrease indomethacin dose.

Lab Effects/Interference:
- May prolong bleeding time.
- Rarely, hemolytic anemia, leukopenia, thrombocytopenia.

Special Considerations:
- Avoid use or use cautiously in the elderly or in patients with epilepsy, Parkinson's disease, renal dysfunction, mental illness.

Potential Toxicities/Side Effects and the Nursing Process

I.   POTENTIAL SENSORY/PERCEPTUAL ALTERATIONS

Defining Characteristics: Dose-related headache occurs in 25–50% of patients (more severe in morning); may be associated with frontal throbbing, vomiting, tinnitus, ataxia, tremor, vertigo, and insomnia. Dizziness, depression, fatigue, and peripheral neuropathy may occur in 3–9% of patients; 1% of patients may have confusion, psychic disturbances, hallucinations, and nightmares. May accentuate epilepsy and Parkinson's disease symptomatology. Blurred vision, corneal and retinal damage, and hearing loss may occur with long-term use.

Nursing Implications: Assess baseline mental and neurologic status. Teach patient to report headache, changes in sensation or perception, and sleep problems. Discuss drug discontinuance with physician if neurologic side effects occur. Patients with visual disturbances or pain, or changes from baseline, should be seen by an ophthalmologist.

II.   ALTERATION IN NUTRITION, LESS THAN BODY REQUIREMENTS, related to GI TOXICITY

Defining Characteristics: Nausea, with or without vomiting and indigestion, heartburn, and epigastric pain occur in ~10% of patients. Diarrhea, abdominal pain/distress, and constipation may occur in ~3%. Other effects occurring in ~1% are anorexia, distension, flatulence, gastroenteritis, rectal bleeding, stomatitis. Severe GI bleeding may occur in 1% of patients, as drug decreases platelet aggregation.

Nursing Implications: Teach patient potential side effects and to self-administer drug with food or antacid. Teach patient to avoid OTC aspirin-containing drugs, alcohol, or steroids, all of which can increase GI toxicity and risk for GI bleeding. Instruct patient to report any signs/symptoms of GI bleeding, abdominal pain immediately, and to stop taking the drug. Guaiac stool for occult blood periodically. If drug must be used, and risk of GI ulceration is high, discuss with physician use of misoprostol to protect the GI mucosa.

III.   POTENTIAL FOR INFECTION, FATIGUE, BLEEDING, related to BONE MARROW INJURY

Defining Characteristics: Although rare (1%), potential toxicities include hemolytic anemia, bone marrow depression (leukopenia, thrombocytopenia), aplastic anemia, thrombocytopenic purpura. Drug inhibits platelet aggregation, but this will reverse to normal within 24 hours of drug discontinuance. May prolong bleeding time, especially in patients with underlying bleeding problems.

Nursing Implications: Assess all medicines the patient is taking and teach patient to avoid OTC aspirin-containing drugs. Teach patient to self-assess and instruct to report signs/symptoms of bleeding, fatigue, and infection.

IV.   POTENTIAL FOR ALTERATION IN ELIMINATION PATTERN related to RENAL DYSFUNCTION

Defining Characteristics: Acute interstitial nephritis with hematuria, proteinuria, nephrotic syndrome may occur in 1% of patients. Patients with renal dysfunction may have worsening of renal function. Increased K+ levels may occur in the elderly or in patients with renal dysfunction. Risk increases with long-term therapy.

Nursing Implications: Assess baseline renal status. Discuss alternate drugs if renal dysfunction. Monitor serum K+, sodium (Na+), especially if receiving other drugs that affect serum K+ level (e.g., amphotericin, diuretics), or in the elderly.

V.   POTENTIAL FOR ALTERATION IN CARDIAC OUTPUT related to CARDIAC EFFECTS

Defining Characteristics: CHF, tachycardia, chest pain, arrhythmias, palpitations, hypertension, and edema may occur in < 1% of patients.

Nursing Implications: Assess baseline cardiovascular status and monitor periodically while receiving the drug. Assess efficacy of antihypertensive medication due to possible drug interaction.

VI.   POTENTIAL FOR INJURY related to DERMATOLOGIC AND SENSITIVITY REACTIONS

Defining Characteristics: Dermatologic effects occur in < 1% of patients and include pruritus, urticaria, rash, exfoliative dermatitis, and Stevens–Johnson syndrome. Allergic reactions occur in < 1%, characterized by asthma in aspirin-sensitive individuals, dyspnea, fever, acute anaphylaxis.

Nursing Implications: Assess baseline dermatologic, pulmonary status, and continue during drug use. Instruct patient to report any adverse reactions immediately.

MANAGEMENT

Drug: ketorolac tromethamine (Toradol)

Class: NSAID.

Mechanism of Action: Inhibits prostaglandin synthesis peripherally to exert analgesic, anti-inflammatory, and antipyretic activity.

Metabolism: Drug completely absorbed following PO or IM administration of the drug, with peak serum levels in 44 and 50 minutes, respectively. Drug is extensively bound to serum protein (99%). Terminal half-life is 2.4–9.2 hours. Excreted by the kidney.

Indication: For the short-term (< 5 days) treatment of acute pain that requires analgesia at the opioid level, usually in the postoperative setting. Therapy should be initiated with IV formulation, followed by tablets to continue treatment, if necessary. Combined use of oral and IV is not to exceed 5 days.

Contraindications: In patients with (1) recent GI bleed or perforation, history of peptic ulcer disease, or GI bleeding; (2) advanced renal impairment or at risk for renal failure due to volume depletion; (3) nursing mothers; (4) hypersensitivity to the drug, or allergy to aspirin or other NSAIDs; (5) as prophylactic analgesia before surgery or intraoperatively; (6) currently taking aspirin or NSAIDs; (7) for neuraxial (epidural or intrathecal) administration; (8) concomitant use of drug with probenecid; (9) in labor and delivery; (10) suspected or confirmed cerebrovascular bleeding, hemorrhagic diathesis, incomplete hemostasis, or at high risk of bleeding.

Dosage/Range:
- Single dose: IM, 60 mg; IV, 30 mg.
- Multiple doses: IM/IV, 30 mg q 6 h (maximum daily dose is 120 mg).
- 50% dose reduction for patients aged ≥ 65 years, renal impaired, or weight < 50 kg (maximum daily dose should not exceed 60 mg).
- Oral: for continuation therapy, never as initial therapy.
- Patients < 65 years old: 20 mg, × 1, then 10 mg q 4–6 h (max 40 mg/24 hours).
- Patients ≥ 65: 10 mg q 4–6 h (max 40 mg/24 hours).
- MAXIMUM USE OF KETOROLAC (oral and parenteral) IS 5 DAYS.

Drug Preparation:
- Store at controlled room temperature of 15–30°C (59–86°F) and protect from light.

Drug Administration:
- PO, IM, or IV.

Drug Interactions:
- Other salicylates: displace ketorolac from protein binding. DO NOT USE together or dose-reduce ketorolac.
- Anticoagulants: possible increase in bleeding time; use with caution and monitor closely.
- Furosemide: decreased diuretic response; need to increase diuretic dose.

- Probenecid: causes prolonged, increased serum ketorolac levels; use cautiously, and reduce dose.
- Lithium, methotrexate: theoretically increased serum levels, so should be dose-reduced if given with ketorolac.
- ACE inhibitors, angiotensin II receptor antagonists: increased risk of renal impairment especially in volume-depleted patients.
- SSRIs: increased risk of GI bleeding.

Lab Effects/Interference:
- None known.

Special Considerations:
- Warnings and Precautions:
  - GI risk (peptic ulcers, GI bleeding or perforation) especially in the elderly. Drug is contraindicated in patients with active peptic ulcer disease or GI bleeding.
  - Cardiovascular thrombotic events may occur in patients receiving NSAIDs. Risk may increase with increased duration of use. Drug is contraindicated in the setting of CABG surgery.
  - Renal risk. Drug is contraindicated in patients with advanced renal impairment or at risk for renal failure due to volume depletion.
  - Risk of bleeding.
  - Hypersensitivity, including anaphylactic shock may rarely occur.
  - Drug should NOT be administered intrathecally or epidurally.
  - Drug should NOT be administered during labor and delivery as may adversely affect fetal circulation and inhibit mother's uterine contractions.
  - Concurrent use with other NSAIDs including aspirin is contraindicated due to risk of additive toxicity.
  - Dose should be reduced in patients aged 65 or older, weighing < 50 kg, patients with moderately elevated serum creatinine; maximum daily dose is 60 mg for these patients.
  - Oral tablets: approved as continuation therapy (combined oral and parenteral not to exceed 5 days); maximum total daily dose is 40 mg.
  - Heart failure and edema may occur in patients receiving NSAIDs.
  - HTN: new or worsening HTN may occur, and patient response to thiazide or loop diuretics may have an impaired response. Monitor BP closely during therapy.
  - Serious skin reaction: exfoliative dermatitis, Stevens–Johnson syndrome, and toxic epidermal necrolysis has occurred. Teach patient to stop drug and report skin changes suggesting of these severe reactions right away.
  - Pregnancy: teach women of reproductive potential to use effective contraception to avoid pregnancy during therapy. Drug may cause premature closure of the ductus arteriosus in the fetus.
  - Hepatotoxicity: use drug cautiously in patients with hepatic impairment. Assess LFTs.
  - Hematologic effect: anemia may rarely occur.
  - Preexisting asthma: use drug cautiously in patients with preexisting asthma, and do not give drug to patients who have aspirin-sensitive asthma.

MANAGEMENT

Potential Toxicities/Side Effects and the Nursing Process

I.   ALTERATION IN NUTRITION, LESS THAN BODY REQUIREMENTS, related to GI SIDE EFFECTS

Defining Characteristics: Dyspepsia, heartburn, nausea, vomiting, anorexia, diarrhea, constipation, stomatitis, bloating, epigastric, and abdominal pain may occur.

Nursing Implications: Assess history of GI symptoms and history of ulcer disease. Teach patient to take NSAID with meals or milk. Teach patient potential side effects and instruct to report them. If symptoms are severe, discuss alternative NSAIDs with physician.

II.   POTENTIAL FOR BLEEDING related to INHIBITION OF PLATELET AGGREGATION

Defining Characteristics: Drug can prolong bleeding time and inhibit platelet aggregation. Peptic ulceration and occult GI bleeding can occur and be life-threatening. Increased risk factors: smoking, alcoholism.

Nursing Implications: Assess risk, history of peptic ulcer disease or GI bleeding. Assess baseline Hgb, HCT and presence/absence of occult bleeding by guaiac of stools. Instruct patient to report signs/symptoms of abdominal pain, black stools, blood per rectum, epistaxis, menorrhagia. If patient at risk for bleeding, discuss with physician use of misoprostol to protect GI mucosa. Teach patient to avoid concurrent use of aspirin, other NSAIDs.

III. POTENTIAL SENSORY/PERCEPTUAL ALTERATIONS related to CNS CHANGES

Defining Characteristics: Dizziness, headache, nervousness, fatigue, drowsiness, malaise/light-headedness, anxiety, confusion, mental depression, and emotional lability may occur. Decreased hearing, visual acuity, changes in color vision, conjunctivitis, diplopia, and cataracts have been reported. In addition, though rare, aseptic meningitis has occurred.

Nursing Implications: Assess baseline neurologic and mental status. Instruct patient to report changes in sensory/perceptual pattern, especially VISUAL CHANGES. If visual changes occur, discuss with physician referral to ophthalmologist as soon as possible. Assess for rare occurrence of aseptic meningitis (fever, coma). Discuss drug continuance with physician for significant symptoms.

IV.   ALTERATION IN NUTRITION, LESS THAN BODY REQUIREMENTS, related to HEPATIC TOXICITY

Defining Characteristics: Severe and sometimes fatal hepatotoxicity has occurred. Jaundice and hepatitis occur rarely. Borderline increase in LFTs occurs in 15% of patients, while values increase by 3 times in 1%.

Nursing Implications: Assess baseline LFTs and monitor periodically during long-term therapy. Instruct patient to report jaundice, abdominal pain. Discuss discontinuance of drug with physician for significant toxicity.

V. ALTERATION IN RENAL ELIMINATION related to INHIBITION OF RENAL PROSTAGLANDINS

Defining Characteristics: Acute renal failure may occur rarely within first few days of treatment in patients with preexisting renal dysfunction. Other signs/symptoms of renal dysfunction that may occur rarely are azotemia, cystitis, hematuria, increased serum BUN and creatinine, and decreased creatinine clearance. Peripheral edema has also been described.

Nursing Implications: Assess baseline renal function. Teach patient to report any changes in urinary function. Monitor periodic serum BUN, creatinine during chronic therapy.

VI. ALTERATION IN SKIN INTEGRITY related to RASH

Defining Characteristics: Rash (urticaria, vesicles, or erythematous macular) may occur, as may Stevens–Johnson syndrome, flushes, alopecia, rectal itching, and acne.

Nursing Implications: Assess baseline skin integrity and presence of lesions. Instruct patient to report abnormalities. Provide symptomatic relief for rashes, pruritus.

VII. POTENTIAL FOR FATIGUE AND INFECTION related to BONE MARROW INJURY

Defining Characteristics: Neutropenia, agranulocytosis, aplastic anemia, hemolytic anemia, and thrombocytopenia may occur rarely.

Nursing Implications: Assess baseline CBC, WBC, differential, and platelet count. Discuss abnormalities with physician. Instruct patient to report severe fatigue, infection, bleeding. Monitor lab values periodically during treatment.

MANAGEMENT

Drug: pregabalin (Lyrica)

Class: Anticonvulsant, analgesic for peripheral neuropathy.

Mechanism of Action: Unknown, but believed to reduce the calcium-dependent release of several neurotransmitters, possibly by modulating the calcium channel function. In neuropathic pain, voltage-gated calcium channels let extra calcium into the neuron ending, which then binds to vesicles containing pain-causing chemicals (neurotransmitters). The vesicles then migrate to the neuronal membrane, and secrete them into the nerve endings.

Pregabalin binds with the alpha-2-delta site (axillary subunit of the voltage-gated calcium channel) in CNS tissues (but not cardiac-related, voltage-gated calcium channels).

Metabolism: Well absorbed from GI tract with peak plasma levels in 1.5 hours; bioavailability is > 90% independent of dose. Drug does not bind to plasma proteins. Steady state is reached in 24–48 hours. Drug is not metabolized in the body, and 90% of intact drug is eliminated in the urine. Because of this, drug elimination rate is proportional to the creatinine clearance, so drug dose must be reduced in patients with renal compromise. Drug crosses blood–brain barrier in laboratory animals, so is presumed to do so in humans. The drug has an elimination half-life of 6 hours.

Indications: For (1) neuropathic pain associated with diabetic peripheral neuropathy; (2) postherpetic neuralgia; (3) adjunctive therapy for adult patients with partial onset seizures; (4) fibromyalgia; and (5) neuropathic pain associated with spinal cord injury.

Contraindications: Known hypersensitivity to drug or any of its components.

Dosage/Range (modify dose for renal impairment (CrCl < 60 mL/min):
- Diabetic peripheral neuropathy: Begin dosing at 50 mg PO tid, and increase to 100 mg PO tid over 1 week, to goal of 300 mg/day within 1 week, with or without food, in patients with creatinine clearance of > 60 mL/minute.
- Postherpetic neuralgia: Begin dosing at 75 mg PO bid or 50 mg PO tid with goal 300 mg/day within 1 week; maximum dose of 600 mg/day.
- Adjunctive therapy for adult patients with partial onset seizures: 2–3 divided doses per day, to a maximum of 600 mg/day.
- Fibromyalgia: 2 divided doses per day, goal 300 mg/day within 1 week; maximum of 450 mg/day.
- Neuropathic pain associated with spinal cord injury: 2 divided doses a day, goal 300 mg/day within 1 week. Maximum dose of 600 mg/day.
- Patients with renal impairment: Dose should be reduced 50% if creatinine clearance is 30–60 mL/minute, another 50% if creatinine clearance is 15–30 mL/minute, and a further 50% if < 15 mL/minute (see package insert).
- If patient is being hemodialyzed, see package insert for supplementary doses.

Drug Preparation:
- Available 25-, 50-, 75-, 100-, 150-, 200-, 225-, 300-mg capsules; 20 mg/mL oral solution (16 fl oz).
- Oral; take with food or on an empty stomach.
- Teach patients to keep medication in a safe place, out of reach of children and pets.

Drug Interactions:
- None.

Lab Effects/Interference:
- Creatine kinase in 2% of patients.
- Platelets (20% below baseline in 3% of patients).
- EKG changes: PR interval prolongation by 3–6 msec.

Special Considerations:
- Most common adverse effects ($\geq$ 5% and 2X placebo): dizziness, somnolence, dry mouth, edema, blurred vision, weight gain, abnormal thinking (decreased ability to concentrate and pay attention).
- Warnings and Precautions:
  - Angioedema (swelling of throat, head, and neck) can occur rarely and be life-threatening. Provide immediate medical assistance and discontinue drug immediately.
  - Hypersensitivity reactions (hives, dyspnea, wheezing) can occur; discontinue drug immediately, and provide ordered medical intervention.
  - Increased seizure activity: As with any antiepileptic drugs, the drug should be withdrawn gradually to minimize the potential of increased seizure frequency in patients with seizure disorders. If discontinued, the drug should be gradually reduced in dose over at least 1 week.
  - Increased risk of suicidal thoughts or behavior.
  - Impaired ability to drive or operate machinery due to dizziness, somnolence.
  - Drug may cause fetal harm. Teach women of reproductive potential to use effective contraception to avoid pregnancy. Breastfeeding is not recommended.
- Abrupt discontinuation of drug may result in insomnia, headache, nausea, and diarrhea (discontinue over a minimum of 1 week).
- Although uncommon, 2% of patients had creatine kinase > 3 times the ULN; patients should be taught to report immediately unexplained muscle pain or tenderness, especially if these muscle symptoms are associated with malaise or fever so that they can be further evaluated, and rhabdomyolysis or myopathy ruled out. Discontinue drug if myopathy is suspected or confirmed, or if patient develops markedly elevated creatine kinase.

Potential Toxicities/Side Effects and the Nursing Process

I.   SENSORY/PERCEPTUAL ALTERATIONS related to CNS CHANGES

Defining Characteristics: The most common side effects are somnolence (22%), dizziness (29%), blurred vision (6%), abnormal thinking (concentration and attention). Somnolence and dizziness start right after the drug is initiated, increase in frequency as the dose is increased, and may persist throughout treatment. Less commonly, ataxia, vertigo, confusion, diplopia, euphoria, incoordination, and amnesia may occur. Increased sleepiness and dizziness if taking concomitant opioids for pain, alcohol, or antianxiety/sedatives.

Nursing Implications: Assess baseline neurologic status and document. Instruct patient of general side effects that may occur, and to report them as well as any changes that may occur, such as reduced visual acuity. Assess for suicidal ideation. If significant CNS changes occur, discuss dose reduction or change to an alternative drug with physician. Instruct patient not to drive a car or to do activities that require mental acuity until full effect of drug is known. If blurred vision, dizziness, or weakness occurs, teach patient to report this immediately.

II.   ALTERATION IN NUTRITION related to GI TOXICITY

Defining Characteristics: Gastroenteritis and increased appetite with weight gain (7% over baseline over 13 weeks) may occur. Weight gain of diabetic patients averaged 1.6 kg. Less commonly, cholecystitis, cholelithiasis, colitis, dysphagia, esophagitis, gastritis, GI hemorrhage, melena, mouth ulceration, pancreatitis, rectal hemorrhage, and tongue edema may occur. Rarely, aphthous stomatitis may occur.

Nursing Implications: Assess patient tolerance of GI side effects. Instruct patient to report side effects. Discuss symptomatic management depending upon symptoms. If patient is also taking rosiglitazone (Avandia) or pioglitazone (Actos), counsel about increased risk of weight gain.

III.   ALTERATION IN SKIN INTEGRITY related to PRURITUS, EDEMA

Defining Characteristics: Pruritus is common; infrequently, patients may develop alopecia, dry skin, eczema, hirsutism, skin ulcer, urticaria, or vesiculobullous rash. Rarely, patients may develop exfoliative dermatitis. Edema, principally peripheral edema, occurs in 6% of patients, especially in diabetic patients taking thiazolidinedione antidiabetic agents (these drugs in and of themselves can cause fluid retention and weight gain).

Nursing Implications: Perform baseline skin assessment, and note any areas that are not intact, are swollen, or itch. Teach patient to self-assess for itching, swelling, other changes, and to report them. If rash develops, instruct patient to notify provider immediately. If itching occurs, discuss symptomatic management.

IV.   ALTERATION IN COMFORT related to ARTHRALGIA, LEG CRAMPS, MYALGIA, EDEMA, PERIPHERAL EDEMA, ECCHYMOSIS, ABDOMINAL PAIN

Defining Characteristics: Although not common, arthralgias, leg cramps, myalgias, ecchymosis, and abdominal pain can occur.

Nursing Implications: Perform baseline comfort assessment, and teach patient to report these side effects if they occur. Develop a plan for symptomatic relief.

OPIOID ANALGESICS

Drug: codeine (as sulfate or phosphate); may be combined with acetaminophen (Phenaphen with Codeine, Tylenol with Codeine, Codaphen [Odalan]), or with aspirin (Empirin with Codeine, Soma Compound with Codeine, Fiorinal with Codeine)

Class: Opioid analgesic (opioid agonist).

Mechanism of Action: Resembles morphine but has milder action; binds to opiate receptors in CNS (limbic system, thalamus, striatum, hypothalamus, midbrain, spinal cord), altering pain perception at level of spinal cord and higher centers, as well as the emotional response to pain. Also suppresses cough reflex.

Metabolism: Well absorbed after oral or parenteral administration. Metabolized by liver; excreted in urine, and small amount in feces.

Indication: Relief of mild-to-moderately severe pain, unrelieved by nonopioid analgesic, where the use of an opioid analgesic is appropriate.

Dosage/Range: Requires opioid Risk Evaluation and Mitigation Strategy (REMS). Mild pain: 30 mg q 4 h (range 15–60 mg), PO, subcutaneous, or IM.

Drug Preparation:
- Store tablets in tight, light-resistant containers at 15–30°C (59–86°F).
- Injection should be protected from light and stored at 15–40°C (59–104°F).
- At home, teach patient to store oral doses in a safe place away from children and pets.

Drug Administration:
- PO, subcutaneous, IM.

Drug Interactions:
- Injection is incompatible with solutions containing aminophylline, ammonium chloride, amobarbital sodium, chlorothiazide sodium, heparin sodium, methicillin sodium, nitrofurantoin, phenobarbital sodium, sodium bicarbonate.
- Alcohol, CNS depressants: additive effects.

Lab Effects/Interference:
- None known.

Special Considerations:
- Risk Evaluation and Mitigation Strategy (REMS) required for use of opioids. Healthcare providers must review REMS-compliant education. In addition, healthcare providers must
  a. Complete a REMS-compliant education program offered by an accredited CE provider or another education program that includes all the elements of the FDA Education Blueprint for Health Care Providers Involved in the Management or Support of Patients with Pain. The blueprint can be found at www.fda.gov/OpioidAnalgesic REMSBlueprint.
  b. Discuss the safe use, serious risks, and proper storage and disposal of opioid analgesics with patients and/or their caregivers every time these medicines are prescribed. The Patient Counseling Guide can be obtained at www.fda.gov/OpioidAnalgesicREMSPCG.
  c. Emphasize to patients and their caregivers the importance of reading the Medication Guide that they will receive from their pharmacist every time an opioid analgesic is dispensed to them.
  d. Consider using other tools to improve patient, household, and community safety, such as patient–prescriber agreements that reinforce patient–prescriber responsibilities.
- Parenteral dose is 2/3 oral dose for equianalgesic effect.

MANAGEMENT

- Onset of action after PO or subcutaneous dose is 15–30 minutes, with duration of analgesia 4–6 hours.
- Addition of acetaminophen or aspirin gives additive analgesia.
- Give smallest effective dose to prevent development of tolerance, physical dependency.
- Reduce dose in debilitated patients, or patients receiving other CNS depressants.
- Use with caution in patients with hepatic or renal dysfunction, hypothyroidism, Addison's disease, severe CNS depression, respiratory depression, head injury, elevated intracranial pressure (ICP).
- If required, naloxone HCl (Narcan) will reverse opiate toxicity (e.g., respiratory depression). However, it is important that acute withdrawal symptoms be prevented by giving only enough naloxone to reverse respiratory depression and that this be continued for opioid drug half-life.
- Teach patient that opioid analgesics may impair the mental and/or physical ability to drive and use machines, and to avoid these activities until the effect of the drug is known.

Potential Toxicities/Side Effects and the Nursing Process

I.   SENSORY/PERCEPTUAL ALTERATIONS related to CNS DEPRESSION

Defining Characteristics: Drowsiness, sedation, mood changes, euphoria, dysphoria, dizziness, mental clouding may occur. At high doses, may cause seizures. Miosis (papillary constriction) may occur.

Nursing Implications: Assess baseline neurologic status. Use cautiously, if at all, in patients with head injury, increased ICP, severe CNS depression, acute alcoholism, or who are elderly or debilitated. Assess other concurrent medications. Use with caution in patients receiving other opioids, tranquilizers, hypnotics, monoamine oxidase (MAO) inhibitors, since increasing CNS depressant effects can occur. Monitor neurologic status closely. Teach patient to avoid driving and operating machinery while taking the medicine, and to AVOID concurrent alcohol.

II.   ALTERATION IN OXYGENATION related to RESPIRATORY DEPRESSION

Defining Characteristics: Opiate agonists directly depress respiratory center in brain stem, causing decreased sensitivity and responsiveness to increased pCO_2 (CO_2 tension in serum). Also may depress deep breathing and reflex to sigh. Tolerance to respiratory depressant effects occurs with chronic use.

Nursing Implications: Assess baseline pulmonary status, and monitor periodically during drug use. Use cautiously in patients with bronchial asthma, chronic obstructive pulmonary disease (COPD), respiratory depression, and monitor closely.

III.   ALTERATION IN ELIMINATION related to CONSTIPATION, ILEUS

Defining Characteristics: Opium agonists bind to opiate receptors in bowel, slowing peristalsis, leading to constipation. Untreated constipation may result in bowel perforation.

MANAGEMENT

Nursing Implications: Assess baseline elimination, fluid intake, diet, and exercise patterns. Teach patient about prevention of constipation: goal is to move bowels at least every 2 days by increasing fluid intake to 3 L/day, following a diet high in fiber (beans, vegetables, fruit), and taking moderate exercise. Assess need for bowel softeners, bulk-forming laxatives, and osmotic cathartics, and discuss prescription with physician. Teach patient self-administration of medications.

IV. ALTERATION IN NUTRITION, LESS THAN BODY REQUIREMENTS, related to GI TOXICITY

Defining Characteristics: Nausea, vomiting, dry mouth may occur. Gastric, biliary, and pancreatic secretions are decreased by opiate agonists; digestion is delayed. Biliary tract muscle tone is increased, and spasm of Oddi's sphincter may occur (morphine > meperidine > codeine).

Nursing Implications: Assess patient tolerance of GI side effects. Teach patient to report side effects. If nausea/vomiting occur, change to another opioid, or premedicate with antiemetic to prevent nausea/vomiting. Assess GI pain, biliary spasm, and consider alternative opioid.

V. ALTERATION IN CARDIAC OUTPUT related to HYPOTENSION, BRADYCARDIA

Defining Characteristics: Orthostatic hypotension, bradycardia due to cholinergic effect, and peripheral vasodilation may occur with rapid IV dosing. There may be histamine-related flushing, pruritus, diaphoresis with chronic drug usage; tolerance develops to this effect.

Nursing Implications: Assess baseline cardiovascular status. Teach patient to change position slowly and to hold onto stable, nearby structure for support as needed. Be careful when giving IV push opioids, and caution patient to remain in supine position for 15–20 minutes after injection. Monitor cardiovascular status after injection.

VI. ALTERATION IN URINE ELIMINATION related to URINARY RETENTION

Defining Characteristics: Increased smooth muscle tone in urinary tract and spasm may occur. Bladder tone is increased and may cause urgency. Vesical sphincter tone may be increased, leading to difficulty urinating. Increased risk of urinary retention in patients with prostatic hypertrophy or urethral stricture.

Nursing Implications: Assess baseline urinary elimination pattern. Teach patient to increase fluids to 3 L/day, and encourage voiding every 2–3 hours. Instruct patient to report problems with urination.

VII. KNOWLEDGE DEFICIT related to DRUG ADMINISTRATION, POTENTIAL FOR TOLERANCE, AND DEPENDENCY

Defining Characteristics: Psychological dependence (addiction) occurs rarely in patients taking opioid agonists for cancer pain (< 1%). Physical dependence (precipitation of withdrawal symptoms) occurs with chronic use of the drug for the relief of chronic cancer pain. In addition, tolerance, or less analgesic effect over time with the same drug dose, occurs and requires increased dosage of drug.

Nursing Implications: Assess baseline knowledge of opioid analgesics, and attitude about their use for cancer pain management. Teach patient about proper self-administration, possible side effects, and self-care measures. Suggest patient maintain diary of pain intensity, precipitating and alleviating factors, drug dose and time taken, and relief. Teach patient to self-administer opioid agonists for relief of chronic cancer pain ATC, not PRN, to prevent pain. Explain use of prescribed short-acting opioid for rescue or to manage BTP. Discuss with physician dose increase or change in frequency of administration if tolerance develops. Teach patient that withdrawal symptoms may occur if chronic, ATC dosing is interrupted. Withdrawal (abstinence) symptoms that may be seen are restlessness, lacrimation, rhinorrhea, yawning, perspiration, gooseflesh, restless sleep, mydriasis in first 24 hours. These are followed by twitching and leg spasm; severe aching of the back, abdomen, and legs; cramping in abdomen and legs; hot/cold flashes; insomnia; nausea/vomiting, diarrhea; severe sneezing; and increased heart rate, BP, and temperature (T), which peak at 36–72 hours. Withdrawal syndrome can be prevented by administration of at least 1/4 of previous opioid dose.

VIII. SEXUAL DYSFUNCTION related to IMPOTENCE, DECREASED LIBIDO

Defining Characteristics: Opiate agonists may suppress gonadotropin, causing impotence and decreased libido.

Nursing Implications: Assess baseline sexual pattern. Discuss potential toxicity and impact on sexuality. Provide information, emotional support, and referral as needed.

Drug: fentanyl buccal tablet (Fentora)

Class: Opioid analgesic (opioid agonist).

Mechanism of Action: Fentanyl is a pure opioid agonist that binds to opioid μ-receptors located in the brain, spinal cord, and smooth muscle. Fentanyl in a buccal tablet is formulated using OraVescent technology so that when the tablet contacts saliva, the resulting reaction releases carbon dioxide and changes the local pH, allowing dissolution and passage of the fentanyl through the buccal membrane. The onset of analgesia is at 15 minutes, with significant decrease in pain intensity at 30 minutes in 50% of patients, and duration of action of 60 minutes.

Metabolism: Approximately 50% of the drug is absorbed through the buccal mucosa. The remaining half of the total dose is absorbed via the GI tract. Absolute bioavailability is 65%. After buccal absorption, there is a steep rise in mean plasma fentanyl concentration, peaking at 46.8 minutes. Drug is highly lipophilic and highly protein-bound (80–85%). Drug is taken up in tissues and eliminated primarily by biotransformation into inactive metabolites in the liver. It is metabolized in the liver primarily and to a lesser extent in the intestinal mucosa to norfentanyl by cytochrome P450 3A4 isoform. In population studies, patients with lower weight have a higher systemic exposure to the drug (men, Japanese subjects). Patients with renal and/or hepatic dysfunction who are receiving high doses of drug may have significantly decreased metabolic elimination of the drug. Four single 100-mcg tablets deliver 12–13% more drug than a single 400-mcg tablet. The dwell time (time tablet takes to disintegrate) does not affect early systemic exposure to fentanyl.

Indication: Indicated for the management of BTP in patients with cancer 18 years or older, who are already receiving and are tolerant to ATC opioid therapy for persistent cancer pain (taking at least 60 mg of oral morphine a day, or 25 mcg of fentanyl per hour, or at least 30 mg of oxycodone daily, or at least 8 mg of hydromorphone daily, or an equianalgesic dose of another opioid, for at least 1 week or longer).

Limitations: Fentora may be dispensed only to patients enrolled in the TIRF REMS Access program.

Contraindications: (1) opioid nontolerant patients; (2) management of acute or postoperative pain including headache, migraine, and dental pain; (3) significant respiratory depression; (4) intolerance or hypersensitivity to fentanyl or its components; (5) acute or severe bronchial asthma in an unmonitored setting or in absence of resuscitative equipment; (6) known or suspected GI obstruction, including paralytic ileus.

Dosage/Range:
- Principles: Patients must require and use ATC opioids when taking this drug. Use the lowest effective dosage for the shortest duration consistent with patient treatment goals. Individualize dosing based on the severity of pain, patient response, prior analgesic experience, and risk factors for addiction, abuse, and misuse. Initial dose is 100 mcg. Initiate titration using multiples of 100 mcg of Fentora tablet. Limit patient access to only one strength of Fentora at one time. Individually titrate to a tolerable dose that provides adequate analgesia using single Fentora 100 mcg tablet. No more than 2 doses per BTP episode. Wait at least 4 hours before treating another episode of BTP with Fentora. Place entire tablet in buccal cavity or under tongue; tablet must not be split, crushed, sucked, chewed, or swallowed whole.
  - Starting dose is 100 mcg; redose with a single BTP episode which may occur 30 minutes after the start of administration of buccal fentanyl using the same dose strength.
  - Prescription is written: place tablet above a rear molar between the upper cheek and gum; one tablet per BTP episode; may repeat once if pain is not relieved after 30 minutes.
  - Titrate to adequate dose by patient diary and discussion with provider to achieve single tablet strength that provides relief; when doses above 100 mcg needed, patient should place one 100-mcg tablet on buccal mucosa on each side of the mouth; if this is ineffective, increase dose by placing two 100-mcg tablets on each side of the mouth, for a total of four 100-mcg tablets.
  - Titrating above 400 mcg: increase dose in 200-mcg increments.
- When converting from oral transmucosal fentanyl (Actiq), a dose of buccal tablet is one-half or less than the Actiq dose (e.g., Actiq 200 or 400 mcg = Fentora 100 mcg; Actiq 600 or 800 mcg = Fentora 200 mcg; Actiq 1,200–1,600 mcg = Fentora 400 mcg).
- The goal is to determine necessary dose in a single tablet.

MANAGEMENT

- After an effective dose has been determined, when the patient requires more than four BTP episodes per day, increase the maintenance (ATC) opioid by an equivalent amount.
- Increase the fentanyl buccal tablet dose when a patient requires more than one dose per BTP episode.
- Drug is available through a restricted distribution program called TIRF REMS Access Program. Outpatients, healthcare professionals who prescribe to outpatients, pharmacies, and distributors are required to enroll in the program.
- Use drug cautiously in patients with renal or hepatic impairment, and monitor closely for toxicity.

Drug Preparation/Administration:
- Available in a carton of seven blister cards with four tablets in each card; blister pack is child-resistant and encased in peelable foil.
- Available in 100-, 200-, 400-, 600-, and 800-mcg fentanyl base tablets.
- Open blister pack immediately before use: tear single blister unit from card, bend blister unit, and peel backing to expose the tablet (do not try to push through the backing).
- Remove tablet from blister unit, and place entire tablet in buccal cavity, usually above a rear molar, between the upper cheek and teeth, or place entire tablet under the tongue; patient should NOT try to split the tablet and/or chew, suck, or swallow the tablet, as this results in lower plasma fentanyl levels.
- Leave the tablet against buccal mucosa until it has fully disintegrated (14–25 minutes).
- After 30 minutes, if tablet remnants remain, the patient can swallow them with a drink of water.
- Teach patient to alternate sides of mouth when administering subsequent doses in the buccal cavity.
- Teach patient that opioid analgesics may impair the mental and/or physical ability to drive and use machines, and to avoid these activities until the effect of the drug is known.
- For patients requiring opioid discontinuation, gradually titrate downward, as it is not known at what level the opioid may be discontinued without causing signs/symptoms of abrupt withdrawal.

Drug Interactions:
- CNS depressants (other opioids, sedatives, hypnotics, general anesthetics, phenothiazines, tranquilizers, skeletal muscle relaxants, sedating antihistamines), potent inhibitors of cytochrome P450 CYP3A4 isoform (erythromycin, ketoconazole, certain protease inhibitors), and alcohol: increased CNS depression, with risk of hypoventilation, hypotension, and profound sedation. Do not coadminister.
- Moderate CYP3A4 inhibitors (aprepitant, diltiazem, grapefruit juice, verapamil): may increase fentanyl plasma levels; use together cautiously.
- MAO inhibitors within 14 days: potentiation of opioid, do not give together.

Lab Effects/Interference:
- None known.

Special Considerations:
- Most common ($\geq$ 10%) adverse reactions: nausea, dizziness, vomiting, fatigue, anemia, constipation, peripheral edema, asthenia, dehydration, headache.

- Warnings and Precautions:
  - Risk Evaluation and Mitigation Strategy (REMS) required for use of opioids. Health-care providers must review REMS-compliant education. In addition, healthcare providers must
    a. Complete a REMS-compliant education program offered by an accredited CE provider or another education program that includes all the elements of the FDA Education Blueprint for Health Care Providers Involved in the Management or Support of Patients with Pain. The blueprint can be found at www.fda.gov/OpioidAnalgesic REMSBlueprint.
    b. Discuss the safe use, serious risks, and proper storage and disposal of opioid analgesics with patients and/or their caregivers every time these medicines are prescribed. The Patient Counseling Guide can be obtained at www.fda.gov/OpioidAnalgesic REMSPCG.
    c. Emphasize to patients and their caregivers the importance of reading the Medication Guide that they will receive from their pharmacist every time an opioid analgesic is dispensed to them.
    d. Consider using other tools to improve patient, household, and community safety, such as patient–prescriber agreements that reinforce patient–prescriber responsibilities.
  - *Life-threatening respiratory depression in patients with chronic pulmonary disease or in elderly, cachectic, or debilitated patients:* can occur, even at approved doses, especially if the patient has an underlying respiratory disorder, is elderly, or is debilitated; is not opioid tolerant; or if the drug is coadministered with other respiratory-depressing drugs. Assess for patient's reduced urge to breathe and decreased respiratory rate, often with a sighing pattern (deep breaths separated by long pauses). Retention of carbon dioxide combined with opioid sedation can lead to accidental overdose. Assess patients at risk closely, especially 24–72 hours within drug initiation or dose change. Ensure proper dosing and titration to prevent respiratory problems
  - *Increased risk of overdose in children due to accidental ingestion or exposure:* Keep unused as well as used dosage units out of reach of children and pets. Review patient self-administration flyer (*Fentora Medication Guide)* in package insert with patient and caregiver.
  - *Risk of concomitant use or discontinuation of cytochrome P450 3A4 inhibitors and inducers:* CYP3A4 inhibitors may increase drug serum level and prolong opioid toxicity, leading to potentially fatal respiratory depression, especially when added after a stable dose has been found. Similarly, the discontinuance of a CYP3A4 inducer may increase serum fentanyl levels and prolong opioid toxicity, including respiratory depression. Conversely, discontinuation of a CYP3A4 inhibitor or addition of a CYP3A4 inducer can reduce fentanyl serum levels resulting in adequate analgesia. Monitor patient very closely, frequently; adjust fentanyl dosage as needed and safe.
  - *Risks from concomitant use with benzodiazepines or other CNS depressants (including alcohol):* Profound sedation, respiratory depression, coma, and death may result. Thus, reserve concomitant use of these drugs only when no alternative exists and monitor patient closely. Assess medication profile and teach patient to avoid alcohol when receiving the drug.

MANAGEMENT

- *Risk of medication errors:* Do not convert a patient to Fentora from any other fentanyl product on a mcg per mcg basis as Fentora is not equivalent to other fentanyl products on a mcg to mcg basis. Fentora is NOT a generic version of other TIRF formulations. Always start opiate tolerant patients at 100 mcg dose and individually titrate to achieve analgesia.
- *Addiction, abuse, and misuse:* Fentora contains fentanyl, a Schedule II–controlled substance. It is an opioid that exposes users to risk of addiction, abuse, and misuse, which can lead to overdose and death. Assess each patient's risk before prescribing, and monitor regularly for evidence of misuse, abuse, or diversion. Addiction is defined as psychological dependence. This is different from physical dependence (goes into withdrawal if drug is abruptly discontinued).
- *Neonatal opioid withdrawal syndrome:* Prolonged use of an opioid during pregnancy can result in neonatal opioid withdrawal syndrome, which may be life-threatening to the newborn if not recognized and treated with expert protocols. If opioid use is required for prolonged periods in a pregnant woman, teach her of the risk of neonatal opioid withdrawal syndrome, and ensure that she understands the newborn must be cared for by a healthcare personnel experienced with the protocols.
- *TIRF REMS Access Program:* (1) Outpatient prescribers must review prescriber educational material, enroll in the program, and comply with the REMS requirements; (2) outpatients must understand the risks and benefits and sign the patient–prescriber agreement; (3) dispensing pharmacies must enroll in the program and agree to comply with the REMS requirements; (4) wholesalers and distributors must enroll in the program and distribute only to authorized pharmacies.
- *Adrenal insufficiency:* Adrenal insufficiency has occurred, especially in patients receiving opioids for >1 month. Signs/symptoms include: nausea, vomiting, anorexia, fatigue, weakness, dizziness, low BP. If adrenal insufficiency is suspected, confirm the diagnosis with lab testing; if confirmed, treat with physiological doses of corticosteroids. Wean the patient off the opioid to allow adrenal function recovery while continuing corticosteroids. Other opioids should be tried.
- *Severe hypotension:* Severe hypotension may occur, including orthostatic hypotension and syncope in ambulatory patients, especially in patients with reduced blood volume, or receiving concurrent certain CNS depressing drugs (e.g., phenothiazines, general anesthetics). Monitor these patients closely for signs/symptoms hypotension after starting drug or dose titration. Do not use Exalgo in patients with circulatory shock.
- *Risk of use in patients with head injury, brain tumor, or increased ICP:* Opioids may obscure clinical course of these patients who are sensitive to the effects of CO_2 retention (respiratory depression). Monitor for sedation and respiratory depression. Avoid use of Fentora in patients with impaired consciousness or coma who are susceptible to the intracranial effects of CO_2 retention.
- *Serotonin syndrome with concomitant use of serotonergic drugs:* Serotonin syndrome (e.g., characterized by mental status changes, autonomic instability, neuromuscular abnormalities, and GI symptoms) has occurred when patients received both fentanyl transdermal patch and serotonergic drugs (e.g., SSRIs, serotonin and norepinephrine reuptake inhibitors [SNRIs] TCAs triptans, 5-HT3 receptor antagonists, drugs that affect the serotonergic neurotransmitter system (e.g., mirtazapine, trazodone, tramadol), and drugs that impair metabolism of serotonin (e.g., MAO inhibitors)).

If serotonin syndrome occurs, onset is usually within several hours to a few days after concomitant use, but may occur later. If serotonin syndrome is suspected, immediately discontinue Fentora if the syndrome is suspected and convert to immediate acting opioids.

- *Risk of use in patients with GI conditions:* Drug is contraindicated if GI obstruction is suspected or known, as well as in patients with preexisting severe GI narrowing as the tablet will not change shape to be accommodated through the narrowing and can become an obstruction (e.g., esophageal motility disorders, small bowel inflammatory disease, short gut syndrome, past history of peritonitis, cystic fibrosis, chronic intestinal pseudo-obstruction, Merkel's diverticulum). Opioids can cause spasm of the sphincter of Oddi, and cause increases in serum amylase; monitor patients with biliary tract disease, including acute pancreatitis, for worsening symptoms.
- *Increased risk of seizures in patients with seizure disorders:* Drug may increase seizure frequency or occurrence in other clinical settings. Monitor patients with a seizure history closely for worsening seizure control when taking this drug.
- *Withdrawal:* Avoid the use of mixed agonist/antagonist (e.g., pentazocine, nalbuphine, butorphanol) analgesics in patients receiving full opioid agonist analgesia as the analgesic effect may be lessened or it may precipitate withdrawal symptoms. When discontinuing the drug, always gradually taper the dose; do NOT abruptly discontinue.
- *Risks of driving and operating machinery:* Drug may impair mental and/or physical abilities of driving or operating machinery. Teach patient to avoid driving and operation of machinery until the effect of the opioid is known.
- *Cardiac disease:* IV fentanyl may produce bradycardia. Use drug cautiously in patients with bradyarrhythmias.
- *Application site reactions:* Application site reactions occurred in 10% of patients in clinical trials (from paresthesia to ulceration and bleeding). Teach patient to report any skin or sensation changes, and to rotate application sites.
- *MAO inhibitors:* Do not use in patients who have used MAO inhibitors within 14 days, because severe and unpredictable potentiation of MAO inhibitors may occur.
- Drug is an opioid and may cause physical dependence and withdrawal if stopped (along with maintenance opioid) abruptly.
  - Fentora is not bioequivalent to other fentanyl products and drug is not interchangeable with Actiq formulation of fentanyl.
  - Accidental ingestion by a child or pet may be fatal. Drug must be safely secured out of the reach of children and pets.
- Teach women of reproductive potential to use effective contraception to avoid pregnancy. The drug is passed in human milk, so mothers should not breastfeed while receiving the drug.

Potential Toxicities/Side Effects and the Nursing Process

I. POTENTIAL ALTERATION IN OXYGENATION related to HYPOVENTILATION

Defining Characteristics: Increased cough and/or dyspnea are rare, but the chief toxicity in naïve patients or if excessive dosing is respiratory depression. Drug may cause bradycardia; thus, use with caution in patients with bradyarrhythmias.

MANAGEMENT

Nursing Implications: Assess baseline pulmonary status. Use with caution in patients with COPD, bradycardia, or renal or hepatic dysfunction, and in the older population. Teach patient to report any pulmonary difficulties immediately. Ensure that patient knows that if respiratory difficulty develops the drug must be removed from mouth and discarded immediately. Ensure that patient understands how to administer drug safely and to keep drug supply out of reach of children and pets.

II. SENSORY/PERCEPTUAL ALTERATIONS related to CNS CHANGES

Defining Characteristics: CNS depression and changes in mental status may occur, characterized by somnolence (9%) or dizziness (13%), confusion (7%), depression (8%), and insomnia (6%). Rarely, hypoesthesia, lethargy, balance problems, anxiety, disorientation, and hallucinations may occur.

Nursing Implications: Assess baseline gait, mental, affective, and neurologic status. Assess medication profile to identify other contributions (i.e., CNS depressants). Instruct patient to report any changes. Assess patient safety, and measures to ensure safety. Teach patient not to take alcohol, sleep aids, or tranquilizers, except as ordered by the oncology provider. Discuss any significant changes with provider.

III. ALTERATION IN COMFORT related to HEADACHE, PAIN, PERIPHERAL EDEMA

Defining Characteristics: Headache occurs in about 10% of patients, abdominal pain (9%), peripheral edema (12%), asthenia (11%), and fatigue (16%). Back pain (5%) and arthralgia (6%) were reported less commonly.

Nursing Implications: Assess baseline comfort. Assess baseline skin integrity, presence of peripheral edema, and weight. Teach patient to report symptoms and manage based on severity, including elevating legs if peripheral edema present. Assess impact on patient's quality of life. If severe, discuss alternative strategies with physician.

IV. ALTERATION IN NUTRITION, LESS THAN BODY REQUIREMENTS, related to NAUSEA/VOMITING

Defining Characteristics: Nausea occurred in 29% of patients, and vomiting occurred in 20% of patients. Dehydration occurred in 11% of patients, anorexia 8%, and hypokalemia 6%.

Nursing Implications: Assess baseline nutritional status, including electrolyte and fluid balance. Teach patient to take antiemetic agents as prescribed, to drink 8–10 ounces of fluid hourly while awake, and to eat small, frequent, calorie-dense foods. Teach patient to report nausea, vomiting, anorexia, and dehydration. Manage symptomatically. Assess severity and impact on quality of life. Discuss severe or unmanaged symptoms with physician.

V.   ALTERATION IN ELIMINATION related to CONSTIPATION OR DIARRHEA

Defining Characteristics: Opium agonists bind to opiate receptors in bowel, slowing peristalsis, leading to constipation. Untreated constipation may result in bowel perforation. Constipation occurred in 12% of patients and diarrhea in 8% of patients.

Nursing Implications: Assess baseline elimination, fluid intake, diet, and exercise patterns. Instruct patient regarding prevention of constipation: goal is to move bowels at least every 2 days by increasing fluids to 3 L/day (drink 8- to 10-ounce glasses of fluid every hour while awake), following a diet high in fiber (beans, vegetables, fruit), and taking moderate exercise. Review bowel regimen, and assess need for additional bowel softeners, bulk-forming laxatives, and osmotic cathartics, and discuss prescription with physician. Teach patient self-administration of medications. However, all patients MUST be started on bowel regimen when receiving an opioid.

Drug: oral fentanyl citrate, oral transmucosal lozenge, oral transmucosal fentanyl citrate (OTFC) [Actiq, generic equivalents]

Class: Opioid analgesic (opioid agonist).

Mechanism of Action: Fentanyl is a pure opioid agonist that binds to opioid μ-receptors located in the brain, spinal cord, and smooth muscle. The oral transmucosal preparation of the drug is a solid formulation of fentanyl citrate placed on a handle so the drug is placed between the cheek and lower gum, with the patient occasionally moving the drug matrix from one side to the other, over a 15-minute period. Sucking the drug dose coats the oral mucosa, through which 25% of the drug is rapidly absorbed, reportedly as fast as IV morphine.

Metabolism: Initial rapid absorption of about 25% of total dose across buccal mucosa, into systemic circulation, and longer prolonged absorption of swallowed fentanyl (75% of dose) from GI tract. One-third of drug escapes first-pass elimination and enters the systemic circulation for a total of 50% of the total dose that is bioavailable. Following absorption, drug is rapidly distributed to brain, heart, lungs, kidneys, and spleen. Plasma binding is 80–85%. The drug is primarily metabolized in the liver, by the CYP3A4 isoenzyme; < 7% of the dose is excreted in the urine. The terminal elimination half-life is ~7 hours.

Indication: Management of BTP in cancer patients 16 years of age and older who are already receiving and who are tolerant to ATC opioid therapy for their underlying persistent cancer pain.

Tolerance to opioids is defined as taking for 1 week or longer, ATC medication consisting of **at least:** 60 mg oral morphine/day; OR 25 mcg fentanyl transdermal/hr; OR 30 mg of oral oxycodone/day; OR 8 mg of oral hydromorphone/day; OR 25 mg oxymorphone/day; OR 60 mg oral hydrocodone/day; OR an equianalgesic dose of another opioid daily for a week or longer. Patients must be on ATC opioids while taking ACTIQ.

Limitations: (1) Not for use in opioid nontolerant patients; (2) not for use in the management of acute or postoperative pain, including headache/migraine, or dental pain; (3) drug can be dispensed ONLY to patients enrolled in the TIRF REMS Access Program.

Contraindications: (1) Opioid-naïve or not tolerant patients; (2) significant respiratory depression; (3) treatment of acute or postoperative pain, including headache/migraine, dental pain; (4) intolerance to or hypersensitivity to fentanyl or any of the components of oral transmucosal fentanyl citrate (OTFC); (5) acute or severe bronchial asthma in an unmonitored setting or in absence of resuscitative equipment; (6) known or suspected GI obstruction, including paralytic ileus. Do not administer to patients who have received MAO inhibitors within 14 days, as unpredictable potentiation of the opioid may occur. Do not administer to nursing mothers.

Dosage/Range: *Adult (16 years of age and older)*
- OTFC is available only through a restricted program. OTFC can be dispensed only to patients enrolled in the TIRF REMS Access Program. OTFC can be prescribed, dispensed, and distributed only by physicians, pharmacists, and vendors enrolled in the TIRF REMS Access Program. To obtain a list of qualified pharmacies/distributors, see www.TIRF-REMSAccess.com, or call 1-866-822-1483.
- Patients must require and use ATC opioids when taking OTFC.
- *Initial dose of OTFC is always 200 mcg.* Patient should have an initial supply of six 200-mcg OTFC units. Patient should use all units before increasing to a higher dose to prevent confusion and possible overdose.
  - For example, patient begins using a 200-mcg unit for BTP and sucks the medicine for 15 minutes. If the pain is unrelieved, the patient waits an additional 15 minutes, and then administers a second 200-mcg unit (now 30 minutes after starting initial dosage unit).
  - The patient should take a maximum of 2 doses of OTFC for any BTP episode. Patient should wait at least 4 hours before treating another episode of BTP with OTFC. To reduce risk of overdosing, patient should only have one strength of OTFC for any BTP episode.
  - Patients should record their usage of OTFC over several episodes of BTP and share this with their provider to determine if a dosage adjustment is needed.
- *Maintenance dosing*: Once an effective dose is reached, patient should use only one OTFC unit of the appropriate strength per pain episode.
  - If the BTP is not relieved in 15 minutes after completion of the OTFC unit, patient can take only 1 additional dose using the same strength for that episode 15 minutes later.
  - Once the dose has been determined that relieves BTP with a single dose, the patient should require only 4 or fewer doses a day.
  - If more than 4 doses are required, then the ATC (long-acting) opioid dose should be evaluated and likely increased.
- Generally, OTFC dose should be increased only when a single administration of the current BTP dose fails to treat the BTP episode effectively for several consecutive episodes.
- The patient should notify the physician if drug is required more than four times per day, so that the long-acting opioid can be increased.

Drug Preparation:

- Drug is available in dosage strengths of 200, 400, 600, 800, 1,200, and 1,600 mcg. Initial dose is always 200 mcg.
- Drug is on a handle, sealed in a child-resistant foil pouch that requires scissors to open. The drug dose is color-coded.
- Trade name Actiq is manufactured by Cephalon, and generic OTFC lozenges are manu-factured by Anesta Corp, Mallinckrodt Inc., and Par Pharmaceutical Companies Inc.

Drug Administration:

- Use scissors to open blister pack immediately before use. Patient should place drug dose unit in the mouth between cheek and lower gum, occasionally moving the drug matrix from one side to the other using the handle. Patient should suck, NOT CHEW, the medication over 15 minutes, as this would result in lower peak concentrations and lower bioavailability.
- If patient has signs of excessive opioid effects before unit is consumed, the dosage unit should be removed from the patient's mouth, disposed of properly, and subsequent doses should be reduced.
- If the patient achieves adequate analgesia or develops excessive side effects, the drug should be removed from the mouth and discarded immediately. The remaining drug is very dangerous if a child or pet ingests it, so maximum precautions must be taken.
- Destroy any medication remaining on the handle by dissolving it under hot water, and place handle out of reach of children and pets. If unable to dispose of remaining drug right away, place in an empty jar, tightly close lid, and place out of reach of children and pets. Dispose of properly as soon as possible.
- Any remaining drug must be disposed of properly. It can be fatal to a child or pet if ingested, so maximum precautions must be taken.
- Keep medication away from patient's eyes, skin, or mucous membranes when not sucking the medication, and the patient should wash hands after discarding unused medication portion.
- At home, teach patient to store oral doses in a safe place away from children and pets.
- Titrate drug cautiously in patients with COPD or preexisting medical conditions predisposing them to respiratory depression and in patients susceptible to intracranial effects of CO_2.
- Teach patient that opioid analgesics may impair the mental and/or physical ability to drive and use machines, and to avoid these activities until the effect of the drug is known.
- If patient requires discontinuance of opioids, a gradual downward titration is recommended to prevent withdrawal symptoms: yawning, sweating, lacrimation, rhinorrhea, anxiety, restlessness, insomnia, dilated pupils, piloerection, chills, tachycardia, hypertension, nausea/vomiting, cramping, abdominal pain, diarrhea, muscle aches, and pains.

Drug Interactions:

- CNS depressants (e.g., other opioids, alcohol, sedatives, hypnotics, general anesthetics, phenothiazines, tranquilizers, skeletal muscle relaxants, sedating antihistamines) may increase CNS depression (hypoventilation, hypotension, profound sedation, especially in opioid nontolerant patients). Patients who require concomitant drugs should be monitored for a change in opioid effects. Consider adjusting the dose of OTFC if needed.

MANAGEMENT

- Strong CYP3A4 inhibitors (e.g., ritonavir, ketoconazole, itraconazole, troleandomycin, clarithromycin, nelfinavir, nefazodone) or moderate inhibitors (e.g., amprenavir, aprepitant, diltiazem, erythromycin, fluconazole, fosamprenavir, verapamil), and grapefruit/grapefruit juice: may result in increased fentanyl serum levels, increasing opioid side effects, including fatal respiratory depression; avoid concomitant administration. If required, carefully monitor patient for an extended period of time. If dosage increase is required, do so very conservatively and carefully.
- Strong CYP3A4 inducers: may decrease serum fentanyl levels, and decrease analgesia. Avoid concomitant administration.
- MAO inhibitors, or within 14 days of discontinuation; do not administer OTFC.

Lab Effects/Interference:
- None known.

Special Considerations:
- Once an effective dose is identified, drug provides rapid relief of BTP.
- Patients should be taught to call nurse or physician if taking two of the same strength units within 60 minutes without relief or if taking drug more than 4 times/day.
- Most common adverse effects (occurring $\geq$ 5%): nausea, dizziness, somnolence, vomiting, asthenia, headache, dyspnea, constipation, anxiety, confusion, depression, rash, and insomnia. The most serious adverse effects reported with all opioids are respiratory depression, circulatory depression, hypotension, and shock.
- Each OTFC unit contains about 2 g of sugar (hydrated dextrates). Diabetic patients should be warned this may affect their blood glucose levels and medication needed to control their diabetes. In addition, dental decay can be accelerated by the sugar content, and may be exacerbated by opioid-induced dry mouth. Postmarketing reports confirmed cases of dental decay. Patients should be told to contact their dentist to ensure they are performing appropriate oral hygiene.
- Warnings and Precautions:
  - Risk Evaluation and Mitigation Strategy (REMS) required for use of opioids. Healthcare providers must review REMS-compliant education. In addition, healthcare providers must
    a. Complete a REMS-compliant education program offered by an accredited CE provider or another education program that includes all the elements of the FDA Education Blueprint for Health Care Providers Involved in the Management or Support of Patients with Pain. The blueprint can be found at www.fda.gov/OpioidAnalgesic REMSBlueprint.
    b. Discuss the safe use, serious risks, and proper storage and disposal of opioid analgesics with patients and/or their caregivers every time these medicines are prescribed. The Patient Counseling Guide can be obtained at www.fda.gov/OpioidAnalgesic REMSPCG.
    c. Emphasize to patients and their caregivers the importance of reading the Medication Guide that they will receive from their pharmacist every time an opioid analgesic is dispensed to them.
    d. Consider using other tools to improve patient, household, and community safety, such as patient–prescriber agreements that reinforce patient–prescriber responsibilities.

- *Life-threatening respiratory depression:* Life-threatening respiratory depression can occur, even at approved doses, Assess patients closely, especially 24–72 hours within drug initiation or dose change. Ensure proper dosing and titration to prevent respiratory problems.
- *Increased risk of overdose in children due to accidental ingestion or exposure:* Keep unused as well as used dosage units out of reach of children and pets. Review patient self-administration flyer (*Actiq Medication Guide)* in package insert with patient and caregiver.
- *Risk of concomitant use or discontinuation of cytochrome P450 3A4 inhibitors and inducers:* CYP3A4 inhibitors may increase drug serum level and prolong opioid toxicity, leading to potentially fatal respiratory depression, especially when added after a stable dose has been found. Similarly, the discontinuance of a CYP3A4 inducer may increase serum fentanyl levels and prolong opioid toxicity, including respiratory depression. Conversely, discontinuation of a CYP3A4 inhibitor or addition of a CYP3A4 inducer can reduce fentanyl serum levels resulting in adequate analgesia. Monitor patient very closely, frequently; adjust fentanyl dosage as needed and safe.
- *Risks from concomitant use with benzodiazepines or other CNS depressants (including alcohol):* Profound sedation, respiratory depression, coma, and death may result. Thus, reserve concomitant use of these drugs only when no alternative exists and monitor patient closely. Assess medication profile and teach patient to avoid alcohol when receiving the drug.
- *Risk of medication errors:* Do not convert a patient to Actiq from any other fentanyl product on a mcg per mcg basis as Fentora is not equivalent to other fentanyl products on a mcg to mcg basis. Actiq is NOT a generic version of other TIRF formulations. Always start opiate tolerant patients at 200-mcg dose and individually titrate to achieve analgesia.
- *Addiction, abuse, and misuse:* Actiq contains fentanyl, a Schedule II–controlled substance. It is an opioid that exposes users to risk of addiction, abuse, and misuse, which can lead to overdose and death. Assess each patient's risk before prescribing, and monitor regularly for evidence of misuse, abuse, or diversion. Addiction is defined as psychological dependence. This is different from physical dependence (goes into withdrawal if drug is abruptly discontinued).
- *Neonatal opioid withdrawal syndrome:* Prolonged use of Actiq during pregnancy can result in neonatal opioid withdrawal syndrome, which may be life-threatening to the newborn if not recognized and treated with expert protocols. If opioid use is required for prolonged periods in a pregnant woman, teach her of the risk of neonatal opioid withdrawal syndrome, and ensure that she understands the newborn must be cared for by a healthcare personnel experienced with the protocols.
- *TIRF REMS Access program:* (1) Outpatient prescribers must review prescriber educational material, enroll in the program, and comply with the REMS requirements; (2) outpatients must understand the risks and benefits and sign the patient–prescriber agreement; (3) dispensing pharmacies must enroll in the program and agree to comply with the REMS requirements; (4) wholesalers and distributors must enroll in the program and distribute only to authorized pharmacies.
- *Life-threatening respiratory depression in patients with chronic pulmonary disease or in elderly, cachectic, or debilitated patients:* Life-threatening respiratory depression

MANAGEMENT

can occur, even at approved doses, especially if the patient has an underlying respiratory disorder, is elderly, or is debilitated; is not opioid tolerant; or if the drug is coadministered with other respiratory-depressing drugs. Assess for patient's reduced urge to breathe and decreased respiratory rate, often with a sighing pattern (deep breaths separated by long pauses). Retention of carbon dioxide combined with opioid sedation can lead to accidental overdose. Assess patients at risk closely, especially 24–72 hours within drug initiation or dose change. Ensure proper dosing and titration to prevent respiratory problems

- *Adrenal insufficiency:* Adrenal insufficiency has occurred, especially in patients receiving opioids for >1 month. Signs/symptoms include: nausea, vomiting, anorexia, fatigue, weakness, dizziness, low BP. If adrenal insufficiency is suspected, confirm the diagnosis with lab testing; if confirmed, treat with physiological doses of corticosteroids. Wean the patient off the opioid to allow adrenal function recovery while continuing corticosteroids. Other opioids should be tried.

- *Severe hypotension:* Severe hypotension may occur, including orthostatic hypotension and syncope in ambulatory patients, especially in patients with reduced blood volume or receiving concurrent certain CNS depressing drugs (e.g., phenothiazines, general anesthetics). Monitor these patients closely for signs/symptoms hypotension after starting drug or dose titration. Do not use Actiq in patients with circulatory shock.

- *Risk of use in patients with head injury, brain tumor, or increased ICP:* Opioids may obscure clinical course of these patients who are sensitive to the effects of CO_2 retention (respiratory depression). Monitor for sedation and respiratory depression. Avoid use of Fentora in patients with impaired consciousness or coma who are susceptible to the intracranial effects of CO_2 retention.

- *Serotonin syndrome with concomitant use of serotonergic drugs:* Serotonin syndrome (e.g., characterized by mental status changes, autonomic instability, neuromuscular abnormalities, and GI symptoms) has occurred when patients received both fentanyl transdermal patch and serotonergic drugs (e.g., SSRIs, SNRIs, TCAs triptans, 5-HT3 receptor antagonists, drugs that affect the serotonergic neurotransmitter system (e.g., mirtazapine, trazodone, tramadol), and drugs that impair metabolism of serotonin (e.g., MAO inhibitors) (Sentanyl, 2016). If serotonin syndrome occurs, onset is usually within several hours to a few days after concomitant use but may occur later. If serotonin syndrome is suspected, immediately discontinue Fentora is the syndrome is suspected and convert to immediate acting opioids.

- *Risk of use in patients with GI conditions:* Drug is contraindicated if GI obstruction is suspected or known, as well as in patients with preexisting severe GI narrowing as the tablet will not change shape to be accommodated through the narrowing and can become an obstruction (e.g., esophageal motility disorders, small bowel inflammatory disease, short gut syndrome, past history of peritonitis, cystic fibrosis, chronic intestinal pseudo-obstruction, Merkel's diverticulum). Opioids can cause spasm of the sphincter of Oddi and cause increases in serum amylase; monitor patients with biliary tract disease, including acute pancreatitis, for worsening symptoms.

- *Increased risk of seizures in patients with seizure disorders:* Drug may increase seizure frequency or occurrence in other clinical settings. Monitor patients with a seizure history closely for worsening seizure control when taking this drug.

- *Risks of driving and operating machinery:* Drug may impair mental and/or physical abilities of driving or operating machinery. Teach patient to avoid driving and operation of machinery until the effect of the opioid is known.
- *Cardiac disease:* IV fentanyl may produce bradycardia. Use drug cautiously in patients with bradyarrhythmias.
- *Application site reactions:* Application site reactions occurred in 10% of patients in clinical trials (from paresthesia to ulceration and bleeding). Teach patient to report any skin or sensation changes and to rotate application sites.
- *MAO inhibitors:* Do not use in patients who have used MAO inhibitors within 14 days, because severe and unpredictable potentiation of MAO inhibitors may occur.
- Fentanyl products are NOT interchangeable. Patients should not be converted in a mcg to mcg manner from one product to OTFC, or OTFC used to replace another fentanyl product. Rate of absorption is different, and may result in overdosage. OTFC is NOT the generic version of Actiq. There are no safe conversion charts. Thus all opioid-tolerant patients must be started on a 200-mcg dose, and the patient individually titrated up to achieve adequate analgesia and comfort.
  - In performing patient teaching, assess whether there are children in the home. **Full and partially consumed OTFC units contain medication that can be fatal if consumed by a child.** Teach patient and caregiver that all units after use disposed of immediately after use, or if a partially consumed unit remains, it must be stored in a secure place and disposed of properly. An OTFC Child Safety Kit is available.
  - Additive CNS depressant effects occur when drug is coadministered with drugs such as other opioids, phenothiazines, hypnotics, general anesthetics, skeletal muscle relaxants, sedating antihistamines, alcohol. Assess medication profile to identify any drugs, which are CNS depressants. Teach patient not to drink alcohol while taking opioids. Assess for hypotension, hypoventilation, profound sedation. Coadministration with potent CYP3A4 inhibitors may increase fentanyl serum levels (e.g., erythromycin, ketoconazole) resulting in increased CNS sedation. Discuss with physician/NP/PA emergent plan to manage decreased CNS if it occurs (e.g., stop coadministered drug, titrate narcan to reverse opiate-induced CNS depression). Discuss need for dose adjustment with physician/NP/PA.
- Drug is an opioid and may cause physical dependence and withdrawal if stopped (along with maintenance opioid) abruptly.
- Teach women of reproductive potential to use effective contraception to avoid pregnancy. The drug is passed in human milk, so mothers should not breastfeed while receiving the drug.

MANAGEMENT

Potential Toxicities/Side Effects and the Nursing Process

I.   ALTERATION IN OXYGENATION related to HYPOVENTILATION

Defining Characteristics: Dyspnea (7–22%) may occur. Patients are also receiving ATC long-acting opioids.

Nursing Implications: Assess baseline pulmonary status. Use with caution in patients with COPD, bradycardia, or renal or hepatic dysfunction, and in the elderly. Teach patient to report any pulmonary difficulties immediately. Ensure that patient knows that if respiratory difficulty develops, the drug must be removed from mouth and discarded immediately; also, the patient must know to suck and not to chew drug. Ensure that patient understands how to handle drug safely to prevent additional absorption of unused drug. Teach patient and family members to call 911 if the patient is very sedated.

II.   SENSORY/PERCEPTUAL ALTERATIONS related to CNS CHANGES

Defining Characteristics: CNS depression and changes in mental status may occur, characterized by somnolence or dizziness (9–16%); abnormal gait, anxiety, confusion, depression, insomnia, hypesthesia, vasodilation (3–10% incidence).

Nursing Implications: Assess baseline gait and mental, affective, and neurologic status. Assess medication profile to identify other contributions, that is, CNS depressants. Instruct patient to report any changes. Assess patient safety, and take measures to ensure safety. Discuss any significant changes with physician. Teach patient that opioid analgesics may impair the mental and/or physical ability to drive a car or operate machinery, so these activities should be avoided until the drug's full effects are known.

III.   ALTERATION IN SELF-CARE, POTENTIAL, related to LACK OF KNOWLEDGE OF SELF-ADMINISTRATION

Defining Characteristics: Instructions regarding self-administration may be confusing to patients, especially if English is not the patient's native language.

Nursing Implications: Ensure that the patient is taking a long-acting opioid (ATC) and has for at least 1 week. Teach patient about OTFC, that it is an opioid with very important self-care administration points, and why it is being recommended for the management of BTP in this patient. Review the medication guide that comes with the OTFC with the patient. Ask if children live or visit at home, and emphasize how important it is to keep the drug out of reach of children and pets. Teach patient that fentanyl can be abused, so it should never be shared with other people. Teach patient that all patients start with a 200-mcg dose and the patient should have only one strength of OTFC at home at one time. OTFC doses should be 4 hours apart, unless the pain is unrelieved by a single dose; in that case, a second dose can be taken 30 minutes after the first. The goal is to need only 4 doses of BTP medication per day, along with the long-acting ATC opioid; the patient must work with the nurse and doctor to find the right dose. The patient should be given a diary to record pain level, time of BTP dose, activity, and relief achieved. Teach patient to call the nurse or physician if the OTFC with a repeated dose in 15 minutes after the end of the dose (total time 30 minutes) does not control the pain, or if the pain gets worse after taking two doses of BTP OTFC, or if the patient requires more than four BTP medication doses a day. It may be necessary to adjust the dose. Teach patient that opioids may cause constipation, and that the goal is to move bowels at least once every 1–2 days. If nausea and vomiting develop, ensure that patient has a prescription for an antiemetic, along with instructions on how to self-administer.

IV. ALTERATION IN COMFORT related to HEADACHE, FEVER

Defining Characteristics: Headache and asthenia are reported in 4–20% and 15–38% of patients respectively who required OTFC.

Nursing Implications: Assess baseline comfort. Teach patient to report symptoms and manage based on severity. Assess impact on patient's quality of life. If severe, discuss alternative strategies with physician.

V. ALTERATION IN NUTRITION, LESS THAN BODY REQUIREMENTS, related to NAUSEA/VOMITING

Defining Characteristics: Nausea occurs in 24–45% and vomiting in 7–31% of patients.

Nursing Implications: Assess baseline nutritional status. Teach patient to report nausea, vomiting, anorexia, dyspepsia. Manage symptomatically. Teach self-administration of antiemetics 30 minutes prior to drug dose, if possible, and as directed. Assess severity and impact on quality of life. Discuss severe or unmanaged symptoms with physician and revise plan. Ensure that patient is taking adequate fluids to keep hydration status normal.

VI. ALTERATION IN ELIMINATION related to CONSTIPATION OR DIARRHEA

Defining Characteristics: Opium agonists bind to opiate receptors in bowel, slowing peristalsis, leading to constipation. Untreated constipation may result in bowel perforation. In long term treatment, constipation occurred in 20% of patients (any dose).

Nursing Implications: Assess baseline elimination, fluid intake, diet, and exercise patterns. Instruct patient regarding prevention of constipation: goal is to move bowels at least every 2 days by increasing fluids to 3 L/day, following a diet high in fiber (beans, vegetables, fruit), and taking moderate exercise. Assess need for bowel softeners, bulk-forming laxatives, and osmotic cathartics, and discuss prescription with physician. Teach patient self-administration of medications. Patient MUST be started on bowel regimen.

Drug: fentanyl nasal spray (Lazanda)

Class: Opioid analgesic (opioid agonist).

Mechanism of Action: Fentanyl is a pure opioid agonist that binds to opioid μ-receptors located in the brain, spinal cord, and smooth muscle, to achieve analgesia.

Metabolism: Fentanyl nasal spray is absorbed from the nasal mucosa, and the T_{max} (maximal concentration) is achieved from 15 to 21 minutes after a single dose. Presence of allergic rhinitis does not affect absorption. Bioavailability of drug is 20% higher than when administered in an oral transmucosal formulation. Drug is highly lipophilic, with 80–85%

MANAGEMENT

plasma binding. Fentanyl is metabolized by the liver and in the intestinal mucosa to norfentanyl by cytochrome P450 CYP3A4 isoform. Fentanyl is excreted (> 90%) by biotransformation into inactive metabolites. Less than 7% of administered dose is excreted unchanged in the urine, and 1% excreted unchanged in the stool.

Indications: Management of BTP in cancer patients aged 18 years and older who are already receiving and who are tolerant to opioid therapy for their underlying persistent cancer pain. Drug is available ONLY through a restricted distribution program called Transmucosal Immediate Release Fentanyl Risk Evaluation and Mitigation Strategy (TIRF REMS) Access Program. Outpatients and healthcare professionals who prescribe to outpatients, pharmacies, and distributors are required to enroll in the program.

Contraindications: (1) Opioid NON-tolerant patients; (2) management of acute or postoperative pain, including headache/migraine, or dental pain; (3) intolerance or hypersensitivity to fentanyl or drug's components; (4) significant respiratory depression; (5) acute or severe bronchial asthma in an unmonitored setting or in absence of resuscitative equipment; (6) known or suspected GI obstruction, including paralytic ileus.

Dosage/Range:
- Opioid-tolerant patients ONLY. Patient must require and use ATC opioids. Outpatient prescriber, patient, dispensing outpatient pharmacy, and supplier must all be enrolled in and comply with the TIRF REMS Access Program.
  - Use the lowest effective dosage for the shortest duration consistent with individual patient treatment goals.
  - Minimize the number of strengths available to patients at any time to prevent confusion and possible overdosage.
  - Initiate the dosing regimen for each patient individually, taking into account the patient's severity of pain, patient response, prior analgesic treatment experience, and risk factors for addiction, abuse, and misuse.
  - Teach patient how to store drug securely and to properly dispose of unused drug.
  - Drug is NOT bioequivalent to other fentanyl products. Do not convert patients on a mcg per mcg basis from ANY other fentanyl products. There are no conversion directions available.
  - Drug is NOT a generic version of any other oral transmucosal fentanyl product.
- Nasal spray, where each spray delivers 100 mcL of solution containing either 100- or 400-mcg fentanyl base. Supplied in a 5-mL bottle containing 8 sprays.
- Individually titrate to an effective dose, from 100 to 200 mcg, to 400 mcg, and up to a maximum of 800 mcg, with tolerable side effects.
  - Initial dose: 100 mcg. Teach patient to administer one spray in ONE nostril.
  - Do not give another spray for this episode; WAIT AT LEAST 2 HOURS BEFORE USING SPRAY FOR THE NEXT EPISODE.
  - Evaluate whether pain relief was adequate after 30 minutes; if yes, use the same dose for the next pain episode, and this will be the successful and usual dose.
  - If no, for the next pain episode, increase to the next higher dose (e.g., 200 mcg, one 100-mcg spray in EACH nostril). If not effective in 30 minutes, in 2 hours use next higher titration level (e.g., 400 mcg, one 400-mcg spray in ONE nostril or two

100-mcg sprays into each nostril [alternate nostrils]). If not effective in 30 minutes, in 2 hours, use final titration level (e.g., 800 mcg, one 400-mcg spray in EACH nostril).
- Confirm apparent successful dose of drug with a second episode of BTP, and review experience with physician/midlevel to determine if that dose is appropriate or whether further adjustment is needed.
- If pain relief at 30 minutes is inadequate following nasal spray, or if BTP occurs again within 2 hours, use rescue medications as directed by healthcare prescriber.

Dosage Readjustment:
- If there is a marked change in response or adverse reaction, you may need to readjust dose. If patient has > 4 episodes of BTP per day, reevaluate dose of the long-acting opioid used for control of persistent underlying cancer pain. If the dose of the long-acting opioid is increased, reevalute and retitrate the fentanyl nasal spray dose.
- Limit use of fentanyl nasal sprays to treat up to 4 episodes of BTP/day. If more than 4 doses of BTP medication are needed, the long-acting opioid dose should be increased.
- Any dose retitration must be carefully monitored by a healthcare professional.

Drug Preparation: Nasal spray: Each spray delivers 100 mcL of solution, containing either 100 or 400 mcg fentanyl base, supplied in a 5-mL bottle containing 8 sprays. Fentanyl nasal spray bottle MUST be stored out of reach of children and pets, in the specially provided child-resistant container.

Drug Administration:
- Prime the device before use by spraying into the pouch (4 sprays in total), following the instructions for use in the *Medication Guide* provided with the REMS Lazanda pack.
- Insert the nozzle of fentanyl nasal spray bottle 1/2 inch (1 cm) into the nose and point toward the bridge of the nose, tilting the bottle slightly.
- Press down firmly on the finger grips until the patient hears a click, and the number in the counting window advances by one; the fine mist spray is not always felt on the nasal mucosal membrane, so the patient should rely on hearing the audible click and the advancement of the dose counter to confirm a spray has been administered.
- When the 8 doses in the bottle have all been given, the patient should dispose of any remaining drug by aiming the bottle into the provided pouch, and discharge the remaining liquid into the pouch by pressing down on the finger grips a total of 4 times to ensure that any remaining liquid is trapped in the pouch. After the 8 therapeutic sprays have been emitted, the patient will not hear a click and the counter will not advance beyond 8 when spraying the residual into the pouch. Then seal the pouch. Place both the empty bottle and sealed pouch into the child-resistant storage container and discard in the trash.
- Patient should be instructed to wash hands with soap and water immediately after handling the pouch.
- If the pouch is lost, use a pouch from another Lazanda pack to prime and dispose of unused medicine from the current bottle, as well as from the next bottle. If the patient does not have an available empty pouch, teach the patient to call 1-866-435-6775 to order and receive a replacement pouch in the mail.
- Teach patient that opioid analgesics may impair the mental and/or physical ability to drive and use machines, and to avoid these activities until the effect of the drug is known.

MANAGEMENT

Drug Interactions:
- Monitor patients who begin therapy with, or increase the dose of, inhibitors of CYP3A4 for signs of opioid toxicity (e.g., indinavir, nelfinavir, ritonavir, clarithromycin, itraconazole, ketoconazole, nefazodone, saquinavir, telithromycin, aprepitant, diltiazem, erythromycin, fluconazole, grapefruit juice, verapamil, or cimetidine). Coadministration may increase or prolong adverse opioid effects, including potentially fatal respiratory depression.
- Monitor patients who stop therapy with, or decrease the dose of, inducers of CYP3A4 (e.g., barbiturates, carbamazepine, efavirenz, glucocorticoids, modafinil, nevirapine, oxcarbazepine, phenobarbital, phenytoin, pioglitazone, rifabutin, rifampin, St. John's wort, troglitazone) for signs of opioid toxicity. Coadministration of an inducer and fentanyl can decrease the fentanyl serum level, so when stopping the CYP3A4 inducer, the patient may experience a sudden increase in the fentanyl plasma concentration. Adjust fentanyl nasal spray dose accordingly.
- Agents used to treat allergic rhinitis: Coadministration of a vasoconstrictive nasal decongestant may cause fentanyl nasal spray to be less effective. In addition, if the patient is experiencing an acute episode of rhinitis and the fentanyl dose is titrated, an incorrect titration may occur so that when the allergic rhinitis drug is stopped, the drug dose is too high. DO NOT COADMINISTER.
- MAO inhibitors within 14 days: Potentiation of opioid; do not give together.
- CNS depressants (e.g., other opioids, sedatives or hypnotics, general anesthetics, phenothiazines, tranquilizers, skeletal muscle relaxants, sedating antihistamines, alcohol): May increase risk for CNS depression (e.g., hypotension, hypoventilation, profound sedation); do not coadminister; if must coadminister, consider reducing fentanyl nasal spray dose.

Lab Effects/Interference: Increased alkaline phosphatase.

Special Considerations:
- Fentanyl nasal spray (Lazanda) is not equivalent to other fentanyl products on a mcg to mcg basis. DO NOT convert from other products. Therefore, for opioid-tolerant patients starting fentanyl nasal spray, the initial dose is 100 mcg. Individually titrate each patient's dose to provide adequate analgesia and minimizing side effects. DO NOT substitute fentanyl nasal spray for any other fentanyl product.
- Lazanda is available only through the restricted Lazanda TIRF REMS program, and healthcare providers who prescribe to outpatients, pharmacies, and distributors are required to enroll in the TIRF REMS Access Program.
- Information for patients and their caregivers must be taught to keep used and unused bottles in their child-resistant container out of reach of children and pets at all times. Partially used bottles put children at risk. When finished using the drug, the bottle should be completely emptied of all solution by spraying the remaining solution into the carbon-lined pouch. Teach them to wash their hands thoroughly after doing this. Drug can be fatal to children and pets.
- Warnings and Precautions:
  - *Life-threatening respiratory depression:* Respiratory depression can occur, even at approved doses, especially if the patient has an underlying respiratory disorder, is elderly, or is debilitated; is not opioid tolerant; or if the drug is coadministered with

other respiratory-depressing drugs. Assess for patient's reduced urge to breathe and decreased respiratory rate, often with a sighing pattern (deep breaths separated by long pauses). Retention of carbon dioxide combined with opioid sedation can lead to accidental overdose. Assess patients at risk closely.

- *Increased risk of overdosage in children due to accidental ingestion or exposure:* Information for patients and their caregivers must be taught to keep used and unused bottles in their child-resistant container out of reach of children and pets at all times. Partially used bottles put children at risk. When finished using the drug, the bottle should be completely emptied of all solution by spraying the remaining solution into the carbon-lined pouch. Teach patient that drug must be kept out of reach of children and pets, as dose can be LETHAL to children and pets. Keep drug in the specially provided child-resistant container. Teach patient and caregiver to wash their hands thoroughly after handling the drug.
- *Risks of concomitant use or discontinuation of CYP3A4 inhibitors and inducers:* (a) Coadministration with potent CYP3A4 inhibitors may increase fentanyl serum levels (e.g., macrolide antibiotics such as erythromycin, azole antifungals such as ketoconazole and proteasome inhibitors such as ritonavir) resulting in increased CNS sedation and risk of respiratory depression, especially when an inhibitor is added when the patient is on a stable opioid dose; (b) discontinuance of a CYP3A4 inducer (e.g., rifampin, carbamazepine, and phenytoin) may increase serum fentanyl concentrations and prolong adverse effects. Monitor patient closely when either (a) or (b) occurs, and consider dose reduction of fentanyl until the drug effects are stable. Conversely, concomitant use of fentanyl nasal spray with CYP3A4 inducers or discontinuation of an CYP3A4 inhibitor could decrease fentanyl serum concentration, decrease opioid efficacy and lead to withdrawal syndrome. Monitor these patients closely and discuss increasing fentanyl dose as needed for efficacy or if signs/symptoms of withdrawal appear.
- *Risks from concomitant use with benzodiazepines or other CNS depressants:* Additive CNS depressant effects occur when drug is coadministered with drugs such as other opioids, phenothiazines, hypnotics, general anesthetics, skeletal muscle relaxants, sedating antihistamines, alcohol. Assess for hypotension, hypoventilation, profound sedation.
- *Risk of medication errors:* Do not convert a patient from another fentanyl product to fentanyl nasal spray on a mcg-per-mcg basis or substitute a fentanyl nasal spray prescription for another fentanyl product, as this may result in a fatal overdose. There is no conversion. Therefore, for all opioid tolerant patients, the initial dose should be ONE 100 mg spray and then titrated individually to provide adequate analgesia with minimal side effects.
- *Addiction, abuse, and misuse:* Drug is an opioid and may cause physical dependence and withdrawal if stopped (along with maintenance opioid) abruptly. In addition, it can lead to psychological dependence (addiction) if inappropriately used.
- *Transmucosal immediate release fentanyl (TIRF) REMS Access Program:* TIRF REMS Access Program has been developed to reduce the risk of abuse, misuse, addiction, and overdose of fentanyl. This program requires
  - Healthcare professionals who prescribe fentanyl nasal spray must review the prescriber educational materials for the TIRF REMS Access program, enroll in the program, and comply with the REMS requirements. If an outpatient, patient must sign a patient–prescriber Agreement showing the patient understands the risks and benefits.

- Pharmacies who dispense the drug must enroll in the program and agree to comply with REMS requirements.
- Wholesalers and distributers of the drug must enroll in the program and distribute only to authorized pharmacies.
- Further information is available at www.tirfremsaccess.com (1-866-822-1483).
- *Neonatal opioid withdrawal syndrome:* Prolonged use of fentanyl nasal spray during pregnancy can result in withdrawal in the neonate, and if not recognized and treated properly may be life threatening for the infant. Teach pregnant women who require prolonged treatment to ensure that there are protocols developed by neonatal experts to implement once her infant is delivered.
- *Life-threatening respiratory depression in patients with chronic pulmonary obstructive disease or in elderly, cachectic, or debilitated patients:* Chronic pulmonary disease: cautiously adjust dose of fentanyl nasal spray in these patients to avoid decreasing respiratory drive. Elderly, cachectic, or debilitated patients are also at risk. Assess closely when adjusting fentanyl dose.
- *Serotonin syndrome with concomitant use of serotonergic drugs:* has been described, such as when fentanyl is used in combination with SSRIs, SNRIs, tricyclic antidepressants, 5HT3 receptor antagonists, drugs that affect the serotonergic neurotransmitter system (e.g., trazodone, tramadol) and drugs that impair serotonin metabolism life MAO inhibitors. MAO inhibitors: the drug should not be used in patients who have received a MAO inhibitor within the last 14 days as fentanyl effect may be potentiated.
- *Adrenal insufficiency:* has been reported with opioid use > 1 month. Assess for nonspecific signs/symptoms such as nausea, vomiting, anorexia, fatigue, weakness, dizziness, and low BP. If adrenal insufficiency suspected, test as soon as possible, and if confirmed, treat with physiologic corticosteroid replacement doses. Wean the patient off the opioid to allow adrenal function to recover, and continue corticosteroids until adrenal function recovers. May try alternative opioid to see if the adverse effect is avoided, but there is no data.
- *Severe hypotension:* Drug may cause orthostatic hypotension and syncope in ambulatory patients, and the risk is increased if the patient has a low circulating blood volume or concurrent administration with certain CNS depressant drugs. When initiating and titrating dose, assess patients for signs/symptoms of hypotension. Avoid use of drug in patients with circulatory shock as the drug will cause further vasodilatation.
- *Risks of use in patients with increased intracranial pressure, brain tumors, head injury, or impaired consciousness:* Head injuries and increased ICP: opioids may obscure clinical course of these patients who are sensitive to the effects of CO_2 retention (respiratory depression).
- *Risks of use in patients with GI conditions:* Drug is contraindicated in patients with known or suspected GI obstruction. If the patient has biliary disease, monitor patient closely as opioids can cause spasm of the sphincter of Oddi and worsen symptoms. Drug may also cause an increase in serum amylase.
- *Increased risk of seizures in patients with seizure disorders:* Monitor patients with a history of seizures for worsened seizure control during fentanyl therapy.
- *Risks of driving and operating machinery:* May impair mental and/or physical ability to drive a car or operate heavy machinery. Suggest the patient have someone drive him/her until the effect of the drug is known on these skills.

- *Cardiac disease:* IV fentanyl may produce bradycardia; use drug cautiously in patients with bradyarrhythmias.
- Fentanyl citrate is not mutagenic but is embryocidal in rats; in addition, it has been shown to impair fertility. DO NOT use drug during labor and delivery, as it may cause respiratory depression in the fetus. Nursing mothers should not use the drug.
- Most common side effects during titration (frequency > 5%): nausea, vomiting, dizziness.
- Most common side effects during maintenance phase (frequency > 5%): vomiting, nausea, pyrexia, constipation.

Potential Toxicities/Side Effects and the Nursing Process

I. POTENTIAL ALTERATION IN OXYGENATION related to HYPOVENTILATION

Defining Characteristics: Increased cough and/or dyspnea are rare, but the chief toxicity in opioid-naïve patients, or if excessive dosing, is respiratory depression. Drug may cause bradycardia; thus, use with caution in patients with bradyarrhythmias.

Nursing Implications: Assess baseline pulmonary status. Use with caution in patients with COPD, bradycardia, or renal or hepatic dysfunction, and in the older population. Drug is contraindicated in opioid-naïve patients. Teach patient to report any pulmonary difficulties immediately. Ensure that patient knows that if respiratory difficulty develops to call the emergency response system (e.g., 911). Ensure that patient understands how to administer drug safely and to keep drug supply out of reach of children and pets in the specially provided secure container.

II. SENSORY/PERCEPTUAL ALTERATIONS related to CNS CHANGES

Defining Characteristics: CNS depression and changes in mental status may occur, characterized by somnolence (9%) or dizziness (6%), confusion, and headache; dysgeusia may also occur.

Nursing Implications: Assess baseline gait, mental, affective, and neurologic status. Assess medication profile to identify other contributions (i.e., CNS depressants). Instruct patient to report any changes. Assess patient safety, and measures to ensure safety. Teach patient not to take alcohol, sleep aids, or tranquilizers, except as ordered by the oncology provider. Discuss any significant changes with provider. Teach patient that drug may impair the mental and/or physical ability to operate a car or heavy machinery, and to avoid doing so while taking the drug.

III. ALTERATION IN COMFORT related to BACK PAIN, PAIN IN EXTREMITY, ARTHRALGIA

Defining Characteristics: Although uncommon, back pain, extremity pain, and arthralgias may occur.

MANAGEMENT

Nursing Implications: Assess baseline comfort. Teach patient to report symptoms and manage based on severity. Assess impact on patient's quality of life. If severe, discuss alternative strategies with physician.

IV.   ALTERATION IN NUTRITION, LESS THAN BODY REQUIREMENTS, related to NAUSEA/VOMITING

Defining Characteristics: Nausea occurred in 7% of patients during both titration and maintenance. Vomiting occurred in 6% during titration and 10% during maintenance. Dysgeusia, dry mouth, dyspepsia, mouth ulcer, proctalgia rarely occurred.

Nursing Implications: Assess baseline nutritional status, including electrolyte and fluid balance. Teach patient to take antiemetic agents as prescribed, to drink 8–10 ounces of fluid hourly while awake, and to eat small, frequent, calorie-dense foods. Teach patient to report nausea, vomiting, anorexia, and dehydration. Manage symptomatically. Assess severity and impact on quality of life. Discuss severe or unmanaged symptoms with physician.

V.   ALTERATION IN ELIMINATION related to CONSTIPATION

Defining Characteristics: Opium agonists bind to opiate receptors in bowel, slowing peristalsis, leading to constipation. Untreated constipation may result in bowel perforation. Constipation occurred in 6% of patients and diarrhea in 8%.

Nursing Implications: Assess baseline elimination, fluid intake, diet, and exercise patterns. Instruct patient regarding prevention of constipation: goal is to move bowels at least every 2 days by increasing fluids to 3 L/day (drink 8- to 10-ounce glasses of fluid every hour while awake), following a diet high in fiber (beans, vegetables, fruit), and taking moderate exercise. Review bowel regimen, and assess need for additional bowel softeners, bulk-forming laxatives, and osmotic cathartics, and discuss prescription with physician. Teach patient self-administration of medications; however, all patients MUST be started on bowel regimen when receiving an opioid.

Drug: fentanyl sublingual tablets (Abstral)

Class: Opioid analgesic (opioid agonist).

Mechanism of Action: Fentanyl is a pure opioid agonist that binds to opioid μ-receptors located in the brain, spinal cord, and smooth muscle, resulting in analgesia.

Metabolism: Orally administered fentanyl undergoes pronounced hepatic and intestinal first-pass effects. Sublingual tablets are absorbed through the oral mucosa. Bioavailability is 54%. Drug is highly lipophilic, and rapidly distributed to the brain, heart, lungs, spleen, and kidneys, followed by a slower redistribution to muscles and fat. Drug is 80–85% plasma bound; it is primarily metabolized by the liver and intestinal mucosa to norfentanyl by cytochrome P450 3A4 isoform. This metabolite is not pharmacologically active. More than 90% of fentanyl is eliminated by biotransformation into inactive metabolites. Less than 7% of intact drug is excreted in the urine and about 1% is excreted in the feces.

Indication: Indicated for the management of BTP in patients who are at least 18 years old and who are already receiving and are tolerant to opioid therapy for their underlying and persistent cancer pain.
- A patient who is considered tolerant is taking at least 60 mg oral morphine/day; or at least 25 mcg transdermal fentanyl/hour; or 30 mg oral oxycodone/day; or 8 mg oral hydromorphone/day; or 25 mg oral oxymorphone/day; or an equianalgesic dose of another opioid for a week or longer.
- Drug is available through a restricted distribution program called TIRF REMS Access Program. Outpatients and healthcare professionals who prescribe to outpatients, pharmacies, and distributors are required to enroll in the program.

Contraindications: (1) Opioid nontolerant patients; (2) management of acute or postoperative pain, including headache/migraine, dental pain, or use in the emergency department; (3) known hypersensitivity to fentanyl or components.

Dosage/Range: Opioid-tolerant patients ONLY.
- As a part of the TIRF REMS Access program, ABSTRAL may be dispensed only to outpatients enrolled in the program. For inpatient administration (e.g., hospitals, hospices, long-term care facilities that are prescribed for inpatient use), patient and prescriber enrollment is not required.
- Patients must require and use ATC opioids when taking Abstral.
- Use the lowest effective dose for the shortest duration consistent with the patient's treatment goals.
- Administer on the floor of the mouth directly under the tongue and allow to completely dissolve.
- Initial dose: 100 mcg.
- No more than 2 doses of fentanyl sublingual tablets should be used to treat an episode of BTP.
- **Individually titrate** to an effective dose, from 100 to 200 mcg, to 400 mcg, to 600 mcg, and up to a maximum of 800 mcg, with tolerable side effects.
  - Evaluate whether pain relief was adequate after 30 minutes; if yes, use the same dose for the next pain episode, and this will be the successful and usual dose.
  - If not, patient may use a second dose after the 30-minute evaluation period as directed by healthcare provider.
  - Wait at least 2 hours before treating another episode of BTP with fentanyl sublingual tablets.
  - If adequate analgesia was not obtained with the first 100-mcg dose, then continue dose escalation in a stepwise manner over consecutive breakthrough episodes until adequate analgesia with tolerable side effects is achieved.
  - Increase the dose by 100-mcg multiples up to 400 mcg as needed (four 100-mcg tablets, two 200-mcg tablets, or one 400-mcg tablet).
  - Limit consumption of to treat ≤ 4 BTP episodes/day once a successful dose is found.

MANAGEMENT

- If adequate analgesia is not achieved at 400-mcg dose, titrate up to 600 mcg (three 200-mcg tablets or one 600-mcg tablet).
- If adequate analgesia is not achieved at 600-mcg dose, titrate up to 800 mcg (four 200-mcg tablets or one 800-mcg tablet).
- If adequate analgesia is not achieved 30 minutes after the dose of sublingual fentanyl, patient may repeat the same dose. No more than 2 doses of the drug should be used to treat an episode of BTP.
- Rescue medication as directed by the healthcare provider can be used if adequate analgesia is not achieved with the two doses of sublingual fentanyl.
- Patients must be supervised by healthcare professionals during dose titration.
- Maintenance: Once the optimal dose has been identified, instruct patient to use only one sublingual fentanyl tablet of the appropriate strength per dose. If patient does not achieve adequate relief, a second dose may be used after 30 minutes (as directed by healthcare provider). Patients should wait at least 2 hours before treating another episode of BTP.
- Dosage readjustment: If there is a marked change in response or adverse reaction, it may be necessary to readjust dose. If patient has more than 4 episodes of BTP per day, reevaluate dose of the long-acting opioid used for control of persistent underlying cancer pain. If the dose of the long-acting opioid is increased, reevaluate and retitrate the fentanyl nasal spray dose.
- Limit use of fentanyl sublingual to treat fewer than 4 episodes of BTP per day once a successful dose is determined.
- When prescribing, do not convert patients on a mcg-per-mcg basis from any other oral transmucosal fentanyl product to Abstral.
- When dispensing, do not substitute with any other fentanyl product.
- Use with CYP3A4 inhibitors may cause fatal respiratory arrest. Assess patient medication profile for CYP3A4 inhibitors and discuss with physician or NP/PA if found.
- Discontinuation: Discontinue if the patient discontinues opioid therapy, consider discontinuing sublingual fentanyl tablets gradually along with a downward dosing of opioids to minimize withdrawal.

Drug Preparation: Available in 100 mcg (marked 1 on tablet), 200 mcg (marked 2 on tablet), 300 mcg (marked 3 on tablet), 400 mcg (marked 4 on tablet), 600 mcg (marked 6 on tablet), and 800 mcg (marked 8 on tablet) tablets; comes in a blister card with four blister units (each containing a tablet). Store at room temperature in the original blister pack; do not remove to store in a temporary container such as a pill box. Teach patient to store oral doses in a safe place away from children and pets, as dose of tablet may be fatal, and to protect from theft.

Drug Administration:
- Discuss with prescriber minimizing the number of strengths of drug the patient is given at any one time to prevent confusion and possible overdose.
- Remove one blister unit from card by tearing at perforation, then peel back the foil and gently remove tablet. DO NOT try to push through the foil as it will damage the tablet.
- Teach patient to place tablet(s) on the floor of the mouth directly under the tongue, immediately after removing the tablet(s) from the blister pack. Do not chew, suck, or swallow the tablet. Allow the tablet to completely dissolve under the tongue, and do not drink or eat

anything until the tablet is completely dissolved. If the patient has a dry mouth, suggest using a small amount of water to moisten the buccal mucosa before taking the tablet(s).
- Teach patient to keep drug in a safe place away from children and pets.
- Teach patient that opioid analgesics may impair the mental and/or physical ability to drive and use machines, and to avoid these activities until the effect of the drug is known.
- Disposal: Dispose of any **unused tablets** by removing from blister pack and flushing down toilet. Do not flush blister cards or cartons down the toilet. See package insert, and review patient education section and *Patient Medication Guide* with patient and caregiver.

Drug Interactions:
- Monitor patients who begin therapy with, or increase the dose of, inhibitors of CYP3A4 for signs of opioid toxicity (e.g., indinavir, nelfinavir, ritonavir, clarithromycin, itraconazole, ketoconazole, nefazodone, saquinavir, telithromycin, aprepitant, diltiazem, erythromycin, fluconazole, grapefruit juice, verapamil, or cimetidine). Coadministration may increase or prolong adverse opioid effects, including potentially fatal respiratory depression.
- Monitor patients who stop therapy with, or decrease the dose of, inducers of CYP3A4 (e.g., barbiturates, carbamazepine, efavirenz, glucocorticoids, modafinil, nevirapine, oxcarbazepine, phenobarbital, phenytoin, pioglitazone, rifabutin, rifampin, St. John's wort, troglitazone) for signs of opioid toxicity. Coadministration of an inducer and fentanyl can decrease the fentanyl serum level, so when stopping the CYP3A4 inducer, the patient may experience a sudden increase in the fentanyl plasma concentration. Adjust fentanyl sublingual tablet dose accordingly.
- CNS depressants (other opioids, sedatives, hypnotics, general anesthetics, phenothiazines, tranquilizers, skeletal muscle relaxants, sedating antihistamines), potent inhibitors of cytochrome P450 CYP3A4 isoform (erythromycin, ketoconazole, certain protease inhibitors), and alcohol: Increased CNS depression, with risk of hypoventilation, hypotension, and profound sedation.
- Moderate CYP3A4 inhibitors (aprepitant, diltiazem, grapefruit juice, verapamil): May increase fentanyl plasma levels; use together cautiously.
- MAO inhibitors with 14 days: Potentiation of opioid, do not give together.

Lab Effects/Interference:
- None known.

Special Considerations:
- Abstral is available only through the restricted Abstral REMS program, and healthcare providers who prescribe to outpatients, pharmacies, and distributors are required to enroll in the program. Further information is available at www.abstralrems.com or by calling 1-888-227-8725.
- DO NOT convert patients to fentanyl sublingual tablets from other fentanyl products on a mcg-per-mcg basis; do not substitute Abstral for any other fentanyl product, as it may result in fatal overdose.
- Warnings and Precautions:
  - Risk Evaluation and Mitigation Strategy (REMS) required for use of opioids. Healthcare providers must review REMS-compliant education. In addition, healthcare providers must

a. Complete a REMS-compliant education program offered by an accredited CE provider or another education program that includes all the elements of the FDA Education Blueprint for Health Care Providers Involved in the Management or Support of Patients with Pain. The blueprint can be found at www.fda.gov/ OpioidAnalgesicREMSBlueprint.

b. Discuss the safe use, serious risks, and proper storage and disposal of opioid analgesics with patients and/or their caregivers every time these medicines are prescribed. The Patient Counseling Guide can be obtained at www.fda.gov/ OpioidAnalgesicREMSPCG.

c. Emphasize to patients and their caregivers the importance of reading the Medication Guide that they will receive from their pharmacist every time an opioid analgesic is dispensed to them.

d. Consider using other tools to improve patient, household, and community safety, such as patient–prescriber agreements that reinforce patient–prescriber responsibilities.

- *Life-threatening respiratory depression:* Life-threatening respiratory depression can occur, even at approved doses. Assess patients closely, especially 24–72 hours within drug initiation or dose change. Ensure proper dosing and titration to prevent respiratory problems.

- *Increased risk of overdose in children due to accidental ingestion or exposure:* Keep unused as well as used dosage units out of reach of children and pets. Review patient self-administration flyer (*Abstral Medication Guide*) in package insert with patient and caregiver.

- *Risk of concomitant use or discontinuation of cytochrome P450 3A4 inhibitors and inducers:* CYP3A4 inhibitors may increase drug serum level and prolong opioid toxicity, leading to potentially fatal respiratory depression, especially when added after a stable dose has been found. Similarly, the discontinuance of a CYP3A4 inducer may increase serum fentanyl levels and prolong opioid toxicity, including respiratory depression. Conversely, discontinuation of a CYP3A4 inhibitor or addition of a CYP3A4 inducer can reduce fentanyl serum levels resulting in adequate analgesia. Monitor patient very closely, frequently; adjust fentanyl dosage as needed and safe.

- *Risks from concomitant use with benzodiazepines or other CNS depressants (including alcohol):* Profound sedation, respiratory depression, coma, and death may result. Thus, reserve concomitant use of these drugs only when no alternative exists and monitor patient closely. Assess medication profile and teach patient to avoid alcohol when receiving the drug.

- *Risk of medication errors*: Do not convert a patient to Abstral from any other fentanyl product on a mcg per mcg basis as Fentora is not equivalent to other fentanyl products on a mcg to mcg basis. Abstral is NOT a generic version of other TIRF formulations. Always start opiate tolerant patients at 200-mcg dose and individually titrate to achieve analgesia.

- *Addiction, abuse, and misuse:* Abstral contains fentanyl, a Schedule II–controlled substance. It is an opioid that exposes users to risk of addiction, abuse, and misuse, which can lead to overdose and death. Assess each patient's risk before prescribing, and monitor regularly for evidence of misuse, abuse, or diversion. Addiction is defined as psychological dependence. This is different from physical dependence (goes into withdrawal if drug is abruptly discontinued).

- *Neonatal opioid withdrawal syndrome:* Prolonged use of Abstral during pregnancy can result in neonatal opioid withdrawal syndrome, which may be life-threatening to the newborn if not recognized and treated with expert protocols. If opioid use is required for prolonged periods in a pregnant woman, teach her of the risk of neonatal opioid withdrawal syndrome, and ensure that she understands the newborn must be cared for by a healthcare personnel experienced with the protocols.
- *TIRF REMS Access Program:* (1) outpatient prescribers must review prescriber educational material, enroll in the program, and comply with the REMS requirements; (2) outpatients must understand the risks and benefits and sign the patient–prescriber agreement; (3) dispensing pharmacies must enroll in the program and agree to comply with the REMS requirements; (4) wholesalers and distributors must enroll in the program and distribute only to authorized pharmacies.
- *Life-threatening respiratory depression in patients with chronic pulmonary disease or in elderly, cachectic, or debilitated patients:* Life-threatening respiratory depression can occur, even at approved doses, especially if the patient has an underlying respiratory disorder, is elderly, or is debilitated; is not opioid tolerant; or if the drug is coadministered with other respiratory-depressing drugs. Assess for patient's reduced urge to breathe and decreased respiratory rate, often with a sighing pattern (deep breaths separated by long pauses). Retention of carbon dioxide combined with opioid sedation can lead to accidental overdose. Assess patients at risk closely, especially 24–72 hours within drug initiation or dose change. Ensure proper dosing and titration to prevent respiratory problems
- *Adrenal insufficiency:* Adrenal insufficiency has occurred, especially in patients receiving opioids for >1 month. Signs/symptoms include: nausea, vomiting, anorexia, fatigue, weakness, dizziness, low BP. If adrenal insufficiency is suspected, confirm the diagnosis with lab testing; if confirmed, treat with physiological doses of corticosteroids. Wean the patient off the opioid to allow adrenal function recovery while continuing corticosteroids. Other opioids should be tried.
- *Severe hypotension:* Severe hypotension may occur, including orthostatic hypotension and syncope in ambulatory patients, especially in patients with reduced blood volume or receiving concurrent certain CNS depressing drugs (e.g., phenothiazines, general anesthetics). Monitor these patients closely for signs/symptoms hypotension after starting drug or dose titration. Do not use Exalgo in patients with circulatory shock.
- *Risk of use in patients with head injury, brain tumor, or increased ICP:* Opioids may obscure clinical course of these patients who are sensitive to the effects of CO_2 retention (respiratory depression). Monitor for sedation and respiratory depression. Avoid use of Fentora in patients with impaired consciousness or coma who are susceptible to the intracranial effects of CO_2 retention.
- *Serotonin syndrome with concomitant use of serotonergic drugs:* Serotonin syndrome (e.g., characterized by mental status changes, autonomic instability, neuromuscular abnormalities, and GI symptoms) has occurred when patients received both fentanyl transdermal patch and serotonergic drugs (e.g., SSRIs, SNRIs, TCAs triptans, 5-HT3 receptor antagonists, drugs that affect the serotonergic neurotransmitter system (e.g., mirtazapine, trazodone, tramadol), and drugs that impair metabolism of serotonin (e.g., MAO inhibitors) (Sentanyl, 2016). If serotonin syndrome occurs, onset is

MANAGEMENT

usually within several hours to a few days after concomitant use but may occur later. If serotonin syndrome is suspected, immediately discontinue Fentora is the syndrome is suspected and convert to immediate acting opioids.

- *Risk of use in patients with GI conditions:* Drug is contraindicated if GI obstruction is suspected or known. Opioids can cause spasm of the sphincter of Oddi and cause increases in serum amylase; monitor patients with biliary tract disease, including acute pancreatitis, for worsening symptoms.
- *Increased risk of seizures in patients with seizure disorders:* Drug may increase seizure frequency or occurrence in other clinical settings. Monitor patients with a seizure history closely for worsening seizure control when taking this drug.
- *Risks of driving and operating machinery:* Drug may impair mental and/or physical abilities of driving or operating machinery. Teach patient to avoid driving and operation of machinery until the effect of the opioid is known.
- *Cardiac disease*: IV fentanyl may produce bradycardia. Use drug cautiously in patients with bradyarrhythmias.
- Use fentanyl sublingual tablets with extreme caution in patients:
  - With hepatic and/or renal dysfunction, head injuries, increased ICP, cardiac disease (especially with bradyarrythmias), and chronic pulmonary disease.
  - With COPD or preexisting medical conditions predisposing them to hypoventilation.
  - Susceptible to intracranial effects of CO_2 retention.
  - Taking other CNS depressants and potent CYP3A4 inhibitors; they may have increased depressant effects, including hypoventilation, hypotension, and profound sedation. Consider dosage adjustments if warranted.
  - Who are elderly; they are more sensitive to opioids.
  - Who are pregnant: fentanyl citrate is not mutagenic but is embryocidal in rats; in addition, it has been shown to impair fertility. If drug must be given to a pregnant woman, benefit must outweigh potential risk to the fetus.
- DO NOT use drug during labor and delivery, as it may cause respiratory depression in the fetus. Nursing mothers should not take the drug.
- Teach patient that drug must be kept out of reach of children and pets, as dose can be LETHAL to children and pets.
- Most common side effects during titration (frequency > 3%): nausea and somnolence.
- Most common side effects during maintenance phase (frequency > 3%): headache, nausea, constipation.

Potential Toxicities/Side Effects and the Nursing Process

I.   POTENTIAL ALTERATION IN OXYGENATION related to HYPOVENTILATION

Defining Characteristics: Increased cough and/or dyspnea are rare, but the chief toxicity in opioid-naïve patients or if excessive dosing is respiratory depression. Drug may cause bradycardia; thus, use with caution in patients with bradyarrhythmias.

Nursing Implications: Assess baseline pulmonary status. Use with caution in patients with COPD, bradycardia, or renal or hepatic dysfunction, and in the older population.

Teach patient to report any pulmonary difficulties immediately. Ensure that patient knows that if respiratory difficulty develops, the drug must be removed from mouth and discarded in the toilet immediately. Ensure that patient understands how to administer drug safely and to keep drug supply out of reach of children and pets. If respiratory distress occurs, teach patient to call 911 or the local emergency number.

II.   SENSORY/PERCEPTUAL ALTERATIONS related to CNS CHANGES

Defining Characteristics: CNS depression and changes in mental status may occur, characterized by somnolence (4%) or dizziness (2%), and headache (2%). Less commonly, dysgeusia, attention disturbance, amnesia, hypoesthesia, lethargy, labile affect, confusion, depression, disorientation, dysphoria, insomnia, change in mental status, paranoia, sleep disorder, tremor, parosmia (distortion in sense of smell) may occur.

Nursing Implications: Assess baseline gait, mental, affective, and neurologic status. Assess medication profile to identify other contributions (i.e., CNS depressants). Instruct patient to report any changes. Assess patient safety, and measures to ensure safety. Teach patient not to take alcohol, sleep aids, or tranquilizers, except as ordered by the oncology provider. Discuss any significant changes with provider.

III.   ALTERATION IN NUTRITION, LESS THAN BODY REQUIREMENTS, related to NAUSEA/VOMITING

Defining Characteristics: During the titration phase, nausea occurred in 6% of patients; in the maintenance phase, nausea (6%), stomatitis (2%), constipation (5%), and dry mouth (2%) occurred. Rare: abdominal discomfort, dyspepsia, gingival ulceration, impaired gastric emptying, lip ulceration, tongue disorder, and stomatitis occurred.

Nursing Implications: Assess baseline nutritional status including fluid balance. Teach patient to take antiemetic agents as prescribed if needed, to drink 8–10 ounces of fluid hourly while awake, and to eat small, frequent, calorie-dense foods. Teach patient to report nausea, vomiting, anorexia, and dehydration. Manage symptomatically. Assess severity and impact on quality of life. Discuss severe or unmanaged symptoms with physician.

IV.   ALTERATION IN ELIMINATION related to CONSTIPATION

Defining Characteristics: Opium agonists bind to opiate receptors in bowel, slowing peristalsis, leading to constipation. Untreated constipation may result in bowel perforation. Constipation occurred in 5% of patients.

Nursing Implications: Assess baseline elimination, fluid intake, diet, and exercise patterns. Instruct patient regarding prevention of constipation: Goal is to move bowels at least every 2 days by increasing fluids to 3 L/day (drink 8- to 10-ounce glasses of fluid every hour while awake), following a diet high in fiber (beans, vegetables, fruit), and taking moderate exercise. Review bowel regimen, and assess need for additional bowel softeners, bulk-forming laxatives, and osmotic cathartics, and discuss prescription with physician. Teach patient self-administration of medications. However, all patients MUST be started on bowel regimen when receiving an opioid.

Drug: fentanyl sublingual spray (Subsys)

Class: Opioid analgesic (opioid agonist).

Mechanism of Action: Fentanyl is a pure opioid agonist that binds to opioid μ-receptors located in the brain, spinal cord, and smooth muscle, to achieve analgesia.

Metabolism: Following a sublingual spray administration of 400 mcg, the mean bioavailability of fentanyl was 76%. The pharmacokinetics are based on how much of the drug is transmucosally absorbed and how much is swallowed. Peak serum levels achieved in 1.5–2 hours. Patients with mucositis had higher AUC drug levels: grade 1: 73% greater maximum plasma concentration (C_{max}) and systemic exposure compared to patients without mucositis, and patients with grades 2 had 4–7 times greater C_{max}. Primarily metabolized by the liver and intestinal microflora to norfentanyl via CYP3A4 microenzyme system. Drug is highly lipophilic, and is rapidly distributed to the brain, heart, lungs, kidneys, and spleen, then more slowly to the muscles and fat. Drug is 80–85% bound to plasma proteins. More than 90% of drug is eliminated as inactive metabolites, with < 7% excreted in urine, and < 1% in feces, as unchanged drug. Terminal half-life after sublingual spray is 5–12 hours.

Indication: Management of BTP in cancer patients 18 years and older who are already receiving and are tolerant to opioid therapy for their underlying persistent cancer pain.
• Patient must remain on ATC opioids when taking Subsys.
• A patient who is considered tolerant is taking **at least** 60 mg oral morphine/day; or 25 mcg transdermal fentanyl/hour; or 30 mg oral oxycodone/day; or 8 mg oral hydromorphone/day; or 25 mg oral oxymorphone/day; or an equianalgesic dose of another opioid for a week or longer.
• Drug is available through a restricted distribution program called TIRF REMS Access Program. Outpatients and healthcare professionals who prescribe to outpatients, pharmacies, and distributors are required to enroll in the program.

Contraindications: (1) Opioid nontolerant patients; (2) management of acute or postoperative pain, including headache/migraine, dental pain, or in the emergency department; (3) acute or severe bronchial asthma in an unmonitored setting or if resuscitation equipment is unavailable; (4) known or suspected GI obstruction, including paralytic ileus; (5) known hypersensitivity to fentanyl, Subsys, or its components.

Dosage/Range:
• Risk Evaluation and Mitigation Strategy (REMS) required for use of opioids. Healthcare providers must review REMS-compliant education (see below). In addition, healthcare providers must
  a. Complete a REMS-compliant education program offered by an accredited CE provider or another education program that includes all the elements of the FDA Education Blueprint for Health Care Providers Involved in the Management

or Support of Patients with Pain. The blueprint can be found at www.fda.gov/OpioidAnalgesicREMSBlueprint.

b. Discuss the safe use, serious risks, and proper storage and disposal of opioid analgesics with patients and/or their caregivers every time these medicines are prescribed. The Patient Counseling Guide can be obtained at www.fda.gov/OpioidAnalgesic REMSPCG.

c. Emphasize to patients and their caregivers the importance of reading the Medication Guide that they will receive from their pharmacist every time an opioid analgesic is dispensed to them.

d. Consider using other tools to improve patient, household, and community safety, such as patient–prescriber agreements that reinforce patient–prescriber responsibilities.

- Patients must require ATC opioids when taking fentanyl sublingual spray.
- Use lowest effective dose for the shortest duration consistent with patient's treatment goals.
- Individualize dosing based on pain severity, patient response, prior analgesic experience, and risk factors for addiction, abuse, and misuse.
- Initial dose is 100 micrograms (mcg); initial prescription should be for 100-mcg spray only (except if already receiving Actiq). If switching from another fentanyl product, the initial dose is still 100 mcg.
- Individually titrate to an effective and tolerable dose using a single sublingual spray breakthrough dose per episode. Avoid prescribing a higher dose until patient has used up all units to prevent confusion and possible overdose.
  - No more than 2 doses can be taken per BTP episode.
  - Wait at least 4 hours before treating another episode of BTP with sublingual fentanyl.
  - Limit consumption to 4 or fewer doses per day once a successful dose is found.
  - When opioid therapy is discontinued, discontinue fentanyl sublingual spray along with other opioids in a gradual taper, rather than abruptly, to minimize chance of withdrawal.
  - Fentanyl sublingual spray is NOT a generic version of any other oral transmucosal fentanyl product.
  - See package insert and patient educational material for titration steps.
- If patient already receiving Actiq: start with dosing schedule below, teach patient to stop using Actiq and how to properly dispose of any remaining units. See package insert.
  - Current Actiq dose: 200 mcg = initial Subsys dose (mcg) 100-mcg spray
  - Current Actiq dose: 400 mcg = initial Subsys dose (mcg) 100-mcg spray
  - Current Actiq dose: 600 mcg = initial Subsys dose (mcg) 200-mcg spray
  - Current Actiq dose: 800 mcg = initial Subsys dose (mcg) 200-mcg spray
  - Current Actiq dose: 1,200 mcg = initial Subsys dose (mcg) 400-mcg spray
  - Current Actiq dose: 1,600 mcg = initial Subsys dose (mcg) 400-mcg spray
- Do not switch patients on a mcg-per-mcg basis from any other oral transmucosal fentanyl product to Subsys.
- To reduce risk of overdosage during titration, patients should have only one strength of Subsys available at any one time.
- Dose modification in patients with oral mucositis: Patients have increased drug exposure and require closer monitoring for respiratory and CNS depression, especially when drug is being started. If patient has grade 2 or higher mucositis, avoid use of SUBSYS unless benefits outweigh the risks.

Drug Preparation:
- Available in 100-, 200-, 400-, 600-, and 800-mcg dosage strengths.

Drug Interactions:
- Mixed agonist/antagonist and partial agonist opioid analgesic: avoid use with fentanyl sublingual spray as they may reduce analgesic effect of the fentanyl sublingual spray or may precipitate withdrawal.
- CYP 3A4 inhibitors: (strong or moderate): may increase depressant effects, including respiratory depression, hypotension, and profound sedation. Consider dosage adjustments if needed.
- CNS depressants: may increase depressant effects, including respiratory depression, hypotension, and profound sedation. Consider dosage adjustments if needed.

Lab Effects/Interference:
- None known.

Special Considerations:
- Warnings and Precautions:
  - *Life-threatening respiratory depression:* Life-threatening respiratory depression can occur, even at approved doses. Assess patients closely, especially 24–72 hours within drug initiation or dose change. Ensure proper dosing and titration to prevent respiratory problems
  - *Increased risk of overdose in children due to accidental ingestion or exposure:* Keep unused as well as used dosage units out of reach of children and pets. Review patient self-administration flyer (*SUBSYS Medication Guide)* in package insert with patient and caregiver. Guide gives important instructions for managing overdosage. Review patient educational material with patient and caregiver, and answer any questions.
  - *Risk of concomitant use or discontinuation of cytochrome P450 3A4 inhibitors and inducers:* CYP3A4 inhibitors may increase drug serum level and prolong opioid toxicity, leading to potentially fatal respiratory depression, especially when added after a stable dose has been found. Similarly, the discontinuance of a CYP3A4 inducer may increase serum fentanyl levels and prolong opioid toxicity, including respiratory depression. Conversely, discontinuation of a CYP3A4 inhibitor or addition of a CYP3A4 inducer can reduce fentanyl serum levels resulting in adequate analgesia. Monitor patient very closely, frequently; adjust fentanyl dosage as needed and safe.
  - *Risks from concomitant use with benzodiazepines or other CNS depressants (including alcohol):* Profound sedation, respiratory depression, coma, and death may result. Thus, reserve concomitant use of these drugs only when no alternative exists and monitor patient closely. Assess medication profile and teach patient to avoid alcohol when receiving the drug.
  - *Risk of medication errors:* Do not convert a patient to SUBSYS from any other fentanyl product on a mcg per mcg basis as Fentora is not equivalent to other fentanyl products on a mcg to mcg basis. SUBSYS is NOT a generic version of other TIRF formulations. Always start opiate tolerant patients at 200-mcg dose and individually titrate to achieve analgesia.
  - *Addiction, abuse, and misuse:* SUBSYS contains fentanyl, a Schedule II–controlled substance. It is an opioid that exposes users to risk of addiction, abuse, and misuse, which can lead to overdose and death. Assess each patient's risk before prescribing, and monitor regularly for evidence of misuse, abuse, or diversion. Addiction

is defined as psychological dependence. This is different from physical dependence (goes into withdrawal if drug is abruptly discontinued).

- *Neonatal opioid withdrawal syndrome:* Prolonged use of SUBSYS during pregnancy can result in neonatal opioid withdrawal syndrome, which may be life-threatening to the newborn if not recognized and treated with expert protocols. If opioid use is required for prolonged periods in a pregnant woman, teach her of the risk of neonatal opioid withdrawal syndrome, and ensure that she understands the newborn must be cared for by a healthcare personnel experienced with the protocols.

- *TIRF REMS Access Program:* (1) Outpatient prescribers must review prescriber educational material, enroll in the program, and comply with the REMS requirements; (2) outpatients must understand the risks and benefits and sign the patient–prescriber agreement; (3) dispensing pharmacies must enroll in the program and agree to comply with the REMS requirements; (4) wholesalers and distributors must enroll in the program and distribute only to authorized pharmacies.

- *Life-threatening respiratory depression in patients with chronic pulmonary disease or in elderly, cachectic, or debilitated patients:* Life-threatening respiratory depression can occur, even at approved doses, especially if the patient has an underlying respiratory disorder, is elderly, or is debilitated; is not opioid tolerant; or if the drug is coadministered with other respiratory-depressing drugs. Assess for patient's reduced urge to breathe and decreased respiratory rate, often with a sighing pattern (deep breaths separated by long pauses). Retention of carbon dioxide combined with opioid sedation can lead to accidental overdose. Assess patients at risk closely, especially 24–72 hours within drug initiation or dose change. Ensure proper dosing and titration to prevent respiratory problems.

- *Adrenal insufficiency:* Adrenal insufficiency has occurred, especially in patients receiving opioids for >1 month. Signs/symptoms include: nausea, vomiting, anorexia, fatigue, weakness, dizziness, low BP. If adrenal insufficiency is suspected, confirm the diagnosis with lab testing; if confirmed, treat with physiological doses of corticosteroids. Wean the patient off the opioid to allow adrenal function recovery while continuing corticosteroids. Other opioids should be tried.

- *Severe hypotension:* Severe hypotension may occur, including orthostatic hypotension and syncope in ambulatory patients, especially in patients with reduced blood volume, or receiving concurrent certain CNS depressing drugs (e.g., phenothiazines, general anesthetics). Monitor these patients closely for signs/symptoms hypotension after starting drug or dose titration. Do not use Exalgo in patients with circulatory shock.

- *Risk of use in patients with head injury, brain tumor, or increased ICP:* Opioids may obscure clinical course of these patients who are sensitive to the effects of CO_2 retention (respiratory depression). Monitor for sedation and respiratory depression. Avoid use of Fentora in patients with impaired consciousness or coma who are susceptible to the intracranial effects of CO_2 retention.

- *Serotonin syndrome with concomitant use of serotonergic drugs:* Serotonin syndrome (e.g., characterized by mental status changes, autonomic instability, neuromuscular abnormalities, and GI symptoms) has occurred when patients received both fentanyl transdermal patch and serotonergic drugs (e.g., SNRIs, TCAs triptans, 5-HT3 receptor antagonists, drugs that affect the serotonergic neurotransmitter system (e.g., mirtazapine, trazodone, tramadol), and drugs that impair metabolism of serotonin (e.g., MAO inhibitors) (Insys Therapeutics, 2016). If serotonin syndrome occurs, onset is usually within several hours to a few days after concomitant use but may occur later. If serotonin syndrome is suspected, immediately discontinue Fentora is the syndrome is suspected and convert to immediate acting opioids.

- *Risk of use in patients with GI conditions:* Drug is contraindicated if GI obstruction is suspected or known. Opioids can cause spasm of the sphincter of Oddi and cause increases in serum amylase; monitor patients with biliary tract disease, including acute pancreatitis, for worsening symptoms.
- *Increased risk of seizures in patients with seizure disorders:* Drug may increase seizure frequency or occurrence in other clinical settings. Monitor patients with a seizure history closely for worsening seizure control when taking this drug.
- *Risks of driving and operating machinery:* Drug may impair mental and/or physical abilities of driving or operating machinery. Teach patient to avoid driving and operation of machinery until the effect of the opioid is known.
- *Cardiac disease:* IV fentanyl may produce bradycardia. Use drug cautiously in patients with bradyarrhythmias.
- Teach patient/caregiver to safely store and dispose of drug as appropriate and to keep it away from children and pets, as drug can be fatal to a child. Full and consumed SUBSYS units contain medication that can be fatal to a child or pet. Ensure proper storage and disposal.
- Most common adverse effects during treatment (> 5%): vomiting, nausea, constipation, dyspnea, somnolence.

Potential Toxicities/Side Effects and the Nursing Process

I.   POTENTIAL ALTERATION IN OXYGENATION related to HYPOVENTILATION

Defining Characteristics: Increased cough and/or dyspnea are rare, but the chief toxicity in opioid-naïve patients or if there is excessive dosing is respiratory depression. Drug may cause bradycardia; thus, use with caution in patients with bradyarrhythmias.

Nursing Implications: Assess baseline pulmonary status. Use with caution in patients with COPD, bradycardia, or renal or hepatic dysfunction, and in the older population. Teach patient to report any pulmonary difficulties immediately. Ensure that patient knows that if respiratory difficulty develops, the drug must be removed from mouth and discarded in the toilet immediately. Ensure that patient understands how to administer drug safely and to keep drug supply out of reach of children and pets. If respiratory distress occurs, teach patient to call 911 or the local emergency number.

II.   SENSORY/PERCEPTUAL ALTERATIONS related to CNS CHANGES

Defining Characteristics: CNS depression and changes in mental status may occur, characterized by somnolence (4%) or dizziness (2%), and headache (2%). Less commonly, dysgeusia, attention disturbance, amnesia, hypoesthesia, lethargy, labile affect, confusion, depression, disorientation, dysphoria, insomnia, change in mental status, paranoia, sleep disorder, tremor, parosmia (distortion in sense of smell) may occur.

Nursing Implications: Assess baseline gait, mental, affective, and neurologic status. Assess medication profile to identify other contributions (i.e., CNS depressants). Instruct patient to report any changes. Assess patient safety, and measures to ensure safety. Teach patient not to take alcohol, sleep aids, or tranquilizers, except as ordered by the oncology provider. Discuss any significant changes with provider.

III. ALTERATION IN NUTRITION, LESS THAN BODY REQUIREMENTS, related to NAUSEA/VOMITING

Defining Characteristics: During the titration phase, nausea occurred in 6% of patients; in the maintenance phase, nausea (6%), stomatitis (2%), constipation (5%), and dry mouth (2%) occurred. Rare: abdominal discomfort, dyspepsia, gingival ulceration, impaired gastric emptying, lip ulceration, tongue disorder, and stomatitis occurred.

Nursing Implications: Assess baseline nutritional status, including fluid balance. Teach patient to take antiemetic agents as prescribed, if needed, to drink 8–10 ounces of fluid hourly while awake, and to eat small, frequent, calorie-dense foods. Teach patient to report nausea, vomiting, anorexia, and dehydration. Manage symptomatically. Assess severity and impact on quality of life. Discuss severe or unmanaged symptoms with physician.

IV. ALTERATION IN ELIMINATION related to CONSTIPATION

Defining Characteristics: Opium agonists bind to opiate receptors in bowel, slowing peristalsis, leading to constipation. Untreated constipation may result in bowel perforation. Constipation occurred in 5% of patients.

Nursing Implications: Assess baseline elimination, fluid intake, diet, and exercise patterns. Instruct patient regarding prevention of constipation: Goal is to move bowels at least every 2 days by increasing fluids to 3 L/day (drink 8- to 10-ounce glasses of fluid every hour while awake), following a diet high in fiber (beans, vegetables, fruit), and taking moderate exercise. Review bowel regimen; assess need for additional bowel softeners, bulk-forming laxatives, and osmotic cathartics; and discuss prescription with physician. Teach patient self-administration of medications. However, all patients MUST be started on bowel regimen when receiving an opioid.

Drug: fentanyl transdermal system (Duragesic)

Class: Opioid analgesic (opioid agonist).

Mechanism of Action: Strong opioid analgesic; 20–30 times more potent than parenteral morphine when given transdermally to opioid-naïve patients. Drug interacts primarily with

MANAGEMENT

opioid μ-receptors, found in the brain, spinal cord, and other tissues, causing analgesia and sedation. Transdermal fentanyl patches provide continuous-released fentanyl from a transdermal reservoir system at a constant amount per unit time. The drug moves from areas of higher concentration (patch) to areas of lower concentration (skin). Initially, the skin under the patch absorbs the fentanyl, and the drug is concentrated in the upper skin layers. The drug gradually enters the systemic circulation, leveling off 2–24 hours later, and remaining fairly constant for the 72-hour application period.

Metabolism: Primarily metabolized by the liver; 75% of IV dose excreted in urine, 9% in feces, and < 10% as unchanged drug. Peak levels occur 24–72 hours after a single application. Half-life is ~17 hours (after system removal, serum fentanyl concentrations fall to 50% in ~17 hours; range, 13–22 hours).

Indication: In opioid-tolerant patients, management of pain severe enough to require daily, ATC, long-term opioid treatment, and for which alternative treatment is inadequate. A patient who is considered tolerant is taking for at least 1 week or longer, at least 60 mg oral morphine/day; or 25 mcg transdermal fentanyl/hour; or 30 mg oral oxycodone/day; or 8 mg oral hydromorphone/day; or 25 mg oral oxymorphone/day; or 60 mg oral hydrocodone/day; or an equianalgesic dose of another opioid for a week or longer.

Limitations of use: Because of risks of addiction, abuse, and misuse of opioids, even at recommended doses, and because of the greater risks of overdose and death with extended-release opioid formulations, Duragesic drug is reserved for use in patients for whom alternative treatment options (e.g., nonopioid analgesics or immediate-release opioids) are ineffective, not tolerated, or would be otherwise inadequate to provide sufficient management of pain.

Contraindications: (1) Opioid nontolerant patients; (2) acute or intermittent pain, postoperative pain, mild pain; (3) significant respiratory depression; (4) acute or severe bronchial asthma in an unmonitored setting or in the absence of resuscitative equipment; (5) known or suspected GI obstruction, including paralytic ileus; (6) known hypersensitivity to fentanyl or any components of transdermal system; (7) as needed (PRN) use.

Dosage/Range:
- Risk Evaluation and Mitigation Strategy (REMS) required for use of opioids. Healthcare providers must review REMS-compliant education. In addition, healthcare providers must
  a. Complete a REMS-compliant education program offered by an accredited CE provider or another education program that includes all the elements of the FDA Education Blueprint for Health Care Providers Involved in the Management or Support of Patients with Pain. The blueprint can be found at www.fda.gov/OpioidAnalgesicREMSBlueprint.
  b. Discuss the safe use, serious risks, and proper storage and disposal of opioid analgesics with patients and/or their caregivers every time these medicines are prescribed. The Patient Counseling Guide can be obtained at www.fda.gov/OpioidAnalgesic REMSPCG.
  c. Emphasize to patients and their caregivers the importance of reading the Medication Guide that they will receive from their pharmacist every time an opioid analgesic is dispensed to them.

   d. Consider using other tools to improve patient, household, and community safety, such as patient–prescriber agreements that reinforce patient–prescriber responsibilities.

- To be prescribed only by healthcare providers knowledgeable in use of potent opioids for management of chronic pain.
- Use the lowest effective dosage for the shortest duration consistent with individual patient treatment goals.
- Individualize dosing based on the severity of pain, patient response, prior analgesic experience, and risk factors for addiction, abuse, and misuse.
- Each transdermal system is intended to be worn for 72 hours. Reduce dose in geriatric patients or if patient has persistent fever.
- Adhere to instructions concerning administration and disposal of transdermal fentanyl patch.
- Do not use in patients with severe hepatic impairment.
- If patient has mild-to-moderate hepatic dysfunction, start with one-half the usual transdermal fentanyl dose; monitor closely for sedation and respiratory depression, initially and with every dosage increase.
- Renal impairment: Avoid transdermal fentanyl if severe renal impairment; if mild or moderate, start with one-half of the usual transdermal fentanyl dose; monitor closely for sedation and respiratory depression, initially and with every dosage increase.
- Do NOT abruptly discontinue fentanyl transdermal patch in a physically dependent patient as this may precipitate withdrawal.
- **Initial doses** for patients currently receiving opioid analgesics who are tolerant can be calculated from information in Tables 1 and 2 of the Duragesic package insert (September 2018).
- DO NOT initiate treatment with fentanyl transdermal patch in opioid nontolerant patients (see contraindications).
- Discontinue all other ATC opioid drugs when fentanyl therapy is started.
- Monitor the patient closely for respiratory depression, especially in the first 24–72 hours of initiating therapy when serum concentration peaks.

Alternatively, for adult and pediatric patients taking opioids or doses not listed in Table 2 in the package insert, use the following methodology and package insert:

1. Calculate the previous 24-hour analgesic requirement.
2. Convert this amount to the equianalgesic oral morphine dose, using a reliable reference. Initiate transdermal fentanyl treatment using the recommended dose (see package insert Table 1) and titrate patients upwards (no more frequently than 3 days after the initial dose and every 6 days thereafter) until effective analgesia is attained.
3. The recommended starting dose when converting from other opioids to fentanyl transdermal is intended to minimize the potential for overdosing with the first dose.

Titration and Maintenance of Therapy:
Individually titrate Duragesic to a dose that gives adequate analgesia and minimizes toxicity. This requires continual reevaluation to assess pain control and incidence of adverse reactions, including frequent telephone calls or communication between prescriber or nurse, the patient, and home-care nurse.

- Dosing interval is 72 hours; do not increase the fentanyl transdermal patch dose for the first time until at least 3 days after initial Duragesic patch is applied.

MANAGEMENT

- Ensure patient has a prescription that is filled for BTP medication and to keep a diary of each time the breakthrough medication is needed and pain intensity.
- Titrate the dose based on the patient's need for supplemental short-acting, BTP medication on days 2 and 3 after application until the next patch is due. It may take up to 6 days for fentanyl levels to reach equilibrium on a new dose. Thus, further titration should wait until two 3-day applications have been made before any further dose increase.
- Base dosage increments on the amount of daily BTP medications needed using the ratio of 45 mg/24 hours of oral morphine to a 12 mcg/hr increase in Duragesic dose (Janssen, 2017).
- Adjust the dose to achieve analgesia and to balance any adverse effects that occur.
- If, once the dose has been stabilized, the patient has increased pain, discuss with the provider ways to identify possible sources of the increased pain before increasing the transdermal fentanyl.

Some patients will require a 48-hour change in Duragesic but an increase in Duragesic dose every 3 days, prior to decreasing the interval to 48 hours. This may occur if the patient has persistent fever, and the patch medication is absorbed after 48 hours. Dosing intervals < every 72 hours has not been studied in children or adolescents.

Drug Preparation:
- Transdermal systems available: 12, 25, 37.5, 50, 75, 100 mcg/hr.

Drug Administration:
- Review patient written instructions from package insert.
- Remove existing transdermal fentanyl patch, and select a different site for new patch. Apply to nonirritated and nonirradiated skin; clip hair (not shave) as needed. May cleanse with water only and allow to dry completely if necessary. Select site that is a flat surface such as the chest, back, flank, or upper arm. In young children and persons with cognitive impairment, monitor that patch is adhering to the skin (upper back preferred location).
  - Apply patch immediately after removal from package (do not cut in any way), and after removal of the outer protective hard plastic liner.
  - Press firmly into place with palm of hand for 10–20 seconds, making sure contact is complete, especially around edges. Patient wears for 72 hours, then changes patch. Some patients may need to reapply new patches every 48 hours especially if febrile.
  - Short-acting opioids must be continued for at least 24 hours until serum fentanyl level achieved to provide BTP analgesia and until correct transdermal fentanyl dose determined.
  - If adhesion is a problem, the edges may be taped, and if problem persists, patch may be overlaid with a transparent adhesive film dressing.
  - If the patch falls off before 72 hours, it should be properly disposed of and a new patch should be applied in a different skin site.
  - If a patient develops fever, or increased core body temperature due to strenuous exertion, the drug may be more quickly absorbed and the patient at risk for increased toxicity; the patient may need dose reduction.
- Patient/Caregiver Teaching:
  - Wash hands with soap and water after applying the patch to prevent accidental exposure to a child or other person (e.g., if hugging). Wash off site of previous patch and wash hands and towel again as drug may be present.

- Store oral doses in a safe place away from children and pets, as accidental ingestion can be fatal.
- Opioid analgesics may impair the mental and/or physical ability to drive and use machines; avoid these activities until the effect of the drug is known.
- Heat can increase fentanyl absorption from the patch, this increasing risk of overdosage, which may be fatal. This can occur when the anatomical location is exposed to direct heat source, such as an electric blanket, heat/tanning lamp, hot bath, sauna, hot tub, heated water bed, or while sunbathing. Teach patient to avoid heat sources to the application site (e.g., hot tub, sunbathing).
- Disposal: at home, patient must fold so adhesive side of system adheres to itself; then flush it down the toilet (Janssen, 2017). In hospital, used patches must be returned to pharmacy for proper disposal. If the patch is unused, the plastic backing should be removed, and sticky side folded together then flushed down the toilet. Care must be used to properly dispose of transdermal patches as it might otherwise result in accidental exposure and death.
- When not converting to another opioid, use a gradual titration downward (e.g., 50% dose reduction every 6 days) while monitoring for signs/symptoms of withdrawal. If the patient develops signs/symptoms, raise the dose to the previous level and taper more slowly (e.g., increase interval between decreases, decreasing the amount of change in dose, or both). Do not abruptly discontinue.
- Pediatric use: safety and efficacy in pediatric patients < 2 years old has not been established. To guard against accidental ingestion by children, use caution when choosing the application site (back is preferred).
- Accidental exposure: teach patients to strictly adhere to recommended handling and disposal instructions.
- **Risks of concomitant use** or discontinuation of CYP3A4 inhibitors: (e.g., macrolide antibiotics, azole-antifungal agents, and protease inhibitors) may increase the serum fentanyl level causing potentially fatal respiratory depression. Avoid if possible, but otherwise monitor closely and frequently. Consider decreasing fentanyl dose if necessary.
- **Risks of concomitant use** or discontinuation of CYP3A4 inducers may decrease fentanyl concentration, decrease opioid efficiency, or lead to withdrawal. When drug is discontinued, serum fentanyl level may increase with toxicity. Monitor patient closely and frequently if an inducer is coadministered or discontinued.

Drug Initiation:
- Assess patient for 24–72 hours and use a consistent pain intensity scale, when serum concentrations from the initial patch will peak. It may take as long as 6 days when the dose is titrated up; therefore, wait for two 72-hour dosing at the new increased dose before further increasing the dose. Continue short-acting, break through medications during this time, and factor their equianalgeic dose in when determining the increase in dose needed. For equivalence, morphine 45 mg/24 hours = 12 mcg/24 hours transdermal fentanyl (Mylan, 2014).
- Discontinue all other long-acting, ATC medications when transdermal fentanyl is initiated.
- It is preferable to underestimate the patient's 24-hour fentanyl requirement and provide rescue medication than to overestimate it and have the patient somnolent.

- Use Dosing Table in package insert (Janssen, 2017).
- Hypotensive effects: monitor BP and pulse during initiation and titration.

Discontinuance of fentanyl transdermal system:
- Significant amounts of fentanyl continue to be absorbed for 24 hours or more once the patch is removed.
- Convert to another opioid: remove transdermal patch and titrate the dose of the new analgesic based upon patient assessment of pain until adequate analgesia achieved-17 hours or more are necessary for a 50% decrease in serum fentanyl concentration. Withdrawal symptoms may occur after conversion or dose adjustment (see package insert). Do not use package insert tables for conversion as this may cause an overdose of the new analgesic.
- When discontinuing transdermal fentanyl without conversion to another opioid, use a gradual downward titration, such as halving the dose every 6 days, in order to reduce the chance of withdrawal symptoms.

Drug Interactions:
- Potentiation of CNS depressant effects, when administered concurrently with other opioids, benzodiazepines, or other CNS depressants.
- Mixed agonist/antagonist and partial opioid analgesics: Do not use together, as they may reduce analgesic effect or precipitate withdrawal symptoms.
- CYP3A4 inhibitors: May result in increased fentanyl plasma concentrations and risk for toxicity. Avoid coadministration.
- CYP3A4 inducer: May decrease fentanyl plasma levels. If they are concomitantly administered, and the CYP3A4 inducer is discontinued, assess for increased fentanyl plasma levels and increased risk for toxicity.
- Monomine oxidase inhibitors (MAOIs): Avoid use with fentanyl transdermal system in these patients or within 14 days of stopping MAOIs.

Lab Effects/Interference:
- None known.

Special Considerations:
- Warnings and Precautions:
  - *Addiction, abuse and misuse:* Drug is a Schedule II–controlled substance with an abuse potential similar to other opioid analgesics. TIRF REMS Access Program has been developed to reduce the risk of abuse, misuse, addiction, and overdose of fentanyl. This program requires training, patient education, and use of a medication guide. Assess patient's likelihood to abuse the drug, or if patient's family members may do so, and develop a plan to provide analgesia while preventing abuse.
- *Opioid Analgesic Risk Evaluation and Mitigation Strategy (REMS):* REMS is now required for use of all opioids. Healthcare providers must review REMS-compliant education. In addition, healthcare providers must
- Complete a REMS-compliant education program offered by an accredited CE provider or another education program that includes all the elements of the FDA Education Blueprint for Health Care Providers Involved in the Management or Support of Patients with Pain. The blueprint can be found at www.fda.gov/OpioidAnalgesicREMSBlueprint.

- Discuss the safe use, serious risks, and proper storage and disposal of opioid analgesics with patients and/or their caregivers every time these medicines are prescribed. The Patient Counseling Guide can be obtained at www.fda.gov/OpioidAnalgesicREMSPCG.
- Emphasize to patients and their caregivers the importance of reading the Medication Guide that they will receive from their pharmacist every time an opioid analgesic is dispensed to them.
- Consider using other tools to improve patient, household, and community safety, such as patient–prescriber agreements that reinforce patient–prescriber responsibilities.
  - *Life-threatening respiratory depression:* Fatal respiratory depression has occurred in patients receiving transdermal fentanyl, but the risk is greatest during initiation of therapy or after a dose increase. Ensure drug is used ONLY in opioid-tolerant patients. Have another clinician double check any conversion calculations, and make sure that the dose is not overestimated. Monitor patient closely for respiratory depression during initiation (within the first 48–72 hours) or following dose increase. Ensure the drug is safely stored so that it is out of reach of children and pets.
  - *Accidental exposure* to discarded fentanyl patches (e.g., child or pet chews the patch) can result in death. Patient and caregivers must STRICTLY follow handling and disposal guidelines to prevent accidental exposure.
  - *Neonatal opioid withdrawal syndrome:* If fentanyl transdermal patches are used for a long time in a pregnant woman, teach her that the baby will be at risk for neonatal opioid withdrawal syndrome, which can be fatal, and requires a special nursery with protocols to manage this syndrome. The syndrome is characterized by irritability, hyperactivity, and abnormal sleep pattern, high-pitched cry, tremor, vomiting, diarrhea, failure to gain weight. The syndrome may have subtle signs and symptoms, so newborn must be cared for at an institution able to provide care for this syndrome. Nursing mothers should make a decision to stop nursing or to stop transdermal fentanyl, taking into account the importance of the drug to the mother's health.
  - *Risks of concomitant use or discontinuation of CYP3A4 inhibitors and inducers:* (a) Coadministration with potent CYP3A4 inhibitors may increase fentanyl serum levels (e.g., macrolide antibiotics, such as erythromycin, azole antifungals, such as ketoconazole, and proteasome inhibitors, such as ritonavir) resulting in increased CNS sedation and risk of respiratory depression, especially when an inhibitor is added when the patient is on a stable opioid dose; (b) discontinuance of a CYP3A4 inducer (e.g., rifampin, carbamazepine, and phenytoin) may increase serum fentanyl concentrations and prolong adverse effects. Monitor patient closely when either (a) or (b) occurs, and consider dose reduction of fentanyl until the drug effects are stable. Conversely, concomitant use of fentanyl with CYP3A4 inducers or discontinuation of an CYP3A4 inhibitor could decrease fentanyl serum concentration, decrease opioid efficacy, and lead to withdrawal syndrome. Monitor these patients closely and discuss increasing fentanyl dose as needed for efficacy or if signs/symptoms of withdrawal appear.
  - *Risk of increased fentanyl absorption with application of external heat:* Heat exposure has resulted in increased release of fentanyl from the patch resulting in increased serum levels and drug exposure. There are reports of overdosage and death as a result of exposure to heat.
  - *Risks from concomitant use with benzodiazepines or other CNS depressants:* When used concurrently, profound sedation, respiratory depression, coma, and death may

MANAGEMENT

result. If necessary to coprescribe, prescribe a lower initial dose of the benzodiazepine/ other CNS depressant than indicated when used alone, and titrate based on clinical response. If the patient is already taking the benzodiazepine/other CNS depressant, prescribe a lower starting opioid analgesic dose. Use with other CNS depressants or moderately strong or strong CYP3A4 inhibitors may increase depressant effects including respiratory depression, hypotension, and profound sedation. Assess patient's use of alcohol or other drugs that affect the CNS. Discuss with physician/NP/PA dose adjustments as necessary. Teach patients not to drive or operate heavy machinery until the effects are known. Warn patients and caregivers of risk of overdose and death associated with the use of additional CNS depressants including alcohol and illicit drugs.

- *Risk of increased fentanyl absorption with elevated body temperature:* Serum fentanyl concentrations increase when a patient has a fever. Models predict serum concentrations by approximately one-third when the body temperature is 40°C (104°F). Monitor patients with fever closely for sedation and respiratory depression; advise patients not to do strenuous exercises that leads to increased core body temperature and possible excessive fentanyl dose.
- *Life-threatening respiratory depression in patients with chronic pulmonary disease or in elderly, cachectic, or debilitated patients* (see package insert): Monitor patients closely, especially initially, when titrating doses, and when adding other drugs.
- *Serotonin syndrome with concomitant use of serotonergic drugs:* Serotonin syndrome (e.g., characterized by mental status changes, autonomic instability, neuromuscular abnormalities, and GI symptoms) has occurred when patients received both fentanyl transdermal patch and serotonergic drugs (e.g., SSRIs, SNRIs, TCAs triptans, 5-HT3 receptor antagonists, drugs that affect the serotonergic neurotransmitter system (e.g., mirtazapine, trazodone, tramadol), and drugs that impair metabolism of serotonin (e.g., MAO inhibitors)) (Janssen, 2018). If serotonin syndrome occurs, onset is usually within several hours to a few days after concomitant use, but may occur later. If serotonin syndrome is suspected, immediately discontinue transdermal fentanyl and convert to immediate acting opioids.
- *Adrenal insufficiency:* Adrenal insufficiency has been reported with opioid use, with onset usually after 1 month of dosing. Signs/symptoms include nausea, vomiting, anorexia, fatigue, weakness, dizziness, and low BP. If suspected, perform lab confirmation, and if confirmed, administer corticosteroids as ordered. Patient should be weaned off opioids allowing adrenal function to recover and continue corticosteroids. Other opioids should be used and evaluated.
- *Risks of use in patients with increased ICP, brain tumors, head injury, or impaired consciousness:* Head Injuries and Increase ICP: opioids may obscure clinical course of these patients who are sensitive to the effects of CO_2 retention (respiratory depression). Opioids may also obscure the clinical course of patients with head injury; drug should be avoided in patients with impaired consciousness or coma.
- *Severe hypotension:* Hypotensive effects may occur, including orthostatic hypotension. Risk is increased in patients with reduced blood volume or who have concurrent administration of CNS depressing drugs (e.g., phenothiazines or general anesthesia). Monitor patients closely when changing dose.
- *Hepatic impairment:* Drug is metabolized by the liver; do not use the drug in patients with severe hepatic impairment. Dose in patients with mild–moderate impairment

should be 50% of the regular dose to begin, and titrated to the patient's response for efficacy and toxicity (Janssen, 2018).

- *Renal impairment*: Do not use the drug in patients with severe renal impairment. Dose in patients with mild-moderate impairment should be 50% of the regular dose to begin, and titrated to the patient's response for efficacy and toxicity (Mylan, 2014).
- *Risks of use in patients with GI conditions*: Use in biliary/pancreatic tract disease: drug may cause spasm in sphincter of Oddi; monitor patient closely for worsening symptoms, including pancreatitis. Serum amylase concentration may increase.
- *Cardiac disease:* Drug may cause bradycardia; assess patients with cardiac disease closely.
- *Avoidance of withdrawal*: Do not coadminister with mixed agonist/antagonist (e.g., pentazocine) or partial agonist (e.g., buprenorphine) analgesics as it may cause patient to go into withdrawal.
- *Increased risk of seizures in patients with seizure disorders:* May increase the frequency of seizures, and risk of seizures occurring in other clinical settings. Monitor patients having a history of seizure disorder for worsened seizure control.
- *Risks of driving and operating machinery:* Teach patients to avoid driving and operating machinery as drug may impair mental and physical ability to drive a car or operate heavy machinery. Teach patient to avoid this until the full effect of the drug is known.
- Use with caution in the following patients, and monitor closely for sedation and respiratory depression:
  - COPD predisposed to hypoventilation
  - Head injuries, brain tumor (very sensitive to effects of CO_2 retention)
  - Cardiac disease (may cause bradyarrhythmias)
  - Hepatic or renal dysfunction
  - Elderly or cachectic, debilitated patients, and those with chronic pulmonary disease
- Interactions with CNS depressants: concomitant use may cause profound sedation, respiratory depression, and death. If must be coadministered, consider dose reduction of one or both drugs.
- Drug may cause fetal harm. Teach women of childbearing potential who become or are planning to become pregnant to talk to their healthcare provider before starting or continuing transdermal fentanyl therapy.
- Most common adverse reactions ($\geq$ 5%) are nausea, vomiting, somnolence, dizziness, insomnia, constipation, hyperhidrosis, fatigue, feeling cold, anorexia, headache, diarrhea.
- Assess each patient's risk for addiction, abuse, or misuse prior to prescribing transdermal fentanyl, and monitor patients for the development of these behaviors.

Potential Toxicities/Side Effects and the Nursing Process

I. ALTERATION IN OXYGENATION related to HYPOVENTILATION, FEVER

Defining Characteristics: Dyspnea, hypoventilation, apnea (3–10% of patients); hemoptysis, pharyngitis, hiccups rare; stertorous breathing, asthma, respiratory dysfunction.

Nursing Implications: Assess baseline pulmonary status. Use with caution in patients with COPD, brain tumors, increased ICP, hepatic failure. NEVER exceed 25 mcg/hr if patient not tolerant to opioids. Must continue to observe patient for 17 hours after dose removed for signs/symptoms of toxicity—same is true if naloxone HCl (Narcan) required to reverse opioid. Theoretically, a temperature of 39°C (102°F) will increase serum fentanyl by 33% due to drug delivery and skin absorption. If patient develops fever, observe for signs/symptoms of overdosage. Elderly patients (> 60–65 years old) may have reduced ability to clear drug, so start at 25 mcg/hr unless already tolerant of > 135 mg morphine sulfate/24 hours.

II. SENSORY/PERCEPTUAL ALTERATIONS related to CNS CHANGES

Defining Characteristics: CNS depression and changes in mental status may occur, characterized by somnolence, confusion, depression, asthenia (> 10%), dizziness, nervousness, hallucinations, anxiety, depression, euphoria (3–10%), tremors, abnormal coordination, speech disorder, abnormal thinking, dreams. Rare: aphasia, vertigo, stupor, hypotonia, hypertonia, hostility.

Nursing Implications: Assess baseline mental, neurologic status. Dose of other opioids and benzodiazepines should be 50%. Use cautiously in substance abusers.

III. ALTERATION IN CARDIAC OUTPUT related to ARRYTHMIA, ANGINA

Defining Characteristics: Arrhythmia, chest pain may occur; IV fentanyl has caused bradyarrhythmias.

Nursing Implications: Assess baseline cardiac status, and monitor during drug use. Instruct patient to report palpitations, chest pain.

IV. ALTERATION IN NUTRITION, LESS THAN BODY REQUIREMENTS, related to NAUSEA, VOMITING

Defining Characteristics: Nausea, vomiting, anorexia, dyspepsia, rare abdominal distension.

Nursing Implications: Assess baseline nutritional status. Instruct patient to report nausea, vomiting, anorexia, dyspepsia.

V. ALTERATION IN ELIMINATION related to CONSTIPATION, ILEUS

Defining Characteristics: Opium agonists bind to opiate receptors in bowel, slowing peristalsis, leading to constipation. Untreated constipation may result in bowel perforation. Opiate receptors in bowel decrease peristalsis.

Nursing Implications: Assess baseline elimination, fluid intake, diet, and exercise patterns. Instruct patient regarding prevention of constipation: goal is to move bowels at least every 2 days, by increasing fluids to 3 L/day, following a diet high in fiber (beans, vegetables, fruit), and taking moderate exercise. Assess need for bowel softeners, bulk-forming laxatives, and osmotic cathartics, and discuss prescription with physician. Teach patient self-administration of medications. MUST be started on bowel regimen.

VI. ALTERATION IN CARDIAC OUTPUT related to HYPOTENSION, BRADYCARDIA

Defining Characteristics: Orthostatic hypotension, bradycardia due to cholinergic effect, and peripheral vasodilation may occur with rapid IV dosing. There may be histamine-related flushing, pruritus, diaphoresis with chronic drug usage; tolerance develops to this effect.

Nursing Implications: Assess baseline cardiovascular status. Teach patient to change position slowly and to hold onto stable, nearby structure for support as needed.
  Be careful when giving IV push opioids, and caution patient to remain in supine position for 15–20 minutes after injection. Monitor cardiovascular status after injection.

VII. ALTERATION IN URINE ELIMINATION related to URINARY RETENTION

Defining Characteristics: Increased smooth muscle tone in urinary tract and spasm may occur. Bladder tone is increased, which may cause urgency. Vesical sphincter tone may be increased, leading to difficulty urinating. Increased risk of urinary retention in patients with prostatic hypertrophy or urethral stricture. Rare bladder pain, oliguria, urinary frequency.

Nursing Implications: Assess baseline urinary elimination pattern. Teach patient to increase fluids to 3 L/day, and encourage voiding every 2–3 hours. Instruct patient to report problems with urination.

VIII. ALTERATION IN SKIN INTEGRITY/COMFORT related to RASH, PRURITUS

Defining Characteristics: Sweating, pruritus, rash; erythema, papules, itching, edema, exfoliative dermatitis, pustules at application site; headache rare.

Nursing Implications: Teach patient proper drug application and to rotate sites.

Drug: hydromorphone (Dilaudid)

Class: Opioid analgesic (opioid agonist).

Mechanism of Action: Hydromorphone is a hydrogented ketone of morphine. Binds to opiate receptors in CNS (limbic system, thalamus, striatum, hypothalamus, midbrain, spinal cord), altering pain perception at level of spinal cord and higher centers, as well as the emotional response to pain. Also suppresses cough reflex.

Metabolism: Well absorbed after oral, rectal, and parenteral administration. Onset of action is 15–30 minutes (more rapid than morphine), with a duration of action of 4–5 hours. Metabolized by liver and excreted in urine.

Indication: For the management of pain in patients where an opioid analgesic is appropriate. Dilaudid-HP (high-potency) is intended for use only in opioid-tolerant patients.

Contraindications: Patients with (1) known hypersensitivity to hydromorphone, (2) respiratory depression in the absence of resuscitative equipment, (3) status asthmaticus, and (4) obstetrical analgesia.

Dosage/Range:
- Requires opioid Risk Evaluation and Mitigation Strategy (REMS).
- Use caution in
  - Patients who have not received opiates before and have not developed tolerance.
  - Elderly patients who may require doses lower than 2–4 mg every 4 hours.
- Moderate pain: oral: 1–6 mg q 4–6 h; subcutaneous or IM: 2–4 mg q 4–6 h, 3 mg rectal suppository.
- Severe pain: oral: 4 mg or more q 4 h; subcutaneous or IM: 4 mg or more, then titrate based on patient response and tolerance.
- Moderate hepatic dysfunction: start at lower dose and monitor closely during dose titration.
- Hydromorphone oral liquid: 2.5–10 mg (2.5–10 mL, or 1/2 to 2 tsp) of 1 mg/1 mL liquid, every 3–6 hours as directed.
- Hydromorphone tablets: 2–4 mg orally, every 4–6 hours as needed for pain.
- Initial dose should be reduced in patients with renal or hepatic impairment.

Drug Preparation:
- Available as hydromorphone oral liquid (1 pint, 473 mL); hydromorphone 2-, 4-, and 8-mg tablets; and Dilaudid IV: 1-, 2-, and 4-mg/mL ampules; and Dilaudid-HP (high-potency) in 10-mg/mL ampules and vials.
- Store tablets in tight, light-resistant containers at 15–30°C (59–86°F).
- Injection should be protected from light and stored at 15–40°C (59–104°F).

Drug Administration:
- PO (liquid or tablet), subcutaneous, IM, IV. Use highly concentrated injectable solution for patients who are tolerant to opiate agonists.
- At home, teach patient to store oral doses in a safe place away from children and pets.
- Teach patient that opioid analgesics may impair the mental and/or physical ability to drive and use machines, and to avoid these activities until the effect of the drug is known.
- Chronic pain: Requires ATC dosing (with hydromorphone at frequent intervals or preferably with a long-acting opiate), with 5–15% of the total daily hydromorphone dosage every 2 hours as BTP medication.
- Continue to reassess pain after initial dosing to ensure adequate pain control through titration.

Drug Interactions:
- Alcohol, CNS depressants: Additive effects.

Lab Effects/Interference:
- None known.

Special Considerations:
- Risk Evaluation and Mitigation Strategy (REMS) required for use of opioids. Healthcare providers must review REMS-compliant education. In addition, healthcare providers must

a. Complete a REMS-compliant education program offered by an accredited CE provider or another education program that includes all the elements of the FDA Education Blueprint for Health Care Providers Involved in the Management or Support of Patients with Pain. The blueprint can be found at www.fda.gov/OpioidAnalgesic REMSBlueprint.

b. Discuss the safe use, serious risks, and proper storage and disposal of opioid analgesics with patients and/or their caregivers every time these medicines are prescribed. The Patient Counseling Guide can be obtained at www.fda.gov/OpioidAnalgesicREMSPCG.

c. Emphasize to patients and their caregivers the importance of reading the Medication Guide that they will receive from their pharmacist every time an opioid analgesic is dispensed to them.

d. Consider using other tools to improve patient, household, and community safety, such as patient–prescriber agreements that reinforce patient–prescriber responsibilities.

- Parenteral dose is 1/5 oral dose for equianalgesic effect.
- Additive benefit when combined with acetaminophen or aspirin.
- Give smallest effective dose to prevent development of tolerance (e.g., takes more drug to provide the same relief over time), physical dependency (e.g., withdrawal symptoms if drug is stopped abruptly). These are separate and distinct from abuse and addiction.
- Drug can lead to drug abuse and addiction if not used for the relief of pain.
- Reduce dose in debilitated patients or patients receiving other CNS depressants.
- Use with caution in patients with hepatic or renal dysfunction, hypothyroidism, Addison's disease, severe CNS depression, respiratory depression, head injury, elevated ICP.
- Most common adverse reactions are lightheadedness, dizziness, sedation, nausea, vomiting, sweating, flushing, dysphoria, euphoria, dry mouth, pruritus, constipation.
- If required, naloxone HCl will reverse opiate toxicity (e.g., respiratory depression). However, it is important that acute withdrawal symptoms be prevented by giving only enough naloxone to reverse respiratory depression and that this be continued for opioid drug half-life.
- Drug should not be used by nursing mothers, and use is contraindicated during labor and delivery.

Potential Toxicities/Side Effects and the Nursing Process

I. SENSORY/PERCEPTUAL ALTERATIONS related to CNS DEPRESSION

Defining Characteristics: Drowsiness, sedation, mood changes, euphoria, dysphoria, dizziness, mental clouding may occur. At high doses, may cause seizures. Miosis (papillary constriction) may occur.

Nursing Implications: Assess baseline neurologic status. Use cautiously, if at all, in patients with head injury, increased ICP, severe CNS depression, acute alcoholism, the elderly, and the debilitated. Assess other concurrent medications. Use with caution in patients receiving other opioids, tranquilizers, hypnotics, MAO inhibitors, since increasing CNS depressant effects can occur. Monitor neurologic status closely. Teach patient to avoid driving and operating machinery while taking the medicine, and to AVOID concurrent alcohol.

II. ALTERATION IN OXYGENATION related to RESPIRATORY DEPRESSION

Defining Characteristics: Opiate agonists directly depress respiratory center in brain stem, causing decreased sensitivity and responsiveness to increased pCO_2. Also may depress deep breathing and reflex to sigh. Tolerance to respiratory depressant effects occurs with chronic use.

Nursing Implications: Assess baseline pulmonary status, and monitor periodically during drug use. Use cautiously in patients with bronchial asthma, COPD, respiratory depression, and monitor closely.

III. ALTERATION IN ELIMINATION related to CONSTIPATION, ILEUS

Defining Characteristics: Opium agonists bind to opiate receptors in bowel, slowing peristalsis, leading to constipation. Untreated constipation may result in bowel perforation.

Nursing Implications: Assess baseline elimination, fluid intake, diet, and exercise patterns. Instruct patient about prevention of constipation: goal is to move bowels at least every 2 days by increasing fluids to 3 L/day, following a diet high in fiber (beans, vegetables, fruit), and taking moderate exercise. Assess need for bowel softeners, bulk-forming laxatives, and osmotic cathartics, and discuss prescription with physician. Teach patient self-administration of medications.

IV. ALTERATION IN NUTRITION related to GI TOXICITY

Defining Characteristics: Nausea, vomiting, and dry mouth may occur. Gastric, biliary, and pancreatic secretions are decreased by opiate agonists; digestion is delayed. Biliary tract muscle tone is increased, and spasm of Oddi's sphincter may occur (morphine $>$ meperidine $>$ codeine).

Nursing Implications: Assess patient tolerance of GI side effects. Teach patient to report side effects. If nausea/vomiting occur, change to another opioid, or premedicate with antiemetic to prevent nausea/vomiting. Assess GI pain, biliary spasm, and consider alternative opioid.

V. ALTERATION IN CARDIAC OUTPUT related to HYPOTENSION, BRADYCARDIA

Defining Characteristics: Orthostatic hypotension, bradycardia due to cholinergic effect, and peripheral vasodilation may occur with rapid IV dosing. There may be histamine-related flushing, pruritus, diaphoresis with chronic drug usage; tolerance develops to this effect.

Nursing Implications: Assess baseline cardiovascular status. Teach patient to change position slowly and to hold onto stable, nearby structure for support as needed. Be careful when giving IV push opioids, and caution patient to remain in supine position for 15–20 minutes after injection. Monitor cardiovascular status after injection.

VI. ALTERATION IN URINE ELIMINATION related to URINARY RETENTION

Defining Characteristics: Increased smooth muscle tone in urinary tract and spasm may occur. Bladder tone is increased, which may cause urgency. Vesical sphincter tone may be increased, leading to difficulty urinating. Increased risk of urinary retention in patients with prostatic hypertrophy or urethral stricture.

Nursing Implications: Assess baseline urinary elimination pattern. Teach patient to increase fluids to 3 L/day, and encourage voiding every 2–3 hours. Instruct patient to report problems with urination.

VII. KNOWLEDGE DEFICIT related to DRUG ADMINISTRATION, POTENTIAL FOR TOLERANCE, AND DEPENDENCY

Defining Characteristics: Psychological dependence (addiction) occurs rarely in patients taking opioid agonists for cancer pain ($> 1\%$). Physical dependence (precipitation of withdrawal symptoms) occurs with chronic use of the drug for the relief of chronic cancer pain. In addition, tolerance, or less analgesic effect over time with the same drug dose, occurs and requires increased dosage of drug.

Nursing Implications: Assess baseline knowledge of opioid analgesics and attitude about their use for cancer pain management. Teach patient about proper self-administration, possible side effects, and self-care measures. Suggest patient maintain diary of pain intensity, precipitating and alleviating factors, drug dose and time taken, and relief. Teach patient to self-administer opioid agonists for relief of chronic cancer pain ATC, not PRN, to prevent pain. Explain use of prescribed short-acting opioid for rescue or to manage BTP. Discuss with physician dose increase or change in frequency of administration if tolerance develops. Teach patient that withdrawal symptoms may occur if chronic, ATC dosing is interrupted. Withdrawal (abstinence) symptoms that may be seen are restlessness, lacrimation, rhinorrhea, yawning, perspiration, gooseflesh, restless sleep, mydriasis in first 24 hours. These are followed by twitching and leg spasm; severe aching of the back, abdomen, and legs; cramping in abdomen and legs; hot/cold flashes; insomnia; nausea/vomiting, diarrhea; severe sneezing; and increased heart rate, BP, T, which peak at 36–72 hours. Withdrawal syndrome can be prevented by administration of at least one-quarter of previous opioid dose.

VIII. SEXUAL DYSFUNCTION related to IMPOTENCE, DECREASED LIBIDO

Defining Characteristics: Opiate agonists may suppress gonadotropin, causing impotence and decreased libido.

Nursing Implications: Assess baseline sexual pattern. Discuss potential toxicity and impact on sexuality. Provide information, emotional support, and referral as needed.

MANAGEMENT

Drug: hydromorphone HCl extended-release tablets (Exalgo)

Class: Opioid analgesic (opioid agonist).

Mechanism of Action: Agonist of mu-opioid receptors, having a weak affinity for K-receptors. Drug binds to the mu-receptor in the CNS (limbic system, thalamus, striatum, hypothalamus, midbrain, spinal cord), altering pain perception at level of spinal cord and higher centers as well as the emotional response to pain. Also suppresses cough reflex by direct effect on the cough center in the medulla. It is 5 times more potent (by weight) than morphine. Respiratory depression occurs via direct action on cerebral respiratory control center (brainstem) and may cause nausea/vomiting by direct stimulation of the chemoreceptor trigger zone (posterior medulla).

Metabolism: Uses OROS push–pull osmotic delivery system so that drug is released at a controlled rate, with gradual increase in drug serum concentrations. After a single dose, plasma concentrations increase gradually over 6–8 hours and are sustained for ~18–24 hours after drug is given. Median T_{max} is 12–16 hours, and mean half-life is about 11 hours (range 8–5 hours). Steady state plasma concentrations approximately twice those observed following the first dose, with steady state reached after 3–4 days of once-daily dosing. Once reached, steady state serum levels maintained with once-daily dosing, within the same concentration range as immediate-release tablets given 4 times daily, but without the peaks and troughs seen with immediate-release drug dosing. Drug absorption is unaffected by food or fluid. Drug has extensive tissue distribution. Twenty-seven percent of drug binds to plasma proteins. Immediate-release formulation undergoes extensive first-pass metabolism, primarily by the liver (glucuronidation), forming hydromorphone in plasma. Seventy-five percent of the administered dose is excreted in the urine, mostly as metabolites; 7% of unchanged drug is excreted in the urine, and 1% in the feces. Females have ~10% higher mean systemic exposure (C_{max}, AUC).

Indication: In opioid-tolerant patients for the management of pain severe enough to require daily, ATC, long-term opioid treatment and for which alternative treatment options are inadequate. A patient who is considered tolerant is taking for 1 week or longer, at least 60 mg oral morphine/day; or 25 mcg transdermal fentanyl/day; or 30 mg of oral oxycodone/day; or 25 mg oral oxymorphone/day; 8 mg oral hydromorphone/day; or an equianalgesic dose of another opioid.

Limitations of use: Because of potential risks of addiction, abuse, and misuse with opioids, the drug should be reserved for use in patients for whom alternative treatment options are ineffective/intolerable. Drug is not indicated as an as-needed (PRN) analgesic.

Contraindications: (1) Opioid nontolerant patients; (2) significant respiratory depression; (3) acute or severe bronchial asthma in an unmonitored setting or in the absence of resuscitative equipment; (4) known or suspected GI obstruction, including paralytic ileus; (5) narrowed or obstructed GI tract; (6) known hypersensitivity to any components, including hydromorphone HCl and sulfites. Drug is NOT indicated as an as-needed PRN analgesic.

Dosage/Range:
- Requires an opioid Risk Evaluation and Mitigation Strategy (REMS).
- Prescribers and pharmacists must know that hydromorphone is available as both immediate release 8 mg tablets, and extended-release 8 mg tablets. These should not be confused.
- Drug should be prescribed only by healthcare professionals who are knowledgeable in the use of potent opioids for the management of chronic pain.
- Drug should be used ONLY in opioid tolerant patients. Discontinue or taper other extended-release opioids when Exalgo therapy initiated. Exalgo should NEVER be the first opioid.
  - Use the lowest effective dosage for the shortest duration consistent with individual patient treatment goals.
  - Initiate drug dosing individually, considering the patient's prior analgesic regimen and risk factors for addiction, abuse, and misuse.
  - Monitor patients closely for respiratory depression, especially within the first 24–72 hours after initiating the drug and after dose increases; adjust dose as needed.
- Once-daily administration; patient must swallow tablets intact. Do NOT crush, chew, or dissolve tablet as this will result in uncontrolled delivery of hydromorphone and can lead to overdose or death.
- Dose must be individualized for each patient and should NEVER be administered as a first opioid (opioid-naïve patient).
  - If taking immediate-release hydromorphone tablets, the starting Exalgo dose is the current 24-hour dose of the immediate-release hydromorphone.
  - To convert to Exalgo from another opioid, use available conversion factors to obtain estimated dose. See Table 1 in package insert. See instructions for calculation of dose (Mallinckrodt, 2016). Table is not an equianalgesic dose table, and starts with 50% of the equianalgesic dose, so rescue (immediate-release) hydromorphone should also be prescribed.
- Dose may be increased in increments of 4–8 mg every 3–4 hours as needed to achieve adequate analgesia.
- *Moderate hepatic impairment:* Start treatment at 25% of the dose of a patient with normal liver function. Monitor closely for respiratory and CNS depression.
- *Moderate and severe renal impairment:* Start treatment of patients with moderate renal impairment at 50% of the dose for patients with normal renal function, and patients with severe renal impairment at 25% of the dose. Monitor closely for respiratory and CNS depression.

Dose Reductions:
- Moderate and severe hepatic dysfunction (fourfold increase in patients with moderate liver impairment) and patients with moderate renal impairment: consider alternate analgesic if severe renal impairment (two- to fourfold increase in plasma concentrations, as well as delayed excretion increasing the terminal half-life to 40 hours). Start patients with moderate hepatic impairment on 25% of the normal dose. Closely monitor patient for respiratory and CNS depression.

MANAGEMENT

- Moderate renal impairment: start patient on 50% of the normal dose; if severe renal impairment, start patient at 25% of the normal dose daily and closely monitor for effect and toxicity.
- Concurrent administration of CNS depressants: assess duration of use of the CNS depressant, patient's response including tolerance to CNS depression, use of alcohol or illicit drugs that can cause CNS depression; if the decision to use Exalgo is made, start with one-third to one-half the calculated starting dose, monitor for signs of sedation and respiratory depression, and consider using a lower dose of the concomitant CNS depressant.
- See conversion chart in package insert and instructions (Mallinckrodt, 2016). When converting from another opioid, calculate a starting dose equivalent to the patient's total daily oral hydromorphone dose, taken once daily. Carefully titrate the dose of extended-release hydromorphone, in increments of 4–8 mg every 3–4 days until adequate pain relief with tolerable side effects is achieved (plasma levels of EXALGO are sustained for 18–24 hours).
- Consider dosage increases of 25–50% of the current daily dose for each titration step. If more than 2 rescue doses of immediate-release analgesic are needed within a 24-hour period for 2 consecutive days, the dose of extended-release hydromorphone may need to be titrated upward. Do not administer extended-release hydromorphone **more than once a day**.
- For patients taking more than one opioid, calculate the approximate oral hydromorphone dose for each opioid and sum the totals to obtain the approximate total hydromorphone daily dose.
- BTP: ensure patient has a prescription for short-acting hydromorphone for rescue, and have patient keep a pain diary. If possible, it is important to try to identify the source of increased pain before increasing the Exalgo dose.
- Maintain frequent contact with the patient/family when titrating dose to assess tolerance and efficacy.
- When the drug is no longer needed, **taper doses gradually**, by 25–50% every 2–3 days down to a dose of 8 mg/day, before discontinuing therapy to prevent symptoms of withdrawal in the physically dependent patient. Signs and symptoms of withdrawal are restlessness, lacrimation, rhinorrhea, yawning, perspiration, chills, piloerection, myalgia, mydriasis, irritability, anxiety, backache, joint pain, weakness, abdominal cramps, insomnia, nausea, anorexia, vomiting, diarrhea, BP, respiratory rate, and heart rate. Infants born to mothers who are physically dependent on opioids will also exhibit respiratory difficulties and withdrawal symptoms.
- Do not give mixed agonist/antagonist with this drug (e.g., pentazocine, nalbuphine, and butorphanol), as it may precipitate withdrawal as well as decrease the analgesic effect.
- Do not abruptly discontinue Exalgo.
- Drug is not to be used for (1) PRN analgesic, (2) pain that is mild or not expected to persist for an extended time, (3) acute pain, (4) postoperative pain, unless already receiving chronic opioid therapy prior to surgery, or if postoperative pain is expected to be moderate to severe and persisting for an extended period of time.

Drug Preparation:
- Oral. Available as 8-, 12-, 16-, or 32-mg strengths. Store at 59–86°F (25–30°C).
- Ensure that pharmacist knows that this drug (extended-release form) is different from immediate-release hydromorphone 8-mg tablets.

Drug Administration:
- Oral, swallowed whole, with adequate water or liquid, once every 24 hours, with or without food.
- Teach patient that drug must not be broken, crushed, dissolved, or chewed before swallowing.
- Discontinue or taper all other extended-release opioids when beginning this drug.
- USE CAUTION WHEN ADMINISTERING, AND ENSURE THAT CORRECT drug and dose are prescribed, as hydromorphone *immediate release* is also available as an 8-mg tablet. When extended-release hydromorphone HCl is no longer needed, unused tablets should be destroyed by flushing them down the toilet (Mallinckrodt, 2015; FDA).
- Teach patient that opioid analgesics may impair the mental and/or physical ability to drive and use machines, and to avoid these activities until the effect of the drug is known.
- Disposal: flush all remaining tablets down the toilet or remit to authorities at a certified drug take-back program.

Drug Interactions:
- CNS depressants (e.g., hypnotics, sedatives, general anesthetics, antipsychotics, alcohol): may cause additive depressant effects and respiratory depression, hypotension, profound sedation, coma; if must use concurrently, reduce dose of one or both agents. Do not take drug when drinking alcohol.
- MAO inhibitors: MAO inhibitors may cause CNS excitation or depression, hypotension, or hypertension if used concurrently. Do not use concurrently, and separate by at least 14 days after stopping the MAO inhibitor.
- Mixed agonist/antagonist opioid analgesics (e.g., buprenorphine, nalbuphine, pentazocine) may reduce analgesic effect by competitive blockade of receptors ± precipitate withdrawal symptoms. Do not use concurrently.
- Anticholinergic drugs may increase the risk of urinary retention and/or severe constipation leading to paralytic ileus.
- Cytochrome P450 enzymes: minimal potential to inhibit CYP3A4, -2C9, -2C19, -2D6, and -4A11.

Lab Effects/Interference:
- None known.

Special Considerations:
- Warnings and Precautions:
  - Risk Evaluation and Mitigation Strategy (REMS) required for use of opioids. Healthcare providers must review REMS-compliant education. In addition, healthcare providers must
    - Complete a REMS-compliant education program offered by an accredited CE provider or another education program that includes all the elements of the FDA Education Blueprint for Health Care Providers Involved in the Management or Support of Patients with Pain. The blueprint can be found at www.fda.gov/OpioidAnalgesicREMSBlueprint.
    - Discuss the safe use, serious risks, and proper storage and disposal of opioid analgesics with patients and/or their caregivers every time these medicines are prescribed. The Patient Counseling Guide can be obtained at www.fda.gov/OpioidAnalgesicREMSPCG.

- Emphasize to patients and their caregivers the importance of reading the Medication Guide that they will receive from their pharmacist every time an opioid analgesic is dispensed to them.
- Consider using other tools to improve patient, household, and community safety, such as patient–prescriber agreements that reinforce patient–prescriber responsibilities.
  - *Addiction, abuse, and misuse:* Exalgo contains hydromorphone, a Schedule II–controlled substance. It is an opioid that exposes users to risk of addiction, abuse, and misuse, which can lead to overdose and death. Assess each patient's risk before prescribing, and monitor regularly for evidence of misuse, abuse, or diversion. Addiction is defined as psychological dependence. This is different from physical dependence (goes into withdrawal if drug is abruptly discontinued).
  - *Serious, life-threatening or fatal respiratory depression* may occur. Monitor patient closely, especially upon initial dosing or after a dose increase. Teach patients to swallow Exalgo tablets whole to avoid exposure to a potentially fatal dose of hydromorphone.
  - Accidental ingestion of Exalgo, especially by children, of a single dose of Exalgo can result in fatal respiratory depression.
  - *Neonatal opioid withdrawal syndrome:* Prolonged use of Exalgo during pregnancy can result in neonatal opioid withdrawal syndrome, which may be life-threatening to the newborn if not recognized and treated with expert protocols. If opioid use is required for prolonged periods in a pregnant woman, teach her of the risk of neonatal opioid withdrawal syndrome, and ensure that she understands the newborn must be cared for by a healthcare personnel experienced with the protocols.
  - *Risk for concomitant use with benzodiazepines or other CNS depressants* (e.g., non-benzodiazepine sedatives/hypnotics, anxiolytics, tranquilizers, muscle relaxants, general anesthetics, antipsychotics, other opioids, alcohol): Use with other CNS depressants may increase depressant effects including respiratory depression, hypotension, and profound sedation. Assess patient's use of alcohol or other drugs that affect the CNS. Discuss with physician/NP/PA dose adjustments as necessary. Teach patient not to drive or operate heavy machinery until the effect of the medication is known.
  - *Life-threatening respiratory depression in patients with chronic pulmonary disease or in elderly, cachectic, debilitated patients:* Monitor closely because of increased risk for life-threatening respiratory depression, especially when starting or changing dose (titration).
  - *Adrenal insufficiency:* Adrenal insufficiency has occurred, especially in patients receiving opioids for >1 month. Signs/symptoms include: nausea, vomiting, anorexia, fatigue, weakness, dizziness, low BP. If adrenal insufficiency is suspected, confirm the diagnosis with lab testing; if confirmed, treat with physiological doses of corticosteroids. Wean the patient off the opioid to allow adrenal function recovery while continuing corticosteroids. Other opioids should be tried.
  - *Severe hypotension:* Severe hypotension may occur, including orthostatic hypotension and syncope in ambulatory patients, especially in patients with reduced blood volume or receiving concurrent certain CNS depressing drugs (e.g., phenothiazines, general anesthetics). Monitor these patients closely for signs/symptoms hypotension after starting drug or dose titration. Do not use Exalgo in patients with circulatory shock.
  - *Risk of use in patients with head injury, brain tumor, or increased ICP:* Opioids may obscure clinical course of these patients who are sensitive to the effects of CO_2

retention (respiratory depression). Monitor for sedation and respiratory depression. Avoid use of Exalgo in patients with impaired consciousness or coma who are susceptible to the intracranial effects of CO_2 retention.

- *Risk of use in patients with GI conditions:* Drug is contraindicated if GI obstruction is suspected or known, as well as in patients with preexisting severe GI narrowing as the tablet will not change shape to be accommodated through the narrowing and can become an obstruction (e.g., esophageal motility disorders, small bowel inflammatory disease, short gut syndrome, past history of peritonitis, cystic fibrosis, chronic intestinal pseudo-obstruction, Merkel's diverticulum). Hydromorphone can cause spasm of the sphincter of Oddi and cause increases in serum amylase; monitor patients with biliary tract disease, including acute pancreatitis, for worsening symptoms.
- *Increased risk of seizures in patients with seizure disorders:* Drug may increase seizure frequency or occurrence in other clinical settings. Monitor patients with a seizure history closely for worsening seizure control when taking this drug.
- *Withdrawal:* Avoid the use of mixed agonist/antagonist (e.g., pentazocine, nalbuphine, butorphanol) analgesics in patients receiving full opioid agonist analgesia as the analgesic effect may be lessened or it may precipitate withdrawal symptoms. When discontinuing the drug, always gradually taper the dose; do NOT abruptly discontinue.
- *Sulfites:* Drug contains sodium metabisulfite that may cause an allergic reaction, including anaphylactic symptoms and life-threatening or less severe asthmatic episodes in susceptible individuals. Sulfite sensitivity is seen more frequently in asthmatic people.
- *Risks of driving and operating machinery:* Drug may impair the mental and/or physical abilities needed to perform potentially hazardous activities (e.g., driving a car, operating machinery). Teach patient not to drive or operate machinery until it is known how the patient will react to Exalgo.
- Individualize dose for each patient when starting dosing regimen. Overestimating the initial dose when converting from another opioid can result in overdosage and death.
  - Balance between pain control and adverse effects.
  - Risk factors for abuse, addiction, or diversion, including a prior history of abuse, addiction, or diversion.
  - Monitor closely for respiratory depression, especially within the first 24–72 hours of starting therapy.
- Drug is not recommended during labor and delivery, pregnancy, or nursing. Prolonged use of the drug during pregnancy can result in neonatal opioid withdrawal syndrome, which may be life-threatening if not recognized and treated by established neonatal protocols.
- **Teach patient/caregiver to keep out of reach of children and pets, as accidental ingestion can result in a fatal overdose.**
- Most common side effects ($> 10\%$) are constipation, nausea, vomiting, somnolence, headache, dizziness.
- Drug should not be abruptly discontinued, as it may precipitate withdrawal symptoms.
- If acute overdosage occurs, respiratory depression, somnolence progressing to stupor or coma, skeletal muscle flaccidity, cold and clammy skin, constricted pupils, sometimes bradycardia, hypotension, and death may occur. Once emergently reversed (e.g., narcan), patient will require continued monitoring for 24–48 hours or more due to delayed peak plasma level, which occurs at 16 hours from time of dose, as well as 11-hour mean elimination half-life.

Potential Toxicities/Side Effects and the Nursing Process

I.   SENSORY/PERCEPTUAL ALTERATIONS related to CNS DEPRESSION

Defining Characteristics: Drowsiness, sedation, mood changes, euphoria, dysphoria, dizziness, mental clouding may occur. At high doses, may cause seizures. Miosis (pupillary constriction) may occur.

Nursing Implications: Assess baseline neurologic status. Use cautiously, if at all, in patients with head injury, increased ICP, severe CNS depression, acute alcoholism, the elderly, and the debilitated. Assess other concurrent medications. Use with caution in patients receiving other opioids, tranquilizers, hypnotics, or MAO inhibitors, since increasing CNS depressant effects can be dangerous. Monitor neurologic status closely. Teach patient to avoid driving and operating machinery while taking the medicine and to AVOID concurrent alcohol. Recall that drug can produce changes in pupillary response, which can obscure neurologic signs of increasing ICP in patients with head injuries.

II.   ALTERATION IN OXYGENATION related to RESPIRATORY DEPRESSION

Defining Characteristics: Opiate agonists directly depress respiratory center in brain stem, causing decreased sensitivity and responsiveness to increased pCO_2. Also may depress deep breathing. Patients have a reduced urge to breathe, a decreased respiratory rate, and often have a "sighing" pattern of breathing (deep breaths separated by abnormal, long pauses). CO_2 retention can also exacerbate opioid sedation. Tolerance to respiratory depressant effects occurs with chronic use. Patients at risk are the elderly, debilitated, suffering from conditions causing hypoxia or hypercapnia. Drug may decrease respiratory drive while simultaneously increasing airway resistance so that apnea occurs in patients at risk. Methadone is challenging, as the drug conversion ratio varies widely based on its long half-life. Consider alternative analgesic in patients with significant COPD, cor pulmonale, or patients with substantially decreased respiratory reserve, hypoxia, hypercapnia, or preexisting respiratory depression.

Nursing Implications: Assess baseline pulmonary status, and monitor periodically during drug use. Ensure that dose calculations when converting patient to drug are conservative, with underdosing and use of rescue medications for BTP preferable to overdosing with increased toxicity. It is easier to dose-increase than to have to dose-reduce given the long drug half-life. Special consideration and close monitoring is needed for (1) patients being converted from methadone, (2) elderly, cachectic, or debilitated patients with COPD, cor pulmonale, or with substantially reduced respiratory reserve, hypoxia, hypercapnia, or preexisting respiratory depression. Monitor patients closely at this time, as well as any change in dose. Interventions include close observation, supportive measures, and use of opioid antagonists to reverse the respiratory depression.

III.   ALTERATION IN ELIMINATION related to CONSTIPATION, ILEUS

Defining Characteristics: Opium agonists bind to opiate receptors in bowel, slowing peristalsis, leading to constipation. Untreated constipation may result in bowel perforation.

Nursing Implications: Assess baseline elimination, fluid intake, diet, and exercise patterns. Instruct patient about prevention of constipation: goal is to move bowels at least every 2 days by increasing fluids to 3 L/day, following a diet high in fiber (beans, vegetables, fruit), and doing moderate exercise. Assess need for bowel softeners, bulk-forming laxatives, and osmotic cathartics, and discuss prescription with physician. Teach patient self-administration of medications.

IV. ALTERATION IN NUTRITION related to GI TOXICITY

Defining Characteristics: Nausea, vomiting, and dry mouth may occur. Gastric, biliary, and pancreatic secretions are decreased by opiate agonists; digestion is delayed. Biliary tract muscle tone is increased and spasm of Oddi's sphincter may occur, increasing biliary tract pressure (morphine > meperidine > codeine).

Nursing Implications: Assess patient tolerance of GI side effects. Teach patient to report side effects. If nausea/vomiting occur, change to another opioid, or premedicate with antiemetic to prevent nausea/vomiting. Assess GI pain, biliary spasm, and consider alternative opioid. The drug must be used cautiously if at all in patients with inflammatory or obstructive bowel disorders, patients with acute pancreatitis secondary to biliary tract disease, and patients about to undergo biliary surgery.

V. ALTERATION IN CARDIAC OUTPUT related to HYPOTENSION, BRADYCARDIA

Defining Characteristics: Orthostatic hypotension, bradycardia due to cholinergic effect, and peripheral vasodilatation may occur. There may be histamine-related flushing, pruritus, and diaphoresis with chronic drug usage; tolerance develops to this effect. Syncope may occur. Risk is increased in patients with reduced blood volume or concomitant administration of some CNS-depressing medications (e.g., phenothiazines, general anesthetics).

Nursing Implications: Assess baseline cardiovascular status. Teach patient to change position slowly and to hold onto stable, nearby structure for support as needed.

Be careful when giving IV push opioids, and caution patient to remain in supine position for 15–20 minutes after injection. Monitor cardiovascular status after injection.

VI. ALTERATION IN URINE ELIMINATION related to URINARY RETENTION

Defining Characteristics: Increased smooth muscle tone in urinary tract and spasm may occur. Bladder tone is increased, which may cause urgency. Vesical sphincter tone may be increased, leading to difficulty urinating. Increased risk of urinary retention in patients with prostatic hypertrophy or urethral stricture.

Nursing Implications: Assess baseline urinary elimination pattern. Teach patient to increase fluids to 3 L/day, and encourage voiding every 2–3 hours. Instruct patient to report problems with urination.

VII.   KNOWLEDGE DEFICIT related to DRUG ADMINISTRATION, POTENTIAL FOR TOLERANCE, AND DEPENDENCY

Defining Characteristics: Psychological dependence (addiction) occurs rarely in patients taking opioid agonists for cancer pain (> 1%). Physical dependence (precipitation of withdrawal symptoms) occurs with chronic use of the drug for the relief of chronic cancer pain. In addition, tolerance, or less analgesic effect over time with the same drug dose, occurs and requires increased dosage of drug.

Nursing Implications: Assess baseline knowledge of opioid analgesics and attitude about their use for cancer pain management. Teach patient about proper self-administration, possible side effects, and self-care measures. Suggest patient maintain diary of pain intensity, precipitating and alleviating factors, drug dose and time taken, and relief. Teach patient to self-administer opioid agonists for relief of chronic cancer pain ATC, not PRN, to prevent pain. Explain use of prescribed short-acting opioid for rescue or to manage BTP. Discuss with physician dose increase or change in frequency of administration if tolerance develops. Teach patient that withdrawal symptoms may occur if chronic, ATC dosing is interrupted. Withdrawal (abstinence) symptoms that may be seen are restlessness, lacrimation, rhinorrhea, yawning, perspiration, gooseflesh, restless sleep, mydriasis in first 24 hours. These are followed by twitching and leg spasm; severe aching of the back, abdomen, and legs; cramping in abdomen and legs; hot/cold flashes; insomnia; nausea/vomiting, diarrhea; severe sneezing; and increased heart rate, BP, and T, which peak at 36–72 hours. Withdrawal syndrome can be prevented by administration of at least 1/4 of previous opioid dose.

VIII.   SEXUAL DYSFUNCTION related to IMPOTENCE, DECREASED LIBIDO

Defining Characteristics: Opiate agonists may suppress gonadotropin, causing impotence and decreased libido.

Nursing Implications: Assess baseline sexual pattern. Discuss potential toxicity and impact on sexuality. Provide information, emotional support, and referral as needed.

Drug: methadone (Dolophine, Methadose)

Class: Opioid analgesic (opioid agonist).

Mechanism of Action: A synthetic opioid agonist, methadone resembles morphine but has milder action; binds to opiate receptors in CNS (limbic system, thalamus, striatum, hypothalamus, midbrain, spinal cord), altering pain perception at level of spinal cord and higher centers, as well as the emotional response to pain. Also suppresses cough reflex.

Metabolism: Well absorbed from GI tract; onset and duration of single dose similar to morphine. Short-term duration of analgesic action is 4–8 hours. With chronic administration, plasma elimination half-life is substantially longer (e.g., 8–59 hours, median 22–48 hours). Peak respiratory depressant effects occur later and persist longer than its peak analgesic effects. With repeated dosing, methadone may be retained in the liver, then slowly released, prolonging the duration of action despite low plasma concentrations. Highly tissue-bound; metabolized by liver, excreted by renal filtration, then is reabsorbed (pH dependent). Steady-state plasma concentrations and full analgesic effects are usually not apparent until 3–5 days after dosing.

Indication: For the treatment of moderate-to-severe pain not responsive to nonopioid analgesics, and for the detoxification treatment of opioid addiction.

Dosage/Range: *For moderate to severe pain:*
- Requires opioid Risk Evaluation and Mitigation Strategy (REMS).
- Because of long half-life with long-term dosing, management is complex and requires meticulous patient assessment to prevent overdosage.
- PO: 5–20 mg q 6–8 h, or more for severe cancer pain.
- Subcutaneous, IM (10 mg/mL): 2.5–10 mg q 3–4 h.

Drug Preparation:
- Store tablets in tight, light-resistant containers at 15–30°C (59–86°F).
- Injection should be protected from light and stored at 15–40°C (59–104°F).
- At home, teach patient to store oral doses in a safe place away from children and pets.

Drug Administration:
- PO, IM, subcutaneous.
- Teach patient that opioid analgesics may impair the mental and/or physical ability to drive and use machines, and to avoid these activities until the effect of the drug is known.

Drug Interactions:
- Injection incompatible with solutions containing aminophylline, ammonium chloride, amobarbital sodium, chlorothiazide sodium, heparin sodium, methicillin sodium, nitrofurantoin, phenobarbital sodium, sodium bicarbonate.
- Alcohol, CNS depressants: additive effects.
- Opioid antagonists, mixed agonist/antagonists, partial agonists: may precipitate withdrawal symptoms and reduce analgesia.
- Anti-retroviral agents (abacavir, amprenavir, efavirenz, nelfinavir, nevirapine, ritonavir, lopinavir + ritonavir combination): increased clearance with decreased methadone plasma levels, and decreased methadone effectiveness. Monitor patient for signs/symptoms of withdrawal and discuss methadone dose adjustment with physician or NP/PA.
- Didanosine and stavudine: methadone decreases the AUC of these drugs.
- Zidovudine: methadone increases the AUC of zidovudine, which can result in increased zidovudine toxicity.
- CYP3A4 inducers (e.g., rifampin, phenytoin, St. John's wort): decrease methadone serum level, increasing the risk for withdrawal and decreased pain relief. Assess patient and discuss methadone dose adjustment with physician or NP/PA. Teach patient NOT to take St. John's wort.

MANAGEMENT

- CYP3A4 inhibitors (e.g., ketoconazole, erythromycin, voriconazole; also sertraline, fluvoxamine): decrease methadone clearance, resulting in increased methadone serum level and risk of toxicity. Monitor patient closely and assess need for dose adjustment if coadministration is medically necessary.
- Monamine oxidase inhibitors (MAOIs): MAO inhibitors may cause CNS excitation or depression, hypotension, or hypertension if used concurrently. Do not use concurrently, and separate by at least 14 days after stopping the MAO inhibitor.

Lab Effects/Interference:
- Prolonged QTc interval.

Special Considerations:
- Risk Evaluation and Mitigation Strategy (REMS) required for use of opioids. Healthcare providers must review REMS-compliant education. In addition, healthcare providers must
  a. Complete a REMS-compliant education program offered by an accredited CE provider or another education program that includes all the elements of the FDA Education Blueprint for Health Care Providers Involved in the Management or Support of Patients with Pain. The blueprint can be found at www.fda.gov/OpioidAnalgesicREMSBlueprint.
  b. Discuss the safe use, serious risks, and proper storage and disposal of opioid analgesics with patients and/or their caregivers every time these medicines are prescribed. The Patient Counseling Guide can be obtained at www.fda.gov/OpioidAnalgesicREMSPCG.
  c. Emphasize to patients and their caregivers the importance of reading the Medication Guide that they will receive from their pharmacist every time an opioid analgesic is dispensed to them.
  d. Consider using other tools to improve patient, household, and community safety, such as patient–prescriber agreements that reinforce patient–prescriber responsibilities.
- Oral dose is twice parenteral dose (equianalgesic effect).
- May produce similar or slightly greater respiratory depression than equivalent doses of morphine.
- Additive benefit when combined with acetaminophen or aspirin.
- Give smallest effective dose to prevent development of tolerance, physical dependency.
- Reduce dose in debilitated patients or patients receiving other CNS depressants.
- Use with caution in patients with hepatic or renal dysfunction, hypothyroidism, Addison's disease, severe CNS depression, respiratory depression, head injury, elevated ICP.
- Drug is Pregnancy Category C and not recommended during pregnancy unless the potential benefit justifies the potential risk to the fetus.
- Drug should not be used by nursing mothers.
- If required, naloxone HCl will reverse opiate toxicity (e.g., respiratory depression). However, it is important that acute withdrawal symptoms be prevented by giving only enough naloxone to reverse respiratory depression and that this be continued for opioid drug half-life.

Potential Toxicities/Side Effects and the Nursing Process

I. SENSORY/PERCEPTUAL ALTERATIONS related to CNS DEPRESSION

Defining Characteristics: Drowsiness, sedation, mood changes, euphoria, dysphoria, dizziness, mental clouding may occur. At high doses, may cause seizures. Miosis (papillary constriction) may occur.

Nursing Implications: Assess baseline neurologic status. Use cautiously, if at all, in the elderly, the debilitated, and patients with head injury, increased ICP, severe CNS depression, acute alcoholism. Assess other concurrent medications. Use with caution in patients receiving other opioids, tranquilizers, hypnotics, MAO inhibitors, since increasing CNS depressant effects can occur. Monitor neurologic status closely. Instruct patient to avoid driving and operating machinery while taking the medicine, and to AVOID concurrent alcohol.

II. ALTERATION IN OXYGENATION related to RESPIRATORY DEPRESSION

Defining Characteristics: Opiate agonists directly depress respiratory center in brain stem, causing decreased sensitivity and responsiveness to increased pCO_2. Also may depress deep breathing and reflex to sigh. Tolerance to respiratory depressant effects occurs with chronic use.

Nursing Implications: Assess baseline pulmonary status, and periodically during drug use. Use cautiously in patients with bronchial asthma, COPD, respiratory depression, and monitor closely.

III. ALTERATION IN ELIMINATION related to CONSTIPATION, ILEUS

Defining Characteristics: Opium agonists bind to opiate receptors in bowel, slowing peristalsis, leading to constipation. Untreated constipation may result in bowel perforation.

Nursing Implications: Assess baseline elimination, fluid intake, diet, and exercise patterns. Instruct patient regarding prevention of constipation: goal is to move bowels at least every 2 days by increasing fluids to 3 L/day, following a diet high in fiber (beans, vegetables, fruit), and taking moderate exercise. Assess need for bowel softeners, bulk-forming laxatives, and osmotic cathartics, and discuss prescription with physician. Teach patient self-administration of medications.

IV. ALTERATION IN NUTRITION, LESS THAN BODY REQUIREMENTS, related to GI TOXICITY

Defining Characteristics: Nausea, vomiting, and dry mouth may occur. Gastric, biliary, and pancreatic secretions are decreased by opiate agonists; digestion is delayed.

MANAGEMENT

Biliary tract muscle tone is increased, and spasm of Oddi's sphincter may occur (morphine > meperidine > codeine).

Nursing Implications: Assess patient tolerance of GI side effects. Instruct patient to report side effects. If nausea/vomiting occur, change to another opioid, or premedicate with antiemetic to prevent nausea/vomiting. Assess GI pain, biliary spasm, and consider alternative opioid.

V.   ALTERATION IN CARDIAC OUTPUT related to HYPOTENSION, BRADYCARDIA

Defining Characteristics: Orthostatic hypotension, bradycardia due to cholinergic effect, and peripheral vasodilation may occur with rapid IV dosing. There may be histamine-related flushing, pruritus, diaphoresis with chronic drug usage; tolerance develops to this effect.

Nursing Implications: Assess baseline cardiovascular status. Teach patient to change position slowly and to hold onto stable, nearby structure for support as needed. Be careful when giving IV push opioids, and caution patient to remain in supine position for 15–20 minutes after injection. Monitor cardiovascular status after injection.

VI.   ALTERATION IN URINE ELIMINATION related to URINARY RETENTION

Defining Characteristics: Increased smooth muscle tone in urinary tract and spasm may occur. Bladder tone is increased, which may cause urgency. Vesical sphincter tone may be increased, leading to difficulty urinating. Increased risk of urinary retention in patients with prostatic hypertrophy or urethral stricture.

Nursing Implications: Assess baseline urinary elimination pattern. Teach patient to increase fluids to 3 L/day, and encourage voiding every 2–3 hours. Instruct patient to report problems with urination.

VII.   KNOWLEDGE DEFICIT related to DRUG ADMINISTRATION, POTENTIAL FOR TOLERANCE, AND DEPENDENCY

Defining Characteristics: Psychological dependence (addiction) occurs rarely in patients taking opioid agonists for cancer pain (> 1%). Physical dependence (precipitation of withdrawal symptoms) occurs with chronic use of the drug for the relief of chronic cancer pain. In addition, tolerance, or less analgesic effect over time with the same drug dose, occurs and requires increased dosage of drug.

Nursing Implications: Assess baseline knowledge of opioid analgesics, and attitude about their use for cancer pain management. Teach patient about proper self-administration, possible side effects, and self-care measures. Suggest patient maintain diary of pain intensity, precipitating and alleviating factors, drug dose and time taken, and relief. Teach patient to self-administer opioid agonists for relief of chronic cancer pain ATC, not PRN, to prevent pain. Explain use of prescribed short-acting opioid for rescue or to manage BTP. Discuss with physician dose increase or change in frequency of administration if tolerance develops.

Teach patient that withdrawal symptoms may occur if chronic, around-the–clock dosing is interrupted. Withdrawal (abstinence) symptoms that may be seen are restlessness, lacrimation, rhinorrhea, yawning, perspiration, gooseflesh, restless sleep, mydriasis in first 24 hours. These are followed by twitching and leg spasm; severe aching of the back, abdomen, and legs; cramping in abdomen and legs; hot/cold flashes; insomnia; nausea/vomiting, diarrhea; severe sneezing; and increased heart rate, BP, T, which peak at 36–72 hours. Withdrawal syndrome can be prevented by administration of at least 1/4 of previous opioid dose.

VIII. SEXUAL DYSFUNCTION related to IMPOTENCE, DECREASED LIBIDO

Defining Characteristics: Opiate agonists may suppress gonadotropin, causing impotence and decreased libido.

Nursing Implications: Assess baseline sexual pattern. Discuss potential toxicity and impact on sexuality. Provide information, emotional support, and referral as needed.

Drug: morphine (Astramorph, Avinza, Duramorph, Infumorph, Kadian Morphine Sulfate Sustained Release, MS Contin, MSIR, Morphelan, Oramorph, Roxanol)

Class: Opioid analgesic (opioid agonist).

Mechanism of Action: Binds to opiate receptors in CNS (limbic system, thalamus, striatum, hypothalamus, midbrain, spinal cord). This opioid agonist alters pain perception at level of spinal cord and higher centers, as well as the emotional response to pain. Also suppresses cough reflex.

Metabolism: Variable absorption from GI tract; increased absorption when taken with food. Peak analgesia 60 minutes (oral), 20–60 minutes (rectal), 50–90 minutes (subcutaneous), 30–60 minutes (IM), 20 minutes (IV). Duration is 4–7 hours. Maximum respiratory depression is 30 minutes (IM), 7 minutes (IV), 90 minutes (subcutaneous). Drug is slowly absorbed into systemic circulation after intrathecal (IT) administration. Peak CSF concentrations occur 60–90 minutes after epidural dose. Metabolized by liver and excreted in urine and, to a small degree, feces.

Indication: For the relief of severe, acute pain or severe, chronic pain (e.g., in terminally ill patients). Used also parenterally for preoperative sedation, as a supplement to anesthesia, and for analgesia during labor. Also used in patients with acute pulmonary edema for its cardiovascular effects and to allay anxiety. Morphine should not be used in the treatment of pulmonary edema resulting from a chemical respiratory irritant. Morphine is the drug of choice in relieving pain of MI.

Contraindications: (1) Known hypersensitivity to the drug; (2) in convulsive states (e.g., status epilepticus, tetanus, and strychnine poisoning), as it has a stimulating effect on the spinal cord; (3) heart failure secondary to chronic lung disease; (4) cardiac arrhythmias; (5) brain tumor; (6) acute alcoholism; (7) delirium tremens; (8) if prior idiosyncratic

MANAGEMENT

reaction to the drug; (9) premature infants, or during delivery when premature infant is anticipated.

Dosage/Range: *For moderate to severe pain:*
- Requires an opioid Risk Evaluation and Mitigation Strategy (REMS).
- Oral: 10–60 mg PO q 3–4 h titrated to pain; 10–240 mg sustained release q 8–12 h, titrated to pain.
- Rectal: 10–60 mg q 4 h.
- Subcutaneous, IM: 4–15 mg q 3–4 h.
- IV: 1–100 mg/h, and higher, titrated to need in physically dependent patients.
- Intrathecal: dose is 1/10 the epidural dose.
- Epidural: 5 mg q 24 h.
- At home, teach patient to store oral doses in a safe place away from children and pets.

Drug Preparation:
- Store tablets in tight, light-resistant containers at 15–30°C (59–86°F).
- Injection should be protected from light, and stored at 15–40°C (59–104°F).

Drug Administration:
- Begin morphine therapy using immediate-release oral preparations and increase dose to control pain; once optimal dose identified, convert to sustained-release formulation by dividing 24-hour total morphine dose by 2, giving 2 (q 12 h) doses.
- Intrathecal or epidural: use preservative-free morphine only, for example, Astramorph PF, Duramorph PF, Infumorph; consult individual policies/procedures for administration.
- Teach patient that opioid analgesics may impair the mental and/or physical ability to drive and use machines, and to avoid these activities until the effect of the drug is known.

Drug Interactions:
- Injection incompatible with solutions containing aminophylline, ammonium chloride, amobarbital sodium, chlorothiazide sodium, heparin sodium, methicillin sodium, nitro-furantoin, phenobarbital sodium, sodium bicarbonate.
- Alcohol, CNS depressants: additive effects.

Lab Effects/Interference:
- None known.

Special Considerations:
- Risk Evaluation and Mitigation Strategy (REMS) required for use of opioids. Healthcare providers must review REMS-compliant education. In addition, healthcare providers must
  a. Complete a REMS-compliant education program offered by an accredited CE pro-vider or another education program that includes all the elements of the FDA Educa-tion Blueprint for Health Care Providers Involved in the Management or Support of Patients with Pain. The blueprint can be found at www.fda.gov/OpioidAnalgesic REMSBlueprint.
  b. Discuss the safe use, serious risks, and proper storage and disposal of opioid analgesics with patients and/or their caregivers every time these medicines are prescribed. The Pa-tient Counseling Guide can be obtained at www.fda.gov/OpioidAnalgesicREMSPCG.

c. Emphasize to patients and their caregivers the importance of reading the Medication Guide that they will receive from their pharmacist every time an opioid analgesic is dispensed to them.

d. Consider using other tools to improve patient, household, and community safety, such as patient–prescriber agreements that reinforce patient–prescriber responsibilities.

- Oral to parenteral dose is 3–6 to 1 (equianalgesic dose).
- Highly concentrated formulations are available and are for use in continuous infusion pumps.
- Do not crush sustained-release formulations (e.g., MS Contin, Oramorph).
- When epidural or intrathecal route is used, refer to institutional policy/procedure for administration and patient monitoring.
- Additive benefit when combined with acetaminophen or aspirin.
- Give smallest effective dose to prevent development of tolerance, physical dependency.
- Reduce dose in debilitated patients, or patients receiving other CNS depressants.
- Ensure that patients and caregivers are taught the dose and amount of opioid analgesic to self-administer. It is reported that a patient misunderstood and thought he was taking a 5-mg dose of morphine = 5 mL, when in fact the formulation the patient had was a solution of 100 mg/5 mL. This resulted in a 20-fold overdose. To prevent further errors, the drug has since been repackaged, and requires a Medication Guide be dispensed to each patient with the drug (Roxane Laboratories, December 2010).
- Use with caution in patients with hepatic or renal dysfunction, hypothyroidism, Addison's disease, severe CNS depression, respiratory depression, head injury, elevated ICP.
- If required, naloxone HCl will reverse opiate toxicity (e.g., respiratory depression). However, it is important that acute withdrawal symptoms be prevented by giving only enough naloxone to reverse respiratory depression and that this be continued for opioid drug half-life.
- Kadian as well as Avinza are sustained-release morphine formulated for once-a-day dosing; available in 20-, 50-, and 100-mg tablets (Kadian) and 30-, 60-, 90-, and 120-mg capsules (Avinza).

Potential Toxicities/Side Effects and the Nursing Process

I. SENSORY/PERCEPTUAL ALTERATIONS related to CNS DEPRESSION

Defining Characteristics: Drowsiness, sedation, mood changes, euphoria, dysphoria, dizziness, mental clouding may occur. At high doses, may cause seizures. Miosis (papillary constriction) may occur.

Nursing Implications: Assess baseline neurologic status. Use cautiously, if at all, in the elderly, the debilitated, and patients with head injury, increased ICP, severe CNS depression, acute alcoholism. Assess other concurrent medications. Use with caution in patients receiving other opioids, tranquilizers, hypnotics, MAO inhibitors, since increasing CNS depressant effects can occur. Monitor neurologic status closely. Instruct patient to avoid driving and operating machinery while taking the medicine, and to AVOID concurrent alcohol.

II.   ALTERATION IN OXYGENATION related to RESPIRATORY DEPRESSION

Defining Characteristics: Opiate agonists directly depress respiratory center in brain stem, causing decreased sensitivity and responsiveness to increased pCO_2. Also may depress deep breathing and reflex to sigh. Tolerance to respiratory depressant effects occurs with chronic use.

Nursing Implications: Assess baseline pulmonary status, and periodically during drug use. Use cautiously in patients with bronchial asthma, COPD, respiratory depression, and monitor closely.

III.   ALTERATION IN ELIMINATION related to CONSTIPATION, ILEUS

Defining Characteristics: Opium agonists bind to opiate receptors in bowel, slowing peristalsis, leading to constipation. Untreated constipation may result in bowel perforation.

Nursing Implications: Assess baseline elimination, fluid intake, diet, and exercise patterns. Instruct patient regarding prevention of constipation: goal is to move bowels at least every 2 days by increasing fluids to 3 L/day, following a diet high in fiber (beans, vegetables, fruit), and taking moderate exercise. Assess need for bowel softeners, bulk-forming laxatives, and osmotic cathartics, and discuss prescription with physician. Teach patient self-administration of medications.

IV.   ALTERATION IN NUTRITION, LESS THAN BODY REQUIREMENTS, related to GI TOXICITY

Defining Characteristics: Nausea, vomiting, and dry mouth may occur. Gastric, biliary, and pancreatic secretions are decreased by opiate agonists; digestion is delayed. Biliary tract muscle tone is increased, and spasm of Oddi's sphincter may occur (morphine > meperidine > codeine).

Nursing Implications: Assess patient tolerance of GI side effects. Teach patient to report side effects. If nausea/vomiting occur, change to another opioid, or premedicate with antiemetic to prevent nausea/vomiting. Assess GI pain, biliary spasm, and consider alternative opioid.

V.   ALTERATION IN CARDIAC OUTPUT related to HYPOTENSION, BRADYCARDIA

Defining Characteristics: Orthostatic hypotension, bradycardia due to cholinergic effect, and peripheral vasodilation may occur with rapid IV dosing. There may be histamine-related flushing, pruritus, diaphoresis with chronic drug usage; tolerance develops to this effect.

Nursing Implications: Assess baseline cardiovascular status. Teach patient to change position slowly and to hold onto stable, nearby structure for support as needed. Be careful when giving IV push opioids, and caution patient to remain in supine position for 15–20 minutes after injection. Monitor cardiovascular status after injection.

VI. ALTERATION IN URINE ELIMINATION related to URINARY RETENTION

Defining Characteristics: Increased smooth muscle tone in urinary tract and spasm may occur. Bladder tone is increased, which may cause urgency. Vesical sphincter tone may be increased, leading to difficulty urinating. Increased risk of urinary retention in patients with prostatic hypertrophy or urethral stricture.

Nursing Implications: Assess baseline urinary elimination pattern. Teach patient to increase fluids to 3 L/day, and encourage voiding every 2–3 hours. Instruct patient to report problems with urination.

VII. KNOWLEDGE DEFICIT related to DRUG ADMINISTRATION, POTENTIAL FOR TOLERANCE, AND DEPENDENCY

Defining Characteristics: Psychological dependence (addiction) occurs rarely in patients taking opioid agonists for cancer pain ($< 1\%$). Physical dependence (precipitation of withdrawal symptoms) occurs with chronic use of the drug for the relief of chronic cancer pain. In addition, tolerance, or less analgesic effect over time with the same drug dose, occurs and requires increased dosage of drug.

Nursing Implications: Assess baseline knowledge of opioid analgesics, and attitude about their use for cancer pain management. Teach patient about proper self-administration, possible side effects, and self-care measures. Suggest patient maintain diary of pain intensity, precipitating and alleviating factors, drug dose and time taken, and relief. Teach patient to self-administer opioid agonists for relief of chronic cancer pain ATC, not PRN, to prevent pain. Explain use of prescribed short-acting opioid for rescue or to manage BTP. Discuss with physician dose increase or change in frequency of administration if tolerance develops. Teach patient that withdrawal symptoms may occur if chronic, ATC dosing is interrupted. Withdrawal (abstinence) symptoms that may be seen are restlessness, lacrimation, rhinorrhea, yawning, perspiration, gooseflesh, restless sleep, mydriasis in first 24 hours. These are followed by twitching and leg spasm; severe aching of the back, abdomen, and legs; cramping in abdomen and legs; hot/cold flashes; insomnia; nausea/vomiting, diarrhea; severe sneezing; and increased heart rate, BP, T, which peak at 36–72 hours. Withdrawal syndrome can be prevented by administration of at least one-quarter of previous opioid dose.

VIII. SEXUAL DYSFUNCTION related to IMPOTENCE, DECREASED LIBIDO

Defining Characteristics: Opiate agonists may suppress gonadotropin, causing impotence and decreased libido.

Nursing Implications: Assess baseline sexual pattern. Discuss potential toxicity and impact on sexuality. Provide information, emotional support, and referral as needed.

MANAGEMENT

Drug: oxycodone HCI (Percodan, Percocet, Endodan, Roxiprin, Roxicodone)

Class: Opioid analgesic (opioid agonist).

Mechanism of Action: A synthetic opioid agonist, oxycodone resembles morphine but has milder action; binds to opiate receptors in CNS (limbic system, thalamus, striatum, hypothalamus, midbrain, spinal cord), altering pain perception at level of spinal cord and higher centers, as well as the emotional response to pain. Drug is relatively selective for the mu receptor, and can interact with other opioid receptors at high doses. Also suppresses cough reflex. Oxecta formulation uses Aversion Technology, which discourages abuse of the drug (e.g., the active ingredient gels when improperly used thus discourage injection, and they irritate the nasal passages to discourage inhalation). However, it still can be abused by crushing, chewing, snorting, or injecting the product.

Metabolism: Onset of analgesia in 10–15 minutes, peaks 30–60 minutes, duration 3–6 hours. Metabolized by liver and kidney; excreted in urine.

Indications: Management of moderate-to-severe pain where the use of an opioid analgesic is appropriate.

Contraindications: (1) Known hypersensitivity to oxycodone, (2) situations where opioids are contraindicated (e.g., significant respiratory depression in unmonitored settings/ absence of resuscitative equipment), (3) patients with acute or severe bronchial asthma or hypercarbia, (4) patient suspected or having paralytic ileus.

Dosage/Range: *For moderate to moderately severe pain:*
• Requires opioid Risk Evaluation and Mitigation Strategy (REMS).
• 5 mg q 6 h (Roxicodone).
• 5 mg q 6 h, combined with acetaminophen: 300 mg (e.g., Oxycet, Percocet, Roxicet caplets), OR 500 mg (e.g., Roxicet caplets, Tylox); OR combined with aspirin: 325 mg (e.g., Percodan, Codoxy, Roxiprin); OR combined with ibuprofen 5 mg/400 mg (e.g., Combunox).
• Oral solution: 5 mg/5 mL (Roxicodone); 20 mg/mL (Roxicodone, Intensol).
• 5 to 15 mg every 4–6 hours as needed for pain (Oxecta, Roxicodone).

Drug Preparation:
• Store tablets in tight, light-resistant containers at 15–30°C (59–86°F) and protect from light.
• At home, teach patient to store oral doses in a safe place away from children and pets.

Drug Administration:
• Oral.
• Percocet: 2.5/325 (2.5 mg oxycodone plus 325 mg acetaminophen); 5/325, 7.5/325, 7.5/500, 10/325, 10/650. Acetaminophen cumulative dose should not exceed 4,000 mg a day.
• Oxycodone HCl: available as 5-, 15-, and 30-mg tablets.
• Teach patient that opioid analgesics may impair the mental and/or physical ability to drive and use machines, and to avoid these activities until the effect of the drug is known.

Drug Interactions:
- Alcohol, CNS depressants: additive CNS depressant effects.
- Anticoagulants, chemotherapy: aspirin-oxycodone combination may increase bleeding risk; AVOID concurrent use.

Lab Effects/Interference:
- None known.

Special Considerations:
- Warnings and Precautions:
  - Risk Evaluation and Mitigation Strategy (REMS) required for use of opioids. Healthcare providers must review REMS-compliant education. In addition, healthcare providers must
    a. Complete a REMS-compliant education program offered by an accredited CE provider or another education program that includes all the elements of the FDA Education Blueprint for Health Care Providers Involved in the Management or Support of Patients with Pain. The blueprint can be found at www.fda.gov /OpioidAnalgesicREMSBlueprint.
    b. Discuss the safe use, serious risks, and proper storage and disposal of opioid analgesics with patients and/or their caregivers every time these medicines are prescribed. The Patient Counseling Guide can be obtained at www.fda.gov/Opioid AnalgesicREMSPCG.
    c. Emphasize to patients and their caregivers the importance of reading the Medication Guide that they will receive from their pharmacist every time an opioid analgesic is dispensed to them.
    d. Consider using other tools to improve patient, household, and community safety, such as patient–prescriber agreements that reinforce patient–prescriber responsibilities.
  - Addiction, abuse and misuse: Assess each patient's risk before prescribing, and monitor regularly for evidence of misuse, abuse, or diversion. Addiction is defined as psychological dependence. This is different from physical dependence (goes into withdrawal if drug is abruptly discontinued, which is a side effect of all opioids).
  - Serious, life-threatening, or fatal respiratory depression may occur. Monitor patient closely, especially upon initial dosing or after a dose increase. Monitor patients and teach them to be careful in self-administration, and to keep the medication in a safe place as accidental ingestion of opiates, especially by children or pets can be fatal.
  - Hypotensive effects: Monitor patient during initiation, or dose change.
  - Patients with head injury or increased ICP: Opioids may obscure clinical course of these patients who are sensitive to the effects of CO_2 retention (respiratory depression). Monitor for sedation and respiratory depression.
  - Patient selection: Use with caution in patients with hepatic or renal dysfunction, hypothyroidism, Addison's disease, severe CNS depression, respiratory depression, head injury, elevated ICP.
  - Use in biliary/pancreatic disease: Oxycodone can cause spasm of the sphincter of Oddi. Use with caution in these patients and assess for this side effect, including elevated serum amylase.
- Adverse effects are milder than morphine.

- Preparations may contain sodium metabisulfite and may cause allergic reactions, including anaphylaxis and severe asthma-like reactions.
- Additive benefit when combined with acetaminophen or aspirin.
- Give smallest effective dose to prevent development of tolerance, physical dependency.
- Reduce dose in debilitated patients or patients receiving other CNS depressants.
- If required, naloxone HCl will reverse opiate toxicity (e.g., respiratory depression). However, it is important that acute withdrawal symptoms be prevented by giving only enough naloxone to reverse respiratory depression and that this be continued for opioid drug half-life.

Potential Toxicities/Side Effects and the Nursing Process

I. SENSORY/PERCEPTUAL ALTERATIONS related to CNS DEPRESSION

Defining Characteristics: Drowsiness, sedation, mood changes, euphoria, dysphoria, dizziness, mental clouding may occur. At high doses, may cause seizures. Miosis (papillary constriction) may occur.

Nursing Implications: Assess baseline neurologic status. Use cautiously, if at all, in the elderly, the debilitated, and patients with head injury, increased ICP, severe CNS depression, acute alcoholism. Assess other concurrent medications. Use with caution in patients receiving other opioids, tranquilizers, hypnotics, MAO inhibitors, since increasing CNS depressant effects can occur. Monitor neurologic status closely. Instruct patient to avoid driving and operating machinery while taking the medicine, and to AVOID concurrent alcohol.

II. ALTERATION IN OXYGENATION related to RESPIRATORY DEPRESSION

Defining Characteristics: Opiate agonists directly depress respiratory center in brain stem, causing decreased sensitivity and responsiveness to increased pCO_2. Also may depress deep breathing and reflex to sigh. Tolerance to respiratory depressant effects occurs with chronic use.

Nursing Implications: Assess baseline pulmonary status, and periodically during drug use. Use cautiously in patients with bronchial asthma, COPD, respiratory depression, and monitor closely.

III. ALTERATION IN ELIMINATION related to CONSTIPATION, ILEUS

Defining Characteristics: Opium agonists bind to opiate receptors in bowel, slowing peristalsis, leading to constipation. Untreated constipation may result in bowel perforation.

Nursing Implications: Assess baseline elimination, fluid intake, diet, and exercise patterns. Instruct patient regarding prevention of constipation: goal is to move bowels at least every 2 days by increasing fluids to 3 L/day, following a diet high in fiber (beans, vegetables, fruit), and taking moderate exercise. Assess need for bowel softeners, bulk-forming laxatives, and osmotic cathartics, and discuss preparation with physician. Teach patient self-administration of medications. Monitor for decreased bowel motility in postoperative patients.

IV. ALTERATION IN NUTRITION, LESS THAN BODY REQUIREMENTS, related to GI TOXICITY

Defining Characteristics: Nausea, vomiting, dry mouth may occur. Gastric, biliary, and pancreatic secretions are decreased by opiate agonists; digestion is delayed. Biliary tract muscle tone is increased, and spasm of Oddi's sphincter may occur (morphine $>$ meperidine $>$ codeine).

Nursing Implications: Assess patient tolerance of GI side effects. Teach patient to report side effects. If nausea/vomiting occur, change to another opioid, or premedicate with antiemetic to prevent nausea/vomiting. Assess GI pain, biliary spasm, and consider alternative opioid.

V. ALTERATION IN CARDIAC OUTPUT related to HYPOTENSION, BRADYCARDIA

Defining Characteristics: Orthostatic hypotension, bradycardia due to cholinergic effect, and peripheral vasodilation may occur with rapid IV dosing. There may be histamine-related flushing, pruritus, diaphoresis with chronic drug usage; tolerance develops to this effect.

Nursing Implications: Assess baseline cardiovascular status. Teach patient to change position slowly and to hold onto stable, nearby structure for support as needed. Teach patient to report dizziness, any falls, or other problems.

VI. ALTERATION IN URINE ELIMINATION related to URINARY RETENTION

Defining Characteristics: Increased smooth muscle tone in urinary tract and spasm may occur. Bladder tone is increased, which may cause urgency. Vesical sphincter tone may be increased, leading to difficulty urinating. Increased risk of urinary retention in patients with prostatic hypertrophy or urethral stricture.

Nursing Implications: Assess baseline urinary elimination pattern. Teach patient to increase fluids to 3 L/day, and encourage voiding every 2–3 hours. Instruct patient to report problems with urination.

VII. KNOWLEDGE DEFICIT related to DRUG ADMINISTRATION, POTENTIAL FOR TOLERANCE, AND DEPENDENCY

Defining Characteristics: Psychological dependence (addiction) occurs rarely in patients taking opioid agonists for cancer pain ($> 1\%$). Physical dependence (precipitation of withdrawal symptoms) occurs with chronic use of the drug for the relief of chronic cancer pain. In addition, tolerance, or less analgesic effect over time with the same drug dose, occurs and requires increased dosage of drug.

Nursing Implications: Assess baseline knowledge of opioid analgesics, and attitude about their use for cancer pain management. Teach patient about proper self-administration, possible side effects, and self-care measures. Suggest patient maintain diary of pain intensity, precipitating and alleviating factors, drug dose and time taken, and relief. Teach patient to self-administer for relief of chronic cancer pain ATC, not PRN, to prevent pain. Explain use of prescribed short-acting opioid for rescue or to manage BTP. Discuss with physician dose increase or change in frequency of administration if tolerance develops. Teach patient that withdrawal symptoms may occur if chronic, ATC dosing is interrupted. Withdrawal (abstinence) symptoms that may be seen are restlessness, lacrimation, rhinorrhea, yawning, perspiration, gooseflesh, restless sleep, mydriasis in first 24 hours. These are followed by twitching and leg spasm; severe aching of the back, abdomen, and legs; cramping in abdomen and legs; hot/cold flashes; insomnia; nausea/vomiting, diarrhea; severe sneezing; and increased heart rate, BP, T, which peak at 36–72 hours. Withdrawal syndrome can be prevented by administration of at least 1/4 of previous opioid dose.

VIII. POTENTIAL FOR INJURY related to DRUG ABUSE

Defining Characteristics: Oxycodone has been significantly abused in the past. Opiate antagonists are sought after by people with addiction disorders and drug abusers. Addiction is a psychological dependence characterized by compulsive use of an opiate for nonmedical purposes, and despite potential harm. "Drug seeking" behavior is common in addicts and drug abusers, and often involves "doctor shopping," or loss of prescriptions. Newer formulations incorporate tamper-proof technology, such as Aversion Technology used in Oxecta. Additives discourage abuse by forming a gel if a user tries to prepare it for injection, and it irritates the nasal passages if a user tries to snort it (Oxecta). In addition, opioids now require REMS education of prescribers and patients.

Nursing Implications: REMS requires healthcare professionals to complete education about the risks and benefits of prescribing controlled-release opiates, and strategies to prevent abuse or illicit use, in addition to a very detailed patient education guide. Some also require patient agreements. Strategies to prevent abuse include careful record-keeping of prescribing information (e.g., quantity, frequency, renewal requests). Patients should be assessed regularly, and repeated requests to obtain a prescription early before it is due should be explored further, along with "lost prescriptions." In the event the patient is abusing the drug, it is important to develop a contract with the patient stating the expected behaviors and sequelae if they are not adhered to.

IX.   SEXUAL DYSFUNCTION related to IMPOTENCE, DECREASED LIBIDO

Defining Characteristics: Opiate agonists may suppress gonadotropin, causing impotence and decreased libido.

Nursing Implications: Assess baseline sexual pattern. Discuss potential toxicity and impact on sexuality. Provide information, emotional support, and referral as needed.

Drug: oxycodone controlled-release formulation (OxyContin)

Class: Opioid analgesic (opioid agonist).

Mechanism of Action: A synthetic mu-receptor opioid agonist, oxycodone resembles morphine but has milder action; binds to opiate receptors in CNS (limbic system, thalamus, striatum, hypothalamus, midbrain, spinal cord), altering pain perception at level of spinal cord and higher centers, as well as the emotional response to pain. Also suppresses cough reflex.

Metabolism: About 60–87% of oral dose of oxycodone reaches the central compartment compared to a parenteral dose. High bioavailability due to low presystemic and/or first pass metabolism. Drug has biphasic absorption pattern with half-lives of 0.6 and 6.9 hours, corresponding to an initial release of oxycodone from the tablet, followed by a prolonged release. Steady-state plasma concentrations are reached within 24–36 hours of initiation of dosing. Food has no significant effect on extent of absorption of oxycodone from OxyContin. Once absorbed, oxycodone is distributed to skeletal muscle, liver, intestinal tract, lungs, spleen, and brain. Drug has been found in breast milk. Oxycodone HCl is extensively metabolized to noroxycodone, primarily via CYP3A4-mediated *N*-demethylation, and to a lesser degree (to oxymorphone) via CYP2D6-mediated, *O*-demethylation oxycodone and its metabolites are excreted primarily via the kidney. The elimination half-life of oxycodone following the administration of OxyContin was 4.5 hours compared to 3.2 hours for immediate-release oxycodone. The elderly have plasma concentrations of oxycodone 15% higher as compared to younger subjects, and females have a plasma concentration 25% higher than males.

Indications: For the management of pain severe enough to require daily, ATC long-term opioid treatment and for which alternative treatment options are inadequate in (1) adults, and (2) opioid-tolerant pediatric patients 11 years of age and older who are already receiving and tolerate a minimum opioid daily dose of at least 20-mg oxycodone orally or its equivalent.

- Opioid tolerance is defined as: taking **at least** 60 mg oral morphine/day; or 25 mcg transdermal fentanyl/hour; or 30 mg oral oxycodone/day; or 8 mg oral hydromorphone/day; or 25 mg oral oxymorphone/day; or an equianalgesic dose of another opioid for a week or longer.

Limitations: (1) Reserve oxycontin, which is extended release, for patients for whom alternative treatment options (e.g., nonopioid analgesics or immediate-release opioids) are ineffective, not tolerated, or otherwise inadequate to treat the patient's pain, as the risks of addiction, abuse, and misuse along with the risk of overdose and death exist; (2) drug is NOT intended for use as a PRN analgesic.

- **Contraindications:** OxyContin is contraindicated in patients with (1) significant respiratory depression, (2) acute or severe bronchial asthma in an unmonitored setting or in absence of resuscitative equipment, (3) risk of obstruction in patients who have difficulty swallowing or have GI disorders that may predispose them to obstruction, including paralytic ileus, (4) hypersensitivity to oxycodone, (5) as a PRN analgesic.

MANAGEMENT

Dosage/Range:
- Requires an opioid Risk Evaluation and Mitigation Strategy (REMS).
- To be prescribed only by healthcare providers knowledgeable in use of potent opioids for management of chronic pain.
- Oxycontin 60 and 80 mg tablets, a single dose > 40 mg, or a total daily dose > 80 mg, are only for use in patients in whom tolerance to an opioid of comparable potency has been established.
- Treatment must be individualized in every case.
- Start on lowest appropriate dose.
- Teach patient to ensure the drug is used only by the patient for whom it is prescribed. Prescribers must complete OxyContin REMS training (www.oxycontinrems.com): Healthcare Professional Letter, Healthcare Provider Training Guide, Education Confirmation Form. Patients and caregivers can go on this site to obtain the OxyContin Medication Guide.

1a. Adult opioid naïve or opioid nontolerant patient:
- 10 mg every 12 hours. See package insert for information on converting from other opioids.
- Do not use OxyContin 60- or 80-mg tablets, a single dose > 40 mg, or a total daily dose > 80 mg, except in patients with demonstrated tolerance to another opioid of comparable potency as these may cause fatal respiratory depression.

1b. Adult patients who are opioid tolerant (e.g., taking for at least 1 week or longer, at a dose of at least 60 mg oral morphine/day, 25 mcg transdermal fentanyl/hour, 30 mg oral oxycodone/day, 8 mg oral hydromorphone/day, 25 mg oral oxymorphone/day, or an equianalgesic dose of another opioid): use standard conversion ratio estimates. Titrate dose to adequate analgesia with minimal/acceptable side effects.
- Calculate 24-hour requirement of opioid, then convert to oxycodone. Standard conversion estimates may be used but are approximate. It is safer to underestimate the equianalgesic dose, and supplement oxycodone for BTP; then calculate the equivalent total daily dose of combined drug, and divide by two, to obtain the 12-hour dose of oxycontin.
- When converting from oxycodone, divide the 24-hour oxycodone dose in half to obtain the twice-a-day (q 12 h) of OxyContin. Round down to a dose that is appropriate for the tablet strengths available.
- Discontinue all other ATC opioid drugs when OxyContin is initiated.
- Close observation and frequent titration are indicated until the patient is stable on the new therapy.

2. **Pediatric patients aged 11 and older:** (a) Patient must be opioid-tolerant, receiving and tolerating opioids for at least 5 consecutive days with a minimum of 20 mg oxycodone or its equivalent for 2 days immediately prior to starting Oxycontin; (b) see package insert for converting from one opioid to another.

3. **Geriatric patients (debilitated, opioid-nontolerant geriatric patients)**: Start at 1/3 to 1/2 the recommended starting dose and titrate carefully.

4. Patients with hepatic impairment: Initiate at 1/3 to 1/2 the recommended starting dose and titrate carefully.

5. Patients currently taking CNS depressants: Initiate at 1/3 to 1/2 the recommended starting dose and titrate carefully.

- In all cases, patients should also receive a short-acting analgesic for BTP.
- To convert transdermal fentanyl to OxyContin, use 10-mg OxyContin every 12 hours for each 25-μg fentanyl transdermal patch. Initiate OxyContin 18 hours after removal of the patch(s). Follow the patient closely for early titration to find the optimal dose, as there are limited clinical data about dose conversion.
  - If patient no longer requires therapy with OxyContin, taper the dose gradually to prevent withdrawal in the physically dependent patient. Do NOT abruptly discontinue OxyContin in a physically dependent patient.

6. Titrating dose: Frequently assess pain relief and opioid side effects, and any behaviors that suggest abuse/misuse. Titrate to adequate effect (usually mild or no pain), with use of no more than 2 doses of rescue or BTP medication per 24 hours.
  - Titrate dosage every 1–2 days, as steady state concentrations are approximated within 24–36 hours. Increase the dose, NOT the dosing frequency, as there are no data about administering the drug any sooner than every 12 hours.
  - In adults, increase the total daily dose of oxycodone by 25–50% of the current daily dose at each increase.
  - For pediatric patients, the total daily dosage can usually be increased by 25% of the total daily dosage every 1–2 days.
  - If signs of excessive opioid-related side effects occur, reduce the next dose; however, if the pain increases, patient should take a supplemental dose of immediate-release oxycodone, or a nonopioid analgesic adjuvant drug.

- Maintain close contact with the patient/family during dose titration to assess tolerance and effect.
- Oxycontin 60-, 80-, 160-mg tablets, or a single dose > 40 mg or a total daily dose > 80 mg, are to be used ONLY in opiate-tolerant patients (see Special Considerations), as they will be tolerant to the respiratory depressant effects of the drug.

Dose Modification:
- Elderly: initial dose may need to be reduced to 1/3 to 1/2 of the usual dose.
- Hepatic impairment: start therapy at 1/3 to 1/2 of the usual dose with careful dose titration.
- Renal impairment (creatinine clearance < 60 mL/min): start therapy conservatively, as plasma concentrations may be 50% higher than in patients with normal renal function.
- Debilitated, nontolerant patients: start at 1/3 to 1/2 of the usual dose with careful dose titration.

Drug Preparation: Available as 10-, 15-, 20-, 30-, 40-, 60-, 80-mg controlled-release tablets.

Drug Administration:
- Ensure REMS implemented and patient understands and agrees to Patient Guide (see Warnings and Precautions 2).
- Oral.
- Patient should be instructed to swallow the tablet intact, and to NOT chew, break, crush, dissolve, cut, soak, lick, or otherwise wet the tablet, as this can cause rapid release of all

drug, overdose, and potentially fatal outcome. Tablets should be taken one tablet at a time with enough water to ensure complete swallowing after placing in mouth.

  • Do not use OxyContin 60- or 80-mg tablets, a single dose > 40 mg, or a total daily dose > 80 mg, except in patients with demonstrated tolerance to another opioid of comparable potency as these may cause fatal respiratory depression.
• Monitor patients closely for respiratory depression, especially within the first 48–72 hours of starting OxyContin therapy.
• When OxyContin is no longer needed, unused tablets should be destroyed by flushing them down the toilet (per FDA).
• Do **not** abruptly discontinue Oxycontin in a physically dependent patient as it may precipitate withdrawal.
• Teach patient that opioid analgesics may impair the mental and/or physical ability to drive and use machines, and to avoid these activities until the effect of the drug is known.

Drug Interactions: All cytochrome P450 3A4 inhibitors (macrolide antibiotics like erythromycin, azole antifungal agents like ketoconazole, protease inhibitors like ritonavir) may decrease oxycodone metabolism and result in an increase in oxycodone plasma concentrations; do not give concurrently if possible; otherwise monitor the patient closely for an extended period of time and with each dosage adjustment.
• CNS depressants (e.g., hypnotics, sedatives, general anesthetics, antipsychotics, alcohol) may cause additive depressant effects and respiratory depression, hypotension, profound sedation, coma; if must use concurrently, reduce dose of one or both agents. Otherwise respiratory depression, hypotension, and profound sedation or coma may occur. Do not take drug when drinking alcohol.
• MAO inhibitors: MAO inhibitors may cause CNS excitation or depression, hypotension, or hypertension if used concurrently. Do not use concurrently, and separate by at least 14 days after stopping the MAO inhibitor.
• OxyContin may enhance the neuromuscular blocking action of skeletal muscle relaxants and produce an increased degree of respiratory depression.
• Mixed agonist/antagonist opioid analgesics (e.g., buprenorphine, nalbuphine, pentazocine) may reduce analgesic effect by competitive blockade of receptors ± precipitate withdrawal symptoms. Do not use concurrently.
• Anticholinergic drugs may increase risk of urinary retention and/or severe constipation leading to paralytic ileus.

Lab Effects/Interference:
• Increased serum amylase level caused by spasm of sphincter of Oddi.
• Standard urine drug testing for oxycodone may not be reliable. If this testing is required, make sure the specificity and sensitivity is appropriate (Purdue, 2015).

Special Considerations:
• Individualize dose for each patient when starting dosing regimen. Overestimating the initial dose when converting from another opioid can result in overdosage and death. Also remember that the drug has a high risk of abuse. In calculating the initial dose, consider:
  • Risk factors for abuse, addiction, or diversion, including a prior history or family history of abuse, addiction, or diversion.

- Age, general condition, medical status of the patient.
- Daily dose, potency, and specific characteristics of the patient's current opioid.
- Reliability of the relative potency estimate used to calculate the equivalent dose of oxycodone needed.
- Patient's degree of opioid exposure and opioid tolerance.
- Concurrent nonopioid analgesics and other medications, such as those with CNS activity.
- Type and severity of the patient's pain.
- The balance between pain control and adverse effects.
- Warnings and Precautions:
  - *Addiction, abuse, and misuse:* Extended-release opioid drug exposes patient to potential for addiction, abuse, and misuse, which can lead to overdose and death. Assess each patient's risk before prescribing and assess regularly for these behaviors. **Addiction is psychological dependence**—that is, taking the drug not for its pain relief effect but for a psychological "high" or sensation. If a patient with cancer takes the opioid regularly for relief of cancer pain, then the patient is not "addicted." Patients will develop physical dependence, which occurs in all people where the removal of the opiate from the patient's system (e.g., abruptly stopping the drug, or giving narcan to a patient on long-term opiates) will result in withdrawal symptoms. This can be a horrible experience for a patient with cancer in pain and should never be allowed to occur. If narcan is required, it should be titrated so that only enough is given to restore respirations, but not enough to totally remove the opiate from the patient with cancer who has been taking opiates for a long time. Tolerance also normally develops over time, where the body is more efficient in clearing the drug from the system, and patients may require a higher dose to achieve the same level of analgesia as before. This also may occur when the tumor progresses so both must be evaluated as possible causes. This is NOT addiction. Unfortunately, opioids are sought by drug abusers and people with addiction disorders. Abuse or misuse of Oxycontin by crushing, chewing, snorting, or injecting the dissolved product will result in uncontrolled delivery of oxycodone and can result in overdose and death (Purdue, 2018).
  - *Opioid Analgsic Risk Evaluation and Mitigation Strategy (REMS):* Required education is given to healthcare providers who must (1) complete a REMS-compliant education program (CE), includes all elements of FDA Education Blueprint for Healthcare providers involved in the management or support of patients with pain; (2) discuss the safe use, serious risks, and proper storage/disposal of opioid analgesics with patients and/or their caregivers every time these medicines are prescribed (patient counseling guide available at www.fda.gov/OpioidAnalgesicREMSPCG; (3) emphasize to patients/caregivers the importance of reading the Medication Guide that their pharmacist will give them every time an opioid analgesic is dispensed to them; (3) consider using other tools to improve patient, household, and community safety such as patient–prescriber agreements that reinforce patient–prescriber responsibilities. FDA Blueprint can be found at www.fda.gov/OpioidAnalgesicREMSBlueprint.
  - *Life-threatening respiratory depression:* Serious, life-threatening, or fatal respiratory depression may occur. Monitor patient closely especially when initiating drug (first 24–72 hours) and escalating dose. Teach patient to swallow tablet whole, do not chew or crush, as this may expose the patient to a potentially fatal overdose.

MANAGEMENT

- *Accidental ingestion* of drug, especially by children can be fatal. Store medicine out of reach of children or pets, and carefully destroy and dispose of unused drug so that neither children nor pets can ingest the drug.
- *Neonatal opioid withdrawal syndrome:* Prolonged use of oxycontin during pregnancy can result in Neonatal Opioid Withdrawal Syndrome, which can be life-threatening to the newborn if not recognized and treated. Ensure mother understands that the newborn will need care in a facility familiar with this syndrome and that has treatment protocols based on current standards.
- *Risks of concomitant use or discontinuation of cytochrome P450 3A4 inhibitors and inducers:* CYP3A4 inhibitors may increase drug serum level and prolong opioid toxicity, leading to potentially fatal respiratory depression, especially when added after a stable dose has been found. Similarly, the discontinuance of a CYP3A4 inducer may increase serum fentanyl levels and prolong opioid toxicity, including respiratory depression. Conversely, discontinuation of a CYP3A4 inhibitor or addition of a CYP3A4 inducer can reduce fentanyl serum levels resulting in adequate analgesia. Monitor patient very closely, frequently; adjust fentanyl dosage as needed and safe.
- *Risks from concomitant use with benzodiazepines or other CNS depressants (including alcohol):* Profound sedation, respiratory depression, coma and death may result. Thus, reserve concomitant use of these drugs only when no alternative exists, and monitor patient closely. Assess medication profile, and teach patient to avoid alcohol when receiving the drug.
- *Life-threatening respiratory depression in patients with chronic pulmonary disease or in elderly, cachectic, or debilitated patients:* Life-threatening respiratory depression can occur, even at approved doses, especially if the patient has an underlying respiratory disorder, is elderly, or is debilitated; is not opioid tolerant; or if the drug is coadministered with other respiratory-depressing drugs. Assess for patient's reduced urge to breathe and decreased respiratory rate, often with a sighing pattern (deep breaths separated by long pauses). Retention of carbon dioxide combined with opioid sedation can lead to accidental overdose. Assess patients at risk closely, especially 24–72 hours within drug initiation or dose change. Ensure proper dosing and titration to prevent respiratory problems.
- *Adrenal insufficiency:* Adrenal insufficiency has occurred, especially in patients receiving opioids for >1 month. Signs/symptoms include: nausea, vomiting, anorexia, fatigue, weakness, dizziness, low BP. If adrenal insufficiency is suspected, confirm the diagnosis with lab testing; if confirmed, treat with physiological doses of corticosteroids. Wean the patient off the opioid to allow adrenal function recovery while continuing corticosteroids. Other opioids should be tried.
- *Severe hypotension:* Severe hypotension may occur, including orthostatic hypotension and syncope in ambulatory patients, especially in patients with reduced blood volume or receiving concurrent certain CNS depressing drugs (e.g., phenothiazines, general anesthetics). Monitor these patients closely for signs/symptoms hypotension after starting drug or dose titration. Do not use Exalgo in patients with circulatory shock.
- *Risk of use in patients with head injury, brain tumor, or increased ICP:* Opioids may obscure clinical course of these patients who are sensitive to the effects of CO_2 retention (respiratory depression). Monitor for sedation and respiratory depression. Avoid

use of opioids in patients with impaired consciousness or coma who are susceptible to the intracranial effects of CO_2 retention.

- *Difficulty swallowing and risk for obstruction in patients at risk for a small GI lumen*: There have been postmarketing reports of difficulty swallowing Oxycontin tablets (e.g., choking, gagging, regurgitation, and tablets stuck in throat) (Purdue, 2016). Teach patient NOT to presoak or otherwise wet Oxycontin tablets prior to placing in mouth, to take 1 tablet at a time, and to swallow completely with sufficient water before taking the next pill. Rare reports also describe intestinal obstruction requiring removal of the tablet, and exacerbation of diverticulitis. Patients with esophageal cancer may have small GI lumens, so are at greater risk, and consideration for alternative opioids should be made.

- *Risk of use in patients with GI conditions*: Oxycontin is contraindicated in patients with known or suspected GI obstruction, including paralytic ileus. Opioids may cause spasm of the sphincter of Oddi. In addition, opioids may cause an increase in serum amylase. Monitor patients with biliary tract disease, including acute pancreatitis, for worsening symptoms.

- *Increased risk of seizures in patients with seizure disorders*: Drug may increase seizure frequency or occurrence in other clinical settings. Monitor patients with a seizure history closely for worsening seizure control when taking this drug.

- *Risks of driving and operating machinery*: Drug may impair mental and/or physical abilities of driving or operating machinery. Teach patient to avoid driving and operation of machinery until the effect of the opioid is known.

- *Withdrawal*: Avoid the use of mixed agonist/antagonist (e.g., pentazocine, nalbuphine, butophanol) or partial agonists (e.g., buprenorphine) analgesics in patients receiving a full opioid agonist analgesic such as Oxycontin. The agonist/antagonist or partial agonist can reduce the analgesic effect of Oxycontin, and may precipitate withdrawal. If Oxycontin is discontinued, gradually taper the dose; DO NOT abruptly discontinue Oxycontin.

- *Laboratory monitoring:* If urine testing for oxycodone is considered, ensure that the sensitivity and specificity of the assay is appropriate and consider the limitations of the testing used when interpreting results.

- Drug is not recommended during labor and delivery, pregnancy, or nursing.
- Most common adverse effects ($> 5\%$) are constipation, nausea, somnolence, dizziness, vomiting, pruritus, headache, dry mouth, asthenia, and sweating.

Potential Toxicities/Side Effects and the Nursing Process

I.   SENSORY/PERCEPTUAL ALTERATIONS related to CNS DEPRESSION

Defining Characteristics: Drowsiness, sedation, mood changes, euphoria, dysphoria, dizziness, alterations in judgment and levels of consciousness, and mental clouding may occur. The respiratory depressant effects of opioids includes CO_2 retention and secondary increase of CSF; it may be magnified in the presence of head injury, intracranial lesions, or other preexisting causes of increased ICP. At high doses, may cause seizures. Miosis (pupillary constriction) may occur. OxyContin can worsen and obscure neurologic signs (e.g., LOC, pupillary) of increasing ICP in patients who are head injured.

MANAGEMENT

Nursing Implications: Assess baseline neurologic status. Use cautiously, if at all, in the elderly, the debilitated, and patients with head injury, increased ICP, severe CNS depression, acute alcoholism. Assess other concurrent medications. Use with caution in patients receiving other opioids, tranquilizers, hypnotics, and MAO inhibitors, because increasing CNS depressant effects can occur. Discuss using a lower initial dose of a CNS depressant when given to a patient receiving OxyContin. Teach patient NOT to use alcohol or illicit drugs while taking OxyContin. Monitor neurologic status closely. Instruct patient to avoid driving and operating machinery while taking the medicine, and to AVOID concurrent alcohol.

II.   ALTERATION IN OXYGENATION related to RESPIRATORY DEPRESSION

Defining Characteristics: Opiate agonists directly depress respiratory center in brain stem, causing decreased sensitivity and responsiveness to increased pCO_2. Also may depress deep breathing and reflex to sigh. Tolerance to respiratory depressant effects occurs with chronic use.

Nursing Implications: Assess baseline pulmonary status, and periodically during drug use. Use with extreme caution in patients with significant COPD or cor pulmonale; patients with decreased respiratory reserve, hypoxia, or hypercapnia; or patients with preexisting respiratory depression or bronchial asthma. Teach patient and family members to report any "breathlessness" or dyspnea. Monitor patients closely as to analgesic benefit and adverse effects.

III.   ALTERATION IN ELIMINATION related to CONSTIPATION, ILEUS

Defining Characteristics: Opium agonists bind to opiate receptors in bowel, slowing peristalsis, leading to constipation. Untreated constipation may result in bowel perforation.

Nursing Implications: Assess baseline elimination, fluid intake, diet, and exercise patterns. Instruct patient regarding prevention of constipation: goal is to move bowels at least every 2 days by increasing fluids to 3 L/day, following a diet high in fiber (beans, vegetables, fruit), and taking moderate exercise. All patients should be on a bowel regimen. Assess need for bowel softeners, bulk-forming laxatives, and osmotic cathartics, and discuss preparation with physician. Teach patient self-administration of medications.

IV.   ALTERATION IN NUTRITION, LESS THAN BODY REQUIREMENTS, related to GI TOXICITY

Defining Characteristics: Nausea, vomiting, dry mouth may occur. Gastric, biliary, and pancreatic secretions are decreased by opiate agonists; digestion is delayed. Biliary tract muscle tone is increased, and spasm of Oddi's sphincter may occur (morphine > meperidine > codeine).

Nursing Implications: Assess patient tolerance of GI side effects. Teach patient to report side effects. If nausea/vomiting occur, change to another opioid, or premedicate with antiemetic to prevent nausea/vomiting. Assess GI pain, biliary spasm, and consider alternative opioid.

V. ALTERATION IN URINE ELIMINATION related to URINARY RETENTION

Defining Characteristics: Increased smooth muscle tone in urinary tract and spasm may occur. Bladder tone is increased, which may cause urgency. Vesical sphincter tone may be increased, leading to difficulty urinating. Increased risk of urinary retention in patients with prostatic hypertrophy or urethral stricture.

Nursing Implications: Assess baseline urinary elimination pattern. Teach patient to increase fluids to 3 L/day, and encourage voiding every 2–3 hours. Instruct patient to report problems with urination.

VI. ALTERATION IN CARDIAC OUTPUT related to HYPOTENSION, BRADYCARDIA

Defining Characteristics: Orthostatic hypotension, bradycardia due to cholinergic effect, and peripheral vasodilitation may occur. Oxycodone may cause orthostatic hypotension in ambulatory patients. There may be histamine-related flushing, pruritus, diaphoresis with chronic drug usage; tolerance develops to this effect.

Nursing Implications: Assess baseline cardiovascular status. Teach patient to change position slowly and to hold onto stable, nearby structure for support as needed. Teach patient to report dizziness, any falls, or other problems. Drug should be administered with caution if at all, in patients in shock as the vasodilitation caused by the drug may further reduce cardiac output and BP.

VII. KNOWLEDGE DEFICIT related to DRUG ADMINISTRATION, POTENTIAL FOR TOLERANCE, AND PHYSICAL DEPENDENCY

Defining Characteristics: Psychological dependence (addiction) occurs rarely in patients taking opioid agonists for cancer pain ($< 1\%$). Physical dependence (precipitation of withdrawal symptoms) occurs with chronic use of the drug for the relief of chronic cancer pain. In addition, tolerance, or less analgesic effect over time with the same drug dose, occurs and requires increased dosage of drug.

Nursing Implications: Assess baseline knowledge of opioid analgesics and attitude about their use for cancer pain management. Teach patient about proper self-administration, possible side effects, and self-care measures. Suggest patient maintain diary of pain intensity, precipitating and alleviating factors, drug dose and time taken, and relief. Teach patient to self-administer opioid agonists for relief of chronic cancer pain ATC, not PRN, to prevent pain. Explain use of prescribed short-acting opioid for rescue or to manage BTP. Discuss with physician dose increase or change in frequency of administration if tolerance develops.

MANAGEMENT

Teach patient that withdrawal symptoms may occur if chronic, ATC dosing is interrupted. Withdrawal (abstinence) symptoms that may be seen are restlessness, lacrimation, rhinorrhea, yawning, perspiration, gooseflesh, restless sleep, mydriasis in first 24 hours. These are followed by twitching and leg spasm; severe aching of the back, abdomen, and legs; cramping in abdomen and legs; hot/cold flashes; insomnia; nausea/vomiting, diarrhea; severe sneezing; and increased heart rate, BP, T, which peak at 36–72 hours. Withdrawal syndrome can be prevented by administration of at least 1/4 of previous opioid dose.

VIII. POTENTIAL FOR INJURY related to DRUG ABUSE

Defining Characteristics: OxyContin has been significantly abused in the past. Opiate antagonists are sought after by people with addiction disorders and drug abusers. Addiction is a psychological dependence characterized by compulsive use of an opiate for nonmedical purposes, and despite potential harm. "Drug seeking" behavior is common in addicts and drug abusers, and often involves "doctor shopping," or loss of prescriptions. The FDA requires that Purdue Pharma use the same REMS as hydromorphone extended-release tablets (see Exalgo).

Nursing Implications: Healthcare professionals must complete education about the risks and benefits of prescribing controlled-release opiates, and strategies to prevent abuse or illicit use, in addition to a very detailed patient education guide. The Purdue Pharma guide is called Medical Education Resource Catalogue Online (MERCO), a Web-based resource, and has, among the many programs, ASAP (Addressing Substance Abuse Prevention). It is found at http://www.purduepharmamededresources.com. Strategies to prevent abuse include careful record-keeping of prescribing information (e.g., quantity, frequency, renewal requests). Patients should be assessed regularly, and repeated requests to obtain a prescription early before it is due should be explored further, along with "lost prescriptions." In the event the patient is abusing the drug, it is important to develop a contract with the patient stating the expected behaviors and sequelae if they are not adhered to.

IX. SEXUAL DYSFUNCTION related to IMPOTENCE, DECREASED LIBIDO

Defining Characteristics: Opiate agonists may suppress gonadotropin, causing impotence and decreased libido.

Nursing Implications: Assess baseline sexual pattern. Discuss potential toxicity and impact on sexuality. Provide information, emotional support, and referral as needed.

Drug: oxymorphone hydrochloride (Opana)

Class: Opioid analgesic (opioid agonist).

Mechanism of Action: A semisynthetic opioid agonist, oxymorphone HCl resembles morphine but has milder action; binds to opiate receptors in CNS (limbic system, thalamus, striatum, hypothalamus, midbrain, spinal cord), altering pain perception at level of spinal cord and higher centers, as well as the emotional response to pain. Also suppresses cough reflex.

Metabolism: Absolute oral bioavailability is about 10%, and steady-state serum levels occurred after 3 days of multiple doses. Food increases absorption by 38%, so it should not be taken with food. Drug is not bound to plasma proteins to any degree (10–12%), and is highly metabolized by the liver by reduction or conjugation with glucuronide into active and inactive metabolites. In studies of drug in extended formulation, bioavailability is higher in patients with hepatic or renal impairment, and plasma levels in the elderly were 40% higher than younger controls. Drug and metabolites are excreted in the urine and feces.

Indication: For the treatment of pain severe enough to require daily, ATC long and opioid analgesic and for which alternative treatments are inadequate.

Limitations of Use: Because of the risks of addiction, abuse, and misuse with opioids, even at recommended doses, reserve oxymorphone hydrochloride for use in patients for whom alternative treatment options [e.g., nonopioid analgesics or opioid combination products] have not been tolerated, are not expected to be tolerated, have not provided adequate analgesia, or are not expected to provide adequate analgesia.

Contraindication: patients with (1) significant respiratory depression; (2) acute or severe bronchial asthma or hypercarbia; (3) known or suspected GI obstruction, including paralytic ileus; (4) moderate or severe hepatic impairment; (5) known hypersensitivity (e.g., anaphylaxis) to oxymorphone or any components in the drug, or hypersensitivity to morphine analogues such as codeine.

Dosage/Range: *BTP*:
- Requires an opioid Risk Evaluation and Mitigation Strategy (REMS).
- Use the lowest effective dosage for the shortest duration consistent with individual patient treatment goals.
- Individualize dosing based on the pain severity, patient response, prior analgesic experience, and risk factors for addiction, abuse, and misuse.
- Usual initial dose in opioid-naïve patients is 5 mg or patients with mild hepatic impairment, renal impairment (CrCl <50 mL/min), or who are elderly; monitor patient closely for efficacy, sedation, and CNS depression.
- Opioid tolerant patients, dose is 10–20 mg PO q 4–6 h PRN. Oral doses higher than 20 mg are not recommended due to side effects.
- Drug MUST be taken on an empty stomach.
- If patient is receiving parenteral oxymorphone, given the 10% bioavailability, multiply the total parenteral dose of morphone by 10, and administer in 4 or 6 equally divided doses.
- Converting from other opioids to oxymorphone, use a conservative approach as there is considerable variability among patients. Refer to published conversion tables, recognizing the ratios are only approximate. In general start oxymorphone therapy by giving half of the calculated total daily dose of oxymorphone in 4–6 equally divided doses, every 4–6 hours. Adjust the initial dose until adequate pain relief with acceptable side effect (Endo Pharmaceuticals, 2018).

MANAGEMENT

- Patients with mild hepatic impairment, renal impairment, or who are elderly: initial dose is 5 mg PO q 4–6 h PRN. Titrate drug dose up carefully, and monitor for signs of respiratory or CNS depression closely.
- Drug is contraindicated in patients with moderate and severe hepatic dysfunction; use cautiously and start at 5 mg dose in patients with mild hepatic dysfunction, and titrate dose up.
- If patient is receiving CNS depressants (sedatives, hypnotics, general anesthetics, phenothiazines, tranquilizers, or alcohol) concurrently, start at 1/3 to 1/2 of the usual dose.
- If opioids are discontinued, drug should be gradually tapered to prevent signs/symptoms of withdrawal.

Drug Preparation:
- Drug available in 5- and 10-mg tablets.
- At home, teach patient to store oral doses in a safe place away from children and pets. See REMS education for patients/caregivers.

Drug Administration:
- Ensure prescribed medicine is **immediate release** as 5-mg or 10-mg tablets (NOT extended release).
- Teach patient and caregiver to give the drug orally on an **empty stomach** (at least 1 hour before or 2 hours after food ingestion). Teach patient NOT to consume alcohol or prescription or nonprescription medications that contain alcohol while taking the drug. Alcohol may increase drug plasma levels and lead to a potentially fatal overdose of oxymorphone.
- Teach patient that opioid analgesics may impair the mental and/or physical ability to drive and use machines, and to avoid these activities until the effect of the drug is known. See additional information in REMS patient guidelines.

Drug Interactions:
- Alcohol, CNS depressants: Additive CNS depressant effects (hypotension, respiratory depression, profound sedation). Do not use together or dose reduce; teach patient not to drink alcohol while taking oxymorphone HCl.
- Mixed agonist/antagonist analgesics (pentazocine, nalbuphine, butorphanol, buprenorphine) should not be given concurrently, as they may reduce the analgesic effect of oxymorphone and/or precipitate withdrawal.

Lab Effects/Interference:
- None known.

Special Considerations:
- Risk Evaluation and Mitigation Strategy (REMS) required for use of opioids. Healthcare providers must review REMS-compliant education. In addition, healthcare providers must
  a. Complete a REMS-compliant education program offered by an accredited CE provider or another education program that includes all the elements of the FDA Education Blueprint for Health Care Providers Involved in the Management or Support of Patients with Pain. The blueprint can be found at www.fda.gov/OpioidAnalgesic REMSBlueprint.

b. Discuss the safe use, serious risks, and proper storage and disposal of opioid analgesics with patients and/or their caregivers every time these medicines are prescribed. The Patient Counseling Guide can be obtained at www.fda.gov/OpioidAnalgesic REMSPCG.

c. Emphasize to patients and their caregivers the importance of reading the Medication Guide that they will receive from their pharmacist every time an opioid analgesic is dispensed to them.

d. Consider using other tools to improve patient, household, and community safety, such as patient–prescriber agreements that reinforce patient–prescriber responsibilities.

e. Further information available at 1-800-503-0784, or at www.opioidanalgesicrems.com.

- Warnings and Precautions:
  - *Addiction, abuse, and misuse:* Assess each patient's risk for opioid addiction, abuse, or misuse prior to prescribing oxymorphone and monitor all patients for the development of these behaviors. Risks are increased in patients with a personal or family history of substance abuse (including drug or alcohol or addiction) or mental illness, such as major depression. The goal is effective pain management, so if patients have risk factors, provide intensive counseling about the risks, proper use of the drug, and intensive monitoring for signs of addiction, abuse, or misuse. Drug should be prescribed in the smallest appropriate quantity, and advise the patient on the proper disposal of unused drug.
  - *Life-threatening respiratory depression.*
  - *Neonatal opioid withdrawal syndrome.*
  - *Risks from concomitant use with benzodiazepines or other CNS depressants:* Concomitant use may result in profound sedation, respiratory depression, and death. If must coadminister, consider dose reduction in one or both agents. Monitor patient closely.
  - *Life-threatening respiratory depression in patients with chronic pulmonary disease or in the elderly, debilitated, or cachectic patients:* Monitor closely as increased risk of life-threatening respiratory depression.
  - *Anaphylaxis, angioedema, other hypersensitivity reactions:* If any of these reactions occur, stop drug immediately and provide ordered medical intervention. Do not re-challenge patient with any other oxymorphone drug.
  - *Adrenal insufficiency:* If occurs, treat with physiologic replacement of corticosteroids, and wean patient off opioid.
  - *Severe Hypotension:* Opioids cause peripheral vasodilation, which may cause hypotension; in addition, may cause the release of histamine, which can further intensify the hypotension. This may result in orthostatic hypotension and syncope in ambulatory patients. (1) Oxymorphone has a lower likelihood of causing histamine release than other opioids. (2) Monitor patient closely during drug initiation and any dose changes.
  - *Risks of use in patients with head injury, increased ICP, or brain tumors:* Monitor patients closely for sedation and respiratory depression. Opioids may obscure the clinical course of a patient with head injury; *avoid* use of drug in patients with impaired consciousness or coma who may be susceptible to intracranial effects of CP2 retention (e.g., increased ICP).

- *Risks of use in patients with GI conditions:* Drug is contraindicated if patient is obstructed or has a paralytic ileus. Opioids may cause spasm of the sphincter of Oddi and cause an increase in serum amylase. Monitor patients with biliary tract disease, including acute pancreatitis, for worsening symptoms. Use caution in administering to patients with swallowing difficulties or underlying GI disorders to avoid obstruction.
- *Increased risk of seizures in patients with seizure disorder.*
- *Withdrawal:* Avoid the use of mixed agonist/antagonists (e.g., pentazocine, nalbuphine, butorphanol) or partial agonist (e.g., buprenorphine) analgesics in patients who are receiving full opioid agonist analgesia as the drug interaction may reduce the analgesic effect and/or precipitate withdrawal symptoms.
- *Risks of driving and operating machinery:* Opioid analgesia may impair the mental or physical abilities, such as driving a car or operating machinery. Teach patients not to drive or operate dangerous machinery unless they are tolerant to the effects of the drug and know how they will react to the medication.
- *Hepatic impairment:* Use drug cautiously in patients with mild hepatic impairment, starting at 5 mg initial dose, and slowly titrating up to provide adequate analgesia with acceptable toxicity. Drug is contraindicated in patients with moderate or severe hepatic impairment.
- Additive benefit when combined with acetaminophen or aspirin.
- Give smallest effective dose to prevent development of tolerance, physical dependency.
- Reduce dose in debilitated patients or patients receiving other CNS depressants.
- If required, naloxone HCl will reverse opiate toxicity (e.g., respiratory depression). However, it is important that acute withdrawal symptoms are prevented by giving only enough naloxone to reverse respiratory depression, and that this be continued for opioid drug half-life.

Potential Toxicities/Side Effects and the Nursing Process

I.   SENSORY/PERCEPTUAL ALTERATIONS related to CNS DEPRESSION

Defining Characteristics: Adverse effects were $< 10\%$: drowsiness, sedation, mood changes, euphoria, dysphoria, dizziness, confusion.

Nursing Implications: Assess baseline neurologic status. Use cautiously in the elderly, and start with lowest dose and titrate up. Use cautiously, if at all, in patients who are debilitated, and patients with head injury, increased ICP, severe CNS depression, or acute alcoholism. Assess other concurrent medications. Use with caution in patients receiving other opioids, tranquilizers, hypnotics, MAO inhibitors, since increasing CNS depressant effects can occur. Monitor neurologic status closely. Instruct patient to avoid driving and operating machinery while taking the medicine, and to AVOID concurrent alcohol.

II.   ALTERATION IN OXYGENATION related to RESPIRATORY DEPRESSION

Defining Characteristics: Opiate agonists directly depress respiratory center in brain stem, causing decreased sensitivity and responsiveness to increased pCO_2. May also depress deep breathing and reflex to sigh. Tolerance to respiratory depressant effects occurs with chronic use.

Nursing Implications: Assess baseline pulmonary status, and periodically during drug use. Use cautiously in patients with bronchial asthma, COPD, respiratory depression, and monitor closely.

III. ALTERATION IN ELIMINATION related to CONSTIPATION, ILEUS

Defining Characteristics: Opium agonists bind to opiate receptors in bowel, slowing peristalsis, leading to constipation. Untreated constipation may result in bowel perforation. Incidence of constipation in clinical trials was 4%.

Nursing Implications: Assess baseline elimination, fluid intake, diet, and exercise patterns. Instruct patient regarding prevention of constipation: goal is to move bowels at least every 2 days by increasing fluids to 3 L/day, following a diet high in fiber (beans, vegetables, fruit), and taking moderate exercise. Assess need for bowel softeners, bulk-forming laxatives, and osmotic cathartics, and discuss preparation with physician. Teach patient self-administration of medications.

IV. ALTERATION IN NUTRITION, LESS THAN BODY REQUIREMENTS, related to GI TOXICITY

Defining Characteristics: Nausea, vomiting, dry mouth may occur. Gastric, biliary, and pancreatic secretions are decreased by opiate agonists; digestion is delayed. Biliary tract muscle tone is increased, and spasm of Oddi's sphincter may occur (morphine > meperidine > codeine).

Nursing Implications: Assess patient tolerance of GI side effects. Teach patient to report side effects. If nausea/vomiting occur, change to another opioid, or premedicate with antiemetic to prevent nausea/vomiting. Assess GI pain, biliary spasm, and consider alternative opioid.

V. ALTERATION IN URINE ELIMINATION related to URINARY RETENTION

Defining Characteristics: Rarely, increased smooth muscle tone in urinary tract and spasm may occur. Bladder tone is increased, which may cause urgency. Vesical sphincter tone may be increased, leading to difficulty urinating. Increased risk of urinary retention in patients with prostatic hypertrophy or urethral stricture.

Nursing Implications: Assess baseline urinary elimination pattern. Teach patient to increase fluids to 3 L/day, and encourage voiding every 2–3 hours. Instruct patient to report problems with urination.

VI. KNOWLEDGE DEFICIT related to DRUG ADMINISTRATION, POTENTIAL FOR TOLERANCE, AND DEPENDENCY

Defining Characteristics: Psychological dependence (addiction) occurs rarely in patients taking opioid agonists for cancer pain (< 1%). Physical dependence (precipitation of withdrawal symptoms when the drug is abruptly stopped) occurs with chronic use of the drug for the relief of chronic cancer pain. In addition, tolerance, or less analgesic effect over time with the same drug dose, occurs and requires increased dosage of drug.

MANAGEMENT

Nursing Implications: Assess baseline knowledge of opioid analgesics, and attitude about their use for cancer pain management. Teach patient about proper self-administration, possible side effects, and self-care measures. Suggest patient maintain a diary of pain intensity, precipitating and alleviating factors, drug dose and time taken, and relief. Teach patient to self-administer opioid agonists for relief of chronic cancer pain around-the-clock, not PRN, to prevent pain. Explain use of prescribed short-acting opioid for rescue or to manage BTP. Discuss with physician dose increase or change in frequency of administration if tolerance develops. Teach patient that withdrawal symptoms may occur if chronic, ATC dosing is abruptly stopped or interrupted. Withdrawal (abstinence) symptoms that may be seen in the first 24 hours are restlessness, lacrimation, rhinorrhea, yawning, perspiration, gooseflesh, restless sleep, mydriasis. These are followed by twitching and leg spasms; severe aching of the back, abdomen, and legs; cramping in abdomen and legs; hot/cold flashes; insomnia; nausea/vomiting, diarrhea; severe sneezing; and increased heart rate, BP, T, which peak at 36–72 hours. Withdrawal syndrome can be prevented by administration of at least 1/4 of previous opioid dose. For example, if the use of an opioid antagonist is necessary, such as narcan, it should be given slowly with just enough of the drug to reverse the respiratory depression or symptom administered, but not enough to precipitate frank opioid withdrawal.

Drug: modafinil (Provigil)

Class: Wakeful promoting agent, symptom management.

Mechanism of Action: Promotes wakefulness without generalized CNS stimulation by an unknown mechanism. Drug acts in selected brain areas thought to regulate normal wakefulness in the hypothalamus: increased neuronal activity in tuberomammillary nucleus (wake-promoting center), which then projects into cerebral cortex; decreases activity in the ventrolateral preoptic area (sleep promoting); does not affect suprachiasmatic nucleus (regulated circadian rhythm). Action is different from amphetamines.

Metabolism: Rapidly absorbed from the GI system with peak plasma concentrations in 2–4 hours. Taking with food delays absorption by 1 hour, but does not affect bioavailability. About 60% protein-bound (albumin), but at steady state does not displace protein binding of warfarin. Metabolized in the liver, with renal excretion of metabolites. Drug clearance may be reduced in the elderly. Drug is a reversible inhibitor of drug-metabolizing enzyme CYP2C19. Elimination half-life 15 hours.

Indication: To improve wakefulness in adult patients with excessive sleepiness associated with narcolepsy, obstructive sleep apnea, and shift work disorder.

Contraindication: Individuals with known hypersensitivity to modafinil.

Dosage/Range:
- 200 mg as a single dose in the morning for OSA and narcolepsy. For shift-work disorder, it should be taken approximately 1 hour prior to the start of the patient's work shift.
- 50% dose reduction in patients with severe liver impairment.

- Consider dose reduction in elderly patients with renal impairment and/or hepatic impairment.

Drug Preparation:
- Oral, available in 100- and 200-mg tablets.

Drug Administration:
- Oral, in the morning, with a glass of water.

Drug Interactions:
- Potentially, due to reversible inhibition of CYP2C19 enzyme system:
  - Diazepam, phenytoin, propranolol: drug may increase serum levels of these drugs; monitor closely for toxicity and dose reduce if needed.
  - Patients with CYP2C19 deficiency: increased serum levels of TCAs, SSRIs; monitor closely for toxicity and dose-reduce if needed.
  - Patients taking drug chronically may have increased induction of metabolism enzyme CYP3A4, resulting in theoretic decreased serum levels of steroidal contraceptives, cyclosporine, theophylline: monitor closely and dose-increase as necessary.
  - Methylphenidate: delays absorption of modafinil by 1 hour when given together.
  - Use in pregnancy or breastfeeding women only if benefit outweighs risk, as drug is potentially teratogenic.

Lab Effects/Interference:
- Unknown.

Special Considerations:
- Use with caution in patients who have had a recent MI or unstable angina.
- Use cautiously in patients with a history of psychosis.
- Women using steroidal contraceptives should use alternative or concomitant methods of contraception while taking the drug and for 1 month following discontinuation of the drug.
- Drug may produce psychoactive and euphoric effects, alterations in mood, perception, thinking, and feelings typical of other CNS stimulants. Drug binds to dopamine reuptake site and causes an increase in extracellular dopamine but no increase in dopamine release. Drug is reinforcing.
- Incidence of insomnia was 3% (placebo 1%).
- Drug is indicated to improve wakefulness in adult patients with excessive sleepiness associated with narcolepsy, obstructive sleep apnea, and shift work disorder. Drug does not cause withdrawal when discontinued.

Potential Toxicities/Side Effects (dose- and schedule-dependent) and the Nursing Process

I.   ALTERATION IN COMFORT related to HEADACHE, NAUSEA, DEPRESSION, NERVOUSNESS, RHINITIS

Defining Characteristics: In controlled clinical trials, headache occurred 10% more frequently than placebo, nausea occurred 9% more than placebo, depression 1% more than placebo, rhinitis 11% (placebo 8%), and nervousness 2% more than placebo. The few patients who discontinued the drug did so due to headache (1%), nausea (1%), depression (1%), and nervousness (1%).

Nursing Implications: Teach patient that these effects are rare but may occur. Teach symptom management strategies and if these do not work, to notify provider. If this occurs, discuss drug discontinuance versus more aggressive symptom management if drug is effective in reducing fatigue.

II.   ALTERATION IN NUTRITION, POTENTIAL, related to NAUSEA, DRY MOUTH, DIARRHEA, ANOREXIA, THIRST

Defining Characteristics: Although rare, these symptoms may occur: nausea occurs in 13% (placebo 4%), diarrhea 8% (placebo 4%), dry mouth 5% (placebo 1%), anorexia 5% (placebo 1%), and thirst 1%.

Nursing Implications: Perform baseline patient nutritional assessment, history of nausea and vomiting, bowel elimination pattern, oral assessment, and usual appetite. Teach patient these are rare, but to report these side effects so that they can be evaluated. Teach patient self-care measures, including dietary modification, local comfort measures as well as pharmacologic management as determined by the nurse/physician team. Teach patient to report symptoms that persist and do not respond to the planned therapy.

Chapter 7
Nausea and Vomiting

If you ask a newly diagnosed patient who will be starting chemotherapy what his/her greatest fear is, it is often nausea and vomiting. To many, this represents the "worst" of chemotherapy. Nausea and/or vomiting can occur commonly during the course of the cancer experience, related to disease, such as liver metastases, or to treatment, such as with chemotherapy or radiation to the abdomen. In addition, if acute nausea and vomiting are not prevented following cancer chemotherapy, delayed (occurs > 24 hours after the chemotherapy dose) nausea and vomiting often follows or anticipatory nausea and vomiting develop where a stimulus (sight or sound or smell) associated with the event of nausea/vomiting precipitates nausea and vomiting without chemotherapy administration. Thus it is imperative that nausea and vomiting be prevented from the outset of therapy. Some providers believe they should see how well a patient does with a new chemotherapy and then ramp up the antiemetics for the next treatment if nausea and/or vomiting is not prevented. The ASCO Antiemetic guidelines (2017) reiterate how it is important to use the most effective antiemetic the first time the patient receives chemotherapy, rather than using a less effective regimen to see how the patient tolerates chemotherapy. This problem continues.

Articles have long documented that nausea is often underreported and underassessed (Wickham, 2003). Although the dates of publication are old, unfortunately the implications

Table 7.1   Types of Nausea and Vomiting related to Chemotherapy

Type	Manifestations
Acute	Occurs within 24 hours and usually resolves within 24 hours. Peak is when chemotherapy peak serum level peaks, usually 5–6 hours after drug administration.
Delayed	Occurs 1–5 days after chemotherapy administration. Common with drugs having delayed excretion, such as cisplatin.
Breakthrough	Occurring despite prophylaxis when blockade is inadequate or other factors increase risk of nausea and vomiting; requires rescue therapy. Can occur during acute or delayed episodes.
Refractory	Inadequate response to antiemetic blockade which occurs after chemotherapy prophylaxis and/or rescue therapy has failed during a cycle of chemotherapy.
Anticipatory	Conditioned response where the sight, smell, or other reminder of prior chemotherapy, which was associated with significant nausea and vomiting, causes nausea or vomiting prior to the next cycle of chemotherapy. Incidence is estimated 25–60%.

Modified from: Bavaru RM. Managing nausea and vomiting in patients with cancer: what works. *Oncology (Williston Park)* 2018; 32(3):121–125; Hesketh PJ, Kris MG, Basch E, et al. Antiemetics: American Society of Clinical Oncology clinical practice guideline update. *J Clin Oncol* 2017; 35:3240; National Comprehensive Cancer Network. *NCCN Antiemesis. Guidelines.* Version 1.2019. Available at https://www.nccn.org/professionals/physician_gls/pdf/antiemesis.pdf. Accessed May 29, 2019.

remain true. A replication of the Coates et al. (1983) study by de Boer-Dennert et al. (1997) showed that patients rated nausea as more distressing than vomiting since much has been done to prevent and control chemotherapy-induced vomiting. In 2003, Hofman et al. showed that fatigue was the top patient concern, followed by nausea, and then sleep disturbance.

Complete control of chemotherapy-induced nausea and vomiting (CINV) has improved greatly with the advent of serotonin 5-hydroxytryptamine type 3 (5-HT$_3$) receptor antagonists used in combination with dexamethasone, bringing complete control to about 70% for patients receiving high-dose cisplatin. This new century of genomics has led to the understanding that the effectiveness of many drugs, and 5-HT$_3$ receptor antagonists in particular, is influenced by the recipient's genotype. This is because the liver's microenzyme system, cytochrome P450, and subtypes are determined by an individual's genotype. If the genotype is an ultrarapid metabolizer, the drug is rapidly cleared and eliminated from the body with decreased effect and undertreatment, while slow or poor metabolizers slowly clear the drug from the body with the risk of overtreatment. A study by Kaiser et al. (2002) evaluated whether patients who vomited after receiving their first cycle of emetogenic chemotherapy with 5-HT$_3$ receptor antagonist protection by either ondansetron or tropisetron were either ultrarapid or slow metabolizers of the P450 subsystem CYP2D6. They found that 30% had nausea and vomiting. The ultrarapid metabolizers had a higher incidence of nausea and vomiting, which was more marked for tropisetron- than ondansetron-receiving patients, and the poor metabolizers had higher serum concentrations and were protected. As we look to the future, not only do we see patients having genotypic evaluation of their tumors for an individualized prescription of anticancer treatment, but it will also include individual prescription of antiemetic dose based on genotype.

Unfortunately it is estimated that 50% of patients receiving cancer chemotherapy experience chemotherapy-induced nausea and/or vomiting (Moradian & Powell, 2015).

CHEMOTHERAPY-INDUCED NAUSEA AND VOMITING

CINV is primarily determined by the type of chemotherapy being administered, including the dose, schedule, and route of administration. For example, patients receiving cisplatin 100 mg/m^2 have been used as clinical subjects in antiemetic studies, as 100% of patients will vomit without antiemetic premedication. The risk of CINV can be predicted by the drug; in general, highly emetogenic drugs have a risk of 90% or higher of causing emesis, moderately emetogenic drugs have a risk of 30–90%, low-risk drugs have a risk of 10–30%, and minimal-risk drugs have < 10% risk. In combination therapy, however, the addition of one with another agent can increase the risk. For example, doxorubicin and cyclophosphamide are both moderately emetogenic, but when combined, the risk increases to highly emetogenic (Hesketh et al., 2016). See Table 7.2. It is much easier to prevent a patient's nausea and vomiting than it is to try to control it afterwards.

CINV appears mediated by multiple pathways. Nausea usually precedes vomiting, and it is controlled by cerebral and autonomic input, with common accompanying signs and symptoms of tachycardia, pallor, and diaphoresis. Vomiting involves the ejection of stomach contents and is a critical protection mechanism that helps the body excrete poisons

Table 7.2 Emetogenic Risk by Antineoplastic Agent

A. Intravenous Agents

High Risk > 90%	Moderate Risk 30–90%	Low Risk 10–30%	Minimal Risk < 10%
AC combination (anthracycline plus cyclophosphamide) Carmustine > 250 mg/m^2 Carboplatin AUC ≥4 Carmustine >250 mg/ m^2	Aldesleukin > 12–15 million IU/m^2 Amifostine > 300 mg/m^2 Arsenic trioxide Azacitidine Bendamustine Busulfan Carboplatin AUC <4 Carmustine ≤ 250 mg/m^2	Ado-trastuzumab emtansine Aldesleukin ≤ 12 million IU/m^2 Amifostine ≤ 300 mg/m^2 Axicabtagene ciloleucel Belinostat Brentuximab vedotin	Alemtuzumab Atezolizumab Avelumab Asparaginase Bevacizumab Bleomycin Blinatumomab Bortezomib Cetuximab Cladribine Cytarabine < 100 mg/m^2
Cisplatin	Clofarabine	Cabazitaxel Carfilzomib Copanlisib Cytarabine 100–200 mg/m^2 (low dose)	Daratumumab Decitabine Dexrazoxane Durvalumab Elotuzumab
Cyclophosphamide > 1,500 mg/m^2 Dacarbazine	Cyclophosphamide ≤ 1,500 mg/m^2	Docetaxel	Fludarabine
		Doxorubicin (liposomal) Eribulin	Interferon alpha ≤ 5 million IU/m^2 Ipilimumab
	Cytarabine > 200 mg/m^2 Dactinomycin Daunorubicin Dual drug liposomal encapsulated daunorubicin and cytarabine Dinutuximab	Etoposide	Methotrexate ≤ 50 mg/m^2 Nelarabine Nivolumab Obinutuzumab Ofatumumab Panitumumab
Doxorubicin ≥ 60 mg/m^2 Epirubicin > 90 mg/m^2 Ifosfamide ≥ 2 g/m^2 per dose	Doxorubicin < 60 mg/m^2	5-Fluorouracil Floxuridine	Pegaspargase Peginterferon Pembrolizumab Pertuzumab
		Gemcitabine Gemtuzumab ozogamicin Inotuzumab ozogamicin Interferon alfa > 5 < 10 million IU/m^2 Irinotecan liposome Ixabepilone	Ramucirumab Rituximab Rituximab and hyaluronidase (SQ) Siltuximab Temsirolimus Trastuzumab

MANAGEMENT

Table 7.2 (Continued)

A. Intravenous Agents

High Risk > 90%	Moderate Risk 30–90%	Low Risk 10–30%	Minimal Risk < 10%
Mechlorethamine	Epirubicin $\leq$ 90 mg/m^2	Methotrexate > 50 mg/m^2 < 250 mg/m^2 Mitomycin C	Valrubicin
Streptozocin	Idarubicin	Mitoxantrone Necitumumab Olaratumab	Vinblastine Vincristine Vincristine (liposomal)
	Ifosfamide < 2 g/m^2 per dose Interferon alfa $\geq$ 10 million IU/m^2	Omacetaxine	Vinorelbine
	Irinotecan Irinotecan liposomal	Paclitaxel Paclitaxel-albumin bound	
	Melphalan Methotrexate $\geq$ 250 mg/m^2	Pemetrexed Pentostatin Pralatrexate	
	Oxaliplatin Temozolomide Trabectedin	Romidepsin Talimogene laherparepvec Thiotepa Tisagenleuleucel Topotecan Ziv-aflibercept	

B. Oral Agents

Moderate-to-High (> 30% frequency of emesis)	Minimal to Low (< 30% frequency of emesis)
Altretamine Busulfan $\geq$ 4 mg/day Ceritinib Crizotnib Cyclophosphamide $\geq$ 100 mg/m^2/day Dabrafenib Enasidenib	Abemaciclib Acalabrutinib Afatinib Alectinib Axitinib Bexarotene Binimetinib Bosutinib Brigatinib Busulfan < 4 mg/day Cabozantinib Capecitabine

(continues)

Table 7.2 (*Continued*)

B. Oral Agents

Moderate-to-High (> 30% frequency of emesis)	Minimal to Low (< 30% frequency of emesis)
Estramustine	Chlorambucil
Etoposide	Cobimetinib
Lenvatinib	Cyclophosphamide
Lomustine (single	< 100 mg/m²/day
day)	Dascomitinib
	Dasatinib
Midostaurin	Duvelisib
Mitotane	Encorafenib
Niraparib	Erlotinib
Olaparib	Everolimus
	Fludarabine
Procarbazine	Gefitinib
Rucaparib	Gilteritinib
	Glasdegib
	Hydroxyurea
	Ibrutinib
	Idelalisib
	Imatinib
	Ixazomib
	Ivosidenib
	Lapatinib
	Larotrectinib
	Lenalidomide
	Lorlatinib
Temozolomide >	Melphalan
75 mg/m²/day	Mercaptopurine
Trifluridine/tipiracil	Methotrexate
	Neratinib
	Nilotinib
	Osimertinib
	Palbociclib
	Panobinostat
	Pazopanib
	Pomalidomide
	Ponatinib
	Regorafenib
	Ribociclib
	Ruxolitinib
	Sonidegib
	Sorafenib
	Sunitinib
	Talazoparib tosylate

MANAGEMENT

Table 7.2   (Continued)

B. Oral Agents	
Moderate-to-High (> 30% frequency of emesis)	**Minimal to Low (< 30% frequency of emesis)**
	Temozolomide ≤ 75 mg/m^2/day
	Thalidomide
	Thioguanine
	Topotecan
	Trametinib
	Tretinoin
	Vandetanib
	Vemurafenib
	Venetoclax
	Vismodegib
	Vorinostat

Key: High: > 90% risk of emesis; moderate: 30–90% risk of emesis; low risk: 10–30% risk of emesis; minimal risk: < 10% risk of emesis.

Modified from National Comprehensive Cancer Network. NCCN Clinical Practice Guidelines in Oncology (NCCN Guidelines®): Antiemesis (v.1.2019). Available at http://www.nccn.org/professionals/physician_gls/pdf/antiemesis. pdf. Accessed May 29, 2019; Multinational Association of Supportive Care in Cancer (MASCC). MASCC/ESMO Antiemetic Guidelines 2016. Available at https://www.mascc.org/antiemetic-guidelines. Accessed May 29, 2019; Grunberg SM, Warr D, Gralla RJ, et al. Evaluation of new antiemetic agents and definition of antineoplastic agent emetogenicity—state of the art. *Support Care Cancer* 2011; 19(Suppl 1): S43–47.

and is a well preserved evolutionary defense mechanism. Most commonly, receptors in the gut enterochromaffin cells are stimulated and release serotonin. Serotonin binds to 5-HT$_3$ receptors, which stimulate the vagus nerve. This leads to stimulation of the chemotherapy trigger zone (CTZ) in the area postrema on the floor of the fourth ventricle of the brain, leading to activation of the vomiting center (VC) in the medulla, or to stimulation of the VC directly. The 5-HT$_3$ receptor antagonists, such as granisetron and ondansetron, block the emetic impulses from reaching the CTZ and VC. In addition, other neuroreceptors in the CTZ can transmit impulses to the VC, such as dopamine, endorphin, and substance P. Other neuroreceptors that are found in the VC and vestibular center and that appear to have a role in emesis are acetylcholine, corticosteroid, histamine, cannabinoid, opiate, and neurokinin-1 (NK$_1$). Dopamine antagonists include phenothiazines and butyrophenones, and substance P/ NK$_1$ receptor antagonist antiemetics include aprepitant and its IV formulation fosaprepitant, netupitant, and fosnetupitant which have been FDA approved. Emotional and cognitive factors can influence the occurrence and severity of CINV through a descending pathway from the cerebral cortex to the VC, such as with anticipatory nausea and vomiting. Here a conditioned response is set up based on 3–4 past episodes of severe nausea and/or vomiting. The benzodiazepine lorazepam has been effective in preventing or lessening this effect through the drug's amnesiac qualities, as has behavioral therapy, including relaxation/systematic desensitization, hypnosis, and cognitive distraction, for some patients.

Dexamethasone has long been known to reduce the incidence of CINV, through a probable anti-inflammatory effect, leading to a closing of spaces in the gut wall that would permit leakage of emetogens into the bloodstream. A large meta-analysis showed that corticosteroids significantly improved protection from both acute and delayed CINV (Ioannidis et al., 2000). However, the exact mechanism is unknown.

Delayed nausea and vomiting are difficult to control but appear to be influenced by slowed gastric emptying. Thus, delayed antiemetic regimens usually include metoclopramide to speed gastric emptying, along with dexamethasone, and a phenothiazine or serotonin antagonist. It has become clear that substance P and its receptor NK$_1$, in the gut and brainstem, are important mediators in delayed CINV. The NK$_1$ receptors are located near the VC, the "final common pathway" for emesis, so it is expected the NK$_1$ receptor antagonists will have broader application. Most substance P/NK$_1$ receptor antagonists are inhibitors of the microenzyme CYP3A4 so that the concurrent dexamethasone dose must be reduced. Rolapritant (Varubi) is a substance P/NK$_1$ receptor antagonist FDA approved for the prevention of delayed nausea and vomiting and is given prior to the chemotherapy dose. It differs from the others in its class as it is not a CYP3A4 inhibitor, and thus full dose dexamethasone can be given. Although great strides have been made in the prevention and control of CINV, even with maximal pharmacologic blockade of known pathways, 100% protection is not always obtained, so it is clear that other pathways await discovery. See Figure 7.1 for a review of pathophysiology of CINV. See Table 7.2 for the emetogenicity of cancer chemotherapy agents, and Table 7.3 for a schematic for antiemetic drugs and doses for CINV.

MANAGEMENT

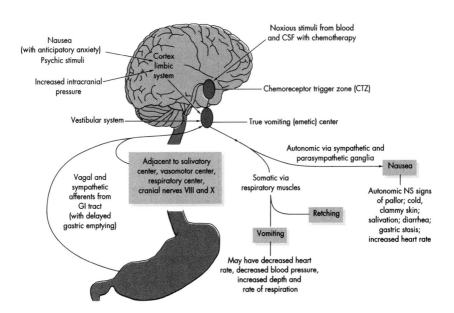

Figure 7.1   The Physiology of Nausea and Vomiting

Table 7.3 Antiemetic Agents Used in CINV

Antiemetic Agent	IV Doses (Acute)	Oral Doses (Acute)	Oral (Delayed)
Serotonin Receptor Antagonists			
Granisetron	0.01 mg/kg or 1 mg IV	1–2 mg oral (total dose) po qd or 3.1 mg/24 h transdermal patch q 7d	1 mg bid delayed
• Ondansetron	0.15 mg/kg q 4 h × 4 h mg/kg q IV per dose	8-16 mg (total dose) PO qd	8 mg bid delayed
• Palonosetron	0.25 mg IV day 1		
Corticosteroids			
• Dexamethasone	20 mg; 12 mg day 1, 8 mg day 2–4 with NK1 receptor antagonists except rolapitant.	20 mg except with NK1 antagonists, when dose is 12 mg or 8 mg.	8 mg bid days 2–4 highly emetogenic, 4–8 mg bid days 2–3 moderately emetogenic
Substance P/NK1 Receptor Antagonist			
• Aprepitant		125 mg PO day 1 with dexamethasone 12 mg PO with serotonin receptor antagonist	80 mg day 2, 3 with dexamethasone 8 mg PO
• Fosaprepitant • Rolapitant		150 mg IV day 1 with dexamethasone 12 mg PO with serotonin receptor antagonist 180 mg PO on day 1, 1–2 hours before chemotherapy, with dexamethasone 20 mg (dose not reduced), and 5-HT$_3$ receptor antagonist	Dexamethasone 8 mg PO/IV day 2, then 8 mg PO/IV bid days 3, 4 • Dexamethasone 8 mg PO/IV bid, on days 2–4
Substance P/NK1 Receptor Antagonist/Serotonin-3 Receptor Antagonist			
• Netupitant/ • palonosetron • (in combination with dexamethasone)	Fosnetupitant 235 mg/ Palonosetron 0.25 mg (fixed product for IV administration) with dexamethasone 12 mg given 30 min before chemotherapy, then 8 mg dexamethasone PO qd × days 2–4.	(A) Highly emetogenic: 300 mg/0.5 mg PO 1 h before chemotherapy with dexamethasone 12 mg PO given 30 min before chemotherapy on day 1	Dexamethasone 8 mg PO days 2–4

(continues)

Table 7.3 *(Continued)*

Antiemetic Agent	IV Doses (Acute)	Oral Doses (Acute)	Oral (Delayed)
Dopamine Receptor Antagonists			
• Metoclo-pramide			20–40 mg PO q 4–6h
• Prochlorpera-zine			10 mg PO or 25 mg PR
Benzodiazepines			
• Lorazepam	0.5–1 mg	1–2 mg	

MANAGEMENT

CINV can occur *acutely*, during the first 24 hours following chemotherapy administration; *delayed*, occurring after the first 24 hours; or *anticipatory*, occurring before chemotherapy, in anticipation of developing nausea and vomiting after a prior bad experience. It can also be refractory to tried antiemetics where blockade failure results in emesis.

Factors that influence the occurrence and severity of CINV include gender (females have higher risk than males), age (younger people have a higher risk than older people), drug dose and emetogenic potential, combination of drugs versus single agent, history of alcohol intake (increased alcohol intake confers protection), and past experience with nausea and vomiting, such as air sickness, which increases risk.

Delayed nausea and vomiting are influenced by the effectiveness of control/prevention of the acute phase of CINV (Blanchard & Hesketh, 2015), as well as the half-life of the antineoplastic agent. For example, the metabolites of cisplatin continue to be excreted for 3–5 days after drug administration, so protection must be provided for that period of time; for cyclophosphamide, the half-life is at least 12 hours, so only half the drug is excreted by that time, and full antiemetic protection must continue for at least 24 hours to prevent delayed nausea and vomiting. Common delayed regimens begin on days 2–4 for highly emetogenic regimens (aprepitant 80 mg PO daily × 2 plus dexamethasone 8 mg PO daily × 3; or a serotonin antagonist such as granisetron 1 mg PO bid or ondansetron 8 mg PO twice daily, plus dexamethasone 8 mg PO daily × 3; or metoclopramide 30–40 mg PO twice daily plus dexamethasone 8 mg PO twice daily × 3 days). For moderately emetogenic regimens, delayed emesis regimens are given on days 2–3 and include a serotonin antagonist, or dexamethasone, or metoclopramide alone or in combination (Grunberg & Siebel, 2007).

Insofar as CINV involves multiple pathways, multiple antiemetics to block these pathways are needed, especially for aggressive antiemesis. Antiemetics must be administered to prevent nausea and vomiting, so the drug(s) should be administered prior to chemotherapy administration in order to block stimulation of the pathways. Oral antiemetics should be administered 30–40 minutes before treatment; rectal (PR) preparations 60 minutes before; intramuscular (IM) injections 20–30 minutes before; and intravenous bolus (IVB) 10–30 minutes prior to chemotherapy.

In order to better identify treatment approaches for CINV, American Society for Clinical Oncology (ASCO) published "Recommendations for the Use of Antiemetics: Evidence-Based Clinical Practice Guidelines" and stated that "at equivalent doses, serotonin-receptor antagonists have equivalent safety and efficacy and can be used inter-changeably based on convenience, availability, and cost" (Hesketh et al., 2017). They listed four agents in this class; three of these agents are commercially available in the United States: dolasetron, granisetron, and ondansetron. This does not include palonosetron, which has a long half-life, and which is effective in preventing delayed as well as acute nausea/vomiting. Finally, key members of the Multinational Association of Supportive Care in Cancer (MASCC/ESMO) have developed consensus and evidence-based antiemetic guidelines (2016).

In addition, the National Comprehensive Cancer Network (NCCN, v1.2019) has developed supportive care guidelines for antiemesis, which identify the following principles of emesis control in patients with cancer:

- The goal is the **prevention** of nausea/vomiting.
- Patients have risk of nausea and vomiting for at least 3 days when receiving highly emetogenic chemotherapy and 2 days for moderately emetogenic chemotherapy after the last dose. They should receive antiemetic protection for the full period of risk.
- Oral and IV antiemetics have equivalent efficacy.
- Use the lowest **fully efficacious** dose before chemotherapy or radiation therapy. Use effective antiemesis to protect against emesis for the **first** chemotherapy administration as failure to do this sets up a pattern of emesis that is hard to break.
- Choose antiemetic(s) based on emetogenicity of the therapy, prior experience with antiemetics, patient factors, and antiemetic(s) potential side effect(s).
- Consider an H_2 blocker or proton pump inhibitor (PPI) to prevent dyspepsia, which can be mistaken for nausea.
- Ensure that other potential causes of emesis in patients with cancer are not overlooked:
  - Partial or complete bowel obstruction.
  - Vestibular dysfunction.
  - Brain metastases.
  - Electrolyte imbalance (hypercalcemia, hyperglycemia, hyponatremia).
  - Uremia.
  - Concomitant drug treatment, including opiates.
  - Gastroparesis (tumor, chemotherapy such as vincristine) or other causes, such as diabetes.
  - Malignant ascites.
  - Psychophysiologic causes (anxiety, anticipatory nausea/vomiting).
- For multi-drug regimens, select antiemetic therapy based on drug with highest emetic risk.
- Lifestyle measures may help to alleviate nausea/vomiting such as eating small, frequent meals, controlling amount of food consumed, and eating foods at room temperature.

Aprepitant (Emend) is the first substance P/NK_1 receptor antagonist indicated for the prevention of acute and delayed nausea and vomiting related to highly emetogenic chemotherapy, in combination with other antiemetic agents. First identified in 1931 and reaching notoriety in 1950 when linked with pain transmission, substance P has continued to be prominent in the symptom management field. Substance P is a member of the tachykinin family of peptides and, together with NK_1 receptors, is found in high concentrations in the CTZ (in the medulla oblongata) and the dorsal horn of the spinal cord (posterior column of gray matter), as well as the gut. Substance P is released from peripheral sensory as well as central sensory nerve endings and plays a key role in transmitting noxious sensory information to the brain. Substance P initiates its activity by binding to the NK_1 receptor, a site distinctly different from the serotonin-mediated $5\text{-}HT_3$ site (Hesketh, 2001).

In an effort to design a serotonin antagonist with a long half-life and activity against delayed CINV, palonosetron (Aloxi) was created and approved for the prevention of CINV. More recently, a hybrid composed of both a serotonin-receptor antagonist (palonosetron) and a substance P/NK_1 receptor antagonist (netupitant) was FDA approved for the prevention of acute and delayed nausea and vomiting associated with initial and repeat courses of cancer chemotherapy. In an effort to provide long antiemetic coverage, as well as avoid the problem of inhibition the metabolism of CYP3A4 drugs such as dexamethasone, rolapitant has been FDA approved and is available for use together with dexamethasone and a $5\text{-}HT_3$ serotonin receptor antagonist (Tesaro, Inc., 2015).

Given these advances, complete protection from CINV should be the standard (Blanchard & Hesketh, 2015); however, there continues to be a minority of patients who have significant nausea and vomiting. The NCCN antiemesis guideline (v1.2019) recommends the following plan for the prevention of IV chemotherapy-induced emesis:

NCCN Recommendations (v1.2019) are shown below for antiemesis.

Highly Emetogenic Parenteral Chemotherapy, Acute and Delayed Emesis Prevention

- Start prior to chemotherapy, using a serotonin ($5\text{-}HT_3$) antagonist, dexamethasone, $\pm$ NK_1 antagonist, $\pm$ olanzapine as detailed below.
  - **Options include 1 of 3 combinations on day 1 (acute), followed by days 2–4 (delayed):** Combination of NK_1 receptor antagonist, dexamethasone, and serotonin ($5\text{-}HT_3$) receptor antagonist OR NK_1 receptor antagonist, $5\text{-}HT_3$ receptor antagonist and olanzapine; OR olanzapine, palonosetron, and dexamethasone regimen.
  - **REGIMEN 1:**
  - DAY 1
    - *Serotonin-receptor antagonist* ($5\text{-}HT_3$): ondansetron 16–24 mg PO $\times$ 1 OR 8–16 mg IV $\times$ 1, day 1; OR granisetron 10 mg SQ $\times$ 1, or 2 mg PO $\times$ 1 or 0.01 mg/kg (max 1 mg) IV $\times$ 1 day 1, or transdermal patch as 3.1 mg/24 hr patch (containing 34.3 mg granisetron total dose) applied 24–48 hours prior to first dose of chemotherapy (maximum duration of patch is 7 days); OR palonosetron 0.25 mg IV day 1 $\times$ 1; OR dolasetron 100 mg PO $\times$ 1; WITH
    - *NK_1 receptor antagonist:* aprepitant 125 mg PO $\times$ 1, or aprepitant injectable emulsion 130 mg IV $\times$ 1; OR fosprepitant 150 mg IV $\times$ 1, OR fosprepitant 150 mg IV $\times$ 1: OR netupitant 300 mg/palonestron 0.5 mg (fixed combination) PO $\times$ 1 OR fosprepitant 235 mg/palonestron 0.25 mg (fixed combination) IV $\times$ 1 OR rolapitant 180 mg PO $\times$ 1; WITH
    - dexamethasone 12 mg PO/IV $\times$ 1
  - **DAYS 2, 3, 4**
    - Aprepitant 80 mg PO qd on days 2, 3 (if aprepitant PO used on day 1)
    - Dexamethason 8 mg PO or IV daily on days 2–4

REGIMEN 2;
DAY 1

- *NK$_1$ receptor antagonist:* aprepitant 125 mg PO × 1, OR aprepitant injectable emulsion 130 mg IV × 1; OR fosprepitant 150 mg IV × 1, OR fosprepitant 150 mg IV × 1: OR netupitant 300 mg/palonestron 0.5 mg (fixed combination) PO × 1 OR fosprepitant 235 mg/palonestron 0.25 mg (fixed combination) IV × 1 OR rolapitant 180 mg PO × 1;
- *Serotonin-receptor antagonist:* ondansetron 16–24 mg PO × 1 OR 8–16 mg IV × 1, day 1; OR granisetron 10 mg SQ × 1, or 2 mg PO × 1 or 0.01 mg/kg (max 1 mg) IV × 1 day 1, or transdermal patch as 3.1 mg/24 hr patch (containing 34.3 mg granisetron total dose) applied 24–48 hours prior to first dose of chemotherapy (maximum duration of patch is 7 days); OR palonosetron 0.25mg IV day 1 × 1; OR dolasetron 100 mg PO × 1; WITH
- Olanzapine 5–10 mg PO × 1 WITH
- Dexamethasone 12 mg PO/IV × 1

DAYS 2, 3, 4

- Aprepitant 80 mg PO qd on days 2, 3 (if aprepitant PO used on day 1)
- Dexamethason 8 mg PO or IV daily on days 2–4
- Olanzapine 5–10 mg PO days 2–4

REGIMEN 3:
DAY 1

- Palonostron 0.25 mg IV × 1
- Olanzapine 5–10 mg PO × 1
- Dexamethasone 12 mg PO/IV × 1

DAYS 2, 3, 4

- Olanzapine 5–10 mg PO days 2–4

Moderate Emetogenic Risk Parenteral Chemotherapy

- **Options include 1 of 3 combinations on day 1 (acute), followed by days 2–3 (delayed):** Combination of (1) serotonin (5-HT$_3$) receptor antagonist and dexamethasone; OR (2) 5-HT$_3$ receptor antagonist, dexamethasone, and olanzapine; OR (3) for patients with additional risk factors or prior treatment failure with a 5-HT$_3$ receptor antagonist, add NK$_1$ receptor antagonist to the 5-HT$_3$ receptor antagonist and dexamethasone.

REGIMEN 1:
DAY 1

- *Serotonin-receptor antagonist (5-HT$_3$):* ondansetron 16–24 mg PO × 1 OR 8–16 mg IV × 1; OR granisetron 10 mg SQ × 1 (preferred), or 2 mg PO × 1 or 0.01 mg/kg (max 1 mg) IV × 1 day 1, or transdermal patch as 3.1 mg/24 hr patch (containing 34.3 mg granisetron total dose) applied 24–48 hours prior to first dose of chemotherapy (maximum duration of patch is 7 days); OR palonosetron 0.25 mg IV day 1 × 1 (preferred); OR dolasetron 100 mg PO × 1; WITH
- Dexamethasone 12 mg PO/IV × 1.

DAYS 2, 3

- Dexamethasone 8 mg PO/IV qd on days 2, 3 montherapy OR
- Serotonin receptor antagonist *(5-HT$_3$)* monotherapy: granisetron 1–2 mg (total dose) PO daily or 0.01 mg/kg (max 1 mg) IV daily on days 2, 3; OR ondansetron 8 mg PO

bid or 16 mg PO daily or 8–16 mg IV daily on days 2, 3 OR dolasetron 100 mg PO daily on days 2, 3.

REGIMEN 2:

DAY 1

- Olanzapine 5–10 mg PO once WITH
- Palonosetron 0.25 mg IV once WITH
- Dexamethasone 12 mg PO/IV once.

DAYS 2, 3

- Olanzapine 5–10 mg PO daily on days 2, 3.

REGIMEN 3 [an NK1 receptor antagonist should be added (to dexamethasone and a 5-HT3 receptor antagonist regimen) for patients who have had nausea/vomiting with dexamethasone and 5HT3 receptor antagonist alone, or if additional risk factors].

DAY 1

- *NK_1 receptor antagonist:* aprepitant 125 mg PO × 1, OR aprepitant injectable emulsion 130 mg IV × 1; OR fosprepitant 150 mg IV × 1, OR netupitant 300 mg/palonestron 0.5 mg (fixed combination) PO × 1 OR fosprepitant 235 mg/palonestron 0.25 mg (fixed combination) IV × 1 OR rolapitant 180 mg PO × 1;
- *Serotonin-receptor antagonist (5HT3):* ondansetron 16–24 mg PO × 1 OR 8–16 mg IV × 1, day 1; OR granisetron 10 mg SQ × 1, or 2 mg PO × 1 or 0.01 mg/kg (max 1 mg) IV × 1 day 1, or transdermal patch as 3.1 mg/24 hr patch (containing 34.3 mg granisetron total dose) applied 24–48 hours prior to first dose of chemotherapy (maximum duration of patch is 7 days); OR palonosetron 0.25mg IV day 1 × 1; OR dolasetron 100 mg PO × 1; WITH
- *Dexamethasone* 12 mg PO/IV × 1.

DAYS 2, 3

- Aprepitant 80 mg PO daily on days 2, 3 (if aprepitant PO used on day 1) +/–
- +/– Dexamethasone 8 mg PO/IV daily on days 2, 3.

Low Emetogenic Chemotherapy:

- Start antiemesis before chemotherapy; repeat daily for multiday doses of chemotherapy.
  - Dexamethasone 8–12 mg PO/IV × 1 OR metoclopramide 10–20 mg PO/IV × 1, OR prochlorperazine 10 mg PO/IV × 1 OR serotonin (5HT3)-receptor antagonist granisetron 1–2 mg (total dose) PO × 1; OR ondansetron 8–16 mg PO × 1; OR dolasetron 100 mg PO × 1.

Minimal Emetogenic Risk Chemotherapy:

- No routine prophylaxis.
- If nausea or emesis occurs within 24 hours, consider using drugs in low emetogenicity category or breakthrough regimen.

Oral Chemotherapy:

High to Moderate Emetic Risk:

- Start before chemotherapy and continue daily.
- Serotonin (5HT3) receptor antagonist: granisetron 1–2 mg (total dose) PO daily OR 3.1 mg/24 hr transdermal patch every 7 days; OR ondansetron 8–16 mg PO (total dose) daily OR dolasetron 100 mg PO daily.

Low to minimal emetic risk: PRN recommended. If nausea/vomiting:
- Start before chemotherapy and continue daily.
  - Metoclopramide 10–20 mg PO and then every 6 hours PRN OR Prochlorperazine 10 mg PO and then every 6 hours PRN (maximum 40 mg/day) OR serotonin (5HT3) receptor antagonist [Granisetron 1–2 mg (total dose) PO daily PRN or Ondansetron 8–16 mg (total dose) PO daily PRN] or dolasetron 100 mg PO daily PRN.

    Rescue or breakthrough emesis management: if breakthrough emesis, consider changing antiemetic regimen to a higher level primary therapy for next cycle. Breakthrough treatment: some patients may require one or several agents utilizing differing mechanisms of action. [NCCN, v.1.2019]:
- Add an additional agent from a different drug class to the current regimen.
  - Atypical antipsychotic: olanzapine 5–10 mg PO daily.
  - Benzodiazepine: lorazepam 0.5–2.0 mg PO/SL/IV every 6 hours.
  - Cannabinoid: dronabinol capsules 5–10 mg or dronabinol oral solution 2.1–4.2 mg/m^2 PO every 3–4 times daily.
  - Other:
    - Haloperidol 0.5–2.0 mg PO/IV every 4–6 hours.
    - Metoclopramide 10–20 mg PO/IV, every 4–6 hr.
    - Scopolamine 1.5 mg transdermal patch 1 patch every 72 hours
  - Phenothiazine:
    - Prochlorperazine 25mg suppository PR every 12 hours or 10 mg PO/IV every 6 hr.
    - Promethazine 25 mg suppository PR every 6 hr or 12.5–25 mg PO every 4–6 hr.
  - Serotonin (5HT3) receptor antagonists:
    - Dolasetron 100 mg PO qd
    - Granisetron 1–2 mg PO daily or 1 mg PO BID or 0.01 mg/kg (maximum 1 mg) IV daily or 3.1 mg/24 h transdermal patch every 7 days.
  - Ondansetron 16–24 mg PO daily or 8–16 mg IV.
    - Corticosteroids: dexamethasone 12 mg PO/IV daily.
- If the patient has dyspepsia, consider antacid therapy (H$_2$ blocker or PPI).
- Ensure adequate hydration or fluid repletion, along with correction of any electrolyte imbalance.
- FOR THE NEXT CYCLE, consider changing the regimen (both day 1 and postchemotherapy regimen) to higher level of primary antiemetic treatment.
- Monitor for dystonic reactions when phenothiazines are used, and administer diphenhydramine as needed to resolve reaction.
- Olanzapine has been shown to be superior to metoclopramide for the treatment of breakthrough emesis in patients receiving highly emetogenic chemotherapy who had also received the highest level of primary antiemesis; dose was olanzapine 10 mg PO × 3 days (Navari et al., 2012).
- Consider anxiolytic therapy to prevent anticipatory emesis (e.g., alprazolam 0.5–1 mg or lorazepam 0.5–2 mg PO) beginning on the night before treatment and then repeated the next day 1–2 hours before chemotherapy begins.
- Consider the transdermal antiemetic route for managing multiday emetogenic chemotherapy regimens.

RADIATION-INDUCED NAUSEA AND VOMITING

Radiation therapy to the gastrointestinal tract usually causes nausea and vomiting. Highest risk (90%) is when total body irradiation (TBI) or external beam radiation is administered to the upper or total abdomen or upper hemithorax. Antiemesis is effective using serotonin antagonists with or without dexamethasone, which should be administered at a time before RT when the drug can be absorbed (NCCN, v.1.2019). NCCN (v1.2019) recommends to protect against upper abdomen/localized sites RT: start pretreatment for each day of RT treatment with granisetron 2 mg PO daily, OR ondansetron 8 mg PO bid, WITH or without dexamethasone 4 mg PO daily prior to RT. Recommended prophylaxis for TBI, starting pretreatment for each day of RT treatment with ondansetron 8 mg PO bid–tid OR granisetron 2 mg PO daily, WITH or without dexamethasone 4 mg PO daily. For breakthrough nausea and vomiting from RT to other sites, use agents described above for breakthrough antiemesis. Antiemesis for patients receiving combined chemotherapy and RT, refer to recommended antiemetics for the chemotherapy agent.

Anticipatory Nausea and Vomiting
Prevent nausea and vomiting so this conditioned response fails to be established. Use the best antiemetic regimen for the chemotherapy agent(s), remembering that combination of moderately emetogenic agents (e.g., doxorubicin and cyclophosphamide) make the combination highly emetogenic. Use behavioral therapy if patient is amenable, between chemotherapy cycles, such as relaxation/systematic desensitization, hypnosis/guided imagery, and music therapy (NCCN, v.1.2019). After patient assessment, consider acupuncture/acupressure, and consider anxiolytic therapy such as alprazolam 0.5–1 mg or lorazepam 0.5–2 mg PO beginning the night before treatment and then repeated the next day 1–2 hours prior to the chemotherapy regimen (NCCN, 2.2016).

DISEASE-INDUCED NAUSEA AND VOMITING

Site of advanced disease is a strong predictor of the risk for nausea and vomiting. Metastases to the liver are often associated with difficult-to-control nausea and vomiting. Pressure from ascites or obstruction of a hollow viscus, as with advanced ovarian cancer, can also lead to intractable nausea and vomiting. A factor here, along with advanced pancreatic cancer, may be delayed gastric emptying, or gastric outlet syndrome. Increased intracranial pressure (ICP) from a malignant brain tumor often causes nausea and vomiting. Other conditions related to disease that cause nausea and vomiting include hypercalcemia, hyperglycemia, electrolyte imbalance, and severe constipation. Strategies to relieve nausea and vomiting in these circumstances vary with the cause; they range from aggressive antiemesis to correction of delayed gastric emptying (metoclopramide) or the obstruction (stent if possible, or if not, release of gastric contents via a gastrostomy tube), to correction of electrolyte abnormalities.

Currently, antiemetics are available as oral, intravenous, rectal suppositories, transdermal, and transmucosal. Some hospitals and hospice pharmacies are also able to compound antiemetic(s) for transdermal absorption.

MANAGEMENT

In summary then, nausea and/or vomiting is preventable. It can arise from treatment or complications of disease. There are a variety of agents useful for blocking a number of neurotransmitter pathways to prevent or control nausea and vomiting in cancer. Specifically, it is known that chemotherapy stimulates nausea and vomiting via multiple pathways and often, therefore, multiple drugs are necessary for the prevention of nausea and vomiting associated with aggressive chemotherapy.

References

Aapro M, Gralla RJ, Herrstedt J, et al. MASCC/ESMO Antiemetic Guideline 2016. Available at http://www.mascc.org/assets/Guidelines-Tools/mascc_antiemetic_guidelines_english_2016_v.1.1.pdf. Accessed May 26, 2016.

American Society of Clinical Oncology. Antiemetics: Clinical Practice Update. July 31, 2017. Available at https://www.asco.org/about-asco/press-center/news-releases/new-recommendations-controlling-nausea-and-vomiting-related. Accessed May 29, 2019.

AbbVie Inc. Marinol (dronabinol) [package insert]. North Chicago, IL. August 2017.

Blanchard EM, Hesketh PJ. Nausea and Vomiting. Chapter 135. In VT DeVita, TS Lawrence, and SA Rosenberg (Eds). *Cancer Principles and Practice of Oncology*, 10th ed. Philadelphia, PA: Wolters Kluwer; 2015: 1976–1984.

Coates A, Abraham S, Kaye SB, et al. On the Receiving End—Patient Perception of the Side-effects of Cancer Chemotherapy. *Eur J Cancer Clin Oncol* 1983; 19:203–208.

Cotanch PM, Stum S. Progressive Muscle Relaxation as Antiemetic Therapy for Cancer Patients. *Oncol Nurs Forum* 1987; 14(1):33–37.

de Boer-Dennert M, de Wit R, Schmitz PIM, et al. Patient Perceptions of the Side-effects of Chemotherapy: The Influence of 5HT3 Antagonists. *Br J Cancer* 1997; 76:1055–1061.

Eisai Inc. Akynzeo (netupitant/palonosetron) [package insert]. Woodcliff Lake, NJ. April 2018.

Eisai Inc. Aloxi (palonestron) [package insert]. Woodcliff Lake, NJ. December 2015.

Food and Drug Administration, et al. 2012; *FDA Drug Safety Communication: New information regarding QT prolongation with ondansetron Zofran* Available at https://www.fda.gov/drugs/drug-safety-and-availability/fda-drug-safety-communication-new-information-regarding-qt-prolongation-ondansetron-zofran. Accessed October 15, 2019.

Genentech, Inc. Kytril (granisetron) [package insert]. South San Francisco, CA. April 2011.

Hellsin Therapeutics (US), Inc. Akynzeo (netupitant and palonosetron capsules). [package insert]. Iselin, NJ. April 2018.

Hellsin Therapeutics (US), Inc. Aloxi (palonosetron HCl) [package insert]. Iselin, NJ. September 2018.

Heron Therapeutics Inc. Cinvanti (aprepitant injectable emulsion) [package insert]. San Diego, CA. February 2019.

Heron Therapeutics Inc. Sustol (granisetron extended-release injection) [package insert]. San Diego, CA. May 2017.

Hesketh PJ, Beck TM, Uhlenhopp M, et al. Adjusting the Dose of Intravenous Ondansetron plus Dexamethasone to the Emetogenic Potential of the Chemotherapy Regimen. *J Clin Oncol* 1995; 13(8):2117–2122.

Hesketh PJ, Kris MG, Basch E et al. Antiemetics: American Society of Clinical Oncology clinical practice guideline update. *J Clin Oncol* 2017; 35:3240–3261.

Hesketh P, Bohlke K, Lyman GH, et al. Antiemetics: American Society of Clinical Oncology Focused Guideline Update. *J Clin Oncol* 2016; 34(4):381–386.

Hesketh P, Rossi G, Rizzi G, et al. Efficacy and safety of NEPA, an oral combination of netupitant and palonosetron, for prevention of chemotherapy-induced nausea and vomiting following highly emetogenic chemotherapy: a randomized dose ranging pivotal study. *Ann Oncol* 2014; 35(7):1340–1346.

Hofman M, Morrow GR, Roscoe JA, et al. Cancer Patients' Expectations of Experiencing Treatment-related Side Effects. *Cancer* 2004; 101(4):851–857.

Hospira, Inc. Metoclopramide [package insert]. Lake Forest, IL. June 2012.

Hospira, Inc. Ondansetron injection. [package insert]. Lake Forest, IL. April 2017.

Insys Therapeutics. Syndros (dronabinol) oral solution, CX [package insert]. Chandler, AZ. July 2016.

Ioannidis JPA, Hesketh P, Lau J. Contribution of Dexamethasone to Control of Chemotherapy-induced Nausea and Vomiting: A Meta-analysis of Randomized Evidence. *J Clin Oncol* 2000; 18:3409–3422.

Kaiser R, Sezer O, Papies A, et al. Patient-tailored Antiemetic Treatment with 5-hydroxytryptamine Type 3 Receptor Antagonists According to Cytochrome P-450 Genotypes. *J Clin Oncol* 2002; 20(12):2805–2811.

Kyowa Kirin Sancuso (granisetron transdermal system) [package insert]. Bedminster NJ. January 2017.

Meda Pharmaceuticals Inc. Cesamet (nabilone) [package insert]. Somerset, NJ. September 2013.

Merck, Sharpe and Dohme Corp. EMEND (aprepitant) [package insert]. Whitehouse Station, NY. January 2019.

Merck, Sharpe and Dohme Corp. EMEND IV (fosprepitant) [package insert]. Whitehouse Station, NY. February 2016.

Midatech Pharma US Inc. Zuplenz (ondansetrol oral soluble film). [package insert]. Raleigh, NC. July 2016.

Moradian S, Powell D. Prevention and Management of Chemotherapy-induced Nausea and Vomiting. *Int J Palliat Nurs* 2015; 21(5):216, 218–224.

Mylan Pharmaceuticals, Inc. Prochlorperazine. [package insert]. Morgantown, WV, November 2016.

National Comprehensive Cancer Network. *Clinical Practice Guideline Antiemesis,* version 1.2019. Available at http://www.nccn.org. Accessed May 29, 2019.

Navari RM. Managing nausea and vomiting in patients with cancer: what works. *Oncology (Williston Park)* 2018; 32(3):121–125.

Navari RM, Nagy CK, Gray SE, et al. The Use of Olanzapine Versus Metoclopramide for the Treatment of Breakthrough Chemotherapy-induced Nausea and Vomiting (CINV) in Patients Receiving Highly Emetogenic Chemotherapy. *J Clin Oncol* 30, 2012 (suppl; abstr 9064).

ProStraken Inc. Sancuso (granisetron transdermal system) [package insert]. Bedminster, NJ. September 2015.

Sagent Pharmaceuticals. Ondansetron. [package insert]. Schaumburg, IL. March 2017.

Sandoz Inc. Aprepitant capsules. [package insert]. Princeton, NJ. June 2017.

Sanofi-aventis. Anzamet (dolasetron) [package insert]. Bridgewater, NJ. October 2015.

Tesaro, Inc. Varubi (rolapitant) [package insert]. Waltham, MA. March 2018.

Teva Pharmaceuticals USA. Granisetron HCl tablets [package insert]. North Wales, PA. August 2014.

Drug: aprepitant (generic oral formulation, Emend)

Class: Substance P/NK$_1$ receptor antagonist. For IV preparation, see the IV aprepitant formulation Cinvanti that follows; also the aprepitant prodrug fosprepitant (Emend).

Mechanism of Action: Selective substance P/NK$_1$ receptor antagonist (high affinity). Drug has no affinity for 5-HT$_3$, dopamine, or corticosteroid receptors. Drug crosses the blood–brain barrier to saturate brain NK$_1$ receptors. Drug increases the activity of serotonin-receptor antagonists and corticosteroids in preventing acute nausea and vomiting, and inhibits both acute and delayed nausea and vomiting related to cisplatin chemotherapy.

Metabolism: Drug is well absorbed after oral administration with 60–65% bioavailability. Drug is 95% bound to plasma proteins and crosses the placenta and blood–brain barrier. Aprepitant undergoes extensive metabolism in the liver by the P450 hepatic microenzyme

MANAGEMENT

system, specifically CYP3A4, and minor metabolism by CYP1A2 and CYP2C19. Seven inactive metabolites have been found in the plasma. The drug is excreted in the urine (57%) and the feces (45%). The terminal half-life of the drug is 9–13 hours.

Indication: (1) Aprepitant (Emend) for oral suspension is indicated in combination with other antiemetic agents in patients 6 months of age or older for the prevention of (a) acute and delayed nausea and vomiting associated with initial and repeat courses of highly emetogenic cancer chemotherapy, including high-dose cisplatin; (b) nausea and vomiting associated with initial and repeat courses of moderately emetogenic cancer chemotherapy; (2) aprepitant (Emend) capsules are indicated in combination with other antiemetic agents, in patients 12 years of age or older, for the prevention of (a) acute and delayed nausea and vomiting associated with initial and repeat courses of highly emetogenic cancer chemotherapy, including high-dose cisplatin; (b) nausea and vomiting associated with initial and repeat courses of moderately emetogenic cancer chemotherapy; (3) prevention of postoperative nausea and vomiting (POVN) in adults.

Aprepitant has not been studied for the treatment of established nausea and vomiting; chronic use is not recommended. Chronic continuous administration is not recommended.

Contraindications: (1) known hypersensitivity; (2) concurrent use with pimozide.

Dosage/Range (see package insert):
- Recommended dose for highly CINV in patients aged 12 and over: Day 1, 125 mg PO 1 hour before chemotherapy, together with a serotonin (HT_3) receptor antagonist on day 1 and dexamethasone (dose reduced to 12 mg day 1, 8 mg days 2, 3, 4); aprepitant on days 2 and 3, 80 mg PO each morning. For children > aged 12 and over: give 50% of adult steroid dose. See package insert for doses in moderately emetogenic chemotherapy as well as steroid use in pediatric patients.
- Recommended dose of aprepitant suspension for the prevention of CINV in pediatric patients aged 6 months to < 12 years old, or pediatric and adult patients unable to swallow capsules: day 1 aprepitant 3 mg/kg (max dose 125 mg) 1 hour prior to chemotherapy, days 2 and 3, aprepitant 2 mg/kg (max dose 80 mg); see package insert for dexamethasone and -5HT-3 receptor antagonist dosing.
- PONV: 40 mg within 3 hours prior to induction of anesthesia.

Drug Preparation:

Available as
- Capsules available in 40-, 80-, and 125-mg strengths. Capsules should be stored at room temperature.
- Oral suspension 125-mg powder in a single-use pouch and preparation kit.
- A health care provider should prepare the aprepitant oral suspension, which is 25 mg/mL, and then can be administered by the patient, parent, or family member.
- Drug is packaged as a kit with one 1 mL dosing dispenser, one 5 mL oral dosing dispenser, one cap and one mixing cup. Fill the cup with room temperature drinking water. Fill the 5 ml oral dosing dispenser with 4.6 mL of water from the cup. **Make sure there is NO air in the dispenser and if found, remove the air.** Remove all remaining water in the cup. Add the 4.6 mL back into the empty cup.

- Pick up aprepitant pouch and hold upright; shake powder down to the bottom. Open the pouch and pour entire contents into cup to be dissolved in the 4.6 mL of water. Gently swirl the contents in the cup around 20 times to dissolve. Wait for foam to dissipate. Fill the dispenser to the ordered dose (see package insert). Use 1 mL dispenser if dose is < 1 mL and the 5 mL dispenser if dose is > 1 mL. If dose is < 1 mL round to the nearest 0.1, if the dose is > 1 mL, round dose to nearest 0.2 mL. Make sure there is no air in the dispenser. Place cap on dispenser until it clicks.
- If not used immediately upon mixing, place dispenser containing dose in refrigerator where it is stable for 72 hours at 2–8°C (36–46°F). When dispensing dose to patient, remind them to put dose in refrigerator until ready to use. When ready to use, can be stored at room temperature for 3 hours. Discard mixing cup and any remaining suspension.

Drug Administration:

- Capsules: Day 1: give 125-mg capsule PO 1 hour before chemotherapy, and then the 80-mg capsule in the morning on days 2 and 3. Give with or without food. Teach patient to swallow whole.
- Suspension: Dose will be prepared by the healthcare provider and dispensed to the patient or caregiver.
- Keep prepared suspension in refrigerator until administered to the patient. The dose can be stored at room temperature for 3 hours before taken.
- Take cap off the dispenser, place dispenser in patient's mouth along the inner cheek (either right or left side) and slowly dispense medicine. The dose must be used within 72 hours of preparation.
  - Discard any remaining doses after 72 hours.

Drug Interactions:

- Drugs that inhibit the CYP3A4 isoenzyme system can increase the serum level of aprepitant: ketoconazole, itraconazole, nefazodone, clarithromycin, ritonavir, nelfinavir; diltiazem (twofold increase in aprepitant plasma concentration), so coadminister cautiously and monitor for aprepitant toxicity or dose-reduce aprepitant.
- Drugs that strongly induce CYP3A4 isoenzyme system can lower aprepitant serum levels: rifampin, carbamazepine, phenytoin; assess for efficacy of aprepitant and need for drug dose increase.
- Drug is a moderate inhibitor of P450 hepatic isoenzyme system CYP3A4, so the plasma concentrations of the following drugs can theoretically be increased if coadministered:
  - Chemotherapy agents are docetaxel, paclitaxel, etoposide, irinotecan, ifosfamide, imatinib, vinorelbine, vinblastine, and vincristine.
  - Dexamethasone (dose-reduce dexamethasone by 50%).
  - Methylprednisolone (dose-reduce 25% if IV, 50% if PO).
  - Benzodiazepines: midazolam, lorazepam, alprazolam, triazolam.
- Drug is an inducer of CYP2C9, and the plasma concentrations of the following drugs can theoretically be decreased if coadministered:
  - Warfarin (34% decrease with 14% decrease in INR; closely monitor INR 7–10 days after 3-day antiemetic regimen, and modify warfarin dose as needed).
  - Phenytoin, tolbutamide, oral contraceptives.

MANAGEMENT

Lab Effects/Interference:
• Decreased INR if patient taking warfarin.

Special Considerations:
• Contraindications: Do not give concomitantly with pimozide, terfenadine, astemizole, or cisapride; do not give if hypersensitive to aprepitant or any of its components; use cautiously if at all during pregnancy or breastfeeding; no studies have been done in patients with severe liver failure.
• Significant drug interactions (see above).
• Drug is well-tolerated with few side effects.
• Warnings and Precautions:
    • *CYP3A4 interactions: aprepitant is a substrate, weak-to-moderate inhibitor and inducer of CYP3A4*:
        • CYP3A4 substrates: coadministration may increase serum level of substrate. Once example is pimozide which is contraindicated. Pimozide is potentially fatal so contraindicated due to risk of prolonged QTc interval.
        • Strong or moderate CYP3A4 inhibitors: may increase serum level of aprepitant and risk of aprepitant toxicity.
        • Strong CYP3A4 inducers: may reduce aprepitant serum level and its efficacy.
    • *Decrease in INR with concurrent warfarin:* Monitor INR closely in the 2-week period, especially on days 7–10 following start of the chemotherapy cycle.
    • *Reduced efficacy of hormonal contraceptives:* Advise patients to use back up methods such as condom and spermicide during treatment and for 1 month after last dose of aprepitant.

Potential Toxicities/Side Effects and the Nursing Process

I. ALTERATION IN NUTRITION, LESS THAN BODY REQUIREMENTS, related to CONSTIPATION, DIARRHEA, NAUSEA, ANOREXIA, HICCUPS

Defining Characteristics: Gastrointestinal side effects may occur but are infrequent with the following incidences: constipation (10.3%), diarrhea (10.3%), nausea (12.7%), vomiting (7.5%), hiccups (10.8%), and anorexia (10.1%).

Nursing Implications: Teach patient that these side effects may occur, and to report them if unrelieved by symptom-management measures. Teach patient self-care measures to manage and prevent symptoms.

II. ALTERATION IN COMFORT related to ASTHENIA/FATIGUE, ABDOMINAL PAIN, HEADACHE

Defining Characteristics: Asthenia/fatigue occurred in 17.8% of patients; abdominal pain 4.6%; headache 8.5%.

Nursing Implications: Teach patient that these side effects may occur and measures to minimize their occurrence. Teach energy-conserving measures, management of abdominal pain and headache. Teach patient to report signs and symptoms that worsen or are unrelieved.

Drug: aprepitant injectable emulsion (Cinvanti)

Class: Substance P/NK$_1$ receptor antagonist.

Mechanism of Action: Crosses blood brain barrier and blocks substance P/NK$_1$ receptors in the brain which help mediate emesis. Augments control of antiemesis when combined with 5-HT$_3$ receptor antagonists and corticosteroids. Fosprepitant is a prodrug of aprepitant.

Metabolism: Greater than 99% protein bound and crosses the blood brain barrier in humans. Extensively metabolized by the CYP3A4 microenzyme system with minor metabolism by CYP1A2 and CYP2C19. Metabolism is primarily oxidation, with the formation of many metabolites, seven of which are found in the serum and are weakly active. Terminal half-life is 9–13 hours. While there were differences when Cmax was calculated based on ethnicity, these were felt to be insignificant.

Indication: In combination with other antiemetic agents, for the prevention of (1) acute and delayed nausea and vomiting associated with initial and repeat courses of highly emetogenic cancer chemotherapy including high-dose cisplatin; (2) nausea and vomiting associated with initial and repeat courses of moderately emetogenic cancer chemotherapy.

Limitations: Drug has not been studied in the treatment of established nausea and vomiting.

Contraindication: in patients who: (1) are hypersensitive to any component of the product as HSRs including anaphylaxis have been reported; (2) are taking pimozide as coadministration with aprepitant could lead to a potentially lethal concentrations of pimozide vis a vis QTc prolongation, a known adverse reaction of pimozide.

Dosage/Range:
- IV administration over 2 minutes or by infusion over 30 minutes.
- Highly emetogenic chemotherapy (single dose regimen): (a) aprepitant 130 mg IV on day 1 only together with (b) dexamethasone 12 mg PO × 1 on day 1, 8 mg PO × 1, and on days 3 and 4: 8 mg PO BID, and (c) 5-HT$_3$ receptor antagonist on day 1.
- Moderately emetogenic chemotherapy (3-day regimen with oral aprepitant on days 2, 3): (a) aprepitant IV 100 mg day 1, followed by aprepitant 80 mg PO on days 2, 3; (c) dexamethasone 12 mg PO × 1 day 1 only; (c) 5-HT$_3$ receptor antagonist on day 1.

Drug Preparation:
- Available as aprepitant injectable emulsion as 130 mg/18 mL (7.2 mg/mL) as an opaque, off-white to amber emulsion, in a single-dose vial.
- IV injection over 2 minutes: aseptically withdraw **18 mL for the 130 mg dose**, and **14 mL for the 100 mg dose**. Do not dilute. Flush line with NS before and after drug administration.
- IV infusion over 30 minutes: (a) aseptically withdraw **18 mL for the 130 mg dose**, and **14 mL for the 100 mg dose** from the vial and transfer it into an infusion bag (**non-DEHP tubing, non-PVC infusion bag**) filled with 100 mL 0.9% sodium chloride injection, USP

MANAGEMENT

or 5% dextrose for injection, USP; (b) gently invert bag to mix (about 4–5 times) but do not shake; (c) inspect bag for particulate matter or discoloration, and do not use if found.
- Diluted solution stable at ambient room temperature for up to 6 hours in 0.9% sodium chloride injection, USP or 12 hours in 5% dextrose for injection, USP, or for up to 72 hours refrigerated in either 0.9% sodium chloride injection, USP or 5% dextrose for injection, USP.
- Drug is incompatible with solutions containing divalent cations such as magnesium or calcium (including Ringer's Lactate and Hartmann's Solution).

Drug Administration:
- IV injection over 2 minutes or as an IV infusion over 30 minutes.
- Flush IV line with normal saline before and after drug is given.

Drug Interactions:
- CYP3A4 inhibitors: strong (e.g., ketoconazole, clarithromycin, protease inhibitors): increase aprepitant toxicity; moderate (e.g., diltizem): avoid concurrent use.
- CYP3A4 inducers (strong): (e.g., rifampin, carbamazepine, phenytoin): decrease serum level of aprepitant, avoid concurrent use.
- CYP3A4 substrates: drug levels of the substrate may be increased:
  - Pimazole: increased pimazole levels; use together is contraindicated.
  - Dexamethasone (dose-reduce dexamethasone by 50%).
  - Methylprednisolone (dose-reduce 25% if IV, 50% if PO). See package insert for specific reductions by chemotherapy regimen.
  - Benzodiazepines: midazolam, lorazepam, alprazolam, triazolam; monitor for adverse effects as benzodiazepine levels may be increased.
  - Chemtherapy agents: vinblastine, vincristine, ifosfamide: monitor for increased chemotherapy toxicity;
  - Hormonal contraceptives: decreased estrogen and progesterone exposure during administration and for 28 days after last dose of aprepitant. Teach patient to use additional contraception such as condoms and spermicides during treatment and for 1 month after last aprepitant dose.
- Drug is an inducer of CYP2C9, and the plasma concentrations of the following drugs can theoretically be decreased if coadministered: Warfarin (34% decrease with 14% decrease in INR; closely monitor INR 7–10 days after 3-day antiemetic regimen and modify warfarin dose as needed).
- Drug is incompatible with solutions containing divalent cations such as magnesium or calcium (including Ringer's Lactate and Hartmann's Solution.

Lab Effects/Interference:
- Decreased INR if patient taking warfarin.

Special Considerations:
- Most common toxicities were fatigue, eructation, headache, and rare infusion site reactions.
- Warnings and Precautions:

- *Clinically significant CYP3A4 drug interactions:* see Drug Interactions.
- *HSRs*: Monitor patient during and after administration for signs of hypersensitivity such as dyspnea, eye swelling, flushing, pruritus, wheezing. If signs/symptoms occur, discontinue drug and do not rechallenge. Implement ordered medical and emergency interventions.
- *Decrease INR with concomitant warfarin:* INR may become decreased with decreased efficacy. Assess INR of patients on chronic warfarin therapy in the 2-week period, especially at 7 to 10 days after the initiation of aprepitant emulsion with each chemotherapy cycle.
- *Risk of reduced hormonal contraceptives:* Teach patients to also use another method of effective contraception such as condom and/or spermicide during treatment and for 1 month after the last aprepitant dose.

Potential Toxicities/Side Effects and the Nursing Process

I. ALTERATION IN COMFORT related to ASTHENIA/FATIGUE, HEADACHE

Defining Characteristics: Asthenia/fatigue and headache may occur.

Nursing Implications: Teach patient that these side effects may occur and measures to minimize their occurrence. Teach energy-conserving measures, as well as management of headache if it occurs. Teach patient to report signs and symptoms that worsen or are unrelieved.

Drug: dexamethasone (Decadron)

Class: Glucocorticoid steroid.

Mechanism of Action: May inhibit prostaglandin release by stabilizing lysosomal membranes, thereby interrupting hypothalamic prostaglandin release and subsequent stimulation of nausea and vomiting. Causes demargination of marginated WBCs, with leukocytosis. Decreases inflammation by suppression of migration of polymorphonuclear leukocytes.

Metabolism: Half-life is 3–4 hours; oral dose peaks in 1–2 hours, with duration of 2 days; IM peaks in 8 hours, with duration of 6 days.

Indication: For management of (1) endocrine disorders (e.g., primary or secondary adrenocortical insufficiency); (2) rheumatic disorders (short-term); (3) collagen diseases; (4) dermatologic diseases; (5) allergic states; (6) ophthalmic diseases; (7) GI diseases (e.g., ulcerative colitis); (8) respiratory diseases; (9) hematologic disorders; (10) neoplastic diseases; (11) edematous states; (12) other diseases or treatments.

Dosage/Range:

Adult (as antiemetic):
- *Oral:* 4 mg q 4 h × 4 doses beginning 1–8 hours before chemotherapy.
- *IV:* 10–20 mg prior to chemotherapy, then q 4–6 h.

MANAGEMENT

Drug Preparation:

- *Oral:* administer with food or milk.
- *IV:* may be given with H_2-antagonist (e.g., ranitidine) to prevent gastric irritation.

Drug Interactions:
- Indomethacin, aspirin: increased GI irritation and bleeding; avoid concurrent administration.
- Barbiturates, phenytoin, rifampin: decreased dexamethasone effect; increase dose as needed.

Lab Effects/Interference:

- Increased WBC may occur due to demargination.
- Increased serum glucose level.
- May cause decreased K.

Special Considerations:
- Contraindicated in patients with psychosis, hypersensitivity, idiopathic thrombocytopenia, acute glomerulonephritis, amebiasis, fungal infections, and nonasthmatic bronchial disease.
- Indicated in the management of inflammation, allergies, neoplasms, cerebral edema, and in combination antiemetic therapy.
- If patient received dexamethasone chronically, drug must be tapered to prevent withdrawal (i.e., signs/symptoms of adrenal insufficiency, rebound weakness, arthralgia, fever, dizziness, orthostatic hypotension, dyspnea, hypoglycemia).

Potential Toxicities/Side Effects and the Nursing Process

I.   ALTERATION IN NUTRITION, LESS THAN BODY REQUIREMENTS, related to GI TOXICITY

Defining Characteristics: Increased appetite, abdominal distension, pancreatitis, GI hemorrhage; diarrhea may occur.

Nursing Implications: Assess baseline nutritional status and monitor throughout therapy. Discuss symptomatic management of diarrhea, abdominal distension, and increased appetite with patient. Assess stool for occult blood and notify physician if positive. Monitor Hgb and HCT values.

II.   ALTERATIONS IN SENSORY/PERCEPTUAL PATTERNS related to CHANGES IN MOOD, VASODILATION, CATARACTS

Defining Characteristics: Euphoria, insomnia, depression, flushing, sweating, headache, mood changes, and cataracts may occur.

Nursing Implications: Assess baseline mental status and monitor during therapy. Discuss symptomatic management or drug discontinuance, based on severity, with physician.

III. ALTERATION IN CARDIAC OUTPUT related to CHF

Defining Characteristics: Congestive heart failure (CHF), hypertension, fluid retention, and edema may occur.

Nursing Implications: Assess baseline vital signs (VS), and monitor during therapy. Discuss hypertension with physician, monitor daily weights, and assess for edema.

IV. ALTERATION IN CARBOHYDRATE METABOLISM related to CARBOHYDRATE INTOLERANCE

Defining Characteristics: May cause hyperglycemia, hypokalemia, and carbohydrate intolerance.

Nursing Implications: Assess baseline blood glucose, K, and monitor during therapy. Teach patient signs/symptoms of hyperglycemia (polyuria, polydipsia), especially if receiving drug for extended period.

Drug: diphenhydramine hydrochloride (Benadryl)

Class: Antihistamine.

Mechanism of Action: Inhibits histamine, and has slight, if any, antiemetic activity by blocking the CTZ and decreasing vestibular stimulation. Acts on blood vessels, GI, respiratory systems by competing with histamine for H1-receptor site; decreases allergic response by blocking histamine.

Metabolism: Biologically transformed in the liver; half-life is 2.4–9.3 hours; 80–85% protein-bound; excreted by the kidney. Metabolized in the liver, crosses placenta, and is excreted in breastmilk.

Indications: Useful in the management of allergic reactions, prevention of allergic reactions, motion sickness, and parkinsonism.

Contraindications: In neonates, nursing mothers, as a local anesthetic and if hypersensitive to the drug or its components.

Dosage/Range:

Adult:
- *Oral:* 25–50 mg q 4 h.
- *IM:* 25–50 mg q 4 h.
- *IV:* 50 mg prior to chemotherapy or 25 mg q 4 h × 4 doses, beginning prior to antiemetic.

Drug Preparation:
- Available forms include 25-, 50-mg capsules; elixir 12.5 mg/mL; syrup 12.5 mg/mL; injection available as 10 and 50 mg/mL.
- Administer IM deep in large muscle mass.

Drug Interactions:
- CNS depressants: increased sedation; monitor patient closely.

Lab Effects/Interference:
- None known.

Special Considerations:

- Useful in treatment or prevention of extrapyramidal side effects (EPS) related to anti-emetics (dopamine antagonists).
- Contraindicated in patients with prior hypersensitivity to H_1-receptor antagonist, acute asthma attack, or lower respiratory tract disease.

Potential Toxicities/Side Effects and the Nursing Process

I. ALTERATIONS IN SENSORY/PERCEPTUAL PATTERNS related to CNS CHANGES

Defining Characteristics: Sedation/drowsiness, dizziness, confusion (especially in the elderly), hyperexcitability, blurred vision/diplopia, tinnitus, dry mouth/nose/throat all may occur.

Nursing Implications: Assess patient's level of consciousness and risk for increased sedation (i.e., elderly, concomitant CNS depressant drugs). Monitor neurologic VS closely if sedated. Instruct patient to avoid alcohol ingestion, operation of equipment, or driving a car while drowsy. Teach strategies to protect safety.

II. ALTERED URINARY ELIMINATION related to URINARY RETENTION, DYSURIA

Defining Characteristics: Urinary retention, dysuria, frequency may occur.

Nursing Implications: Assess baseline urinary elimination pattern. Teach patient potential side effects and instruct to report them. Use drug cautiously in men with prostatic hypertrophy; if side effects occur, instruct patient not to take drug and discuss with physician.

III. ALTERATION IN COMFORT related to RASH

Defining Characteristics: Rash, urticaria, photosensitivity, hypotension, palpitations may occur.

Nursing Implications: Assess baseline drug allergy history. Instruct patient to report rash, itching, and to avoid sunlight while taking the drug. Assess VS and monitor patient closely for hypotension, especially if patient is elderly, sedated, or taking other sedating drugs.

IV.   POTENTIAL FOR INJURY related to BONE MARROW DEPRESSION

Defining Characteristics: Thrombocytopenia, agranulocytosis, hemolytic anemia may occur rarely.

Nursing Implications: Assess baseline CBC, platelet count. Discuss abnormalities with physician.

Drug: dronabinol (Marinol, Syndros)

Class: Cannabinoid.

Mechanism of Action: Active ingredient is d-9-tetrahydrocannabinol (THC). Probably depresses CNS and may disrupt higher cortical input, inhibit prostaglandin synthesis, or bind to opiate receptors in the brain to indirectly block the VC.

Metabolism: Metabolized by the liver.

Indication: For the treatment of (1) anorexia associated with weight loss in patients with AIDS, and (2) nausea and vomiting associated with cancer chemotherapy in patients who have failed to respond adequately to conventional antiemetic treatments.

Contraindications: Marinol: Hypersensitivity to the drug or any of its ingredients.

Syndros: Contraindicated in patients with (1) sensitivity to dronabinol or alcohol; (2) history of hypersensitivity reaction to alcohol; (3) who are receiving, or who have received disulfiram or metronidazole-containing products within the past 14 days.

Dosage/Range:

Adult:
- CINV
  - *Oral:*
    - Marinol: 5 mg given 1–3 hours prior to chemotherapy, then 4 hours postchemotherapy for a total of 3–4 doses/day.
    - Syndros: 4.2 mg/m^2 1–3 hours prior to chemotherapy, then every 2–4 hours after chemotherapy for a total of 4–6 doses a day. See package insert for dose titration. Maximum dose 12.6 mg/m^2 per dose for 4–6 doses/day.
  - If ineffective at above dose and no significant toxicity, dose may be increased. Concurrent use with a phenothiazine increases effect without added toxicity.
- *Appetite Stimulation:*
Marinol: Begin with 2.5 mg PO before lunch and 2.5 mg PO before dinner.
  - If CNS effects occur (e.g., high, confusion), they usually resolve in 1–3 days of continued dosing. If CNS effects are severe, reduce dose to a single bedtime dose.
  - If adverse effects are absent or are mild, increase the dose to 2.5 mg PO before lunch and 5 mg PO before dinner.

MANAGEMENT

Syndros: Starting dose 2.1 mg PO bid, 1 hour before lunch and dinner. See package insert for dose titration. Maximum dosage 8.4 mg bid.

Drug Preparation:
- Marinol Available in 2.5-, 5-, or 10-mg gel capsules that harden under refrigeration.
- Syndros: oral solution 5 mg/mL. Use calibrated oral dosing syringe that comes with medication.

Drug Administration:
- Oral.
    - Marinol: Teach patient to self-administer oral gel capsules.
    - Sandros: Oral. Teach patient to use calibrated oral dosing syringe, and to take dose with a full glass of water (6–8 oz). **See full prescribing information** for dose titration to manage adverse reactions and to achieve desired therapeutic effect.
    - For anorexia/weight loss: Take dose bid, 1 hour before lunch and dinner.
    - For antiemetic use: Administer first dose on an empty stomach at least 30 minutes before eating; subsequent doses can be taken without regard to meals.

Drug Interactions:
- CNS depressants: increased sedation; avoid concurrent use.

Lab Effects/Interference:

- Syndros:
    - Disulfiram and metronidazole: may cause disulfiram-like reaction. Discontinue disulfiram or metronidazole 14 days before starting Syndros and do not administer 7 days after treatment with Syndros.
    - Inhibitors and inducers of CYP2C9 and CYP3A4: may alter dronabinol systemic exposure; monitor for dronabinol-related adverse reactions or loss of efficacy.
    - Highly protein-bound drugs: potential for displacement of other drugs from plasma proteins; monitor for adverse reactions to concomitant narrow therapeutic index drugs (e.g., warfarin, cyclosporine, amphotericin B) when initiating or increasing the dosage of Syndos.

Special Considerations:
- Warnings and Precautions:
    - Teach patient not to drive a car, operate heavy machinery, or engage in any hazardous activity until the drug effect on the patient and how the patient tolerates the effect, is known.
    - Seizure and seizure-like activity; use cautiously in patients with a history of seizures, and stop the drug if a seizure occurs. A full medical evaluation should be performed on the patient.
    - Drug should be used cautiously in patients with hypo or hypertension, syncope, or tachycardia. Avoid use in patients receiving other drugs with similar side effects or hemodynamic changes.
    - Drug should be used cautiously in patients with a history of substance abuse, include alcohol dependency. Use cautiously in patients with a history of mania, depression,

or schizophrenia as drug may exacerbate symptoms; patient should have close psychiatric monitoring while drug is being used. Syndros: avoid use in patients with psychiatric history.

- Elderly, as they may be more sensitive to the neurological, psychoactive, and postural hypotensive effects of the drug.
- Pregnant women, nursing mothers, pediatric patients, as drug has not been studied in these patient populations.
- Syndros:
  - Seizure and seizure-like activity: weigh the potential risk versus benefit before administering Syndros to patients with a history of seizures, or with other factors that lower seizure threshold; monitor patient and discontinue drug if seizures occur.
  - Multiple substance abuse: assess for risk of abuse; monitor patient for development of associated behaviors or conditions.
  - Paradoxical nausea, vomiting, or abdominal pain: consider dose reduction or discontinuation, if worsening symptoms of drug.
  - Toxicities related to propylene glycol in preterm neonates: drug safety has not been established in pediatrics. Avoid use in preterm neonates in the immediate postnatal period.
  - Drug may cause fetal harm; women should not breastfeed while receiving the drug and for 9 days after the last dose (Syndros), or use during pregnancy.
- More effective than placebo and, in some instances, may be better than prochlorperazine. Can produce physical and psychological dependency.
- May increase appetite; may produce dry mouth.
- Contains sesame oil, so should not be used by patients allergic to sesame oil.

Potential Toxicities/Side Effects and the Nursing Process

I. ALTERATIONS IN SENSORY/PERCEPTUAL PATTERNS related to CNS CHANGES

Defining Characteristics: Mood changes, disorientation, drowsiness, muddled thinking, dizziness, and brief impairment of perception, coordination, and sensory functions may occur. Increased toxicity in elderly (up to 35%).

Nursing Implications: Explain to patient these changes may occur to decrease anxiety, fear. Assess baseline mental status, and monitor during therapy. Assess patient safety and implement measures to ensure this. Avoid use in the elderly.

II. ALTERATION IN CARDIAC OUTPUT related to TACHYCARDIA

Defining Characteristics: Tachycardia, orthostatic hypotension may occur.

Nursing Implications: Assess baseline VS, and monitor during therapy. If hypotension occurs, notify physician and anticipate increasing rate of IV fluids to increase BP.

Drug: fosaprepitant dimeglumine (Emend for injection)

Class: Substance P/NK$_1$ receptor antagonist. For oral formulation, see aprepitant.

Mechanism of Action: Drug is a prodrug of aprepitant. Selective substance P/NK$_1$ (NK$_1$) receptor antagonist (high affinity). Drug has no affinity for 5-HT$_3$, dopamine, or corticosteroid receptors. Drug crosses the blood–brain barrier to saturate brain NK$_1$ receptors. Drug increases the activity of serotonin-receptor antagonists and corticosteroids in preventing acute nausea and vomiting and inhibits both acute and delayed nausea and vomiting related to cisplatin chemotherapy.

Metabolism: Drug is rapidly converted to aprepitant after IV administration, and the pro-drug is negligible 30 minutes following administration. The mean aprepitant serum concentrations at 24 hours postdose were similar between a 125-mg oral dose and a 115-mg IV fosaprepitant dose. Aprepitant is 95% bound to plasma proteins and crosses the placenta and blood–brain barrier. Aprepitant undergoes extensive metabolism in the liver by the P450 hepatic microenzyme system, specifically CYP3A4, and minor metabolism by CYP1A2 and CYP2C19. Seven inactive metabolites have been found in the plasma. The drug is excreted in the urine (57%) and the feces (45%). The terminal half-life of the drug is 9–13 hours. The C_{max} is 16% higher for females than males, and the half-life of aprepitant is lower in females than males; however, this is not believed to be clinically important. No dosage adjustment necessary for patients with renal insufficiency or requiring dialysis or patients with mild to moderate hepatic insufficiency.

Indication: In adults and pediatric patients aged 6 months and older, in combination with other antiemetic agents, for the prevention of (a) acute and delayed nausea and vomiting associated with initial and repeat courses of highly emetogenic cancer chemotherapy, including high-dose cisplatin, and (b) delayed nausea and vomiting associated with moderately emetogenic cancer chemotherapy.

Fosprepitant has not been studied in the treatment of established nausea and vomiting.

Contraindications: (1) Patients hypersensitive to drug or any of its components; (2) patients taking pimozide as aprepitant inhibits CYP3A4 which can significantly increase the serum levels of pimozide.

Dosage/Range:

Adults
- *Highly emetogenic chemotherapy:* Day 1: 150-mg IV infusion over 20–30 minutes, started 30 minutes before chemotherapy, together with a serotonin- (HT$_3$-) receptor antagonist and dexamethasone 12 mg PO on day 1, 8 mg PO day 2, and 8 mg PO bid on days 3 and 4.
- *Moderately emetogenic chemotherapy:* Day 1: fosaprepitant 150-mg IV as a 20–30-minute infusion 30 minutes before chemotherapy. serotonin-receptor antagonist day 1; dexamethasone 12 mg PO day 1 only (50% dose reduction).

Pediatrics (weighing at least 6 kg)

- Use a central line for administration; (a) as a 60-minute infusion for patients 6 months to 12 years, and a 30-minute infusion for those aged 12 years to 17 years, completing the infusion 30 minutes before chemotherapy.
- *Single-dose chemotherapy regimen:* Day 1 **Aged 12–17 years** = **150 mg** IV over 30 min; if **2 years old to <12 years** = **4 mg/kg** (maximum dose 150 mg) IV over 60 minutes; **6 months–<2 years old** = **5 mg/kg** (maximum 150 mg) IV infusion over 20–30 minutes, started 30 minutes before chemotherapy, together with a serotonin- (HT_3-) receptor antagonist and dexamethasone 12 mg PO on day 1, 8 mg PO day 2, and 8 mg PO bid on days 3 and 4. Together with an 5-HT3 receptor antagonist plus a corticosteroid such as dexamethasone (50% of the recommended corticosteroids dose on days 1 and 2). See package insert.
- *Multi-day chemotherapy regimen:* Children weighing at least 6 kg. Fosprepitant given on days 1, 2, 3 with day 1 given via a central venous catheter, and days 2 and 3 as capsules or oral suspension.
- *3-day dosing for either a single or multi-day regimen of highly emetogenic or moderately emetogenic chemotherapy:* Day 1 **Aged 12–17 years** = **115 mg** IV over 30 min, days 2 and 3 = 80 mg PO; day 1 if **6 months–<12 years old** = **3 mg/kg** (maximum 115 mg) IV infusion over 60 minutes, and on days 2 and 3 = 2 mg/kg PO (maximum 80 mg), started 30 minutes before chemotherapy, together with a serotonin- (HT_3-) receptor antagonist and dexamethasone 12 mg PO on day 1 = 8 mg PO day 2, and 8 mg PO bid on days 3 and 4, together with an 5-HT3 receptor antagonist +/– a corticosteroid such as dexamethasone (50% of the recommended corticosteroids dose on days 1 through 4). See package insert.

Drug Preparation:

- IV formulation supplied as single dose of 150-mg lyophilized white to off-white solid formulation. Vial should be stored at 2–8°C (36–46°F). Aseptically add 5-mL 0.9% sodium chloride for injection USP, into the vial by injecting onto the vial wall to prevent foaming; gently swirl the contents until dissolved (do not shake or jet the diluent into the vial).
- Aseptically prepare an infusion bag filled with 145 mL of 0.9% sodium chloride for injection USP.
- Aseptically withdraw entire vial contents and add 150-mg dose to a 145-mL infusion bag of 0.9% sodium chloride infusion bag bringing the volume up to 150 mL. This results in a final concentration of 1 mg/mL. Gently invert bag to mix 2–3 times.
- Determine the volume to be administered from the prepared infusion bag: (a) adults, entire 150-mL bag; (b) pediatrics based on patient's age and weight.
- For volumes < 150 mL, transfer the calculated volume to an appropriately sized bag or syringe prior to administration by infusion.
- Before administration, inspect the bag for particulate matter or discoloration, and do not use if found. Do not use IV solutions containing divalent cations such as calcium or magnesium, including Lactated Ringer's Solution and Hartmann's Solution.
- Once prepared, the solution is stable for 24 hours at room temperature (at or below 77°F).

MANAGEMENT

Drug Administration:

Administer IV over 20–30 minutes about 30 minutes prior to chemotherapy. Prepare and administer ordered dexamethasone and 5-HT$_3$ receptor antagonist.

Drug Interactions:

- Drugs that inhibit the CYP3A4 isoenzyme system can increase the serum level of aprepitant: ketoconazole, itraconazole, nefazodone, clarithromycin, ritonavir, nelfinavir; diltiazem (twofold increase in aprepitant plasma concentration); thus, coadminister cautiously and monitor for aprepitant toxicity or dose-reduce aprepitant.
- Drugs that strongly induce CYP3A4 isoenzyme system can lower aprepitant serum levels: rifampin, carbamazepine, phenytoin; assess for efficacy of aprepitant and need for drug dose increase.
- Drug is a moderate inhibitor of P450 hepatic isoenzyme system CYP3A4; thus, the plasma concentrations of the following drugs can theoretically be increased if coadministered:
  - Chemotherapy agents are docetaxel, paclitaxel, etoposide, irinotecan, ifosfamide, imatinib, vinorelbine, vinblastine, and vincristine.
  - Dexamethasone (dose-reduce dexamethasone by 50%).
  - Methylprednisolone (dose-reduce 25% if IV, 50% if PO).
  - Pimozide, terfenadine, astemizole: do not use together.
  - Benzodiazepines: midazolam, lorazepam, alprazolam, triazolam.
- Drug is an inducer of CYP2C9, and the plasma concentrations of the following drugs can theoretically be decreased if coadministered:
  - Warfarin (34%) decrease with 14% decrease in INR; closely monitor during 2 weeks following antiemetic treatment, especially as the INR and PT 7–10 days after 3-day antiemetic regimen may be significantly lowered; assess INR, PT frequently and manage warfarin dose closely).
  - Phenytoin, tolbutamide serum levels can be decreased.
- Hormonal contraceptives can become ineffective during and for 28 days following last dose of fosaprepitant or aprepitant; alternative or backup methods of contraception should be used.

Lab Effects/Interference:

- Decreased INR, PT if patient taking warfarin.

Special Considerations:

- Warnings and Precautions:
  - *Clinically significant CYP3A4 drug interactions*: **See package insert for complete discussion.** Fosaprepitant, a prodrug of aprepitant, is a weak inhibitor of CYP3A4, and aprepitant is a substrate, inhibitor, and inducer of CYP3A4.
    - Use of aprepitant with other drugs that are CYP3A4 substrates, may result in increased plasma concentration of the concomitant drug.
    - Use of aprepitant with strong or moderate CYP3A4 inhibitors (e.g., ketoconazole, diltiazem) may increase plasma concentrations of aprepitant and result in an increased risk of adverse reactions related to aprepitant.

- Use of aprepitant with strong CYP3A4 inducers (e.g., rifampin) may result in a reduction in aprepitant plasma concentrations and decreased efficacy of aprepitant.
- *Hypersensitivity reactions* during fosprepitant infusion may occur characterized by flushing, dyspnea, erythema, and rarely anaphylaxis. If symptoms occur, stop the drug, and provide medical support as ordered. Do not restart the infusion in patients with these symptoms during first-time use.
- *Infusion site reactions:* have been reported, especially when administered with concomitant vesicant (chemotherapy) administration. Necrosis has been described in these situations when associated with extravastion. Most occurred with the first, second, or third exposure to single doses of EMEND IV, and in some cases, reaction persisted for 2 or more weeks. Do not infuse EMEND for injection into small veins or through a butterfly catheter. If a severe infusion site reaction occurs, stop the infusion and administer appropriate therapy as ordered.
- *Decreased INR when aprepitant used with warfarin* (CYP2C9 substrate)*:* Monitor the patient's INR closely, especially during the 2 weeks after aprepitant therapy, especially on days 7–10.
- *Reduced efficacy of hormonal contraceptives:* When coadministered, the hormonal contraceptive may not be effective during aprepitant administration and for 28 days after the last aprepitant dose.
- Most common side effects: hiccups, asthenia/fatigue, increased AST/ALT, headache, constipation, anorexia, dyspepsia, diarrhea, eructation, infusion-site reactions.

Potential Toxicities/Side Effects and the Nursing Process

I. ALTERATION IN NUTRITION, LESS THAN BODY REQUIREMENTS, related to CONSTIPATION, DIARRHEA, NAUSEA, ANOREXIA, HICCUPS

Defining Characteristics: Gastrointestinal side effects may occur but are infrequent with the following incidences: constipation (10.3%), diarrhea (10.3%), nausea (12.7%), vomiting (7.5%), hiccups (10.8%), and anorexia (10.1%).

Nursing Implications: Teach patient that these side effects may occur and to report them if unrelieved by symptom management measures. Teach patient self-care measures to manage and prevent symptoms.

II. ALTERATION IN COMFORT related to ASTHENIA/FATIGUE, ABDOMINAL PAIN, HEADACHE

Defining Characteristics: Asthenia/fatigue occurred in 17.8% of patients; abdominal pain 4.6%; headache 8.5%.

Nursing Implications: Teach patient that these side effects may occur and measures to minimize their occurrence. Teach energy-conserving measures and management of abdominal pain and headache. Teach patient to report signs and symptoms that worsen or are unrelieved.

MANAGEMENT

Drug: granisetron hydrochloride (Kytril)

Class: Serotonin-receptor antagonist.

Mechanism of Action: Binds to vagal afferents (serotonin receptors) adjacent to the enterochromaffin cells in the GI mucosa, thus preventing the stimulation of afferent fibers that would otherwise stimulate the VC and CTZ. In addition, granisetron inhibits a positive feedback loop located on the enterochromaffin cells that normally responds to high levels of serotonin released from chemotherapy injury to the gut mucosa by releasing a surge of additional serotonin. Thus, granisetron blocks two pathways of serotonin release to prevent CINV.

Metabolism: Rapidly and extensively metabolized by the liver using the P450 cytochrome enzymes; 12% of unchanged drug is eliminated in the urine at 48 hours. The half-life of IV granisetron in cancer patients is 9 hours.

Indication: *Oral formulation* indicated for (1) prevention of nausea and/or vomiting associated with initial and repeat courses of emetogenic cancer chemotherapy, including high-dose cisplatin; and (2) prevention of nausea and vomiting associated with radiation, including TBI and fractionated abdominal radiation. *IV formulation* indicated for (1) prevention of nausea and/or vomiting associated with initial and repeat courses of emetogenic cancer chemotherapy, including high-dose cisplatin; and (2) prevention and treatment of PONV in adults.

Contraindication: hypersensitivity to the drug or any of its components.

Dosage/Range:
- CINV: *IV*
  - *Adults and pediatric patients aged 2–16:* Day 1 10-mcg/kg IV over 5 minutes, beginning within 30 minutes prior to chemotherapy.
    - PONV: 1-mg IV undiluted over 30 seconds before anesthesia induction or immediately before reversal of anesthesia.
    - Treatment of PONV: 1-mg IV undiluted over 30 seconds.
- *Oral:*
  - CINV: 2 mg PO or 1 mg bid (q 12 h) beginning up to 1 hour before chemotherapy on day 1.
- RT: 2 mg PO once daily taken within 1 hour of radiation.

Drug Preparation:
- IV available as injection 1 mg/mL (free-base) and 0.1 mg/mL (free base).
- Prepare as IVP or dilute in 20–50 mL 0.9% sodium chloride or 5% dextrose.
- PO available as 1-mg tablets.

Drug Administration:
- IV infusion over 5 minutes.
- Drug can also be given IV push over 30 seconds.

Drug Interactions:

• None known; however, because the drug is metabolized by the P450 cytochrome enzymes, drugs that induce or inhibit this may theoretically change the drug serum levels and half-life.

• Coadministration with drugs that prolong the QTc interval or which may cause arrhythmias may result in "clinical consequences" (Genentech, 2011).

Lab Effects/Interference:

• Rarely, increased AST, ALT.

Special Considerations:

• Most common adverse reactions were (CINV): headache, constipation; and for (PONV), were headache, pain, fever, abdominal pain, increased hepatic enzymes.

• Warnings and Precautions:

  • Granisetron does not stimulate gastric or intestinal peristalsis and should not be used instead of NG suction.

  • QT prolongation has been reported. Use cautiously in patients with preexisting arrhythmia or cardiac conduction disorders.

  • Hypersensitivity reactions, including SOB, hypotension, urticarial, and anaphylaxis may occur, especially if the patient has had prior hypersensitivity to other selective 5-HT$_3$ receptor antagonists.

  • IV formulation contains benzyl alcohol.

• Both IV and tablet formulation are indicated for the prevention of nausea and vomiting associated with initial and repeat courses of emetogenic chemotherapy, including cisplatin.

Potential Toxicities/Side Effects and the Nursing Process

I. ALTERATION IN COMFORT related to HEADACHE, ASTHENIA, SOMNOLENCE

Defining Characteristics: Side effects are uncommon but may include headache, asthenia, and somnolence.

Nursing Implications: Teach patient that side effects may occur. Headache is usually relieved by OTC analgesics such as acetaminophen.

II. ALTERATION IN ELIMINATION related to CONSTIPATION OR DIARRHEA

Defining Characteristics: A small percentage of patients may experience constipation or diarrhea.

Nursing Implications: Assess baseline elimination pattern. Instruct patient to report alterations. Identify patients at risk, such as those receiving narcotic analgesics for cancer pain, who may develop constipation. Assist patient in modifying bowel regimen.

MANAGEMENT

Drug: granisetron hydrochloride extended-release injection (Sustol)

Class: Serotonin-receptor antagonist.

Mechanism of Action: Binds to vagal afferents (serotonin receptors) adjacent to the enterochromaffin cells in the GI mucosa, thus preventing the stimulation of afferent fibers that would otherwise stimulate the VC and CTZ. In addition, granisetron inhibits a positive feedback loop located on the enterochromaffin cells that normally responds to high levels of serotonin released from chemotherapy injury to the gut mucosa by releasing a surge of additional serotonin. Thus, granisetron blocks two pathways of serotonin release to prevent CINV.

Metabolism: Rapidly and extensively metabolized by the liver using the P450 cytochrome enzymes CYP1A1 and CYP3A4; 12% of unchanged drug is eliminated in the urine at 48 hours. The half-life of IV granisetron in cancer patients is 9 hours.

Indication: indicated, with other antiemetics in adults, for (1) prevention of acute and delayed nausea and vomiting associated with initial and repeat courses of moderately emetogenic cancer chemotherapy, or (2) anthracycline and cyclophosphamide (AC) combination chemotherapy regimen.

Contraindication: Hypersensitivity to the drug or any of its components, or to other 5-HT$_3$ receptor antagonists.

Dosage/Range: For subcutaneous (SQ) injection only.

- 10 mg SQ × 1 at least 30 minutes before the start of emetogenic chemotherapy on day 1.
- DO NOT administer any more frequently than every 7 days.
- Do not use for successive chemotherapy cycles lasting >6 months.
- Recommended dexamethasone dose for moderately emetogenic chemotherapy: 8 mg IV on day 1 only.
- Recommended dexamethasone dose for anthracycline/cyclophosphamide chemotherapy: 20 mg IV on day 1, followed by 8 mg PO BID on days 2–4.
- Dose adjustment for renal impairment (CrCl 30–59 mL/min), administer drug on day 1 of chemotherapy no more frequently than every 14 days. DO NOT administer to patients with CrCl <30 mL/min.

Drug Preparation:

- Available as 10 mg/0.4 mL in a single-dose pre-filled syringe with a refrigerated kit. It also contains a special thin-walled 18 gauge 5/8 inch needle, two syringe warming pouches, and a Point Lok needle protection device. See package insert for complete instructions. DO NOT substitute non-kit components.
- At least 60 minutes prior to administration, remove the drug kit from the refrigerator. Allow all contents including syringe to warm to room temperature.
- Activate one of the syringe-warming pouches, and wrap the pre-filled syringe in it for 5–6 minutes to warm the drug to body temperature.

- Prior to administration inspect the syringe contents for particulate matter or discoloration, and if found, do not use. Do not use if the tip cap is missing or has been tampered with or if the Luer fitting is missing or dislodged.

Drug Administration:
- Should be administered by a healthcare provider only.
- Administer in the skin of the back of the upper arm or in the skin of the abdomen at least 1 inch away from the umbilicus; avoid areas where skin has been burned, hardened, inflamed, swollen, or otherwise compromised.
- Viscous solution, so administration requires a slow, sustained injection over 20–30 seconds. Pushing the plunger harder will NOT inject drug faster.
- If needed, use topical anesthetic at the injection site prior to administration.
- Teach patient that injection site reactions may occur including bruising, infection, bleeding, pain, tenderness, and nodules.
  - Infections, bruising, and hematoma may occur up to 2 weeks of more after the injection.
  - Seek immediate medical care for signs of infection at the injection site or injection site bleeding that is severe or lasts >1 day.
  - Tell healthcare provider if s/he develop (a) pain or tenderness severe enough to require pain medication or if it interferes with daily activity; (b) bruising and/or hematoma or a persistent nodule at the injection site.
- Teach patient that an allergic reaction may occur up to 7 days or longer after the injection; teach patient if s/he develops a swollen face or throat, big tongue, difficulty breathing, hives, or chest pain, or any other serious new symptom to seek emergency medical care right away.
- Assess bowel elimination status at each visit as drug may cause constipation. Teach patient self-care measures to prevent or relieve constipation (e.g., diet, hydration, cathartics if needed).

Drug Interactions:
- None known; however, because the drug is metabolized by the P450 cytochrome enzymes, drugs that induce or inhibit this may theoretically change the drug serum levels and half-life.
- Coadministration with drugs that prolong the QTc interval or which may cause arrhythmias may result in "clinical consequences," QTc prolongation potential is a class effect.
- Serotoninergic drugs (e.g., SSRIs, SNRIs): increased risk of serotonin syndrome. See Warnings and Precautions.

Lab Effects/Interference: None known.

Special Considerations:

- Most common adverse effects ($\geq$ 3%) are injection site reactions, constipation, fatigue, headache, diarrhea, abdominal pain, insomnia, dyspepsia, dizziness, asthenia, and gastroesophageal reflux.
- Warnings and Precautions:
  - *Injection Site Reactions (ISRs):* can occur, and can be complicated by (a) infection: incidence in clinical trials was rare (0.4%), with a median time of onset of 9 days after drug administration. All resolved with antibiotic therapy; (b) bruising and/or

MANAGEMENT

hematoma occurred in 38% of patients with a median time of onset of 2 days; 15% of patients had delayed onset of 5 days or more after administration; patients receiving anticoagulants or antiplatelet medication were at greatest risk for severe bruising/hematoma; (c) bleeding occurred in 4% of patients, and bleeding for 5 days was reported in 1% of patients; (d) pain and tenderness occurred in 20% of patients, and 11% more reported tenderness without pain; reaction was severe in 2%; median duration was 5 days, and pain lasting > 7 days occurred in 6% of patients; (e) nodules occurred in 18% of patients in clinical trials, persisted for a median of 15 days, but 6% had nodules persist for > 21 days. An 18 gauge needle is used for drug injection. Management may occur up to 2 weeks or longer after drug injection. If the patient is receiving anticoagulant or antiplatelet therapy, consider this before selecting SQ antiemetic. If the ISR persists, ensure the drug is administered at a site distant from the affected area.

- *GI disorders:* (a) constipation may occur in 13–15% of patients. Monitor patients bowel elimination status, as the drug is slow released over 7 days, especially if the patient is also receiving opioid analgesics. Teach patient bowel elimination management to prevent constipation; (b) progressive ileus and gastric distention may occur and may mask a progressive ileus. Assess patients carefully who have just had abdominal surgery and monitor for decreased bowel activity.

- *HSRs:* HSRs may occur up to 7 days or longer after drug administration because of the extended-release properties. Teach patients that this may rarely occur to report any signs/symptoms of rash, or if more severe HSR occur (e.g., swollen face, swollen throat or tongue, difficulty breathing, hives) to seek emergency medical care right away.

- *Serotonin syndrome:* has been reported with serotonin receptor antagonists used for antiemesis. Most instances develop from the concomitant use of serotonergic drugs such as SSRIs or SNRIs, MAO inhibitors, mirtazapine, fentanyl or lithium. If a patient is taking another serotoninergic drug, closely assess for symptoms: mental status changes (e.g., agitation, hallucinations, delirium, coma), autonomic instability (e.g., tachycardia, labile BP, dizziness, diaphoresis, flushing, hyperthermia), neuromuscular symptoms (e.g., tremor, rigidity, myoclonus, hyperreflexia, incoordination), seizures, with or without GI symptoms (e.g., nausea, vomiting, diarrhea). If serotonin syndrome occurs, drug should be stopped right away and supportive measures instituted. Teach patients to self-assess and report any signs/symptoms.

Potential Toxicities/Side Effects and the Nursing Process

I.   ALTERATION IN COMFORT related to HEADACHE, ASTHENIA, SOMNOLENCE

Defining Characteristics: Side effects are uncommon but may include headache, asthenia, and somnolence.

Nursing Implications: Teach patient that side effects may occur. Headache is usually relieved by OTC analgesics such as acetaminophen.

II.   ALTERATION IN ELIMINATION related to CONSTIPATION OR DIARRHEA

Defining Characteristics: A small percentage of patients may experience constipation or diarrhea.

Nursing Implications: Assess baseline elimination pattern. Instruct patient to report alterations. Identify patients at risk, such as those receiving narcotic analgesics for cancer pain, who may develop constipation. Assist patient in modifying bowel regimen.

Drug: granisetron hydrochloride transdermal (Sancuso)

Class: Serotonin-receptor antagonist.

Mechanism of Action: Drug, in a transdermal patch, is delivered via the transdermal route. Granisetron binds to vagal afferents (serotonin receptors) adjacent to the enterochromaffin cells in the GI mucosa, thus preventing the stimulation of afferent fibers that would otherwise stimulate the VC and CTZ. In addition, granisetron inhibits a positive feedback loop located on the enterochromaffin cells that normally responds to high levels of serotonin released from chemotherapy injury to the gut mucosa by releasing a surge of additional serotonin. Thus, granisetron blocks two pathways of serotonin release to prevent CINV.

Metabolism: Drug contains 34 mg of drug and delivers drug over 5 days. Once absorbed, drug is rapidly and extensively metabolized by the liver using the P450 cytochrome enzymes; 12% of unchanged drug is eliminated in the urine at 48 hours. The half-life of IV granisetron in cancer patients is 9 hours.

Indication: For the prevention of nausea and vomiting in patients receiving moderately and/or highly emetogenic chemotherapy for up to 5 consecutive days.

Contraindication: hypersensitivity to granisetron or to any of the components of the patch.

Dosage/Range:
• 34.3-mg transdermal patch providing antiemesis for 7 days, delivering 3.1 mg/24 hours.

Drug Preparation:
• None.

Drug Administration:
• Remove plastic backing and apply to clean, dry skin.
• Apply to the upper outer arm a minimum of 24 hours and a maximum of 48 hours before chemotherapy. Remove the patch a minimum of 24 hours after completion of chemotherapy. The patch can be worn up to 7 days depending upon the duration of the chemotherapy regimen.

Drug Interactions:
• None known, but because the drug is metabolized by the P450 cytochrome enzymes, drugs that induce or inhibit this may theoretically change the drug serum levels and half-life.

MANAGEMENT

Lab Effects/Interference:
- Rarely, increased AST, ALT.

Special Considerations:

- Warnings and Precautions:
  - *GI:* can mask a progressive ileus and/or gastric distention caused by the underlying condition.
  - *Serotonin syndrome* has been reported with 5-HT$_3$ receptor antagonists alone, but also when used concomitantly with serotoninergic drugs, such as SSRIs, SNRIs, MAO inhibitors, fentanyl, others. If a patient is taking another serotoninergic drug, closely assess for symptoms: mental status changes (e.g., agitation, hallucinations, delirium, coma), autonomic instability (e.g., tachycardia, labile BP, dizziness, diaphoresis, flushing, hyperthermia), neuromuscular symptoms (e.g., tremor, rigidity, myoclonus, hyperreflexia, incoordination), seizures, with or without GI symptoms (e.g., nausea, vomiting, diarrhea). If serotonin syndrome occurs, drug should be stopped right away and supportive measures instituted. Teach patients to self-assess and report any signs/symptoms.
  - *Skin reaction:* skin reactions from patch were reported as mild during clinical trials. If severe or generalized (e.g., allergic rash, including erythematous, macular, papular rash, or pruritis), patch must be removed.
  - *External heat source:* Do not apply a heating pad over patch or in vicinity of patch as this increases systemic absorption of drug.
  - *Exposure to sunlight*: Teach patients to cover the patch application site with clothing to prevent sunlight exposure and for 10 days after its removal as there may be a skin reaction.
- In a non-inferiority trial, transdermal formulation was as good as oral granisetron in the management of patients with cancer receiving first cycle of multiday (3–5 days), moderate or highly emetogenic chemotherapy (Grundberg et al., 2007). This phase III trial was a randomized, double-blind, multinational (nine countries) trial that enrolled 641 patients. Complete protection was achieved in 60.2% of patients receiving the transdermal granisetron and 64.9% of those receiving oral granisetron. Ninety percent of the patients in the transdermal granisetron arm had > 75% patch adherence. Side effects were identical (constipation and headache were most common), and there was no significant irritation at the patch site.

Potential Toxicities/Side Effects and the Nursing Process

I.   ALTERATION IN COMFORT related to HEADACHE, ASTHENIA, SOMNOLENCE

Defining Characteristics: Side effects are uncommon but may include headache, asthenia, and somnolence.

Nursing Implications: Teach patient that side effects may occur. Headache is usually relieved by OTC analgesics such as acetaminophen.

II. ALTERATION IN ELIMINATION related to CONSTIPATION OR DIARRHEA

Defining Characteristics: A small percentage of patients may experience constipation or diarrhea.

Nursing Implications: Assess baseline elimination pattern. Instruct patient to report alterations. Identify patients at risk, such as those receiving narcotic analgesics for cancer pain, who may develop constipation. Assist patient in modifying bowel regimen.

Drug: haloperidol (Haldol)

Class: Butyrophenone.

Mechanism of Action: Tranquilizer that depresses cerebral cortex, hypothalamus, limbic system (controls activity and aggression); appears to block dopamine receptors in CTZ, giving antiemetic activity.

Metabolism: Metabolized by the liver, excreted in the urine, bile, and crosses placenta. Enters breastmilk. Half-life is 21 hours.

Indication: For the management of manifestations of psychotic disorders; control of tics and vocal utternaces of Tourette's disorder in children and adults. May be useful in the management of CINV refractory to other agents.

Dosage/Range:

Adult:
- *Oral:* 3–5 mg q 2 h × 3–4 doses, beginning 30 minutes before chemotherapy.
- *IM:* 0.5–2 mg (dose-reduce in older patients).

Drug Preparation:
- Available as 0.5-, 1-, 2-, 5-, 10-, 20-mg tablets; injection: 5 mg/mL.

Drug Interactions:
- *Epinephrine:* reversal of vasopressor effects; avoid concurrent use.
- *CNS depressants:* increased sedation; monitor patient closely.

Lab Effects/Interference:
- Rarely, increased alk phos, bili, serum transaminases (AST, ALT).
- Rarely, decreased PT (if patient on warfarin).
- Rarely, decreased serum cholesterol.
- Prolongs QTc interval on ECG.

Special Considerations:
- Indicated for the management of psychotic disorders, short-term treatment of hyperactive children showing excessive motor activity, schizophrenia; may be used in the management of nausea and vomiting.

MANAGEMENT

- Contraindicated in severe toxic CNS depression or comatose states; individuals with hypersensitivity; patients with Parkinson's disease, blood dyscrasias, brain damage, bone marrow depression, and alcohol or barbiturate withdrawal states.
- Shown to be equivalent to THC and superior to phenothiazines when tested as an antiemetic.

Potential Toxicities/Side Effects and the Nursing Process

I. ALTERATIONS IN SENSORY/PERCEPTUAL PATTERNS related to TARDIVE DYSKINESIA

Defining Characteristics: With chronic use, tardive dyskinesia syndrome occurs, characterized by involuntary, dyskinetic movements; sedation, EPS may occur when used as an antiemetic.

Nursing Implications: Assess baseline level of consciousness and monitor during therapy. Assess for signs/symptoms of EPS (dystonia, tongue protrusion, trismus, opisthotonus), and administer diphenhydramine as ordered.

II. ALTERATION IN OXYGENATION related to LARYNGOSPASM

Defining Characteristics: Laryngospasm and respiratory depression occur rarely.

Nursing Implications: Assess baseline pulmonary status, and monitor during therapy. Identify risk factors (concomitant narcotics, CNS depressants). Notify physician, and **hold** drug if respiratory depression occurs or is suspected. Be prepared to institute respiratory support if necessary and to reverse opiate.

III. ALTERATION IN CARDIAC OUTPUT/PERFUSION related to ORTHOSTATIC HYPOTENSION

Defining Characteristics: Orthostatic hypotension may occur and may precipitate angina; also, tachycardia, EKG changes, and rare cardiac arrest may occur.

Nursing Implications: Assess VS baseline, and monitor during therapy. If hypotension occurs, notify physician and anticipate increasing rate of IV fluids to increase BP. Epinephrine should NOT be used because the drug reverses vasopressor effect; rather, metaraminol or norepinephrine should be used.

Drug: metoclopramide hydrochloride (Reglan)

Class: Substituted benzamide.

Mechanism of Action: Procainamide derivative without cardiac effects. Acts both centrally and peripherally. Acts peripherally to enhance the action of acetylcholine at muscarinic synapses and in the CNS to antagonize dopamine. Is primarily a dopamine antagonist blocking the CTZ; also stimulates upper GI tract motility, thus increasing gastric emptying, and opposes retrograde peristalsis of retching.

Metabolism: Metabolized by the liver, excreted in the urine, with a half-life of 4 hours.

Indication: *Oral:* for the (1) prevention and management of acute and recurrent diabetic gastroparesis; (2) short-term therapy of symptomatic, documented gastroesophageal reflux disease in adults who fail to respond to conventional therapy. *IV:* (1) prevention of nausea and vomiting associated with emetogenic cancer chemotherapy; (2) prevention of PONV when nasogastric suction is undesirable; (3) facilitation of small bowel intubation when tube does not pass pylorus with conventional maneuvers; (4) acute and recurrent diabetic gastric stasis; (5) stimulation of gastric emptying and intestinal transit or barium where delayed emptying interferes with radiological examination of the stomach and/or small intestines.

Contraindication: Patients with (1) GI hemorrhage, mechanical obstruction or perforation; (2) pheochromocytoma (drug may cause hypertensive crisis); (3) known sensitivity or intolerance of the drug; (4) epilepsy as drug may cause extrapyramidal reactions and enhance those of drugs taken by the patient.

Dosage/Range:

Adult:
- *Oral:* 10 mg qid (gastroparesis) administered 30 minutes before each meal and at bedtime for 2–8 weeks.
- *IV:* Highly emetogenic chemotherapy: 2 mg/kg q 2 h × 3–5 doses OR 3 mg/kg q 2 h × 2 doses, beginning 30 minutes prior to chemotherapy. Dose-reduce 50% renal insufficiency (CrCl < 40 mL/min). Moderately emetogenic chemotherapy: 1 mg/kg given 30 minutes before beginning cancer chemotherapy, and repeat every 2 hours × 2 doses, then every 3 hours × 3 doses.
- *IM:* PONV: 10–20 mg IM near end of surgery.

Drug Preparation:
- *IV:* available as 5 mg/mL; further dilute in 50 mL 0.9% sodium chloride or 5% dextrose and administer over 15 minutes.

Drug Interactions:
- Digoxin: may decrease absorption; monitor digoxin effectiveness and modify dose as needed.
- Aspirin, acetaminophen, tetracycline, ethanol, levodopa, diazepam: may increase absorption; monitor for drug toxicity.
- CNS depressants: increased depressant effects; monitor patient closely.

Lab Effects/Interference:
- None known.

Special Considerations:

- Warnings and Precautions:
  - Rare neuroleptic malignant syndrome (hyperthermia, muscle rigidity, altered LOC, and autonomic instability (e.g., irregular heart rate or BP, tachycardia, diaphoresis, cardiac arrhythmias). If this occurs, stop drug immediately and implement medical orders.
  - Extrapyramidal Symptoms (EPS) including (1) acute dystonic reactions, tardive dyskinesia (involuntary movement of face, tongue, extremities). Drug should be discontinued if tardive dyskinesia occurs; (2) Parkinsonian-like symptoms; (3) depression.
- Increased incidence of dystonic reactions in men under 35 years old. Consider diphenhydramine q 4 h or lorazepam and dexamethasone to minimize dystonic reactions.
- Efficacy as an antiemetic: 60% complete protection against high-dose cisplatin, and increased to 66% with the addition of corticosteroid and lorazepam.
- Contraindicated in patients with prior hypersensitivity to this drug, procaine, or procainamide; patients with seizure disorder, pheochromocytoma, GI obstruction.
- Use cautiously in patients with breast cancer, as may increase prolactin levels, and in patients with renal insufficiency.

Potential Toxicities/Side Effects and the Nursing Process

I.   ALTERATIONS IN SENSORY/PERCEPTUAL PATTERNS related to SEDATION, EPS

Defining Characteristics: Sedation, akathisia (restlessness), adverse dystonic, or extrapyramidal effects may occur; increased risk in patients < 30 years old.

Nursing Implications: Assess baseline neurologic status, and monitor during therapy. Protect patient safety, and keep all necessary patient equipment at the bedside (e.g., commode). Assess for EPS, and administer diphenhydramine as ordered. In addition, lorazepam administered as part of combination antiemetics helps to decrease akathisia.

II.   POTENTIAL FOR ALTERED BOWEL ELIMINATION related to DIARRHEA

Defining Characteristics: Increase in both esophageal sphincter pressure and gastric emptying, leading to diarrhea with high doses. Action antagonized by narcotics.

Nursing Implications: Assess baseline bowel elimination status. Teach patient to report diarrhea, and administer kaolin/pectin as ordered, or other antidiarrheals. Arrange for commode at the bedside if bathroom far from bed. Also, diarrhea may be prevented by administration of dexamethasone as part of antiemetic regimen.

III.   ALTERATION IN COMFORT related to DRY/MOUTH, RASH

Defining Characteristics: Dry mouth, rash, urticaria, hypotension may occur.

Nursing Implications: Assess baseline comfort. Teach patient to report rash, urticaria, and treat symptomatically. Monitor VS, and slow infusion rate if hypotensive, as well as replace IV fluids per physician's order.

Drug: nabilone (Cesamet)

MANAGEMENT

Class: Cannabinoid antiemetic.

Mechanism of Action: Drug interacts with the cannabinoid receptors CB1 and CB2, which are involved in regulating nausea and vomiting. CB1 and CB2 receptors are found throughout the human body.

Metabolism: After oral administration, drug and its carbinol metabolite achieve peak plasma levels in 2 hours, but this amount represents only 10–20% of total drug. Plasma half-life of nabilone is about 2 hours, while that of the total radiocarbon dose was 35 hours. Drug is highly protein-bound. Drug is primarily metabolized by direct enzymatic oxidation in the liver (first pass), and excreted via the biliary system. Drug and its metabolites are excreted primarily in the feces (65%), with 20% excreted in the urine.

A substantial number of patients experience disturbing psychotomimetic reactions not experienced with other antiemetic agents (Cesamet package insert, 2010). Use of nabilone requires close supervision of the patient during initiation and dose adjustments. It is not intended to be used PRN or as the first antiemetic agent the patient has been prescribed.

Indication: treatment of nausea and vomiting from cancer chemotherapy in patients who have failed to respond adequately to standard antiemetic therapy.

Contraindication: hypersensitivity to the drug or any other cannabinoid.

Dosage/Range:
- 1 or 2 mg PO bid, beginning 1–3 hours before planned chemotherapy; beginning with the lower dose is recommended, with dose increase as needed. Some patients have benefited from a beginning dose the night before chemotherapy.
- Give drug during the entire course of each cycle of chemotherapy, and if needed, for 48 hours after the last dose of each cycle of chemotherapy.
- The maximum daily dose is 6 mg, given orally in divided doses 3 times a day.

Drug Preparation:
- None, oral capsule. Available in 1-mg capsules.

Drug Administration:
- Teach patients that they:
  - May experience mood changes and other adverse behavioral effects, so they should not become alarmed when it occurs; patients should be with a responsible (supervisory) person while using the drug, especially initially and during dose adjustments.
  - Should not drive, operate machinery, or engage in any hazardous activity while receiving nabilone.
  - Should not take other substances or drugs that depress the CNS (e.g., alcohol, benzodiazepines, barbiturates).

Drug Interactions:
- Additive CNS depressant effects with alcohol, sedatives, hypnotics, or other psychotomimetic substances. DO NOT give concomitantly.
- Diazepam: significantly impairs psychomotor function; DO NOT give concurrently.

- Amphetamines, cocaine, other sympathomimetic agents: additive HTN, tachycardia, possible cardiotoxicity.
- Atropine, scopolamine, antihistamines, other anticholinergic agents: additive or super-additive tachycardia, drowsiness.
- Amitriptyline, amoxapine, desipramine, and other tricyclic antidepressants: additive tachycardia, HTN, drowsiness.
- Disulfiram: reversible hypomanic reaction possible.
- Opioids: cross-tolerance and mutual potentiation.
- Naltrexone: oral THC effects were enhanced by opioid receptor blockade (THC is active ingredient in marijuana).
- Alcohol: increase in the positive subjective mood effects of smoked marijuana.

Lab Effects/Interference:
- Leukopenia.

Special Considerations:
- Common side effects are unsteadiness, dizziness, difficulty concentrating, drowsiness, mouth dryness, and/or headache.
- Warnings and Precautions:
  - Nabilone drug effects may persist for an unpredictable length of time after oral administration. Adverse psychiatric reactions can last 48–72 hours after last dose of treatment.
  - Drug may affect the CNS, causing dizziness, drowsiness, euphoria "high," ataxia, anxiety, disorientation, depression, hallucinations, and psychosis.
  - Drug can cause tachycardia and orthostatic hypotension. Use cautiously in elderly patients with hypertension or heart disease, as drug elevates supine and standing heart rates; it also causes postural hypotension, as well as tachycardia.
  - Drug should not be taken with alcohol, sedatives, hypnotics, or other psychotomimetic substances.
  - Should not drive, operate machinery, or engage in any hazardous activity while receiving nabilone until its CNS effects are known and how well the patient tolerates the effects.
  - Use cautiously, if at all, in patients with severe liver or renal dysfunction.
  - Use cautiously in patients with a substance abuse history. Drug is a controlled substance; monitor patients for signs of excessive use, abuse, and misuse.
  - Use cautiously in patients with a history of current or previous psychiatric disorders, including bipolar disorder, depression, and schizophrenia, as the symptoms of these disease states may be unmasked by the use of cannabinoids.
- Drug should not be used during pregnancy, in nursing mothers, or in pediatric patients, as safety has not been established.

Potential Toxicities/Side Effects and the Nursing Process

I.   ALTERATIONS IN SENSORY/PERCEPTUAL PATTERNS related to SEDATION, EPS

Defining Characteristics: Frequency of symptoms was drowsiness (66%), psychological high (39%), depression (14%), ataxia (13%), blurred vision (13%), sensation disturbance

(12%), euphoria (4%), and hallucinations (2%). Rarely, syncope, nightmares, distortion in the perception of time, confusion, disassociation, dysphoria, psychotic reactions, and seizures occurred in < 1% of patients. Anxiety, insomnia, and emotional lability may all occur. Increased toxicity in the elderly.

Nursing Implications: Explain to patient these changes may occur and give strategies to decrease anxiety, fear. Assess baseline mental status, and monitor during therapy. Assess patient's comfort and ability to cope with side effects that occur. Assess patient safety and implement measures to ensure this. Teach patient to avoid driving a car and operating machinery until effect of drug is known and safety assured. Develop safety plan for home care, and involve family or significant caregiver in plan. Avoid use of drug in the elderly. Teach patient to notify physician or NP immediately if patient experiences changes in mood (depression, anxiety), confusion, difficulty breathing, fainting, irregular heartbeats, tremors, hallucinations, and increased blood pressure, as they may indicate an overdose.

If psychotic episodes occur, manage patient conservatively if possible. If moderate episode or anxiety reaction, provide verbal support and comforting. If severe, discuss need for antipsychotic drugs, although this has not been studied. Monitor patient closely for additive CNS depressant effects if antipsychotic therapy is used. Protect patient's airway, and support ventilation and perfusion. Consider administration of activated charcoal to decrease GI absorption of drug and to hasten drug elimination.

II. ALTERATION IN CARDIAC OUTPUT related to TACHYCARDIA, ORTHOSTATIC HYPOTENSION

Defining Characteristics: Tachycardia, syncope, orthostatic hypotension may rarely occur.

Nursing Implications: Assess baseline VS, and monitor during therapy. Teach patient to change position from lying to sitting gradually and from sitting to standing so that dizziness is minimized. If hypotension occurs, notify physician and anticipate increasing IV fluids to increase BP during chemotherapy administration.

Drug: netupitant/palonosetron (Akynzeo)

Class: Antiemetic. Netupitant is a substance P/NK_1 receptor antagonist, and palonosetron is a serotonin-3 (5-HT_3) receptor antagonist.

Mechanism of Action: Drug is a fixed combination of netupitant, a substance P/neurokinin 1 (NK1) receptor antagonist, and palonosetron, a serotonin-3 (5-HT_3) receptor antagonist. It blocks the mechanism by which chemotherapy causes nausea and vomiting: (1) blocks the release of serotonin from enterochromaffin cells in the small intestines, which is stimulated by chemotherapy, thereby preventing stimulation of serotonin-3 (5-HT_3) receptors on vagal efferents, and preventing stimulation of the VC; (2) prevents delayed antiemesis by blocking substance P activation of tachykinin family NK_1 receptors in the central and peripheral nervous systems.

Metabolism: After oral administration, the peak plasma concentration for each drug is achieved in approximately 5 hours. Netupitant and its metabolites are highly plasma protein bound. Once absorbed, netupitant is extensively metabolized to three active, major metabolites primarily by CYP3A4, and to a lesser degree by CYP2C9 and CYP2D6. Netupitant is eliminated primarily in the feces (70.7%) and urine (3.95%), with an elimination half-life of 80 ± 29 hours. Palonosetron is metabolized by CYP2D6 and others, with 50% metabolized to two primary, nonactive metabolites (< 1%). Palonosetron is eliminated via the urine (85–93%), with an elimination half-life of 48 ± 19 hours.

Indication: Indicated for the prevention of acute and delayed nausea and vomiting in adults associated with (1) CAPSULES: initial and repeat courses of cancer chemotherapy, including, but not limited to, highly emetogenic chemotherapy, in combination with dexamethasone; (2) INJECTION: initial and repeat courses of highly emetogenic cancer chemotherapy in adults, in combination with dexamethasone.

Limitations of use: has not been studied for the prevention of nausea and vomiting associated with anthracycline plus cyclophosphamide chemotherapy.

[Oral palonosetron prevents nausea and vomiting during the acute phase, and netupitant prevents nausea and vomiting during both the acute and delayed phases.]

Contraindication: None. Avoid use in patients with severe hepatic impairment, and avoid use in patients with severe renal impairment or ESRD.

Dosage/Range:
- **Oral: 300 mg netupitant/0.5 mg palonosetron** (1 capsule) PO 1 hour prior to the start of chemotherapy.
    - **Highly emetogenic chemotherapy**, including cisplatin-based chemotherapy: One capsule administered 1 hour prior to the start of chemotherapy, with dexamethasone 12 mg administered PO 30 minutes prior to chemotherapy on day 1, and 8 mg PO administered on days 2–4.
    - **Anthracycline- and cyclophosphamide-based chemotherapy and chemotherapy not considered highly emetogenic:** One capsule administered 1 hour prior to the start of chemotherapy, with dexamethasone 12 mg PO administered 30 minutes prior to chemotherapy on day 1 only. Dexamethasone on days 2–4 is not necessary.
- The drug can be taken with or without food.
- **IV: Fosnetupitant 235 mg/palonosetron 0.25 mg,** as a lyophilized powder in a single-dose vial for reconstitution.
- **Highly emetogenic chemotherapy**, including cisplatin-based chemotherapy: Fosnetupitant 235 mg/palonosetron 0.25 mg (1 vial) infused over 30 min starting 30 min before chemotherapy, with dexamethasone 12 mg IV/PO 30 min before chemotherapy day 1, then dexamethasone 8 mg PO/IV once daily days 2–4.
- The drug should *not* be used in patients with severe hepatic or renal impairment.

Drug Preparation:
- Oral capsule: 300 mg netupitant/0.5 mg palonosetron.

- IV: Fosnetupitant 235 mg/palonosetron 25 mg, as a lyophilized powder in a single-dose vial for reconstitution.
  - Aseptically inject 20 mL 5% Dextrose Injection USP or 0.9% Sodium Chloride Injection USP into the vial. Ensure the solvent is added to the vial along the vial wall and not jetted in order to prevent foaming. Swirl the vial gently.
  - Aseptically prepare an infusion vial or bag filled with 30 mL 5% Dextrose Injection USP or 0.9% Sodium Chloride Injection USP.
  - Aseptically withdraw the entire volume of reconstituted solution from the vial and transfer it into the infusion vial or bag containing 30 mL of 5% Dextrose Injection USP or 0.9% Sodium Chloride Injection USP to yield a total volume of 50 mL.
  - Gently invert the vial or bag until completely dissolved.
  - Before administration, inspect final diluted solution for any particulate matter and discoloration; do not use if found, and discard. Total time from reconstitution to start of the infusion should not exceed 3 hours. Store the reconstituted solution and final diluted solution/bag at room temperature.
  - Drug for injection is incompatible with any solution containing divalent cations (e.g., calcium or magnesium), such as Lactated Ringers solution.

Drug Administration:
- Capsule: Teach the patient to take the capsule 1 hour before the start of chemotherapy, and to take it either with or without food. Teach patient about dexamethasone, and self-administration with food.
- IV: If IV line used for multiple administrations, flush the line with IV solution used in drug preparation **prior** to administration; **administer** over 30 minutes as an IV infusion. **At end of infusion, flush line** with same IV solution used in preparation to ensure complete drug is administered. Infusion should start within 3 hours of drug reconstitution.
- Review the patient's medication profile for potential serotonergic drugs (e.g., selective serotonin reuptake inhibitors [SSRIs] and serotonin and noradrenaline reuptake inhibitors [SNRIs], dextromethorphan, fentanyl, linezolid, tramadol); discuss changing serotonergic drugs to alternative agents, to prevent possible serotonin syndrome. Teach the patient to *not* take any cold medication (over the counter) that contains dextromethorphan.
- Teach the patient that two rare, potentially life-threatening reactions may occur, and the patient should get emergency help **right away if either occurs**:
  - An allergic, or hypersensitivity reaction, including anaphylaxis: If hives, swollen face, trouble breathing, or chest pain occurs.
  - Serotonin syndrome: Happens when drugs that block serotonin are given with drugs that increase serotonin levels, such as certain antidepressants and cough medicine ingredients. Signs and symptoms include the following:
    - Altered mental status (e.g., agitation, hallucinations, delirium, coma)
    - Autonomic instability (e.g., tachycardia, labile BP, dizziness, diaphoresis, flushing, hyperthermia)
    - Neuromuscular symptoms (e.g., tremor, rigidity, myoclonus, hyperreflexia, incoordination)
    - Seizures, with or without GI symptoms (e.g., nausea, vomiting, diarrhea)

MANAGEMENT

- Serotonin syndrome has been described in patients taking a 5-HT$_3$ receptor antagonist and a serotonergic drug (e.g., SSRIs and SNRIs).
  - If either hypersensitivity or serotonin syndrome occurs, discontinue netupitant/ palonosetron and provide immediate supportive/emergency care.
- Teach the patient not to start any new medication, such as SSRIs or SNRIs, if prescribed by another physician, until after discussing it with the provider.
- Assess geriatric patients closely, as they may have more hepatic or renal impairment, cardiac issues, concomitant disease, or other drug therapy.
- Pregnancy Category C: Drug may be fetotoxic. Teach women of reproductive potential to use effective contraception during treatment.
- It is unknown if the drug is excreted in human milk; a decision should be made whether to discontinue nursing or to discontinue the drug, taking into account the importance to the mother.

Drug Interactions:
Netupitant is a moderate inhibitor of CYP3A4.

- **CYP3A4 substrates** (e.g., dexamethasone; midazolam; chemotherapy agents— docetaxel, paclitaxel, etoposide, irinotecan, cyclophosphamide, ifosfamide, imatinib, vinorelbine, vinblastine, vincristine): Inhibition of CYP3A4 by netupitant can result in increased plasma concentrations of the concomitant drug lasting at least 4 days; use with caution and monitor patient closely postchemotherapy.
- Effects of other drugs on netupitant/palonosetron.
- **CYP3A4 inducers** (e.g., rifampin): Decreased plasma concentrations of netupitant; avoid concomitant use.
- **CYP3A4 inhibitors** (e.g., ketoconazole): Can result in significantly increased plasma concentrations of netupitant; no dosage adjustment necessary for a single dose.

Serotonergic drugs (e.g., SSRIs, SNRIs, dextromethorphan, fentanyl, linezolid, tramadol): Serotonin syndrome may occur; do not use together concomitantly. Serotonin syndrome may occur in patients who take 5-HT$_3$ receptor antagonists and serotonergic drugs. Review the patient's medication profile for concomitant administration of an SSRI or SNRI, and discuss changing the antidepressant.

IV preparation incompatible with solutions containing divalent cations (e.g., calcium, magnesium as in Lactated Ringer's Solution).

Lab Effects/Interference: Increased transaminases (ALT, AST), total bilirubin.

Special Considerations:
- Most common adverse reactions (incidence $\geq$ 3% and greater than that with palonosetron alone): headache, asthenia, dyspepsia, fatigue, constipation, erythema.
- Avoid use of the drug in patients with severe hepatic or renal impairment including ESRD.
- Warnings and Precautions:
  - *Hypersensitivity reactions*, including anaphylaxis, have been reported in patients taking palonosetron. Monitor the patient closely. See Drug Administration.
  - *Serotonin syndrome* may occur in patients who take 5-HT$_3$ receptor antagonists and serotonergic drugs. See Drug Administration. If patient also taking SSRI, SNRI, or MAO inhibitor, monitor closely for signs/symptoms of serotonin syndrome.

Potential Toxicities/Side Effects and the Nursing Process

I. ALTERATION IN COMFORT related to HEADACHE, ASTHENIA, FATIGUE, OR DYSPEPSIA

Defining Characteristics: Headache occurs in 9% of patients. Dyspepsia occurs in 4%, fatigue in 4–7%, and asthenia in 8%.

Nursing Implications: Teach the patient that these symptoms may occur, offer self-care strategies to use, and tell them to report symptoms that do not resolve.

II. ALTERATION IN BOWEL ELIMINATION related to CONSTIPATION

Defining Characteristics: Constipation occurs in approximately 3% of patients.

Nursing Implications: Assess baseline bowel elimination status. Teach patients that constipation may occur, and suggest the use usual strategies to prevent constipation. If constipation occurs, teach the patient to use bowel softeners and laxatives, and to report if these measures are ineffective.

MANAGEMENT

Drug: ondansetron hydrochloride (zofran)

Class: Serotonin-receptor antagonist.

Mechanism of Action: Selective 5-HT$_3$ (serotonin) receptor antagonist and may block 5-HT$_3$ receptors found peripherally on the vagus nerve terminals and centrally in the CTZ, thus preventing chemotherapy-induced vomiting.

Metabolism: Extensively metabolized, with only 5% of parent compound found in urine. Metabolized by hepatic cytochrome P-450 enzymes CYP3A4, CYP2D6, and CYP1A2.

Indication: *IV:* (1) Prevention of nausea and vomiting associated with initial and repeat courses of emetogenic cancer chemotherapy, including high-dose cisplatin; and (2) prevention of postoperative nausea and/or vomiting. *Oral:* (1, 2) Prevention of nausea and vomiting associated with highly and moderately emetogenic cancer chemotherapy; (3) prevention of nausea and vomiting associated with radiotherapy in patients receiving either TBI, single high-dose fraction to the abdomen, or daily fractions to the abdomen; (4) prevention of PONV.

Contraindications: (1) Concomitant use of apomorphine (causes profound hypotension and loss of consciousness), and (2) in patients with a known hypersensitivity to ondansetron.

Dosage/Range:

CINV: *Adult and pediatric patients (6 months to 18 years):*

- *IV:* 0.15 mg/kg (max 16 mg/dose) in 50 mL 5% dextrose or 0.9% sodium chloride injection USP given over 15 min q 4 h × 3 doses, beginning 30 minutes prior to chemotherapy.

- *Oral:*
  - Adult, highly emetogenic chemo: 24 mg PO 30 minutes before chemotherapy. This dose has not been studied in children.
  - Adult, children age 12 and older: Moderately emetogenic chemotherapy: 8 mg PO twice daily, starting 30 minutes before chemotherapy, the second dose given 8 hours later; one 8-mg tablet PO bid (every 12 hours) for 1–2 days after chemotherapy.
  - Children age 4–11 years: Moderately emetogenic chemotherapy: 4-mg tablet PO 3 times a day, the first 30 minutes before chemotherapy, then doses at 4 and 8 hours after the first dose. One 4-mg tablet PO every 8 hours for 1–2 days after chemotherapy.
- *Radiation therapy (RT):* Ondansetron 8 mg PO tid.
  - TBI: Give 8-mg tablet 1–2 hours prior to each fraction of radiation each day.
  - Single high-dose fraction: 8 mg 1–2 hours prior to RT, then every 8 hours after the first dose for 1–2 days after completion of RT.
  - Daily fractionated RT to abdomen: 8 mg PO 1–2 hours prior to RT, with subsequent doses every 8 hours after first dose for each day RT is given.

PONV: *Adult and pediatric patients (age 1 month and older for IV):*

- *IV Adults:* 4 mg IVP (undiluted) over > 30 seconds before induction of anesthesia, or postoperatively if patient did not receive prophylactic antiemetics and experiences nausea and/or vomiting occurring within 2 hours of surgery; may also be given IM.
- *IV Pediatric* (age 1 month–12 years): weight < 40 kg is 0.1-mg/kg single dose or if > 40 kg, a single 4-mg IV dose, IV over 2–5 minutes (at least 30 seconds) immediately prior to or following anesthesia induction, or postoperatively if no previous prophylactic antiemetics and patient experiences nausea.
- *Oral Adults:* 16 mg (two 8-mg tablets or ODT) 1 hour before induction of anesthesia.

Patients with severe hepatic dysfunction (Child-Pugh score $\geq$ 10): maximum total daily dose of 8 mg.

Drug Preparation:

- The 4- and 8-mg doses of Zofran oral solution or Zofran oral disintegrating tablet (ODT) are bioequivalent to corresponding doses of Zofran tablets and may be used interchangeably. One Zofran 24-mg tablet is bioequivalent to and interchangeable with three 8-mg Zofran tablets.
- IV available as 2 mg/mL as single- or multi-dose vial; mix prescribed dose in 50 mL 5% dextrose or 0.9% sodium chloride and infuse over 15 minutes.
- Tablets available as either regular tablet or ODT (oral disintegrating tablet), which is freeze-dried and dissolves instantly on the tongue, available in 4- and 8-mg strengths.
- Zofran ODT available as 4- and 8-mg disintegrating tablets in unit packs of 30 tabs.
- Zofran oral solution available as 5 mg of ondansetron HCL dihydrate, equivalent to 4 mg of ondansetron/5 mL, in glass bottles of 50 mL with child-resistant closures. Protect from light and store bottles upright.

Drug Administration:

- *IV*: Infuse over 15–30 minutes as above, or IVP in prevention of postoperative nausea/ vomiting.
- *PO*: Administer per dosing above.
- Orally disintegrating tablet (Zofran ODT): with dry hands, peel back the foil backing of 1 blister and gently remove the tablet; immediately place the tablet on top of the tongue where it will dissolve in seconds; then swallow with saliva. Administer per dosing above.
- Oral solution: Available as an oral solution, 4 mg/5 mL; 10 mL (2 tsp) is equivalent to one 8-mg Zofran tablet. Administer per dosing section above.
- Rarely, hypersensitivity reactions, including anaphylaxis and bronchospasm, have been reported in patients taking serotonin-receptor antagonists. Teach patient to stop taking drug and notify healthcare provider right away, or seek immediate medical help if reaction serious.

Drug Interactions:

- Apomorphine: concurrent use may result in profound hypotension and loss of consciousness; DO NOT give concurrently (contraindicated).
- Potent inducers of CYP3A4 (e.g., phenytoin, carbamazepine, rifampin): decrease serum levels of ondansetron but no dosage changes recommended for ondansetron.
- Tramadol: potential decreased analgesic effect when drugs are coadministered.
- Alkaline IV solutions: precipitate may form.

Lab Effects/Interference:

- Rarely, increased LFTs.

Special Considerations:

- Warnings and Precautions:
  - Hypersensitivity reported in patients hypersensitive to other 5-HT$_3$ receptor antagonists.
  - ECG changes including prolonged QTc interval as well as torsades de pointes have occurred in patients taking ondansetron. Avoid ondansetron in patients with congenital long QTc syndrome. Monitor and correct electrolyte abnormalities (e.g., hypokalemia, hypomagnesemia) and monitor ECGs in patients at risk for QTc interval prolongation: patients with electrolyte abnormalities, CHF, bradyarrhythmias, or taking other medicines that prolong the QTc interval.
  - Serotonin syndrome: Most reports have been in patients also taking serotonergic drugs (e.g., SSRIs, SNRIs, monoamine oxidase inhibitors, mirtazapine, lithium, tramadol, and IV methylene blue). Assess for signs/symptoms of tremor, rigidity, monoclonus, hyperreflexia, hyperthermia, with or without GI symptoms of nausea, vomiting, diarrhea. Promptly discontinue drug if this occurs, and implement medical orders to manage patient.
  - Ondansetron does not increase gastric or intestinal peristalsis, so the drug should not be used in place of NG-suction.

MANAGEMENT

Maximum IV dose is 16 mg. No larger dose should be given, as there is a dose-related increased risk of prolongation of QTc with potential for torsades de pointes.

- Avoid drug in patients with congenital long QT syndrome. Use ECG to monitor patients with electrolyte abnormalities (e.g., hypomagnesemia, hypokalemia), CHF, bradyarrhythmias, or patients taking other medication that prolongs the QT interval.
- Does not affect the dopamine system, so does not cause EPS.
- Drug is excreted in breastmilk; use caution if administering to a woman who is nursing. Drug should be used during pregnancy only if clearly needed.
- Drug can mask a progressive ileus and gastric distention; drug does not stimulate gastric or intestinal peristalsis.

Potential Toxicities/Side Effects and the Nursing Process

I.   ALTERATION IN ELIMINATION related to DIARRHEA OR CONSTIPATION

Defining Characteristics: Patients may experience diarrhea (22%) or constipation (11%).

Nursing Implications: Assess baseline elimination status. Teach patient to report alterations, and treat symptomatically.

II.   ALTERATION IN COMFORT related to HEADACHE

Defining Characteristics: Headache may occur (16%).

Nursing Implications: Assess comfort level. Teach patient to report headache. Administer acetaminophen as ordered.

III.   ALTERATION IN NUTRITION, LESS THAN BODY REQUIREMENTS, related to LFTs

Defining Characteristics: Transient increases in LFTs may occur (5%).

Nursing Implications: Assess LFTs baseline, and monitor during therapy.

Drug: ondansetron oral soluble film (Zuplenz)

Class: Serotonin-receptor antagonist.

Mechanism of Action: Selective $5\text{-}HT_3$ (serotonin) receptor antagonist and may block $5\text{-}HT_3$ receptors found peripherally on the vagus nerve terminals and centrally in the CTZ, thus preventing chemotherapy-induced vomiting. Novel formulation.

Metabolism: Extensively metabolized, with only 5% of parent compound found in urine.

Indication: FDA-indicated for (1) prevention of nausea and vomiting associated with highly emetogenic cancer chemotherapy; (2) prevention of nausea and vomiting associated with initial and repeat courses of moderately emetogenic cancer chemotherapy; (3) prevention of nausea and vomiting associated with radiotherapy in patients receiving TBI, single high-dose fraction to abdomen, or daily fractions to the abdomen; (4) prevention of postoperative nausea and/or vomiting.

Contraindications: Patients hypersensitive to ondansetron, or concomitant use of apomorphine.

Dosage/Range:

Adult:
- *Prevention of nausea and vomiting associated with **highly emetogenic** cancer chemotherapy (adults):* 24 mg given as successive 8-mg films, administered 30 minutes before the start of single-day highly emetogenic chemotherapy. Allow each oral soluble film to dissolve completely before administering the next film.
- *Prevention of nausea and vomiting associated with **moderately emetogenic** cancer chemotherapy:*
  - Adults and pediatric patients 12 years of age and older: One 8-mg film administered 30 minutes before start of emetogenic chemotherapy, with a subsequent dose 8 hours after the first dose. One 8-mg oral soluble film should be administered twice daily (every 12 hours) for 1–2 days after completion of chemotherapy.
  - Pediatric patients aged 4–11 years: One 4-mg film administered three times a day, with the first dose 30 minutes before start of emetogenic chemotherapy, and subsequent doses 4 and 8 hours after the first dose. Administer one 4-mg film 3 times a day (every 8 hours) for 1–2 days after completion of chemotherapy.
- *Prevention of nausea and vomiting associated with radiotherapy:* One 8-mg film given 3 times a day.
- *Prevention of postoperative nausea and/or vomiting:* 16 mg given successively as two 8-mg films 1 hour before induction of anesthesia. Allow the first oral soluble film to dissolve completely before administering the second film.
- *Dosage adjustment for patients with impaired hepatic function (Child-Pugh score > 10):* Do not exceed a total daily dose of 8 mg.

Drug Preparation:
- Available in 4- and 8-mg oral soluble films, labeled with the dose, in a pouch package.

Drug Administration:
- With dry hands, fold the pouch along the dotted line to expose the tear notch. While still folded, tear the pouch carefully along the edge and remove the oral soluble film for the pouch. Immediately place the film on the top of the tongue, where it will dissolve in 4–20 seconds. Once dissolved, have the patient swallow with or without liquid. Wash hands after administering or taking the oral soluble film.
- Teach patient self-administration: see package insert and patient teaching tool.
- Rarely, hypersensitivity reactions, including anaphylaxis and bronchospasm, have been reported in patients taking serotonin-receptor antagonists. Teach patient to stop taking drug, and notify healthcare provider right away or seek immediate medical help if serious reaction occurs.

MANAGEMENT

Drug Interactions:
- Apomorphine: profound hypotension and loss of consciousness.
- Phenytoin, carbamazepine, rifampicin: these are potent inducers of CYP3A4, and ondansetron clearance is significantly increased, with lower ondansetron serum levels. However, there are no data to show the soluble film dose should be increased.
- Tramadol: concomitant use may reduce analgesic activity of tramadol.

Lab Effects/Interference:
- Rarely, increased LFTs.

Special Considerations:
- Does not affect the dopamine system, so does not cause EPS.
- Warnings and Precautions:
  - Hypersensitivity reactions, including anaphylaxis and bronchospasm, have been reported in patients with hypersensitivity to other selective 5-HT$_3$ receptor antagonists.
  - Transient ECG changes, including QT interval prolongation, have been reported rarely, predominantly with IV ondansetron.
  - The use of ondansetron in patients following abdominal surgery or in patients with CINV may mask a progressive ileus and/or gastric distention.
  - Serotonin syndrome: Serotonin syndrome: most reports have been in patients also taking serotonergic drugs (e.g., SSRIs, SNRIs, monoamine oxidase inhibitors, mirtazapine, lithium, tramadol, fentanyl, and IV methylene blue). However, overdosage of ondansetron or other 5-HT$_3$ receptor antagonists have also resulted in the syndrome. Assess for signs/symptoms of agitation, hallucinations, delirium, tremor, rigidity, monoclonus, hyperreflexia, hyperthermia, with or without GI symptoms of nausea, vomiting, diarrhea. Promptly discontinue drug if this occurs, and implement medical orders to manage patient.
  - Ondansetron does not increase gastric or intestinal peristalsis, so the drug should not be used in place of NG-suction.
- The most common adverse drug reactions (> 5%) in chemotherapy- or radiotherapy-induced nausea and vomiting in trials were headache, mailaise/fatigue, constipation, and diarrhea.
- The most common adverse drug reaction (> 5%) in PONV trials was headache.

Potential Toxicities/Side Effects and the Nursing Process

I. ALTERATION IN ELIMINATION related to DIARRHEA OR CONSTIPATION

Defining Characteristics: Patients may experience diarrhea (3–6%) or constipation (6–9%).

Nursing Implications: Assess baseline elimination status. Teach patient to report alterations, and treat symptomatically.

II.   ALTERATION IN COMFORT related to HEADACHE

Defining Characteristics: Headache may occur (11–27%).

Nursing Implications: Assess comfort level. Teach patient to report headache, and administer acetaminophen as ordered.

III.   ALTERATION IN NUTRITION, LESS THAN BODY REQUIREMENTS, related to LFTs

Defining Characteristics: Rare, transient increases in LFTs may occur, especially in patients receiving cyclophosphamide-based chemotherapy (1–2%).

Nursing Implications: Assess LFTs baseline, and monitor during therapy.

Drug: palonosetron (Aloxi)

Class: Serotonin subtype 3 (5-HT$_3$) receptor antagonist antiemetic.

Mechanism of Action: Selective serotonin antagonist with strong binding affinity to receptor.

Metabolism: Drug is excreted via renal and metabolic pathways.

Indication: *Adults:* for (1) moderately emetogenic cancer chemotherapy-prevention of acute and delayed nausea and vomiting associated with initial and repeat courses; (2) highly emetogenic cancer chemotherapy-prevention of acute and delayed nausea and vomiting associated with initial and repeat courses; (3) prevention of PONV for up to 24 hours after surgery. Efficacy beyond 24 hours has not been demonstrated. *Pediatrics:* (1) Patients aged 1 month to < 17 years: prevention of acute nausea and vomiting associated with initial and repeat courses of emetogenic cancer chemotherapy, including highly emetogenic chemotherapy.

Contraindication: Patients known to have hypersensitivity to drug or any of its components.

Dosage/Range:
- *CINV:*
    - *Adults*: single 0.25-mg IV over 30 **seconds**, given 30 minutes before the start of chemotherapy. Give once every 7 days.
    - *Pediatrics (1 month to < 17 years old):* 20 micrograms/kg (max 1.5 mg) $\times$ 1; infuse over 15 **minutes** beginning approximately 30 minutes before the start of chemotherapy.
- *Postoperative nausea and vomiting, Adult (PONV, Adult):*
    - A single 0.075-mg dose given IV over 10 **seconds** immediately before the induction of anesthesia.

MANAGEMENT

Drug Preparation:
- Available at a concentration of 0.05 mg/mL (50 mcg/mL) and supplied as a single-use sterile glass vial that provides 0.25 mg/5mL (free base) and 0.075 mg/1.5 mL (free base).
- Draw up in a syringe to administer IVP, or draw up prescribed dose and place in appropriate pediatric pump for slow infusion over 15 minutes.

Drug Administration:
- Inspect drug for particulate matter and discoloration, and do not use if found. Drug should be colorless without particulate matter.
- *Adult:* IV over 30 seconds (CINV) or 10 seconds (PONV) as above dosage section; flush line with normal saline prior to and after drug administration.
- *Pediatric:* IV infuse over 15 minutes as above dosage section; flush line with normal saline prior to and after drug administration.
- Assess for hypersensitivity reaction, including anaphylaxis, which has been reported in patients with or without known hypersensitivity to other selective 5-HT$_3$ receptor antagonists.

Drug Interactions:
- None known.

Lab Effects/Interference:
- Rare prolongation of QTc interval on ECG (> 500 msec, changes > 60 msec from baseline).

Special Considerations:
- Warnings and Precautions:
  - *Hypersensitivity reactions*, including anaphylaxis. Rarely, patients hypersensitive to other HT$_3$ receptor antagonists may be hypersensitive to palonosetron.
  - *Serotonin syndrome* has been reported with 5-HT$_3$ receptor antagonists alone, but especially when coadministered with concomitant use of serotonergic drugs (e.g., SSRI, SNRI, MAO inhibitor).
- Palonosetron has greater potency, higher binding affinity to the 5-HT$_3$ receptor, and has a longer half-life (40 hours) than any of the first-generation serotonin-receptor antagonists.
- Most common side effects are:
  - CINV (occurring in > 5%): headache, constipation.
  - PONV (occurring in > 2%): QT prolongation, bradycardia, headache, constipation.

Potential Toxicities/Side Effects and the Nursing Process

I.   ALTERATION IN COMFORT related to HEADACHE

Defining Characteristics: Headache occurs in 3.7% (capsule) 0–9% (IV) of patients.

Nursing Implications: Teach patients that this may occur, and to take acetaminophen to relieve headache if it occurs.

II.   ALTERATION IN BOWEL ELIMINATION related to CONSTIPATION

Defining Characteristics: Constipation occurs in about 0.6% (capsule) to 5% (injection) of patients.

Nursing Implications: Assess baseline bowel elimination status. Teach patients that constipation may occur, and to use usual strategies to prevent constipation. If constipation occurs, teach patient to use bowel softeners, laxatives as needed, and to increase oral fluids, fiber, and exercise to promote peristalsis.

III.   ALTERATION IN OXYGENATION related to RARE CARDIAC EVENTS

Defining Characteristics: Cardiovascular events are rare and occur in 1% of patients. These include nonsustained tachycardia, bradycardia, hypotension or hypertension, sinus arrhythmia, supraventricular extrasystoles, sinus tachycardia, and QT prolongation. The relationship to palonosetron was not clear in all instances. In nonclinical studies, palonosetron has the ability to block ion channels involved in ventricular depolarization and repolarization and to prolong action potential duration.

Nursing Implications: Assess baseline cardiac status, and monitor closely during therapy. Teach patient to notify the provider if any abnormalities occur, such as rapid or slow heartbeat.

MANAGEMENT

Drug: prochlorperazine (Compazine)

Class: Phenothiazine.

Mechanism of Action: Blocks dopamine receptors in CTZ; also decreases vagal stimulation of VC by peripheral afferents.

Metabolism: Metabolized by liver, excreted in kidney, crosses placenta, excreted in breastmilk. Onset of action for oral is 30–40 minutes, duration 3–4 hours; extended release 30–40 minutes with duration 10–13 hours; PR onset 60 minutes, duration 3–4 hours; and IM onset 10–20 minutes, duration 12 hours.

Indication: (1) For the control of severe nausea and vomiting; and (2) treatment of schizophrenia.

Contraindication: Do not use (1) in patients with known hypersensitivity to phenothiazines; (2) in patients with comatose states or in the presence of large amounts of CNS depressants (e.g., alcohol, barbiturates, opioids); (3) in pediatric surgery; (4) in pediatric patients < 2 years of age or weighing < 20 lbs, or in children with conditions for which dosage has not been established. Drug is NOT indicated for the treatment of elderly patients with dementia-related psychosis treated with antipsychotic drugs, as there is an increased mortality in these patients.

Dosage/Range:

Adult:

- *Oral:* 5–25 mg q 4–6 h; slow-release: 10–75 mg q 12 h.
- *IM/IV:* 5–40 mg q 3–4 h; dilute in 50 mL 5% dextrose or 0.9% sodium chloride and administer IV over 20–30 minutes.
- *PR:* 25 mg q 4–6 h.

Drug Preparation:
- Store in tight, light-resistant containers. Administer IM injection deep into large muscle mass.

Drug Interactions:

- Antacids: decreased prochlorperazine absorption; take 2 hours before or after antacid.
- Antidepressants: increased parkinsonian symptoms; avoid concomitant use or use cautiously.
- Barbiturates: decreased prochlorperazine effect; may need to increase dose of prochlorperazine.

Lab Effects/Interference:
- Rarely, may cause increased LFTs.

Special Considerations:

- Increased risk of dystonic reactions in men under 35 years old. Consider diphenhydramine or lorazepam and decadron q 4 h to minimize risk of dystonia.
- Dose-reduce in the elderly.
- Use cautiously in combination with CNS depressants.

Potential Toxicities/Side Effects and the Nursing Process

I.   ALTERATIONS IN SENSORY PERCEPTUAL PATTERN related to SEDATION, EPS

Defining Characteristics: Sedation, blurred vision, EPS reactions may occur, especially dystonia; also, seizure threshold may be lowered.

Nursing Implications: Assess baseline mental status. Teach patient to report signs/symptoms of EPS and assess for them during treatment (tongue protrusion, trismus, akathisia or restlessness, tremor, insomnia, dizziness). Administer diphenhydramine as ordered to reverse reaction. Diphenhydramine may be ordered prior to drug to prevent EPS.

II.   ALTERATION IN NUTRITION related to CONSTIPATION, APPETITE, CHOLESTATIC JAUNDICE

Defining Characteristics: Dry mouth, constipation, increased appetite and weight gain, cholestatic jaundice may occur.

Nursing Implications: Assess baseline nutritional patterns, moistness of mucous membranes, and elimination pattern. Assess baseline liver function, and monitor during therapy.

III.   ALTERATION IN SKIN INTEGRITY related to RASH

Defining Characteristics: Mild photosensitivity, rash, urticaria, and, rarely, exfoliative dermatitis may occur.

Nursing Implications: Assess baseline skin integrity. Teach patient to report any changes.

IV.   ALTERATION IN CARDIAC OUTPUT related to ORTHOSTATIC HYPOTENSION

Defining Characteristics: Orthostatic hypotension, tachycardia, and EKG changes may occur.

Nursing Implications: Assess baseline VS prior to and during IV infusions, especially with high doses. Discuss with physician and anticipate increasing IV fluid rate if hypotensive.

MANAGEMENT

Drug: Rolapitant (Varubi)

Class: Substance P/NK$_1$ receptor antagonist.

Mechanism of Action: Selective and competitive antagonist of human substance P/NK$_1$ receptors.

Metabolism: Drug crosses BBB and occupies NK$_1$ receptors. Drug is measurable in the plasma between 30 minutes and 4 hours, the time of peak plasma concentrations (C_{max}). Food does not affect absorption or pharmacokinetics. Drug is primarily metabolized by CYP3A4 and forms a major metabolite with a half-life of 158 hours. Drug and metabolite are excreted primarily by biliary/hepatic route. See package insert for discussion of decreased hepatic metabolism in patients with moderate hepatic dysfunction, and impaired renal dysfunction.

Indication: In adults, prevention of delayed nausea and vomiting associated with initial and repeat courses of emetogenic chemotherapy, including highly emetogenic chemotherapy.

Contraindication: (1) hypersensitivity (HSR) to the drug or any drug component, (2) concurrent use with pimozide or thioridazine, a CYP2D6 substrate, as potentially fatal QTc prolongation may occur.

Dosage/Range: 180 mg PO 1–2 hours prior to start of chemotherapy. It is given with dexamethasone and a 5-HT$_3$ receptor antagonist. Dose of dexamethasone does NOT need to be adjusted as with other NK1 inhibitors.

Drug Preparation: Tablets available as 90 mg of rolapitant.

Drug Administration:

- Highly emetogenic chemotherapy: Rolapitant 180 mg PO 1–2 hours before chemotherapy day 1; in combination with dexamethasone 20 mg given 30 minutes prior to chemotherapy on day 1, then 8 mg bid given on days 2, 3, 4.
- Moderately emetogenic chemotherapy (e.g., combination of anthracycline and cyclophosphamide): Rolapitant 180 mg PO 1–2 hours before chemotherapy day 1; in combination with dexamethasone 20 mg given 30 minute prior to chemotherapy on day 1, and a 5-HT$_3$ receptor antagonist (see drug information for specific agent used).
- Teach patient to take 2 tablets 1–2 hours prior to chemotherapy administration, but not to take more that this dose every 14 days.

Drug Interactions:

- Breast cancer resistance protein (BCRP) and P-glycoprotein (P-gp) substrates with a narrow therapeutic window: rolapitant inhibits BCRP and P-gp which can increase the plasma concentration of the concomitant drug and increase risk for toxicity.
- Strong CYP3A4 inducers (rifampin): significantly reduced plasma concentrations with decreased rolapitant efficacy; avoid using rolapitant if the other drug is medically necessary and must be continued.

Lab Effects/Interference: None known.

Special Considerations:

- Most common adverse reactions ($\geq 5\%$):
  - Cisplatin-based highly emetogenic chemotherapy: neutropenia, hiccups.
  - Moderately emetogenic and combinations of anthracycline and cyclophosphamide: decreased appetite, neutropenia, dizziness.
- Warnings and Precautions:
  - *Interaction with CYP2D6 substrates with a narrow therapeutic index* (e.g., pimozide which is contraindicated). The inhibitory effect of a single dose of rolapitant on CYP2D6 lasts at least 7 days, and perhaps longer. Avoid coadministration. Monitor for adverse effects if must be used concomitantly with other CYP2D6 substrates with a narrow therapeutic index.
  - *HSR:* serious HSRs have been reported including anaphylaxis and anaphylactic shock which occurred during the first few minutes, during or soon after the drug was administered. Monitor closely for signs/symptoms of anaphylaxis such as swelling of face or throat, hives, facial flushing, itching, abdominal cramping, abdominal pain, vomiting, back pain or chest pain, hypotension, or shock. If this occurs, stop infusion and implement ordered emergency medical interventions.

Potential Toxicities/Side Effects and the Nursing Process

I. KNOWLEDGE DEFICIT, POTENTIAL, related to SELF-ADMINISTRATION OF ROLAPITANT

Defining Characteristics: Patients may be confused about the dosing.

Nursing Implications: Review patient education, and use package insert education or other tools to reinforce directions are (1) when to take the rolapitant tablets 1–2 hours prior to chemotherapy, and (2) the patient will also receive two other medications prior to chemotherapy (dexamethasone and serotonin-receptor antagonist; (3) to tell the doctor/ nurse/NP/PA/pharmacist all the medications the patient is taking as there may be some interactions.

Drug: scopolamine transdermal patch (Transderm Scop, The Travel Patch)

Class: Anti-muscarinic; used as an antiemetic.

Mechanism of Action: Appears to prevent nausea/vomiting associated with motion sickness by blocking cholinergic impulses, thus preventing stimulation of the VC.

Metabolism: Drug is well-absorbed percutaneously behind the ear, and circulating plasma levels detectable at 4 hours, and peak levels within 24 hours. Drug crosses placenta and blood–brain barrier, and may be reversibly bound to plasma proteins. Drug is extensively metabolized and conjugated, with < 10% of total dose excreted in the urine over 108 hours. Half-life of drug after patch removal is 9.5 hours.

Indication: In adults (1) for the prevention of nausea and vomiting associated with motion sickness; and (2) recovery from anesthesia and surgery. The patch should be applied only to the skin in the postauricular area.

Contraindication: For patients (1) who are hypersensitive to the drug scopolamine, to other belladonna alkaloids, or to other component ingredients in the drug or delivery system; and (2) with angle-closure (narrow-angle) glaucoma.

Dosage/Range:

Adult:
- Patch: transdermal patch 1.5 mg every 72 hours.
- Drug releases 1 mg scopolamine over 3 days.

Drug Preparation:
- Available as a tan-colored circular patch, 2.5 cm^2 on a clear, oversized hexagonal peel strip, which is removed prior to use.
- Each patch contains 1.5 mg scopolamine and is programmed to deliver 1.0 mg scopolamine over 3 days.
- Available in packages of 4 patches, each individually wrapped.

Drug Administration:
- Apply 4 hours prior to time protection is needed.
- To prevent postoperative nausea/vomiting, the patch should be applied the night before scheduled surgery.
- Apply to clean and dry hairless area behind ear; remove clear plastic cover, exposing adhesive layer; apply directly to skin behind ear and press firmly; wash hands.
- If patch falls off, wash area; then reapply new patch in another location behind the ear.
- If therapy is required for > 3 days, the first patch should be removed and a fresh one placed on the hairless area behind the other ear.
- For perioperative use, the patch should be kept in place for 24 hours after surgery, then removed and discarded.
- If patient needs an MRI, patch should be removed to avoid skin burns (patch contains aluminum).

Drug Interactions:
- None significant.

Lab Effects/Interference:
- None known.

Special Considerations:
- Wash hands after handling patch to prevent exposure to scopolamine.
- Use cautiously in:
  - Elderly patients with urinary bladder-neck obstruction.
  - Patients with history of seizures or psychosis, as drug can potentially aggravate both disorders.
  - Patients with impaired liver or renal function; there is increased likelihood of CNS effects.
  - Patients with chronic, open-angle glaucoma; monitor closely, as mydriatic effect of drug may increase intraocular pressure.
- Drug should not be used in children and should be used with caution in the elderly.
- Teach patients that drowsiness, disorientation, and confusion may occur with this drug, and to avoid activities that require mental alertness, such as driving a motor vehicle or operating dangerous machinery.
- Rarely, idiosyncratic reactions have occurred, including acute toxic psychosis, confusion, agitation, rambling speech, hallucinations, paranoid behaviors, and delusions.

Potential Toxicities/Side Effects and the Nursing Process

I.   ALTERATION IN MUCOUS MEMBRANE INTEGRITY related to DRY MOUTH

Defining Characteristics: Dry mouth occurs in 67% of patients.

Nursing Implications: Teach patient this may occur. Suggest patient suck ice chips, sugar-free candy, or practice usual oral hygiene regimen more frequently.

II.   ALTERATIONS IN SENSORY/PERCEPTUAL PATTERNS related to DROWSINESS, BLURRED VISION

Defining Characteristics: Drowsiness, blurred vision, mydriasis may occur; rarely, disorientation, restlessness, confusion may occur.

Nursing Implications: Assess baseline mental status. Instruct patient to report changes in vision or feeling state. Assess patient safety needs, and provide safe environment.

MANAGEMENT

Chapter 8
Anorexia and Cachexia

Anorexia and weight loss may be presenting symptoms of cancer, or symptoms of advanced disease. No other symptoms may cause more powerful distress to a patient than being confronted with weight loss and inability to eat due to anorexia (Jatoi, 2015). Consequences of severe anorexia include nutritional depletion and further weight loss, which result in decreased functional status, diminished treatment responses to chemotherapy, and apparent decreased quality of life. Primary cachexia, or wasting syndrome, occurs in at least two-thirds of patients with advanced cancer or human immunodeficiency virus (HIV) disease. The associated extreme weakness and fatigue lead to incapacity, dependency, social isolation, and again, apparent diminished quality of life.

Anorexia and cachexia can be terrifying and frustrating to family members. The patient's spouse may be used to nurturing the patient and preparing meals, and feel rejected and frightened by a loved one's inability to eat. This may symbolize personal failure on the part of the spouse, as well as failure of current treatment to reverse the disease process and a poor prognosis.

Loprinzi and Jatoi (2019) state that "cancer-related anorexia/cachexia syndrome is characterized by anorexia together with loss of body weight associated with reduced muscle mass and adipose tissue." Contrary to expectation, resting energy can be higher related to muscle protein breakdown and lipolysis (Loprinzi and Jatoi, 2019). Fearon et al. (2011) report on international consensus development of definition and classification: a multifactorial syndrome defined an ongoing loss of skeletal muscle mass (with or without loss of fat mass) that cannot be fully reversed by traditional nutritional support interventions, and it leads to progressive functional impairment. Pathophysiology was attributed to negative protein and energy balance related to abnormal metabolism and decreased food intake. Diagnostic criterion for cachexia was a weight loss > 5% over the preceding 6 months, or weight loss > 2% in patients already depleted (BMI < 20 kg/m^2 or decreased skeletal muscle mass [sarcopenia]). The group also identified that the cachexia syndrome can progress through stages: from precachexia to cachexia to refractory cachexia. Precachexia was defined as weight loss ≤ 5%, with other risk factors such as anorexia or impaired glucose tolerance. Cachexia was defined as a weight loss > 5% or other characteristics of the diagnostic criteria. Refractory cachexia was defined as patients who no longer were responsive to cancer treatment with a low performance status (PS) score and a life expectancy of < 3 months. Historically, the North Central Cancer Treatment Group defined cancer cachexia as a 5-lb weight loss in the preceding 2 months and/or estimated caloric intake of < 20 calories/kg, patient desire to increase appetite and gain weight, physician's opinion that weight gain would be beneficial to the patient (Jatoi, 2015). Today, with the advent of molecular targeted therapy, it is possible that the drug is causing changes in body composition (Jatoi, 2015). For example, Artoun et al. (2010) studied the muscle wasting resulting from sorafenib treatment of patients with advanced renal cell cancer.

The development of anorexia and cachexia is influenced by many factors, most principally the tumor, but also by effects of cancer treatment and less well-defined psychosocial issues. In the literature, metabolically, cachexia appears to result from chronic, systemic inflammation with the release of acute-phase proteins and orchestration by cytokines such as tumor necrosis factor, IL-1 and IL-6 (Laviano et al., 2002). Morley et al. (2006) suggest that other potential mediators of cachexia are testosterone, insulin-like growth factor I deficiency, excess myostatin, and excess glucocorticoids. This leads to the preferential breakdown of skeletal muscle protein and body fat, resulting in the profound wasting syndrome characterized by anorexia, early satiety, weight loss, decreased function, and death. Secondary cachexia is simple starvation from decreased food intake or defective nutrient absorption, and results from situations such as nausea, vomiting, and anorexia due to chemotherapy. As expected, patients responding to chemotherapy will show a weight gain.

Pharmacologic agents used to stimulate appetite are varied in mechanism of action, efficacy, and strength of evidence. Corticosteroids have been tried for many years, with usual effect within 1–3 weeks (Ottery et al., 1998; Loprinzi et al., 1999). However, side effects, such as insomnia, muscle catabolism, and hyperglycemia, have limited their usefulness. When compared with megestrol acetate 800 mg/day, dexamethasone (0.75 mg 4 times daily) patients had similar responses but different toxicities: megestrol acetate caused thromboembolism, whereas dexamethasone caused myopathy, peptic ulcers, and problems related to Cushingoid side effects (Loprinzi et al., 1999). Of the studies of pharmacologic agents in the treatment of anorexia and cachexia in cancer, megestrol acetate has shown statistical improvement in nonfluid weight gain (Ottery, 1998). Mantovani et al. (1998) suggest that megestrol acetate, in fact, downregulates cytokine production, resulting in increased appetite and anabolism. There appears to be a dose-response effect, and Loprinzi et al. (1992) showed optimal weight gain at a dose of 800 mg/day. Patients showed increased appetite, increased food intake, weight gain, and less nausea and vomiting. The incidence of thrombophlebitis was 6%. Loprinzi et al. also demonstrated that the weight gain resulting from megestrol acetate is increased fat and lean body mass, not water gain (i.e., edema, ascites).

Metoclopramide, at low doses for stimulation of GI motility, has been shown to decrease early satiety and postprandial fullness, and may be helpful for some patients (Kris et al., 1985). Cannabinoid derivatives, such as δ-9-tetrahydrocannabinol (THC) and dronabinol, appear to stimulate appetite and possible weight gain in some patients (Beal et al., 1997; Kaplan et al., 1998; Klausner et al., 1996; Jatoi, 2006). Dronabinol and nabilone have each been FDA approved for treatment of HIV-related anorexia associated with weight loss in patients with AIDS. Eicosapentaenoic acid (EPA) (fish oil, thought to stabilize acute phase proteins) in a nutritional supplement was compared with megestrol acetate or a combination of both; megestrol acetate was found more effective in stimulating appetite (Jatoi et al., 2004). Studies continue to explore whether other agents, such as melatonin (regulation of circadian rhythm), can be of benefit (Cunningham, 2003).

The ONS Putting Evidence into Practice (PEP) cards for anorexia recommend for practice, based on strong evidence from rigorously conducted studies, corticosteroids (reserved for those with anorexia with advanced disease or who may have disease regression, where a short-term benefit is needed), and progestins. In addition, they point out that dietary counseling is likely to be effective, as individual dietary counseling has been shown to improve nutritional intake and body weight. They point out that effectiveness is not established for cyproheptadine, EPA, erythropoietin, ghrelin, metoclopramide, oral branched chain amino acids, pentoxifylline, and thalidomide. Effectiveness is unlikely with cannabinoids, hydrazine sulfate, and melatonin (Adams et al., 2008). Studies with ghrelin and mimetics were initially promising, but results were not reproducible (Garcia et al., 2010). A Cochrane systematic review of randomized control trials of ghrelin showed that there was insufficient evidence to demonstrate that ghrelin increased food intake, or alone or in combination, made any difference in body weight (Khatib et al., 2017).

It is exciting to think that perhaps nutritional stimulation might improve the patient's ability to tolerate aggressive therapy or in some way improve efficacy of the treatment; however, a randomized, double-blind, controlled trial compared megestrol acetate or placebo together with chemotherapy and radiation therapy for newly diagnosed patients with extensive small cell lung cancer (SCLC), and there was no difference in patient response (efficacy), quality of life, or overall survival between the two groups (Loprinzi & Jatoi, 2007). In an earlier study (1999) with chemotherapy only, patients receiving megestrol acetate had more thromboembolic events and edema, and inferior response to chemotherapy and survival (Rowland et al., 1996).

Psychologically, patients with anorexia and cachexia may also be depressed, as this syndrome is characteristic of a number of advanced solid tumors. In addition to assessment of physical factors, assessment of psychosocial issues is very important as well in developing a plan of care for the patient experiencing cancer anorexia and cachexia.

This complex metabolic problem continues to challenge clinicians; however, continued success in cancer therapy and ensuring access to all patients, will help to reduce the incidence of the problem.

References

AbbieVie Inc. Marinol (dronabinol) [package insert]. North Chicago, IL. August 2017.

Adams L, Cunningham R, Caruso RA, Norling M, Shepard N. *Anorexia: What Interventions Are Effective in Managing Anorexia in People with Cancer.* Pittsburgh, PA: Oncology Nursing Society; 2008.

Artoun S, Birdsell L, Sawyer MB, et al. Association of Skeletal Muscle Wasting with Treatment with Sorafenib in Patients with advanced Renal Cell Carcinoma: Results from a Placebo-controlled Study. *J Clin Oncol* 2010; 28:1054–1060.

Beal JE. Long-term Efficacy and Safety of Dronabinol for Acquired Immunodeficiency Syndrome-associated Anorexia. *J Pain Symptom Manage* 1997; 14(1):7–14.

Cunningham RS. (2014). The Cancer Cachexia Syndrome, Chapter 17. In Yarbro CH, Wujuk D, Gobel BH (eds), *Cancer Symptom Management*, 4th ed. Burlington, MA: Jones & Bartlett Learning; 351–384.

Fearon K, Strasser F, Anker SD, et al. Definition and classification of cancer cachexia: An international consensus. *Lancet Oncol* 2011; 12(5):489–495.

Garcia JM, Friend J, Allen S. Therapeutic Potential of anamorelin, a Novel, Oral Ghrelin Mimetic, in Patients with Cancer-related Cachexia: A Multicenter, Randomized, Double-blind, Crossover, Pilot Study. *Support Care Cancer* 2013; 21:129–137.

MANAGEMENT

Insys Therapeutics. Syndros (dronabinol) oral solution [package insert]. Chandler, AZ. September 2018.

Jatoi A, Rowland K, Loprinzi CL, et al. An Eicosapentaenoic Acid Supplement Versus Megestrol Acetate Versus Both for Patients with Cancer-Associated Wasting: A North Central Cancer Treatment Group and National Cancer Institute of Canada Collaborative Effort. *J Clin Oncol* 2004; 22:2469–2476.

Jatoi A. Anorexia and Cachexia. *Cancer Network* June 1, 2015. Available at http://www.cancernetwork .com/cancer-management/anorexia-and-cachexia. Accessed May 31, 2016.

Jatoi A. Pharmacologic Therapy for the Cancer Anorexia/Weight Loss Syndrome: A Data Driven, Practical Approach. *J Support Oncol* 2006; 4(10):499–502.

Khatib M, Shankar AH, Kirubakaran R et al. Gherlin for the management of cachexia associated with cancer. *Cochrane Database of Systemic Reviews* 2018; 2(CD012229). DOI: 10.1002/144651858. CD912228.pub2.

Klausner JD, Makonkawkeyoon S, Akarasewi P, et al. The Effect of Thalidomide on the Pathogenesis of Human Immunodeficiency Virus Type 1 and *M. tuberculosis* Infection. *J Acquir Immune Defic Syndr Hum Retrovirology* 1996; 11:247–257.

Laviano A, Russo M, Freda F, et al. Neurochemical Mechanisms for Cancer Cachexia. *Nutrition* 2002; 18:100–105.

Loprinzi C, Jatoi A. Anorexia and Cachexia. In Pazdur R, Coia LR, Hoskins WJ, Wagman LD (eds), *Cancer Management: A Multidisciplinary Approach*, 12th ed. Lawrence, KS: CMP Healthcare Media LLC; 2009.

Loprinzi CL and Jatoi A. Pharmacologic management of cancer anorexia/cachexia. *Up-to-Date, 2019.* Available at https://www.uptodate.com/contents/pharmacologic-management-of-cancer-anorexia-cachexia. Accessed May 31, 2019.

Loprinzi CL, Ellison NM, Schard OJ, et al. Controlled Trial of Megestrol Acetate for the Treatment of Cancer Anorexia and Cachexia. *J Natl Cancer Inst* 1990; 82:1127–1132.

Loprinzi CL, Jensen M, Burnham N, et al. Body Composition Changes in Cancer Patients Who Gain Weight from Megestrol Acetate. *Proc Am Soc Clin Oncol* 1992; 11:378.

Loprinzi CL, Kugler JW, Sloan JA, et al. Randomized Comparison of Megestrol Acetate Versus Dexamethasone Versus Fluoxymesterone for the Treatment of Cancer Anorexia/Cachexia. *J Clin Oncol* 1999; 17:3299–3306.

Loprinzi CL, Mailliard J, Schaid D, et al. Dose/Response Evaluation of Megestrol Acetate for the Treatment of Cancer Anorexia/Cachexia: A Mayo Clinic and North Central Cancer Treatment Group Trial. *Proc Am Soc Clin Oncol* 1992; 11:378.

Mantovani G, Maccio A, Paola L, et al. Cytokine Activity in Cancer-related Anorexia/Cachexia: Role of Megestrol Acetate and Medroxyprogesterone Acetate. *Semin Oncol* 1998; 25 (suppl): 45–52.

Morley JE, Thomas DR, Wilson MMG. Cachexia: Pathophysiology and Relevance. *Am J Clin Nutr* 2006; 83:735–743.

Ottery FD, Walsh D, Strawford A. Pharmacologic Management of Anorexia/Cachexia. *Semin Oncol* 1998; 25 (suppl):35–44.

Rowland KM, Loprinzi CL, Shaw EG, et al. Randomized Double Blind Placebo Controlled Trial of Cisplatin and Etoposide Plus Megestrol Acetate/Placebo in Extensive-Stage Small Cell Lung Cancer: A North Central Cancer Treatment Group Study. *J Clin Oncol* 1996; 14:135–141.

Turcott JG, Del Rocio Guillen Nunez M, Flores-Estrada D et al. The effect of nabilone on appetite, nutritional status, and quality of life in lung cancer patients: a randomized double-blind clinical trial. *Support Care Cancer* 2018; 26(9):3029–3038.

Drug: dronabinol (Marinol, Syndros)

Class: Cannabinoid.

Mechanism of Action: Stimulates appetite in acquired immunodeficiency syndrome (AIDS) patients, leading to trends toward improved body weight and mood.

Metabolism: 90–95% absorption after oral dose, but because of first-pass effect of the liver and high lipid solubility, only about 20% of the dose reaches the systemic circulation. Large area of distribution so that drug continues to be excreted for a long period of time. The appetite stimulation effect may persist for 24 hours from a single dose.

Indication: For the treatment of (1) anorexia associated with weight loss in patients with AIDS; and (2) nausea and vomiting associated with cancer chemotherapy in patients who have failed to respond adequately to conventional antiemetic treatments.

Contraindications: Marinol: Hypersensitivity to the drug or any of its ingredients.

Syndros: Contraindicated in patients with (1) sensitivity to dronabinol or alcohol; (2) history of hypersensitivity reaction to alcohol; (3) who are receiving, or who have received disulfiram or metronidazole-containing products within the past 14 days.

Dosage/Range:

Marinol
- Anorexia: 2.5 mg bid before lunch and supper, or if patient is intolerant, a single 2.5-mg dose may be taken in the evening or at bedtime.
- If clinically indicated and if no significant adverse effects, dose may be gradually increased to a maximum of 20 mg/day.
- CINV in adult patients who failed conventional antiemetics: 5 mg/m^2 PO 1–3 hours before chemotherapy administration, then every 2–4 hours after chemotherapy for a total of 4–6 doses per day. Administer first dose on an empty stomach at least 30 minutes prior to eating; subsequent doses can be taken without regard to meals.

Syndros
- Anorexia: Starting dose 2.1 mg PO bid, 1 hour before lunch and dinner. See package insert for dose titration.
- Maximum dosage 8.4 mg bid.
- CINV adult patients who failed conventional antiemetics: starting dose is 4.2 mg/m^2 administered 1–3 hours prior to chemotherapy, then every 2–4 hours after chemotherapy for a total of 4–6 doses per day. Administer first dose on an empty stomach at least 30 minutes prior to eating; subsequent doses can be taken without regard to meals. See package insert for dose titration.
- Administration via silicone enteral feeding tube (size ≥ 14 French) such as nasogastric tube, gastrostomy tube, percutaneous endoscopic gastrostomy tube (PEG), or gastrojejunostomy tube (GJ-tube). Do not use polyurethane feeding tubes.

MANAGEMENT

Drug Preparation:
- **Marinol:** Available in 2.5-, 5-, or 10-mg gel capsules that harden under refrigeration.
- **Syndros:** Oral solution 5 mg/mL. Use calibrated oral dosing syringe that comes with medication.

Drug Administration:
- Oral.
  - Marinol: Teach patient to self-administer oral gel capsules.
  - Syndros: Oral. Teach patient to use calibrated oral dosing syringe, and to take dose with a full glass of water (6–8 oz). **See full prescribing information** for dose titration to manage adverse reactions and to achieve desired therapeutic effect.
    - For anorexia/weight loss: Take dose bid, 1 hour before lunch and dinner.
    - For antiemetic use: Administer first dose on an empty stomach at least 30 minutes before eating; subsequent doses can be taken without regard to meals.
- Syndros Feeding tube: Administration via silicone enteral feeding tube (size $\geq$ 14 French) such as nasogastric tube, gastrostomy tube, percutaneous endoscopic gastrostomy tube (PEG), or gastrojejunostomy tube (GJ-tube). Do not use polyurethane feeding tubes.
  - Draw up prescribed dose with calibrated dosing syringe packaged with Syndros.
  - If the prescribed dose is $>$ 5 mg, the total dose will need to be divided and drawn up in 2 or more portions using the oral syringe.
  - Using the calibrated dosing syringe, administer the dose via the feeding tube.
  - Use a catheter-tip syringe to flush the feeding tube with 30 mL water.

Drug Interactions:
- Amphetamines, cocaine: additive hypertension, tachycardia.
- Atropine, scopolamine: tachycardia, drowsiness.
- Amitriptyline, tricyclic antidepressants: additive tachycardia, hypertension.
- Barbiturates, CNS depressants, buspirone: drowsiness and additive CNS depression.
- Theophylline: increased metabolism.
- Syndros:
  - Disulfiram and metronidazole: may cause disulfiram-like reaction. Discontinue disulfiram or metronidazole 14 days before starting Syndros and do not administer 7 days after treatment with Syndros.
  - Inhibitors and inducers of CYP2C9 and CYP3A4: may alter dronabinol systemic exposure; monitor for dronabinol-related adverse reactions or loss of efficacy.
  - Highly protein-bound drugs: potential for displacement of other drugs from plasma proteins; monitor for adverse reactions to concomitant narrow therapeutic index drugs (e.g., warfarin, cyclosporine, amphotericin B) when initiating or increasing the dosage of Syndros.

Lab Effects/Interference:
- None known.

Special Considerations:
- Marinol contains sesame oil, so should not be used by patients allergic to sesame oil.
- Can produce physical and psychological dependency.
- Can cause dry mouth.

- Warnings and Precautions:
  - *Neuropsychiatric adverse reactions:* Teach patient not to drive, operate machinery, or engage in hazardous activity until it is clear they can tolerate the drug and perform these tasks.
  - *Hemodynamic instability:* Patients with cardiac disorders are at risk as occasional hypotension, HTN, syncope, and/or tachycardia may occur. Review medication profile to ensure the patient is not taking other drugs with similar effects (e.g., sympathomimetic drugs); monitor patient closely for hemodynamic changes after starting or increasing the dosage of the drug.
  - *Seizures and seizure-like activity:* have occurred while taking this drug. Physicians should weigh the risk vs benefits in patients with a history of seizures or who are taking antiepileptic drugs or who otherwise have a lower seizure threshold before starting patient on the drug. Monitor patients at risk closely.
  - *Multiple substance abuse:* Before prescribing dronabinol in patients who have a history of substance abuse or dependence, assess the patient's risk for abuse or misuse of the drug. Monitor patient closely for behaviors suggesting drug abuse or misuse.
  - *Paradoxical nausea, vomiting, or abdominal pain:* If symptoms develop, assess need to reduce dronabinol dose or discontinue drug.
  - Use cautiously and only if benefit outweighs risk in patients with:
    - Seizure disorder, as drug may lower seizure threshold.History of substance abuse, as drug has abuse potential.
    - History of mania, depression, schizophrenia, as drug may exacerbate these conditions; monitor patients closely.
    - Patients receiving concomitant CNS depressants (e.g., sedatives, hypnotics, other psychoactive drugs), as CNS effects may be additive or synergistic.
    - Elderly, as they may be more sensitive to the neurological, psychoactive, and postural hypotensive effects of the drug.

Syndros:
- *Neuropsychiatric adverse reactions:* (1) cognitive adverse reactions such as cognitive impairment and altered mental status; if this occurs, reduce the drug dose or discontinue the drug; (2) hazardous activities: Teach patient not to drive, operate machinery, or engage in hazardous activity until it is clear they can tolerate the drug and perform these tasks.
- *Hemodynamic instability:* Patients with cardiac disorders are at risk as occasional hypotension, HTN, syncope, and/or tachycardia may occur. Review medication profile to ensure the patient is not taking other drugs with similar effects (e.g., sympathomimetic drugs); monitor patient closely for hemodynamic changes after starting or increasing the dosage of the drug.
- *Interaction with disulfiram and metronidazole:* Syndros contains 50% dehydrated alcohol and 5.5% propylene glycol. Use of Syndros may cause a disulfiram-like reaction, characterized by abdominal cramps, nausea, vomiting, headaches, and flushing. Discontinue disulfiram or metronidazole at least 14 days before starting treatment with Syndros and do not administer either of these drugs within 7 days of completing treatment with Syndros.

- *Seizure and seizure-like activity:* weigh the potential risk versus benefit before administering Syndros to patients with a history of seizures, or with other factors that lower seizure threshold; monitor patient and discontinue drug if seizures occur.
- *Multiple substance abuse:* assess for risk of abuse; monitor patient for development of associated behaviors or conditions.
- *Paradoxical nausea, vomiting or abdominal pain:* consider dose reduction or discontinuation, if worsening of symptoms on drug.
- *Toxicity in Preterm neonates:* Ethanol in the drug competitively inhibits the metabolism of propylene glycol, leading to potentially higher serum propylene glycol levels. Neonates are at risk of propylene glycol adverse effects as they have a decreased ability to metabolize propylene glycol. Drug is not indicated in pediatrics and should not be given to neonates. In the postnatal period. Propylene glycol adverse effects include hyperosmolarity with or without lactic acidosis, renal toxicity, CNS depression (stupor, coma, apnea), seizures, hypotonia, cardiac arrythmias, ECG changes, and hemolysis.
- *Embryo-fetal toxicity:* Drug may cause fetal harm. Teach women of reproductive potential to use effective contraception while taking the drug. Teach nursing mothers not to breastfeed while receiving the drug and for 9 days after the last dose (Syndros) or use during pregnancy.
- Toxicities related to propylene glycol in preterm neonates: drug safety has not been established in pediatrics. Avoid use in preterm neonates in the immediate postnatal period
- Drug has antiemetic qualities.

Potential Toxicities/Side Effects and the Nursing Process

I.   ALTERATIONS IN SENSORY/PERCEPTUAL PATTERNS related to CNS CHANGES

Defining Characteristics: Drug can cause changes in mood, cognition, memory, and perception. In addition, nervousness, anxiety, confusion, dizziness, depersonalization, euphoria, paranoid reaction, somnolence, and thinking abnormalities can occur. Drug has abuse potential.

Nursing Implications: Assess appropriateness of drug for patient, as this would not be the drug of choice for a substance abuser, either one who is actively using or who has withdrawn and is abstaining because of abuse potential. Teach patient of possible side effects, as well as self-care strategies to avoid heightened fear or anxiety.

II.   POTENTIAL FOR ALTERATION IN OXYGENATION related to SYMPATHOMIMETIC EFFECTS

Defining Characteristics: Tachycardia and conjunctival infection may occur. Drug interactions may cause hypertension.

Nursing Implications: Review patient medication profile to identify any possible drug interactions. Monitor appetite stimulation effects, and weigh these against any sympathomimetic changes.

Drug: megestrol acetate oral suspension (Megace OS)

Class: Synthetic progestin.

Mechanism of Action: Alters malignant cell environment in hormonally sensitive tumors, discouraging tumor cell proliferation; appears to stimulate appetite and weight gain in cancer cachexia directly or indirectly through antagonism of TNF. Designated as orphan drug by FDA for management of anorexia, cachexia, or weight loss > 10% of baseline. Approved for AIDS-related cachexia.

Metabolism: Well-absorbed from GI tract. Metabolized in liver and excreted by kidneys.

Indication: Treatment of anorexia, cachexia, or an unexplained, significant weight loss in patients with a diagnosis of AIDS.

Contraindication: Megace ES: known hypersensitivity, known or suspected pregnancy.

Dosage/Range:
- Optimal dose for management of cachexia is 800 mg/day in a single dose.
- Studies showed that daily doses of 400 and 800 mg a day were found to be clinically effective.
- Available in:
  - Megace OS 40 mg/mL.
  - Megace ES formulation (concentrated suspension) delivering 625 mg (125 mg/mL), which has been shown equivalent to the 800 mg of Megace oral suspension (40 mg/mL) (in volunteers under federally approved conditions).

Drug Preparation:
- Store in tight container at temperature 15–25°C (59–77°F).
- Available in bottles of 240 mL (8 fl oz).
- Oral administration: shake container well before using.

Drug Administration:
- 20 mL Megase OS (800 mg) PO once a day; OR
- 5 mL of Megace ES (625 mg) once a day.

Drug Interactions:
- None.

Lab Effects/Interference:
- May increase glucose, lactic dehydrogenase (LDH).
- Rare leukopenia.

Special Considerations:
- One-third of patients with metastatic cancer gain weight.
- Weight gain appears to be from increased fat stores rather than from water gain (Loprinzi et al., 1992).
- Warnings and Precautions:
  - Drug can cause fetal harm. Teach women to avoid pregnancy; if used during pregnancy, the patient should be apprised of the potential hazard to the fetus.

MANAGEMENT

- Drug is not intended for prophylactic use to avoid weight loss.
- Drug has glucocorticoid activity and may exacerbate or lead to new onset diabetes mellitus; care should be taken if the drug is stopped to prevent adrenal insufficiency (slowly withdraw drug).
  - Use cautiously in diabetics and patients with a history of thromboembolic disease.
- Breakthrough vaginal bleeding may occur in women.
- Women of reproductive age who are sexually active should use effective contraception to avoid pregnancy.
- Nursing mothers should make a decision to stop nursing or stop the drug, taking into consideration the importance of the drug to the mother's health.
- Most common adverse events in > 5% of patients receiving 800 mg/20 mL Megace OS in two clinical efficacy trials were nausea, diarrhea, impotence, rash, flatulence, HTN, and asthenia.

Potential Toxicities/Side Effects and the Nursing Process

I. ALTERATIONS IN PERFUSION related to DEEP VEIN THROMBOSIS

Defining Characteristics: Rarely, 6% of patients may experience deep vein thrombosis (DVT) or pulmonary emboli.

Nursing Implications: Assess baseline peripheral vascular status and monitor during therapy. Teach patient to report immediately pain in calf, erythema, shortness of breath, chest pain.

II. ALTERATION IN NUTRITION related to HYPERGLYCEMIA

Defining Characteristics: Hyperglycemia is uncommon but may be significant if it occurs.

Nursing Implications: Assess baseline FBS, and monitor during therapy. Teach patient signs and symptoms of hyperglycemia and to report them (polydipsia, polyuria, polyphagia).

III. ALTERATION IN COMFORT related to CARPAL TUNNEL SYNDROME, NAUSEA AND VOMITING, TUMOR FLARE

Defining Characteristics: Carpal tunnel syndrome, nausea, vomiting, tumor flare may occur rarely.

Nursing Implications: Instruct patient to report any signs/symptoms. Discuss with patient, physician symptomatic measures.

IV. ANXIETY related to ABNORMAL UTERINE BLEEDING

Defining Characteristics: Breakthrough vaginal bleeding, discharge often occur in females, and can cause anxiety.

Nursing Implications: Teach female patient that this is an expected side effect. Encourage patient to verbalize feelings, provide patient with emotional support and information about cause and management.

Chapter *9*
Anxiety and Depression

It is estimated that approximately 20% of patients with cancer experience depression, and 10% anxiety (Pitman, 2018). Anxiety and depression in response to uncertainty and hopelessness are frequently associated with the cancer experience. Studies have shown that anxiety increases with the cancer diagnosis and remains elevated to some degree throughout treatment, regardless of modality or setting (Baron, 2016). Drugs such as central nervous system (CNS) stimulants, psychotropics, steroids, and caffeine may cause anxiety (Rucker & Gobel, 2014). The American Society of Clinical Oncology (ASCO) (Andersen et al., 2014; Li et al., 2016) promulgates screening, assessment, and care of anxiety and depressive symptoms in adult patients with cancer, using available evidence-based tools, which can be found on their Website. These include management algorithms for both anxiety and depression. The ASCO/Oncology Nursing Society (ONS) Chemotherapy Administration Safety Standards (2016) include assessment of psychosocial concerns, including distress, which encompasses anxiety and depression, and need for support, with action taken as needed. The National Comprehensive Cancer Network (NCCN) has published Distress Management guidelines that are very helpful to the clinician in assessing and managing anxiety and depression in patients with cancer (NCCN, v3, 2019).

Nursing efforts are aimed at anxiety-reducing strategies, such as helping the patient explore the anxiety and find anxiety-reducing activities (e.g., relaxation exercises, verbalization of feelings). Nurses can also refer patients for specialized support if necessary, and, as appropriate, teach patients and their families about prescribed anxiolytic medications. Depression is an often expected response to the cancer experience, to an actual or perceived loss of health, role, and life. The reported incidence of depression in hospitalized cancer patients is 25–42% (Trask, 2004). It may also be associated with chronic cancer pain and can clearly adversely affect quality of life. Prominent features may be perceived loss of self-esteem, worthlessness, hopelessness, guilt, and sadness. There is a continuum of depression, ranging from everyday sadness to severe, debilitating depression with physical and/or psychological symptoms that constitute a major depressive disorder (Valentine, 2007).

Pyter et al. (2009) postulated that malignant tumors released substances that contribute to depression. Although the study was conducted with rats, it showed that these animals were less eager to eat and had increased levels of cytokines in both blood and the hippocampus, compared to healthy rats. Certain antineoplastic medications can be associated with depression, such as docetaxel, interferon-alpha, interleukin-2, leuprolide, paclitaxel, and tamoxifen (Fulcher, 2014). Most commonly in practice, nurses assess patient symptoms of changes in appetite, sleeplessness, lethargy, and social withdrawal. Nurses use caring and compassion to help patients who are depressed acknowledge and explore their feelings. Through patient teaching and supportive counseling, short-term realistic and achievable goals can often be negotiated by patient and nurse. Now, nurses are helping patients to make the "mountain" more manageable.

Patients cope individually with the multiple threats that cancer brings. Patients with depression may have a variety of symptoms that fall within one or more categories of functioning, with symptoms that may include (Andersen et al., 2014):

- Mood symptoms: feelings of sadness, helplessness, hopelessness; irritability; feelings of guilt or worthlessness.
- Cognitive symptoms: decreased ability to concentrate, decreased memory, suicidal thoughts.
- Physical symptoms: fatigue or low energy, poor appetite, inability to experience pleasure.
- Behavioral symptoms: social withdrawal, crying spells, loss of interest in activities or hobbies, decreased sex drive.

In 2007, the Institute of Medicine published a report called *Cancer Care for the Whole Patient,* and proposed a model based on the NCCN model of psychosocial care that should be incorporated into routine cancer care: screening for distress and psychosocial needs, making a treatment plan to address the needs and implementing it, referring to specialists/services as needed, and reevaluating and revising the plan as needed (IOM, 2007). Nurses have been using the nursing process to do this routinely, but now it has become a team responsibility. Long thought to be an integral component in the clinical management of cancer patients, today, national organizations committed to outstanding oncology care have developed standards to ensure that the consistent assessment of patient's psychosocial issues is routinely performed during the cancer experience, such as NCCN, The Joint Commission, and Quality Oncology Performance Initiative (QOPI, ASCO's quality arm) (NCCN, 2012). In Canada, emotional distress is called the 6th vital sign that is routinely assessed (Bultz et al., 2011). ASCO (2014) developed guidelines as reported by Andersen et al. (2014) for the screening, assessment, and care of anxiety and depressive symptoms in adults with cancer. This validates the importance for the entire healthcare team to assess and identify anxiety and depression issues in patients. ASCO's rationale is that "failure to identify and treat anxiety and depression" in the patients with cancer that we provide care for, "increases the risk for poor quality of life and potential disease-related morbidity and mortality."

Of course, pharmacotherapy is also very important. It is generally accepted that depression results from a deficiency in key neurotransmitters, resulting in either an overexpression or underexpression of neurotransmitters that control the release or breakdown of the neurotransmitters (Barsevick & Much, 2003).

The tricyclic antidepressant (TCA) medications once were the cornerstone of managing cancer-related depression, partially because of their ability to improve sleeplessness and to enhance analgesia. These drugs include amitriptyline (Elavil). However, these drugs also have undesirable side effects, such as dry mouth, constipation, and blurred vision related to their anticholinergic, α-adrenergic–blocking, and antihistamine properties (Valentine, 2007). Selective serotonin antagonist reuptake inhibitors (SSRIs) raise serotonin levels and include citalopram (Celexa), Escitalopram (Lexapro), Fluoxetine, (Prozac), Paroxetine (Paxil), Sertraline (Zoloft), and Vilazodone (Viibryd). Common side effects include dry mouth, dizziness, sedation, orthostasis, and rarely priapism in men. Monoamine oxidase inhibitors (MAOIs) are not used often because of the many drug interactions that can occur. These drugs are phenelzine (Nardil) and tranylcypromine (Parnate) and prevent the breakdown of neurotransmitters, thus increasing their levels. Side effects include insomnia and orthostasis.

Newer antidepressant medications are more commonly used and have found a firm niche in oncology care. The selective serotonin reuptake inhibitors (SSRIs) are quite effective for many patients and have few side effects, together with a short half-life. In addition, they differ from the TCAs in that they are generally less lethal if a patient accidentally overdoses (except citalopram hydrobromide). They also do not possess anticholinergic or α-adrenergic–blocking properties and thus are safer in medically complex patients (Valentine, 2007). These agents block serotonin reuptake, and thus, more serotonin is available as a neurotransmitter; they include fluoxetine (Prozac), sertraline (Zoloft), citalopram (Celexa), escitalopram (Lexapro), paroxetine (Paxil), fluvoxamine (Luvox), and Vilazodone (Viibryd). Common side effects are nausea, insomnia, headache, and sexual problems. The serotonin-norepinephrine reuptake inhibitors (SNRIs) increase the levels of norepinephrine as well as serotonin to act as neurotransmitters. Drugs in this category are venlafaxine (Effexor), duloxetine (Cymbalta), levomilnacipran (Fetzima), and mirtazapine (Remeron), and common side effects are nausea, dry mouth, headache, and sedation. Another SNRI, desvenlafaxine (Pristiq) is a synthetic form of the active metabolite of venlafaxine that is being studied as a nonhormonal treatment for menopausal symptoms.

Because of an increased risk of suicidality (suicidal thinking and behavior) in young adults 18–24 years old during the initial treatment (first 1–2 months), the FDA (2007) has required that all antidepressant drugs indicate this risk as a black box warning.

Massie and Popkin (1998) suggest principles to guide antidepressant therapy in patients with cancer: start with a lower dose, slowly increase the dose, as the therapeutic dose may be lower than that in noncancer patients, and monitor very carefully for side effects, as there may be overlapping toxicity in organ systems (with chemotherapy, the malignancy).

In addition, it is important to do a thorough assessment of herbs used in the management of anxiety and depression, as these may be interacting with anticancer drug therapy. For example, St. John's wort is both an inducer and/or inhibitor of the key metabolic CYP3A4, CYP2C9, and CYP2D6 pathways. It induces the metabolism of irinotecan primary active metabolite SN-38 via the cytochrome P450 CYP3A4 subsystem, lowering serum levels by up to 42% with an effect lasting up to 3 weeks (Mathijssen et al., 2002). Table 9.1 depicts antianxiety and antidepressant agents commonly prescribed.

Table 9.1   Agents Commonly Used in the Management of Anxiety and Depression in Patients with Cancer

Drug	Dose Range (Oral)	Half-Life or Onset of Therapeutic Effect	Common Side Effects	Comments
Antianxiety				
Alprazolam (Xanax)	0.25–1.0 mg PO every 6–24 hours	10–15 hours half-life	Sedation, confusion, motor incoordination, somnolence	Short half-life; rapid onset; tolerance may develop rapidly

(continues)

Table 9.1 *(Continued)*

Drug	Dose Range (Oral)	Half-Life or Onset of Therapeutic Effect	Common Side Effects	Comments
Clonazepam (Klonopin)	0.5–2.0 PO every 6–24 hours	Peak serum level 1–2 hours; half-life 18–60 hours, median 30–40 hours	Drowsiness, dizziness, motor incoordination, orthostasis, ↓ mental alertness	Increased CNS depressant effects when combined with CNS depressants
Chlorazepate (Tranxene)	15–30 mg a day, maximum 60 mg/day	48 hours	Dizziness, blurred vision, insomnia, nausea, muscle weakness, amnesia	Long half-life leads to accumulation of active metabolites
Diazepam (Valium, Valrelease)	2–10 mg every 6–24 hours PO, IM, IV	20–70 hours half-life	Drowsiness, fatigue, lethargy, weakness, rash, vivid dreams, feeling "hung over"	Long half-life, so accumulation of active metabolites; fast absorption; difficult to use in older patients
Lorazepam (Ativan)	0.5–2.0 mg PO, IM, IV every 4–12 hours	10–20 hours half-life	Drowsiness, fatigue, lethargy, weakness, rash, vivid dreams	Short half-life with intermediate absorption; continuous IV infusion in severe cases
Oxazepam (Serax)	30–120 mg/day (usual max dose 60 mg/day)	5–15 hours	Drowsiness, fatigue, lethargy, weakness, rash, vivid dreams	Short half-life
Antidepressants SSRIs				
Paroxetine (Paxil)	20 mg to start PO (morning) to 50 mg every day 62.5 mg if paroxetine CR	Onset 3–10 days	Nausea, dry mouth, rash, headache, drowsiness, loss of libido, postural hypotension, mild nausea, anxiety; sedation	Caution in elderly, patients with renal or hepatic dysfunction, suicidal ideation; dose ↑ if needed after 2–3 weeks; if renal or hepatic dysfunction, begin with one-half to one-fourth of the normal starting dose to start
Sertraline (Zoloft)	50 PO to start (morning), up to 200 mg every day	Onset 7 days	Same as paroxetine, except, no sedation, sexual dysfunction	Same
Fluoxetine (Prozac)		Onset 2–4 weeks	Same as paroxetine; sexual dysfunction	Same
Escitalopram (Lexapro)	10 mg PO daily; if ↑ to 20 mg daily, do so after at least 1 week	Half-life of 27–32 hours; steady-state plasma levels in 1 week	Same as paroxetine, no sedation	Same

Table 9.1 *(Continued)*

Drug	Dose Range (Oral)	Half-Life or Onset of Therapeutic Effect	Common Side Effects	Comments
Citalopram hydro-bromide (Celexa)	20 mg PO to start (morning); 40 mg PO daily after at least 1 week	Terminal half-life of 25 hours; steady state in 1 week	Same as paroxetine, except may be fatal if overdosed	Same
TCAs				
Amitripty-line (Elavil)	25–250 mg	Onset 4–6 weeks	Anticholinergic (urinary retention, dry mouth, thirst, blurred vision, sedation) and antihistaminic (sedation); tachycardia, orthostatic hypotension, arrhythmia; withdrawal reaction	Caution in patients with suicidal ideation, cardiac/renal or hepatic dysfunction; don't stop drug abruptly; do baseline EKG and assess toxicity
Desipramine (Norpramin)	25–150 mg	4–6 weeks	Same as amitriptyline	Same as amitriptyline; serum level correlates with therapeutic effect
Doxepin (Sinequan)	50–150 mg	4–6 weeks	Same as amitriptyline	Same as amitriptyline
Imipramine (Tofranil)	25–150 mg	4–6 weeks	Same as amitriptyline	Same as amitriptyline; serum level correlates with therapeutic effect
Nortriptyline (Pamelor)	50–150 mg	4–6 weeks	Same as amitriptyline	Same as amitriptyline; serum level correlates with therapeutic effect
Trazodone (Dyseril)	50–250 mg	1–4 weeks	Same as amitriptyline	Same as amitriptyline
SNRI				
Venlafax-ine HCl (Effexor)	75–225 mg/day	1–4 weeks	Emotional lability, vertigo, trismus, nausea	Use cautiously in elderly, patients with cardiac/renal or hepatic dysfunction; also helpful with hot flashes
Nefazo-done HCl (Serzone)	200–600 mg/day	1–4 weeks	Dizziness, drowsiness, dry mouth, headache	Use cautiously in elderly, patients with cardiac/renal or hepatic dysfunction
Duloxetine (Cymbalta)	40 mg daily to start, ↑ to 60 mg PO daily	Half-life of 12 hours, steady state achieved in 3 days	Nausea, dry mouth, constipation, diarrhea, insomnia, decreased appetite, somnolence	Contraindicated if narrow angle glaucoma; indicated in patients with peripheral neuropathic pain

MANAGEMENT

(continues)

Table 9.1 (Continued)

Drug	Dose Range (Oral)	Half-Life or Onset of Therapeutic Effect	Common Side Effects	Comments
Mirtazapine (Remeron)	15 mg PO daily to start; ↑ to 45 mg PO daily after 2–4 weeks if needed	Elimination half-life of 20–40 hours; steady state in 3–4 days	↑ appetite, weight gain, peripheral edema; CNS effects, drowsiness, orthostasis	Use cautiously and monitor closely hepatic or renal insufficiency, epilepsy, organic brain syndrome, heart disease, BPH, acute narrow angle glaucoma, DM; rare BMD
Desvenlafaxine (Pristiq)	50 mg recommended dose; may slowly ↑ dose to 400 mg in clinical trials	Elimination half-life 11 hours; time to steady state 4–5 days	Nausea, headache, dry mouth, sweating, dizziness, insomnia	Dose reduction for severe renal impairment; use cautiously in older persons or in patients with cardiac/renal or hepatic dysfunction
Atypical (Unknown MOA)				
Bupropion hydrochloride (Wellbutrin)	100 mg PO twice daily for at least 3 days, may ↑ to 100 mg 3 times daily; after 4 weeks may ↑ to 150 mg 3 times daily if needed	Half-life of 14 hours	Weight loss, restlessness, agitation, insomnia, dizziness, tachycardia, changes in BP, dry mouth, anorexia, nausea, vomiting, urinary retention	Drug increases activity, so useful if psychomotor slowing; rare sexual dysfunction; may cause seizures; contraindicated if history of seizures, bulimia, anorexia nervosa

BPH: benign prostatic hypertrophy, DM: diabetes mellitus, BMD: bone marrow depression.

References

Adler NE, Page NEK, Institute of Medicine (IOM). *Cancer Care for the Whole Patient: Meeting Psychosocial Health Needs.* Available at http://www.nationalacademies.org/hmd/Reports /2007/Cancer-Care-for-the-Whole-Patient-Meeting-Psychosocial-Health-Needs.aspx. Accessed August 21, 2016.

Andersen BL, DeRubeis RJ, Berman BS, et al. Screening, Assessment, and Care of Anxiety and Depressive Symptoms in Adults with Cancer: An American Society of Clinical Oncology guideline adaptation. *J Clin Oncol* 2014; 32(15):1605–1619.

Baron RH. Psychosocial Management. In Gobel BH, Triest-Robertson S, Vogel W (eds.). *Advanced Oncology Nursing Certification Review and Resource Manual*, 2nd ed. Pittsburgh, PA: Oncology Nursing Society; 2016: 737–773.

Bultz BD, Groff SL, Fitch M, et al. Implementing Screening Distress, The 6th Vital Sign: A Canadian Strategy for Changing Practice. *Psychooncology* 2011; 20:463–469.

Federal Drug Administration. *FDA Proposes New Warnings About Suicidal Thinking, Behavior in Young Adults Who Take Antidepressant Medications.* Available at https://www.fda.gov /drugs/postmarket-drug-safety-information-patients-and-providers/suicidality-children-and -adolescents-being-treated-antidepressant-medications. Accessed October 15, 2019.

Fulcher CD. Depression, chapter 31. In Yarbro CH, Wujuk D, and Gobel BH (eds.). *Cancer Symptom Management*, 4th ed. Burlington, MA: Jones & Bartlett Learning; 2014: 655–673.

Lacouture ME, Anadkat MJ, Bensadoun RJ, et al. Clinical practice guidelines for the prevention and treatment of EGFR inhibitor-associated dermatologic toxicities. *Support Care Cancer* 2011; 19: 1079–1095.

Li M, Kennedy EB, Byrne N et al. Management of depression in patients with cancer: a clinical practice guideline. *J Oncology Practice* 2016; 12(8):747–756.

Loprinzi CL, Sloan J, Stearns V, et al. New Antidepressants and Gabapentin for Hot Flashes: An Individual Patient Pooled Analysis. *J Clin Oncol* 2009; 27(17):2831–2837.

Massie MJ, Popkin MK. Depressive Disorders, *Chapter 10*. In Holland JC. *Psycho-Oncology*. New York, NY: Oxford University Press; 1998: 518–540.

Mathijssen RH, Verweij J, de Bruijn P, et al. Effects of St. John's Wort on Irinotecan Metabolism. *J Natl Cancer Inst* 2002; 94(16):1247–1249.

Merck and Co., Inc. Remeron (mirtazapine) [package insert]. Whitehouse Station, NY. May 2018.

Mylan Pharmaceuticals Inc. Buspirone HCl [package insert]. Morgantown, WV. December 2016.

Mylan Pharmaceuticals Inc. Citalopram [package insert]. Morgantown, WV. January 2019.

Mylan Pharmaceuticals Inc. Clonazepam [package insert]. Morgantown, WV. May 2018.

Mylan Pharmaceuticals Inc. Paroxetine hydrochloride [package insert]. Morgantown, WV. August 2017.

National Comprehensive Cancer Network (NCCN). *Distress management*, v.3, 2019. Available at https://www.nccn.org/professionals/physician_gls/pdf/distress.pdf. Accessed May 31, 2019.

Neuss MN, Polovich M, McNiff K, et al. Updated American Society of Clinical Oncology/Oncology Nursing Society Chemotherapy Administration Safety Standards Including Standards for the Safe Administration and Management of Oral Chemotherapy. *J Oncology Practice* 2013; 9(2s): 5s–13s. 2016

Neuss MN, Gilmore TR, Belderson KM et al. Updated American Society of Clinical Oncology/Oncology Nursing Society Chemotherapy Administration Safety Standards Including Standards for Pediatric Oncology. *J Oncology Practice* 12(12):1262–1271.

Pfizer Inc. Xanax (alprazolam). [package insert]. New York, NY. December 2016.

Pfizer Inc. Pristique ER (deslenlafaxine) [package insert]. New York, NY. November 2018.

Pfizer Inc. Zoloft (sertraline HCL) [package insert]. New York, NY. April 2019.

Pitman A. Depression and anxiety in patients with cancer. *BMJ* 2018; 361: k1415. Doi: 10.1136/bmj. k1415.

Pyter LM, Pineros V, Galang JA. Peripheral Tumors Induce Depressive-like Behaviors and Cytokine Production and Alter Hypothalamic-Pituitary-Adrenal Axis Regulation. *Proc Natl Acad Sci* 2009; 106:9069–9074.

Rucker Y, Gobel BH. Anxiety, chapter 29. In Yarbro CH, Wujuk D, Gobel BH (eds.). *Cancer Symptom Management*, 4th ed. Burlington, MA: Jones & Bartlett Learning; 2014: 619–637.

Smith EM, Pang H, Cirrincione C, et al. Effect of duloxetine on pain, function, and quality of life among patients with chemotherapy-induced painful peripheral neuropathy. *JAMA* 2013; 309(13): 1359–1367.

Valeant Pharmaceuticals North America LLC. Wellbutrin XL (bupropion HCL extended-release tablets) [package insert]. Bridgewater, NJ. May 2017.

Drug: alprazolam (Xanax)

Class: Benzodiazepine (anxiolytic).

Mechanism of Action: Binds to benzodiazepine receptors in the CNS (limbic and cortical areas, cerebellum, brain stem, and spinal cord), resulting in the following effects: anxiolytic, ataxia, anticonvulsant, muscle relaxation. Appears to potentiate the effects of γ-aminobutyric acid (GABA).

Metabolism: Well absorbed from GI tract. Widely distributed in body tissues and fluids, including CSF. Crosses placenta and is excreted in breastmilk. Highly bound to plasma proteins. Metabolized in liver and excreted in urine. Short elimination time; half-life of 12–15 hours. May produce psychological and physical dependence. Indicated for management of anxiety, the short-term relief of anxiety associated with depression, and panic disorder.

Indication: For the management of patients with (1) anxiety disorder; (2) panic disorder, with or without agoraphobia.

Contraindications: In (1) patients with known sensitivity to the drug or other benzodiazepines; (2) in combination with ketoconazole or itraconaxole, as these drugs impair metabolism of alprazolam.

Dosage/Range:

Adult:
• Anxiety: 0.25–0.5 mg PO tid (may gradually increase dose q 3–4 days over time to maximum 4 mg/day in divided doses).
• Elderly/debilitated: 0.25 mg PO bid.
• Discontinue drug by decreasing dose by 0.25–0.5 mg q 3–7 days.
• Drug should be used for short-term use only (< 4 months).
• Panic: optimal dosage not determined; titrate dose and increase slowly.

Drug Preparation:
• Available in 0.25-, 0.50-, and 1-mg tablets.
• Store in tight, light-resistant containers at 15–30°C (59–86°F).

Drug Administration:
• Orally, in divided doses.
• May take with food if stomach upset occurs.

Drug Interactions:
• CNS depressants (alcohol, anticonvulsants, phenothiazines, opiates): additive CNS depression; avoid concurrent use or use cautiously and monitor carefully.
• Smoking: may decrease alprazolam serum level by up to 50%.

- CYP3A potent inhibitors (e.g., ketoconazole, itraconazole, nefazodone, fluvoxamine, erythromycin): increase alprazolam serum levels by decreasing drug metabolism; avoid coadministration or monitor closely for toxicity.
- CYP3A inducers (e.g., cabamazepine, HIV protease inhibitors such as ritonivir): may decrease alprazolam serum levels by inducing metabolism of the drug.
- TCAs: increased serum levels of antidepressant possible; use together cautiously.
- Digoxin: may decrease renal excretion of digoxin; monitor for overdosage; may need to decrease digoxin.

Lab Effects/Interference:
- No consistent pattern of interaction between benzodiazepines and laboratory tests.

Special Considerations:

- Wide margin of safety between therapeutic and toxic doses.
- May impair ability to perform activities requiring mental alertness (e.g., driving a car, operating machinery).
- May produce psychological and physical dependence.
- Administer cautiously in patients with liver or renal impairment.
- Use cautiously in patients with chronic pulmonary disease or sleep apnea.
- Contraindicated in patients with depressive neuroses, psychotic reactions (without prominent anxiety), acute alcoholic intoxication (with depressed VS), known hypersensitivity to the drug, or acute angle-closure glaucoma.
- May cause fetal damage so should not be used during pregnancy or if the mother is breastfeeding.
- Withdrawal symptoms (including seizure, delirium) can occur with rapid drug discontinuance in patients taking high or chronic doses.
- If manic episodes or hyperactivity occur soon after drug started, drug should be discontinued.
- Drug should not be used to manage "everyday stress."

Potential Toxicities/Side Effects and the Nursing Process

I. ALTERATIONS IN SENSORY/PERCEPTUAL PATTERNS related to CNS DEPRESSION

Defining Characteristics: CNS depressant effects include drowsiness, fatigue, lethargy, confusion, weakness, headache, which may occur initially and resolve with continued therapy or dose reduction. Vivid dreams, suicidal ideation, and bizarre behavior also may occur. Patient risk factors: elderly, debilitated, liver dysfunction, low serum albumin.

Nursing Implications: Assess baseline neurologic status and risk factors, and monitor during treatment. Instruct patient to report signs/symptoms and discuss drug modification with physician. Evaluate patient satisfaction with drug efficacy. If patient expresses suicidal ideation (more common in panic disorders), refer patient for psychiatric evaluation and drug modification. Instruct patient to avoid alcohol while taking drug. Teach patient prescribed schedule for discontinuing drug when used chronically: assess for signs/symptoms of withdrawal (increased anxiety, rebound insomnia; may also include agitation, dysphoria, nausea/vomiting, irritability, muscle cramps, hallucinations, seizures).

II.   ALTERATION IN NUTRITION, LESS THAN BODY REQUIREMENTS, related to GI SIDE EFFECTS

Defining Characteristics: Nausea, vomiting, weight increase or decrease, dry mouth, constipation may occur; also, elevated serum LFTs.

Nursing Implications: Assess baseline nutrition and elimination patterns and LFTs, and monitor during therapy. Discuss abnormalities and drug modification with physician. Teach patient to self-administer prescribed antiemetics as appropriate.

III.   POTENTIAL FOR INJURY related to DECREASE IN MENTAL ALERTNESS, PHYSICAL COORDINATION

Defining Characteristics: Drug may cause drowsiness, dizziness, and impair physical coordination, mental alertness.

Nursing Implications: Assess other medications that may increase risk (e.g., opiates, phenothiazines) and response to drug. Instruct patient to avoid potentially hazardous activities, including driving a car, operating machinery.

IV.   ALTERATIONS IN CARDIAC OUTPUT related to RHYTHM DISTURBANCES, VASODILATION

Defining Characteristics: Drug may cause bradycardia, tachycardia, hyper-or hypotension, palpitations, edema.

Nursing Implications: Assess baseline VS, and monitor during therapy. Discuss abnormalities with physician. Instruct patient to report dizziness on standing or other changes.

V.   ALTERATIONS IN SKIN INTEGRITY related to RASH

Defining Characteristics: Urticaria, pruritus, rash (morbilliform, urticarial, or maculopapular) may occur.

Nursing Implications: Assess baseline skin integrity, and instruct patient to report changes. Teach symptomatic skin management, and discuss drug discontinuance with physician if severe.

Drug: amitriptyline hydrochloride (Elavil)

Class: Tricyclic antidepressant.

Mechanism of Action: Blocks reuptake of neurotransmitters at neuronal membrane, thus increasing available serotonin and norepinephrine in CNS, and potentiating their effects. Appears to have analgesic effect separate from antidepressant action. May increase bioavailability of morphine. Indicated in the treatment of depressive (affective) mood disorders. Also used as an adjuvant analgesic in cancer pain management.

Metabolism: Well absorbed from GI tract. Distributed to lungs, heart, brain, liver; highly bound to plasma, proteins. Plasma half-life of 10–50 hours. Metabolized in liver, excreted in urine and, to a lesser degree, in bile and feces.

Indication: For the relief of symptoms of depression.

Dosage/Range:

Adult:

- Oral: 25–100 mg PO hs divided or single dose; may increase to 200–300 mg/day (300 mg maximum).
- Cancer pain: 25 mg/day hs; may increase by 25 mg of 1–2 days to 75–150 mg, when desired relief level is reached; may start at 10 mg in elderly.
- Elderly: 30 mg/day in divided doses.
- Intramuscular (IM): 20–30 mg qid or as single dose at bedtime.

Drug Preparation:

- Oral: store in well-closed containers at 15–30°C (59–86°F); store Elavil 10-mg capsules away from light. Administer as a single bedtime dose.
- IM: administer IM in large muscle mass; change to oral as soon as possible.

Drug Interactions:

- MAOIs: increased excitation, hyperpyrexia, seizures; use together cautiously (especially if high dose is used).
- CNS depressants (alcohol, sedatives, hypnotics): increase CNS depression; use together cautiously.
- Sympathomimetic (epinephrine, amphetamines): increased hypertension; AVOID concurrent use.
- Cimetidine methylphenidate: increased amitriptyline levels, increased toxicity; use cautiously and monitor for increased toxicity.
- Warfarin: may increase PT; monitor closely and decrease dose of warfarin as needed.

Lab Effects/Interference:

- None known; bone marrow depression uncommon.

MANAGEMENT

Special Considerations:

- Antidepressant effect may take 2 weeks or longer.
- Adjuvant analgesic useful in cancer pain management.
- May also decrease depression associated with chronic cancer pain and promote improved sleep.
- Contraindicated in patients with myocardial infarction, seizure disorder, or benign prostatic hypertrophy.
- Use cautiously in patients with urine retention, narrow-angle glaucoma, hyperthyroidism, hepatic dysfunction, or suicidal ideation.
- Drug should be gradually discontinued rather than abruptly withdrawn to prevent anxiety, malaise, dizziness, nausea/vomiting.
- May be helpful in treating hiccups.
- Increased anticholinergic side effects in older persons.
- Teach all patients/families to call provider right away if thoughts of suicide or dying; attempts to commit suicide; new or worsening depression; new or worsening anxiety; feeling very agitated or restless; panic attacks; trouble sleeping (insomnia); new or worsening irritability; aggressive, angry, or violent behavior; acting on dangerous impulses; extreme increase in activity or talking (mania); any unusual changes in behavior or mood.

Potential Toxicities/Side Effects and the Nursing Process

I.   ALTERATIONS IN SENSORY/PERCEPTUAL PATTERNS related to DROWSINESS, FATIGUE, EPS

Defining Characteristics: Drowsiness, dizziness, weakness, lethargy, and fatigue are common; confusion, disorientation, hallucinations may occur in the elderly. Extrapyramidal symptoms may occur (fine tremor, rigidity, dystonia, dysarthria, dysphagia), as may peripheral neuropathy and blurred vision.

Nursing Implications: Assess baseline gait, neurologic and mental status, and monitor during therapy. Instruct patient to report signs/symptoms; discuss benefit/risk ratio with physician. Assess for signs/symptoms of suicidal ideation; if they occur, refer for psychiatric evaluation. Inform patient that drowsiness, dizziness will resolve after 1–2 weeks; instruct to avoid hazardous activities while drowsy (e.g., driving a car, operating machinery).

II.   ALTERATION IN CARDIAC OUTPUT related to POSTURAL HYPOTENSION, TACHYCARDIA

Defining Characteristics: Postural hypotension, EKG changes, tachycardia, hypertension may occur.

Nursing Implications: Assess baseline orthostatic BP, heart rate, and monitor during therapy. Instruct patient to report abnormalities, including postural dizziness, palpitations. Drug should be stopped several days before surgery to prevent hypertensive crisis, especially if high dose.

III. ALTERATION IN NUTRITION, LESS THAN BODY REQUIREMENTS, related to GI SIDE EFFECTS

Defining Characteristics: Dry mouth, anorexia, nausea, vomiting, diarrhea, abdominal cramping may occur; also, elevated LFTs.

Nursing Implications: Assess baseline nutrition and elimination patterns and LFTs, and monitor during therapy. Discuss abnormalities with physician, and discuss drug modification. Teach patient to self-administer prescribed antiemetics as appropriate. LFTs should be repeated, and if still elevated, the drug should be discontinued. Teach patient to take full dose at bedtime. Suggest patient use sugar-free hard candy, frequent ice chips, or artificial saliva for dry mouth.

IV. ALTERATION IN URINARY ELIMINATION related to URINARY RETENTION

Defining Characteristics: Urinary retention may occur. Increased risk if patient has history of urinary retention.

Nursing Implications: Assess baseline urinary elimination pattern and risk. Assess for urinary retention, and instruct patient to report signs/symptoms. Discuss alternative drug with physician if this occurs.

V. ALTERATIONS IN SKIN INTEGRITY related to ALLERGY

Defining Characteristics: Urticaria, erythema, rash, and photosensitivity may occur.

Nursing Implications: Assess baseline drug allergy history and skin integrity. Instruct patient to report skin changes. If angioedema of face or tongue develops, discuss drug discontinuance with physician. Instruct patient to avoid sunlight or to use sunblock protection.

Drug: bupropion hydrochloride (Wellbutrin)

Class: Aminoketone antidepressant.

Mechanism of Action: Unknown. Does block reuptake of serotonin, norepinephrine, and dopamine weakly; does not inhibit MAO; has CNS stimulant effects.

Metabolism: Peak plasma level 2 hours after oral administration, and it appears that only a small percentage of the dose reaches the systemic circulation. Half-life about 14 hours (8–24 hours average). Four major metabolites, with significantly longer elimination half-lives. Primarily excreted in the urine (87%) and to a lesser extent in the feces (10%).

Indication: For the treatment of major depressive disorder.

Contraindications: (1) Seizure disorder; (2) current or prior diagnosis of bulimia or anorexia nervosa; (3) abrupt discontinuation of alcohol, benzodiazepines, barbiturates, antiepileptic drugs; (4) MAOIs during or within 14 days of stopping treatment with buproprion

HCL, or within 14 days of stopping an MAOI intended to treat psychiatric disorders; (5) patients being treated with linezolid or IV methylene blue; (6) known hypersensitivity to drug or other ingredients.

Dosage/Range:

Adult:
- Initial dose: 100 mg bid (200 mg/day) for at least 3 days.
- After 3 days, may increase dose to 100 mg PO 3 times daily (300 mg/day) with at least 6 hours between doses. Usual target dose is 300 mg/day in 3 divided doses.
- Maximum dose is 450 mg/day given as 150 mg 3 times a day.
- Gradually titrate dose to reduce seizure risk.
- Periodically reassess the dose and need for maintenance treatment.
- Mild-to-moderate hepatic impairment: reduce dose and/or frequency of dosing.
- Renal impairment: reduce dose and/or frequency.
- If after 4 weeks of treatment there is no clinical response, may increase to a maximum of 450 mg/day (150 mg tid).

Drug Preparation:
- Available in 75- and 100-mg tablets.
- Protect tablets from light and moisture.
- Ensure at least 6 hours between doses (optimally, give in morning and evening).

Drug Interactions:
- Because of extensive drug metabolism by liver, when given with other drugs that have hepatic metabolism may have decreased effect of that drug (e.g., carbamazepine, cimetidine, phenobarbital, phenytoin).
- MAOIs may increase drug toxicity.
- Use cautiously in patients receiving L-dopa, starting with small initial dose, and slowly increasing dose.
- Use cautiously in patients receiving other seizure-threshold-lowering drugs, starting with a small initial dose, and slowly and gradually increasing dose.
- Bupropion (Zyban; smoking cessation aid): DO NOT USE TOGETHER, as will increase risk of seizures.

Lab Effects/Interference:
- Rarely, anemia and pancytopenia.

Special Considerations:
- Warnings and Precautions:
  - Seizure risk is dose-related; minimize risk by gradually increasing dose and limiting dose to 450 mg/day. Discontinue if seizures occur.
  - Hypertension: can occur; monitor BP before starting treatment and periodically during treatment.
  - Activation of mania/hypomania: screen patients for bipolar disorder and monitor for these symptoms.

- Psychosis and other neuropsychiatric reactions: Teach patient to contact a healthcare professional right away if this occurs.
- Teach patient to avoid alcohol when taking drug.
- Use cautiously, if at all, in individuals:
  - Who are underweight, as drug may cause weight loss of at least 2.25 kg (5 lb) (28% of patients), and most patients do not gain weight (only 9% of patients gain weight).
  - With a recent history of myocardial infarction or unstable heart disease.
- Drug contains same ingredient found in bupropion, which is used in smoking cessation. DO NOT USE TOGETHER.
- Teach all patients/families to call provider right away if thoughts of suicide or dying; attempts to commit suicide; new or worsening depression; new or worsening anxiety; feeling very agitated or restless; panic attacks; trouble sleeping (insomnia); new or worsening irritability; aggressive, angry, or violent behavior; acting on dangerous impulses; extreme increase in activity or talking (mania); any unusual changes in behavior or mood.

Potential Toxicities/Side Effects and the Nursing Process

I.   ALTERATIONS IN SENSORY/PERCEPTUAL PATTERNS related to RESTLESSNESS, AGITATION, INSOMNIA

Defining Characteristics: Many patients experience increased restlessness, agitation, anxiety, and insomnia, especially after initiation of therapy. This may be severe enough to require treatment with sedative/hypnotic or drug discontinuation. Restlessness, agitation, hostility, decreased concentration, ataxia, incoordination, confusion, paranoia, anxiety, manic episodes in bipolar manic depressives, migraine, insomnia, euphoria, and psychoses may occur. Akathisia, dyskinesia, dystonia, muscle spasms, bradykinesia, and sensory disturbances may occur.

Nursing Implications: Assess baseline gait, neurologic and mental status, and monitor during therapy. Teach patient to report signs/symptoms; discuss benefit/risk ratio with physician. Assess for signs/symptoms of suicidal ideation; if they occur, refer for psychiatric evaluation. Inform patient that drowsiness, dizziness will resolve after 1–2 weeks; instruct to avoid hazardous activities while drowsy (e.g., driving a car, operating machinery). Instruct patient to avoid alcohol ingestion, as this may precipitate seizures.

II.   ALTERATION IN CARDIAC OUTPUT related to CHANGES IN BP, HR

Defining Characteristics: Dizziness, tachycardia, hypertension or hypotension, palpitations, edema, syncope, and cardiac arrhythmias may occur.

Nursing Implications: Assess baseline orthostatic BP, heart rate, presence of peripheral edema, and monitor during therapy. Patient should have a baseline EKG. Instruct patient to report abnormalities including postural dizziness, palpitations. Discuss any significant changes with physician, and discuss interventions. If the patient has had a recent myocardial infarction, expect that dose of drug may be reduced.

MANAGEMENT

III. ALTERATION IN NUTRITION, LESS THAN BODY REQUIREMENTS, related to GI SIDE EFFECTS

Defining Characteristics: Dry mouth, anorexia, nausea, vomiting, diarrhea, constipation, weight loss of up to 2.25 kg (5 lb), dyspepsia, weight gain and increased appetite, increased salivation, taste changes, stomatitis may occur rarely.

Nursing Implications: Assess baseline nutrition and elimination patterns, weight, and monitor during therapy. Discuss abnormalities with physician, and discuss drug modification. Teach patient to self-administer prescribed antiemetics as appropriate. Suggest patient use sugar-free hard candy, frequent ice chips, or artificial saliva for dry mouth.

IV. ALTERATION IN URINARY ELIMINATION related to URINARY RETENTION

Defining Characteristics: Urinary retention, frequency, and nocturia may occur. Increased risk in patients with history of urinary retention.

Nursing Implications: Assess baseline urinary elimination pattern and risk. Assess for urinary retention, and instruct patient to report signs/symptoms. Discuss alternative drug with physician if this occurs.

V. ALTERATIONS IN SKIN INTEGRITY related to ALLERGY

Defining Characteristics: Urticaria, erythema, rash, pruritus may occur.

Nursing Implications: Assess baseline drug allergy history and skin integrity. Instruct patient to report skin changes. If angioedema of face or tongue develops, tell patient to stop drug and discuss drug discontinuance with physician.

VI. POTENTIAL SEXUAL DYSFUNCTION related to IMPOTENCE, IRREGULAR MENSES

Defining Characteristics: Impotence in men and irregular menses in women may occur.

Nursing Considerations: Assess baseline sexual functioning. Inform patient that alterations may occur, and instruct to report them. If severe, discuss dysfunction with physician, and whether another antidepressant would provide equal benefit with less dysfunction.

Drug: buspirone hydrochloride (BuSpar)

Class: Antianxiety agent.

Mechanism of Action: Unclear; drug is considered a midbrain modulator and affects many neurotransmitters (serotonin, dopamine, and cholinergic and noradrenergic systems).

Metabolism: Rapid and complete GI absorption. Food may delay absorption but does not affect total serum drug level. Distributed to body tissues and fluids, especially brain. Metabolized in liver and excreted in urine.

Indication: For the management of anxiety disorders or the short-term relief of symptoms of anxiety.

Dosage/Range:

Adult:
- Oral: 10–15 mg in 2–3 divided doses.
- May be increased in 5-mg increments every 2–4 days to achieve goal (maximum 60 mg/day).
- Maintenance: usual is 5–10 mg tid.

Drug Preparation:
- Store tablets in tight, light-resistant containers at < 30°C (86°F).
- Administer with food.

Drug Interactions:
- MAOIs: increased BP; AVOID CONCURRENT USE.
- Haloperidol: increased haloperidol serum levels; AVOID CONCURRENT USE or reduce haloperidol dose.
- Alcohol: may increase fatigue, drowsiness, dizziness; AVOID CONCURRENT USE.
- Other CNS depressants (analgesics, sedatives): may increase fatigue, drowsiness, dizziness; AVOID CONCURRENT USE.

Lab Effects/Interference:
- None known.

Special Considerations:
- Selective anxiolytic; causes little sedation or psychomotor dysfunction.
- Anxiolytic effect comparable to oral diazepam.
- Onset slower, so patients should be told to expect full anxiolytic effect in 3–4 weeks.
- Use with caution if renal insufficiency; dose-reduce in anuric patients.

Potential Toxicities/Side Effects and the Nursing Process

I.   ALTERATIONS IN SENSORY/PERCEPTUAL PATTERNS related to DIZZINESS, DROWSINESS

Defining Characteristics: Far less sedation than with other anxiolytics. May cause dizziness, drowsiness, headache in 10% of patients; fatigue, nightmares, weakness, paresthesia occur less frequently.

Nursing Implications: Assess baseline neurologic status, and monitor during therapy. Instruct patient to report signs/symptoms, and discuss drug modification with physician. Instruct patient to avoid alcohol while taking drug.

II.   ALTERATION IN NUTRITION, LESS THAN BODY REQUIREMENTS, related to GI SIDE EFFECTS

Defining Characteristics: Nausea occurs in 8% of patients; less common is dry mouth, vomiting, diarrhea, or constipation.

Nursing Implications: Assess baseline nutrition and elimination patterns, and monitor during therapy. Instruct patient to report signs/symptoms.

Drug: citalopram hydrobromide (Celexa)

Class: Antidepressant.

Mechanism of Action: SSRI with unique structure unlike other antidepressants (racemic bicyclic phthalane derivative). Drug inhibits the reuptake of neurotransmitter serotonin in the CNS, thus potentiating serotonin activity in the CNS and relieving depressive symptoms.

Metabolism: Steady-state plasma level reached in 1 week. Bioavailability is 80% following single daily dose, unaffected by food intake, and peak plasma level is reached in 4 hours. Metabolism is primarily hepatic, with a terminal half-life of 25 hours. Renal excretion accounts for 20% of drug excretion. In the elderly, drug is more slowly cleared, with increases in area under the curve (AUC) by 23% and half-life by 30%. Patients with hepatic dysfunction have reduced drug clearance (37%), with half-life of drug extended to 8 hours.

Indication: For the treatment of depression.

Contraindication: (1) concurrent use or within 14 days of using a MAO inhibitor; (2) concurrent use of pimozide; (3) hypersensitivity to citalopram or any of its component elements.

Dosage/Range:

Adult:
- 20 mg daily, increased to 40 mg daily after at least 1 week.
- Patients with hepatic dysfunction, CYP2C19 poor metabolizers, or elderly: 20 mg daily.
- If changing to or from MAOIs therapy, wait at least 14 days between drugs.
- No dose modification for mild or moderate renal impairment; use with caution if at all in patients with severe renal impairment.

Drug Preparation:
- Oral: available in 20-mg (pink) and 40-mg (white) oval, scored tablets.

Drug Administration:
- Administer orally in morning or evening, without regard to food.

Drug Interactions (see package insert):

- MAOIs: potential for serious, sometimes fatal interactions (hyperthermia, rigidity, myoclonus, autonomic instability, mental status changes, including coma). DO NOT USE TOGETHER, and if changing to/from citalopram HBr, drugs MUST be separated by at least 14 days.
- Alcohol: possible potentiation of depression of cognitive and motor function; DO NOT USE TOGETHER.
- Cimetidine: increases AUC of citalopram HBr by 43%. Use together with caution, if at all; assess for toxicity and reduce dose as needed if must use together.
- Lithium: use together cautiously, and monitor serum lithium levels if used together.
- Warfarin: monitor INR, PT closely.
- Carbamazepine, ketoconazole, itraconazole, fluconazole, erythromycin: possible increase in clearance of citalopram HBr, monitor drug effectiveness and increase dose as needed.
- Metoprolol: may increase metoprolol levels; monitor BP and HR.
- TCAs (e.g., imipramine): possible increases in plasma TCA level; use together cautiously, if at all.

Lab Effects/Interference:
- Infrequently, increased liver function tests, alk phos, and abnormal glucose tolerance test.
- Rarely, bilirubinemia, hypokalemia, and hypoglycemia.

Special Considerations:
- At high doses in animals, drug is teratogenic, and, in some tests, mutagenic and carcinogenic (> 20 times the human maximum dose). DO NOT give to pregnant women or nursing mothers.
- Most responses occur within 1–4 weeks of therapy, but if no benefit has yet occurred, patients should be taught to continue taking medicine as prescribed.
- Use cautiously in patients with a seizure disorder, and monitor closely during therapy.
- Teach all patients/families to call provider right away if thoughts of suicide or dying; attempts to commit suicide; new or worsening depression; new or worsening anxiety; feeling very agitated or restless; panic attacks; trouble sleeping (insomnia); new or worsening irritability; aggressive, angry, or violent behavior; acting on dangerous impulses; extreme in activity or talking (mania); any unusual changes in behavior or mood.
- Warnings (see package insert):
  - *Clinical worsening with suicide risk*
  - *QT-prolongation and Torsades de Pointes:* may occur as drug prolongs QTc. Do not administer to patients with congenital long QTc, bradycardia, hypomagnesemia, hypokalemia, recent MI, or uncompensated heart failure. Do not coadminster with drugs that prolong the QTc: certain antiarrythymics, antipsychotic medication, antibiotics (see package insert).
  - *Screening for bipolar disorder*
  - *Serotonin syndrome*
  - *Angle closure glaucoma*

MANAGEMENT

Potential Toxicities/Side Effects and the Nursing Process

I. ALTERATION IN NUTRITION related to GI SIDE EFFECTS

Defining Characteristics: Nausea (21%) and dry mouth (20%) are common. Less common are diarrhea (8%), dyspepsia (5%), vomiting (4%), and abdominal pain (3%). Infrequent are gastritis, stomatitis, erructation, dysphagia, teeth grinding, change in weight, and gingivitis. The following were rare: colitis, cholecystitis, gastroesophageal reflux, diverticulitis, and hiccups.

Nursing Implications: Assess baseline nutrition and elimination patterns, and monitor during therapy. Discuss abnormalities with physician, and discuss drug modification. Teach patient to self-administer prescribed antiemetics as appropriate. Suggest patient use sugar-free hard candy, frequent ice chips, or artificial saliva for dry mouth.

II. ALTERATION IN CARDIAC OUTPUT, POTENTIAL, related to CHANGES IN BLOOD PRESSURE

Defining Characteristics: Tachycardia, postural hypotension, and hypotension are common. The following are infrequent: hypertension, bradycardia, peripheral edema, angina, arrhythmias, flushing, and cardiac failure. Rarely, transient ischemic attacks, phlebitis, changes in cardiac conduction (atrial fibrillation, bundle branch block), and cardiac arrest.

Nursing Implications: Assess baseline orthostatic BP, heart rate, and monitor during therapy. Teach patient to report abnormalities, including postural dizziness, palpitations. Discuss significant changes with physician. If patient has orthostatic hypotension, teach patient to change position slowly and to hold on to support.

III. SENSORY/PERCEPTUAL ALTERATIONS related to CHANGES IN MENTAL STATUS

Defining Characteristics: The following may occur: somnolence (18%), insomnia (15%), agitation (3%), impaired concentration, amnesia, apathy, confusion, taste perversion, abnormal ocular accommodation, and possibly worsening depression and suicide attempt. Infrequently, increased libido, aggressive reaction, depersonalization, hallucination, euphoria, paranoia, emotional lability, and panic reaction may occur.

Nursing Implications: Assess baseline gait, neurologic, affective, and mental status, and monitor during therapy. Teach patient to report signs and symptoms; discuss benefit/risk ratio with physician. Assess for signs and symptoms of suicidal ideation; if they occur, refer for psychiatric evaluation. Teach patient that drowsiness may occur, and teach to avoid hazardous activities while drowsy (e.g., driving a car, operating machinery).

IV.   POTENTIAL FOR INJURY related to DRUG OVERDOSE

Defining Characteristics: Although rare, drug overdoses have resulted in fatalities (total drug 3,920 mg and 2,800 mg in two cases resulting from this drug only) while other total doses of 6,000 have not resulted in death. Symptoms resulting from overdose include dizziness, sweating, nausea, vomiting, tremor, somnolence, sinus tachycardia, amnesia, confusion, coma, convulsions, hyperventilation, cyanosis, rhabdomyolysis, and EKG changes (QT interval prolongation, nodal rhythm, and ventricular arrhythmias).

Nursing Implications: Teach patient self-administration schedule and to keep drug in tightly closed container out of reach of children and pets. Teach patient not to double doses if a dose is missed. Give prescriptions in smallest number of pills possible (e.g., 1 month's worth at a time). In the event of an overdosage, teach patient to come to nearest emergency department where focus is on maintaining a patent airway and oxygenation, gastric evacuation by lavage and use of activated charcoal, and close monitoring of cardiac and overall status. Because of large area of drug distribution, dialysis is unlikely to be beneficial.

V.   ALTERATIONS IN SKIN INTEGRITY related to RASH, SKIN CHANGES

Defining Characteristics: Rash and pruritus may occur. Less commonly, photosensitivity, urticaria, eczema, acne, dermatitis, alopecia, and dry skin may occur. Rarely, angioedema, epidermal necrolysis, erythema multiforme have been reported.

Nursing Implications: Assess baseline skin integrity. Teach patient to report skin changes. If angioedema of face or tongue develops, discuss drug discontinuance with physician. Assess impact of changes on patient and discuss strategies to minimize distress and preserve skin integrity and comfort.

VI.   SEXUAL DYSFUNCTION, POTENTIAL, related to ↓ LIBIDO, IMPOTENCE, ANORGASMIA

Defining Characteristics: While difficult to separate from sexual dysfunction related to depression, the following have been reported in men: decreased ejaculation disorder (6.1%), decreased libido (3.8%), and impotence (2.8%); and in women: decreased libido (1.3%) and anorgasmia (1.1%). Dysmenorrhea and amenorrhea may occur in female patients.

Nursing Implications: Assess baseline sexual functioning. Teach patient that alterations may occur and to report them. If severe, discuss dysfunction with physician and whether an antidepressant other than an SSRI would provide equal benefit with less dysfunction.

MANAGEMENT

VII.   ALTERATION IN URINE ELIMINATION related to CHANGES IN PATTERNS

Defining Characteristics: Polyuria is common. Less commonly, the following may occur: urinary frequency, incontinence, retention, and dysuria. Rarely, hematuria, liguria, pyelonephritis, renal calculus, and renal pain have been reported.

Nursing Implications: Assess baseline urinary elimination pattern and risk for alterations. Assess for changes in urinary elimination and teach patient to report signs and symptoms. Discuss alternative drug with physician if severe or bothersome symptoms occur.

Drug: clonazepam (Klonopin)

Class: Benzodiazepine.

Mechanism of Action: Appears to enhance the activity of GABA, which inhibits neurotransmitter activity in the CNS. Drug is able to suppress absence seizures (petit mal) and decrease the frequency, amplitude, and duration of minor motor seizures. Unclear mechanism in relieving panic episodes.

Metabolism: Completely absorbed after oral administration, with peak plasma levels of 1–2 hours. Drug half-life is 18–60 hours (typically 30–40 hours), and therapeutic serum level is 20–80 ng/mL; 80% protein-bound, metabolized by the liver via the P450 cytochrome enzyme system, and inactive metabolites are excreted in the urine.

Indication: (1) Alone or as an adjunct in the treatment of Lennox–Gastaut syndrome (petit mal), akinetic and myoclonic seizures; (2) panic disorder.

Dosage/Range:

Adult (panic attacks):
- Initial: 0.25 mg bid.
- May increase as needed to target dose of 1 mg/day after at least 3 days on the previous dose. Some individuals may require doses of up to 4 mg/day in divided doses, and dose is titrated up to that dose in increments of 0.125–0.25 mg bid every 3 days until panic disorder is controlled or as limited by side effects.
- Withdrawal of treatment must be gradual, with a decrease of 0.125 mg bid every 3 days until drug is completely withdrawn.

Adult (seizure disorders):
- Initial dose: 1.5 mg/day in 3 divided doses.
- Dosage may be increased in increments of 0.5–1 mg every 3 days until seizures are controlled or as limited by side effects.
- Maximum recommended daily dose is 20 mg/day.

Drug Preparation:
- Oral.
- Available in 0.5-, 1-, and 2-mg tablets.

- Discontinuance of drug when used for panic attacks: gradually discontinue, by 0.125 mg bid every 3 days, until drug is completely withdrawn.

Drug Interactions:
- CNS depressants (narcotics, barbiturates, hypnotics, anxiolytics, phenothiazines): potentiation of CNS depressive effects; use together cautiously, if at all, and monitor patient closely.
- Alcohol: potentiates CNS depressant effects; DO NOT use together.
- Phenobarbital: increases hepatic metabolism of clonazepam so that decreased serum levels lead to decreased clonazepam effect; assess patient for drug efficacy and need for increased drug dose.
- Phenytoin: increased hepatic metabolism of clonazepam so that decreased serum levels lead to decreased clonazepam effect; assess patient for drug efficacy and need for increased drug dose.
- Valproic acid: increased risk of absence seizure activity.

Lab Effects/Interference:
- Rarely, anemia, leukopenia, thrombocytopenia, eosinophilia.
- Transient elevation of liver function studies (serum transaminases and alk phos).

Special Considerations:
- Contraindicated during pregnancy, for breastfeeding mothers, and patients with severe liver dysfunction or acute narrow-angle glaucoma.
- May cause psychological and physical dependency.
- Warnings (see package insert)
  - *Risk from concomitant use with opioids*
  - *Interference with cognitive and motor performance*
  - *Suicidal behavior and ideation*
  - *Withdrawal symptoms*

Potential Toxicities/Side Effects and the Nursing Process

I.   ALTERATIONS IN SENSORY/PERCEPTUAL PATTERNS related to CNS DEPRESSION

Defining Characteristics: CNS depressant effects include drowsiness (37%), and, less commonly, dizziness (8%); abnormal coordination (6%); ataxia (5%); dysarthria (2%); depression (7%); memory disturbance (4%); nervousness (3%); decreased intellectual ability (2%); emotional lability; confusion; paresthesia; feeling of drunkenness; paresis; tremor; head fullness; hyperactivity, or hypoactivity. Rarely, suicidal ideation.

Nursing Implications: Assess baseline gait, neurologic status, affects, and monitor during treatment. Instruct patient to report signs/symptoms, and discuss drug modification with physician. Evaluate patient satisfaction with drug efficacy. Instruct patient to avoid alcohol while taking drug. Instruct patient-prescribed schedule for discontinuing drug when used chronically: assess for signs/symptoms of withdrawal. Assess patient risk for suicide, and if at risk, refer to psychiatry for supportive counseling.

MANAGEMENT

II.   ALTERATION IN NUTRITION, LESS THAN BODY REQUIREMENTS, related to GI SIDE EFFECTS

Defining Characteristics: Constipation (1%), decreased appetite (1%), and less commonly, abdominal pain, flatulence, increased salivation, dyspepsia, decreased appetite; also elevated serum transaminases and alk phos.

Nursing Implications: Assess baseline nutrition and elimination patterns and serum transaminases, alk phos, and monitor during therapy. Assess degree of discomfort and interference with nutrition. Discuss significant abnormalities with physician and discuss drug modification.

III.   INJURY related to DECREASE IN MENTAL ALERTNESS, PHYSICAL COORDINATION

Defining Characteristics: Drug may cause drowsiness, dizziness, and impair physical coordination, mental alertness.

Nursing Implications: Assess other medications that may increase risk (e.g., opiates, phenothiazines) and response to drug. Instruct patient to avoid potentially hazardous activities, including driving a car, operating machinery. Instruct patient to avoid alcohol.

IV.   ALTERATIONS IN CARDIAC OUTPUT related to POSTURAL HYPOTENSION

Defining Characteristics: Drug may cause postural hypotension, palpitations, chest pain, edema.

Nursing Implications: Assess baseline VS, and monitor during therapy. Discuss abnormalities with physician. Instruct patient to report dizziness on standing or other changes, and to change position slowly and hold on to support if this occurs.

V.   ALTERATIONS IN SKIN INTEGRITY related to SKIN DISORDERS

Defining Characteristics: Acne flare, xeroderma, contact dermatitis, pruritus, skin disorders may occur.

Nursing Implications: Assess baseline skin integrity, and instruct patient to report changes. Teach symptomatic skin management, and discuss drug discontinuance with physician if severe.

VI.   SEXUAL DYSFUNCTION related to CHANGES IN LIBIDO, MENSTRUAL IRREGULARITIES

Defining Characteristics: Loss or increase in libido, menstrual irregularities in women; decreased ejaculation in men.

Nursing Implications: Assess baseline sexual functioning. Inform patient that alterations may occur, and instruct to report them. If severe, discuss dysfunction with physician, and whether another antidepressant would provide equal benefit with less dysfunction.

VII. ALTERATION IN ELIMINATION, URINARY, related to DYSURIA, BLADDER DYSFUNCTION

Defining Characteristics: Dysuria, polyuria, cystitis, urinary incontinence, bladder dysfunction, urinary retention, urine discoloration, and urinary bleeding may occur uncommonly.

Nursing Implications: Assess baseline urinary elimination pattern. Instruct patient to report any changes. Discuss impact on patient, and severity, and discuss significant problems with physician.

Drug: desipramine hydrochloride (Norpramin, Pertofrane)

Class: TCA.

Mechanism of Action: Blocks reuptake of neurotransmitters at neuronal membrane, thus increasing available serotonin and norepinephrine in CNS, and potentiating their effects. Appears to have analgesic effect separate from antidepressant action. May increase bioavailability of morphine. Indicated in the treatment of depressive (affective) mood disorders. Also used as an adjuvant analgesic in cancer pain management.

Metabolism: Well absorbed from GI tract. Highly protein-bound. Plasma half-life of 7–60 hours. Metabolized in liver, and primarily excreted in urine.

Indication: For the treatment of depression.

Dosage/Range:

Adult:
- Oral: 75–150 mg hs, or in divided doses.
- May be gradually increased to 300 mg/day if needed.
- Elderly: 25–50 mg/day, maximum 150 mg/day.

Drug Preparation:
- Store in tight containers at < 40°C (104°F).
- Administer as a single bedtime dose.

Drug Interactions:
- MAOIs: increased excitation, hyperpyrexia, seizures; use together cautiously (especially if high dose used).
- Sympathomimetic (epinephrine, amphetamines): increased hypertension; AVOID concurrent use.

- Cimetidine methylphenidate: increased amitriptyline levels, increased toxicity; use cautiously and monitor for increased toxicity.
- Warfarin: may increase PT; monitor closely and decrease dose of warfarin as needed.
- Barbiturates: may decrease desipramine serum level; monitor for decreased antidepressant effect; may need increased dose.
- Alcohol: may antagonize antidepressant effects; AVOID CONCURRENT USE.

Lab Effects/Interference:
- Rarely, altered liver function studies.
- Rarely, increased or decreased serum glucose levels.
- Rarely, increased pancreatic enzymes.
- Rarely, bone marrow depression with agranulocytosis, eosinophilia, purpura, thrombocytopenia.

Special Considerations:
- Antidepressant effect may take 2 weeks or longer.
- Adjuvant analgesic useful in cancer pain management.
- May also decrease depression associated with chronic cancer pain and promote improved sleep.
- Contraindicated in patients with myocardial infarction, seizure disorder, or benign prostatic hypertrophy.
- Use cautiously in patients with urine retention, narrow-angle glaucoma, hyperthyroidism, hepatic dysfunction, or suicidal ideation.
- Drug should be gradually discontinued rather than abruptly withdrawn to prevent anxiety, malaise, dizziness, nausea/vomiting.
- May be helpful in treating hiccups.
- Increased anticholinergic side effects in elderly.
- Teach all patients/families to call provider right away if thoughts of suicide or dying; attempts to commit suicide; new or worsening depression; new or worsening anxiety; feeling very agitated or restless; panic attacks; trouble sleeping (insomnia); new or worsening irritability; aggressive, angry, or violent behavior; acting on dangerous impulses; extreme increase in activity or talking (mania); any unusual changes in behavior or mood.

Potential Toxicities/Side Effects and the Nursing Process

I.   ALTERATIONS IN SENSORY/PERCEPTUAL PATTERNS related to DROWSINESS, EPS

Defining Characteristics: Drowsiness, dizziness, weakness, lethargy, fatigue are common; confusion, disorientation, hallucinations may occur in the elderly. Extrapyramidal symptoms may occur (fine tremor, rigidity, dystonia, dysarthria, dysphagia), as may peripheral neuropathy and blurred vision. Less sedation than amitriptyline.

Nursing Implications: Assess baseline gait, neurologic and mental status, and monitor during therapy. Instruct patient to report signs/symptoms; discuss benefit/risk ratio with physician. Assess for signs/symptoms of suicidal ideation; if they occur, refer for psychiatric evaluation. Inform patient that drowsiness, dizziness will resolve after 1–2 weeks; instruct to avoid hazardous activities while drowsy (e.g., driving a car, operating machinery).

II. ALTERATION IN CARDIAC OUTPUT related to POSTURAL HYPOTENSION, TACHYCARDIA

Defining Characteristics: Postural hypotension, EKG changes, tachycardia, hypertension may occur. Less severe than with other tricyclics.

Nursing Implications: Assess baseline orthostatic BP, heart rate, and monitor during therapy. Instruct patient to report abnormalities, including postural dizziness, palpitations. Drug should be stopped several days before surgery to prevent hypertensive crisis, especially if high dose is used.

III. ALTERATION IN NUTRITION, LESS THAN BODY REQUIREMENTS, related to GI SIDE EFFECTS

Defining Characteristics: Dry mouth, anorexia, nausea, vomiting, diarrhea, abdominal cramping may occur; also, elevated LFTs.

Nursing Implications: Assess baseline nutrition and elimination patterns and LFTs, and monitor during therapy. Discuss abnormalities with physician, and discuss drug modification. Teach patient to self-administer prescribed antiemetics as appropriate. LFTs should be repeated, and if still elevated, the drug should be discontinued. Instruct patient to take full dose at bedtime. Suggest patient use sugar-free hard candy, frequent ice chips, or artificial saliva for dry mouth.

IV. ALTERATION IN URINARY ELIMINATION related to URINARY RETENTION

Defining Characteristics: Urinary retention may occur. Increased risk in patients with history of urinary retention.

Nursing Implications: Assess baseline urinary elimination pattern and risk. Assess for urinary retention, and instruct patient to report signs/symptoms. Discuss alternative drug with physician if this occurs.

V. ALTERATIONS IN SKIN INTEGRITY related to ALLERGY

Defining Characteristics: Urticaria, erythema, rash, and photosensitivity may occur.

Nursing Implications: Assess baseline drug allergy history and skin integrity. Instruct patient to report skin changes. If angioedema of face or tongue develops, discuss drug discontinuance with physician. Instruct patient to avoid sunlight or to use sunblock protection.

MANAGEMENT

Drug: desvenlafaxine succinate extended release (Pristiq)

Class: SNRI antidepressant.

Mechanism of Action: Drug is synthetic active metabolite of venlafaxine. It appears to potentiate neurotransmitter activity by inhibiting neuronal serotonin and norepinephrine reuptake.

Metabolism: Drug is well absorbed after oral administration (80% bioavailability, with mean time to peak plasma level of 7.5 hours after the dose). With once-daily dosing, steady state is reached in 4–5 days. The terminal half-life is 11 hours. Drug is 30% protein-bound. Metabolized primarily by conjugation (UGT isoforms) and to a minor extent through oxidation (CYP3A4); 45% of the drug is excreted unchanged in the urine 72 hours after oral administration. Elimination half-lives significantly prolonged in severe renal dysfunction or end-stage renal disease (ESRD), and thus, dose should be adjusted in this population.

Indication: For the treatment of major depressive disorder.

Contraindication: (1) hypersensitivity to drug, or its excipients, or to venlafaxine HCL; (2) use of MAOIs with drug, or within 7 days of stopping desvenlafaxine succinate due to risk of serotonin syndrome; (d) starting desvenlafaxine succinate in a patient who is being treated with MAOIs such as linezolid or IV methylene blue. Not approved for pediatric use.

Dosage/Range:
- Adult (indicated for the treatment of depression): extended-release tablet 50 mg daily, with or without meals.
- In clinical studies, doses 50–400 mg daily were used. There is no evidence a dose higher than 50 mg daily offers increased benefit.
- Patients with moderate to severe hepatic dysfunction: 50 mg/day. Do not escalate dose > 100 mg.
- Patients with renal impairment:
  - Mild (CrCl 50–80 mL/min): no dose adjustment.
  - Moderate (CrCl 30–50 mL/min) dysfunction: Maximum 50 mg PO daily but do not escalate dose.
  - Severe renal dysfunction (CrCl M 30 mL/min) or ESRD, 50 mg PO every other day; do not escalate dose. Do not give supplemental doses after hemodialysis.
- In older patients, ensure renal function when considering dose.
- Maintenance/continuation/extended treatment: periodically assess need for continued therapy.
- If discontinuing drug, gradually decrease dose to prevent discontinuation symptoms. The 25 mg PO dose is to be used for this for weaning.
- Switching to or from a MAO inhibitor to/from desvenlafaxine succinate: 14 days must separate time of MAOI discontinuation to starting desvenlafaxine succinate, and give at least 7 days after stopping desvenlafaxine succinate before starting the MAOI.
- Use of desvenlafaxine succinate with other MAOIs such as linezolid or methylene blue: see package insert.

Drug Preparation:
- XL capsule available in 25-, 50-, and 100-mg strengths.
- Administer PO daily with or without food at about the same time each day; tablets must be swallowed whole (DO NOT dissolve, crush, divide, or chew).
- Drug can cause HTN: monitor BP and correct HTN before initiating treatment, and monitor BP during therapy.
- When changing from an MAOI to venlafaxine HCl, wait at least 14 days after MAOI is stopped; when stopping desvenlafaxine and beginning an MAOI, wait at least 7 days.
- If drug is discontinued, taper with gradual dose reduction if possible (e.g., decrease frequency).

Drug Interactions:
- MAOIs: tremor, myoclonus, diaphoresis, nausea, vomiting, flushing, dizziness, hyperthermia resembling neuroleptic malignant syndrome, and may be fatal. DO NOT USE TOGETHER. See Administration section.
- CNS-active agents: concomitant use has not been studied; use cautiously and monitor closely if required.
- Serotonergic drugs: use cautiously together if at all, and monitor closely.
- Drugs interfering with hemostasis (aspirin, NSAIDs, warfarin): serotonin important in hemostasis, and when reuptake blocked, risk of upper GI bleeding increased.
  - Aspirin, NSAIDs: increased risk of bleeding; do not use together concomitantly if possible.
  - Warfarin: altered anticoagulant effects, including increased bleeding; monitor INR and signs/symptoms bleeding closely, especially when drug started or stopped.
- Ethanol: no increased impairment, but because of CNS-active drug interaction, patients should be instructed not to drink alcohol.
- Venlafaxine: desvenlafaxine is the active metabolite in venlafaxine, and thus, the patient will overdose; do not coadminister.
- Inhibitors of CYP3A4 (e.g., ketoconazole increases AUC of desvenlafaxine by 43%): may increase serum level of desvenlafaxine, and thus, do not coadminister if possible.
- Drugs metabolized by CYP2D6: concomitant administration with desvenlafaxine may increase concentration of that drug.

Lab Effects/Interference:
- Elevated cholesterol, low-density lipids (LDL), and triglycerides: monitor baseline and throughout therapy.
- Hyponatremia.
- Rare abnormal LFTs, increased prolactin serum level.

Special Considerations:
- Drug is indicated for the treatment of patients with major depressive disorder.
- Avoid drug use during pregnancy and in nursing mothers. Drug exposure to fetus in third trimester resulted in neonates developing complications requiring prolonged hospitalization with respiratory support and tube feedings.
- Contraindicated in patients hypersensitive to desvenlafaxine succinate, venlafaxine HCl, or any excipients of drug; patients receiving MAO inhibitors (see Administration).

- Warnings (see package insert):
  - *Suicidal thoughts and behaviors* in pediatric and young adult patients; screen all patients. Screen for bipolar disorder.
  - Serotonin syndrome: Monitor all patients for the emergence of serotonin syndrome (mental status changes, autonomic instability, neuromuscular symptoms, seizures, and GI symptoms). If symptoms occur, discontinue desvenlafaxine succinate and any concomitant serotonergic agents immediately and manage symptoms as ordered.
  - *Elevated BP:* Use caution and monitor patients closely who have preexisting HTN, cardiovascular or cerebrovascular conditions. Monitor patient BP during therapy.
  - *Increased risk of bleeding:* Concomitant use of aspirin, NSAIDs, warfarin, or other anticoagulants increase the risk. Teach patient to report any bleeding, which is uncommon. If patient is on warfarin, monitor INR closely when starting this desvenlafaxine succinate, titrating, or discontinuing desvenlafaxine succinate.
  - *Angle closure glaucoma:* Avoid drug in patients with untreated narrow angles.
  - Drug can *activate mania/hypomania states.* Use cautiously in patients with bipolar disorder; screen patients initially for bipolar disorder, as drug is not approved for treatment of related depression. The risk of mania is 0.1%. Use cautiously in patients with a history of or family history of mania or hypomania and inform about the risk of activation of mania/hypomania.
  - *Discontinuation syndrome:* Nausea, sweating, dysphoric mood, irritability, agitation, dizziness and other symptoms can occur with abrupt drug cessation. Wean patient off drug to discontinue.
  - *Seizures:* Rarely seizures can occur: use cautiously in patients with a history of seizures.
  - *Hyponatremia* may occur. Monitor patients for this, especially the elderly and patients taking diuretics. Drug may need to be stopped if hyponatremia severe. Teach patients to report symptoms: headache, difficulty concentrating, memory impairment, confusion, weakness, and unsteadiness and increased falls risk. If severe, hallucinations, syncope, seizure, coma, respiratory arrest, or death may occur.
  - Rarely *interstitial lung disease and eosinophilic pneumonia* can occur; if patients develop progressive dyspnea, cough, or chest discomfort, stop drug and fully evaluate patient's pulmonary status.
- Monitor for clinical worsening and suicide risk. Teach all patients/families to call provider right away if thoughts of suicide or dying; attempts to commit suicide; new or worsening depression; new or worsening anxiety; feeling very agitated or restless; panic attacks; trouble sleeping (insomnia); new or worsening irritability; aggressive, angry, or violent behavior; acting on dangerous impulses; extreme increase in activity or talking (mania); any unusual changes in behavior or mood.

Potential Toxicities/Side Effects and the Nursing Process

I.   ALTERATION IN OXYGENATION, POTENTIAL, related to CHANGES IN BP, TACHYCARDIA, HYPERLIPIDEMIA

Defining Characteristics: At all doses, some patients experienced sustained hypertension defined as a treatment-emergent diastolic BP of ≥ 90 and ≥ 10 mm Hg above baseline for three consecutive visits. This occurred at all doses with the following incidence: placebo 0.5%, 50 mg/day: 1.3%, 100 mg/day: 0.7%, 200 mg/day, 1.1%, and 400 mg/day 2.3%. Orthostatic hypotension also occurred. Rarely, small increases in heart rate occurred in patients during clinical studies (incidence 1–2%). Patients with a history of MI, unstable heart disease, uncontrolled HTN were excluded from studies. Dose-related increases in LDL, total serum cholesterol, and triglycerides were seen during clinical studies, affecting 3–10% of patients depending on dose.

Nursing Implications: Assess baseline weight, cardiac status and BP at each visit. If BP elevated, reassess × 3, and if patient has three successive episodes as defined previously here, discuss dose reduction or change to another antidepressant with physician. Teach patient to change position slowly as risk of orthostatic hypotension. Instruct patient to report any headache, edema, palpitations, chest pain, or any changes in condition. Discuss any symptoms with the physician depending on severity. Monitor baseline cholesterol, LDL, and triglycerides, and monitor during therapy.

II. ALTERATIONS IN SENSORY/PERCEPTUAL PATTERNS related to DIZZINESS, INSOMNIA, SOMNOLENCE, ANXIETY

Defining Characteristics: Infrequently, dizziness, fatigue, or somnolence can occur. Insomnia occurs in 9–15% of patients depending on dose. Anxiety occurs in 3–5% of patients. Rarely, blurred vision, mydriasis (2% incidence at 50-mg dose and 6% at 400-mg dose), tinnitus, taste perversion, irritability, manic or hypomanic reaction, seizure, depersonalization, syncope, extrapyramidal disorder, and abnormal dreams may occur.

Nursing Implications: Assess baseline neurologic status, affective state, and risk factors, and monitor during treatment. Instruct patient to avoid alcohol while taking drug. Assess effect on older persons and/or patients with hepatic or renal dysfunction. Assess for symptoms at each visit, and instruct patient to report changes. If symptoms occur, discuss strategies to ensure patient safety and comfort.

III. ALTERATION IN NUTRITION, LESS THAN BODY REQUIREMENTS, related to GI SIDE EFFECTS, HYPONATREMIA

Defining Characteristics: Nausea (22–41% of patients), vomiting (3–9% compared with 3% placebo), dry mouth (11–25%), diarrhea (11%), constipation (9–14%), and decreased appetite (5–10%). Hyponatremia is rare and appears related to syndrome of inappropriate antidiuretic hormone (SIADH). Rarely, cases of serum sodium < 110 mmol/L have occurred. Patients at risk are older persons who are volume-depleted or on diuretic therapy.

Nursing Implications: Assess baseline nutrition and gastrointestinal functional status, and instruct the patient to report any GI disturbances or changes. Discuss measures to reduce nausea and/or stimulate appetite. Assess baseline serum sodium and risk factors for developing hyponatremia (SIADH), and monitor closely during therapy. Teach patients at risk signs and symptoms (headache, difficulty concentrating, memory impairment, confusion,

MANAGEMENT

weakness and unsteadiness; severe signs and symptoms are hallucination, syncope, seizure, coma) and to call their provider (mild) or to come to the emergency room or clinic right away (severe) if they occur.

IV.   SEXUAL DYSFUNCTION, POTENTIAL, related to EJACULATORY DISTURBANCES

Defining Characteristics: Anorgasmia occurred in 0% at the 50-mg dose, 3% at the 100-mg dose, 5% at 200-mg dose, and 8% at 400-mg dose; decreased libido in 3–6% of patients, abnormal orgasm in 1–3%, and delayed ejaculation in 1–7% of patients; and ejaculation dysfunction in 3–11% of patients depending on the dose. Women rarely experienced anorgasmia (1–3%).

Nursing Implications: Assess baseline sexual functioning. Inform patient that alterations may occur, and instruct to report them. If severe, discuss dysfunction with physician and whether another antidepressant would provide equal benefit with less dysfunction.

V.   ALTERATION IN COMFORT related to HYPERHIDROSIS, HEADACHE

Defining Characteristics: Hyperhidrosis (excessive sweating) occurs in 10% at a 50-mg dose, 18% at 200-mg dose, and 21% at a 400-mg dose. Headache may occur uncommonly.

Nursing Implications: Assess baseline comfort level. Instruct patient to report any changes in comfort, and discuss strategies to reduce discomfort. If hyperhidrosis is severe, teach patient to change clothes frequently to see if this increases comfort.

Drug: diazepam (Valium)

Class: Benzodiazepine (anxiolytic).

Mechanism of Action: Binds to benzodiazepine receptors in the CNS (limbic and cortical areas, cerebellum, brain stem, and spinal cord), resulting in the following effects: anxiolytic, ataxia, anticonvulsant, muscle relaxation. Appears to potentiate the effects of GABA.

Metabolism: Well absorbed from GI tract. Widely distributed in body tissues and fluids, including CSF. Crosses placenta and is excreted in breastmilk. Highly bound to plasma proteins. Metabolized in liver and excreted in urine. Half-life of 20–80 hours. May produce psychological and physical dependence. Indicated for management of anxiety, the relief of reflex spasm or spasticity, and as an anticonvulsant for termination of status epilepticus.

Indication: (1) Management of anxiety disorders or for the short-term relief of anxiety symptoms; (2) acute alcohol withdrawal; (3) relief of skeletal muscle spasm due to reflex spasm; (4) adjunctive in the management of convulsive disorders.

Dosage/Range:

Adult:
- Oral: 2–10 mg tid–qid or 15–30 mg/day extended-release preparation.
- Intravenous (IV) (tension): 5–10 mg IV, maximum 30 mg/8 hours.
- IV (seizures): 5–10 mg IV, maximum 30 mg; may repeat in 2–4 hours if needed.
- IV (status epilepticus): 5–20 mg slow IV push (IVP) (2–5 mg/min), q 5–10 minutes, maximum 60 mg.
- IV (elderly, debilitated): 2–5 mg slow IVP.

Drug Preparation:
- Oral: protect tablets from light and store at 15–30°C (59–86°F).
- IV: Do not administer with other drugs; drug may absorb to sides of plastic syringe or to plastic IV bag and tubing if added to IV infusion bag; consult hospital pharmacist for IV infusion protocol; administer IVP slowly 2–5 mg/min; have emergency equipment available.

Drug Interactions:
- CNS depressants (alcohol, anticonvulsants, phenothiazines, opiates): additive CNS depression; avoid concurrent use or use cautiously and monitor carefully.
- Oral contraceptives, isoniazid, ketoconazole, or cimetidine: decrease plasma clearance of diazepam so may increase effect (e.g., sedation); monitor patient closely.
- TCAs: increased serum levels of antidepressant possible; use together cautiously.
- Digoxin: may decrease renal excretion of digoxin; monitor for overdosage; may need to decrease digoxin.
- Levodopa: may decrease levodopa effect; monitor patient response; may have to increase levodopa dose.

Lab Effects/Interference:
- Rarely, altered liver function studies.
- Rarely, neutropenia.

Special Considerations:
- Wide margin of safety between therapeutic and toxic doses.
- May impair ability to perform activities requiring mental alertness (e.g., driving a car, operating machinery).
- May produce psychological and physical dependence.
- Administer cautiously in patients with liver or renal impairment.
- Use cautiously in patients with chronic pulmonary disease or sleep apnea.
- Contraindicated in patients with depressive neuroses, psychotic reactions (without prominent anxiety), acute alcoholic intoxication (with depressed VS), known hypersensitivity to the drug, or acute angle-closure glaucoma.
- May cause fetal damage, so should not be used during pregnancy or if the mother is breastfeeding.
- Withdrawal symptoms (including seizure, delirium) can occur with rapid drug discontinuance in patients taking high or chronic doses.

MANAGEMENT

Potential Toxicities/Side Effects and the Nursing Process

I.   ALTERATIONS IN SENSORY/PERCEPTUAL PATTERNS related to CNS DEPRESSION

Defining Characteristics: CNS depressant effects include drowsiness, fatigue, lethargy, confusion, weakness, headache, which may occur initially and resolve with continued therapy or dose reduction. Vivid dreams, visual disturbances, slurred speech, "hangover," and bizarre behavior may also occur. Patient risk factors: elderly, debilitated, liver dysfunction, low serum albumin.

Nursing Implications: Assess baseline neurologic status and risk factors, and monitor during treatment. Instruct patient to report signs/symptoms and discuss drug modification with physician. Evaluate patient satisfaction with drug efficacy. Instruct patient to avoid alcohol while taking drug. Teach patient prescribed schedule for discontinuing drug when used chronically: assess for signs/symptoms of withdrawal (increased anxiety, rebound insomnia; may also include agitation, dysphoria, nausea/vomiting, irritability, muscle cramps, hallucinations, seizures).

II.   ALTERATION IN NUTRITION, LESS THAN BODY REQUIREMENTS, related to GI SIDE EFFECTS

Defining Characteristics: Nausea, vomiting, abdominal discomfort may occur; also, elevated LFTs.

Nursing Implications: Assess baseline nutrition and elimination patterns and LFTs, and monitor during therapy. Discuss abnormalities with physician and discuss drug modification. Teach patient to self-administer prescribed antiemetics as appropriate.

III.   INJURY related to DECREASE IN MENTAL ALERTNESS, PHYSICAL COORDINATION

Defining Characteristics: Drug may cause drowsiness, dizziness, and impair physical coordination, mental alertness.

Nursing Implications: Assess other medications that may increase risk (e.g., opiates, phenothiazines) and response to drug. Instruct patient to avoid potentially hazardous activities, including driving a car, operating machinery.

IV.   ALTERATIONS IN PERFUSION related to CARDIOPULMONARY COMPROMISE

Defining Characteristics: Drug may cause transient hypotension, bradycardia, cardiovascular collapse, respiratory depression.

Nursing Implications: Assess baseline VS; have resuscitation equipment nearby. Monitor q 5–15 min and before IV dose of drug. Discuss abnormalities with physician.

V. ALTERATIONS IN SKIN INTEGRITY related to RASH

Defining Characteristics: Urticaria, rash may occur; also phlebitis, pain at injection site.

Nursing Implications: Assess baseline skin integrity, and instruct patient to report changes. Teach symptomatic skin management, and discuss drug discontinuance with physician if severe. Assess IV site for evidence of pain, phlebitis, and change site; apply heat as needed.

Drug: doxepin hydrochloride (Sinequan)

Class: Antidepressant of the dibenzoxepine tricyclic class.

Mechanism of Action: Appears to exert adrenergic effect at the synapses, preventing deactivation of norepinephrine by reuptake into the nerve terminals.

Metabolism: Metabolized in the liver by the P450 enzyme system, into active metabolite. Effective serum level of doxepin and metabolite is 100–200 mg/mL. Takes 2–8 days to reach steady state.

Indication: For the relief of depression; relief of insomnia.

Dosage/Range:

Adult:
- Initial dose of 75 mg/day is recommended; in elderly, dose should start at 25–50 mg/day.
- Dose may be titrated up or down based on response. Usual dose is 75–150 mg/day. Patients with mild symptoms may require only 25–50 mg/day.
- Patients with severe symptoms may require gradual titration up to 300 mg/day.

Drug Preparation:
- Oral, taken in a single dose (maximum 150-mg dose) or in divided doses. Single dose given at bedtime enhances sleep.
- Available in 10-, 25-, 50-, 75-, 100-, and 150-mg capsules.
- If changing a patient from MAOI to doxepin HCl, wait at least 14 days before the careful initiation of doxepin.

Drug Interactions:
- Alcohol: do not use concomitantly, as increases drug toxicity.
- MAOI: severe reaction, including death may occur; DO NOT USE TOGETHER.
- Cimetidine: increased serum levels of drug and anticholinergic side effects (severe dry mouth, urinary retention, blurred vision); avoid concurrent use.
- Tolazamide: may cause severe hypoglycemia; monitor patient's serum glucose carefully.

Lab Effects/Interference:

- Rarely, eosinophilia, bone marrow depression (e.g., agranulocytosis, leukopenia, thrombocytopenia, purpura).
- Increased or decreased blood glucose levels.

Special Considerations:

- Contraindicated in patients with glaucoma or urinary retention.
- Antianxiety effect appears before the antidepressant effect, which takes 2–3 weeks.
- Most sedating of antidepressants, so useful in enhancing sleep, and single dose (up to 150 mg) should be taken at bedtime.
- Recommended for the treatment of depression accompanied by anxiety and insomnia, depression associated with organic illness or alcohol, psychotic depressive disorders with associated anxiety.
- Teach all patients/families to call provider right away if thoughts of suicide or dying; attempts to commit suicide; new or worsening depression; new or worsening anxiety; feeling very agitated or restless; panic attacks; trouble sleeping (insomnia); new or worsening irritability; aggressive, angry, or violent behavior; acting on dangerous impulses; extreme increase in activity or talking (mania); any unusual changes in behavior or mood.
- Doxepin has been studied, and it has been found to reduce pruritis from EGFRI rash (Lacouture et al., 2011).

Potential Toxicities/Side Effects and the Nursing Process

I. ALTERATIONS IN SENSORY/PERCEPTUAL related to DROWSINESS, EPS

Defining Characteristics: Drowsiness, which may disappear as therapy continues. Rarely, dizziness, confusion, disorientation, hallucinations, numbness, paresthesia, ataxia, extrapyramidal symptoms, seizures, blurred vision, tardive dyskinesia, tremor may occur.

Nursing Implications: Assess baseline gait, neurologic, affective and mental status, and monitor during therapy. Instruct patient to report signs/symptoms; discuss benefit/risk ratio with physician and measures to reduce extrapyramidal side effects if they occur. Assess for signs/symptoms of suicidal ideation; if they occur, refer for psychiatric evaluation. Inform patient that drowsiness will decrease after 1–2 weeks, and instruct to avoid hazardous activities while drowsy (e.g., driving a car, operating machinery). Instruct patient to avoid alcohol while taking drug.

II. ALTERATION IN CARDIAC OUTPUT related to BLOOD PRESSURE CHANGES

Defining Characteristics: Hypotension or hypertension, tachycardia may occur.

Nursing Implications: Assess baseline orthostatic BP, heart rate, and monitor during therapy. Instruct patient to report abnormalities, including postural dizziness, palpitations.

III. ALTERATION IN NUTRITION, LESS THAN BODY REQUIREMENTS, related to GI SIDE EFFECTS

Defining Characteristics: Dry mouth, anorexia, nausea, vomiting, diarrhea, indigestion, taste changes, aphthous stomatitis may occur rarely.

Nursing Implications: Assess baseline nutrition and elimination patterns. Discuss abnormalities with physician, and discuss drug modification. Teach patient to self-administer prescribed antiemetics as appropriate. Instruct patient to take full dose at bedtime (if 150 mg or less). Suggest patient to use sugar-free hard candy, frequent ice chips, or artificial saliva for dry mouth.

IV. ALTERATION IN URINARY ELIMINATION related to URINARY RETENTION

Defining Characteristics: Urinary retention may occur. Increased risk in patients with history of urinary retention.

Nursing Implications: Assess baseline urinary elimination pattern and risk. Assess for urinary retention, and instruct patient to report signs/symptoms. Discuss alternative drug with physician if this occurs.

V. ALTERATIONS IN SKIN INTEGRITY related to ALLERGY

Defining Characteristics: Urticaria, erythema, rash, and photosensitivity may occur.

Nursing Implications: Assess baseline drug allergy history and skin integrity. Instruct patient to report skin changes. If severe changes occur, discuss drug discontinuance with physician. Instruct patient to avoid sunlight or to use sunblock protection.

VI. SEXUAL DYSFUNCTION related to CHANGES IN LIBIDO

Defining Characteristics: Increased or decreased libido, testicular swelling, gynecomastia in males; enlargement of breasts and galactorrhea in women.

Nursing Implications: Assess baseline sexual functioning. Inform patient that alterations may occur, and instruct to report them. If severe, discuss dysfunction with physician and whether another antidepressant would provide equal benefit with less dysfunction.

Drug: duloxetine hydrochloride (Cymbalta)

Class: Antidepressant.

Mechanism of Action: Selective serotonin and norepinephrine uptake inhibitor (SSNRI), resulting in potentiation of serotonergic and noradrenergic activity in the CNS, and antidepressant, central pain inhibition, and anxiolytic qualities.

MANAGEMENT

Metabolism: After oral ingestion, drug undergoes extensive metabolism, but metabolites do not appear to contribute to the drug effect. The drug is highly protein-bound. Elimination half-life is about 12 hours, achieving steady-state plasma levels in 3 days of dosing. When taken with food, the time to reach peak concentration increases from 6 to 10 hours and reduces absorption by about 10%. When the drug is taken in the evening, there is a 3-hour delay in absorption and a 33% increase in drug clearance compared with taking the drug in the morning. The drug is metabolized by the CYP1A2 and CYP2D6P450 hepatic enzymes. Metabolites are excreted in the urine primarily (70%) with 20% excreted in the feces. Drug AUC is about 25% higher, and the half-life of the drug about 4 hours longer in older women. Smoking reduces the bioavailability by 33%, but the manufacturer does not recommend dose modification in smokers. Drug is not recommended for patients with severe renal impairment (urinary creatinine clearance < 30 mL/min), including patients on dialysis or patients with hepatic insufficiency.

Indication: (1) Major depressive disorder; (2) generalized anxiety disorder; (3) diabetic peripheral neuropathic pain; (4) fibromyalgia; (5) chronic musculoskeletal pain.

Dosage/Range:

Adult (depression):
- 20 mg orally twice daily to 60 mg/day (given either once a day or as 30 mg twice daily) without regard to meals.

Adult (diabetic peripheral neuropathy):
- 60 mg orally once daily without regard to meals (start with a lower dose if renal impairment and gradually increase dose).

Adult (generalized anxiety disorder):
- 60 mg orally once daily without regard to meals.

Drug Preparation:
- Oral, available as delayed release capsules in 20-, 30-, and 60-mg strengths.
- When discontinuing fluoxetine, the drug should be gradually reduced in dose (tapered), as otherwise, discontinuation symptoms such as dizziness, nausea, headache, paresthesia, vomiting, irritability, nightmares, insomnia, diarrhea, anxiety, hyperhidrosis, and vertigo may occur.
- Allow at least 14 days between stopping an MAOI and beginning fluoxetine; when stopping fluoxetine to begin an MAOI, wait at least 5 days after stopping fluoxetine before beginning the MAOI.

Drug Interactions:
- CYP1A2 inhibitors (cimetidine, ciprofloxacin, levofloxacin, enoxacin): increased serum levels and terminal half-life of duloxetine; avoid concurrent administration.
- CYP2D6 inhibitors (paroxetine, quinidine): increased duloxetine serum levels by 60%; avoid concurrent use.
- Drugs metabolized by CYP1A2: no effect on the other drugs.
- Drugs metabolized by CYP2D6 (TCAs, phenothiazines, type 1C antiarrhythmics such as propafenone and flecainide): increased serum levels of these drugs; use together

cautiously if at all and monitor TCA serum levels; do not give concurrently with thioridazine as increased risk of ventricular arrhythmias and sudden death.

- Alcohol: DO NOT USE CONCOMITANTLY, as this may increase the risk of hepatic injury in heavy alcohol imbibers.
- CNS-acting drugs: use together cautiously, if at all.
- Serotonergic drugs (triptans, linezolid, lithium, tramadol, St. John's wort): increased risk for serotonin syndrome (mental status changes such as agitation, hallucinations, coma); autonomic instability such as tachycardia, labile BP, hyperthermia; neuromuscular aberrations such as hyperreflexia, incoordination; and/or GI symptoms such as nausea, vomiting, diarrhea. DO NOT use concurrently.
- Drugs that affect gastric acidity: drug requires a pH of 5.5 to dissolve the enteric coating. No effect with magnesium or aluminum containing antacids, but caution advised in patients with slow gastric emptying (diabetics). It is not known whether concurrent administration with proton-pump inhibitors affects drug absorption.
- MAOIs: when drug is given concomitantly or within a short time period, severe, potentially life-threatening interactions may occur, including symptoms resembling neuroleptic malignant syndrome. DO NOT GIVE TOGETHER, AND END SEPARATELY, as stated in the Administration section.

Lab Effects/Interference:
- Increased liver transaminases.
- Rare anemia, leucopenia, thrombocytopenia.
- Rare hypercholesteremia, hyperlipidemia, hypoglycemia, dyslipidemia, hypertriglyceridemia.
- Rare increased serum creatinine.

Special Considerations:
- Duloxetine significantly reduced painful chemotherapy-induced peripheral neuropathy compared to placebo (Smith et al., 2013).
- FDA-approved for the treatment of major depressive disorder, the management of neuropathic pain associated with diabetic peripheral neuropathy, and the treatment of generalized anxiety disorder (associated with at least three symptoms such as restlessness, easy fatigability, difficulty concentrating, irritability, muscle tension, and/or sleep disturbance).
- Contraindicated in patients who are (1) taking MAOIs, (2) have uncontrolled narrow-angle glaucoma, (3) have ESRD or severe renal impairment (urinary creatinine clearance < 30 mL/min), (4) have hepatic insufficiency, and (5) nursing mothers.
- Women who are pregnant in the third trimester: neonates exposed to SSRIs, SNRIs developed complications requiring prolonged hospitalization; must consider risk versus benefit, and consider tapering drug during third trimester.
- Increased risk of suicidality (thinking and behavior) in young adults aged 18–24 years, as well as children and adolescents, especially during the first 2 months of treatment; monitor closely for signs/symptoms of suicidality (emergency of agitation, irritability, unusual changes in behavior, emergence of suicidality).
- Teach all patients/families to call provider right away if thoughts of suicide or dying; attempts to commit suicide; new or worsening depression; new or worsening anxiety; feeling very agitated or restless; panic attacks; trouble sleeping (insomnia); new or worsening irritability; aggressive, angry, or violent behavior; acting on dangerous impulses; extreme increase in activity or talking (mania); any unusual changes in behavior or mood.

MANAGEMENT

Potential Toxicities/Side Effects and the Nursing Process

I.   ALTERATIONS IN SENSORY/PERCEPTUAL PATTERNS related to CNS EFFECTS

Defining Characteristics: Blurred vision, vertigo, lethargy, dizziness, somnolence, tremor, paresthesia/hypoesthesia, hot flushes, agitation, anxiety, nervousness, nightmare/abnormal dreams, sleep disorder may occur in at least 1 of 100 patients. Patients aged 18–24 years are at risk for suicide, or others at risk for suicide may commit suicide during initial period of treatment.

Nursing Implications: Assess baseline neurologic status and risk factors, and monitor during treatment. Instruct patient to report signs/symptoms, and discuss drug modification with physician. Evaluate patient satisfaction with drug efficacy. Instruct patient to avoid alcohol while taking drug. Assess suicide risk, and if at high risk, monitor closely and provide supportive counseling and referral to a psychiatrist. The patient should receive only a small number of pills to prevent overdose.

II.   ALTERATION IN NUTRITION, LESS THAN BODY REQUIREMENTS, related to GI SIDE EFFECTS

Defining Characteristics: Nausea and less commonly vomiting, diarrhea, constipation, dry mouth, dyspepsia, anorexia, abdominal discomfort, flatulence, taste changes, and gastroenteritis may occur.

Nursing Implications: Assess baseline nutrition and elimination patterns. Discuss abnormalities with physician and discuss drug modification. Teach patient to self-administer prescribed antiemetics as appropriate. If patient is losing weight, instruct patient to report this and involve nutritionist in care.

III.   SEXUAL DYSFUNCTION, POTENTIAL, related to IMPOTENCE

Defining Characteristics: Sexual dysfunction and anorgasmia and erectile dysfunction in men can occur uncommonly.

Nursing Implications: Assess baseline sexual functioning. Inform patient that alterations may rarely occur and that they should be reported. If severe, discuss dysfunction with a physician and whether another antidepressant would provide equal benefit with less dysfunction.

Drug: escitalopram oxalate (Lexapro)

Class: Antidepressant.

Mechanism of Action: Selective inhibitor of neuronal reuptake of serotonin (SSRI) in the CNS, resulting in potentiation of serotonin activity in the CNS; has minimal effect on reuptake of norepinephrine or dopamine.

Metabolism: After oral administration, 80% of the drug is absorbed, with peak plasma levels in 5 hours and steady-state plasma concentrations in about 1 week. Drug is 56% bound to plasma proteins. The terminal half-life of the drug is 27–32 hours. Drug undergoes hepatic biotransformation, with CYP3A4 and CYP2C19 liver microsomes primarily involved in drug metabolism. Bioavailability of tablet is the same as the oral solution.

Indication: For the acute and maintenance treatment of major depressive disorder; acute treatment of generalized anxiety disorder.

Dosage/Range:
- Recommended dose is 10 mg/day orally (20 mg daily has not shown improved benefit); however, if dose is increased to 20 mg daily, wait at least 1 week before increasing the dose.

Drug Preparation:
- Available in 5-, 10-, and 20-mg tablets, as well as 5-mg/5-mL oral solution.
- May be given in morning or evening and with or without food.
- When discontinuing drug, the dose should be gradually tapered rather than abruptly stopped.

Drug Interactions:
- CYP1A2 inhibitors (cimetidine): increased serum levels of escitalopram oxalate by 43%; avoid concurrent administration.
- Drugs metabolized by CYP2D6 (TCAs, phenothiazines, metoprolol): possible, increased serum levels of these drugs; use together cautiously and monitor TCA serum levels.
- Alcohol: DO NOT USE CONCOMITANTLY, as this may increase the risk of hepatic injury in heavy alcohol imbibers.
- CNS-acting drugs: use together cautiously, if at all.
- Serotonergic drugs (triptans, linezolid, lithium, tramadol, St. John's wort): increased risk for serotonin syndrome (mental status changes such as agitation, hallucinations, coma); autonomic instability such as tachycardia, labile BP, hyperthermia; neuromuscular aberrations such as hyperreflexia, incoordination; and/or GI symptoms such as nausea, vomiting, diarrhea. DO NOT use concurrently.
- Drugs that interfere with hemostasis (NSAIDs, aspirin, warfarin): increased risk of upper-GI bleeding; use cautiously, if at all, and monitor closely.
- MAOIs: when drug is given concomitantly or within a short time period, severe, potentially life-threatening interactions may occur, including symptoms resembling neuroleptic malignant syndrome. DO NOT GIVE TOGETHER AND END SEPARATELY, as stated in the Administration section.
- Lithium: enhanced serotonergic effects, monitor patient closely; monitor lithium levels.
- Pimozide: increased QTc by 10 msec; avoid concurrent use.
- Sumatriptan: weakness, hyperreflexia, and incoordination; avoid concurrent use.

Lab Effects/Interference:
- None known.

Special Considerations:
- FDA approved for the treatment of major depressive disorder, the management of neuropathic pain associated with diabetic peripheral neuropathy, and the treatment of

generalized anxiety disorder (associated with at least three symptoms, such as restlessness, easy fatigability, difficulty concentrating, irritability, muscle tension, and/or sleep disturbance).

- Contraindicated in patients who are (1) taking MAOIs, (2) have uncontrolled narrow-angle glaucoma, (3) have ESRD or severe renal impairment (urinary creatinine clearance < 30 mL/min), (4) have hepatic insufficiency, and (5) nursing mothers.
- Women who are pregnant in the third trimester: neonates exposed to SSRIs, SNRIs developed complications requiring prolonged hospitalization; must consider risk versus benefit and consider tapering drug during third trimester.
- Increased risk of suicidality (thinking and behavior) in young adults aged 18–24, as well as children and adolescents, especially during the first 2 months of treatment; monitor closely for signs/symptoms of suicidality (emergency of agitation, irritability, unusual changes in behavior, emergence of suicidality).
- Teach all patients/families to call provider right away if thoughts of suicide or dying; attempts to commit suicide; new or worsening depression; new or worsening anxiety; feeling very agitated or restless; panic attacks; trouble sleeping (insomnia); new or worsening irritability; aggressive, angry, or violent behavior; acting on dangerous impulses; extreme increase in activity or talking (mania); any unusual changes in behavior or mood.

Potential Toxicities/Side Effects and the Nursing Process

I.   ALTERATIONS IN SENSORY/PERCEPTUAL PATTERNS related to CNS EFFECTS

Defining Characteristics: Somnolence (13%), insomnia (12%), abnormal dreaming (3%), lethargy (3%), and dizziness (2%) may occur. Patients age 18–24 years are at risk for suicide, or others at risk for suicide may commit suicide during initial period of treatment.

Nursing Implications: Assess baseline neurologic status, sleep patterns, and risk factors, and monitor during treatment. Instruct patient to report signs/symptoms, and discuss drug modification with physician. Evaluate patient satisfaction with drug efficacy. Instruct patient to avoid alcohol while taking drug. Assess suicide risk, and if at high risk, monitor closely and provide supportive counseling and referral to a psychiatrist. The patient should receive only a small number of pills to prevent overdose.

II.   ALTERATION IN NUTRITION, LESS THAN BODY REQUIREMENTS, related to GI SIDE EFFECTS

Defining Characteristics: Nausea (18%), dry mouth (9%), diarrhea (8%), constipation (5%), indigestion (3%), vomiting (3%), and rarely abdominal discomfort and flatulence may occur. Weight changes were no different from placebo group.

Nursing Implications: Assess baseline nutrition and elimination patterns. Discuss abnormalities with physician, and discuss drug modification. Teach patient to self-administer prescribed antiemetics as appropriate. If patient is losing weight, instruct patient to report this and involve nutritionist in care.

III. SEXUAL DYSFUNCTION, POTENTIAL, related to IMPOTENCE

Defining Characteristics: Sexual dysfunction, including ejaculation disorder (primarily ejaculatory delay), decreased libido, and impotence in men and decreased libido and anorgasmia in women can occur uncommonly. SSRIs have a rare incidence of priapism.

Nursing Implications: Assess baseline sexual functioning. Inform patient that alterations may rarely occur and should be reported. If severe, discuss dysfunction with physician and whether another antidepressant would provide equal benefit with less dysfunction.

Drug: fluoxetine hydrochloride (Prozac)

Class: Antidepressant.

Mechanism of Action: Inhibits CNS neuronal uptake of serotonin.

Metabolism: Well absorbed after oral administration, and peak serum levels occur in 6–8 hours. Peak plasma concentrations are 15–55 mg/mL. Time to steady state in serum level is 2–4 weeks; 94.5% protein-bound. Drug is extensively metabolized in the liver to norfluoxetine and other metabolites using P450 enzyme pathway; inactive metabolites are excreted in the urine. Elimination half-life is 1–3 days when administered acutely, and 4–6 days with chronic administration.

Indication: For the treatment of (1) major depressive disorder; (2) panic disorder.

Dosage/Range:

Adult (for depression):
- 20 mg/day initially.
- After several weeks of therapy, if no response, may increase dose gradually to a maximum dose of 80 mg/day.
- Patients with hepatic dysfunction, elderly, or patients with concurrent diseases: start at lower dose or give less frequently.
- Weekly 90-mg tablets: begin 7 days after last 20-mg daily dose.

Drug Preparation:
- Give orally with or without food in the morning; with higher doses, for example, 80 mg/ day, may give 2 doses, 1 in the morning and 1 at noon.
- Available in pulvules of 10 and 20 mg; liquid/oral solution available as 20 mg/5 mL; weekly 90-mg tablets.
- Allow at least 14 days between stopping an MAOI and beginning fluoxetine; when stopping fluoxetine to begin an MAOI, wait at least 5 weeks before beginning the MAOI.

Drug Interactions:
- Alcohol: DO NOT USE CONCOMITANTLY, as increases impaired judgment, thinking, and motor skills.

MANAGEMENT

- TCAs: decreased metabolism and increased serum levels of TCA; monitor for increased toxicity and dose-reduce TCA as necessary when drug is given concomitantly with fluoxetine.
- MAOIs: when drug is given concomitantly or within a short time period, severe, potentially life-threatening interactions may occur, including symptoms resembling neuroleptic malignant syndrome. DO NOT GIVE TOGETHER, AND END SEPARATELY, as stated in Administration section.
- Buspirone: reduced effects of buspirone; assess need to increase dose.
- Carbamazepine: increased serum levels of carbamazepine, with potential increased toxicity; monitor closely and dose-reduce as necessary.
- Cyproheptadine: decreased fluoxetine serum levels, so that effect was reduced or reversed; avoid concomitant administration if possible.
- Dextromethorphan: increased risk of hallucinations.
- Diazepam: increased diazepam half-life with increased circulating serum levels, leading to increased toxicity (e.g., excessive sedation or impaired psychomotor skills); dose-reduce diazepam or avoid concurrent administration.
- Digoxin: displaces fluoxetine from plasma protein binding, leading to increased fluoxetine serum levels and effect; monitor for toxicity and dose reduce as necessary.
- Lithium: increased lithium serum levels leading to possible increased neurotoxicity; monitor patient closely, and reduce lithium dose as needed.
- Phenytoin: increased phenytoin serum levels; monitor effect and serum levels, and modify dose accordingly.
- Tamoxifen: study indicates that taking this drug with tamoxifen may negate the benefit of tamoxifen; do not use together. Tamoxifen is a prodrug that requires metabolism by the CYP2D6 enzymes, which are inhibited by SSRIs including fluoxetine hydrochloride.
- Thioridazine: DO NOT administer together. Discontinue fluoxetine at least 5 weeks before starting thioridazine.
- Tryptophan: increased risk of CNS toxicity (e.g., headache, sweating, dizziness, agitation, aggressiveness) and peripheral toxicity (e.g., nausea, vomiting); use together cautiously if at all; avoid if possible.
- Warfarin: displaces fluoxetine from plasma protein binding sites, leading to increased fluoxetine serum levels, and effect; monitor for toxicity and dose-reduce as necessary.
- Teach all patients/families to call provider right away if thoughts of suicide or dying; attempts to commit suicide; new or worsening depression; new or worsening anxiety; feeling very agitated or restless; panic attacks; trouble sleeping (insomnia); new or worsening irritability; aggressive, angry, or violent behavior; acting on dangerous impulses; extreme increase in activity or talking (mania); any unusual changes in behavior or mood.

Lab Effects/Interference:
- None known.

Special Considerations:
- Weekly dosing is for patients whose depression is stable on daily dosing. Diarrhea and cognitive changes are more common with weekly dosing.
- May take up to 4 weeks of therapy before benefit is seen.

- Possibility of suicide attempt may exist in depression and persist until depression managed by drug; monitor high-risk patients closely and give smallest prescription of tablets possible to ensure frequent follow-up and reduce the risk of overdosage.
- Has slight-to-no anticholinergic, sedative, or orthostatic hypotensive side effects.
- Avoid use in women who are pregnant or breastfeeding.
- Drug is also indicated for treatment of obsessive-compulsive disorder and bulimia disorder.

Potential Toxicities/Side Effects and the Nursing Process

I. ALTERATIONS IN SKIN INTEGRITY related to RASH

Defining Characteristics: Urticaria, rash may occur (7%). In initial trials, in one-third of patients developing rash, rash was associated with fever, leukocytosis, arthralgias, edema, carpal tunnel syndrome, respiratory distress, lymphadenopathy, proteinuria, and/or mildly elevated liver transaminase levels that required drug discontinuation, which largely resolved symptoms.

Nursing Implications: Assess baseline skin integrity, and instruct patient to report rash immediately. Discuss drug discontinuance with physician if severe or associated with other symptoms as above. Teach symptomatic skin management.

II. ALTERATIONS IN SENSORY/PERCEPTUAL PATTERNS related to CNS EFFECTS

Defining Characteristics: CNS effects include headache and, less commonly, activation of mania or hypomania, insomnia, anxiety, decreased ability to concentrate, tremor, sensory disturbances, abnormal dreams, nervousness, dizziness, fatigue, sedation, lightheadedness, blurred vision. Rarely, seizures may occur. Patients at risk for suicide may commit suicide during initial period of treatment.

Nursing Implications: Assess baseline neurologic status and risk factors, and monitor during treatment. Instruct patient to report signs/symptoms, and discuss drug modification with physician. Evaluate patient satisfaction with drug efficacy. Instruct patient to avoid alcohol while taking drug. Assess suicide risk, and if at high risk, monitor closely, provide supportive counseling, and prescribe only small numbers of pills to prevent overdosage. May take up to 4 weeks for therapeutic effect to be seen.

III. ALTERATION IN NUTRITION, LESS THAN BODY REQUIREMENTS, related to GI SIDE EFFECTS

Defining Characteristics: Nausea and, less commonly, vomiting, diarrhea, constipation, dry mouth, dyspepsia, anorexia, abdominal discomfort, flatulence, taste changes, gastroenteritis, and increased hunger may occur. Significant weight loss can occur in underweight, depressed patients.

Nursing Implications: Assess baseline nutrition and elimination patterns. Discuss abnormalities with physician and discuss drug modification. Teach patient to self-administer prescribed antiemetics as appropriate. If patient is losing weight, instruct patient to report this immediately, and discuss benefit of continuation of drug with physician.

IV.   INJURY related to DECREASE IN MENTAL ALERTNESS, PHYSICAL COORDINATION

Defining Characteristics: Drug may cause drowsiness, dizziness, and impair physical co-ordination, mental alertness.

Nursing Implications: Assess other medications that may increase risk (e.g., opiates, phenothiazines) and response to drug. Instruct patient to avoid potentially hazardous activities, including driving a car, operating machinery.

V.   SEXUAL DYSFUNCTION, POTENTIAL, related to IMPOTENCE

Defining Characteristics: Sexual dysfunction, impotence, anorgasmia may occur.

Nursing Implications: Assess baseline sexual functioning. Inform patient that alterations may occur, and instruct to report them. If severe, discuss dysfunction with physician, and whether another antidepressant would provide equal benefit with less dysfunction.

VI.   ALTERATION IN OXYGENATION, POTENTIAL, related to ALTERED BREATHING PATTERNS

Defining Characteristics: Bronchitis, upper respiratory infections, pharyngitis, cough, dyspnea, rhinitis, nasal congestion, and sinusitis may occur infrequently.

Nursing Implications: Assess baseline respiratory status, and instruct patient to report any changes. Discuss serious changes with physician, and interventions necessary.

VII.   ALTERATION IN COMFORT, POTENTIAL, related to PAIN

Defining Characteristics: Pain in muscles, joints, or back may occur; flu-like symptoms are infrequent, as are asthenia, chest pain, and limb pain.

Nursing Implications: Assess baseline comfort level; instruct patient to report any changes. Discuss symptom management strategies, unless severe, and then discuss benefit of changing to another antidepressant medicine.

Drug: imipramine pamoate (Tofranil-PM)

Class: TCA.

Mechanism of Action: Blocks reuptake of neurotransmitters at neuronal membrane, thus increasing available serotonin and norepinephrine in CNS, and potentiating their effects.

Appears to have analgesic effect separate from antidepressant action. May increase bioavailability of morphine. Indicated in the treatment of depressive (affective) mood disorders. Also used as an adjuvant analgesic in cancer pain management.

Metabolism: Completely absorbed from GI tract; highly protein-bound. Plasma half-life is 8–16 hours. Metabolized in liver; excreted in urine and, to lesser degree, in bile and feces.

Indication: For the relief of symptoms of depression.

Dosage/Range:

Adult:
- Oral: 75–100 mg/day (may increase on patient response, to maximum 300 mg; reduce dose in elderly, 30–40 mg/day, to maximum 100 mg).
- IM: used only when oral route cannot be used.

Drug Preparation:
- Oral: store in well-closed containers at 15–30°C (59–86°F). Administer as a single bedtime dose.
- IM: administer IM in large muscle mass; change to oral as soon as possible.

Drug Interactions:
- MAOIs: increased excitation, hyperpyrexia, seizures; use together cautiously (especially if high dose is used).
- CNS depressants (alcohol, sedatives, hypnotics): increase CNS depression; use together cautiously.
- Sympathomimetic (epinephrine, amphetamines): increased hypertension; AVOID concurrent use.
- Cimetidine methylphenidate: increased imipramine levels, increased toxicity; use cautiously and monitor for increased toxicity.
- Warfarin: may increase PT; monitor closely and decrease dose of warfarin as needed.
- Barbiturates: may decrease imipramine level; monitor patient response; may need to increase dose.

Lab Effects/Interference:
- Increased metanephrine (Pisano test).
- Decreased urinary 5-HIAA.

Special Considerations:
- Antidepressant effect may take 2 weeks or longer.
- Adjuvant analgesic useful in cancer pain management.
- May also decrease depression associated with chronic cancer pain and promote improved sleep.
- Contraindicated in patients with myocardial infarction, seizure disorder, or benign prostatic hypertrophy.
- Use cautiously in patients with urine retention, narrow-angle glaucoma, hyperthyroidism, hepatic dysfunction, or suicidal ideation.
- Drug should be gradually discontinued rather than abruptly withdrawn to prevent anxiety, malaise, dizziness, nausea/vomiting.

MANAGEMENT

- May be helpful in treating hiccups.
- Increased anticholinergic side effects in elderly.
- Some preparations may contain sodium bisulfite, which can cause allergic reactions, including anaphylaxis, in hypersensitive individuals. Check ingredients. Assess allergy history.
- Teach all patients/families to call provider right away if thoughts of suicide or dying; attempts to commit suicide; new or worsening depression; new or worsening anxiety; feeling very agitated or restless; panic attacks; trouble sleeping (insomnia); new or worsening irritability; aggressive, angry, or violent behavior; acting on dangerous impulses; extreme increase in activity or talking (mania); any unusual changes in behavior or mood.

Potential Toxicities/Side Effects and the Nursing Process

I.   ALTERATIONS IN SENSORY/PERCEPTUAL PATTERNS related to DROWSINESS, CNS EFFECT

Defining Characteristics: Drowsiness, dizziness, weakness, lethargy, fatigue are common; confusion, disorientation, hallucinations may occur in the elderly. Extrapyramidal symptoms may occur (fine tremor, rigidity, dystonia, dysarthria, dysphagia), as may peripheral neuropathy and blurred vision.

Nursing Implications: Assess baseline gait, neurologic and mental status, and monitor during therapy. Instruct patient to report signs/symptoms; discuss benefit/risk ratio with physician. Assess for signs/symptoms of suicidal ideation; if they occur, refer for psychiatric evaluation. Inform patient that drowsiness, dizziness will resolve after 1–2 weeks; instruct to avoid hazardous activities while drowsy (e.g., driving a car, operating machinery).

II.   ALTERATION IN CARDIAC OUTPUT related to POSTURAL HYPOTENSION, TACHYCARDIA

Defining Characteristics: Postural hypotension, EKG changes, tachycardia, hypertension may occur.

Nursing Implications: Assess baseline orthostatic BP, heart rate, and monitor during therapy. Instruct patient to report abnormalities, including postural dizziness, palpitations. Drug should be stopped several days before surgery to prevent hypertensive crisis (especially if high dose is used).

III.   ALTERATION IN NUTRITION related to GI SIDE EFFECTS

Defining Characteristics: Dry mouth, anorexia, nausea, vomiting, diarrhea, and abdominal cramping may occur; also, elevated LFTs.

Nursing Implications: Assess baseline nutrition and elimination patterns and LFTs, and monitor during therapy. Discuss abnormalities with physician, and discuss drug modification. Teach patient to self-administer prescribed antiemetics as appropriate. LFTs should be repeated, and if still elevated, the drug should be discontinued. Instruct patient to take full dose at bedtime. Suggest patient use sugar-free hard candy, frequent ice chips, or artificial saliva for dry mouth.

IV. ALTERATION IN URINARY ELIMINATION related to URINARY RETENTION

Defining Characteristics: Urinary retention may occur. Increased risk in patients with history of urinary retention.

Nursing Implications: Assess baseline urinary elimination pattern and risk. Assess for urinary retention, and instruct patient to report signs/symptoms. Discuss alternative drug with physician if this occurs.

V. ALTERATIONS IN SKIN INTEGRITY related to ALLERGY

Defining Characteristics: Urticaria, erythema, rash, photosensitivity may occur.

Nursing Implications: Assess baseline drug allergy history and skin integrity. Instruct patient to report skin changes. If angioedema of face or tongue develops, discuss drug discontinuance with physician. Instruct patient to avoid sunlight or to use sunblock protection.

Drug: lorazepam (Ativan)

Class: Benzodiazepine (anxiolytic).

Mechanism of Action: Binds to benzodiazepine receptors in the CNS (limbic and cortical areas, cerebellum, brain stem, and spinal cord), resulting in the following effects: anxiolytic, ataxia, anticonvulsant, muscle relaxation. Appears to potentiate the effects of GABA.

Metabolism: Well absorbed from GI tract. Widely distributed in body tissues and fluids, including CSF. Crosses placenta and is excreted in breastmilk. Highly bound to plasma proteins. Metabolized in liver and excreted in urine. Short half-life of 10–20 hours. May produce psychological and physical dependence. Indicated for management of anxiety and short-term relief of anxiety associated with depression.

Indication: (1) Treatment of status epilepticus; (2) preanesthetic in adult patients.

Dosage/Range:

Adult:
Oral: 1–6 mg/day in divided doses (maximum 10 mg/day).
- IM: 0.044 mg/kg or 2 mg, whichever is smaller (initial dose).
- IV: 0.044 mg/kg (up to 2 mg) given 15–20 minutes prior to surgery; 1.4 mg/m^2 given 30 minutes prior to chemotherapy; or 0.05 mg/kg (maximum 4 mg) if perioperative amnesia is desired.
- Use maximum dose (2 mg) in patients > 50 years old.

MANAGEMENT

Drug Preparation:
- Oral: may administer with food to decrease stomach upset; has been given sublingually for more rapid onset (investigational).
- IM and IV: store drug in refrigerator until use.
- IM: administer undiluted, deep IM in large muscle mass (e.g., gluteus maximus).
- IV: dilute in equal volume of 0.9% sodium chloride or 5% dextrose for IVP administration (administer slowly; not > than 2 mg/min) OR dilute in 50 mL 0.9% sodium chloride or 5% dextrose immediately prior to administering IVB over 15 minutes.

Drug Interactions:
- CNS depressants (alcohol, anticonvulsants, phenothiazines, opiates): additive CNS depression; avoid concurrent use or use cautiously and monitor carefully.
- Oral contraceptives, isoniazid, ketoconazole: decrease plasma clearance of lorazepam so may increase effect (e.g., sedation); monitor patient closely.
- TCAs: increased serum levels of antidepressant possible; use together cautiously.
- Digoxin: may decrease renal excretion of digoxin; monitor for overdosage; may need to decrease digoxin.

Lab Effects/Interference:
- Rarely, leukopenia, elevated LDH.
- Less frequently, elevated liver function studies.

Special Considerations:
- Wide margin of safety between therapeutic and toxic doses.
- May impair ability to perform activities requiring mental alertness (e.g., driving a car, operating machinery).
- May produce psychological and physical dependence.
- Administer cautiously in patients with liver or renal impairment.
- Use cautiously in patients with chronic pulmonary disease or sleep apnea.
- Contraindicated in patients with depressive neuroses, psychotic reactions (without prominent anxiety), acute alcoholic intoxication (with depressed VS), known hypersensitivity to the drug, or acute angle-closure glaucoma.
- May cause fetal damage, so should not be used during pregnancy or if the mother is breastfeeding.
- Withdrawal symptoms (including seizure, delirium) can occur with rapid drug discontinuance in patients taking high or chronic doses.
- If manic episodes or hyperactivity occur soon after drug started, drug should be discontinued.
- Drug should not be used to manage "everyday stress."
- Causes anterograde amnesia.

Potential Toxicities/Side Effects and the Nursing Process

I.   ALTERATIONS IN SENSORY/PERCEPTUAL PATTERNS related to CNS DEPRESSION

Defining Characteristics: CNS depressant effects include drowsiness, fatigue, lethargy, confusion, weakness, headache, which may occur initially and resolve with continued therapy or dose reduction. Vivid dreams, suicidal ideation, and bizarre behavior may also occur. Patient risk factors: elderly, debilitated, liver dysfunction, low serum albumin.

Nursing Implications: Assess baseline neurologic status and risk factors, and monitor during treatment. Instruct patient to report signs/symptoms and discuss drug modification with physician. Evaluate patient satisfaction with drug efficacy. If patient expresses suicidal ideation (more common in panic disorders), refer patient for psychiatric evaluation and drug modification. Instruct patient to avoid alcohol while taking drug. Teach patient prescribed schedule for discontinuing drug when used chronically; assess for signs/symptoms of withdrawal (increased anxiety, rebound insomnia; may also include agitation, dysphoria, nausea/vomiting, irritability, muscle cramps, hallucinations, seizures).

II. ALTERATION IN NUTRITION, LESS THAN BODY REQUIREMENTS, related to GI SIDE EFFECTS

Defining Characteristics: Nausea, vomiting, weight increase or decrease, dry mouth, constipation may occur; also elevated serum LFTs.

Nursing Implications: Assess baseline nutrition and elimination patterns and LFTs, and monitor during therapy. Discuss abnormalities with physician and discuss drug modification. Teach patient to self-administer prescribed antiemetics as appropriate.

III. INJURY related to DECREASE IN MENTAL ALERTNESS, PHYSICAL COORDINATION

Defining Characteristics: Drug may cause drowsiness, dizziness, and impair physical coordination, mental alertness. Sedation, amnesia may last hours, impaired thinking and coordination 24–48 hours, and longer in the elderly.

Nursing Implications: Assess other medications that may increase risk (e.g., opiates, phenothiazines) and response to drug. Instruct patient to avoid potentially hazardous activities, including driving a car, operating machinery. For 8 hours following IV injection, assess level of consciousness and instruct patient to call nurse for assistance in ambulating if needed. Instruct patient to avoid alcohol for 24–48 hours after drug injection.

IV. ALTERATIONS IN CARDIAC OUTPUT related to CHANGES IN BP, HR

Defining Characteristics: Drug may cause bradycardia, tachycardia, hypertension or hypotension, palpitations, edema.

Nursing Implications: Assess baseline VS, and monitor during therapy. Discuss abnormalities with physician. Instruct patient to report dizziness upon standing or other changes.

MANAGEMENT

V.   ALTERATIONS IN SKIN INTEGRITY related to RASH

Defining Characteristics: Urticaria, pruritus, rash (morbilliform, urticarial, or maculopapular) may occur.

Nursing Implications: Assess baseline skin integrity, and instruct patient to report changes. Teach symptomatic skin management, and discuss drug discontinuance with physician if severe.

Drug: mirtazapine (Remeron)

Class: Antidepressant.

Mechanism of Action: Centrally active presynaptic α_2-antagonist, which increases central noradrenergic and serotonergic neurotransmission (via 5-HTs$_1$ receptors). Drug also blocks 5-HT$_2$ and 5-HT$_3$ receptors that contribute to antidepressant action. Thus, drug increases brain levels of both serotonin and norepinephrine. Antagonizes histamine H$_1$ causing some sedation but has limited anticholinergic or cardiovascular effects.

Metabolism: Active ingredient mirtazapine is rapidly absorbed from the GI tract with > 50% bioavailability. Peak plasma level is reached in about 2 hours, with approximately 85% of drug protein-bound. Mean elimination half-life is 20–40 hours with rare variation (up to 65 hours vs. shorter in young men). Steady state reached in 3–4 days. Drug extensively metabolized (demethylation, oxidation, conjugation) and eliminated via urine and feces in a few days. Renal or hepatic insufficiency can delay drug clearance.

Indication: For the treatment of major depressive disorder.

Contraindications: (1) Hypersensitivity to the drug or any of its components; (2) concurrent administration of MAOIs or within 14 days of stopping treatment with m mirtazapine because of an increased risk of serotonin syndrome; (3) concurrent administration with linezolid or IV methylene blue for the same reason.

Dosage/Range:

Adults:
- 15 mg PO daily to start, increasing in 2–4 weeks to a maximum of 45 mg daily if no response.
- If no response at maximal dose in 2–4 weeks, stop drug.
- Monitor elderly patients during dose titration. Use lowest dose, and monitor patients with renal or hepatic insufficiency closely due to reduced drug clearance.
- Response should be seen in 2–4 weeks of treatment at optimal dose.
- Once a response is obtained, drug is usually continued until the patient is symptom free for 4–6 months, and then the drug is gradually discontinued.

Drug Preparation:
- Tablets available in 15-, 30-, and 45-mg strengths, as well as in SolTab Orally Disintegrating Tablets (ODT), which dissolve on the tongue within 30 seconds.
- Administer tablets in a single daily dose at bedtime or in two divided doses (morning and evening).
- Administer SolTab ODT with or without water, to be chewed or allowed to disintegrate on the tongue.
- Store drug in the dark at 2–30°C.

Drug Interactions:
- Alcohol: AVOID concurrent use as potentiation of CNS depressant effects.
- MAOIs: AVOID concurrent use; DO NOT start mirtazapine until at least 2 weeks after the cessation of MAOI, and do not start an MAOI until at least 2 weeks after cessation of mirtazapine.
- Benzodiazepines: Potentiate CNS depressant effects of drug. Use together cautiously, if at all.

Lab Effects/Interference:
- Transient increase in hepatic transaminases (SGOT/AST and SGPT/ALT).

Special Considerations: (see package insert for full discussion or Warnings and Precautions)
- Rarely, granulocytopenia or agranulocytosis may occur, usually after 4–6 weeks of treatment.
- Possibility of suicide attempt may exist in depression and persist until depression is managed by drug. Monitor high-risk patients closely and give smallest prescription of tablets to ensure frequent follow-up and reduce the risk of overdosage.
- Avoid use in women who are pregnant or breastfeeding.
- Discontinue the drug if jaundice develops.
- Abrupt termination of drug after long-term therapy can result in nausea, headache, and malaise; when drug is discontinued, taper the dose to avoid an abrupt discontinuation syndrome.
- Drug at low doses enhances sleep.
- Patients requiring close monitoring for toxicity include those with epilepsy or organic brain syndrome; hepatic or renal insufficiency; heart disease, including conduction disturbances, and angina pectoris, or history of myocardial infarction; hypotension; prostatic hypertrophy or other voiding (micturition) disturbances; acute narrow-angle glaucoma; and diabetes mellitus.
- Teach all patients/families to call provider right away if thoughts of suicide or dying; attempts to commit suicide; new or worsening depression; new or worsening anxiety; feeling very agitated or restless; panic attacks; trouble sleeping (insomnia); new or worsening irritability; aggressive, angry, or violent behavior; acting on dangerous impulses; extreme increase in activity or talking (mania); any unusual changes in behavior or mood.

Potential Toxicities/Side Effects and the Nursing Process

I.   ALTERATION IN NUTRITION, MORE THAN BODY REQUIREMENTS, related to INCREASED APPETITE, WEIGHT GAIN, EDEMA

Defining Characteristics: Increased appetite and weight gain are common. Peripheral edema may occur, resulting in increased weight. Drug may be chosen for its appetite stimulation in patients with advanced cancer who are depressed and losing weight.

Nursing Implications: Assess baseline nutrition pattern and weight, and monitor during therapy. Assess baseline fluid status and presence of edema, and monitor during therapy. Teach patient that these side effects may occur and to report them, especially edema. If patient develops significant edema, assess cardiopulmonary status (heart rate, orthostatic blood pressure, respiratory rate at rest and with activity, oxygen saturation). Discuss significant edema with physician.

II.   ALTERATIONS IN SENSORY/PERCEPTUAL PATTERNS related to CNS EFFECTS

Defining Characteristics: CNS effects include drowsiness and sedation, especially during the first few weeks of treatment. Rarely, seizure, tremor, or myoclonus may occur. Worsening of psychotic symptoms may occur in patients with schizophrenia or other psychotic disturbances, and paranoid thoughts may become intensified. Mania may become activated in patients with manic depressive psychosis. Patients at risk for suicide may attempt/commit suicide during initial period of treatment.

Nursing Implications: Assess baseline neurologic status and risk factors, and monitor during treatment. Instruct patient to report signs/symptoms, and discuss drug modification with physician. Evaluate patient satisfaction with drug efficacy. Teach patient to avoid alcohol while taking drug, and to avoid benzodiazepines unless physician feels benefits outweigh risks. Assess suicide risk, and if at high risk, monitor closely, provide supportive counseling, and prescribe only a small number of pills to prevent overdosage. May take up to 4 weeks for therapeutic effect to be seen.

III.   POTENTIAL FOR INJURY related to DECREASE IN MENTAL ALERTNESS, PHYSICAL COORDINATION, ORTHOSTATIC HYPOTENSION

Defining Characteristics: Drug may cause drowsiness, decreased mental alertness, and orthostatic hypotension.

Nursing Implications: Assess other medications patient is taking that may increase the risk (e.g., opiates, phenothiazines) and response to drug. Instruct patient to avoid potentially hazardous activities, such as driving a car or other vehicle, and operating machinery. Assess baseline orthostatic blood pressure and heart rate, and monitor during therapy.

Teach patient that orthostatic hypotension may occur, and to report symptoms such as dizziness when changing position. Teach patient self-care measures to minimize risk of injury, such as changing position slowly over the course of 5 minutes, going from lying to sitting, and then from sitting to standing positions, holding on to walls or fixed railings when walking, and removing scatter rugs from walkways.

IV. POTENTIAL FOR INFECTION, BLEEDING, AND FATIGUE, related to RARE BONE MARROW DEPRESSION

Defining Characteristics: Rare granulocytopenia or agranulocytosis may occur, usually after 4–6 weeks of treatment. If it occurs, it is usually reversible following drug discontinuance.

Nursing Implications: Teach patient that this rare side effect may occur. Instruct patient to stop the drug and to report signs and symptoms of infection, such as fever, sore throat, productive cough, or dysuria right away. If the patient develops any signs and symptoms of infection, the drug should be stopped and a complete blood count with differential checked. Assess baseline CBC/differential, and periodically during therapy, especially at 4–6 weeks after drug initiated.

V. POTENTIAL ALTERATION IN SKIN INTEGRITY related to EXANTHEMA

Defining Characteristics: Rarely, skin rash resembling chickenpox, measles, or rubella may develop.

Nursing Implications: Assess baseline skin integrity, and instruct patient to report rash immediately. Discuss drug cessation or discontinuance with physician. Teach patient symptomatic skin management.

Drug: nefazodone HCl (Serzone)

Class: Antidepressant, synthetically derived phenylpiperazine.

Mechanism of Action: Appears to inhibit neuronal uptake of serotonin and norepinephrine. Drug occupies central serotonin (5-HT$_2$) receptors and acts as an antagonist. In addition, it antagonizes α-adrenergic receptors that may explain the associated postural hypotension.

Metabolism: Rapidly and completely absorbed after oral administration, but extensively metabolized by the liver using the P450 cytochrome enzyme system. Food delays absorption and decreases bioavailability by 20%. Peak plasma concentrations occur at 1 hour, and half-life of the drug is 2–4 hours. Drug is extensively protein-bound (> 99%). Time to steady state is 4–5 days. Only 1% of drug is excreted unchanged in the urine.

Indication: For the treatment of depression.

MANAGEMENT

Dosage/Range:

Adult:
- Initial: 200 mg/day, administered in 2 divided doses.
- If no or slight response, increase dose by 100–200 mg/day in 2 divided doses after at least 1 week at the previous dose; usual dose requirements are 300–600 mg/day in 2 divided doses.
- Elderly (especially women) or debilitated patients: begin at 50% of dose or 100 mg/day in 2 divided doses, and titrate up to therapeutic dose very slowly and gradually.

Drug Preparation:
- Oral, total dose given in 2 divided, bid doses on an empty stomach.
- Available in 100-, 150-, 200-, and 250-mg tablets.
- If changing from an MAOI to nefazodone HCl, allow at least 14 days after discontinuance of the MAOI before starting nefazodone; if changing from nefazodone to an MAOI, allow at least 7 days after stopping nefazodone before starting the MAOI.

Drug Interactions:
- Terfenadine, astemizole, cisapride: are metabolized by the P450 hepatic enzyme system; nefazodone can inhibit their metabolism, resulting in QT elongation and potential cardiac arrest; DO NOT GIVE CONCOMITANTLY WITH NEFAZODONE.
- MAOIs: may cause symptoms resembling neuroleptic malignant syndrome, including death. DO NOT USE CONCURRENTLY. See Administration guidelines when changing from/to MAOIs.
- Alprazolam: increased serum levels of alprazolam; monitor effect and toxicity, and determine need for dose reduction.
- Digoxin: increased plasma levels of digoxin; assess effect and toxicity, and need for dose reduction of digoxin.
- Propranolol: decreased plasma levels of propranolol; assess effect and need for increased dosage.
- Triazolam: increased plasma levels of triazolam; assess effect, toxicity, and need for dosage reduction.

Lab Effects/Interference:
- Rarely, increased AST, ALT, LDH.
- Rarely, decreased HCT, anemia, leukopenia.
- Rarely, hypercholesterolemia, hypoglycemia.

Special Considerations:
- Contraindications: coadministration with terfenadine, astemizole, cisapride, or MAOIs.
- Drug produces slight anticholinergic effects, moderate sedation, and slight orthostatic hypotension.
- May take several weeks until therapeutic effect is known.
- Use with caution in patients recovering from myocardial infarction, who have unstable heart disease and are taking digoxin, and patients with a history of mania.
- Monitor patients at risk for suicide carefully, as attempts may be made during initial period before significant antidepressant effects of the drug are seen.
- Avoid use during pregnancy or in nursing mothers.

• Teach all patients/families to call provider right away if thoughts of suicide or dying; attempts to commit suicide; new or worsening depression; new or worsening anxiety; feeling very agitated or restless; panic attacks; trouble sleeping (insomnia); new or worsening irritability; aggressive, angry, or violent behavior; acting on dangerous impulses; extreme increase in activity or talking (mania); any unusual changes in behavior or mood.

Potential Toxicities/Side Effects and the Nursing Process

I. ALTERATIONS IN SENSORY/PERCEPTUAL PATTERNS related to DROWSINESS, DIZZINESS

Defining Characteristics: Dizziness (17% incidence), drowsiness (25%), insomnia (17%), lightheadedness (10%), activation of mania or hypomania, agitation, blurred vision (9%), confusion (7%), decreased concentration (3%), memory impairment (4%), paresthesia (4%), ataxia (2%), incoordination (2%), psychomotor retardation (2%), tremor (1%), hypertonia (1%), vertigo, twitching, hallucinations, abnormal dreams (3%), and paranoia may occur. Neuroleptic malignant syndrome is rare (e.g., hyperthermia, seizures).

Nursing Implications: Assess baseline gait, neurologic and mental status, and monitor during therapy. Instruct patient to report signs/symptoms; depending upon severity and dysfunction, discuss benefit/risk ratio with physician. Assess for signs/symptoms of suicidal ideation; if they occur, refer for psychiatric evaluation. Inform patient that drowsiness, dizziness will resolve after 1–2 weeks; instruct to avoid hazardous activities while drowsy (e.g., driving a car, operating machinery).

II. ALTERATION IN CARDIAC OUTPUT related to POSTURAL HYPOTENSION, TACHYCARDIA

Defining Characteristics: Infrequent postural hypotension (4% incidence), hypotension (2%), tachycardia, hypertension, syncope, ventricular ectopic beats, angina pectoris, and CVA may occur rarely.

Nursing Implications: Assess baseline orthostatic BP, heart rate, and monitor during therapy. Instruct patient to report abnormalities, including postural dizziness, palpitations. If patient has orthostatic hypotension, teach patient to change position slowly and to hold on to supportive structure. If symptoms are significant, discuss changing to another antidepressant with physician.

III. ALTERATION IN NUTRITION, LESS THAN BODY REQUIREMENTS, related to GI SIDE EFFECTS

Defining Characteristics: Dry mouth (25% incidence), nausea (22%), vomiting (rare), diarrhea (5%), constipation (14%), dyspepsia (9%), and rarely eructation, gastritis, stomatitis, peptic ulceration, rectal hemorrhage have been reported.

MANAGEMENT

Nursing Implications: Assess baseline nutrition and elimination patterns and LFTs, and monitor during therapy. Discuss abnormalities with physician, and discuss drug modification. Teach patient to self-administer prescribed antiemetics, and other symptom management interventions, as ordered. Suggest patient use sugar-free hard candy, frequent ice chips, or artificial saliva for dry mouth.

IV.   ALTERATION IN URINARY ELIMINATION related to URINARY FREQUENCY

Defining Characteristics: Infrequently (2% incidence), urinary frequency, urinary retention, and urinary tract infections may occur.

Nursing Implications: Assess baseline urinary elimination pattern and risk. Assess for urinary frequency, retention, and infection, and instruct patient to report signs/symptoms. Discuss alternative drug with physician if this occurs.

V.   ALTERATION IN COMFORT related to HEADACHE

Defining Characteristics: Headache (36% incidence), asthenia (11%), arthralgia (1%) may occur.

Nursing Implications: Assess baseline comfort. Instruct patient to report unrelieved symptoms, and consider symptom-management strategies. Discuss severe discomfort that is unrelieved with physician and consider alternative antidepressant therapy.

Drug: nortriptyline hydrochloride (Aventyl, Pamelor)

Class: TCA.

Mechanism of Action: Blocks reuptake of neurotransmitters at neuronal membrane, thus increasing available serotonin and norepinephrine in CNS, and potentiating their effects. May increase bioavailability of morphine. Indicated in the treatment of depressive (affective) mood disorders. Also used as an adjuvant analgesic in cancer pain management.

Metabolism: Distributed to lungs, heart, brain, liver; highly bound to plasma, proteins. Plasma half-life is 16–90 hours. Metabolized in liver, excreted in urine, and, to a lesser degree, in bile and feces.

Indication: For the relief of depressive symptoms.

Dosage/Range:

Adult:
- Oral: 75–100 mg/day (maximum 100 mg or serum levels should be monitored; therapeutic dose: 50–150 mg/mL).
- Elderly: 30–50 mg/day.

Drug Preparation:
- Store oral solution in tight, light-resistant containers; store tablets in tight containers; keep at temperature of 15–30°C (59–86°F).
- Administer in single bedtime dose.

Drug Interactions:
- MAOIs: increased excitation, hyperpyrexia, seizures; use together cautiously (especially if high dose is used).
- CNS depressants (alcohol, sedatives, hypnotics): increase CNS depression; use together cautiously.
- Sympathomimetic (epinephrine, amphetamines): increased hypertension; AVOID concurrent use.
- Cimetidine methylphenidate: increased nortriptyline levels, increased toxicity; use cautiously and monitor for increased toxicity.
- Warfarin: may increase PT; monitor closely and decrease dose of warfarin as needed.
- Barbiturates: may decrease nortriptyline levels; monitor patient response; may need to increase dose.

Lab Effects/Interference:
- Rarely, bone marrow depression (agranulocytosis, eosinophilia, purpura, thrombocytopenia).
- Rarely, increased or decreased serum glucose levels.

Special Considerations:
- Antidepressant effect may take 2 weeks or longer.
- Adjuvant analgesic useful in cancer pain management.
- May also decrease depression associated with chronic cancer pain and promote improved sleep.
- Contraindicated in patients with myocardial infarction, seizure disorder, or benign prostatic hypertrophy.
- Use cautiously in patients with urine retention, narrow-angle glaucoma, hyperthyroidism, hepatic dysfunction, or suicidal ideation.
- Drug should be gradually discontinued rather than abruptly withdrawn to prevent anxiety, malaise, dizziness, nausea/vomiting.
- May be helpful in treating hiccups.
- Increased anticholinergic side effects in elderly.
- Some preparations may contain sodium bisulfite, which can cause allergic reactions, including anaphylaxis, in hypersensitive individuals. Check ingredients and assess allergy history.
- Teach all patients/families to call provider right away if thoughts of suicide or dying; attempts to commit suicide; new or worsening depression; new or worsening anxiety; feeling very agitated or restless; panic attacks; trouble sleeping (insomnia); new or worsening irritability; aggressive, angry, or violent behavior; acting on dangerous impulses; extreme increase in activity or talking (mania); any unusual changes in behavior or mood.

MANAGEMENT

Potential Toxicities/Side Effects and the Nursing Process

I. ALTERATIONS IN SENSORY/PERCEPTUAL PATTERNS related to DROWSINESS, DIZZINESS

Defining Characteristics: Drowsiness, dizziness, weakness, lethargy, fatigue are common; confusion, disorientation, hallucinations may occur in the elderly. Extrapyramidal symptoms may occur (fine tremor, rigidity, dystonia, dysarthria, dysphagia), as may peripheral neuropathy and blurred vision.

Nursing Implications: Assess baseline gait, neurologic and mental status, and monitor during therapy. Instruct patient to report signs/symptoms; discuss benefit/risk ratio with physician. Assess for signs/symptoms of suicidal ideation; if they occur, refer for psychiatric evaluation. Inform patient that drowsiness, dizziness will resolve after 1–2 weeks; instruct to avoid hazardous activities while drowsy (e.g., driving a car, operating machinery).

II. ALTERATION IN CARDIAC OUTPUT related to POSTURAL HYPOTENSION, TACHYCARDIA

Defining Characteristics: Low incidence of postural hypotension; EKG changes, tachycardia, and hypertension may occur.

Nursing Implications: Assess baseline orthostatic BP, heart rate, and monitor during therapy. Instruct patient to report abnormalities, including postural dizziness, palpitations. Drug should be stopped several days before surgery to prevent hypertensive crisis (especially if high dose is used).

III. ALTERATION IN NUTRITION, LESS THAN BODY REQUIREMENTS, related to GI SIDE EFFECTS

Defining Characteristics: Dry mouth, anorexia, nausea, vomiting, diarrhea, abdominal cramping may occur; also, elevated LFTs.

Nursing Implications: Assess baseline nutrition and elimination patterns and LFTs, and monitor during therapy. Discuss abnormalities with physician, and discuss drug modification. Teach patient to self-administer prescribed antiemetics as appropriate. LFTs should be repeated, and if still elevated, the drug should be discontinued. Instruct patient to take full dose at bedtime. Suggest patient use sugar-free hard candy, frequent ice chips, or artificial saliva for dry mouth.

IV. ALTERATION IN URINARY ELIMINATION related to URINARY FREQUENCY

Defining Characteristics: Urinary retention may occur. Increased risk if history of urinary retention.

Nursing Implications: Assess baseline urinary elimination pattern and risk. Assess for urinary retention, and instruct patient to report signs/symptoms. Discuss alternative drug with physician if this occurs.

V.   ALTERATIONS IN SKIN INTEGRITY related to ALLERGY

Defining Characteristics: Urticaria, erythema, rash, photosensitivity may occur.

Nursing Implications: Assess baseline drug allergy history and skin integrity. Instruct patient to report skin changes. If angioedema of face or tongue develops, discuss drug discontinuance with physician. Instruct patient to avoid sunlight or to use sunblock protection.

Drug: oxazepam (Serax)

Class: Benzodiazepine (anxiolytic).

Mechanism of Action: Binds to benzodiazepine receptors in the CNS (limbic and cortical areas, cerebellum, brain stem, and spinal cord), resulting in the following effects: anxiolytic, ataxia, anticonvulsant, muscle relaxation. Appears to potentiate the effects of GABA.

Metabolism: Well absorbed from GI tract. Widely distributed in body tissues and fluids, including CSF. Crosses placenta and is excreted in breastmilk. Highly bound to plasma proteins. Metabolized in liver and excreted in urine. Short half-life of 5–20 hours. May produce psychological and physical dependence. Indicated for management of anxiety, the short-term relief of anxiety associated with depression, and alcohol withdrawal.

Indication: Management of (1) anxiety disorders or for the short-term relief of symptoms of anxiety; (2) alcoholics with acute tremulousness, confusional state, or anxiety associated with alcohol withdrawal.

Dosage/Range:

Adult:
- Oral: 10–30 mg tid–qid.
- Elderly: 10 mg tid OR 15 mg tid–qid.

Drug Preparation:
- Store tablets in tight container at < 40°C (104°F).

Drug Interactions:
CNS depressants (alcohol, anticonvulsants, phenothiazines, opiates): additive CNS depression; avoid concurrent use or use cautiously and monitor carefully.
- Oral contraceptives, isoniazid, ketoconazole, or cimetidine: decrease plasma clearance of oxazepam, so may increase effect (e.g., sedation); monitor patient closely.
- TCAs: increased serum levels of antidepressant possible; use together cautiously.
- Digoxin: may decrease renal excretion of digoxin; monitor for overdosage; may need to decrease digoxin.

MANAGEMENT

Lab Effects/Interference:
- Rarely, leukopenia.
- Rarely, altered liver function studies.

Special Considerations:
- Wide margin of safety between therapeutic and toxic doses.
- May impair ability to perform activities requiring mental alertness (e.g., driving a car, operating machinery).
- May produce psychological and physical dependence.
- Administer cautiously in patients with liver or renal impairment.
- Use cautiously in patients with chronic pulmonary disease or sleep apnea.
- Contraindicated in patients with depressive neuroses, psychotic reactions (without prominent anxiety), acute alcoholic intoxication (with depressed VS), known hypersensitivity to the drug, or acute angle-closure glaucoma.
- May cause fetal damage, so should not be used during pregnancy or if the mother is breastfeeding.
- Withdrawal symptoms (including seizure, delirium) can occur with rapid drug discontinuance in patients taking high or chronic doses.
- If manic episodes or hyperactivity occur soon after drug started, drug should be discontinued.
- Drug should not be used to manage "everyday stress."
- Serax 15-mg tablet contains dye tartrazine, which may cause allergic reactions in sensitive individuals, especially if sensitive to aspirin.

Potential Toxicities/Side Effects and the Nursing Process

I.   ALTERATIONS IN SENSORY/PERCEPTUAL PATTERNS related to CNS DEPRESSION

Defining Characteristics: CNS depressant effects include drowsiness, fatigue, lethargy, weakness. Cumulative effects are less, as there is a short plasma half-life. Risk factors: elderly, debilitated, liver dysfunction, low serum albumin.

Nursing Implications: Assess baseline neurologic status and risk factors, and monitor during treatment. Instruct patient to report signs/symptoms. Instruct patient to avoid alcohol while taking drug. Teach patient prescribed schedule for discontinuing drug when drug is used chronically.

II.   ALTERATION IN NUTRITION, LESS THAN BODY REQUIREMENTS, related to GI SIDE EFFECTS

Defining Characteristics: Nausea, vomiting, weight increase or decrease, dry mouth, constipation may occur; also, elevated LFTs.

Nursing Implications: Assess baseline nutrition and elimination patterns and LFTs, and monitor during therapy. Discuss abnormalities with physician and discuss drug modification. Teach patient to self-administer prescribed antiemetics as appropriate.

III. INJURY related to DECREASE IN MENTAL ALERTNESS, PHYSICAL COORDINATION

Defining Characteristics: Drug may cause drowsiness, dizziness, and impair physical coordination, mental alertness.

Nursing Implications: Assess other medications that may increase risk (e.g., opiates, phenothiazines) and response to drug. Instruct patient to avoid potentially hazardous activities, including driving a car, operating machinery.

IV. ALTERATIONS IN CARDIAC OUTPUT related to TRANSIENT HYPOTENSION

Defining Characteristics: Transient hypotension may occur.

Nursing Implications: Assess baseline VS, and monitor during therapy. Discuss abnormalities with physician. Instruct patient to report dizziness on standing or other changes.

V. ALTERATIONS IN SKIN INTEGRITY related to RASH

Defining Characteristics: Urticaria, pruritus, rash (morbilliform, urticarial, or maculopapular) may occur.

Nursing Implications: Assess baseline skin integrity, and instruct patient to report changes. Teach symptomatic skin management, and discuss drug discontinuance with physician if severe.

Drug: paroxetine hydrochloride (Paxil)

Class: Antidepressant with mechanism of action different from SSRIs, tricyclic, or tetracyclic antidepressants.

Mechanism of Action: Appears to potentiate serotonergic activity of the CNS by potent and selective inhibition of serotonin reuptake by the neurons.

Metabolism: Completely absorbed after oral administration and metabolized to some degree by the P450 hepatic enzyme system. Distributed throughout the body, including the CNS, and is extensively protein-bound (95%). Increased serum levels occur in patients with hepatic or renal dysfunction (twofold), and in elderly patients. Time to peak plasma levels 5.2 hours, and time to reach steady state is 10–24 days. Largely excreted in the urine (64%) over a 10-day period, and approximately 36% is excreted in the feces.

Indication: For the treatment of (1) major depressive disorder; (2) obsessive and compulsive disorder; (3) panic disorder; (4) social anxiety disorder.

Contraindications: (1) concurrent use with MAOIs or within 14 days of stopping paroxetine; (2) the use of paroxetine within 14 days of stopping an MAOI; (3) concurrent use with linezolid or IV methylene blue; (4) concurrent use with thioridazine or pimozide; (5) hypersensitivity to paroxetine or its components.

Dosage/Range:

Adult (depression):
- Initial: 20 mg/day PO in the morning. Initial response may be delayed; if no response, may increase dose in 10-mg/day increments after an interval of at least 1 week, to a maximum of 50 mg/day.
- Patients who are elderly, or who have severe hepatic or renal dysfunction: initial dose of 10 mg/day, with increased dose adjustments made after at least 1 week, in 10-mg/day increments up to a maximum of 40 mg/day.

Drug Preparation:
- Oral, available in 10-, 20-, 30-, and 40-mg tablets.
- Administer as a single daily dose, usually in the morning.
- Allow at least 14 days when changing from an MAOI to paroxetine, or when changing from paroxetine to an MAOI.

Drug Interactions:
- Tryptophan: when administered concomitantly, headache, nausea, sweating, and dizziness may occur; avoid concomitant administration.
- MAOIs: reactions including death have occurred (hyperthermia, rigidity, myoclonus, autonomic instability, mental status changes including delirium/coma); allow at least 14 days between changing to or from paroxetine to an MAOI.
- Warfarin: increased bleeding despite a normal PT; give together cautiously, if at all.
- Sumatriptan: may cause hyperreflexia, weakness; incoordination may occur; monitor patient closely.
- Drugs inhibiting the P450 cytochrome hepatic metabolic pathway (e.g., cimetidine): paroxetine serum levels may be increased by up to 50%; assess response and toxicity carefully and need to decrease paroxetine dosage.
- Drugs inducing the P450 cytochrome hepatic metabolic pathway (e.g., phenobarbital, phenytoin): paroxetine serum levels may be reduced by up to 25–50%; assess response and need to increase paroxetine dosage.
- Drugs metabolized by the P450 cytochrome hepatic metabolic pathway (other antidepressant medications, phenothiazines, type 1C antiarrhythmics): paroxetine may inhibit the metabolism of these drugs, resulting in increased toxicity.
- TCAs should be given together with caution, and the dose of the TCA may need to be reduced.
- Drugs that are highly bound to plasma proteins: paroxetine may displace the other drug from serum proteins, thus increasing the serum level of the other drug, resulting in toxicity. Give together cautiously and monitor/reduce drug as needed.
- Alcohol: avoid concurrent administration.
- Lithium, digoxin: use together cautiously; digoxin levels may be reduced.
- Procyclidine: increased anticholinergic effects possible; decrease dose of procyclidine if necessary to coadminister.

- Tamoxifen: study indicates that taking this drug with tamoxifen may negate the benefit of tamoxifen; do not use together. Tamoxifen is a prodrug that requires metabolism by the CYP2D6 enzymes, which are inhibited by SSRIs including fluoxetine hydrochloride. See *tamoxifen* in *Chapter 1*.
- Theophylline: may elevate serum theophylline levels; monitor and adjust dose accordingly.

Lab Effects/Interference:
- None known.

Special Considerations (see package insert for Warnings and Precautions):
- Drug excreted in breastmilk; drug should be administered cautiously, if at all, in breast-feeding mothers.
- Drug is teratogenic, so women of childbearing age should use contraception if sexually active.
- Drug indicated for the treatment of depression, panic disorder, obsessive–compulsive disorder.
- Teach all patients/families to call provider right away if thoughts of suicide or dying; attempts to commit suicide; new or worsening depression; new or worsening anxiety; feeling very agitated or restless; panic attacks; trouble sleeping (insomnia); new or worsening irritability; aggressive, angry, or violent behavior; acting on dangerous impulses; extreme increase in activity or talking (mania); any unusual changes in behavior or mood.

MANAGEMENT

Potential Toxicities/Side Effects and the Nursing Process

I. ALTERATIONS IN SENSORY/PERCEPTUAL PATTERNS related to DIZZINESS, SOMNOLENCE

Defining Characteristics: Somnolence, dizziness, insomnia, tremor, nervousness, and asthenia occur in more than 5% of patients. Less common are headache, agitation, seizures, anxiety, activation of mania or hypomania, paresthesia, confusion, impaired concentration, emotional lability, depression.

Nursing Implications: Assess baseline neurologic status, affective state, and risk factors, and monitor during treatment. Instruct patient to avoid alcohol while taking drug. Assess effect on elderly and/or patients with hepatic or renal dysfunction. Inform patient that daytime drowsiness may occur, and instruct to use caution if driving or operating heavy machinery. Assess for symptoms at each visit, and instruct patient to report changes. If symptoms occur, discuss strategies to ensure patient safety and comfort.

II. ALTERATION IN NUTRITION, LESS THAN BODY REQUIREMENTS, related to GI SIDE EFFECTS

Defining Characteristics: Nausea and decreased appetite may occur.

Nursing Implications: Assess baseline nutrition status, and instruct patient to report any nausea or loss of appetite. Discuss measures to reduce nausea and/or stimulate appetite.

III. ALTERATION IN COMFORT related to SWEATING

Defining Characteristics: Sweating may occur.

Nursing Implications: Inform patient that this may occur, and assess impact on patient and need for intervention.

IV. SEXUAL DYSFUNCTION, POTENTIAL, related to EJACULATORY DISTURBANCES

Defining Characteristics: Incidence of ejaculatory disturbances is 13%; other disorders may occur (10%), including erectile difficulties, delayed ejaculation/orgasm, impotence, and other sexual dysfunction.

Nursing Implications: Assess baseline sexual functioning. Inform patient that alterations may occur, and instruct to report them. If severe, discuss dysfunction with physician, and whether another antidepressant would provide equal benefit with less dysfunction.

Drug: sertraline hydrochloride (Zoloft)

Class: Antidepressant.

Mechanism of Action: Inhibits CNS neuronal uptake of serotonin.

Metabolism: Undergoes extensive first-pass metabolism by the liver and is excreted in the urine (45% by 9 days) and the feces (40–45%). Time to peak plasma levels is 4.5–8.4 hours, and peak plasma levels are 20–55 mg/mL. Food reduces time to reach peak serum levels. Highly protein-bound (98%). Time to steady-state plasma levels is 7 days but is increased to 2–3 weeks in the elderly.

Indication: For the treatment of (1) major depressive disorder in adults; (2) obsessive–compulsive disorder; (3) panic disorder; (4) post-traumatic stress disorder; (5) premenstrual dysphoria disorder; (6) social anxiety disorder.

Contraindication: (1) concomitant use of MAOIs or use within 14 days of stopping MAOIs; (2) concomitant use of pimozide; (3) known hypersensitivity to sertraline or excipients; (4) oral solution only: concomitant use with disulfiram.

Dosage/Range (see package insert for dosages for other indications):

Adult (Major Depressive Disorder):
- Initial: 50 mg/day. If no response after a period of 1–2 weeks, may titrate gradually up to a maximum dose of 200 mg/day.

Drug Preparation:
- Oral, once daily in morning or evening.
- Available in 25-, 50-, and 100-mg tablets; oral solution 20 mg/mL (must be diluted before administration).

- When changing from an MAOI to sertraline HCl, wait at least 14 days after stopping the MAOI before initiating sertraline; when changing from sertraline HCl to an MAOI, wait at least 14 days after stopping sertraline before beginning the MAOI.
- **Drug Administration:** Screen for bipolar disorder prior to starting sertraline.
- Dose modify for hepatic dysfunction: (a) mild hepatic impairment: 50% starting and maximum doses; (b) moderate or severe: drug not recommended.
- When discontinuing drug, reduce gradually and wean patient so discontinuance syndrome avoided.

Drug Interactions:
- MAOIs: Severe reactions, similar to neuroleptic malignant syndrome, including death may occur; DO NOT ADMINISTER CONCURRENTLY; see Administration section.
- Alcohol: DO NOT give concurrently.
- Benzodiazepines: Decreased metabolism of benzodiazepine drugs, which are metabolized by the P450 enzyme system in the liver, resulting in increased serum levels and toxicity; monitor for toxicity and adjust dose accordingly.
- Tamoxifen: Study indicates that taking this drug with tamoxifen may negate the benefit of tamoxifen; do not use together. Tamoxifen is a prodrug that requires metabolism by the CYP2D6 enzymes, which are inhibited by SSRIs including fluoxetine hydrochloride.
- Tolbutamide: Decreased clearance with increased serum levels; monitor blood-sugar levels closely.
- Warfarin: Increased PT and delayed normalization of same; monitor PT values closely.
- CNS-active drugs: Monitor effects closely and modify drug doses accordingly (e.g., lithium).

Lab Effects/Interference:
- Increased AST or ALT, total cholesterol, triglycerides.
- Decreased serum uric acid.

Special Considerations:
- Warnings and Precautions (see package insert for details and discussion):
  - *Serotonin syndrome:* increased risk when coadministered with other serotonergic drugs (e.g., SSRIs, SNRIs, triptans) but also when taken alone. If it occurs, discontinue sertraline and manage symptoms.
  - *Increased risk of bleeding:* Concomitant use of aspirin, NSAIDs, other antiplatelet drugs, warfarin, and other anticoagulants increase risk. Monitor patient INR when starting drug, titrating, and stopping drug. Teach patient to report any bleeding.
  - *Activation of mania/hypomania:* Screen patients for bipolar disorder.
  - *Seizures*: Use with caution in patients with seizure disorder.
  - *Angle closure glaucoma:* Avoid drug in patients with untreated anatomically narrow angles.
  - *QTc prolongation:* Use with caution in patients with risk factors for QTc prolongation.
- Teach all patients/families to call provider right away if thoughts of suicide or dying; attempts to commit suicide; new or worsening depression; new or worsening anxiety; feeling very agitated or restless; panic attacks; trouble sleeping (insomnia); new or worsening irritability; aggressive, angry, or violent behavior; acting on dangerous impulses; extreme increase in activity or talking (mania); any unusual changes in behavior or mood.

Potential Toxicities/Side Effects and the Nursing Process

I. ALTERATIONS IN SENSORY/PERCEPTUAL PATTERNS related to HEADACHE, INSOMNIA

Defining Characteristics: Commonly, headache, insomnia. Less commonly, drowsiness, dizziness, agitation, nervousness, anxiety, tremor, fatigue, impaired concentration, paresthesia, yawning, hypoesthesia, twitching, confusion, abnormal coordination (ataxia), abnormal gait, hyperesthesia, hyperkinesia, abnormal dreams, amnesia, apathy, hallucinations. Suicidal ideation or attempt is uncommon, but patients at risk may attempt suicide during initial treatment before therapeutic effects of drug are felt.

Nursing Implications: Assess baseline gait, neurologic, affective, and mental status, and monitor during therapy. Instruct patient to report signs/symptoms; discuss benefit/risk ratio with physician. Assess for signs/symptoms of suicidal ideation; if they occur, refer for psychiatric evaluation. Inform patient that drowsiness may occur, and instruct to avoid hazardous activities while drowsy (e.g., driving a car, operating machinery).

II. ALTERATION IN CARDIAC OUTPUT, POTENTIAL, related to CHANGES IN BP

Defining Characteristics: Rarely, palpitations, edema, hypertension or hypotension, peripheral ischemia, postural hypotension, tachycardia, and syncope may occur.

Nursing Implications: Assess baseline orthostatic BP, heart rate, and monitor during therapy. Instruct patient to report abnormalities, including postural dizziness, palpitations. Discuss significant changes with physician. If patient has orthostatic hypotension, teach patient to change position slowly and to hold on to support.

III. ALTERATION IN NUTRITION, LESS THAN BODY REQUIREMENTS, related to GI SIDE EFFECTS

Defining Characteristics: Nausea and diarrhea are common. Less common are dry mouth, constipation, dyspepsia, increased or decreased appetite, vomiting, increased salivation, abdominal pain, gastroenteritis, dysphagia, eructation, taste changes; also, elevated LFTs.

Nursing Implications: Assess baseline nutrition and elimination patterns and LFTs, and monitor during therapy. Discuss abnormalities with physician, and discuss drug modification. Teach patient to self-administer prescribed antiemetics as appropriate. Suggest patient use sugar-free hard candy, frequent ice chips, or artificial saliva for dry mouth.

IV. ALTERATION IN URINARY ELIMINATION related to URINARY FREQUENCY

Defining Characteristics: Urinary frequency, dysuria, urinary incontinence, nocturia, polyuria may occur.

Nursing Implications: Assess baseline urinary elimination pattern and risk. Assess for changes in urinary elimination, and instruct patient to report signs/symptoms. Discuss alternative drug with physician if this occurs.

V.   ALTERATIONS IN SKIN INTEGRITY related to RASH

Defining Characteristics: Maculopapular rash, acne, facial edema, pruritus, excessive sweating, alopecia, and dry skin may occur rarely.

Nursing Implications: Assess baseline skin integrity. Instruct patient to report skin changes. If angioedema of face or tongue develops, discuss drug discontinuance with physician. Assess impact of changes on patient and discuss strategies to minimize distress.

VI.   SEXUAL DYSFUNCTION, POTENTIAL, related to MENSTRUAL IRREGULARITY, ↓ LIBIDO

Defining Characteristics: Menstrual disorders, dysmenorrhea, intermenstrual bleeding, sexual dysfunction, decreased libido may occur.

Nursing Implications: Assess baseline sexual functioning. Inform patient that alterations may occur, and instruct to report them. If severe, discuss dysfunction with physician, and whether another antidepressant would provide equal benefit with less dysfunction.

MANAGEMENT

Drug: trazodone hydrochloride (Desyrel, Trialodine)

Class: Antidepressant.

Mechanism of Action: Appears to selectively inhibit the uptake of serotonin by brain synaptosomes and potentiates the behavioral changes induced by the serotonin precursor, 5-hydroxytryptophan.

Metabolism: Well absorbed after oral administration, with peak plasma levels occurring at 1 hour when taken on an empty stomach and at 2 hours when taken with food. Metabolized by the liver and excreted in the urine and feces. Time to steady state is 3–7 days. Elimination half-life initially is 3–6 hours, followed by slower phase with a half-life of 5–9 hours.

Indication: For the treatment of major depressive disorder in adults.

Dosage/Range:

Adult:
- Initial dose of 150 mg in divided doses.
- Increase dose by 50 mg/day q 3–4 days (maximum outpatient dosage is 300 mg/day, and inpatient is 600 mg/day in divided doses).

Maintenance:
- Lowest possible dose; once therapeutic effect reached, may be able to gradually reduce dose.

Elderly:
- 75 mg/day in divided doses; increase dose as needed and tolerated, every 3–4 days.

Drug Preparation:
- Oral administration, shortly after a meal or light snack, in divided doses.
- If drowsiness, may take majority of dose at bedtime.

Drug Interactions:
- Alcohol, CNS depressants: increased CNS depression; DO NOT GIVE TOGETHER.
- Antihypertensives: additive hypotension; evaluate and modify dose of antihypertensive as needed.
- Barbiturates: increased CNS depression; avoid concomitant use.
- Clonidine: reduced effect of clonidine; assess need for increased clonidine dosage.
- Digoxin: trazodone may increase serum digoxin levels; assess effects, and need to decrease digoxin dosage.
- MAOIs: initiate combined therapy cautiously and monitor patient for toxicity.
- Phenytoin: serum phenytoin levels may be increased; monitor levels and therapeutic effect and need for reduced phenytoin dosage.

Lab Effects/Interference:
- Occasional decreased WBC and neutrophil count.

Special Considerations:
- 75% of patients will respond within 2 weeks of therapy, and the remainder within 2–4 weeks.
- Drug causes moderate sedative effects and orthostatic hypotension, with slight anticholinergic effects.
- Contraindicated in patients during recovery from myocardial infarction, or patients receiving electroshock therapy.
- Elderly may be more vulnerable to sedative and hypotensive effects of drug.
- Teach all patients/families to call provider right away if thoughts of suicide or dying; attempts to commit suicide; new or worsening depression; new or worsening anxiety; feeling very agitated or restless; panic attacks; trouble sleeping (insomnia); new or worsening irritability; aggressive, angry, or violent behavior; acting on dangerous impulses; extreme increase in activity or talking (mania); any unusual changes in behavior or mood.

Potential Toxicities/Side Effects and the Nursing Process

I.   SEXUAL DYSFUNCTION related to PRIAPISM

Defining Characteristics: Priapism (prolonged or inappropriate penile erection) may occur, and has required surgical intervention in some cases, and in others there was permanent dysfunction.

Nursing Implications: Teach male patients that this may occur. If it does, patient should immediately discontinue the drug and call physician. Make certain the patient understands the instructions and knows how to contact the physician. If priapism has persisted for 24 hours or more, a urologist should be consulted.

II. ALTERATIONS IN SENSORY/PERCEPTUAL PATTERNS related to CNS DEPRESSION

Defining Characteristics: CNS depressant effects include drowsiness, fatigue, nightmares, confusion, anger, excitement, decreased ability to concentrate, disorientation, insomnia, nervousness, impaired memory, dizziness, lightheadedness; rarely, hallucinations, impaired speech, hypomania, incoordination, tremors, paresthesias may occur.

Nursing Implications: Assess baseline gait, neurologic status, affective state, and risk factors, and monitor during treatment. Instruct patient to report worsening depression, and assess for any suicidal ideation. Instruct patient to avoid alcohol while taking drug. Assess effect on elderly and/or debilitated patients (cognition, motor function, other sensitivities). Assess effect of drug side effects on patient, and weigh against benefit. Inform patient that daytime drowsiness may occur, and instruct to use caution if driving or operating heavy machinery. If sleep problems, have patient take majority of dose at bedtime to enhance sleep.

III. ALTERATION IN NUTRITION, LESS THAN BODY REQUIREMENTS, related to GI SIDE EFFECTS

Defining Characteristics: Diarrhea, nausea, vomiting, flatulence may occur rarely.

Nursing Implications: Assess baseline nutrition status, and instruct the patient to report any nausea or vomiting. If required, discuss with physician antiemetic to manage symptoms. If severe, discuss alternative antidepressant medications.

IV. INJURY related to DECREASE IN MENTAL ALERTNESS, PHYSICAL COORDINATION

Defining Characteristics: Drug may cause drowsiness, dizziness, blurred vision, and impair physical coordination, mental alertness.

Nursing Implications: Assess baseline mental alertness, and teach patient to assess tolerance of medication before driving a car or operating heavy machinery. Assess medication profile to identify other medications that may increase risk (e.g., opiates, phenothiazines) and response to drug.

V. ALTERATION IN OXYGENATION, POTENTIAL, related to CHANGES IN BP, SYNCOPE

Defining Characteristics: Rarely, hypotension or hypertension, syncope, palpitations, tachycardia, shortness of breath, and chest pain may occur.

Nursing Implications: Assess baseline cardiovascular status, and vital signs, and monitor during therapy at each visit. Instruct patient to report any palpitations, chest pain, or any changes in condition. Discuss significant symptoms with the physician. If patient is hypotensive and receiving antihypertensive medication, discuss with physician discontinuing or dose-reducing the antihypertensive medication. Prior to elective surgery, because interaction with anesthesia is unknown, temporarily discontinue drug.

Drug: venlafaxine hydrochloride (Effexor, Effexor XR)

Class: SNRI antidepressant.

Mechanism of Action: Appears to potentiate neurotransmitter activity by inhibiting neuronal serotonin and norepinephrine reuptake.

Metabolism: Well absorbed after oral administration, and eliminated via the kidneys; time to reach steady state is 3–4 days. Drug and metabolite half-lives are 5 ± 2 and 11 ± 2 hours. Increased drug serum levels in patients with renal or hepatic dysfunction.

Indications: XR: treatment of (1) major depressive disorder; (2) generalized anxiety disorder; (3) social anxiety disorder; (4) panic disorder. Immediate release: treatment of (1) major depressive disorder; (2) hot flashes.

Dosage/Range:

Adult (indicated for the treatment of depression and generalized anxiety disorder):
- Initial (extended-release capsule): 75 mg once a day, at the same time each day; if indicated, can start dose at 37.5 mg once daily for 4–7 days, increasing to 75-mg capsule strength; if no response after adequate trial at 75 mg/day, may increase dose in 75-mg increments after at least a 4-day trial at the previous dose, up to a maximum of 225 mg per day in a single dose.
- Initial (immediate-release tablets): 75 mg/day in 2 or 3 divided doses.
- If little or no response, dose may be increased in dose increments of up to 75 mg/day after at least 4 days at the previous dose, to 150 mg/day, and up to a maximum of 225 mg/day for moderately depressed patients. Severely depressed patients may need up to 350–375 mg/day in three divided doses.
- Patients with hepatic dysfunction: daily dose should be reduced at least 50%.
- Patients with renal impairment: Mild to moderate dysfunction: reduce daily dose by 25%; patients receiving hemodialysis: 50% dose reduction; dose is given after dialysis.

Drug Preparation:
- Effexor XR tablets available in a 225-mg dose (uses Osmodex controlled-release technology).
- XL capsule available in 37.5-, 75-, and 150-mg strengths.
- Immediate-release tablets available as 25-, 37.5-, 50-, 75-, and 100-mg tablets.
- Drug should be administered orally with food in a single dose in morning or at night (same time every day) for extended-release capsule, or in 2–3 divided doses for tablets.

- When changing from an MAOI to venlafaxine HCl, wait at least 14 days after MAOI is stopped; when stopping venlafaxine HCl and beginning an MAOI, wait at least 7 days.
- When discontinuing drug after > 1 week of therapy, taper dose. If more than 6 weeks of therapy, taper over 2 weeks.

Drug Interactions:
- MAOIs: tremor, myoclonus, diaphoresis, nausea, vomiting, flushing, dizziness, hyperthermia resembling neuroleptic malignant syndrome, and may be fatal. DO NOT USE TOGETHER. See Administration section.
- Cimetidine: may increase venlafaxine HCl serum levels that are significant in patients with existing hypertension, hepatic dysfunction, or who are elderly; use with caution in these patients and monitor closely.
- Haloperidol: may increase haloperidol serum levels; monitor patient when drugs are administered concomitantly.

Lab Effects/Interference:
- Infrequent increased alk phos, creatinine, transaminases AST, ALT.
- Infrequent hyperglycemia with glycosuria, hyperlipemia, bilirubinemia, hyperuricemia, hypercholesterolemia, hypoglycemia, hypokalemia, hyperkalemia, hyperphosphatemia, hyponatremia, hypophosphatemia, hypoproteinemia, uremia, albuminuria.

Special Considerations:
- Avoid drug use during pregnancy and in nursing mothers.
- Dose-reduce in patients with hepatic or renal dysfunction.
- Use caution in patients with mania.
- Use for more than 4–6 weeks has not been evaluated.
- Contraindicated in patients receiving MAOIs.
- Studies have shown equal efficacy to fluoxetine (Costa, 1998; Silverstone & Ravindran, 1999).
- Drug has been shown to reduce hot flashes (vasomotor symptoms) (Loprinzi et al., 2009).
- Serious adverse reactions have occurred in patients changing from MAOIs to venlafaxine HCl or from venlafaxine to an MAOI. It is imperative to wait 14 days changing from MAOIs to venlafaxine HCl or 7 days after stopping venlafaxine before starting an MAOI.
- Teach all patients/families to call provider right away if thoughts of suicide or dying; attempts to commit suicide; new or worsening depression; new or worsening anxiety; feeling very agitated or restless; panic attacks; trouble sleeping (insomnia); new or worsening irritability; aggressive, angry, or violent behavior; acting on dangerous impulses; extreme increase in activity or talking (mania); any unusual changes in behavior or mood.

Potential Toxicities/Side Effects and the Nursing Process

I.   ALTERATION IN OXYGENATION, POTENTIAL, related to CHANGES IN BP

Defining Characteristics: Rarely, hypertension, vasodilation, tachycardia, postural hypotension, angina, extrasystoles, syncope, thrombophlebitis, peripheral edema occur. Migraine headaches are frequent.

MANAGEMENT

Nursing Implications: Assess baseline weight, presence of peripheral edema, cardiac status and vital signs, and monitor during therapy at each visit. Instruct patient to report any edema, palpitations, chest pain, or any changes in condition. Discuss any symptoms with the physician depending on severity.

II. ALTERATIONS IN SENSORY/PERCEPTUAL PATTERNS related to EMOTIONAL LABILITY, VERTIGO

Defining Characteristics: Emotional lability, trismus, vertigo occur frequently; infrequently, apathy, ataxia, circumoral paresthesia, CNS stimulation, euphoria, hallucinations, hostility, blurred vision, abnormal accommodation, photophobia, tinnitus, taste perversion, manic reaction, psychosis, sleep disturbance, abnormal dreams, and stupor may occur.

Nursing Implications: Assess baseline neurologic status, affective state, and risk factors, and monitor during treatment. Instruct patient to avoid alcohol while taking drug. Assess effect on elderly and/or patients with hepatic or renal dysfunction. Assess for symptoms at each visit, and instruct patient to report changes. If symptoms occur, discuss strategies to ensure patient safety and comfort.

III. ALTERATION IN NUTRITION, LESS THAN BODY REQUIREMENTS, related to GI SIDE EFFECTS

Defining Characteristics: Nausea (37% of patients), anorexia (11%), constipation (15%) may occur. Less commonly, dry mouth, diarrhea, dyspepsia, flatulence, dysphagia, melena, gastroenteritis, and eructation may occur.

Nursing Implications: Assess baseline nutrition and gastrointestinal functional status, and instruct the patient to report any GI disturbances or changes. Discuss measures to reduce nausea and/or stimulate appetite.

IV. SEXUAL DYSFUNCTION, POTENTIAL, related to EJACULATORY DISTURBANCES

Defining Characteristics: Incidence of ejaculatory disturbances is 12%, and other disorders may occur (1–6%), including erectile difficulties, delayed ejaculation/orgasm, impotence, and other sexual dysfunction. Rarely, women with uterine fibroids may develop enlargement, uterine hemorrhage, or vaginal hemorrhage; in addition, women may develop vaginitis and metrorrhagia and, rarely, amenorrhea.

Nursing Implications: Assess baseline sexual functioning. Inform patient that alterations may occur, and instruct to report them. If severe, discuss dysfunction with physician, and whether another antidepressant would provide equal benefit with less dysfunction.

V.   ALTERATION IN COMFORT related to PAIN

Defining Characteristics: Malaise, neck pain, hangover-like effect, arthritis, bone pain may occur infrequently.

Nursing Implications: Assess baseline comfort level. Instruct patient to report any changes in comfort, and discuss strategies to reduce discomfort.

VI.   ALTERATION IN OXYGENATION, POTENTIAL, related to ALTERED BREATHING PATTERNS

Defining Characteristics: Bronchitis, dyspnea may occur frequently; infrequently, asthma, chest congestion, hyperventilation, laryngitis may occur.

Nursing Implications: Assess baseline respiratory status, and instruct patient to report any changes. Discuss serious changes with physician, and interventions necessary.

VII.   ALTERATION IN SKIN INTEGRITY, POTENTIAL, related to RASH

Defining Characteristics: Infrequently, acne, alopecia, brittle nails, contact dermatitis, dry skin, maculopapular rash, urticaria, and herpes simplex and zoster may occur.

Nursing Implications: Assess baseline skin integrity, and instruct patient to report any changes. Discuss serious changes with the physician, and need for changing to another antidepressant depending on severity.

VIII.   POTENTIAL FOR INJURY related to EFFECTS ON BLOOD CELL ELEMENTS

Defining Characteristics: Frequently, ecchymosis may occur; less commonly, anemia, leucocytosis, leukopenia, lymphadenopathy, lymphocytosis, thrombocytopenia, thrombocythemia may occur.

Nursing Implications: Assess baseline CBC and presence of bruising on skin. Instruct patient to report any bleeding, bruising, infection, or any changes in condition. Check CBC as indicated and discuss any changes with physician.

IX.   ALTERATION IN URINARY ELIMINATION related to DYSURIA

Defining Characteristics: Frequently, dysuria, hematuria, metrorrhagia, impaired urination, or vaginitis may occur. Infrequently, albuminuria, kidney calculus, cystitis, nocturia, bladder pain, kidney pain, polyuria, prostatitis, pyelonephritis, pyuria, incontinence, urinary urgency may occur.

Nursing Implications: Assess baseline urinary status. Instruct patient to report any changes, and discuss interventions with physician.

MANAGEMENT

Drug: zolpidem tartrate (Ambien)

Class: Benzodiazepine-like hypnotic.

Mechanism of Action: Despite a chemical structure unlike the benzodiazepines, it selectively binds to one of the GABA complexes that the benzodiazepines non-selectively bind to, producing deep sleep (stages 3 and 4) without muscle relaxant or anticonvulsant properties.

Metabolism: Well absorbed from GI tract, with 70% of drug reaching the systemic circulation. Absorption and distribution affected by food intake. Widely distributed in body tissues and fluids, including CSF. Crosses placenta and is excreted in breastmilk. Highly bound to plasma proteins. Metabolized in liver and excreted in urine, bile, and feces. Onset of action in 7–27 minutes, with a peak of 0.5–2.3 hours, and duration of 6–8 hours. Elimination half-life is 1.7–2.5 hours.

Indication: For the short-term treatment of insomnia characterized by difficulties with sleep initiation. Ambien has been shown to decrease sleep latency for up to 35 days.

Dosage/Range:

Adult (for insomnia):
- Oral: 10–20 mg PO at hs.
- Elderly or debilitated individuals: 5 mg PO.

Drug Preparation:
- Store tablets in tight container at $< 40°C$ (104°F).
- Administer on an empty stomach immediately before bedtime.

Drug Interactions:
- CNS depressants (e.g., alcohol, phenothiazines): additive CNS depression; avoid concurrent use or use cautiously and monitor carefully.

Lab Effects/Interference:
- None.

Special Considerations:
- Indicated for the short-term treatment of insomnia, generally 7–10 days of use.
- Contraindications: nursing mothers.
- Administer cautiously in patients with liver or renal dysfunction, pregnancy, pulmonary compromise, or who are depressed.
- May cause increased depression in patients who are already depressed.

Potential Toxicities/Side Effects and the Nursing Process

I. ALTERATIONS IN SENSORY/PERCEPTUAL PATTERNS related to CNS DEPRESSION

Defining Characteristics: CNS depressant effects include drowsiness, fatigue, lethargy, drugged feeling, depression, anxiety, irritability.

Nursing Implications: Assess baseline neurologic status, affective state, and risk factors, and monitor during treatment. Instruct patient to report worsening depression, and assess for any suicidal ideation. Instruct patient to avoid alcohol while taking drug. Assess effect on elderly and/or debilitated patients (cognition, motor function, other sensitivities). Assess effect of drug side effects on patient, and weigh against benefit. Inform patient that daytime drowsiness may occur, and instruct to use caution if driving or operating heavy machinery.

II. ALTERATION IN NUTRITION, LESS THAN BODY REQUIREMENTS, related to GI SIDE EFFECTS

Defining Characteristics: Nausea, vomiting, dyspepsia may occur.

Nursing Implications: Assess baseline nutrition status, and instruct the patient to report any nausea or vomiting.

III. INJURY related to DECREASE IN MENTAL ALERTNESS, PHYSICAL COORDINATION

Defining Characteristics: Drug may cause drowsiness, dizziness, diplopia, and impair physical coordination, mental alertness. At doses > 10 mg, patients may experience anterograde amnesia or memory impairment.

Nursing Implications: Assess other medications that may increase risk (e.g., opiates, phenothiazines) and response to drug. Instruct patient to avoid potentially hazardous activities, including driving a car, operating machinery.

MANAGEMENT

Section 3
Complications

Chapter *10*
Managing Tumor-Related Skeletal Events and Hypercalcemia

Metastases to bone can significantly alter a patient's quality of life related to pain, disability, hypercalcemia, and complications such as fracture (Roodman, 2004). Fortunately, there has been significant progress in the management of tumor-related skeletal events as the biology underlying metastases to bone is better understood. To review, bones normally undergo constant remodeling where osteoclasts break down bone cells (a process called resorption), followed by the building of new bone by osteoblasts. The process is tightly regulated by the body, and osteoclastic activity—as well as osteoblastic activity—is controlled by both systemic and local factors. For example, osteoclasts (breakdown) are stimulated by the parathyroid hormone-related peptide (PTHrP) hormone, 1,25-dihydroxyvitamin D_3, and thyroxine (T_4). This happens by inducing the bone marrow stromal cells and the osteoblasts to express the receptor activator of nuclear factor-kB ligand (RANKL, or osteoclast differentiation factor). RANKL is also important in immune function, as it is a survival factor for dendritic cells, and RANKL has an important role in cell migration to bone and in specific metastatic behaviors of cancer cells (Jones et al., 2008). Locally, osteoblasts secrete interleukin-6 (IL-6), IL-1, prostaglandin Es, and colony-stimulating factors (CSFs), which lead to the formation of osteoclasts. Epidermal growth factor (EGF) and tumor necrosis factor (TNF) stimulate osteoclastic activity, as do thymocyte-dependent lymphocytes (T-cells), which produce IL-17. The microenvironment of the bone includes the stromal cells, which produce macrophage CSF and RANKL, as do osteoblasts. This stimulates monocyte-macrophage precursors to produce osteoclasts. The systemic factors upregulate or increase the expression of RANKL on the marrow stromal cells and the osteoblasts. RANKL binds to the RANK receptor on the osteoclast precursors made by the monocyte-macrophage precursors.

Osteoclastic activity can be halted by local and systemic factors, such as corticosteroids (which kill osteoblasts) and osteoprotegerin (called osteoclastogenesis inhibitory factor, a member of the TNF superfamily). These inhibit the differentiation of macrophages into osteoclasts, and osteoprotegerin binds to RANKL on osteoblast/stromal cells and osteoclast precursor cells. Thus, it is the balance between RANKL and osteoprotegerin that moves osteoclast activity. The osteoclasts act on the trabecular bone surface and break down the minerals and matrix by releasing proteases that dissolve the matrix, leaving small holes in the bone trabecula or framework of bone on the surface. Then the osteoclasts undergo apoptosis. Now the scales favor osteoblastic activity, and the osteoblasts fill the bone holes with new bone that still needs to be mineralized or calcified. Mesenchymal stem cells produce the osteoblasts and a transcription factor called Runx-2, which turns on the genes responsible for the differentiation or maturation of the osteoblasts. Systemic factors (e.g., parathyroid hormone [PTH], prostaglandins, cytokines, platelet-derived growth factor [PDGF]) and local factors that are released from the bone matrix (e.g., bone morphogenetic proteins [BMPs]), insulin-like growth factor (IGF), fibrocyte growth factor, vascular endothelial growth factor (VEGF), and prostate-specific antigen (PSA) all increase osteoblastic proliferation and differentiation. Old bone is replaced systematically, so building and tearing down of bone are always balanced without damaging the integrity of the skeleton. As women get older and reach menopause, the osteoblastic process (buildup) lags behind osteoclastic (breakdown) activity, so these women are at risk for osteoporosis. In addition, women being treated with hormones for breast cancer with selective estrogen receptor modulators (SERMs) are at risk for bone density loss and are thus advised to take calcium and vitamins, and to exercise regularly. Patients with cancers that metastasize to bone are at risk for skeletal lesions: patients with breast cancer have primarily osteoblastic with about 15–20% having osteolytic, and patients with prostate cancer have largely osteoblastic lesions. Patients with multiple myeloma have only osteoblastic bone lesions. Only osteoblastic processes (active bone formation) show on bone scans (Roodman, 2004).

As more is understood about the process of bone resorption and metastases, agents are targeted against the malignant pathways, such as denosumab (Xgeva), a human monoclonal antibody that blocks RANKL. Osteoclast differentiation, activation, and survival are regulated by three molecules: receptor activator of nuclear factor kB (RANK), the cytokine RANKL, and osteoprotegerin, a soluble decoy receptor of RANKL, which can turn off RANKL to stop bone loss (Body et al., 2006; Mirrakhimov, 2015). RANKL binds to RANK on premature and mature osteoclasts and regulates their differentiation, function, and survival (Body et al., 2006). The seed and soil hypothesis suggests that breast or prostate cancer cells are the "seeds," which secrete substances that create a microenvironment in the skeleton (bone), where various cytokines and growth factors make a very rich "soil" that attracts circulating tumor cells and fosters tumor growth in the bone. RANKL appears to regulate cancer cell migration and bone metastases in cells that express the receptor RANK, such as breast cancer cells (Jones et al., 2006). RANK is also expressed by prostate cancer cells where again RANKL has been found to act directly on RANK-expressing prostate tumor cells, guiding tumor cell migration to bone, and expressing tumor metastases genes that further stimulate tumor growth (Armstrong et al., 2008). Bisphosphonates have been shown to directly inhibit tumor growth in laboratory studies of human breast cancer cell lines. In addition, disseminated tumor cells in the bone marrow in early-stage breast cancer are reduced with treatment by zoledronic acid (Zometa) (Rack et al., 2007).

In 2013, Xgeva was FDA approved for the treatment of adults and skeletally mature adolescents with giant cell tumor of bone that is unresectable or where surgical resection will likely be disfiguring. Although now being used as an anti-tumor treatment, it has been left in this chapter as the mechanism of action, and the drug's other uses are best described here.

Hypercalcemia is a metabolic complication of malignant disease and is evidenced by a serum calcium of > 10.5 mg/dL. Potentially fatal, hypercalcemia occurs in 10–20% of patients with cancer, principally in patients with breast cancer; multiple myeloma; squamous cell cancers of head, neck, and esophagus; prostate cancer; and adult T-cell lymphoma. Hypercalcemia is compounded by problems of advanced disease, such as immobility and dehydration. Hypercalcemia of malignancy is either humoral or related to tumor invasion of bone. In humoral hypercalcemia, osteoclasts are activated and break down bone (resorption) as a result of tumor-released factors, such as PTH-related protein, as shown in Figure 10.1. This type may occur in patients with squamous-cell malignancies of the lung, head and neck, or with genitourinary cancers, such as renal cell or ovarian cancer. This group of patients in most cases does not have bony involvement by tumor. In contrast, patients with bony metastases in which a tumor has invaded the bone have tumors that release local substances that cause the bone to undergo resorption by osteoclasts (bone is broken down) with the release of calcium. Malignancies commonly associated with this type of hypercalcemia are breast cancer and multiple myeloma.

In reviewing normal calcium homeostasis, calcium is found primarily in bone. As such, 99% of the body's calcium is in the form of insoluble crystals, giving the human skeleton strength and durability. The remaining 1% is distributed between the body's intracellular and extracellular fluids: 45% is ionized in the serum, 45% is bound by protein, and 10% is found in insoluble complexes.

The ionized fraction of calcium is necessary for excitation of nerves, voluntary skeletal muscle, cardiac muscle, and involuntary muscles in the gut. If the body has too much ionized calcium, there is decreased excitability of these tissues. For instance, symptoms of

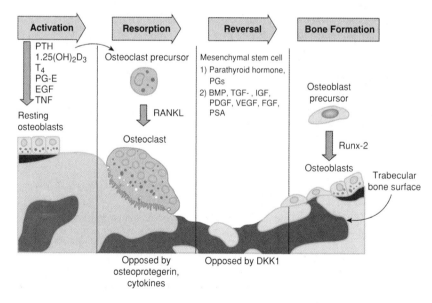

Figure 10.1   Process of Bone Building and Breakdown

Data from Loberg RD, Logothetis CJ, Keller ET, Pienta KJ. Pathogenesis and treatment of prostate cancer bone metastases: Targeting the lethal phenotype. *J Clin Oncol* 2005; 23(32):8232–8241; Logothetis CJ, Lin SH. Osteoblasts in prostate cancer metastasis to bone. *Nat Rev Cancer* 2005; 5(1):21–28; Roodman GD. Mechanisms of bone metastasis. *N Engl J Med* 2004; 350(16):1655–1664.

early hypercalcemia (calcium of 10–12 mg/dL) are fatigue, lethargy, constipation, anorexia, nausea and vomiting, and polyuria. Later symptoms, when the calcium is > 12 mg/dL, are altered mental status, coma, decreased deep tendon reflexes, increased cardiac contractility, and oliguric renal failure. In contrast, if there is too little ionized calcium in the body, there is increased excitability of nerves and muscle. The body attempts to regain more calcium to raise the level of ionized calcium by "raiding" the bone matrix.

Because 45% of the calcium outside of bone is bound to albumin, it is important to correct the value of ionized calcium in the serum if the albumin is low (normally bound calcium is now free in the serum, and the serum level may actually be higher than the laboratory value). The formula to determine ionized serum calcium, corrected for low serum albumin is:

$$\text{Corrected serum calcium} = \text{measured total serum calcium (mg/dL)}$$
$$+ [4.0 - \text{serum albumin (g/dL)}] \times 0.8$$

For example, a patient has a serum calcium of 10.0 mg/dL but has a serum albumin of 2.2 (normal is 3.5–5.5 g/dL). The corrected serum calcium is 10.0 mg/dL + (4.0 − 2.2 = 1.8 g/dL) $\times$ 0.8 + 10.0 + 1.44 = 11.44 mg/dL. Thus, a serum calcium level that appears normal may be abnormal (high) in the presence of a low serum albumin level.

The human skeleton undergoes constant remodeling, where there is an exquisite balance between bone formation and bone resorption (breakdown). Bone formation is mediated by osteoblasts and bone resorption by osteoclasts. Calcium balance is maintained by a number of factors. First, PTH released by the parathyroid gland increases serum calcium levels by stimulating bone resorption, increasing renal absorption of calcium, and stimulating the production of $1,25(OH)_2D_3$, which increases the intestinal absorption of calcium. In contrast, calcitonin balances these effects by reducing serum calcium: it inhibits bone resorption (breakdown) and decreases renal absorption of calcium. Normally, intestinal absorption of calcium is balanced by an approximately equal loss of calcium through urinary excretion. In most individuals before midlife, bone formation balances bone resorption.

There are many potential causes of hypercalcemia of malignancy. These include:

- Secretion of parathyroid-related protein by tumor.
- Secretion of other bone-resorbing substances by tumor (i.e., cytokines, transforming growth factor [TGF-α], IL-1, TNF).
- Conversion of 25-hydroxyvitamin D_3 to 1,25-dihydroxyvitamin D_3 by tumor.
- Local effects of osteolytic bony metastasis.

Therapeutic efforts to lower serum calcium in hypercalcemia of malignancy are based on rehydration to restore glomerular filtration and excretion of calcium (normally up to 600 mg/day), and drugs that promote calcium excretion or inhibit osteoclastic bone resorption. Today, bisphosphonate agents have been shown to decrease the development of osteoclastic bone lesions from breast and prostate cancer metastases and multiple myeloma. For patients with advanced disease, general management principles are based on palliation of symptoms. Diet restriction of calcium is not necessary, as calcium absorbed from the gut is often less than normal and patients are malnourished. Patients with T-cell lymphoma, who have increased 1,25-dihydroxyvitamin D_3, are an exception to this rule. These patients have high levels of 1,25-dihydroxyvitamin D_3 and should avoid intake of dairy products. It is important for patients to bear weight if possible, since immobility increases osteoclastic activity and decreases osteoblastic activity. Since calcium is a potent diuretic, patients are often dehydrated with the loss of sodium and water. Further, as the serum calcium increases, the distal renal tubules become less able to retain sodium, and there is further sodium loss from the kidneys. Patients are usually rehydrated with 3–4 L/day of 0.9% sodium chloride over 48 hours to restore fluid volume. Loop diuretics are administered, such as furosemide (Lasix), which increase calcium excretion. Thiazide diuretics are avoided, since they increase tubular reabsorption of calcium. This usually provides symptomatic improvement, but it is important to monitor the patient closely for possible fluid overload on the one hand, or intravascular dehydration with electrolyte imbalance on the other.

A number of drugs inhibit osteoclastic bone activity. The bisphosphonates have potent hypocalcemic activity, binding tightly to the calcified bone matrix. Some of the drugs inhibit lymphokine-and prostaglandin-mediated bone resorption, and the drugs vary in their inhibition of bone mineralization. Pamidronate (Aredia) and zoledronic acid (Zometa) inhibit bone resorption at low doses without decreasing mineralization and normalizing serum calcium in 80–90% of patients within 48–96 hours (Fitton & McTavish, 1991). Pamidronate and zolendronic acid are effective in reducing pain from bony metastases and decrease the incidence of bone metastasis in patients with multiple myeloma or breast cancer. Zolendronic acid was shown to reduce skeletal events in patients with prostate cancer (Berenson et al., 2001). More recently, studies have determined that bone resorption markers such as N-telopeptide of type I collagen (NTX) correlate with the extent of bone metastases and reflect the extent of bony metastases in patients (Lipton et al., 2007). Furthermore, studies have suggested that the normalization of NTX as a result of bisphosphonate therapy results in decreased progression of bony metastases and lower incidence of fractures (Brown et al., 2005).

Lipton et al. (2007) demonstrated in a retrospective subset analysis of a phase III randomized controlled trial patients with breast cancer that early normalization of elevated baseline NTX through zolendronic acid therapy was associated with higher event-free survival (e.g., fewer fractures) and higher overall survival. Similarly, Hirsch et al. (2008) found statistically significant correlations between zolendronic acid and increased survival compared to placebo in patients with high baseline NTX levels. Well, what about prevention of bony metastases and improved survival in the adjuvant breast cancer setting? In a very exciting presentation, Ghant (2009) reported that in a randomized, open-label phase III trial of patients with early premenopausal breast cancer, there was improved outcome when zoledronic acid was added to endocrine therapy (either tamoxifen or anastrozole) (Austrian Breast and Colorectal Cancer Study Group, ABCSG-12). Adjuvant zolendronic acid was included in the study, both to counter the significant bone loss associated with ovarian suppression (goserelin) and to see whether the antitumor effects seen in the metastatic setting would be seen in the adjuvant setting as well as measured by time to disease recurrence and overall survival. At a median follow-up of 60 months, patients receiving zolendronic acid had improved disease-free survival ($p = 0.011$), as evidenced by less contralateral breast cancer, distant metastases, and local regional recurrence, as well as longer relapse-free survival ($p = 0.014$) and a trend toward improved overall survival ($p = 0.001$). However, in the final analysis, there was no significant difference in overall survival. There were no reported renal toxicity or confirmed osteonecrosis of the jaw during the study. Although the initial study report from the ABCSG-12 trial (Ghant et al., 2009) showed that zolendronic acid reduced breast cancer recurrence and breast cancer death by 33%, the *Adjuvant Zoledronic Acid to Reduce Recurrence* (AZURE) study reported in 2010 showed no effect on breast cancer recurrence or suvival overall (Coleman et al., 2010). However, a subset analysis did show that in postmenopausal women ($>$ 5 years menopausal), zolendronic acid did show a significant benefit on overall survival, reducing the risk for death by 29% (p = 0.017). There was no benefit in younger ($<$ 5 years postmenopausal) or premenopausal women. Studies are ongoing to further define the role of bisphosphonates on cancer recurrence (NSABP B-34, SWOG SO307), and adjuvant treatment of breast cancer with zolendronic acid is not recommended at this time.

A class effect of bisphosphonates is potential renal insufficiency (zolendronic acid $>$ pamidronate) and also rarely osteonecrosis of the jaw. Patients should have a serum creatinine assessed before each treatment, as well as serial urinalyses for protein. In addition, patients should have a baseline oral exam by a dentist or oral surgeon, and patients at highest risk for osteonecrosis of the jaw (e.g., poor dental health) should be seen regularly. As more patients are treated with bisphosphonates, and for longer periods of time, osteonecrosis of the jaw is emerging as a more significant problem. Dental surgery appears to be a risk factor so that a dental screening with necessary extractions and implants should be done prior to beginning bisphosphonate therapy. The risk of developing osteonecrosis of the jaw increases the longer a patient is on therapy. Oncology nurses should continue to assess patients for any signs or symptoms of dental problems during bisphosphonate therapy.

Table 10.1 shows staging and recommendations from the American Association of Oral and Maxillofacial Surgeons.

Other hypocalcemic agents include the following, but are less often used. Oral phosphates inhibit bone resorption and stimulate bone formation, as well as precipitate calcium. However, the side effect of diarrhea limits their usefulness. Glucocorticoids have an unpredictable effect, and their value is limited by side effects of high drug doses. However, they are often used in steroid-responsive malignancies such as multiple myeloma and lymphoma. Calcitonin inhibits bone resorption and promotes urinary calcium excretion with a rapid, but brief, response (2–3 days). Plicamycin (mithramycin) inhibits osteoclastic bone resorption by killing the osteoclasts. It is potent, lowering calcium in 24–72 hours, but rebound hypercalcemia often occurs within 1 week. The high toxicity of the drug prevents wide usage.

After symptomatic hypercalcemia is resolved, the malignant disease is treated if appropriate to prevent recurrence (e.g., with chemotherapy or radiotherapy to lytic bone lesions). Nursing implications revolve around management of the patient receiving aggressive hydration and hypocalcemic medications. Patient education is prominent, as patients and their families are taught about the disease, as well as self-assessment of signs and symptoms of hypercalcemia, fluid balance, activity, and oral care. For patients receiving bisphosphonates for the prevention of bony metastases, nursing priorities include assessment of renal function before each treatment, oral assessment and patient education about potential, albeit rare, osteonecrosis of the jaw, and teaching patients about self-administration of calcium and vitamin D supplements to prevent osteoporosis.

Table 10.1   Staging and Recommendations for Treatment of Bisphosphonate-Related Osteonecrosis of the Jaw

Stage	Recommended Treatment
At risk: No apparent necrotic bone in patients who have been treated with either oral or IV bisphosphonates	Teach patient about risk and close need for monitoring; no treatment indicated
Stage 0: No clinical evidence of necrotic bone, but non-specific clinical findings and symptoms	Systemic management, including the use of analgesics and antibiotics
Stage 1: Exposed and necrotic bone in patients who are asymptomatic and have no evidence of infection	Antibacterial mouth rinse, clinical follow-up on a quarterly basis, patient education, and review of indications for continued bisphosphate therapy
Stage 2: Exposed and necrotic bone associated with infection, as evidenced by pain and erythema in the region of exposed bone with or without purulent discharge	Symptomatic treatment with oral antibiotics, oral antibacterial mouth rinses, pain control, and superficial debridement to relieve soft-tissue irritation
Stage 3: Exposed and necrotic bone in patients with pain, infection, and one or more of the following: exposed and necrotic bone extending beyond the region of the alveolar bone; pathologic fracture; extra-oral fistulae; oral-antral or oral-nasal communication; or osteolysis extending to the inferior border of the mandible of the sinus floor	Antibacterial mouth rinse, antibiotic therapy and pain control, and surgical debridement/resection for longer-term palliation of infection and pain

Data from American Association of Oral and Maxillofacial Surgeons, Position Paper, January 2009.

References

American Association of Oral and Maxillofacial Surgeons. *Position Paper on Bisphosphonate-Related Osteonecrosis of the Jaw, 2014 Update.* Available at https://www.joms.org/article /S0278-2391(14)00463-7/pdf. Accessed October 15, 2019.

Amgen. Xgeva (denosumab) [package insert]. Thousand Oaks, CA. May 2019.

Amgen. Sensipar (cinacalcet) tablets [package insert]. Thousand Oaks, CA. March 2019.

Armstrong AP, Miller RE, Jones JC, Zhang J, Keller ET, Dougall WC. RANKL Acts Directly on RANK-expressing Prostate Tumor Cells and Mediates Migration and Expression of Tumor Metastasis Genes. *Prostate* 2008; 68(1):92–104.

Berenson JR, Rosen LS, Howell A. Zoledronic Acid Reduces Skeletal-related Events in Patients with Osteolytic Metastases. A Double-blind, Randomized Dose-response Study. *Cancer* 2001; 91: 144–154.

Blum RH, Novetsky D, Shasha D, Fleishman S. The Multidisciplinary Approach to Bone Metastases. *Oncology* 2003; 17:845–857.

Body JJ, Facon T, Coleman RE, et al. A Study of the Biological Receptor Activator of Nuclear Factor kB-ligand Inhibitor, Denosumab, in Patients with Multiple Myeloma or Bone Metastases from Breast Cancer. *Clin Cancer Res* 2006; 12:1221–1228.

Bone HG, Bolognese MA, Yuen CK, Kendler DL, Wang H, Liu Y, San Martin J. Effects of Denosumab on Bone Mineral Density and Bone Turnover in Postmenopausal Women. *J Clin Endocrinol Metabolism* 2008; 93(6):2149–2157.

Coleman R, Coleman R, Thorpe H, et al. Adjuvant Treatment with Zoledronic Acid in Stage II/III Breast Cancer. The AZURE trial (BIG 01/04). *Cancer Res* 2010; 70(24 suppl): Abstract S4–5.

Ghant M, Mlineritsch B, Schippinger W, et al. Adjuvant Ovarian Suppression Combined with Tamoxifen or Anastrozole, Alone or in Combination with Zoledronic Acid, in Premenopausal Women with Hormone-responsive, Stage I and II Breast Cancer: First Efficacy Results from ABCSG-12. *J Clin Oncol* 2008 (May 20 suppl: abstract LBA4); 26.

Ghant M, Mlineritsch B, Schippinger W, et al. Endocrine Therapy Plus Zoledronic Acid in Premenopausal Breast Cancer *N Engl J Med* 2009; 360:679–691.

Hirsch V, Major PP, Lipton A, et al. Zoledronic Acid and Survival in Patients with Metastatic Bone Disease from Lung Cancer and Elevated Markers of Osteoclast Activity. *Thorac Oncol* 2008; 3(3):228–236.

Hospira Inc. Pamidronate [package insert]. Lake Forest, IL. September 2009.

Jones DH, Nakashima T, Sanchez OH, et al. Regulation of Cancer Cell Migration and Bone Metastasis by RANKL. *Nature* 2006; 440(7084):692–696.

Lipton A, Cook RJ, Major P, Smith MR, Coleman RE. Zoledronic Acid and Survival in Breast Cancer Patients with Bone Metastases and Elevated Markers of Osteoclast Activity. *Oncologist* 2007; 12:1035–1043.

Lipton A, Steger GG, Figueroa J, et al. Randomized Active Controlled Phase II Study of Denosumab Efficacy and Safety in Patients with Breast Cancer Related Bone Metastases. *J Clin Oncol* 2007; 25(28):4431–4437.

Mirrakhimov AE. Hypercalcemia of malignancy: An update on pathogenesis and management. *N Am J Med Sci* 2015; 7(11):483–493.

Mylan Institutional LLC. Pamidronate [package insert]. Rockford IL. December 2015.

Novartis Pharmaceuticals Corp. Zometa (zoledronic acid) [package insert]. East Hanover, NJ. December 2018.

Rack BK, Jueckstock J, Genss E-M, et al. *Effect of zoledronate on persisting isolated tumor cells in the bone marrow of patients without recurrence of early breast cancer.* Presented at the 30th San Antonio Breast Cancer Symposium, San Antonio, TX; December 13–16, 2007, Abstract 511.

Reich CD. Advances in the Treatment of Bone Metastases. *Clin J Oncol Nurs* 2003; 7:641–646.

Roodman GD. Mechanisms of Bone Metastases. *N Engl J Med* 2004; 350(16):1655–1664.

Drug: cinacalcet HCl (Sensipar)

Class: Hypocalcemic agent.

Mechanism of Action: The calcium-sensing receptor on the surface of the chief cell of the parathyroid gland regulates PTH secretion. PTH is responsible for telling the bones to break down bone (osteoclastic) and release calcium into the blood when it is needed. Cinacalcet HCl is a calcium-sensing receptor agonist, which directly decreases PTH levels by increasing the sensitivity of calcium-sensing receptors to activation by extracellular calcium. As PTH levels decrease, the level of calcium in the blood decreases.

Metabolism: Oral drug is well absorbed, and maximum plasma levels are achieved in 2–6 hours. Drug AUC levels are increased 82% when ingested with a high-fat meal. Drug is metabolized by CYP3A4, CYP2D6, and CYP1A2 enzymes of the P450 microenzyme system. Drug is excreted in the urine (80%) primarily, and to a lesser degree in the feces (15%). Drug is poorly excreted in patients with moderate-to-severe hepatic impairment, with a half-life prolonged 33 and 70%, respectively. Drug is highly protein-bound so hemodialysis does not treat overdosage.

Indication: Calcium-sensing receptor agonist indicated for (1) secondary hyperparathyroidism (HPT) in patients with chronic kidney disease on dialysis; (2) hypercalcemia in adult patients with parathyroid carcinoma (PC); (3) hypercalcemia in adult patients with primary HPT for whom parathyroidectomy is indicated, who are unable to undergo the procedure.

Contraindication: Patients with serum calcium is < LLN range. NOT indicated for pediatric patients. NOT indicated for patients with CKD NOT on dialysis.

Dosage/Range:
- *Secondary HPT in patients with CKD on dialysis*: starting dose is 30 mg PO qd, titrated every 2–4 weeks through sequential doses of 30 mg PO qd, then 60 mg PO qd, then 90 mg PO qd, 120, PO qd, and then to 180 mg PO once daily as necessary to achieve targeted intact parathyroid hormone (iPTH). Monitor response at least **12 hours after dose**.
- Target iPTH level: 150–300 pg/mL.
- Drug can be used alone or in combination with vitamin D and/or phosphate binders.
- If hypocalcemia develops during titration, correct with calcium repletion.
- If serum calcium falls < 8.4 mg/dL but remains > 7.5 mg/dL, or if symptoms of hypocalcemia occur, calcium-containing phosphate binders and/or vitamin D sterols can be used to raise serum calcium. If serum calcium falls < 7.5 mg/dL, or if symptoms of hypocalcemia persist and the dose of Vitamin D cannot be increased, hold cinacalcet administration until serum calcium reaches 8.0 mg/dL and/or symptoms of hypocalcemia have resolved. Restart cinacalcet using the next lowest dose of cinacalcet.
- *Hypercalcemia in patients with PC or hypercalcemia in patients with primary PTH:* start at 30 mg PO bid; titrate every 2–4 weeks through sequential doses of 30 mg PO bid, then 60 mg PO bid, then 90 mg PO bid, and then 90 mg tid or qid as necessary to normalize serum calcium levels. Monitor serum calcium within 1 week after initiation or dose adjustment.
- Once maintenance dose has been established, monitor serum calcium levels monthly (secondary HPT) and every 2 months for patients with PC or primary HPT.
- If switching from Parsabiv (etelcalcetide) to cinacalcet: discontinue etelcalcetide for at least 4 weeks prior to starting cinacalcet; ensure corrected serum calcium is at or above the LLN prior to starting cinacalcet.
- Monitor patients with moderate or severe hepatic impairment closely.
- Do not administer if serum calcium is less than the LLN range (e.g., < 8.4 mg/dL).
- Monitor calcium levels frequently during dose titration.

Drug Preparation:
- Drug available in 30-, 60-, and 90-mg tablets.
- Administer with food or shortly after a meal.

Drug Administration:

Teach patient to
- Take tablet(s) with a meal or shortly after one.
- Take whole, do not divide, chew, or crush.
- Review with nurse schedule for follow-up and blood test monitoring.

COMPLICATIONS

Drug Interactions:
- Drug is a potent inhibitor of CYP2D6: Dosage adjustment may be needed for drugs primarily metabolized by CYP2D6 (e.g., flecainide, vinblastine, thioridazine, tricyclic antidepressants).
- Strong CYP3A4 inhibitor: Coadministration may increase cinacalcet HCl serum levels (e.g., ketoconazole: increased cinacalcet HCl AUC by 2.3 times). Dosage adjustments may be needed; monitor iPTH, serum phosphorus, and serum calcium.

Lab Effects/Interference:
- Hypocalcemia.
- Hyperphosphatemia.

Special Considerations:
- Most common adverse reactions were nausea and vomiting.
- Drug should not be used by pregnant or breastfeeding mothers, unless benefit outweighs risk.
- Drug is NOT indicated in pediatric patients.
- Warnings and Precautions:
  - *Hypocalcemia*: life-threatening events may occur: hypocalcemia prolongs QT interval, lowers the threshold for seizures and can cause hypotension, worsening heart failure, and/or arrhythmia as well as paresthesias, myalgias, muscle spasms, and tetany. Monitor serum calcium carefully for the occurrence of hypocalcemia during treatment. Closely monitor patients with a PMH of (1) congenital long QT syndrome, QT interval prolongation or are taking medications that prolong the QT interval; (2) seizure disorder; (3) receiving other therapies that lower serum calcium. Teach patients that if low calcium blood levels develop, the patient will need to receive supplemental calcium and to contact a healthcare provider if they develop any symptoms of hypocalcemia (e.g., paresthesias, myalgias, muscle spasms, and tetany). Calcium supplementation with calcium, calcium-containing phosphate binders, and/or vitamin D sterols, or increase in dialysate calcium, if needed, and drug dose reduced or drug discontinued.
  - *Upper GI bleeding:* Patients with known gastritis, esophagitis, ulcers, or severe vomiting may be at risk. Monitor patients for worsening GI adverse effects (e.g., nausea and vomiting) and for any signs/symptoms of upper GI bleeding and ulceration. Patient should be promptly evaluated if GI bleeding is suspected.
  - *Hypotension, worsening heart failure, and/or arrhythmias*: isolated instances of hypotension, worsening heart failure and/or arrhythmias have been reported.
  - *Adynamic bone disease*: may develop if iPTH levels are suppressed below 100 pg/mL. If iPTH levels decrease < 150 pg/mL in patients receiving cinacalcet, reduce dose of cinacalcet and/or vitamin D sterols, or cinacalcet therapy discontinued.
  - Hepatic impairment: AUC is increased in patients with moderate and severe hepatic impairment; monitor patient's serum calcium, phosphorus, and iPTH levels closely throughout treatment.

Potential Toxicities/Side Effects and the Nursing Process

I   POTENTIAL FOR INJURY related to HYPOCALCEMIA

Defining Characteristics: Drug lowers serum calcium. Signs and symptoms of hypocalcemia are paresthesia, myalgias, cramping, tetany, and seizures.

Nursing Implications: Assess baseline serum calcium, phosphate, magnesium levels, as well as PTH level. Develop a plan for titration with the patient, and frequency of laboratory monitoring. Teach patient symptoms of hypocalcemia, and to report them right away if they occur. Serum calcium should be assessed within 1 week after initiation or dose adjustment. Once dose has been established, serum calcium should be assessed every month. If serum calcium > 7.5 mg/dL but < 8.4 mg/dL, or if symptoms of hypocalcemia occur, discuss with physician the addition of calcium-containing phosphate binders and/or vitamin D sterols to raise the serum calcium. If the serum calcium falls to < 7.5 mg/dL or if symptoms of hypocalcemia persist, stop drug until serum calcium level reaches 8.0 mg/dL and/or symptoms resolve. Resume dose per physician, at next lowest dose of drug.

II   ALTERATION IN NUTRITION, LESS THAN BODY REQUIREMENTS, related to GI SIDE EFFECTS

Defining Characteristics: Nausea (31%) and vomiting (27%) are most common adverse effects, but diarrhea may also occur (21%).

Nursing Implications: Assess baseline nutritional and elimination status, and monitor during treatment. Ensure adequate hydration and urinary output of 2 L/day. Teach patient to administer oral antiemetics prior to taking drug, and as needed between drug doses. Assess food preferences, and suggest small, frequent feedings. Teach patient to report symptoms that worsen or do not resolve with supportive care.

III   ALTERATION IN COMFORT related to MYALGIA AND DIZZINESS

Defining Characteristics: Myalgia affects about 15% of patients and dizziness 10% of patients.

Nursing Implications: Assess baseline hydration, comfort status, and teach patient that these side effects may occur. Teach patient to change position slowly if dizziness occurs, and to notify nurse or physician if dizziness worsens or does not resolve. Teach patient symptom-management strategies, such as local application of heat for myalgias, and to notify provider if myalgias worsen.

Drug: denosumab (Xgeva)

Class: Inhibitor of osteoclastic bone resorption via inhibition of RANKL; RANK ligand (RANKL) inhibitor.

Mechanism of Action: Human monoclonal antibody (IgG_2) with specificity and affinity for RANKL, so it binds to RANKL, thus preventing RANKL from activating its receptor RANK on the surface of osteoclasts and their precursors. This inhibits or turns off osteoclast formation, function, and survival, and decreases bone resorption. Increased osteoclast activity (bone resorption), stimulated by RANKL, is a mediator of bony metastases in solid tumors. It mimics the effect of the RANK modulator osteoprotegerin. The end result

COMPLICATIONS

is increased bone mass and strength in both cortical and trabecular bone. Giant cell bone tumors consist of stromal cells expressing RANKL, and osteoclast-like giant cells express the RANK receptors. Cell signaling through the RANK receptor enhances osteolysis and tumor growth. Denosumab (Xgeva) prevents RANKL from activating the RANK receptor on osteoclasts, their precursors, and osteoclast-like giant cells so they cannot break down bone.

Metabolism: After subcutaneous dosing, bioavailability of denosumab is 62%, and multiple dosing of 120 mg every 4 weeks resulted in up to a 2.8-fold accumulation of denosumab concentration, with steady state reached by 6 months. The mean elimination half-life is 28 days. Drug clearance and volume of distribution is proportional to body weight: 48% higher in a 100-lb. (45-kg) person, and 46% lower in a 265-lb. (120-kg) person, compared to the 145-lb. (66-kg) person. Renal impairment did not affect drug pharmacokinetics, and no studies were done to evaluate the effect of hepatic impairment.

Indication: For (1) prevention of skeletal-related events in patients with multiple myeloma and in patients with bone metastases from solid tumors; (2) treatment of adults and skeletally mature adolescents with giant cell tumor of bone that is unresectable or where surgical resection is likely to result in severe morbidity; (3) hypercalcemia of malignancy refractory to bisphosphonate therapy.

Contraindications: (1) hypocalcemia; (2) known clinically significant hypersensitivity.

Dosage/Range (subcutaneously only):
- *Prevention of skeletal-related events in patients with multiple myeloma or with bone metastases from solid tumors*: 120 mg SQ every 4 weeks.
- *Treatment of adults and skeletally mature adolescents with giant cell tumor of bone*: 120 mg SQ every 4 weeks, with additional 120-mg doses on days 8 and 15 of the first month of treatment.
- Administer calcium and vitamin D to treat or prevent hypocalcemia.
- *Hypercalcemia of Malignancy*: 120 mg SQ every 4 weeks with additional 120-mg doses on days 8 and 15 of the first month of treatment.

Drug Preparation:
- Drug is available as 120 mg/1.7 mL (70 mg/mL) single-use vial. Drug should be refrigerated at 36–46°F (2–8°C) in its original carton. Do not freeze. Once removed from the refrigerator, drug must not be exposed to temperatures above 25°C (77°F) or direct light, and it must be used within 14 days. Protect from direct light and heat.
  - Prior to administration, remove drug from refrigerator and bring to room temperature, 25°C (77°F), by letting it stand in the original container for 15–30 minutes. Do not warm any other way.
  - Inspect drug for particulate matter or discoloration, and discard if found. Solution should be clear, colorless to pale yellow, and it may contain trace amounts of proteinaceous particles ranging from translucent to white.
  - Using a 27-gauge needle, aseptically draw up entire contents of vial; do not reenter vial. Discard the empty vial.

Drug Administration:
- Administer subcutaneously in the upper arm, upper thigh, or abdomen. Rotate sites. Administer calcium and vitamin D as necessary to treat or prevent hypocalcemia.
- Drug is contraindicated in patients with clinically significant hypersensitivity to drug or its components.
- Same active ingredient in Prolia, so patient should not take Prolia when taking Xgeva.

Drug Interactions:
- No studies have been carried out. There are no identified drug interactions with standard chemotherapy or hormonal therapy.
- Drugs causing hypocalcemia: increased risk for hypocalcemia.

Lab Effects/Interference:
- Hypocalcemia, hypercholesterolemia, hypophosphatemia.

Special Considerations:
- Most common adverse reactions (> 25%) were fatigue/asthenia, hypophosphatemia, nausea (in patients with bone metastases), (> 10% in patients with giant cell tumor): arthralgia, headache, nausea, back pain, fatigue, and extremity pain; and (> 20% in patients with hypercalcemia of malignancy) nausea, dyspepsia, decreased appetite, headache, peripheral edema, vomiting, anemia, constipation, diarrhea.
- If the patient becomes pregnant while receiving the drug, Amgen has a Pregnancy Surveillance Program. RANKL and RANK function in other body processes, and thus, the long-term effects of antagonism of this cytokine are unclear.
- Drug is not recommended in pediatric patients, as it may impair bone growth in children with open growth plates, as well as inhibit teeth eruption.
- Warnings and Precautions:
  - *Drug products with same active ingredient*: Prolia contains denosumab. Patients taking Xgeva should not take Prolia.
  - *Hypersensitivity*, including anaphylaxis, has been rarely reported. Reactions may include hypotension, dyspnea, upper airway edema, lip swelling, rash, pruritus, and urticaria. If anaphylactic or other significant allergic reaction occurs, provide emergency intervention as ordered; drug should be permanently discontinued.
  - *Severe hypocalcemia* may occur; preexisting hypocalcemia should be corrected prior to starting denosumab.
    - Monitor calcium levels prior to each treatment. Patients with renal impairment (creatinine clearance < 30 mL/min or receiving dialysis) are at increased risk.
    - Patients MUST take adequate calcium and vitamin D supplements, as well as magnesium, as prescribed by their physician or nurse practitioner.
    - Teach patient to report signs/symptoms of hypocalcemia (abdominal cramping, irregular heartbeat, depression, irritability, lethargy or sluggishness, muscle spasms, seizures).
  - *Osteonecrosis of the jaw (ONJ)* may develop.
    - ONJ is characterized by jaw pain, osteomyelitis, osteitis, bone erosion, tooth or periodontal infection, toothache, gingival ulceration or gingival erosion, delayed healing of mouth or jaw after dental surgery.

COMPLICATIONS

- Patient should have an oral exam prior to starting denosumab, have any dental work completed prior to starting the drug, and be monitored closely for symptoms with periodic dental exams. Patient should avoid invasive dental procedures during treatment with denosumab.
- If ONJ develops, patient should be referred to a dentist or oral surgeon; however, extensive oral surgery may exacerbate the condition.
- Risk factors of ONJ are associated with tooth extraction and/or local infection with delayed healing, as well as immunosuppression, treatment with angiogenesis inhibitors, systemic corticosteroids, diabetes, and gingival infections.
- Teach patients to report any dental or jaw issues, such as pain, right away during therapy. Teach patient to practice good oral hygiene regularly during drug therapy. Consider discontinuance of drug therapy if ONJ develops based on individual patient assessment, and patients should be evaluated and treated by a dentist or oral surgeon.

- *Atypical subtrochanteric and diaphyseal femoral fracture*: Drug may cause atypical femoral fracture, occurring anywhere in the femoral shaft from just below the lesser trochanter to above the supracondylar flare, which may be transverse or short oblique, without communication.
  - Fracture is not usually associated with trauma, or it may occur with minimal trauma to the area. Fractures may be bilateral and patients may report prodromal pain (e.g., dull, aching thigh pain) prior to the diagnosis, weeks to months before complete fracture occurs.
  - Concomitant administration of corticosteroids may increase risk. Teach patients to report any new or unusual thigh, hip, or groin pain immediately. Evaluate patients for incomplete fracture. Also assess patient for signs and symptoms of fracture in the contralateral limb. Consider interrupting denosumab therapy pending a risk/benefit assessment.

- *Hypercalcemia following treatment discontinuation in patients with Giant Cell tumor of bone, and in patients with growing skeletons:* may happen within weeks to months after last dose. Monitor and treat hypercalcemia if it develops after drug discontinuation.
- *Multiple vertebral fractures (MVF) following treatment discontinuation*: Increased risk in patients at risk for, or with a PMH of osteoporosis. When discontinuing denosumab, assess patient risk for MVF and monitor closely.
- *Embryo-fetal toxicity*: Teach women of reproductive potential to use effective contraception to avoid pregnancy during treatment and for at least 5 months after last dose of denosumab. Patient should contact physician if pregnancy is suspected. It is not known if the drug is excreted in human milk, so patients who are nursing should discontinue nursing or discontinue the drug.

Potential Toxicities/Side Effects and the Nursing Process

I.   ALTERATIONS IN ELECTROLYTES related to HYPOCALCEMIA

Defining Characteristics: Denosumab may cause severe hypocalcemia. In clinical trials, hypocalcemia was reported in 18% (3.1% severe), with hypophosphatemia in 32% (severe in 15.4%). Drug is contraindicated in patients who are hypocalcemic. Drug may worsen hypocalcemia, especially if the patient has severe renal impairment (creatinine clearance < 30 mL/min or receiving dialysis). Patients must take calcium and vitamin D supplements, as well as magnesium, as needed and prescribed. Patients at risk for hypocalcemia are those taking other concomitant drugs that reduce serum calcium, or with a history of hypoparathyroidism, thyroid surgery, parathyroid surgery, malabsorption syndromes, excision of small intestine, or severe renal impairment as above. Post-marketing reports have documented severe symptomatic hypocalcemia, including fatal cases.

Nursing Implications: Assess serum calcium, phosphorus, and magnesium baseline and prior to each treatment. Consider monitoring patients with renal impairment, those who are receiving concomitant drugs that may cause hypocalcemia, or those with other risk for hypocalcemia more closely during therapy. Prior to drug administration, hypocalcemia must be corrected. Teach patient importance of daily calcium and vitamin D supplements and assess adherence (recommended daily calcium 1,000-mg and at least 400-mg vitamin D supplements). Assess for signs/symptoms of hypocalcemia (muscle twitching, spasm tetany, seizures), and teach patient to report any symptoms right away (spasms, twitches, muscle stiffness, or cramps in muscles, numbness or tingling in fingers, toes, or around the mouth).

II.   POTENTIAL FOR INJURY related to ONJ

Defining Characteristics: Patients receiving denosumab are at risk for ONJ, which is associated with RANKL inhibitor and bisphosphonate therapy. The incidence in denosumab clinical trials was 2.2%; of those who developd ONJ, 79% had a history of tooth extraction, poor oral hygiene, or use of a dental appliance, tooth extraction, and/or local infection with delayed healing. Patients at risk for ONJ are those who have had invasive dental procedures, a cancer diagnosis, concomitant therapies with corticosteroids, poor oral hygiene, and preexisting periodontal or dental disease. Patients on clinical trials also had pain in the back, musculoskeleton, and abdomen that was not significantly higher than placebo. Patient symptoms were jaw pain, osteomyelitis, osteitis, bone erosion, tooth or periodontal infection, toothache, gingival ulceration, and gingival erosion.

Nursing Implications: Ensure that patient has a thorough oral exam and dental history prior to starting drug, and periodically during therapy. If the patient has risk factors such as invasive dental procedures (e.g., tooth extraction, dental implants, oral surgery, cancer diagnosis, concomitant therapies such as chemotherapy and corticosteroids, poor oral hygiene, periodontal and/or other preexisting dental disease, anemia, coagulopathy, infection, ill-fitting dentures), patient should have a dental exam with necessary preventive dentistry prior to starting the drug. Any outstanding oral or dental issues must be referred to a dentist or oral surgeon for preventive work prior to starting the drug. Assess patient's baseline oral hygiene practices and ensure that they are effective. Teach patient to practice good oral hygiene consistently, and to report to the nurse or physician any problems that arise in the oral cavity or teeth. Monitor patients at risk closely. If ONJ does develop, consult a dentist or oral surgeon. Unfortunately, extensive dental surgery to treat ONJ may exacerbate the condition. If a patient is suspected to have, or has ONJ, patient should receive care by a dentist or oral surgeon (e.g., extensive dental surgery to treat ONJ may exacerbate it).

COMPLICATIONS

III.   ALTERATIONS IN NUTRITION, LESS THAN BODY REQUIREMENTS, related to NAUSEA, DIARRHEA

Defining Characteristics: Nausea occurred in > 25% of patients, while diarrhea occurred less.

Nursing Implications: Assess baseline nutritional and elimination status, and monitor during treatment. Instruct patient to report nausea and diarrhea, and discuss appropriate antiemetic with physician or nurse practitioner. Discuss bowel elimination plan. Teach patient to report any abdominal discomfort.

Drug: pamidronate disodium (Aredia)

Class: Bisphosphonate; hypocalcemic agent.

Mechanism of Action: Probably inhibits osteoclast activity in bone (bone breakdown) and may also block dissolution of minerals (hydroxyapatite) in bone, thus preventing calcium release from bone. Does not inhibit bone formation or bone mineralization. Indicated for the treatment of hypercalcemia of malignancy, in conjunction with adequate hydration, as well as prevention of osteolytic lesions in breast cancer and multiple myeloma.

Metabolism: Excreted by kidneys.

Indication: (1) Treatment of moderate or severe hypercalcemia associated with malignancy, with or without bone metastases; (2) treatment of moderate to severe Paget's disease of bone; (3) in conjunction with standard antineoplastic therapy, for the treatment of osteolytic bone metastases of breast cancer and osteolytic lesions of multiple myeloma.

Contraindications: Patients with clinically significant hypersensitivity to pamidronate disodium or other bisphosphonates. Do not administer to patients with severe renal impairment (e.g., serum creatinine > 3.0 mg/dL or CrCl < 30 mL/min).

Dosage/Range:

Adult (hypercalcemia of malignancy):
- IV (moderate hypercalcemia, 12–13.5 mg/dL corrected): 60–90 mg as single IV infusion dose over 2–24 hours; infusions > 2 hours may reduce risk of renal dysfunction.
- IV (severe hypercalcemia > 13.5 mg/dL): 90 mg as single-dose IV infusion over 2–24 hours. Infusions > 2 hours may reduce risk of renal dysfunction especially in patients with preexisting renal insufficiency.
- If retreatment required, wait a minimum of 7 days between treatments to allow for full response to initial dose.

Osteolytic bone metastases of breast cancer:
- 90 mg IV via 2-hour infusion every 3–4 weeks.
- *Assess serum creatinine baseline and prior to each treatment, and hold drug as follows: (a) patients with normal baseline creatinine, increase of 0.5 mg/dL; (b) patients with abnormal baseline creatinine, increase of 1.0 mg/dL. Osteolytic lesions of multiple myeloma:*

- 90 mg IV infusion over 4-hours every month.
- Assess serum creatinine baseline and prior to each treatment, and hold drug as follows: (a) patients with normal baseline creatinine, increase of 0.5 mg/dL; (b) patients with abnormal baseline creatinine, increase of 1.0 mg/dL.
- *Paget's Disease (moderate to severe):* 30 mg daily as a 4-hour infusion on 3 consecutive days for a total dose of 90 mg.

Drug Preparation:
- DO NOT exceed a dose of 90 mg pamidronate.
- Reconstitute by adding 10 mL sterile water for injection to 30-mg vial. Further dilute in 250 mL–1 L 0.0.45–9% sodium chloride or 5% dextrose injection as per manufacturer's directions.
- DO NOT mix with calcium-containing infusion solutions, such as Ringer's Lactate. Use separate IV solution and line from any other drug.
- Inspect parenteral drug products for particulate matter and discoloration, and do not use if found.

Drug Administration:
- Assess serum creatinine prior to each treatment as drug is excreted intact by the kidneys and risk of renal impairment exists if patients have renal insufficiency. If renal function is deteriorating, drug should be withheld until renal function returns to baseline.
- Infuse over 2–24 hours via infusion pump or rate controller via its own IV line.
- When drug is given to prevent lytic lesions in the bone, patients should take an oral calcium supplement of 500 mg and a multivitamin containing 400 IU of vitamin D daily.

Drug Interactions:
- Use caution with other potentially nephrotoxic drugs.
- Increased risk of renal function deterioration in multiple myeloma patients also receiving thalidomide.

Lab Effects/Interference:
- Decreased calcium.
- Decreased K+, decreased Mg, decreased P (phosphate).
- Increased serum creatinine, urinary excretion of protein (proteinuria).

Special Considerations:
- Most common adverse effects:
- Warnings and Precautions:
  - *Alteration in hypercalcemia-related metabolic parameters:* Monitor serum levels of calcium, phosphate, magnesium, and potassium baseline, after drug initiation, and carefully monitor during therapy. Monitor patients closely, especially patients with a history of thyroid surgery who may have relative hypoparathyroidism that would predispose to hypocalcemia when treated with pamidronate.
  - *Deterioration in renal function:* Use cautiously when combined with renally toxic drugs, such as aminoglycoside antibiotics or loop diuretics. Use cautiously in patients who have aspirin-sensitive asthma. Monitor serum creatinine and urine for protein prior to each treatment. Hold the drug for increased serum creatinine or proteinuria.

See package insert for holding drug based on renal function. Saline hydration to maintain urinary output of 2 L/day should be maintained during treatment for hypercalcemia.

- *Pregnancy category D*: Teach women of reproductive potential to use effective contraception to avoid pregnancy.
- *Osteonecrosis of the jaw*: The drug may rarely cause osteonecrosis of the jaw, often in conjunction with a dental procedure, such as tooth extraction. Patients should have an oral examination and preventive dentistry completed before starting bisphosphonate therapy and periodically during treatment if high risk or symptoms arise. Patients should avoid dental work being done while receiving bisphosphonate therapy.
- *Laboratory Monitoring:* Serum creatinine prior to each treatment; closely monitor serum calcium, electrolytes, phosphate, magnesium, and CBC/differential. Patients with preexisting anemia, leukopenia, or thrombocytopenia should be monitored closely for 2 weeks after pamidronate disodium treatment.
- *Drug Interactions:* Use drug cautiously when giving other potentially nephrotoxic drugs and monitor patient's renal function closely. Multiple myeloma patients may have an increased risk of renal dysfunction when pamidronate is used in combination with thalidomide.
- *Carcinogenesis, mutagenesis, impairment of fertility:* Rats developed adrenal pheochromocytoma and decreased fertility; however the drug was not carcinogenic.
- *Embryo-fetal toxicity:* Pregnancy category D. Teach female patients of reproductive potential to use effective contraception during treatment with palmidronate. It is unknown if drug is secreted in human milk.

- Clinical studies show 64% of patients have corrected serum calcium levels by 24 hours after beginning therapy, and after 7 days 100% of the 90-mg group had normal corrected levels. For some (33–53%), normal or partially corrected calcium levels in 60-mg and 90-mg groups persisted $\times$ 14 days.
- Drug may cause atypical femoral fracture, occurring anywhere in the femoral shaft from just below the lesser trochanter to above the supracondylar flare, which may be transverse or short oblique, without communication. Fracture is not usually associated with trauma, or may occur with minimal trauma to the area. Fractures may be bilateral, and patients may report prodromal pain (e.g., dull, aching thigh pain) prior to the diagnosis, weeks to months before complete fracture occurs.
  - Concomitant administration of corticosteroids may increase risk.
  - Teach patients to report any new or unusual thigh, hip, or groin pain immediately. Evaluate patients for incomplete fracture, and suspect atypical fracture in any patient who has/is receiving bisphosphonate therapy and presents with thigh or groin pain without trauma. Also assess patient for signs and symptoms of fracture in the contralatateral limb.
  - Consider discontinuing pamidronate therapy pending a risk/benefit assessment. It is unknown if the atypical femur fracture continues after therapy is stopped. Poor healing of the atypical fracture has been reported.
- Has been shown to reduce bony metastasis in patients with multiple myeloma and to reduce pain.

Potential Toxicities/Side Effects and the Nursing Process

I ALTERATIONS IN NUTRITION, LESS THAN BODY REQUIREMENTS, related to GI SIDE EFFECTS

Defining Characteristics: Nausea, vomiting, abdominal discomfort, constipation, and anorexia may occur rarely.

Nursing Implications: Assess baseline nutritional and elimination status and monitor during treatment. Ensure adequate hydration and urinary output of 2 L/day. Administer ordered antiemetics. Administer oral phosphates as cathartics if ordered. Assess food differences and offer small, frequent feedings.

II. ALTERATION IN ELECTROLYTES related to HYPOCALCEMIA, HYPERCALCEMIA

Defining Characteristics: Rarely, if drug is very effective, hypocalcemia may occur; conversely, if drug is ineffective, hypercalcemia may occur. Hypokalemia, hypomagnesemia, hypophosphatemia may occur. Women with breast cancer taking the drug to prevent lytic lesions are at risk for developing osteoporosis.

Nursing Implications: Monitor serum calcium closely. Assess for signs/symptoms of hypocalcemia (muscle twitching, spasm tetany, seizures) and hypercalcemia (bone pain, nausea, vomiting, polyuria, polydipsia, constipation, bradycardia, lethargy, muscle weakness, psychosis). Notify physician, recheck serum calcium immediately, and institute corrective measures as ordered. Monitor serum potassium, magnesium, phosphate levels and notify physician of abnormalities. Women receiving drug to prevent lytic lesions should receive calcium and vitamin D supplements and should be encouraged to exercise. If a smoker, she should be encouraged to stop smoking to reduce the risk of osteoporosis.

III. ALTERATIONS IN COMFORT related to LOCAL VEIN IRRITATION

Defining Characteristics: Transient fever (1°C or 3°F elevation) may occur 24–48 hours after drug administration (27% of patients); local reactions (pain, irritation, phlebitis) are common with 90-mg dose.

Nursing Implications: Assess baseline temperature, and monitor during and after infusion. Administer antipyretics as ordered. Assess IV site and restart new IV as needed for 90-mg dose in large vein where drug can be rapidly diluted. Apply warm packs as needed to site.

IV. ALTERATIONS IN FLUID BALANCE related to AGGRESSIVE HYDRATION

Defining Characteristics: Patients receive aggressive saline hydration to ensure urinary output of 2 L/day. Hypertension may occur. Patients with history of heart disease or renal insufficiency are at risk for fluid overload.

COMPLICATIONS

Nursing Implications: Assess baseline hydration status, total body fluid balance; monitor q 4 h. Discuss with physician need for diuretics once hydrated to keep body fluid balance equal (I = O). Monitor vital signs q 4 h during hydration, and notify physician of changes.

Drug: zoledronic acid (Zometa)

Class: Bisphosphonate.

Mechanism of Action: Inhibits bone resorption. Inhibits tumor-related osteoclast activity in bone (bone breakdown), promotes apoptosis of osteoclasts, and blocks dissolution of minerals (hydroxyapatite) in bone, thus preventing calcium release from bone, as well as osteoclastic resorption of cartilage. It also inhibits osteoclast activity and the release of calcium from the bones that is caused by tumor-related stimulatory factors. It does not inhibit bone formation or bone mineralization. Drug is very rapidly taken up in the bone, but very slowly released. Drug appears to inhibit endothelial cell proliferation and to inhibit the beta fibroblast growth factor (bFGF)–mediated angiogenesis. The drug is 100–850 times more potent than pamidronate.

Metabolism: Drug is primarily eliminated intact via the kidney. Long terminal half-life in plasma of 167 hours. Rapid injection results in 30% increase in serum drug concentration and renal damage.

Indication: Treatment of (1) hypercalcemia of malignancy; (2) patients with multiple myeloma and patients with documented bone metastases from solid tumors, in conjunction with standard antineoplastic therapy.

Limitation: the safety and efficacy of Zometa has not been established for use in hyperparathyroidism or nontumor-related hypercalcemia.

Contraindication: Hypersensitivity to any component of zoledronic acid.

Dosage/Range:
- Patient should be adequately hydrated (vigorously with IV saline) before treatment to encourage a urinary output of 2 L/day throughout treatment.
- Monitor renal function closely, baseline and prior to each treatment.
- *Hypercalcemia of malignancy* (corrected calcium ≥ 12 mg/dL): 4-mg (maximum) IV over at least 15 minutes; if retreatment required, wait at least 7 days before administering again and monitor renal function closely.
  - Vigorous saline IV hydration, with urinary output of 2 L/day.
  - Dose modification not necessary for mild-to-moderate renal impairment (serum creastinine < 4.5 mg/dL).
  - Mild or asymptomatic hypercalcemia may be treated more conservatively (saline hydration +/– loop diuretics).
- Multiple myeloma and metastatic bone lesions from solid tumors with urinary creatinine clearance of at least 60 mL/min is 4-mg IV over at least 15 minutes every 3–4 weeks.
  - Assess serum creatinine prior to EACH DOSE:
    - If patient has a normal serum creatinine prior to treatment but has an increase of 0.5 mg/dL within 2 weeks of next dose, hold zoledronic acid until the serum creatinine is at least within 10% of baseline value.

- If patient has an abnormal serum creatinine prior to treatment but has an increase of 1.0 mg/dL within 2 weeks of next dose, zoledronic acid should be withheld until the serum creatinine is at least within 10% of baseline value.
  - *Dose reductions for renal insufficiency if urinary creatinine clearance (CrCl) is (4-mg dose for normal Cr Cl > 60 mL/min):*
    - 50–60 mL/min: dose is 3.5 mg.
    - 40–49 mL/min: dose is 3.3 mg.
    - 30–39 mL/min: dose is 3.0 mg.
- Single doses should NOT exceed 4 mg, and duration of infusion should be at least 15 minutes, as otherwise increases risk of renal dysfunction.
- Coadminister oral calcium supplements of 500 mg and a multivitamin containing 400 IU of vitamin D daily.

Drug Preparation:
- Drug is available in 4-mg/100-mL single-use, ready-to-use bottle, or 4-mg/5-mL single-use vial of concentrate.
- Do not mix with calcium or other divalent cation-containing infusion solutions (e.g., Lactated Ringer's).
- **4-mg/100-mL single-use, ready-to-use bottle** (contains overfill so can you can withdraw entire 4-mg dose as 100 mL): Administer 4 mg (100 mL) without further dilution for full dose. To prepare reduced doses for patients with decreased CrCl, aseptically remove the specified volume from the vial and discard: 12 mL to make a 3.5-mg dose, 18 mL to make a 3.3-mg dose, and 25 mL to make a 3.0-mg dose. Replace the 0.9% sodium chloride or 5% dextrose injection in the same volume that was withdrawn into the vial, bringing the volume back to 100 mL.
- Preparation of Reduced Doses Zometa Ready-to-Use bottles:
  - Dose 3.5 mg = remove and discard 12 mL from Zometa ready-to-use bottle
  - Dose 3.3 mg = remove and discard 18 mL from Zometa ready-to-use bottle
  - Dose 3.0 mg = remove and discard 25 mL from Zometa ready-to-use bottle
- **4-mg/5-mL single-use vial of concentrate**: Withdraw 4-mg (5-mL) dose and immediately dilute in 100 mL 5% dextrose injection, USP or 0.9% sodium chloride injection, USP. DO NOT use any other IV solution, such as lactated Ringer's solution. Administer full dose as ordered over at least 15 minutes. To prepare reduced doses for patients with decreased baseline CrCl, withdraw the specified volume from the vial and then immediately dilute in 100 mL 5% dextrose injection, USP or 0.9% sodium chloride injection, USP: 3.5-mg dose = 4.4-mL, 3.3-mg dose = 4.1-mL, and 3.0-mg dose = 3.8 mL.
- Preparation of Reduced Doses from Zometa 4 mg/5 mL single-dose vial for dilution:
  - Dose 3.5 mg = remove and USE 4.4 mL from Zometa diluted vial
  - Dose 3.3 mg = remove and USE 4.1 mL from Zometa diluted vial
  - Dose 3.0 mg = remove and USE 3.8 mL from Zometa diluted vial
  - Add removed volume from vial to a 100 mL bag of sterile 0.9% Sodium Chloride USP or 5% Dextrose Injection USP.
- If not used immediately, drug may be refrigerated at 2–8°C (36–46°F) for up to 24 hours (make sure the drug mixing time/date are clear on the label, as the nurse must complete administration within 24 hours of the initial dilution).

COMPLICATIONS

Drug Administration:
- Assess serum creatinine results and patient hydration status.
- Administer as a single IV dose over *at least* 15 minutes. Use a separate, vented infusion line from all other drugs; do not allow drug to come into contact with any calcium or divalent cation-containing solutions.
- Do not exceed 4-mg dose.
- *Hypercalcemia of malignancy:*
  - Assure that patient has been adequately rehydrated prior to drug administration and that the BUN and creatinine are WNL. Monitor electrolytes during treatment.
  - Dose adjustments are not necessary in patients presenting with mild-to-moderate renal impairment prior to starting zolendronic acid (serum creatinine $<$ 400 µM/L or 4.5 mg/dL).
- Multiple myeloma and metastatic bone lesions of solid tumors:
  - For patients who require retreatment and who have had altered renal status after receiving the drug, here are manufacturer's recommendations for patients with:
    - Normal serum creatinine before receiving drug, but have an increase of 0.5 mg/dL within 2 weeks of next dose: hold drug until serum creatinine is at least within 10% of baseline value.
    - Abnormal serum creatinine before receiving drug, but have an increase of 1.0 mg/dL within 2 weeks of next dose: drug should be held until serum creatinine is at least within 10% of baseline value.
    - See dose reductions based on serum creatinine.
- Patients should take an oral calcium supplement of 500 mg and a multivitamin containing 400 IU of vitamin D daily.

Drug Interactions:
- Incompatible with calcium-containing fluids, such as lactated Ringer's, or divalent-cation-containing solutions.
- Use cautiously together with aminoglycoside antibiotics, as there may be an additive effect resulting in hypocalcemia for prolonged periods, as well as renal toxicity.
- Use cautiously together with loop diuretics, as the risk of hypocalcemia and nephrotoxicity may be increased.
- Reclast: patients should NOT take both Zometa (zoledronic acid) and Reclast (also contains zoledronic acid).
- Nephrotoxic drugs: use with caution.
- Thalidomide: combination in patients with multiple myeloma may increase risk of renal dysfunction.

Lab Effects/Interference:
- Hypocalcemia.
- Hypophosphatemia.
- Hypomagnesemia.
- Increased BUN and serum creatinine.

Special Considerations:
- Most common ($>$ 25%): nausea, fatigue, anemia, bone pain, constipation, fever, vomiting, and dyspnea.

- Warnings and Precautions:
  - *Drugs with same active ingredient or in the same drug class:* Patients treated with zoledronic acid should not be treated with Reclast (zoledronic acid).
  - *Hydration and electrolyte monitoring:* Adequately rehydrate patients with hypercalcemia of malignancy before administering zoledronic acid, and monitor electrolytes during treatment. Loop diuretics should not be used until patient is adequately rehydrated and should be used with caution to avoid hypocalcemia. Carefully monitor baseline, before each dose, and as needed: serum calcium, phosphate, magnesium, creatinine. Replete as needed for hypocalcemia, hypophosphatemia, or hypomagnesemia.
  - *Renal Impairment:* Renal toxicity may be greater in patients with renal impairment.
    - DO NOT use doses > 4 mg.
    - Treatment in patients with hypercalcemia of malignancy: severe renal impairment (serum creatinine > 4.5 mg/dL), zoledronic acid treatment not recommended.
    - Treatment in patients with bone metastases with severe renal impairment: do not give zoledronic acid if serum crasetinine > 3.0 mg/dL.
    - Monitor serum creatinine before each dose.
  - *Osteonecrosis of the jaw* may occur. Preventative dental exams should be performed before starting zoledronic acid. Avoid invasive dental procedures while receiving drug if possible.
  - *Musculoskeletal Pain:* Severe, incapacitating bone, joint, muscle pain may occur. Zoledronic acid should be discontinued if severe symptoms occur.
  - *Embryo-fetal toxicity:* Zoledronic acid can cause fetal harm. Teach women of reproductive potential to use effective contraception to avoid pregnancy during and after zoledronic acid use. It is not known if drug is excreted in breast milk.
  - *Atypical femoral fracture* may occur, occurring anywhere in the femoral shaft from just below the lesser trochanter to above the supracondylar flare, which may be transverse or short oblique, without communication. Fracture is not usually associated with trauma, or may occur with minimal trauma to the area. Fractures may be bilateral, and patients may report prodromal pain (e.g., dull, aching thigh pain) prior to the diagnosis, weeks to months before complete fracture occurs.
    - Concomitant administration of corticosteroids may increase risk. Teach patients to report any new or unusual thigh, hip, or groin pain immediately. Evaluate patients for incomplete fracture; assess patient also for signs and symptoms of fracture in the contralateral limb. Consider discontinuing Zometa therapy pending a risk/benefit assessment.
    - It is unknown whether the atypical femur fracture will continue after therapy is stopped. Poor healing of the atypical fracture has been reported.
  - *Hypocalcemia:* Initially, correct hypocalcemia before starting zoledronic acid. Ensure patient receives adequate calcium and vitamin D supplementation. Monitor serum calcium closely when other drugs that can cause hypocalcemia are administered with zoledronic acid.
  - *Hepatic Impairment:* Limited data exists about risks of administration of drug to patients with hepatic insufficiency.
  - *Patients with Asthma:* postmarketing reports of bronchoconstriction in aspirin-sensitive patients receiving bisphosphonates has occurred.

COMPLICATIONS

- Use cautiously when combined with renally toxic drugs, such as aminoglycoside antibiotics or loop diuretics. Use drug cautiously in patients who have aspirin-sensitive asthma, as well as in older patients.
- Laboratory Monitoring: Monitor serum creatinine before each dose and closely assess geriatric patients; monitor serum electrolytes, magnesium, phosphate, and hematocrit/hemoglobin baseline and regularly during treatment. Discuss abnormal values with physician, as risk must be weighed against benefit. Risk factors for deteriorating renal function, possibly renal failure are (1) impaired renal function and (2) multiple cycles of bisphosphonate therapy.
- Compared with pamidronate in the management of hypercalcemia of malignancy, zoledronic acid had a 45.3% response rate by day 4 and an 82.6% response rate by day 7, as compared with a 33.3% response rate and a 63.6% response rate, respectively, when pamidronate was given. Time to relapse was 30 days with zoledronic acid and 17 days with pamidronate.

Potential Toxicities/Skin Effects and the Nursing Process

I.   ALTERATION IN COMFORT, related to FEVER, NAUSEA AND VOMITING, INSOMNIA, AND FLU-LIKE SYMPTOMS

Defining Characteristics: Fever occurred in 44% of patients during clinical trials. Flu-like symptoms of chills, bone pain, and/or arthralgias and myalgias may occur less commonly. Nausea occurred in 29% of patients, and vomiting 14%. Insomnia affects 15%. The symptom frequency was similar to the pamidronate and placebo groups.

Nursing Implications: Assess baseline comfort and temperature. Teach patient that these side effects may occur and to report them. Administer or teach patient self-administration of acetaminophen or over-the-counter NSAIDs as appropriate to manage fever, arthralgias, or myalgias if they occur. Teach patient to report if symptoms do not resolve. Administer antiemetics as ordered to minimize nausea and vomiting.

II.   ALTERATION IN BOWEL ELIMINATION PATTERN related to CONSTIPATION, DIARRHEA, ABDOMINAL PAIN, AND ANOREXIA

Defining Characteristics: Diarrhea affected 24% (vs. 18% placebo) of patients in clinical trials, while 31% developed constipation (compared to 38% in placebo). Fouteen percent of patients developed abdominal pain (vs. 11% in placebo), and 22% anorexia (compared to 23% in placebo).

Nursing Implications: Assess baseline bowel elimination status, and teach patient to report alterations. Teach patient to use diet modifications depending upon changes, and over-the-counter antidiarrheals or laxatives as necessary. Teach patient to report persistent diarrhea or constipation (lasting more than 24 hours), presence of blood, abdominal cramping, or pain.

III. ALTERATION IN ACTIVITY TOLERANCE related to ANEMIA, FATIGUE

Defining Characteristics: Anemia occurred in 33% of patients (compared to 23% in placebo arm) during clinical trials.

Nursing Implications: Assess baseline hemoglobin and hematocrit. Teach patient to report fatigue, and discuss strategies to conserve energy, such as alternating rest and activity. Discuss with physician transfusion if symptoms are severe.

IV. ALTERATION IN FLUID AND ELECTROLYTE BALANCE related to CHANGES IN RENAL EXCRETION

Defining Characteristics: Drug will cause renal dysfunction with rise in serum creatinine if drug is given rapidly or in less than 15 minutes. Hypophosphatemia occurred in 13% of patients during clinical trials, hypokalemia in 12%, and hypomagnesemia in 10%.

Nursing Implications: Assess baseline renal function and electrolytes prior to initial therapy, post-therapy, and prior to any additional therapy as needed. Dose reduction necessary in patients with renal insufficiency. Hold drug if renal abnormalities do not correct, as indicated in Administration section.

V. POTENTIAL FOR INJURY related to OSTEOPOROSIS, OSTEONECROSIS OF THE JAW (ONJ)

Defining Characteristics: Women with breast cancer and men with prostate cancer are at risk for osteoporosis from various cancer treatments, including hormonal manipulation. ONJ may occur rarely, and it is associated with recent dental procedures, such as tooth extraction.

Nursing Implications: Teach patient to take calcium and vitamin D supplements (or multivitamin) while receiving bisphosphonates, and encourage patient to exercise regularly. If a smoker, encourage the patient to stop smoking to reduce the risk of osteoporosis. Teach patient to have a dental exam and preventive dental work before starting therapy, and to practice excellent oral hygiene.

COMPLICATIONS

Chapter *11*
Infection

According to the Centers for Disease Control (CDC), there are more than 650,000 cancer patients receiving chemotherapy yearly. These patients are susceptible to infections related to their treatments. Many standard cancer chemotherapy regimens cause neutropenia resulting in delays or reductions in dosages of chemotherapy for patients that may result in higher mortality rates, longer hospitalizations, and higher costs of care. Chemotherapy, radiation therapy, and even the malignancy itself can result in immunosuppression and infection risk. This risk for infection results from damage to bone marrow and stem cells. Additionally, cancer patients receiving intensive treatments, such as hematopoietic stem cell transplant, and those receiving high-dose corticosteroids, purine analogues, and alemtuzumab are at risk for life-threatening infection.

Febrile neutropenia is a serious and life-threatening condition resulting from a decreased white blood cell (WBC) count and from patients' inability to fight infection. Leukocytes, or WBCs, are divided into cells that contain granules in the cytoplasm (granulocytes) and cells that do not (agranulocytes). WBCs containing granules include neutrophils, basophils, and eosinophils, while the agranulocytes (mononuclear leukocytes) include lymphocytes, monocytes, and macrophages. Neutrophils fight against invading microorganisms by migrating to the site of infection. The type and amount of neutrophils are key indicators of both infection and risk associated with infection, especially for the patient with cancer. See Figure 11.1 for maturation of the formed blood cell elements.

The risk of infection is related to the degree and duration of neutropenia, as shown in Table 11.1. The absolute neutrophil count (ANC), the number of neutrophils in the body, determines the risk for infection. This calculation is shown in Table 11.2.

Assessing the risk of infection includes: treatment intent (curative therapy, adjuvant therapy, prolonged survival, better health-related quality of life, symptom management), chemotherapy regimen risk (high, moderate, low) and treatment-related factors (type and kind of myelosuppressive agents, history of surgery, chemotherapy and/or radiation therapy, relative dose intensity), and patient-related factors (age, nutritional status, performance status, immune function, active infection, history of infection or febrile neutropenia, stage and type of cancer, hemoglobin and albumin levels, comorbidities).

In non-neutropenic, immunocompromised patients, the level of risk may be more difficult to quantify. Yet, we know that the frequency and severity of infection are inversely proportional to the neutrophil count. Therefore, the patient's rate of decline and the length of neutropenic time results in greater risk of infection. Infection and fever in a neutropenic patient represent a medical emergency, and, if untreated, can result in sepsis and death. Neutropenia-related infections can be life threatening and require aggressive treatment with antibiotic, antifungal, and/or antiviral agents. Additionally, an estimated 8.5% of all cancer deaths in the United States are associated with severe sepsis at a cost of $3.4 billion or more annually.

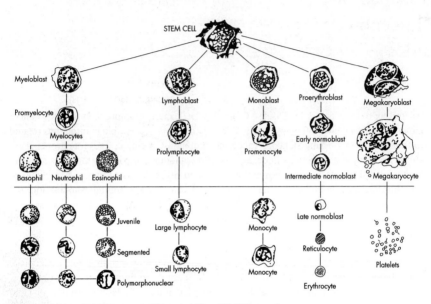

Figure 11.1   Development of Formed Blood Cell Elements

Table 11.1   Relative Risk of Infection

Risk	Number/Neutrophils
No significant risk	1,500–2,000/mm³
Minimal risk	1,000–1,500/mm³
Moderate risk	500–1,000/mm³
Severe risk	< 500/mm³

Table 11.2   Calculation of Absolute Neutrophil Count

Patient Example	Normal Values
1. Lab results: total white blood count (WBC) = 4,000/mm³	5,000–10,000/mm³
neutrophils = 40	50–70%
lymphocytes = 50	20–40%
monocytes = 6	2–6%
eosinophils = 1	0.5–1%
bands = 2	
2. Total WBC × % (neutrophils + bands)	2,500–7,000/mm³
4,000 × % (40 + 2) =	
4,000 × 42/100 =	
4,000 × 0.42 = 1,680/mm³	

Gram-negative bacilli are responsible for the high incidence of life-threatening infections (*Escherichia coli, Klebsiella* spp., *Proteus* spp., and *Pseudomonas aeruginosa*). However, gram-positive organisms such as *Staphylococcus epidermis* and streptococci have increased as a result of decreasing gram-negative sepsis that is treated promptly with empiric antimicrobial therapy. Healthcare-associated infections (HAIs) stem from central line—associated bloodstream infections (CLABSI), catheter-associated urinary tract infections (CAUTI), selected surgical-site infections (SSI), hospital-onset *Clostridium difficile* infections, and hospital-onset methicillin-resistant *Staphylococcus aureus* (MRSA) bacteremia.

CENTRAL LINE INFECTIONS

Central venous catheters are common in the oncology patient population. A central line is a catheter that tip terminates in a great vessel, such as aorta, pulmonary artery, superior vena cava, inferior vena cava, brachiocephalic veins, internal jugular veins, subclavian veins, external iliac veins, and common femoral veins. The CDC *Guidelines for the Prevention of Intravascular Catheter-related Infections* (2011, http://www.cdc.gov/hicpac/pdf/guidelines/bsi-guidelines-2011.pdf) estimated 250,000 cases of central line–associated bloodstream infections (BSIs) occur in hospitals in the United States. Catheter-related bloodstream infections (CRBSI/CLABSI) independently increase hospital costs and length of stay, but have not been shown to independently increase mortality. While 80,000 CRBSIs occur in ICUs each year, the total of 250,000 cases of BSIs are estimated to occur annually. By several analyses, costs of these infections are substantial, both in terms of morbidity and expenditure of financial resources. Mortality from *Staphylococcus aureus* CLABSI can be as high as 25–30% in oncology settings (Wilson, 2018). To improve patient outcomes and reduce healthcare costs, there is considerable interest by healthcare providers, insurers, regulators, and patient advocates in reducing the incidence of these infections (CDC, 2011).

Yet, vascular access is necessary for patients undergoing intensive or cyclic chemotherapy. The risk of infection varies by device used, duration of placement, and extent of the patient's immunosuppression (CDC, 2011; NCCN, v.2.2015). According to NCCN, infections are categorized as entry- or exit-site infections, tunnel or port-pocket infections, septic phlebitis, or catheter-associated bloodstream infections. These infections tend to be caused by gram-positive organisms with coagulase-negative staphylococci being cultured most frequently. Catheter-associated bloodstream infections usually respond without the need for catheter removal except if the causal microorganism is yeast or nontuberculosis mycobacterium. Bloodstream infections caused by Bacillus organisms, *Candida, S. aureus, Acinetobacter, C. jeikeium, P. aeruginosa, S. maltophilia,* and vancomycin-resistant enterococci (VRE) may be difficult to eradicate with antimicrobial therapy alone, making removal of the catheter imperative (NCCN, v.2.2015).

In addition to a course of antibacterial therapy, research suggests that administering antibiotics into lumens of central venous catheters, using catheters impregnated with minocycline and rifampin or silver-chlorhexidine, and using vancomycin-lock solution may reduce vascular access infections. However, studies are not definitive and data are inconclusive to

COMPLICATIONS

recommend any of these interventions. Instead, hand hygiene, maximal barrier precautions during insertion, using transparent dressings and chlorhexidine, and changing the needle-less system device and end cap on a routine basis according to manufacturer guidelines can help minimize the risk of venous access device infections.

INFECTIOUS ORGANISMS

Disease-related immunosuppression is associated with defects in cell-mediated immunity (thymus-dependent lymphocytes), such as with certain lymphomas. This leads to an increased risk for bacterial infections (*Mycobacterium, Nocardia asteroides, Legionella, Salmonella*), as well as infections caused by fungi (*Cryptococcus, Histoplasma, Candida, Aspergillus*), parasites (*Pneumocystis carinii* pneumonia, *Toxoplasma gondii*), and viruses (varicella zoster, cytomegalovirus). Other malignancies may have defects in the humoral immune system (B lymphocytes), as in multiple myeloma and chronic lymphocytic leukemia (CLL). Patients with these malignancies are at risk for infection from bacteria (*Streptococcus pneumoniae, Haemophilus influenzae, Neisseria meningitidis, Klebsiella pneumoniae,* and *S. aureus*) and certain enteroviruses. Antibiotic resistance, such as VRE and MRSA, is a concern for cancer patients.

Since 1989, U.S. hospitals report a rapid increase in the incidence of infection and colonization from VRE. This increase poses important problems, including (a) the lack of available antimicrobial therapy for VRE infections, since most VRE infections are resistant to drugs previously used to treat these infections (e.g., aminoglycosides and ampicillin); and (b) the possibility that vancomycin-resistant genes present in VRE can be transferred to other gram-positive microorganisms (e.g., *S. aureus*). Recommendations regarding management of multidrug-resistant organisms are found in *Guideline for the Management of Multidrug-resistant Organisms in Healthcare Settings* (CDC, 2006), http://www.cdc.gov /hicpac/pdf/guidelines/MDROGuideline2006.pdf. This document remains an important resource despite its publication date.

Increased risk for VRE infection and colonization is associated with previous vancomycin and/or multi-antimicrobial therapy, severe underlying disease or immunosuppression, and intra-abdominal surgery. Enterococci are found in normal gastrointestinal and female genital tracts, thus most enterococcal infections are attributed to endogenous sources. Whenever possible, empiric antimicrobial therapy should be modified based on culture and sensitivity results.

Methicillin-resistant *S. aureus* (MRSA), a bacterial infection, is highly resistant to antibiotics. The MRSA infections are grouped into types: community-acquired MRSA (CA-MRSA) and hospital-or healthcare-acquired MRSA (HA-MRSA). HA-MRSA infections occur in people who are or have recently been in a hospital or other healthcare facility. Those who have been hospitalized or had surgery within the past year are at increased risk. The MRSA bacteria are responsible for a large percentage of hospital-acquired staph infections. Community-acquired MRSA infections occur in otherwise healthy people who have not recently been in the hospital. Infections occur among athletes sharing equipment or personal items (such as towels or razors) and children in daycare facilities. Members of the military and those who get tattoos are at risk, and the number of CA-MRSA cases is on the rise.

Recently the CDC has been tracking the drug-resistant fungus called *Candida auris* (*C. auris*) that has been linked to the death of patients with serious underlying conditions. There has been a long-standing concern about the spread of antibiotic-resistant bacterial infections as mentioned previously. However, this fungus is relatively new, is found world-wide, and can be spread in hospitals. Hospitalized cancer patients are at risk since many of them are treated with antibiotics that kill healthy bacteria that usually protect the patient from disease. Identifying *C. auris* is difficult requiring special laboratory methods, yet treating this fungus is even more difficult since fungal samples have been resistant to current antifungal therapy. Prevention is the key until drugs are developed to treat this organism. Hospitals should clean rooms thoroughly after discharging a patient who has been diagnosed with a fungal infection.

ANTIMICROBIAL AGENTS

Antimicrobial medications kill or inhibit the growth of organisms without harming the patient. Antimicrobial agents may be bacteriostatic (inhibit growth of organisms) or bactericidal (kill microorganisms). Drug activity varies so that at low concentrations a drug may be bacteriostatic but bactericidal in higher concentrations. Antimicrobial medications used to treat infections in patients with cancer are considered antibacterial, antiviral, and antifungal. These drugs target specific cellular mechanisms of the infectious agent. For example, sulfonamide antibiotics inhibit para-aminobenzoic acid, an essential requirement for nucleic acid synthesis in many bacteria but not in humans. Penicillins and cephalosporins contain a β-lactam ring that disrupts the synthesis of peptidoglycan. Peptidoglycan gives shape and strength to the bacterial cell wall. Table 11.3 provides an overview of antibacterial agents including penicillins, cephalosporins, streptogramins, oxazolidinones, macrolides, lipopeptides, and ketolides.

Making minor modifications to an existing class of drugs has largely developed newer antibiotics. Daptomycin is a cyclic lipopeptide. Its mode of action kills gram-positive bacteria rapidly by disrupting multiple aspects of bacterial membrane function. Telithromycin, a first-in-class antibiotic group called ketolide, is structurally related to macrolide antibiotics; the newest drug of the macrolide antibiotic class is fidaxomicin, which is specifically designed to offer optimal spectrum activity for first-line treatment of upper-and lower-respiratory tract infections. Fidaxomicin is approved for *C. difficile* infections, along with bezlotoxumab.

Polyketides are a large family of structurally diverse, natural products with a broad range of biologic activities, including antibiotic and pharmacologic properties. Many important antibiotics are polyketides, such as tetracyclines, erythromycin, adriamycin, monensin, rifamycin, and avermectins. Glycylcyclines are structurally similar to tetracyclines and tigecycline is the first agent in this class to be FDA-approved for treatment of MRSA. There are a growing number of MRSA-resistant agents, including colistimethate.

Work is beginning on a general strategy for biosynthesis of polyketides through cloning gene clusters. This fundamentally new strategy for treating infectious disease is being bioengineered in the laboratory. One such proposed treatment would modulate the host's immune responses to enhance clearance of infectious agents. Antimicrobial host defense

COMPLICATIONS

Table 11.3   Comparison of Antibiotic Categories

Antibacterial Category	Examples	Mechanism of Action, Including Differences among or between Categories or Unique Characteristics
Penicillins		Penicillins are derived from the fungus *Penicillium* and contain a β-lactam ring.
Natural penicillins	• penicillin V • penicillin G	The first group comprises natural penicillins, which are active against many aerobic gram-positive cocci (*S. aureus, Streptococcus*), gram-negative aerobic cocci (*N. meningitidis,* some *H. influenzae*), and some spirochetes. However, they are resistant to *Pseudomonas,* most *Enterobacter,* and to bacteria that produce the enzyme penicillinase, which inactivates the penicillin molecule.
Penicillinase-resistant penicillins	• cloxacillin • dicloxacillin • nafcillin • oxacillin	The second group contains the penicillinase-resistant penicillins. These are semisynthetic drugs that can withstand the action of the enzyme penicillinase and continue to exert their antibiotic action. They are primarily used to treat *S. aureus* and *S. epidermidis* strains that secrete penicillinase; they also have some activity against gram-negative bacteria and spirochetes.
Aminopenicillins	• amoxicillin • ampicillin • bacampicillin	The third group includes the aminopenicillins; this group has heightened activity against gram-negative bacteria as compared to the first two groups. These drugs are resistant to penicillinase-producing bacteria.
Extended-spectrum penicillins	• carbenicillin • mezlocillin • piperacillin • ticarcillin	The fourth group is composed of the extended-spectrum penicillins; drugs in this group have enhanced activity against gram-negative bacilli, both aerobic and nonaerobic.
Cephalosporins		The cephalosporins are derived from cephalosporin C (produced by a fungus) and have broad bactericidal activity. They contain a β-lactam ring and may also be referred to as β-lactam antibiotics. Bacterial resistance can develop, and a major mechanism is the development by the bacteria of an enzyme, β-lactamase, which inactivates the cephalosporin antibiotic by destroying the β-lactam ring.
First-generation cephalosporins	• cefadroxil • cephalothin • cefazolin • cephalexin • cephapirin • cephradine	First-generation cephalosporins are active against gram-positive cocci (*Staphylococcus* and *Streptococcus*) and have only limited activity against gram-negative bacteria (e.g., *E. coli*); they have no activity against enterococci.

Table 11.3   *(Continued)*

Antibacterial Category	Examples	Mechanism of Action, Including Differences among or between Categories or Unique Characteristics
Second-generation cephalosporins	• cefaclor • cefamandole • cefmetazole • cefonicid • ceforanide • cefotetan • cefoxitin • cefprozil • cefuroxime • cefuroxime axetil	Second-generation cephalosporins are active against the same organisms as the first-generation drugs but are slightly more active against gram-negative bacteria. In addition, they are active against *H. influenzae*.
Third-generation cephalosporins	• cefdinir • cefixime • cefoperazone • cefotaxime • cefpodoxime • ceftazidime • ceftibuten • ceftizoxime • ceftriaxone • loracarbef	Third-generation cephalosporins are less active against gram-positive organisms but have broader activity against gram-negative organisms than either first- or second-generation drugs.
Fourth-generation cephalosporins	• cefepime • ceftaroline • fosamil	Fourth-generation cephalosporins are projected to have many attributes, including: • Extended spectrum of activity for gram-negative and gram-positive organisms (different from third-generation cephalosporins) • Minimal β-lactamase activity due to rapid periplasmic penetration and high penicillin-binding protein (PBP) access • Spectrum of activity to include gram-negative organisms with multiple drug resistance patterns (*Enterobacter* and *Klebsiella*)
Streptogramins	• quinupristin • dalfopristin	This new class of antibiotics, the streptogramin group, is a separate family of antimicrobials. Synercid is an intravenous combination of two semisynthetic, water-soluble derivatives of naturally occurring pristinamycin. The two distinct compounds are quinupristin and dalfopristin, derived from pristinamycin I and pristinamycin II. These two compounds work synergistically to kill susceptible bacteria through a two-pronged attack on protein synthesis in bacterial cells. Each component of the drug binds irreversibly to different sites on the bacterial cell's ribosomal subunit to form a stable quinupristin-ribosome—dalfopristin complex, which disables the cell's ability to make cellular protein. Without the ability to manufacture new proteins, the bacterial cell dies.

COMPLICATIONS

(Continued)

Table 11.3   *(continued)*

Antibacterial Category	Examples	Mechanism of Action, Including Differences among or between Categories or Unique Characteristics
Oxazolidinones	• linezolid	Inhibits initiation of protein synthesis by binding to a site on bacterial 23S ribosomal RNA of the 50S subunit. This mechanism of inhibiting protein synthesis is not shared by other antibacterials. Cross-resistance is unlikely.
Macrolides	• azithromycin • clarithromycin • erythromycin • fidaxomicin	Binds to 50S ribosomal subunit, resulting in inhibition of protein synthesis. In some cases, the drug metabolite is twice as active as the parent compound.
Lipopeptides	• daptomycin	Derived from the fermentation of *Streptomyces roseosporus*. The mechanism of action is not fully understood. Binds to bacterial membranes and causes a rapid depolarization of membrane potential. This loss of membrane potential leads to inhibition of protein, DNA, and RNA synthesis resulting in bacterial cell death.
Ketolides	• telithromycin	Similar to that of macrolides and is related to the 50S-ribosomal subunit binding with inhibition of bacterial protein synthesis. Telithromycin appears to have greater affinity for the ribosomal binding site than macrolides. It concentrates in phagocytes, where it exhibits activity against intracellular respiratory pathogens.
Glycylcyclines	• tigecycline	Glycylcyclines are a new class of antibiotics derived from tetracycline. These tetracycline analogues are specifically designed to overcome two common mechanisms of tetracycline resistance, namely resistance mediated by acquired efflux pumps and/or ribosomal protection.

peptides are being investigated for their potential as a new class of antimicrobial drug (Easton et al., 2009). This work has shown promise in the laboratory and, if actualized, modulation of innate immunity by synthetic variants of host defense peptides might be protective without direct antimicrobial action.

Another newer class of antimicrobial agents, echinocandins or glucan synthesis inhibitors, is an option available for treating opportunistic fungal infections. Caspofungin inhibits the synthesis of a key component of the fungal cell wall. Caspofungin demonstrates fungicidal activity against *Candida* species; it is indicated for treatment of invasive *Aspergillus* in patients who are refractory to, or intolerant of, other therapies. Caspofungin appears to be well-tolerated. Another drug, Micafungin, inhibits synthesis of 1, 3-b-D-glucan, an essential component of fungal cell walls. Micafungin is indicated for treatment of patients with esophageal candidiasis and as prophylaxis for *Candida* infections in patients undergoing hematopoietic stem cell transplantation.

The latest echinocandin, anidulafungin, was FDA-approved for treatment of candidemia and esophageal candidiasis. All three echinocandins are well-tolerated and have some use in febrile neutropenia. There are anecdotal reports regarding use of these agents to treat less common fungal infections and limited use as a component of antifungal therapy. The echinocandins are an important addition to the antifungal armamentarium for treating fungal infections in immunocompromised patients.

Posaconazole, a broad-spectrum triazole, is another drug used for treatment and prevention of invasive fungal infections. It is a lipophilic antifungal triazole similar to other members in this class and effective against *Candida* species, *Cryptococcus neoformans, Aspergillus* species, *Fusarium* species, zygomycetes, and endemic fungi. The compound is available as an oral suspension and appears to be well-tolerated, even in long-term courses of treatment. Tablets are also available but they are pharmacokinetically different from suspension. Another new agent is isavuconazole.

The latest options in the anti-infective area are combinations of drugs, such as ceftazidime/avibactam (Avycaz) and ceftolozane/tazobactam (Zerbaxa). These drugs use a two-pronged approach for treating infection. Ceftazidime/avibactam combines a next-generation non-beta-lactam beta-lactamase inhibitor and third-generation antipseudomonal cephalosporin antibiotic. Ceftolozane/tazobactam is a combination of a cephalosporin-class antibacterial and a beta-lactamase inhibitor. They are primarily reserved for treatment of highly resistant gram-negative infections.

There is a new drug, bezlotoxumab (Zinplava), used to treatment *Clostridium difficile* toxin B infection (CDI). Bezlotoxumab is not an antibacterial drug and should only be used in conjunction with antibacterial treatment of CDI. Bezlotoxumab is a human monoclonal antibody that binds to *C. difficile* toxicin B, inhibits the binding of toxin B, and prevents/neutralizes its effects. Bezlotoxumab does not bind to *C. difficile* toxin A. It is indicated to reduce the recurrence of CDI in patients 18 years of age and older who are receiving antibacterial drug treatment for CDI and who are at high risk for CDI recurrence. This new use of monoclonal antibodies may be the way to treating infections in the future.

On the horizon are some agents that are newly discovered and now in development as anti-infective agents, such as platensimycin, a previously unknown class of antibiotics produced by *Streptomyces platensis*. It remains to be seen whether this new class of antibiotics will be effective against microorganisms in humans.

It was mentioned previously that *Candida auris* is a dangerous form of yeast that is resistant to antifungal drugs. Some strains of *C. auris* are resistant to all three major classes of antifungal drugs: triazoles, polyenes, and echinocandins. This type of multidrug resistance has not been seen before in other species of *Candida*. Of concern is the fact that *C. auris* can persist on surfaces in healthcare environments and spread between patients in healthcare facilities, unlike most *Candida* species. The CDC has developed Interim Recommendations to help prevent the spread of *C. auris*. These recommendations can be found at https://www.cdc.gov /fungal/diseases/candidiasis/recommendations.html.

Bacteriophage therapy to treat bacterial infections offers a new approach built on top of an old idea. There is growing interest in bacteriophages as treatment for infection, especially in light of growing antibiotic resistance (Kutateladze & Adamia, 2010; Lu & Koeris, 2011). This treatment is underutilized in the United States but is growing in popularity in other parts of the world. However, advances in biotechnology, bacterial diagnostics, macromolecular delivery, and synthetic biology are providing opportunities to overcome clinical development issues. Some of these issues include regulation, limited host range, bacterial resistance to phages, manufacturing challenges, side effects of bacterial lysis, and delivery mechanisms.

COMPLICATIONS

EVIDENCE-BASED GUIDELINES

Patients diagnosed with cancer are at higher risk of bacterial, viral, or fungal infections as a result of the cancer itself or the treatments. Infections in patients with cancer are a topic of interest beyond the treatment of infections. Preventing infection or early treatment is a key factor in minimizing sequelae for neutropenic cancer patients. There are an ever-expanding number of prevention and treatment evidence-based guidelines. The National Comprehensive Cancer Network (NCCN), the Oncology Nursing Society (ONS), Putting Evidence into Practice (PEP), the American Society of Clinical Oncologists (ASCO), the Multinational Association for Supportive Care in Cancer (MASCC), and the CDC report and/or update evidence-based guidelines regularly. Many healthcare institutions including hospitals have developed neutropenia protocols based on these guidelines and the best available evidence.

The NCCN Prevention and Treatment of Cancer-related Infections, Version 2.2015, offers comprehensive evidence-based guidelines to prevent and treat cancer-related infections. The guidelines delineate prevention, diagnosis, and treatment of major common and opportunistic infections, highlighting the risk of infection for cancer patients, presenting fever and neutropenia risk, and recommending antimicrobial prophylaxis. The NCCN Guidelines can be found at http://www.nccn.org.

The ONS PEP Guidelines focus on nursing-sensitive patient outcomes (NSPOs), which are outcomes that are attained through or are significantly impacted by nursing interventions. The interventions must be within the scope of nursing practice and integral to the processes of nursing care. The specific ONS PEP Guidelines are available at https://www.ons.org/search?search_api_views_fulltext=research%20pep. These NSPOs validate the value and effectiveness of nursing practice and help nurses demonstrate their contribution to quality patient care.

The ASCO Guidelines focus on how and when to prevent and treat infection in patients receiving outpatient chemotherapy. Guidelines focus on febrile neutropenia and provide advice on identifying patients who have both neutropenia and fever but are at low risk for complications and can be treated at home. The ASCO Guidelines can be found at http://www.asco.org/sites/www.asco.org/files/fn_adult_guideline.pdf.

Interestingly, the problem of infections in cancer patients is an international issue as well. The MASCC Guidelines focus on use of granulocyte-colony stimulating factors and WBC growth factors in reducing febrile neutropenia. This organization validated a risk assessment tool for febrile neutropenia. The Immunocompromised Host Society and MASCC produced a set of guidelines on methodology for clinical trials involving patients with febrile neutropenia. The MASCC Guidelines can be found in detail at http://www.mascc.org.

Institutions have begun instituting a "clean protocol" in an effort to decrease pathogens within healthcare organizations. Microbiologically contaminated surfaces within institutions may be reservoirs of potential pathogens. However environmental surfaces carry the least risk of disease transmission and can be safely decontaminated using less rigorous methods than those used on medical instruments and devices. Environmental surfaces are not directly associated with transmission of infections to either staff or patients. Transferral of microorganisms from environmental surfaces to patients is largely via hand contact with the surface. Hand hygiene is imperative to minimize the incidence of healthcare-associated infections. Recently updated in 2019, additional guidance on "clean protocols" can be found at https://www.cdc.gov/infection control/guidelines/environmental/index.html.

Finally, the CDC has ongoing initiatives related to HAIs and antibiotic resistance. Several guidelines have been developed concerning various aspects of HAIs, including evidence-based guidelines, infection rates, and economic impact of HAIs to the healthcare system. Most recently the CDC allotted $21 million for the expansion of its antibiotic-resistant bacteria monitoring program, including the purchase of more-sensitive equipment for screening samples from hospitals. More information about this program and the CDC guidelines can be found at http://www.cdc.gov/HAI.

As more and more antibiotic, antibacterial, antiviral, and antifungal agents are discovered, the cost for these drugs continues to rise. It is through the use of the guidelines mentioned above that we can provide evidence-based care to cancer patients while attempting to maintain the costs of health care in today's environment.

References

Agency for Healthcare Research and Quality. *Research Activities*, 2008; 339 (November) 1. Available at http://www.ahrq.gov/. Accessed June 2012.

American Thoracic Society. Guidelines for the Management of Adults with Hospital-acquired, Ventilatory-associated and Health Care-associated Pneumonia. *Am J Respiratory Crit Care* 2005; 171:388–416.

Ampicillin Sodium/Sulbactam Sodium. Available at http://hcunviweb05/mdxcgi/quiklocn.exe?CTL=E :/Mdx/mdxcgi/MEGAT.SYS&SET=1C573/. Accessed June 2005.

APP Pharmaceuticals, LLC. NebuPent (pentamidine isethionate) [package insert]. Schaumburg, IL: Available at http://editor.fresenius-kabi.us/PIs/NebuPent_45847C_Feb_08.pdf. Accessed May 2016.

Aventis Pharmaceutical Inc. Ketek [product information]. March 2004. Avycaz [package insert]. Available at http://pi.actavis.com/data_stream.asp?product_group=1957&p=pi&language=E. Accessed May 2015.

Avycaz. Available at http://www.avycaz.com. Accessed May 2015.

Avycaz. Available at http://www.drugs.com/cdi/avycaz.html. Accessed May 2015.

Avycaz. Available at http://www.drugs.com/history/avycaz.html. Accessed May 2015.

Baden LR, Bensinger W, Angarone M, Casper C, et al. *NCCN Prevention and Treatment of Cancer-related Infections v.1.2013*. Available at http://www.nccn.org/professionals/physician_gls/pdf/infections .pdf. Accessed June 2013.

BioCryst Pharmaceuticals, Inc. RAPIVAB (peramivir IV) [package insert]. Durham, NC: Available at http://labeling.cslbehring.com/PI/US/Rapivab/EN/Rapivab-Prescribing-Information.pdf. Accessed May 2016.

Brungs SM, Render ML. Using Evidence-based Practice to Reduce Central Line Infections. *Clin J Oncol Nurs* 2006; 10(6):723–725.

Center for Disease Control and Prevention. *Guidelines for Environmenetal Infection Control in Health-Care Facilties. Recommendations of CDC and the Healthcare Infection Control Practices Advisory Committee (HICPAC)*. (July 2019). Available at https://www.cdc.gov/infection-control/guidelines/environmental/index.html.

Centers for Disease Control and Prevention. *Candida auris*. (June 2019). Available at https://www.cdc.gov/fungal/candida-auris/candida-auris-quanda.html.

COMPLICATIONS

Centers for Disease Control and Prevention. *Basic Infection Control and Prevention Plan Outpatient Oncology Settings*. (November 2011). Available at http://www.cdc.gov/HAI/settings/outpatient /basic-infection-control-prevention-plan-2011/.

Centers for Disease Control and Prevention. Guidelines for Preventing Opportunistic Infections among Hematopoietic Stem Cell Transplant Recipients: Recommendations of CDC, the Infection Disease Society of America, and the American Society of Blood and Marrow Transplant. *Morbidity Mortality Weekly Rep* 2000; 49 (RR-10): 1–126.

Centers for Disease Control and Prevention. *Guidelines for the Prevention of Intravascular Catheter-related Infections*. Available at http://www.cdc.gov/hicpac/pdf/guidelines/bsi-guidelines-2011.pdf.

Centers for Disease Control and Prevention. *Guide to Infection Prevention in Outpatient Settings: Minimum Expectations for Safe Care* (May 2011). Available at http://www.cdc.gov/HAI/settings /outpatient/outpatient-care-guidelines.html.

Centers for Disease Control and Prevention. *Management of Multi-drug Resistant Organisms in Healthcare Settings*. Available at http://www.cdc.gov/hicpac/pdf/guidelines/MDROGuideline 2006.pdf.

Centers for Disease Control and Prevention. *Candida auris* Interim Recommendations for Healthcare Facilities and Laboratories. Available at https://www.cdc.gov/fungal/diseases/candidiasis /recommendations.html.

Center Watch. *Drug Information: Baxdela (delafloxacin)*. Available at https://www.centerwatch.com/ drug-information/fda-approvals/drug/delafloxacin. Accessed May 15, 2018.

Center Watch. *Drug Information: Nuzyra (omadacycline)*. Available at https://www.centerwatch.com/ drug-information/fda-approvals/drug/100264/nuzyra. Accessed May 15, 2019.

Center Watch. *Drug Information: Recarbrio (imipenem, cilastatin, and relebactam)*. Available at https://www.centerwatch.com/drug-information/fda-approvals/drug/100398/recarbrio. Accessed May 15, 2019.

Center Watch. *Drug Information: Telavancin*. Available at http://www.centerwatch.com/drug-information /fda-approvals/drug-details.aspx?DrugID=1055. Accessed November 1, 2010.

Center Watch. *Drug Information: Xerava (eravacycline)*. Available at https://www.centerwatch.com/ drug-information/fda-approvals/drug/100298/xerava. Accessed May 1, 2019.

Center Watch. *Drug Information: Xofluza (baloxavir marboxil)*. Available at https://www.centerwatch. com/drug-information/fda-approvals/drug/xofluza. Accessed May 15, 2019.

Colistimethate Injection. Drugs.com. Drug Information Online. Available at http://www.drugs.com /MTM/colistimethate.html. Accessed June 2010.

Cooper MA, Shales D. Fix the Antibiotics Pipeline. *Nature* 2011; 472:7.

Courtney R, Pai S, Laughlin M, Lim J, Batra V. Pharmacokinetics, Safety, and Tolerability of Oral Posaconazole Administered in Single and Multiple Doses in Healthy Adults. *Antimicrobial Agents Chemotherapy* 2003; 47(9):2788–2795.

Cresemba [package insert]. Available at http://www.astellas.us/docs/cresemba.pdf. Accessed May 2015.

Cresemba New FDA Drug Approval. *Center Watch*. Available at http://www.centerwatch.com /drug-information/fda-approved-drugs. Accessed May 2015.

Cresemba. Available at http://www.drugs.com/cresemba.html. Accessed May 2015.

Crawford, J, Dale, DC, Kuderer, NM, et al. Risk and Timing of Neutropenic Events in Adult Cancer Patients Receiving Chemotherapy: The Results of a Prospective Nationwide Study of Oncology Practice. *J Natl Compr Canc Netw* 2008; 6:109–118.

Cubist Pharmaceutical Inc. Cubicin [product information]. Lexington, MA. September 2003.

Dalvance [package insert]. Available at http://content.stockpr.com/duratatherapeutics/files/docs /Dalvance+APPROVED+USPI.PDF. Accessed May 2015.

Dalvance new FDA drug approval. *Center Watch*. Available at http://www.centerwatch.com/drug -information/fda-approved-drugs. Accessed May 2015.

Dalvance. Available at http://www.drugs.com/sfx/dalvance-side-effects.html. Accessed May 2015.

Daptomycin. Drugs.com. Drug Information Online. Available at http://www.drugs.com/MTM /daptomycin.html. Accessed June 2004.

Declomycin. Available at http://www.rxmed.com/b.main/b2.pharmaceutical/b2.1monographs /CPS-Monographs. Accessed June 2004.

Declomycin [product information]. *Lederle Pharmaceutical Division, American Cynamid Co.* Pearl River, NY: 2003.

Doripenem Monograph. *National PBM Drug Monograph, January 2008. VHA Pharmacy Benefits Management Services and the Medical Advisory Panel.* Available at http://www.pbm.va.gov. Accessed June 2010.

Doripenem. Drugs.com. Drug Information Online. Available at http://www.drugs.com/MTM /doripenem .html. Accessed June 2010 and 2011.

Easton DM, Nijnik A, Mayer ML, Hancock REW. Potential of Immunomodulatory Host Defense Peptides as Novel Anti-infectives. *Trends Biotechnol.* 2009; 27(10):582–590.

Facta Farmaceutici S.p.A. Nucleo Industriale. TEFLARO® (ceftaroline fosamil) [package insert]. Teramo, Italy, 2011.

Facta Farmaceutici, S.P.A., Teramo, Italy and Melinta Therapeutics, Inc. Vabomere [product information]. Lincolnshire, Il. April 2018.

Flowers CR, Seidenfeld J, Bow EJ, Karten C, Gleason C, Hawley DK, Kuderer NM, Langston AA, Marr KA, Rolston KVI, Ramsey SD. Antimicrobial Prophylaxis and Outpatient Management of Fever and Neutropenia in Adults Treated for Malignancy: American Society of Clinical Oncology Clinical Practice Guidelines. *J Clin Oncol* 2013; 31(6 February 20): 794–810.

Freifeld AG, Bow EJ, Sepkowitz KA, Boeckh MJ, Ito JI, Mullen CA, Raad II, Rolston KV, Young JH, Wingard JR. Clinical Practice Guideline for the Use of Antimicrobial Agents in Neutropenic Patients with Cancer: 2010 Update by the Infectious Diseases Society of America. *Clin Infect Dis* 2011; 52: e56–e93 or 427–431.

Fujisawa Pharmaceutical Company LTD. Mycamine [package insert]. Osaka, Japan. 2005.

Gemifloxacin Mesylate [package insert]. Available at http://hcunviweb05/mdxcgi/quiklocn.exe?CTL =E:/Mdx/mdxcgi/ MEGAT.SYS&SET=1C573. June 2005.

Genentech, Inc. TAMIFLU® (oseltamivir phosphate) [package insert]. San Francisco, CA. June 2016.

Genetech USA, Inc. Valganciclovir [package insert]. San Francisco, CA. Available at http://www.gene.com/gene/products/information/valcyte/pdf/pi.pdf. Accessed August 2010.

Genentech USA, San Francisco, CA and Shionogi & Co., Ltd. Xofluza [product information]. Osaka, Japan. 2018.

GlaxoSmithKline. RELENZA (zanamivir) [package insert]. Research Triangle Park, NC: Available at https://www.gsksource.com/pharma/content/dam/GlaxoSmithKline/US /en/Prescribing_Information/Relenza/pdf/RELENZA-PI-PIL-COMBINED.PDF. Accessed May 2016.

Goh KP. Management of Hyponatremia. *AM Fam Phys* 2004; 69(10)2387–2394.

Hernandez-Aponte C, Silva-Sanchez J, Quintero-Hernandez V, Rodriguez-Romera A, Balderas C, Possani LD, Gurrola GB. Vejovine, A New Antibiotic from the Scorpion Venom of Vaejovis mexicanus. *Toxicon* 2011; 57:84–92.

Irwin M, Erb C, Williams C, Wilson BJ, Zitella LJ. *Putting Evidence into Practice (PEP): Improving Oncology Patient Outcomes. Prevention of Infection.* Pittsburgh, PA: Oncology Nursing Society; 2013.

Kutateladze M, Adamia R. Bacteriophages as Potential New Therapeutics to Replace or Supplement Antibiotics. *Trends Biotechnol.* 2010; 28(12):591–595.

Lu TK, Koeris MS. The Next Generation of Bacteriophage Therapy. *Curr Opin Microbiol.* 2011; 14: 524–531.

COMPLICATIONS

Malpiedi PJ, Peterson KD, Soe M, Edwards JE, Scott RD, Wise ME, Baggs J, Yi SH, Dudeck MA, Arnold KE, Weiner LM, Rebmann CA, Srinivasan A, Fridkin SK, McDonald LC. *2011 National and State Healthcare-Associated Infection Standardized Infection Ratio Report.* Published February 22, 2013. Available at http://www.cdc.gov/hai/national-annual-sir/index.html.

Medline. *Drug Information: Daptomycin.* Available at http://www.nlm.nih.gov/medline. Accessed June 2004.

Medline Plus. *Drug Information: Colistimethate Injection.* Available at http://www.nlm.nih.gov /medlineplus/print/druginfo/meds/a682860.html. Accessed June 2010.

Medline Plus. *Drug Information: Doripenem.* Available at http://www.nlm.nih.gov/medlineplus /print/ druginfo/meds/a608015.html. Accessed June 2010.

Medline Plus. *Drug Information: Norfloxacin.* Available at http://www.nlm.nih.gov/medlineplus/print /druginfo/meds/a687006.html. Accessed June 2010.

Melinta Therapeutics, Inc. Baxdela [product information]. Lincolnshire, IL. June 2017.

Merck & Co., Inc. Bezlotoxumab [package insert]. Whitehouse Station, NJ. Available at http://www .merck.com/product/usa/pi_circulars/z/zinplava/zinplava_pi.pdf. Accessed May 2017.

Merck & Co. Inc. Norfloxacin [product information]. September 2008.

Merck & Co. Inc. Prevymis [product information]. Whitehouse Station, NJ. 2017.

Merck & Co. Inc. Recarbrio [product information]. Whitehouse Station, NJ. 2019.

Meropenem [package insert]. http://hcunviweb05/mdxcgi/quiklocn.exe?CTL=E:/Mdx/mdxcgi/ MEGAT .SYS&SET=1C573. Accessed June 2005.

National Comprehenisve Cancer Network. *Prevention and Treatment of Cancer-related Infections.* Available at http://www.nccn.org/professionals/physician_gls/pdf/infections.pdf. Accessed May 2016.

Norfloxacin. Drugs.com. Drug Information Online. Available at http://www.drugs.com/MTM /norfloxacin.html. Accessed June 2010.

Optimer Pharmaceuticals, Inc., Dificid [product information]. San Diego, CA. 2011.

Orbactiv [package insert]. Available at http://www.themedicinescompany.com/app/webroot/img /orbactiv -prescribing-information.pdf. Accessed May 2015.

Orbactiv. Available at http://www.drugs.com/mtm/orbactiv.html. Accessed May 2015.

Orbactiv. Available at http://www.drugs.com/pro/orbactiv.html. Accessed May 2015.

Orbactiv. Available at http://www.drugs.com/sfx/orbactiv-side-effects.html. Accessed May 2015.

Orbactiv. Available at http://www.drugs.com/cdi/orbactiv.html. Accessed May 2015.

Paratek Pharmaceuticals, Inc. Nuzyra [product information]. Boston, MA. June 2019.

Raad II, Graybill JR, Bustamante AB, et al. Safety of Long-Term Oral Posaconazole Use in the Treatment of Refractory Invasive Fungal Infections. *Clin Infect Dis* 2006; 42(15 June): 1726–1734.

Rifaximin [package insert]. Available at http://hcunviweb05/mdxcgi/quiklocn.exe?CTL=E:/Mdx /mdxcgi/MEGAT.SYS&SET=1C573. June 2005.

Scott RD. *The Direct Medical Cost of Healthcare-Associated Infections in U.S. Hospitals and the Benefits of Prevention.* Atlanta, GA: Centers for Disease Control; 2009.

Sivextro [package insert]. Available at http://sivextro.com/pdf/sivextro-prescribing-info.pdf. Accessed May 2015.

Spellberg, B. New Antibiotic Development: Barriers and Opportunities in 2012 in Confronting Today's Crisis in Antibiotic Development. *The Alliance for the Prudent Use of Antibiotics (APUA) Newsletter* 2012; 30(1): 8–10.

Colistin/Polymyxin B for Injection (Colistimethate Sodium/Polymyxin B, sulfate) [package insert]. X-GEN Pharmaceuticals, Inc., PO Box 445, Big Flats, NY 14814.

TAJ Pharmaceuticals, 434, Laxmi Plaza, Laxmi Ind. Estate, New Link Road, Andheri (W), Mumbai, India 400 053.

Telithromycin. Available at http://www.centerwatch.com/patient/drugs/dru853.html. Accessed June 2004.

Telithromycin. Thompson Center Watch. *Clinical Trials Listing Service. Drugs Approved by the FDA.* Available at http://www.mcromedex.com/products/updates/drugdex_updates/de/ tilithromycin-full .html. Accessed June 2004.

Torres HA, Hachem RY, Chemaly RF, et al. Posaconazole: A Broad Spectrum Triazole Antifungal. *Lancet Infect Dis* 2005; 5(12):775–785.

United States Pharmacopeia Drug Information for Health Care Professionals, 18th ed. Rockville, MD.

Tetraphase Pharmaceuticals, Inc. Xerava [product information]. Watertown, MA. 2018.

The U.S. Pharmacopeial Convention. Available at http://www.usp.org/about-usp. Accessed May 2016.

Vasquez JA, Sobel JD. Anidulafungin: A Novel Echinocandin. *Clin Infect Dis* 2006; 43:215–222.

VHA Pharmacy Benefits Management Strategic Healthcare Group and Medical Advisor Panel. *Daptomycin.*

Warner-Lambert Co. Omnicef [package insert]. Morris Plains, NJ. 1998.

Williams, MD, Braun, LA, Cooper, LM, et al. Hospitalized Cancer Patients with Severe Sepsis: Analysis of Incidence, Mortality, and Associated Costs of Care. *Critical Care* 2004; 8: R291-R298 (doi:10.1186/cc2893). Available at http://ccforum.com/content/8/5/R291. Accessed June 2014.

Wilson, BJ, Zitella, LJ, Erb, CH, Foster, J, Peterson, M, Wood, SK. Prevention of Infection: A Systematic Review of Evidence-based Practice Interventions for Management in Patients with Cancer. *Clinical Journal of Oncology Nursing* 2018; 22:A1–A12.

Wyeth Pharmaceuticals, Inc. Tygacil [package insert]. Philadelphia, PA. 2005.

X-GEN Pharmaceuticals, Inc. Colistin/Polymyxin B for Injection (Colistimethate Sodium/Polymyxin B, sulfate) [package insert]. Big Flats, NY.

Zerbaxa [package insert]. Available at http://www.zerbaxa.com/pdf/PrescribingInformation.pdf. Accessed May 2015.

Zerbaxa. Available at http://www.drugs.com/mtm/zerbaxa.html. Accessed May 2015.

Zerbaxa. Available at http://www.drugs.com/pro/zerbaxa.html. Accessed May 2015.

Zerbaxa. Available at http://www.drugs.com/sfx/zerbaxa-side-effects.html. Accessed May 2015.

ANTIBIOTICS

Drug: amikacin sulfate (Amikin)

Class: Aminoglycoside antibacterial antibiotic.

Mechanism of Action: Synthetic antibiotic derived from kanamycin; bactericidal, most probably by inhibition of protein synthesis. Active against aerobic microorganisms: many sensitive gram-negative organisms (including *Acinetobacter, Citrobacter, Enterobacter, E. coli, Klebsiella, Proteus, Pseudomonas, Salmonella, Serratia,* and *Shigella*), and some sensitive gram-positive organisms (*S. aureus* and *S. epidermidis*). Over time bacterial resistance may develop, either naturally or acquired.

Metabolism: Well-absorbed following parenteral administration, but variability in absorption after IM injection (peak serum level 0.5–2 hours, duration 8–12 hours). Widely distributed into body fluids. Minimally protein-bound. Readily crosses placenta and found in breastmilk. Drug excreted unchanged in the urine.

Indication: For the treatment of infections caused by susceptible strains of microorganisms, especially gram-negative bacteria.

COMPLICATIONS

Dosage/Range:
• 15 mg/kg/day given in 8-, 12-, or 24-hour doses IV
• Desired peak serum concentration is 15–30 mg/mL, and trough serum concentration is 4–10 mg/mL.

Drug Preparation:
• Store injectable at < 40°C (104°F).
• Potency not affected by pale yellow color that may develop.
• Stable for 24 hours at concentrations of 0.25 and 5 mg/mL in 0.9% sodium chloride, 5% dextrose.

Drug Administration:
• IV: in 100–200 mL IV fluid (e.g., 0.9% sodium chloride or 5% dextrose injection), infused over 30–60 minutes.

Drug Interactions:
• Increased risk of toxicity with other ototoxic drugs: acyclovir, other aminoglycosides, amphotericin B, bacitracin, cephalosporins, colistin, cisplatin, ethacrynic acid, furosemide, vancomycin.
• Potentiation of neuromuscular blockade when given concurrently with general anesthetics (succinylcholine, tubocurarine)—use cautiously; observe for signs/symptoms of respiratory depression.
• Synergism with extended-spectrum penicillins but must be administered separately.

Lab Effects/Interference:
• Serum ALT, serum alk phos, serum AST, serum bilirubin, and serum LDH values all may be increased.
• BUN and serum creatinine values may be increased.
• Serum Ca+, serum Mg+, serum K+, and serum Na+ concentrations may be decreased.

Special Considerations:
• Used as first-line treatment in short-term treatment of serious gram-negative infections (e.g., septicemia, respiratory tract infections).
• Use against gram-positive organisms only as second-line treatment.
• Use in pregnancy only if infection is life-threatening and no safer drug exists; drug crosses placenta and may cause fetal toxicity.
• Do not use in Myasthenia Gravis.

Potential Toxicities/Side Effects and the Nursing Process

I.   ALTERATIONS IN SENSORY/PERCEPTUAL PATTERNS related to OTOTOXICITY

Defining Characteristics: Damage to eighth cranial nerve (auditory) may result in dizziness, nystagmus, vertigo, ataxia (vestibular damage), and less commonly, tinnitus, roaring sound in ears, and impaired hearing (auditory damage). Hearing loss usually begins with high-frequency loss, followed by clinical hearing loss, then permanent hearing loss if damage continues. Increased risk in elderly or renally impaired patients.

Nursing Implications: Assess baseline hearing (ability to hear spoken voice) and continue during therapy. Teach patient potential side effects, and instruct patient to report any hearing/perceptual problems (e.g., tinnitus, vertigo, decreased hearing). Discuss drug discontinuance and audiogram with physician to confirm hearing dysfunction if symptoms arise. Assess for increased risk if given concurrently with other ototoxic medications (e.g., cisplatin, furosemide).

II. ALTERATION IN URINARY ELIMINATION related to NEPHROTOXICITY

Defining Characteristics: Renal damage characterized by tubular necrosis with increased serum BUN, creatinine; decreased urine creatinine clearance and specific gravity; proteinuria and casts in urine. Azotemia usually not associated with oliguria. Rarely, electrolyte wasting with hypomagnesemia, hypocalcemia, and hypokalemia may occur. Renal dysfunction usually reversible after drug discontinuance. Increased risk in elderly and in patients with preexisting renal dysfunction. Risk is low in well-hydrated patients with normal renal function when normal doses are given.

Nursing Implications: Assess baseline renal function and electrolytes, and monitor periodically during therapy. Discuss any abnormalities with physician, as drug should be dose-reduced or discontinued if renal dysfunction develops. Assess baseline total body fluid balance, weight, and monitor periodically during antibiotic therapy. Monitor hydration status to keep patient well hydrated. Assess drug peak and trough levels as ordered so that drug dosage is correctly titrated. Increased risk of toxicity if peak serum concentration > 30–35 mg/mL. Draw blood for peak drug concentration 30 minutes after completion of 30-minute infusion or at the end of a 60-minute infusion; draw trough immediately before next dose.

III. ALTERATIONS IN SENSORY/PERCEPTUAL PATTERNS related to CNS EFFECTS, NEUROMUSCULAR BLOCKADE

Defining Characteristics: Headache, tremor, lethargy may occur. Peripheral neuropathy or encephalopathy (numbness, skin-tingling, muscle-twitching) may occur rarely. Neuromuscular blockade is dose related, self-limiting, and uncommon: risk is greater with topical application or when drug is administered to patient with neuromuscular disease (myasthenia gravis) or hypocalcemia.

Nursing Implications: Assess baseline neurologic status. Assess coexisting risk factors, neuroblockade medications. Teach patient about side effects, and instruct to report headache, tremor, and lethargy. Observe for respiratory depression. If signs/symptoms arise, discuss drug discontinuance with physician.

IV. POTENTIAL FOR INJURY related to HYPERSENSITIVITY

Defining Characteristics: Rash, urticaria, pruritus, fever, and eosinophilia have occurred rarely. CROSS-SENSITIVITY between AMINOGLYCOSIDES exists.

COMPLICATIONS

Nursing Implications: Assess for drug allergies to any aminoglycoside—amikacin, gentamicin, kanamycin, neomycin, netilmicin, streptomycin, tobramycin—prior to drug administration. Instruct patient to report any allergic reactions. Assess for signs/symptoms of allergic reaction after drug dose.

V.   ALTERATION IN NUTRITION, LESS THAN BODY REQUIREMENTS, related to GI SIDE EFFECTS

Defining Characteristics: Nausea, vomiting, and anorexia have occurred rarely. Also, transient hepatomegaly with elevated LFTs—AST, ALT, LDH, alk phos—has occurred.

Nursing Implications: Assess baseline nutritional status, preexisting nausea/vomiting, and anorexia. Assess baseline LFTs and monitor periodically during treatment. Instruct patient to report side effects. Provide symptomatic interventions if side effects occur; discuss with physician use of alternative drug(s).

VI.   POTENTIAL FOR FATIGUE, INFECTION, AND BLEEDING related to BONE MARROW INJURY

Defining Characteristics: Anemia, leukopenia, granulocytopenia, and thrombocytopenia may occur. Also, patients receiving antibiotics are at risk for overgrowth of nonsusceptible microorganisms, such as fungi (superinfection). Rare.

Nursing Implications: Assess baseline CBC, differential, and monitor periodically during treatment. Instruct patient to report signs/symptoms of fatigue, infection, or bleeding immediately. Assess for signs/symptoms of superinfection. Discuss any adverse effects with physician.

Drug: amoxicillin (Amoxil, Polymox, Trimox, Wymox; amoxicillin plus potassium clavulanate is Augmentin)

Class: Penicillin (aminopenicillin antibiotic); β-lactam.

Mechanism of Action: Semisynthetic antibiotic prepared from fungus *Penicillium*. Contains β-lactam ring and is bactericidal by inhibiting cell wall synthesis. Aminopenicillins have increased activity against gram-negative bacilli (*H. influenzae, E. coli*), as well as some activity against gram-positive bacilli (*Streptococci* and *Staphylococci*).

Metabolism: Well-absorbed from GI tract; rate of absorption slowed by food, but total amount of drug absorbed remains unchanged. Widely distributed in body tissues and fluids. Crosses placenta and is found in breastmilk. Excreted in urine and bile.

Indication: For the treatment of infections of upper and lower respiratory tract, genito-urinary (GU) tract, and skin caused by sensitive organisms. Infections, such as tonsillitis, bronchitis, pneumonia, and gonorrhea, and infections of ear, nose, throat, skin, or urinary tract. Sometimes used in combination with clarithromycin (Biaxin) to treat stomach ulcers caused by *Helicobacter pylori.*

Dosage/Range:

Adult:

- 125–500 mg PO q 8 h 48–72 hours after infection eradicated; for uncomplicated urinary tract infection, may use single dose of 3 g PO.
- Drug dose should be reduced if severe renal failure occurs.
- Augmentin dose: mild to moderate infection: 500 mg PO bid; severe infection: 875 mg PO bid.

Drug Preparation:
- Store capsules in tight container at 15–30°C (59–86°F).
- Administer on empty stomach.

Drug Interactions:
- Aminoglycosides (e.g., gentamicin): incompatible when mixed together; administer at separate sites at different times. Penicillinase-resistant penicillins can inactivate aminoglycoside serum samples from patients receiving both drugs.
- Rifampin: possible antagonism, only at high doses of penicillin.
- Probenecid: increased serum level of penicillin; may be coadministered to exert this effect.
- Methotrexate: avoid concomitant use or decrease methotrexate dose.
- Clavulanic acid (β-lactamase inhibitor): synergistic bactericidal effect. Amoxicillin plus potassium clavulanate = Augmentin.

Lab Effects/Interference:

Major clinical significance:
- Urine glucose: high urinary concentrations of a penicillin may produce false-positive or falsely elevated test results with copper-reduction tests (Benedict's, Clinitest, or Fehling's); glucose enzymatic tests (Clinistix or Tes-Tape) are not affected.

Clinical significance:
- Coombs' tests: false-positive result may occur during therapy with any penicillin.
- ALT, alk phos, AST, serum bilirubin, and serum LDH values may be increased.
- Estradiol, total-conjugated estriol, estriol-glucuronide, or conjugated estrone concentrations may be transiently decreased in pregnant women following administration of amoxicillin.
- WBC: leukopenia or neutropenia is associated with the use of all penicillins; the effect is more likely to occur with prolonged and severe hepatic function impairment.

Special Considerations:
- Contraindicated in patients with prior hypersensitivity to penicillins. Use with caution in patients sensitive to other β-lactams (e.g., cephalosporins) since partial cross-allergenicity exists.
- Obtain ordered specimen and send for culture and sensitivity prior to first antibiotic dose.

COMPLICATIONS

- Consider alternative antibiotic therapy if eosinophilia, drug fever or rash, arthralgia, hematuria, or unexplained rise in BUN and serum creatinine occur.
- Monitor electrolytes and renal, hepatic, and hematologic laboratory parameters during extended treatment periods.
- Use with caution in pregnancy or with nursing women.
- Amoxicillin rash may occur that is distinct from drug-allergic rash; increased risk if concurrent use of allopurinol.
- Lower incidence of diarrhea as a GI side effect than ampicillin.
- May cause false-positive with Clinitest glucose testing.

Potential Toxicities/Side Effects and the Nursing Process

I.   POTENTIAL FOR INJURY related to HYPERSENSITIVITY REACTION

Defining Characteristics: Urticaria, pruritus, rash (maculopapular or erythematous), fever and chills, eosinophilia, myalgia, edema, erythema, angioedema, Stevens–Johnson syndrome, and exfoliative skin reactions occur in 5% of patients. Increased risk in individuals allergic to cephalosporin antibiotics. A nonimmunologic rash may occur 3–14 days after drug started, characterized as a generalized erythematous/maculopapular rash, and worse over pressure areas of elbows and knees. Rash usually subsides in 6–14 days, even if drug is continued. If drug is stopped, resolves in 1–7 days.

Nursing Implications: Assess allergy to cephalosporin antibiotics and penicillin: if patient states "yes," determine actual response (e.g., "swollen lips = angioedema"). If angioedema, patient should not receive drug. Discuss other patient responses with physician to determine whether drug should be given. Assess baseline skin condition, including integrity and allergy history to drugs. Instruct patient to report rash, itching, other skin changes. Teach patient skin care and symptomatic measures as appropriate. If skin rash develops, discuss drug discontinuance with physician. If rash progresses, drug should be discontinued, as fatal Stevens–Johnson syndrome may develop. Be prepared to treat severe acute hypersensitivity reactions with airway management, oxygen, epinephrine, corticosteroids, and antihistamines as ordered.

II.   ALTERATION IN NUTRITION, LESS THAN BODY REQUIREMENTS, related to GI SIDE EFFECTS

Defining Characteristics: Nausea, vomiting, diarrhea, and anorexia may occur; rarely, pseudomembranous colitis caused by *C. difficile* resistant to the antibiotic occurs. Rarely, transient increases in LFTs—AST, ALT, alk phos, bilirubin—may occur.

Nursing Implications: Assess baseline nutritional status. Instruct patient to report GI disturbances. Administer and instruct patient to self-administer antiemetics as needed and as ordered. Teach patient importance of nutritious diet and suggest small, frequent, high-calorie, high-protein meals as appropriate. Assess baseline LFTs and monitor periodically during treatment. Discuss abnormalities and drug interruption with physician.

III. FUNGAL SUPERINFECTION related to OVERGROWTH OF ENDOGENOUS MICROORGANISMS

Defining Characteristics: Vaginal candidiasis, vaginitis may occur as endogenous bacteria are eliminated and normal fungal population expands.

Nursing Implications: Teach female patient to report vaginal itching or discharge. Discuss appropriate antifungal treatment with physician. Teach perineal hygiene and symptomatic management.

IV. ALTERATIONS IN PROTECTIVE MECHANISMS (RARE) related to TRANSIENT LEUKOPENIA

Defining Characteristics: Rarely, transient leukopenia, lymphocytosis, anemia, eosinophilia may occur. Prolonged PT, prolonged activated partial thromboplastin time (aPTT), and hypoprothrombinemia have occurred rarely, especially in elderly or debilitated patients or in individuals with vitamin K deficiency.

Nursing Implications: Assess baseline laboratory parameters and monitor periodically during treatment. Assess patient for response to antibiotics. Discuss abnormalities with physician.

V. KNOWLEDGE DEFICIT related to SELF-ADMINISTRATION OF MEDICATION

Defining Characteristics: Increased compliance when patient is instructed in self-care activities.

Nursing Implications: Assess knowledge regarding infection and planned treatment. Teach drug action, potential side effects, and when and how to take drug (take medication as directed, 1 hour before or 2 hours after food). Instruct patient to report any possible drug side effects that occur.

COMPLICATIONS

Drug: ampicillin sodium/sulbactam sodium (Unasyn)

Class: Penicillin (aminopenicillin antibiotic).

Mechanism of Action: Semisynthetic antibiotic prepared from fungus *Penicillium*. Contains β-lactam ring and is bactericidal by inhibiting cell wall synthesis. Aminopenicillins have increased activity against gram-negative bacilli (*H. influenzae, E. coli*), as well as some activity against gram-positive bacilli (*Streptococci* and *Staphylococci*). Although sulbactam alone possesses little useful antibacterial activity, whole organism studies have shown that sulbactam restores ampicillin activity against beta lactamase-producing strains of bacteria.

Metabolism: Widely distributed in body tissues and fluids. Crosses placenta and is found in breastmilk. Excreted in urine and bile.

Indication: For treatment of infections of the skin, intra-abdominal infections, and gynecologic infections caused by sensitive organisms. In combination with sulbactam, there is irreversible inhibition of beta lactamases, thus making ampicillin effective against beta lactamase bacteria that would otherwise be resistant to it.

Dosage/Range:

Adult:
- Dose modification necessary if renal impairment occurs. See manufacturer's package insert.
- Unasyn: 1.5–3 g ampicillin and 0.5–1 g sulbactam IV/IM every 6 hours (dose not to exceed 4 g sulbactam a day).

Drug Preparation:
- IV dilute with normal saline only; give over 10–30 minutes.
- IM: reconstitute per manufacturer's directions and use within 1 hour after reconstitution.

Drug Interactions:
- Aminoglycosides (e.g., gentamicin): incompatible when mixed together; administer at separate sites at different times. Also, penicillinase-resistant penicillins can inactivate aminoglycoside serum samples from patients receiving both drugs.
- Rifampin: possible antagonism, only at high doses of ampicillin.
- Probenecid: decreases renal tubular secretion of ampicillin and sulbactam.
- Oral contraceptives: may decrease efficacy of contraceptive and increase incidence of breakthrough bleeding. Suggest additional use of barrier contraception.
- Sulbactam: broadens antibacterial coverage of ampicillin against resistant β-lactamase-producing microorganisms.
- Concurrent administration of allopurinol and ampicillin increases the incidence of rashes.

Lab Effects/Interference:
- Urine glucose: high urinary concentrations of penicillin may produce false-positive or falsely elevated test results with copper-reduction tests (Benedict's Clinitest, or Fehling's); glucose enzymatic tests (Clinistix or Tes-Tape) are not affected.
- Estradiol, total conjugated estriol, estriol-glucuronide or conjugated estrone concentrations may be transiently decreased in pregnant women following administration of ampicillin.
- Increased AST (SGOT), ALT (SGPT), alkaline phosphatase, and LDH.
- Decreased serum albumin and total protein.
- WBC: leukopenia or neutropenia is associated with the use of all penicillins; the effect is more likely to occur with prolonged and severe hepatic function impairment.
- BUN and serum creatinine: increased concentrations have been associated with ampicillin.

Special Considerations:

- Contraindicated in patients with prior hypersensitivity to penicillins. Use with caution in patients sensitive to other β-lactams (e.g., cephalosporins) since partial cross-allergenicity exists.
- Obtain ordered specimen and send for culture and sensitivity prior to first antibiotic dose.
- Consider alternative antibiotic therapy if eosinophilia, drug fever or rash, arthralgia, hematuria, or unexplained rise in BUN and serum creatinine occur.

- Monitor electrolytes and renal, hepatic, and hematologic laboratory parameters during extended treatment periods.
- Use with caution in pregnancy or with nursing women.
- Renal dysfunction: Unasyn dose must be reduced.

Potential Toxicities/Side Effects and the Nursing Process

I. POTENTIAL FOR INJURY related to HYPERSENSITIVITY REACTION AND LOCAL REACTIONS (pain at injection site and thrombophlebitis)

Defining Characteristics: Urticaria, pruritus, rash (maculopapular or erythematous), fever and chills, eosinophilia, myalgia, edema, erythema, angioedema, Stevens–Johnson syndrome, and exfoliative skin reactions occur in 5% of patients. Increased risk in individuals allergic to cephalosporin antibiotics.

Nursing Implications: Assess allergy to cephalosporin antibiotics and penicillin: if patient states "yes," determine actual response (e.g., "swollen lips = angioedema"). If angioedema, patient should not receive drug. Discuss other patient responses with physician to determine whether drug should be given. Assess baseline skin condition including integrity and allergy history to drugs. Instruct patient to report rash, itching, other skin changes. Teach patient skin care and symptomatic measures as appropriate. If skin rash develops, discuss drug discontinuance with physician. If rash progresses, drug should be discontinued, as fatal Stevens–Johnson syndrome may develop. Be prepared to treat severe acute hypersensitivity reactions with airway management, oxygen, epinephrine, corticosteroids, and antihistamines as ordered.

II. ALTERATION IN NUTRITION, LESS THAN BODY REQUIREMENTS, related to GI SIDE EFFECTS

Defining Characteristics: Nausea, vomiting, diarrhea may occur; rarely, pseudomembranous colitis caused by *C. difficile* resistant to the antibiotic occurs. Rarely, transient increases in LFTs—AST, ALT, alk phos, bilirubin—may occur.

Nursing Implications: Assess baseline nutritional status. Instruct patient to report GI disturbances. Administer and teach patient to self-administer antiemetics as needed and as ordered. Teach patient importance of nutritious diet and suggest small, frequent, high-calorie, high-protein meals as appropriate. Assess baseline LFTs, and monitor periodically during treatment. Discuss abnormalities and drug interruption with physician.

III. FUNGAL SUPERINFECTION related to REDISTRIBUTION OF ENDOGENOUS MICROORGANISMS

Defining Characteristics: Vaginal candidiasis, vaginitis may occur as endogenous bacteria are eliminated and normal fungal population expands.

COMPLICATIONS

Nursing Implications: Instruct female patient to report vaginal itching or discharge. Discuss appropriate antifungal treatment with physician. Teach perineal hygiene and symptomatic management.

IV.   KNOWLEDGE DEFICIT related to SELF-ADMINISTRATION OF MEDICATION

Defining Characteristics: Increased compliance when patient is instructed in self-care activities.

Nursing Implications: Assess knowledge regarding infection and planned treatment. Teach about drug action, potential side effects, and when and how to take drug. (Take medication as directed, 1 hour before or 2 hours after food.) Instruct patient to report any possible drug side effects.

Drug: azithromycin (Zithromax)

Class: Antibacterial (macrolide).

Mechanism of Action: Azithromycin binds to the 50S ribosomal subunit of the 70S ribosome of susceptible organisms, thereby inhibiting RNA-dependent protein synthesis. Bactericidal for *S. pyogenes, S. pneumoniae,* and *H. influenzae.* It is bacteriostatic for staphylococci and most aerobic gram-negative species.

Metabolism: Rapidly and widely distributed throughout the body; concentrates intracellularly, resulting in tissue concentrations 10–100 times those in plasma and serum. Rapidly absorbed with decreased absorption when given with food. Azithromycin is highly concentrated in phagocytes and fibroblasts. Over 50% of the dose is eliminated through biliary excretion as unchanged drug; approximately 4.5% of the dose is excreted unchanged in the urine within 72 hours.

Indication: For treatment of many different types of infections caused by bacteria, such as respiratory infections, skin infections, ear infections, and sexually transmitted diseases.

Dosage/Range:
- Oral: loading dose of 500 mg as a single dose on day 1, then 250 mg once a day on days 2–5. Treatment of 500 mg for 3 days is also an option.
- No adjustment in dose is required in patients with mild renal function impairment. No data available for patients with more severe renal function impairment.
- IV: if indicated, 500 mg may be given daily × 1–2 days, then followed by oral therapy 250 mg to complete course.

Drug Preparation:
- Reconstitute 500-mg vial with 4.8 mL sterile water for concentration of 100 mg/mL.
- Further dilute to a concentration of 1–3 mg/mL prior to administration. Compatible with NS, D5W, and Ringers lactated solution.

Drug Administration:
- Oral: give at least 1 hour before and 2 hours after meals. Give at least 1 hour before and 2 hours after aluminum-and magnesium-containing antacids. The extended-release suspension (Zmax(R)) may be taken with antacids.
- IV: infuse 500 mg/500 mL over 3 hours and 500 mg/250 mL over 1 hour.

Drug Interactions:
- Concurrent use with antacids has decreased peak serum concentration by approximately 24%.

Lab Effects/Interference:
- Serum SGPT, serum SGOT values may be increased.
- Creatinine clearance. Can be used in pts with GFR >10 mL/min.

Special Considerations:
- Do not use when there is a known hypersensitivity to erythromycins or other macrolides.
- QT prolongation reported in pts at risk.
- Avoid Class 1 A, Class 3 antiarrhythmics due to risk of QT prolongation and torsades.
- Use with caution in patients with severe, impaired hepatic function.

Potential Toxicities/Side Effects and the Nursing Process

I.   POTENTIAL FOR INJURY related to HYPERSENSITIVITY

Defining Characteristics: Rarely, serious allergic reactions such as anaphylaxis and angioedema have been known to occur. Fever, joint pain, skin rash, urticaria, pruritus, difficulty breathing, swelling of face, mouth, neck, hands, and feet have occurred rarely.

Nursing Implications: Assess for drug allergies to erythromycin or macrolide antibiotic prior to drug administration. Teach patient to report any allergic reactions. Assess for signs/symptoms of allergic reaction after drug dose.

II.   ALTERATION IN NUTRITION related to GI SIDE EFFECTS

Defining Characteristics: Abdominal pain, diarrhea, nausea, and vomiting have occurred rarely.

Nursing Implications: Assess baseline nutritional status, preexisting nausea/vomiting, and anorexia. Assess baseline LFTs and monitor periodically during treatment. Teach patient to report side effects. Provide symptomatic interventions if side effects occur; discuss with physician use of alternative drug(s).

III.   ALTERATION IN URINARY ELIMINATION related to ACUTE INTERSTITIAL NEPHRITIS

Defining Characteristics: Risk is low, but patient may manifest symptoms of acute interstitial nephritis—fever, joint pain, skin rash.

COMPLICATIONS

Nursing Implications: Assess baseline renal function and electrolytes, and monitor periodically during therapy. Monitor hydration status to keep patient well hydrated.

IV. SENSORY/PERCEPTUAL ALTERATIONS related to CNS EFFECTS OF DIZZINESS AND HEADACHE

Defining Characteristics: Dizziness and headache may occur.

Nursing Implications: Assess baseline neurologic status. Teach patient about side effects and to report dizziness or headache. If signs/symptoms arise, discuss drug discontinuance with physician.

Drug: aztreonam (Azactam)

Class: Antibacterial (systemic).

Mechanism of Action: Bactericidal by inhibition of cell wall synthesis, which results in cell wall disintegration, lysis, and cell death. Narrow spectrum of activity against aerobic, gram-negative microorganisms (*Enterobacteriaceae* and *P. aeruginosa*).

Metabolism: Given IV. Widely distributed in body tissue and fluids, including CSF and peritoneal fluid. Crosses placenta and is excreted in breastmilk. Infant risk is minimal, compatible with breastfeeding. Partially metabolized and excreted primarily in urine.

Indication: For treatment of gram-negative infections of urinary and lower respiratory tract, septicemia, and gynecologic and intra-abdominal infections. Drug improves breathing symptoms in cystic fibrosis (CF) patients with lung infections caused by *P. aeruginosa*.

Dosage/Range:
- Given IV or IM (IV preferred for doses > 1 g, and for serious infections).
- Adults: 500 mg–2 g IV/IM q 6–12 h (maximum 8 g/day).
- Dose modification needed for renal dysfunction (creatinine clearance < 30 mL/min); may need to modify dosage in hepatic impairment.

Drug Preparation:
- IV: reconstitute by adding 10 mL sterile water for injection or compatible IV fluid. Further dilute by adding to a volume of IV fluid (50 mL for each gram of drug) so final concentration is < 20 mg/mL. Administer over 20–60 minutes. Flush line with plain IV fluid before and after drug infusion to prevent incompatibilities.
- IM: reconstitute drug with 3 mL for each gram of drug using sterile or bacteriostatic water for injection, or 0.9% sodium chloride. Do not mix with local anesthetics. Administer deep IM in large muscle mass (e.g., gluteus maximus).

Drug Interactions:
- Magnesium, calcium: incompatible in IV fluid.

Lab Effects/Interference:
- Serum ALT, serum alk phos, serum AST, and serum LDH values may be transiently increased during therapy.
- Serum creatinine concentrations may be transiently increased during therapy.

Special Considerations:
- Obtain and send specimen for culture and sensitivity prior to first drug dose.
- May cause false-positive Clinitest glucose result.
- Use with caution in patients with renal or hepatic dysfunction.
- Drug crosses placenta and is excreted in breastmilk. Use with caution if patient is pregnant; weigh potential risks and benefits carefully if lactating; compatible with breastfeeding.
- Use cautiously if prior immediate hypersensitivity reaction to penicillins or cephalosporins; little risk of cross-allergenicity, but monitor patient closely.

Potential Toxicities/Side Effects and the Nursing Process

I.   ALTERATIONS IN SKIN INTEGRITY related to ALLERGY HYPERSENSITIVITY REACTION

Defining Characteristics: 1–2% incidence of rash that is mild, transient, pruritic, and/or erythematous. Less than 1% of patients develop purpura, erythema multiforme, urticaria, or exfoliative dermatitis. Less than 1% incidence occurs of immediate hypersensitivity reaction characterized by angioedema, bronchospasm, severe shock. Little cross-allergenicity with penicillins, cephalosporins (less than 1%).

Nursing Implications: Assess baseline skin integrity and presence of drug allergies; if anaphylactic reaction to penicillins or cephalosporins, monitor patient closely during drug infusions. Instruct patient to report immediately signs/symptoms of rash, pruritus, shortness of breath, and adverse sensation. Teach patient skin care and symptomatic measures as appropriate. If skin rash develops, discuss drug discontinuance with physician. If rash progresses, especially in HIV-infected patients, drug should be discontinued, as fatal Stevens–Johnson syndrome may develop. Be prepared to treat severe acute hypersensitivity reactions with airway management, oxygen, epinephrine, corticosteroids, antihistamines as ordered.

II. ALTERATION IN NUTRITION, LESS THAN BODY REQUIREMENTS, related to GI SIDE EFFECTS

Defining Characteristics: Nausea, vomiting, diarrhea, and anorexia may occur; rarely, pseudomembranous colitis caused by *C. difficile* resistant to the antibiotic occurs. Rarely, transient increases in LFTs—AST, ALT, alk phos—may occur. May develop taste alteration and halitosis.

Nursing Implications: Assess baseline nutritional status. Instruct patient to report GI disturbances. Administer and teach patient to self-administer antiemetics as needed and as ordered. Teach patient importance of nutritious diet and suggest small, frequent, high-calorie, high-protein meals as appropriate. Assess baseline LFTs and monitor periodically during treatment. Discuss abnormalities and drug interruption with physician. Encourage oral hygiene after meals and at bedtime.

III.   FUNGAL SUPERINFECTION related to REDISTRIBUTION OF ENDOGENOUS MICROORGANISMS

Defining Characteristics: Vaginal candidiasis, vaginitis may occur as endogenous bacteria are eliminated and normal fungal population expands.

Nursing Implications: Instruct female patient to report vaginal itching or discharge. Discuss appropriate antifungal treatment with physician. Teach perineal hygiene and symptomatic management.

IV.   ALTERATIONS IN PROTECTIVE MECHANISMS (RARE) related to PANCYTOPENIA

Defining Characteristics: Pancytopenia, neutropenia, thrombocytopenia, anemia, leukocytosis, or thrombocytosis may occur rarely. Eosinophilia occurs in 11% of patients. May have slight prolongation of bleeding time with high doses (e.g., 2-g IV q 6 h).

Nursing Implications: Assess baseline laboratory parameters, and monitor periodically during treatment. Assess patient for response to antibiotics. Discuss abnormalities with physician. Assess for signs/symptoms of bleeding. If taking anticoagulants, assess for increased PT, signs/symptoms of bleeding.

V.   ALTERATIONS IN SENSORY/PERCEPTUAL PATTERNS related to DIZZINESS, SOMNOLENCE

Defining Characteristics: Dizziness, headache, somnolence, or seizures occur rarely.

Nursing Implications: Assess baseline neurologic function and comfort, and monitor during treatment. Instruct patient to report any changes. Discuss any abnormalities with physician.

VI.   ALTERATIONS IN COMFORT related to LOCAL INJECTION IRRITATION

Defining Characteristics: Two to three percent incidence of phlebitis and thrombophlebitis when administering IV; 3% incidence of pain and swelling at injection site when given IM.

Nursing Implications: Rotate IM injection sites and administer drug deep IM in large muscle mass (e.g., gluteus maximus). Use IM injection when IV administration is not possible. Change IV sites q 48 h and assess for signs/symptoms of phlebitis prior to each administration. Administer drug slowly. Apply warm packs to increase comfort.

VII. ALTERATIONS IN CARDIAC OUTPUT related to CARDIOVASCULAR CHANGES

Defining Characteristics: Rare, ~1% incidence of hypotension, transient EKG changes (e.g., premature ventricular contractions), bradycardia, flushing, and chest pain.

Nursing Implications: Assess baseline heart rate and BP; monitor during therapy, at least with initial dose.

Drug: cefaclor (Ceclor)

Class: Second-generation cephalosporin antibiotic.

Mechanism of Action: Semisynthetic derivative of cephalosporin C (produced by fungus); contains β-lactam ring and is related to penicillins and cephamycins (e.g., cefoxitin). Bactericidal through inhibition of cell wall synthesis with resulting cell wall instability and cell lysis.

Metabolism: Well-absorbed from GI tract; delayed GI absorption if taken with food but total amount of drug absorption is the same. Widely distributed in body tissues, fluids except CSF; readily crosses placenta and is excreted in breastmilk. Unchanged drug rapidly excreted by the kidneys.

Indication: For treatment of certain infections caused by bacteria, such as pneumonia and infections of the ears, lungs, throat, urinary tract, and skin. Active against organisms causing lower respiratory tract infections (*H. influenzae, Klebsiella, Proteus, S. aureus, S. pneumoniae*); urinary tract infections (*Enterobacter, E. coli*); skin and soft-tissue infections (*S. aureus, E. coli*); septicemia; and biliary infections.

Dosage/Range:
• Oral: 250–500 mg q 8 h (maximum total 4 g/day).

Drug Preparation:
• Store in tight container at 15–30°C (59–86°F).

Drug Interactions:
• Probenecid: increased serum concentrations of cefaclor, but does not usually require dose reduction of antibiotic.

Lab Effects/Interference:

Major clinical significance:

• Coombs' (antiglobulin) tests: a positive reaction frequently appears in patients who receive large doses of cephalosporins; hemolysis rarely occurs, but it has been reported; test may be positive in neonates whose mothers received cephalosporins before delivery.

COMPLICATIONS

- Urine glucose: cefaclor may produce false-positive or falsely elevated test results with copper sulfate tests (Benedict's, Clinitest, or Fehling's); glucose enzymatic tests (Clinistix or Tes-Tape) are not affected.
- PT: may be prolonged; cephalosporins may inhibit vitamin K synthesis by suppressing gut flora.

Clinical significance:
- Serum ALT, serum alk phos, serum AST, serum bili, or serum LDH values may be increased.
- BUN and serum creatinine concentrations may be increased.
- CBC or platelet count: transient leukopenia, neutropenia, agranulocytosis, thrombocytopenia, eosinophilia, lymphocytosis, and thrombocytosis have been seen on rare occasions.

Special Considerations:
- Use cautiously if renal impairment is present.
- Contraindicated if hypersensitive to other cephalosporins, or if has had angioedema response to penicillin.
- Urine glucose testing with Clinitest may result in false-positive.

Potential Toxicities/Side Effects and the Nursing Process

I.   POTENTIAL FOR INJURY related to HYPERSENSITIVITY REACTION

Defining Characteristics: Urticaria, pruritus, rash (maculopapular or erythematous), fever and chills, eosinophilia, myalgia, edema, erythema, angioedema, Stevens–Johnson syndrome, and exfoliative skin reactions occur in 5% of patients. Increased risk in individuals allergic to penicillin.

Nursing Implications: Assess allergy to cephalosporin antibiotics and penicillin: if patient states "yes," determine actual response (e.g., "swollen lips = angioedema"). If angioedema, patient should not receive drug. Discuss other patient responses with physician to determine whether drug should be given. Assess baseline skin condition including integrity and allergy history to drugs. Instruct patient to report rash, itching, or other skin changes. Teach patient skin care and symptomatic measures as appropriate. If skin rash develops, discuss drug discontinuance with physician. If rash progresses, drug should be discontinued, as fatal Stevens–Johnson syndrome may develop. Be prepared to treat severe acute hypersensitivity reactions with airway management, oxygen, epinephrine, corticosteroids, antihistamines as ordered.

II.   ALTERATION IN NUTRITION, LESS THAN BODY REQUIREMENTS, related to GI SIDE EFFECTS

Defining Characteristics: Nausea, vomiting, diarrhea, and anorexia may occur; rarely, pseudomembranous colitis caused by *C. difficile* resistant to the antibiotic occurs. May cause transient increases in LFTs.

Nursing Implications: Assess baseline nutritional status. Instruct patient to report GI disturbances. Administer and teach patient to self-administer antiemetics as needed and as ordered. Teach patient importance of nutritious diet and suggest small, frequent, high-calorie, high-protein meals as appropriate. Assess baseline LFTs and monitor periodically during treatment. Discuss abnormalities and drug interruption with physician.

III. FUNGAL SUPERINFECTION related to REDISTRIBUTION OF ENDOGENOUS MICROORGANISMS

Defining Characteristics: Vaginal candidiasis, vaginitis may occur as endogenous bacteria are eliminated and normal fungal population expands.

Nursing Implications: Instruct female patient to report vaginal itching or discharge. Discuss appropriate antifungal treatment with physician. Teach perineal hygiene and symptomatic management.

IV. ALTERATIONS IN PROTECTIVE MECHANISMS (RARE) related to CHANGES IN BLOOD CELL ELEMENTS, CLOTTING FACTOR

Defining Characteristics: Rarely, transient leukopenia, lymphocytosis, anemia, eosinophilia may occur. Prolonged PT, prolonged aPTT, and hypoprothrombinemia have occurred rarely, especially in elderly or debilitated patients, or in individuals with vitamin K deficiency.

Nursing Implications: Assess baseline laboratory parameters and monitor periodically during treatment. Assess patient for response to antibiotics. Discuss abnormalities with physician.

V. ALTERATIONS IN SENSORY/PERCEPTUAL PATTERNS related to DIZZINESS, SOMNOLENCE

Defining Characteristics: Dizziness, headache, or somnolence occur rarely.

Nursing Implications: Assess baseline neurologic function and comfort and monitor during treatment. Instruct patient to report any changes. Discuss any abnormalities with physician.

VI. KNOWLEDGE DEFICIT related to SELF-ADMINISTRATION OF MEDICATION

Defining Characteristics: Increased compliance when patient is instructed in self-care activities.

Nursing Implications: Assess knowledge regarding infection and planned treatment. Teach about drug action, potential side effects, and when and how to take drug. Instruct patient to report any possible side effects that occur.

COMPLICATIONS

Drug: cefadroxil (Duracef)

Class: First-generation cephalosporin antibacterial.

Mechanism of Action: Semisynthetic derivative of cephalosporin contains β-lactam ring and is related to penicillins and cephamycins. Bactericidal through inhibition of cell wall synthesis by binding to one or more of the PBPs that in turn inhibit final transpeptidation step of peptidoglycan synthesis in bacterial cell walls, thus inhibiting cell wall biosynthesis. Bacteria eventually lyse due to ongoing activity of cell wall autolytic enzymes (autolysins and murein hydrolases) while cell wall assembly is arrested.

Metabolism: Well-absorbed from GI tract; delayed GI absorption if taken with food but total amount of drug absorption is the same. Widely distributed in body tissues, fluids except cerebrospinal fluid; readily crosses placenta and is excreted in breastmilk. Unchanged drug rapidly excreted by the kidneys.

Indication: For treatment of certain infections caused by bacteria, such as skin, throat, and urinary tract infections.

Dosage/Range:
- Adults: 1–2 g/day every 12 hours.
- Dose: reduce if creatinine clearance is reduced per manufacturer's recommendations.

Drug Preparation:
- Store suspension in refrigerator, discard after 14 days.
- Oral administration.

Drug Interactions:
- Coumadin
- Contraceptives
- Probenecid may decrease cephalosporin elimination and increase effect.

Lab Effects/Interference:
- Serum SGPT, serum alk phos, serum SGOT, serum bilirubin, or serum LDH—values may be increased.

Special Considerations:
- Use with caution in patients with renal dysfunction—dose reduction required if severe impairment exists.
- Contraindicated in patients hypersensitive to other cephalosporin antibiotics.
- Use cautiously if sensitive to penicillin; contraindicated if angioedema reaction to penicillin.
- Obtain ordered specimen and send for culture and sensitivity prior to first drug dose, if applicable.

Potential Toxicities/Side Effects and the Nursing Process

I. POTENTIAL FOR INJURY related to HYPERSENSITIVITY REACTION

Defining Characteristics: Urticaria, pruritus, rash (maculopapular or erythematous), fever and chills, eosinophilia, myalgia, edema, erythema, or angioedema. Increased risk in individuals allergic to penicillin.

Nursing Implications: Assess allergy to cephalosporin antibiotics and penicillin: if patient states "yes," determine actual response (e.g., "swollen lips = angioedema"). If angioedema, patient should not receive drug. Discuss other patient responses with physician to determine whether drug should be given. Assess baseline skin condition including integrity and allergy history to drugs. Teach patient to report rash, itching, other skin changes. Teach patient skin care and symptomatic measures as appropriate. If skin rash develops, discuss drug discontinuance with physician.

II. ALTERATION IN NUTRITION, LESS THAN BODY REQUIREMENTS, related to GI SIDE EFFECTS

Defining Characteristics: Nausea and vomiting, diarrhea, and anorexia may occur. Rarely, transient increases in LFTs—AST (SGOT), ALT (SGPT), ALK PHOS, bilirubin—may occur.

Nursing Implications: Assess baseline nutritional status. Teach patient to report GI disturbances. Administer and teach patient to self-administer medication as needed and as ordered. Teach patient importance of nutritious diet and suggest small, frequent, high-calorie, high-protein meals as appropriate. Assess baseline LFTs and monitor periodically during treatment. Discuss abnormalities and drug interruption with physician.

III. FUNGAL SUPERINFECTION related to REDISTRIBUTION OF ENDOGENOUS MICROORGANISMS

Defining Characteristics: Vaginal moniliasis or vaginitis may occur as endogenous bacteria are eliminated and normal fungal population expands.

Nursing Implications: Teach female patient to report vaginal itching or discharge. Discuss appropriate antifungal treatment with physician. Teach perineal hygiene and symptomatic management.

Drug: cefazolin sodium (Ancef)

Class: First-generation cephalosporin antibacterial.

Mechanism of Action: Semisynthetic derivative of cephalosporin C (produced by fungus); contains β-lactam ring and is related to penicillins and cephamycins (e.g., cefoxitin).

COMPLICATIONS

Bactericidal through inhibition of cell wall synthesis, with resulting cell wall instability and cell lysis.

Metabolism: Not absorbed from GI tract, so must be given IV or IM. Widely distributed to body tissues and fluids, including bile; 74–86% bound to serum proteins. Excreted unchanged in urine. Crosses placenta and is excreted in breastmilk.

Indication: For the treatment of biliary tract infections caused by susceptible *E. coli, Klebsiella, P. mirabilis, S. aureus*, or various streptococci. Active against many gram-positive aerobic cocci (*S. aureus*, groups A and B streptococci); some susceptible gram-negative organisms (*E. coli, H. influenzae, Klebsiella, Proteus*); and gram-negative organisms causing intra-abdominal and biliary infections.

Dosage/Range:
- IV is same as IM.
- Adults: 250 mg–1.5 g q 6–8 h (maximum 12 g/day in life-threatening infections).
- May give loading dose of 500 mg.

CrCl (mL/min)	Dosage
55 or greater	Full dose
35–54	Full dose with at least 8-hour intervals
11–34	1/2 usual dose at 12-hour intervals
Less than 10	1/2 usual dose at 18-to 24-hour intervals

Drug Preparation:
- Store powder at < 40°C (104°F) and protect from light. Is available as frozen solution that should be stored at $T < -20°C$ (– 4°F).
- Reconstitute powder with sterile water for injection, bacteriostatic water for injection, or 0.9% sodium chloride; solution stable for 24 hours at room temperature or 96 hours at 5°C (41°F).
- Further dilute in 50–100 mL 0.9% sodium chloride or 5% dextrose for IV administration.
- For IM administration, reconstitute with 2–2.5 mL sterile or bacteriostatic water for injection or 0.9% sodium chloride injection. Administer deep IM in large muscle mass (e.g., gluteus maximus).

Drug Interactions:
- Probenecid: increased serum concentrations of antibiotic; monitor and decrease dose if needed.

Lab Effects/Interference:

Major clinical significance:
- Coombs' (antiglobulin) tests: a positive reaction frequently appears in patients who receive large doses of cephalosporins; hemolysis rarely occurs but it has been reported; test may be positive in neonates whose mothers received cephalosporins before delivery.
- Urine glucose: cefazolin may produce false-positive or falsely elevated test results with copper sulfate tests (Benedict's, Clinitest, or Fehling's); glucose enzymatic tests (Clinistix or Tes-Tape) are not affected.
- PT may be prolonged; cephalosporins may inhibit vitamin K synthesis by suppressing gut flora.

Clinical significance:
- Serum ALT, serum alk phos, serum AST, serum bili, or serum LDH values may be increased.
- BUN and serum creatinine concentrations may be increased.
- CBC or platelet count: transient leukopenia, neutropenia, agranulocytosis, thrombocytopenia, eosinophilia, lymphocytosis, thrombocytosis have been seen on rare occasions.

Special Considerations:
- Used in treatment of serious infections of respiratory tract, urinary tract, skin and soft tissues, and biliary tree.
- Use with caution in patients with renal dysfunction—dose reduction required if severe impairment exists.
- Use cautiously if history of colitis exists.
- Contraindicated in patients hypersensitive to other cephalosporin antibiotics.
- Use cautiously if sensitive to penicillin; contraindicated if angioedema reaction to penicillin.
- Obtain ordered specimen and send for culture and sensitivity prior to first drug dose.
- May cause false-positive direct Coombs' test.
- May cause false-positive Clinitest glucose result.

Potential Toxicities/Side Effects and the Nursing Process

I. POTENTIAL FOR INJURY related to HYPERSENSITIVITY REACTION

Defining Characteristics: Urticaria, pruritus, rash (maculopapular or erythematous), fever and chills, eosinophilia, myalgia, edema, erythema, angioedema, Stevens–Johnson syndrome, and exfoliative skin reactions occur in 5% of patients. Increased risk in individuals allergic to penicillin.

Nursing Implications: Assess allergy to cephalosporin antibiotics and penicillin: if patient states "yes," determine actual response (e.g., "swollen lips = angioedema"). If angioedema, patient should not receive drug. Discuss other patient responses with physician to determine whether drug should be given. Assess baseline skin condition including integrity and allergy history to drugs. Instruct patient to report rash, itching, or other skin changes. Teach patient skin care and symptomatic measures as appropriate. If skin rash develops, discuss drug discontinuance with physician. If rash progresses, drug should be discontinued, as fatal Stevens–Johnson syndrome may develop. Be prepared to treat severe acute hypersensitivity reactions with airway management, oxygen, epinephrine, corticosteroids, antihistamines as ordered.

COMPLICATIONS

II. ALTERATION IN NUTRITION, LESS THAN BODY REQUIREMENTS, related to GI SIDE EFFECTS

Defining Characteristics: Nausea, vomiting, diarrhea, and anorexia may occur; rarely, pseudomembranous colitis caused by *C. difficile* resistant to the antibiotic occurs. Rarely, transient increases in LFTs—AST, ALT, alk phos, bili—may occur.

Nursing Implications: Assess baseline nutritional status. Instruct patient to report GI disturbances. Administer and teach patient to self-administer antiemetics as needed and as ordered. Teach patient importance of nutritious diet and suggest small, frequent, high-calorie, high-protein meals as appropriate. Assess baseline LFTs and monitor periodically during treatment. Discuss abnormalities and drug interruption with physician.

III.   FUNGAL SUPERINFECTION related to REDISTRIBUTION OF ENDOGENOUS MICROORGANISMS

Defining Characteristics: Vaginal candidiasis, vaginitis may occur as endogenous bacteria are eliminated and normal fungal population expands.

Nursing Implications: Teach female patient to report vaginal itching or discharge. Discuss appropriate antifungal treatment with physician. Teach perineal hygiene and symptomatic management.

IV.   ALTERATIONS IN PROTECTIVE MECHANISMS (RARE) related to CHANGES IN FORMED BLOOD CELL ELEMENTS

Defining Characteristics: Rarely, transient leukopenia, lymphocytosis, anemia, eosinophilia may occur. Prolonged PT, prolonged aPTT, and hypoprothrombinemia have occurred rarely, especially in elderly or debilitated patients, or in individuals with vitamin K deficiency.

Nursing Implications: Assess baseline laboratory parameters and monitor periodically during treatment. Assess patient for response to antibiotics. Discuss abnormalities with physician. Assess for signs/symptoms of bleeding. If they occur, especially in elderly or debilitated patients, discuss vitamin K administration with physician. Instruct patient to avoid aspirin. If taking oral anticoagulants, assess for increased PT, signs/symptoms of bleeding.

V.   ALTERATIONS IN SENSORY/PERCEPTUAL PATTERNS related to DIZZINESS, SOMNOLENCE

Defining Characteristics: Dizziness, headache, or somnolence occur rarely.

Nursing Implications: Assess baseline neurologic function and comfort and monitor during treatment. Teach patient to report any changes. Discuss any abnormalities with physician.

VI.   ALTERATIONS IN COMFORT related to LOCAL INJECTION IRRITATION

Defining Characteristics: Pain, induration, sterile abscesses may form in IM injection sites; phlebitis may develop in IV sites.

Nursing Implications: Rotate IM injection sites, and administer drug deep IM in large muscle mass (e.g., gluteus maximus). Use IM injection when IV administration is not possible. Change IV sites q 48 h, and assess for signs/symptoms of phlebitis prior to each administration. Administer drug slowly. Apply warm packs to increase comfort.

Drug: cefdinir (Omnicef)

Class: Third-generation cephalosporin broad-spectrum antibiotic.

Mechanism of Action: Inhibits cell wall synthesis, thus destroying microorganisms. Stable in presence of some β-lactamase enzymes, so active against many microorganisms that are resistant to the penicillins and other cephalosporin antibiotics. Cefdinir developed to enhance activity against both gram-positive and gram-negative organisms relative to other oral cephalosporins

Metabolism: Well-absorbed from the GI tract following oral dosing, with maximal plasma concentration in 2–4 hours. Drug largely unmetabolized and eliminated by the kidneys. Mean plasma half-life is 1.7 hours. Dose must be adjusted in patients with severe renal dysfunction or who receive hemodialysis.

Indication: For treatment of moderate infections caused by certain bacteria.

Dosage/Range:

Indication	Dosage (mg)	Route	Interval/Duration
Community-acquired pneumonia	300	PO	q 12 h for 5–10 days
Acute exacerbation of chronic bronchitis	300	PO	q 12 h
	600	PO	q 24 h × 10 days
Acute maxillary sinusitis	300	PO	q 12 hr
	600	PO	q 24 h × 10 days
Pharyngitis/tonsillitis	300	PO	q 12 h × 5–10 days
	600	PO	q 24 h × 10 days
Uncomplicated skin/skin structures	300	PO	q 12 h × 10 days
Patients with renal insufficiency	300	PO	q 24 h
Hemodialysis	300	PO	Every other day with additional doses of 300 mg given at end of each dialysis

Drug Preparation:
• Oral, available as 300-mg tablets or oral suspension that, when reconstituted as directed, results in 125 mg/5 mL in 60- or 100-mL bottles.

Drug Administration:
• Take orally without regard to meals or food intake.

Drug Interactions:
• Antacids containing magnesium or aluminum decrease absorption of cefdinir; take cefdinir at least 2 hours before or after the antacid.
• Iron or iron supplements decrease absorption by up to 80%; separate drugs by at least 2 hours.
• Probenecid inhibits the renal excretion of cefdinir, increasing peak plasma levels by 54% and prolonging half-life by 50%; decrease cefdinir dose if must use together.

Lab Effects/Interference:
• False-positive reaction for ketones in testing using nitroprusside.
• False-positive test for glucose in the urine using Clinitest, Benedict's solution, or Fehling's solution (suggest using Clinistix or Tes-Tape).
• False-positive Coombs' test (rare).
• Increased gamma glutamyltransferase (1%); rarely other liver function tests.

Special Considerations:
• Indicated for the treatment of adults with mild-to-moderate infections.
• Community-acquired pneumonia caused by *H. influenzae* (including β-lactamase–producing strains), penicillin-susceptible strains of *S. pneumoniae, Moraxella catarrhalis* (including β-lactamase–producing strains).
• Acute exacerbation of chronic bronchitis caused by *H. influenzae* (including β-lactamase–producing strains), penicillin-susceptible strains of *S. pneumoniae, M. catarrhalis* (including β-lactamase–producing strains).
• Acute maxillary sinusitis caused by *H. influenzae* (including β-lactamase–producing strains), penicillin-susceptible strains of *S. pneumoniae, M. catarrhalis* (including β-lactamase–producing strains).
• Pharyngitis/tonsillitis caused by *S. pyogenes.*
• Uncomplicated skin and skin structure infections caused by *S. aureus* (including β-lactamase–producing strains) and *S. pyogenes.*
• Contraindicated in patients with an allergy to the cephalosporin class of antibiotics as well as penicillin (cross-sensitivity in 10% of patients).
• Use cautiously, if at all, in patients with a history of colitis.
• Use in pregnancy only when benefits outweigh risks.
• If patient has severe renal dysfunction as evidenced by creatinine clearance < 30 mL/min, the dose should be reduced to 300 mg q day.
• Diabetic patients should know that the oral suspension has 2.86 g of sucrose per teaspoon.

Potential Toxicities/Side Effects and the Nursing Process

I.   ALTERATION IN NUTRITION related to GI SIDE EFFECTS

Defining Characteristics: Diarrhea occurs in approximately 16% of patients, and nausea in 3%. Less common are abdominal discomfort (1%), vomiting < 1%, and anorexia (< 1%).

The following rarely occur: dyspepsia, flatulence, constipation, abnormal stools (red-colored in patients taking iron). As with all antibiotics, pseudomembranous colitis may occur, ranging in severity from mild to life threatening. Treatment with antibiotics changes the intestinal microflora, so *C. difficile* bacteria may overgrow. Once diagnosis is made, mild diarrhea may stop with cessation of drug; if moderate to severe, it will require, in addition, hydration, electrolyte replacement, nutritional support, and antibacterial coverage against *C. difficile.*

Nursing Implications: Assess baseline nutritional and elimination status. Teach patient to report GI disturbances. Teach patient to report diarrhea immediately, consider whether this is pseudomembranous colitis, and send stool specimen for *C. difficile;* if positive, discuss drug discontinuance with physician. Administer and teach patient to self-administer antiemetics, antidiarrheals as needed and as ordered. Teach patient importance of nutritious diet and suggest small, frequent, high-calorie, high-protein meals as appropriate. Assess baseline LFTs and monitor periodically during treatment. Discuss abnormalities and drug interruption with physician.

II. SENSORY/PERCEPTUAL ALTERATIONS related to CNS EFFECTS

Defining Characteristics: Headaches occur in 2% of patients, and less common (< 1%) are dizziness, asthenia, insomnia, and somnolence.

Nursing Implications: Assess baseline neurologic function and comfort and monitor during treatment. Teach patient to report any changes. Teach patient how to manage symptoms. If unrelieved or persistent, discuss any abnormalities with physician.

III. ALTERATION IN SKIN INTEGRITY related to ALLERGY/HYPERSENSITIVITY

Defining Characteristics: Uncommonly (< 1%), rash and pruritus may occur; other manifestations include eosinophilia, urticaria, flushing, fever, chills, photosensitivity, or angioedema. Rarely, Stevens–Johnson syndrome reaction, toxic epidermal necrolysis, and exfoliative dermatitis have occurred. Anaphylactic reactions have occurred rarely.

Nursing Implications: Assess baseline skin condition including integrity and drug allergy history. Teach patient to report rash, itching, other skin changes. Teach patient skin care and symptomatic measures as appropriate. If skin rash develops, discuss drug discontinuance with physician. If rash progresses, drug should be discontinued, as fatal Stevens–Johnson syndrome may develop. Be prepared to treat severe acute hypersensitivity reactions with airway management, oxygen, epinephrine, corticosteroids, or antihistamines as ordered.

IV. FUNGAL SUPERINFECTION related to REDISTRIBUTION OF ENDOGENOUS MICROORGANISMS

Defining Characteristics: Vaginal moniliasis or vaginitis may occur as endogenous bacteria are eliminated and normal fungal population expands.

COMPLICATIONS

Nursing Implications: Teach female patient to report vaginal itching or discharge. Discuss appropriate antifungal treatment with physician. Teach perineal hygiene and symptomatic management.

Drug: cefditoren pivoxil (Spectracef)

Class: Cephalosporin antibacterial.

Mechanism of Action: Semisynthetic derivative of cephalosporin C, contains β-lactam ring, and is related to penicillins and cephamycins. Bactericidal through inhibition of cell wall synthesis, with resulting cell wall instability and cell lysis.

Metabolism: Well-absorbed from GI tract.

Indication: For treatment of infections caused by susceptible bacteria.

Dosage/Range:
• Oral (adult 12 years and older): 200–400 mg q 12 hours.
• Dose modification if renal impairment:

CrCl (mL/min/1.73 m²)	Dosage (mg/kg)
30 to 49	200 mg 2× daily
Less than 30	200 mg 1× daily
ESRD	No data

• Hepatic impairment: no adjustment necessary with mild or moderate hepatic impairment (Child-Pugh Class A or B); no data for severe hepatic impairment (Child-Pugh Class C).

Drug Preparation:
• Take with food.

Drug Interactions:
• Probenecid: increased serum concentrations of antibiotic; monitor and decrease dose if needed.
• Histamine H_2 antagonists: Famotidine decreases oral absorption; concomitant use should be avoided.
• Nephrotoxic drugs: may increase risk of renal dysfunction; avoid if possible.
• Magnesium-and aluminum-containing antacids decrease oral absorption; concomitant use should be avoided.

Lab Effects/Interference:
• Serum ALT (SGPT), serum alk phos, serum AST (SGOT), and serum bilirubin—values may be increased.
• BUN and serum creatinine—concentrations may be increased.

Special Considerations:
- Use cautiously if renal impairment is present.
- Contraindicated if hypersensitive to other cephalosporins, or has had angioedema response to penicillin.
- Milk protein hypersensitivity; tablets contain sodium caseinate.

Potential Toxicities/Side Effects and the Nursing Process

I. POTENTIAL FOR INJURY related to HYPERSENSITIVITY REACTION

Defining Characteristics: Urticaria, pruritus, rash (maculopapular or erythematous), fever and chills, eosinophilia, myalgia, edema, erythema, or angioedema. Increased risk in individuals allergic to penicillin.

Nursing Implications: Assess allergy to cephalosporin antibiotics and penicillin: if patient states "yes," determine actual response (e.g., "swollen lips = angioedema"). If angioedema, patient should not receive drug. Discuss other patient responses with physician to determine whether drug should be given. Assess baseline skin condition including integrity and allergy history to drugs. Teach patient to report rash, itching, or other skin changes. Teach patient skin care and symptomatic measures as appropriate. If skin rash develops, discuss drug discontinuance with physician.

II. ALTERATION IN NUTRITION, LESS THAN BODY REQUIREMENTS, related to GI SIDE EFFECTS

Defining Characteristics: Nausea, vomiting, diarrhea, and anorexia may occur.

Nursing Implications: Assess baseline nutritional status. Teach patient to report GI disturbances. Administer and teach patient to self-administer antiemetics as needed and as ordered. Teach patient importance of nutritious diet and suggest small, frequent, high-calorie, high-protein meals as appropriate. Discuss abnormalities and drug interruption with physician.

III. FUNGAL SUPERINFECTION related to REDISTRIBUTION OF ENDOGENOUS MICROORGANISMS

Defining Characteristics: Vaginal moniliasis or vaginitis may occur as endogenous bacteria are eliminated and normal fungal population expands.

Nursing Implications: Teach female patient to report vaginal itching or discharge. Discuss appropriate antifungal treatment with physician. Teach perineal hygiene and symptomatic management.

COMPLICATIONS

Drug: cefepime (Maxipime)

Class: Fourth-generation cephalosporin antibiotic.

Mechanism of Action: Exerts bactericidal action by inhibiting cell wall synthesis. Highly resistant to hydrolysis by β-lactamases, and exhibits rapid penetration into gram-negative bacterial cells.

Metabolism: Given intramuscularly and parenterally. Widely distributed into body tissues and fluids. Serum protein binding is less than 19% and is independent of its concentration in the serum. Excreted in urine. The average elimination half-life is approximately 2 hours.

Indication: For treatment of moderate-to-severe nosocomial pneumonia, infections caused by multiple drug-resistant microorganisms (e.g., *P. aeruginosa*) and empirical treatment of febrile neutropenia. Drug is used for treatment of infections in lower respiratory tract, skin, abdomen, and urinary tract. Active against gram-negative and gram-positive organisms. Spectrum of activity includes gram-negative organisms with multiple drug resistance patterns (*Enterobacter* and *Klebsiella*).

Dosage/Range:

Adult:
• IV and IM are similar.

Indication	Dosage (g)	Route	Interval/Duration
Mild-moderate UTI	0.5–1	IV or IM	q 12 h for 7–10 days
Severe UTI, *K. pneumoniae*	2	IV	q 12 h × 10 days
Moderate-to-severe pneumonia	1–2	IV	q 12 h × 10 days
Febrile neutropenia	2	IV	q 8 h × 7 days or neutrophil recovery

Drug Preparation:
• IV or IM: add diluent recommended by manufacturer into vial.

Drug Interactions:
• Solutions of cefepime should not be added to solutions of metronidazole, vancomycin hydrochloride, gentamicin sulfate, tobramycin sulfate, or netilmicin sulfate and aminophylline because of potential side effects. If necessary, administer each drug separately.

Lab Effects/Interference:

Major clinical significance:
• Coombs' (antiglobulin) tests: a positive reaction has appeared in clinical trials without evidence of hemolysis.
• PT or PTT: may be prolonged; cephalosporins may inhibit vitamin K synthesis by suppressing gut flora.

Clinical significance:
- Serum SGPT, serum alk phos, serum SGOT, serum bilirubin, or serum LDH: values may be increased.
- BUN and serum creatinine: concentrations may be increased.
- CBC or platelet count: transient leukopenia, neutropenia, agranulocytosis, thrombocytopenia, eosinophilia, lymphocytosis, and thrombocytosis have been seen on rare occasions.

Special Considerations:
- Contraindicated in patients hypersensitive to other cephalosporin antibiotics.
- Use cautiously if sensitive to penicillin; contraindicated if angioedema reaction to penicillin.
- Obtain specimen and send for culture and sensitivity prior to first drug dose.
- May cause false-positive Clinitest glucose result.

Potential Toxicities/Side Effects and the Nursing Process

I. POTENTIAL FOR INJURY related to HYPERSENSITIVITY REACTION

Defining Characteristics: Urticaria, pruritus, rash (maculopapular or erythematous), fever and chills, eosinophilia, myalgia, edema, erythema, angioedema, Stevens–Johnson syndrome, and exfoliative skin reactions occur in 5% of patients. Increased risk in individuals allergic to penicillin.

Nursing Implications: Assess allergy to cephalosporin antibiotics and penicillin: if patient states "yes," determine actual response (e.g., "swollen lips = angioedema"). If angioedema, patient should not receive drug. Discuss other patient responses with physician to determine whether drug should be given. Assess baseline skin condition including integrity and allergy history to drugs. Teach patient to report rash, itching, or other skin changes. Teach patient skin care and symptomatic measures as appropriate. If skin rash develops, discuss drug discontinuance with physician. If rash progresses, drug should be discontinued, as fatal Stevens–Johnson syndrome may develop. Be prepared to treat severe acute hypersensitivity reactions with airway management, oxygen, epinephrine, corticosteroids, or antihistamines as ordered.

II. ALTERATION IN NUTRITION, LESS THAN BODY REQUIREMENTS, related to GI SIDE EFFECTS

Defining Characteristics: Nausea, vomiting, diarrhea, constipation, abdominal pain, and dyspepsia may occur; rarely, pseudomembranous colitis caused by *C. difficile* resistant to the antibiotic occurs. Rarely, transient increases in LFTs—AST (SGOT), ALT (SGPT), alk phos, bilirubin—may occur.

Nursing Implications: Assess baseline nutritional status. Teach patient to report GI disturbances. Administer and teach patient to self-administer antiemetics, antidiarrheals as needed and as ordered. Teach patient importance of nutritious diet and suggest small, frequent, high-calorie, high-protein meals as appropriate. Assess baseline LFTs and monitor periodically during treatment. Discuss abnormalities and drug interruption with physician.

III.   FUNGAL SUPERINFECTION related to REDISTRIBUTION OF ENDOGENOUS MICROORGANISMS

Defining Characteristics: Vaginal moniliasis, vaginitis may occur as endogenous bacteria are eliminated and normal fungal population expands.

Nursing Implications: Teach female patient to report vaginal itching or discharge. Discuss appropriate antifungal treatment with physician. Teach perineal hygiene and symptomatic management.

IV.   ALTERATIONS IN PROTECTIVE MECHANISMS (RARE) related to CHANGES IN FORMED BLOOD CELL ELEMENTS

Defining Characteristics: Rarely, transient leukopenia, lymphocytosis, anemia, or eosinophilia may occur. Prolonged PT, prolonged aPTT, and hypoprothrombinemia have occurred rarely, especially in elderly or debilitated patients, or in individuals with vitamin K deficiency.

Nursing Implications: Assess baseline laboratory parameters and monitor periodically during treatment. Assess patient for response to antibiotics. Discuss abnormalities with physician. Assess for signs and symptoms of bleeding. If they occur, especially in elderly or debilitated patients, discuss vitamin K administration with physician. Teach patient to avoid aspirin. If taking oral anticoagulants, assess for increased PT, signs and symptoms of bleeding.

V.   SENSORY/PERCEPTUAL ALTERATIONS related to DIZZINESS, SOMNOLENCE

Defining Characteristics: Dizziness, headache, or somnolence occur rarely.

Nursing Implications: Assess baseline neurologic function and comfort and monitor during treatment. Teach patient to report any changes. Discuss any abnormalities with physician.

Drug: cefixime (Suprax)

Class: Third-generation cephalosporin antibacterial.

Mechanism of Action: Semisynthetic derivative of cephalosporin C (produced by fungus); contains β-lactam ring and is related to penicillins and cephamycins (e.g., cefoxitin). Bactericidal through inhibition of cell wall synthesis, with resulting cell wall instability and cell lysis.

Metabolism: Thirty to fifty percent absorbed from GI tract; rate of absorption slowed by food but does not affect total dose absorbed; 65–70% protein-bound. Eliminated unchanged in urine and to a lesser degree in bile and feces.

Indication: For treatment of infections caused by bacteria, such as pneumonia, bronchitis, gonorrhea; and ear, lung, throat, and urinary infections. Active against a wide spectrum of bacteria such as *S. aureus, S. pyogenes, M. catarrhalis, E. coli, P. mirabilis, Salmonella, Shigella, Neisseria gonorrhoeae,* and sensitive gram-negative bacteria (e.g., urinary tract infections caused by *E. coli, Proteus, H. influenzae*), as well as *S. pneumoniae* and *H. influenzae* related to acute bronchitis and acute exacerbations of chronic bronchitis.

Dosage/Range:

Adult:
- 400 mg/day PO (single, or two divided doses q 12 h).
- Duration: 5–10 days for uncomplicated urinary tract infection or upper respiratory infection; 10–14 days for lower respiratory tract infections.
- Dose modification if renal impairment:

CrCl (mL/min)	Dosage Adjustment	Route
60 or greater	Not necessary	Oral suspension
21–59	Adjust oral suspension dose to 6.5 mL daily of 200 mg/5 mL concentration OR	
	2.6 mL daily of 500 mg/5 mL concentration	
20 or less	Adjust oral suspension dose to 8.6 mL daily of 100 mg/5 mL concentration OR	Oral suspension Tablets or chewable tablets
	4.4 mL daily of 200 mg/5 mL concentration OR	
	1.8 mL daily of 500 mg/5 mL concentration	
Hemodialysis	Adjust oral suspension dose to 6.5 mL daily of 200 mg/5 mL concentration OR	Oral suspension
	2.6 mL daily of 500 mg/5 mL concentration	

Drug Preparation:
- Store tablets in tight container at 15–30°C (59–86°F).
- Oral administration.

Drug Interactions:
- Probenecid: increased serum concentrations of antibiotic; monitor and decrease dose if needed.

Lab Effects/Interference:

Major clinical significance:
- Coombs' (antiglobulin) tests: a positive reaction frequently appears in patients who receive large doses of cephalosporins; hemolysis rarely occurs, but it has been reported; test may be positive in neonates whose mothers received cephalosporins before delivery.

COMPLICATIONS

- PT: may be prolonged; cephalosporins may inhibit vitamin K synthesis by suppressing gut flora.

Clinical significance:
- Serum ALT, serum alk phos, serum AST, serum bili, or serum LDH values may be increased.
- BUN and serum creatinine concentrations may be increased.
- CBC or platelet count: transient leukopenia, neutropenia, agranulocytosis, thrombocytopenia, eosinophilia, lymphocytosis, and thrombocytosis have been seen on rare occasions.

Special Considerations:
- Use with caution in patients with renal dysfunction; dose reduction required if severe impairment exists.
- Use cautiously if history of colitis exists.
- Contraindicated in patients hypersensitive to other cephalosporin antibiotics.
- Use cautiously if sensitive to penicillin; contraindicated if angioedema reaction to penicillin.
- Obtain ordered specimen and send for culture and sensitivity prior to first drug dose.
- May cause false-positive direct Coombs' test.
- May cause false-positive Clinitest glucose result.

Potential Toxicities/Side Effects and the Nursing Process

I.   POTENTIAL FOR INJURY related to HYPERSENSITIVITY REACTION

Defining Characteristics: Urticaria, pruritus, rash (maculopapular or erythematous), fever and chills, eosinophilia, myalgia, edema, erythema, angioedema, Stevens–Johnson syndrome, and exfoliative skin reactions occur in 5% of patients. Increased risk in individuals allergic to penicillin.

Nursing Implications: Assess allergy to cephalosporin antibiotics and penicillin: if patient states "yes," determine actual response (e.g., "swollen lips = angioedema"). If angioedema, patient should not receive drug. Discuss other patient responses with physician to determine whether drug should be given. Assess baseline skin condition including integrity and allergy history to drugs. Instruct patient to report rash, itching, or other skin changes. Teach patient skin care and symptomatic measures as appropriate. If skin rash develops, discuss drug discontinuance with physician. If rash progresses, drug should be discontinued, as fatal Stevens–Johnson syndrome may develop. Be prepared to treat severe acute hypersensitivity reactions with airway management, oxygen, epinephrine, corticosteroids, or antihistamines as ordered.

II.   ALTERATION IN NUTRITION, LESS THAN BODY REQUIREMENTS, related to GI SIDE EFFECTS

Defining Characteristics: Nausea, vomiting, diarrhea, and anorexia may occur; rarely, pseudomembranous colitis caused by *C. difficile* resistant to the antibiotic occurs. Rarely, transient increases in LFTs—AST, ALT, alk phos, bili—may occur.

Nursing Implications: Assess baseline nutritional status. Instruct patient to report GI disturbances. Administer and teach patient to self-administer antiemetics as needed and as ordered. Teach patient importance of nutritious diet and suggest small, frequent, high-calorie, high-protein meals as appropriate. Assess baseline LFTs and monitor periodically during treatment. Discuss abnormalities and drug interruption with physician.

III. FUNGAL SUPERINFECTION related to REDISTRIBUTION OF ENDOGENOUS MICROORGANISMS

Defining Characteristics: Vaginal candidiasis or vaginitis may occur as endogenous bacteria are eliminated and normal fungal population expands.

Nursing Implications: Teach female patient to report vaginal itching or discharge. Discuss appropriate antifungal treatment with physician. Teach perineal hygiene and symptomatic management.

IV. ALTERATIONS IN PROTECTIVE MECHANISMS (RARE) related to TRANSIENT LEUKOPENIA

Defining Characteristics: Rarely, transient leukopenia, lymphocytosis, anemia, or eosinophilia may occur. Prolonged PT, prolonged aPTT, and hypoprothrombinemia have occurred rarely, especially in elderly or debilitated patients, or in individuals with vitamin K deficiency.

Nursing Implications: Assess baseline laboratory parameters and monitor periodically during treatment. Assess patient for response to antibiotics. Discuss abnormalities with physician. Assess for signs/symptoms of bleeding. If they occur, especially in elderly or debilitated patients, discuss vitamin K administration with physician. Instruct patient to avoid aspirin. If taking oral anticoagulants, assess for increased PT, signs/symptoms of bleeding.

V. ALTERATIONS IN SENSORY/PERCEPTUAL PATTERNS related to DIZZINESS, SOMNOLENCE

Defining Characteristics: Dizziness, headache, or somnolence occur rarely.

Nursing Implications: Assess baseline neurologic function and comfort and monitor during treatment. Instruct patient to report any changes. Discuss any abnormalities with physician.

COMPLICATIONS

Drug: cefoperazone sodium (Cefobid)

Class: Third-generation cephalosporin antibacterial.

Mechanism of Action: Semisynthetic derivative of cephalosporin C, contains β-lactam ring, and is related to penicillins and cephamycins. Bactericidal through inhibition of cell wall synthesis, with resulting cell wall instability and cell lysis.

Metabolism: Not absorbed from GI tract so must be given IV or IM. Widely distributed in body fluids, including bile and cerebrospinal fluid at high doses, and body tissues. Metabolized by liver and excreted by kidneys into urine.

Indication: For treatment of susceptible infections, such as respiratory tract infection, infections of the skin, and skin structures, urinary tract infections, pelvic inflammatory disease, endometritis, and other infections. Commonly used against gram-negative bacteria.

Dosage/Range:
- IV route when possible, but IV and IM doses are the same.
- Adults: 2–12 g q 6–12 h IM/IV; MAX 16 g/day.
- Pediatrics: 100–150 mg/kg/day q 8–12 hours IV; MAX 6 g/day.

Dosage adjustment:
- No dosage adjustment for renal function
- Dose of cefoperazone should not exceed 1–2 g/day without close monitoring of serum concentrations in patients with both HEPATIC DYSFUNCTION and significant RENAL DISEASE.

Drug Preparation:
- Store vial containing powder at < 30°C (86°F).
- IV: Reconstitute with sterile water for injection, and further dilute in 50–100 mL of 0.9% sodium chloride or 5% dextrose injection and infuse over 15–30 minutes at maximum concentration of 50 mg/mL.
- IM: Reconstitute by adding sterile or bacteriostatic water for injection. Depending on dose, divide dose and give in separate IM sites; may need to administer large doses to avoid discomfort. Administer IM injections deeply into large muscle (e.g., gluteus maximus).

Drug Interactions:
- Probenecid: increased serum concentrations of antibiotic; monitor and decrease dose if needed.
- Heparin and warfarin-cephalosporins may inhibit vitamin K synthesis by suppressing gut flora.
- Typhoid vaccine.

Lab Effects/Interference:
- PT: may be prolonged; cephalosporins may inhibit vitamin K synthesis by suppressing gut flora.
- Serum SGPT, serum alk phos, serum SGOT, serum bilirubin, or serum LDH: values may be increased.
- BUN and serum creatinine: concentrations may be increased.

Special Considerations:
- Use with caution in patients with renal and hepatic dysfunction; dose reduction required if severe impairment exists.
- Contraindicated in patients hypersensitive to other cephalosporin antibiotics.
- Use cautiously if sensitive to penicillin; contraindicated if angioedema reaction to penicillin.

- Obtain ordered specimen and send for culture and sensitivity prior to first drug dose.
- Alcohol consumption: disulfiram-like reactions after alcohol consumption within 72 hours of cefoperazone administration

Potential Toxicities/Side Effects and the Nursing Process

I.   POTENTIAL FOR INJURY related to HYPERSENSITIVITY REACTION

Defining Characteristics: Urticaria, pruritus, rash (maculopapular or erythematous), fever and chills, eosinophilia, myalgia, edema, erythema, and angioedema. Increased risk in individuals allergic to penicillin.

Nursing Implications: Assess allergy to cephalosporin antibiotics and penicillin: if patient states "yes," determine actual response (e.g., "swollen lips = angioedema"). If angioedema, patient should not receive drug. Discuss other patient responses with physician to determine whether drug should be given. Assess baseline skin condition including integrity and allergy history to drugs. Teach patient to report rash, itching, or other skin changes. Teach patient skin care and symptomatic measures as appropriate. If skin rash develops, discuss drug discontinuance with physician.

II.   ALTERATION IN NUTRITION, LESS THAN BODY REQUIREMENTS, related to GI SIDE EFFECTS

Defining Characteristics: Diarrhea or anorexia may occur.

Nursing Implications: Assess baseline nutritional status. Teach patient to report GI disturbances. Administer and teach patient to self-administer antidiarrheal agent as needed and as ordered.

III.   FUNGAL SUPERINFECTION related to REDISTRIBUTION OF ENDOGENOUS MICROORGANISMS

Defining Characteristics: Vaginal moniliasis, vaginitis may occur as endogenous bacteria are eliminated and normal fungal population expands.

Nursing Implications: Teach female patient to report vaginal itching or discharge. Discuss appropriate antifungal treatment with physician. Teach perineal hygiene and symptomatic management.

IV.   ALTERATIONS IN PROTECTIVE MECHANISMS (RARE)

Defining Characteristics: Prolonged PT, prolonged aPTT, and hypoprothrombinemia have occurred rarely, especially in elderly, debilitated patients, or in individuals with vitamin K deficiency.

COMPLICATIONS

Nursing Implications: Assess baseline laboratory parameters, and monitor periodically during treatment. Assess patient for response to antibiotics. Discuss abnormalities with physician. Assess for signs/symptoms of bleeding. If they occur, especially in elderly or debilitated patients, discuss vitamin K administration with physician. Teach patient to avoid aspirin. If taking oral anticoagulants, assess for increased PT, signs/symptoms of bleeding.

V.   ALTERATIONS IN COMFORT related to LOCAL INJECTION IRRITATION

Defining Characteristics: Pain, induration, and sterile abscesses may form in IM injection sites; phlebitis may develop in IV sites.

Nursing Implications: Rotate IM injection sites, and administer drug deep IM in large muscle mass (e.g., gluteus maximus). Use IM injection when IV administration is not possible. Change IV sites q 48 hours, and assess for signs/symptoms of phlebitis prior to each administration. Administer drug slowly. Apply warm packs to increase comfort.

Drug: cefotaxime sodium (Claforan)

Class: Third-generation cephalosporin antibacterial.

Mechanism of Action: Semisynthetic derivative of cephalosporin C (produced by fungus); contains β-lactam ring and is related to penicillins and cephamycins (e.g., cefoxitin). Bactericidal through inhibition of cell wall synthesis, with resulting cell wall instability and cell lysis.

Metabolism: Not absorbed from GI tract, so must be given IV or IM. Widely distributed in body fluids, including bile and CSF at high doses, and body tissues. Crosses placenta and is excreted in breastmilk. Metabolized by liver and excreted by kidneys into urine.

Indication: For treatment of infections of lower respiratory tract, including pneumonia; urinary tract; skin and skin structures; peritonitis; gynecological infections, including pelvic inflammatory disease, endometritis, and pelvic cellulitis caused by susceptible strains of specific microorganisms; perioperative prophylaxis. Active against gram-negative cocci (*Enterobacter,* some strains of *Pseudomonas, E. coli, Klebsiella, Serratia*), as well as gram-positive *S. aureus* and *S. epidermidis,* and *S. pneumoniae.* Used to treat serious lower respiratory tract, urinary tract, gynecologic, CNS, blood, and skin infections caused by sensitive bacteria.

Dosage/Range:
- IV route when possible, but IV and IM doses are the same.
- Adults: 1–2 g q 6–8 h (severe, 2 g q 4 h) × 48–72 hours after infection eradicated.
- Renal dosing in renal impairment: estimated CrCl less than 20 mL/min/1.73 m^2, reduce dose by 50%.

Drug Preparation:
- Store vial containing powder at < 30°C (86°F).
- Frozen injection should be stored at < 20°C (4°F).

- IV: reconstitute with 10 mL sterile water for injection, and further dilute in 50–100 mL of 0.9% sodium chloride or 5% dextrose injection and infuse over 20–30 minutes.
- IM: reconstitute by adding 2–5 mL sterile or bacteriostatic water for injection. Depending on dose, divide dose and give in separate IM sites; may need to administer large doses (2 g) IV to avoid discomfort. Administer IM injections deeply into large muscle (e.g., gluteus maximus).

Drug Interactions:
- Probenecid: increased serum concentrations of antibiotic; monitor and decrease dose if needed.
- Aminoglycosides, penicillins: may have synergistic antibacterial effect against some organisms.
- Nephrotoxic drugs (aminoglycosides, colistin, vancomycin): may increase risk of renal dysfunction; avoid if possible.

Lab Effects/Interference:

Major clinical significance:
- Coombs' (antiglobulin) tests: a positive reaction frequently appears in patients who receive large doses of cephalosporins; hemolysis rarely occurs, but it has been reported, test may be positive in neonates whose mothers received cephalosporins before delivery.
- PT: may be prolonged; cephalosporins may inhibit vitamin K synthesis by suppressing gut flora.

Clinical significance:
- Serum ALT, serum alk phos, serum AST, serum bili, or serum LDH values may be increased.
- BUN and serum creatinine concentrations may be increased.
- CBC or platelet count: transient leukopenia, neutropenia, agranulocytosis, thrombocytopenia, eosinophilia, lymphocytosis, and thrombocytosis have been seen on rare occasions.

Special Considerations:
- Use with caution in patients with renal dysfunction; dose reduction required if severe impairment exists.
- Use cautiously if history of colitis exists.
- Contraindicated in patients hypersensitive to other cephalosporin antibiotics.
- Use cautiously if sensitive to penicillin; contraindicated if angioedema reaction to penicillin.
- Obtain ordered specimen and send for culture and sensitivity prior to first drug dose.
- May cause false-positive direct Coombs' test.

COMPLICATIONS

Potential Toxicities/Side Effects and the Nursing Process

I. POTENTIAL FOR INJURY related to HYPERSENSITIVITY REACTION

Defining Characteristics: Urticaria, pruritus, rash (maculopapular or erythematous), fever and chills, eosinophilia, myalgia, edema, erythema, angioedema, Stevens–Johnson syndrome, and exfoliative skin reactions occur in 5% of patients. Increased risk in individuals allergic to penicillin.

Nursing Implications: Assess allergy to cephalosporin antibiotics and penicillin: if patient states "yes," determine actual response (e.g., "swollen lips = angioedema"). If angioedema, patient should not receive drug. Discuss other patient responses with physician to determine whether drug should be given. Assess baseline skin condition including integrity and allergy history to drugs. Instruct patient to report rash, itching, or other skin changes. Teach patient skin care and symptomatic measures as appropriate. If skin rash develops, discuss drug discontinuance with physician. If rash progresses, drug should be discontinued, as fatal Stevens–Johnson syndrome may develop. Be prepared to treat severe acute hypersensitivity reactions with airway management, oxygen, epinephrine, corticosteroids, or antihistamines as ordered.

II.   ALTERATION IN NUTRITION, LESS THAN BODY REQUIREMENTS, related to GI SIDE EFFECTS

Defining Characteristics: Nausea, vomiting, diarrhea, and anorexia may occur; rarely, pseudomembranous colitis caused by *C. difficile* resistant to the antibiotic occurs. Rarely, transient increases in LFTs—AST, ALT, alk phos, bili—may occur.

Nursing Implications: Assess baseline nutritional status. Instruct patient to report GI disturbances. Administer and teach patient to self-administer antiemetics as needed and as ordered. Teach patient importance of nutritious diet and suggest small, frequent, high-calorie, high-protein meals as appropriate. Assess baseline LFTs, and monitor periodically during treatment. Discuss abnormalities and drug interruption with physician.

III.   FUNGAL SUPERINFECTION related to REDISTRIBUTION OF ENDOGENOUS MICROORGANISMS

Defining Characteristics: Vaginal candidiasis or vaginitis may occur as endogenous bacteria are eliminated and normal fungal population expands.

Nursing Implications: Instruct female patient to report vaginal itching or discharge. Discuss appropriate antifungal treatment with physician. Teach perineal hygiene and symptomatic management.

IV.   ALTERATIONS IN PROTECTIVE MECHANISMS (RARE) related to TRANSIENT LEUKOPENIA

Defining Characteristics: Rarely, transient leukopenia, lymphocytosis, anemia, eosinophilia may occur. Prolonged PT, prolonged aPTT, and hypoprothrombinemia have occurred rarely, especially in elderly or debilitated patients, or in individuals with vitamin K deficiency.

Nursing Implications: Assess baseline laboratory parameters, and monitor periodically during treatment. Assess patient for response to antibiotics. Discuss abnormalities with physician. Assess for signs/symptoms of bleeding. If they occur, especially in elderly or debilitated patients, discuss vitamin K administration with physician. Instruct patient to avoid aspirin. If taking oral anticoagulants, assess for increased PT, signs/symptoms of bleeding.

V. ALTERATIONS IN SENSORY/PERCEPTUAL PATTERNS related to DIZZINESS, SOMNOLENCE

Defining Characteristics: Dizziness, headache, or somnolence occur rarely.

Nursing Implications: Assess baseline neurologic function and comfort and monitor during treatment. Instruct patient to report any changes. Discuss any abnormalities with physician.

VI. ALTERATIONS IN COMFORT related to LOCAL INJECTION IRRITATION

Defining Characteristics: Pain, induration, and sterile abscesses may form in IM injection sites; phlebitis may develop in IV sites.

Nursing Implications: Rotate IM injection sites, and administer drug deep IM in large muscle mass (e.g., gluteus maximus). Use IM injection when IV administration is not possible. Change IV sites q 48 h, and assess for signs/symptoms of phlebitis prior to each administration. Administer drug slowly. Apply warm packs to increase comfort.

Drug: cefotetan (Cefotan)

COMPLICATIONS

Class: Second-generation cephalosporin antibiotic with anaerobic activity.

Mechanism of Action: Semisynthetic derivative of cephalosporin C; contains β-lactam ring, and is related to penicillins and cephamycins. Bactericidal through inhibition of cell wall synthesis by binding to one or more of the PBPs that in turn inhibit the final transpeptidation step of peptidoglycan synthesis in bacterial cell walls, thus inhibiting cell wall biosynthesis. Bacteria eventually lyse due to ongoing activity of cell wall autolytic enzymes (autolysins and murein hydrolases) while cell wall assembly is arrested.

Metabolism: Widely distributed in body tissues, fluids except cerebrospinal fluid; readily crosses placenta and is excreted in breastmilk. Unchanged drug rapidly excreted by the kidneys.

Indication: For treatment of infections of the lungs, skin, bones, joints, stomach area, blood, female reproductive organs, and urinary tract. Used before surgery to prevent infections. Abdominal infections.

Dosage/Range:
- Oral (adult): 1–6 g/day in divided doses every 12 hours, usual dose: 1–2 g every 12 hours for 5–10 days; 1–2 g may be given every 24 hours for urinary tract infection.

• Dose modification if renal impairment:

CrCl (mL/min)	Dosage Adjustment
Greater than 30	Usual dose and interval
10–30	Usual dose q 24 h
	OR
	1/2 usual dose q 12 h
Less than 10	Usual dose q 48 h
	OR
	1/4 usual dose q 12 h
Hemodialysis	1/4 usual dose q 24 h on days between dialysis
	AND
	1/2 usual dose on day of dialysis

Drug Preparation:
• Refrigerate suspension.

Drug Interactions:
• Probenecid: increased serum concentrations of cefotetan but does not usually require dose reduction of antibiotic.
• Disulfiram-like reaction has been reported when taken within 72 hours of ethanol consumption.

Lab Effects/Interference:
• Serum ALT (SGPT), serum alk phos, serum AST (SGOT), and serum bilirubin—values may be increased.
• BUN and serum creatinine—concentrations may be increased.

Special Considerations:
• Use cautiously if renal impairment is present.
• Contraindicated if hypersensitive to other cephalosporins, or if has had angioedema response to penicillin.

Potential Toxicities/Side Effects and the Nursing Process

I.   POTENTIAL FOR INJURY related to HYPERSENSITIVITY REACTION

Defining Characteristics: Urticaria, pruritus, rash (maculopapular or erythematous), fever and chills, eosinophilia, myalgia, edema, erythema, or angioedema. Increased risk in individuals allergic to penicillin.

Nursing Implications: Assess allergy to cephalosporin antibiotics and penicillin: if patient states "yes," determine actual response (e.g., "swollen lips = angioedema"). If angioedema, patient should not receive drug. Discuss other patient responses with physician to determine whether drug should be given. Assess baseline skin condition including integrity and allergy history to drugs. Teach patient to report rash, itching, or other skin changes. Teach patient skin care and symptomatic measures as appropriate. If skin rash develops, discuss drug discontinuance with physician.

I. ALTERATION IN NUTRITION, LESS THAN BODY REQUIREMENTS, related to GI SIDE EFFECTS

Defining Characteristics: Nausea, vomiting, diarrhea, and anorexia may occur. May cause transient increases in LFTs.

Nursing Implications: Assess baseline nutritional status. Teach patient to report GI disturbances. Administer and teach patient to self-administer antiemetics as needed and as ordered. Teach patient importance of nutritious diet and suggest small, frequent, high-calorie, high-protein meals as appropriate. Assess baseline LFTs and monitor periodically during treatment. Discuss abnormalities and drug interruption with physician.

II. FUNGAL SUPERINFECTION related to REDISTRIBUTION OF ENDOGENOUS MICROORGANISMS

Defining Characteristics: Vaginal moniliasis or vaginitis may occur as endogenous bacteria are eliminated and normal fungal population expands.

Nursing Implications: Teach female patient to report vaginal itching or discharge. Discuss appropriate antifungal treatment with physician. Teach perineal hygiene and symptomatic management.

III. KNOWLEDGE DEFICIT related to SELF-ADMINISTRATION OF MEDICATION

Defining Characteristics: Increased compliance when patient is instructed in self-care activities.

Nursing Implications: Assess knowledge regarding infection and planned treatment. Teach about drug action, potential side effects, and when and how to take drug. Teach patient to report any possible side effects that occur.

COMPLICATIONS

Drug: cefoxitin sodium (Mefoxin)

Class: Considered second-generation cephalosporin based on activity spectrum; technically, a cephamycin antibacterial.

Mechanism of Action: β-lactam antibiotic that inhibits bacterial cell wall synthesis, leading to cell lysis.

Metabolism: Not absorbed from GI tract, so must be administered IV or IM.

Indication: For treatment of infections of the lower respiratory tract, urinary tract, skin and skin structures, bone and joint, intra-abdominal infections, gynecological infections, septicemia caused by susceptible microorganisms, and perioperative prophylaxis. Active against sensitive gram-negative bacteria causing lower respiratory infections (*H. influenzae, E. coli, Klebsiella*); GU infections (*E. coli, Klebsiella, Proteus*); septicemia; pelvic infections (*E. coli, N. gonorrhoeae*); or skin infections (*E. coli, Klebsiella*). Also, some gram-positive infections, including lower respiratory tract infections (*S. aureus, S. pneumoniae,* streptococci).

Dosage/Range:
- IV route preferred; IV and IM dosages the same.
- Adult: 1–2 g q 6–8 h (maximum 12 g/day in divided doses).
- Dose-reduce for renal compromise (based on manufacturer's package insert).

Drug Preparation:
- Store sterile powder at < 30°C (86°F); frozen injection should be stored at < 20°C (4°F).
- IV: reconstitute drug by adding 10 mL sterile water for injection. Further dilute in 50–100 mL 0.9% sodium chloride or 5% dextrose injection and infuse over 30–60 minutes.
- IM: reconstitute drug by adding 2 mL sterile water for injection or 0.5 or 1% lidocaine HCl injection without epinephrine to 1 g of cefoxitin. Administer IM deeply into large muscle mass (e.g., gluteus maximus). Using proper technique, ensure that injection is not into blood vessel. (Make certain patient is NOT ALLERGIC to lidocaine.)

Drug Interactions:
- Probenecid: increased serum concentrations of antibiotic; monitor and decrease dose if needed.
- Magnesium, calcium: incompatible in IV fluid.
- Oral anticoagulants, aspirin: may increase risk of bleeding.
- Alcohol: disulfiram-like reaction (flushing, throbbing headache, dyspnea, nausea, vomiting, diaphoresis, chest pain, palpitation, hyperventilation, tachycardia, hypertension, syncope, weakness, blurred vision) when alcohol ingested within 48–72 hours of cefoxitin; does not occur if alcohol ingested prior to first antibiotic dose. If no alcohol prior to first dose, avoid alcohol for 72 hours after last dose.

Lab Effects/Interference:

Major clinical significance:
- Coombs' (antiglobulin) tests: a positive reaction frequently appears in patients who receive large doses of cephalosporins; hemolysis rarely occurs, but it has been reported; test may be positive in neonates whose mothers received cephalosporins before delivery.
- Urine glucose: some cephalosporins (cefoxitin) may produce false-positive or falsely elevated test results with copper sulfate tests (Benedict's, Fehling's, or Clinitest); glucose enzymatic tests (Clinistix and Tes-Tape) are not affected.
- PT: may be prolonged; cephalosporins may inhibit vitamin K synthesis by suppressing gut flora.

Clinical significance:
- Serum and urine creatinine may falsely elevate test values when the Jaffe reaction is used; serum samples should not be obtained within 2 hours of administration.

- Serum ALT, serum alk phos, serum AST, serum bili, or serum LDH values may be increased.
- BUN and serum creatinine concentrations may be increased.
- CBC or platelet count: transient leukopenia, neutropenia, agranulocytosis, thrombocytopenia, eosinophilia, lymphocytosis, and thrombocytosis have been seen on rare occasions.

Special Considerations:
- Use with caution in patients with renal dysfunction; dose reduction required if severe impairment exists.
- Use cautiously if history of colitis exists.
- Contraindicated in patients hypersensitive to other cephalosporin antibiotics.
- Use cautiously if sensitive to penicillin; contraindicated if angioedema reaction to penicillin.
- Obtain ordered specimen and send for culture and sensitivity prior to first drug dose.
- May cause false-positive direct Coombs' test.
- May cause false-positive Clinitest glucose result.

Potential Toxicities/Side Effects and the Nursing Process

I.   POTENTIAL FOR INJURY related to HYPERSENSITIVITY REACTION

Defining Characteristics: Urticaria, pruritus, rash (maculopapular or erythematous), fever and chills, eosinophilia, myalgia, edema, erythema, angioedema, Stevens–Johnson syndrome, and exfoliative skin reactions occur in 5% of patients. Increased risk in individuals allergic to penicillin.

Nursing Implications: Assess allergy to cephalosporin antibiotics and penicillin: if patient states "yes," determine actual response (e.g., "swollen lips = angioedema"). If angioedema, patient should not receive drug. Discuss other patient responses with physician to determine whether drug should be given. Assess baseline skin condition including integrity and allergy history to drugs. Instruct patient to report rash, itching, or other skin changes. Teach patient skin care and symptomatic measures as appropriate. If skin rash develops, discuss drug discontinuance with physician. If rash progresses, drug should be discontinued, as fatal Stevens–Johnson syndrome may develop. Be prepared to treat severe acute hypersensitivity reactions with airway management, oxygen, epinephrine, corticosteroids, or antihistamines as ordered.

II.   ALTERATION IN NUTRITION, LESS THAN BODY REQUIREMENTS, related to GI SIDE EFFECTS

Defining Characteristic: Nausea, vomiting, diarrhea, or anorexia may occur; rarely, pseudomembranous colitis caused by *C. difficile* resistant to the antibiotic occurs. Rarely, transient increases in LFTs—AST, ALT, alk phos, bilirubin—may occur.

Nursing Implications: Assess baseline nutritional status. Instruct patient to report GI disturbances. Administer and teach patient to self-administer antiemetics as needed and

COMPLICATIONS

as ordered. Teach patient importance of nutritious diet, and suggest small, frequent, high-calorie, high-protein meals as appropriate. Assess baseline LFTs and monitor periodically during treatment. Discuss abnormalities and drug interruption with physician.

III. FUNGAL SUPERINFECTION related to REDISTRIBUTION OF ENDOGENOUS MICROORGANISMS

Defining Characteristics: Vaginal candidiasis or vaginitis may occur as endogenous bacteria are eliminated and normal fungal population expands.

Nursing Implications: Instruct female patient to report vaginal itching or discharge. Discuss appropriate antifungal treatment with physician. Teach perineal hygiene and symptomatic management.

IV. ALTERATIONS IN PROTECTIVE MECHANISMS (RARE) related to TRANSIENT LEUKOPENIA

Defining Characteristics: Rarely, transient leukopenia, lymphocytosis, anemia, eosinophilia may occur. Prolonged PT, prolonged aPTT, and hypoprothrombinemia have occurred rarely, especially in elderly or debilitated patients, or in individuals with vitamin K deficiency.

Nursing Implications: Assess baseline laboratory parameters, and monitor periodically during treatment. Assess patient for response to antibiotics. Discuss abnormalities with physician. Assess for signs/symptoms of bleeding. If they occur, especially in elderly or debilitated patients, discuss vitamin K administration with physician. Instruct patient to avoid aspirin. If taking oral anticoagulants, assess for increased PT, signs/symptoms of bleeding.

V. ALTERATIONS IN SENSORY/PERCEPTUAL PATTERNS related to DIZZINESS, SOMNOLENCE

Defining Characteristics: Dizziness, headache, somnolence occur rarely.

Nursing Implications: Assess baseline neurologic function and comfort and monitor during treatment. Instruct patient to report any changes. Discuss any abnormalities with physician.

VI. ALTERATIONS IN COMFORT related to LOCAL INJECTION IRRITATION

Defining Characteristics: Pain, induration, or sterile abscesses may form in IM injection sites; phlebitis may develop in IV sites.

Nursing Implications: Rotate IM injection sites and administer drug deep IM in large muscle mass (e.g., gluteus maximus). Use IM injection when IV administration is not possible. Change IV sites q 48 h, and assess for signs/symptoms of phlebitis prior to each administration. Administer drug slowly. Apply warm packs to increase comfort.

Drug: cefpodoxime proxetil (Vantin)

Class: Cephalosporin antibacterial.

Mechanism of Action: Semisynthetic derivative of cephalosporin C; contains β-lactam ring and is related to penicillins and cephamycins. Bactericidal through inhibition of cell wall synthesis, with resulting cell wall instability and cell lysis.

Metabolism: Well-absorbed from GI tract.

Indication: For treatment of infections of the respiratory tract, urinary tract, skin and skin structures, and treatment of sexually transmitted diseases caused by susceptible strains of specific microorganisms.

Dosage/Range:

Indication	Dosage	Route	Interval/Duration
Adult 13 years and older	100–400 mg	Oral	q 12 h
Gonorrhea indication	200 mg single dose	Oral	Single dose
Child 6 months to 12 years	10 mg/kg/daily (MAX 400 mg/day)	Oral	BID daily
Renal impairment: CrCl less than 30 mL/min	100–400 mg	Oral	Increase dosing interval to q 24 h

Drug Preparation:
• Take with food.

Drug Interactions:
• Probenecid: increased serum concentrations of antibiotic; monitor and decrease dose if needed.
• Magnesium, calcium, and aluminum.
• Warfarin—increased risk of bleeding.

Lab Effects/Interference:
• Serum ALT (SGPT), serum alk phos, serum AST (SGOT), and serum bilirubin: values may be increased.
• BUN and serum creatinine: concentrations may be increased.

Special Considerations:
• Contraindicated if hypersensitive to other cephalosporins, or if has had angioedema response to penicillin.
• Colitis; use caution.

Potential Toxicities/Side Effects and the Nursing Process

I. POTENTIAL FOR INJURY related to HYPERSENSITIVITY REACTION

Defining Characteristics: Urticaria, pruritus, rash (maculopapular or erythematous), fever and chills, eosinophilia, myalgia, edema, erythema, or angioedema. Increased risk in individuals allergic to penicillin.

COMPLICATIONS

Nursing Implications: Assess allergy to cephalosporin antibiotics and penicillin: if patient states "yes," determine actual response (e.g., "swollen lips = angioedema"). If angioedema, patient should not receive drug. Discuss other patient responses with physician to determine whether drug should be given. Assess baseline skin condition including integrity and allergy history to drugs. Teach patient to report rash, itching, or other skin changes. Teach patient skin care and symptomatic measures as appropriate. If skin rash develops, discuss drug discontinuance with physician.

II.   ALTERATION IN NUTRITION, LESS THAN BODY REQUIREMENTS, related to GI SIDE EFFECTS

Defining Characteristics: Nausea, vomiting, diarrhea, and anorexia may occur.

Nursing Implications: Assess baseline nutritional status. Teach patient to report GI disturbances. Administer and teach patient to self-administer antiemetics as needed and as ordered. Teach patient importance of nutritious diet and suggest small, frequent, high-calorie, high-protein meals as appropriate. Discuss abnormalities and drug interruption with physician.

III.   FUNGAL SUPERINFECTION related to REDISTRIBUTION OF ENDOGENOUS MICROORGANISMS

Defining Characteristics: Vaginal moniliasis or vaginitis may occur as endogenous bacteria are eliminated and normal fungal population expands.

Nursing Implications: Teach female patient to report vaginal itching or discharge. Discuss appropriate antifungal treatment with physician. Teach perineal hygiene and symptomatic management.

Drug: cefprozil (Cefzil)

Class: Second-generation cephalosporin antibiotic.

Mechanism of Action: Semisynthetic derivative of cephalosporin C; contains β-lactam ring, and is related to penicillins and cephamycins. Bactericidal through inhibition of cell wall synthesis, with resulting cell wall instability and cell lysis.

Metabolism: Well-absorbed from GI tract; delayed GI absorption if taken with food, but total amount of drug absorption is the same. Widely distributed in body tissues and fluids, except cerebrospinal fluid; readily crosses placenta and is excreted in breastmilk. Unchanged drug rapidly excreted by the kidneys.

Indication: For treatment of certain infections caused by bacteria, such as bronchitis and infections of the ears, throat, sinuses, and skin.

Dosage/Range:
• Oral (adult 13 years and older): 250–500 mg q 12–24 hours.

Drug Preparation:
• Refrigerate suspension.
• Discard after 14 days.

Drug Interactions:
• Probenecid: increased serum concentrations of cefprozil but does not usually require dose reduction of antibiotic.
• Oral contraceptives decrease effectiveness.
• Typhoid vaccine.

Lab Effects/Interference:
• Serum ALT (SGPT), serum alk phos, serum AST (SGOT), and serum bilirubin: values may be increased.
• BUN and serum creatinine: concentrations may be increased.

Special Considerations:
• Contraindicated if hypersensitive to other cephalosporins, or if has had angioedema response to penicillin.
• Cefprozil oral suspension contains phenylalanine; use with caution in patients with phenylketonuria.

Potential Toxicities/Side Effects and the Nursing Process

I. POTENTIAL FOR INJURY related to HYPERSENSITIVITY REACTION

Defining Characteristics: Urticaria, pruritus, rash (maculopapular or erythematous), fever and chills, eosinophilia, myalgia, edema, erythema, or angioedema. Increased risk in individuals allergic to penicillin.

Nursing Implications: Assess allergy to cephalosporin antibiotics and penicillin: if patient states "yes," determine actual response (e.g., "swollen lips = angioedema"). If angioedema, patient should not receive drug. Discuss other patient responses with physician to determine whether drug should be given. Assess baseline skin condition, including integrity and allergy history to drugs. Teach patient to report rash, itching, or other skin changes. Teach patient skin care and symptomatic measures as appropriate. If skin rash develops, discuss drug discontinuance with physician.

II. ALTERATION IN NUTRITION, LESS THAN BODY REQUIREMENTS, related to GI SIDE EFFECTS

Defining Characteristics: Nausea, vomiting, diarrhea, and anorexia may occur. May cause transient increases in LFTs.

Nursing Implications: Assess baseline nutritional status. Teach patient to report GI disturbances. Administer and teach patient to self-administer antiemetics as needed and as ordered. Teach patient importance of nutritious diet and suggest small, frequent, high-calorie, high-protein meals as appropriate. Assess baseline LFTs and monitor periodically during treatment. Discuss abnormalities and drug interruption with physician.

III.   FUNGAL SUPERINFECTION related to REDISTRIBUTION OF ENDOGENOUS MICROORGANISMS

Defining Characteristics: Vaginal moniliasis or vaginitis may occur as endogenous bacteria are eliminated and normal fungal population expands.

Nursing Implications: Teach female patient to report vaginal itching or discharge. Discuss appropriate antifungal treatment with physician. Teach perineal hygiene and symptomatic management.

IV.   KNOWLEDGE DEFICIT related to SELF-ADMINISTRATION OF MEDICATION

Defining Characteristics: Increased compliance when patient is instructed in self-care activities.

Nursing Implications: Assess knowledge regarding infection and planned treatment. Teach about drug action, potential side effects, and when and how to take drug. Teach patient to report any possible side effects that occur.

Drug: ceftaroline fosamil (Teflaro)

Class: Fifth-generation cephalosporin antibacterial.

Mechanism of Action: Semisynthetic, broad-spectrum, prodrug antibacterial of cephalosporin class of β-lactams; contains β-lactam ring and is related to penicillins and cephamycins (e.g., cefoxitin). Bactericidal through inhibition of cell wall synthesis, with resulting cell wall instability and cell lysis.

Metabolism: Widely distributed in body fluids, including bile and CSF at high doses, and body tissues. Not known whether ceftaroline fosamil is excreted in breastmilk. Because many drugs are excreted in breastmilk, caution should be exercised when ceftaroline fosamil is administered to a nursing woman. Metabolized by liver and excreted by kidneys into urine. The risk of adverse reactions may be greater in patients with impaired renal function. Because elderly patients are more likely to have decreased renal function, care should be taken in dose selection in this age group; monitor renal function. Elderly subjects had greater ceftaroline fosamil exposure relative to nonelderly subjects when administered the same single dose. Higher exposure in elderly subjects attributed to age-related changes in renal function. Dosage adjustment for elderly patients should be based on renal function.

Indication: For treatment of patients with acute bacterial skin and skin structure infections (ABSSSI) caused by susceptible isolates of the following gram-positive and gram-negative microorganisms: *S. aureus,* including methicillin-susceptible and -resistant isolates (MRSA; also known as oxacillin-resistant *S. aureus*, ORSA), *S. pyogenes* (group A beta-hemolytic streptococci)*, Streptococcus agalactiae* (group B streptococci)*, E. coli, K. pneumoniae*, and *Klebsiella oxytoca.*

It is also indicated for treatment of community-acquired bacterial pneumonia (CABP) caused by susceptible isolates of gram-positive and gram-negative microorganisms: *S. pneumonia,* including cases with concurrent bacteremia, *S. aureus* (methicillin-susceptible isolates only), *H. influenzae, K. pneumoniae, K. oxytoca,* and *E. coli.*

Dosage/Range:
- The recommended dosage of Teflaro is 600 mg administered every 12 hours by intravenous (IV) infusion over 1 hour in patients > 18 years of age. The duration of therapy guided by severity and site of infection and patient's clinical and bacteriological progress. Recommended dosage and administration by infection are described in the table below:

Indication	Dosage (mg)	Route	Infusion Time (hours)	Interval/Duration
Acute Bacterial Skin and Skin Structure Every Infection (ABSSSI)	600	IV	1	q 12 h × 5–14 days
Community-Acquired Bacterial Pneumonia (CABP)	600	IV	1	q 12 h × 5–7 days

- Dose modification for renal impairment:

CrCl (mL/min)	Dosage Adjustment (mg)	Route	Interval/Duration
Greater than 30–50	400	IV	5–60 minutes q 12 h
15–30	300	IV	5–60 minutes q 12 h
ESRD Less than 15 OR hemodialysis	200	IV	5–60 minutes q 12 h; administer after hemodialysis on hemodialysis days

COMPLICATIONS

Drug Preparation:
- Supplied in single-use, clear glass vials containing either 600 or 400 mg of sterile ceftaroline fosamil powder. Constituted solution further diluted in 250 mL before infusion. Resulting solution administered IV over approximately 1 hour.
- Appropriate infusion solutions include:
  - 0.9% sodium chloride injection, USP (normal saline).
  - 5% dextrose injection, USP.
  - 2.5% dextrose injection, USP.
  - 0.45% sodium chloride injection.
- Lactated Ringer's injection.

Drug Interactions:
- No clinical drug–drug interaction studies conducted with ceftaroline fosamil.
- Minimal potential for drug–drug interactions between ceftaroline fosamil and CYP450 substrates, inhibitors, or inducers; drugs known to undergo active renal secretion; and drugs that may alter renal blood flow.
- Safety and effectiveness in pediatric patients not established.

Lab Effects/Interference:
- Coombs' (antiglobulin) tests: a positive reaction frequently appears in patients who receive large doses of cephalosporins.
- If anemia develops during or after therapy, a diagnostic workup for drug-induced hemolytic anemia should be performed; consideration given to discontinuation of Ceftaroline fosamil.

Special Considerations:
- Known serious hypersensitivity to ceftaroline fosamil or other members of the cephalosporin class. Serious hypersensitivity (anaphylactic) reactions have been reported with β-lactam antibiotics, including ceftaroline fosamil.
- Caution in patients with known hypersensitivity to β-lactam antibiotics.
- *Clostridium difficile*-associated diarrhea (CDAD) reported with nearly all systemic antibacterial agents, including ceftaroline fosamil. Evaluate if diarrhea occurs.
- Use with caution in patients with renal dysfunction.
- Contraindicated in patients hypersensitive to other cephalosporin antibiotics.
- Use cautiously if sensitive to penicillin; contraindicated if angioedema reaction to penicillin.
- Obtain ordered specimen and send for culture and sensitivity prior to first drug dose.
- May cause false-positive direct Coombs' test.

Potential Toxicities/Side Effects and the Nursing Process

I.   POTENTIAL FOR INJURY related to HYPERSENSITIVITY REACTION

Defining Characteristics: Urticaria, pruritus, rash (maculopapular or erythematous), fever and chills, eosinophilia, myalgia, edema, erythema, and angioedema have been known to occur. Increased risk in individuals allergic to penicillin.

Nursing Implications: Assess allergy to cephalosporin antibiotics and penicillin: if patient states "yes," determine actual response (e.g., "swollen lips = angioedema"). If angioedema, patient should not receive drug. Discuss other patient responses with physician to determine whether drug should be given. Assess baseline skin condition, including integrity and allergy history to drugs. Instruct patient to report rash, itching, or other skin changes. Teach patient skin care and symptomatic measures as appropriate. If skin rash develops, discuss drug discontinuance with physician. If rash progresses, drug should be discontinued, as fatal Stevens–Johnson syndrome may develop. Be prepared to treat severe acute hypersensitivity reactions with airway management, oxygen, epinephrine, corticosteroids, or antihistamines as ordered.

II. ALTERATION IN NUTRITION, LESS THAN BODY REQUIREMENTS, related to GI SIDE EFFECTS

Defining Characteristics: Nausea, vomiting, diarrhea, and anorexia may occur; rarely, pseudomembranous colitis caused by *C. difficile* resistant to the antibiotic occurs.

Nursing Implications: Assess baseline nutritional status. Instruct patient to report GI disturbances. Administer and teach patient to self-administer antiemetics as needed and as ordered. Teach patient importance of nutritious diet, and suggest small, frequent, high-calorie, high-protein meals as appropriate. Assess baseline LFTs, and monitor periodically during treatment. Discuss abnormalities and drug interruption with physician.

III. FUNGAL SUPERINFECTION related to REDISTRIBUTION OF ENDOGENOUS MICROORGANISMS

Defining Characteristics: Vaginal candidiasis or vaginitis may occur as endogenous bacteria are eliminated and normal fungal population expands.

Nursing Implications: Instruct female patient to report vaginal itching or discharge. Discuss appropriate antifungal treatment with physician. Teach perineal hygiene and symptomatic management.

IV. ALTERATIONS IN PROTECTIVE MECHANISMS (RARE) related to TRANSIENT LEUKOPENIA

Defining Characteristics: Rarely, transient leukopenia, lymphocytosis, anemia, or eosinophilia may occur. Prolonged PT, prolonged aPTT, and hypoprothrombinemia have occurred rarely, especially in elderly or debilitated patients, or in individuals with vitamin K deficiency.

Nursing Implications: Assess baseline laboratory parameters, and monitor periodically during treatment. Assess patient for response to antibiotics. Discuss abnormalities with physician. Assess for signs/symptoms of bleeding. If they occur, especially in elderly or debilitated patients, discuss vitamin K administration with physician. Instruct patient to avoid aspirin. If taking oral anticoagulants, assess for increased PT, signs/symptoms of bleeding.

COMPLICATIONS

Drug: ceftazidime (Fortaz, Tazicef, Tazidime)

Class: Third-generation cephalosporin antibacterial.

Mechanism of Action: Semisynthetic derivative of cephalosporin C (produced by fungus); contains β-lactam ring and is related to penicillins and cephamycins (e.g., cefoxitin). Bactericidal through inhibition of cell wall synthesis, with resulting cell wall instability and cell lysis.

Metabolism: Not absorbed from GI tract so must be administered parenterally. Small degree of protein binding (5–24%). Widely distributed in body fluids (including CSF and bile) and body tissues. Crosses placenta and is excreted unchanged in urine.

Indication: For treatment of infections caused by susceptible strains of organisms in lower respiratory tract, skin and skin structures, urinary tract, bacterial septicemia, bone and joint infections, gynecologic infections, intra-abdominal infections including peritonitis, and central nervous system infections including meningitis. Active against sensitive microorganisms causing lower respiratory tract, urinary tract, skin, bone and joint, gynecologic, and intra-abdominal infections. These include primarily gram-negative bacteria (*Enterobacter, E. coli, Klebsiella, Proteus, Serratia,* and *Pseudomonas*) and, to a lesser degree, some gram-positive bacteria (*S. aureus, S. epidermidis,* streptococci).

Dosage/Range:
- IV and IM doses are the same.
- Adult: maximum 6 g/day

Indication	Dosage	Route	Interval/Duration
Uncomplicated pneumonia, skin/structure infections	0.5–1 g	IV	q 8 h
Bone, joint infection	2 g	IV	q 12 h
Severe GYN, abdominal infections or febrile neutropenia	2 g	IV	q 8 h
Lung infection by pseudomonas in patients with cystic fibrosis	30–50 mg/kg	IV	q 8 h

- Dose should be reduced in renal insufficiency according to manufacturer's package insert.
- (Adult) Give initial 1 g loading dose; (Pediatric) Modify dose frequency consistent with adult recommendations.

CrCl (mL/min)	Dosage (g)	Route	Interval/Duration
31–50	1 g	IV	q 12 h
16–30	1 g	IV	q 24 h
6–15	0.5g	IV	q 24 h
Less than 5	0.5 g	IV	q 48 h
Hemodialysis	1 g	IV	After each hemodialysis period
Peritoneal dialysis	0.5 g	IV	q 24 h OR add 250 mg to 2 L of dialysis fluid

Drug Preparation:
- Store sterile powder vials at 15–30°C (59–86°F) and protect from light; frozen injection containers should be stored at < 20°C (4°F).
- IV: reconstitute according to manufacturer's package insert, as some preparations contain sodium carbonate. Further dilute in 100 mL of 0.9% sodium chloride or 5% dextrose and infuse over 30–60 minutes.
- IM: reconstitute according to manufacturer's package insert, which may suggest the addition of 0.5–1% lidocaine HCl to decrease discomfort. Make certain patient is NOT ALLERGIC to lidocaine. Administer deep IM in large muscle mass (e.g., gluteus maximus).

Drug Interactions:
- Probenecid: increased serum concentrations of antibiotic; monitor and decrease dose if needed.
- Warfarin: increased bleeding risk.
- Sodium bicarbonate: incompatible; DO NOT administer concurrently through same IV site.
- Typhoid vaccine.
- Contraceptives.

Lab Effects/Interference:

Major clinical significance:
- Coombs' (antiglobulin) tests: a positive reaction frequently appears in patients who receive large doses of cephalosporins; hemolysis rarely occurs, but it has been reported; test may be positive in neonates whose mothers received cephalosporins before delivery.
- PT: may be prolonged; cephalosporins may inhibit vitamin K synthesis by suppressing gut flora.

Clinical significance:
- Serum ALT, serum alk phos, serum AST, serum bilirubin, or serum LDH values may be increased.
- BUN and serum creatinine concentrations may be increased.
- CBC or platelet count: transient leukopenia, neutropenia, agranulocytosis, thrombocytopenia, eosinophilia, lymphocytosis, and thrombocytosis have been seen on rare occasions.

Special Considerations:
- Empiric use in management of febrile neutropenic patient appears to be as effective as combination antibiotic regimens; vancomycin may need to be added to ceftazidime to better cover gram-positive bacteria (e.g., *S. epidermidis*).
- Has excellent coverage against *P. aeruginosa.*
- Use with caution in patients with renal dysfunction; dose reduction required if severe impairment exists.
- Use cautiously if history of colitis exists.
- Contraindicated in patients hypersensitive to other cephalosporin antibiotics.
- Use cautiously if sensitive to penicillin; contraindicated if angioedema reaction to penicillin.
- Obtain specimen and send for culture and sensitivity prior to first drug dose.
- May cause false-positive direct Coombs' test.
- May cause false-positive Clinitest glucose result.

COMPLICATIONS

Potential Toxicities/Side Effects and the Nursing Process

I.   POTENTIAL FOR INJURY related to HYPERSENSITIVITY REACTION

Defining Characteristics: Urticaria, pruritus, rash (maculopapular or erythematous), fever and chills, eosinophilia, myalgia, edema, erythema, angioedema, Stevens–Johnson syndrome, and exfoliative skin reactions occur in 5% of patients. Increased risk in individuals allergic to penicillin.

Nursing Implications: Assess allergy to cephalosporin antibiotics and penicillin: if patient states "yes," determine actual response (e.g., "swollen lips = angioedema"). If angioedema, patient should not receive drug. Discuss other patient responses with physician to determine whether drug should be given. Assess baseline skin condition including integrity and allergy history to drugs. Instruct patient to report rash, itching, or other skin changes. Teach patient skin care and symptomatic measures as appropriate. If skin rash develops, discuss drug discontinuance with physician. If rash progresses, drug should be discontinued, as fatal Stevens–Johnson syndrome may develop. Be prepared to treat severe acute hypersensitivity reactions with airway management, oxygen, epinephrine, corticosteroids, or antihistamines as ordered.

II.   ALTERATION IN NUTRITION, LESS THAN BODY REQUIREMENTS, related to GI SIDE EFFECTS

Defining Characteristics: Nausea, vomiting, diarrhea, and anorexia may occur; rarely, pseudomembranous colitis caused by *C. difficile* resistant to the antibiotic occurs. Rarely, transient increases in LFTs—AST, ALT, alk phos, bilirubin—may occur.

Nursing Implications: Assess baseline nutritional status. Instruct patient to report GI disturbances. Administer and teach patient to self-administer antiemetics as needed and as ordered. Teach patient importance of nutritious diet and suggest small, frequent, high-calorie, high-protein meals as appropriate. Assess baseline LFTs, and monitor periodically during treatment. Discuss abnormalities and drug interruption with physician.

III.   FUNGAL SUPERINFECTION related to REDISTRIBUTION OF ENDOGENOUS MICROORGANISMS

Defining Characteristics: Vaginal candidiasis or vaginitis may occur as endogenous bacteria are eliminated and normal fungal population expands.

Nursing Implications: Instruct female patient to report vaginal itching or discharge. Discuss appropriate antifungal treatment with physician. Teach perineal hygiene and symptomatic management.

IV.   ALTERATIONS IN PROTECTIVE MECHANISMS (RARE) related to TRANSIENT LEUKOPENIA

Defining Characteristics: Rarely, transient leukopenia, lymphocytosis, anemia, or eosinophilia may occur. Prolonged PT, prolonged aPTT, and hypoprothrombinemia have occurred rarely, especially in elderly or debilitated patients, or in individuals with vitamin K deficiency.

Nursing Implications: Assess baseline laboratory parameters, and monitor periodically during treatment. Assess patient for response to antibiotics. Discuss abnormalities with physician.

V.   ALTERATIONS IN SENSORY/PERCEPTUAL PATTERNS related to DIZZINESS, SOMNOLENCE

Defining Characteristics: Dizziness, headache, or somnolence occur rarely.

Nursing Implications: Assess baseline neurologic function and comfort and monitor during treatment. Instruct patient to report any changes. Discuss any abnormalities with physician.

VI.   ALTERATIONS IN COMFORT related to LOCAL INJECTION IRRITATION

Defining Characteristics: Pain, induration, sterile abscesses may form in IM injection sites; phlebitis may develop in IV sites.

Nursing Implications: Rotate IM injection sites and administer drug deep IM in large muscle mass (e.g., gluteus maximus). Use IM injection when IV administration is not possible. Change IV sites q 48 h, and assess for signs/symptoms of phlebitis prior to each administration. Administer drug slowly. Apply warm packs to increase comfort.

Drug: ceftazidime/avibactam (Avycaz)

Class: Antibacterial—third generation with beta-lactamase inhibitor.

Mechanism of Action: An antibacterial combination product consisting of the semisynthetic cephalosporin ceftazidime pentahydrate and the beta-lactamase inhibitor avibactam sodium for intravenous administration.

Metabolism: Ceftazidime is mostly (80–90% of the dose) eliminated as unchanged drug. No metabolism of avibactam was observed in liver microsomes and hepatocytes. Avibactam was found in human plasma. Both ceftazidime and avibactam are excreted mainly by the kidneys.

Indications: Complicated intra-abdominal infections (cIAI), used in combination with metronidazole; complicated urinary tract infections (cUTI), including pyelonephritis.

As only limited clinical safety and efficacy data for ceftazidime/avibactam are currently available, reserve use for patients who have limited or no alternative treatment options.

To reduce the development of drug-resistant bacteria and maintain the effectiveness of this and other antibacterial drugs, ceftazidime/avibactam should be used only to treat infections that are proven or strongly suspected to be caused by susceptible bacteria.

Dosage/Range: The recommended dosage is 2.5 g (2 g ceftazidime and 0.5 g avibactam) administered every 8 hours by IV infusion over 2 hours in patients 18 years or older. For treatment of cIAI, metronidazole should be given concurrently. Guidelines for dosage in patients with normal renal function are listed below:

COMPLICATIONS

Dosage of Ceftazidime-Avibactam by Indication

Indication	Dosage	IV Infusion Time (h)	Interval/Duration
Complicated IAI (used in combination with metronidazole)	2.5 g (2 g/0.5 g)	2	q 8 h × 5–14 days
Complicated UTI including pyelonephritis	2.5 g (2 g/0.5 g)	2	q 8 h × 7–14 days

Drug Preparation:
- Ceftazidime/avibactam for injection is available in single-use vials containing 2 g ceftazidime and 0.5 g avibactam.
- Constitute powder in 10 mL of sterile water for injection, USP; 0.9% of sodium chloride injection, USP (normal saline); 5% of dextrose injection, USP; all combinations of dextrose injection and sodium chloride injection, USP, containing up to 2.5% dextrose, USP; and 0.45% sodium chloride, USP, or lactated Ringer's injection, USP.
- Mix gently. With same diluent used for constitution of powder (except sterile water for injection), dilute reconstituted solution further to achieve a total volume of 50–250 mL before infusion.
- Mix gently and ensure that contents are dissolved completely. Visually inspect diluted solution (for administration) for particulates and discoloration prior to administration (color of infusion solution for administration ranges from clear to light yellow).
- Use diluted solution in infusion bags within 12 hours when stored at room temperature. Diluted solution in infusion bags may be stored under refrigeration at 2–8°C (36–46°F) up to 24 hours following dilution; use within 12 hours of subsequent storage at room temperature.

Drug Interactions: As a potent OAT (organic anion transport) inhibitor, probenecid inhibits OAT uptake of avibactam by 56–70% in vitro and has potential to decrease elimination of avibactam when coadministered. Because a clinical interaction the study of avibactam alone with probenecid has not been conducted, coadministration of avibactam with probenecid is not recommended. There are drug interactions with warfarin, chloramphenicol, typhoid vaccine, and contraceptives.

Lab Effects/Interference:
- Administration of ceftazidime may result in a false-positive reaction for glucose in urine with certain methods. Recommend glucose tests based on enzymatic glucose oxidase reaction.

Special Considerations:
- Ceftazidime/avibactam is contraindicated in patients with known serious hypersensitivity to avibactam-containing products, ceftazidime, or other members of the cephalosporin class.
- Drug has decreased efficacy in patients with baseline CrCl of 30–50 mL/min. Monitor CrCl at least daily in patients with changing renal function and adjust the dose of ceftazidime/avibactam accordingly.

- Hypersensitivity reactions include: anaphylaxis and serious skin reactions. Cross-hypersensitivity may occur in patients with history of penicillin allergy. If an allergic reaction occurs, discontinue drug.
- CDAD: CDAD has been reported with nearly all systemic antibacterial agents, including ceftazidime/avibactam. Evaluate if diarrhea occurs.
- Central nervous system reactions: Seizures and other neurologic events may occur, especially in patients with renal impairment. Adjust dose in patients with renal impairment.

Potential Toxicities/Side Effects and the Nursing Process

I.   POTENTIAL FOR INJURY related to HYPERSENSITIVITY REACTION

Defining Characteristics: Urticaria, pruritus, rash (maculopapular or erythematous), fever and chills, eosinophilia, myalgia, edema, erythema, angioedema, Stevens–Johnson syndrome, and exfoliative skin reactions occur in 5% of patients. Increased risk in individuals allergic to penicillin.

Nursing Implications: Assess allergy to cephalosporin antibiotics and penicillin; if patient states "yes," determine actual response (e.g., "swollen lips angioedema"). If angioedema is present, patient *should not* receive drug. Discuss other patient responses with physician to determine whether drug should be given. Assess baseline skin condition, including integrity, and allergy history to drugs. Instruct patient to report rash, itching, or other skin changes. Teach patient skin care and symptomatic measures as appropriate. If skin rash develops, discuss drug discontinuance with physician. If rash progresses, drug should be discontinued, as fatal Stevens–Johnson syndrome may develop. Be prepared to treat severe acute hypersensitivity reactions with airway management, oxygen, epinephrine, corticosteroids, or antihistamines as ordered.

II.   ALTERATION IN NUTRITION, LESS THAN BODY REQUIREMENTS, related to GI SIDE EFFECTS

Defining Characteristics: Nausea, vomiting, diarrhea, and anorexia may occur; rarely, pseudomembranous colitis caused by *C. difficile* resistant to the antibiotic occurs.

Nursing Implications: Assess baseline nutritional status. Instruct patient to report GI disturbances. Administer, and teach patient to self-administer, antiemetics as needed and as ordered. Teach patient importance of a nutritious diet, and suggest small, frequent, high-calorie, high-protein meals as appropriate. Assess baseline LFTs, and monitor periodically during treatment. Discuss abnormalities and drug interruption with physician.

III.   FUNGAL SUPERINFECTION related to REDISTRIBUTION OF ENDOGENOUS MICROORGANISMS

Defining Characteristics: Vaginal candidiasis or vaginitis may occur as endogenous bacteria are eliminated and normal fungal population expands.

COMPLICATIONS

Nursing Implications: Instruct female patients to report vaginal itching or discharge. Discuss appropriate antifungal treatment with physician. Teach perineal hygiene and symptomatic management.

IV.   ALTERATIONS IN COMFORT related to LOCAL INJECTION-SITE IRRITATION

Defining Characteristics: Pain or phlebitis may develop in IV sites.

Nursing Implications: Change IV sites every 48 hours, and assess for signs and symptoms of phlebitis prior to each administration. Administer drug slowly. Apply warm packs to increase comfort.

Drug: ceftibuten (Cedax)

Class: Third-generation cephalosporin antibacterial.

Mechanism of Action: Semisynthetic derivative of cephalosporin C, contains β-lactam ring, and is related to penicillins and cephamycins. Bactericidal through inhibition of cell wall synthesis, with resulting cell wall instability and cell lysis.

Metabolism: Well-absorbed from GI tract; delayed GI absorption if taken with food, but total amount of drug absorption is the same. Widely distributed in body tissues and fluids, except cerebrospinal fluid; readily crosses placenta and is excreted in breastmilk. Unchanged drug rapidly excreted by the kidneys.

Indication: For treatment of certain mild to moderate infections caused by susceptible bacteria, such as bronchitis and ear and throat infections caused by *S. pyogenes* (Group A beta-hemolytic streptococci).

Dosage/Range:
- Adults: 400 mg orally daily × 10 days.
- Dose modification for renal impairment:

CrCl (mL/min)	Dosage Adjustment
30–49	200 mg q 24 h OR 4.5 mg/kg q 24 h
5–29	100 mg q 24 h OR 2.25 mg/kg q 24 h
Hemodialysis	Single dose of 400 mg OR 9 mg/kg at end of each hemodialysis session

Drug Preparation:
- Store suspension in refrigerator; discard after 14 days.
- Oral administration.

Drug Interactions:
- Aminoglycosides, penicillins: may have synergistic antibacterial effect against some organisms.
- Typhoid vaccine.

Lab Effects/Interference:
- Serum SGPT, serum alk phos, serum SGOT, serum bilirubin, or serum LDH: values may be increased.
- BUN and serum creatinine: concentrations may be increased.

Special Considerations:
- Use with caution in patients with renal dysfunction; dose reduction required if severe impairment exists.
- Contraindicated in patients hypersensitive to other cephalosporin antibiotics.
- Use cautiously if sensitive to penicillin; contraindicated if angioedema reaction to penicillin.
- Obtain ordered specimen and send for culture and sensitivity prior to first drug dose.

Potential Toxicities/Side Effects and the Nursing Process

I. POTENTIAL FOR INJURY related to HYPERSENSITIVITY REACTION

Defining Characteristics: Urticaria, pruritus, rash (maculopapular or erythematous), fever and chills, eosinophilia, myalgia, edema, erythema, or angioedema. Increased risk in individuals allergic to penicillin.

Nursing Implications: Assess allergy to cephalosporin antibiotics and penicillin: if patient states "yes," determine actual response (e.g., "swollen lips = angioedema"). If angioedema, patient should not receive drug. Discuss other patient responses with physician to determine whether drug should be given. Assess baseline skin condition including integrity and allergy history to drugs. Teach patient to report rash, itching, or other skin changes. Teach patient skin care and symptomatic measures as appropriate. If skin rash develops, discuss drug discontinuance with physician.

II. ALTERATION IN NUTRITION, LESS THAN BODY REQUIREMENTS, related to GI SIDE EFFECTS

Defining Characteristics: Nausea, vomiting, diarrhea, and anorexia may occur. Rarely, transient increases in LFTs—AST (SGOT), ALT (SGPT), alk phos, bilirubin—may occur.

Nursing Implications: Assess baseline nutritional status. Teach patient to report GI disturbances. Administer and teach patient to self-administer medication as needed and as ordered. Teach patient importance of nutritious diet and suggest small, frequent, high-calorie,

COMPLICATIONS

high-protein meals as appropriate. Assess baseline LFTs and monitor periodically during treatment. Discuss abnormalities and drug interruption with physician.

III. FUNGAL SUPERINFECTION related to REDISTRIBUTION OF ENDOGENOUS MICROORGANISMS

Defining Characteristics: Vaginal moniliasis or vaginitis may occur as endogenous bacteria are eliminated and normal fungal population expands.

Nursing Implications: Teach female patient to report vaginal itching or discharge. Discuss appropriate antifungal treatment with physician. Teach perineal hygiene and symptomatic management.

Drug: ceftolozane/tazobactam (Zerbaxa)

Class: Antibacterial.

Mechanism of Action: Combination product consisting of a cephalosporin-class antibacterial drug and a beta-lactamase inhibitor.

Metabolism: Ceftolozane is eliminated in urine unchanged and does not appear to be metabolized to any appreciable extent. The beta-lactam ring of tazobactam is hydrolyzed to form a pharmacologically inactive tazobactam metabolite M1. Ceftolozane and tazobactam metabolite M1 are eliminated by kidneys.

Indications: Treatment of cIAI, used in combination with metronidazole caused by gram-negative and gram-positive microorganisms—*E. cloacae, E. coli, K. oxytoca, K. pneumoniae, Proteus mirabilis, Pseudomonas aeruginosa, Bacteroides fragilis, Streptococcus anginosus, Streptococcus constellatus,* and *Streptococcus salivarius.* Treatment of cUTI, including pyelonephritis, caused by gram-negative microorganisms—*E. coli, K. pneumoniae, P. mirabilis,* and *P. aeruginosa.*

Dosage/Range:
- Ceftolozane 1 g and tazobactam 0.5 g (Zerbaxa 1.5 g) for injection, every 8 hours, by IV infusion administered over 1 hour, for patients 18 years or older with creatinine clearance (CrCl) greater than 50 mL/min.
- Dose modification for renal impairment:

CrCl (mL/min)	Dosage Adjustment
30–50	Ceftolozane and tazobactam 750 mg (500 and 250 mg) intravenously every 8 hours
15–29	Ceftolozane and tazobactam 375 mg (250 and 125 mg) intravenously every 8 hours
End-stage renal disease (ESRD) on hemodialysis (HD)	A single loading dose of ceftolozane and tazobactam 750 mg (500 and 250 mg), followed by ceftolozane and tazobactam 150 mg (100 and 50 mg) maintenance dose administered IV every 8 hours, for remainder of treatment period (on hemodialysis days, administer dose at earliest possible time following completion of dialysis)

*CrCl estimated using Cockcroft-Gault formula.
**All doses of ceftolozane and tazobactam are administered over 1 hour.

Drug Preparation:
- Does not contain a bacteriostatic preservative. Aseptic technique must be followed in preparing infusion solution.
- Preparation of doses: Constitute the vial with sterile water for injection or 0.9% sodium chloride for injection, USP and gently shake to dissolve. Final volume is approximately 11.4 mL.
- Caution: The **constituted solution is not for direct injection**.
- To prepare required dose, withdraw appropriate volume per manufacturer's prescribing information. Add the withdrawn volume to an infusion bag containing 0.9% sodium chloride for injection USP or 5% dextrose injection USP.

Drug Interactions:
- No significant drug–drug interactions are anticipated between ceftolozane and tazobactam and substrates, inhibitors, and inducers of cytochrome P450 enzymes (CYPs).
- Drug interacts with probenecid.

Lab Effects/Interference:
- Serum ALT (SGPT), serum alkaline phosphatase, serum AST (SGOT), and serum bilirubin values may be increased. BUN and serum creatinine: concentrations may be increased.

Special Considerations:
- Contraindicated in patients with known serious hypersensitivity to ceftolozane and tazobactam, piperacillin/tazobactam, or other members of beta-lactam class.
- Decreased efficacy in patients with baseline CrCl of 30–50 mL/min. Monitor CrCl at least daily in patients with changing renal function and adjust dose accordingly.
- Serious hypersensitivity (anaphylactic) reactions have been reported with beta-lactam antibacterial drugs. Exercise caution in patients with known hypersensitivity to beta-lactam antibacterial drugs.
- CDAD has been reported with nearly all systemic antibacterial agents. Evaluate if diarrhea occurs.
- Most common adverse reactions ($\geq$ 5% in either indication) are nausea, diarrhea, headache, and pyrexia.
- Drug has not been studied in pediatric patients.
- Dosage adjustment is required in patients with moderately or severely impaired renal function and in patients with end-stage renal disease on hemodialysis.
- Higher incidence of adverse reactions was observed in patients aged 65 years and older. In cIAI, cure rates were lower in patients aged 65 years and older.
- Renal: Decreased efficacy has been reported in patients with baseline creatinine clearance of 30 to less than or equal to 50 mL/min; monitoring recommended. Increased risk of adverse effects in patients with moderate or severe renal impairment and those with ESRD on hemodialysis; monitoring recommended and dose adjustments required.

Potential Toxicities/Side Effects and the Nursing Process

I.   POTENTIAL FOR INJURY related to HYPERSENSITIVITY REACTION

Defining Characteristics: Urticaria, pruritus, rash (maculopapular or erythematous), fever and chills, eosinophilia, myalgia, edema, erythema, or angioedema. Increased risk exists in individuals allergic to penicillin cephalosporin antibiotics.

COMPLICATIONS

Nursing Implications: Assess allergy to cephalosporin antibiotics and penicillin; if patient states "yes," determine actual response (e.g., "swollen lips angioedema"). If angioedema is present, patient *should not* receive drug. Discuss other patient responses with physician to determine whether drug should be given. Assess baseline skin condition, including integrity, and allergy history to drugs. Teach patient to report rash, itching, or other skin changes. Teach patient skin care and symptomatic measures as appropriate. If skin rash develops, discuss drug discontinuance with physician.

II.   ALTERATION IN NUTRITION, LESS THAN BODY REQUIREMENTS, related to GI SIDE EFFECTS

Defining Characteristics: Nausea, vomiting, diarrhea, and anorexia may occur. Drug may cause transient increases in LFTs.

Nursing Implications: Assess baseline nutritional status. Teach patient to report GI disturbances. Administer, and teach patient to self-administer, antiemetics as needed and as ordered. Teach patient importance of a nutritious diet; suggest small, frequent, high-calorie, high-protein meals as appropriate. Assess baseline LFTs and monitor periodically during treatment. Discuss abnormalities and drug interruption with physician.

III.   FUNGAL SUPERINFECTION related to REDISTRIBUTION OF ENDOGENOUS MICROORGANISMS

Defining Characteristics: Vaginal candidiasis and vaginitis may occur as endogenous bacteria are eliminated and normal fungal population expands.

Nursing Implications: Instruct female patients to report vaginal itching or discharge. Discuss appropriate antifungal treatment with physician. Teach perineal hygiene and symptomatic management.

IV.   ALTERATIONS IN PROTECTIVE MECHANISMS (RARE) related to RARE LEUKOPENIA

Defining Characteristics: Rarely, hemolytic anemia, leukopenia, or thrombocytopenia may occur.

Nursing Implications: Assess baseline laboratory parameters, and monitor periodically during treatment. Assess patient for response to antibiotics. Discuss abnormalities with physician.

V.   ALTERATIONS IN COMFORT related to LOCAL INJECTION-SITE IRRITATION

Defining Characteristics: Pain and phlebitis may develop in IV sites.

Nursing Implications: Change IV sites every 48 hours and assess for signs and symptoms of phlebitis prior to each administration. Administer drug slowly. Apply warm packs to increase comfort.

VI.   KNOWLEDGE DEFICIT related to SELF-ADMINISTRATION OF MEDICATION

Defining Characteristics: Increased compliance when patient is instructed in self-care activities.

Nursing Implications: Assess knowledge regarding infection and planned treatment. Teach about drug action, potential side effects, and when and how to take drug. Teach patient to report any possible side effects that occur.

Drug: ceftriaxone sodium (Rocephin)

Class: Third-generation cephalosporin antibacterial.

Mechanism of Action: Semisynthetic derivative of cephalosporin C (produced by fungus); contains β-lactam ring and is related to penicillins and cephamycins (e.g., cefoxitin). Bactericidal through inhibition of cell wall synthesis, with resulting cell wall instability and cell lysis.

Metabolism: Not absorbed from GI tract and must be given parenterally. Widely distributed into body tissues and fluids, including bile and CSF. Crosses placenta and excreted in breastmilk. Protein binding depends on drug concentration, and varies from 58 to 96%. Excreted in urine and feces to a lesser extent. Has a long half-life.

Indication: For treatment of acute bacterial otitis media, infections in lower respiratory tract, skin, bone and joint, abdomen, urinary tract, and pelvis (gonorrhea), as well as for treatment of meningitis and sepsis and as preoperative prophylaxis. Active primarily against gram-negative cocci (*H. influenzae, Enterobacter, E. coli, Klebsiella, Proteus, Pseudomonas*) and, to a lesser degree, gram-positive cocci (*S. aureus* and streptococci).

Dosage/Range:
- IV and IM doses same 1 g q 24 h for most infections.
- CNS infections may require maximum recommended of 4 g/day in divided doses.

Dose Adjustment: None

Drug Preparation:
- Store vial of sterile drug powder at ≤ 25°C (77°F) and protect from light. Frozen injection containers should be stored at ≤ 20°C (4°F).
- IV: Add diluent recommended by manufacturer into vial, then further dilute in 100 mL 0.9% sodium chloride or 5% dextrose. Infuse over 30–60 minutes.
- IM: Add 0.9–7.2 mL of sterile or bacteriostatic water for injection, or 1% lidocaine HCl without epinephrine to appropriate vial, resulting in 250 mg/mL. Administer deep IM into large muscle mass (e.g., gluteus maximus). Make certain patient is NOT ALLERGIC to lidocaine.

Drug Interactions:
- Probenecid: increased serum concentrations of antibiotic; monitor and decrease dose if needed.
- Lactated Ringer's: precipitation occurs.

COMPLICATIONS

- Calcium Acetate: precipitation occurs.
- Warfarin.
- Ceftriaxone.
- Typhoid vaccine.

Lab Effects/Interference:

Major clinical significance:
- Coombs' (antiglobulin) tests: a positive reaction frequently appears in patients who receive large doses of cephalosporins; hemolysis rarely occurs, but it has been reported; test may be positive in neonates whose mothers received cephalosporins before delivery.
- PT: may be prolonged; cephalosporins may inhibit vitamin K synthesis by suppressing gut flora.

Clinical significance:
- Serum ALT, serum alk phos, serum AST, serum bili, or serum LDH values may be increased.
- BUN and serum creatinine concentrations may be increased.
- CBC or platelet count: transient leukopenia, neutropenia, agranulocytosis, thrombocytopenia, eosinophilia, lymphocytosis, and thrombocytosis have been seen on rare occasions.

Special Considerations:
- Use cautiously if history of colitis exists.
- Contraindicated in patients hypersensitive to other cephalosporin antibiotics.
- Use cautiously if sensitive to penicillin; contraindicated if angioedema reaction to penicillin.
- Obtain specimen and send for culture and sensitivity prior to first drug dose.
- May cause false-positive direct Coombs' test.
- May cause false-positive Clinitest glucose result.
- Hematologic: Hemolytic anemia, including fatal cases, has been reported; discontinue if condition occurs.
- Hematologic: Use caution in patients with impaired vitamin K synthesis or low vitamin K stores due to risk of rare prothrombin time alteration.
- Administration: Do not concurrently administer calcium-containing IV solutions in same IV line, including continuous calcium-containing infusions such as parenteral nutrition via a Y-site; may be administered sequentially in patients other than neonates with thorough flushing of lines with compatible fluid between administrations.

Potential Toxicities/Side Effects and the Nursing Process

I.   POTENTIAL FOR INJURY related to HYPERSENSITIVITY REACTION

Defining Characteristics: Urticaria, pruritus, rash (maculopapular or erythematous), fever and chills, eosinophilia, myalgia, edema, erythema, angioedema, Stevens–Johnson syndrome, and exfoliative skin reactions occur in 5% of patients. Increased risk in individuals allergic to penicillin.

Nursing Implications: Assess allergy to cephalosporin antibiotics and penicillin: if patient states "yes," determine actual response (e.g., "swollen lips = angioedema"). If angioedema, patient should not receive drug. Discuss other patient responses with physician to determine whether drug should be given. Assess baseline skin condition including integrity and allergy history to drugs. Instruct patient to report rash, itching, or other skin changes. Teach patient skin care and symptomatic measures as appropriate. If skin rash develops, discuss drug discontinuance with physician. If rash progresses, drug should be discontinued, as fatal Stevens–Johnson syndrome may develop. Be prepared to treat severe acute hypersensitivity reactions with airway management, oxygen, epinephrine, corticosteroids, or antihistamines as ordered.

II. ALTERATION IN NUTRITION, LESS THAN BODY REQUIREMENTS, related to GI SIDE EFFECTS

Defining Characteristics: Nausea, vomiting, diarrhea, and anorexia may occur; rarely, pseudomembranous colitis caused by *C. difficile* resistant to the antibiotic occurs. Rarely, transient increases in LFTs—AST, ALT, alk phos, bili—may occur.

Nursing Implications: Assess baseline nutritional status. Instruct patient to report GI disturbances. Administer and teach patient to self-administer antiemetics, antidiarrheals as needed and as ordered. Teach patient importance of nutritious diet and suggest small, frequent, high-calorie, high-protein meals as appropriate. Assess baseline LFTs and monitor periodically during treatment. Discuss abnormalities and drug interruption with physician.

III. FUNGAL SUPERINFECTION related to REDISTRIBUTION OF ENDOGENOUS MICROORGANISMS

Defining Characteristics: Vaginal candidiasis or vaginitis may occur as endogenous bacteria are eliminated and normal fungal population expands.

Nursing Implications: Instruct female patient to report vaginal itching or discharge. Discuss appropriate antifungal treatment with physician. Teach perineal hygiene and symptomatic management.

IV. ALTERATIONS IN PROTECTIVE MECHANISMS (RARE) related to TRANSIENT LEUKOPENIA

Defining Characteristics: Rarely, transient leukopenia, lymphocytosis, anemia, or eosinophilia may occur. Prolonged PT, prolonged aPTT, and hypoprothrombinemia have occurred rarely, especially in elderly or debilitated patients, or in individuals with vitamin K deficiency.

Nursing Implications: Assess baseline laboratory parameters, and monitor periodically during treatment. Assess patient for response to antibiotics. Discuss abnormalities with

COMPLICATIONS

physician. Assess for signs/symptoms of bleeding. If they occur, especially in elderly or debilitated patients, discuss vitamin K administration with physician. Instruct patient to avoid aspirin. If taking oral anticoagulants, assess for increased PT, signs/symptoms of bleeding.

V.   ALTERATIONS IN SENSORY/PERCEPTUAL PATTERNS related to DIZZINESS, SOMNOLENCE

Defining Characteristics: Dizziness, headache, or somnolence occur rarely.

Nursing Implications: Assess baseline neurologic function and comfort and monitor during treatment. Instruct patient to report any changes. Discuss any abnormalities with physician.

VI.   ALTERATIONS IN COMFORT related to LOCAL INJECTION IRRITATION

Defining Characteristics: Pain, induration, and sterile abscesses may form in IM injection sites; phlebitis may develop in IV sites.

Nursing Implications: Rotate IM injection sites, and administer drug deep IM in large muscle mass (e.g., gluteus maximus). Use IM injection when IV administration is not possible. Change IV sites q 48 h, and assess for signs/symptoms of phlebitis prior to each administration. Administer drug slowly. Apply warm packs to increase comfort.

Drug: cefuroxime (Ceftin, Kefurox, Zinacef)

Class: Second-generation cephalosporin antibiotic.

Mechanism of Action: Semisynthetic derivative of cephalosporin C; contains β-lactam ring and is related to penicillins and cephamycins. Bactericidal through inhibition of cell wall synthesis by binding to one or more of the PBPs that in turn inhibit the final transpeptidation step of peptidoglycan synthesis in bacterial cell walls, thus inhibiting cell wall biosynthesis. Bacteria eventually lyse due to ongoing activity of cell wall autolytic enzymes (autolysins and murein hydrolases) while cell wall assembly is arrested.

Metabolism: Widely distributed in body tissues, fluids; crosses blood–brain barrier; therapeutic concentrations achieved in cerebro-spinal fluid even when meninges are not inflamed; readily crosses placenta and is excreted in breastmilk. Unchanged drug rapidly excreted by the kidneys.

Indication: For treatment of certain bacterial infections such as gonorrhea, Lyme disease, and infections of the ears, throat, sinuses, urinary tract, and skin. Active against a wide variety of bacteria, such as *S. aureus, S. pneumoniae, H. influenza, E. coli, N. gonorrhea,* and many others.

Dosage/Range:

Route	Dosage	Interval/Duration
Oral (Adult)	250–500 mg	2x daily for 10 days
IM and IV (Adult)	750 mg to 1.5 g/dose	q 8 h
	100–150 mg/kg/day in divided doses; maximum dose is 6 g/24 h	q 6–8 h

Drug Preparation:
- Refrigerate suspension; solution stable for 48 hours.
- IV infusion in NS or D_5W solution stable for 7 days when refrigerated.

Drug Interactions:
- Probenecid: increased serum concentrations of cefotetan, but does not usually require dose reduction of antibiotic.
- Drug interacts with Coumadin and contraceptives.

Lab Effects/Interference:
- Serum ALT (SGPT), serum alk phos, serum AST (SGOT), and serum bilirubin—values may be increased.
- BUN and serum creatinine—concentrations may be increased.

Special Considerations:
- Use cautiously if renal impairment is present.
- Contraindicated if hypersensitive to other cephalosporins or had angioedema response to penicillin.

Potential Toxicities/Side Effects and the Nursing Process

I. POTENTIAL FOR INJURY related to HYPERSENSITIVITY REACTION

Defining Characteristics: Urticaria, pruritus, rash (maculopapular or erythematous), fever and chills, eosinophilia, myalgia, edema, erythema, or angioedema. Increased risk in individuals allergic to penicillin.

Nursing Implications: Assess allergy to cephalosporin antibiotics and penicillin: if patient states "yes," determine actual response (e.g., "swollen lips = angioedema"). If angioedema, patient should not receive drug. Discuss other patient responses with physician to determine whether drug should be given. Assess baseline skin condition including integrity and allergy history to drugs. Teach patient to report rash, itching, or other skin changes. Teach patient skin care and symptomatic measures as appropriate. If skin rash develops, discuss drug discontinuance with physician.

II. ALTERATION IN NUTRITION, LESS THAN BODY REQUIREMENTS, related to GI SIDE EFFECTS

Defining Characteristics: Nausea, vomiting, diarrhea, and anorexia may occur. May cause transient increases in LFTs.

COMPLICATIONS

Nursing Implications: Assess baseline nutritional status. Teach patient to report GI disturbances. Administer and teach patient to self-administer antiemetics as needed and as ordered. Teach patient importance of nutritious diet and suggest small, frequent, high-calorie, high-protein meals as appropriate. Assess baseline LFTs and monitor periodically during treatment. Discuss abnormalities and drug interruption with physician.

III.   FUNGAL SUPERINFECTION related to REDISTRIBUTION OF ENDOGENOUS MICROORGANISMS

Defining Characteristics: Vaginal moniliasis or vaginitis may occur as endogenous bacteria are eliminated and normal fungal population expands.

Nursing Implications: Teach female patient to report vaginal itching or discharge. Discuss appropriate antifungal treatment with physician. Teach perineal hygiene and symptomatic management.

IV.   KNOWLEDGE DEFICIT related to SELF-ADMINISTRATION OF MEDICATION

Defining Characteristics: Increased compliance when patient is instructed in self-care activities.

Nursing Implications: Assess knowledge regarding infection and planned treatment. Teach about drug action, potential side effects, and when and how to take drug. Teach patient to report any possible side effects that occur.

Drug: cephalexin (Biocef, Keflex, Keftab)

Class: First-generation cephalosporin antibacterial.

Mechanism of Action: Semisynthetic derivative of cephalosporin C, contains β-lactam ring, and is related to penicillins and cephamycins. Bactericidal through inhibition of cell wall synthesis by binding to one or more of the PBPs that in turn inhibits the final transpeptidation step of peptidoglycan synthesis in bacterial cell walls, thus inhibiting cell wall biosynthesis. Bacteria eventually lyse due to ongoing activity of cell wall autolytic enzymes (autolysins and murein hydrolases) while cell wall assembly is arrested.

Metabolism: Well-absorbed from GI tract; delayed GI absorption if taken with food, but total amount of drug absorption is the same. Widely distributed in body tissues, fluids except cerebrospinal fluid; readily crosses placenta and is excreted in breastmilk. Unchanged drug rapidly excreted by the kidneys.

Indication: For treatment of bacterial infections of the upper respiratory tract, otitis media, skin infections, and urinary tract infections. Active against *S. aureus, S. pneumoniae, H. influenza, E. coli*, and several other bacteria.

Dosage/Range:
- Adults: 250–1,000 mg every 6 hours, maximum—4 g/day.
- Dose modification for renal impairment:

CrCl (mL/min)	Dosage (mg)	Interval/Duration
30–59	No dose modification	Do not exceed 1 g/day
15–29	250	q 8 h or q 12 h
5–14 AND not on dialysis	250	q 24 h
1–4 AND not on dialysis	250	q 48 or 60 h

Drug Preparation:
- Store suspension in refrigerator, discard after 14 days.
- Oral administration.

Drug Interactions:
- Probenecid may decrease cephalosporin elimination and increase effect.

Lab Effects/Interference:
- Serum SGPT, serum alk phos, serum SGOT, serum bilirubin, or serum LDH—values may be increased.
- BUN and serum creatinine—concentrations may be increased.

Special Considerations:
- Use with caution in patients with renal dysfunction—dose reduction required if severe impairment exists.
- Contraindicated in patients hypersensitive to other cephalosporin antibiotics.
- Use cautiously if sensitive to penicillin; contraindicated if angioedema reaction to penicillin.
- Obtain ordered specimen and send for culture and sensitivity prior to first drug dose.
- Hematologic: Longer prothrombin time may occur, especially in patients with hepatic or renal impairment, poor nutritional state, a protracted course of antimicrobial therapy, or treated with anticoagulant therapy; monitoring recommended.

Potential Toxicities/Side Effects and the Nursing Process

I.   POTENTIAL FOR INJURY related to HYPERSENSITIVITY REACTION

Defining Characteristics: Urticaria, pruritus, rash (maculopapular or erythematous), fever and chills, eosinophilia, myalgia, edema, erythema, or angioedema. Increased risk in individuals allergic to penicillin.

COMPLICATIONS

Nursing Implications: Assess allergy to cephalosporin antibiotics and penicillin: if patient states "yes," determine actual response (e.g., "swollen lips = angioedema"). If angioedema, patient should not receive drug. Discuss other patient responses with physician to determine whether drug should be given. Assess baseline skin condition including integrity and allergy history to drugs. Teach patient to report rash, itching, or other skin changes. Teach patient skin care and symptomatic measures as appropriate. If skin rash develops, discuss drug discontinuance with physician.

II.   ALTERATION IN NUTRITION, LESS THAN BODY REQUIREMENTS, related to GI SIDE EFFECTS

Defining Characteristics: Nausea, vomiting, diarrhea, and anorexia may occur. Rarely, transient increases in LFTs—AST (SGOT), ALT (SGPT), alk phos, bilirubin—may occur.

Nursing Implications: Assess baseline nutritional status. Teach patient to report GI disturbances. Administer and teach patient to self-administer medication as needed and as ordered. Teach patient importance of nutritious diet and suggest small, frequent, high-calorie, high-protein meals as appropriate. Assess baseline LFTs and monitor periodically during treatment. Discuss abnormalities and drug interruption with physician.

III.   FUNGAL SUPERINFECTION related to REDISTRIBUTION OF ENDOGENOUS MICROORGANISMS

Defining Characteristics: Vaginal moniliasis, vaginitis may occur as endogenous bacteria are eliminated and normal fungal population expands.

Nursing Implications: Teach female patient to report vaginal itching or discharge. Discuss appropriate antifungal treatment with physician. Teach perineal hygiene and symptomatic management.

Drug: ciprofloxacin (Cipro)

Class: Fluoroquinolone.

Mechanism of Action: Anti-infective; appears to inhibit DNA replication in susceptible bacteria.

Metabolism: Well-absorbed from GI tract; rate decreased by food but not extent of absorption. Widely distributed in body tissues and fluids with highest concentrations in organs, such as liver, kidneys, and lungs. Partially metabolized in liver; excreted in urine and feces. Crosses placenta and is excreted in breastmilk.

Indication: For treatment of different types of bacterial infections. Has a broad spectrum and is active against most gram-negative bacteria (e.g., *Enterobacter, Pseudomonas*), some gram-positive organisms (e.g., methicillin-resistant staphylococci), and some mycobacteria. Also used to treat people who have been exposed to anthrax.

Dosage/Range:
- PO: 250–750 mg q 12 h × 1–2 weeks.
- IV: 200–400 mg q 12–8 h × 1–2 weeks (IV used if patient unable to take oral formulation).
- Dose modification necessary if renal impairment exists—Formal recommendation.

Drug Preparation:
- Oral: Take drug with a large glass of fluid, preferably 2 hours after meal/food. Encourage oral fluids of 2–3 qt/day.
- IV: Further dilute drug in 0.9% sodium chloride or 5% dextrose in water to final concentration of < 2 mg/mL. Administer over 60 minutes.

Drug Interactions:
- Antacids (containing magnesium, aluminum, or calcium) also sucralfate and iron preparation: decrease oral ciprofloxacin serum level; do not administer concurrently. If must administer antacids, administer at least 2 hours apart.
- There are many drug interactions with QT prolonging medications, including zolpidem, mycophenolate, among others.
- Probenecid: 50% increase in ciprofloxacin serum levels; decrease ciprofloxacin dose if given concurrently.
- Theophylline: increases theophylline serum level; avoid if possible, since fatal reactions have occurred. Otherwise, monitor theophylline level very closely and decrease theophylline dose as needed.
- Use with steroids increases tendon rupture.
- Drug interacts with phenytoin and sildenafil.
- Caffeine: delays caffeine clearance from body. Instruct patient to limit coffee, tea, and soft drinks, especially if CNS side effects.

Lab Effects/Interference:
- Serum ALT, serum alk phos, serum AST, and serum LDH values may be increased. May result in false-positive urine opiate tests.

Special Considerations:
- Used in the treatment of infections of urinary and lower respiratory tract, skin, bone and joint, and GI tract, as well as gonorrhea.
- Contraindicated in pregnancy and in women who are breastfeeding.
- Obtain ordered specimen for culture and sensitivity prior to first drug dose.
- Use cautiously in patients with seizure disorders.
- Use cautiously in patients receiving concurrent theophylline, as cardiopulmonary arrest has occurred.

COMPLICATIONS

Potential Toxicities/Side Effects and the Nursing Process

I.   ALTERATION IN NUTRITION, LESS THAN BODY REQUIREMENTS, related to GI SIDE EFFECTS

Defining Characteristics: 2–10% incidence of nausea, vomiting, abdominal discomfort, diarrhea, and anorexia.

Nursing Implications: Assess baseline nutritional and elimination status. Instruct patient to report GI disturbances. Administer and teach patient to self-administer antiemetics, antidiarrheals as needed and as ordered. Teach patient importance of nutritious diet and suggest small, frequent, high-calorie, high-protein meals as appropriate. Assess baseline LFTs and monitor periodically during treatment. Discuss abnormalities and drug interruption with physician. Assess whether taking other hepatotoxic drugs. (See Special Considerations section.)

II.   ALTERATIONS IN SENSORY/PERCEPTUAL PATTERNS related to CNS EFFECTS

Defining Characteristics: One to two percent incidence of headache, restlessness. Dizziness, hallucinations, and seizures may also occur. Exacerbated by caffeine, as ciprofloxacin delays caffeine excretion.

Nursing Implications: Assess baseline neurologic function and comfort and monitor during treatment. Instruct patient to report any changes. Discuss any abnormalities with physician. Teach patient to limit or restrict all caffeine-containing fluids, medications, for example, tea, coffee, soft drinks containing caffeine.

III.   ALTERATION IN SKIN INTEGRITY related to ALLERGY/HYPERSENSITIVITY

Defining Characteristics: One to four percent incidence of rash; other manifestations include eosinophilia, urticaria, flushing, fever, chills, photosensitivity, angioedema. Fatal hypersensitivity reactions have occurred rarely. Direct exposure to sunlight can cause sunburn (moderate to severe phototoxicity).

Nursing Implications: Assess baseline skin condition, including integrity and drug allergy history. Instruct patient to report rash, itching, or other skin changes. Teach patient skin care and symptomatic measures as appropriate. If skin rash develops, discuss drug discontinuance with physician. If rash progresses, especially in HIV-infected patients, drug should be discontinued as fatal Stevens–Johnson syndrome may develop. Be prepared to treat severe acute hypersensitivity reactions with airway management, oxygen, epinephrine, corticosteroids, antihistamines as ordered. Instruct patient to avoid excessive sun exposure and to use skin protection factor (SPF) 15 or higher.

IV. ALTERATION IN URINARY ELIMINATION related to RENAL TOXICITY

Defining Characteristics: Increased BUN and creatinine, crystal and stone formation in urine, interstitial nephritis, and renal failure may occur.

Nursing Implications: Assess baseline renal function; expect that drug dose will be decreased in presence of renal dysfunction. Instruct patient to take drug with at least 8 oz (240 mL) of water, and to increase oral fluids to 2–3 qt/day.

V. ALTERATION IN COMFORT related to IV ADMINISTRATION

Defining Characteristics: Drug may cause pain, inflammation, and rare thrombophlebitis at IV site.

Nursing Implications: Change IV site q 48 h. Assess for phlebitis, discomfort, and IV patency prior to each administration. Administer drug slowly over 60–90 minutes in large volume of 5% dextrose (see Drug Preparation). Apply heat to promote comfort.

VI. FUNGAL SUPERINFECTION related to REDISTRIBUTION OF ENDOGENOUS MICROORGANISMS

Defining Characteristics: Vaginal candidiasis or vaginitis may occur as endogenous bacteria are eliminated and normal fungal population expands.

Nursing Implications: Instruct female patient to report vaginal itching or discharge. Discuss appropriate antifungal treatment with physician. Teach perineal hygiene and symptomatic management.

VII. TENDONITIS AND TENDON RUPTURE

Black box warning: Fluoroquinolones are associated with an increased risk of tendinitis and tendon rupture in all ages. Risk further increases with age over 60 years, concomitant steroid therapy, and kidney, heart, or lung transplants. Fluoroquinolones may exacerbate muscle weakness in persons with myasthenia gravis. Avoid in patients with known history of myasthenia gravis.

COMPLICATIONS

Drug: clarithromycin (Biaxin, Biaxin XL)

Class: Antibacterial (macrolide).

Mechanism of Action: Clarithromycin exerts its antibacterial action by binding to 50S ribosomal subunit resulting in inhibition of protein synthesis. The 14-OH metabolite of clarithromycin is twice as active as the parent compound against certain organisms.

Metabolism: Rapidly and widely distributed throughout the body. Highly stable in presence of gastric acid (unlike erythromycin); food delays but does not affect extent of absorption. Widely distributed in body tissues but does not cross blood-brain barrier into CSF. Metabolized by liver and excreted by kidneys into urine.

Indication: For treatment of certain bacterial infections such as pneumonia, bronchitis, infections of the ears, sinuses, skin, and throat. Used to treat and prevent disseminated *Mycobacterium avium* complex (MAC), a lung infection that often affects people with HIV. May be used in combination to eliminate *H. pylori*.

Dosage/Range:
- Adults: Usual dosage 250–500 mg every 12 hours or 1,000 mg (two 500-mg extended-release tablets) once daily for 7–14 days.
- Renal: severe renal impairment: CrCl less than 30 mL/min, dose should be reduced 50%.

Drug Preparation:
- Store tablets and granules for oral suspension at controlled room temperature.
- Reconstituted oral suspension should not be refrigerated because it might gel.
- Microencapsulated particles of clarithromycin in suspension are stable for 14 days when stored at room temperature.

Drug Interactions:
- Alfentanil (and possible other narcotic analgesics): Serum levels may be increased by clarithromycin—monitor for increased effect.
- Astemizole: Concomitant use is contraindicated—may lead to QT prolongation or torsades de pointes.
- Benzodiazepines (those metabolized by CYP3A4, including alprazolam and triazolam): Serum levels may be increased by clarithromycin—somnolence and confusion have been reported.
- Bromocriptine: Serum levels may be increased by clarithromycin—monitor for increased effect.
- Buspirone: Serum levels may be increased by clarithromycin—monitor.
- Calcium channel blockers (felodipine, verapamil, and potentially others metabolized by CYP3A4): Serum levels may be increased by clarithromycin—monitor.
- Carbamazepine: Serum levels may be increased by clarithromycin—monitor.
- Cisapride: Serum levels may be increased by clarithromycin—monitor.
- Cilostazol: Serum levels may be increased by clarithromycin—monitor.
- Clozapine: Serum levels may be increased by clarithromycin—monitor.
- Cyclosporine: Serum levels may be increased by clarithromycin—monitor serum levels.
- Delavirdine: Serum levels may be increased by clarithromycin.
- Digoxin: Serum levels may be increased by clarithromycin; digoxin toxicity and potentially fatal arrhythmias have been reported; monitor digoxin levels.
- Disopyramide: Serum levels may be increased by clarithromycin—monitor.
- Ergot alkaloids: Concurrent use may lead to acute ergot toxicity (severe peripheral vasospasm and dysesthesia).

- Fluconazole: Increases clarithromycin levels and AUC by approximately 25%.
- Indinavir: Serum levels may be increased by clarithromycin—monitor.
- Loratadine: Serum levels may be increased by clarithromycin—monitor.
- Neuromuscular-blocking agents: May be potentiated by clarithromycin (case reports).
- Oral contraceptives: Serum levels may be increased by clarithromycin—monitor.
- Phenytoin: Serum levels may be increased by clarithromycin; other evidence suggests phenytoin levels may be decreased in some patients—monitor.
- Pimozide: Serum levels may be increased, leading to malignant arrhythmias; concomitant use is contraindicated.
- Quinolone antibiotics (ciprofloxacin, levofloxacin, or moxifloxacin): Concomitant use may increase the risk of malignant arrhythmias—avoid concomitant use.
- Rifabutin: Serum levels may be increased by clarithromycin—monitor.
- Ritonavir: Concurrent use results in a 77% increase in clarithromycin levels (100% increase in metabolite levels); may be given together without dosage adjustment in patients with normal renal function; dosage of clarithromycin must be decreased in renal impairment.
- Sildenafil: Serum levels may be increased by clarithromycin—monitor.
- Tacrolimus: Serum levels may be increased by clarithromycin—monitor serum concentrations.
- Terfenadine: Serum levels may be increased by clarithromycin; may lead to QT prolongation, ventricular tachycardia, ventricular fibrillation or torsades de pointes; concomitant use is contraindicated.
- Theophylline: Serum levels may be increased by clarithromycin (by as much as 20%)—monitor.
- Valproic acid (and derivatives): Serum levels may be increased by clarithromycin—monitor.
- Warfarin: Effects may be potentiated—monitor INR closely and adjust warfarin dose as needed or choose another antibiotic.
- Zidovudine: Peak levels (but not AUC) of zidovudine may be increased—other studies suggest levels may be decreased.
- St. John's wort: May decrease clarithromycin levels.
- CYP3A3/4 enzyme substrate—CYP1A2 and CYP3A3/4 enzyme inhibitor.

Lab Effects/Interference:
- PT/INR—may be prolonged.
- Serum SGPT, serum alk phos, serum SGOT, serum bilirubin, or serum LDH—values may be increased.
- BUN and serum creatinine—concentrations may be increased.

Special Considerations:
- Use with caution in patients with renal dysfunction—dose reduction required if severe impairment exists.
- Do not use when there is known hypersensitivity to erythromycins or other macrolides.
- Obtain ordered specimen and send for culture and sensitivity prior to first drug dose.

COMPLICATIONS

Potential Toxicities/Side Effects and the Nursing Process

I.   POTENTIAL FOR INJURY related to HYPERSENSITIVITY REACTION

Defining Characteristics: Urticaria, pruritus, rash (maculopapular or erythematous), fever and chills, eosinophilia, myalgia, edema, erythema, or angioedema.

Nursing Implications: Assess allergy to erythromycin: if patient states "yes," determine actual response (e.g., "swollen lips = angioedema"). If angioedema, patient should not receive drug. Discuss other patient responses with physician to determine whether drug should be given. Assess baseline skin condition including integrity and allergy history to drugs. Teach patient to report rash, itching, or other skin changes. Teach patient skin care and symptomatic measures as appropriate. If skin rash develops, discuss drug discontinuance with physician.

II.   ALTERATION IN NUTRITION, LESS THAN BODY REQUIREMENTS, related to GI SIDE EFFECTS

Defining Characteristics: Abdominal pain, diarrhea, nausea, and vomiting may occur.

Nursing Implications: Assess baseline nutritional status, preexisting nausea/vomiting, and anorexia. Assess baseline LFTs and monitor periodically during treatment. Teach patient to report GI disturbances. Administer and teach patient to self-administer symptomatic interventions if side effects occur; discuss with physician use of alternative drug(s).

III.   FUNGAL SUPERINFECTION related to REDISTRIBUTION OF ENDOGENOUS MICROORGANISMS

Defining Characteristics: Vaginal moniliasis or vaginitis may occur as endogenous bacteria are eliminated and normal fungal population expands.

Nursing Implications: Teach female patient to report vaginal itching or discharge. Discuss appropriate antifungal treatment with physician. Teach perineal hygiene and symptomatic management.

IV.   ALTERATIONS IN PROTECTIVE MECHANISMS (RARE)

Defining Characteristics: Prolonged PT, prolonged INR, and hypoprothrombinemia have occurred rarely, especially in elderly or debilitated patients, or in individuals with vitamin K deficiency.

Nursing Implications: Assess baseline laboratory parameters and monitor periodically during treatment. Assess patient for response to antibiotics. Discuss abnormalities with physician. Assess for signs/symptoms of bleeding. If they occur, especially in elderly or debilitated patients, discuss vitamin K administration with physician. Teach patient to avoid aspirin. If taking oral anticoagulants, assess for increased PT, signs/symptoms of bleeding.

Drug: clindamycin phosphate (Cleocin)

Class: Antibacterial (systemic); antiprotozoal.

Mechanism of Action: Bacteriostatic or bactericidal depending on drug concentration or when used against highly susceptible organisms; binds to bacterial ribosomes and prevents peptide bond formation, thus inhibiting protein synthesis.

Metabolism: Well-absorbed (90% of dose) from GI tract. Food may delay absorption but does not affect amount absorbed. Widely distributed in body tissues and fluids, including bile. Crosses placenta and is excreted in breastmilk. Excreted in urine, bile, and feces.

Indication: For treatment of acute otitis media caused by penicillin-resistant *S. pneumoniae* and to be used in individuals with penicillin hypersensitivity; bone and joint infections including acute hematogenous osteomyelitis caused by *S. aureus* and as adjunct in surgical treatment of chronic bone and joint infections; gynecologic infections (endometritis, nongonococcal tubo-ovarian abscess, pelvic cellulitis, postsurgical vaginal cuff infections), including pelvic inflammatory disease; and intra-abdominal infections (peritonitis, intra-abdominal abscess). Clindamycin is an alternative treatment for pharyngitis and tonsillitis caused by susceptible *S. pyogenes* (group A beta-hemolytic streptococci) in patients who cannot receive beta-lactam anti-infectives and have infections caused by macrolide-resistant *S. pyogenes*. Respiratory tract infections, septicemia, and skin structures caused by susceptible anaerobes, *S. pneumoniae, S. pyogenes*, other streptococci, or *S. aureus*. Actinomycosis caused by *Actinomyces israelii*; Babesiosis caused by *Babesia microti*; diarrheal-type food poisoning caused by *Bacillus cereus*; bacterial vaginosis; Capnocytophaga infections caused by *Capnocytophaga canimorsus*; clostridial myonecrosis (gas gangrene) caused *Clostridium perfringens* or other Clostridium; malaria caused by chloroquine-resistant *Plasmodium falciparum*; pneumocystis jiroveci (*Pneumocystis carinii*) pneumonia; toxoplasmosis in immunocompromised adults, adolescents, or children (including HIV-infected patients); and anthrax. Active against gram-positive cocci (e.g., staphylococci, streptococci) and many anaerobic gram-positive and gram-negative bacilli (e.g., clostridia, mycobacteria). Prevention of bacterial endocarditis, perinatal group B streptococcal disease, and perioperative prophylaxis.

Dosage/Range:

Adult:
- Oral: 150–450 mg PO q 6 h; IM/IV: 300 mg q 6–12 h (maximum 2.7 g/day). Doses up to 900 have been used.

Drug Preparation:
- Oral: Administer with 8 oz (240 mL) of water to prevent esophageal irritation.
- IM: Single dose should not exceed 600 mg.
- Further dilute in 0.9% sodium chloride or 5% dextrose in water to final concentration < 12 mg/mL, and infuse over 20 minutes (600-mg dose) or 30–40 minutes (1.2-g dose). Maximum 1.2 g in single 1-hour period. May be given as continuous infusion.

COMPLICATIONS

Drug Interactions:
- Neuromuscular-blocking agents (tubocurarine, ether, pancuronium): may increase neuromuscular blockade; use concurrently with caution.
- Erythromycin: decreases bactericidal activity of clindamycin.
- Kaolin: decreases GI absorption of clindamycin. Avoid concurrent administration, or administer at least 2 hours apart.
- QT prolonging drugs: colchicine, fluconazole, select 3A4 substrates, simvastatin, among others.

Lab Effects/Interference:
- Serum ALT, serum alk phos, and serum AST concentrations may be increased.

Special Considerations:
- Contraindicated in patients with hypersensitivity to clindamycin or lincomycin; contraindicated in patients with history of colitis.
- Can cause severe, sometimes fatal colitis. Stop drug if diarrhea develops, or if necessary, continue only under close monitoring and endoscopy. Can cause severe diarrhea and GI upset.
- Used in the treatment of serious infections of respiratory tract, skin/soft tissues, female pelvic/genital tract. May be used investigationally with other drugs in treatment of MAC; also may be used to treat *P. carinii* pneumonia, cryptosporidiosis, and toxoplasmosis in AIDS patients.
- Also used for prophylaxis of bacterial endocarditis in penicillin-allergic, erythromycin-intolerant patients.
- DO NOT GIVE rapid IVB: cardiopulmonary arrest has occurred.
- Avoid use in pregnant or breastfeeding women.

Potential Toxicities/Side Effects and the Nursing Process

I.   ALTERATION IN NUTRITION, LESS THAN BODY REQUIREMENTS, related to GI SIDE EFFECTS

Defining Characteristics: Nausea, vomiting, diarrhea, abdominal pain, and tenesmus may occur. Flatulence, bloating, anorexia, and esophagitis may occur as well. Fatal pseudomembranous colitis has occurred, characterized by severe diarrhea, abdominal cramping, and melena. Usually begins 2–9 days after drug is initiated.

Nursing Implications: Assess elimination and nutrition pattern, baseline and during therapy. Instruct patient to report diarrhea and/or abdominal pain immediately. Discuss drug discontinuance with physician if diarrhea occurs. Guaiac stool for occult blood, and notify physician if positive. If severe diarrhea develops, discuss management plan including endoscopy, and fluid and electrolyte replacement. Do not administer antiperistaltic agents such as opiates and diphenoxylate with atropine (Lomotil), since it may worsen condition. Assess for nausea/vomiting, and administer prescribed antiemetic medications. Encourage small, frequent feedings as tolerated. Instruct patient to take oral dose with a full glass of water.

II.   ALTERATION IN SKIN INTEGRITY related to HYPERSENSITIVITY

Defining Characteristics: Maculopapular rash, urticaria may occur. Rarely, erythema multiforme may occur. Increased risk of allergic reaction in asthma patients. Anaphylaxis may rarely occur.

Nursing Implications: Assess baseline allergy history. Assess baseline skin integrity. Instruct patient to report rash, pruritus. Teach patient symptomatic management of rash, pruritus. Assess for hypersensitivity reaction; if it occurs, monitor vital signs (VS), discontinue drug, notify physician, and institute supportive measures.

III.   ALTERATIONS IN COMFORT related to LOCAL ADMINISTRATION EFFECTS

Defining Characteristics: IM administration may cause pain, induration, sterile abscesses, and transient increase in creatine phosphokinase (CPK) due to muscle injury. IV administration may cause erythema, pain, swelling, and thrombophlebitis.

Nursing Implications: Administer maximum 600-mg dose IM deeply in large muscle mass (e.g., gluteus maximus). Rotate sites. Assess IV site prior to each dose for phlebitis or swelling, and change site at least q 48 h. Administer dose slowly: 300–600 mg in 50 mL over 20–30 minutes, and 900–1,200-mg dose in 100-mL IV over 40–60 minutes. Apply heat to painful IV sites as ordered.

IV.   ALTERATION IN HEPATIC FUNCTION related to TRANSIENT INCREASES IN LFTs

Defining Characteristics: Transient increases in serum bili, AST, alk phos have occurred.

Nursing Implications: Assess baseline LFTs, and monitor during therapy.

V.   FUNGAL SUPERINFECTION related to REDISTRIBUTION OF ENDOGENOUS MICROORGANISMS

Defining Characteristics: Vaginal candidiasis or vaginitis may occur as endogenous bacteria are eliminated and normal fungal population expands.

Nursing Implications: Instruct female patient to report vaginal itching or discharge. Discuss appropriate antifungal treatment with physician. Teach perineal hygiene and symptomatic management.

COMPLICATIONS

Drug: colistimethate (Colistin/Polymyxin B)

Class: Antibiotic.

Mechanism of Action: Colistimethate sodium is a cyclic polypeptide antibiotic derived from Bacillus polymyxa var. colistinus and belongs to the polymyxin group. The polymyxin antibiotics are cationic surface-active agents that work by damaging the cell membrane. The resulting physiological effects are lethal to the bacterium. Polymyxins are selective for gram-negative bacteria that have a hydrophobic outer membrane. **Metabolism:** When given by nebulization, variable absorption has been reported that may depend on the aerosol particle size, nebulizer system and lung status. Studies in healthy volunteers and patients with various infections have reported serum levels from nil to potentially therapeutic concentrations of 4 mg/L or more. Therefore, the possibility of systemic absorption should always be borne in mind when treating patients by inhalation.

Indications: Treatment infections for susceptible bacteria: Intravenous administration for infections caused by gram-negative bacteria, including lower respiratory tract and urinary tract. Treatment by inhalation of *P. aeruginosa* lung infection in patients with cystic fibrosis.

Contraindications: Colistin/polymyxin B is contraindicated in patients with known hypersensitivity to colistimethate sodium (colistin) or to polymyxin B and in patients with myasthenia gravis.

Dosage/Range:
- Given as 50 mL intravenous infusion over 30 minutes.
- Patients with totally implantable venous access device (TIVAD) may tolerate bolus injection of up to 2 million units in 10 mL given over 5 minutes or more. Minimum of 5 days treatment is recommended. For respiratory exacerbations in cystic fibrosis, treatment should continue for up to 12 days.

Indication	Dosage	Route	Interval/Duration
Up to 60 kg	50,000 units/kg/day to a maximum of 75,000 units/kg/day	IV	Total daily dose divided into 3 doses given at 8-hour intervals
Over 60 kg	1–2 million units 3 times a day	IV	The maximum dose is 6 million units in 24 hours.

Dose Modification for Renal Impairment: Grade	Cr Cl (mL/min)	Over 60 kg Body weight
Mild	20–50	1–2 million units every 8 hours
Moderate	10–20	1 million units every 12–18 hours
Severe	< 10	1 million units every 18–24 hours

Drug Preparation: For local treatment of lower respiratory tract infections, dissolve powder in 2–4 mL of water for injections or 0.9% sodium chloride intravenous infusion for use in a nebulizer attached to an air/oxygen supply.

Stabile for 28 days at 4°C. Use solutions immediately and no longer than 24 hours at 2–8°C, unless reconstituted and diluted under controlled and validated aseptic conditions.

Solutions for nebulization have similar in-use stability and should be treated as above. Patients self-treating with nebulized antibiotic should be advised to use solutions immediately after preparation. If this is not possible, solutions should not be stored for longer than 24 hours in a refrigerator.

Drug Interactions:
- Concomitant use with other neurotoxic and/or nephrotoxic potential should be avoided including aminoglycoside antibiotics (gentamicin, amikacin, netilmicin, tobramycin).
- Increased risk of nephrotoxicity if given concomitantly with cephalosporin antibiotics.
- Neuromuscular: blocking drugs and ether should be used with extreme caution in patients receiving colistimethate sodium.
- Renal Impairment: Use with caution in renal impairment.
- Hepatic Impairment: No data available.
- Pregnancy: No adequate data.
- Lactation: Colistimethate sodium is secreted in breastmilk.
- Geriatric Use: Elderly patients are more likely to have decreased renal function, hence care should be taken in dose selection and it may be useful to monitor renal function.

Lab Effects/Interference:
- None reported.

Special Considerations:
- Mixing drugs in infusions, injections, and nebulizer solutions involving colistimethate sodium should be avoided.
- Adding of other antibiotics (erythromycin, tetracycline, cephalothin) to solutions may lead to precipitation.

Potential Toxicities/Side Effects and the Nursing Process

I. ALTERATIONS IN SKIN INTEGRITY related to ALLERGY HYPERSENSITIVITY REACTION

Defining Characteristics: Incidence of rash that is mild, transient, pruritic, and/or erythematous. Incidence of immediate hypersensitivity reaction characterized by angioedema, bronchospasm, severe shock. Little cross-allergenicity with penicillins, cephalosporins (less than 1%).

Nursing Implications: Assess baseline skin integrity and presence of drug allergies; if anaphylactic reaction to penicillins or cephalosporins, monitor patient closely during drug infusions. Instruct patient to report immediately signs/symptoms of rash, pruritus, shortness of breath, and adverse sensation. Teach patient skin care and symptomatic measures as appropriate. If skin rash develops, discuss drug discontinuance with physician. If rash progresses, especially in HIV-infected patients, drug should be discontinued, as fatal Stevens–Johnson syndrome may develop. Be prepared to treat severe acute hypersensitivity reactions with airway management, oxygen, epinephrine, corticosteroids, antihistamines as ordered.

II. ALTERATION IN NUTRITION, LESS THAN BODY REQUIREMENTS, related to GI SIDE EFFECTS

Defining Characteristics: Nausea, vomiting, diarrhea, and anorexia may occur; rarely, pseudomembranous colitis caused by *C. difficile* resistant to the antibiotic occurs. Rarely, transient increases in LFTs—AST, ALT, alk phos—may occur.

COMPLICATIONS

Nursing Implications: Assess baseline nutritional status. Instruct patient to report GI disturbances. Administer and teach patient to self-administer antiemetics as needed and as ordered. Teach patient importance of nutritious diet and suggest small, frequent, high-calorie, high-protein meals as appropriate. Assess baseline LFTs and monitor periodically during treatment. Discuss abnormalities and drug interruption with physician. Encourage oral hygiene after meals and at bedtime.

III. FUNGAL SUPERINFECTION related to REDISTRIBUTION OF ENDOGENOUS MICROORGANISMS

Defining Characteristics: Vaginal candidiasis or vaginitis may occur as endogenous bacteria are eliminated and normal fungal population expands.

Nursing Implications: Instruct female patient to report vaginal itching or discharge. Discuss appropriate antifungal treatment with physician. Teach perineal hygiene and symptomatic management.

IV. ALTERATIONS IN SENSORY/PERCEPTUAL PATTERNS related to DIZZINESS, SOMNOLENCE

Defining Characteristics: Tingling of extremities and tongue, slurred speech, dizziness, vertigo, and paresthesia have occurred.

Nursing Implications: Assess baseline neurologic function and comfort and monitor during treatment. Instruct patient to report any changes. Discuss any abnormalities with physician.

Drug: colistimethate injection (Coly-Mycin M)

Class: Antibacterial (systemic).

Mechanism of Action: Colistimethate sodium is a surface-active agent that penetrates into and disrupts the bacterial cell membrane.

Metabolism: Partially metabolized, and excreted primarily in urine.

Indication: For treatment of bacterial infections in many different parts of the body, including most strains of aerobic gram-negative microorganisms *E. aerogenes*, *E. coli*, *K. pneumoniae,* and *P. aeruginosa.*

Dosage/Range:
• Given IV or IM (IV preferred for doses > 1 g, and for serious infections).

Renal Function Status	Body Weight (Adult)	Dosage	Interval/Duration
Normal	Normal	Max daily dose—not exceed 5 mg/kg/day (2.3 mg/lb)	2–4 divided doses of 2.5–5 mg/kg/day, depending on infection severity
Normal	Obese	Should be based on ideal body weight	N/A

- Dose modification for renal and hepatic impairment:

Impaired Renal Function.

Acute Bacterial Exacerbation	Chronic Bronchitis, Community-Acquired	Pneumonia, Acute Maxillary Sinusitis, Uncomplicated Skin Infections
CrCl 20–49 mL/min	500 mg	250 mg q 24 h
CrCl 10–19 mL/min	500 mg	250 mg q 48 h
Hemodialysis	500 mg	250 mg q 48 h
CAPD	500 mg q 48 h	250 mg q 48 h
Uncomplicated UTI/Acute Pyelonephritis		
CrCl 10–19 mL/min	250 mg	250 mg q 48 h

Drug Preparation:

- The 150-mg vial should be reconstituted with 2 mL sterile water for injection, USP. The reconstituted solution provides colistimethate sodium at a concentration equivalent to 75 mg/mL colistin base activity.
- During reconstitution swirl gently to avoid frothing.
- Parenteral drug products should be inspected visually for particulate matter and discoloration prior to administration, whenever solution and container permit. If these conditions are observed, the product should not be used.
- *Direct intermittent administration:* Slowly inject one-half of the total daily dose over a period of 3–5 minutes every 12 hours.
- *Continuous infusion:* Slowly inject one-half of the total daily dose over 3–5 minutes. Add the remaining half of the total daily dose of colistimethate for injection, USP, to one of the following: 0.9% NaCl; 5% dextrose in 0.9% NaCl; 5% dextrose in water; 5% dextrose in 0.45% NaCl; 5% dextrose in 0.225% NaCl; lactated Ringer's solution; 10% invert sugar solution.
- Insufficient data to recommend usage of colistimethate for injection, USP, with other drugs or other than the previously listed infusion solutions.
- Administer the second half of the total daily dose by slow IV infusion, starting 1–2 hours after the initial dose, over the next 22–23 hours.
- In the presence of impaired renal function, reduce the infusion rate depending on the degree of renal impairment. The choice of IV solution and the volume to be employed are dictated by the requirements of fluid and electrolyte management.

COMPLICATIONS

- Any infusion solution containing colistimethate sodium should be freshly prepared and used for no longer than 24 hours.

Drug Interactions:
- Curariform muscle relaxants (e.g., tubocurarine) and other drugs, including ether, succinylcholine, gallamine, decamethonium, and sodium citrate, potentiate the neuromuscular blocking effect and should be used with extreme caution in patients being treated with colistimethate.
- Aminoglycosides and penicillins have been reported to interfere with nerve transmission at the neuromuscular junction. They should not be given with colistimethate.
- Nephrotoxic drugs (aminoglycosides, colistin, vancomycin) may increase risk of renal dysfunction; avoid if possible.

Lab Effects/Interference:
- None, well-documented.

Special Considerations:
- The use of colistimethate for injection, USP, is contraindicated for patients with a history of sensitivity to the drug or any of its components.
- Transient neurologic disturbances may occur. These include circumoral paresthesia or numbness, tingling or formication of the extremities, generalized pruritus, vertigo, dizziness, and slurring of speech. For these reasons, patients should be warned not to drive vehicles or use hazardous machinery while on therapy. Reduction of dosage may alleviate symptoms. Therapy need not be discontinued, but such patients should be observed with particular care.
- Nephrotoxicity can occur and is probably a dose-dependent effect of colistimethate sodium. These manifestations of nephrotoxicity are reversible following discontinuation of the antibiotic—not always.
- Respiratory arrest has been reported following IM administration of colistimethate sodium. Impaired renal function increases the possibility of apnea and neuromuscular blockade following administration of colistimethate sodium. Follow recommended dosing guidelines.
- Obtain and send specimen for culture and sensitivity prior to first drug dose.
- Use cautiously if prior immediate hypersensitivity reaction to penicillins or cephalosporins; little risk of cross-allergenicity, monitor patient closely.
- Can also be given as inhalation but can cause respiratory failure.
- Use with caution in patients with renal or hepatic dysfunction.

Potential Toxicities/Side Effects and the Nursing Process

I.   ALTERATIONS IN SKIN INTEGRITY related to ALLERGY HYPERSENSITIVITY REACTION

Defining Characteristics: Incidence of rash that is mild, transient, pruritic, and/or erythematous. Incidence of immediate hypersensitivity reaction characterized by angioedema, bronchospasm, severe shock. Little cross-allergenicity with penicillins, cephalosporins (less than 1%).

Nursing Implications: Assess baseline skin integrity and presence of drug allergies; if anaphylactic reaction to penicillins or cephalosporins, monitor patient closely during drug infusions. Instruct patient to report immediately signs/symptoms of rash, pruritus, shortness of breath, and adverse sensation. Teach patient skin care and symptomatic measures as appropriate. If skin rash develops, discuss drug discontinuance with physician. If rash progresses, especially in HIV-infected patients, drug should be discontinued, as fatal Stevens–Johnson syndrome may develop. Be prepared to treat severe acute hypersensitivity reactions with airway management, oxygen, epinephrine, corticosteroids, or antihistamines as ordered.

II. ALTERATION IN NUTRITION, LESS THAN BODY REQUIREMENTS, related to GI SIDE EFFECTS

Defining Characteristics: Nausea, vomiting, diarrhea, and anorexia may occur; rarely, pseudomembranous colitis caused by *C. difficile* resistant to the antibiotic occurs. Rarely, transient increases in LFTs—AST, ALT, alk phos—may occur.

Nursing Implications: Assess baseline nutritional status. Instruct patient to report GI disturbances. Administer and teach patient to self-administer antiemetics as needed and as ordered. Teach patient importance of nutritious diet and suggest small, frequent, high-calorie, high-protein meals as appropriate. Assess baseline LFTs, and monitor periodically during treatment. Discuss abnormalities and drug interruption with physician. Encourage oral hygiene after meals and at bedtime.

III. FUNGAL SUPERINFECTION related to REDISTRIBUTION OF ENDOGENOUS MICROORGANISMS

Defining Characteristics: Vaginal candidiasis or vaginitis may occur as endogenous bacteria are eliminated and normal fungal population expands.

Nursing Implications: Instruct female patient to report vaginal itching or discharge. Discuss appropriate antifungal treatment with physician. Teach perineal hygiene and symptomatic management.

IV. ALTERATIONS IN SENSORY/PERCEPTUAL PATTERNS related to DIZZINESS, SOMNOLENCE

Defining Characteristics: Tingling of extremities and tongue, slurred speech, dizziness, vertigo, and paresthesia have occurred.

Nursing Implications: Assess baseline neurologic function and comfort and monitor during treatment. Instruct patient to report any changes. Discuss any abnormalities with physician.

COMPLICATIONS

V.   ALTERATIONS IN COMFORT related to LOCAL INJECTION IRRITATION

Defining Characteristics: Potential for incidence of phlebitis and thrombophlebitis when administering IV; potential incidence of pain and swelling at injection site when given IM.

Nursing Implications: Rotate IM injection sites and administer drug deep IM in large muscle mass (e.g., gluteus maximus). Use IM injection when IV administration is not possible. Change IV sites q 48 h and assess for signs/symptoms of phlebitis prior to each administration. Administer drug slowly. Apply warm packs to increase comfort.

Drug: co-trimoxazole; trimethoprim and sulfamethoxazole (Bactrim, Bactrim DS, Cotrim, Septra)

Class: Sulfonamide antibacterial (systemic); antiprotozoal.

Mechanism of Action: Bactericidal by preventing folic acid synthesis so microorganism cannot undergo cell division (sequential inhibition of folic acid synthesis, first by sulfamethoxazole, then by trimethoprim).

Metabolism: Rapidly absorbed from GI tract. Widely distributed into body tissues and fluids; crosses the placenta and is excreted in breastmilk. Highly protein-bound. Metabolized by the liver and excreted in the urine.

Indication: For treatment of many bacterial infections, such as pneumonia, bronchitis (*S. pneumoniae, H. influenzae, Legionella micdadei, L. pittsburgensis, or L. pneumoniae*), infections of the urinary tract (*E. coli, Klebsiella, Enterobacter, Morganella morganii, P. mirabilis, or P. vulgaris*), ears (*S. pneumoniae or H. influenza*), and intestines (susceptible enterotoxigenic *E. coli*, enteroinvasive *E. coli*, *Shigella flexneri* or *Shigella sonnei*, *Yersinia enterocolitica*, *Yersinia pseudotuberculosis*). Active against gram-positive bacteria (streptococci, *S. aureus, Nocardia*), gram-negative bacteria (*Enterobacter, E. coli, Proteus, Klebsiella, Shigella*), and protozoa (*P. carinii*).

Dosage/Range: Dose is usually based on trimethoprim component and needs to be specified.

Adult:
- Oral: Trimethoprim 160 mg and sulfamethoxazole 800 mg (double-strength tablet DS) q 12 h × 7–14 days (depending on infection).

Indication	Dosage (mg)	Route	Interval/Duration
P. carinii for pneumonia prophylaxis	1 DS tablet	Oral	2× daily 2 days/week (typically consecutive) OR 1 DS tablet q other day
P. carinii pneumonia in AIDS patients	10–20 mg/kg in 2 to 4 divided doses	IV	q 6–8 h (usually 21 days for *P. carinii* pneumonia in AIDS patients)

Dose modification for renal impairment:

CrCl (mL/min)	Dose Adjustment
Greater than 30	Give usual dose
15–30	Give 1/2 usual dose
Less than 15	Do not administer

Drug Preparation:
- Oral tablets should be stored in tight, light-resistant containers; vials of powder for injection and suspension should be stored at 15–30°C (59–86°F).

Drug Administration:
- Oral: Administer with full (8 oz or 240 mL) glass of water.
- IV: Add each 5 mL of drug to 125 mL of 5% dextrose in water ONLY. Stable for 6 hours. If patient is fluid restricted, can mix each 5 mL in 75 mL of 5% dextrose immediately prior to administration and give within 2 hours. DO NOT REFRIGERATE. Administer over 60–90 minutes.

Drug Interactions:
- Warfarin: increases PT. Monitor PT closely and decrease dose of warfarin as needed.
- Sulfonylureas: increases hypoglycemic effect. Monitor blood glucose closely and reduce sulfonylurea dose as needed.
- Phenytoin: increases and prolongs serum levels. Monitor serum phenytoin level closely and reduce dose as needed.
- Thiazide diuretics (in elderly): increases toxicity (thrombocytopenia with purpura). AVOID CONCURRENT USE.
- Cyclosporine: decreases cyclosporine effect; increases risk of nephrotoxicity. AVOID CONCURRENT USE when possible.
- Methotrexate: increases methotrexate level and potential toxicity (e.g., bone marrow depression). Monitor levels or decrease methotrexate dose as needed.
- Oral contraceptives: decreases contraceptive effect. Monitor for breakthrough bleeding and counsel patient to use barrier contraceptive in addition during antibiotic therapy.
- Ammonium chloride or ascorbic acid: causes antibiotic drug precipitation in kidneys. AVOID CONCURRENT USE.

Lab Effects/Interference:
- Jaffe alkaline picrate reaction overestimation of creatinine by 10%.

Special Considerations:
- Drug is teratogenic, so should not be used in pregnant women if avoidable.
- Drug is excreted in breastmilk and can cause kernicterus in infants. Alternative drug should be used or mother should interrupt breastfeeding during drug use.
- Contraindicated if patient has porphyria.
- Contraindicated in patients with hypersensitivity to sulfites, sulfonamides, or to trimethoprim.
- Contraindicated if severe renal failure (creatinine clearance < 15 mL/min).

COMPLICATIONS

- Use with caution at reduced dosage in patients with glucose-6-phosphate dehydrogenase deficiency (G6PD); hemolysis may occur. Also, use with caution in patients with impaired renal or hepatic function, severe allergy, bronchial asthma, and blood dyscrasias.
- Use cautiously in patients with known hypersensitivity to sulfonamide-derivative drugs such as thiazides, acetazolamide, tolbutamide.
- Increased incidence of adverse side effects in AIDS patients, especially allergic, hematologic reactions. Monitor closely for toxicity.
- Send specimen for culture and sensitivity prior to initial drug dose, as appropriate.

Potential Toxicities/Side Effects and the Nursing Process

I.   ALTERATION IN SKIN INTEGRITY related to HYPERSENSITIVITY REACTION

Defining Characteristics: Skin reactions ranging from mild maculopapular rash with urticaria, pruritus to erythema multiforme, exfoliative dermatitis, and Stevens–Johnson syndrome. Risk for rash is increased in AIDS patients; usually occurs 7–14 days after beginning drug. Other allergic manifestations include fever, chills, photosensitivity, angioedema, and anaphylaxis.

Nursing Implications: Assess for prior hypersensitivity to drug. Assess for signs/symptoms of drug allergy. Instruct patient to report rash, allergic reaction immediately. Discuss any drug continuance with physician if rash appears. Teach patient symptomatic management of discomfort and skin irritation. Be prepared to treat severe acute hypersensitivity reactions with airway management, oxygen, epinephrine, corticosteroids, or antihistamines as ordered.

II.   POTENTIAL FOR INFECTION, BLEEDING, AND FATIGUE related to HEMATOLOGIC TOXICITY

Defining Characteristics: Leukopenia, neutropenia, and thrombocytopenia are common in AIDS patients. Agranulocytosis, aplastic and megaloblastic anemia, thrombocytopenia, hemolytic anemia, neutropenia, hypoprothrombinemia, and eosinophilia may occur less commonly. Increased risk exists in folate-deficient patients: elderly, alcoholic, malnourished; also, patients receiving folate antimetabolites, for example, phenytoin, methotrexate, or thiazide diuretics; or in patients with renal dysfunction.

Nursing Implications: Assess baseline risk, CBC, and monitor CBC periodically during treatment. Assess for and teach patient to monitor signs/symptoms of infection, bleeding, fatigue, and to report these. If side effects occur, discuss with physician use of folinic acid (leucovorin).

III.   ALTERATION IN NUTRITION, LESS THAN BODY REQUIREMENTS, related to GI TOXICITY

Defining Characteristics: Nausea, vomiting, and anorexia are most common; pseudomembranous colitis, glossitis, stomatitis, abdominal pain, or diarrhea may occur.

Nursing Implications: Assess GI function. Teach patient to assess for and instruct to report GI side effects and to administer prescribed antiemetics or antidiarrheals as needed. Assess oral mucosa, and if stomatitis develops, discuss with physician use of leucovorin (folinic acid). Teach patient oral hygiene. Take drug with 8 oz (240 mL) water to prevent esophageal ulcerations. Discuss food preferences, use of spices, and suggest small, frequent meals if anorexia develops.

IV. SENSORY/PERCEPTUAL DYSFUNCTION related to FATIGUE, WEAKNESS

Defining Characteristics: Headache, vertigo, insomnia, fatigue, weakness, mental depression, seizures, and hallucinations may occur.

Nursing Implications: Assess baseline neurologic function and comfort and monitor during treatment. Instruct patient to report any changes. Discuss any abnormalities with physician.

V. ALTERATION IN URINARY ELIMINATION related to RENAL TOXICITY

Defining Characteristics: Increased BUN and creatinine, crystal and stone formation in urine, interstitial nephritis, and renal failure may occur.

Nursing Implications: Assess baseline renal function; expect that drug dose will be decreased in presence of renal dysfunction. Instruct patient to take drug with at least 8 oz water and to increase oral fluids to 2–3 qt/day.

VI. ALTERATION IN COMFORT related to IV ADMINISTRATION

Defining Characteristics: Drug may cause pain, inflammation, and rare thrombophlebitis at IV site.

Nursing Implications: Change IV site q 48 h. Assess for phlebitis, discomfort, and IV patency prior to each administration. Administer drug slowly over 60–90 minutes in large volume of 5% dextrose (see Drug Administration). Apply heat to promote comfort.

VII. FUNGAL SUPERINFECTION related to REDISTRIBUTION OF ENDOGENOUS MICROORGANISMS

Defining Characteristics: Vaginal candidiasis or vaginitis may occur as endogenous bacteria are eliminated and normal fungal population expands.

Nursing Implications: Instruct female patient to report vaginal itching or discharge. Discuss appropriate antifungal treatment with physician. Teach perineal hygiene and symptomatic management.

COMPLICATIONS

Drug: delafloxacin (Baxdela)

Class: Fluoroquinolone.

Mechanism of Action: Antibacterial activity due to inhibition of both bacterial topoisomerase II and IV enzymesrequired for DNA replication, transcription, repair, and recombination.

Metabolism: Well-absorbed from GI tract; rate decreased by food but not extent of absorption. Widely distributed in body tissues and fluids with highest concentrations in organs, such as liver, kidneys, and lungs. Partially metabolized in liver; excreted in urine and feces.

Indication: For treatment of acute bacterial skin infections and skin structure infections (ABSSSI). Has a broad spectrum and is active against gram-negative bacteria (e.g., *Enterobacter, Pseudomonas, Klebseilla,* and *E. coli*), and certain gram-positive organisms (e.g., MRSA, MSSI, various strains of *Streptococcus*), and some mycobacteria.

Dosage/Range:
- PO 450 mg q 12 h × 1–2 weeks.
- IV: 300–450 mg q 12 h × 1–2 weeks (IV used if patient unable to take oral formulation).
- Dosage for patients with renal impairment is based on eGFR. Not recommended with ESRD.

Drug Preparation:
- Oral: Drug can be taken with meal/food.
- IV: Reconstitute drug in 0.9% sodium chloride or 5% dextrose in water to final concentration of 25 mg/mL. Further dilute to a total volume of 250 mL. Administer over 60 minutes.

Drug Interactions:
- Antacids (containing magnesium or aluminum) also sucralfate and iron preparation or multivitamins containing iron or zinc: decrease oral delafloxacin serum level; do not administer concurrently. If must administer antacids, administer at least 2 hours before and 6 hours after antacids.
- Use with steroids increases tendon rupture.
- Theophylline: increases theophylline serum level; avoid if possible, since fatal reactions have occurred. Otherwise, monitor theophylline level very closely and decrease theophylline dose as needed.
- Caffeine: delays caffeine clearance from body. Instruct patient to limit coffee, tea, soft drinks, especially if CNS side effects.

Lab Effects/Interference:
- Serum ALT, serum alk phos, serum AST, and serum LDH values may be increased.

Special Considerations:
- Black Box Warning: Fluoroquinolones associated with disabling, potentially serious adverse reactions, such as: tendinitis, tendon rupture, peripheral neuropathy, and CNS effects.

- Contraindicated in pregnancy and in women who are breastfeeding.
- Obtain ordered specimen for culture and sensitivity prior to first drug dose.
- Use cautiously in patients with seizure disorders.

Potential Toxicities/Side Effects and the Nursing Process

I.   ALTERATION IN NUTRITION, LESS THAN BODY REQUIREMENTS, related to GI SIDE EFFECTS

Defining Characteristics: common side effect is diarrhea.

Nursing Implications: Assess baseline nutritional and elimination status. Instruct patient to report GI disturbances. Administer and teach patient to self-administer antidiarrheals as needed and as ordered. Teach patient importance of nutritious diet and suggest small, frequent, high-calorie, high-protein meals as appropriate.

II.   ALTERATIONS IN SENSORY/PERCEPTUAL PATTERNS related to CNS EFFECTS

Defining Characteristics: Dizziness, hallucinations, and seizures may occur. Peripheral neuropathies have occurred with delafloxacin.

Nursing Implications: Assess baseline neurologic function and comfort and monitor during treatment. Instruct patient to report any changes. Discuss any abnormalities with physician. Teach patient to contact provider if they experience headache or restlessness. Assess for symptoms of peripheral neuropathies. If symptoms of peripheral neuropathy such as pain, burning, tingling, numbness, or weakness develop, discontinue immidately.

III.   ALTERATION IN SKIN INTEGRITY related to ALLERGY/HYPERSENSITIVITY

Defining Characteristics: Fatal hypersensitivity reactions have occurred rarely.

Nursing Implications: Assess baseline skin condition, including integrity and drug allergy history. Instruct patient to report rash, itching, other skin changes. Teach patient skin care and symptomatic measures as appropriate. If skin rash develops, discuss drug discontinuance with physician. If rash progresses, especially in HIV-infected patients, drug should be discontinued as fatal Stevens-Johnson syndrome may develop. Be prepared to treat severe acute hypersensitivity reactions with airway management, oxygen, epinephrine, corticosteroids, antihistamines as ordered.

IV.   FUNGAL SUPERINFECTION related to REDISTRIBUTION OF ENDOGENOUS MICROORGANISMS

Defining Characteristics: Vaginal candidiasis, vaginitis may occur as endogenous bacteria are eliminated and normal fungal population expands.

COMPLICATIONS

Nursing Implications: Instruct female patient to report vaginal itching or discharge. Discuss appropriate antifungal treatment with physician. Teach perineal hygiene and symptomatic management.

V.   TENDONITIS AND TENDON RUPTURE

Defining Characteristics: Black box warning: Fluoroquinolones are associated with an increased risk of tendinitis and tendon rupture in all ages. Risk further increases with age over 60 years, concomitant steroid therapy, and kidney, heart, or lung transplants. Fluoroquinolones may exacerbate muscle weakness in persons with myasthenia gravis. Avoid in patients with known history of myasthenia gravis.

Nursing Implications: Need to warn about tendon ruptures and myasthenia gravis (black box warning). Contact healthcare provider if they experience pain, swelling, inflammation of the tendon or inability to move joint/s or muscle weakness. The risk is higher in people over the age of 60 years.

Drug: dalbavancin (Dalvance)

Class: Antibacterial (systemic).

Mechanism of Action: Semisynthetic lipoglycopeptide, interferes with cell wall synthesis, thereby preventing cross-linking. Dalbavancin is bactericidal in vitro against *S. aureus* and *S. pyogenes*.

Metabolism: Drug is not a substrate, inhibitor, or inducer of CYP450 isoenzymes. A minor metabolite of dalbavancin (hydroxy-dalbavancin) has been observed in urine. A small percentage (20% of dose) is excreted in feces. An average 33% of the administered dose is excreted in urine as unchanged dalbavancin; 12% of administered dose is excreted in urine as metabolite hydroxy-dalbavancin. Elimination half-life is 8.5 days.

Indications: ABSSSI caused by designated susceptible strains of gram-positive microorganisms—*S. aureus* (including methicillin-susceptible and-resistant strains), *S. pyogenes*, *S. agalactiae*, and *S. anginosus* group (including *S. anginosus*, *Streptococcus intermedius*, and *S. constellatus*).

Dosage/Range:
- Two-dose regimen: 1,000 mg, followed 1 week later by 500 mg.
- Dosage adjustment for patients with creatinine clearance less than 30 mL/min and not receiving regularly scheduled hemodialysis: 750 mg, followed 1 week later by 375 mg.
- Administer by IV infusion over 30 minutes.

Drug Preparation:
- Reconstituted vials may be stored either refrigerated at 2–8°C (36–46°F), or at controlled room temperature (20–25°C [68–77°F]). Do not freeze.

- Aseptically transfer required dose of reconstituted dalbavancin solution from vial(s) to an IV bag or bottle containing 5% dextrose injection, USP. The diluted solution must have a final dalbavancin concentration of 1–5 mg/mL. Discard any unused portion of the reconstituted solution.
- Once diluted into an IV bag or bottle, drug may be stored either refrigerated at 2–8°C (36–46°F) or at controlled room temperature (20–25°C [68–77°F]). Do not freeze.
- Total time from reconstitution to dilution to administration should not exceed 48 hours.
- Inspect visually for particulate matter prior to infusion. If particulate matter is identified, do not use.
- Administered via IV infusion, using a total infusion time of 30 minutes.
- Do not coinfuse with other medications or electrolytes. Saline-based infusion solutions may cause precipitation and should not be used. Compatibility with intravenous medications, additives, or substances other than 5% dextrose injection, USP has not been established.
- If a common IV line is being used to administer other drugs, line should be flushed with 5% dextrose injection, USP before and after each dalbavancin infusion.

Drug Interaction: No clinical drug–drug interaction studies have been conducted. There is minimal potential for drug–drug interactions between dalbavancin and cytochrome P450 (CYP450) substrates, inhibitors, or inducers.

Lab Effects/Interference:
- Drug–lab test interactions have not been reported.

Special Considerations:
- Most common adverse reactions in patients treated with dalbavancin were nausea (5.5%), headache (4.7%), and diarrhea (4.4%).
- Hypersensitivity to dalbavancin is possible.
- Serious hypersensitivity (anaphylactic) and skin reactions have been reported with glycopeptide antibacterial agents, including dalbavancin; exercise caution in patients with known hypersensitivity to glycopeptides.
- Rapid IV infusion of glycopeptide antibacterial agents can cause reactions.
- ALT elevations with dalbavancin treatment were reported in clinical trials.
- CDAD is reported with nearly all systemic antibacterial agents, including dalbavancin. Evaluate if diarrhea occurs.

COMPLICATIONS

Potential Toxicities/Side Effects and the Nursing Process

I.   POTENTIAL FOR INJURY related to HYPERSENSITIVITY REACTION

Defining Characteristics: Urticaria, pruritus, rash (maculopapular or erythematous), fever and chills, eosinophilia, myalgia, edema, erythema, and angioedema.

Nursing Implications: Assess allergy to cephalosporin antibiotics and penicillin; if patient states "yes," determine actual response (e.g., "swollen lips angioedema"). If angioedema is present, patient *should not* receive drug. Discuss other patient responses with physician to determine whether drug should be given. Assess baseline skin condition, including integrity, and allergy history to drugs. Instruct patient to report rash, itching, or other skin changes. Teach patient skin care and symptomatic measures as appropriate. If skin rash develops, discuss drug discontinuance with physician. If rash progresses, drug should be discontinued, as fatal Stevens–Johnson syndrome may develop. Be prepared to treat severe acute hypersensitivity reactions with airway management, oxygen, epinephrine, corticosteroids, or antihistamines as ordered.

II.   ALTERATION IN NUTRITION, LESS THAN BODY REQUIREMENTS, related to GI SIDE EFFECTS

Defining Characteristic: Nausea, vomiting, diarrhea, and anorexia may occur; rarely, pseudomembranous colitis caused by *C. difficile* resistant to the antibiotic occurs.

Nursing Implications: Assess baseline nutritional status. Instruct patient to report GI disturbances. Administer, and teach patient to self-administer, antiemetics as needed and as ordered. Teach patient importance of a nutritious diet; suggest small, frequent, high-calorie, high-protein meals as appropriate. Assess baseline LFTs and monitor periodically during treatment. Discuss abnormalities and drug interruption with physician.

III.   FUNGAL SUPERINFECTION related to REDISTRIBUTION OF ENDOGENOUS MICROORGANISMS

Defining Characteristics: Vaginal candidiasis or vaginitis may occur as endogenous bacteria are eliminated and normal fungal population expands.

Nursing Implications: Instruct female patients to report vaginal itching or discharge. Discuss appropriate antifungal treatment with physician. Teach perineal hygiene and symptomatic management.

IV.   ALTERATIONS IN COMFORT related to LOCAL INJECTION-SITE IRRITATION

Defining Characteristics: Pain and phlebitis may develop in IV sites.

Nursing Implications: Change IV sites every 48 hours, and assess for signs and symptoms of phlebitis prior to each administration. Administer drug slowly. Apply warm packs to increase comfort.

V.   ALTERATIONS IN COMFORT related to HEADACHE

Defining Characteristics: Headache has occurred in some patients.

Nursing Implications: Assess baseline hearing (ability to hear spoken voice) and continue to assess during therapy. Teach patient potential side effects, and instruct patient to report any hearing/perceptual problems (e.g., tinnitus, vertigo, decreased hearing). Discuss drug discontinuance and audiogram with physician to confirm hearing dysfunction if symptoms arise. Assess for increased risk if given concurrently with other ototoxic medications (e.g., cisplatin, furosemide).

Drug: daptomycin (Cubicin)

Class: Cyclic lipopeptide antibiotic.

Mechanism of Action: This antibiotic is the first in a new structural class. It is derived from the fermentation of *S. roseosporus*. The mechanism of action is not fully understood. Daptomycin binds to bacterial membranes and causes a rapid depolarization of membrane potential. This loss of membrane potential leads to inhibition of protein, DNA, and RNA synthesis resulting in bacterial cell death. It acts against gram-positive bacteria, and retains in vitro potency against isolates resistant to methicillin, vancomycin, and linezolid.

Metabolism: Excreted by the kidney. Renal excretion is primary route of elimination.

Indication: For treatment of complicated skin and skin structure infections (cSSSI) and septicemias including right-sided endocarditis.

Dosage/Range:

Adult:
• 4 mg/kg by IV infusion q d for 7–14 days.
• Drug dose should be reduced or adjusted in patients with severe renal insufficiency.

Drug Preparation:
• 0.9% sodium chloride injection.
• Administer over 30 minutes.

Drug Interactions:
• Tobramycin: interaction between daptomycin and tobramycin is unknown. Caution is warranted when daptomycin is coadministered with tobramycin.
• Warfarin: anticoagulant activity in patients receiving daptomycin and warfarin should be monitored for the first several days.
• HMG-CoA reductase inhibitors.

Lab Effects/Interference:
• No reported drug-laboratory test interactions. Dapto may falsely prolong INR.

Special Considerations:
• Contraindicated in patients with known hypersensitivity to daptomycin.
• Can cause myopathy and CPK elevations.
• Obtain ordered specimen and send for culture and sensitivity prior to first antibiotic dose.
• Consider alternative antibiotic therapy if anemia, drug rash or fever, arthralgia, or unexplained rise in BUN and serum creatinine occur.

COMPLICATIONS

Potential Toxicities/Side Effects and the Nursing Process

I.   ALTERATION IN NUTRITION, LESS THAN BODY REQUIREMENTS, related to GI SIDE EFFECTS

Defining Characteristics: Constipation, nausea, diarrhea, vomiting, or dyspepsia.

Nursing Implications: Assess baseline nutritional status, preexisting nausea/vomiting, and anorexia. Assess baseline bowel pattern. Administer symptomatic interventions if side effects occur; discuss with physician use of alternative drug(s).

II.   POTENTIAL FOR INJURY related to HYPERSENSITIVITY REACTION

Defining Characteristics: Rash, urticaria, pruritus, and fever can occur in individuals with hypersensitivity to daptomycin.

Nursing Implications: Assess for drug allergies prior to drug administration. Instruct patient to report any allergic reactions. Assess for signs/symptoms of allergic reaction after drug dose.

III.   SENSORY/PERCEPTUAL ALTERATIONS related to CNS EFFECTS OF DIZZINESS AND HEADACHE

Defining Characteristics: Dizziness, headache, and insomnia may occur.

Nursing Implications: Assess baseline neurologic status. Teach patient about side effects and to report dizziness or headache. If signs/symptoms arise, discuss drug discontinuance with physician.

Drug: demeclocycline hydrochloride (Declomycin)

Class: Antibacterial (systemic); tetracycline; antiprotozoal.

Mechanism of Action: Bacteriostatic but may be bactericidal at high concentrations. Binds to bacterial ribosomes and prevents protein synthesis.

Metabolism: Absorbed from the GI tract. Widely distributed into body tissues and fluids. Crosses placenta and is excreted in breastmilk. Concentrated in the liver, excreted into the bile. The rate of demeclocycline hydrochloride clearance is less than half that of tetracycline.

Indication: For treatment of a broad range of gram-negative and gram-positive organisms. Demeclocycline hydrochloride may also be used in special cases of fluid retention (SIADH). A syndrome of polyuria, polydipsia, and weakness has been shown to be nephrogenic, dose-dependent, and reversible on discontinuation of therapy.

Dosage/Range:

Adult:
• Oral: 150 mg q 6 h or 300 mg q 12 h.
• Duration of therapy depends on indication.

- As treatment for hyponatremia: 600–1200 mg daily.
- Tetracyclines including demeclocycline should be avoided when possible in hepatic disease because of their catabolic or antianabolic effects, which may yield an endogenous nitrogen load requiring hepatic metabolism. One-third to two-thirds of patients with pre-existing hepatic disease will develop increased fat in liver cells while receiving tetracyclines. These effects may be reversed after discontinuing the drug.
- Demeclocycline should be avoided in patients with renal failure, as further deterioration of renal function may occur.

Drug Preparation:
- Oral: Take 1 hour before meals or 2 hours after meals.

Drug Interactions:
- Oral anticoagulants: increase PT. Monitor patient closely and decrease anticoagulant dose as needed.
- Concurrent use of tetracyclines with oral contraceptives may render oral contraceptives less effective. Advise patient to use barrier contraceptive as well during a course of tetracycline therapy.
- Methoxyflurane: fatal renal toxicity has been reported with concurrent use.
- Iron preparations: decreases oral absorption. Administer iron preparations 3 hours after or 2 hours before any tetracycline.
- Antacids and antidiarrheals: may decrease absorption of tetracyclines. Avoid concurrent use—can space it out.

Lab Effects/Interference:
- No reported drug-laboratory test interactions.
- SGPT, alk phos, amylase, SGOT, and bilirubin: serum concentrations may be increased.

Special Considerations:
- Avoid use in pregnant or lactating women.
- Children younger than 8 years: avoid—risk for permanent discoloration of the teeth; photosensitivity may occur; discontinue use if erythema occurs
- Long-term therapy; nephrogenic, dose-dependent, and reversible diabetes insipidus syndrome (polyuria, polydipsia, and weakness) has occurred.
- Contraindicated in patients with known hypersensitivity to tetracyclines.
- Obtain ordered specimen and send for culture and sensitivity prior to first antibiotic dose.

COMPLICATIONS

Potential Toxicities/Side Effects and the Nursing Process

I. ALTERATION IN NUTRITION related to GI SIDE EFFECTS

Defining Characteristics: Anorexia, nausea, vomiting, diarrhea, glossitis, dysphagia, enterocolitis, or pancreatitis.

Nursing Implications: Assess baseline nutritional status. Assess for and teach patient to report any symptoms. Administer and teach patient self-administration of prescribed antiemetic or antidiarrheal medication as appropriate. Administer and teach to self-administer oral dose with at least 8 oz of water at least 1 hour before or 2 hours after a meal or sleep.

II.   ALTERATION IN SKIN INTEGRITY related to RASH, PHOTOSENSITIVITY

Defining Characteristics: Maculopapular and erythematous rash may occur. Photosensitivity risk (exaggerated sunburn) persists 1–2 days after completion of drug therapy.

Nursing Implications: Teach patient about potential side effects, to avoid sunlight during drug therapy, and to report rash and other abnormalities. Teach symptomatic skin care as appropriate.

III.   INJURY related to HYPERSENSITIVITY

Defining Characteristics: Urticaria, angioneurotic edema, anaphylaxis may occur; also fever, arthralgias, eosinophilia, and pericarditis.

Nursing Implications: Assess drug allergy history. Assess baseline allergy history. Assess baseline skin integrity. Teach patient to report rash, pruritus. Teach patient symptomatic management of rash, pruritus. Assess for hypersensitivity reaction; if it occurs, monitor VS, discontinue drug, notify physician, and institute supportive measures.

IV.   FUNGAL SUPERINFECTION related to REDISTRIBUTION OF ENDOGENOUS MICROORGANISMS

Defining Characteristics: Vaginal moniliasis or vaginitis may occur as endogenous bacteria are eliminated and normal fungal population expands.

Nursing Implications: Teach female patient to report vaginal itching or discharge. Discuss appropriate antifungal treatment with physician. Teach perineal hygiene and symptom management.

Drug: dicloxacillin sodium (Dycill, Dynapen, Pathocil)

Class: Penicillin antibacterial.

Mechanism of Action: Semisynthetic antibiotic prepared from fungus *Penicillium*. Contains β-lactam ring and is bactericidal by inhibiting cell wall synthesis.

Metabolism: Well-absorbed from GI tract, but food decreases rate and extent of absorption. Widely distributed through body tissues and fluids; crosses placenta and is excreted in breastmilk; 95–99% bound to serum proteins. Excreted in urine and bile.

Indication: For treatment of, and active against, penicillin-resistant staphylococci that produce penicillinase. Used to treat upper and lower respiratory tract and skin infections.

Dosage/Range:
- Adult: 125–500 mg PO q 6 h × 14 days (depends on severity of infection).

Drug Preparation:
• Store in tight containers at < 40°C (104°F).

Drug Administration:
• Oral: administer at least 1 hour before or 2 hours after meals.
• **Drug interacts with** methotrexate, warfarin, tetracyclines, bupropion, donepezil, and typhoid vaccine.
• Probenecid: increased serum level of penicillin; may be coadministered to exert this effect.

Lab Effects/Interference:

Major clinical significance:
• Urine glucose: high urinary concentrations of a penicillin may produce false-positive or falsely elevated test results with copper sulfate tests (Benedict's, Clinitest, or Fehling's); glucose enzymatic tests (Clinistix or Tes-Tape) are not affected.

Clinical significance:
• Coombs' (direct antiglobulin) test: false-positive result may occur during therapy with any penicillin.
• ALT, alk phos, AST, serum LDH values may be increased.
• WBC: leukopenia or neutropenia is associated with the use of all penicillins; the effect is more likely to occur with prolonged therapy and severe hepatic function impairment.

Special Considerations:
• Contraindicated in patients with prior hypersensitivity to penicillins. Use with caution in patients sensitive to other β-lactams (e.g., cephalosporins) since partial cross-allergenicity exists.
• Obtain ordered specimen and send for culture and sensitivity prior to first antibiotic dose.
• Consider alternative antibiotic therapy if eosinophilia, drug fever or rash, arthralgia, hematuria, or unexplained rise in BUN and serum creatinine occur.
• Monitor electrolytes and renal, hepatic, and hematologic laboratory parameters during extended treatment periods.
• Use with caution in pregnancy or with nursing women.

COMPLICATIONS

Potential Toxicities/Side Effects and the Nursing Process

I. POTENTIAL FOR INJURY related to HYPERSENSITIVITY REACTION

Defining Characteristics: Urticaria, pruritus, rash (maculopapular or erythematous), fever and chills, eosinophilia, myalgia, edema, erythema, angioedema, Stevens–Johnson syndrome, and exfoliative skin reactions occur in 5% of patients. Increased risk exists in individuals allergic to cephalosporin antibiotics.

Nursing Implications: Assess allergy to cephalosporin antibiotics and penicillin: if patient states "yes," determine actual response (e.g., "swollen lips = angioedema"). If angioedema, patient should not receive drug. Discuss other patient responses with physician to determine whether drug should be given. Assess baseline skin condition including integrity and allergy history to drugs. Instruct patient to report rash, itching, or other skin changes. Teach patient skin care and symptomatic measures as appropriate. If skin rash develops, discuss drug discontinuance with physician. If rash progresses, drug should be discontinued, as fatal Stevens–Johnson syndrome may develop. Be prepared to treat severe acute hypersensitivity reactions with airway management, oxygen, epinephrine, corticosteroids, or antihistamines as ordered.

II.   ALTERATION IN NUTRITION, LESS THAN BODY REQUIREMENTS, related to GI SIDE EFFECTS

Defining Characteristics: Nausea, vomiting, or diarrhea may occur; rarely, pseudomembranous colitis caused by *C. difficile* resistant to the antibiotic occurs. Rarely, transient increases in LFTs—AST, ALT, alk phos, bili—may occur.

Nursing Implications: Assess baseline nutritional status. Instruct patient to report GI disturbances. Administer and teach patient to self-administer antiemetics as needed and as ordered. Teach patient importance of nutritious diet and suggest small, frequent, high-calorie, high-protein meals as appropriate. Assess baseline LFTs, and monitor periodically during treatment. Discuss abnormalities and drug interruption with physician.

III.   FUNGAL SUPERINFECTION related to REDISTRIBUTION OF ENDOGENOUS MICROORGANISMS

Defining Characteristics: Vaginal candidiasis or vaginitis may occur as endogenous bacteria are eliminated and normal fungal population expands.

Nursing Implications: Instruct female patient to report vaginal itching or discharge. Discuss appropriate antifungal treatment with physician. Teach perineal hygiene and symptomatic management.

IV.   ALTERATIONS IN PROTECTIVE MECHANISMS (RARE) related to TRANSIENT LEUKOPENIA

Defining Characteristics: Rarely, transient leukopenia, lymphocytosis, anemia, or eosinophilia may occur. Prolonged PT, prolonged aPTT, and hypoprothrombinemia have occurred rarely, especially in elderly or debilitated patients, or in individuals with vitamin K deficiency.

Nursing Implications: Assess baseline laboratory parameters, and monitor periodically during treatment. Assess patient for response to antibiotics. Discuss abnormalities with physician.

V. KNOWLEDGE DEFICIT related to SELF-ADMINISTRATION OF MEDICATION

Defining Characteristics: Increased compliance when patient is instructed in self-care activities.

Nursing Implications: Assess knowledge about infection and planned treatment. Teach about drug action, potential side effects, and when and how to take drug (take medication as directed, 1 hour before or 2 hours after food). Instruct patient to report any possible drug side effects that occur.

Drug: doripenem (Doribax)

Class: Antibacterial. Doripenem is a β-lactam antibiotic, carbapenem type.

Mechanism of Action: Bactericidal through inhibition of cell wall synthesis, with resulting cell wall instability and cell lysis.

Metabolism: Metabolized to an inactive ring-opened metabolite by dehydropeptidase-I. Doripenem is not a substrate for hepatic CYP450 enzymes. Within 48 hours, approximately 70% is excreted unchanged by the kidneys and 15% as the ring-opened metabolite. Less than 1% excreted in feces after 1 week. Pharmacokinetics are linear over a dose range of 500- to 1,000-mg IV over 1 hour. Following a single 1-hour IV infusion of 500 mg, the mean plasma C_{max} and AUC are 23 μg/mL and 36.3 μg h/mL, respectively. Dosage adjustment is necessary in patients with moderate and severe renal function impairment. Hepatic function impairment: Not established; however, because doripenem does not undergo hepatic *metabolism,* the pharmacokinetics are not expected to be affected by hepatic function impairment.

Indication: For treatment of cIAI and cUTI, including pyelonephritis, caused by susceptible strains of specific microorganisms. Active against most anaerobic and aerobic gram-positive and gram-negative organisms. Doripenem demonstrates more potent activity against *P. aeruginosa* than imipenem.

Dosage/Range:

Indication	Dosage (mg)	Route	Interval/Duration
Intra-abdominal infection	500	IV	Administer over 1 h; q 8 h for 5–14 days
UTI, including pyelonephritis	500	IV	Administer over 1 h; q 8 h for 10 days May extend to 14 days for bacteremia
Renal function impairment— CrCl 30–50 mL/min or less	250	IV	Administer over 1 h; q 8 h
Renal function impairment— CrCl greater than 10 to less than 30 mL/min	250	IV	Administer over 1 h; q 12 h

COMPLICATIONS

Drug Preparation:
- Store vial at 59–86°F. Constituted suspension in vial may be stored for 1 hour prior to dilution in infusion bag. Infusion solution prepared in normal saline may be stored at room temperature for 8 hours (includes infusion time) or under refrigeration for 24 hours (includes infusion time). Infusion solution prepared in dextrose 5% may be stored at room temperature for 4 hours (includes infusion time) or under refrigeration for 24 hours (includes infusion time).
- Product does not contain a bacteriostatic preservative.
- To prepare 500-mg dose: constitute with 10 mL of sterile water for injection or sodium chloride 0.9% injection, gently shaking vial to form a suspension (concentration, 50 mg/mL). Withdraw suspension and add to infusion bag containing normal saline 100 mL or dextrose 5%, gently shaking until clear (concentration, 4.5 mg/mL).
- To prepare 250-mg dose: constitute with 10 mL of sterile water for injection or sodium chloride 0.9% injection, gently shaking vial to form a suspension (concentration, 50 mg/mL). Withdraw suspension and add to infusion bag containing normal saline 100 mL or dextrose 5%, gently shaking until clear (concentration, 4.5 mg/mL). Remove 55 mL of this solution from bag and discard. Infuse remaining solution (concentration, 4.5 mg/mL).
- Do not mix product with or physically add to solutions containing other drugs.
- Consider a switch to appropriate oral therapy after at least 3 days of parenteral therapy, once clinical improvement has been demonstrated.

Drug Interactions:
- Probenecid: Doripenem plasma levels may be increased and prolonged because of interference with active tubular secretion by probenecid.
- Valproic acid: Valproic acid serum concentrations may be reduced to subtherapeutic levels, resulting in loss of seizure control. If serum valproic acid levels cannot be maintained in the therapeutic range or if seizures occur, consider alternative antibacterial or anticonvulsant therapy.

Lab Effects/Interference:
- None well-documented.

Special Considerations:
- Lactation: Undetermined.
- Hypersensitivity: Serious and occasionally fatal anaphylactic and serious skin reactions have been reported in patients receiving β-lactam antibiotics. These reactions are more likely to occur in individuals with a history of sensitivity to multiple allergens.
- Superinfection: May result in bacterial or fungal overgrowth of nonsusceptible organisms.
- Pseudomembranous colitis: Consider possibility in patients with diarrhea.
- **Contraindicated in patients hypersensitive to doripenem,** and serious skin reactions have been reported in patients receiving β-lactam antibiotics. Use cautiously in patients sensitive to penicillin or other β-lactams, as partial cross-allergenicity exists.
- Drug dosage needs to be reduced if moderate to severe renal insufficiency.

Potential Toxicities/Side Effects and the Nursing Process

I.   POTENTIAL FOR INJURY related to HYPERSENSITIVITY REACTION

Defining Characteristics: Urticaria, pruritus, rash (maculopapular or erythematous), fever and chills, eosinophilia, myalgia, edema, erythema, angioedema, Stevens–Johnson syndrome, and exfoliative skin reactions occur in 5% of patients. Increased risk in individuals allergic to penicillin.

Nursing Implications: Assess allergy to cephalosporin antibiotics and penicillin: if patient states "yes," determine actual response (e.g., "swollen lips = angioedema"). If angioedema, discuss with physician risk versus benefit prior to drug administration, as there is partial cross-allergenicity. Discuss other patient responses with physician to determine whether drug should be given. Assess baseline skin condition, including integrity and allergy history to drugs. Instruct patient to report rash, itching, or other skin changes. Teach patient skin care and symptomatic measures as appropriate. If skin rash develops, discuss drug discontinuance with physician. If rash progresses, drug should be discontinued, as fatal Stevens–Johnson syndrome may develop. Be prepared to treat severe acute hypersensitivity reactions with airway management, oxygen, epinephrine, corticosteroids, or antihistamines as ordered.

II.   ALTERATION IN NUTRITION, LESS THAN BODY REQUIREMENTS, related to GI SIDE EFFECTS

Defining Characteristics: Nausea, vomiting occurs more frequently than diarrhea and anorexia; rarely, pseudomembranous colitis caused by *C. difficile* resistant to the antibiotic occurs. Rarely, transient increases in LFTs—AST, ALT, alk phos, bili—may occur.

Nursing Implications: Assess baseline nutritional status. Instruct patient to report GI disturbances. Administer and teach patient to self-administer antiemetics as needed and as ordered. Teach patient importance of nutritious diet and suggest small, frequent, high-calorie, high-protein meals as appropriate. Assess baseline LFTs and monitor periodically during treatment. Discuss abnormalities and drug interruption with physician.

III.   FUNGAL SUPERINFECTION related to REDISTRIBUTION OF ENDOGENOUS MICROORGANISMS

Defining Characteristics: Vaginal candidiasis or vaginitis may occur as endogenous bacteria are eliminated and normal fungal population expands.

Nursing Implications: Instruct female patient to report vaginal itching or discharge. Discuss appropriate antifungal treatment with physician. Teach perineal hygiene and symptomatic management.

COMPLICATIONS

IV.   ALTERATIONS IN PROTECTIVE MECHANISMS (RARE) related to ANEMIA

Defining Characteristics: Rarely, anemia may occur.

Nursing Implications: Assess baseline laboratory parameters, and monitor periodically during treatment. Assess patient for response to antibiotics. Discuss abnormalities with physician.

V.   ALTERATIONS IN SENSORY/PERCEPTUAL PATTERNS related to HEADACHE AND SEIZURES

Defining Characteristics: Headache, somnolence, and seizures occur rarely. Most seizures have occurred in patients with preexisting CNS problems, those who had received higher-than-recommended IV doses, the elderly, and patients with impaired renal function.

Nursing Implications: Assess baseline neurologic function and comfort, and monitor during treatment. Instruct patient to report any changes. Discuss any abnormalities with physician. Institute seizure precautions. If seizures occur, discuss with physician anticonvulsant therapy or discontinuance of antibiotic.

VI.   ALTERATIONS IN COMFORT related to LOCAL INJECTION IRRITATION

Defining Characteristics: Phlebitis may develop in IV sites.

Nursing Implications: Change IV sites q 48 h, and assess for signs/symptoms of phlebitis prior to each administration. Administer drug slowly. Apply warm packs to increase comfort.

Drug: doxycycline hyclate (Vibramycin, Doryx, Monodox)

Class: Antibacterial (systemic); antiprotozoal.

Mechanism of Action: Bacteriostatic but may be bactericidal at high concentrations. Binds to bacterial ribosomes and prevents protein synthesis.

Metabolism: Absorbed (60–80%) from GI tract. Widely distributed into body tissues and fluids. Crosses placenta and is excreted in breastmilk. Excreted unchanged in urine.

Indication: Drug is used for treatment of a broad range of gram-positive and gram-negative bacteria, *Chlamydia,* and *Mycoplasma.* It may be used to treat acne, certain amoeba infections, and as a preventive for malaria and anthrax.

Dosage/Range:

Adult:

Route	Induction Dosage	Maintenance Dosage (mg)	Interval	Duration of Therapy
Oral	100 mg for first day	100–200 OR 50–100	1× daily q 12 h	Depends on indication
IV	200 mg for first day OR 100 mg q 12 h for first day	100–200 OR 50–100	Daily OR q 12 h	

Drug Preparation:
- Oral: may be taken with food, water, milk, or carbonated beverages.
- IV: add 10 mL sterile water for injection to 100-mg vial or 20 mL to each 200-mg vial. Further dilute in 100–1,000 mL or in 200–2,000 mL, respectively, of lactated Ringer's injection or 5% dextrose and lactated Ringer's injection. Infuse over 1–4 hours.
- CONCENTRATIONS LESS THAN 100 MICROGRAMS/ML OR GREATER THAN 1 MG/ML ARE NOT RECOMMENDED.
- AVOID RAPID ADMINISTRATION.
- Solution stable for 6 hours, so use after mixing. Avoid exposure to heat or sunlight. Convert to oral preparation as soon as possible, as there is risk of thrombophlebitis.
- DO NOT ADMINISTER INTRAMUSCULARLY OR SUBCUTANEOUSLY.

Drug Interactions:
- Hepatotoxic drugs: may increase hepatotoxicity if given concurrently. Assess baseline and periodically during treatment.
- Iron preparations: decrease oral and possibly IV absorption. Administer iron preparations 3 hours after or 2 hours before any tetracycline.
- Oral anticoagulants: increase PT. Monitor patient closely and decrease anticoagulant dose as needed.
- Antidiarrheals (containing kaolin, pectate, or bismuth): may decrease absorption of tetracyclines. Avoid concurrent use.
- Oral contraceptives: decreased effectiveness of contraceptive and increased incidence of breakthrough bleeding. Advise patient to use barrier contraceptive as well during a course of tetracycline therapy.
- Lithium: may decrease lithium levels. Monitor serum levels and increase dose as needed.

Lab Effects/Interference:
- Urine catecholamine determinations: may produce false elevations of urinary catecholamines because of interfering fluorescence in the Hingerty method.
- SGPT, alk phos, amylase, SGOT, and bilirubin: serum concentrations may be increased.

COMPLICATIONS

Special Considerations:
- Use cautiously in patients with myasthenia gravis: may increase muscle weakness.
- Avoid use in pregnant or lactating women.
- Obtain ordered specimen for culture and sensitivity prior to first dose.
- IV preparation contains ascorbic acid and may cause false-positive result using Clinitest, or false-negative result when using Clinistix and Tes-Tape.
- Drug has affinity for ischemic, necrotic tissue, and may localize in tumors.
- Concomitant use: Avoid isotretinoin use.
- Concomitant use: Avoid penicillin use.
- Sunlight or ultraviolet light exposure increases risk for photosensitivity; discontinue if skin erythema occurs.
- Intracranial hypertension (IH) has been reported, especially in women of childbearing age who are overweight or have a history of IH, and may result in permanent vision loss; if symptoms occur, monitoring recommended.

Potential Toxicities/Side Effects and the Nursing Process

I. ALTERATION IN NUTRITION related to GI SIDE EFFECTS

Defining Characteristics: Nausea, vomiting, diarrhea, anorexia, abdominal discomfort, epigastric burning and distress, glossitis, or black, hairy tongue may occur.

Nursing Implications: Assess baseline nutritional status. Assess for and teach patient to report any symptoms. Administer and teach patient self-administration of prescribed antiemetic or antidiarrheal medication as appropriate. Administer and teach patient to self-administer oral dose with at least 8 oz of water taken at least 1 hour before lying down for sleep.

II. ALTERATION IN SKIN INTEGRITY related to RASH, PHOTOSENSITIVITY

Defining Characteristics: Maculopapular and erythematous rashes may occur. Rarely, exfoliative dermatitis, onycholysis, and nail discoloration. Photosensitivity risk (exaggerated sunburn) persists 1–2 days after completion of drug therapy.

Nursing Implications: Teach patient about potential side effects, to avoid sunlight during drug therapy, and to report rash, other abnormalities. Teach symptomatic skin care as appropriate.

III. INJURY related to HYPERSENSITIVITY

Defining Characteristics: Urticaria, angioneurotic edema, or anaphylaxis may occur; also, fever, rash, arthralgias, eosinophilia, and pericarditis.

Nursing Implications: Assess drug allergy history. Assess baseline allergy history. Assess baseline skin integrity. Teach patient to report rash, pruritus. Teach patient symptomatic management of rash, pruritus. Assess for hypersensitivity reaction; if it occurs, monitor VS, discontinue drug, notify physician, and institute supportive measures.

IV. FUNGAL SUPERINFECTION related to REDISTRIBUTION OF ENDOGENOUS MICROORGANISMS

Defining Characteristics: Vaginal moniliasis or vaginitis may occur as endogenous bacteria are eliminated and normal fungal population expands.

Nursing Implications: Teach female patient to report vaginal itching or discharge. Discuss appropriate antifungal treatment with physician. Teach perineal hygiene and symptomatic management.

V. ALTERATION IN HEPATIC FUNCTION

Defining Characteristics: Associated with high IV doses (> 2 g/day): hepatotoxicity and cholestasis may occur.

Nursing Implications: Assess baseline LFTs and monitor during therapy.

VI. INFECTION AND BLEEDING related to NEUTROPENIA, THROMBOCYTOPENIA

Defining Characteristics: Neutropenia, leukocytosis, leukopenia, atypical lymphocytes, thrombocytopenia, thrombocytopenic purpura, or hemolytic anemia occur rarely with long-term therapy.

Nursing Implications: Assess baseline WBC, hematocrit, and platelets, and monitor periodically during long-term therapy.

VII. ALTERATIONS IN COMFORT related to LOCAL ADMINISTRATION EFFECTS

Defining Characteristics: IM administration may cause pain, induration due to muscle injury. IV administration may cause erythema, pain, swelling, and thrombophlebitis.

Nursing Implications: Rotate sites. Apply ice as ordered to painful buttock. Assess IV site prior to each dose for phlebitis or swelling and change site at least q 48 h. Apply heat to painful IV sites as ordered.

VIII. SENSORY/PERCEPTUAL ALTERATION

Defining Characteristics: Lightheadedness, dizziness, or headache may occur.

Nursing Implications: Assess baseline neurologic status. Teach patient to report any changes and discuss them with physician.

COMPLICATIONS

Drug: eravacycline (Xerava)

Class: Synthetic tetracycline-class antibacterial

Mechanism of Action: Eravacycline is an fluorocycline antibacterial within the tetracycline class of antibacterial drugs. Bacteriostatic but may be bactericidal at high concentrations. Binds to bacterial ribosomes and prevents protein synthesis.

Metabolism: Eravacycline metabolized primarily by CYP3A4- and FMO-mediated oxidation. Widely distributed into body tissues and fluids. Crosses placenta and is excreted in breastmilk. Excreted unchanged in urine (34%) and feces (47%).

Indication: Drug is used for complicated intra-abdominal infections (cIAI) in patients 18 years and older. Examples of susceptible organisms are *E. coli, K. pneumoniae, E. faecium, Streptococcus anginosus* group, *C. perfringens*, and *Parabacteroids distasonis*.

Dosage/Range:

Adult:
- IV: 1 mg/kg every 12 hours. Administer over 60 minutes every 12 hours. Duration of therapy for cIAI is 4 to 14 days.
- Patients with severe hepatic impairment: Administer 1 mg/kg every 12 hours day 1; 1 mg/kg every 24 hours day 2 for a total duration of 4 to 14 days. No dose adjustment with mild to moderate hepatic impairment.
- Patients with concomitant use of strong CYP3A inducer: Administer 1.5 mg/kg every 12 hours for a total of 4 to 14 days. No dose adjustment is warranted in patients with concomitant use of a weak or moderate CYP3A inducer.

Drug Preparation:
- IV: Reconstitute with 5 mL sterile water for injection. Further dilute 0.9% sodium chloride injection. Target concentration in IV bag should be 0.3 mg/kg. Infuse over 60 minutes.
- AVOID RAPID ADMINISTRATION.
- DO NOT ADMINISTER INTRAMUSCULARLY OR SUBCUTANEOUSLY.

Drug Interactions:
- Eravacycline compatibility with other drugs and infusion solutions has not been established.
- Hepatotoxic drugs: may increase hepatotoxicity if given concurrently. Assess baseline and periodically during treatment.
- Oral anticoagulants: increase PT. Monitor patient closely and decrease anticoagulant dose as needed.
- Antidiarrheals (containing kaolin, pectate, or bismuth): may decrease absorption of tetracyclines. Avoid concurrent use.
- Oral contraceptives: decreased effectiveness of contraceptive and increased incidence of breakthrough bleeding. Advise patient to use barrier contraceptive as well during a course of tetracycline therapy.

Lab Effects/Interference:
- SGPT, alk phos, amylase, SGOT, and bilirubin: serum concentrations may be increased.

Special Considerations:
- Use cautiously in patients with myasthenia gravis: may increase muscle weakness.
- Avoid use in pregnant or lactating women.
- Obtain ordered specimen for culture and sensitivity prior to first dose.
- Sunlight or ultraviolet light exposure increases risk for photosensitivity; discontinue if skin erythema occurs

Potential Toxicities/Side Effects and the Nursing Process

I. ALTERATION IN NUTRITION related to GI SIDE EFFECTS

Defining Characteristics: Nausea, vomiting, diarrhea, anorexia, abdominal discomfort, epigastric burning and distress, glossitis may occur.

Nursing Implications: Assess baseline nutritional status. Assess for and teach patient to report any symptoms. Administer and teach patient self-administration of prescribed antiemetic or antidiarrheal medication as appropriate. Administer and teach patient to self-administer oral dose with at least 8 oz of water taken at least 1 hour before lying down for sleep.

II. ALTERATION IN SKIN INTEGRITY related to RASH, PHOTOSENSITIVITY

Defining Characteristics: Maculopapular and erythematous rashes may occur. Rarely, exfoliative dermatitis, onycholysis, and nail discoloration. Photosensitivity risk (exaggerated sunburn) persists 1–2 days after completion of drug therapy.

Nursing Implications: Teach patient about potential side effects, to avoid sunlight during drug therapy, and to report rash, other abnormalities. Teach symptomatic skin care as appropriate.

III. INJURY related to HYPERSENSITIVITY

Defining Characteristics: Urticaria, angioneurotic edema, anaphylaxis may occur; also, fever, rash, arthralgias, eosinophilia, and pericarditis.

Nursing Implications: Assess drug allergy history. Assess baseline allergy history. Assess baseline skin integrity. Teach patient to report rash, pruritus. Teach patient symptomatic management of rash, pruritus. Assess for hypersensitivity reaction; if it occurs, monitor VS, discontinue drug, notify physician, and institute supportive measures.

IV. FUNGAL SUPERINFECTION related to REDISTRIBUTION OF ENDOGENOUS MICROORGANISMS

Defining Characteristics: Vaginal moniliasis, vaginitis may occur as endogenous bacteria are eliminated and normal fungal population expands.

COMPLICATIONS

Nursing Implications: Teach female patient to report vaginal itching or discharge. Discuss appropriate antifungal treatment with physician. Teach perineal hygiene and symptomatic management.

V.   TETRACYCLINE CLASS ADVERSE REACTIONS

Defining Characteristics: Omadacycline is similar to tetracycline-class antibacterial drugs and may have similar adverse reactions. In addition to photosensitivity, tetracycline-class adverse reaction include pseudotumor cerebri, anti-anabolic action (increased BUN, azotemia, hyperphosphatemia, pancreatitis, abnormal liver function tests).

Nursing Implications: Teach patients to be aware of tooth discoloration and enamel hypoplasia Drug may cause permanent discoloration of teeth (yellow-gray-brown) especially during last half of pregnancy. May cause reversible inhibition of bone growth if used during the second and third trimesters of pregnancy.

VI.   ALTERATIONS IN COMFORT related to LOCAL ADMINISTRATION EFFECTS

Defining Characteristics: IV administration may cause erythema, pain, swelling, and thrombophlebitis.

Nursing Implications: Assess IV site prior to each dose for phlebitis or swelling and change site at least q 48 hours. Apply heat to painful IV sites as ordered.

Drug: ertapenem sodium (Invanz)

Class: Antibiotic, carbapenem.

Mechanism of Action: The bactericidal activity results from the inhibition of cell wall synthesis. Penetrates the cell wall of most gram-positive and gram-negative bacteria to reach PBP targets.

Metabolism: Widely distributed in body tissues and fluids, excreted in urine.

Indication: For treatment of gynecologic infections (*S. agalactiae* [group B streptococci], *E. coli, B. fragilis, Porphyromonas asaccharolytica, Peptostreptococcus*, or *Prevotella bivia*); intra-abdominal infections (*E. coli, Clostridium clostridioforme, Eubacterium lentum, Peptostreptococcus, B. fragilis, B. distasonis, B. ovatus, B. thetaiotaomicron, B. uniformis*); respiratory tract infections (penicillin-susceptible *S. pneumoniae*, non-beta-lactamase–producing strains of *H. influenzae, M. catarrhalis*); skin and skin structures (oxacillin-susceptible [methicillin-susceptible] strains of *S. aureus, S. agalactiae*, group A beta-hemolytic *S. pyogenes, E. coli, K. pneumoniae, P. mirabilis, B. fragilis, Peptostreptococcus* species, *P. asaccharolytica*, or *P. bivia*); urinary tract infections (*E. coli, K. pneumoniae*).

Dosage/Range:

Adult:

Indication	Dosage (g)	Route	Interval/Duration
Acute pelvic infection	1	IV or IM	1× daily for 3–10 days
Community-acquired pneumonia	1	IV or IM	1× daily for 10–14 days
Intra-abdominal infection	1	IV or IM	1× daily for 5–14 days
Skin/skin structure infections	1	IV or IM	1× daily for 7–14 days
Urinary tract infections	1	IV or IM	1× daily for 10–14 days
Diabetic foot infections	1	IV or IM	1× daily for 7–14 days
Renally impaired patients with CrCl of 30 mL/min/1.73 m² or less May be at risk for seizures	Dose adjustment recommended		

- Adjust dose in patients with renal impairment and on hemodialysis.

Drug Administration:
- IV infusion for up to 14 days.
- IM injection for up to 7 days.
- DO NOT DILUTE WITH diluents containing dextrose.

Drug Interactions:
- Probenecid competes with ertapenem for active tubular secretion; increasing AUC by 25% and reducing the plasma and renal clearances by 20 and 35%, respectively.
- Drug interacts with valproic acid and tacrolimus (increase in tacrolimus levels).

Lab Effects/Interference:
- Ertapenem possesses the characteristic low toxicity of the β-lactam group of antibiotics.
- Periodically assess organ system function: renal, hepatic, and hematopoietic.

Potential Toxicities/Side Effects and the Nursing Process

I.   POTENTIAL FOR INJURY related to HYPERSENSITIVITY REACTION AND LOCAL REACTIONS (pain at injection site)

Defining Characteristics: Urticaria, pruritus, rash (maculopapular or erythematous), fever and chills, eosinophilia, myalgia, edema, erythema, angioedema.

Nursing Implications: Assess allergy to cephalosporin antibiotics and penicillin; if patient states "yes," determine actual response (e.g., "swollen lips = angioedema"). If angioedema, patient SHOULD NOT receive drug. Discuss other patient responses with physician to determine whether drug should be given. Assess baseline skin condition including integrity and allergy history to drugs. Instruct patient to report rash, itching, or other skin changes. Teach patient skin care and symptomatic measures as appropriate. If skin rash develops,

COMPLICATIONS

discuss drug discontinuance with physician. Be prepared to treat severe acute hypersensitivity reactions with airway management, oxygen, epinephrine, corticosteroids, or antihistamines as ordered.

II. ALTERATION IN NUTRITION, LESS THAN BODY REQUIREMENTS, related to GI SIDE EFFECTS

Defining Characteristics: Nausea, vomiting, and diarrhea may occur; rarely, pseudomembranous colitis caused by antibiotic resistance occurs.

Nursing Implications: Assess baseline nutritional status. Instruct patient to report GI disturbances. Administer and teach patient to self-administer antiemetics as needed and as ordered. Teach patient importance of nutritious diet and suggest small, frequent, high-calorie, high-protein meals as appropriate. Assess baseline LFTs, and monitor periodically during treatment. Discuss abnormalities and drug interruption with physician.

III. FUNGAL SUPERINFECTION related to REDISTRIBUTION OF ENDOGENOUS MICROORGANISMS

Defining Characteristics: Vaginal candidiasis or vaginitis may occur as endogenous bacteria are eliminated and normal fungal population expands.

Nursing Implications: Instruct female patient to report vaginal itching or discharge. Discuss appropriate antifungal treatment with physician. Teach perineal hygiene and symptomatic management.

Drug: erythromycin (ERYC, E-Mycin, Ilotycin, Erythrocin)

Class: Antibacterial (macrolide).

Mechanism of Action: Erythromycin is a bacteriostatic macrolide antibiotic. It may be bactericidal in high concentrations or when used against highly susceptible organisms. It is thought to penetrate the bacterial cell membrane and to reversibly bind to the 50S ribosomal subunit. It does not directly inhibit peptide formation; rather, it inhibits the translocation of peptides from the acceptor site on the ribosome to the donor site, inhibiting subsequent protein synthesis. Effective against actively dividing organisms.

Metabolism: 90% of the drug is metabolized by the liver; may accumulate in patients with severe hepatic disease. Primarily excreted into the bile. Between 2% and 5% is excreted unchanged by the kidneys following oral administration; 12–15% excreted unchanged following IV administration. Erythromycins cross the placental barrier in pregnancy; can be found in breastmilk.

Indication: For treatment of bacterial infections, such as bronchitis, diphtheria, Legionnaires' disease, pertussis, pneumonia, rheumatic fever, venereal disease, and ear, intestine, lung, urinary tract, and skin infections. Erythromycin is a broad-spectrum antibiotic with activity against gram-positive and gram-negative bacteria, and other infectious agents, including *Chlamydia trachomatis,* mycoplasmas (*Mycoplasma pneumoniae* and *Ureaplasma urealyticum*), and spirochetes (*Treponema pallidum* and *Borrelia* species). Erythromycin has good activity against *S. pyogenes, S. pneumoniae* (group A beta-hemolytic streptococci), and *S. aureus*.

Dosage/Range:

Route	Dosage (mg)	Interval/Duration
Oral	250 OR	q 6 h for 10 days
	500 OR	q 6 h for 10 days
	333	q 8 h for 10 days
IV	500	q 6 h
	Up to 1,000	q 6 h for Legionnaires' disease

Drug Preparation:
- Further dilute in 0.9% sodium chloride to a concentration of 1–5 mg/mL (500 mg/100 mL, 1,000 mg/250 mL).
- Reconstitute 500-mg or 1-g vials with 10 or 20 mL, respectively, of sterile water for injection only (no preservatives).

Drug Administration:
- Must not be given IV push.
- Intermittent IV infusion over 1 hour is appropriate.

Drug Interactions:
- Use of alcohol concurrently with IV erythromycin increases peak blood alcohol concentrations by 40%; this is thought to be related to rapid gastric emptying, less exposure to alcohol dehydrogenase in the gastric mucosa, and slower small intestine transit time.
- Concurrent use of astemizole or terfenadine with erythromycins is contraindicated and may increase risk of cardiotoxicity, such as torsades de pointes, ventricular tachycardia, and death—other medications can prolong QT.
- Erythromycins may inhibit carbamazepine and valproic acid metabolism, resulting in increased anticonvulsant plasma concentration and toxicity.
- Concurrent use of chloramphenicol, lincomycins, and erythromycins is not recommended due to their antagonizing effects. It is best to avoid concurrent use of bactericidal and bacteriostatic drugs until culture and sensitivity results are determined.
- Erythromycin can increase cyclosporin plasma concentrations and may increase the risk of nephrotoxicity.
- Erythromycins inhibit the metabolism of ergotamine and increase the vasospasm associated with ergotamines.
- Simultaneous administration of erythromycin and lovastatin should be used with caution since concurrent use may increase the risk of rhabdomyolysis.

COMPLICATIONS

- Concurrent use of midazolam and triazolam with erythromycins can increase the pharmacologic effect of these drugs.
- Erythromycins may cause prolonged prothrombin time and increased risk of hemorrhage, especially in the elderly.
- Use of erythromycins and xanthines (i.e., aminophylline, caffeine, oxtriphylline, and theophylline) may lead to increased serum levels of xanthines and toxicity.
- Drug interactions occur with warfarin, fentanyl and other QT prolonging drugs, idelalisib, nintedanib, quinolones, darunavir, afatinib, fluoxetine, and lopinavir.

Lab Effects/Interference:
- Serum SGPT, serum SGOT, serum bilirubin, and alkaline phosphatase—values may be increased by all erythromycins.
- Urinary catecholamines may produce false-positive results when patient is on erythromycin.

Special Considerations:
- Do not use when there is a known hypersensitivity to erythromycins.
- Use with caution in patients with impaired hepatic function.
- Patients with a history of hearing loss may be at risk of further hearing loss, especially if hepatic or renal function is present, or if on high-dose erythromycins, or if patient is elderly.

Potential Toxicities/Side Effects and the Nursing Process

I.   ALTERATION IN NUTRITION related to GI SIDE EFFECTS

Defining Characteristics: Nausea, vomiting, and anorexia have occurred frequently. Also, transient increase LFTs—AST (SGOT), ALT (SGPT), LDH, alk phos, bili—has occurred. Hepatotoxicity (fever, nausea, skin rash, stomach pain, severe and unusual tiredness or weakness, yellow eyes or skin, and vomiting) has occurred less frequently. Pancreatitis (severe abdominal pain, nausea, and vomiting) has occurred but is rare.

Nursing Implications: Assess baseline nutritional status, preexisting nausea/vomiting, and anorexia. Assess baseline LFTs and monitor periodically during treatment. Teach patient to report side effects. Provide symptomatic interventions if side effects occur; discuss with physician use of alternative drug(s).

II.   POTENTIAL FOR INJURY related to HYPERSENSITIVITY REACTION

Defining Characteristics: Urticaria, pruritus, rash (maculopapular or erythematous), fever and chills, eosinophilia, myalgia, edema, erythema, angioedema.

Nursing Implications: Assess for drug allergies to erythromycin or macrolide antibiotic prior to drug administration. Teach patient to report any allergic reactions. Assess for signs/symptoms of allergic reaction after drug dose. Assess baseline skin integrity and presence of drug allergies; monitor patient closely during drug infusions. Teach patient to report immediately signs/symptoms of rash, pruritus, shortness of breath, any adverse sensation. Teach patient skin care and symptomatic measures as appropriate. If skin rash develops, discuss drug discontinuance with physician. If rash progresses, especially in human immunodeficiency virus (HIV)–infected patients, drug should be discontinued, as fatal Stevens–Johnson syndrome may develop. Be prepared to treat severe acute hypersensitivity reactions with airway management, oxygen, epinephrine, corticosteroids, or antihistamines as ordered.

III. ALTERATIONS IN COMFORT related to LOCAL INJECTION IRRITATION

Defining Characteristics: Incidence of phlebitis, thrombophlebitis, and pain when administering IV.

Nursing Implications: Change IV sites q 48 hours, and assess for signs/symptoms of phlebitis prior to each administration. Administer drug slowly. Apply warm packs to increase comfort.

IV. ALTERATIONS IN CARDIAC OUTPUT related to CARDIOVASCULAR CHANGES

Defining Characteristics: Rare incidence of cardiac arrhythmias, EKG changes (e.g., QT prolongation), torsades de pointes (irregular or slow heart rate, recurrent fainting, sudden death).

Nursing Implications: Assess baseline heart rate and blood pressure; monitor during therapy, at least with initial dose.

V. SENSORY/PERCEPTUAL ALTERATIONS related to OTOTOXICITY

Defining Characteristics: Damage to eighth cranial nerve (auditory) may result in dizziness, nystagmus, vertigo, ataxia (vestibular damage), and more commonly tinnitus, roaring sound in ears, and impaired hearing (auditory damage). Hearing loss usually begins with high-frequency loss, followed by clinical hearing loss, then permanent hearing loss if damage continues. Increased risk in elderly, renally, hepatically impaired patients.

Nursing Implications: Assess baseline hearing (ability to hear spoken voice) and continue to assess during therapy. Teach patient potential side effects, and instruct patient to report any hearing/perceptual problems (e.g., tinnitus, vertigo, decreased hearing). Discuss drug discontinuance and audiogram with physician to confirm hearing dysfunction if symptoms arise. Assess for increased risk if given concurrently with other ototoxic medications (e.g., cisplatin, furosemide).

COMPLICATIONS

VI.   FUNGAL SUPERINFECTION related to REDISTRIBUTION OF ENDOGENOUS MICROORGANISMS

Defining Characteristics: Vaginal candidiasis (sore mouth or tongue; white patches in mouth and/or tongue); vaginitis (vaginal candidiasis); vaginal itching and discharge may occur as endogenous bacteria are eliminated and normal fungal population expands.

Nursing Implications: Teach female patient to report vaginal itching or discharge. Discuss appropriate antifungal treatment with physician. Teach perineal hygiene and symptomatic management.

Drug: fidaxomicin (Dificid)

Class: Antibacterial (macrolide).

Mechanism of Action: Fidaxomicin is a fermentation product obtained from the Actinomycete *Dactylosporangium aurantiacum*. Active primarily against species of clostridia, including *C. difficile*. Bactericidal against *C. difficile* in vitro, inhibiting RNA synthesis by RNA polymerases. Bactericidal for CDAD. Since there is minimal systemic absorption of fidaxomicin, Dificid is not effective for treatment of systemic infections. Demonstrates no invitro cross-resistance with other classes of antibacterial drugs. Fidaxomicin and its main metabolite OP-1118 do not exhibit any antagonistic interaction with other classes of antibacterial drugs.

Metabolism: Fidaxomicin is primarily transformed by hydrolysis at the isobutyryl ester to form its main and microbiologically active metabolite, OP-1118. Metabolism of fidaxomicin and formation of OP-1118 are not dependent on cytochrome P450 (CYP) enzymes. Fidaxomicin acts locally in the gastrointestinal tract on *C. difficile*. Fidaxomicin has minimal systemic absorption following oral administration, with plasma concentrations of fidaxomicin and OP-1118 in the ng/mL range at the therapeutic dose. Fidaxomicin is mainly confined to the gastrointestinal tract following oral administration. Mainly excreted in feces.

Indication: For treatment of diarrhea caused by *C. difficile* (*C. difficile*–associated diarrhea).

Dosage/Range:
- The recommended dose is one 200-mg Dificid tablet orally twice daily for 10 days with or without food.

Drug Interactions:
- Fidaxomicin and its main metabolite, OP-1118, are substrates of the efflux transporter, P-glycoprotein (P-gp), which is expressed in the gastrointestinal tract.
- Cyclosporine: is an inhibitor of multiple transporters, including P-gp. Plasma concentrations of fidaxomicin and OP-1118 were significantly increased but remained in the ng/mL range. Concentrations of fidaxomicin and OP-1118 may decrease at the site of action (i.e., gastrointestinal tract) via P-gp inhibition; however, concomitant P-gp inhibitor use

had no attributable effect on safety or treatment outcome of fidaxomicin-treated patients in controlled clinical trials. Fidaxomicin may be coadministered with P-gp inhibitors, and no dose adjustment is recommended.

Lab Effects/Interference:
- None.

Special Considerations:
- Do not use when there is a known hypersensitivity to erythromycins or other macrolides.
- Use during pregnancy only if clearly needed.
- It is not known whether fidaxomicin is excreted in breastmilk. Because many drugs are excreted in breastmilk, caution should be exercised when Dificid is administered to a nursing woman.
- The safety and effectiveness of Dificid in patients less than 18 years of age have not been established.

Potential Toxicities/Side Effects and the Nursing Process

I.   ALTERATION IN NUTRITION related to GI SIDE EFFECTS

Defining Characteristics: Nausea (11%), vomiting (7%), abdominal pain (6%), and gastrointestinal hemorrhage (4%).

Nursing Implications: Assess baseline nutritional status, preexisting nausea/vomiting, and anorexia. Assess baseline LFTs and monitor periodically during treatment. Teach patient to report side effects. Provide symptomatic interventions if side effects occur; discuss with physician use of alternative drug(s).

II.   INFECTION, BLEEDING related to BONE MARROW DEPRESSION (rare)

Defining Characteristics: Neutropenia and anemia occur in 2% of patients, respectively.

Nursing Implications: Assess baseline WBC, ANC, and platelet count; monitor throughout therapy (every other day initially, then 3 times/week). Hold ganciclovir if ANC $< 500/mm^3$, platelet count $< 25,000/mm^3$. Assess for signs/symptoms of infection or bleeding; instruct patient in signs/symptoms of infection and bleeding, and instruct to report these immediately. Teach patient self-care measures to minimize risk of infection, bleeding, including avoidance of OTC aspirin-containing medicines. Administer or teach patient to self-administer prescribed G-CSF or GM-CSF. Assess Hgb/HCT and signs/symptoms of fatigue. Instruct patient to alternate rest and activity periods.

III.   FUNGAL SUPERINFECTION related to REDISTRIBUTION OF ENDOGENOUS MICROORGANISMS

Defining Characteristics: Vaginal candidiasis (sore mouth or tongue; white patches in mouth and/or tongue); vaginitis (vaginal candidiasis); vaginal itching and discharge may occur as endogenous bacteria are eliminated and normal fungal population expands.

Nursing Implications: Teach female patient to report vaginal itching or discharge. Discuss appropriate antifungal treatment with physician. Teach perineal hygiene and symptomatic management.

Drug: gentamicin sulfate (Gentamicin)

Class: Aminoglycoside antibacterial.

Mechanism of Action: Derived from *Micromonospora;* bactericidal, most probably by inhibition of protein synthesis.

Metabolism: Well-absorbed following IV administration, but variability in absorption after IM injection (peak serum level 0.5–2 hours, duration 8–12 hours). Widely distributed into body fluids. Minimally protein-bound. Readily crosses placenta and into breastmilk. Drug excreted unchanged in the urine.

Indication: For treatment of serious infections caused by susceptible bacteria. Active against aerobic microorganisms: many sensitive gram-negative organisms (including *Acinetobacter, Brucella, Citrobacter, Enterobacter, E. coli, Klebsiella, Proteus, Pseudomonas, Salmonella, Serratia,* and *Shigella*) and some sensitive gram-positive organisms (*S. aureus* and *S. epidermidis*). Over time, bacterial resistance may develop, either naturally or acquired.

Dosage/Range:
- Desired peak serum concentration 4–10 mg/mL, and trough serum concentration is less than 1–2 mg/mL.

Route	Loading Dose	Maintenance Dose	Interval/ Duration	Dose Modification for Renal Impairment
IM or IV	2 mg/kg	3 to 6 mg/kg/day	In 1 daily dose OR 2 equal doses q 8 h	For once daily dose, refer to Hartford nomogram for aminoglycoside dosing
IT	4–8 mg (preservative-free)			

Drug Preparation:
- Store injectable at < 40°C (104°F). Stable for 24 hours at room temperature in 0.9% sodium chloride or 5% dextrose.

Drug Administration:
- Do not mix with other drugs.
- IV: Mix in 50–200 mL 0.9% sodium chloride or 5% dextrose injection and infuse over 30 minutes to 2 hours. Can also be given IM.

Drug Interactions:
- Increased risk of toxicity with other ototoxic/nephrotoxic drugs: acyclovir, other aminoglycosides, amphotericin B, bacitracin, cephalosporins, colistin, cisplatin, ethacrynic acid, furosemide, vancomycin.

- Potentiation of neuromuscular blockade when given concurrently with general anesthetics (succinylcholine, tubocurarine); use cautiously, observe for signs/symptoms of respiratory depression.

Lab Effects/Interference:
- Serum ALT, serum alk phos, serum AST, serum bili, and serum LDH values may be increased.
- BUN and serum creatinine concentrations may be increased.
- Serum Ca^{++}, serum Mg^{++}, serum K^+, and serum Na^+ concentrations may be decreased.

Special Considerations:
- Used as treatment in short-term treatment of serious gram-negative infections (e.g., septicemia, respiratory tract infections).
- Use against gram-positive organisms only as second-line treatment.
- Use in pregnancy only if infection is life-threatening and no safer drug exists; drug crosses placenta and may cause fetal toxicity.

Potential Toxicities/Side Effects and the Nursing Process

I. ALTERATIONS IN SENSORY/PERCEPTUAL PATTERNS related to OTOTOXICITY

Defining Characteristics: Damage to eighth cranial nerve (auditory) may result in dizziness, nystagmus, vertigo, ataxia (vestibular damage), and more commonly tinnitus, roaring sound in ears, and impaired hearing (auditory damage). Hearing loss usually begins with high-frequency loss, followed by clinical hearing loss, then permanent hearing loss if damage continues. Increased risk in elderly or renally impaired patients.

Nursing Implications: Assess baseline hearing (ability to hear spoken voice) and continue to access during therapy. Teach patient potential side effects and instruct patient to report any hearing/perceptual problems (e.g., tinnitus, vertigo, decreased hearing). Discuss drug discontinuance and audiogram with physician to confirm hearing dysfunction if symptoms arise. Assess for increased risk if given concurrently with other ototoxic medications (e.g., cisplatin, furosemide).

II. ALTERATION IN URINARY ELIMINATION related to NEPHROTOXICITY

Defining Characteristics: Renal damage characterized by tubular necrosis with increased serum BUN, creatinine; decreased urine creatinine clearance and specific gravity; proteinuria and casts in urine. Azotemia usually not associated with oliguria. Rarely, electrolyte wasting with hypomagnesemia, hypocalcemia, and hypokalemia may occur. Renal dysfunction is usually reversible after drug discontinuance. Increased risk exists in elderly and if preexisting renal dysfunction. Risk low in well-hydrated patients with normal renal function when normal doses given.

COMPLICATIONS

Nursing Implications: Assess baseline renal function and electrolytes, and monitor periodically during therapy. Discuss any abnormalities with physician, as drug should be dose-reduced or discontinued if renal dysfunction develops. Assess baseline total body fluid balance, weight, and monitor periodically during antibiotic therapy. Monitor hydration status to keep patient well hydrated. Assess drug peak and trough levels as ordered so that drug dosage is correctly titrated. Increased risk of toxicity if peak serum concentration > 10–12 mg/mL. Draw blood for peak drug concentration 30 minutes after end of 30-minute infusion or at the end of a 60-minute infusion; draw trough immediately before next dose.

III.   ALTERATIONS IN SENSORY/PERCEPTUAL PATTERNS related to CNS EFFECTS, NEUROMUSCULAR BLOCKADE

Defining Characteristics: Headache, tremor, lethargy may occur. Peripheral neuropathy or encephalopathy (numbness, skin tingling, muscle twitching) may occur rarely. Neuromuscular blockade is dose-related, self-limiting, and uncommon; risk is greater with topical application or when drug is administered to patient with neuromuscular disease (myasthenia gravis) or hypocalcemia.

Nursing Implications: Assess baseline neurologic status. Assess coexisting risk factors, neuromuscular blockade medications. Teach patient about side effects and to report headache, tremor, lethargy. Observe for respiratory depression. If signs/symptoms arise, discuss drug discontinuance with physician.

IV.   POTENTIAL FOR INJURY related to HYPERSENSITIVITY

Defining Characteristics: Rash, urticaria, pruritus, fever, and eosinophilia have occurred rarely. CROSS-SENSITIVITY between AMINOGLYCOSIDES exists.

Nursing Implications: Assess for drug allergies to any aminoglycoside—amikacin, gentamicin, kanamycin, neomycin, netilmicin, streptomycin, tobramycin—prior to drug administration. Instruct patient to report any allergic reactions. Assess for signs/symptoms of allergic reaction after drug dose.

V.   ALTERATION IN NUTRITION, LESS THAN BODY REQUIREMENTS, related to GI SIDE EFFECTS

Defining Characteristics: Nausea, vomiting, and anorexia have occurred rarely. Also, transient hepatomegaly with increased LFTs—AST, ALT, LDH, alk phos, bili—has occurred.

Nursing Implications: Assess baseline nutritional status, preexisting nausea/vomiting, and anorexia. Assess baseline LFTs and monitor periodically during treatment. Instruct patient to report side effects. Provide symptomatic interventions if side effects occur; discuss with physician use of alternative drug(s).

VI. POTENTIAL FOR FATIGUE, INFECTION, AND BLEEDING, related to BONE MARROW INJURY

Defining Characteristics: Anemia, leukopenia, granulocytopenia, and thrombocytopenia may occur. Also, patients receiving antibiotics are at risk for overgrowth of nonsusceptible microorganisms, such as fungi (superinfection); rare.

Nursing Implications: Assess baseline CBC, differential, and monitor periodically during treatment. Instruct patient to report signs/symptoms of fatigue, infection, or bleeding immediately. Assess for signs/symptoms of superinfection. Discuss any adverse effects with physician.

Drug: imipenem/cilastatin sodium/relebactam (Recarbrio)

Class: Antibacterial.

Mechanism of Action: Imipenem is a β-lactam antibiotic, carbapenem type. Cilastatin inhibits an enzyme in the kidneys that breaks down imipenem, increasing drug potency and protecting kidneys. Relebactam is a diazabicyclooctane beta lactamase inhibitor.

Semisynthetic derivative of cephalosporin C (produced by fungus); contains β-lactam ring and is related to penicillins and cephamycins (e.g., cefoxitin). Bactericidal through inhibition of cell wall synthesis, with resulting cell wall instability and cell lysis.

Metabolism: Not well-absorbed from GI tract, so must be given IV. Incompletely absorbed after IM injection. Widely distributed in body tissues and fluids, including bile; does not result in significant CSF drug levels. Crosses placenta and is excreted in breastmilk. Cilastatin decreases renal metabolism of imipenem; drugs are excreted in urine, and to a lesser degree in feces.

Indication: For treatment of complicated urinary tract infections (cUTI), including pyelonephritis. Active against gram-negative organisms. These include *E. coli, P. aeruginosa,* and *Klebsiella.* Resists hydrolysis by β lactamase enzymes produced by microorganisms, so resistance to these organisms is much less than other β-lactam antibiotics (e.g., cephalosporins, penicillins).

Dosage/Range:

Adult:
- IV: 1.2 g infused over 30 minutes q 6 h in patients 18 years and older. Dose reduce in patients with renal impairment.

Drug Preparation:
- IV: Reconstitute according to manufacturer's package insert and further dilute in 100 mL 0.9% sodium chloride or 5% dextrose injection.

COMPLICATIONS

Drug Interactions:
• Probenecid: increases serum concentrations of imipenem. DO NOT USE CONCURRENTLY.
• Aminoglycosides: may have synergistic antimicrobial effect.
• There should not be a duplication of therapy, using several betalactams together may induce seizures. However there have been rare cases where it was a necessity due to nature of infection.
• Ganciclovir: may decrease seizure threshold. Do not use concurrently unless critical for life-saving treatment.

Lab Effects/Interference:
• Serum ALT, serum alk phos, and serum AST values may be transiently increased.

Clinical Significance:
• Serum bili, BUN concentrations, and serum creatinine concentrations may be transiently increased.

Special Considerations:
• Contraindicated in patients hypersensitive to imipenem or cilastatin. Use cautiously in patients sensitive to penicillin or other β-lactams, as partial cross-allergenicity exists.
• Ensure specimen sent for culture and sensitivity prior to first antibiotic dose.
• Central nervous system events, including seizures, confusional states, and myoclonic activity, have been reported, especially when recommended dosages were exceeded or patients had CNS disorders (e.g., brain lesions, seizure history) or compromised renal function.
• Drug dosage needs to be reduced if severe renal insufficiency.

Potential Toxicities/Side Effects and the Nursing Process

I.   POTENTIAL FOR INJURY related to HYPERSENSITIVITY REACTION

Defining Characteristics: Urticaria, pruritus, rash (maculopapular or erythematous), fever and chills, eosinophilia, myalgia, edema, erythema, angioedema, Stevens–Johnson syndrome, and exfoliative skin reactions occur in 5% of patients. Increased risk in individuals allergic to penicillin.

Nursing Implications: Assess allergy to cephalosporin antibiotics and penicillin: if patient states "yes," determine actual response (e.g., "swollen lips = angioedema"). If angioedema, discuss with physician RISK versus benefit prior to drug administration, as there is partial cross-allergenicity. Discuss other patient responses with physician to determine whether drug should be given. Assess baseline skin condition, including integrity and allergy history to drugs. Instruct patient to report rash, itching, other skin changes. Teach patient skin care and symptomatic measures as appropriate. If skin rash develops, discuss drug discontinuance with physician. If rash progresses, drug should be discontinued, as fatal Stevens–Johnson syndrome may develop. Be prepared to treat

---

severe acute hypersensitivity reactions with airway management, oxygen, epinephrine, corticosteroids, antihistamines as ordered.

II. ALTERATION IN NUTRITION, LESS THAN BODY REQUIREMENTS, related to GI SIDE EFFECTS

Defining Characteristics: Nausea, vomiting occurs more frequently than diarrhea, anorexia; rarely, pseudomembranous colitis caused by *C. difficile* resistant to the antibiotic occurs. Rarely, transient increases in LFTs—AST, ALT, alk phos, bili—may occur.

Nursing Implications: Assess baseline nutritional status. Instruct patient to report GI disturbances. Administer and teach patient to self-administer antiemetics as needed and as ordered. Teach patient importance of nutritious diet and suggest small, frequent, high-calorie, high-protein meals as appropriate. Assess baseline LFTs and monitor periodically during treatment. Discuss abnormalities and drug interruption with physician.

III. FUNGAL SUPERINFECTION related to REDISTRIBUTION OF ENDOGENOUS MICROORGANISMS

Defining Characteristics: Vaginal candidiasis, vaginitis may occur as endogenous bacteria are eliminated and normal fungal population expands.

Nursing Implications: Instruct female patient to report vaginal itching or discharge. Discuss appropriate antifungal treatment with physician. Teach perineal hygiene and symptomatic management.

IV. ALTERATIONS IN SENSORY/PERCEPTUAL PATTERNS related to DIZZINESS, SOMNOLENCE

Defining Characteristics: Dizziness, headache, somnolence, seizures occur rarely. Most seizures have occurred in patients with preexisting CNS problems, those who had received higher-than-recommended IV doses, the elderly, and patients with impaired renal function.

Nursing Implications: Assess baseline neurologic function and comfort and monitor during treatment. Instruct patient to report any changes. Discuss any abnormalities with physician. Institute seizure precautions. If seizures occur, discuss with physician anticonvulsant therapy or discontinuance of antibiotic.

VI. ALTERATIONS IN COMFORT related to LOCAL INJECTION IRRITATION

Defining Characteristics: Pain, induration, phlebitis may develop in IV sites.

Nursing Implications: Change IV sites q 48 h and assess for signs/symptoms of phlebitis prior to each administration. Administer drug slowly. Apply warm packs to increase comfort.

COMPLICATIONS

Drug: levofloxacin (Levaquin)

Class: Fluoroquinolone antibiotic.

Mechanism of Action: Drug is a synthetic, broad-spectrum antibacterial agent. Inhibits DNA gyrase (bacterial topoisomerase II), which is necessary for DNA replication, transcription, and repair. Has activity against a wide range of gram-negative and gram-positive bacteria, as well as against some bacteria resistant to β-lactam antibiotics.

Metabolism: Drug is well-absorbed from the GI tract without regard to food, with 99% bioavailability; peak serum levels occur in 1–2 hours. Steady state is reached in 48 hours. Drug is not extensively metabolized, with 87% of drug excreted largely unchanged in the urine at 48 hours. Terminal half-life is 6–8 hours.

Indication: For treatment of bacterial infections such as pneumonia, chronic bronchitis and sinus, urinary tract, kidney, prostate, and skin infections.

Dosage/Range:

Indication	Dosage (mg)	Route	Interval/Duration
Acute bacterial exacerbation of chronic bronchitis	500	PO	Daily × 7 days
Uncomplicated skin and skin structure infection	500	PO	Daily × 7 to 10 days
Acute maxillary sinusitis	500	PO	Daily × 10 to 14 days
Uncomplicated UTI, acute pyelonephritis	500	PO	Daily × 10 days
Community acquired pneumonia	750	IV or PO	Every 24 hours × 5 days

Drug Preparation:
- Oral Solution: 500 mg/20 mL, 25 mg/1 mL, 250 mg/10 mL
- Oral Syrup: 25 mg/1 mL
- Oral Tablet: 250, 500, 750 mg
- IV: Administer over 60 min to prevent hypotension; IV available in premixed 250- or 500-mg bags, or 20-mL vial containing 500 mg that is further diluted in 5% dextrose, 0.9% sodium chloride.

Drug Administration:
- Administer without regard to food.
- Dose-reduce if renal compromise (see Special Considerations section).
- Administer oral doses at least 2 hours before or 2 hours after antacids containing magnesium or aluminum, as well as sucralfate, medications such as iron, and multivitamins containing zinc.

Drug Interactions:
- Antacids containing magnesium or aluminum, sucralfate, iron, multivitamins containing zinc: may decrease serum levels of levofloxacin; take any of these agents at least 2 hours before or 2 hours after levofloxacin.

- Theophylline: possible increase in theophylline serum levels; monitor levels and change dose accordingly.
- Warfarin: theoretically could enhance effects of oral anticoagulants; monitor INR closely and modify dose accordingly.
- NSAIDs: possible increase in the risk of CNS stimulation and seizures; assess patient risk for seizures, and use cautiously if at all in patients at risk.
- Antidiabetic agents: changes in glucose (hyper-or hypoglycemia); monitor blood sugar closely, and modify dose accordingly.
- Drug interacts with QT prolonging medications and steroids.

Lab Effects/Interference:
- Decreased glucose, decreased lymphocytes.

Special Considerations:
- Indicated for the treatment of acute maxillary sinusitis due to *S. pneumoniae, H. influenzae,* or *M. catarrhalis*; acute bacterial exacerbation of chronic bronchitis due to *S. aureus, S. pneumoniae, H. influenzae, H. parainfluenzae,* or *M. catarrhalis;* community-acquired pneumonia due to *S. aureus, S. pneumoniae, H. influenzae, H. parainfluenzae, K. pneumoniae, M. catarrhalis, Chlamydia pneumoniae, Legionella pneumophila,* or *M. pneumoniae.*
- Active against the above as well as aerobic gram-positive *Enterococcus faecalis* and *S. pyogenes* and aerobic gram-negative microorganisms *Enterobacter cloacae, E. coli, P. mirabilis,* and *P. aeruginosa.*
- Dose modifications for renal impairment:

Acute Bacterial Exacerbation:	Chronic Bronchitis, Community-Acquired	Pneumonia, Acute Maxillary Sinusitis, Uncomplicated Skin Infections
CrCl 20–49 mL/min	500 mg	250 mg q 24 h
CrCl 10–19 mL/min	500 mg	250 mg q 48 h
Hemodialysis	500 mg	250 mg q 48 h
CAPD	500 mg q 48 h	250 mg q 48 h
Uncomplicated UTI/Acute Pyelonephritis		
CrCl 10–19 mL/min	250 mg	250 mg q 48 h

- Use drug cautiously, if at all, in the following patients: (1) known or suspected CNS or seizure disorder (e.g., severe cerebral arteriosclerosis or epilepsy); (2) possess factors lowering seizure threshold (e.g., renal dysfunction, other drug therapy); (3) pregnant or nursing mothers; (4) children < 18 years old.
- Obtain ordered specimen for culture and sensitivity prior to first drug dose.
- Black box warning: Fluoroquinolones, including levofloxacin, are associated with an increased risk of tendinitis and tendon rupture in all ages. Risk further increases with age over 60 years, concomitant steroid therapy, and kidney, heart, or lung transplants. Fluoroquinolones, including levofloxacin, may exacerbate muscle weakness in persons with myasthenia gravis. Avoid in patients with known history of myasthenia gravis.

COMPLICATIONS

Potential Toxicities/Side Effects and the Nursing Process

I.   ALTERATION IN NUTRITION related to GI SIDE EFFECTS

Defining Characteristics: 0.1–3.0% incidence of nausea, vomiting, abdominal discomfort, diarrhea, and anorexia. As with all antibiotics, pseudomembranous colitis may occur, ranging in severity from mild to life-threatening. Treatment with antibiotics changes the intestinal microflora, so *C. difficile* bacteria may overgrow. Once diagnosis is made, mild diarrhea may stop with cessation of drug; if moderate to severe, it will require hydration, electrolyte replacement, nutritional support, and antibacterial coverage against *C. difficile*.

Nursing Implications: Assess baseline nutritional and elimination status. Teach patient to report GI disturbances. Teach patient to report diarrhea immediately, and consider whether this is pseudomembranous colitis and send stool specimen for *C. difficile*; if positive, discuss drug discontinuance with physician. Administer and teach patient to self-administer antiemetics, antidiarrheals as needed and as ordered. Teach patient importance of nutritious diet, and suggest small, frequent, high-calorie, high-protein meals as appropriate. Assess baseline LFTs and monitor periodically during treatment. Discuss abnormalities and drug interruption with physician.

II.   SENSORY/PERCEPTUAL ALTERATIONS related to CNS EFFECTS

Defining Characteristics: One to two percent incidence of insomnia, dizziness, taste perversion, headache, nervousness, anxiety, tremors, and seizures may also occur.

Nursing Implications: Assess baseline neurologic function and comfort, and monitor during treatment. Teach patient to report any changes. Discuss any abnormalities with physician. Teach patient to avoid caffeine-containing fluids, medications (e.g., tea, coffee, soft drinks).

III.   ALTERATION IN SKIN INTEGRITY related to ALLERGY/HYPERSENSITIVITY

Defining Characteristics: One to four percent incidence of rash; other manifestations include eosinophilia, urticaria, flushing, fever, chills, photosensitivity, angioedema. Fatal hypersensitivity reactions have occurred rarely. Direct exposure to sunlight can cause sunburn (moderate-to-severe phototoxicity).

Nursing Implications: Assess baseline skin condition, including integrity and drug allergy history. Teach patient to report rash, itching, other skin changes. Teach patient skin care and symptomatic measures as appropriate. If skin rash develops, discuss drug discontinuance with physician. If rash progresses, especially in HIV-infected patients, drug should be discontinued, as fatal Stevens–Johnson syndrome may develop. Be prepared to treat severe acute hypersensitivity reactions with airway management, oxygen, epinephrine, corticosteroids, or antihistamines as ordered. Teach patient to avoid excessive sun exposure and to use SPF 15 or higher.

IV. FUNGAL SUPERINFECTION related to REDISTRIBUTION OF ENDOGENOUS MICROORGANISMS

Defining Characteristics: Vaginal moniliasis or vaginitis may occur as endogenous bacteria are eliminated and normal fungal population expands.

Nursing Implications: Teach female patient to report vaginal itching or discharge. Discuss appropriate antifungal treatment with physician. Teach perineal hygiene and symptomatic management.

Drug: linezolid (Zyvox)

Class: Oxazolidinone class of antibiotic.

Mechanism of Action: Linezolid inhibits initiation of protein synthesis by preventing the formation of the fmet-tRNA:mRNA:30S subunit ternary complex. Oxazolidinones bind to the 50S subunit in a region shared with the peptidyl transferase inhibitor chloramphenicol. Oxazolidinones are not peptidyl transferase inhibitors, and it is not known which specific ribosome reaction is inhibited by 50S subunit binding.

Metabolism: Primarily metabolized by oxidation of the morpholine ring, resulting in two inactive carboxylic acid metabolites. Only about 30% of a dose is excreted unchanged in the urine.

Indication: Linezolid has a specific mechanism of action against bacteria resistant to other antibiotics, including MRSA, multiresistant strains of *S. pneumoniae*, and VRE. The drug is used to treat nosocomial and community-acquired pneumonia, septicemias, and complicated and uncomplicated skin and skin structure infections caused by susceptible strains of specific organisms.

Dosage/Range:
- Oral: 600 mg q 12 h for 10–14 days.
- IV: 600 mg q 12 h for 10–14 days.
- Duration is based on infection (complicated vs. uncomplicated).
- Longer duration is associated with myelosuppression.

Drug Preparation:
- Available in single-use, ready-to-use infusion bags.

Drug Administration:
- IV infusion over 30–120 minutes.
- Linezolid has the potential to interact with adrenergic (phenylpropanolamine, pseudoephedrine) and serotonergic agents since it is a reversible, nonselective monoamine oxidase inhibitor.
- Large quantities of foods or beverages with high tyramine content should be avoided.

Lab Effects/Interference:
• Thrombocytopenia has been seen when this drug is administered long term (up to 28 days).

Special Considerations:
• IV and PO doses are the same.

Potential Toxicities/Side Effects and the Nursing Process

Nurses need to be aware of serotonin syndrome with long-term use.

I.   ALTERATION IN NUTRITION related to GI SIDE EFFECTS

Defining Characteristics: Nausea, vomiting, and anorexia have occurred frequently.

Nursing Implications: Assess baseline nutritional status, preexisting nausea/vomiting, and anorexia. Teach patient to report side effects. Provide symptomatic interventions if side effects occur; discuss with physician use of alternative drug(s).

II.   POTENTIAL FOR INJURY related to HYPERSENSITIVITY REACTION

Defining Characteristics: Urticaria, pruritus, rash (maculopapular or erythematous), fever and chills, eosinophilia, myalgia, edema, erythema, and angioedema.

Nursing Implications: Assess for drug allergies to erythromycin or macrolide antibiotic prior to drug administration. Teach patient to report any allergic reactions. Assess for signs/symptoms of allergic reaction after drug dose. Assess baseline skin integrity and presence of drug allergies; monitor patient closely during drug infusions. Teach patient to report immediately signs/symptoms of rash, pruritus, shortness of breath, any adverse sensation. Teach patient skin care and symptomatic measures as appropriate. If skin rash develops, discuss drug discontinuance with physician. If rash progresses, especially in human immunodeficiency virus (HIV)–infected patients, drug should be discontinued, as fatal Stevens–Johnson syndrome may develop. Be prepared to treat severe acute hypersensitivity reactions with airway management, oxygen, epinephrine, corticosteroids, or antihistamines as ordered.

III.   ALTERATIONS IN COMFORT related to HEADACHE

Defining Characteristics: Headache has occurred in some patients.

Nursing Implications: Assess baseline hearing (ability to hear spoken voice) and continue to assess during therapy. Teach patient potential side effects, and instruct patient to report any hearing/perceptual problems (e.g., tinnitus, vertigo, decreased hearing). Discuss drug discontinuance and audiogram with physician to confirm hearing dysfunction if symptoms arise. Assess for increased risk if given concurrently with other ototoxic medications (e.g., cisplatin, furosemide).

IV.   FUNGAL SUPERINFECTION related to REDISTRIBUTION OF ENDOGENOUS MICROORGANISMS

Defining Characteristics: Vaginal or oral candidiasis (sore mouth or tongue; white patches in mouth and/or tongue); vaginitis (vaginal candidiasis); vaginal itching and discharge may occur as endogenous bacteria are eliminated and normal fungal population expands. Nurses need to be aware of myelosuppression with long-term use.

Nursing Implications: Teach female patient to report vaginal itching or discharge. Discuss appropriate antifungal treatment with physician. Teach perineal hygiene and symptomatic management.

Drug: meropenem (Merrem)

Class: Antibiotic, carbapenem.

Mechanism of Action: The bactericidal activity results from the inhibition of cell wall synthesis. Penetrates cell wall of most gram-positive and gram-negative bacteria to reach PBP targets.

Metabolism: Widely distributed in body tissues and fluids, excreted in urine.

Indication: Drug is used as empiric anti-infective therapy of presumed bacterial infections in febrile neutropenia patients. It is also used to treat severe infections of the skin and skin structures (beta-lactamase–producing strains [but not oxacillin-resistant (methicillin-resistant) strains of *S. aureus*; group A beta-hemolytic streptococci of *S. pyogenes*; group B streptococci of *S. agalactiae*; *viridans streptococci*; non-vancomycin-resistant strains of *Enterococcus faecalis*; *P. aeruginosa*; *E. coli*; *P. mirabilis*; *B. fragilis*; *Peptostreptococcus*), respiratory tract (CAP caused by *S. pneumoniae*, *P. aeruginosa, Klebsiella*, or other gram-negative bacteria; nosocomial pneumonia), gastrointestinal tract (susceptible *viridans streptococci*; *E. coli*; *Klebsiella pneumoniae*; *P. aeruginosa*; *B. fragilis*; *B. thetaiotaomicron; Peptostreptococcus*), bacterial meningitis (*S. pneumoniae*; *H. influenzae*; *Enterobacter; Citrobacter; Serratia marcescens*). Other infections include urinary tract infections, Acinetobacter infections, anthrax, bacillus, Burkholderia, Campylobacter, Capnocytophaga, Nocardia, and Rhodococcus infections.

Dosage/Range:

Adult:

Indication	Dosage (g)	Route	Interval/Duration
Intra-abdominal infection	1	IV	q 8 h
Meningitis	2	IV	q 8 h

COMPLICATIONS

Dose modification for renal impairment:

CrCl (mL/min)	Dosage Adjustment	
Renal impairment CrCl greater than 25 to less than 50 mL/min		Increase dosing interval to q 12 h
Renal impairment, CrCl 10–25 mL/min	1/2 recommended dose depending on type of infection	Increase dosing interval to q 12 h
Renal impairment, CrCl less than 10 mL/min	1/2 recommended dose depending on type of infection	Increase dosing interval to q 24 h hemodialysis; an additional dose following hemodialysis session is recommended

An additional dose following hemodialysis session is recommended.

Drug Preparation:
- IV bolus, dilute with 5–20 mL. Sterile water for injection and give over 3–5 minutes.
- IV infusion dilute with D_5W or normal saline, infuse over 15–30 minutes, maximum concentration 50 mg/mL.

Drug Interactions:
- Valproic acid.
- Probenecid competes with meropenem for active tubular secretion and thus inhibits the renal excretion of meropenem.
- Meropenem may reduce serum levels of valproic acid to subtherapeutic levels.

Lab Effects/Interference:
- Meropenem possesses the characteristic low toxicity of the β-lactam group of antibiotics.
- Periodically assess organ system function; renal, hepatic, and hematopoietic.

Potential Toxicities/Side Effects and the Nursing Process

I. POTENTIAL FOR INJURY related to HYPERSENSITIVITY REACTION AND LOCAL REACTIONS (pain at injection site)

Defining Characteristics: Urticaria, pruritus, rash (maculopapular or erythematous), fever and chills, eosinophilia, myalgia, edema, erythema, and angioedema.

Nursing Implications: Assess allergy to cephalosporin antibiotics and penicillin: if patient states "yes," determine actual response (e.g., "swollen lips = angioedema"). If angioedema, patient SHOULD NOT receive drug. Discuss other patient responses with physician to determine whether drug should be given. Assess baseline skin condition, including integrity and allergy history to drugs. Instruct patient to report rash, itching, or other skin changes. Teach patient skin care and symptomatic measures as appropriate. If skin rash develops, discuss drug discontinuance with physician. Be prepared to treat severe acute hypersensitivity reactions with airway management, oxygen, epinephrine, corticosteroids, or antihistamines as ordered.

II. ALTERATION IN NUTRITION, LESS THAN BODY REQUIREMENTS, related to GI SIDE EFFECTS

Defining Characteristics: Nausea, vomiting, or diarrhea may occur; rarely, pseudomembranous colitis caused by antibiotic resistance occurs. Patient may be susceptible to *C. difficile* infection.

Nursing Implications: Assess baseline nutritional status. Instruct patient to report GI disturbances. Administer and teach patient to self-administer antiemetics as needed and as ordered. Teach patient importance of nutritious diet, and suggest small, frequent, high-calorie, high-protein meals as appropriate. Assess baseline LFTs, and monitor periodically during treatment. Discuss abnormalities and drug interruption with physician.

III. FUNGAL SUPERINFECTION related to REDISTRIBUTION OF ENDOGENOUS MICROORGANISMS

Defining Characteristics: Vaginal candidiasis or vaginitis may occur as endogenous bacteria are eliminated and normal fungal population expands.

Nursing Implications: Instruct female patient to report vaginal itching or discharge. Discuss appropriate antifungal treatment with physician. Teach perineal hygiene and symptomatic management.

Drug: meropenem/vaborbactam (Vabomere)

Class: Combination of a penem antibacterial agent and a beta-lactamase inhibitor.

Mechanism of Action: The bactericidal activity results from the inhibition of cell wall synthesis. Penetrates the cell wall of most gram-positive and gram-negative bacteria to reach penicillin-binding protein (PBP) targets.

Metabolism: Widely distributed in body tissues and fluids, excreted in urine.

Indication: Drug is used for treatment of patients 18 years and older with complicated UTIs, including pyelonephritis caused by *E. coli*; *Klebiella pneumoniae*; *Enterobacter cloacae species complex.*

Dosage/Range:

Adult:
- 4 g IV every 8 hours infused over 3 hours.
- Dosage adjustment renal impairment:
  - Adults, CrCl 30 to 49 mL/min: decrease dose to 2 g every 8 hours
  - Adults, CrCl 15 to 29 mL/min: decrease dose to 2 g every 12 hours
  - Adults, CrCl less than 15 mL/min: 1 g every 12 hours

COMPLICATIONS

Drug Preparation:
- IV infusion reconsitute with 0.9% sodium chloride injection, dilute in sodium chloride and infuse over NOT MORE THAN 4 hours, maximum concentration 21.3 mg/mL.

Drug Interactions:
- Probenecid competes with meropenem for active tubular secretion and thus inhibits the renal excretion of meropenem.
- Meropenem coadministered with valproic acid or divalproex sodium reduces serum concentration levels of valproic acid to subtherapeutic levels followed by breakthough seizures.

Lab Effects/Interference:
- Meropenem possesses the characteristic low toxicity of the β-lactam group of antibiotics.
- Periodically assess organ system function; renal, hepatic, and hematopoietic.

Potential Toxicities/Side Effects and the Nursing Process

I.   POTENTIAL FOR INJURY related to HYPERSENSITIVITY REACTION AND LOCAL REACTIONS (pain at injection site)

Defining Characteristics: Urticaria, pruritus, rash (maculopapular or erythematous), fever and chills, eosinophilia, myalgia, edema, erythema, angioedema.

Nursing Implications: Assess allergy to cephalosporin antibiotics and penicillin: if patient states "yes," determine actual response (e.g., "swollen lips = angioedema"). If angioedema, patient SHOULD NOT receive drug. Discuss other patient responses with physician to determine whether drug should be given. Assess baseline skin condition, including integrity and allergy history to drugs. Instruct patient to report rash, itching, and other skin changes. Teach patient skin care and symptomatic measures as appropriate. If skin rash develops, discuss drug discontinuance with physician. Be prepared to treat severe acute hypersensitivity reactions with airway management, oxygen, epinephrine, corticosteroids, antihistamines as ordered.

II.   ALTERATION IN NUTRITION, LESS THAN BODY REQUIREMENTS, related to GI SIDE EFFECTS

Defining Characteristics: *C. difficile* diarrhea may occur; rarely, pseudomembranous colitis caused by antibiotic resistance occurs.

Nursing Implications: Assess baseline nutritional status. Instruct patient to report GI disturbances. Administer and teach patient to self-administer anti-diarrheal agents as needed and as ordered. Teach patient importance of nutritious diet and suggest small, frequent, high-calorie, high-protein meals as appropriate. Assess baseline LFTs and monitor periodically during treatment. Discuss abnormalities and drug interruption with physician.

III.   FUNGAL SUPERINFECTION related to REDISTRIBUTION OF ENDOGENOUS MICROORGANISMS

Defining Characteristics: Vaginal candidiasis, vaginitis may occur as endogenous bacteria are eliminated and normal fungal population expands.

Nursing Implications: Instruct female patient to report vaginal itching or discharge. Discuss appropriate antifungal treatment with physician. Teach perineal hygiene and symptomatic management. In cancer patients there is a higher than normal risk of *C. difficile*. Patient should be taught about this condition.

IV. SEIZURE POTENTIAL

Defining Characteristics: Dizziness, headache, neuromuscular irritability, and seizures may occur with high drug serum levels.

Nursing Implications: Assess baseline neurologic function and comfort and monitor during treatment. Instruct patient to report any changes. Discuss any abnormalities with physician. Institute seizure precautions.

Drug: minocycline hydrochloride (Minocin)—Only Minocin IV is marketed brand in United States

Class: Antibacterial (systemic); antiprotozoal.

Mechanism of Action: Bacteriostatic, but may be bactericidal at high concentrations. Binds to bacterial ribosomes and prevents protein synthesis.

Metabolism: Absorbed (60–80%) from GI tract. Widely distributed into body tissues and fluids. Crosses placenta and is excreted in breastmilk. Excreted unchanged in urine.

Indication: For treatment of a broad range of gram-positive and gram-negative bacteria and a variety of bacterial infections.

Dosage/Range:

Adult:
• IV: 200 mg initially, then 100 mg q 12 h for 5–15 days depending on indications.
• Dose modification necessary if renal dysfunction exists.

Drug Preparation:
• Oral: may be taken with food, water, or milk.
• IV: add 5–10 mL sterile water for injection to 100-mg vial. Further dilute in 500–1,000 mL of 0.9% sodium chloride injection, dextrose injection, dextrose and sodium chloride injections, Ringer's injection, or lactated Ringer's injection. Do not use other calcium-containing solutions, since precipitate may form.

COMPLICATIONS

- AVOID RAPID ADMINISTRATION.
- Solution stable for 24 hours at room temperature. Avoid exposure to heat or sunlight. Convert to oral preparation as soon as possible, as there is risk of thrombophlebitis.
- DO NOT ADMINISTER INTRAMUSCULARLY OR SUBCUTANEOUSLY.

Drug Interactions:
- Hepatotoxic drugs: may increase hepatotoxicity if given concurrently. Assess baseline and periodically during treatment.
- Iron preparations: decrease oral and possibly IV absorption. Administer iron preparations 3 hours after or 2 hours before any tetracycline.
- Oral anticoagulants: increase PT. Monitor patient closely and decrease anticoagulant dose as needed.
- Antidiarrheals (containing kaolin, pectate, or bismuth): may decrease absorption of tetracyclines. Avoid concurrent use.
- Oral contraceptives: decreased effectiveness of contraceptive and increased incidence of breakthrough bleeding. Advise patient to use barrier contraceptive as well during a course of tetracycline therapy.
- Lithium: may decrease lithium levels. Monitor serum levels and increase dose as needed.
- Other drug interactions include: Atazanavir, digoxin, retinoids, antacids, certain antidiabetic agents.

Lab Effects/Interference:
- Urine catecholamine determinations: may produce false elevations of urinary catecholamines because of interfering fluorescence in the Hingerty method.
- SGPT, alk phos, amylase, SGOT, and bilirubin: serum concentrations may be increased.

Special Considerations:
- May cause dizziness, lightheadedness, or unsteadiness (CNS toxicity). Advise patient to avoid driving or using hazardous machines until drug effects are realized due to dizziness, vertigo, and lightheadedness.
- Pigmentation of skin and mucous membranes may occur.
- Warn male and female patients to avoid pregnancy. Additional form of birth control recommended due to potential for decreased effectiveness of oral contraceptives.
- Use cautiously in patients with myasthenia gravis: may increase muscle weakness.
- Avoid use in pregnant or lactating women.
- Subgingival side effects: may include local sensitivity, dental pain, or stomatitis.
- Obtain ordered specimen for culture and sensitivity prior to first dose.
- IV preparation contains ascorbic acid and may cause false-positive result using Clinitest, or false-negative when using Clinistix and Tes-Tape.
- Drug has affinity for ischemic, necrotic tissue, and may localize in tumors.

Potential Toxicities/Side Effects and the Nursing Process

I.   ALTERATION IN NUTRITION related to GI SIDE EFFECTS

Defining Characteristics: Nausea, vomiting, diarrhea, anorexia, abdominal discomfort, epigastric burning and distress, glossitis, or black, hairy tongue may occur.

Nursing Implications: Assess baseline nutritional status. Assess for and teach patient to report any symptoms. Administer and teach patient self-administration of prescribed antiemetic or antidiarrheal medication as appropriate. Administer and teach patient to self-administer oral dose with at least 8 oz of water taken at least 1 hour before lying down for sleep.

II.   ALTERATION IN SKIN INTEGRITY related to RASH, PHOTOSENSITIVITY

Defining Characteristics: Maculopapular and erythematous rashes may occur. Rarely, exfoliative dermatitis, onycholysis, and nail discoloration. Photosensitivity risk (exaggerated sunburn) persists 1–2 days after completion of drug therapy. Hyperpigmentation in many organs, including nails, bone, skin, eyes, thyroid, visceral tissue, oral cavity (teeth, mucosa, bone), sclera, and heart valves, has been reported with tetracycline therapy. Tissue pigmentation, other than skin and oral hyperpigmentation, has been reported only after prolonged use of tetracyclines.

Nursing Implications: Teach patient about potential side effects to avoid sunlight during drug therapy and to report rash, other abnormalities. Teach symptomatic skin care as appropriate.

III.   INJURY related to HYPERSENSITIVITY

Defining Characteristics: Urticaria, angioneurotic edema, or anaphylaxis may occur; also, fever, rash, arthralgias, eosinophilia, and pericarditis.

Nursing Implications: Assess drug allergy history. Assess baseline allergy history. Assess baseline skin integrity. Teach patient to report rash, pruritus. Teach patent symptomatic management of rash, pruritus. Assess for hypersensitivity reaction; if it occurs, monitor VS, discontinue drug, notify physician, and institute supportive measures.

IV.   FUNGAL SUPERINFECTION related to REDISTRIBUTION OF ENDOGENOUS MICROORGANISMS

Defining Characteristics: Vaginal moniliasis or vaginitis may occur as endogenous bacteria are eliminated and normal fungal population expands.

Nursing Implications: Teach female patient to report vaginal itching or discharge. Discuss appropriate antifungal treatment with physician. Teach perineal hygiene and symptomatic management.

V.   ALTERATION IN HEPATIC FUNCTION

Defining Characteristics: Associated with high IV doses (> 2 g/day): hepatotoxicity and cholestasis may occur.

Nursing Implications: Assess baseline LFTs and monitor during therapy.

COMPLICATIONS

VI.   INFECTION AND BLEEDING related to NEUTROPENIA, THROMBOCYTOPENIA

Defining Characteristics: Neutropenia, leukocytosis, leukopenia, atypical lymphocytes, thrombocytopenia, thrombocytopenic purpura, hemolytic anemia occur rarely with long-term therapy.

Nursing Implications: Assess baseline WBC, HCT, and platelets, and monitor periodically during long-term therapy.

VII.   ALTERATION IN COMFORT related to LOCAL ADMINISTRATION EFFECTS

Defining Characteristics: IM administration may cause pain, induration due to muscle injury. IV administration may cause erythema, pain, swelling, and thrombophlebitis.

Nursing Implications: Rotate sites. Apply ice as ordered to painful buttock. Assess IV site prior to each dose for phlebitis or swelling and change site at least q 48 h. Apply heat to painful IV sites as ordered.

VIII.   SENSORY/PERCEPTUAL ALTERATION

Defining Characteristics: Lightheadedness, dizziness, or headache may occur.

Nursing Implications: Assess baseline neurologic status. Teach patient to report any changes and discuss them with physician.

Drug: moxifloxacin (ABC Pack; Avelox)

Class: Antibiotic; quinolone.

Mechanism of Action: Acts intracellularly by inhibiting DNA gyrase and bacterial topoisomerase IV. DNA gyrase is required for DNA replication and transcription, DNA repair, recombination, and transposition; inhibition is bactericidal.

Metabolism: Widely distributed to most body fluids and tissues with highest concentrations in organs, such as kidneys, gallbladder, lungs, liver, gynecologic tissue, prostatic tissue, phagocytic cells, urine, sputum, and bile. Well-absorbed from GI tract. Metabolized in liver; excreted in urine and feces. Crosses placenta and is excreted in breastmilk.

Indication: For treatment of different types of bacterial infections of the complicated and uncomplicated skin and skin structures, sinuses, lungs (bronchitis and CAP), and cIAI. Moxifloxacin is a broad-spectrum anti-infective, active against a wide range of aerobic gram-positive and gram-negative organisms.

Dosage/Range:
- 400 mg PO or IV daily.

Drug Preparation:

- Oral: Take drug with large glass of water, preferably 2 hours after meal/food. Encourage oral fluids of 2–3 qt/day.
- IV: Further dilute drug in 0.9% sodium chloride or 5% dextrose in water to final concentration of 2 mg/mL. Administer over 60 minutes; do not infuse by rapid or bolus IV infusion.
- Do not refrigerate.

Drug Interactions:

- Antacids (containing magnesium, aluminum, or calcium) and iron decrease absorption of serum level of moxifloxacin; do not administer concurrently. If must administer antacids or iron, administer at least 4 hours apart. The administration of antacids containing aluminum, magnesium, calcium, sucralfate, zinc, or iron may substantially reduce the absorption of moxifloxacin; do not administer concurrently.
- Serum digoxin concentrations should be monitored; moxifloxacin may raise serum levels in some patients.
- Probenecid: decreases the renal tubular secretion of moxifloxacin, resulting in a prolonged elimination half-life and increased risk of toxicity.
- Moxifloxacin may have the potential to prolong the QT interval of the EKG in some patients. Moxifloxacin should not be used in patients with prolonged QT interval; patients with uncorrected hypokalemia; and patients on quinidine, procainamide, amiodarone, and sotalol (antiarrhythmic agents).
- Increased intracranial pressure and psychosis has been reported along with CNS stimulation.
- Hypersensitivity reactions have been reported.

Lab Effects/Interference:
- Serum SGPT, serum alk phos, serum SGOT, and serum LDH—values may be increased.

Special Considerations:

- Used in the treatment of respiratory tract infections (acute bacterial exacerbation of chronic bronchitis, acute bacterial sinusitis, and commonly acquired pneumonia).
- Used in the treatment of uncomplicated infections of the skin and skin structures.
- Contraindicated in pregnancy or women who are breastfeeding.
- Obtain ordered specimen for culture and sensitivity prior to first drug dose.
- Use cautiously in patients with seizure disorders.
- Black box warning: Fluoroquinolones, including levofloxacin, are associated with an increased risk of tendinitis and tendon rupture in all ages. Risk further increases with age over 60 years, concomitant steroid therapy, and kidney, heart, or lung transplants. Fluoroquinolones, including levofloxacin, may exacerbate muscle weakness in persons with myasthenia gravis. Avoid in patients with known history of myasthenia gravis.

COMPLICATIONS

Potential Toxicities/Side Effects and the Nursing Process

I.   ALTERATION IN NUTRITION related to GI SIDE EFFECTS

Defining Characteristics: Incidence of nausea, vomiting, abdominal discomfort, diarrhea, and anorexia.

Nursing Implications: Assess baseline nutritional and elimination status. Teach patient to report GI disturbances. Administer and teach patient to self-administer antiemetics, antidiarrheals as needed and as ordered. Teach patient importance of nutritious diet, and suggest small, frequent, high-calorie, high-protein meals as appropriate. Assess baseline LFTs and monitor periodically during treatment. Discuss abnormalities and drug interruption with physician.

II.   SENSORY/PERCEPTUAL ALTERATIONS related to CNS EFFECTS

Defining Characteristics: Incidence of headache, restlessness. Dizziness, hallucinations, and seizures may occur. Exacerbated by caffeine as quinolones delay caffeine excretion.

Nursing Implications: Assess baseline neurologic function and comfort, and monitor during treatment. Teach patient to report any changes. Discuss any abnormalities with physician. Teach patient to limit or restrict all caffeine-containing fluids, medications (e.g., tea, coffee, soft drinks).

III.   ALTERATION IN SKIN INTEGRITY related to ALLERGY/HYPERSENSITIVITY

Defining Characteristics: Incidence of rash; other manifestations include eosinophilia, urticaria, flushing, fever, chills, photosensitivity, and angioedema. Fatal hypersensitivity reactions have occurred rarely. Direct exposure to sunlight can cause sunburn (moderate-to-severe phototoxicity).

Nursing Implications: Assess baseline skin condition, including integrity and drug allergy history. Teach patient to report rash, itching, or other skin changes. Teach patient skin care and symptomatic measures as appropriate. If skin rash develops, discuss drug discontinuance with physician. Be prepared to treat severe acute hypersensitivity reactions with airway management, oxygen, epinephrine, corticosteroids, antihistamines as ordered. Teach patient to avoid excessive sun exposure and to use SPF 15 or higher. If rash progresses, especially in HIV-infected patients, drug should be discontinued, as fatal Stevens–Johnson syndrome may develop.

IV.   FUNGAL SUPERINFECTION related to REDISTRIBUTION OF ENDOGENOUS MICROORGANISMS

Defining Characteristics: Vaginal moniliasis or vaginitis may occur as endogenous bacteria are eliminated and normal fungal population expands.

Nursing Implications: Teach female patient to report vaginal itching or discharge. Discuss appropriate antifungal treatment with physician. Teach perineal hygiene and symptomatic management.

V.   ALTERATION IN URINARY ELIMINATION related to RENAL TOXICITY

Defining Characteristics: Increased BUN and creatinine, crystal and stone formation in urine, interstitial nephritis, and renal failure may occur.

Nursing Implications: Assess baseline renal function; expect that drug dose will be decreased in presence of renal dysfunction. Teach patient to take drug with at least 8 oz of water, and to increase oral fluids to 2–3 qt/day.

VI.   ALTERATION IN COMFORT related to LOCAL ADMINISTRATION

Defining Characteristics: Drug may cause pain, inflammation, and rare thrombophlebitis at IV site.

Nursing Implications: Change IV site q 48 hours. Assess for phlebitis, discomfort, and IV patency prior to each administration. Administer drug slowly over 60–90 minutes in large volume of 5% dextrose (see Drug Preparation). Apply heat to promote comfort.

Drug: nafcillin sodium (Unipen)

Class: Antibacterial (systemic).

Mechanism of Action: Semisynthetic antibiotic. Contains β-lactam ring and is bactericidal by inhibiting cell wall synthesis. Penicillinase-resistant penicillin; active against penicillin-resistant staphylococci that produce the enzyme penicillinase.

Metabolism: Incompletely absorbed from GI tract; rapidly absorbed when given IM or IV. Widely distributed in body tissues and fluid, including bile. Crosses placenta and is excreted in breastmilk; 70–90% bound to serum proteins. Metabolized in liver excreted in bile, to a lesser degree in the urine.

Indication: For treatment of infections caused by, or suspected of being caused by, susceptible penicillinase-producing staphylococci, including respiratory tract; skin and skin structures; bone and joint; urinary tract infections; meningitis; and bacteremia.

Dosage/Range:

Adult:

Route	Dosage	Interval/Duration	Dose Adjustment
Oral	500 mg to 1 g	q 6 h	Reduce usual dose by 50% if severe renal and hepatic impairment
IM/IV	500 mg to 2 g	q 4 h	

Drug Preparation:
- Oral: Reconstitute per manufacturer's recommendation or by capsules or tablets. Administer 1 hour before meals or 2 hours after meals.

COMPLICATIONS

- IM: Reconstitute with sterile or bacteriostatic water for injection and give deep IM in large muscle (e.g., gluteus maximus).
- IV: Reconstitute with sterile water for injection or 0.9% sodium chloride for injection according to manufacturer's package insert. Further dilute in 100-mL IV solution and infuse over 40–60 minutes.

Drug Interactions:
- Aminoglycosides (e.g., gentamicin): incompatible when mixed together; administer at separate sites at different times. Also, penicillinase-resistant penicillins can inactivate aminoglycoside serum samples from patients receiving both drugs.
- Rifampin: possible antagonism, only at high doses of penicillin.
- Concurrent use of CYCLOSPORINE and NAFCILLIN may result in decreased CYCLOSPORINE concentrations
- Concurrent use of NAFCILLIN and WARFARIN may result in decreased INR/prothrombin time and anticoagulant effectiveness.
- Concurrent use of PENICILLINS and TETRACYCLINES may result in decreased antibacterial effectiveness.
- Nafcillin may decrease effectiveness of CYP4503A4 substrates (Nifedipine, clarithromycin, etc.).

Lab Effects/Interference:

Major clinical significance:
- Urine glucose: high urinary concentrations of a penicillin may produce false-positive or falsely elevated test results with copper sulfate tests (Benedict's, Clinitest, or Fehling's); glucose enzymatic tests (Clinistix or Tes-Tape) are not affected.

Clinical significance:
- Coombs' (direct antiglobulin) test: false-positive result may occur during therapy with any penicillin.
- ALT, alk phos, AST, serum LDH: values may be increased.
- WBC: leukopenia or neutropenia is associated with the use of all penicillins; the effect is more likely to occur with prolonged therapy and severe hepatic function impairment.

Special Considerations:
- Contraindicated in patients with prior hypersensitivity to penicillins. Use with caution in patients sensitive to other β-lactams (e.g., cephalosporins) since partial cross-allergenicity exists.
- Hypersensitivity to corn or corn products; dextrose solutions may precipitate an allergic reaction
- Obtain ordered specimen and send for culture and sensitivity prior to first antibiotic dose.
- Consider alternative antibiotic therapy if eosinophilia, drug fever or rash, arthralgia, hematuria, or unexplained rise in BUN and serum creatinine occur.
- Monitor electrolytes and renal, hepatic, and hematologic laboratory parameters during extended treatment periods.
- Use with caution in pregnancy or with nursing women.

Potential Toxicities/Side Effects and the Nursing Process

I. POTENTIAL FOR INJURY related to HYPERSENSITIVITY REACTION

Defining Characteristics: Urticaria, pruritus, rash (maculopapular or erythematous), fever and chills, eosinophilia, myalgia, edema, erythema, angioedema, Stevens–Johnson syndrome, and exfoliative skin reactions occur in 5% of patients. Increased risk in individuals allergic to cephalosporin antibiotics.

Nursing Implications: Assess allergy to cephalosporin antibiotics and penicillin: if patient states "yes," determine actual response (e.g., "swollen lips = angioedema"). If angioedema, patient should not receive drug. Discuss other patient responses with physician to determine whether drug should be given. Assess baseline skin condition, including integrity and allergy history to drugs. Instruct patient to report rash, itching, or other skin changes. Teach patient skin care and symptomatic measures as appropriate. If skin rash develops, discuss drug discontinuance with physician. If rash progresses, drug should be discontinued, as fatal Stevens–Johnson syndrome may develop. Be prepared to treat severe acute hypersensitivity reactions with airway management, oxygen, epinephrine, corticosteroids, antihistamines as ordered.

II. ALTERATION IN NUTRITION, LESS THAN BODY REQUIREMENTS, related to GI SIDE EFFECTS

Defining Characteristics: Nausea, vomiting, or diarrhea may occur; rarely, pseudomembranous colitis caused by *C. difficile* resistant to the antibiotic occurs. Rarely, transient increases in LFTs—AST, ALT, alk phos, bili—may occur.

Nursing Implications: Assess baseline nutritional status. Instruct patient to report GI disturbances. Administer and teach patient to self-administer antiemetics, antidiarrheals as needed and as ordered. Teach patient importance of nutritious diet, and suggest small, frequent, high-calorie, high-protein meals as appropriate. Assess baseline LFTs and monitor periodically during treatment. Discuss abnormalities and drug interruption with physician.

III. FUNGAL SUPERINFECTION related to REDISTRIBUTION OF ENDOGENOUS MICROORGANISMS

Defining Characteristics: Vaginal candidiasis or vaginitis may occur as endogenous bacteria are eliminated and normal fungal population expands.

Nursing Implications: Instruct female patient to report vaginal itching or discharge. Discuss appropriate antifungal treatment with physician. Teach perineal hygiene and symptomatic management.

COMPLICATIONS

IV.   ALTERATIONS IN PROTECTIVE MECHANISMS (RARE) related to TRANSIENT LEUKOPENIA

Defining Characteristics: Rarely, transient leukopenia, lymphocytosis, anemia, or eosinophilia may occur. Prolonged PT, prolonged aPTT, and hypoprothrombinemia have occurred rarely, especially in elderly or debilitated patients, or in individuals with vitamin K deficiency.

Nursing Implications: Assess baseline laboratory parameters, and monitor periodically during treatment. Assess patient for response to antibiotics. Discuss abnormalities with physician.

V.   ALTERATIONS IN COMFORT related to PHLEBITIS

Defining Characteristics: Phlebitis and thrombophlebitis may occur with IV administration. Increased risk in elderly.

Nursing Implications: Assess IV site prior to each dose for phlebitis, erythema, and swelling, and change site at least q 48 h. Apply heat to painful IV site as ordered.

Drug: omadacycline (Nuzyra)

Class: Antibacterial (systemic); modernized tetracycline specifically designed to overcome tetracycline resistance.

Mechanism of Action: Omadacycline is an aminomethylcycline antibacterial within the tetracycline class of antibacterial drugs. Bacteriostatic but may be bactericidal at high concentrations. Binds to bacterial ribosomes and prevents protein synthesis.

Metabolism: Absorbed (60–80%) from GI tract. Widely distributed into body tissues and fluids. Crosses placenta and is excreted in breastmilk. Excreted unchanged in urine.

Indication: Drug is used for specific infections: community-acquired bacterial pneumonia and acute bacterial skin and skin structure infections (ABSSSI).

Dosage/Range:

Adult:
- Oral: 450 mg once day 1 and 2 (loading dose); then 300 mg once daily. Duration of therapy depends on indication.
- IV: 200 mg over 60 minutes day 1 or 100 mg over 30 minutes twice day 1; then 100 mg over 30 minutes daily. Duration of therapy depends on indication.

Drug Preparation:
- Oral: take on an empty stomach with water and no food or drink (except water) for 2 hours afterwards. Do not take with dairy products, antacids, or multivitamins for 4 hours.

- IV: add 5 mL sterile water, 0.9% sodium chloride injection, or 5% dextrose injection to 100-mg vial. Further dilute in 100 mL (nominal volume) of 0.9% sodium chloride injection or 5% dextrose injection. Infuse over 30 minutes for 100 mg dose and 60 minutes for 200 mg dose.
- AVOID RAPID ADMINISTRATION.
- DO NOT ADMINISTER INTRAMUSCULARLY OR SUBCUTANEOUSLY.

Drug Interactions:
- Hepatotoxic drugs: may increase hepatotoxicity if given concurrently. Assess baseline and periodically during treatment.
- Iron preparations: decrease oral and possibly IV absorption. Administer iron preparations 3 hours after or 2 hours before any tetracycline.
- Oral anticoagulants: increase PT. Monitor patient closely and decrease anticoagulant dose as needed.
- Antidiarrheals (containing kaolin, pectate, or bismuth): may decrease absorption of tetracyclines. Avoid concurrent use.
- Oral contraceptives: decreased effectiveness of contraceptive and increased incidence of breakthrough bleeding. Advise patient to use barrier contraceptive as well during a course of tetracycline therapy.

Lab Effects/Interference:
- Urine catecholamine determinations: may produce false elevations of urinary catecholamines because of interfering fluorescence in the Hingerty method.
- SGPT, alk phos, amylase, SGOT, and bilirubin: serum concentrations may be increased.

Special Considerations:
- Use cautiously in patients with myasthenia gravis: may increase muscle weakness.
- Avoid use in pregnant or lactating women.
- Obtain ordered specimen for culture and sensitivity prior to first dose.
- Sunlight or ultraviolet light exposure increases risk for photosensitivity; discontinue if skin erythema occurs.

Potential Toxicities/Side Effects and the Nursing Process

I. ALTERATION IN NUTRITION related to GI SIDE EFFECTS

Defining Characteristics: Nausea, vomiting, diarrhea, anorexia, abdominal discomfort, epigastric burning and distress, glossitis may occur.

Nursing Implications: Assess baseline nutritional status. Assess for and teach patient to report any symptoms. Administer and teach patient self-administration of prescribed antiemetic or antidiarrheal medication as **appropriate**. Administer and teach patient to self-administer oral dose with at least 8 oz of water taken at least 1 hour before lying down for sleep.

II.   ALTERATION IN SKIN INTEGRITY related to RASH, PHOTOSENSITIVITY

Defining Characteristics: Maculopapular and erythematous rashes may occur. Rarely, exfoliative dermatitis, onycholysis, and nail discoloration. Photosensitivity risk (exaggerated sunburn) persists 1–2 days after completion of drug therapy.

Nursing Implications: Teach patient about potential side effects, to avoid sunlight during drug therapy, and to report rash, other abnormalities. Teach symptomatic skin care as appropriate.

III.   INJURY related to HYPERSENSITIVITY

Defining Characteristics: Urticaria, angioneurotic edema, anaphylaxis may occur; also, fever, rash, arthralgias, eosinophilia, and pericarditis.

Nursing Implications: Assess drug allergy history. Assess baseline allergy history. Assess baseline skin integrity. Teach patient to report rash, pruritus. Teach patient symptomatic management of rash, pruritus. Assess for hypersensitivity reaction; if it occurs, monitor VS, discontinue drug, notify physician, and institute supportive measures.

IV.   FUNGAL SUPERINFECTION related to REDISTRIBUTION OF ENDOGENOUS MICROORGANISMS

Defining Characteristics: Vaginal moniliasis, vaginitis may occur as endogenous bacteria are eliminated and normal fungal population expands.

Nursing Implications: Teach female patient to report vaginal itching or discharge. Discuss appropriate antifungal treatment with physician. Teach perineal hygiene and symptomatic management.

V.   TETRACYCLINE CLASS ADVERSE REACTIONS

Defining Characteristics: Omadacycline is similar to tetracycline-class antibacterial drugs and may have similar adverse reactions.

Nursing Implications: Teach patients to be aware of tooth discoloration and enamel hypoplasia Drug may cause permanent discoloration of teeth (yellow-gray-brown) especially during last half of pregnancy. May cause reversible inhibition of bone growth if used during the second and third trimesters of pregnancy.

VI.   ALTERATIONS IN COMFORT related to LOCAL ADMINISTRATION EFFECTS

Defining Characteristics: IM administration may cause pain, in duration due to muscle injury. IV administration may cause erythema, pain, swelling, and thrombophlebitis.

Nursing Implications: Rotate sites. Apply ice as ordered to painful buttock. Assess IV site prior to each dose for phlebitis or swelling and change site at least q 48 hours. Apply heat to painful IV sites as ordered.

Drug: oritavancin (Orbactiv)

Class: Antibacterial.

Mechanism of Action: Lipoglycopeptide antibacterial drug indicated for treatment of adult patients with ABSSSI caused, or suspected to be caused, by gram-positive microorganisms.

Metabolism: Oritavancin is bound to plasma proteins and is excreted unchanged in feces and urine.

Indications: Treatment of adult patients with ABSSSI caused by susceptible gram-positive microorganisms—*S. aureus* (including methicillin-susceptible and -resistant isolates), *S. pyogenes*, *S. agalactiae*, *Streptococcus dysgalactiae*, *S. anginosus* group (including *S. anginosus*, *S. intermedius*, and *S. constellatus*), and *E. faecalis* (vancomycin-susceptible isolates only).

Dosage/Range: A 1,200-mg single dose is administered by IV infusion over 3 hours.

Drug Preparation:
- Oritavancin is intended for IV infusion, only after reconstitution and dilution.
- Aseptic technique should be used to reconstitute oritavancin vials. Reconstitute per manufacturer package insert instructions with sterile water for injection.
- Gently swirl to avoid foaming and ensure powder is completely reconstituted in solution. Inspect vial visually for particulate matter after reconstitution. Fluid should be clear, colorless to pale yellow solution.
- Dilution: Use *only* 5% dextrose in sterile water (D_5W) for dilution. Do *not* use normal saline for dilution, as it is incompatible with oritavancin and may cause precipitation of drug.
- Because no preservative or bacteriostatic agent is present in this product, aseptic technique must be used in preparing the final IV solution.
- Diluted IV solution in an infusion bag should be used within 6 hours when stored at room temperature, or used within 12 hours when refrigerated at 2–8°C (36–46°F). Combined storage time (reconstituted solution in vial and diluted solution in bag) and 3-hour infusion time should not exceed 6 hours at room temperature or 12 hours if refrigerated.

Drug Interaction: In vitro studies with human liver microsomes showed that oritavancin inhibited the activities of cytochrome P450 (CYP) enzymes 1A2, 2B6, 2D6, 2C9, 2C19, and 3A4. The observed inhibition of multiple CYP isoforms by oritavancin in vitro is likely to be reversible, and the mechanism of inhibition is probably noncompetitive. In vitro studies indicate that oritavancin is neither a substrate nor an inhibitor of the efflux transporter P-glycoprotein (P-gp).

COMPLICATIONS

- Heparin: concurrent use of HEPARIN and ORITAVANCIN may result in falsely elevated aPTT test results.
- Warfarin: concurrent use of ORITAVANCIN and WARFARIN may result in increased warfarin exposure.

Lab Effects/Interference:
- Concomitant warfarin use: Coadministration of oritavancin and warfarin may result in higher exposure of warfarin, which may increase risk of bleeding. Use oritavancin in patients on chronic warfarin therapy only when the benefits can be expected to outweigh the risk of bleeding.
- Coagulation test interference: Oritavancin has been shown to artificially prolong aPTT for up to 48 hours, and may prolong PT and INR for up to 24 hours.
- Use of intravenous unfractionated heparin sodium is contraindicated for 48 hours after oritavancin administration.

Special Considerations:
- Hypersensitivity reactions have been reported with use of antibacterial agents including oritavancin. Discontinue infusion if signs of acute hypersensitivity occur. Monitor patients with known hypersensitivity to glycopeptides.
- Infusion-related reactions have been reported. Slow infusion rate or interrupt infusion if an infusion reaction develops.
- *C. difficile*–associated colitis: Evaluate patients if diarrhea occurs.

Potential Toxicities/Side Effects and the Nursing Process

I.   POTENTIAL FOR INJURY related to HYPERSENSITIVITY REACTION

Defining Characteristics: Urticaria, pruritus, rash (maculopapular or erythematous), fever and chills, eosinophilia, myalgia, edema, erythema, and angioedema.

Nursing Implications: No cross allergenicity to PCN and CEF antibiotics is noted. However, previous sensitivity to glycopeptides may be a concern. Assess allergy to cephalosporin antibiotics and penicillin; if patient states "yes," determine actual response (e.g., "swollen lips = angioedema"). If angioedema is present, patient *should not* receive drug. Discuss other patient responses with physician to determine whether drug should be given. Assess baseline skin condition, including integrity, and allergy history to drugs. Instruct patient to report rash, itching, or other skin changes. Teach patient skin care and symptomatic measures as appropriate. If skin rash develops, discuss drug discontinuance with physician. If rash progresses, drug should be discontinued. Be prepared to treat severe acute hypersensitivity reactions with airway management, oxygen, epinephrine, corticosteroids, and antihistamines as ordered.

II.   ALTERATION IN NUTRITION, LESS THAN BODY REQUIREMENTS, related to GI SIDE EFFECTS

Defining Characteristics: Nausea, vomiting, diarrhea, and anorexia may occur; rarely, pseudomembranous colitis caused by *C. difficile* resistant to the antibiotic occurs.

Nursing Implications: Assess baseline nutritional status. Instruct patient to report GI disturbances. Administer, and teach patient to self-administer, antiemetics as needed and as ordered. Teach patient about importance of a nutritious diet; suggest small, frequent, high-calorie, high-protein meals as appropriate. Assess baseline LFTs and monitor periodically during treatment. Discuss abnormalities and drug interruption with physician.

III. FUNGAL SUPERINFECTION related to REDISTRIBUTION OF ENDOGENOUS MICROORGANISMS

Defining Characteristics: Vaginal candidiasis and vaginitis may occur as endogenous bacteria are eliminated and normal fungal population expands.

Nursing Implications: Instruct female patients to report vaginal itching or discharge. Discuss appropriate antifungal treatment with physician. Teach perineal hygiene and symptomatic management.

IV. ALTERATIONS IN PROTECTIVE MECHANISMS (RARE) related to TRANSIENT LEUKOPENIA

Defining Characteristics: Rarely, transient leukopenia, lymphocytosis, anemia, and eosinophilia may occur. Prolonged PT, prolonged aPTT, and hypoprothrombinemia have occurred rarely, especially in elderly or debilitated patients or in individuals with vitamin K deficiency.

Nursing Implications: Assess baseline laboratory parameters, and monitor periodically during treatment. Assess patient for response to antibiotics. Discuss abnormalities with physician. Assess for signs and symptoms of bleeding. If they occur, especially in elderly or debilitated patients, discuss vitamin K administration with physician. Instruct patient to avoid aspirin. If taking oral anticoagulants, assess for increased PT and signs and symptoms of bleeding.

V. ALTERATIONS IN COMFORT related to LOCAL INJECTION-SITE IRRITATION

Defining Characteristics: Pain and phlebitis may develop in IV sites.

Nursing Implications: Change IV sites every 48 hours, and assess for signs and symptoms of phlebitis prior to each administration. Administer drug slowly. Apply warm packs to increase comfort.

COMPLICATIONS

Drug: oxacillin sodium (Bactocill, Prostaphlin)

Class: Antibacterial (systemic).

Mechanism of Action: Semisynthetic antibiotic. Contains β-lactam ring and is bactericidal by inhibiting cell wall synthesis. Penicillinase-resistant penicillin and active against penicillin-resistant staphylococci, which produce the enzyme penicillinase.

Metabolism: Incompletely absorbed from GI tract; rapidly absorbed when given IM or IV. Widely distributed in body tissues and fluid, including bile. Crosses placenta and is excreted in breastmilk; 89–94% bound to serum proteins. Metabolized in liver, excreted in urine.

Indication: For treatment of infections caused by penicillinase-producing staphylococci; initial therapy of suspected staphylococcal infections eliminating bacteria that cause infections, including pneumonia, meningitis, urinary tract, skin, bone, joint, blood, and heart valve infections.

Dosage/Range:

Adult:

Route	Dosage	Interval/Duration	Dose Adjustment
Oral	500 mg to 1 g	q 4 to 6 h	Renal adjustment not necessary
IM/IV	500 mg to 2 g	q 4 h	

Drug Preparation:
- Oral: Reconstitute per manufacturer's package insert or by capsules or tablets. Administer 1 hour before meals or 2 hours after meals.
- IM: Reconstitute with sterile or bacteriostatic water for injection, and give deep IM in large muscle (e.g., gluteus maximus).
- IV: Reconstitute with sterile water for injection or 0.9% sodium chloride for injection according to manufacturer's package insert. Further dilute in 100-mL IV solution and infuse over 40–60 minutes.

Drug Interactions:
- Aminoglycosides (e.g., gentamicin): incompatible when mixed together; administer at separate sites at different times. Also, penicillinase-resistant penicillins can inactivate aminoglycoside serum samples from patients receiving both drugs.
- Tetracyclines may result in decreased antibacterial effectiveness.
- Warfarin may result in decreased INR/prothrombin time and anticoagulant effectiveness.
- Drug interacts with bupropion; donepezil lower seizure threshold.
- Typhoid vaccine.

Lab Effects/Interference:

Major clinical significance:
- Urine glucose: high urinary concentrations of a penicillin may produce false-positive or falsely elevated test results with copper sulfate tests (Benedict's, Clinitest, or Fehling's); glucose enzymatic tests (Clinistix or Tes-Tape) are not affected.

Clinical significance:
- Coombs' (direct antiglobulin) test: false-positive result may occur during therapy with any penicillin.
- ALT, alk phos, AST, serum LDH values may be increased.
- WBC: leukopenia or neutropenia is associated with the use of all penicillins; the effect is more likely to occur with prolonged therapy and severe hepatic function impairment.

Special Considerations:
- Take oral tabs on empty stomach.
- Contraindicated in patients with prior hypersensitivity to penicillins. Use with caution in patients sensitive to other β-lactams (e.g., cephalosporins) since partial cross-allergenicity.
- Obtain ordered specimen and send for culture and sensitivity prior to first antibiotic dose.
- Consider alternative antibiotic therapy if eosinophilia, drug fever or rash, arthralgia, hematuria, or unexplained rise in BUN and serum creatinine occur.
- Monitor electrolytes and renal, hepatic, and hematologic laboratory parameters during extended treatment periods.
- Use with caution in pregnant or nursing women.

Potential Toxicities/Side Effects and the Nursing Process

I.   POTENTIAL FOR INJURY related to HYPERSENSITIVITY REACTION

Defining Characteristics: Urticaria, pruritus, rash (maculopapular or erythematous), fever and chills, eosinophilia, myalgia, edema, erythema, angioedema, Stevens–Johnson syndrome, and exfoliative skin reactions occur in 5% of patients. Increased risk in individuals allergic to cephalosporin antibiotics.

Nursing Implications: Assess allergy to cephalosporin antibiotics and penicillin: if patient states "yes," determine actual response (e.g., "swollen lips = angioedema"). If angioedema, patient should not receive drug. Discuss other patient responses with physician to determine whether drug should be given. Assess baseline skin condition, including integrity and allergy history to drugs. Instruct patient to report rash, itching, or other skin changes. Teach patient skin care and symptomatic measures as appropriate. If skin rash develops, discuss drug discontinuance with physician. If rash progresses, drug should be discontinued, as fatal Stevens–Johnson syndrome may develop. Be prepared to treat severe acute hypersensitivity reactions with airway management, oxygen, epinephrine, corticosteroids, or antihistamines as ordered.

II.   ALTERATION IN NUTRITION, LESS THAN BODY REQUIREMENTS, related to INCREASED LFTs

Defining Characteristics: Oral lesions may occur, as may hepatitis (rare) and increased LFTs.

Nursing Implications: Assess baseline oral mucosa, and LFTs—AST, ALT, alk phos, bili. Teach patient to practice oral hygiene after meals and at bedtime, and instruct to report any oral lesions. Monitor LFTs periodically during treatment, and discuss abnormalities with physician.

III.   FUNGAL SUPERINFECTION related to REDISTRIBUTION OF ENDOGENOUS MICROORGANISMS

Defining Characteristics: Vaginal candidiasis or vaginitis may occur as endogenous bacteria are eliminated and normal fungal population expands.

COMPLICATIONS

Nursing Implications: Instruct female patient to report vaginal itching or discharge. Discuss appropriate antifungal treatment with physician. Teach perineal hygiene and symptomatic management.

IV. ALTERATIONS IN PROTECTIVE MECHANISMS (RARE) related to TRANSIENT LEUKOPENIA

Defining Characteristics: Rarely, transient leukopenia, lymphocytosis, anemia, or eosinophilia may occur. Prolonged PT, prolonged aPTT, and hypoprothrombinemia have occurred rarely, especially in elderly or debilitated patients, or in individuals with vitamin K deficiency.

Nursing Implications: Assess baseline laboratory parameters, and monitor periodically during treatment. Assess patient for response to antibiotics. Discuss abnormalities with physician.

V. ALTERATIONS IN COMFORT related to PHLEBITIS

Defining Characteristics: Phlebitis and thrombophlebitis may occur with IV administration. Increased risk in elderly.

Nursing Implications: Assess IV site prior to each dose for phlebitis, erythema, and swelling, and change site at least q 48 h. Apply heat to painful IV site as ordered.

VI. ALTERATIONS IN URINARY ELIMINATION related to RENAL DAMAGE

Defining Characteristics: Interstitial nephritis, transient proteinuria, or hematuria may occur rarely.

Nursing Implications: Assess baseline liver, renal function tests (e.g., serum BUN, creatinine, and urinalysis), and monitor during therapy.

VII. ALTERATIONS IN SENSORY/PERCEPTUAL PATTERNS related to NEUROPATHY

Defining Characteristics: Neuropathy, seizures, or neuromuscular irritability may occur rarely.

Nursing Implications: Assess baseline neurologic function and comfort, and monitor during treatment. Instruct patient to report any changes. Discuss any abnormalities with physician.

Drug: penicillin G (PenG potassium, PenG sodium intravenous; PenVK oral preparation)

Class: Natural penicillin.

Mechanism of Action: Produced by fermentation of *Penicillium chrysogenum*.

Metabolism: Decreased oral absorption, but IM or IV absorption is quite rapid and complete. Widely distributed in body tissues and fluids; 45–68% bound to proteins. Eliminated in urine and bile.

Indication: This drug is used to treat a variety of bacterial infections. Active against many gram-positive bacteria (streptococci, staphylococci) but resistant to *S. aureus* and *S. epidermidis* strains that produce penicillinases. Also active against some gram-negative bacteria (*Neisseria, H. influenzae*), and spirochetes.

Dosage/Range:

- Oral: 250–500 mg qid.
- IV: 200,000–4 million U q 4 h.
- Dose modification for renal impairment:

CrCl (mL/min/1.73 m²)	Induction Dosage (mg/kg)	Maintenance Dosage (mg/kg)
Less than 10	Administer full-loading dose	1/2 loading dose q 8–10 h
Greater than 10 with uremia	Administer full-loading dose	1/2 loading dose q 4–5 h

- With hepatic impairment, additional dosage adjustments may be necessary; specific recommendations not provided
- Geriatric: initiate at lower end of dosing range

Drug Preparation:
- Oral: Administer at least 1 hour before or 2 hours after meals.
- IM: Reconstitute drug as directed. Administration of greater than 100,000 U is likely to result in some discomfort. Give IM deep in large muscle mass.
- IV: Reconstitute drug as directed. Further dilute in 0.9% sodium chloride or 5% dextrose in water, and administer over 1–2 hours.

Drug Interactions:
- Aminoglycosides (e.g., gentamicin): incompatible when mixed together; administer at separate sites at different times. Also, penicillinase-resistant penicillins can inactivate aminoglycoside serum samples from patients receiving both drugs.
- Rifampin: possible antagonism, only at high doses of penicillin.
- Probenecid: increased serum level of penicillin; may be coadministered to exert this effect.

COMPLICATIONS

- Warfarin: increased risk of bleeding.
- Methotrexate: increased risk of toxicity.
- Drug interacts with bupropion; donepezil: lower seizure threshold; typhoid vaccine; and contraceptives: loss of efficacy.

Lab Effects/Interference:

Major clinical significance:
- Urine glucose: high urinary concentrations of a penicillin may produce false-positive or falsely elevated test results with copper sulfate tests (Benedict's, Clinitest, or Fehling's); glucose enzymatic tests (Clinistix or Tes-Tape) are not affected.

Clinical significance:
- Coombs' (direct antiglobulin) test: false-positive result may occur during therapy with any penicillin.
- ALT, alk phos, AST, serum LDH values may be increased.
- Serum K+: hyperkalemia may occur following administration of parenteral penicillin G potassium because of the high potassium content.
- Serum Na+: hypernatremia may occur following administration of large doses of parenteral penicillin G sodium because of the high sodium content.
- WBC: leukopenia or neutropenia is associated with the use of all penicillins; the effect is more likely to occur with prolonged therapy and severe hepatic function impairment.

Special Considerations:
- Contraindicated in patients with prior hypersensitivity to penicillins. Use with caution in patients sensitive to other β-lactams (e.g., cephalosporins) since partial cross-allergenicity exists.
- Obtain ordered specimen and send for culture and sensitivity test prior to first antibiotic dose.
- Consider alternative antibiotic therapy if eosinophilia, drug fever or rash, arthralgia, hematuria, or unexplained rise in BUN and serum creatinine occur.
- Monitor electrolytes and renal, hepatic, and hematologic laboratory parameters during extended treatment periods.
- Hyperkalemia may occur with high-dose therapy: monitor serum K+.
- Use with caution in pregnant or nursing women.
- Penicillin G benzathine should never be given IV (suspension); give IM only.

Potential Toxicities/Side Effects and the Nursing Process

I.   POTENTIAL FOR INJURY related to HYPERSENSITIVITY REACTION

Defining Characteristics: Urticaria, pruritus, rash (maculopapular or erythematous), fever and chills, eosinophilia, myalgia, edema, erythema, angioedema, Stevens–Johnson syndrome, and exfoliative skin reactions occur in 5% of patients. Increased risk exists in individuals allergic to cephalosporin antibiotics.

Nursing Implications: Assess allergy to cephalosporin antibiotics and penicillin: if patient states "yes," determine actual response (e.g., "swollen lips = angioedema"). If angioedema, patient should not receive drug. IF patient is allergic to pcn, they should not receive it. Discuss other patient responses with physician to determine whether drug should be given. Assess baseline skin condition, including integrity and allergy history to drugs. Instruct patient to report rash, itching, or other skin changes. Teach patient skin care and symptomatic measures as appropriate. If skin rash develops, discuss drug discontinuance with physician. If rash progresses, drug should be discontinued, as fatal Stevens–Johnson syndrome may develop. Be prepared to treat severe acute hypersensitivity reactions with airway management, oxygen, epinephrine, corticosteroids, antihistamines as ordered.

II. ALTERATION IN NUTRITION, LESS THAN BODY REQUIREMENTS, related to GI SIDE EFFECTS

Defining Characteristics: Rarely, nausea, vomiting, diarrhea, and pseudomembranous colitis caused by *C. difficile* resistant to the antibiotic may occur. Rarely, transient increases in LFTs—AST, ALT, alk phos, bili—may occur.

Nursing Implications: Assess baseline nutritional status. Instruct patient to report GI disturbances. Administer and teach patient to self-administer antiemetics as needed and as ordered. Teach patient importance of nutritious diet, and suggest small, frequent, high-calorie, high-protein meals as appropriate. Assess baseline LFTs and monitor periodically during treatment. Discuss abnormalities and drug interruption with physician.

III. FUNGAL SUPERINFECTION related to REDISTRIBUTION OF ENDOGENOUS MICROORGANISMS

Defining Characteristics: Vaginal candidiasis; vaginitis may occur as endogenous bacteria are eliminated and normal fungal population expands.

Nursing Implications: Instruct female patient to report vaginal itching or discharge. Discuss appropriate antifungal treatment with physician. Teach perineal hygiene and symptomatic management.

IV. ALTERATIONS IN PROTECTIVE MECHANISMS (RARE) related to RARE LEUKOPENIA

Defining Characteristics: Rarely, hemolytic anemia, leukopenia, thrombocytopenia may occur.

Nursing Implications: Assess baseline laboratory parameters, and monitor periodically during treatment. Assess patient for response to antibiotics. Discuss abnormalities with physician.

COMPLICATIONS

V.   ALTERATIONS IN SENSORY/PERCEPTUAL PATTERNS related to NEUROPATHY

Defining Characteristics: Neuropathy, seizures may occur with high doses.

Nursing Implications: Assess baseline neurologic function and comfort, and monitor during treatment. Instruct patient to report any changes. Discuss any abnormalities with physician.

VI.   ALTERATIONS IN COMFORT related to LOCAL INJECTION IRRITATION

Defining Characteristics: Pain, induration may form in IM injection sites; phlebitis may develop in IV sites.

Nursing Implications: Rotate IM injection sites, and administer drug deep IM in large muscle mass (e.g., gluteus maximus). Use IM injection when IV administration is not possible. Change IV sites q 48 h, and assess for signs/symptoms of phlebitis prior to each administration. Administer drug slowly. Apply warm packs to increase comfort.

Drug: piperacillin sodium (Pipracil); combined with tazobactam sodium (Zosyn)

Class: Antibacterial (systemic) (extended-spectrum penicillin).

Mechanism of Action: Semisynthetic antibiotic prepared from fungus *Penicillium*. Contains β-lactam ring and is bactericidal by inhibiting cell wall synthesis.

Metabolism: Poorly absorbed from GI tract, so must be given parenterally. Widely distributed in body tissues and fluids. Crosses placenta and is excreted in breastmilk. Excreted via urine and bile.

Indication: For treatment of intra-abdominal, urinary tract, gynecologic, lower respiratory tract infections; septicemia; skin and skin structures infections; bone and joint infections; gonococcal urethritis; and treatment of infections caused by susceptible microorganisms. Active against most gram-positive (except penicillinase-producing strains) and most gram-negative bacilli. Used in the treatment of serious gram-negative infections, especially *P. aeruginosa*–related infections of lower respiratory tract, urinary tract, and skin. When combined with tazobactam sodium, which inhibits β-lactamases, piperacillin sodium is effective against resistant bacteria.

Dosage/Range:
• IV route
      Moderate-to-severe pneumonia caused by piperacillin-resistant *S. aureus* that produces B-lactamase: 3.375 g IV q 6 h plus aminoglycoside × 7–10 days.
      Dose modification necessary if severe renal insufficiency exists. (There are several ways to dose adjust for renal dysfunction, depending on the dose.)

Adult:
Piperacillin sodium: not used by itself.
- IV: 3–4 g q 4–6 h (maximum 24 g, but higher doses may be used in severe infection); IM: maximum 2 g/dose.

Zosyn:
- 3 g piperacillin and 0.375 g tazobactam (3.375 g)–4 g piperacillin and 0.50 g tazobactam (4.50 g) q 6 h IV × 7–10 days. Also 4.5 gm q 6–8 h given. Can be given as continuous infusion.
- Moderate-to-severe pneumonia caused by piperacillin-resistant *S. aureus* that produces β-lactamase: 3.375 g IV q 6 h plus aminoglycoside × 7–10 days.
- Dose modification necessary if severe renal insufficiency exists. (There are several ways to dose adjust for renal dysfunction, depending on the dose.)

Drug Preparation:
- IV: Reconstitute each gram of drug with at least 5 mL of sterile or bacteriostatic water. Further dilute in 50–100 mL 0.9% sodium chloride or 5% dextrose injection and infuse over 30 minutes.
- IM: Reconstitute with 2 mL of sterile or bacteriostatic water, or 0.5–1.0% lidocaine HCl (without epinephrine), with final concentration 1 g/2.5 mL. Administer as deep IM injection in large muscle mass (e.g., gluteus maximus). Make certain patient is NOT ALLERGIC to lidocaine.

Drug Interactions:
- Aminoglycosides (e.g., gentamicin): incompatible when mixed together; administer at separate sites at different times. Also, penicillinase-resistant penicillins can inactivate aminoglycoside serum samples from patients receiving both drugs.
- Probenecid: increased serum level of piperacillin; may be coadministered to exert this effect.
- Tazobactam: inhibits β-lactamase, thus broadening drug's antimicrobial effectiveness.
- Drug interacts with warfarin: increased risk of bleeding; methotrexate: increased risk of toxicity; bupropion; donepezil: lower seizure threshold; and typhoid vaccine.

Lab Effects/Interference:

Major clinical significance:
- Urine glucose: high urinary concentrations of a penicillin may produce false-positive or falsely elevated test results with copper sulfate tests (Benedict's, Clinitest, or Fehling's); glucose enzymatic tests (Clinistix or Tes-Tape) are not affected.
- PTT and PT: an increase has been associated with IV piperacillin.
- May result in false-positive galactomannan detection due to mechanism unknown.

Clinical significance:
- Coombs' (direct antiglobulin) test: false-positive result may occur during therapy with any penicillin.
- Urine protein: high urinary concentrations of piperacillin may produce false-positive protein reactions (pseudoproteinuria) with the sulfosalicylic acid and boiling test; bromophenol blue reagent test strips (Multistix) are reportedly unaffected.

COMPLICATIONS

- ALT, alk phos, AST, serum LDH values may be increased.
- Serum bili: an increase has been associated with piperacillin.
- BUN and serum creatinine: increased concentrations have been associated with piperacillin.
- Serum K+: hypokalemia may occur following administration of parenteral piperacillin, which may act as a nonreabsorbable anion in the distal tubules; this may cause an increase in pH and result in increased urinary potassium loss: the risk of hypokalemia increases with use of larger doses.
- WBC: leukopenia or neutropenia is associated with the use of all penicillins; the effect is more likely to occur with prolonged therapy and severe hepatic function impairment.

Special Considerations:
- Contraindicated in patients with prior hypersensitivity to penicillins. Use with caution in patients sensitive to other β-lactams (e.g., cephalosporins), since partial cross-allergenicity exists.
- Obtain ordered specimen and send for culture and sensitivity test prior to first antibiotic dose.
- Consider alternative antibiotic therapy if eosinophilia, drug fever or rash, arthralgia, hematuria, or unexplained rise in BUN and serum creatinine occur.
- Monitor electrolytes and renal, hepatic, and hematologic laboratory parameters during extended treatment periods.
- Use with caution in pregnant or nursing women.
- Low Na+ content: 1.98 mEq/g of drug.
- Increased activity against *P. aeruginosa*.

Potential Toxicities/Side Effects and the Nursing Process

I.   POTENTIAL FOR INJURY related to HYPERSENSITIVITY REACTION

Defining Characteristics: Urticaria, pruritus, rash (maculopapular or erythematous), fever and chills, eosinophilia, myalgia, edema, erythema, angioedema, Stevens–Johnson syndrome, and exfoliative skin reactions occur in 5% of patients. Increased risk exists in individuals allergic to cephalosporin antibiotics.

Nursing Implications: Assess allergy to cephalosporin antibiotics and penicillin: if patient states "yes," determine actual response (e.g., "swollen lips = angioedema"). If angioedema, patient should not receive drug. Discuss other patient responses with physician to determine whether drug should be given. Assess baseline skin condition, including integrity and allergy history to drugs. Instruct patient to report rash, itching, or other skin changes. Teach patient skin care and symptomatic measures as appropriate. If skin rash develops, discuss drug discontinuance with physician. If rash progresses, drug should be discontinued, as fatal Stevens–Johnson syndrome may develop. Be prepared to treat severe acute hypersensitivity reactions with airway management, oxygen, epinephrine, corticosteroids, antihistamines as ordered.

II. ALTERATION IN NUTRITION, LESS THAN BODY REQUIREMENTS, related to GI SIDE EFFECTS

Defining Characteristics: Nausea, vomiting, diarrhea may occur; rarely, pseudomembranous colitis caused by *C. difficile* resistant to the antibiotic occurs. Rarely, transient increases in LFTs—AST, ALT, alk phos, bili—may occur.

Nursing Implications: Assess baseline nutritional status. Instruct patient to report GI disturbances. Administer and teach patient to self-administer antiemetics as needed and as ordered. Teach patient importance of nutritious diet, and suggest small, frequent, high-calorie, high-protein meals as appropriate. Assess baseline LFTs and monitor periodically during treatment. Discuss abnormalities and drug interruption with physician.

III. FUNGAL SUPERINFECTION related to REDISTRIBUTION OF ENDOGENOUS MICROORGANISMS

Defining Characteristics: Vaginal candidiasis; vaginitis may occur as endogenous bacteria are eliminated and normal fungal population expands.

Nursing Implications: Instruct female patient to report vaginal itching or discharge. Discuss appropriate antifungal treatment with physician. Teach perineal hygiene and symptomatic management.

IV. ALTERATIONS IN PROTECTIVE MECHANISMS (RARE) Related to HEMATOLOGIC ABNORMALITIES

Defining Characteristics: Rarely, transient leukopenia, lymphocytosis, anemia, eosinophilia may occur. Prolonged PT, prolonged aPTT, and hypoprothrombinemia have occurred rarely, especially in elderly or debilitated patients, or in individuals with vitamin K deficiency.

Nursing Implications: Assess baseline laboratory parameters, and monitor periodically during treatment. Assess patient for response to antibiotics. Discuss abnormalities with physician. Assess for signs/symptoms of bleeding.

V. ALTERATIONS IN SENSORY/PERCEPTUAL PATTERNS related to DIZZINESS, SOMNOLENCE

Defining Characteristics: Dizziness, headache, somnolence occur rarely. Neuromuscular irritability and seizures may occur with high drug serum levels.

Nursing Implications: Assess baseline neurologic function and comfort, and monitor during treatment. Instruct patient to report any changes. Discuss any abnormalities with physician. Institute seizure precautions.

COMPLICATIONS

VI.   ALTERATIONS IN COMFORT related to LOCAL INJECTION IRRITATION

Defining Characteristics: Vein irritation (pain, erythema), phlebitis, and thrombophlebitis may occur at IV administration site.

Nursing Implications: Change IV sites q 48 h, and assess for signs/symptoms of phlebitis prior to each administration. Administer drug slowly. Apply warm packs to increase comfort. Discuss central line with patient and physician to facilitate administration.

VII.   ALTERATION IN FLUID AND ELECTROLYTE BALANCE related to HYPOKALEMIA AND INCREASED SODIUM INTAKE

Defining Characteristics: Prolonged therapy may cause hypokalemia; also, drug is prepared as sodium salt. Frequent IV infusions increase fluid intake.

Nursing Implications: Assess baseline electrolytes, fluid balance, weight, and monitor throughout therapy. Monitor renal function studies, especially if patient has preexisting renal dysfunction.

Drug: plazomicin (Zemdri)

Class: Aminoglycoside antibacterial

Mechanism of Action: Bactericidal, most probably by inhibition of protein synthesis.

Metabolism: Plazomicin does not appear to be metabolized to any appreciable extent. Excreted from the kidneys. Well-absorbed following IV administration, widely distributed into body fluids. Minimally protein-bound. Probabaly crosses placenta and into breastmilk. Drug excreted unchanged in the urine.

Indication: For the treatment of patients 18 and older with complicated urinary tract infections (cUTI) including pyelonephritis. For treatment of serious infections caused by susceptible bacteria. Over time, bacterial resistance may develop, either naturally or acquired.

Dosage/Range: Administer 15 mg/kg every 24 hours over 30 minutes by IV infusion. Continue therapy based on patient status up to 7 days. Dose adjust based on renal function.

Drug Preparation: Reconsitute in sterile water for injection for a concentration of 50 mg/ml. Further dilute in 0.9% sodium chloride injection or lactated ringer's injection for a final volume of 50 ml.

Drug Interactions:
- Increased risk of toxicity with other ototoxic/nephrotoxic drugs: acyclovir, other aminoglycosides, amphotericin B, bacitracin, cephalosporins, colistin, cisplatin, ethacrynic acid, furosemide, vancomycin.
- Potentiation of neuromuscular blockade when given concurrently with general anesthetics (succinylcholine, tubocurarine); use cautiously, observe for signs/symptoms of respiratory depression.

Lab Effects/Interference:
- Serum ALT, serum alk phos, serum AST, serum bili, and serum LDH values may be increased.
- BUN and serum creatinine concentrations may be increased.
- Serum Ca++, serum Mg++, serum K+, and serum Na+ concentrations may be decreased.

Special Considerations:
- Use in pregnancy only if infection is life-threatening and no safer drug exists; drug crosses placenta and may cause fetal toxicity.

Potential Toxicities/Side Effects and the Nursing Process

I.   ALTERATIONS IN SENSORY/PERCEPTUAL PATTERNS related to OTOTOXICITY

Defining Characteristics: Damage to eighth cranial nerve (auditory) may result in dizziness, nystagmus, vertigo, ataxia (vestibular damage), and more commonly tinnitus, roaring sound in ears, and impaired hearing (auditory damage). Hearing loss usually begins with high-frequency loss, followed by clinical hearing loss, then permanent hearing loss if damage continues. Increased risk in elderly or renally impaired patients.

Nursing Implications: Assess baseline hearing (ability to hear spoken voice) and continue to access during therapy. Teach patient potential side effects and instruct patient to report any hearing/perceptual problems (e.g., tinnitus, vertigo, decreased hearing). Discuss drug discontinuance and audiogram with physician to confirm hearing dysfunction if symptoms arise. Assess for increased risk if given concurrently with other ototoxic medications (e.g., cisplatin, furosemide).

II.   ALTERATION IN URINARY ELIMINATION related to NEPHROTOXICITY

Defining Characteristics: Renal damage characterized by tubular necrosis with increased serum BUN, creatinine; decreased urine creatinine clearance and specific gravity; proteinuria and casts in urine. Azotemia usually not associated with oliguria. Rarely, electrolyte wasting with hypomagnesemia, hypocalcemia, and hypokalemia may occur. Renal dysfunction is usually reversible after drug discontinuance. Increased risk exists in elderly and if preexisting renal dysfunction. Risk low in well-hydrated patients with normal renal function when normal doses given.

Nursing Implications: Assess baseline renal function and electrolytes and monitor periodically during therapy. Discuss any abnormalities with physician, as drug should be dose-reduced or discontinued if renal dysfunction develops. Assess baseline total body fluid balance, weight, and monitor periodically during antibiotic therapy. Monitor hydration status to keep patient well hydrated. Assess drug peak and trough levels as ordered so that drug dosage is correctly titrated. Increased risk of toxicity if peak serum concentration > 10–12 mg/mL. Draw blood for peak drug concentration 30 minutes after end of 30-minute infusion or at the end of a 60-minute infusion; draw trough immediately before next dose.

COMPLICATIONS

III.   ALTERATIONS IN SENSORY/PERCEPTUAL PATTERNS related to CNS EFFECTS, NEUROMUSCULAR BLOCKADE

Defining Characteristics: Headache, tremor, lethargy may occur. Peripheral neuropathy or encephalopathy (numbness, skin tingling, muscle twitching) may occur rarely. Neuromuscular blockade is dose-related, self-limiting, and uncommon; risk is greater with topical application or when drug is administered to patient with neuromuscular disease (myasthenia gravis) or hypocalcemia.

Nursing Implications: Assess baseline neurologic status. Assess coexisting risk factors, neuromuscular blockade medications. Teach patient about side effects and to report headache, tremor, lethargy. Observe for respiratory depression. If signs/symptoms arise, discuss drug discontinuance with physician.

IV.   POTENTIAL FOR INJURY related to HYPERSENSITIVITY

Defining Characteristics: Rash, urticaria, pruritus, fever, and eosinophilia have occurred rarely. CROSS-SENSITIVITY between AMINOGLYCOSIDES exists.

Nursing Implications: Assess for drug allergies to any aminoglycoside—amikacin, gentamicin, kanamycin, neomycin, netilmicin, streptomycin, tobramycin—prior to drug administration. Instruct patient to report any allergic reactions. Assess for signs/symptoms of allergic reaction after drug dose.

V.   ALTERATION IN NUTRITION, LESS THAN BODY REQUIREMENTS, related to GI SIDE EFFECTS

Defining Characteristics: Nausea, vomiting, and anorexia have occurred rarely. Also, transient hepatomegaly with increased LFTs—AST, ALT, LDH, alk phos, bili—has occurred.

Nursing Implications: Assess baseline nutritional status, preexisting nausea/vomiting, and anorexia. Assess baseline LFTs and monitor periodically during treatment. Instruct patient to report side effects. Provide symptomatic interventions if side effects occur; discuss with physician use of alternative drug(s).

VI.   POTENTIAL FOR FATIGUE, INFECTION, AND BLEEDING related to BONE MARROW INJURY

Defining Characteristics: Anemia, leukopenia, granulocytopenia, and thrombocytopenia may occur. Also, patients receiving antibiotics are at risk for overgrowth of nonsusceptible microorganisms, such as fungi (superinfection); rare.

Nursing Implications: Assess baseline CBC, differential, and monitor periodically during treatment. Instruct patient to report signs/symptoms of fatigue, infection, or bleeding immediately. Assess for signs/symptoms of superinfection. Discuss any adverse effects with physician.

Drug: quinupristin/dalfopristin (Synercid)

Class: Macrolide-lincosamide-streptogramin (MLS) class of antibiotic.

Mechanism of Action: Synercid inhibits bacterial protein synthesis by each component irreversibly binding to different sites on the 50S bacterial ribosome subunit to form stable quinupristin-ribosome-dalfopristin tertiary complex. Quinupristin inhibits peptide chain formation and results in early termination, while dalfopristin directly interferes with peptidyl transferase and inhibits peptide chain elongation.

Metabolism: Quinupristin and dalfopristin are rapidly converted in the liver to several active metabolites. Quinupristin is broken down into two active metabolites: one glutathione-conjugated metabolite and one cysteine-conjugated metabolite. Dalfopristin has one active metabolite formed by drug hydrolysis. Elimination half-life is approximately 0.9 and 0.75 hours for quinupristin and dalfopristin, respectively. Protein binding for quinupristin ranges from 55 to 78%, and from 11 to 26% for dalfopristin. Excreted in feces (75–77%) and urine (15% of quinupristin and 19% dalfopristin).

Indication: For treatment of serious or life-threatening infections associated with VREG; treatment of cSSSI caused by *S. aureus* (methicillin-susceptible) or *S. pyogenes*. Active against gram-positive aerobic microorganisms (e.g., *Enterococcus faecium*), including vancomycin- and teicoplanin-resistant organisms and vancomycin-resistant, but teicoplanin-susceptible organisms; staphylococci; streptococci; some anaerobes and respiratory pathogens.

Dosage/Range:
- Recommended dose is 7.5 mg/kg of actual body weight in D_5W over 60 minutes q 8–12 h, depending upon the type and severity of infection.

Drug Preparation:
- Reconstitute single-dose vial by slowly adding 5 mL of solution or preservative-free sterile water for injection. CAUTION: FURTHER DILUTION IS REQUIRED PRIOR TO ADMINSTRATION.
- According to patient weight, Synercid solution should be added to 250 mL of D_5W solution within 30 minutes of initial reconstitution.
- Stability of the prepared infusate is 5 hours at room temperature or 54 hours under refrigeration at 2–8°C (36–46°F).
- Drug is NOT compatible with 0.9% sodium chloride or heparin-containing solutions.
- Desired dose should be administered IV over 60 minutes. If drug is administered through a common IV line, flush with 5% dextrose prior to and following administration.

Drug Interactions:
- Synercid should not be physically mixed with or added to other drugs since compatibility has not been established.
- Drugs metabolized by CYP3A4 isoenzyme system: isoenzymes and is an inhibitor of CYP3A4, and thus may increase the serum concentrations of drugs metabolized by this isoenzyme, for example, nifedipine, cyclosporin. Use together with caution and assess for toxicity.
- Tacrolimus, statins, vincristine, taxol.

COMPLICATIONS

Lab Effects/Interference:

- Eosinophils, BUN, GGT (gamma glutamyl transferase), LDH, CPK, AST, ALT, blood glucose, alk phos, and creatinine: concentrations may be increased.
- Hemoglobin and hematocrit: may be decreased.
- Serum K+ and platelet count: may be increased or decreased.

Special Considerations:

- Infusion via central line preferred to decrease incidence of local infusion reactions.

Potential Toxicities/Side Effects and the Nursing Process

I.   ALTERATION IN NUTRITION related to GI SIDE EFFECTS

Defining Characteristics: Nausea, vomiting, diarrhea, constipation, abdominal pain, dyspepsia, stomatitis, and pseudomembranous enterocolitis may occur.

Nursing Implications: Assess elimination and nutrition pattern, baseline and during therapy. Teach patient to report diarrhea and/or abdominal pain immediately. Discuss drug discontinuance with physician if diarrhea occurs. Guaiac stool for occult blood, and notify physician if positive. If severe diarrhea develops, discuss management plan, including endoscopy, fluid and electrolyte replacement. Assess for nausea/vomiting, and administer prescribed antiemetic medications. Encourage small, frequent feedings as tolerated.

II.   ALTERATION IN SKIN INTEGRITY related to HYPERSENSITIVITY

Defining Characteristics: Maculopapular rash and urticaria may occur. Allergic reactions (anaphylactic-like) may rarely occur.

Nursing Implications: Assess baseline allergy history. Assess baseline skin integrity. Teach patient to report rash, pruritus. Teach patient symptomatic management of rash, pruritus. Assess for hypersensitivity reaction; if it occurs, monitor VS, discontinue drug, notify physician, and institute supportive measures.

III.   ALTERATION IN COMFORT related to LOCAL ADMINISTRATION EFFECTS

Defining Characteristics: IV administration may cause erythema, pain, swelling, and thrombophlebitis.

Nursing Implications: Assess IV site prior to each dose for phlebitis or swelling, and change site at least q 48 h. Administer dose slowly over 60 minutes. Apply heat to painful IV sites as ordered. Infuse via central line if possible.

IV.   ALTERATION IN COMFORT

Defining Characteristics: Myalgias and arthralgias may occur.

Nursing Implications: Assess baseline T, VS, neurologic status, and comfort level, and monitor q 4–6 h if patient in hospital. Teach patient self-care measures, including use of prescribed medications, as well as use of heat or cold for myalgias and arthralgias.

V. ALTERATION IN HEPATIC FUNCTION

Defining Characteristics: Transient increases in serum BR, AST (SGOT), alk phos have occurred.

Nursing Implications: Assess baseline LFTs and monitor during therapy.

VI. FUNGAL SUPERINFECTION related to REDISTRIBUTION OF ENDOGENOUS MICROORGANISMS

Defining Characteristics: Vaginal moniliasis, vaginitis, and oral moniliasis may occur as endogenous bacteria are eliminated and normal fungal population expands.

Nursing Implications: Teach female patient to report vaginal itching or discharge. Discuss appropriate antifungal treatment with physician. Teach perineal hygiene and symptomatic management.

Drug: rifaximin (Xifaxan)

Class: Anti-infective, antidiarrheals, gastrointestinal, rifamycin.

Mechanism of Action: Acts by binding to the beta-subunit of bacterial DNA-dependent RNA polymerase resulting in inhibition of bacterial RNA synthesis. Structural analog of rifampin.

Metabolism: Well-absorbed following PO administration. Poorly absorbed from the gastrointestinal tract. Drug excreted unchanged in the feces.

Indication: For treatment of bacterial infections only in the intestines. Active against *E. coli* (enterotoxigenic and enteroaggregative strains).

Dosage/Range:
• Traveler's diarrhea: 200 mg orally 3 times daily for 3 days.
• Prophylaxis: hepatic encephalopathy and irritable bowel syndrome 550 mg BID.

Drug Preparation:
• Oral preparation.

Drug Administration:
• May be taken with or without food.

Drug Interactions:
• Rifaximin has not been shown to significantly affect intestinal or hepatic CYP3A4 activity.

COMPLICATIONS

- Rifaximin has not been shown to affect contraceptives containing ethinyl estradiol and norgestimate.

Lab Effects/Interference:
- None reported.

Special Considerations:
- Rifaximin was teratogenic in animal studies. There are no adequate and well-controlled studies in pregnant women.

Potential Toxicities/Side Effects and the Nursing Process

I.   ALTERATION IN NUTRITION related to GI SIDE EFFECTS

Defining Characteristics: Gas, abdominal pain, nausea, vomiting, constipation, and pseudomembranous enterocolitis may occur.

Nursing Implications: Assess elimination and nutrition pattern, baseline and during therapy. Teach patient to report changes in diarrhea and/or abdominal pain immediately. Guaiac stool for occult blood, and notify physician if positive. Discuss management plan, including fluid and electrolyte replacement. Assess for nausea/vomiting, and administer prescribed antiemetic medications. Encourage small, frequent feedings as tolerated.

Drug: tedizolid phosphate (Sivextro)

Class: Antibacterial; tedizolid belongs to the oxazolidinone class of antibacterial drugs.

Mechanism of Action: Tedizolid phosphate, a phosphate prodrug, is converted to tedizolid in the presence of phosphatases. Tedizolid is mediated by binding to the 50S subunit of the bacterial ribosome, resulting in inhibition of protein synthesis. Tedizolid inhibits bacterial protein synthesis through a mechanism of action different from that of nonoxazolidinone antibacterial agents.

Metabolism: Tedizolid accounts for approximately 95% of the total circulating metabolites in plasma. The majority of its elimination occurs via the liver, 82% recovered in feces and 18% in urine.

Indications: Oxazolidinone-class antibacterial drugs are indicated in adults for treatment of ABSSSI caused by susceptible gram-positive microorganisms—*S. aureus* (including MRSA and MSSA isolates), *S. pyogenes*, *S. agalactiae*, *S. anginosus* group (including *S. anginosus*, *S. intermedius*, and *S. constellatus*), and *E. faecalis*.

Dosage/Range:
- Recommended dosage is 200 mg administered once daily for 6 days either orally (with or without food) or as an IV infusion in patients 18 years or older.
- No dose adjustment is necessary when changing from IV to oral formulation.

- If patients miss a dose, they should take it as soon as possible, anytime up to 8 hours prior to their next scheduled dose. If less than 8 hours remains before the next dose, wait until the next scheduled dose to resume administration.

Drug Preparation:
- Supplied as a sterile, lyophilized powder for injection in single-use vials.
- Reconstitute with sterile water for injection, USP and subsequently dilute only with 0.9% sodium chloride injection, USP. Vials contain no antimicrobial preservatives and are intended for single use only. Vials should be reconstituted using aseptic technique. Reconstitute the tedizolid phosphate with sterile water for injection.
- Minimize foaming. *Avoid* vigorous agitation or shaking of vial during or after reconstitution. Gently swirl contents, then let vial stand until powder is completely dissolved and any foam disperses.
- Inspect vial to ensure solution contains no particulate matter and no cake or powder remains. If necessary, invert vial to dissolve any remaining powder and swirl gently to prevent foaming. Reconstituted solution should be clear and colorless to pale yellow in color. Total storage time should not exceed 24 hours at either room temperature or under refrigeration at 2–8°C (36–46°F).
- Reconstituted solution must be further diluted in 0.9% sodium chloride injection, USP. Invert the bag gently to mix contents. Do *not* shake bag, as this may cause foaming.
- Administer as IV infusion only. Do not administer as IV push or bolus. Do not mix tedizolid phosphate with other drugs when administering. Drug is not intended for intra-arterial, intramuscular, intrathecal, intraperitoneal, or subcutaneous administration.
- The IV bag containing reconstituted and diluted IV solution should be inspected visually for particulate matter prior to administration. Discard if visible particles are observed. Resulting solution should be clear and colorless to pale yellow in color.
- After reconstitution and dilution, administer via IV infusion using a total time of 1 hour.
- Total time from reconstitution to administration should not exceed 24 hours at room temperature or under refrigeration at 2–8°C (36–46°F).

Drug Interaction:
- Neither tedizolid phosphate nor tedizolid detectably inhibited or induced the metabolism of selected CYP enzyme substrates. No potential drug interactions with tedizolid were identified in vitro CYP inhibition or induction studies. These results suggest that drug–drug interactions based on oxidative metabolism are unlikely.
- Drug combination studies with tedizolid and aztreonam, ceftriaxone, ceftazidime, imipenem, rifampin, trimethoprim/sulfamethoxazole, minocycline, clindamycin, ciprofloxacin, daptomycin, vancomycin, gentamicin, amphotericin B, ketoconazole, and terbinafine demonstrated neither synergy nor antagonism.
- Consideration should be made for drugs able to cause serotonin syndrome.

Lab Effects/Interference:
- Has not been documented in prescribing materials.

Special Considerations:
- Most common adverse reactions in patients treated with tedizolid phosphate were nausea (8%), headache (6%), diarrhea (4%), vomiting (3%), and dizziness (2%).

COMPLICATIONS

Potential Toxicities/Side Effects and the Nursing Process

I.   ALTERATION IN NUTRITION related to GI SIDE EFFECTS

Defining Characteristics: Nausea, vomiting, and anorexia have occurred frequently.

Nursing Implications: Assess baseline nutritional status, preexisting nausea/vomiting, and anorexia. Teach patient to report side effects. Provide symptomatic interventions if side effects occur; discuss with physician use of alternative drug(s). Nurses should be aware of serotonin syndrome.

II.   ALTERATIONS IN COMFORT related to HEADACHE AND DIZZINESS

Defining Characteristics: Headache has occurred in some patients.

Nursing Implications: Assess baseline hearing (ability to hear spoken voice) and continue to assess during therapy. Teach patient about potential side effects, and instruct patient to report any hearing/perceptual problems (e.g., tinnitus, vertigo, decreased hearing). Discuss drug discontinuance and audiogram with physician to confirm hearing dysfunction if symptoms arise. Assess for increased risk if drug is given concurrently with other ototoxic medications (e.g., cisplatin, furosemide).

III.   FUNGAL SUPERINFECTION related to REDISTRIBUTION OF ENDOGENOUS MICROORGANISMS

Defining Characteristics: Vaginal or oral candidiasis (sore mouth or tongue; white patches in mouth and/or tongue), vaginitis (vaginal candidiasis), and vaginal itching and discharge may occur as endogenous bacteria are eliminated and normal fungal population expands.

Nursing Implications: Teach female patients to report vaginal itching or discharge. Discuss appropriate antifungal treatment with physician. Teach perineal hygiene and symptomatic management.

Drug: telavancin (Vibativ)

Class: Lipopeptide antibiotic.

Mechanism of Action: Inhibits bacterial cell wall synthesis by interfering with the polymerization and cross-linking of peptidoglycan. Telavancin binds to the bacterial membrane and disrupts membrane barrier function.

Metabolism: Excreted by the kidney. Renal excretion is primary route of elimination.

Indication: Is used to treat severe skin infections, hospital-acquired, and ventilator-acquired pneumonia. It acts against gram-positive bacteria, including *S. aureus* (methicillin-susceptible and methicillin-resistant isolates) and *E. faecalis* (vancomycin-susceptible isolates only).

Dosage/Range:

Adult:
- IV: 10 mg/kg administered over a 60-minute period by IV infusion once every 24 hours for 7–14 days.
- Dose modification for renal impairment:

CrCl (mL/min)	Dosage Adjustment
30–50	7.5 mg/kg q 24 h
30–10	10 mg/kg q 48 h

Drug Preparation:
- Reconstitute 250-mg vial with 15 mL of dextrose 5% injection, sterile water for injection, or sodium chloride 0.9% injection; reconstitute the 750-mg vial with 45 mL of dextrose 5% injection, sterile water for injection, sodium chloride 0.9% injection. The resultant solution has a concentration of 15 mg/mL.
- Administer over a period of no less than 60 minutes by IV infusion.
- Discard the vial if the vacuum did not pull the diluent into the vial.
- If the same IV line is used for sequential infusion of additional medications, the line should be flushed before and after infusion of telavancin with dextrose 5% injection, sodium chloride 0.9% injection, or lactated Ringer's injection.

Drug Interactions:
- *Drugs affecting kidney function (e.g., ACE inhibitors, loop diuretics, NSAIDs):* risk of renal adverse events may be increased. Use with caution. Observe the patient for adverse renal events. Monitor renal function.
- *QT-prolonging drugs (e.g., amiodarone, pimozide, ziprasidone):* possible additive effects with other drugs that prolong the QT interval. Use with caution.

Lab Effects/Interference:
- Telavancin does not interfere with coagulation; however, it interferes with certain tests used to monitor coagulation, including activated *clotting* time, aPTT, coagulation-based factor Xa tests, INR, and PT. No evidence of increased risk of bleeding has been observed. Telavancin interferes with urine qualitative dipstick protein assays and quantitative dye methods (e.g., pyrogallol red-molybdate). However, microalbumin assay is not affected and can be used to monitor urinary protein excretion during telavancin treatment.

Special Considerations:
- Contraindicated in patients with known hypersensitivity to telavancin.
- Obtain ordered specimen and send for culture and sensitivity prior to first antibiotic dose.
- Consider alternative antibiotic therapy if anemia, drug rash or fever, arthralgia, or unexplained rise in BUN and serum creatinine occur.

COMPLICATIONS

Potential Toxicities/Side Effects and the Nursing Process

I.   ALTERATION IN NUTRITION, LESS THAN BODY REQUIREMENTS, related to GI SIDE EFFECTS

Defining Characteristics: Constipation, nausea, diarrhea, vomiting, dyspepsia.

Nursing Implications: Assess baseline nutritional status, preexisting nausea/vomiting, and anorexia. Assess baseline bowel pattern. Administer symptomatic interventions if side effects occur; discuss with physician use of alternative drug(s).

II.   POTENTIAL FOR INJURY related to HYPERSENSITIVITY REACTION

Defining Characteristics: Rash, urticaria, pruritus, and fever can occur in individuals with hypersensitivity to telavancin.

Nursing Implications: Assess for drug allergies prior to drug administration. Instruct patient to report any allergic reactions. Assess for signs/symptoms of allergic reaction after drug dose.

III.   SENSORY/PERCEPTUAL ALTERATIONS related to CNS EFFECTS OF DIZZINESS AND HEADACHE

Defining Characteristics: Dizziness, headache, and insomnia may occur.

Nursing Implications: Assess baseline neurologic status. Teach patient about side effects and to report dizziness or headache. If signs/symptoms arise, discuss drug discontinuance with physician.

IV.   ALTERATIONS IN COMFORT related to LOCAL INJECTION IRRITATION

Defining Characteristics: Pain or phlebitis may develop in IV sites.

Nursing Implications: Change IV sites q 48 h, and assess for signs/symptoms of phlebitis prior to each administration. Administer drug slowly. Apply warm packs to increase comfort.

Drug: tigecycline (Tygacil)

Class: Antimicrobial agent. This antibiotic is the first in a new class called glycylcyclines. This novel IV antibiotic has a broad spectrum of antimicrobial activity, including activity against the drug-resistant bacteria MRSA.

Mechanism of Action: Inhibits protein transplantation in bacteria by binding to the 30S ribosomal subunit and blocking entry of amino-acyl tRNA molecules into the A site of the ribosome.

Metabolism: Is not extensively metabolized. Eliminated by multiple pathways: 7% of the dose is excreted unchanged by biliary and/or intestinal secretion; 59% of the dose is excreted unchanged in bile/feces and 33% of the dose is excreted in the urine. May accumulate in patients with severe hepatic disease.

Indication: For treatment of CABP, cSSSI, and cIAI caused by susceptible strains of specific microorganisms. Demonstrated efficacy against MRSA, *E. coli, E. faecalis* (vancomycin-resistant isolates), *S. anginosus, S. intermedius, S. constellatus, B. fragilis, B. thetaiotaomicron, B. uniformis, B. vulgatus, Clostridium perfringens*, and *Peptostreptococcus micros.*

Dosage/Range:

Adult:
- Initial dose 100 mg IV, followed by 50 mg every 12 hours.
- Duration of therapy depends on indication.
- Tigecycline has an orphan drug status for treatment of AML—doses are completely different.
- Drug dose should be reduced or adjusted in patients with severe hepatic insufficiency.

Drug Preparation:
- IV injection should be administered over 30–60 minutes every 12 hours.

Drug Interactions:
- Monitor prothrombin time if administered with warfarin.
- Diclofenac: increased diclofenac exposure.
- Concurrent use of antibacterial drugs with oral contraceptives may render the oral contraceptives less effective.

Lab Effects/Interference:
- No reported drug-laboratory test interactions. SGPT, alk phos, amylase, SGOT, and bilirubin: serum concentrations may be increased in patients with preexisting hepatic disease.

Special Considerations:
- Black box warning: An increase in all-cause mortality has been reported with tigecycline versus comparator antibiotics, especially in ventilator-associated pneumonia (unapproved use), with deaths usually resulting from worsening infection, complications of infection, or underlying comorbidities; reserve use for situations when alternatives are not suitable.
- Gastrointestinal: Acute pancreatitis, including fatal cases, been reported including in patients without known risk factors; consider discontinuing use if suspected
- Hepatic: Hepatic failure and significant hepatic dysfunction during treatment and dysfunction after discontinuation have been reported; monitoring recommended
- Avoid use in pregnant or lactating women.
- Contraindicated in patients with known hypersensitivity.
- Obtain ordered specimen and send for culture and sensitivity prior to first antibiotic dose.

COMPLICATIONS

Potential Toxicities/Side Effects and the Nursing Process

I.   ALTERATION IN NUTRITION related to GI SIDE EFFECTS

Defining Characteristics: Anorexia, nausea, vomiting, diarrhea, glossitis, dysphagia, gastroenteritis, gastritis, constipation.

Nursing Implications: Assess baseline nutritional status. Assess for and teach patient to report any symptoms. Administer and teach patient self-administration of prescribed antiemetic or antidiarrheal medication as appropriate.

II.   POTENTIAL FOR INJURY related to HYPERSENSITIVITY REACTION

Defining Characteristics: Urticaria, pruritus, rash (maculopapular or erythematous), fever and chills, eosinophilia, myalgia, edema, erythema, angioedema, Stevens–Johnson syndrome, and exfoliative skin reactions occur.

Nursing Implications: Assess allergy to antibiotics: if patient states "yes," determine actual response (e.g., "swollen lips = angioedema"). If angioedema, patient should not receive drug. If patients allergic to tetracyclines do NOT administer. Discuss other patient responses with physician to determine whether drug should be given. Assess baseline skin condition, including integrity and allergy history to drugs. Instruct patient to report rash, itching, or other skin changes. Teach patient skin care and symptomatic measures as appropriate. If skin rash develops, discuss drug discontinuance with physician. If rash progresses, drug should be discontinued, as fatal Stevens–Johnson syndrome may develop. Be prepared to treat severe acute hypersensitivity reactions with airway management, oxygen, epinephrine, corticosteroids, and antihistamines as ordered.

III.   ALTERATIONS IN COMFORT related to LOCAL INJECTION IRRITATION

Defining Characteristics: Vein irritation (pain, erythema), phlebitis, and thrombophlebitis may occur at IV administration site.

Nursing Implications: Change IV sites q 48 h, and assess for signs/symptoms of phlebitis prior to each administration. Administer drug slowly. Apply warm packs to increase comfort. Discuss central line with patient and physician to facilitate administration.

IV.   FUNGAL SUPERINFECTION related to REDISTRIBUTION OF ENDOGENOUS MICROORGANISMS

Defining Characteristics: Vaginal moniliasis, vaginitis may occur as endogenous bacteria are eliminated and normal fungal population expands.

Nursing Implications: Teach female patient to report vaginal itching or discharge. Discuss appropriate antifungal treatment with physician. Teach perineal hygiene and symptom management.

Drug: tobramycin sulfate (Nebcin, Tobi (nebulized))

Class: Aminoglycoside antibacterial (systemic).

Mechanism of Action: Synthetic antibiotic derived from *Streptomyces*; bactericidal, most probably by inhibition of protein synthesis.

Metabolism: Well-absorbed following parenteral administration, but variability in absorption after IM injection (peak serum level 0.5–2 hours, duration 8–12 hours). Widely distributed into body fluids. Minimally protein-bound. Readily crosses placenta and excreted in breastmilk. Drug excreted unchanged in the urine.

Indication: For treatment of a variety of bacterial infections, including bone and joint infections, bacterial meningitis and other central nervous system infections, respiratory tract infections, septicemia, skin and skin structure infections, urinary tract infections, and empiric treatment of febrile neutropenia. Active against aerobic microorganisms: many sensitive gram-negative (including *Acinetobacter, Citrobacter, Enterobacter, E. coli, Klebsiella, Proteus, Pseudomonas, Salmonella, Serratia,* and *Shigella*) and some sensitive gram-positive organisms (*S. aureus* and *S. epidermidis*). Over time, bacterial resistance may develop, either naturally or acquired.

Dosage/Range:
- Desired peak serum concentration is 4–10 mg/mL, and trough serum concentration is 1–2 mg/mL.

Indication	Dosage
Usual	3 mg/kg day given in equally divided doses q 8 h
Life-threatening infections	5–6 mg/kg/day in 3 equally divided doses; if loading dose required, 2 mg/kg; usual dosing q 8 h, but q 12 or 24 dosing may also be used
Inhalation solution	300 mg (1 ampule) inhaled via nebulizer 2× daily q 12 h (28 days on, 28 days off); do not take less than 6 h apart
Inhalation powder	112 mg (4 capsules) inhaled via Podhaler ™ 2× daily q 12 h (28 days on, 28 days off); do not take less than 6 h apart

- DOSE-REDUCE IF RENAL IMPAIRMENT: Depending on schedule used but Hartford Nomogram is useful in this regard for once daily.

Drug Preparation:
- Store unreconstituted vials at 15–30°C (59–86°F).
- Store injections at 25°C (77°F).
- Store reconstituted solution (using sterile water for injection, with final concentration 40 mg/mL) at room temperature (stable 24 hours) or in refrigerator at 2–8°C (36–46°F) (stable 96 hours).

Drug Administration:
- IV: further dilute by adding dose to 50–100 mL in 0.9% sodium chloride and administer over 30–60 minutes.

Drug Interactions:
- Increased risk of toxicity with other ototoxic drugs: acyclovir, other aminoglycosides, amphotericin B, bacitracin, cephalosporins, colistin, cisplatin, ethacrynic acid, furosemide, vancomycin.
- Potentiation of neuromuscular blockade when given concurrently with general anesthetics (succinylcholine, tubocurarine); use cautiously; observe for signs/symptoms of respiratory depression.
- Synergism with extended-spectrum penicillins, but must be administered separately.

Lab Effects/Interference:
- Serum ALT, serum alk phos, serum AST, serum bili, and serum LDH values may be increased.
- BUN and serum creatinine concentrations may be increased.
- Serum Ca++, serum Mg++, serum K+, and serum Na+ concentrations may be decreased.

Special Considerations:
- Not first line treatment
- Only synergy in some cases.
- Neuromuscular: Neuromuscular disorders (e.g., myasthenia gravis or Parkinson disease); aminoglycosides may aggravate muscle weakness
- Use in pregnancy only if infection is life-threatening and no safer drug exists; drug crosses placenta and may cause fetal toxicity.

Potential Toxicities/Side Effects and the Nursing Process

I.   ALTERATIONS IN SENSORY/PERCEPTUAL PATTERNS related to OTOTOXICITY

Defining Characteristics: Damage to eighth cranial nerve (auditory) may result in dizziness, nystagmus, vertigo, ataxia (vestibular damage), and more commonly, tinnitus, roaring sound in ears, and impaired hearing (auditory damage). Hearing loss usually begins with high-frequency loss, followed by clinical hearing loss, then permanent hearing loss if damage continues. Increased risk in elderly or renally impaired patients.

Nursing Implications: Assess baseline hearing (ability to hear spoken voice) and continue during therapy. Teach patient potential side effects, and instruct patient to report any hearing/perceptual problems (e.g., tinnitus, vertigo, decreased hearing). Discuss drug discontinuance and audiogram with physician to confirm hearing dysfunction if symptoms arise. Assess for increased risk if given concurrently with other ototoxic medications (e.g., cisplatin, furosemide).

II.   ALTERATION IN URINARY ELIMINATION related to NEPHROTOXICITY

Defining Characteristics: Risk of nephrotoxicity is multifactorial and rather depends on other factors, concomitant medication, ICU stay, hypoperfusion, rather than the aminoglycoside choice). Renal damage characterized by tubular necrosis with increased serum BUN, creatinine; decreased urine creatinine clearance and specific gravity; proteinuria and casts in urine. Azotemia usually not associated with oliguria. Rarely, electrolyte wasting with hypomagnesemia, hypocalcemia, and hypokalemia may occur. Renal dysfunction is usually reversible after drug discontinuance. Increased risk exists in elderly and if there is preexisting renal dysfunction. Risk is lower in well-hydrated patients with normal renal function when normal doses given.

Nursing Implications: Assess baseline renal function and electrolytes, and monitor periodically during therapy. Discuss any abnormalities with physician, as drug should be dose-reduced or discontinued if renal dysfunction develops. Assess baseline total body fluid balance, weight, and monitor periodically during antibiotic therapy. Monitor hydration status to keep patient well hydrated. Assess drug peak and trough levels as ordered so that drug dosage is correctly titrated. Peak and trough levels: follow troughs for toxicity, peaks for efficacy. Draw blood for peak drug concentration 30 minutes after end of 30-minute infusion or at the end of a 60-minute infusion; draw trough immediately before next dose.

III.   ALTERATIONS IN SENSORY/PERCEPTUAL PATTERNS related to CNS EFFECTS, NEUROMUSCULAR BLOCKADE

Defining Characteristics: Headache, tremor, lethargy may occur. Peripheral neuropathy or encephalopathy (numbness, skin tingling, muscle twitching) may occur rarely. Neuromuscular blockade is dose-related, self-limiting, and uncommon. Risk is greater with topical application or when drug is administered to patient with neuromuscular disease (myasthenia gravis) or hypocalcemia.

Nursing Implications: Assess baseline neurologic status. Assess coexisting risk factors, neuromuscular blockade medications. Teach patient about side effects, and instruct to report headache, tremor, lethargy. Observe for respiratory depression. If signs/symptoms arise, discuss drug discontinuance with physician.

IV.   POTENTIAL FOR INJURY related to HYPERSENSITIVITY

Defining Characteristics: Rash, urticaria, pruritus, fever, eosinophilia have occurred rarely. CROSS-SENSITIVITY between AMINOGLYCOSIDES exists!

COMPLICATIONS

Nursing Implications: Assess for drug allergies to any aminoglycoside—amikacin, gentamicin, kanamycin, neomycin, netilmicin, streptomycin, tobramycin—prior to drug administration. Instruct patient to report any allergic reactions. Assess for signs/symptoms of allergic reaction after drug dose.

V.   ALTERATION IN NUTRITION, LESS THAN BODY REQUIREMENTS, related to GI SIDE EFFECTS

Defining Characteristics: Nausea, vomiting, and anorexia have occurred rarely. Also, transient hepatomegaly with increased LFTs—AST, ALT, LDH, alk phos—has occurred.

Nursing Implications: Assess baseline nutritional status, preexisting nausea/vomiting, and anorexia. Assess baseline LFTs and monitor periodically during treatment. Instruct patient to report side effects. Provide symptomatic interventions if side effects occur; discuss with physician use of alternative drug(s).

VI.   POTENTIAL FOR FATIGUE, INFECTION, AND BLEEDING related to BONE MARROW INJURY

Defining Characteristics: Anemia, leukopenia, granulocytopenia, and thrombocytopenia may occur. Also, patients receiving antibiotics are at risk for overgrowth of nonsusceptible microorganisms, such as fungi (superinfection). Rare.

Nursing Implications: Assess baseline CBC, differential, and monitor periodically during treatment. Instruct patient to report signs/symptoms of fatigue, infection, or bleeding immediately. Assess for signs/symptoms of superinfection. Discuss any adverse effects with physician.

Drug: vancomycin hydrochloride (Vancocin)

Class: Antibacterial (systemic).

Mechanism of Action: Derived from cultures of *Streptomyces orientalis*; drug is bactericidal by binding to bacterial cell wall, thus blocking protein polymerization and cell wall synthesis. Also damages cell membrane and acts at a different site than the penicillins. Bacteriostatic for enterococci.

Metabolism: It's a large molecule and does not cross the gastrointestinal lining. For treatment of CDAD it is used as an oral version, specifically for that reason, to become concentrated at the site of infection. IV vancomycin cannot be used for CDAD, as it will not be effective. For systemic infection, IV should be used,

Effective when administered IV and is widely distributed in body tissues and fluid, including bile. Crosses placenta; unknown whether drug is excreted in breastmilk; 52–60% bound to plasma proteins. IV dose excreted primarily by kidneys and, to a small degree, in bile; oral dose excreted in feces.

Indication: For treatment of *C. difficile*–associated diarrhea and staphylococcal enterocolitis. Active against many gram-positive organisms (staphylococci, group A b-hemolytic streptococci, *S. pneumoniae, C. difficile,* enterococci, *Corynebacterium, Clostridium*).

Dosage/Range (Adult):

Dosage	Route	Interval/Duration
125 mg	Oral (for use with *Clostridium Difficile* Associated Disease (CDAD))	q 6 hrs × 10 to 14 days
Up to 500 mg	Oral (for severe complicated infections)	q 6 h
500 mg in 100 mL NS	Rectal	q 6 h
500 mg to 1 g OR Weight-based dosage 10–30 mg/kg	IV	q 12 h 2 divided doses

- Trough serum concentration is 5–20 mg/mL.
- Dose reduction necessary if renal dysfunction; see manufacturer's package insert.

Drug Preparation:
- Oral dose for treatment of *C. difficile.* Oral dose not recommended for treating systemic infections.
- Reconstituted by adding 10 mL of sterile water to 500-mg vial (20 mL to 1-g vial). Further dilute in at least 100 mL 0.9% sodium chloride or 5% dextrose in water, and infuse over 1 hour (central line).
- For peripheral lines, further dilution in 250 mL is recommended.
- Causes tissue necrosis if given IM; DO NOT ADMINISTER IM.

Drug Interactions:
- Nephrotoxic drugs (aminoglycoside antibiotics, amphotericin B, cisplatin, colistin): increased risk of nephrotoxicity; avoid concurrent use if possible.

Lab Effects/Interference:
- BUN and creatinine concentrations may be increased; follow serum levels.

Special Considerations:
- Use cautiously in patients with renal dysfunction.
- DO NOT USE in patients with hearing loss. Cannot reduce doses, may loose effectiveness.
- Contraindicated in patients with known hypersensitivity.
- Obtain ordered specimen for culture and sensitivity prior to first antibiotic dose.
- Use with caution in pregnancy, as fetal effects are unknown, and in lactating mothers, as drug may be excreted in breastmilk.

Potential Toxicities/Side Effects and the Nursing Process

I.   ALTERATIONS IN SENSORY PERCEPTUAL PATTERNS related to OTOTOXICITY

Defining Characteristics: IV drug appears to damage eighth cranial nerve (auditory). First symptom of ototoxicity is tinnitus and may progress to deafness; may also be associated with vertigo and dizziness (vestibular branch). High risk exists in patients with renal impairment who are receiving concurrent ototoxic drugs (e.g., cisplatin) or prolonged therapy, or those whose age > 60 years old.

Nursing Implications: Assess baseline hearing (ability to hear spoken voice) or audiogram if patient is at high risk—both at baseline and throughout therapy. Monitor serum drug concentrations during therapy if at high risk. Teach patient potential side effects, and instruct patient to report any hearing/perceptual problems (e.g., tinnitus, decreased hearing, vertigo). Discuss drug discontinuance with physician if symptoms arise.

II.   ALTERATION IN URINARY ELIMINATION related to NEPHROTOXICITY

Defining Characteristics: Renal damage may occur, characterized by transient increases in serum BUN or creatinine, hyaline casts, and albuminuria. May cause acute interstitial nephritis. High risk in patients with renal impairment who are receiving concurrent nephrotoxic drugs (e.g., cisplatin) or prolonged therapy, or those whose age > 60 years.

Nursing Implications: Assess baseline renal function and electrolytes, and monitor periodically during therapy. Discuss any abnormalities with physician, as drug should be dose-reduced or discontinued if renal dysfunction develops. Assess baseline hydration status, including urinary output, total body balance, daily weights; keep patient well hydrated.

III.   ALTERATION IN COMFORT related to LOCAL TISSUE EFFECTS

Defining Characteristics: Vesicant if given IM (causing tissue necrosis). Irritating to veins when given IV, causing pain and thrombophlebitis.

Nursing Implications: Administer drug IV, *NOT* IM. Assess IV site prior to each dose and at completion of dose; instruct patient to report pain or burning; change IV site if irritation, phlebitis develop. Change site at least q 48 h and consider central line for prolonged therapy. AVOID EXTRAVASATION.

IV.   ALTERATION IN CARDIAC OUTPUT related to RAPID IV INFUSION

Defining Characteristics: Rapid IV administration may cause histamine release and "red-neck" syndrome, characterized by rapid onset of hypotension, flushing, and erythematous or maculopapular rash of neck, face, chest. May be associated with wheezing, dyspnea, angioedema, urticaria, pruritus. Rarely, seizures and cardiac arrest may occur. Syndrome occurs minutes after beginning infusion, but may occur at end; usually resolves spontaneously over 2+ hours, but may require antihistamines, corticosteroids, or IV fluids. Rare when drug is administered over at least 1 hour/g.

Nursing Implications: Monitor temperature, VS at baseline, 5 minutes into IV administration, and at end of infusion, at least with the initial dose; infuse over at least 1 hour, using infusion controller if necessary. Observe patient during first 5 minutes, and instruct patient to report rash, wheezing, itching immediately. If reaction occurs, stop infusion, assess VS, and notify physician. Patient may be treated with antihistamine or IV fluids, or both. Completion of dose and subsequent doses may be ordered at very slow rate. Document episode in medical record and update care plan/medication sheet to reflect change in drug administration.

V.   INJURY related to BONE MARROW SUPPRESSION

Defining Characteristics: Rarely, leukopenia, thrombocytopenia, agranulocytosis may occur, especially with cumulative doses > 25 g.

Nursing Implications: Monitor baseline and periodic WBC, differential, platelet count, especially if receiving other bone marrow-suppressive drugs. Discuss abnormalities with physician.

VI.   INFECTION related to OVERGROWTH OF NONSUSCEPTIBLE MICROORGANISMS

Defining Characteristics: Normal microflora populations altered by drug, with possible overgrowth by nonsusceptible microorganisms, that is, fungi, gram-negative bacteria.

Nursing Implications: Assess for signs/symptoms of other infections of skin, mucous membranes. Instruct patient to report signs/symptoms. Discuss further antimicrobial therapy with physician.

ANTIFUNGALS

Drug: amphotericin B (deoxycholate) (Fungizone); amphotericin B lipid complex (Abelcet); amphotericin B cholesteryl sulfate complex (Amphotec); liposomal amphotericin B (AmBisome)

Class: Antifungal (systemic); antiprotozoal.

Mechanism of Action: Produced by *Streptomyces*; Amphotericin B binds primarily to ergosterol in cell membranes of sensitive fungi, causing changes in membrane permeability that result in leakage of intracellular contents and cell death is fungistatic (prevents replication at normal doses) and fungicidal (kills fungi at high doses).

Metabolism: Poorly absorbed from GI tract so must be given IV. Crosses BBB and the placenta; 90–95% bound to serum proteins. Single-dose elimination half-life is 24 hours, while following long-term administration is 15 days.

Indication: For treatment of progressive and potentially life-threatening fungal infections. It may be used to treat protozoal infections. Active against systemic fungal infections

(*Aspergillus, Candida, Cryptococcus, Histoplasma capsulatum*); used to treat fungal meningitis and *Leishmania* (protozoan) infections.

Dosage/Range:

Adult:

Amphotericin B (deoxycholate): requires premedication
- Initial: 0.25 mg/kg IV (or first dose of 1 mg IV) over 6-hour period (may use 2–4 hours). Gradual increase in daily dosage (e.g., over 1 week) to dose of 0.5–1 mg/kg/day or 1.5 mg/kg on alternate days (maximum 1.5 mg/kg/day).
- If dose is interrupted for > 1 week, reinstitute at 0.25 mg/kg/day and titrate up.
- Intrathecal: 25 mg (0.1 mL diluted with 10–20 mL CSF) biw–tiw.
- Oral: oral candida: amphotericin B oral suspension: 1 mL (100 mg) qid.

Lipid-based amphotericin B (infection refractory or pt has renal impairment):
- Amphotec: test dose 1.6–8.3 mg/10 mL IV over 15–30 minutes, 3–4 mg/kg/day prepared as a 0.6 mg/mL infusion IV at 1 mg/kg/hr.
- Abelcet: 5 mg/kg/day (1–2 mg/mL) IV at 2.5 mg/kg/hr; if infusion time > 2 hours shake to remix q 2 h.
- AmBisome: 3–5 mg/kg/day IV (1–2 mg/mL) over 1–2 hours.
- Bladder irrigation: 50 mg/mL solution given into bladder intermittently or as a continuous irrigation × 5–20 days.
- Dosage adjustment: No data exists with regards to adequate dose adjustment in renal failure. Adjust in severe renal failure.

Drug Preparation:

Amphotericin B deoxycholate:
- Use sterile water for injection (NO PRESERVATIVES) to reconstitute drug; for peripheral line only further dilute to a concentration of 0.1 mg/mL using 500 mL of 5% dextrose injection. Manufacturer recommends protecting from light but appears to be stable for 24 hours in room light.

Drug Administration:
- Administer slowly over 2–6 hours.
- If an inline filter is used, it must have a mean pore diameter of ≥ 1 mm or drug will be filtered out; no filter for Amphotec, Abelcet.
- Protect from light during infusion.

Drug Interactions:
- Additive nephrotoxic effects when combined with other nephrotoxic drugs: aminoglycosides, cisplatin, cyclosporine, pentamidine, vancomycin, so concurrent administration should be avoided.
- Enhanced hypokalemic effects when combined with other drugs that lower serum potassium: corticosteroids.
- Enhanced digitoxin: toxicity related to amphotericin-induced hypokalemia.
- Synergism with flucytosine with increased drug effect.

- Antagonism with miconazole: do not use together.
- Nitrogen mustard: increases toxicity (renal, bronchospasm, hypotension) avoid concurrent administration.
- Cyclosporine toxicity (cholestasis, paresthesias) increased
- Granulocyte transfusions: acute pulmonary dysfunction may occur if given concurrently or close together. Time administration far apart and monitor pulmonary function.

Lab Effects/Interference:
- Increased AST, ALT, alk phos, creatinine, BUN.
- Hypomagnesemia, hypokalemia, hypocalcemia.
- Hypoglycemia, hyperglycemia.
- Falsely elevated serum phosphate levels.

Special Considerations:
- Use with caution in patients with renal dysfunction.
- Contraindicated if hypersensitive to amphotericin.
- Safety in pregnancy has not been established—use with caution and only if benefits outweigh risks.
- Drug encapsulation in liposome decreases toxicity, including renal toxicity. Amphotericin B lipid complex injection is approved for the treatment of aspergillosis in patients refractory or intolerant to conventional amphotericin B.

Potential Toxicities/Side Effects and the Nursing Process

I.   POTENTIAL FOR INJURY related to DRUG ADMINISTRATION

Defining Characteristics: Headache, hypotension, malaise, myalgias, tachypnea, cramping, nausea, and vomiting may occur. Fever and chills usually begin 1–3 hours after infusion is started, and tolerance develops with subsequent doses. Rapid IV administration may cause hypertension and shock, hypokalemia, and arrhythmias. Anaphylaxis can occur.

Nursing Implications: Assess baseline comfort level, temperature, VS. Teach patient potential side effects, and instruct to report any changes. Discuss premedication with physician, such as ibuprofen (inhibits prostaglandin PGE_2) and/or hydrocortisone. Discuss with physician use of IV meperidine HCl (Demerol) for management of rigor if it develops. Administer test dose (e.g., 1 mg/250 mL 5% dextrose IV over 1–4 hours) and monitor temperature, heart rate, BP, respiratory rate during infusion. Administer drug slowly (over 2–6 hours) and escalate dose slowly. Administer antiemetic agents as needed, then prophylactically.

II.   ALTERATION IN URINARY ELIMINATION related to NEPHROTOXICITY

Defining Characteristics: 80% incidence; multiple toxic effects (vasoconstriction, lytic action on renal tubular cell membranes, calcium deposits in distal nephron); hypokalemia may precede azotemia with increased BUN and creatinine, decreased creatinine clearance, and increased excretion of K+, uric acid, and protein. Renal tubular acidosis may occur. Renal impairment usually diminishes after drug discontinuance, but some degree of impairment may be permanent.

Nursing Implications: Assess baseline renal function and electrolytes; monitor every other day during dosage escalation, then at least weekly. Discuss any abnormalities with physician. Drug should be dose-reduced if renal dysfunction develops. Slowly administer initial test dose, then gradually increase doses over first week. Assess fluid status and total body balance closely to keep patient well hydrated. Assess for signs/symptoms of hypokalemia: arthralgia, myalgia, muscle weakness. Administer potassium and magnesium replacements as ordered.

III. FATIGUE related to ANEMIA

Defining Characteristics: High incidence of reversible normocytic, normochromic anemia that rarely requires transfusion.

Nursing Implications: Assess baseline CBC, HCT; monitor Hgb and HCT during treatment. Instruct patient to report fatigue, shortness of breath, headache. Transfuse red blood cells as needed and ordered by physician.

IV. ALTERATION IN COMFORT, PAIN related to PAIN AT INJECTION SITE

Defining Characteristics: Drug may cause pain at injection site, phlebitis, thrombophlebitis; extravasation causes local irritation.

Nursing Implications: Select veins for IV administration distally and then more proximally, avoiding phlebitic veins or small veins. Apply heat to increase comfort. Administer drug slowly.

V. ALTERATION IN CARDIAC OUTPUT related to CARDIOPULMONARY DYSFUNCTION

Defining Characteristics: Rarely, hypertension, ventricular fibrillation, cardiac arrest, failure, pulmonary edema may occur. Pulmonary hypersensitivity may occur with bronchospasm, wheezing, or pulmonary pneumonitis.

Nursing Implications: Monitor VS closely, noting heart rate and rhythm, BP, breath sounds at baseline and during infusion. Instruct patient to report dyspnea, other changes in breathing pattern, or general feeling state ASAP. Discuss any changes, abnormalities with physician. Administer granulocyte transfusions as far apart from amphotericin administration as possible, and monitor pulmonary status closely. Be prepared to provide basic life support/resuscitation if needed.

VI. ALTERATIONS IN SENSORY/PERCEPTUAL PATTERNS related to PERIPHERAL AND CNS DYSFUNCTION

Defining Characteristics: Rarely, hearing loss, tinnitus, transient vertigo, blurred vision or diplopia, peripheral neuropathy, and seizures may occur. Following intrathecal drug administration: headache, lumbar nerves, arachnoiditis, and visual changes may occur.

Nursing Implications: Assess baseline neurologic function and monitor during drug administration and over time, especially when drug is given intrathecally. Notify physician if abnormalities occur. Discuss with physician coadministration of small doses of intrathecal corticosteroids to decrease CNS irritation.

VII. ALTERATION IN NUTRITION, LESS THAN BODY REQUIREMENTS related to GI TOXICITY

Defining Characteristics: Anorexia, nausea, vomiting, dyspepsia, cramping, epigastric pain, and diarrhea may occur. Rarely, melena and hemorrhagic gastroenteritis may occur. Elevated LFTs may occur.

Nursing Implications: Assess baseline nutritional status, including weight and usual weight. Administer antiemetics as ordered and needed, then prophylactically prior to infusion if nausea and/or vomiting develop. Administer antidiarrheal medicine as ordered and needed. Instruct patient to report any symptoms; teach/reinforce importance of high-calorie, high-protein diet; suggest family/significant other bring in favorite foods from home as appropriate. Assess LFT results at baseline and periodically during treatment as elevated serum aminotransferase, bili, and alk phos may occur. Discuss abnormalities with physician. Encourage patient to eat favorite foods, especially those high in calories, protein, potassium, and magnesium. Monitor daily weight during treatment, and discuss weight loss with dietitian, patient, and physician to revise nutritional plan.

VIII. ALTERATION IN PROTECTIVE MECHANISMS related to BONE MARROW INJURY

Defining Characteristics: Rarely, thrombocytopenia, leukopenia, agranulocytosis, and coagulation defects may occur.

Nursing Implications: Assess baseline CBC, differential. Assess for any signs/symptoms of bleeding or infection, and discuss with physician if they occur. Teach patient general self-assessment guidelines, such as taking temperature and reporting any changes from baseline condition.

COMPLICATIONS

Drug: anidulafungin (Eraxis)

Class: Antifungal.

Mechanism of Action: Semisynthetic lipopeptide synthesized from fermentation products of *Aspergillus nidulans*. Fungistatic by damaging fungal cell membrane increasing permeability, altering cell metabolism, and inhibiting cell growth. Fungicidal at high concentrations. Inhibits the synthesis of β(1,3)-D-glucan synthase, resulting in selective inhibition of the synthesis of glucan, an integral component of the fungal cell wall.

Metabolism: Unique among echinocandins because it slowly degrades in human plasma, undergoing a process of biotransformation rather than metabolism. Degradation products pass into the feces via the biliary tree.

Indication: For treatment of certain types of fungal infections, including esophageal candidiasis, candidemia, and other forms of *Candida* infections (intra-abdominal abscess and peritonitis).

Dosage/Range:
- Esophageal candidiasis: 100 mg/day (loading dose), followed by 50 mg/day $\times$ 14 days or $\times$ 7 days after resolution of symptoms.
- Candidemia and other deep-tissue *Candida* infections: 200 mg on day 1, followed by 100 mg/day $\times$ 14 days after the last positive blood culture.

Drug Preparation:
- Do not mix or coinfuse with other medications.
- No dose adjustment is required in patients based on age, sex, weight, disease state, concomitant drug therapy, or renal or hepatic insufficiency.
- IV: Use manufacturer's suggested dilution guideline.
- Infuse slowly; histamine-mediated reactions have been observed related to infusion rate.

Drug Interactions:
- Contraindications: hypersensitivity to anidulafungin, other echinocandins, or any component of the formulation.
- Anidulafungin was found to be safe and was not affected by concomitant treatment with substrates, inhibitors, or inducers of the cytochrome P450 metabolic pathway, including rifampin and cyclosporine in clinical trials—Eraxis can cause increase in cyclosporine levels

Lab Effects/Interference:

Major clinical significance:
- Elevated liver function tests, hepatitis, and worsening hepatic failure have been reported.

Special Considerations:
- Used in treatment of fungal infections.
- On the basis of a lack of interactions with amphotericin B and voriconazole, anidulafungin is well suited to be used in combination with other antifungal agents.

- Histamine-mediated reactions (urticaria, flushing, hypotension) have been observed related to infusion rate.
- Hepatitis, hepatic failure, and significant hepatic dysfunction have been reported; monitoring recommended.

Potential Toxicities/Side Effects and the Nursing Process

I. POTENTIAL FOR INJURY related to INFUSION-RELATED ADVERSE EVENTS

Defining Characteristics: Infusion-related adverse events occurred in 1.3% (N = 6) of the patients in clinical trials. Hypotension with tachycardia, dyspnea, rash, urticaria, flushing, pruritus, dyspnea, hypotension, and dizziness may occur.

Nursing Implications: Assess baseline VS and monitor throughout infusion. Instruct patient to report signs/symptoms immediately. Assess for signs/symptoms: nausea, generalized itching, crampy abdominal pain, chest tightness, anxiety, agitation, sense of impending doom, wheezing, and dizziness.

II. ALTERATION IN NUTRITION, LESS THAN BODY REQUIREMENTS, related to GI SIDE EFFECTS

Defining Characteristics: Nausea, vomiting, diarrhea, and anorexia may occur.

Nursing Implications: Assess baseline nutritional and elimination status. Instruct patient to report GI disturbances. Administer and teach patient to self-administer antiemetics, antidiarrheals as needed and as ordered. Teach patient importance of nutritious diet, and suggest small, frequent, high-calorie, high-protein meals as appropriate.

III. ALTERATIONS IN SENSORY/PERCEPTUAL PATTERNS related to CNS, ENDOCRINE EFFECTS

Defining Characteristics: Dizziness, headache, and somnolence may occur. Hypokalemia occurs in 3% of patients.

Nursing Implications: Assess baseline neurologic function and comfort, and monitor during treatment. Instruct patient to report any changes. Discuss any abnormalities with physician.

COMPLICATIONS

Drug: caspofungin (Cancidas)

Class: Echinocandin; glucan synthesis inhibitor.

Mechanism of Action: Caspofungin inhibits the synthesis of $\beta(1,3)$-D-glucan, an integral component of the fungal cell wall of susceptible filamentous fungi.

Metabolism: Caspofungin is slowly metabolized by hydrolysis and N-acetylation. Elimination route is via feces and urine.

Indication: For treatment of invasive aspergillosis in patients refractory to or intolerant of other antifungal therapies; empirical treatment for presumed fungal infections in febrile neutropenia, treatment of esophageal candidiasis, and treatment of candidemia and the following *Candida* infections: intra-abdominal abscess, peritonitis and pleural space infections. Drug has demonstrated activity in regions of active cell growth of *Aspergillus fumigatus*.

Dosage/Range:
- The recommended dose of caspofungin is a 70-mg loading dose on the first day, followed by 50 mg/daily.
- No dosage adjustment is necessary for the elderly.
- No dosage adjustment is necessary for patients with renal insufficiency. Caspofungin is not dialyzable.
- No dosage adjustment is recommended for patients with mild hepatic insufficiency (Child-Pugh score 5–6). In those with moderate hepatic insufficiency (Child-Pugh score 7–9), a daily dose of 35 mg after the 70-mg loading dose is recommended.

Drug Administration:
- Caspofungin should be given as a slow IV infusion in 250 mL 0.9% sodium chloride over 1 hour.
- Caspofungin is not compatible with dextrose-containing solutions.

Drug Interactions:
- Transient increase in AST and ALT have been observed when caspofungin and cyclosporine are coadministered. Therefore, concomitant use of these two agents is not recommended unless the potential benefit outweighs the potential risk.
- Drug interactions with tacrolimus, rifampin, nevirapine, dexamethasone, efavirenz, phenytoin, carbamazepine. Increased levels; reduce caspofungin levels.

Potential Toxicities/Side Effects and the Nursing Process

I. ALTERATIONS IN COMFORT related to LOCAL VEIN IRRITATION (IV ADMINISTRATION)

Defining Characteristics: Erythema, irritation, pain, swelling, phlebitis may occur at injection site. Consider use of central line.

Nursing Implications: Assess IV site for patency, irritation prior to each dose. Change IV site at least q 48 h. Apply warmth/heat to painful area as needed.

II. POTENTIAL FOR INJURY related to HYPERSENSITIVITY REACTION

Defining Characteristics: Fever and erythema. Increased risk in allergic individuals.

Nursing Implications: Assess allergy/allergic potential to drug. Discuss other patient responses with physician to determine whether drug should be given. Assess baseline skin condition including integrity and allergy history to drugs. Teach patient to report rash, itching, or other skin changes. Teach patient skin care and symptomatic measures as appropriate. If reaction occurs, discuss drug discontinuance with physician.

III. ALTERATION IN NUTRITION, LESS THAN BODY REQUIREMENTS, related to GI SIDE EFFECTS

Defining Characteristics: Nausea and vomiting may occur. Rarely, transient increases in LFTs—AST (SGOT), ALT (SGPT), alk phos, bili—may occur with coadministration of cyclosporine.

Nursing Implications: Assess baseline nutritional status. Teach patient to report GI disturbances. Administer and teach patient to self-administer antiemetics as needed and as ordered. Teach patient importance of nutritious diet and suggest small, frequent, high-calorie, high-protein meals as appropriate. Assess baseline LFTs and monitor periodically during treatment. Discuss abnormalities and drug interruption with physician.

IV. SENSORY/PERCEPTUAL ALTERATIONS

Defining Characteristics: Headache.

Nursing Implications: Assess baseline neurologic function and comfort and monitor during treatment. Teach patient to report any changes. Discuss any abnormalities with physician.

Drug: clotrimazole (Canesten)

Class: Clotrimazole is an imidazole derivative with a broad spectrum antimycotic activity

Mechanism of Action: Clotrimazole acts against fungi by inhibiting ergosterol synthesis. Inhibition of ergosterol synthesis leads to structural and functional impairment of the cytoplasmic membrane

Metabolism: Studies of urinary excretion have shown that less than 0.5% of dermally applied clotrimazole cream appears in the urine over a 5-day period of observation. Fecal excretion, the route by which most of the absorbed drug is likely to be eliminated, has not been studied.

Indication: Vaginal Creams: clotrimazole vaginal creams indicated for topical treatment of vulvovaginal candidiasis. Vaginal Tablets (Compressed Pessaries): clotrimazole vaginal pessaries indicated for topical treatment of vaginal candidiasis.

Composite Pack: clotrimazole composite pack is indicated for treatment of candidal infections of vagina and vulvovaginal as well as for sexual partner.

COMPLICATIONS

Dosage/Range:
- 5 mg/day × 1, 3–6 days (candidiasis)
   No dosage adjustment is necessary in patients with renal or hepatic impairment due to limited systemic absorption following topical or vaginal application.

Drug Preparation:
- Store < 25°C

Drug Administration:
- Single dose vaginally.

Drug Interactions: None

Lab Effects/Interference: None

Special Considerations:
- Known hypersensitivity to clotrimazole, cetostearyl alcohol and/or to any other excipients.
- Immune system disorders: allergic reaction (syncope, hypotension, dyspnea, urticaria).
- Reproductive system and breast disorders: genital peeling, pruritus, rash, edema, discomfort, burning, irritation, pelvic pain
- Gastrointestinal disorders: abdominal pain

Potential Toxicities/Side Effects and the Nursing Process

I.   ALTERATION IN NUTRITION, LESS THAN BODY REQUIREMENTS, related to GI SIDE EFFECTS

Defining Characteristics: Nausea, vomiting is seen in 3–10% of patients. Diarrhea, abdominal pain, flatulence, constipation may occur less frequently. Increased LFTs may occur: AST, ALT, alk phos. Hepatotoxicity is less common, is usually reversible, and is rarely fatal.

Nursing Implications: Assess baseline nutritional and elimination status. Instruct patient to report GI disturbances. Administer and teach patient to self-administer antiemetics, antidiarrheals as needed and as ordered. Teach patient importance of nutritious diet, and suggest small, frequent, high-calorie, high-protein meals as appropriate. Assess baseline LFTs and monitor periodically during treatment. Discuss abnormalities and drug interruption with physician. Assess whether taking other hepatotoxic drugs (see Special Considerations section). Assess for increased fatigue, jaundice, dark urine, pale stools (signs of hepatotoxicity), and discuss drug discontinuance immediately with physician.

II.   ALTERATION IN SKIN INTEGRITY related to ALLERGIC REACTION

Defining Characteristics: Rash, dermatitis, purpura, urticaria occur in 1% of patients; rarely, anaphylaxis may occur.

Nursing Implications: Assess baseline skin condition and integrity. Teach patient to report itch, rash, and other skin changes. Teach patient skin care and symptomatic measures.

If rash or dermatitis progresses, discuss drug discontinuance with physician. Assess for signs/symptoms of anaphylaxis.

III. ALTERATIONS IN SENSORY/PERCEPTUAL PATTERNS related to CNS EFFECTS

Defining Characteristics: Dizziness, headache, nervousness, insomnia, lethargy, somnolence, and paresthesia have occurred in approximately 1% of patients.

Nursing Implications: Assess baseline neurologic function and comfort and monitor during treatment. Instruct patient to report any changes. Discuss any abnormalities with physician.

Drug: fluconazole (Diflucan)

Class: Azole, antifungal (systemic).

Mechanism of Action: Fungistatic; causes increased permeability of fungal cell membrane, so intracellular nutrients leak out (potassium, amino acids) and cell is unable to take in nutrients to make DNA (precursors for purine, pyrimidines).

Metabolism: Drug is rapidly and highly absorbed from GI tract, with > 90% of drug bioavailable. GI absorption is unaffected by food or gastric pH. Steady-state plasma levels achieved in 5–10 days, or by second day if loading dose given. Widely distributed in body tissues and fluids, including CSF. There is minimal protein binding. It is unknown whether drug crosses the placenta or is excreted in human milk; 60–80% of drug is excreted unchanged in the urine. Renal dysfunction results in higher circulating serum levels with prolonged drug effect and potential toxicity. Drug elimination in elderly clients may be decreased.

Indication: For treatment of most fungi, including yeast.

Dosage/Range:
• Oral and parenteral dosages are the same; IV dosage recommended for patients unable to take oral form. Dose is a single daily dose.

Indication	Induction Dosage	Maintenance Dosage
Oropharyngeal or esophageal candidiasis	200 mg day 1	followed by 100 mg/day (may titrate based on patient's response up to 400 mg/day) × 2 weeks (oropharyngeal) OR × 3 weeks or at least × 2 weeks after symptoms resolve (esophageal)
Systemic candidiasis	400–800 mg day 1	followed by 200 to 400 mg/day × 4 weeks at least THEN × 2 weeks after symptoms resolve (esophageal)
Cryptococcal infections	400 mg day 1	followed by 200–400 mg/day × 10–12 weeks after CSF cultures for *Cryptococcus* are negative
AIDS patients		200 mg/day indefinitely
Vaginal Candidiasis	150 mg PO/IV × 1	

COMPLICATIONS

• Dose modification for renal impairment:

CrCl (mL/min)	Dosage Reduction Percentage (%)
20–50	Reduce by 50%
11–20	Reduce by 75%

Drug Preparation:
• Oral: store in tight containers at < 30°C (86°F).
• Parenteral: glass vials for injection should be stored at 5–30°C (41–86°F); protect from freezing. Plastic containers should be stored at 5–25°C (41–77°F). Inspect for any discoloration, particulate matter, or leaks in plastic bags. If found, do not use.

Drug Administration:
• Oral: once daily without regard to food intake.
• IV: once daily at a rate ≤ 200 mg/h. DO NOT ADD ADDITIVES. DO NOT ADMINISTER IV IN SERIES THAT COULD INTRODUCE AIR EMBOLISM.

Drug Interactions:
• Coumarin anticoagulants: increased PT; monitor PT closely.
• Cyclosporine: increased cyclosporine serum levels; monitor closely and adjust dose.
• Phenytoin: increased phenytoin serum level; monitor closely and reduce phenytoin dose as needed.
• Rifampin: decreased fluconazole serum level; increase fluconazole dose when given concurrently.
• Sulfonylurea antidiabetic agents (tolbutamide, glyburide, glipizide): increased drug serum levels; monitor blood glucose levels closely and decrease dose as needed.
• Thiazide diuretics: increased fluconazole serum level; do not appear to increase fluconazole toxicity so dose adjustment not necessary.
• Rifampin, isoniazid, phenytoin, valproic acid, oral sulfonylurea: increased risk of elevated hepatic transaminases exists.
• Prolonging drugs (methadone, mesoridazine, tacrolimus, clarithromycin, saquinavir, voriconazole, pazopanib, netdetanib, toremifene, nilotinib, amifampridine, ritonavir, solifenacin, sparfloxacin, sunitinib, lomitapide, atazanavir, thioridazine, quetiapine, sorafenib, trazodone, ivabradine, propafenone, donepezil, panobinostat, dasatinib).
• Dronedarone—increased risk of torsades.
• Drug interacts with CYP3A4 substrates.

Lab Effects/Interference:

Major clinical significance:
• ALT, alk phos, AST, and serum bili values may be elevated.

Special Considerations:
• Drug is being studied as a prophylactic antifungal agent in patients at risk for neutropenia and fungal infections (cancer patients receiving myelosuppressive chemotherapy, bone marrow transplant patients).

- Use cautiously in patients with renal dysfunction; dose reduction based on creatinine clearance (see Dosage/Range section).
- Absorption NOT affected by gastric pH or food intake.
- Risk of drug toxicity may be higher in patients with HIV infection.

Potential Toxicities/Side Effects and the Nursing Process

I. ALTERATION IN NUTRITION, LESS THAN BODY REQUIREMENTS, related to GI SIDE EFFECTS

Defining Characteristics: 2–8% incidence of mild-to-moderate nausea, vomiting, abdominal pain, diarrhea is seen; anorexia, dyspepsia, dry mouth, flatus, bloating occur rarely; 5–7% incidence of mild, transient increases in LFTs, which are reversible with drug discontinuance.

Nursing Implications: Assess baseline nutritional and elimination status. Instruct patient to report GI disturbances. Administer and teach patient to self-administer antiemetics, antidiarrheals as needed and as ordered. Teach patient importance of nutritious diet and suggest small, frequent, high-calorie, high-protein meals as appropriate. Assess baseline LFTs and monitor periodically during treatment. Discuss abnormalities and drug interruption with physician. Assess whether patient is taking other hepatotoxic drugs (see Special Considerations section).

II. ALTERATION IN SKIN INTEGRITY related to ALLERGY/HYPERSENSITIVITY

Defining Characteristics: 5% incidence is seen of rash, often diffuse, associated with eosinophilia and pruritus; rarely, exfoliative dermatitis and Stevens–Johnson syndrome may occur in patients receiving multiple drugs.

Nursing Implications: Assess baseline skin condition, including integrity and drug allergy history. Instruct patient to report rash, itching, or other skin changes. Teach patient skin care and symptomatic measures as appropriate. If skin rash develops, discuss drug discontinuance with physician. If rash progresses, especially in HIV-infected patients, drug should be discontinued, as fatal Stevens–Johnson syndrome may develop. Be prepared to treat severe acute hypersensitivity reactions with airway management, oxygen, epinephrine, corticosteroids, antihistamines as ordered.

III. ALTERATIONS IN SENSORY/PERCEPTUAL PATTERNS related to CNS EFFECTS

Defining Characteristics: Dizziness and headache occur in 2% of patients. Rarely, somnolence, delirium/coma, dysesthesia, malaise, fatigue, seizure, and psychiatric disturbance may occur.

COMPLICATIONS

Nursing Implications: Assess baseline neurologic function and comfort, and monitor during treatment. Instruct patient to report any changes. Discuss any abnormalities with physician.

Drug: flucytosine (Ancobon)

Class: Antifungal (systemic).

Mechanism of Action: Nonantibiotic antifungal; enters fungal cell and undergoes deamination to fluorouracil, which acts as an antimetabolite, preventing RNA and protein synthesis; may also interfere with DNA synthesis.

Metabolism: Oral preparation well-absorbed from GI tract; decreased rate of absorption when taken with food. Widely distributed into body tissues and fluids, including CSF; 75–90% of dose excreted unchanged by kidneys, with increased serum levels and toxicity in patients with renal dysfunction.

Indication: For treatment of *Cryptococcus*.

Dosage/Range:
- Oral: 50–150 mg/kg/day in four equally divided doses given q 6 h × weeks or months until fungal studies are negative. Dose may be 150–250 mg/kg/day in *Cryptococcus* meningitis.
- Dose modification if renal impairment
- Dose may be determined by creatinine clearance.

CrCl (mL/min)	Dosing Interval (hr)
10–50	12–24
Less than 10	24–48
20–40	q 12 h
10–20	q 24 h
Less than 10	24–48

Drug Preparation:
- Store in tight, light-resistant container at < 40°C (104°F).
- Oral.

Drug Interactions:
- Amphotericin can increase toxicity
- Drug interacts with levomethadyl, tegafur, zidovudine, cytarabine.

Lab Effects/Interference:
- Rare anemia, leukopenia, agranulocytosis, thrombocytopenia, pancytopenia, eosinophilia.

Special Considerations
- Can cause hallucinations, cardiotoxicity, renal failure.
- Use only in severe infections, as drug is toxic.

- Theoretically synergistic with amphotericin, but some studies do not show significant benefit of combination.
- Therapeutic response (negative fungal cultures) may take weeks to months.
- Drug has no antineoplastic activity.
- Drug is teratogenic, capable of causing fetal malformations when given to pregnant women. Risks and benefits should be carefully considered before drug is used in a pregnant patient.

Potential Toxicities/Side Effects and the Nursing Process

I. POTENTIAL FOR INFECTION, BLEEDING, AND FATIGUE, related to BONE MARROW DEPRESSION

Defining Characteristics: Anemia, leukopenia, thrombocytopenia may occur; agranulocytosis and aplastic anemia occur rarely. Increased risk exists with increased serum flucytosine levels (100 mg/mL), especially in patients with renal compromise or those receiving concurrent amphotericin B.

Nursing Implications: Assess baseline CBC, differential, BUN, and creatinine, and monitor closely during therapy, especially if receiving concurrent amphotericin B. Assess for signs/symptoms of bleeding, fatigue, infection during therapy. Teach patient to self-assess for signs/symptoms of infection, bleeding, and instruct to report them immediately. Discuss dose with physician; dose modification is needed if renal dysfunction occurs. Monitor flucytosine therapeutic levels (to maintain level of 25–100 mg/mL).

II. ALTERATION IN NUTRITION, LESS THAN BODY REQUIREMENTS, related to MUCOSITIS, NAUSEA, VOMITING

Defining Characteristics: Frequently dividing epithelial cells of GI mucosa are damaged, leading to diarrhea and possible bowel perforation (rare). Nausea, vomiting, anorexia, abdominal bloating may also occur. Elevated LFTs may occur, but are dose-related and reversible; liver enlargement may occur.

Nursing Implications: Assess elimination and nutritional status, baseline and throughout treatment. Assess baseline LFTs. Instruct patient to report diarrhea, nausea, vomiting immediately, and teach self-administration of prescribed antiemetics and antidiarrheal medication. Monitor weight, and teach patient importance of high-protein, high-calorie diet. Instruct patient to administer dose over 15 minutes to decrease nausea and vomiting. If weight loss occurs/persists, refer to dietitian/nutritionist. Monitor LFTs during treatment: AST, ALT, bili, and alk phos.

III. INJURY related to ANAPHYLAXIS

Defining Characteristics: Rare anaphylaxis has occurred in patients with AIDS, characterized by diffuse erythema, pruritus, injection of conjunctiva, fever, tachycardia, hypotension, edema, and abdominal pain.

COMPLICATIONS

Nursing Implications: Instruct AIDS patients to report any signs/symptoms of rash, pruritus, conjunctivitis, abdominal pain immediately. Use drug cautiously in AIDS patients. Monitor any adverse sensations over time. Assess for signs/symptoms.

IV.   ALTERATION IN SENSORY/PERCEPTUAL PATTERNS related to CNS CHANGES

Defining Characteristics: Confusion, sedation, hallucinations, and headaches occur infrequently.

Nursing Implications: Assess baseline mental status. Instruct patient to report headaches, abnormal thoughts, mental status changes. Discuss alternative drug if mental status changes occur.

Drug: isavuconazonium sulfate (Cresemba)

Class: Isavuconazonium sulfate is an azole antifungal indicated for patients 18 years of age and older.

Mechanism of Action: Prodrug of isavuconazole, an azole antifungal drug.

Metabolism: Isavuconazole is extensively distributed and is highly protein bound (greater than 99%), predominantly to albumin. Isavuconazonium sulfate was recovered in both feces and urine. Renal excretion of isavuconazole itself was less than 1% of the dose administered.

Indications: Treatment of invasive aspergillosis and invasive mucormycosis.

Dosage/Range:

	Dosage/Range (mg)	Interval/Duration	Route
Loading Dose	372 (equivalent to 200 of isavuconazole)	q 8 h for 6 doses (48 h)	Oral or IV administration
Maintenance Dose	372 (equivalent to 200 of isavuconazole) 1× daily	Once daily starting 12–24 h after the last loading dose	Oral or IV administration

- Capsules can be taken with or without food; swallow capsules whole. Do not chew, crush, dissolve, or open capsules.
- Switching between intravenous and oral formulations of isavuconazonium sulfate is acceptable as bioequivalence has been demonstrated; a loading dose is not required when switching between formulations.
- Dose adjustment: not needed for renal impairment and mild or moderate hepatic impairment Hepatic impairment (severe, Child-Pugh class C): Use only if benefits outweigh potential risks; monitoring recommended.

Drug Preparation:
- Aseptic technique must be strictly observed in all handling, no preservative or bacteriostatic agent is present in isavuconazonium sulfate or in materials specified for its reconstitution.
- Isavuconazonium sulfate is water soluble, preservative free, sterile, and nonpyrogenic.
- Reconstitute drug by adding water for injection, USP per package insert. Gently shake to dissolve powder completely. Visually inspect reconstituted solution for particulate matter and discoloration.
- Reconstituted isavuconazonium sulfate should be clear and free of visible particulates. Reconstituted solution may be stored below 25°C for a maximum of 1 hour prior to preparation of patient infusion solution.
- IV formulation may form insoluble particulates following reconstitution. Isavuconazonium sulfate for injection must be administered via an infusion set with an in-line filter (pore size, 0.2–1.2 micron). Flush IV lines with 0.9% sodium chloride injection, USP or 5% dextrose injection, USP prior to and after infusion of isavuconazonium sulfate.
- Infuse IV formulation over a minimum of 1 hour in 250 mL of a compatible diluent, to reduce risk of infusion-related reactions. Do not administer as an IV bolus injection. Do not infuse isavuconazonium sulfate with other IV medications.
- After dilution of IV formulation, avoid unnecessary vibration or vigorous shaking of solution. Do not use a pneumatic transport system.

Drug Interactions:
- CYP3A4 inhibitors or inducers may alter plasma concentrations of isavuconazole. Appropriate therapeutic drug monitoring and dose adjustment of immunosuppressants (i.e., tacrolimus, sirolimus, cyclosporine, phenytoin, carbamazepine, primidone, phenobarbital, rifampin, mitotane, rifabutin, oxcarbazepine, fosphenytoin, St. John's wort, rifapentine, efavirenz, enzalutamide) may be necessary when coadministered with isavuconazonium sulfate. Drugs with a narrow therapeutic window that are P-gp substrates, such as digoxin, may require dose adjustment when administered concomitantly with isavuconazonium sulfate.
- Several drugs may significantly alter isavuconazole concentrations. Coadministration of strong CYP3A4 inhibitors, such as ketoconazole or high-dose ritonavir (400 mg every 12 hours), with isavuconazonium sulfate is contraindicated because strong CYP3A4 inhibitors can increase plasma concentration of isavuconazole (i.e. ketoconazole, clarithromycin, itraconazole, nefazodone, saquinavir, indinavir, delavirdine, nelfinavir, voriconazole, tipranavir, imatinib, telithromycin, conivaptan, posaconazole, boceprevir, telaprevir, cobicistat, atazanavir, idelalisib)
- Isavuconazole may alter concentrations of several drugs. Coadministration of strong CYP3A4 inducers, such as rifampin, carbamazepine, St. John's wort, or long-acting barbiturates, with isavuconazonium sulfate is contraindicated because strong CYP3A4 inducers can decrease plasma concentration of isavuconazole.

Lab Effects/Interference: Serious hepatic reactions have been reported. Evaluate liver-related lab tests at beginning and during course of isavuconazonium sulfate therapy.

COMPLICATIONS

Special Considerations:
- Infusion-related reactions have been reported during IV administration of isavuconazonium sulfate. Discontinue infusion if an infusion-related reaction occurs.
- Do not administer drug to pregnant women unless the benefit to the mother outweighs the risk to the fetus. Inform pregnant patients of potential hazards.
- Isavuconazonium sulfate is contraindicated in persons with known hypersensitivity to isavuconazole. Serious hypersensitivity and severe skin reactions, such as anaphylaxis and Stevens–Johnson syndrome, have been reported during treatment with other azole antifungal agents. Discontinue isavuconazonium sulfate if patient develops an exfoliative cutaneous reaction.
- Isavuconazonium sulfate has been shown to shorten the QTc interval. It is contraindicated in patients with familial short QT syndrome.

Potential Toxicities/Side Effects and the Nursing Process

I.   ALTERATION IN SKIN INTEGRITY related to ALLERGY/HYPERSENSITIVITY

Defining Characteristics: Rash, often diffuse, associated with eosinophilia and pruritus, has been reported. Rarely, exfoliative dermatitis and Stevens–Johnson syndrome may occur in patients receiving multiple drugs.

Nursing Implications: Assess patient's baseline skin condition, including integrity, and drug allergy history. Instruct patient to report rash, itching, or other skin changes. Teach patient skin care and symptomatic measures as appropriate. If skin rash develops, discuss drug discontinuance with physician. If rash progresses, drug should be discontinued, as fatal Stevens–Johnson syndrome may develop. Be prepared to treat severe acute hypersensitivity reactions with airway management, oxygen, epinephrine, corticosteroids, or antihistamines, as ordered. Assess baseline VS. Instruct patient to report signs and symptoms immediately. Assess for nausea, generalized itching, crampy abdominal pain, chest tightness, anxiety, agitation, sense of impending doom, wheezing, and dizziness.

II.   ALTERATION IN COMFORT related to PRURITUS, PHLEBITIS, SKIN ERUPTIONS AND FEVER

Defining Characteristics: Phlebitis and pruritus with or without rash may occur.

Nursing Implications: Assess temperature, skin integrity, and comfort prior to drug administration, and monitor throughout treatment. Discuss with physician use of diphenhydramine to decrease itching. Change IV sites every 48 hours to decrease phlebitis, or discuss use of a central line with patient and physician. If rash and pruritus worsen, discuss drug discontinuance with physician.

III. ALTERATION IN NUTRITION, LESS THAN BODY REQUIREMENTS, related to GI SIDE EFFECTS

Defining Characteristics: Nausea, vomiting, diarrhea, constipation, and anorexia; mild, transient increases in LFTs.

Nursing Implications: Assess patient's baseline nutritional and elimination status. Instruct patient to report GI disturbances. Administer, and teach patient to self-administer, anti-emetics and antidiarrheals as needed and as ordered. Teach patient importance of a nutritious diet; suggest small, frequent, high-calorie, high-protein meals as appropriate. Assess baseline LFTs and monitor periodically during treatment. Discuss abnormalities and drug interruption with physician. Assess whether patient is taking other hepatotoxic drugs.

Drug: itraconazole (Sporanox)

Class: Azole; antifungal.

Mechanism of Action: Fungistatic; may be fungicidal, depending on concentration; azole antifungals interfere with cytochrome P450 activity, which is necessary for the demethylation of 14-a-methylsterols to ergosterol. Ergosterol, the principal sterol in the fungal cell membrane, becomes depleted. This damages the cell membrane, producing alterations in membrane function and permeability. In *C. albicans,* azole antifungals inhibit transformation of blastospores into invasive mycelial form.

Metabolism: Rapidly absorbed from GI tract in acid environment. Decreased absorption in patients with gastric hypochlorhydria or achlorhydria or in patients taking medications that raise pH (antacids, H_2 antagonists). There are itraconazole levels that can be ordered to measure absorption.

Indication: For treatment of fungal infections.

Dosage/Range:
- Oral: 100–200 mg/day $\times$ 7–14 days (candidiasis); longer for other infections (400 mg/day in severe infections).
- Although studies did not provide a loading dose, in life-threatening situations a loading dose of 200 mg 3 times a day (600 mg/day) for the first 3 days is recommended, based on pharmacokinetic data.
- Doses above 200 mg/day should be given in 2 divided doses.

Drug Preparation:
- Store in tightly closed container at < 40°C (104°F).
- Itraconazole injection must be diluted prior to IV infusion. The entire 250-mg ampule should be diluted in the 50-mL bag of 0.9% sodium chloride provided by the manufacturer. The final concentration of the solution is 3.33 mg/mL (250 mg/75 mL).

COMPLICATIONS

Drug Administration:
- Orally in single or split dose, depending on total daily dose.
- Should take with meals to increase absorption of medication.
- Oral solution should be taken on an empty stomach to increase absorption of the medication.
- To administer a 200-mg dose of itraconazole, 60 mL should be given by IV infusion over 60 minutes. The infusion should be given using a controlled infusion device, the manufacturer-provided infusion set, and a dedicated IV line. When the infusion is complete, the manufacturer recommends that the infusion set be flushed via the two-way stopcock using 15–20 mL of 0.9% sodium chloride over 30 seconds to 15 minutes. The entire IV line should then be discarded.

Drug Interactions:
- Drugs that increase gastric pH: antacids, anticholinergics/antispasmodics, histamine H_2-receptor antagonists, or omeprazole will decrease the absorption of itraconazole.
- Didanosine contains a buffer to increase its absorption; this will decrease the absorption of itraconazole, since itraconazole needs an acidic environment.
- Dug interacts with CYP3A4 inhibitors (strong inhibitors are contraindicated) and substrates and QT prolonging medications.
- Use with oral antidiabetic agents has increased the plasma concentration of these sulfonylurea agents, leading to hypoglycemia.
- Use with carbamazepine may decrease itraconazole plasma concentrations, leading to clinical failure or relapse.
- Itraconazole may increase digoxin concentrations, leading to digoxin toxicity.
- Use with lovastatin or simvastatin may increase the plasma concentrations of these cholesterol-lowering agents and may increase the risk of rhabdomyolysis.
- Use with midazolam or triazolam may potentiate the hypnotic and sedative effects of these benzodiazepines.

Lab Effects/Interference:

Major clinical significance:
- ALT, alk phos, AST, serum bili values may be elevated.
- Serum K+: hypokalemia has occurred in approximately 2–6% of patients treated with itraconazole and has resulted in ventricular fibrillation, especially in higher doses.

Special Considerations:
- High failure rate in HIV-infected patients due to achlorhydria.

Potential Toxicities/Side Effects and the Nursing Process

I.   ALTERATION IN NUTRITION, LESS THAN BODY REQUIREMENTS, related to GI SIDE EFFECTS

Defining Characteristics: Increased LFTs may occur: AST, ALT, alk phos. Hepatotoxicity is less common, is usually reversible, and is rarely fatal.

Nursing Implications: Assess baseline nutritional and elimination status. Instruct patient to report GI disturbances. Administer and teach patient to self-administer antiemetics, antidiarrheals as needed and as ordered. Teach patient importance of nutritious diet, and suggest small, frequent, high-calorie, high-protein meals as appropriate. Assess baseline LFTs and monitor periodically during treatment. Discuss abnormalities and drug interruption with physician. Assess whether taking other hepatotoxic drugs (see Special Considerations section). Assess for increased fatigue, jaundice, dark urine, pale stools (signs of hepatotoxicity), and discuss drug discontinuance immediately with physician.

II. ALTERATION IN SKIN INTEGRITY related to ALLERGIC REACTION

Defining Characteristics: Rash, dermatitis, purpura, urticaria occur; rarely, anaphylaxis may occur.

Nursing Implications: Assess baseline skin condition and integrity. Instruct patient to report itch, rash, and other skin changes. Teach patient skin care and symptomatic measures. If rash or dermatitis progresses, discuss drug discontinuance with physician. Assess for signs/symptoms of anaphylaxis.

Drug: ketoconazole (Nizoral)

Class: Azole; antifungal (systemic).

Mechanism of Action: Fungistatic by damaging fungal cell membrane and increasing permeability, altering cell metabolism, and inhibiting cell growth. Fungicidal in high concentrations.

Metabolism: Rapidly absorbed from GI tract in acid environment. Decreased absorption in patients with gastric hypochlorhydria (25% of all AIDS patients) or in patients taking medications that raise pH (antacids, H_2 antagonists). Distributed widely but cerebrospinal penetration is unpredictable. Drug is approximately 90% protein-bound. Partially metabolized in liver and mostly excreted in the feces via bile.

Indication: For treatment of histoplasmosis, coccidioidomycosis, and blastomycosis for treatment of Tinea pedis, cruris, corporis.

Dosage/Range:
- Oral: 200 mg/day × 7–14 days (candidiasis); longer for other infections (400 mg/day in severe infections).

Drug Preparation:
- Store in tightly closed container at < 40°C (104°F).

Drug Administration:
- Orally in single dose.
- May take with meals to decrease GI side effects (unclear if food increases absorption).

- In patients with gastric achlorhydria, patient may be instructed to dissolve ketoconazole in 4-mL aqueous solution of 0.2 N hydrochloric acid and drink through a straw; follow with 4 oz (120 mL) of water.

Drug Interactions:
- Drugs that increase gastric pH: antacids, cimetidine, ranitidine, famotidine, sucralfate decrease ketoconazole absorption; give these drugs at least 2 hours after ketoconazole.
- Other hepatotoxic drugs: use cautiously and monitor liver function studies closely.
- Rifampin or rifampin plus isoniazid: decreased ketoconazole levels especially if isoniazid is taken as well. Increase ketoconazole dose.
- Acyclovir: synergism and increased antiviral action against herpes simplex virus.
- Norfloxacin: theoretically increases antifungal action of ketoconazole, but studies are inconsistent.
- Coumarin anticoagulants: increased PT; monitor patient closely and decrease anticoagulant dose accordingly.
- Cyclosporine: increased cyclosporine serum level; monitor serum level and decrease cyclosporine dose accordingly.
- Phenytoin: may have altered serum levels of phenytoin or ketoconazole; monitor serum levels of each and adjust dosages accordingly.
- Theophylline: may decrease theophylline serum concentrations; monitor serum levels and increase dosage accordingly.
- Corticosteroids: may increase corticosteroid serum level; may need to decrease dosage.
- Drug interacts with medications that prolong QT interval and Colchicine.

Lab Effects/Interference:

Major clinical significance:
- ALT, alk phos, AST, and serum bili values may be elevated.
- ACTH-induced serum corticosteroid concentrations and serum testosterone concentrations may be decreased by doses of 800 mg/day of ketoconazole; serum testosterone concentrations are abolished by values of 1.6 g/day of ketoconazole but return to baseline values when ketoconazole is discontinued.

Special Considerations:
- Monitor liver function studies.
- High failure rate in HIV-infected patients due to achlorhydria.
- **Cardiovascular:** Cardiac dysrhythmia, prolonged QT interval, torsades de pointes, ventricular arrhythmia.
- **Hepatic:** Hepatotoxicity.
- Anaphylaxis.

Potential Toxicities/Side Effects and the Nursing Process

I. ALTERATION IN NUTRITION, LESS THAN BODY REQUIREMENTS, related to GI SIDE EFFECTS

Defining Characteristics: Nausea, vomiting is seen in 3–10% of patients. Diarrhea, abdominal pain, flatulence, constipation may occur less frequently. Increased LFTs may occur: AST, ALT, alk phos. Hepatotoxicity is less common, is usually reversible, and is rarely fatal.

Nursing Implications: Assess baseline nutritional and elimination status. Instruct patient to report GI disturbances. Administer and teach patient to self-administer antiemetics, antidiarrheals as needed and as ordered. Teach patient importance of nutritious diet, and suggest small, frequent, high-calorie, high-protein meals as appropriate. Assess baseline LFTs and monitor periodically during treatment. Discuss abnormalities and drug interruption with physician. Assess whether taking other hepatotoxic drugs (see Special Considerations section). Assess for increased fatigue, jaundice, dark urine, pale stools (signs of hepatotoxicity), and discuss drug discontinuance immediately with physician.

II.   ALTERATION IN COMFORT related to GYNECOMASTIA AND BREAST TENDERNESS

Defining Characteristics: Breast enlargement and tenderness may occur in some men, lasting weeks to duration of therapy.

Nursing Implications: Assess for occurrence in male patients. Assess comfort level, degree of tenderness, and self-care measures used to increase comfort. Assess impact on body image.

III.   ALTERATION IN SKIN INTEGRITY related to ALLERGIC REACTION

Defining Characteristics: Rash, dermatitis, purpura, and urticaria occur in 1% of patients; rarely, anaphylaxis may occur.

Nursing Implications: Assess baseline skin condition and integrity. Teach patient to report itch, rash, and other skin changes. Teach patient skin care and symptomatic measures. If rash or dermatitis progresses, discuss drug discontinuance with physician. Assess for signs/ symptoms of anaphylaxis.

IV.   ALTERATIONS IN SENSORY/PERCEPTUAL PATTERNS related to CNS EFFECTS

Defining Characteristics: Dizziness, headache, nervousness, insomnia, lethargy, somnolence, and paresthesia have occurred in approximately 1% of patients.

Nursing Implications: Assess baseline neurologic function and comfort and monitor during treatment. Instruct patient to report any changes. Discuss any abnormalities with physician.

COMPLICATIONS

Drug: metronidazole hydrochloride (Flagyl)

Class: Antibacterial (systemic); antiprotozoal.

Mechanism of Action: Disrupts DNA, inhibits nucleic acid synthesis in susceptible organisms.

Metabolism: Well-absorbed after oral administration; rate affected by food, but not amount absorbed. Oral and IV serum levels are similar. Widely distributed in body tissues and fluids, including CSF, placenta, and breastmilk. Excreted in urine (60–80%) and feces.

Indication: For treatment of parasitic and bacterial infections. This drug is active against anaerobic gram-negative (*Bacteroides*) and gram-positive bacilli (*Clostridium*), and protozoa (*Trichomonas, Giardia*).

Dosage/Range:

Adults:

Indication	Dosage	Route	Interval/Duration
Trichomoniasis	250–750 mg	Oral	3×/day for 7–10 days
	2 g	Oral	Single dose
C. difficile-associated diarrhea Mild to Moderate Initial episode or first recurrence	500 mg	Oral	3x/day for 10–14 days
C. difficile-associated diarrhea	Loading dose: 15 mg/kg (1 g)	IV	over 1 hour
	Maintenance dose: 7.5 mg/kg (500 mg) (maximum 4 g/day)	IV	q 8 h (max 1 g/day)

Drug Preparation:
- Oral: Store in light-resistant container at < 30°C (86°F).
- IV: Protect from light and freezing. Reconstitute according to manufacturer's package insert. Further dilute with 0.9% sodium chloride or 5% dextrose to concentration of ≤ 8 mg/mL. Do not use aluminum needles. Administer over 30–60 minutes. May be given as continuous or intermittent infusion.

Drug Interactions:
- Coumarin anticoagulants: increase anticoagulant effect. Avoid concurrent use if possible; otherwise, monitor PT closely and decrease anticoagulant drug dose as needed.
- Alcohol: inhibits alcohol metabolism, causing a disulfiram-like reaction (flushing, headache, nausea, vomiting, abdominal cramps, diaphoresis). Avoid alcohol and alcohol-containing medications for 48 hours after last metronidazole dose.
- Disulfiram: causes acute psychoses and confusion. Avoid concurrent use and separate use by 2 weeks.
- Phenobarbital/phenytoin: decrease metronidazole activity. Monitor effectiveness and increase metronidazole dose as needed.
- Cimetidine: increases metronidazole levels with potential for increased toxicity. Avoid concurrent administration.
- Drug interacts with amprenavir, QT prolonging medications, tacrolimus, Busulfan, Bupropion decrease seizure threshold, Lithium, Cyclosporine, Carbamazepine, Ergot alkaloids.

Lab Effects/Interference:
- Serum ALT, serum AST, and LDH: metronidazole has a high absorbance at the wavelength at which NADH is determined; therefore, elevated liver enzyme concentrations may appear to be suppressed by metronidazole when measured by continuous-flow methods based on endpoint decrease.

Special Considerations:
- Carcinogenic in rodents, so drug is used only when necessary.
- Contraindicated in first trimester of pregnancy and administered only as salvage therapy in second and third trimesters when other agents have failed; lactating mothers should interrupt breastfeeding during treatment with drug.
- Use with caution in patients with a history of blood dyscrasias, CNS disorders/dysfunction, hepatic dysfunction, or alcoholism.
- Total and differential leukocyte counts: before and after therapy in patients with current or past blood dyscrasias, or who require prolonged or repeated treatment.
- May interfere with laboratory determinations of LFTs (AST, ALT, LDH).

Potential Toxicities/Side Effects and the Nursing Process

I.   ALTERATION IN NUTRITION, LESS THAN BODY REQUIREMENTS, related to GI SIDE EFFECTS

Defining Characteristics: Nausea (with/without headache), anorexia, dry mouth, metallic taste in mouth have occurred; less frequently, vomiting, diarrhea, epigastric distress, or constipation. Rare pseudomembranous colitis.

Nursing Implications: Assess baseline nutritional and elimination status. Instruct patient to report GI disturbances. Administer and teach patient to self-administer antiemetics, antidiarrheals as needed and as ordered. Teach patient importance of nutritious diet, and suggest small, frequent, high-calorie, high-protein meals as appropriate. Assess baseline LFTs and monitor periodically during treatment. Discuss abnormalities and drug interruption with physician. Assess whether taking other hepatotoxic drugs (see Special Considerations section). Instruct patient to avoid alcohol and alcohol-containing medications for 48 hours after last drug dose.

II.   ALTERATIONS IN SENSORY/PERCEPTUAL PATTERNS related to PERIPHERAL NEUROPATHY

Defining Characteristics: Peripheral neuropathy (numbness, tingling, paresthesia) is reversible with drug discontinuance. Headache, dizziness, ataxia, confusion, and mood changes have also occurred.

Nursing Implications: Assess baseline neurologic function and comfort, and monitor during treatment. Instruct patient to report any changes. Discuss abnormalities and drug discontinuance with physician.

COMPLICATIONS

III.   ALTERATIONS IN SKIN INTEGRITY related to SENSITIVITY REACTIONS

Defining Characteristics: Urticaria, erythematous rash, pruritus, flushing, or transient joint pain may occur.

Nursing Implications: Assess drug allergy history. Assess baseline skin integrity. Instruct patient to report rash, pruritus. Teach patient symptomatic management of rash, pruritus.

IV.   ALTERATIONS IN URINARY ELIMINATION related to DYSURIA

Defining Characteristics: Urethral burning, dysuria, cystitis, polyuria, incontinence, and sensation of pelvic pressure may occur with oral dose. Urine may be dark or reddish-brown.

Nursing Implications: Assess baseline elimination status. Instruct patient to report side effects, and to increase oral fluids to 2–3 qt/day. Reassure patient urine color change is related to drug and will disappear when drug therapy is completed.

V.   ALTERATIONS IN SEXUALITY related to DECREASED LIBIDO, DYSPAREUNIA

Defining Characteristics: Decreased libido, dyspareunia, and dryness of vagina and vulva may occur.

Nursing Implications: Assess pattern of sexuality. Inform patient and partner that these effects, if they occur, are temporary. Suggest frequent perineal hygiene as needed to relieve dryness and use of lubricants during intercourse.

VI.   FUNGAL SUPERINFECTION related to REDISTRIBUTION OF ENDOGENOUS MICROORGANISMS

Defining Characteristics: Vaginal candidiasis or vaginitis may occur as endogenous bacteria are eliminated and normal fungal population expands.

Nursing Implications: Instruct female patient to report vaginal itching or discharge. Discuss appropriate antifungal treatment with physician. Teach perineal hygiene and symptomatic management.

VII.   ALTERATIONS IN COMFORT related to PHLEBITIS

Defining Characteristics: Phlebitis and thrombophlebitis may occur with IV administration.

Nursing Implications: Assess IV site prior to each dose for phlebitis, erythema, and swelling, and change site at least q 48 h. Apply heat to painful IV site as ordered.

Drug: micafungin sodium (Mycamine)

Class: Antifungal.

Mechanism of Action: Fungistatic by damaging fungal cell membrane, increasing permeability, altering cell metabolism, and inhibiting cell growth. Inhibits the synthesis of 1,3-β-D-glucan, an integral component of the fungal cell wall.

Metabolism: Metabolized by liver and excreted in urine.

Indication: For treatment of fungal infections in cancer patients; it is fungicidal at high concentrations.

Dosage/Range:
- 100–150 mg/day × 15 days.
- Prophylaxis 50 mg/day.

Drug Preparation:
- Do not mix or coinfuse with other medications. Micafungin has been shown to precipitate when mixed directly with a number of other commonly used medications.
- No dose adjustment is required with concomitant use of mycophenolate mofetil, cyclosporine, tacrolimus, prednisolone, sirolimus, nifedipine, fluconazole, ritonavir, or rifampin.
- A loading dose is not required; typically, 85% of the steady state is achieved after 3 daily doses.
- IV: Dilute in 0.9% sodium chloride, USP (without a bacteriostatic agent) or 5% dextrose injection, USP.
- Infuse over 1 hour. Stable × 24 hours at room temperature.

Drug Interactions:
- Coumarin anticoagulants: increased PT. Monitor patient closely and decrease anticoagulant dose accordingly.
- Cyclosporine: increased cyclosporine serum level. Monitor serum level and decrease cyclosporine dose accordingly.

Lab Effects/Interference:

Major clinical significance:
- ALT, alk phos, AST, or serum bilirubin values may be elevated.

Special Considerations:
- Used in treatment of fungal infections.
- Monitor HCT, Hgb, serum electrolytes, and lipids, as changes may occur during treatment.

Potential Toxicities/Side Effects and the Nursing Process

I.   POTENTIAL FOR INJURY related to ANAPHYLAXIS

Defining Characteristics: Anaphylaxis with tachycardia, arrhythmias, and cardiac arrest may occur.

Nursing Implications: Assess baseline VS and monitor throughout infusion. Instruct patient to report signs/symptoms immediately. Assess for signs/symptoms: nausea, generalized itching, crampy abdominal pain, chest tightness, anxiety, agitation, sense of impending doom, wheezing, and dizziness.

II.   ALTERATION IN COMFORT related to PRURITUS, PHLEBITIS, SKIN ERUPTIONS, FEVER

Defining Characteristics: Phlebitis, pruritus with or without rash may occur.

Nursing Implications: Assess temperature, skin integrity, and comfort prior to drug administration, and monitor throughout treatment. Discuss with physician use of diphenhydramine to decrease itching. Change IV sites q 48 h to decrease phlebitis, or discuss with patient and physician use of central line. If rash and pruritus worsen, discuss with physician drug discontinuance.

III.   ALTERATION IN NUTRITION, LESS THAN BODY REQUIREMENTS, related to GI SIDE EFFECTS

Defining Characteristics: Nausea, vomiting, diarrhea, and anorexia may occur.

Nursing Implications: Assess baseline nutritional and elimination status. Instruct patient to report GI disturbances. Administer and teach patient to self-administer antiemetics, antidiarrheals as needed and as ordered. Teach patient importance of nutritious diet, and suggest small, frequent, high-calorie, high-protein meals as appropriate.

IV.   ALTERATIONS IN SENSORY/PERCEPTUAL PATTERNS related to CNS, ENDOCRINE EFFECTS

Defining Characteristics: Dizziness, headache, and somnolence may occur.

Nursing Implications: Assess baseline neurologic function and comfort and monitor during treatment. Instruct patient to report any changes. Discuss any abnormalities with physician.

Drug: miconazole nitrate (Monistat)

Class: Azole; antifungal (systemic).

Mechanism of Action: Fungistatic by damaging fungal cell membrane and increasing permeability, altering cell metabolism and inhibiting cell growth.

Metabolism: Cream or suppository is used topically.

Indication: Used as a vaginal cream for candidal vulvovaginitis and for Tinea.

Dosage/Range:

Route	Dosage
Suppository	200 mg intravaginally at bedtime for 3 days OR 100 mg intravaginally at bedtime for 7 days OR 1,200 mg intravaginally as a one-time dose
2% cream	Insert 1 applicatorful (5 g) intravaginally daily for 7 days
4% cream	Insert 1 applicatorful (5 g) intravaginally daily for 3 days

• (FDA and guideline dosage)

Drug Interactions:
• None.

Lab Effects/Interference:
• None known.

Special Considerations:
• Concomitant use of other vaginal products (e.g., tampons, douches, spermicides) not recommended during therapy (vaginal).

Potential Toxicities/Side Effects and the Nursing Process

I.   POTENTIAL FOR INJURY related to ANAPHYLAXIS

Defining Characteristics: Anaphylaxis with tachycardia, arrhythmias, and cardiac arrest may occur on first IV dose, probably related to suspension medium of drug (castor oil).

Nursing Implications: Ensure first dose is given in inpatient setting with resuscitation equipment and physician available. Assess baseline VS and monitor throughout infusion. Instruct patient to report signs/symptoms immediately. Assess for signs/symptoms: nausea, generalized itching, crampy abdominal pain, chest tightness, anxiety, agitation, sense of impending doom, wheezing, and dizziness.

II.   ALTERATION IN COMFORT related to PRURITUS, PHLEBITIS, SKIN ERUPTIONS, FEVER

Defining Characteristics: Phlebitis, pruritus with or without rash may occur.

Nursing Implications: Assess temperature, skin integrity, and comfort prior to drug administration and monitor throughout treatment. Discuss with physician use of diphenhydramine to decrease itching. Change IV sites q 48 h to decrease phlebitis, or discuss with patient and physician use of central line. If rash and pruritus worsen, discuss with physician drug discontinuance.

COMPLICATIONS

Drug: nystatin (Mycostatin, Nilstat)

Class: Antifungal.

Mechanism of Action: Binds to sterol molecule in fungi cell membrane, increasing permeability so that potassium and other intracellular ions are lost.

Metabolism: Drug is not absorbed from intact skin, mucous membranes, and is poorly absorbed from GI tract. Excreted as unchanged drug in feces.

Indication: Active against yeast and fungi, especially *Candida*.

Dosage/Range:
- Oral: (for treatment of oral or intestinal candidiasis): 500,000–1 million U tid; continue therapy for 48 hours after clinical remission to prevent recurrence.
- Tablet: 1 to 2 tablets (500,000–1,000,000 units) ORALLY 3 times/day; continue treatment for at least 48 hours after clinical cure.
- Powder: topical for *Candida* rash infections.
- Vaginal: 100,000 U as vaginal tablet inserted into vagina daily or bid × 14 days.

Drug Preparation:
- Oral suspension and tablets should be stored in tight, light-resistant containers < 40°C (104°F).

Drug Administration:
- Oral suspension. Instruct patient to:
  - Rinse mouth with oral hygiene solution to clean food debris.
  - Hold suspension in mouth and swish for 1–2 minutes, then swallow or spit solution.
  - Do not rinse mouth or eat for 15–30 minutes.

Drug Interactions:
- None.

Lab Effects/Interference:
- None known.

Special Considerations:
- For patients with oral thrush who have difficulty taking oral suspension:
  - Oral suspension can be frozen in medicine cups so it is easier to administer if the patient has stomatitis.
  - Vaginal suppository may be sucked, as this increases mucosal contact with drug.
  - Cannot be used to treat systemic infections.
  - Adverse effects are infrequent.

Potential Toxicities/Side Effects and the Nursing Process

I.   ALTERATION IN NUTRITION, LESS THAN BODY REQUIREMENTS, related to GI SIDE EFFECTS

Defining Characteristics: High oral doses may cause nausea, vomiting, or diarrhea.

Nursing Implications: Assess baseline nutritional status. Instruct patient to report GI disturbances. Administer and teach patient to self-administer antiemetics, antidiarrheals as needed and as ordered. Teach patient importance of nutritious diet and suggest small, frequent, high-calorie, high-protein meals as appropriate.

II. KNOWLEDGE DEFICIT related to SELF-ADMINISTRATION OF MEDICATION

Defining Characteristics: Increased compliance when patient is instructed in self-care activities.

Nursing Implications: Assess knowledge about infection and planned treatment. Teach about drug action, potential side effects, and when and how to take drug. Instruct patient to rinse mouth with saline gargle (or other rinse) to remove food debris prior to taking nystatin suspension; solution should be swished in mouth 1–2 minutes, then swallowed or spit out. Patient should not eat or rinse mouth for 15–30 minutes.

Drug: pentamidine isethionate (Nebupent)

Class: Antifungal.

Mechanism of Action: pentamidine isethionate is a nonpyrogenic lyophilized product. Studies suggest that the pentamidine isethionate interferes with microbial nuclear metabolism by inhibition of DNA, RNA, phospholipids and protein synthesis. However, the mode of action is not fully understood.

Metabolism: Drug is not absorbed from intact skin, mucous membranes, and is poorly absorbed from GI tract. Excreted as unchanged drug in feces.

Indication: Pentamidine isethionate is indicated for prevention of *Pneumocystis jiroveci* pneumonia (PJP) in high-risk, HIV-infected patients defined by one or both of the following criteria:
• a history of one or more episodes of PJP
• a peripheral CD4+ (T4 helper/inducer) lymphocyte count less than or equal to 200/mm^3.

Dosage/Range:
• Recommended adult dosage of Pentamidine isethionate for prevention of *P. jiroveci* pneumonia is 300 mg once every 4 weeks administered via the Respirgard® II nebulizer.
• Dose delivered until nebulizer chamber is empty (approximately 30–45 minutes).
• Flow rate should be 5–7 L/minute from a 40–50 pounds per square inch (PSI) air or oxygen source.
• Alternatively a 40–50 PSI air compressor can be used with flow limited by setting the flowmeter at 5–7 L/minute or by setting the pressure at 22–25 PSI.
• Low pressure (less than 20 PSI) compressors should not be used.

Drug Preparation:
Contents of one vial (300 mg) must be dissolved in 6 mL sterile water for injection, USP.

COMPLICATIONS

Drug Administration:
- Place the entire reconstituted contents of the vial into the Respirgard II nebulizer reservoir for administration.
- Freshly prepared solutions for aerosol use are recommended.
- After reconstitution with sterile water, solution is stable for 48 hours in the original vial at room temperature if protected from light.

Drug Interactions:
- Specific studies on drug interactions have not been conducted.
- Majority of patients in clinical trials received concomitant medications, including zidovudine, with no reported interactions.
- Because nephrotoxic effects may be additive, concomitant or sequential use of pentamidine and other nephrotoxic drugs (aminoglycosides, amphotericin B, cisplatin, foscarnet, or vancomycin) should be closely monitored and avoided, if possible.

Lab Effects/Interference:
- None known.

Special Considerations:
- Pentamidine isethionate is contraindicated in patients with a history of an anaphylactic reaction to inhaled or parenteral pentamidine isethionate.

Potential Toxicities/Side Effects and the Nursing Process

I.   KNOWLEDGE DEFICIT related to SELF-ADMINISTRATION OF MEDICATION

Defining Characteristics: Increased compliance when patient is instructed in self-care activities.

Nursing Implications: Assess knowledge about infection and planned treatment. Teach about drug action, potential side effects, and when and how to take drug.

Drug: posaconazole (Noxafil)

Class: Triazole; antifungal (systemic).

Mechanism of Action: Fungistatic; inhibits fungi by blocking ergosterol synthesis through inhibition of the enzyme lanosterol 14 alpha-demethylase (CYP51). Ergosterol depletion coupled with accumulation of methylated sterol precursors results in inhibition of fungal cell growth, fungal death by damaging fungal cell membrane and increasing permeability, altering cell metabolism, and inhibiting cell growth. Fungicidal at high concentrations.

Metabolism: Absorbed from GI tract when administered as an oral suspension. Partially metabolized in liver and mostly excreted in the feces via bile.

Indication: Active against invasive *Candida* species, *Aspergillus* species, non-*Aspergillus* hyalohyphomycetes, phaeohyphomycetes, zygomycetes, and endemic fungi.

Dosage/Range:

Route	Loading Dose	Maintenance Dose
Oral Suspension	200 mg q 8–6 hrs for 7 days	400 mg q 12 h daily Dose may not be increased beyond 800 mg as absorption is saturable
Oral (Delayed-release) Tablet	300 mg orally 2× daily on day 1	300 orally 1× daily starting on day 2
IV (Injection)	300 mg as IV infusion 2× daily on day 1	300 mg as IV infusion 1× daily on day 2

• Oral tablet and suspension are not interchangeable.

Drug Preparation:
• Drug is given orally and IV.

Drug Administration:
• Oral Suspension. May take 1 hour before meals or 1 hour after meals.
• Absorption of suspension enhanced by coadministration with food and nutritional supplements.
• Extended release tablet should not be crushed.
• IV Posaconazole: accumulation of vehicle can occur when renal dysfunction.
• Posaconazole levels can be monitored to ensure absorption, compliance.

Drug Interactions:
• Drugs that increase gastric pH: antacids, cimetidine, ranitidine, and sucralfate have minor or no significant effect on posaconazole.
• Hepatotoxic drugs: use cautiously, and monitor liver function studies closely.
• Coumarin anticoagulants: increases PT; monitor patient closely and decrease anticoagulant dose accordingly.
• Do not administer to persons with known hypersensitivity to posaconazole or other azole antifungal agents.
• Do not coadminister Noxafil with the following drugs. Noxafil increases concentrations of:
  • Sirolimus: can result in sirolimus toxicity
  • CYP3A4 substrates (pimozide, quinidine): can result in QTc interval prolongation and cases of TdP
  • HMG-CoA reductase inhibitors primarily metabolized through CYP3A4: can lead to rhabdomyolysis
  • Ergot alkaloids: can result in ergotism
• Potential interactions could occur with concomitant use of posaconazole and cisapride, astemizole, terfenadine, quinidine, pimozide, bepridil, sertindole, dofetilide, and halofantrine.
• Well-tolerated in pediatric and elderly patients.
• Contraindicated with increased myopathy, QT prolonging medications, and CYP3A medications.

COMPLICATIONS

Lab Effects/Interference:

Major clinical significance:
• ALT, alk phos, AST, or serum bilirubin values may be elevated.

Special Considerations:
• Monitor liver function studies.

Potential Toxicities/Side Effects and the Nursing Process

I.   ALTERATION IN NUTRITION, LESS THAN BODY REQUIREMENTS, related to GI SIDE EFFECTS

Defining Characteristics: Nausea, vomiting is seen in 18% of patients. Diarrhea, abdominal pain, flatulence, constipation may occur less frequently. Increased LFTs may occur: AST, ALT, alk phos. Hepatotoxicity is less common, is usually reversible, and is rarely fatal.

Nursing Implications: Assess baseline nutritional and elimination status. Instruct patient to report GI disturbances. Administer and teach patient to self-administer antiemetics, antidiarrheals as needed and as ordered. Teach patient importance of nutritious diet and suggest small, frequent, high-calorie, high-protein meals as appropriate. Assess baseline LFTs and monitor periodically during treatment. Discuss abnormalities and drug interruption with physician. Assess whether taking other hepatotoxic drugs (see Special Considerations section). Assess for increased fatigue, jaundice, dark urine, pale stools (signs of hepatotoxicity), and discuss drug discontinuance immediately with physician.

II.   ALTERATION IN SENSORY/PERCEPTUAL PATTERNS related to HEADACHE

Defining Characteristics: Treatment-related disturbances are common (17%). Generally mild and rarely result in discontinuing treatment.

Nursing Implications: Assess for occurrence. Assess comfort level. Educate patient about this side effect. Assess impact on body image.

III.   ALTERATION IN COMFORT related to PRURITUS, DRY SKIN, AND FLUSHING

Defining Characteristics: Rash, dry skin, and flushing.

Nursing Implications: Assess temperature, skin integrity, and comfort before drug administration and monitor throughout course of treatment. Discuss with physician use of diphenhydramine to decrease itching and cream or lotions to smooth skin and maintain skin integrity. If rash and skin condition worsens, discuss with physician drug discontinuance.

Drug: voriconazole (Vfend)

Class: Triazole; antifungal (systemic).

Mechanism of Action: Fungistatic by damaging fungal cell membrane and increasing permeability, altering cell metabolism, and inhibiting cell growth.

Metabolism: Rapidly absorbed from GI tract in acid environment. Partially metabolized in liver and mostly excreted in the feces via bile.

Indication: For treatment of fungal infections in cancer patients. It is fungicidal at high concentrations. Active against invasive *A. fumigatus, Fusarium* spp. infection, and *Scedosporium apiospermum* infection.

Dosage/Range:
- Oral: 200 mg q 12 h for 7–14 days; dose may be increased if there is an inadequate response to infections (300 mg q 12 h).
- IV preparation is available. Dose 6 mg/kg q 12 h $\times$ 2 load, then 4 mg/kg maintenance q 12 h.
- Final voriconazole preparation must be infused over 1–2 hours at a maximum rate of 3 mg/kg/hr.
- Levels can be monitored for efficacy and toxicity.
- Dose adjustment: No dosage for renal dysfunction, IV preparation contains diluent (cyclodextrin), which can accumulate if CrCl < 30.

Drug Preparation:
- Once reconstituted, drug should be used immediately, or it can be stored for no longer than 24 hours at 2–8°C (37–46°F).

Drug Administration:
- Orally. May take 1 hour before meals or 1 hour after meals.
- The final voriconazole preparation must be infused over 1–2 hours at a maximum rate of 3 mg/kg/hr.

Drug Interactions:
- St. John's wort, sirolimus, tacrolimus, efavirenz, rifabutin, statins, QT prolonging medications, barbiturates, nevirapine, glimepiride, sildenafil, vincristine.
- Drugs that increase gastric pH: antacids, cimetidine, ranitidine have minor or no significant effect on voriconazole.
- Hepatotoxic drugs: use cautiously and monitor liver function studies closely.
- Rifampin decreases the steady state of voriconazole.
- Coumarin anticoagulants: increases PT; monitor patient closely and decrease anticoagulant dose accordingly.
- Cyclosporine: increases cyclosporine serum level; monitor serum level and decrease cyclosporine dose accordingly.

COMPLICATIONS

- Phenytoin: may have altered serum levels of phenytoin or ketoconazole; monitor serum levels of each and adjust dosages accordingly.
- Carbamazepine and long-acting barbiturates and macrolide antibiotics reduce the efficacy of voriconazole.

Lab Effects/Interference:

Major clinical significance:
- ALT, alk phos, AST, or serum bili values may be elevated.

Special Considerations:
- Monitor liver function studies, and serum levels to assess toxicity, compliance, and absorption.

Potential Toxicities/Side Effects and the Nursing Process

I.   ALTERATION IN NUTRITION, LESS THAN BODY REQUIREMENTS, related to GI SIDE EFFECTS

Defining Characteristics: Nausea, vomiting is seen in 3–10% of patients. Diarrhea, abdominal pain, flatulence, constipation may occur less frequently. Increased LFTs may occur: AST, ALT, alk phos. Hepatotoxicity is less common, is usually reversible, and is rarely fatal.

Nursing Implications: Assess baseline nutritional and elimination status. Instruct patient to report GI disturbances. Administer and teach patient to self-administer antiemetics, antidiarrheals as needed and as ordered. Teach patient importance of nutritious diet, and suggest small, frequent, high-calorie, high-protein meals as appropriate. Assess baseline LFTs and monitor periodically during treatment. Discuss abnormalities and drug interruption with physician. Assess whether taking other hepatotoxic drugs (see Special Considerations section). Assess for increased fatigue, jaundice, dark urine, pale stools (signs of hepatotoxicity), and discuss drug discontinuance immediately with physician.

II.   ALTERATION IN SENSORY/PERCEPTUAL PATTERNS related to VISUAL DISTURBANCES

Defining Characteristics: Treatment-related visual disturbances are common (30%). Generally mild and rarely result in discontinuing treatment.

Nursing Implications: Assess for occurrence. Assess comfort level. Educate patient about this side effect. Assess impact on body image.

III.   ALTERATION IN SKIN INTEGRITY related to ALLERGIC REACTION

Defining Characteristics: Rash, dermatitis, purpura, urticaria occur in 6% of patients.

Nursing Implications: Assess baseline skin condition and integrity. Teach patient to report itch, rash, and other skin changes. Teach patient skin care and symptomatic measures. If rash or dermatitis progresses, discuss drug discontinuance with physician. Assess for signs/ symptoms of anaphylaxis.

ANTIVIRALS

Drug: acyclovir (Zovirax)

Class: Antiviral (systemic).

Mechanism of Action: Interferes with DNA synthesis so that viral replication cannot occur.

Metabolism: Variable GI absorption; unaffected by food. Widely distributed in body tissue and fluids, including CSF. Variable protein-binding (9–33%). Crosses placenta and is excreted in breastmilk.

Indication: Active against herpes simplex virus (HSV-1, HSV-2), varicella-zoster virus (VZV) (shingles), Epstein-Barr virus (EBV), and cytomegalovirus (CMV).

Dosage/Range:

Adult:
- Oral: 200 mg PO q 4 h (genital herpes) to 800 mg PO 5 ×/day (acute herpes zoster).
- IV (initial/recurrent infections in immunocompromised patients): 5–10 mg/kg q 8 h × 7 days; 5 mg/kg q 8 h × 7–14 days (herpes simplex); 10 mg/kg q 8 h × 7–14 days (herpes zoster, herpes encephalitis).
- Use ideal body weight for dose calculation.
- Avoid doses greater than 1,000 mg/dose.
- Dose modification is required if renal dysfunction is present.

Drug Preparation:
- Oral: store in tight, light-resistant containers at 15–25°C (59–77°F).
- IV: reconstitute with sterile water for injection per manufacturer's directions and further dilute in 50–100 mL IV fluid; a final concentration of 7 mg/mL or less is recommended to minimize the incidence of phlebitis; infuse over 1 hour.

Drug Interactions:
- Foscarnet and other nephrotoxic agents.
- Zidovudine: potentiates antiretroviral activity of zidovudine but may cause increased neurotoxicity (drowsiness, lethargy) in AIDS patients. Monitor for increased neurotoxicity.
- Probenecid: may increase plasma half-life. Monitor for increased acyclovir toxicity.
- Antifungals: potential antiviral synergy.
- Interferon: potential synergistic antiviral effect, potential increased neurotoxicity. Use together with caution.
- Drug interacts with mycophenolate, phenytoin, and meperidine.
- Methotrexate (intrathecal): possible increased neurotoxicity. Use together with caution.

COMPLICATIONS

Lab Effects/Interference:

Major clinical significance:
- BUN and serum creatinine concentrations required prior to and during therapy, since IV acyclovir may be nephrotoxic; if acyclovir is given by rapid IV injection or its urine solubility is exceeded, precipitation of acyclovir crystals may occur in renal tubules; renal tubular damage may occur and may progress to acute renal failure.

Clinical significance:
- Pap test: although clear association has not been shown to date, patients with genital herpes may be at increased risk of developing cervical cancer. Pap test should be done at least once a year to detect early cervical changes.

Special Considerations:
- Use cautiously in patients with preexisting renal dysfunction or dehydration; underlying neurologic dysfunction or neurologic reactions to cytotoxic drugs, intrathecal methotrexate, or interferon and in patients with hepatic dysfunction.
- It is imperative that patients be well hydrated, with adequate urine output prior to and for up to 2 hours after IV dosing.
- Administer with caution if patient is receiving other nephrotoxic drugs.
- Contraindicated in patients hypersensitive to drug.
- Minimal injury to normal cells, so few adverse effects exist.
- Monitor for renal toxicity, especially in elderly and with higher doses.

Potential Toxicities/Side Effects and the Nursing Process

I. ALTERATION IN URINARY ELIMINATION related to RENAL TOXICITY

Defining Characteristics: Transient increase is seen in renal function tests (serum BUN, creatinine) and decreased urine creatinine clearance, as drug may precipitate in renal tubules during dehydration or rapid IV drug administration. Increased risk exists if preexisting renal disease or concurrent administration of nephrotoxic drugs.

Nursing Implications: Assess baseline renal function and monitor periodically during therapy. Notify physician of any abnormalities before administering next dose. Ensure adequate hydration and urine output prior to and for 2 hours after IV drug administration. Administer IV drug slowly over 1 hour.

II. ALTERATIONS IN SENSORY/PERCEPTUAL PATTERNS related to ENCEPHALOPATHY

Defining Characteristics: IV administration: encephalopathy (lethargy, tremors, confusion, agitation, seizures, dizziness) may occur rarely. Oral: headache occurs in 13% of patients receiving chronic suppressive treatment.

Nursing Implications: Assess baseline neurologic function and comfort, and monitor during treatment. Instruct patient to report any changes. Discuss any abnormalities with physician.

III.   ALTERATIONS IN COMFORT related to LOCAL VEIN IRRITATION (IV ADMINISTRATION)

Defining Characteristics: Erythema, irritation, pain, swelling, and phlebitis may occur at injection site.

Nursing Implications: Assess IV site for patency, irritation prior to each dose. Change IV site at least q 48 h. Apply warmth/heat to painful area as needed.

IV.   ALTERATION IN NUTRITION, LESS THAN BODY REQUIREMENTS, related to GI SIDE EFFECTS (ORAL DOSAGE)

Defining Characteristics: Nausea, vomiting, and diarrhea occur in 2–5% of patients receiving chronic therapy.

Nursing Implications: Assess history of nausea/vomiting, diarrhea, and instruct patient to report any occurrence. Teach patient self-medication of prescribed antinausea or antidiarrheal medicines. Discuss drug discontinuance with physician if symptoms are severe.

V.   ALTERATION IN SKIN INTEGRITY related to RASH

Defining Characteristics: Rash, urticaria, or pruritus may occur.

Nursing Implications: Assess baseline history of drug allergy and skin integrity. Instruct patient to report any occurrence of rash, pruritus. Teach symptomatic management measures unless severe; if severe, discuss drug discontinuance with physician.

VI.   KNOWLEDGE DEFICIT related to (ORAL) DRUG ADMINISTRATION

Defining Characteristics: Patient may not realize drug does not cure viral infection, nor does it prevent spread of virus to others. Prodrome of tingling, itching, or pain can herald mucocutaneous herpes.

Nursing Implications: Teach patient about herpetic infection and goal of therapy to suppress infection. When used to treat recurrent episodes of chronic infection, teach patient to recognize prodromal symptoms and to take prescribed drug then or within 2 days of onset of lesions. Teach patient about routes of viral spread and instruct to avoid contacts with others that may lead to viral spread.

Drug: baloxavir marboxil (Xofluza)

Class: Antiviral drug with activity against influenza virus.

Mechanism of Action: Polymerase acidic (PA) endonuclease inhibitor, an influenza virus-specific enzyme in the viral RNA polymerase complex required for gene transcription, resulting in inhibition of influenza virus replication.

COMPLICATIONS

Metabolism: Baloxavir is a prodrug that is almost completely converted to its active metabolite, baloxavir, following oral administration.

Indication: For the treatment of acute uncomplicated influenza in patients 12 years of age and older who have been symptomatic for no more than 48 hours.

Dosage/Range: Take a single dose orally within 48 hours of symptom onset with or without food. Total dose depends upon weight of patient.

Drug Preparation: 20 mg or 40 mg tablets

Drug Administration: Oral

Drug Interactions: Avoid coadministration with dairy products, calcium-fortified beverages, polyvalent cation-containing laxatives, antacids, or oral supplements (e.g. calcium, iron, magnesium, selenium, or zinc).

Lab Effects:

Special Consideration: Contraindicated in patients with a history of hypersentivity to baloxavir marboxil or any of its ingredients.

I.   ALTERATION IN NUTRITION, LESS THAN BODY REQUIREMENTS, related to GI SIDE EFFECTS (ORAL DOSAGE)

Defining Characteristics: Nausea, vomiting, and diarrhea occur in 2–5% of patients receiving chronic therapy.

Nursing Implications: Assess history of nausea/vomiting, diarrhea, and instruct patient to report any occurrence. Teach patient self-medication of prescribed antinausea or antidiarrheal medicines. Discuss drug discontinuance with physician if symptoms are severe.

II.   ALTERATION IN SKIN INTEGRITY related to RASH

Defining Characteristics: Rash, urticaria, pruritus may occur.

Nursing Implications: Assess baseline history of drug allergy and skin integrity. Instruct patient to report any occurrence of rash, pruritus. Teach symptomatic management measures unless severe; if severe, discuss drug discontinuance with physician.

III.   KNOWLEDGE DEFICIT related to (ORAL) DRUG ADMINISTRATION

Defining Characteristics: Patient may not realize drug does not cure viral infection; nor does it prevent spread of virus to others. Prodrome of tingling, itching, or pain can herald mucocutaneous herpes.

Nursing Implications: Teach patient about herpetic infection and goal of therapy to suppress infection. When used to treat recurrent episodes of chronic infection, teach patient to recognize prodromal symptoms and to take prescribed drug then or within 2 days of onset of lesions. Teach patient about routes of viral spread and instruct to avoid contacts with others that may lead to viral spread.

Drug: cidofovir (Vistide)

Class: Antiviral (systemic).

Mechanism of Action: Suppresses CMV replication by selective inhibition of viral DNA synthesis.

Metabolism: Less than 6% bound to plasma proteins. Renal clearance is reduced with the concomitant administration of probenecid.

Indication: For treatment of viral infections in cancer patients.

Dosage/Range: Given with probenecid and saline hydration.
- Weekly induction regimen: 5 mg/kg infused every week $\times$ 2 weeks.
- Twice-monthly maintenance regimen: 5 mg/kg infused every other week.

Drug Preparation:
- Requires chemotherapy safety handling (drug is mutagenic, tumorigenic, embryotoxic).
- Reconstitute drug (single use, nonpreserved); vial contains 75 mg/mL.
- Further dilute in 100 mL 0.9% sodium chloride.

Drug Administration:
- Administer 2 g probenecid (four 500-mg tabs) 3 hours prior to drug infusion.
- Infuse 1 L of 0.9% sodium chloride over 1–2 hours immediately prior to drug infusion.
- Infuse IV drug over 1 hour.
- As ordered by physician, may administer second liter of 0.9% sodium chloride at the start of the drug infusion and continue for 1–3 hours.
- Two hours after end of drug infusion, administer 1 g probenecid (two 500-mg tabs).
- Eight hours after end of the drug infusion, administer 1 g probenecid (two 500-mg tabs).

Drug Interactions:
- Drug interacts with foscarnet, pentamidine IV, and tobramycin.
- Probenecid: interacts with the metabolism or renal tubular excretion of acetaminophen, acyclovir, angiotensin-converting enzyme (ACE) inhibitors, barbiturates, NSAIDs, theophylline, and zidovudine.
- Increased nephrotoxicity when combined with other nephrotoxic drugs.

Lab Effects/Interference:
- Serum creatinine levels may be elevated.

Special Considerations:
- Indicated for the treatment of AIDS patients who have newly diagnosed or relapsed CMV retinitis.
- Dose-limiting toxicity is nephrotoxicity evidenced by proteinuria and increased serum creatinine.

COMPLICATIONS

- Treatment requires prehydration and posthydration use of concomitant probenecid.
- Drug contraindicated in patients with baseline serum creatinine > 1.5 mg/dL, creatinine clearance ≤ 55 mL/min, proteinuria ≥ 3+, past severe hypersensitivity to probenecid or other sulfa-containing medications, hypersensitivity to cidofovir, and patients who are pregnant or breastfeeding.

Dose Reductions:

a. Patients with baseline normal renal function: (changes during therapy) reduce maintenance dose to 3 mg/kg for an increase in serum creatinine of 0.3–0.4 mg/dL above baseline; discontinue therapy for an increase of 0.5 mg/dL or greater above baseline or development of 3+ or greater proteinuria.

Renal Abnormality	Cidofovir Dosage
Serum creatinine 0.3–0.4 mg/dL > baseline	3 mg/kg
Serum creatinine 0.5 mg/dL above baseline	discontinue cidofovir
Proteinuria ≥ 3+	discontinue cidofovir

b. Patients with baseline renal impairment: renal impairment: (preexisting) contraindicated in patients with a serum creatinine greater than 1.5 mg/dL, a calculated CrCl of 55 mL/min or less, or a urine protein of 100 mg/dL or more (equivalent to greater than or equal to 2+ proteinuria).

Creatinine Clearance (mL/min)	Induction (mg/kg) (Once a Week × 2 weeks)	Maintenance (mg/kg) (Once Every 2 weeks)
41–55	2.0	2.0
30–40	1.5	1.1
20–29	1.0	1.0
≤ 19	0.5	0.1

- Patient teaching:
  - Encourage increased oral intake of fluids to 1–3 L as tolerated.
  - Return to clinic for appointments (induction: weekly × 2 weeks, maintenance every other week).
  - Report side effects immediately.
  - Ophthalmologic appointments as scheduled for intraocular pressure (IOP), visual acuity monitoring.

Potential Toxicities/Side Effects and the Nursing Process

I.   POTENTIAL FOR INJURY related to NEUTROPENIA

Defining Characteristics: Neutropenia (< 750/mm^2) may occur in 28% of patients, and < 500/mm^3 occurred in 20% of patients. Infections occurred in 25% of patients.

Nursing Implications: Monitor WBC and ANC prior to each drug dose, and hold treatment if neutropenic. Discuss with physician use of G-CSF. If the patient is receiving zidovudine, the zidovudine should be temporarily discontinued or dose decreased by 50% on days of probenecid therapy. Instruct patient to monitor temperature and to report fever > 101°F immediately. Discuss use of G-CSF with physician as needed (up to 34% required G-CSF in clinical trials).

II. ALTERATION IN NUTRITION, LESS THAN BODY REQUIREMENTS, related to NAUSEA/VOMITING

Defining Characteristics: Nausea/vomiting occur in about 65% of patients.

Nursing Implications: Encourage patients to eat food prior to each dose of probenecid. Discuss antiemetic prior to the first dose of probenecid and then during period of probenecid therapy.

III. ALTERATION IN COMFORT related to FEVER, CHILLS, RASH, HEADACHE FROM PROBENECID

Defining Characteristics: Fever occurs in up to 57% of patients, rash in 30%, headache in 27%, chills in 24%. Asthenia (46% incidence), diarrhea (27%), alopecia (25%), anorexia (22%), dyspnea (22%), abdominal pain (17%), and anemia (20%). In clinical trials, 25% of patients withdrew from treatment due to adverse events.

Nursing Implications: Assess baseline comfort, and instruct patient to report symptoms. Discuss symptom management with physician, such as antihistamine and/or antipyretic (acetaminophen) for fever, and then use prophylactically in subsequent doses.

IV. ALTERATION IN ELIMINATION related to RENAL TOXICITY

Defining Characteristics: Creatinine elevations to > 1.5 mg/dL occur in approximately 17% of patients, proteinuria in 80% of patients, and decreased serum bicarbonate in > 5% of patients.

Nursing Implications: Encourage patients to increase their daily oral fluid intake to 2–3 L. Closely monitor renal function; patients who have received foscarnet are at increased risk for nephrotoxicity. Ensure that patient receives prehydration and posthydration, and is able to take oral fluids. Discuss dose reductions based on alterations in renal function with physician. Check urine for protein. If positive, discuss additional hydration and rechecking of urine for blood with physician.

V. ALTERATIONS IN SENSORY/PERCEPTUAL PATTERNS related to OCULAR HYPOTONY

Defining Characteristics: OCULAR HYPOTONY occurs rarely, may be increased risk for patients with concomitant diabetes mellitus.

Nursing Implications: Patients should see ophthalmologist for IOP assessments and visual acuity periodically.

COMPLICATIONS

VI. METABOLIC ACIDOSIS related to DECREASED SERUM BICARBONATE

Defining Characteristics: Occurs rarely (2%).

Nursing Implications: Assess for decreases in serum bicarbonate < 16 mEq/L associated with evidence of renal tubular damage (incidence 9%). Serious metabolic acidosis in association with liver failure, mucormycosis, Aspergillus, and disseminated MAC has occurred, with subsequent death in one patient. Monitor baseline chemistries, and review results prior to each treatment.

Drug: famciclovir (Famvir)

Class: Antiviral (systemic).

Mechanism of Action: Rapidly transformed into antiviral penciclovir, which inhibits herpes simplex types HSV-1, HSV-2, or VZV by inhibiting HSV-2 polymerase. Herpes viral DNA synthesis and viral replication are selectively inhibited.

Metabolism: Oral bioavailability is 77%, with peak plasma levels 30–90 minutes after dosing. Plasma half-life is 2.3 hours. In the virus, the active form of the drug has a long intracellular half-life. Low protein binding and rapid and complete elimination in the urine (73%) and feces (27%).

Indication: For treatment of viral infections in cancer patients.

Dosage/Range:
- Herpes zoster (Shingles or varicella): 500 mg q 8 h × 5–10 days.
- Genital herpes simplex: 125 mg bid × 5 days. 250 mg orally 3 times daily for 7–10 days; may extend duration if healing is incomplete after 10 days of therapy (HIV-infected) 500 mg orally twice daily for 5–14 days.
- HIV infection—Recurrent genital herpes simplex, immune suppression: 500 mg ORALLY twice daily.
- 1,500 mg ORALLY as a single dose; initiate at earliest sign or symptom of a cold sore.
- (HIV-infected) 500 mg ORALLY twice daily for 5–10 days (guideline dosing) or for 7 days (manufacturer dosing); initiate at earliest sign or symptom of a cold sore.

Drug Preparation:
- Available in 125-, 250-, 500-mg tablets.

Drug Administration:
- Oral, without regard to meals.

Drug Interactions:
- None.

Lab Effects/Interference:
- None known.

Special Considerations:

- Treatment of herpes zoster: viral shedding stopped 50% faster than with placebo, with full crusting in < 1 week, and shorter time to relief from acute pain. In addition, drug significantly reduces the duration of postherpetic neuralgia by 2 months compared to placebo.
- Dose modification for renal impairment:

CrCl (mL/min)	Treatment Herpes Zoster	Treatment Recurrent Genital Herpes	Treatment Suppression of Recurrent Genital Herpes	Treatment Recurrent Herpes Labialis	Treatment Recurrent Orolabial or Genital Herpes in HIV-Infected Patients
60 or greater	Usual dose	Usual dose	Usual dose	Usual dose	Usual dose
40–59	500 mg q 12 h	500 mg q 12 h for 1 day	Usual dose	750 mg as single dose	Usual dose
20–39	500 mg q 24 h	500 mg as a single dose	125 mg q 12 h	500 mg as single dose	500 mg q 24 h
Less than 20	250 mg q 24 h	250 mg as a single dose	125 mg q 24 h	250 mg as a single dose	250 mg q 24 h
Hemodialysis	250 mg following each dialysis	250 mg as a single dose following dialysis	125 mg following each dialysis	250 mg as a single dose following dialysis	250 mg following each dialysis

- Hepatic impairment (mild to moderate): no dosage adjustment necessary.

Potential Toxicities/Side Effects and the Nursing Process

I.   ALTERATION IN COMFORT related to HEADACHE, NAUSEA

Defining Characteristics: Headache occurred in approximately 22% of patients. Nausea occurred in 12% of patients.

Nursing Implications: Teach patient that side effects may occur and are usually mild. Instruct patient to report headache that does not resolve with acetaminophen, or nausea that does not resolve with diet modification.

Drug: foscarnet sodium (Foscavir)

Class: Antiviral (systemic).

Mechanism of Action: Inhibits binding sites on virus-specific DNA polymerases and reverse transcriptases without affecting cellular DNA polymerases. Thus, prevents viral replication of all known herpes viruses: CMV, HSV-1, HSV-2, EBV, and VZV.

COMPLICATIONS

Metabolism: Fourteen to seventeen percent bound to plasma proteins and excreted into urine 80–90% unchanged by kidneys. Variable penetration into CSF.

Indication: For treatment of CMV retinitis in AIDS patients. Foscarnet sodium is active against resistant herpes simplex viruses that are resistant via thymidine kinase deficiency.

Dosage/Range:

Adult (normal renal function):

CrCl (ml/min)/kg	HSV	Treatment CMV/HHV-6	Maintenance CMV/HHV-6
Normal Dose	40 mg/kg q 12 h	90 mg/kg q 12 h	90 mg/kg q 24 h
> 1 to 1.4	30 mg/kg q 12 h	70 mg/kg q 12 h	70 mg/kg q 24 h
> 0.8 to 1	20 mg/kg q 12 h	50 mg/kg q 12 h	50 mg/kg q 24 h
> 0.6 to 0.8	35mg/kg q 24 h	80 mg/kg q 24 h	80 mg/kg q 48 h
> 0.5 to 0.6	25 mg/kg q 24 h	60 mg/kg q 24 h	60 mg/kg q 48 h
≥ 0.4 to 0.5	20 mg/kg q 24 h	50 mg/kg q 24 h	50 mg/kg q 48 h
< 0.4	Not recommended	Not recommended	Not recommended

- Dose modification is necessary if renal insufficiency.

Drug Preparation:
- Add drug solution (24 mg/mL) to 0.9% sodium chloride or 5% dextrose to achieve a final concentration = 12 mg/mL.

Drug Administration:
- Administer via rate controller or infusion pump over 1 hour (induction) or 2 hours (maintenance) via peripheral or central vein.
- Do not administer or give concurrently with other drugs or solutions.

Drug Interactions:
- Incompatible with D30W, amphotericin B, lactated Ringer's, total parenteral nutrition (TPN), acyclovir, ganciclovir, trimetrexate, pentamidine, vancomycin, trimethoprim/ sulfamethoxazole, diazepam, digoxin, phenytoin, leucovorin, prochlorperazine.
- Pentamidine: potentially fatal HYPOCALCEMIA; seizures have occurred; AVOID CONCURRENT USE.
- Nephrotoxic drugs (amphotericin B, aminoglycosides): additive nephrotoxicity; AVOID CONCURRENT USE.
- Hypocalcemic agents: additive hypocalcemia; AVOID CONCURRENT USE.
- Zidovudine: increased anemia; monitor patient closely and transfuse with red blood cells as ordered.

Lab Effects/Alterations:

Major clinical significance:
- Serum calcium (ionized), serum calcium (total), and serum phosphate: concentrations of phosphate may be increased or decreased; concentrations of total calcium may be

decreased; although the total calcium concentration may also appear normal, the level of ionized calcium may be decreased and result in symptomatic hypocalcemia.
- Serum creatinine concentrations may be increased.
- Serum Mg++ concentrations may be decreased.
- Renal: Acute renal failure has been reported in patients with underlying renal disease following inappropriately high doses for level of renal function; dose reduction recommended.

Clinical significance:
- ALT, alk phos, AST, and serum bilirubin values may be increased.
- Serum K+ concentrations may be decreased.

Special Considerations:
- Contraindicated in patients hypersensitive to foscarnet.
- DO NOT administer concomitantly with IV pentamidine.
- Avoid use during pregnancy; lactating women should interrupt breastfeeding while receiving the drug.
- Regular monitoring of renal function IMPERATIVE; dose modifications must be made if renal insufficiency exists.
- Use measures for safe handling of cytotoxic drugs (see *Appendix 1*).

Potential Toxicities/Side Effects and the Nursing Process

I. ALTERATION IN URINARY ELIMINATION related to RENAL TOXICITY

Defining Characteristics: Abnormal renal function occurs commonly; increased serum creatinine, decreased creatinine clearance, and acute renal failure may occur.

Nursing Implications: Assess baseline elimination pattern and renal function studies, and monitor closely throughout treatment. Manufacturer suggests creatinine clearance be calculated biw–tiw (induction) and q 1–2 weeks (maintenance). Creatinine clearance can be calculated from modified Cockcroft and Gault equation:

$$\text{For male: } \frac{140 - \text{age}}{\text{serum creatineine} \times 72}$$

$$\text{For female: } \frac{140 - \text{age}}{\text{serum creatineine} \times 72} \times 0.085$$

Discuss dose modifications with physician if renal dysfunction occurs. Ensure adequate hydration and urinary output prior to and following dose; administer drug slowly over 1–2 hours, at no more than 1 mg/kg/min. Teach patient to increase oral fluids as tolerated to clear drug from kidneys.

II. ALTERATION IN ELECTROLYTE BALANCE related to METABOLIC ABNORMALITIES

Defining Characteristics: Hypocalcemia, hypophosphatemia, hyperphosphatemia, hypomagnesemia, and hypokalemia occur. Transient decreased ionized calcium may not appear

COMPLICATIONS

in serum total calcium value. Tetany and seizures may occur, especially in patients receiving foscarnet and IV pentamidine. Increased risk exists if renal impairment or neurologic impairment.

Nursing Implications: Assess baseline calcium, phosphorus, magnesium, potassium, and concurrent drugs that might affect these values. Assess patient for signs/symptoms of hypocalcemia, such as perioral tingling, numbness, or paresthesias during or after infusion. Instruct patient to report these signs/symptoms immediately. If signs/symptoms occur, stop infusion, notify physician, and evaluate serum electrolyte, renal studies. Administer ordered electrolyte repletion.

III. ALTERATIONS IN SENSORY/PERCEPTUAL PATTERNS related to NEUROLOGIC CHANGES

Defining Characteristics: Headache, paresthesia, dizziness, involuntary muscle contractions, hypoesthesia, neuropathy, and seizures (including grand mal) have occurred. Increased risk exists of hypocalcemia (ionized $Ca++$) and renal insufficiency.

Nursing Implications: Assess baseline risk factors and neurologic status, and monitor during treatment. Assess for and instruct patient to report signs/symptoms. Discuss abnormalities with physician, and possible drug discontinuance.

IV. FATIGUE related to ANEMIA

Defining Characteristics: Anemia occurs in 33% of patients and in 60% of patients receiving concomitant zidovudine.

Nursing Implications: Assess baseline HCT/Hgb, activity tolerance, cardiopulmonary status, and monitor during therapy. Instruct patient to report increasing fatigue, headache, irritability, shortness of breath, chest pain. Transfuse RBCs as ordered by physician. Discuss with clinic patient self-care ability; refer for home health assistance as needed.

V. ALTERATION IN NUTRITION, LESS THAN BODY REQUIREMENTS, related to GI SIDE EFFECTS

Defining Characteristics: Nausea, vomiting, and diarrhea are common; anorexia and abdominal pain may also occur.

Nursing Implications: Assess baseline nutrition and liver function, and monitor during therapy. Instruct patient to report GI side effects. Administer or teach patient to self-administer prescribed antiemetic or antidiarrheal medications. Encourage adequate oral or IV hydration. Notify physician of abnormal LFTs. If anorexia occurs, encourage favorite foods and small, frequent meals as tolerated.

VI. INFECTION related to NEUTROPENIA

Defining Characteristics: May occur in 17% of patients; increased risk when receiving concurrent zidovudine.

Nursing Implications: Assess baseline WBC, ANC, and temperature; monitor during therapy. Assess for signs/symptoms of infection and discuss these with physician. Instruct patient to report signs/symptoms of infection.

VII. ALTERATIONS IN COMFORT related to LOCAL VEIN IRRITATION (IV ADMINISTRATION)

Defining Characteristics: Erythema, irritation, pain, swelling, or phlebitis may occur at injection site. Consider use of central line.

Nursing Implications: Assess IV site for patency, irritation prior to each dose. Change IV site at least q 48 h. Apply warmth/heat to painful area as needed.

VIII. ALTERATION IN SKIN INTEGRITY related to RASH

Defining Characteristics: Rash, sweating may occur. Also, rarely, local irritation and ulcerations of penile epithelium in males, and vulvovaginal mucosa in females has occurred—perhaps related to drug in urine.

Nursing Implications: Assess skin integrity baseline and during treatment. Instruct patient to report any irritation or lesions. Teach patient to perform frequent perineal hygiene.

Drug: ganciclovir (Cytovene)

Class: Antiviral (systemic).

Mechanism of Action: Interferes with DNA synthesis so that viral replication cannot occur.

Metabolism: Poorly absorbed from GI tract. Appears to be widely distributed, concentrates in kidneys, and is well distributed to the eyes. Crosses BBB. Drug crosses placenta and is excreted in breastmilk in animals. Excreted unchanged in urine.

Indication: Active against CMV infections, especially in the retina.

Dosage/Range:

Adult:
- IV induction: 5 mg/kg IV q 12 h × 14–21 days.
- Maintenance: 5 mg/kg IV 7 days/week or 6 mg/kg/day × 5 days/week.

COMPLICATIONS

- Prophylaxis of CMV disease 5 mg/kg once daily, or 6 mg/kg once daily 5 days/week until day 100 posttransplant.
- Intravitreous by ophthalmologist (investigational).
- Dose modification for renal impairment:

CrCl (mL/min)	Induction Dosage	Maintenance Dosage
70 or greater	5 mg/kg q 12 h	5 mg/kg q 24 h
50–69	2.5 mg/kg q 12 h	2.5 mg/kg q 24 h
25–49	2.5 mg/kg q 24 h	1.25 mg/kg q 24 h
10–24	1.25 mg/kg q 24 h	0.625 mg/kg q 24 h
Less than 10	1.25 mg/kg 3×/week following hemodialysis	0.625 mg/kg q 24 h
Hemodialysis	1/25 mg/kg 3×/week following hemodialysis	0.625 mg/kg 3×/week following hemodialysis

- Geriatric: Use care when selecting dosage in patients over 65 years due to possibility of renal dysfunction
- Hemodialysis: Induction dosage, 1.25 mg/kg 3 times/week following hemodialysis; do not exceed this dosage
- Hemodialysis: Maintenance dosage, 0.625 mg/kg 3 times per week following hemodialysis

Drug Preparation:
- Drug is CARCINOGENIC and TERATOGENIC: use chemotherapy handling precautions (see *Appendix 1*) when preparing and administering ganciclovir.
- Administer only if ANC is > 500 cells/mm^3 and platelet count > 25,000/mm^3.
- Add 10 mL of sterile water for injection to 500-mg vial. Further dilute dose in 50–250 mL of IV fluid and infuse over at least 1 hour.

Drug Interactions:
- Zidovudine: increased hematologic toxicity (neutropenia, anemia); do not use together if possible.
- Consider didanosine (ddI) instead of zidovudine (AZT) or concomitant use of neutrophil growth factor (e.g., G-CSF or GM-CSF).
- Foscarnet: additive or synergistic antiviral activity.
- Probenecid: may increase ganciclovir serum levels. Monitor closely and decrease ganciclovir dose as needed.
- Immunosuppressant (corticosteroids, cyclosporine, azathioprine): increased bone marrow suppression; dose-reduce or hold immunosuppressants during ganciclovir treatment.
- Interferon: potent synergism against herpes virus, VZV.
- Imipenem/cilastatin: increase neurotoxicity with seizures. AVOID CONCURRENT USE.
- Cytotoxic antineoplastic agents: additive toxicity in bone marrow, gonads, GI epithelium/mucosa.
- Other cytotoxic drugs (dapsone, pentamidine, flucytosine, amphotericin B, trimethoprim-sulfamethoxazole): increase toxicity. Use cautiously if unable to avoid concurrent use.

Lab Effects/Interference:
- Serum ALT, serum alk phos, serum AST, and serum bili values may be increased.
- BUN and serum creatinine values may be increased.

Special Considerations:
- Do not use in pregnancy.
- Patient should be well hydrated; use with caution at reduced doses if renal insufficiency exists.
- Drug is mutagenic; patient should use barrier contraceptive.
- CMV retinitis patient should see ophthalmologist at least every 6 weeks during ganciclovir therapy.
- Administer over at least 1 hour.
- Monitor blood counts frequently.
- Neutropenia, ANC less than 500/mcL: Do not administer.
- Thrombocytopenia, platelets less than 25,000/mcL: Do not administer.

Potential Toxicities/Side Effects and the Nursing Process

I. INFECTION, BLEEDING related to BONE MARROW DEPRESSION

Defining Characteristics: Neutropenia ($< 1,000/\text{mm}^3$) occurs in 25–50% of patients, especially in patients with AIDS or those undergoing bone marrow transplant. Thrombocytopenia ($< 50,000/\text{mm}^3$) occurs in 20% of patients. Anemia occurs in 1% of patients.

Nursing Implications: Assess baseline WBC, ANC, and platelet count; monitor throughout therapy (every other day initially, then 3 × per week). Hold ganciclovir if ANC $< 500/\text{mm}^3$, platelet count $< 25,000/\text{mm}^3$. Assess for signs/symptoms of infection or bleeding; instruct patient in signs/symptoms of infection and bleeding, and instruct to report these immediately. Teach patient self-care measures to minimize risk of infection, bleeding, including avoidance of OTC aspirin-containing medicines. Administer or teach patient to self-administer prescribed G-CSF or GM-CSF. Assess Hgb/HCT and signs/symptoms of fatigue. Instruct patient to alternate rest and activity periods.

II. ALTERATIONS IN SENSORY/PERCEPTUAL PATTERNS related to SENSORY CHANGES

Defining Characteristics: Retinal detachment may occur in 30% of patients treated for CMV retinitis. Local reactions (foreign body sensation, conjunctival or vitreal hemorrhage) may occur with intravitreal injection. CNS effects include headache, confusion, altered dreams, ataxia, and dizziness, affecting 5–17% of patients.

Nursing Implications: Assess baseline neurologic status, including vision, and monitor during treatment. Patient should see ophthalmologist at least every 6 weeks. Instruct patient to report any abnormalities and discuss them with physician.

COMPLICATIONS

III.   ALTERATION IN NUTRITION, LESS THAN BODY REQUIREMENTS, related to GI SIDE EFFECTS

Defining Characteristics: Nausea, vomiting, diarrhea, and anorexia may occur in 2% of patients. Elevated LFTs may occur due to drug, but may be difficult to distinguish from CMV infection of liver or biliary tree.

Nursing Implications: Assess baseline nutrition, liver function, and monitor during therapy. Instruct patient to report GI side effects. Administer or teach patient to self-administer prescribed antiemetic or antidiarrheal medications. Encourage adequate oral or IV hydration. Notify physician of abnormal LFTs. If anorexia occurs, encourage favorite foods and small, frequent meals as tolerated.

IV.   ALTERATION IN URINARY ELIMINATION related to RENAL TOXICITY

Defining Characteristics: Two percent of patients have increased serum BUN, creatinine, hematuria. Increased risk exists in elderly or patients with renal insufficiency.

Nursing Implications: Ensure adequate hydration with urinary output prior to drug administration and infuse drug over at least 1 hour. Dose should be reduced in patients with decreased renal function.

V.   ALTERATIONS IN COMFORT related to LOCAL VEIN IRRITATION (IV ADMINISTRATION)

Defining Characteristics: Inflammation, phlebitis, pain occur often at IV infusion site due to high pH of drug.

Nursing Implications: Assess IV site for patency, irritation prior to each dose. Change IV site at least q 48 h. Apply warmth/heat to painful area as needed. Assess need for tunneled central line. Avoid drug extravasation.

VI.   ALTERATION IN CARDIAC OUTPUT related to CHANGES IN BP

Defining Characteristics: Rarely, hypotension, or hypertension, arrhythmia, myocardial infarction, and arrest occur.

Nursing Implications: Assess baseline VS and monitor throughout treatment. Notify physician of any changes from baseline.

VII.   ALTERATION IN SEXUALITY/REPRODUCTIVE PATTERNS related to REPRODUCTIVE HAZARD

Defining Characteristics: Drug is carcinogenic, mutagenic, and teratogenic; may produce infertility in males. It is unknown whether drug crosses placenta and is excreted in breastmilk.

Nursing Implications: Assess sexuality/reproductive patterns. Teach patient and partner about reproductive hazards; offer contraceptive counseling or refer for counseling as barrier contraceptive should be used by patient.

Drug: letermovir (Prevymis)

Class: Antiviral

Mechanism of Action: Antiviral drug against CMV. Letermovir inhibits the CMV DNA terminase complex.

Metabolism: Majority (93%) excreted in feces

Indications: CMV infection and disease in adult CMVseropositive recipients of an allogeneic hematopoietic stem cell transplant (HSCT).

Dosage/Range:
Oral: 480 mg once a day between day 0 and day 28 post-transplanation (before or after engraftment). Continue through day 100 post-transplant.
   IV: 480 mg once a day between day 0 and day 28 post-transplanation (before or after engraftment). Continue through day 100 post-transplant. **This preparation should be taken only when unable to take oral preparation and transitioned to oral preparation as soon as patient is able to take oral medications.**

Drug Preparation:
Oral: Tablets come in 240-mg and 480-mg packaging,
   IV: Add one single dose vial to 250 ml IV bag of 0.9% sodium chloride injection or 5% dextrose injection.

Lab Effects/Interferences:
Monitor CBC and creatine regularly.

Special Considerations:
Amiodarone: Monitor for adverse effects when coadministered.
   Warfarin: Monitor INR when coadministered.
   Phenytoin: Monitor phenytoin concentrations when coadministered.
   Cyclosporine: When coadministered Do NOT USE repaglinide.
   Monitor glucose concentrations with coadministration of repaglinide, glyburide, or rosiglitazone
   Voriconizole: Monitor closely for reduced effectiveness—if concomitant administration is necessary.
   Rifampin: Not receoommended to coadminister.
   Pimozide: Contrainindicated due to risk of QT prolongation and torsades de pointes.
   Ergotamine: Contraindicated.
   Atorvastatin: DO not exceed atorvastin dose of 20 mg daily. When cyclosporine is co-administered DO NOT use atorvastin.

Pitavastin/simvastin: Not recommended to coadminister. When coadministered with cyclosporine use of either pitavastin or simavastin is contraindicated due to increase concentrations of pitavastin and simavastin and risk of myopathy or rhabdomyolysis.

Cyclosporine: Decrease dose to letermovir to 240 mg once daily. Monitor whole blood concentrations of cyclosporine.

Sirolimus: When coadministered with cyclospone and sirolimus refer to prescribing information for specific dosing recommendations. Monitor whole blood concentrations of sirolimus.

Omeprazole: Monitor and dose adjust if necessary.

Pantoprazole: Monitor and dose adjust if necessary.

CYP3A substrates: Refer to prescribing information for specific dosing recommendations. Pimozide and ergot alkaloids are contraindicated

Potential Toxicities/Side Effects and the Nursing Process

I.   ALTERATION IN NUTRITION, LESS THAN BODY REQUIREMENTS, related to NAUSEA/VOMITING/DIARRHEA

Defining Characteristics: Nausea/vomiting/diarrhea occurs in some patients.

Nursing Implications: Encourage patients to eat food prior to dose. Discuss antiemetic prior to the first dose and then during period of therapy. Consider antidiarrheals. Discuss with healthcare provider.

II.   ALTERATION IN ELIMINATION related to RENAL TOXICITY

Defining Characteristics: Creatinine elevations to > 1.5 mg/dL occur in approximately 17% of patients, proteinuria in 80% of patients, and decreased serum bicarbonate in $> 5\%$ of patients.

Nursing Implications: Encourage patients to increase their daily oral fluid intake to 2–3 L. Closely monitor renal function; patients who have received foscarnet are at increased risk for nephrotoxicity. Ensure that patient receives prehydration and posthydration and is able to take oral fluids. Discuss dose reductions based on alterations in renal function with physician. Check urine for protein. If positive, discuss additional hydration and rechecking of urine for blood with physician.

III.   INJURY related to HYPERSENSITIVITY

Defining Characteristics: Urticaria, angioneurotic edema, anaphylaxis may occur; also, fever, rash, arthralgias, eosinophilia, and pericarditis.

Nursing Implications: Assess drug allergy history. Assess baseline allergy history. Assess baseline skin integrity. Teach patient to report rash, pruritus. Teach patient symptomatic management of rash, pruritus. Assess for hypersensitivity reaction; if it occurs, monitor VS, discontinue drug, notify physician, and institute supportive measures.

Drug: oseltamivir phosphate (Tamiflu)

Class: Antiviral.

Mechanism of Action: Oseltamivir is an antiviral drug. Oseltamivir carboxylate is an inhibitor of influenza virus neuraminidase affecting release of viral particles.

Metabolism: Oseltamivir is readily absorbed from the gastrointestinal tract after oral administration of oseltamivir phosphate and is extensively converted predominantly by hepatic esterases to oseltamivir carboxylate. At least 75% of an oral dose reaches the systemic circulation as oseltamivir carboxylate.

Indication: Oseltamivir phosphate is an influenza neuraminidase inhibitor indicated for treatment of acute, uncomplicated influenza in patients 2 weeks of age and older who have been symptomatic for no more than 2 days; and prophylaxis of influenza in patients 1 year and older.

Contraindications:
- Most common adverse reactions:
  - Treatment studies—Nausea, vomiting.
  - Prophylaxis studies—Nausea, vomiting, diarrhea, abdominal pain.
- Patients with known serious hypersensitivity to oseltamivir.
  - Serious skin/hypersensitivity reactions such as Stevens–Johnson syndrome, toxic epidermal necrolysis, and erythema multiforme.
  - Neuropsychiatric events: Patients may be at an increased risk of confusion or abnormal behavior early in their illness. Monitor for signs of abnormal behavior.
- Live attenuated influenza vaccine intranasal:
  - Do not administer until 48 hours following cessation.
  - Do not administer oseltamivir phosphate until 2 weeks following administration of the live attenuated influenza vaccine, unless medically indicated.

Dosage/Range:
- Treatment of influenza
  - Adults and adolescents (13 years and older): 75 mg twice daily for 5 days.
- Prophylaxis of influenza
  - Adults and adolescents (13 years and older): 75 mg once daily for at least 10 days.
  - Community outbreak: 75 mg once daily for up to 6 weeks. Children dose based on weight once daily for up to 6 weeks.

CrCl (mL/min)	Treatment of Influenza	Prophylaxis of Influenza
Greater than 30–60	Reduce to 30 mg 2× daily for 5 days	Reduce to 30 mg 1× daily
Greater than 10–30	Reduce to 30 mg 1× daily for 5 days	Reduce to 30 mg 1× every other day
ESRD patients on hemodialysis	Reduce to 30 mg after every hemodialysis cycle. Treatment duration not exceed 5 days	Reduce to 30 mg after alternate hemodialysis cycles for the recommended duration of prophylaxis
ESRD patients on CAPD	Reduce to single 30-mg dose administered immediately after a dialysis exchange	Reduce to 30 mg 1× weekly immediately after dialysis exchange for the recommended duration of prophylaxis

COMPLICATIONS

Drug Preparation:
- Capsules: 30, 45, 75 mg.
- Powder for oral suspension: 360 mg oseltamivir base (constituted to a final concentration of 6 mg/mL).

Drug Administration: This is an oral and inhaled drug.

Drug Interactions:
- Clinically important drug interactions involving competition for renal tubular secretion are unlikely due to the known safety margin for most of these drugs, the elimination characteristics of oseltamivir carboxylate (glomerular filtration and anionic tubular secretion) and the excretion capacity of these pathways.
- Coadministration of probenecid results in an approximate two-fold increase in exposure to oseltamivir carboxylate due to a decrease in active anionic tubular secretion in the kidney.
- No pharmacokinetic interactions have been observed when coadministering oseltamivir with amoxicillin, acetaminophen, aspirin, cimetidine, antacids (magnesium and aluminum hydroxides and calcium carbonates), or warfarin.

Special Considerations: Due to safety margin, no dose adjustments required when coadministering with probenecid.

Potential Toxicities/Side Effects and the Nursing Process

I.   POTENTIAL FOR INJURY related to HYPERSENSITIVITY REACTION

Defining Characteristics: Urticaria, pruritus, rash (maculopapular or erythematous), fever and chills, eosinophilia, myalgia, edema, erythema, angioedema, Stevens–Johnson syndrome, and exfoliative skin reactions occur in 5% of patients. Increased risk in allergic individuals.

Nursing Implications: Assess allergy potential: if patient states "yes," determine actual response (e.g., "swollen lips = angioedema"). If angioedema, patient SHOULD NOT receive drug. Discuss other patient responses with physician to determine whether drug should be given. Assess baseline skin condition, including integrity and allergy history to drugs. Instruct patient to report rash, itching, or other skin changes. Teach patient skin care and symptomatic measures as appropriate. If skin rash develops, discuss drug discontinuance with physician. If rash progresses, drug should be discontinued, as fatal Stevens–Johnson syndrome may develop. Be prepared to treat severe acute hypersensitivity reactions with airway management, oxygen, epinephrine, corticosteroids, or antihistamines as ordered.

Drug: peramivir injection (Rapivab)

Class: Antiviral.

Mechanism of Action: Peramivir is an antiviral drug.

Metabolism: Peramivir is not significantly metabolized in humans. The elimination half-life following IV administration to healthy subjects of 600 mg as a single dose is approximately 20 hours. The major route of elimination is via the kidney. Renal clearance of unchanged peramivir accounts for approximately 90% of total clearance.

Indication: Peramivir is an influenza virus neuraminidase inhibitor indicated for the treatment of acute uncomplicated influenza in patients 18 years and older who have been symptomatic for no more than two days.

Limitations of Use:
- Efficacy based on clinical trials in which the predominant influenza virus type was influenza A; a limited number of subjects infected with influenza B virus were enrolled.
- Consider available information on influenza drug susceptibility patterns and treatment effects when deciding whether to use.
- Efficacy could not be established in patients with serious influenza requiring hospitalization.

Contraindications:
- None.

Dosage/Range:
- Administer as a single dose within 2 days of onset of influenza symptoms.
- Recommended dose is 600 mg, administered by intravenous infusion for a minimum of 15 minutes.
- Renal Impairment: Recommended dose for patients with creatinine clearance 30–49 mL/min is 200 mg and recommended dose for patients with creatinine clearance 10–29 mL/min is 100 mg.
- Hemodialysis: Administer after dialysis.
- Must be diluted prior to administration.

Drug Preparation: Use aseptic technique during the preparation. There is no preservative or bacteriostatic agent present in the solution.

- Follow the steps below to prepare a diluted solution:
  - Visually inspect for particulate matter and discoloration prior to administration.
  - Dilute appropriate dose in 0.9% or 0.45% sodium chloride, 5% dextrose, or lactated Ringer's to a maximum volume of 100 mL.
  - Administer diluted solution via intravenous infusion for 15–30 minutes.
  - Discard unused diluted solution after 24 hours.
  - Once a diluted solution has been prepared, administer immediately or store under refrigerated conditions (2–8°C or 36–46°F) for up to 24 hours.
- If refrigerated, allow the diluted solution to reach room temperature then administer immediately.

Drug Administration: This is an intravenous drug only

Drug Interactions: Live attenuated influenza vaccine (LAIV), intranasal: Avoid use of LAIV within 2 weeks before or 48 hours after administration of peramivir injection, unless medically indicated.

COMPLICATIONS

Special Considerations:
- Allergic Reactions: Serious skin/hypersensitivity reactions such as Stevens–Johnson syndrome and erythema multiforme have occurred.
- Neuropsychiatric Events: Patients with influenza may be at an increased risk of seizures, confusion, or abnormal behavior early in their illness.
- Most common adverse reaction (incidence >2%) is diarrhea.

Potential Toxicities/Side Effects and the Nursing Process

I.   POTENTIAL FOR INJURY related to HYPERSENSITIVITY REACTION

Defining Characteristics: Urticaria, pruritus, rash (maculopapular or erythematous), fever and chills, eosinophilia, myalgia, edema, erythema, angioedema, Stevens–Johnson syndrome, and exfoliative skin reactions occur in 5% of patients. Increased risk in allergic individuals.

Nursing Implications: Assess allergy potential: if patient states "yes," determine actual response (e.g., "swollen lips = angioedema"). If angioedema, patient should not receive drug. Discuss other patient responses with physician to determine whether drug should be given. Assess baseline skin condition, including integrity and allergy history to drugs. Instruct patient to report rash, itching, or other skin changes. Teach patient skin care and symptomatic measures as appropriate. If skin rash develops, discuss drug discontinuance with physician. If rash progresses, drug should be discontinued, as fatal Stevens–Johnson syndrome may develop. Be prepared to treat severe acute hypersensitivity reactions with airway management, oxygen, epinephrine, corticosteroids, or antihistamines as ordered.

Drug: valacyclovir hydrochloride (Valtrex)

Class: Antiviral (systemic).

Mechanism of Action: Drug is well-absorbed and rapidly converted to acyclovir. Drug interferes with DNA synthesis so that viral replication cannot occur. A pro-drug of acyclovir.

Metabolism: Widely distributed in body tissues and fluids including the CNS.

Indication: For treatment of viral infections in cancer patients. It is active against HSV-1, HSV-2, VZV (shingles), EBV, and CMV.

Dosage/Range:
- Herpes zoster and Bell's palsy: 1 g tid × 7 days.
- Genital herpes simplex, initial and recurrent episodes:
  - Initial episode: 1 g orally twice daily for 10 days; most effective when started within 48 hours of signs and symptoms.
  - Recurrent episode: 500 mg orally twice daily for 3 days; start within 24 hours of onset of signs and symptoms (FDA dosage).

- Recurrent episode: 1 g once daily for 5 days OR 500 mg orally twice daily for 3 days; initiate treatment preferably within 1 day of lesion onset or during preceding prodrome (guideline dosage).
- Genital herpes simplex, initial and recurrent episodes; HIV infection
  - 1 g ORALLY twice daily for 5–14 days
- Herpes labialis
  - 2 g ORALLY twice daily for 1 day; separate doses by 12 hours; start at the earliest onset of symptoms
  - 1 g ORALLY twice daily for 5–10 days

Drug Preparation:
- Available in 500-mg caplets.
- Oral, without regard to meals.

Drug Interactions:
- Cimetidine and probenecid decrease renal clearance of valacyclovir.
- Avoid foscarnet.

Lab Effects/Interference:
- None known.

Special Considerations:
- Dose-reduce for renal impairment:

Creatinine Clearance (cc/min) Zoster	Dose
≥ 50	Usual dose
30–49	1 g q 12 h
10–29	1 g q 24 h
< 10	500 mg q 24 h

Renal impairment, genital herpes: (initial episode) CrCl 30 mL/min or greater, usual dose; CrCl 10 to 29 mL/min, 1 g every 24 hours; CrCl less than 10 mL/min, 0.5 g every 24 hours

- Treatment should be started within 48 hours of rash onset.
- AVOID DRUG IN IMMUNOCOMPROMISED PATIENTS, as patients with advanced HIV infection, and those undergoing bone marrow and renal transplants, have developed thrombotic thrombocytopenic purpura/hemolytic uremic syndrome (TTP/HUS).

Potential Toxicities/Side Effects and the Nursing Process

I.   ALTERATION IN COMFORT related to HEADACHE, NAUSEA

Defining Characteristics: Headache occurred in approximately 22% of patients. Nausea occurred in 12% of patients.

Nursing Implications: Teach patient that side effects may occur and are usually mild. Patient should report headache that does not resolve with acetaminophen or nausea that does not resolve by diet modification.

COMPLICATIONS

Drug: valganciclovir hydrochloride (Valcyte)

Class: Antiviral (systemic).

Mechanism of Action: Valganciclovir is an antiviral drug. Interferes with DNA synthesis so that viral replication cannot occur. Valganciclovir is a cytomegalovirus (CMV) nucleoside analogue DNA polymerase inhibitor. Valganciclovir is metabolized to ganciclovir. There are pediatric indications for use also; see package insert for the specific pediatric indications.

Metabolism: Appears to be widely distributed, concentrates in kidneys, and is well-distributed to the eyes. Crosses BBB. Drug crosses placenta and is excreted in breastmilk in animals. Excreted unchanged in urine. The bioavailability of ganciclovir from valganciclovir is significantly higher than from ganciclovir capsules. Valganciclovir tablets cannot be substituted for ganciclovir capsules on a one-to-one basis.

Indication: Active against CMV retinitis in patients with acquired immunodeficiency syndrome (AIDS) and prevention of CMV disease in kidney, heart, or kidney–pancreas transplant in adults. It is also active against CMV infections, especially in the retina.

Contraindications:
- Valganciclovir is not indicated for use in either adult or pediatric liver transplant patients.
- The safety and efficacy of valganciclovir has not been established for:
  - Prevention of CMV disease in solid organ transplants other than those indicated and prevention of CMV disease in pediatric solid organ transplant patients less than 4 months of age.
  - Treatment of congenital CMV disease.

Dosage/Range:

Adult:
- Tablets: 450 mg and tablets should be taken with food.
- Oral solution: 50 mg/mL and must be prepared by the pharmacist prior to dispensing to the patient.

Drug Preparation:
- Drug is CARCINOGENIC, TERATOGENIC, IMPAIRS FERTILITY, and is TOXIC to the blood forming organs; use chemotherapy handling precautions (see *Appendix 1*) when preparing and administering ganciclovir.
- Valganciclovir tablets should not be broken or crushed.
- Valganciclovir for oral solution and tablets cannot be substituted for ganciclovir capsules on a one-to-one basis.
- Adult patients should use valganciclovir tablets, not valganciclovir for oral solution.
- Administer only if ANC is > 500 cells/mm^3 and platelet count > 25,000/mm^3.
- Add 10 mL of sterile water for injection to 500-mg vial. Further dilute dose in 50–250 mL of IV fluid and infuse over at least 1 hour.

Drug Administration:
- AIDS—Cytomegaloviral retinitis.
- Induction, 900 mg ORALLY twice daily for 14–21 days, followed by 900 mg ORALLY once daily for chronic maintenance therapy; for immediate sight-threatening lesions, use in combination with ganciclovir intraocular implant (guideline dosing).
- Induction, 900 mg ORALLY twice daily for 21 days, followed by maintenance, 900 mg ORALLY once daily (manufacturer dosing).
- Cytomegalovirus infection, in high-risk kidney, heart, or kidney-pancreas transplant patients; prophylaxis.
- Tablets, 900 mg ORALLY once a day with food; begin therapy within 10 days of transplantation, continue through day 100 posttransplantation in heart or kidney–pancreas transplant patients, and through day 200 posttransplantation in kidney transplant patients.
- Oral solution is not recommended in adults.
- Dose modification for renal impairment:

CrCl (mL/min)	Induction Dosage	Maintenance Dosage
60 or greater	Usual dose	Usual dose
40–59	450 mg 2× daily	450 mg 1× daily
25–39	450 mg 1× daily	450 mg × 2 days
10–24	450 mg × 2 days	450 mg 2× weekly
Less than 10	Not recommended	Not recommended

- Hemodialysis: not recommended.

Drug Interactions:
- Zidovudine: increased hematologic toxicity (neutropenia, anemia); do not use together if possible. Monitor with frequent tests of WBC counts with differential and hemoglobin levels.
- Didanosine: may increase didanosine concentrations. Monitor for didanosine (ddI) toxicity.
- Probenecid: may increase ganciclovir serum levels. Monitor closely for ganciclovir toxicity; decrease dose as needed.
- Mycophenolate mofetil (MMF): may increase ganciclovir concentrations and levels of MMF metabolites in patients with renal impairment. Monitor for ganciclovir and MMF toxicity.
- Tacrolimus—nephrotoxicity.

Special Considerations:
- Hypersensitivity to valganciclovir or ganciclovir.
- Most common adverse events and laboratory abnormalities (reported in at least one indication by > 20% of patients) are diarrhea, pyrexia, nausea, tremor, neutropenia, graft rejection, thrombocytopenia, and vomiting.
- Do not use in pregnancy.
- Patient should be well-hydrated.
- Drug is mutagenic; patient should use barrier contraceptive for 90 days.
- Monitor blood counts frequently.
- Black Box Warning:
  - WARNING: HEMATOLOGIC TOXICITY, CARCINOGENICITY, TERATOGENICITY, AND IMPAIRMENT OF FERTILITY

- Clinical toxicity of valganciclovir, which is metabolized to ganciclovir, includes granulocytopenia, anemia, and thrombocytopenia.
- In animal studies, ganciclovir was carcinogenic, teratogenic, and caused aspermatogenesis.

Potential Toxicities/Side Effects and the Nursing Process

I.   INFECTION, BLEEDING related to BONE MARROW DEPRESSION

Defining Characteristics: Severe leukopenia, neutropenia, anemia, thrombocytopenia, pancytopenia, bone marrow aplasia, and aplastic anemia have been reported in patients treated with valganciclovir or ganciclovir. Valganciclovir should not be administered if the ANC is less than 500 cells/μL, the platelet count is less than 25,000/μL, or the hemoglobin is less than 8 g/dL. Valganciclovir should also be used with caution in patients with preexisting cytopenias, or who have received or who are receiving myelosuppressive drugs or irradiation.

Nursing Implications: Assess baseline WBC, ANC, and platelet count; monitor throughout therapy (every other day initially, then 3 times/week). Hold valganciclovir if ANC < 500/mm³, platelet count < 25,000/mm³. Assess for signs/symptoms of infection or bleeding; instruct patient in signs/symptoms of infection and bleeding, and instruct to report these immediately. Teach patient self-care measures to minimize risk of infection, bleeding, including avoidance of OTC aspirin-containing medicines. Administer or teach patient to self-administer prescribed G-CSF or GM-CSF. Assess Hgb/HCT and signs/symptoms of fatigue. Instruct patient to alternate rest and activity periods.

II.   ALTERATION IN NUTRITION, LESS THAN BODY REQUIREMENTS, related to GI SIDE EFFECTS

Defining Characteristics: Nausea, vomiting, diarrhea, and anorexia may occur in 2% of patients. Elevated LFTs may occur due to drug, but may be difficult to distinguish from CMV infection of liver or biliary tree.

Nursing Implications: Assess baseline nutrition, liver function, and monitor during therapy. Instruct patient to report GI side effects. Administer or teach patient to self-administer prescribed antiemetic or antidiarrheal medications. Encourage adequate oral or IV hydration. Notify physician of abnormal LFTs. If anorexia occurs, encourage favorite foods and small, frequent meals as tolerated.

III.   ALTERATION IN URINARY ELIMINATION related to RENAL TOXICITY

Defining Characteristics: 2% of patients have increased serum BUN, creatinine, hematuria. Increased risk of acute renal failure may occur in elderly patients with or without reduced renal function, patients who have concomitant nepthrotoxic drugs, or inadequately hydrated patients.

Nursing Implications: Ensure adequate hydration with urinary output prior to drug administration. Dose should be reduced in patients with decreased renal function. Use with caution in elderly patients or those taking nephrotoxic drugs, reduce dosage in patients with renal impairment, and monitor renal function.

IV. ALTERATION IN CARDIAC OUTPUT related to CHANGES IN BP

Defining Characteristics: Rarely, hypotension, or hypertension, arrhythmia, myocardial infarction, or arrest occurs.

Nursing Implications: Assess baseline VS and monitor throughout treatment. Notify physician of any changes from baseline.

V. ALTERATION IN SEXUALITY/REPRODUCTIVE PATTERNS related to REPRODUCTIVE HAZARD

Defining Characteristics: Drug is carcinogenic, mutagenic, and teratogenic; may produce temporary or permanent inhibition of spermatogenesis and infertility in males. It is unknown whether drug crosses placenta and is excreted in breastmilk.

Nursing Implications: Assess sexuality/reproductive patterns. Teach patient and partner about reproductive hazards; offer contraceptive counseling or refer for counseling, as barrier contraceptive should be used by patient.

Drug: zanamivir (Relenza)

Class: Antiviral.

Mechanism of Action: Zanamivir is an antiviral drug.

Metabolism: Zanamivir is renally excreted as unchanged drug. No metabolites have been detected in humans. The serum half-life of zanamivir following administration by oral inhalation ranges from 2.5 to 5.1 hours. It is excreted unchanged in the urine with excretion of a single dose completed within 24 hours. Total clearance ranges from 2.5 to 10.9 L/h. Unabsorbed drug is excreted in the feces.

Indication: Zanamivir is an influenza neuraminidase inhibitor indicated for:
• Treatment of influenza in patients aged 7 years and older who have been symptomatic for no more than 2 days.
• Prophylaxis of influenza in patients aged 5 years and older.
• Limitations: not recommended for treatment or prophylaxis of influenza in individuals with underlying airways disease.
• Not proven effective for treatment in individuals with:
  • Underlying airways disease.
  • Prophylaxis in nursing home residents.
  • Not a substitute for annual influenza vaccination.

Contraindications:
• Do not use in patients with history of allergic reaction to any ingredient of zanamivir including milk proteins.

COMPLICATIONS

Dosage/Range:

Indication	Dose
Treatment of Influenza	10 mg 2× daily for 5 days
Prophylaxis:	
Household Setting	10 mg 2× daily for 10 days
Community Outbreaks	10 mg 2× daily for 28 days

Drug Preparation: Blister for oral inhalation: 5 mg. Four 5-mg blisters of powder on a ROTADISK for oral inhalation via DISKHALER. Packaged in carton containing 5 ROTA-DISKs (total of 10 doses) and 1 DISKHALER inhalation device.

Drug Administration: This is an oral and inhaled drug.

Drug Interactions: Zanamivir is not a substrate nor does it affect cytochrome P450 (CYP) isoenzymes (CYP1A1/2, 2A6, 2C9, 2C18, 2D6, 2E1, and 3A4) in human liver microsomes. No clinically significant pharmacokinetic drug interactions are predicted based on data from in vitro studies.

Special Considerations:

• Allergic Reactions: Bronchospasm: Serious, sometimes fatal, cases have occurred. Not recommended in individuals with underlying airways disease.
• Neuropsychiatric Events: Patients with influenza, particularly pediatric patients, may be at an increased risk of seizures, confusion, or abnormal behavior early in their illness.
• High-risk: Underlying medical conditions as safety and effectiveness have not been demonstrated in these patients.

Potential Toxicities/Side Effects and the Nursing Process

I.   POTENTIAL FOR INJURY related to HYPERSENSITIVITY REACTION

Defining Characteristics: Urticaria, pruritus, rash (maculopapular or erythematous), fever and chills, eosinophilia, myalgia, edema, erythema, angioedema, Stevens–Johnson syndrome, and exfoliative skin reactions occur in 5% of patients. Increased risk in allergic individuals.

Nursing Implications: Assess allergy potential: if patient states "yes," determine actual response (e.g., "swollen lips = angioedema"). If angioedema, patient should not receive drug. Discuss other patient responses with physician to determine whether drug should be given. Assess baseline skin condition, including integrity and allergy history to drugs. Instruct patient to report rash, itching, or other skin changes. Teach patient skin care and symptomatic measures as appropriate. If skin rash develops, discuss drug discontinuance with physician. If rash progresses, drug should be discontinued, as fatal Stevens–Johnson syndrome may develop. Be prepared to treat severe acute hypersensitivity reactions with airway management, oxygen, epinephrine, corticosteroids, or antihistamines as ordered.

Chapter *12*
Constipation

Constipation may be defined differently by patients and providers, but practically speaking it is decreased frequency of defecation that is difficult. Constipation is multifactorial, and can be related to diet and nutrition, changes in routine, metabolic and endocrine conditions, or problems in the colon and rectum, to name a few. Drugs can frequently cause constipation, such as opioids, anticholinergics (e.g., H_1 antihistamines), antihypertensives, the serotonin (5-HT$_3$) receptor antagonist antiemetics (e.g., ondansetron), chemotherapeutic drugs such as vincristine, molecular targeted therapy (e.g., axitinib, crizotinib), and immunotherapy agents such as thalidomide. Levy (1992) reports five causes of constipation in cancer patients:

- Disease itself: primary bowel cancers, paraneoplastic autonomic neuropathy.
- Disease sequelae: dehydration, paralysis, immobility, alterations in bowel elimination patterns.
- Prior history of laxative abuse, hemorrhoids/anal fissures, other diseases.
- Cancer therapy: chemotherapy (vinca alkaloids, e.g., vincristine, vinblastine); bowel surgery.
- Medications used to manage symptoms: opioids, antihistamines, tricyclic antidepressants, aluminum antacids.

Complications of constipation can be severe (i.e., bowel perforation) and extremely painful. Psychologically, it can compromise quality of life (Sanchez & Bercik, 2011). Nurses play an enormous role in preventing morbidity from constipation in patients with cancer.

The National Comprehensive Cancer Network (NCCN) Palliative Care guidelines suggest that management includes (1) identifying the cause of constipation, and (2) assess for impaction and obstruction. If the patient is unobstructed then it is important to proceed with laxative and prokinetic therapy. Clinically, the nurse assesses the patient's previous and current nutrition and elimination patterns, along with assessment of probable etiology of constipation. Once constipation is relieved, the nurse teaches the patient/family about constipation management and prevention. Teaching should include dietary modifications to include high-fiber intake (fruits, vegetables, or nutritional supplements high in fiber); fluid intake of 3 L/day; and moderate exercise as tolerated. Patients receiving drugs (i.e., opioids) that are likely to be constipating should ALWAYS receive a bowel regimen to prevent constipation along with it. Combinations of opioid antagonists can help alleviate opioid-induced constipation, such as methylnaltrexone (Relistor). Available types of laxatives include the following types:

- *Bulk-forming laxatives* cause the stool to retain water, and thus increase peristalsis (fiber, bran, psyllium, methylcellulose).
- *Lubricants* coat and soften the stool so it can move more smoothly through the intestines (mineral oil).

- *Saline laxatives* pull water into the gut and into the stool, increasing peristalsis (magnesium citrate, sodium biphosphate, magnesium hydroxide).
- *Osmotic laxatives* work through colonic bacteria that metabolize osmotic laxatives causing increased osmotic pressure gradient, pulling water into the gut and then into the stool, thus increasing peristalsis (lactulose, sorbitol, polyethylene glycol).
- *Detergent laxatives* reduce surface tension of the colonic cells, so water and fats enter the stool; in addition, electrolyte and water absorption is decreased (docusate salts).
- *Stimulant laxatives* irritate the gut, increasing gut motility (bisacodyl).
- *Anthraquinone laxatives* are activated by gut bacteria degradation (senna, casanthrol, cascara).
- *Suppositories* cause local irritation and stimulate rectal emptying (glycerin, bisacodyl, senna).

Other approaches to opioid-induced constipation prevention and management include the use of opioid antagonists, such as methylnaltrexone (Relistor) and naloxegol (Movantik).

References

AstraZeneca Pharmaceuticals, LP. Movantik (naloxegol) [package insert]. Wilmington, DE. February 2018.

Levy MH. Constipation and Diarrhea in Cancer Patients, Part I. *Prim Care Center* 1992; 12(4):11–18.

National Comprehensive Cancer Network (NCCN). *Palliative Care* v.2, 2019. Available at https://www .nccn.org/professionals/physician_gls/pdf/palliative.pdf. Accessed May 31, 2019.

Salix Pharmaceuticals. Relistor (methylnaltrexone bromide) [package insert]. Bridgewater, NJ. November 2018.

Sanchez MIP, Bercik P. Epidemiology and Burden of Chronic Constipation. *Canadian J of Gastroenterol* 2011; 25(suppl B):11B–15B.

Drug: bisacodyl (Dulcolax)

Class: Stimulant laxative.

Mechanism of Action: Stimulates/irritates smooth muscle of intestines, increasing peristalsis; increases fluid accumulation in colon and small intestines. Indicated for relief of constipation and bowel preparation prior to bowel surgery.

Metabolism: Minimal oral absorption. Evacuation occurs in 6–10 hours when taken orally, or within 15 minutes to 1 hour when administered rectally.

Indication: For relief of constipation, preparation for diagnostic procedures (e.g., colonoscopy), and in preoperative and postoperative treatment when constipation occurs.

Dosage/Range:

Adult:
- Oral: 5–15 mg at bedtime or early morning. Bowel preparation may use up to 30 mg.
- Suppository: 10 mg PR.

Drug Preparation:
• Administer oral tablet > 1 hour after antacids or milk.
• Insert suppository as high as possible against wall of rectum.

Drug Interactions:
• None.

Lab Effects/Interference:
• None known.

Special Considerations:
• Contraindicated in patients with signs/symptoms of acute abdomen (nausea, vomiting, abdominal pain), intestinal obstruction, fecal impaction, or ulcerative bowel lesions.

Potential Toxicities/Side Effects and the Nursing Process

I.   ALTERATIONS IN BOWEL ELIMINATION related to CHRONIC USE

Defining Characteristics: Removes defecation reflexes when used chronically (laxative dependence). Narcotic analgesics and vinca alkaloid chemotherapy may predispose to constipation.

Nursing Implications: Assess baseline elimination pattern. Teach patient how to self-administer laxative. Encourage patient to normalize bowel habits through adequate fluid intake (2–3 L/day), diet high in fiber and bulk (bran, cereals, fruits, and vegetables), and exercise as tolerated. Teach patient bowel regimen when on narcotics or vinca alkaloids to promote regular evacuation.

II.   ALTERATION IN NUTRITION, LESS THAN BODY REQUIREMENTS, related to GI SIDE EFFECTS

Defining Characteristics: Constipation or drug may cause nausea, vomiting, abdominal pain; rectal suppository may cause burning in rectum as it is absorbed.

Nursing Implications: Assess comfort level and GI distress related to constipation. Encourage patient to drink cold fluids or ginger ale as tolerated. Encourage patient to try resting in different positions; warm packs may decrease abdominal pain. Teach patient to expect burning sensation with suppository use; reassure that it will resolve in 5–10 minutes.

III.   ALTERATION IN FLUID AND ELECTROLYTE BALANCE related to LAXATIVE ABUSE

Defining Characteristics: Diarrhea resulting from laxative abuse can deplete fluid volume, nutrients, and electrolytes.

Nursing Implications: Teach patient regular bowel regimen when receiving constipating drugs (narcotics, vinca alkaloids). Teach patient to replace lost fluids and electrolytes (encourage chicken soup, sports drink).

COMPLICATIONS

Drug: docusate calcium, docusate potassium, docusate sodium (Dioctyl Calcium Sulfosuccinate, Dioctyl Potassium Sulfosuccinate, Dioctyl Sodium Sulfosuccinate, Colace, Diocto-K, Diosuccin, DOK-250, Doxinate, Duosol, Laxinate 100, Regulax SS, Stulex)

Class: Stool softener.

Mechanism of Action: The calcium, sodium, and potassium salts of docusate soften stool by decreasing surface tension, emulsification, and wetting action, thus increasing stool absorption of water in the bowel.

Metabolism: Appears to be absorbed somewhat in the duodenum and jejunum, and excreted in bile. Stool softening occurs in 1–3 days.

Indication: To soften stool.

Dosage/Range:

Adult:
• Oral: 50–360 mg/day, in single or divided doses, depending on stool-softening response.

Drug Preparation:
• Oral: store gelatin capsule in tight container; store syrup in light-resistant containers.
• Rectal: according to manufacturer's package insert.

Drug Interactions:
• Mineral oil: increased mineral oil absorption; AVOID CONCURRENT USE.

Lab Effects/Interference:
• None known.

Special Considerations:
• Useful in prevention of straining-at-stool in patients receiving narcotics; when combined with other agents/laxatives, prevents constipation in these patients.
• Does not increase intestinal peristalsis; stop drug if severe abdominal cramping occurs.
• Is effective only in prevention of constipation, not in treating constipation.

Potential Toxicities/Side Effects and the Nursing Process

I. KNOWLEDGE DEFICIT related to BOWEL ELIMINATION

Defining Characteristics: Oncology patients who are receiving narcotic analgesics, vinca alkaloid chemotherapy (vincristine, vinblastine, vindesine), or who are dehydrated or hypercalcemic are at increased risk of constipation.

Nursing Implications: Assess baseline elimination pattern. Teach patient need for bowel movement at least every other day, depending on usual pattern. Teach patient importance of adequate fluid intake (2–3 L/day), diet high in fiber and bulk (bran, cereals, fruits, vegetables, and supplements with fiber), and exercise as tolerated. Teach self-administration of stool softeners and prescribed laxatives.

Drug: glycerin suppository (Fleet Babylax, Sani-Supp)

Class: Hyperosmotic laxative.

Mechanism of Action: Local irritant, with hyperosmotic action, drawing water from tissues into feces and stimulating fecal evacuation within 15–30 minutes.

Metabolism: Poorly absorbed from rectum.

Indication: To relieve constipation.

Dosage/Range:

Adult:
• Rectal suppository: 2–3 g PR.
• Enema: 5–15 mL PR.

Drug Preparation:
• Rectal administration must be retained for 15 minutes.

Drug Interactions:
• None.

Lab Effects/Interference:
• None known.

Special Considerations:
• Contraindicated in patients with undiagnosed abdominal pain, intestinal obstruction.

Potential Toxicities/Side Effects and the Nursing Process

I.   ALTERATIONS IN BOWEL ELIMINATION related to CHRONIC USE

Defining Characteristics: Removes defecation reflexes when used chronically (laxative dependence). Narcotic analgesics and vinca alkaloid chemotherapy may predispose to constipation.

Nursing Implications: Assess baseline elimination pattern. Teach patient how to self-administer laxative. Encourage patient to normalize bowel habits through adequate fluid intake (2–3 L/day), diet high in fiber and bulk (bran, cereals, fruits, and vegetables), and exercise as tolerated. Teach patient bowel regimen when on narcotics or vinca alkaloids to promote regular evacuation.

COMPLICATIONS

II. ALTERATION IN FLUID AND ELECTROLYTE BALANCE related to LAXATIVE ABUSE

Defining Characteristics: Diarrhea resulting from laxative abuse can deplete fluid volume, nutrients, and electrolytes.

Nursing Implications: Teach patient regular bowel regimen when receiving constipating drugs (narcotics, vinca alkaloids). Teach patient to replace lost fluids and electrolytes (encourage chicken soup, sports drink).

III. ALTERATION IN COMFORT related to CRAMPING PAIN, RECTAL IRRITATION, OR DISCOMFORT

Defining Characteristics: Cramping pain, rectal irritation, and inflammation or discomfort may occur.

Nursing Implications: Teach patient this may occur. If discomfort is not self-limited, suggest sitz bath, warm or cold packs, and position changes.

Drug: magnesium citrate

Class: Saline laxative.

Mechanism of Action: Draws water into small intestinal lumen, stimulating peristalsis and evacuation in 3–6 hours.

Metabolism: 15–30% absorbed, excreted in urine.

Indication: For relief of occasional constipation (generally produces bowel movement in 1/2–6 hours).

Dosage/Range:

Adult:
• Oral: 11–25 g (5–10 oz or 150–300 mL)/day as single or divided dose at bedtime.

Drug Preparation:
• Refrigerate and serve with ice. Taste can be masked by adding small amount of juice.

Drug Interactions:
• None.

Lab Effects/Interference:
• None known.

Special Considerations:
• Contraindicated in patients with signs/symptoms of acute abdomen (nausea, vomiting, abdominal pain), intestinal obstruction, fecal impaction, or ulcerative bowel lesions.
• Contraindicated in patients with rectal fissures, myocardial infarction, renal disease.

Potential Toxicities/Side Effects and the Nursing Process

I.   ALTERATIONS IN BOWEL ELIMINATION related to CHRONIC USE

Defining Characteristics: Removes defecation reflexes when used chronically (laxative dependence). Narcotic analgesics and vinca alkaloid chemotherapy may predispose to constipation.

Nursing Implications: Assess baseline elimination pattern. Teach patient how to self-administer laxative. Encourage patient to normalize bowel habits through adequate fluid intake (2–3 L/day), diet high in fiber and bulk (bran, cereals, fruits, and vegetables), and exercise as tolerated. Teach patient bowel regimen when on narcotics or vinca alkaloids to promote regular evacuation.

II.   ALTERATION IN NUTRITION, LESS THAN BODY REQUIREMENTS, related to GI SIDE EFFECTS

Defining Characteristics: Constipation or drug may cause nausea and abdominal pain.

Nursing Implications: Assess comfort level and GI distress related to constipation. Encourage patient to drink cold fluids or ginger ale as tolerated. Encourage patient to try resting in different positions; warm packs may decrease abdominal pain.

III.   ALTERATION IN FLUID AND ELECTROLYTE BALANCE related to LAXATIVE ABUSE

Defining Characteristics: Diarrhea resulting from laxative abuse can deplete fluid volume, nutrients, and electrolytes.

Nursing Implications: Teach patient regular bowel regimen when receiving constipating drugs (narcotics, vinca alkaloids). Teach patient to replace lost fluids and electrolytes (encourage chicken soup, sports drink).

COMPLICATIONS

Drug: methylcellulose (Citrucel)

Class: Bulk-producing laxative.

Mechanism of Action: Absorbs water; bulk expansion stimulates peristalsis and evacuation in 12–24 hours. May also be used to slow diarrhea.

Metabolism: Not absorbed by GI tract.

Indication: For relief of constipation.

Dosage/Range:

Adult:
• Oral: up to 6 g/day PO in 2–3 divided doses.

Drug Preparation:
- Administer each dose with at least 250 mL of water or juice.

Drug Interactions:
- None.

Lab Effects/Interference:
- None known.

Special Considerations:
- Safest and most physiologically normal laxative.

Potential Toxicities/Side Effects and the Nursing Process

I.   ALTERATIONS IN BOWEL ELIMINATION related to CHRONIC USE

Defining Characteristics: Removes defecation reflexes when used chronically (laxative dependence). Narcotic analgesics and vinca alkaloid chemotherapy may predispose to constipation.

Nursing Implications: Assess baseline elimination pattern. Teach patient how to self-administer laxative. Encourage patient to normalize bowel habits through adequate fluid intake (2–3 L/day), diet high in fiber and bulk (bran, cereals, fruits, and vegetables), and exercise as tolerated. Teach patient bowel regimen when on narcotics or vinca alkaloids to promote regular evacuation.

II.   ALTERATION IN NUTRITION, LESS THAN BODY REQUIREMENTS, related to GI SIDE EFFECTS

Defining Characteristics: Constipation or drug may cause nausea, vomiting, cramps.

Nursing Implications: Assess comfort level and GI distress related to constipation. Encourage patient to drink cold fluids or ginger ale as tolerated. Encourage patient to try resting in different positions; warm packs may decrease abdominal pain. Teach patient laxative effect may take 12–24 hours, and assess need for other cathartic(s).

Drug: methylnaltrexone bromide (Relistor)

Class: Selective, peripherally acting opioid antagonist.

Mechanism of Action: Mu opioid antagonist that competes with opioid analgesics for opioid receptors in the periphery, such as in the gut, but not in the CNS, as it is unable to cross the blood–brain barrier. Thus, it does not interfere with opioid pain relief, which is centrally mediated. Drug inhibits opioid-induced delayed intestinal transit time.

Metabolism: Absorbed rapidly with peak serum level in 30 minutes. Drug is metabolized in the liver and is excreted by the kidneys (about 50%) and in the feces; 85% of the drug is excreted intact. The terminal half-life is 8 hours.

Indication: For treatment of (1) opioid-induced constipation in adult patients with chronic noncancer pain, including patients with chronic pain related to prior cancer or its treatment who do not require frequent (e.g., weekly) opioid dose escalation; (2) opioid-induced constipation in patients with advanced illness or pain caused by cancer who require opioid dose escalation for palliative care.

Limitation of use: treatment beyond 4 months has not been studied.

Contraindication: Patients with known or suspected mechanical GI obstruction or at risk for recurrent obstruction.

Dosage Range Available as tablets or subcutaneous injection:
• Methylnaltrexone bromide SQ: Prefilled syringes contain 8 mg or 12 mg doses; use the vial for other dosage amounts.
  Opioid-induced constipation in patients with chronic noncancer pain.
    • Methylnaltrexone bromide tablets: 450 mg PO once daily in the morning.
    • Methylnaltrexone bromide 12 mg SQ once daily.
  Opioid-induced constipation in adult patients with advanced illness
    • Weight <38 kg: 0.15 mg/kg SQ every other day (calculate injection volume by multiplying patient weight in kg by 0.0075 and then rounding to the nearest 0.1 mL).
    • 38–62 kg [84–136 lbs]: 8 mg SQ every other day (volume 0.4 mL) 62 kg to 114 kg [136–251 lbs)]: 12 mg SQ every other day (volume 0.6 mL)
    • >114 kg: 0.15 mg/kg SQ every other day (calculate injection volume by multiplying weight in kg by 0.0075, and round up the volume to the nearest 0.1 mL).
    • If needed more frequently than every other day, maximum frequency is once every 24 hours.
• ***Renal Impairment****:* Moderate or severe renal impairment: CrCl < 60 mL/min as estimated by Cockcroft-Gault.
  Chronic noncancer pain:
    • Methylnaltrexone bromide tablets: 150 mg PO once daily in the morning.
    • Methylnaltrexone bromide injection: 6 mg SQ once daily (use vial).
  Adult patients with advanced illness:
    • Weight < 38 kg: 0.075 mg/kg SQ once every other day (calculate injection volume by multiplying weight in kg by 0.00375 and round up the volume to the nearest 0.1 mL).
    • 38 kg to < 62 kg: 4 mg SQ once every other day (volume 0.2 mL).
    • 62–114 kg: 6 mg SQ once every other day (volume 0.3 mL).
    • >114 kg: 0.075 mg/kg SQ once every other day (calculate injection volume by multiplying weight in kg by 0.00375 and round up the volume to the nearest 0.1 mL).
• ***Hepatic Impairment (severe) [Child-Pugh Class B or C]***
  Chronic noncancer pain (PO):
    • Methylnaltrexone bromide tablets: 150 mg PO once daily in the morning.

COMPLICATIONS

Chronic noncancer pain (SQ):
- Weight < 38 kg: 0.075 mg/kg SQ once every day (calculate injection volume by multiplying weight in kg by 0.00375 and round up the volume to the nearest 0.1 mL).
- 38 kg to < 62 kg: 4 mg SQ once every day (volume 0.2 mL).
- 62–114 kg: 6 mg SQ once every day (volume 0.3 mL).
- >114 kg: 0.075 mg/kg SQ once every day (calculate injection volume by multiplying weight in kg by 0.00375 and round up the volume to the nearest 0.1 mL).

- If severe or persistent diarrhea occurs during treatment, advise patients to discontinue therapy and contact their physician.
- Use cautiously in patients with known or suspected lesions of GI tract, as drug may rarely cause GI perforation.
- Drug is contraindicated in patients with known or suspected mechanical GI obstruction.
- Safety and efficacy of drug in pediatric patients has not been established.

Drug Preparation:
- Drug is available as tablets or injection.
  Tablets: available as 150 mg methylnaltrexone bromide.
  Injection
  - Single-dose vials containing 12 mg in 0.6 mL for subcutaneous administration, **for use** with a 27-gauge × 1/2-inch needle and 1-mL syringe.
  - Single-use **prefilled syringe** containing (1) 8 mg in 0.4-mL solution for subcutaneous administration, with a 29-gauge × 1/2-inch fixed needle and a needle guard, and (2) 12 mg in 0.6-mL solution for subcutaneous administration with a 29-gauge × 1/2-inch fixed needle and needle guard. Select prefilled syringe for exact dose.
- Once drawn up, if not used right away, may be stored at ambient room temperature for 24 hours.
- Store vial at controlled room temperature and protect from light.
- Do not remove prefilled syringe from tray until ready to use.
- Inspect solution for particulate matter or discoloration and if found, do not use. Color should be colorless to pale yellow.

Drug Administration:
- Teach patient to be near a toilet once administered.
- Discontinue drug if opioid analgesic medication discontinued.
- Opioid-induced constipation in **chronic, noncancer pain**: (1) discontinue maintenance laxative therapy before starting methylnaltrexone bromide; patient may resume after taking methylnaltrexone bromide for 3 days if suboptimal response; (2) have patient near bathroom or commode after injection; (3) patients receiving opioids for < 4 weeks may be less responsive; (4) re-evaluate need for methylnaltrexone bromide when opioid regimen changed to avoid adverse reactions; (5) teach patient to take tablets with water on an empty stomach at least 30 minutes before the first meal of the day.
- Subcutaneous injection (8-mg dose is 0.4 mL and 12-mg dose is 0.6 mL) in upper arm, abdomen, or thigh. Rotate injection sites.

Drug Interactions:
- Weak inhibitor of cytochrome P450 isozyme CYP2D6 activity, but did not interact with dextromethorphan.

Special Considerations:
- Approved only for adult use. Drug has not been studied in patients with peritoneal catheters.
- Most common side effects in patients with opioid induced constipation from:
  - Chronic noncancer pain: (1) tablets (>/=2%): abdominal pain, diarrhea, headache, abdominal distension, vomiting, hyperhidrosis (excessive sweating), anxiety, muscle spasms, rhinorrhea, and chills; (2) injection (>/=1%): abdominal pain, nausea, diarrhea, hyperhidrosis, hot flush, tremor, chills.
  - Advanced illness: injection (>//= 5%): abdominal pain, flatulence, nausea, dizziness, diarrhea.
- Postmarketing reports include cramping, perforation, vomiting, diaphoresis, flushing, malaise, pain.
- No difference in efficacy or safety profile in older patients.
- Warnings and Precautions:
  - *GI perforation* has been reported. Use drug cautiously in patients with known or suspected lesions of the GI tract, e.g. diverticular disease, Crohn's disease. Teach patients to notify provider right away if they develop severe, persistent, or worsening abdominal symptoms. Discontinue drug if this occurs and implement appropriate intervention.
  - *Severe or persistent diarrhea*; discontinue therapy and discuss with physician.
  - *Opioid withdrawal* has occurred characterized by hyperhidrosis, chills, diarrhea, abdominal pain, anxiety, and yawning. Patients with disruption in blood–brain barrier are at risk for withdrawal symptoms. Assess adequacy of analgesia as well as relief of constipation.
  - Pregnancy: may precipitate opioid withdrawal in the fetus.
  - Breastfeeding not recommended.
  - Thirty percent of patients have laxation within 30 minutes of drug administration, and 48–62% have laxation within 4 hours of first dose.

Potential Toxicities/Side Effects and the Nursing Process

I.   ALTERATION IN NUTRITION, POTENTIAL, related to GI SIDE EFFECTS

Defining Characteristics: Drug may cause nausea (11.5%), abdominal pain (28.5%), flatulence (13.3%), and diarrhea (5.5%).

Nursing Implications: Assess comfort level and GI distress related to constipation. Encourage patient to drink cold fluids or ginger ale as tolerated. Encourage patient to try resting in different positions; warm packs may decrease abdominal pain. Teach patient to call nurse or physician if abdominal pain, nausea, or vomiting become more severe or if new symptoms develop. If patient develops persistent or severe diarrhea, stop drug and discuss with physician.

COMPLICATIONS

Drug: mineral oil (Fleet Mineral Oil)

Class: Lubricant laxative.

Mechanism of Action: Lubricates intestine, preventing fecal fluid from being absorbed in colon; water retention distends colon, stimulating peristalsis and evacuation in 6–8 hours.

Metabolism: Minimal GI absorption occurs following oral or rectal administration.

Indication: For relief of constipation.

Dosage/Range:

Adult:
• Oral: 15–45 mL PO in single or divided doses.
• Rectal enemas: 120 mL PR as a single dose.

Drug Preparation:
• Administer plain mineral oil at bedtime on an empty stomach.
• Administer mineral oil emulsion with food if desired at bedtime.
• May mix with juice to mask taste.

Drug Interactions:
• Docusate salts: increase mineral oil absorption; DO NOT ADMINISTER CONCURRENTLY.
• Fat-soluble vitamins: decrease absorption with chronic mineral oil administration.

Lab Effects/Interference:
• Decreased fat-soluble vitamins (e.g., vitamins A, D, E, K) with chronic drug administration.

Special Considerations:
• Contraindicated in patients with signs/symptoms of acute abdomen (nausea, vomiting, abdominal pain), intestinal obstruction, fecal impaction, or ulcerative bowel lesions.
• Do not use for more than 1 week.

Potential Toxicities/Side Effects and the Nursing Process

I.   ALTERATIONS IN BOWEL ELIMINATION related to CHRONIC USE

Defining Characteristics: Removes defecation reflexes when used chronically (laxative dependence). Narcotic analgesics and vinca alkaloid chemotherapy may predispose to constipation.

Nursing Implications: Assess baseline elimination pattern. Teach patient how to self-administer laxative. Encourage patient to normalize bowel habits through adequate fluid intake (2–3 L/day), diet high in fiber and bulk (bran, cereals, fruits, and vegetables), and exercise as tolerated. Teach patient bowel regimen when on narcotics or vinca alkaloids to promote regular evacuation.

II. ALTERATION IN NUTRITION, LESS THAN BODY REQUIREMENTS, related to GI SIDE EFFECTS

Defining Characteristics: Constipation or drug may cause nausea, vomiting, cramps.

Nursing Implications: Assess comfort level and GI distress related to constipation. Encourage patient to drink cold fluids or ginger ale as tolerated. Encourage patient to try resting in different positions; warm packs may decrease abdominal pain. Teach patient to expect burning sensation with suppository use; reassure that it will resolve in 5–10 minutes.

Drug: naloxegol (Movantik)

Class: Opioid antagonist.

Mechanism of Action: Naloxegol is mu-opioid receptor antagonist, and blocks GI mu-opioid receptor binding, thereby decreasing the constipating effect of opioid analgesics. It results in slowed GI motility and transit time. The drug does not cross the blood–brain barrier at recommended doses due to PEGylation, although it is a naloxone derivative.

Metabolism: Following oral administration, peak concentration occurs in less than 2 hours, with a secondary peak occurring 0.4–3 hours after the first peak. Consuming a high-fat meal increases the extent and rate of absorption. Naloxegol is metabolized by the CYP3A microenzyme system. The rug is primarily excreted in the feces (68%), and to a lesser degree in the urine (16%). Half-life of therapeutic doses ranges from 6 to 11 hours.

Indication: Treatment of opioid-induced constipation in adults with chronic noncancer pain, including patients with chronic pain related to prior cancer and its treatment who do not require frequent opioid dosage escalation. The drug has shown efficacy in patients receiving opioids for at least 4 weeks.

Contraindications:
- Known or suspected GI obstruction, or patient at increased risk of recurrent obstruction.
- Concomitant use with strong CYP3A4 inhibitors (e.g., clarithromycin, ketoconazole).
- Known serious or severe hypersensitivity reaction to naloxegol or its excipients.

Dosage/Range:
- 25 mg PO once daily in the morning; if not tolerated, reduce dose to 12.5 mg once daily, on an empty stomach.
  - If unable to swallow tablet, crush tablet into a powder, mix with 4 oz (120 mL) water and have patient drink immediately.
  - Refill the glass with 4 oz water to rinse any remaining drug, stir, and have patient drink.
  - Can also be administered via nasogastric tube (NG): (1) flush NG tube with 30 mL water using a 60 mL syringe; (2) crush the tablet to a powder in a container and mix with about 2 oz (60 mL) water; (3) draw up mixture using the 60 mL syringe and administer contents through NG tube; (4) add 2 oz (60 mL) water to the same container used to prepare the dose; (5) draw up the water into the 60 mL syringe, and use to flush the NG tube and inject any remaining drug into the NG tube.

- If **renal impairment** (CrCl < 60 mL/min, moderate, severe, or ESRD): 12.5 mg once daily; if tolerated by constipation continues, increase to 25 mg once daily if tolerated and monitor for adverse reactions.
- **Concomitant use of moderate CYP3A4 inhibitor drugs** (e.g., diltiazem, erythromycin, verapamil): if concurrent use unavoidable, reduce naloxegol dose to 12.5 mg once daily and monitor for adverse effects.
- Stop maintenance laxative therapy before starting naloxegol; may resume if the patient develops opioid-induced constipation symptoms after taking naloxegol for 3 days.
- Discontinue treatment if opioid analgesic is also discontinued.

Drug Preparation: Available in 12.5- and 25-mg tablets.

Drug Administration:
- Teach the patient to take the tablet on an empty stomach at least 1 hour before the first meal of the day or 2 hours after the meal.
- The patient should swallow the tablets whole; do not crush or chew them.
- Avoid grapefruit juice or eating grapefruit.
- Discontinue naloxegol if the opioid analgesic is discontinued.

Drug Interactions:
- Naloxegol is metabolized primarily by CYP3A and is a substrate of the P-glycoprotein transporter. It is contraindicated in patients who must take strong CYP3A4 inhibitors.
- Moderate CYP3A4 inhibitors (e.g., diltiazem, erythromycin, verapamil): Increased naloxegol concentrations. Avoid coadministration; if it is unavoidable, reduce the naloxegol dose to 12.5 mg once daily, and monitor for adverse reactions.
- Strong CYP3A4 inducers (e.g., rifampin, carbamazepine, St. John's wort): Decreased concentration of naloxegol. Do not use concomitantly. Teach patients not to take St. John's wort when receiving naloxegol.
- Other opioid antagonists: There is a potential for an additive effect and increased risk of opioid withdrawal. Do not use concomitantly.

Lab Effects/Interference: None known.

Special Considerations:
- Most common adverse reactions in clinical trials with an incidence of 3% or greater: abdominal pain, diarrhea, nausea, flatulence, vomiting, headache.
- Warnings and Precautions:
  - *GI perforation* may occur rarely, in patients with loss of structural integrity (e.g., peptic ulcer disease, Ogilvie's syndrome, diverticular disease, infiltrative GI malignancies or peritoneal metastases). Weigh the relative risk against the potential benefit. Monitor the patient closely for development of severe, persistent, or worsening abdominal pain, and discontinue the drug immediately if it occurs.
  - *Opioid withdrawal* may occur rarely (< 1%); it is characterized by hyperhidrosis, chills, diarrhea, abdominal pain, anxiety, irritability, and yawning. Risk for opioid withdrawal may be higher in patients (1) receiving methadone for pain or (2) having a disruption of the blood–brain barrier, in which case they may also be at risk for

reduced analgesia. Weigh the relative risk against the potential benefit. Monitor the patient closely for opioid withdrawal.

- *Severe abdominal pain and/or diarrhea:* uncommon, but may occur, and is more likely in patients taking the 25 mg dose. Onset within a few days of starting the drug. Monitor patients for development of abdominal pain and/or diarrhea, and discontinue drug if severe symptoms occur. Consider restarting drug at 12.5 mg if appropriate.
- Use in pregnancy may precipitate opioid withdrawal in the fetus.
- Nursing mothers should make a decision to discontinue nursing or the drug, taking into account the importance to the mother.

Potential Toxicities/Side Effects and the Nursing Process

I. ALTERATION IN NUTRITION, LESS THAN BODY REQUIREMENTS, related to GI SIDE EFFECTS, HEADACHE

Defining Characteristics: Incidence of symptoms in patients in the clinical trials (for opioid-induced constipation and noncancer pain) at doses of 25 and 12.5 mg naloxegol, respectively, was as follows: abdominal pain (21%, 21%; 7% placebo), diarrhea (9%, 6%; 5% placebo), nausea (8%, 7%; 5% placebo), flatulence (6%, 3%; 3% placebo), vomiting (5%, 3%; 4% placebo), and headache (4%, 4%; 3% placebo).

Nursing Implications: Assess the patient's comfort level and GI distress related to constipation as well as the potential side effects of naloxegol. Teach the patient strategies to manage symptoms, and to report symptoms that persist. Encourage the patient to drink cold fluids or ginger ale as tolerated. Encourage the patient to try resting in different positions; warm packs may decrease abdominal pain.

Drug: polyethylene glycol 3350, NF powder (Miralax)

Class: Osmotic cathartic.

Mechanism of Action: Drug is an osmotic agent that pulls water into the intestines with the stool, softening the stool and causing peristalsis and evacuation in 2–4 days.

Metabolism: Is not fermented by colonic microflora and does not affect intestinal absorption or secretion of glucose or electrolytes.

Indication: For relief of constipation.

Dosage/Range:
- 17 g (1 heaping T) (product comes with a measuring cup).

Drug Preparation:
- Mix in 8 oz of water and take orally once a day.

COMPLICATIONS

Drug Administration:
- Oral. Available in 14- and 26-oz containers.
- Store at room temperature.

Drug Interactions:
- None.

Lab Effects/Interference:
- None.

Special Considerations:
- Contraindicated in patients with bowel obstruction.
- Indicated for the treatment of occasional constipation for up to 2 weeks.
- Use during pregnancy only if clearly needed.
- Excessive or frequent use or use > 2 weeks may result in electrolyte imbalance and dependence on laxatives.

Potential Toxicities/Side Effects and the Nursing Process

I.   ALTERATIONS IN BOWEL ELIMINATION related to CHRONIC USE

Defining Characteristics: Removes defecation reflexes when used chronically (laxative dependence). Narcotic analgesics and vinca alkaloid chemotherapy may predispose to constipation.

Nursing Implications: Assess baseline elimination pattern. Teach patient how to self-administer laxative. Encourage patient to normalize bowel habits through adequate fluid intake (2–3 L/day), diet high in fiber and bulk (bran, cereals, fruits, and vegetables), and exercise as tolerated. Teach patient bowel regimen when on narcotics or vinca alkaloids to promote regular evacuation.

II.   ALTERATION IN NUTRITION related to GI SIDE EFFECTS

Defining Characteristics: Constipation or drug may cause nausea, cramps, abdominal bloating, flatulence. High doses may cause diarrhea, especially in the elderly. Continued use beyond 2 weeks may cause electrolyte imbalance.

Nursing Implications: Assess comfort level and GI distress related to constipation. Encourage patient to drink cold fluids or ginger ale as tolerated. Encourage patient to try resting in different positions; warm packs may decrease abdominal pain. Teach patient laxative effect may take 2–4 days, and assess need for other cathartic(s).

Drug: senna (Senexon, Senokot)

Class: Irritant/stimulant laxative.

Mechanism of Action: Stimulates/irritates smooth muscle of intestines, increasing peristalsis; increases fluid accumulation in colon and small intestines. Indicated for relief of constipation or bowel preparation prior to bowel surgery.

Metabolism: Minimal oral absorption occurs. Evacuation occurs in 6–10 hours when taken orally.

Indication: For the relief of, and prevention of, constipation.

Dosage/Range:
• Senexon: 2 tablets at bedtime (187 mg senna).
• Senokot: 2–4 tablets bid (187 mg senna); 1–2 tsp granules bid (326 mg senna); 1 suppository at bedtime, repeat PRN in 2 hours (652 mg senna).
• Black-Draught: 2 tablets (600 mg senna) or 1/4 to 1/2 level tsp granules (1.65 g senna).

Drug Preparation:
• Store in a tightly closed bottle.

Drug Interactions:
• None.

Lab Effects/Interference:
• None known.

Special Considerations:
• Contraindicated in patients with signs/symptoms of acute abdomen (nausea, vomiting, abdominal pain), intestinal obstruction, fecal impaction, or ulcerative bowel lesions.
• Senna is very effective as part of bowel regimen for patients receiving narcotic analgesic medication.

Potential Toxicities/Side Effects and the Nursing Process

I.   ALTERATIONS IN BOWEL ELIMINATION related to CHRONIC USE

Defining Characteristics: Removes defecation reflexes when used chronically (laxative dependence). Narcotic analgesics and vinca alkaloid chemotherapy may predispose to constipation.

Nursing Implications: Assess baseline elimination pattern. Teach patient how to self-administer laxative. Encourage patient to normalize bowel habits through adequate fluid intake (2–3 L/day), diet high in fiber and bulk (bran, cereals, fruits, and vegetables), and exercise as tolerated. Teach patient bowel regimen when on narcotics or vinca alkaloids to promote regular evacuation.

II.   ALTERATION IN NUTRITION, LESS THAN BODY REQUIREMENTS, related to GI SIDE EFFECTS

Defining Characteristics: Constipation or drug may cause nausea, vomiting, abdominal pain; rectal suppository may cause burning in rectum as it is absorbed.

COMPLICATIONS

Nursing Implications: Assess comfort level and GI distress related to constipation. Encourage patient to drink cold fluids or ginger ale as tolerated. Encourage patient to try resting in different positions; warm packs may decrease abdominal pain. Teach patient to expect burning sensation with suppository use; reassure that it will resolve in 5–10 minutes.

III.   ALTERATION IN FLUID AND ELECTROLYTE BALANCE related to LAXATIVE ABUSE

Defining Characteristics: Diarrhea resulting from laxative abuse can deplete fluid volume, nutrients, and electrolytes.

Nursing Implications: Teach patient regular bowel regimen when receiving constipating drugs (narcotics, vinca alkaloids). Teach patient to replace lost fluids and electrolytes (encourage chicken soup, sports drink).

Drug: sorbitol

Class: Hyperosmotic laxative.

Mechanism of Action: Local irritant, with hyperosmotic action, drawing water from tissues into feces and stimulating fecal evacuation within 15–30 minutes.

Metabolism: Poorly absorbed from GI tract.

Indication: For the relief of constipation.

Dosage/Range:

Adult:
• Oral: 15 mL of 70% solution repeated until diarrhea starts.
• Rectal: 120 mL if a 25–30% solution is used.

Drug Preparation:
• Keep stored in tightly closed bottle.

Drug Interactions:
• None.

Lab Effects/Interference:
• None known.

Special Considerations:
• Contraindicated in patients with undiagnosed abdominal pain, intestinal obstruction.
• Oral 70% sorbitol may be as effective as lactulose in relieving constipation.

Potential Toxicities/Side Effects and the Nursing Process

I.   ALTERATIONS IN BOWEL ELIMINATION related to CHRONIC USE

Defining Characteristics: Removes defecation reflexes when used chronically (laxative dependence). Narcotic analgesics and vinca alkaloid chemotherapy may predispose to constipation.

Nursing Implications: Assess baseline elimination pattern. Teach patient how to self-administer laxative. Encourage patient to normalize bowel habits through adequate fluid intake (2–3 L/day), diet high in fiber and bulk (bran, cereals, fruits, and vegetables), and exercise as tolerated. Teach patient bowel regimen when on narcotics or vinca alkaloids to promote regular evacuation.

II.   ALTERATION IN FLUID AND ELECTROLYTE BALANCE related to LAXATIVE ABUSE

Defining Characteristics: Diarrhea resulting from laxative abuse can deplete fluid volume, nutrients, and electrolytes.

Nursing Implications: Teach patient regular bowel regimen when receiving constipating drugs (narcotics, vinca alkaloids). Teach patient to replace lost fluids and electrolytes (encourage chicken soup, sports drink).

III.   ALTERATION IN COMFORT related to CRAMPING PAIN, RECTAL IRRITATION, OR DISCOMFORT

Defining Characteristics: Cramping pain, rectal irritation, and inflammation or discomfort may occur.

Nursing Implications: Teach patient this may occur. If discomfort is not self-limited, suggest sitz bath, warm or cold packs, and position changes.

COMPLICATIONS

Chapter *13*
Diarrhea

Diarrhea continues to challenge patients and their nurses and may be caused by disease, such as diarrhea related to carcinoid syndrome, or treatment. Diarrhea is one of the most common side effects of chemotherapy and radiation therapy (Shaw & Taylor, 2012). Diarrhea can be debilitating and result in dehydration, fluid and electrolyte imbalance, altered nutritional status, increased risk for falls, and rarely patient death.

Rutledge and Engleking (1998) define diarrhea as an abnormal increase in liquidity and frequency, occurring as acute (within 24–48 hours of a stimulus, resolving in 7–14 days) or chronic (late onset, lasting > 2–3 weeks). Diarrhea occurring in patients with cancer is most often related to osmotic, absorptive, secretory, exudative, or motility dysfunction, or is chemotherapy-induced (Muehlbauer & Christine-Lopez, 2014).

- *Osmotic diarrhea* occurs as a result of hyperosmolar or nonabsorbable substances, which draw large volumes of fluid into the intestines, producing watery stools that usually resolve with removal of the cause. Causative factors include high-osmolality tube feedings, lactulose or sorbitol, and gastrointestinal hemorrhage.
- *Malabsorptive diarrhea* results from changes in mucosal integrity, causing changes in membrane permeability; or loss of absorptive surfaces, resulting in diarrhea that is large-volume, frothy, and foul-smelling (steatorrhea). Causes include deficiency of an enzyme responsible for digestion of fats (lactose intolerance, pancreatic insufficiency) or surgical resection or removal of the intestines.
- *Secretory diarrhea* results from intestinal hypersecretion of large volumes (> 1 L/day) of watery stool with an osmolality equal to that in the plasma. Causes are endocrine tumors (VIPoma and carcinoid), enterotoxin-producing pathogens such as *Clostridium difficile*, acute graft-versus-host disease, and short gut syndrome.
- *Exudative diarrhea* is caused by inflammation or ulceration of the bowel mucosa, resulting in stools containing mucus, blood, and serum protein; the patient experiences frequent stooling, although the total volume is usually < 1 L/day. Unfortunately, this type of diarrhea is associated with hypoalbuminemia and anemia. Causes are radiation to the bowel (radiation enteritis) or opportunistic infection in the denuded bowel, such as with neutropenic typhlitis.
- *Dysmotility-associated diarrhea* is related to factors that increase or decrease normal peristalsis, such as with irritable bowel syndrome, the ingestion of food or medication that affects peristalsis, or psychological factors such as anxiety or fear that cause parasympathetic stimulation. Diarrhea of this type is usually semisolid to liquid, small, and frequent.

- *Chemotherapy-induced diarrhea* occurs as a result of chemotherapy-induced cell death of the intestinal mucosa, causing overstimulation of intestinal water and electrolyte secretion. The patient experiences frequent watery to semisolid stools within 24–96 hours of chemotherapy administration. With irinotecan chemotherapy, acute diarrhea occurs initially during or soon after administration related to cholinergic stimulation, and then delayed diarrhea occurs about 9–12 days later. In combination with 5-fluorouracil, the delayed diarrhea can lead to dehydration, and together with neutropenia, sepsis. Some of the most common drugs causing diarrhea are: (1) chemotherapy: capecitabine, 5-FU, irinotecan, methotrexate; (2) targeted therapy (especially protein kinase inhibitors): lapatinib, cabozantinib, pazopanib, crizotinib; (3) immunotherapy: high dose interleukin-2 (IL-2), and the immune checkpoint inhibitors that can cause immune-related adverse effects (irAEs): such as colitis (ipilumumab and ipilumumab plus nivolumab combination therapy). Nurses play a very important role in teaching patients about the potential life-threatening diarrhea that may occur from chemotherapy and immunotherapy, self-administration of antidiarrheal medicines or administration of corticosteroids and other medications for irAEs, increased fluid and diet modifications, and triage if these efforts are not effective. Nurses understand that there is a significant difference between diarrhea caused by methotrexate and the potentially life-threatening colitis caused by ipilumomab or combined with nivolumab (irAE colitis).

Grading is important in diarrhea assessment as drug doses may need to be modified or interrupted. See *Chapter 4* for staging of irAE diarrhea and colitis. The NCCN Palliative Care guideline (v21, 2019) and NCI CTCAE version 4.0 (June 2010) is as follows, based on the number of stools over baseline:

Grade 1: Increase of < 4 stools over baseline, mild increase in ostomy output compared to baseline.

Grade 2: Increase of 4–6 stools over baseline, moderate increase in ostomy output compared to baseline.

Grade 3: Increase of 7 or more stools over baseline, incontinence, hospitalization indicated; severe increase in ostomy output compared to baseline; limiting self-care; interferes with ability to do activities of daily living.

Grade 4: Life-threatening consequences; urgent intervention indicated.

Additional classifications can be made as to (1) the *duration of diarrhea*: (a) acute: 1–2 days, and resolves on its own; (b) persistent: lasting 2–4 weeks; (c) chronic: lasting at least 4 weeks; (2) *intensity of diarrhea* and whether it is (a) uncomplicated (e.g., grade 1–2 without other symptoms); or (b) complicated (e.g., grade 3 or 4, or grade 1–2 with symptoms of cramping, dehydration, sepsis (if diarrhea related to chemotherapy occurs at time of neutrophil nadir/ neutropenia), decreased performance status, nausea, vomiting).

Nurses are key in the management of diarrhea. Nurses play a significant role in patient assessment and patient/family teaching. Assessment of the patient's previous and current nutrition and elimination patterns, as well as assessment of probable etiology of diarrhea, are critical, as is patient/family teaching about the management and prevention of diarrhea. If the patient has no likely cause for diarrhea and it is persistent, then the nurse needs to discuss ruling out a microorganism cause, such as *C. difficile* in a patient who is receiving antibiotics.

Patient teaching includes (Muehlbauer & Christine-Lopez, 2014):

- Fluids: Increase fluid intake to at least 8-oz fluid replacement per episode of diarrhea; goal is at least 8–10 (8-oz) glasses of fluid per day. Drink fluids at room temperature.
- Diet modification:
  - Eat 5–6 small, frequent meals instead of 3 large meals.
  - Eat foods high in soluble fiber (e.g., applesauce, oatmeal, bananas, cooked carrots, peeled potatoes, rice); foods low in insoluble fiber (e.g., rice, noodles, well-cooked eggs, bananas, white toast, canned or cooked fruit without skin, skinned turkey or chicken, fish, mashed potatoes); foods and fluids that are high in electrolytes (e.g., sodium and potassium) to replace those lost in diarrhea (broths and soups, bananas, peach nectar, oranges, peeled potatoes).
  - Avoid foods high in insoluble fiber (e.g., raw fruit and vegetables, whole grain bread, nuts, popcorn, skins, seeds, legumes), greasy, fried, and/or high-fat foods; spicy foods; foods and beverages containing lactose or supplements with lactase enzyme; hyperosmotic liquids (e.g., fruit juice, sweetened fruit drinks); caffeinated beverages; alcohol.
- Care of irritated skin, mucosa in perirectal area; critical in neutropenic or immunocompromised patients.
- Self-administration of prescribed antidiarrheal medication(s).
- Need for blood tests to assess electrolyte imbalance and hydration if diarrhea is severe.
- See *Chapter 4* for discussion of assessment of immune checkpoint inhibitor-induced diarrhea, its management, and nursing care plan (ASCO, 2018; NCCN, 2019).

Diarrhea can lead to severe fluid and electrolyte imbalance, as well as significant patient discomfort. Common electrolyte imbalances related to diarrhea include metabolic acidosis, hypokalemia, hyperchloremia, hypocalcemia, and hypomagnesemia. Signs and symptoms of dehydration include fever; poor skin turgor; pallor; dry mucous membranes; thick saliva; lethargy; confusion; dizziness; rapid, weak, thready pulse; hypotension; and decreased urinary output. These increase the patient's risk of injury and should be prevented. If dehydration occurs, rehydration and correction of electrolyte imbalance is key.

Ippoliti (1998) describes antidiarrheal agents as:

- *Intraluminal agents:* Decrease water in gut by absorption, increasing bulk of the stool, and protecting intestinal mucosa; includes absorbents such as activated charcoal and mucilloid preparations, and adsorbents such as psyllium, kaolin, and pectate; less commonly used as more effective agents available without possible drug interactions or difficulty ingesting them.
- *Intestinal transit inhibitors:* Primarily anticholinergic (atropine sulfate and scopolamine) and opiate agonists (DTO and the synthetic opioids diphenoxylate and loperamide), which slow down intestinal peristalsis and increase fluid absorption.
- *Proabsorptive agents:* Intraluminal absorbent agents as above.
- *Antisecretory agents:* Octreotide (Sandostatin) is a synthetic somatostatin analogue that inhibits the secretion of gut hormones like serotonin and motilin, and thus slows transit time and improves regulation of water and electrolyte movement in the gut. Bismuth subsalicylate (Pepto-Bismol) also works to decrease gut mucosal inflammation and hypermotility by binding to toxins and inhibiting prostaglandin synthesis.

COMPLICATIONS

In addition,

- *Anti-inflammatory corticosteroids:* are used in the management of immune-related colitis and diarrhea caused by immune checkpoint inhibitors (see *Chapter 4*).
- As more knowledge is gained as to mechanisms of disease, targeted treatments may be developed. Approximately 78% of patients with carcinoid syndrome develop a watery diarrhea related to increased serotonin levels. Telotristat ethyl (Xermelo®), a tryptophan hydroxylase inhibitor, has been FDA approved in combination with a somatostatin analogue to treat patients with carcinoid syndrome diarrhea who have an inadequate response to somatostatin analogue therapy. Telotristat ethyl (Xermelo®) inhibits the biosynthesis of serotonin within the tumor cell by blocking the rate limiting enzyme tryphtophan hydroxylase; this then blocks the synthesis of serotonin and its subsequent release into the systemic circulation. Patients with high-circulating serum levels of serotonin are associated with severe carcinoid syndrome, carcinoid heart disease, and a poor prognosis (Kulke et al., 2017).

References

American Society of Clinical Oncology. Management of Immune-Related Adverse Events in Patients Treated with Immune Checkpoint Inhibitor Therapy: American Society of Clinical Oncology Clinical Practice Guidelines. *J Clin Oncol* 2018; 36(17):1714–1768.

Bulloch M. Diarrhea: A New Indication Contributing to the Opioid Epidemic? *Pharmacy Times* July 10, 2018. Available at https://www.pharmacytimes.com/contributor/marilyn-bulloch-pharmd-bcps/2018/07/diarrhea-a-new-indication-contributing-to-the-opioid-epidemic. Accessed May 31, 2019.

Kulke MH, Horsch D, Caplin ME et al. Telotristat Ethyl, A Tryptophan Hydroxylase Inhibitor for Treatment of Carcinoid Syndrome. *J Clin Oncol* 2017; 35(1):14–23.

Lexicon Pharmaceuticals, Inc. Xermelo (telotristat ethyl) package insert. The Woodlands, TX. February 2017.

Muehlbauer PM, Christine-Lopez R. Diarrhea. Chapter 10 in Yarbro CH, Wujuk D, Gobel BH (Eds.), *Cancer Symptom Management*, 4th ed. Burlington, MA: Jones & Bartlett Learning; 2014: 185–213. National Cancer Center.

National Institutes of Health. *Common Toxicity Criteria of Adverse Effects*. Version 4.03, June 10, 2010. Available at http://evs.nci.nih.gov/ftp1/CTCAE/CTCAE_4.03_2010-06-14_QuickReference_5x7.pdf. Accessed May 31, 2019.

National Comprehensive Cancer Network. *Palliative Care Guideline*. Version 2, 2019. Available at https://www.nccn.org/professionals/physician_gls/pdf/palliative.pdf. Accessed May 31, 2019.

National Comprehensive Cancer Network. *NCCN Guidelines Version 2. 2019 (April 8, 2019) Management of Immunotherapy-related Toxicities*. Available at https://www.nccn.org/professionals/physician_gls/pdf/immunotherapy.pdf. Accessed May 3, 2019.

Novartis Pharmaceuticals Corporation. Sandostatin LAR Depot (octreotide acetate for injectable suspension) [package insert]. East Hanover, NJ: Novartis Pharmaceuticals Corporation; April 2019.

Rutledge D, Engleking C. Cancer-Related Diarrhea: Selected Findings of a National Survey of Oncology Nurse Experiences. *Oncol Nurs Forum* 1998; 25:861–878.

Shaw C, Taylor L. Treatment-related diarrhea in patients with cancer. *Clin J Oncol Nurs* 2012; 16(4):413–417.

Teva Pharmaceuticals, Inc. USA. Loperamide HCl [package insert]. North Wales, PA. November 2016.

Drug: deodorized tincture of opium (DTO, Laudanum)

Class: Opium antidiarrheal agent.

Mechanism of Action: Increases GI smooth muscle tone and inhibits GI motility, delaying movement of intestinal contents; water is absorbed from fecal contents, decreasing diarrhea.

Metabolism: Variable absorption from GI tract; metabolized by liver and excreted in urine.

Indication: For the relief of diarrhea in adults.

Dosage/Range:

Adult:
- Oral: 0.3–1 mL qid (maximum 6 mL/day).

Drug Preparation:
- Store in tight, light-resistant bottle. Administer with water or juice.

Drug Interactions:
- None.

Lab Effects/Interference:
- None known.

Special Considerations:
- DTO contains 25 times more morphine than paregoric.
- Physical dependence may develop if drug is used chronically (e.g., colitis).
- Controlled substance.
- May be used in combination with kaolin and pectin mixtures.
- Do not use in diarrhea that results from poisoning until poison is removed (e.g., by lavage or cathartics).

Potential Toxicities/Side Effects and the Nursing Process

I. ALTERATION IN NUTRITION, LESS THAN BODY REQUIREMENTS, related to GI SIDE EFFECTS

Defining Characteristics: Nausea, vomiting may occur.

Nursing Implications: Assess baseline nutrition, GI status. If nausea/vomiting appears to follow dose administration, administer DTO with juice to disguise taste.

Drug: diphenoxylate hydrochloride and atropine (Lomotil)

Class: Antidiarrheal agent.

COMPLICATIONS

1948   *Chapter   13   Diarrhea*
Mechanism of Action: Diphenoxylate is a synthetic opiate agonist that inhibits intestinal smooth muscle activity, thereby slowing peristalsis so that excess water is absorbed from feces. Atropine discourages deliberate overdosage.
Metabolism: Well absorbed from GI tract. Metabolized in liver. Excreted principally via feces in bile. Onset of action 45 minutes to 1 hour; duration 3–4 hours.
Indication: For the relief of diarrhea.

Dosage/Range:

Adult:
- Oral: 5 mg PO qid then titrate to response × 2 days (if no response in 48 hours, drug ineffective).

Drug Preparation:
- Oral: one tablet contains 2.5 mg diphenoxylate HCl and 0.025 mg atropine sulfate.

Drug Interactions:
- CNS depressants (alcohol, barbiturates): potentiate CNS depressant action; use together cautiously.
- MAOIs: may cause hypertensive crisis (similar structure to meperidine); use together cautiously.

Lab Effects/Interference:
- None known.

Special Considerations:
- May be habit-forming when used in high doses (40–60 mg); physical dependence.
- Use with extreme caution in patients with hepatic cirrhosis, as drug may precipitate hepatic coma, and in patients with acute ulcerative colitis.
- Contraindicated in patients with jaundice, diarrhea resulting from poisoning or pseudomembranous colitis caused by antibiotics.

Potential Toxicities/Side Effects and the Nursing Process

I.   ALTERATION IN NUTRITION, LESS THAN BODY REQUIREMENTS, related to GI SIDE EFFECTS

Defining Characteristics: Nausea, vomiting, abdominal distension or discomfort, anorexia, mouth dryness, and (rarely) paralytic ileus may occur.

Nursing Implications: Assess baseline nutrition and elimination status. Instruct patient to report signs and symptoms. Discuss drug discontinuance with physician. Instruct patient that drug should be used for 2 days and physician notified if diarrhea persists.

II. ALTERATIONS IN SENSORY/PERCEPTUAL PATTERNS related to SEDATION

Defining Characteristics: Sedation, dizziness, lethargy, restlessness or insomnia, headache, paresthesia occur rarely with higher doses and prolonged therapy. Blurred vision may occur due to mydriasis.

Nursing Implications: Teach patient that drug is for short-term relief of diarrhea. Assess for and instruct patient to report signs/symptoms. Discuss drug discontinuance with physician if symptoms are severe.

III. ALTERATION IN SKIN INTEGRITY related to RASH, SENSITIVITY

Defining Characteristics: Pruritus, angioedema (swelling of lips, face, gums), giant urticaria may occur.

Nursing Implications: Assess for and instruct patient to report signs/symptoms immediately. Drug should be discontinued if angioedema or giant urticaria occurs.

Drug: kaolin/pectin (Kaodene, K-P, Kaopectate, K-Pek)

Class: Antidiarrheal agent.

Mechanism of Action: Drug acts as absorbent and protectant; decreases stool fluidity but not total amount of fluid excreted.

Metabolism: Not absorbed from GI tract and excreted in stool.

Indication: For the relief of diarrhea.

Dosage/Range:

Adult:
• Oral: 60–120 mL regular or 45–90 mL concentrated suspension after each loose bowel movement < 48 hours.

Drug Preparation:
• Shake well prior to administration.

Drug Interactions:

• Oral lincomycin: decreases lincomycin absorption; administer kaolin/pectin at least 2 hours before or 3–4 hours after lincomycin dose.
• Oral digoxin: decreases digoxin absorption; administer kaolin/pectin 2 hours after digoxin dose.

COMPLICATIONS

Lab Effects/Interference:
• None known.

Special Considerations:
• Few adverse effects.
• Used for temporary relief of diarrhea.

Potential Toxicities/Side Effects and the Nursing Process

I.   KNOWLEDGE DEFICIT related to SELF-ADMINISTRATION

Defining Characteristics: Transient constipation may occur.

Nursing Implications: Assess understanding of medication and self-administration schedule. Instruct patient in self-administration and to notify nurse/physician if diarrhea persists beyond 48 hours or fever develops. Reinforce need to drink fluids, especially in elderly or debilitated patients, to prevent constipation.

Drug: loperamide hydrochloride (Imodium)

Class: Antidiarrheal agent.

Mechanism of Action: Slows intestinal motility by inhibiting peristalsis (direct effect on circular and longitudinal intestinal muscles); increases stool bulk and viscosity.

Metabolism: Well absorbed from GI tract. Metabolized by cytochrome P450 hepatic and feces as intact drug. If given concurrently with CYP3A4 inhibitors (e.g., ketoconazole) or CYP2C8 inhibitors (e.g. gemfibrozil) or inhibitors of P-glycoprotein (e.g., quinidine, ritonavir), loperamide serum levels will be elevated.

Indication: For the control and symptomatic relief of (1) acute nonspecific diarrhea in patients aged 2 and older; and (2) chronic diarrhea associated with inflammatory bowel disease; (3) reducing volume of ileostomy drainage.

Contraindications: Contraindicated in patients with (1) pediatric patients < 2 years old; (2) known hypersensitivity to loperamide or its components; (3) abdominal pain in the absence of diarrhea; (4) acute dysentery (blood in stool and high fever); (5) acute ulcerative colitis; (6) bacterial entercolitis caused by invasive microorganisms such as *Salmonella, Shigella, Camylobacter;* (7) pseudomembranous colitis (e.g., *C. difficile)* associated with broad-spectrum antibiotic use.

Dosage/Range: Acute Diarrhea

• Adults and pediatric patients aged 13 and older): 4 mg (2 capsules) followed by 2 mg (1 capsule) after each unformed stool (maximum 16 mg); higher dose if under direction of a physician such as for irinotecan induced diarrhea.

- Pediatric patients aged 2 through 12 years old: Use oral solution for patients aged 2–5 years.
  - First day doses
    - Age 2–5 (13–20 kg): 1 mg PO tid (3 mg total dosage)
    - Aged 6–8 (20–30 kg): 2 mg PO bid (4 mg total dosage)
    - Aged 8 through 12 (>30 kg): 2 mg tid (6 mg total dosage)
  - Subsequent daily dosing
    - Give loperamide HCl only after a loose stool: 1 mg/kg body weight. Do not exceed total doses shown on day 1.
- Chronic diarrhea
  - Adults: 4 mg (2 capsules) followed by 2 mg (1 capsule) after each unformed stool until diarrhea controlled, after which then dose should be PRN.
  - Elderly, patients with impaired hepatic or renal function: no studies done. No modification necessary for renal dysfunction, but use drug with caution in patients with hepatic dysfunction.

Drug Preparation:
- Oral.
- Available as 2-mg capsules and oral solution

Drug Interactions:
- CYP3A4 inhibitors (e.g., itraconazole): avoid coadministration if possible due to increased loperamide serum levels; if unavoidable, monitor patients closely for cardiac adverse effects.
- CYP2C8 inhibitors (e.g., gemfibrozil): avoid coadministration if possible due to increased loperamide serum levels; if unavoidable, monitor patients closely for cardiac adverse effects.
- P-glycoprotein inhibitors (e.g., quinidine, ritonavir): avoid coadministration if possible due to increased loperamide serum levels; if unavoidable, monitor patients closely for cardiac adverse effects.
- Effects of loperamide on saquinavir: decreased saquinavir serum level by 54%. Monitor patient for saquinavir efficacy if concurrent use unavoidable.

Lab Effects/Interference:
- None known.

Special Considerations:
- Most common adverse effects: constipation, dizziness.
- Drug has abuse potential: It is a mu-opioid agonist and has greater CNS opioid effects when taken at higher than recommended doses. It can be abused by drug users who wish to prevent withdrawal, and overdosage can result in life-threatening cardiac, CNS, and respiratory adverse effects (Bulloch, 2018). Assess patients for risk of abusing or misusing the drug.
- Warnings and Precautions:
  - *Cardiac adverse reactions including torsades de pointes and sudden death:* Prolongation of the QTc interval can be prolonged and has been reported in patients taking

excessive doses (e.g., misuse and abuse to prevent opioid withdrawal as drug is an opioid). Syncope and ventricular tachycardia were reported. Significant risk including respiratory depression have occurred in pediatric patients < 2 years of age so that is why drug is contraindicated in this population. Do NOT use drug in combination with other drugs or herbal products known to prolong the QTc (certain antiarrythymics, antipsychotics, some antibiotics, others: see package insert).

- *Dehydration:* Requires hydration and electrolyte replacement in addition to treatment with Imodium to stop diarrhea.
- *GI disorders:* Do not use drug if peristalsis is inhibited as this can lead to ileus, megacolon, etc. Discontinue drug use promptly when constipation, ileus, or abdominal distention occurs.
- *Variability in pediatric response:* Dehydration in children < 6 years of age may increase variability; keep children well hydrated.
- *Allergic reaction:* Extremely rare but anaphylaxis and anaphylactic shock have been reported. Extremely rare reports or rash, which should be evaluated for erythema multiforme (EM), Stevens-Johnson Syndrome (SJS), or toxic epidermal necrolysis (TEN).
- *Hepatic impairment:* Not studied. Use drug cautiously in this population as systemic exposure may be higher due to decreased liver function and metabolism of drug. Monitor patients at risk for CNS toxicity.
- *Renal impairment:* Dose modification not required.
- *Geriatric use:* Elderly patients are more likely to take other medications; do not in combination with drugs that can prolong the QTc (e.g., Class IA or III antiarrythymics). Review patient medication profile for interacting drugs and discuss alternatives with physician and pharmacist.
- Reduces electrolyte and fluid loss from intestines; may be used to reduce volume of ileostomy drainage. Two to three times more potent than diphenoxylate.
- Intended for self-medication × 48 hours; patients should be taught to notify nurse/physician if symptoms persist or fever occurs.
- Pregnancy category C: avoid use in pregnancy; teach patients of reproductive potential to use effective contraception during use with Imodium. Nursing mothers should not breastfeed while receiving the drug.
- Use cautiously in pregnant or nursing women.

Potential Toxicities/Side Effects and the Nursing Process

I.   ALTERATION IN NUTRITION, LESS THAN BODY REQUIREMENTS, related to GI SIDE EFFECTS

Defining Characteristics: Less frequent adverse reactions occur than with diphenoxylate/atropine. Nausea, vomiting, abdominal pain, and distension may occur.

Nursing Implications: Assess baseline nutrition and elimination status. Instruct patient to report signs and symptoms. Discuss drug discontinuance with physician. Instruct patient that drug should be used for 2 days and physician notified if diarrhea persists.

II. ALTERATIONS IN SENSORY/PERCEPTUAL PATTERNS related to DROWSINESS

Defining Characteristics: Drowsiness, dizziness, fatigue may occur.

Nursing Implications: Teach patient that drug is for short-term relief of diarrhea. Assess for and instruct patient to report signs/symptoms. Discuss drug discontinuance with physician if symptoms are severe.

III. ALTERATION IN SKIN INTEGRITY related to RASH, SENSITIVITY

Defining Characteristics: Rarely, rash may develop.

Nursing Implications: Assess baseline skin integrity. Instruct patient to report rash. Discuss drug discontinuance with physician.

Drug: octreotide acetate (Sandostatin)

Class: Cyclic octapeptide that mimics the pharmacologic actions of the natural hormone somatostatin and is long-acting. It is a somatostatin analogue.

Mechanism of Action: Drug is a more potent inhibitor than somatostatin of growth hormone, glucagon, insulin; also suppresses LH (luteinizing hormone) response to GnRH (gonadotropin-releasing hormone); decreases splanchnic blood flow; and inhibits release of serotonin, gastrin, vasoactive intestinal peptide (VIP), secretin, motilin, and pancreatic-polypeptide–like somatostatin. Stimulates fluid and electrolyte absorption from GI tract, and lengthens transit time of intestinal contents. Controls symptoms associated with carcinoid syndrome (e.g., flushing, levels of serotonin metabolite 5-HIAA), and VIP-secreting adenomas (e.g., watery diarrhea).

Metabolism: Absorbed rapidly and completely after injection, with peak concentrations after 24 minutes. Protein binding 65%, and eliminated from plasma with a half-life of 1.7 hours (natural hormone is 1–3 minutes). Duration of action approximately 12 hours, depending upon tumor type. Excreted in urine, with decreased clearance by 26% in the elderly. LAR Depot consists of biodegradable microspheres that slowly release octreotide from the injection site over 4 weeks. After IM injection, serum octreotide concentration reaches a transient initial peak within 1 hour, then declines over the next 3–5 days, then slowly increases to plateau 2–3 weeks, post-injection. Steady state is reached by the third monthly injection.

Indication: (1) Acromegaly: Reduce blood levels of growth hormone and IGF-I (somatomedin C) in acromegaly patients who have had an inadequate response to or cannot be treated with surgical resection, pituitary irradiation, and bromocriptine mesylate at maximally tolerated doses; (2) Carcinoid tumors: symptomatic treatment of patients with metastatic carcinoid tumors where it suppresses or inhibits the severe diarrhea and flushing

COMPLICATIONS

episodes associated with the disease; (3) Vasoactive intestinal peptide tumors (VIPomas): treatment of profuse, watery diarrhea associated with vasoactive intestinal peptide tumors.

Limitations of Use: In patients with carcinoid syndrome or VIPomas, the effect of octreotide injection (immediate release), and LAR depot (Sandostatin LAR depot) on tumor size, growth rate, and development of metastases has not been studied.

Dosage/Range:

Long acting depot (LAR depot) should be administered by a trained healthcare provider.
Indicated Usage (patients not currently receiving octreotide injection subcutaneously):
- Acromegaly: 50 micrograms 3 daily Sandostatin injection subcutaneously for at least 2 weeks, after assessment of GH and IGF-1 levels to assess response, followed by Sandostatin LAR Depot 20 mg intragluteally every 4 weeks for 3 months.
- Carcinoid tumors and VIPomas: Sandostatin injection subcutaneously 100–600 micrograms/day in 2–4 divided doses for 2 weeks, followed by Sandostatin LAR Depot 20 mg intragluteally every 4 weeks for 2 months.
- VIPomas.

Indicated Usage (patients currently receiving Sandostatin injection subcutaneously):
- Acromegaly: 20 mg Sandostatin LAR intragluteally every 4 weeks for 3 months.
- Carcinoid and VIPomas: 20 mg Sandostatin LAR intragluteally every 4 weeks for 2 months.
- Renal impairment, patients on dialysis: 10 mg Sandostatin LAR every 4 weeks.
- Hepatic impairment, cirrhosis: 10 mg Sandostatin LAR every 4 weeks.

Other Usage (octreotide) (Sandostatin LAR Depot):
- Renal failure: drug half-life may be increased, requiring dosage adjustment.

Carcinoid Tumors and VIPomas:
- If patient is not currently on octreotide acetate, begin therapy with immediate-release dosing for 2 weeks: Carcinoid: 100–600 μg/day SQ in 2–4 divided doses (mean daily dose 300 μg), although some patients may require up to 1,500 μg/day; VIPoma: 200–300 μg/day SQ in 2–4 divided doses (range 150–750 μg), and dosage may be individualized to control symptoms, but usually does not exceed 450 μg/day.
- For patients who respond to the initial 2-week therapy, switch to Sandostatin LAR Depot 20 mg IM q 4 weeks × 2 months. In addition, since it will take at least 2 weeks to achieve steady state, the patient should ALSO continue to receive Sandostatin immediate-release dosing SQ for at least 2 weeks at the same dose as in the first 2 weeks. After 2 months of Sandostatin LAR Depot 20 mg, the dose may be increased to 30 mg q 4 weeks if symptoms are not controlled. Some patients who have their symptoms controlled on 20 mg q 4 weeks may be decreased to 10 mg q 4 weeks. Do not exceed a 30-mg dose.
- Some patients may have exacerbation of symptoms and require temporary additional immediate release, in addition to the LAR Depot, to control the increase in symptoms.

Acromegaly:
- If patient is not currently on octreotide acetate, begin therapy with immediate-release dosing q 8 h at an initial dose of 50 μg tid, and gradually increase as needed (based on growth hormone [GH] levels), as the goal is to normalize GH and IGF-1 (somatomedin

C) levels. After 2 weeks, tolerability and response should be evident, so that patient can be changed to LAR Depot at a dose of 20 mg q 4 weeks if effective and well tolerated.

- For patients currently on octreotide, they can be changed directly to LAR Depot q 4 weeks, and at the end of 3 months, the LAR Depot dose should be titrated based on growth hormone level:
  - GH ≤ 2.5 ng/mL, IGF-1 (somatomedin C) normal and controlled symptoms, 20 mg IM (intragluteally) q 4 weeks.
  - GH > 2.5 ng/mL, IGF-1 elevated and/or uncontrolled symptoms, increase dose to 30 mg IM q 4 weeks.
  - GH ≤ 1 ng/mL, IGF-1 normal and controlled symptoms, reduce dose to 10 mg IM q 4 weeks.

Drug Preparation:
- Available in 1-mL (50-, 100-, 500-μg) ampules, and 5-mL (200- and 1,000-micrograms/mL) multidose vials. Stable in solution in 0.9% sodium chloride or 5% dextrose in water for 24 hours; dilute drug in 50–200 mL of 0.9% sodium chloride or 5% dextrose for IV infusions over 15–30 minutes.
- Patient may develop pain, stinging, tingling, or burning sensation at injection site, with redness and swelling.

LAR Depot:
- Available in (5-mL) vials containing 10-, 20-, or 30-mg octreotide-free peptide; injection kit includes a syringe containing 2.5 mL of diluent, two sterile 1.5-inch 19-gauge needles, and two alcohol wipes, as well as instruction booklet.
- Allow drug vial and diluent-filled syringe to reach room temperature (30–60 minutes) prior to preparation of drug suspension.
- Drug must be administered immediately after mixing.
- Tap vial to ensure drug has settled to bottom of vial; aseptically inject diluent slowly down the inside wall of the vial while rotating the vial to evenly distribute the diluent using one of the needles. Allow to sit for 5 minutes or longer to assure full saturation of the drug powder; once saturated, swirl the vial gently for 30–60 seconds until a milky uniform suspension appears (DO NOT shake vigorously or invert the vial). Aseptically withdraw the ordered dose, holding the vial at 45 degrees. There will be some remaining suspension as the vial has overfill. Add a small amount of air into the syringe, and gently rock back and forth until the patient is given the injection (DO NOT invert syringe). Eliminate air from the syringe.
- Replace needle with second needle, and aseptically administer drug immediately.

Drug Administration:
- Immediate-release injection: administer SQ, IV over 15–30 minutes, or IVP over 3 minutes.
- LAR: Administer IM in gluteal muscle, as other sites are too painful (never give IV or SC) q 28 days.
- Record injection site and rotate sites.
- Teach patients the importance of adhering closely to scheduled return visits for next injection so symptoms do not become exacerbated.

COMPLICATIONS

Drug Interactions:
- May affect absorption of orally administered drugs.
- Cyclosporine: decreased serum levels of cyclosporine, resulting in transplant rejection.
- Insulin, oral hypoglycemic agents: octreotide inhibits insulin and glucagon secretion. Monitor serum glucose level and adjust antidiabetic therapy dose PRN.
- Beta-blockers: ↓ heart rate; assess patient response and need for dosage adjustment of these drugs.
- Bromocriptine: bromocriptine availability.
- Drugs metabolized by CYP3A4 with narrow therapeutic window (e.g., quinidine): use together cautiously and monitor closely.

Lab Effects/Interference:
- Hypoglycemia or hyperglycemia; monitor during therapy.
- Suppression of TSH may result in hypothyroidism and decreased total/free T_4.
- Decreased vitamin B_{12} levels (Shilling's test); monitor during therapy.

Special Considerations:
- Sandostatin LAR Depot is indicated for patients in whom initial treatment with Sandostatin injection has been shown to be effective and tolerated: (1) carcinoid tumors: the long-term treatment of severe diarrhea and flushing episodes, (2) VIPomas: long-term treatment of profuse watery diarrhea, (3) acromegaly: long-term maintenance therapy that requires medical treatment.
- Octreotide acetate is appropriate when other conventional antidiarrheal medications have failed, and other treatable causes of diarrhea have been excluded (e.g., obstruction, infection).
- Patient should be taught sterile SQ injection technique for immediate-release preparations.
- Laboratory test monitoring (efficacy) based on treatment intent:
  - Carcinoid: 5-HIAA (urinary 5-hydroxyindoleacetic acid), plasma substance P, and serotonin.
  - VIPoma: VIP (plasma vasoactive intestinal peptide) baseline and periodic total and/ or free T_4.
  - Acromegaly: growth hormone (GH), IGF-1 (somatomedin C).
- Adverse reactions of diabetes mellitus, hypothyroidism, and cardiovascular disease occur in patients treated for acromegaly.
- May change to long-acting depot if already controlled on immediate-release preparation, or in a new patient, after response is assessed after 2 weeks of immediate-release dosing.
- Warnings and Precautions:
  - *Cholelithiasis and complications of cholelithiasis:* Drug inhibits gallbladder contraction and decreases bile secretion, which may lead to gallstones and biliary sludge. Monitor periodically.
  - Drug may rarely cause alterations in hormonal levels, so patients receiving long-term therapy should be monitored baseline and periodically during treatment: glucose, glucose tolerance in patients receiving antidiabetic drugs, thyroid function (TSH, total and/or free T_4), B_{12} level, and zinc level in patients receiving TPN.
  - *Hypoglycemia or hyperglycemia* may occur. Monitor glucose closely, and antidiabetic treatment may need to be adjusted.

- *Thyroid function abnormalities:* Drug may significantly suppress thyroid-stimulating hormone (TSH), causing hypothyroidism; monitor thyroid levels (TSH, total and/or free T4) periodically during therapy.
- *Cardiac function abnormalities*: In patients with acromegaly or carcinoid, drug may rarely cause cardiac abnormalities such as bradycardia (HR < 50 bpm), QT prolongation, nonspecific ST segment changes, and worsening of CHF; use drug cautiously in patients with cardiac risk factors.
- *Nutrition*: Octreotide may alter absorption of dietary fats; vitamin B12 levels may occur and should be monitored during therapy. If patient receiving TPN, serum zinc may rise excessively; monitor serum zinc in these patients.
- Monitoring laboratory tests (1) acromegaly: GH, IGF-1; (2) carcinoid: 5-HIAA (urinary 5-hydroxyindole acetic acid), plasma serotonin, plasma Substance P; (3) VI-Poma: plasma vasoactive intestinal peptide (VIP) baseline and total and/or free T4 periodically during chronic therapy.
- *Drug Interactions*: may have effect on absorption of orally administered drugs as octreotide may alter GI absorption. Concomitant administration with cyclosporine may decrease blood levels of cyclosporine.

Potential Toxicities/Side Effects (Dose-and Schedule-Dependent) and the Nursing Process

I.   ALTERATION IN NUTRITION, LESS THAN BODY REQUIREMENTS, related to CARBOHYDRATE METABOLISM

Defining Characteristics: Rarely, transient hypoglycemia or hyperglycemia due to altered balance between hormones regulating serum glucose (insulin, glucagon, growth hormone). Rarely, diarrhea, nausea and vomiting, abdominal pain, or discomfort. Incidence 3–10%. Drug may alter absorption of dietary fats.

Nursing Implications: Assess baseline nutritional balance. Instruct patient to report any changes, and assess for hyperglycemia (drowsiness, dry mouth, flushing, dry skin, fruity breath, polyuria, polydipsia, polyphagia, weight loss, stomach ache, nausea/vomiting, fatigue), hypoglycemia (anxiety, chills, cool/pale skin, difficulty concentrating, headache, hunger, shakiness, diaphoresis, fatigue, weakness, nausea). If patient is hypoglycemic, teach patient to carry candy. Monitor serum glucose, and discuss alterations with physician. Treat nausea and vomiting symptomatically, and discuss need for antiemetic if significant.

II.   ALTERATION IN COMFORT related to HEADACHE, FLUSHING

Defining Characteristics: Rarely (1–3%) patient may experience lightheadedness, dizziness, fatigue, pedal edema, headache, flushing of the face, weakness. Back and abdominal pain may also occur, as can injection-site pain.

Nursing Implications: Assess baseline comfort, and instruct patient to report any changes. Assess safety, and manage symptoms symptomatically. If unrelieved or significant, discuss with physician. Rotate injection sites, and teach patient local comfort measures at injection site.

COMPLICATIONS

Drug: Telotristat ethyl (Xermelo)

Classification: Tryptophan hydroxylase inhibitor

Mechanism of Action: Telotristat is the active metabolite of telotristat ethyl, and is 29 times more powerful than telotristat ethyl in blocking tryptophan hydroxylase (TPH). TPH is the rate limiting step in serotonin biosynthesis, and by inhibiting TPH, serotonin synthesis within the tumor cell is halted. Carcinoid syndrome is characterized by excessive serotonin synthesis and release by tumor cells, and may be associated with severe carcinoid syndrome, carcinoid heart disease, and a poor prognosis (Kulke et al., 2017). Serotonin is a neurotransmitter that mediates bowel secretion, motility, inflammation and sensation (Lexicon, 2017). Through TPH inhibition, peripheral serotonin production is reduced with a subsequent reduction in frequency of carcinoid syndrome related diarrhea. Telotristat is complimentary to somatostatin analogues that work by blocking external cell receptors for serotonin. Telotristat does not cross the blood brain barrier; this is important because serotonin is also a CNS neurotransmitter that regulates mood.

Metabolism: After oral dosing, telotristat ethyl is absorbed and metabolized to its active metabolite telotristat; peak plasma concentrations (C_{max}) occur for telotristat ethyl in 0.5–2 hours, and that of telotristat within 1–3 hours. Taking the drug with a high fatty meal, C_{max} is increased 112% and the area under the curve (AUC) increased 264% higher than if given without food. Both telotristat and its active metabolite are 99% protein bound to plasma proteins. Elimination half-life for telotristat ethyl is 0.6 hours, and 5 hours for telotristat. Telotristat is further metabolized, and 93.2% of telotristat ethyl dose is recovered in 10 days (92.8% in feces, and < 0.4% in the urine). It is unknown whether severe renal impairment (CrCl < 20 mL/hr) or moderate to severe hepatic impairment affect drug metabolism or excretion.

Indications: Treatment of adult patients with carcinoid syndrome who have inadequate control of diarrhea with somatostatin analogue (SSA) therapy alone; telotristat ethyl is given in combination with SSA therapy.

Contraindication: None.

Dosage Range:
- 250 mg tablet PO three times a day, taken with food.
- Drug should be discontinued if severe constipation develops.

Drug Preparation: Oral, none. Available as 250 mg of telotristat ethyl.

Drug Administration:
- Teach patient to take tablet 3 times a day with food. Teach patient if a dose is missed, take the next dose at the regular time (do not take 2 doses to make up for the missed dose).
- If short-acting octreotide (as opposed to a long-acting) is used, administer octreotide at least 30 minutes after telotristat ethyl administration.
- Teach patient to monitor for constipation and to notify healthcare provider if this occurs. Drug should be stopped if severe constipation occurs.

Drug Interactions:
- **CYP3A4 substrates** (e.g., midazolam): decreased midazolam C_{max} and AUC. Use caution when coadministering and assess for decreased midazolam effect. Modify midazolam dosage accordingly.
- **Short-acting (SA) octreotide:** telotristat ethyl C_{max} and AUC reduced by 86 and 81% respectively; telotristat mean C_{max} reduced 79% and AUC by 68% when coadministered. Give SA octreotide at least 30 minutes after telotristat ethyl dose.

Laboratory Effects/Interference:
- **5-HIAA** (metabolite of serotonin) is increased in patients with carcinoid syndrome; with treatment, 5-HIAA should be reduced.

Special Considerations:
- Most common adverse reactions (>/=5%): nausea, headache, increased serum GGT, depression, flatulence, decreased appetite, peripheral edema, and pyrexia.
- Black Box Warning: Constipation is an uncommon but is significant side effect. Assess for and monitor patient for constipation, and discontinue drug for severe constipation.

Potential Toxicities/Side Effects and the Nursing Process

I. POTENTIAL ALTERATION IN ELIMINATION, CONSTIPATION

Defining Characteristics: Telotristat ethyl decreases the number of bowel movements a patient has. In the clinical trial, in a 36-week extension period, 8.6% of patients developed constipation. Of the patients with severe constipation, one patient developed intestinal perforation, and one bowel obstruction.

Nursing Implications: Assess bowel function, number of daily stools, and whether nocturnal diarrhea occurs. Teach patient to keep a diary to assess response. Teach patient that constipation may occur and to stop drug and notify healthcare provider if this occurs. Drug should be discontinued for severe constipation.

COMPLICATIONS

Appendix 1
Occupational Exposure to Hazardous Drugs

Since the first Occupational Safety and Health Administration (OSHA) recommendations for the safe handling of hazardous drugs in 1986, updated in 2016, together with the National Institute for Occupational Safety and Health (NIOSH) recommendations of 2004 to 2016, some oncology nurses continue to ignore recommendations. NIOSH establishes a list of hazardous drugs which is updated every two years. Not all oncology nurses consistently comply with the guidelines, especially in regard to using personal protective equipment (PPE); the guidelines are not enforceable by state or federal statute. This has been shown in a number of nursing research studies, including that by Friese et al. (2019). This cluster randomized controlled trial measured improvement in personal protective equipment (PPE) use when one group of oncology nurses received a one-hour educational module on PPE use with quarterly reminders (the control) compared to a second group of oncology nurses who received the control intervention plus tailored messages that attempted to address perceived barriers, together with quarterly data gathered on hazardous drug spills. The authors found that prior to the study, use of PPEs was suboptimal, and after the study, the suboptimal use of PPEs persisted (no significant change between groups). To change practice and enforce compliance with the updated recommendations, the USP <800> guideline, issued by the U.S. Pharmacopeial Convention, expands the existing guideline for compounding and administration of hazardous drugs, is enforceable, and will go into effect nationwide in December 2019. In addition, the American Society of Clinical Oncology (ASCO) has released a 2019 standard on safe handling of hazardous drugs, and this will potentially be included in the ASCO Quality Oncology Practice Initiative (Celano et al., 2019). For oncology nurses, despite having the knowledge of the potential risks of exposure to hazardous drugs, such as reproductive issues, oncology nurses often choose to ignore the recommendations of OSHA and NIOSH. For more detailed discussion, please see Polovich 2019, and other references.

Hazardous drugs

Hazardous drugs are defined as drugs that are capable of inducing one or more of the following adverse effects in animals or humans, such as carcinogenicity, teratogenicity or fetal developmental toxicity, reproductive toxicity, organ toxicity at low doses, genotoxicity. Drugs that are similar structurally or with similar toxicity to drugs classified as hazardous, are also considered hazardous drugs (Polovich, 2019).

   USP<800> Recommendations (selected) [Eisenberg, 2018; US Pharmacopeial Convention, 2019].

   In December 2019, healthcare organizations are required to have a specific hazardous drug program in place (Eisenberg, 2018) with policies and procedures specifically identifying handling of hazardous drugs from the time the drug is received by the institution, through pharmacy preparation, nurse administration, disposal after administration, and management of spills. This applies to oral as well as parenterally administered hazardous drugs, including those administered in the operating room, cystoscopy suite, intraperitoneally in the clinic, or administered to a nononcology patient on a nononcology setting. The nurse must be educated on the safe handling of hazardous drugs before being able to administer them and must have a competency determination annually. This already is established in many institutions. Education must be provided in a systematic way for spill management to appropriate personnel as hazardous drugs may be handled by nurses, housekeepers, or others depending upon where the spill occurs. Policies and procedures established by the institution/practice should also provide for alternative duty for workers who are actively trying to conceive, are pregnant, or are breastfeeding.

Specific statements include:

- Double chemotherapy gloves for all patients receiving hazardous drugs.
- Use disposable gowns demonstrated to resist chemotherapy (long sleeves, elastic knit cuffs, closed front, no seams or closures that would permit exposure).
- Full face chemical cartridge respirator or PAPR if risk of respirator exposure or when cleaning a hazardous drug that exceeds that which could be contained with a spill kit or if a known or suspected airborne exposure to powder or vapors occurs.
- Face shields and goggles for risk of spills such as working above eye level, cleaning spills, administering chemotherapy during surgery.
- Place used PPEs in a special container designated for hazardous drugs.
- Closed system transfer device (CSTD) required for administration of hazardous drug when route allows.
- Education required before handling hazardous drugs, and annually thereafter.
- System of medical surveillance for all employees handling hazardous drugs, with specific recommendations.

Next steps

As the USP <800> is fully implemented nationally, it will be important to evaluate compliance of oncology nurses in their practice. Not only will nurses need to have the knowledge (e.g., such as a chemotherapy provider card through ONS) but also demonstrate continued competence in safe handling of hazardous drugs. To ensure the safe handling of hazardous drugs, pharmacy, nursing, and physicians will need to collaborate and expect compliance. If ASCO makes their safe handling guideline.

References

Celano P, Fausel CA, Kennedy EB et al. Safe handling of hazardous drugs: ASCO standards. *J Clin Oncol* 2019; 37(7):598–609.

Eisenberg S. Hazardous drugs and USP<800>: Implications for nursing. *Clin J Oncol Nurs* 2018; 21(2):179–187.

Friese CR, Yang J, Mendelsohn-Victor K, and McCullagh MC. Randomized controlled trial of an intervention to improve nurses' hazardous drug handling. *Onc Nurs Forum* 10`9; 46(2):248–255.

National Institute for Occupational Safety and Health. (2016a). Hierarchy of controls. Available at http://www.cdc.gov/niosh/topics/hierarchy. Accessed June 15, 2019.

National Institute for Occupational Safety and Health. (2016b). *NIOSH list of antineoplastic and other hazardous drugs in healthcare settings, 2016* (DHHS [NIOSH] Publication No. 2016-161). Available at http://www.cdc.gov/niosh/docs/2016-161/default.html. Accessed June 15, 2019.

Occupational Safety and Health Administration. (2016). Controlling occupational exposure to hazardous drugs. Available at www.osha.gov/SLTC/hazardousdrugs/controlling_occexhazardousdrugs.html. Accessed June 15, 2019.

Polovich M. Safe handling of hazardous drugs. Chapter 12 in (Eds) Olsen MM, LeFebvre KB, Brassil KJ. Chemotherapy and immunotherapy guidelines and recommendations for practice. Pittsburgh, PA. Oncology Nursing Society, 2019, pp. 235–247.

U.S. Pharmacopeial Convention. (2017). USP General Chapter <800> Hazardous drugs—Handling in healthcare. *The United States Pharmacopeia–National Formulary* (USP 40–NF 35, Second Supplement). Available at http://www.usp.org/sites/default/files/usp/document/our-work/health-care-quality-safety/general-chapter-800.pdf. Accessed June 15, 2019.

This appendix provides a summary of the OSHA recommendations for minimizing exposure to hazardous drugs.

Occupational Exposure to Hazardous Drugs

A. Introduction

In response to numerous inquiries,[1] the Occupational Safety and Health Administration (OSHA) published guidelines for the management of cytotoxic (antineoplastic) drugs in the workplace in 1986.[106] At that time, surveys indicated little standardization in the use of engineering controls and personal protective equipment (PPE).[56, 73] Although practices have improved in subsequent years, problems still exist.[111] In addition, the occupational management of these chemicals has been further clarified. These trends, in conjunction with many information requests, have prompted OSHA to revise its recommendations for hazardous drug (HD) handling. In addition, some of these agents are covered under the Hazard Communication Standard (HCS) (29 CFR 1910.1200).[107] In order to provide recommendations consistent with current scientific knowledge, this informational guidance document has been expanded to cover HDs, in addition to the cytotoxic drugs (CDs) that were covered in the 1986 guidelines. The recommendations apply to all settings where employees are occupationally exposed to HDs, such as hospitals, physicians' offices, and home healthcare agencies. This review will:

- Provide criteria for classifying drugs as hazardous.
- Summarize the evidence supporting the management of HDs as an occupational hazard.
- Discuss the equipment and worker education recommended, as well as the legal requirements of standards, for the protection of workers exposed and potentially exposed to HDs.
- Update the important aspects of medical surveillance.
- List some common HDs currently in use.

Anesthetic agents have not been considered in this review. However, exposure to some of these agents is a recognized health hazard,[104] and they have been considered in a separate Technical Manual Chapter.

B. Categorization of Drugs as Hazardous

The purpose of this section is to describe the biologic effects of those pharmaceuticals that are considered hazardous. A number of pharmaceuticals in the healthcare setting may pose occupational risk to employees through acute and chronic workplace exposure. Past attention focused on drugs used to treat cancer. However, it is clear that many other agents also have toxicity profiles of concern. This recognition prompted the American Society of Hospital Pharmacists (ASHP) to define a class of agents as "HDs."[3] That report specified concerns about antineoplastic and nonantineoplastic HDs in use in most institutions throughout the country. OSHA shares this concern. The ASHP Technical Assistance Bulletin (TAB) described four drug characteristics, each of which could be considered hazardous:

- Genotoxicity.
- Carcinogenicity.
- Teratogenicity or fertility impairment.
- Serious organ or other toxic manifestation at low doses in experimental animals or treated patients.

Table A.1 lists some common drugs that are considered hazardous by the above criteria. There is no standardized reference for this information, nor is there complete consensus

Table A.1   Some Common Drugs Considered Hazardous

Chemical/Generic Name	Source*
ALTRETAMINE	C
AMINOGLUTETHIMIDE	A
AZATHIOPRINE	ACE
L-ASPARAGINASE	ABC
BLEOMYCIN	ABC
BUSULFAN	ABC
CARBOPLATIN	ABC
CARMUSTINE	ABC
CHLORAMBUCIL	ABCE
CHLORAMPHENICOL	E
CHLOROTRIANISENE	B
CHLOROZOTOCIN	E
CISPLATIN	ABCE
CYCLOSPORIN	E
CYCLOPHOSPHAMIDE	ABCE
CYTARABINE	ABC
DACARBAZINE	ABC
DACTINOMYCIN	ABC
DAUNORUBICIN	ABC
DIETHYLSTILBESTROL	BE
DOXORUBICIN	ABCE
ESTRADIOL	B
ESTRAMUSTINE	AB
ETHINYL ESTRADIOL	B
ETOPOSIDE	ABC

Chemical/Generic Name	Source*
FLOXURIDINE	AC
FLUOROURACIL	ABC
FLUTAMIDE	BC
GANCICLOVIR	AD
HYDROXYUREA	ABC
IDARUBICIN	AC
IFOSFAMIDE	ABC
INTERFERON-α	BC
ISOTRETINOIN	D
LEUPROLIDE	BC
LEVAMISOLE	C
LOMUSTINE	ABCE
MECHLORETHAMINE	BC
MEDROXYPROGESTERONE	B
MEGESTROL	BC
MELPHALAN	ABCE
MERCAPTOPURINE	ABC
METHOTREXATE	ABC
MITOMYCIN	ABC
MITOTANE	ABC
MITOXANTRONE	ABC
NAFARELIN	C
PIPOBROMAN	C
PLICAMYCIN	BC
PROCARBAZINE	ABCE
RIBAVIRIN	D
STREPTOZOCIN	AC
TAMOXIFEN	BC
TESTOLACTONE	BC
THIOGUANINE	ABC
THIOTEPA	ABC
URACIL MUSTARD	ACE
VIDARABINE	D
VINBLASTINE	ABC
VINCRISTINE	ABC
ZIDOVUDINE	D

Sources:
A The National Institutes of Health, Clinical Center Nursing Department
B Antineoplastic drugs in the *Physicians' Desk Reference*
C American Hospital Formulary, Antineoplastics
D Johns Hopkins Hospital
E International Agency for Research on Cancer

on all agents listed. Professional judgment by personnel trained in pharmacology/toxicology is essential in designating drugs as hazardous, and Reference 65 provides information regarding the development of such a list at one institution. Some drugs, which have a long history of safe use in humans despite in vitro or animal evidence to toxicity, may be excluded by the institution's experts by considerations such as those used to formulate GRAS (generally regarded as safe) lists by the FDA under the Food, Drug, and Cosmetics Act.

Table A.1 is not all-inclusive, should not be construed as complete, and represents an assessment of some, but not all, marketed drugs at a fixed point in time. Table A.1 was developed through consultation with institutions that have assembled teams of pharmacists and other healthcare personnel to determine which drugs should be used with caution. These teams reviewed product literature and drug information when considering each product.

Sources for this appendix are the *Physicians' Desk Reference,* Section 10:00 in the American Hospital Formulary Service Drug Information,[68] IARC publications (particularly Volume 50),[43] the Johns Hopkins Hospital, and the National Institutes of Health, Clinical Center Nursing Department. No attempt to include investigational drugs was made, but they should be prudently handled as HDs until adequate information becomes available to exclude them. Any determination of the hazard status of drugs should be periodically reviewed and updated as new information becomes available. Importantly, new drugs should routinely undergo a hazard assessment.

List of Abbreviations

ANSI	American National Standards Institute
ASHP	American Society of Hospital Pharmacists
BSC	Biological safety cabinet
CD	Cytotoxic drug
EPA	Environmental Protection Agency
HCS	Hazard communication standard
HD	Hazardous drug
HEPA	High-efficiency particulate air
IARC	International Agency for Research on Cancer
MSDS	Material safety data sheet
NIOSH	National Institute for Occupational Safety and Health
NTP	National Toxicology Program
OSHA	Occupational Safety and Health Administration
PPE	Personal protective equipment

In contrast, investigational drugs are new chemicals for which there is often little information on potential toxicity. Structure or activity relationships with similar chemicals and in vitro data can be considered in determining potential toxic effects. Investigational drugs should be prudently handled as HDs unless adequate information becomes available to exclude them.

Some major considerations by professionals trained in pharmacology/toxicology[65] in designating a drug as hazardous are:

- Is the drug designated as Therapeutic Category 10:00 (Antineoplastic Agent) in the American Hospital Formulary Service Drug Information?[68]
- Does the manufacturer suggest the use of special isolation techniques in its handling, administration, or disposal?
- Is the drug known to be a human mutagen, carcinogen, teratogen, or reproductive toxicant?
- Is the drug known to be carcinogenic or teratogenic in animals? (Drugs known to be mutagenic in multiple bacterial systems or animals should also be considered hazardous.)
- Is the drug known to be acutely toxic to an organ system?

C. Background: Hazardous Drugs as Occupational Risk

Preparation, administration, and disposal of HDs may expose pharmacists, nurses, physicians, and other healthcare workers to potentially significant workplace levels of these chemicals. The literature establishing these agents as occupational hazards deals primarily with CDs; however, documentation of adverse exposure effects from other HDs is rapidly accumulating.[15,40–43,59] The degree of absorption that takes place during work and the significance of secondary early biologic effects on each individual encounter are difficult to assess and may vary depending on the HD. As a result, it is difficult to set safe levels of exposure on the basis of current scientific information.

However, there are several lines of evidence supporting the toxic potential of these drugs if handled improperly. Therefore, it is essential to minimize exposure to all HDs. Summary tables of much of the data presented below can be found in Sorsa[95] and Rogers.[84]

1. Mechanism of Action

Most HDs either bind directly to genetic material in the cell nucleus or affect cellular protein synthesis. CDs may not distinguish between normal and cancerous cells. The growth and reproduction of the normal cells are often affected during treatment of cancerous cells.

2. Animal Data

Numerous studies document the carcinogenic, mutagenic, and teratogenic effects of HD exposure in animals. They are well summarized in the pertinent IARC publications.[37–43] Alkylating agents present the strongest evidence of carcinogenicity (e.g., cyclophosphamide, mechlorethamine hydrochloride [nitrogen mustard]). However, other classes, such as some antibiotics, have been implicated as well. Extensive evidence for mutagenic and reproductive effects can be found in all antineoplastic classes. The antiviral agent *ribavirin* has additionally been shown to be teratogenic in all rodent species tested.[31,49] The ASHP recommends that all pharmaceutical agents that are animal carcinogens be handled as if human carcinogens.

3. Human Data at Therapeutic Levels

Many HDs are known human carcinogens, for which there is no safe level of exposure. The development of secondary malignancies is a well-documented side effect of chemotherapy treatment.[52,86,90,115] Leukemia has been most frequently observed. However, other secondary malignancies, such as bladder cancer and lymphoma, have been documented in patients treated for other, usually solid, primary malignancies.[52,114] Chromosomal aberrations can result from chemotherapy treatment as well. One study, on *chlorambucil*, reveals chromosomal damage in recipients to be cumulative and related to both dose and duration of therapy.[77]

Numerous case reports have linked chemotherapeutic treatment to adverse reproductive outcomes.[7,88,91,98] Testicular and ovarian dysfunction, including permanent sterility, have occurred in male and female patients who have received CDs either singly or in combination.[14] In addition, some antineoplastic agents are known or suspected to be transmitted to infants through breastmilk.[79]

The literature also documents the effects of these drugs on other organ systems. Extravasation of some agents can cause severe soft-tissue injury, consisting of necrosis and sloughing of exposed areas.[23,78,87] Other HDs, such as *pentamidine* and *zidovudine* (formerly AZT), are known to have significant side effects (i.e., hematologic abnormalities) in treated patients.[4,33] Serum transaminase elevation has also been reported in treated patients.[4,33]

4. Occupational Exposure—Airborne Levels

Monitoring efforts for CDs have detected measurable air levels when exhaust biological safety cabinets (BSCs) were not used for preparation or when monitoring was performed inside the BSC.[50,73]

Concentrations of *fluorouracil* ranging from 0.12 to 82.26 ng/m^3 have been found during monitoring of drug preparation without a BSC implying an opportunity for respiratory exposure.[73] Elevated concentrations of *cyclophosphamide* were found by these authors as well. Cyclophosphamide has also been detected on the HEPA filters of flow hoods used in HD preparation, demonstrating aerosolization of the drug and an exposure opportunity mitigated by effective engineering controls.[81]

A recent study has reported wipe samples of cyclophosphamide, one of the Class I IARC carcinogens, on surfaces of work stations in an oncology pharmacy and outpatient treatment areas (sinks and countertops). Concentrations ranged from 0.005 to 0.03 μg/cm^2, documenting opportunity for dermal exposure.[60]

Administration of drugs via aerosolization can lead to measurable air concentrations in the breathing zone of workers providing treatment. Concentrations up to 18 μg/m^3 have been found by personal air sampling of workers administering *pentamidine*.[67] Similar monitoring for *ribavirin* has found concentrations as high as 316 μg/m.[3,31]

5. Occupational Exposure—Biologic Evidence of Absorption
Urinary Mutagenicity

Falck et al. were the first to note evidence of mutagenicity in the urine of nurses who handled CDs.[26] The extent of this effect increased over the course of the workweek.

With improved handling practices, a decrease in mutagenic activity was seen.[27] Researchers have also studied pharmacy personnel who reconstitute antineoplastic drugs. These employees showed increasingly mutagenic urine over the period of exposure; when they stopped handling the drugs, activity fell within 2 days to the level of unexposed controls.[5,76] They also found mutagenicity in workers using horizontal laminar flow BSCs that decreased to control levels with the use of vertical flow containment BSCs.[76] Other studies have failed to find a relationship between exposure and urine mutagenicity.[25] Sorsa[95] summarizes this information and discusses the factors, such as differences in urine collection timing and variations in the use of PPE, which could lead to disparate results. Differences may also be related to smoking status; smokers exposed to CDs exhibit greater urine mutagenicity than exposed nonsmokers or control smokers, suggesting contamination of the work area by CDs and some contribution of smoking to their mutagenic profile.[9]

Urinary Thioethers

Urinary thioethers are glutathione-conjugated metabolites of alkylating agents that have been evaluated as an indirect means of measuring exposure. Workers who handle CDs have been reported to have increased levels compared to controls and also have increasing thioether levels over a 5-day work week.[44,48] Other studies of nurses who handle CDs and of treated patients have yielded variable results that could be due to confounding by smoking, PPE, and glutathione-S-transferase activity.[11]

Urinary Metabolites

Venitt[112] assayed the urine of pharmacy and nursing personnel handling cisplatin and found platinum concentrations at or below the limit of detection for both workers and controls. Hirst[35] found *cyclophosphamide* in the urine of two nurses who handled the drug, documenting worker absorption. (Hirst also documented skin absorption in human volunteers by using gas chromatography after topical application of the drug.) Urinary *pentamidine* recovery has also been reported in exposed healthcare workers.[94]

6. Occupational Exposure—Human Effects
Cytogenetic Effects

A number of studies have examined the relationship of exposure to CDs in the workplace to chromosomal aberrations. These studies have looked at a variety of markers for damage, including sister chromatid exchanges (SCE), structural aberrations (e.g., gaps, breaks, translocations), and micronuclei in peripheral blood lymphocytes. The results have been somewhat conflicting. Several authors found increases in one or more markers.[74,75,88,113] Increased mutilation frequency has been reported as well.[17] Other studies have failed to find a significant difference between workers and controls.[99,101] Some researchers have found higher individual elevations[28] or a relationship between number of drugs handled and SCEs.[8] These disparate results are not unexpected. The difficulties in quantitating exposure have resulted in different exposure magnitudes between studies; workers in several negative studies appear to have a lower overall exposure.[10] In addition, differences in the use of PPE and work technique will alter absorption of CDs and resultant biologic effects.

Finally, techniques for SCE measurement may not be optimal. A recent study that looked at correlation of phosphoramide-induced SCE levels with duration of anticancer drug handling found a statistically significant correlation coefficient of 0.[63,66]

Taken together, the evidence indicates an excess of markers of mutagenic exposure in unprotected workers.

Reproductive Effects

Reproductive effects associated with occupational exposure to CDs have been well documented. Hemminki et al.[32] found no difference in exposure between nurses who had spontaneous abortions and those who had normal pregnancies. However, the study group consisted of nurses who were employed in surgical or medical floors of a general hospital. When the relationship between CD exposure and congenital malformations was explored, the study group was expanded to include oncology nurses, among others, and an odds ratio of 4:7 was found for exposures of more than once per week. This observed odds ratio is statistically significant. Selevan et al.[39] found a relationship between CD exposure and spontaneous abortion in a case-control study of Finnish nurses. This well-designed study reviewed the reproductive histories of 568 women (167 cases) and found a statistically significant odds ratio of 2:3. Similar results were obtained in another large case-control study of French nurses,[102] and a study of Baltimore area nurses found a significantly higher proportion of adverse pregnancy outcomes when exposure to antineoplastic agents occurred during the pregnancy.[85] The nurses involved in these studies usually prepared and administered the drugs. Therefore, workplace exposure of these groups of professionals to such products has been associated with adverse reproductive outcomes in several investigations.

Other Effects

Hepatocellular damage has been reported in nurses working in an oncology ward; the injury appeared to be related to intensity and duration of work exposure to CDs.[96] Symptoms such as lightheadedness, dizziness, nausea, headache, and allergic reactions have also been described in employees after the preparation and administration of antineoplastic drugs in unventilated areas.[22,96] In occupational settings, these agents are known to be toxic to the skin and mucous membranes, including the cornea.[69,82]

Pentamidine has been associated with respiratory damage in one worker who administered the aerosol. The injury consisted of a decrease in diffusing capacity that improved after exposure ceased.[29] The onset of bronchospasm in a pentamidine-exposed worker has also been reported.[22] Employees involved in the aerosol administration of *ribavirin* have noted symptoms of respiratory tract irritation.[55] A number of medications including *psyllium* and various antibiotics are known respiratory and dermal sensitizers. Exposure in susceptible individuals can lead to asthma or allergic contact dermatitis.

D. Work Areas

Risks to personnel working with HDs are a function of the drugs' inherent toxicity and the extent of exposure. The main routes of exposure are: inhalation of dusts or aerosols, dermal absorption, and ingestion. The primary means of ingestion is contact with contaminated food or cigarettes. Opportunity for exposure to HDs may occur at many points in the handling of these drugs.

1. Pharmacy or Other Preparation Areas

In large oncology centers, HDs are usually prepared in the pharmacy. However, in small hospitals, outpatient treatment areas, and physicians' offices they have been prepared by physicians or nurses without appropriate engineering controls and protective apparel.[16,20] Many HDs must be reconstituted, transferred from one container to another, or manipulated before administration to patients. Even if care is taken, opportunity for absorption through inhalation or direct skin contact can occur.[35,36,73,116] Examples of manipulations that can cause splattering, spraying, and aerosolization include:

- Withdrawal of needles from drug vials.
- Drug transfer using syringes and needles or filter straws.
- Breaking open of ampoules.
- Expulsion of air from a drug-filled syringe.

Evaluation of these preparation techniques, using fluorescent dye solutions, has shown contamination of gloves and the sleeves and chest of gowns.[97]

Horizontal airflow workbenches provide an aseptic environment for the preparation of injectable drugs. However, these units provide a flow of filtered air originating at the back of the workspace and exiting toward the employee using the unit. Thus, they increase the likelihood of drug exposure for both the preparer and other personnel in the room. As a result, the use of horizontal BSCs is contraindicated in the preparation of HDs. Smoking, drinking, applying cosmetics, and eating where these drugs are prepared, stored, or used also increase the chance of exposure.

2. Administration of Drugs to Patients

Administration of drugs to patients is generally performed by nurses or physicians. Drug injection into the IV line, clearing of air from the syringe or infusion line, and leakage at the tubing, syringe, or stopcock connection present opportunities for skin contact and aerosol generation. Clipping used needles and crushing used syringes can produce considerable aerosolization as well.

Such techniques where needles and syringes are contaminated with blood or other potentially infectious material are prohibited by the Bloodborne Pathogens Standard.[109] Prohibition of clipping or crushing of any needle or syringe is sound practice.

Excreta from patients who have received certain antineoplastic drugs may contain high concentrations of the drug or its hazardous metabolites. For example, patients receiving *cyclophosphamide* excrete large amounts of the drug and its mutagenic metabolites.[46,92] Patients treated with *cisplatin* have been shown to excrete potentially hazardous amounts of the drug.[112] Unprotected handling of urine or urine-soaked sheets by nursing or housekeeping personnel poses a source of exposure.

3. Disposal of Drugs and Contaminated Materials

Contaminated materials used in the preparation and administration of HDs, such as gloves, gowns, syringes, and vials, present a hazard to support and housekeeping staff. The use of properly labeled, sealed, and covered disposal containers, handled by trained and protected personnel, should be routine and is required under the Bloodborne Pathogens Standard[109] if such items are contaminated with blood or other potentially infectious materials. HDs and contaminated materials should be disposed of in accordance with federal, state, and local laws. Disposal of some of these drugs is regulated by the EPA. Those drugs that are unused commercial chemical products and are considered by the EPA to be toxic wastes must be disposed of in accordance with 40 CFR Part 261.33.[24] Spills can also represent a hazard; the employer should ensure that all employees are familiar with appropriate spill procedures.

4. Survey of Current Work Practices

Surveys of U.S. cancer centers and oncology clinics reveal wide variation in work practices, equipment, or training for personnel preparing CDs.[56,73] This lack of standardization results in a high prevalence of potential occupational exposure to CDs. One survey found that 40% of hospital pharmacists reported a skin exposure to CDs at least once a month, and only 28% had medical surveillance programs in their workplace.[16] Nurses, particularly those in outpatient settings, were found to be even less well protected than pharmacists.[111] Such findings emphasize current lack of protection for all personnel who risk potential exposure to HDs.

E. Prevention of Employee Exposure

1. Hazardous Drug Safety and Health Plan

Where HDs, as defined in this review, are used in the workplace, sound practice would dictate that a written Hazardous Drug Safety and Health Plan be developed. Such a plan assists in:

- Protecting employees from health hazards associated with HDs.
- Keeping exposures as low as reasonably achievable.

When a Hazardous Drug Safety and Health Plan is developed, it should be readily available and accessible to all employees, including temporary employees, contractors, and trainees.

The ASHP recommends that the plan include each of the following elements and indicate specific measures that the employer is taking to ensure employee protection[3]:

- Standard operating procedures relevant to safety and health considerations to be followed when healthcare workers are exposed to HDs.
- Criteria that the employer uses to determine and implement control measures to reduce employee exposure to HDs including engineering controls, the use of PPE, and hygiene practices.
- A requirement that ventilation systems and other protective equipment function properly, and specific measures to ensure proper and adequate performance of such equipment.
- Provision for information and training.
- The circumstances under which the use of specific HDs (i.e., FDA investigational drugs) require prior approval from the employer before implementation.

- Provision for medical examinations of potentially exposed personnel.
- Designation of personnel responsible for implementation of the Hazardous Drug Safety and Health Plan, including the assignment of a Hazardous Drug Officer (who is an industrial hygienist, nurse, or pharmacist health and safety representative); and, if appropriate, establishment of a Hazardous Drug Committee or a joint Hazardous Drug Committee/Chemical Committee.

The ASHP further recommends that specific consideration of the following provisions be included where appropriate:

- Establishment of a designated HD handling area.
- Use of containment devices such as BSCs.
- Procedures for safe removal of contaminated waste.
- Decontamination procedures.

The ASHP recommends that the Hazardous Drug Safety and Health Plan be reviewed and its effectiveness reevaluated at least annually and updated as necessary.

A comparison of OSHA 200 log entries to employee medical clinic appointment or visit rosters can be made[3] to establish if there is evidence of disorders that could be related to HD.

Previous health and safety inspections by local health departments, fire departments, regulatory or accrediting agencies may be helpful for the facility's planning purposes, as well as any OSHA review of hazards and programs in the facility. Joint Commission on Accreditation of Healthcare Organizations (JCAHO) or College of American Pathologists (CAP) review of facilities may contain information on HDs used in the facility.

2. Drug Preparation Precautions
Work Area
The ASHP recommends that HD preparation be performed in a restricted, preferably centralized, area. Signs restricting the access of unauthorized personnel are to be prominently displayed. Eating, drinking, smoking, chewing gum, applying cosmetics, and storing food in the preparation area should be prohibited.[71] The ASHP recommends that procedures for spills and emergencies, such as skin or eye contact, be available to workers, preferably posted in the area.[3]

Biological Safety Cabinets
Class II or III BSCs that meet the current National Sanitation Foundation Standard 49[70,72] should minimize exposure to HDs during preparation. Although these cabinets are designed for biohazards, several studies have documented reduced urine mutagenicity in CD-exposed workers or reduce environmental levels after the institution of BSCs.[5,51,61] If a BSC is unavailable—for example, in a private practice office—accepted medical practice is the sharing of a cabinet (e.g., several medical offices share a cabinet) or sending the patient to a center where HDs can be prepared in a BSC. Alternatively, preparation can be performed in a facility with a BSC and the drugs transported to the area of administration. Use of a dedicated BSC, where only HDs are prepared, is prudent medical practice.

Types of BSCs

Four main types of Class II BSCs are available. They all have downward airflow and HEPA filters. They are differentiated by the amount of air recirculated within the cabinet, whether this air is vented to the room or the outside, and whether contaminated ducts are under positive or negative pressure. These four types are:

- Type A cabinets recirculate approximately 70% of cabinet air through HEPA filters back into the cabinet; the rest is discharged through a HEPA filter into the preparation room. Contaminated ducts are under positive pressure.
- Type B1 cabinets have higher velocity air inflow, recirculate 30% of the cabinet air, and exhaust the rest to the outside through HEPA filters. They have negative pressure contaminated ducts and plenums.
- Type B2 systems are similar to type B1 except that no air is recirculated.
- Type B3 cabinets are similar to type A in that they recirculate approximately 70% of cabinet air. However, the other 30% is vented to the outside and the ducts are under negative pressure.

　　Class III cabinets are totally enclosed with gas-tight construction. The entire cabinet is under negative pressure, and operations are performed through attached gloves. All air is HEPA-filtered.

　　Class II, type B, or Class III BSCs are recommended since they vent to the outside.[3] Those without air recirculation are the most protective. If the BSC has an outside exhaust, it should be vented away from air intake units.

　　The blower on the vertical airflow hood should be on at all times. If the BSC is turned off, it should be decontaminated and covered in plastic until airflow is resumed.[3,72] Each BSC should be equipped with a continuous monitoring device to allow confirmation of adequate air flow and cabinet performance. The cabinet should be in an area with minimal air turbulence; this will reduce leakage to the environment.[6,70] Additional information on design and performance testing of BSCs can be found in papers by Avis and Levchuck,[6] Bryan and Marback,[10] and the National Sanitation Foundation.[70] Practical information regarding space needs and conversion possibilities is contained in the ASHP's 1990 technical assistance bulletins.[3]

　　Ventilation and BSCs installed should be maintained and evaluated for proper performance in accordance with the manufacturer's instructions.

Decontamination

The cabinet should be cleaned according to the manufacturer's instructions. Some manufacturers have recommended weekly decontamination as well as whenever spills occur or when the cabinet requires moving, service, or certification.

　　Decontamination should consist of surface cleaning with water and detergent, followed by thorough rinsing. The use of detergent is recommended because there is no single accepted method of chemical deactivation for all agents involved.[13,45] Quaternary ammonium cleaners should be avoided due to the possibility of vapor buildup in recirculated air.[3] Ethyl alcohol or 70% isopropyl alcohol may be used with the cleaner if the contamination is soluble only in alcohol.[3] Alcohol vapor buildup has also been a concern, so the use of alcohol should be avoided in BSCs where air is recirculated.[3] Spray cleaners should also be avoided due to the risk of spraying the HEPA filter. Ordinary decontamination procedures, which include fumigation with a germicidal agent, are inappropriate in a BSC used for HDs because such procedures do not remove or deactivate the drugs.

Removable work trays, if present, should be lifted in the BSC, so the back and the sump below can be cleaned. During cleaning, the worker should wear PPE similar to that used for spills. *Ideally, the sash should remain down during cleaning; however, a NIOSH-approved respirator appropriate for the hazard must be worn by the worker if the sash will be lifted during the process.* The exhaust fan/blower should be left on. Cleaning should proceed from least to most contaminated areas. The drain spillage trough area should be cleaned twice since it can be heavily contaminated. All materials from the decontamination process should be handled as HDs and disposed of in accordance with federal, state, and local laws.

Service and Certification

The ASHP recommends that BSCs be serviced and certified by a qualified technician every 6 months or any time the cabinet is moved or repaired.[3,71] Technicians servicing these cabinets or changing the HEPA filters should be aware of HD risk through hazard communication training from their employers and should use the same PPE as recommended for large spills. Certification of the BSC includes performance testing as outlined in the procedures of the National Sanitation Foundation's Standard Number 49.[70] Helpful information on such testing can be found in the ASHP 1990 technical assistance bulletins,[3] the BSC manufacturer's equipment manuals, and Bryan and Marback's paper.[10] HEPA filters should be changed when they restrict air flow or if they are contaminated by an accidental spill. They should be bagged in plastic and disposed of as HDs. Any time the cabinet is turned off or transported, it should be sealed with plastic.

Personal Protective Equipment

1. Gloves

Research indicates that the thickness of gloves used in handling HDs is more important than the type of material, since all materials tested have been found to be permeable to some HDs.[3,19,53] The best results are seen with latex gloves. Therefore, latex gloves should be used for the preparation of HDs unless the drug-product manufacturer specifically stipulates that some other glove provides better protection.[19,53,72,93,100] Thicker, longer latex gloves that cover the gown cuff are recommended for use with HDs. *Individuals with latex allergy should consider the use of vinyl or nitrile gloves or glove liners.* Gloves with minimal or no powder are preferred since the powder may absorb contamination.[3,104]

The sources referenced here have noted great variability in permeability within and between glove lots. Therefore, double gloving is recommended if it does not interfere with an individual's technique.[3] Because all gloves are permeable to some extent and their permeability increases with time, they should be changed regularly (hourly) or immediately if they are torn, punctured, or contaminated with a spill. Hands should always be washed before gloves are put on and after they are removed. Employees need thorough training in proper methods for contaminated glove removal.

2. Gowns

A protective disposable gown made of lint-free, low-permeability fabric with a closed front, long sleeves, and elastic or knit closed cuff should be worn. The cuffs should be tucked under the gloves. If double gloves are worn, the outer glove should be over the gown cuff and the inner glove should be under the gown cuff. When the gown is removed, the inner glove should be removed last. Gowns and gloves in use in the HD preparation area should not be used outside the HD preparation area.[3]

As with gloves, there is no ideal material. Research has found nonporous Tyvek and Kaycel to be more permeable than Saranex-laminated Tyvek and polyethylene-coated Tyvek after 4 hours of exposure to the CDs tested.[54] However, little airflow is allowed with the latter materials. As a result, manufacturers have produced gowns with Saranex or polyethylene reinforced sleeves and front in an effort to decrease permeability in the most exposure-prone areas, but little research exists on decreasing exposure.

3. Respiratory Protection

A BSC is essential for the preparation of HDs. Where a BSC is not currently available, a *NIOSH-approved respirator** *appropriate for the hazard must be worn to afford protection until the BSC is installed.* The use of respirators must comply with OSHA's Respiratory Protection Standard,[105] which outlines the aspects of a respirator program, including selection, fit testing, and worker training. Surgical masks are *not appropriate*, since they *do not prevent* aerosol inhalation. Permanent respirator use, in lieu of BSCs, is imprudent practice and should not be a substitute for engineering controls.

4. Eye and Face Protection

Whenever splashes, sprays, or aerosols of HDs may be generated, which can result in eye, nose, or mouth contamination, chemical barrier face and eye protection must be provided and used in accordance with 29 CFR 1910.133. Eyeglasses with temporary side shields are inadequate protection.

When a respirator is used to provide temporary protection as described here, and splashes, sprays, or aerosols are possible, employee protection should be either:

- A respirator with a full face piece, or
- A plastic face shield or splash goggles complying with ANSI standards[2] when using a respirator of less than full face piece design.
- Eyewash facilities should also be made available.

5. PPE Disposal and Decontamination

All gowns, gloves, and disposable materials used in preparation should be disposed of according to the hospital's HD waste procedures and as described under this review's section on Waste Disposal. Goggles, face shields, and respirators may be cleaned with mild detergent and water for reuse.

---

*NIOSH recommendation at the time of this publication is for a respirator with a high-efficiency filter, preferably a powered air-purifying respirator.

Work Equipment

NIH has recommended the work with HDs be carried out in a BSC on a disposable, plastic-backed paper liner. The liner should be changed after preparation is completed for the day, or after a shift, whichever comes first. Liners should also be changed after a spill.[103]

Syringes and IV sets with Luer-Lok fittings should be used for HDs. Syringe size should be large enough so that they are not full when the entire drug dose is present.

A covered disposable container should be used to contain excess solution. A covered sharps container should be in the BSC.

The ASHP recommends that HD-labeled plastic bags be available for all contaminated materials (including gloves, gowns, and paper liners), so that contaminated material can be immediately placed in them and disposed of in accordance with ASHP recommendations.[3]

Work Practices

Correct work practices are essential to worker protection. *Aseptic technique* is assumed as a standard practice in drug preparation. The general principles of aseptic technique, therefore, will not be detailed here. It should be noted, however, that BSC benches differ from horizontal flow units in several ways that require special precautions. Manipulations should not be performed close to the work surface of a BSC. Unsterilized items, including liners and hands, should be kept downstream from the working area. Entry and exit of the cabinet should be perpendicular to the front. Rapid lateral hand movements should be avoided. Additional information can be found in the National Sanitation Foundation Standard 49 for Class II (Laminar Flow) Biohazard Cabinetry[70] and Avis and Levchuck's paper.[6] All operators should be trained in these containment-area protocols.

All PPE should be donned before work is started in the BSC. All items necessary for drug preparation should be placed within the BSC before work is begun. Extraneous items should be kept out of the work area.

1. Labeling

In addition to standard pharmacy labeling practices, all syringes and IV bags containing HDs should be labeled with a distinctive warning label such as:

SPECIAL HANDLING/Disposal Precautions

In addition, those HDs covered under HCS must have labels in accordance with section (f) of the standard to warn employees handling the drug(s) of the hazards.

2. Disposing of Needles

The ASHP recommends that all syringes and needles used in the course of preparation be placed in medical waste-disposal (sharps) containers for disposal without being crushed, clipped, or capped.[3,103]

3. Priming

Prudent practice dictates that drug administration sets be attached and primed within the BSC prior to addition of the drug. This eliminates the need to prime the set in a less well-controlled environment and ensures that any fluid that escapes during priming contains no drug. If priming must occur at the site of administration, the intravenous line should be primed with nondrug-containing fluid, or a backflow closed system should be used.[3]

4. Handling Vials

Extremes of positive and negative pressure in medication vials should be avoided, for example, attempting to withdraw 10 mL of fluid from a 10-mL vial, or placing 10 mL of a fluid into an air-filled 10-mL vial. The use of large-bore needles, #18 or #20, avoids *high-pressure syringing* of solutions. However, some experienced personnel believe that large-bore needles are more likely to drip. Multi-use dispensing pins are recommended to avoid these problems.

Venting devices such as filter needles or dispensing pins permit outside air to replace the withdrawn liquid. Proper worker education is essential before using these devices.[3] Although venting devices are recommended, another technique is to add diluent slowly to the vial by alternately injecting small amounts and allowing displaced air to escape into the syringe. When all diluent has been added, a small amount of additional air may be withdrawn to create a slight negative pressure in the vial. This should not be expelled into room air because it may contain drug residue. It should either be injected into a vacuum vial or remain in the syringe to be discarded.

If any negative pressure must be applied to withdraw a dosage from a stoppered vial and handling safety is compromised, an air-filled syringe should be used to equalize pressure in the stoppered vial. The volume of drug to be withdrawn can be replaced by injecting small amounts of air into the vial and withdrawing equal amounts of liquid until the required volume is withdrawn. The drug should be cleared from the needle and hub (neck) of the syringe before separating to reduce spraying on separation.

5. Handling Ampules

Prudent practice requires that ampules with dry material should be *gently tapped down* before opening to move any material in the top of the ampule to the bottom quantity. A sterile gauze pad should be wrapped around the ampule neck before breaking the top.[3] This can protect against cuts and catch airborne powder or aerosol. If diluent is to be added, it should be injected slowly down the inside wall of the ampule. The ampule should be tilted gently to ensure that all the powder is wet before agitating it to dissolve the contents.

After the solution is withdrawn from the ampule with a syringe, the needle should be cleared of solution by holding it vertically with the point upwards; the syringe should be tapped to remove air bubbles. Any bubbles should be expelled into a closed container.

6. Packaging HDs for Transport

The outside of bags or bottles containing the prepared drug should be wiped with moist gauze.

Entry ports should be wiped with moist alcohol pads and capped. Transport should occur in sealed plastic bags and in containers designed to avoid breakage.

HDs that are shipped and that are subject to EPA regulation as hazardous waste are also subject to Department of Transportation (DOT) regulations as specified in 49 CFR Part 172.101.

7. Handling Nonliquid HDs

The handling of nonliquid forms of HDs requires special precautions as well. Tablets that may produce dust or potential exposure to the handler should be counted in a BSC. Capsules (i.e., gel caps or coated tablets) are unlikely to produce dust unless broken in handling.

These are counted in a BSC on equipment designated for HDs only, because even manual counting devices may be covered with dust from the drugs handled. Automated counting machines should not be used unless an enclosed process isolates the hazard from the employee(s).

Compounding should also occur in a BSC. A gown and gloves should be worn. *(If a BSC is unavailable, an appropriate NIOSH-approved respirator must be worn.)*

Drug Administration

1. Personal Protective Equipment

The National Study Commission on Cytotoxic Exposure has recommended that personnel administering HDs wear gowns, latex gloves, and chemical splash goggles or equivalent safety glasses as described under the PPE Section, Preparation.[71] *NIOSH-approved respirators should be worn when administering aerosolized drugs.*

2. Administration Kit

Protective and administration equipment may be packaged together and labeled as an HD administration kit. Such a kit should include:

- Personal protective equipment.
- Gauze (4 × 4) for cleanup.
- Alcohol wipes.
- Disposable plastic-backed absorbent liner.
- Puncture-resistant container for needles and syringes.
- Thick sealable plastic bag (with warning label).
- Accessory warning labels.

3. Work Practices

Safe work practices when handling HDs should include:

- Hands should be washed before donning and after removing gloves. Gowns or gloves that become contaminated should be changed immediately. Employees should be trained in proper methods to remove contaminated gloves and gowns. After use, gloves and gowns should be disposed of in accordance with ASHP recommendations.
- Infusion sets and pumps, which should have Luer-Lok fittings, should be observed for leakage during use. A plastic-backed absorbent pad should be placed under the tubing during administration to catch any leakage. Sterile gauze should be placed around any push sites; IV tubing connection sites should be taped.
- Priming IV sets or expelling air from syringes should be carried out in a BSC. If done at the administration site, ASHP recommends that the line be primed with nondrug-containing solution or that a backflow closed system be used. IV containers with venting tubes should not be used.[3]

- Syringes, IV bottles and bags, and pumps should be wiped clean of any drug contamination with sterile gauze. Needles and syringes should not be crushed or clipped. They should be placed in a puncture-resistant container and then into the HD disposal bag with all other HD-contaminated materials. Administration sets should be disposed of intact. Disposal of the waste bag should follow HD disposal requirements. Unused drugs should be returned to the pharmacy.
- Protective goggles should be cleaned with detergent and properly rinsed. All protective equipment should be disposed of upon leaving the patient care area.
- Nursing stations where these drugs will be administered should have spill and emergency skin and eye decontamination kits available and relevant MSDSs for guidance. The HCS requires MSDSs to be readily available in the workplace to all employees working with hazardous chemicals.
- PPE should be used during the administration of oral HDs if splashing is possible.

A large number of investigational HDs are under clinical study in healthcare facilities. Personnel not directly involved in the investigation should not administer these drugs unless they have received adequate instructions regarding safe handling procedures. Literature regarding potential toxic effects of investigational drugs should be evaluated prior to the drug's introduction into the workplace.[65]

The increased use of HDs in the home environment necessitates special precautions. Employees involved in home care delivery should follow the above work practices, and employers should make administration and spill kits available. Home healthcare workers should have emergency protocols with them, as well as phone numbers and addresses, in the event emergency care becomes necessary.[3] Waste disposal for drugs delivered for home use and other home-contaminated material should also be considered by the employer and should follow applicable regulations.

4. Aerosolized Drugs

The administration of aerosolized HDs requires special engineering controls to prevent exposure to healthcare workers and others in the vicinity. In the case of *pentamidine*, these controls include treatment booths with local exhaust ventilation designed specifically for its administration. A variety of ventilation methods have also been used for the administration of *ribavirin*. These include isolation rooms with separate HEPA-filtered ventilation systems and administration via endotracheal tube.[30,47] Engineering controls used to manage employee exposure to anesthetic gases is a traditional example of occupational chemical management. Both isolation and ventilation are used for these volatile HDs.

Caring for Patients Receiving HDs

In accordance with the Bloodborne Pathogens Standard, universal precautions must be observed to prevent contact with blood or other potentially infectious materials. Under circumstances in which differentiation between body fluid types is difficult or impossible, all body fluids should be considered potentially infectious materials and must be managed as dictated in the Bloodborne Pathogens Standard.[109]

1. Personal Protective Equipment

Personnel dealing with excreta, primarily urine, from patients who have received HDs in the last 48 hours should be provided with and wear latex or other appropriate gloves and disposable gowns, to be discarded after each use or whenever contaminated, as detailed under Waste Disposal. Eye protection should be worn if splashing is possible. Such excreta contaminated with blood, or other potentially infectious materials as well, should be managed according to the Bloodborne Pathogen Standard. Hands should be washed after removal of gloves or after contact with the above substances.

2. Linen
Linen contaminated with HDs or excreta from patients who have received HDs in the past 48 hours is a potential source of exposure to employees. Linen soiled with blood or other potentially infectious materials, as well as contaminated with excreta, must also be managed according to the Bloodborne Pathogens Standard.[109] Linen contaminated with HDs should be placed in specially marked laundry bags and then placed in a labeled, impervious bag. The laundry bag and its contents should be prewashed, and then the linens added to other laundry for a second wash. Laundry personnel should wear latex gloves and gowns while handling prewashed material.

3. Reusable Items
Glassware or other contaminated reusable items should be washed twice with detergent by a trained employee wearing double latex gloves and a gown.

Waste Disposal
1. Equipment
Thick, leakproof plastic bags, colored differently from other hospital trash bags, should be used for routine accumulation and collection of used containers, discarded gloves, gowns, and any other disposable material. Bags containing hazardous chemicals (as defined by Section C of HCS), shall be labeled in accordance with Section F of the Hazard Communication Standard where appropriate. Where the Hazard Communication Standard does not apply, labels should indicate that bags contain HD-related wastes.

Needles, syringes, and breakable items not contaminated with blood or other potentially infectious materials should be placed in a waste-disposal (sharps) container before they are stored in the waste bag. Such items that are contaminated with blood or other potentially infectious material *must* be placed in a sharps container. Similarly, needles should not be clipped or capped nor syringes crushed. If contaminated by blood or other potentially infectious material, such needles/syringes *must not* be clipped, capped, or crushed (except in a rare instance where a *medical* procedure requires recapping). The waste bag should be kept inside a covered waste container clearly labeled "HD Waste Only." At least one such receptacle should be located in every area where the drugs are prepared or administered. Waste should not be moved from one area to another. The bag should be sealed when filled and the covered waste container taped.

2. Handling
Prudent practice dictates that every precaution be taken to prevent contamination of the exterior of the container. Personnel disposing of HD waste should wear gowns and protective gloves when handling waste containers with contaminated exteriors. Prudent practice further dictates that such a container with a contaminated exterior be placed in a second container in a manner that eliminates contamination of the second container. HD waste handlers should also receive hazard communication training as discussed in Section H.

3. Disposal

HD-related wastes should be handled separately from other hospital trash and disposed of in accordance with applicable EPA, state, and local regulations for hazardous waste.[24,110] This disposal can occur at either an incinerator or a licensed sanitary landfill for toxic wastes, as appropriate. Commercial waste disposal is performed by a licensed company. While awaiting removal, the waste should be held in a secure area in covered, labeled drums with plastic liners.

Chemical inactivation traditionally has been a complicated process that requires specialized knowledge and training. The MSDS should be consulted regarding specific advice on cleanup (IARC[13]) and Lunn et al.[56] have validated inactivation procedures for specific agents that are effective. However, these procedures vary from drug to drug and may be impractical for small amounts. Care must be taken because of unique problems presented by the cleanup of some agents, such as byproduct formation.[57] Serious consideration should be given to alternative disposal methods.

Spills

Emergency procedures to cover spills or inadvertent release of HDs should be included in the facility's overall health and safety program.

Incidental spills and breakages should be cleaned up immediately by a properly protected person trained in the appropriate procedures. The area should be identified with a warning sign to limit access to the area. Incident reports should be filed to document the spill and those exposed.

1. Personnel Contamination

Contamination of protective equipment or clothing, or direct skin or eye contact should be treated by:

- Immediately removing the gloves or gown.
- Immediately cleansing the affected skin with soap and water.
- Flooding an affected eye at an eyewash fountain or with water or isotonic eyewash designated for that purpose for at least 15 minutes, for eye exposure.
- Obtaining medical attention. (Protocols for emergency procedures should be maintained at the designated sites for such medical care. Medical attention should also be sought for inhalation of HDs in powder form.)
- Documenting the exposure in the employee's medical record.

2. Cleanup of Small Spills

The ASHP considers small spills to be those less than 5 mL. The 5-mL volume of material should be used to categorize spills as large or small. Spills of less than 5 mL or 5 mg outside a BSC should be cleaned up immediately by personnel wearing gowns, double latex gloves, and splash goggles. *An appropriate NIOSH-approved respirator should be used for either powder or liquid spills where airborne powder or aerosol is or has been generated.*

- Liquids should be wiped with absorbent gauze pads; solids should be wiped with wet absorbent gauze. The spill areas should then be cleaned three times using a detergent solution followed by clean water.

- Any broken glass fragments should be picked up using a small scoop (never the hands) and placed in a sharps container. The container should then go into an HD disposal bag, along with used absorbent pads and any other contaminated waste.
- Contaminated reusable items (e.g., glassware and scoops) should be treated as outlined under Reusable Items.

3. Cleanup of Large Spills
When a large spill occurs, the area should be isolated and aerosol generation avoided. For spills larger than 5 mL, liquid spread is limited by gently covering with absorbent sheets or spill-control pads or pillows. If a powder is involved, damp cloths or towels should be used. Specific individuals should be trained to clean up large spills.

- As with small spills, protective apparel and respirators should be used when there is any suspicion of airborne powder or that an aerosol has been or will be generated. Most CDs are not volatile; however, this may not be true for all HDs. The volatility of the drug should be assessed in selecting the type of respiratory protection.
- As discussed under Waste Disposal, chemical inactivation should be avoided in this setting.
- All contaminated surfaces should be thoroughly cleaned three times with detergent and water.
- All contaminated absorbent sheets and other materials should be placed in the HD disposal bag.

4. Spills in BSCs
Extensive spills within a BSC necessitate decontamination of all interior BSC surfaces after completion of the spill cleanup. The ASHP[3] recommends this action for spills larger than 150 mL or the contents of one vial. If the HEPA filter of a BSC is contaminated, the unit should be labeled and sealed in plastic until the filter can be changed and disposed of properly by trained personnel wearing appropriate protective equipment.

5. Spill Kits
Spill kits, clearly labeled, should be kept in or near preparation and administrative areas. The MSDSs include sections on emergency procedures, including appropriate PPE. The ASHP recommends that kits include chemical splash goggles, two pairs of gloves, utility gloves, a low-permeability gown, two sheets (12″ × 12″) of absorbent material, 250-mL and liter spill-control pillows, a waste-disposal (sharps) container, a small scoop to collect glass fragments, and two large HD waste-disposal bags.[3]

    Prior to cleanup, appropriate protective equipment should be used. Absorbent sheets should be incinerable. Protective goggles and respirators should be cleaned with mild detergent and water after use.

Storage and Transport
1. Storage Areas
Access to areas where HDs are stored should be limited to authorized personnel with signs restricting entry.[72] A list of drugs covered by HD policies and information on spill and emergency contact procedures should be posted or easily available to employees. Facilities

used for storing HDs should not be used for other drugs and should be designed to prevent containers from falling to the floor (e.g., bins with barrier fronts). Warning labels should be applied to all HD containers, as well as the shelves and bins where these containers are permanently stored.

2. Receipt of Damaged HD Packages

Damaged shipping cartons should be opened in an isolated area or a BSC by a designated employee wearing double gloves, a gown, goggles, and appropriate respiratory protection. Individuals must be trained to process damaged packages as well.

The ASHP recommends that broken containers and contaminated packaging mats be placed in a waste-disposal (sharps) container and then into HD disposal bags.[3] The bags should then be closed and placed in receptacles as described under Waste Disposal.

The appropriate protective equipment and waste-disposal materials should be kept in the area where shipments are received, and employees should be trained in their use and the risks of exposure to HDs.

3. Transport

HDs should be securely capped or sealed, placed in sealed clear plastic bags, and transported in containers designed to avoid breakage.

Personnel involved in transporting HDs should be trained in spill procedures, including sealing off the contaminated area and calling for appropriate assistance.

All HD containers should be labeled as noted in Drug Preparation Work Practices. If transport methods are used that produce stress on contents, such as the use of pneumatic tubes, guidance from the OSHA clarification of 1910.1030 with respect to transport (M.4.b.8[c]) should be followed. This clarification provides for use of packaging material inside the tube to prevent breakage. These recommendations that pertain to the Bloodborne Pathogens Standard are prudent practice for HDs (e.g., padded inserts for carriers).

F. Medical Surveillance

Workers who are potentially exposed to chemical hazards should be monitored in a systematic program or medical surveillance intended to prevent occupational injury and disease.[3,7] The purpose of surveillance is to identify the earliest reversible biologic effects so that exposure can be reduced or eliminated before the employee sustains irreversible damage. The occurrence of exposure-related disease or other adverse health effects should prompt immediate reevaluation of primary preventive measures (e.g., engineering controls, PPE). In this manner, medical surveillance acts as a check on the appropriateness of controls already in use.[62]

For detection and control of work-related health effects, *job-specific* medical evaluations should be performed:

- Before job placement.
- Periodically during employment.
- Following acute exposures.
- At the time of job termination or transfer (exit examination).

This information should be collected and analyzed in a systematic fashion to allow early detection of disease patterns in individual workers and groups of workers.

1. Preplacement Medical Examinations

Sound medical practice dictates that employees who will be working with HDs in the workplace have an initial evaluation consisting of a history, physical exam, and laboratory studies. The employer should make the following information available to the examining physician:

- Description of the employee's duties as they relate to the employee's exposure.
- Employee's exposure levels or anticipated exposure levels.
- Description of any PPE used or to be used.
- Information from previous medical examinations of the employee that is not readily available to the examining physician.

The history details the individual's medical and reproductive experience with emphasis on potential risk factors, such as past hematopoietic, malignant, or hepatic disorders. It also includes a complete occupational history with information on extent of past exposures (including environmental sampling data, if possible) and use of protective equipment. Surrogates for worker exposure, in the absence of environmental sampling data, include:

- Records of drugs and quantities handled.
- Hours spent handling these drugs per week.
- Number of preparations/administrations per week.

The physical examination should be complete, but the skin, mucous membranes, cardiopulmonary, lymphatic system, and liver should be emphasized. An evaluation for respirator use must be performed in accordance with 29 CFR 1910.134, if the employee will wear a respirator. The laboratory assessment may include a complete blood count with differential, liver function tests, blood urea nitrogen, creatinine, and a urine dipstick. Other aspects of the physical and laboratory evaluation should be guided by known toxicities of the HD of exposure. Due to poor reproducibility, interindividual variability, and lack of prognostic value regarding disease development, no biologic monitoring tests (e.g., genotoxic markers) are currently recommended for routine use in employee surveillance. Biologic marker testing should be performed only within the context of a research protocol.

2. Periodic Medical Examinations

Recognized occupational medicine experts in the HD area recommend these exams to update the employee's medical, reproductive, and exposure histories. They are recommended on a yearly basis or every 2–3 years. The interval between exams is a function of the opportunity for exposure, duration of exposure, and possibly the age of the worker at the discretion of the occupational medicine physician, guided by the worker's history. Careful documentation of an individual's routine exposure and any acute accidental exposures are made. The physical examination and laboratory studies follow the format outlined in the preplacement examination.[54]

3. Postexposure Examinations

Postexposure evaluation is tailored to the type of exposure (e.g., spills or needle sticks from syringes containing HDs). An assessment of the extent of exposure is made and included in the confidential database (discussed in the Exposure/Health Outcome Linkage section) and in an incident report. The physical examination focuses on the involved area as well as other organ systems commonly affected (i.e., for CDs the skin and mucous membranes; for aerosolized HDs the pulmonary system). Treatment and laboratory studies follow as indicated and should be guided by emergency protocols.

4. Exit Examinations

The exit examination completes the information on the employee's medical, reproductive, and exposure histories. Examination and laboratory evaluation should be guided by the individual's history of exposures and follow the outline of the periodic evaluation.

5. Exposure/Health Outcome Linkage

Exposure assessment of all employees who have worked with HDs is important, and the maintenance of records is required by 29 CFR 1910.20. The use of previously outlined exposure surrogates is acceptable, although actual environmental or employee monitoring data are preferable. An MSDS can serve as an exposure record. Details of the use of PPE and engineering controls present should be included. A confidential database should be maintained with information regarding the individual's medical and reproductive history, with linkage to exposure information to facilitate epidemiologic review.

6. Reproductive Issues

The examining physician should consider the reproductive status of employees and inform them regarding relevant reproductive issues. The reproductive toxicity of HDs should be carefully explained to all workers who will be exposed to these chemicals, and is required for those chemicals covered by the HCS. Unfortunately, no information is available regarding the reproductive risks of HD handling with the current use of BSCs and PPE. However, as discussed earlier, both spontaneous abortion and congenital malformation excesses have been documented among workers handling some of these drugs without currently recommended engineering controls and precautions. The facility should have a policy regarding reproductive toxicity of HDs and worker exposure in male and female employees and should follow that policy.

G. Hazard Communication

> *This section is for informational purposes only and is not a substitute for the requirements of the Hazard Communication Standard.*

The Hazard Communication Standard (HCS),[107] is applicable to some drugs. It defines a hazardous chemical as *any chemical that is a physical hazard or a health hazard.*

Physical hazard refers to characteristics such as combustibility or reactivity. A health hazard is defined as *a chemical for which there is statistically significant evidence based on at least one study conducted in accordance with established scientific principles that acute or chronic health effects may occur in exposed employees.* Appendixes A and B of the HCS outline the criteria used to determine whether an agent is hazardous.

According to HCS Appendix A, agents with any of the following characteristics would be considered hazardous:

- Carcinogens.
- Corrosives.
- Toxic or highly toxic agents (defined on the basis of median lethal doses).
- Irritants.
- Sensitizers.
- Target organ effectors, including reproductive toxins, hepatotoxins, nephrotoxins, neurotoxins, agents that act on the hematopoietic system, and agents that damage the lungs, skin, eyes, or mucous membranes.

Both human and animal data are to be used in this determination. HCS Appendix C lists sources of toxicity information.

As a result of the February 21, 1990, Supreme Court decision,[21] all provisions of the Hazard Communication Standard (29 CFR 1910.1200)[107] are now in effect for all industrial segments. This includes the coverage of drugs and pharmaceuticals in the nonmanufacturing sector. On February 9, 1994, OSHA issued a revised Hazard Communication Final Rule with technical clarification regarding drugs and pharmaceutical agents.

The Hazard Communication Standard (HCS) requires that drugs posing a health hazard (with the exception of those in solid, final form for direct administration to the patient, i.e., tablets or pills) be included on lists of hazardous chemicals to which employees are exposed.[107] Their storage and use locations can be confirmed by reviewing purchasing office records of currently used and past used agents such as those in Table A.1. Employee exposure records, including workplace monitoring, biologic monitoring, and MSDSs, as well as employee medical records related to drugs posing a health hazard, must be maintained and access to them provided to employees in accordance with 29 CFR 1910.20. Training required under the HCS should include all employees potentially exposed to these agents, not only healthcare professional staff, but also physical plant, maintenance, or support staff.

MSDSs are required to be prepared and transmitted with the initial shipment of all hazardous chemicals including covered drugs and pharmaceutical products. This excludes drugs defined by the Federal Food, Drug, and Cosmetic Act, which are in solid, final form for direct administration to the patient (e.g., tablets, pills, or capsules) or which are packaged for sale to consumers in a retail establishment. Package inserts and the *Physicians' Desk Reference* are not acceptable in lieu of requirements of MSDSs under the Standard. Items mandated by the Standard will use the term *shall* instead of *should*.

1. Written Hazard Communication Program

Employers shall develop, implement, and maintain at the workplace, a written hazard communication program for employees handling or otherwise exposed to chemicals, including drugs that represent a health hazard to employees. The written program will describe how the criteria specified in the standard concerning labels and other forms of warning, MSDSs, and employee information and training will be met. This also includes the following:

- List of the covered HDs known to be present using an identity that is referenced on the appropriate MSDS.
- Methods the employer will use to inform employees of the hazards of nonroutine tasks in their work areas.
- Methods the employer will use to inform employees of other employers of hazards at the worksite.

The employer shall make the written hazard communication program available, upon request, to employees, their designated representatives, and the assistant secretary of OSHA in accordance with requirements of the HCS.

2. MSDSs

In accordance with requirements in the Hazard Communication Standard, the employer must maintain MSDSs accessible to employees for all covered HDs used in the hospital. Specifics regarding MSDS content are contained in the Standard. Essential information includes health hazards, primary exposure routes, carcinogenic evaluations, acute exposure treatment, chemical inactivators, solubility, stability, volatility, PPE-required, and spill procedures for each covered HD. MSDSs shall also be made readily available upon request to employees, their designated representatives, or the Assistant Secretary of OSHA.

H. Training and Information Dissemination

In compliance with the Hazard Communication Standard, all personnel involved in any aspect of the handling of covered HDs (physicians, nurses, pharmacists, housekeepers, employees involved in receiving, transport, or storage) must receive information and training to apprise them of the hazards of HDs present in the work area.[71] Such information should be provided at the time of an employee's initial assignment to a work area where HDs are present and prior to assignments involving new hazards. The employer should provide annual refresher information and training.

The National Study Commission on Cytotoxic Exposure has recommended that knowledge and competence of personnel be evaluated after the first orientation or training session, and then yearly, or more often if a need is perceived.[71] Evaluation may involve direct observation of an individual's performance on the job. In addition, non-HD solutions should be used for evaluation of preparation technique; quinine, which will fluoresce under ultraviolet light, provides an easy mechanism for evaluation of technique.

1. Employee Information

Employees must be informed of the requirements of the Hazard Communication Standard, 29 CFR 1910.1200:

- Any operation/procedure in their work area where drugs that present a hazard are present.
- The location and availability of the written hazard communication program.

In addition, they should be informed regarding:

- Any operations or procedure in their work area where other HDs are present.
- The location and availability of any other plan regarding HDs.

2. Employee Training

Employee training must include at least:

- Methods of observations that may be used to detect the presence or release of an HCS-covered HD in the work area (such as monitoring conducted by the employer, continuous monitoring devices, visual appearance, or odor of covered HDs being released).
- Physical and health hazards of the covered HDs in the area.
- Measures employees can take to protect themselves from these hazards, including specific procedures that the employer has implemented to protect the employees from exposure to such drugs, such as identification of covered drugs and those to be handled as hazardous, appropriate work practices, emergency procedures (for spills or employee exposure), and PPE.
- Details of the hazard communication program developed by the employer, including an explanation of the labeling system and the MSDS, and how employees can obtain and use the appropriate hazard information.

It is essential that workers understand the carcinogenic potential and reproductive hazards of these drugs. Both females and males should understand the importance of avoiding exposure, especially early in pregnancy, so they can make informed decisions about the hazards involved. In addition, the facility's policy regarding reproductive toxicity of HDs should be explained to workers. Updated information should be provided to employees on a regular basis and whenever their jobs involve new hazards. Medical staff and other personnel who are not hospital employees should be informed of hospital policies and of the expectation that they will comply with these policies.

I. Record Keeping

Any workplace-exposure record created in connection with HD handling shall be kept, transferred, and made available for at least 30 years, and medical records shall be kept for the duration of employment plus 30 years in accordance with the Access to Employee Exposure and Medical Records Standard (29 CFR 1910.20).[108] In addition, sound practice dictates that training records should include the following information:

- Dates of the training sessions.
- Contents or a summary of the training sessions.
- Names and qualifications of the persons conducting the training.
- Names and job titles of all persons attending the training sessions.

Training records should be maintained for 3 years from the date on which the training occurred.

Position Statement

For the handling of cytotoxic agents by women who are pregnant, attempting to conceive, or breastfeeding, there are substantial data regarding the mutagenic, teratogenic, and abortifacient properties of certain cytotoxic agents both in animals and humans who have received therapeutic doses of these agents. Additionally, the scientific literature suggests a possible association of occupational exposure to certain cytotoxic agents during the first trimester of pregnancy with fetal loss or malformation. These data suggest the need for caution when women who are pregnant, or attempting to conceive, handle cytotoxic agents. Incidentally, there is no evidence relating male exposure to cytotoxic agents with adverse fetal outcome. There are no studies that address the possible risk associated with the occupational exposure to cytotoxic agents and the passage of these agents into breastmilk. Nevertheless, it is prudent that women who are breastfeeding should exercise caution in handling cytotoxic agents.

If all procedures for safe handling, such as those recommended by the Commission, are complied with, the potential for exposure will be minimized. Personnel should be provided with information to make an individual decision. This information should be provided in written form, and it is advisable that a statement of understanding be signed. It is essential to refer to individual state right-to-know laws to ensure compliance.

Approved by the National Study Commission on Cytotoxic Exposure, September 1987.

References

1. American Medical Association Council on Scientific Affairs. Guidelines for handling parenteral antineoplastics. *JAMA* 1985; 253:1590–1592.
2. American National Standards Institute. Occupational and educational eye and face protection. *ANSI* 1968; Z87 1.
3. American Society of Hospital Pharmacists. ASHP technical assistance bulletin on handling cytotoxic and hazardous drugs. *Am. J. Hosp. Pharm.* 1990; 47:1033–1049.
4. Andersen R, Boedicker M, Ma M, Goldstein EJC. Adverse reactions associated with pentamidine isethionate in AIDS patients: recommendations for monitoring therapy. *Drug Intell. Clin. Pharm.* 1986; 20:862–868.
5. Anderson RW, Puckett WH, Dana WJ, et al. Risk of handling injectable antineoplastic agents. *Am. J. Hosp. Pharm.* 1982; 39:188–1887.
6. Avis KE, Levchuck JW. Special considerations in the use of vertical laminar flow workbenches. *Am. J. Hosp. Pharm.* 1984; 41:81–87.
7. Barber RK. Fetal and neonatal effects of cytotoxic agents. *Obstet. Gynecol.* 1981; 51:41S–47S.
8. Benhamou S, Pot-Deprun J, Sancho-Garnier H, Chouroulinkov I. Sister chromatid exchanges and chromosomal aberrations in lymphocytes of nurses handling cytostatic drugs. *Int. J. Cancer* 1988; 41:350–353.
9. Bos RP, Leenars AO, Theuws JL, Henderson PT. Mutagenicity of urine from nurses handling cytostatic drugs, influence of smoking. *Int. Arch. Occ. Envir. Health* 1982; 50:359–369.
10. Bryan D, Marback RC. Laminar-airflow equipment certification: what the pharmacist needs to know. *Am. J. Hosp. Pharm.* 1984; 41:1343–1349.
11. Burgaz S, Ozdamar YN, Karakaya AE. A signal assay for the detection of toxic compounds: application on the urines of cancer patients on chemotherapy and of nurses handling cytotoxic drugs. *Human Toxicol.* 1988; 7:557–560.

12. California Department of Health Services Occupational Health Surveillance and Evaluation Program. *Health Care Worker Exposure to Ribavirin Aerosol: Field Investigation FI-86-009.* Berkeley: California Department of Health Services, 1986.

13. Castegnaro M, Adams J, Armour MA, eds, et al. Laboratory decontamination and destruction of carcinogens in laboratory wastes: some antineoplastic agents. International Agency for Research on Cancer. Scientific Publications No. 73. Lyons, France: IARC 1985.

14. Chapman RM. Effect of cytotoxic therapy on sexuality and gonadal function. Perry MC, Yarbro JW (eds), *Toxicity of Chemotherapy.* Orlando: Grune & Stratton, 1984: 343–363.

15. Chen CH, Vazquez-Padua M, Cheng YC. Effect of antihuman immunodeficiency virus nucleoside analogs on mDNA and its implications for delayed toxicity. *Mol. Pharm.* 1990; 39:625–628.

16. Christensen CJ, Lemasters GK, Wakeman MA. Work practices and policies of hospital pharmacists preparing antineoplastic agents. *J. Occup. Med.* 1990; 32:508–512.

17. Chrysostomou A, Morley AA, Seshadri R. Mutation frequency in nurses and pharmacists working with cytotoxic drugs. *Aust. N. Z. J. Med.* 1984; 14:381–834.

18. Connor JD, Hintz M, Van Dyke R. Ribavirin pharmacokinetics in children and adults during therapeutic trials. Smith RA, Knight V, Smith JAD (eds), In *Clinical Applications of Ribavirin.* Orlando: Academic Press, 1984.

19. Connor TH, Laidlaw JL, Theiss JC, et al. Permeability of latex and polyvinyl chloride gloves to carmustine. *Am. J. Hosp. Pharm.* 1984; 41:676–679.

20. Crudi CB. A compounding dilemma: I've kept the drug sterile but have I contaminated myself? *Nat. Intra. Therapy J.* 1980; 3:77–80.

21. Dole V. United Steelworkers. 1990; 494 U.S.26.

22. Doll C. Aerosolised pentamidine. *Lancet* 1989; ii 1284–1285.

23. Duvall E, Baumann B. An unusual accident during the administration of chemotherapy. *Cancer Nurse.* 1980; 3:305–306.

24. Environmental Protection Agency. *Discarded commercial chemical products, off specification species, container residues, and spill residues thereof.* 40 CFR 1991; 261.33(f).

25. Everson RB, Ratcliffe JM, Flack PM, et al. Detection of low levels of urinary mutagen excretion by chemotherapy workers, which was not related to occupational drug exposures. *Cancer Res.* 1985; 45:6487–6497.

26. Falck K, Grohn P, Sorsa M, et al. Mutagenicity in urine of nurses handling cytostatic drugs. *Lancet* 1979; i 1250–1251.

27. Falck K, Sorsa M, Vainio H. Use of the bacterial fluctuation test to detect mutagenicity in urine of nurses handling cytostatic drugs (abstract). *Mutat. Res.* 1981; 85:236–237.

28. Ferguson LR, Everts R, Robbie MA, et al. The use within New Zealand of cytogenetic approaches to monitoring of hospital pharmacists for exposure to cytotoxic drugs: report of a pilot study in Auckland. *Aust. J. Hosp Pharm.* 1988; 18:228–233.

29. Gude JK. Selective delivery of pentamidine to the lung by aerosol. *Am. Rev. Resp. Dis.* 1989; 139:1060.

30. Guglielmo BJ, Jacobs RA, Locksley RM. The exposure of healthcare workers to ribavirin aerosol. *JAMA* 1989; 261:1880–1881.

31. Harrison R, Bellows J, Rempel D, et al. Assessing exposures of healthcare personnel to aerosols of ribavirin-California. *Morbidity & Mortality Weekly Rep.* 1988; 37:560–563.

32. Hemminki K, Kyyronen P, Lindbohm ML. Spontaneous abortions and malformations in the offspring of nurses exposed to anaesthetic gases, cytostatic drugs, and other potential hazards: in hospitals, based on registered information of outcome. *J. Epidem. Comm. Health* 1985; 39 141–147.

33. Henderson DK, Gerberding JL. Prophylactic zidovudine after occupational exposure to the human immunodeficiency virus: An interim analysis. *J. Infectious Dis.* 1989; 160:321–327.

34. Hillyard IW. The preclinical toxicology and safety of ribavirin. Smith RA, Kirkpatrick W (eds), *In Ribavirin: a broad spectrum antiviral agent*. New York: Academic Press 1980.

35. Hirst M, Tse S, Mills DG, et al. Occupational exposure to cyclophosphamide. *Lancet* 1984; i 186–188.

36. Hoy RH, Stump LM. Effect of an air-venting filter device on aerosol production from vials. *Am. J. Hosp. Pharm.* 1984; 41:324–326.

37. International Agency for Research on Cancer. *IARC Monographs on the Evaluation of the Carcinogenic Risk of Chemicals to Man: Some Aziridines, N-, S-, and O-mustards and selenium*. Lyons, France. 1975; Vol. 9.

38. International Agency for Research on Cancer. *IARC Monographs on the Evaluation of the Carcinogenic Risk of Chemicals to Man: Some naturally occurring substances*. Lyons, France: IARC. 1976; Vol. 10.

39. International Agency for Research on Cancer. *IARC Monographs on the Evaluation of the Carcinogenic Risk of Chemicals to Humans: Some Antineoplastic and Immunosuppressive Agents*. Lyons, France: IARC. 1981; Vol. 26.

40. International Agency for Research on Cancer. *IARC Monographs on the Evaluation of the Carcinogenic Risk of Chemicals to Humans: Chemicals, Industrial Processes and Industries Associated with Cancer in Humans*. Lyons, France: IARC. 1982; Vol. 1–29 (Suppl. 4).

41. International Agency for Research on Cancer. *IARC Monographs on the Evaluation of the Carcinogenic Risk of Chemicals to Humans: Genetic and related effects: An updating of selected IARC Monographs from Volumes 1–42*. Lyons, France: IARC. 1987; Vol. 1–42 (Suppl. 6).

42. International Agency for Research on Cancer. *IARC Monographs on the Evaluation of the Carcinogenic Risk of Chemicals to Humans; Overall evaluations of carcinogenicity: An updating of IARC Monographs Volumes 1 to 42*. Lyons, France: IARC. 1987; Vol. 1–42 (Suppl. 7).

43. International Agency for Research on Cancer. *IARC Monographs on the Evaluation of the Carcinogenic Risk of Chemicals to Humans: Pharmaceutical Drugs*. Lyons, France: IARC.

44. Jagun O, Ryan M, Waldron HA. Urinary thioether excretion in nurses handling cytotoxic drugs. *Lancet* 1982; i:443–444.

45. Johnson EG, Janosik JE. Manufacturer's recommendations for handling spilled antineoplastic agents. *Am. J. Hosp. Pharm.* 1989; 46:318–319.

46. Juma FD, Rogers HJ, Trounce JR, Bradbrook ID. Pharmacokinetics of intravenous cyclophosphamide in man, estimated by gas-liquid chromatography. *Cancer Chemother. Pharmacol.* 1978; 1:229–231.

47. Kacmarek RM. Ribavirin and pentamidine aerosols: caregiver beware! *Respiratory Care* 1990; 35:1034–1036.

48. Karakaya AE, Burgaz S, Bayhan A. The significance of urinary thioethers as indicators of exposure to alkylating agents. *Arch. Toxicol.* 1989; 13 (suppl): 117–119.

49. Kilham L, Ferm VH. Congenital anomalies induced in hamster embryos with ribavirin. *Science* 1977; 195:413–414.

50. Kleinberg ML, Quinn MJ. Airborne drug levels in a laminar-flow hood. *Am. J. Hosp. Pharm.* 1981; 38:1301–1303.

51. Kolmodin-Hedman B, Hartvig P, Sorsa M, Falck K. Occupational handling of cytostatic drugs. *Arch. Toxicol.* 1983; 54:25–33.

52. Kyle RA. Second malignancies associated with chemotherapy. Perry MC, Yarbro JW (eds), *Toxicity of Chemotherapy*. Orlando: Grune & Stratton, 1984: 479–506.

53. Laidlaw JL, Connor TH, Theiss JC, et al. Permeability of latex and polyvinyl chloride gloves to 20 antineoplastic drugs. *Am. J. Hosp. Pharm.* 1984; 41:2618–2623.

54. Laidlaw JL, Connor TH, Theiss JC, et al. Permeability of four disposable protective clothing materials to seven antineoplastic drugs. *Am. J. Hosp. Pharm.* 1985; 42:2449–2454.

55. Lee SB. Ribavirin-exposure to healthcare workers. *Am. Ind. Hyg. Assoc.* 1988; 49:A13–A14.

56. LeRoy ML, Roberts MJ, Theisen JA. Procedures for handling antineoplastic injections in comprehensive cancer centers. *Am. J. Hosp. Pharm.* 1983; 40:601–603.
57. Lunn G, Sansone EB. Validated methods for handling spilled antineoplastic agents. *Am. J. Hosp. Pharm.* 1989; 46:1131.
58. Lunn G, Sansone EB, Andrews AW, Hellwig LC. Degradation and disposal of some antineoplastic drugs. *J. Pharm. Sciences* 1989; 78:652–659.
59. Matthews T, Boehme R. Antiviral activity and mechanism of action of ganciclovir. *Rev. Infect. Diseases* 1988; 10 (suppl 3) S490–94.
60. McDevitt JJ, Lees PSJ, McDiarmid MA. Exposure of hospital pharmacists and nurses to anti-neoplastic agents. *J. Occup. Med.* 1993; 35:57–60.
61. McDiarmid MA, Egan T, Furio M, et al. Sampling for airborne fluorouracil in a hospital drug preparation area. *Am. J. Hosp. Pharm.* 1988; 43:1942–1945.
62. McDiarmid MA, Emmett EA. Biological monitoring and medical surveillance of workers exposed to antineoplastic agents. *Seminars in Occup. Med.* 1987; 2:109–117.
63. McDiarmid MA, Jacobson-Kram D. Aerosolized pentamidine and public health. *Lancet* 1989; ii 863.
64. McDiarmid MA. Medical surveillance for antineoplastic-drug handlers. *Am. J. Hosp. Pharm.* 1990; 47:1061–1066.
65. McDiarmid MA, Gurley HT, Arrington D. Pharmaceuticals as hospital hazards: Managing the risks. *J. Occup. Med.* 1991; 33:155–158.
66. McDiarmid MA, Kolodner K, Humphrey F, et al. Baseline and phosphoramide mustard-induced sister chromatid exchanges in pharmacists handling anti-cancer drugs. *Mutat. Res.* 1992; 279: 199–204.
67. McDiarmid MA, Schaefer J, Richard CL, Chaisson RE, Tepper BS. Efficacy of engineering controls in reducing occupational exposure to aerosolized pentamidine. *Chest* 1992; 102:1764–1766.
68. McEvoy GK, ed. *American Hospital Formulary Service Drug Information.* Bethesda: American Society of Hospital Pharmacists, 1993.
69. McLendon BF, Bron AF. Corneal toxicity from vinblastine solution. *Br. J. Ophthalmol.* 1978; 62:97–99.
70. National Sanitation Foundation. *Standard No. 49 for Class II (Laminar Flow) Biohazard Cabinetry.* Ann Arbor: National Sanitation Foundation, 1990.
71. National Study Commission on Cytotoxic Exposure. Louis P Jeffrey Sc. D, Chairman, (ed), *Recommendations for Handling Cytotoxic Agents.* Providence, Rhode Island: Rhode Island Hospital, 1983.
72. National Study Commission on Cytotoxic Exposure. Louis P Jeffrey Sc. D, (ed), *Consensus Responses to Unresolved Questions Concerning Cytotoxic Agents.* Providence, Rhode Island: Chairman, Rhode Island Hospital, 1984.
73. Neal AD, Wadden RA, Chiou WL. Exposure of hospital workers to airborne antineoplastic agents. *Am. J. Hosp. Pharm.* 1983; 40:597–601.
74. Nikula E, Kiviniitty K, Leisti J, Taskinen P. Chromosome aberrations in lymphocytes of nurses handling cytostatic agents. *Scand. J. Work Environ. Health* 1984; 10:71–74.
75. Norppa H, Sorsa M, Vainio H, et al. Increased sister chromatid exchange frequencies in lymphocytes of nurses handling cytostatic drugs. *Scand. J. Work Environ. Health* 1980; 6:299–301.
76. Nguyen TV, Theiss JC, Matney TS. Exposure of pharmacy personnel to mutagenic antineoplastic drugs. *Cancer Res.* 42:4792–4796.
77. Palmer RG, Dore CJ, Denman AM. Chlorambucil-induced chromosome damage to human lymphocytes is dose-dependent and cumulative. *Lancet* 1984; i: 246–249.
78. Perry MC, Yarbro JW (eds). *Toxicity of Chemotherapy.* Orlando, FL: Grune & Stratton, 1984.
79. Physicians' Desk Reference. Barnhart ER (eds). *Physicians' Desk Reference,* 45th ed. Oradell, New Jersey: Medical Economics Data, 1991: 730.

80. Pohlova H, Cerna M, Rossner P. Chromosomal aberrations, SCE and urine mutagenicity in workers occupationally exposed to cytostatic drugs. *Mutat. Res.* 1986; 174:213–217.

81. Pyy L, Sorsa M, Hakala E. Ambient monitoring of cyclophosphamide in manufacture and hospitals. *Am. Ind. Hyg. Assoc. J.* 1988; 49:314–317.

82. Reich SD, Bachur NR. Contact dermatitis associated with adriamycin (NSC-123127) and daunorubicin (NSC-82151). *Cancer Chemotherap. Rep.* 1975; 59:677–678.

83. Reynolds RD, Ignoffo R, Lawrence J, et al. Adverse reactions to AMSA in medical personnel. *Cancer Treat. Rep.* 1982; 66:1885.

84. Rogers B. Health hazards to personnel handling antineoplastic agents. *Occupational Med. State Art Rev.* 1987; 2:513–524.

85. Rogers B, Emmett EA. Handling antineoplastic agents: urine mutagenicity in nurses. *IMAGE J. Nurs. Scholarship.* 1987; 19:108–113.

86. Rosner F. Acute leukemia as a delayed consequence of cancer chemotherapy. *Cancer* 1976; 37: 1033–1036.

87. Rudolph R, Suzuki M, Luce JK. Experimental skin necrosis produced by adriamycin. *Cancer Treat. Rep.* 1979; 63:529–537.

88. Schafer AI. Teratogenic effects of antileukemic therapy. *Arch. Int. Med.* 1981; 141:514–515.

89. Selevan SG, Lindbolm ML, Homung RW, Hemminki K. A study of occupational exposure to antineoplastic drugs and fetal loss in nurses. *New Engl. J. Med.* 1985; 313:1173–1178.

90. Sieber SM. Cancer chemotherapeutic agents and carcinogenesis. *Cancer Chemotherapy Rep.* 1975; 59:915–918.

91. Sieber SM, Adamson RH. Toxicity of antineoplastic agents in man: chromosomal aberrations, antifertility effects, congenital malformations, and carcinogenic potential. *Adv. Cancer Res.* 1975; 22:57–155.

92. Siebert D, Simon U. Cyclophosphamide: pilot study of genetically active metabolites in the urine of a treated human patient. *Mutat. Res.* 1973; 19:65–72.

93. Slevin ML, Ang LM, Johnston A, Turner P. The efficiency of protective gloves used in the handling of cytotoxic drugs. *Cancer Chemo. Pharmacol.* 1984; 12:151–153.

94. Smaldone GC, Vincicuerra C, Marchese J. Detection of inhaled pentamidine in healthcare workers. *New Engl. J. Med.* 1991; 325:891–892.

95. Sorsa M, Hemminki K, Vanio H. Occupational exposure to anticancer drugs—potential and real hazards. *Mutat. Res.* 1985; 154:135–149.

96. Sotaniemi EA, Sutinen S, Arranto AJ, et al. Liver damage in nurses handling cytostatic agents. *Acta Med. Scand.* 1983; 214:181–189.

97. Stellman JM. The spread of chemotherapeutic agents at work: assessment through stimulation. *Cancer Invest.* 1987; 5:75–81.

98. Stephens JD, Golbus MS, Miller TR, et al. Multiple congenital abnormalities in a fetus exposed to 5-fluorouracil during the first trimester. *Am. J. Obstet. Gynecol.* 1980; 137:747–749.

99. Stiller A, Obe G, Bool I, Pribilla W. No elevation of the frequencies of chromosomal aberrations as a consequence of handling cytostatic drugs. *Mutat. Res.* 1983; 121:253–259.

100. Stoikes ME, Carlson JD, Farris FF, Walker PR. Permeability of latex and polyvinyl chloride gloves to fluorouracil and methotrexate. *Am. J. Hosp. Pharm.* 1987; 44:1341–1346.

101. Stucker I, Hirsch A, Doloy T, et al. Urine mutagenicity, chromosomal abnormalities, and sister chromatid exchanges in lymphocytes of nurses handling cytostatic drugs. *Int. Arch. Occup. Environ. Health* 1986; 57:195–205.

102. Stucker I, Caillard JF, Collin R, et al. Risk of spontaneous abortion among nurses handling antineoplastic drugs. *Scand. J. Work Environ. Health* 1990; 16:102–107.

103. U.S. Department of Health and Human Services. Public Health Service. National Institutes of Health. *Recommendations for the Safe Handling of Cytotoxic Drugs.* NIH Publication No. 92–2621. 1992.

104. U.S. Department of Health and Human Services. Public Health Service. Centers for Disease Control. National Institute for Occupational Safety and Health. *Guidelines for Protecting the Safety and Health of Health Care Workers.* DHHS (NIOSH) Publication No. 88–119. 1988.

105. U.S. Department of Labor, Occupational Safety and Health Administration. Respiratory Protection Standard. 1984; 29 CFR 1910.134.

106. U.S. Department of Labor, Occupational Safety and Health Administration. Work practice guidelines for personnel dealing with cytotoxic (antineoplastic) drugs. OSHA Publication #8-1.1. 1986.

107. U.S. Department of Labor, Occupational Safety and Health Administration. *Hazard Communication Standard.* 1989; 29 CFR 1910.1200, as amended February 9, 1994.

108. U.S. Department of Labor, Occupational Safety and Health Administration. *Access to Employee and Medical Records Standard.* 1990; 29 CFR 1910. 20.

109. U.S. Department of Labor, Occupational Safety and Health Administration. *Occupational Exposure to Bloodborne Pathogens Standard.* 1991; 29 CFR 1910. 1030.

110. Vaccari FL, Tonat K, DeChristoforo R, et al. Disposal of antineoplastic waste at the NIH. *Am. J. Hosp. Pharm.* 1984; 41:87–92.

111. Valanis B, Vollmer WM, Labuhn K, Glass A, Corelle C. Antineoplastic drug handling protection after OSHA guidelines: comparison by profession, handling activity, and work site. *J. Occup. Med.* 1992; 34:149–155.

112. Venitt S, Crofton-Sleigh C, Hunt J, et al. Monitoring exposure of nursing and pharmacy personnel to cytotoxic drugs. Urinary mutation assays and urinary platinum as markers of absorption. *Lancet* 1984; i: 74 6.

113. Waksvik H, Klepp O, Brogger A. Chromosome analyses of nurses handling cytostatic agents. *Cancer Treat. Rep.* 1981; 65:607–610.

114. Wall RL, Clausen KP. Carcinoma of the urinary bladder in patients receiving cyclophosphamide. *New Engl. J. Med.* 1975; 293:271–273.

115. Weisburger JH, Griswold DP, Prejean JD, et al. Tumor induction by cytostatics. The carcinogenic properties of some of the principal drugs used in clinical cancer chemotherapy. *Recent Results Cancer Res.* 1975; 52:1–17.

116. Zimmerman PF, Larsen RK, Barkley EW, Gallelli JF. Recommendations for the safe handling of injectable antineoplastic drug products. *Am. J. Hosp. Pharm.* 1981; 38:1693–1695.

Appendix 2
Common Terminology Criteria for Adverse Events (CTCAE)

Rather than include the entire CTCAE, the following gives the highlights of the resource. The CTCAE can be found online at http://evs.nci.nih.gov/ftp1/CTCAE/CTCAE_4.03_2010-06-14_QuickReference_5x7.pdf

Version 4.0
Published: May 28, 2009 (v4.03: June 14, 2010)
U.S. DEPARTMENT OF HEALTH AND HUMAN SERVICES
National Institutes of Health
National Cancer Institute

Common Terminology Criteria for Adverse Events v4.0 (CTCAE)
Publish Date: May 28, 2009 (v4.03 June 14, 2010)

Quick Reference

The NCI Common Terminology Criteria for Adverse Events is a descriptive terminology that can be utilized for Adverse Event (AE) reporting. A grading (severity) scale is provided for each AE term.

Components and Organization
CTCAE Terms

An Adverse Event (AE) is any unfavorable and unintended sign (including an abnormal laboratory finding), symptom, or disease temporally associated with the use of a medical treatment or procedure that may or may *not* be considered related to the medical treatment or procedure. An AE is a term that is a unique representation of a specific event used for medical documentation and scientific analyses. Each CTCAE v4.0 term is a MedDRA LLT (Lowest Level Term).

Definitions

A brief definition is provided to clarify the meaning of each AE term.

Grades

Grade refers to the severity of the AE. The CTCAE displays grades 1 through 5 with unique clinical descriptions of severity for each AE based on this general guideline:

Grade 1:
Mild; asymptomatic or mild symptoms; clinical or diagnostic observations only; intervention not indicated.

Grade 2:
Moderate; minimal, local, or noninvasive intervention indicated; limiting age-appropriate instrumental ADL (e.g., preparing meals, shopping for groceries or clothes, using the telephone, managing money).

Grade 3:
Severe or medically significant but not immediately life-threatening; hospitalization or prolongation of hospitalization indicated; disabling; limiting self-care ADL (e.g., bathing, dressing and undressing, feeding self, using toilet, taking medications, and not bedridden).

Grade 4:
Life-threatening consequences; urgent intervention indicated.

Grade 5:
Death related to AE.

Not all grades are appropriate for all AEs. Therefore, some AEs are listed with fewer than five options for grade selection.

Index

Note: Generic names are indicated by boldface type.
Figures and tables are indicated by *f* and *t*, respectively, following the page number.

Lorazepam (Ativan), 1566*t*, 1611–1614
Lorbrena (**lorlatinib**), 717–722
Lorlatinib (Lorbrena), 717–722
L-PAM (**melphalan hydrochloride**), 3, 13*t*, 296–300
L-phenylalanine mustard (**melphalan hydrochloride**), 3, 296–300
L-sarcolysin (**melphalan hydrochloride**), 3, 296–300
Lubricant laxatives, 1923
Lung cancer
    genomics and, 15
    hypercalcemia and, 1645
    metastasis and, 480
Lung toxicity, 3
Lupron Depot (**leuprolide acetate for depot suspension**), 285–289
Lymphocytes, 491–492
Lymphoma
    immunosuppression and, 1669
    molecular targeted therapies and, 476, 484–485, 490
    skeletal-related conditions and, 1645–1646, 1648
    topoisomerase and, 15
Lynparza (**olaparib**), 497*t*, 744–748
Lyrica (**pregabalin**), 1389–1392
Lysodren (**mitotane**), 318–320

M

MAbs (monoclonal antibodies), 429, 460, 472, 478, 877, 887–893, 894, 1298
Macrolides, 1676*t*
Magnesium citrate, 1928–1929
Malabsorptive diarrhea, 1943
Malignant transformation, 469*f*, 472. *See also* Metastasis
Mammalian target of rapamycin (mTOR), 463–464, 659–660, 819–820
MAOIs (monamine oxidase inhibitors), 1436, 1456
Marinol (**dronabinol**), 1513–1515, 1557–1560
Matrix metalloproteinases (MMPs), 481
Matulane (**procarbazine hydrochloride**), 370–373
Maxipime (**cefepime**), 1710–1712
Mechanism of action of chemotherapy drugs, 3, 4*f*, 12*t*–13*t*
Mechlorethamine hydrochloride (Mustargen, Nitrogen mustard, HN₂), 293–296
Meda Cap (**acetaminophen**), 1361–1362, 1392–1396
Medicare, 884, 929
Medroxyprogesterone acetate (Depo-Provera, Provera), 19*t*

Mefoxin (**cefoxitin sodium**), 1723–1726
Megace OS (**megestrol acetate oral suspension**), 1561–1562
Megestrol acetate oral suspension (Megace OS), 1561–1562
Mekinist (**trametinib**), 826–833
Mektovi® (**binimetinib**), 548–553
Melanoma, 463, 867–870
Melatonin, 1554
Melphalan hydrochloride (Alkeran, L-phenylalanine mustard, L-PAM, L-sarcolysin), 3, 13*t*, 296–300
Melphalan for injection (evomela), 300–304
Mercaptopurine (Purixan oral suspension Purinethol, 6-MP), 304–308
Meropenem (Merrem), 1811–1813
Meropenem/vaborbactam (Vabomere), 1813–1815
Merrem (**meropenem**), 1811–1813
Mesenchymal cells, 458, 473, 489
Mesna for injection (Mesnex), 449–451
Mesnex (**mesna for injection**), 449–451
Messenger RNA (mRNA), 462, 465
Metastasis, 214, 313, 343, 456, 464, 472–473, 473*f*, 480, 482, 488–490, 576, 840, 851, 980, 983, 986, 987, 1008, 1172, 1174, 1257, 1643–1648
Methadone (Dolophine, Methadose), 1454–1459
Methadose (**methadone**), 1454–1459
Methicillin-resistant *Staphylococcus aureus* (MRSA), 1671, 1672
Methotrexate (Amethopterin, Folex, Mexate), 3, 308–314
Methylation, 475–476
Methylcellulose (Citrucel), 1929–1930
Methylnaltrexone bromide (Relistor), 1930–1933
Methylprednisolone, 48–51
Metoclopramide hydrochloride (Reglan), 1528–1530
Metronidazole hydrochloride (Flagyl), 1881–1884
Mexate (**methotrexate**), 3, 308–314
Micafungin sodium (Mycamine), 1885–1887
Miconazole nitrate (Monistat), 1886–1887
Midol 200 (**ibuprofen**), 1375–1378
Midostaurin (Rydapt), 476, 495*t*, 722–725
Mineral oil (Fleet Mineral Oil), 1934–1935
Minocin (**minocycline hydrochloride**), 1815–1818
Minocycline hydrochloride (Minocin), 1815–1818
Miralax (**polyethylene glycol 3350, NF powder**), 1937–1938
Mirtazapine (Remeron), 1614–1617
Mithramycin, 1648